FOR INSTRUCTORS

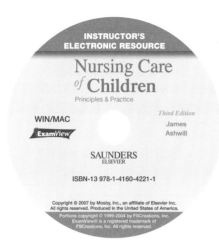

Instructor's Electronic Resource

978-1-4160-4221-1

Available in CD and online formats, this helpful instructor's package provides all of the tools needed to quickly and consistently develop lectures and student assignments and evaluate student comprehension. The *Instructor's Manual* includes learning objectives, teaching strategies, supplemental resources, curriculum guides for courses of various lengths, and open-book quizzes. The ExamView *test bank* contains questions in NCLEX® format and an answer key with page references to the text, rationales, and NCLEX® coding. Also included are a full-color *Image Collection* and *PowerPoint Lecture Slides* for building presentations and developing lectures.

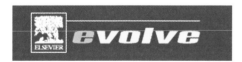

Evolve Course Management System

http://evolve.elsevier.com/James/ncoc/

Evolve is an interactive teaching and learning environment that works in coordination with *Nursing Care of Children, 3rd edition*, providing Internet-based course content that reinforces and expands on the concepts that instructors deliver in class. In addition to the resources available to students, instructors are able to access all of the components of the *Instructor's Electronic Resource*, including the computerized test bank and PowerPoint slides. Instructors can also use Evolve to: publish class syllabi, outline, and lecture notes; set up "virtual office hours" and email communication; share important dates and information through the online class *Calendar*; and encourage student participation through *Chat Rooms* and *Discussion Boards*. Instructors are encouraged to contact their sales representative for more information about integrating Evolve into their curriculum.

CONTENTS

COMPANION CD

ANIMATIONS

Abdominal Anatomy (Ch. 9)
Adrenal Function (Ch. 27)
Asthma (Ch. 21)
Bag Ventilation (Ch. 10)
Band Formation (Ch. 23)
Brain Lobes (Ch. 28)
Central Venous Access via Jugular Vein (Ch. 14)
CPR, Pediatric (Ch. 10)
Cranial Nerve Examination (Ch. 28)
Cranial Nerves (Ch. 9)
Hemophilia A (Ch. 23)
Intubation (Ch. 21)
Intubation in Children (Ch. 21)
IV Line Placement (Ch. 14)
Organ Systems 3-D Tour (Ch. 9)
Passage of Food Through Digestive Tract (Ch. 19)
PICC Line Placement (Ch. 14)
Seizure, Generalized (Ch. 28)
Sickle Cell Anemia (Ch. 23)
Spine Structure (Ch. 26)
Structure of the Heart (Ch. 22)
Subaortic Stenosis (Ch. 22)
Umbilical Vein Catheter Placement (Ch. 22)
Ventriculoperitoneal Shunt (Ch. 28)
Volvulus, Pediatric (Ch. 19)

AUDIO GLOSSARY (WITH ENGLISH AND SPANISH PRONUNCIATIONS)

NCLEX REVIEW QUESTIONS

PEDIATRIC ASSESSMENT VIDEO CLIPS

General Assessment

1. Evaluation: Head Circumference—Male Neonate (Ch. 9)
2. Palpation: Lymph Nodes, Head and Neck—Female Child (Ch. 9)
3. Inspection and Palpation: Head and Neck—Male Infant (Ch. 9)
4. Inspection: Oropharynx, Teeth and Tongue—Female Child (Ch. 9)
5. Inspection: Ear Canal—Male Toddler (Ch. 9)
6. Evaluation: Eye Fixation Using the Cover/Uncover Test—Female Child (Ch. 9)
7. Inspection: Chest and Lungs, Posterior—Male Child (Ch. 9)
8. Auscultation: Breath Sounds, Anterior Chest—Male Child (Ch. 9)
9. Auscultation: Heart, Anterior Chest—Male Neonate (Ch. 9)
10. Palpation: Pedal Pulses—Male Neonate (Ch. 9)
11. Inspection and Palpation: Abdomen, Umbilicus—Male Infant (Ch. 5)
12. Palpation: Liver—Female Adolescent (Ch. 9)
13. Inspection: External Genitalia—Female Neonate (Ch. 5)
14. Inspection: Muscle Strength, Upper Extremities—Male Child (Ch. 9)
15. Evaluation: Muscle Strength, Neck, Shoulders, and Tongue: Cranial Nerve VII, XI, XII—Male Child (Ch. 9)
16. Inspection: Fine Motor Coordination, Upper Extremities—Female Adolescent (Ch. 9)

Newborn

17. Inspection: Male Genitalia, Circumcision—Male Neonate (Ch. 5)
18. Evaluation: Cremasteric Reflex—Male Neonate (Ch. 5)
19. Evaluation: Barlow-Ortolani Maneuvers (Ch. 26)
20. Evaluation: Symmetry of Gluteal Folds—Male Infant (Ch. 5)

Infant

21. Evaluation: Motor Development (Rolling Over)—Male Infant (Ch. 5)
22. Evaluation: Motor Development (Head Control)—Male Infant (Ch. 5)
23. Evaluation: Babinski Reflex—Male Infant (Ch. 5)

Toddler and Preschooler

24. Evaluation: Crawling to Standing—Female Toddler (Ch. 6)
25. Evaluation: Fine Motor Skills—Male Child (Ch. 6)

School-Age

26. Evaluation: Muscular Development—Male Child (Ch. 7)
27. Evaluation: Balance Using Heel-to-Toe Walking—Male Child (Ch. 7)
28. Inspection and Palpation: Spine for Alignment—Male Child (Ch. 26)

Adolescent

29. Inspection: Female Breasts (Sitting Position)—Female Child (Ch. 8)
30. Inspection and Palpation: Capillary Refill, Upper Extremities—Female Adolescent (Ch. 22)

PEDIATRIC SKILLS

Administering Oral Medications (Ch. 14)
Admitting Child to the Health Care System (Ch. 11)
Calculating Safe Dosages for Children (Ch. 14)
Car Seat Safety (Ch. 5)
Communicating with Children (Ch. 3)
Fostering Healthy Sleep Patterns in Children (Ch. 6)
Implementing Seizure Precautions (Ch. 28)
Infant Bathing (Ch. 13)
Infant Feeding (Ch. 5)
Instructing Families in Child Safety (Ch. 6)
Managing Pain (Ch. 15)
Measuring Body Temperature (Ch. 13)
Measuring Oxygen Saturation (Ch. 13)
Measuring Physical Growth (Ch. 9)
Monitoring Neurovascular Status (Ch. 26)
Preparing the Child for Procedures (Ch. 13)
Preparing the Child for Surgery (Ch. 11)
Providing Culturally-Sensitive Care (Ch. 2)
Therapeutic Play (Ch. 11)
Urine Specimen Collection (Ch. 13)

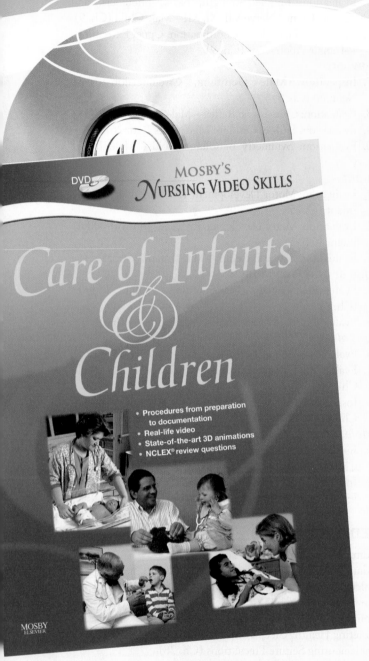

Nursing Care *of* Children

Principles & Practice

Third Edition

Susan Rowen James, RN, PhD(c)
Associate Professor
Curry College Division of Nursing
Milton, Massachusetts

Jean Weiler Ashwill, MSN, RN
Director of Undergraduate Student Services
School of Nursing
University of Texas at Arlington
Arlington, Texas

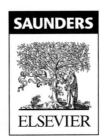

SAUNDERS

ELSEVIER

SAUNDERS
ELSEVIER

11830 Westline Industrial Drive
St. Louis, Missouri 63146

Nursing Care of Children: Principles & Practice, Third Edition

ISBN: 978-1-4160-3084-3

Notice

Knowledge and best practice in this field are constantly changing. As new research and experience broaden our knowledge, changes in practice, treatment and drug therapy may become necessary or appropriate. Readers are advised to check the most current information provided (i) on procedures featured or (ii) by the manufacturer of each product to be administered, to verify the recommended dose or formula, the method and duration of administration, and contraindications. It is the responsibility of the practitioner, relying on their own experience and knowledge of the patient, to make diagnoses, to determine dosages and the best treatment for each individual patient, and to take all appropriate safety precautions. To the fullest extent of the law, neither the Publisher nor the Authors assume any liability for any injury and/or damage to persons or property arising out or related to any use of the material contained in this book.

The Publisher

NCLEX, NCLEX-RN, and NCLEX-PN are registered trademarks and servicemarks of the National Council of State Boards of Nursing, Inc.

ISBN: 978-1-4160-3084-3

Acquisitions Editor: Catherine Jackson
Managing Editor: Michele D. Hayden
Publishing Services Manager: Deborah L. Vogel
Senior Project Manager: Steve Ramay
Designer: Paula Ruckenbrod

Printed in Canada

Last digit is the print number: 9 8 7 6 5 4 3 2 1

To my sister Anne, outstanding mother and grandmother. Your continuing positive outlook and commitment to overcoming what appear to be insurmountable life events have been a source of inspiration for me. God bless you as you continue to achieve all of your goals.

Susan Rowen James

To my friends and colleagues who have mentored me throughout my professional life. In love and thanksgiving for my family, especially my husband Vince, my children Vin, Amy, and Heidi, and their children Avery, Liam, Katie, Patrick, Charlie, and Andrew, who are the joy of my life.

Jean Weiler Ashwill

CONTRIBUTORS

Mary Jane Piskor Ashe, RN, MA, CNS
Assistant Director
Undergraduate Student Services
School of Nursing
The University of Texas at Arlington
Arlington, Texas
Chapter 27: The Child With an Endocrine or Metabolic Alteration

Karen Samper Bernardy, RN, MSN
Child Health Consultant
Conyers, Georgia
Chapter 19: The Child With a Gastrointestinal Alteration

Cam Brandt, RN, MS
Education Coordinator, Emergency Services
Cook Children's Health Care System
Fort Worth, Texas
Chapter 10: Emergency Care of the Child

Debra L. Calligaro-Wharton, RN, MS
Clinical Nurse Specialist
Murphy, Texas
Chapter 28: The Child With a Neurologic Alteration

Sheryl A. Cifrino, RN, BS, MA, MSN
Nursing Instructor
Curry College
Milton, Massachusetts
Chapter 11: The Ill Child in the Hospital and Other Care Settings

Dolores W. Clark, RN, MSN, FNP, PNP
Pediatric Nurse Practitioner
Cook Children's Physician Network
Fort Worth, Texas;
Consultant
University of Texas at Arlington
School of Nursing
Arlington, Texas
Chapter 9: Physical Assessment of Children

Wrennah L. Gabbert, RN, MSN, CPNP, FNP-C, PhD(c)
Professional Specialist, Nursing Faculty
Angelo State University
San Angelo, Texas
Chapter 16: The Child With an Infectious Disease

Judy L. LeFlore, RNC, PhD, NNP, CPNP-PC, CPNP-AC
Associate Clinical Professor and Director
Pediatric and Acute Care Pediatric Nurse Practitioner Program
The University of Texas at Arlington
School of Nursing
Arlington, Texas;
Neonatal and Pediatric Nurse Practitioner
Children's Medical Center of Dallas
Dallas, Texas
Chapter 22: The Child With a Cardiovascular Alteration

Melissa A. LeMoine, RN, MSN, CPNP
Pediatric Nurse Practitioner, Pediatric Nephrology Services
Cook Children's Health Care System
Fort Worth, Texas
Chapter 20: The Child With a Genitourinary Alteration

Madoka Lightfoot, RN, MSN, CS, PMHNP
Psychiatric Mental Health Nurse Practitioner
The Holiner Psychiatric Group
Dallas, Texas
Chapter 29: The Child With a Psychosocial Disorder
Chapter 30: The Child With a Cognitive Impairment

Mary Mallory, RN, MS, ACRN, APRN-BC
Pediatric Nurse Practitioner
ARMS Clinic
Children's Medical Center—Dallas
University of Texas Southwestern Medical Center
Dallas, Texas
Chapter 17: The Child With an Immunologic Alteration

Victoria Mannion, RN, MSN, FNP-C
Family Nurse Practitioner
Children's Clinic
Wilmington, North Carolina
Chapter 26: The Child With a Musculoskeletal Alteration

Gwendolyn T. Martin, RN, MS, CNS, CPN
Assistant Clinical Professor
Texas Woman's University
Dallas, Texas
Chapter 12: The Child With a Chronic Condition or Terminal Illness
Chapter 15: Pain Management for Children

Sharon M. McLeod, MS, CCLS, CTRS
Senior Clinical Director
Division of Child Life
Cincinnati Children's Hospital Medical Center
Cincinnati, Ohio
Chapter 3: Communicating With Children and Families

Patricia Newcomb, RN, PhD, CPNP
Assistant Professor
Harris School of Nursing
Texas Christian University;
Pediatric Nurse Practitioner
Cook Children's Health Care System
Fort Worth, Texas
Chapter 25: The Child With an Integumentary Alteration

Sharon A. Ransom, RN, BSN, MHA, CPN
Education Coordinator
Cook Children's Health Care System
Fort Worth, Texas
Chapter 18: The Child With a Fluid and Electrolyte Alteration

James P. Riddel, Jr., RN, MS, CPNP
Pediatric Nurse Practitioner
Division of Hematology
Children's Hospital and Research Center—Oakland
Oakland, California;
Doctoral Student
Department of Physiological Nursing
University of California, San Francisco
San Francisco, California
Chapter 23: The Child With a Hematologic Alteration

Jennifer Walsh Treseler, RN, MSN
Staff Nurse II, Intermediate Care Program
Children's Hospital
Boston, Massachusetts
Chapter 21: The Child With a Respiratory Alteration

Kathleen M. White, RN, MSN, CPNP
Assistant Professor
Tarrant County College;
Pediatric Nurse Practitioner
Cook Children's Health Care System
Fort Worth, Texas
Chapter 24: The Child With Cancer

INSTRUCTOR'S MANUAL, OPEN-BOOK QUIZZES, CURRICULUM GUIDES

Betty W. Hamlisch, RN, MS
Professor of Nursing
Tompkins Cortland Community College
Dryden, New York

POWERPOINT LECTURE SLIDES

Myra K. Goldman, RN, MSN, ARNP
Family Nurse Practitioner
Louisville, Kentucky

TEST BANK

Amy Zlomek Hedden, RN, MS, NP
Associate Professor
California State University—Bakersfield
Department of Nursing
Pediatric and Neonatal Intensive Care Departments
Bakersfield Memorial Hospital
Pediatric Content Expert and Team Leader
Bakersfield, California

NCLEX REVIEW QUESTIONS

Karen Clark Griffith, RN, BSN, MA, PhD
Clinical Assistant Professor
The University of Iowa
College of Nursing
Iowa City, Iowa

REVIEWERS

Sharon M. Coyer, RN, PhD, CPNP, APN
Assistant Professor
Northern Illinois University
School of Nursing
DeKalb, Illinois

Richard E. Dumont, RN, MSN
Manager
Prisma Mental Health Center
Waalwijk, The Netherlands

Marilyn L. Greer, RN, MS
Associate Professor
Department of Nursing
Rockford College
Rockford, Illinois

Carey Hovestol, RN, BSN
Pediatric Nurse
Longmont United Hospital
Longmont, Colorado

Charlotte A. Kuss, RN, MSN
Nurse Educator
Okaloosa-Walton College
Niceville, Florida

Brenda Kay Lenz, RN, PhD
Assistant Professor
Department of Nursing Science
St. Cloud State University
St. Cloud, Minnesota

Donna McBrien, RN, MSN
Nursing Instructor
Vinal Tech Practical Nurse Program
Middletown, Connecticut

Marion E. McRae, RN, BC, MSN, CCRN, CCN, APRN, BC
Acute Care Nurse Practitioner
Cardiac Surgery
Toronto General Hospital
Toronto, Canada

Ronald Napier, LVN
Children's Hospital—Central California
Madera, California

Melanie S. Percy, RN, PhD, CPNP, FAAN
Assistant Professor
New York University
College of Nursing
New York, New York

Marcia L. Scott, RN, MSN
Professor of Nursing
Polk Community College
Winter Haven, Florida

PREFACE

Children are precious gifts. Two of the most satisfying nursing roles are being a resource to children and families as they develop their own unique identities and comforting them in times of illness and stress. Holding a child, talking softly, or entering into imaginary play—all are parts of nursing children. Hugging or sitting quietly with a parent, explaining a procedure or a disease, or providing reassurance through quiet, competent care can literally change the way a parent views the child's experience of illness.

High-quality nursing care of children combines compassion with the most up-to-date clinical knowledge grounded in basic theoretical principles of nursing care. This third edition of *Nursing Care of Children: Principles & Practice* emphasizes evidence-based nursing care throughout. This scientific base is demonstrated in the narrative and features in which the nursing process is applied. Nursing process elements incorporate both Nursing Outcomes Classification (NOC) and Nursing Interventions Classifications (NIC) terminology. Physiologic and pathophysiologic processes are presented in a format that assists the student to understand why health problems occur and how to derive appropriate nursing care. Current references provide the student with the latest information that applies to the clinical area. National standards and guidelines, such as those from the American Nurses Association and the Society of Pediatric Nurses, have been incorporated where applicable.

This text addresses contemporary changes in health care, recognizing that health care costs have led to shorter hospital stays and a shift to health care provided in the community and the home. The third edition of *Nursing Care of Children* includes a strong focus on the growing and changing roles of nurses caring for children in varied settings. To expand and enhance its community emphasis, the text incorporates both the *Healthy People 2010* national objectives and material from the *Bright Futures* health promotion guidelines project. In addition, adaptation of principles to the home, community, and school settings is illustrated throughout and has been increased in this edition.

The text's emphasis on health and wellness is found in a comprehensive unit covering growth and development, with anticipatory guidance for families. This unit is organized around the recommended schedule of well visits as described by the American Academy of Pediatrics. Health Promotion boxes assist students with information needed to understand developmental milestones, health promotion activities, and anticipatory guidance for infants and children of specific ages and developmental levels.

Legal and ethical issues add to the complexity of practice for today's nurse. The first chapter of our book discusses the ethical and legal obligations of nurses who work with children and how to meet these obligations while providing optimum client care. Issues such as including children in research, what constitutes a mature minor, and the care of technology-dependent children are discussed where applicable throughout the book.

Contemporary nursing students have time demands from work, family, and community activities in addition to their nursing education. A significant number of students use English as a second language. With those realities in mind, we have written a text to effectively convey essential information that focuses on critical elements and that is concise without unnecessarily complex language. Important items are defined on the first page of each chapter for ready access as the student studies. Teaching guidelines in the form of Want to Know boxes and other material are written in language that will assist students to teach parents and children about home care, self-care, preventive care, and follow-up care.

In keeping with the focus of incorporating Evidence-Based Practice as a thread throughout most nursing curricula, this edition includes a new feature, Using Research to Improve Practice, which facilitates critical thinking about how research could be used in a practice setting.

CONCEPTS

Several conceptual threads are interwoven throughout the text.

Family—The nurse must care for the child within the context of the family. In this text, emphasis is placed on the importance of focusing on the family when caring for children of all ages and in many different settings. Changing family structure and diversity in types of families are considered. Special sections are devoted to the needs of siblings.

Growth and development within the concept of health promotion—Concepts of health promotion and anticipatory guidance are organized around a developmental framework. A general chapter on health promotion for developing children describes the various developmental assessment areas—parameters of growth; factors influencing growth and development; developmental milestones, including a description of the Denver Developmental Screening Test II; play; nutrition; immunizations; and safety. Each of the subsequent growth and development chapters discusses these areas as they apply to the infant, child, or adolescent of a specific age or developmental level. Each also provides a review of physical and psychosocial changes unique to that age-group and emphasizes the nurse's role with children of specific ages and at varying developmental levels.

Child advocacy—Legal and ethical responsibilities of nurses are identified and explained in such areas as violence, abuse, neglect, drug abuse, and access to health care.

Communication—Communicating appropriately with children can be a challenge. The third edition includes special Communication Cues and describes techniques to enhance therapeutic communication with children and families. An entire chapter is devoted to communicating with children and families.

Culture—Cultural variety characterizes nursing practice today as the lines between individual nations become more blurred. The nurse must assess for the child's and family's unique cultural needs and incorporate them in care as much as possible to promote the acceptance of nursing intervention. Cultural influences are examined in many ways in our text, and principles of culturally sensitive care are incorporated throughout as an important thread.

TEXT ORGANIZATION

Similar to the second edition, the text uses an objective-oriented approach that makes it easy for students to understand and retain important material. Nursing care sections are organized around nursing process because of the ability to teach easily using a problem-solving method. The text begins with an overview of contemporary nursing of children, including general principles of care. Comprehensive growth and development chapters follow. Principles for adapting care of well children to those requiring admission to an emergency or hospital setting precede the final chapters, which cover care of children with specific health alterations. Narrative coverage of important childhood disorders is consistently organized in a nursing process format, again with NANDA diagnoses, expected outcomes, and evaluation questions. Less common disorders are grouped and discussed in tables in each body system chapter.

FEATURES

Visual appeal characterizes many features in the text. Beautiful full-color illustrations and photographs convey clinical information and also capture the essence of nursing care of children. Illustrations reinforce knowledge of growth and development, explain pathophysiology, make learning procedures easier, show manifestations of diseases and disorders, and provide models of interactions with patients and families.

Learning Objectives

Learning Objectives provide direction for the reader to understand what is important to glean from the chapter. Many objectives ask that the learner use critical thinking and apply the nursing process—two crucial components of professional nursing.

Health Promotion Boxes

Health Promotion boxes summarize needed information to perform a comprehensive assessment of well infants and children at various ages. Organized around the AAP-recommended schedule for well child visits, examples are given of questions designed to elicit developmental and behavioral information from parent and child. These boxes also include what the student might expect to see for health screening or immunization and review specific topics for anticipatory guidance.

Nursing Process

Although all steps of the nursing process are used consistently in nursing process sections, nursing process appears in two different formats throughout the text. The different formats show the student that there is more than one way to communicate nursing process. Nursing process can be applied to care of children with the most common childhood conditions through an *in-text discussion* that demonstrates how the process relates to a typical child with a specific condition. Nursing process for children with more complex nursing problems is illustrated through the use of a *care plan format*, which encompasses focused assessment, nursing diagnoses, expected outcomes, interventions, rationales, and evaluation criteria. This format helps the nursing instructor teach students how to individualize care for their specific clients based on a generic plan of care.

Critical Thinking Exercises

Critical thinking is encouraged in multiple ways throughout *Nursing Care of Children*, but specific Critical Thinking Exercises are included in all chapters in the text. These present scenarios of real-life situations or issues and ask the student to solve nursing care problems that are not always obvious. Answers are given at the end of each chapter, so the students can check solutions to these problems.

Critical to Remember Boxes

Students always want to know, "Will this be on the test?" The authors cannot answer that question, but Critical to Remember boxes provide a condensed summary of very important information needed to deliver safe nursing care.

Want to Know Boxes

Because teaching is an essential part of nursing care, we give students teaching guidelines for common client needs in terms that most lay people can understand. The Want to Know boxes provide sample answers for questions that children or parents are most likely to ask.

Clinical Reference Pages

This edition continues the popular Clinical Reference pages, which are a resource for the student when reviewing basic anatomy and physiology and differences between children and adults as they pertain to the body system being discussed. They also include diagnostic studies, laboratory values, and nursing care associated with these procedures.

Pathophysiology Boxes

Pathophysiology boxes give the student a brief overview of how various illnesses occur. The boxes provide a scientific basis for understanding the therapeutic management of the illness and its nursing care.

Photo Stories

"A picture is worth a thousand words" applies to the Photo Stories. These help the student visualize well child examinations, developmental assessments, and other experiences of nursing care.

Procedure Boxes

Clinical skills are presented in Procedures boxes throughout the text. The text includes two chapters that describe step-by-step general and medication procedures used when caring for children. Many of these procedures have expanded to include home adaptations.

Drug Guide Boxes

Drug information is generally presented through Drug Guide boxes. Drug guides for specific, commonly used medications provide the student nurse with detailed information.

Key Concepts

Key Concepts summarize important points of each chapter. They provide a general review for the material just presented to help the student identify areas in which more study is needed.

ACKNOWLEDGMENTS

We would first like to thank our families and friends who supported us in this endeavor by understanding when we were unavailable and encouraging us when we were overwhelmed.

We express our sincere appreciation to the clinicians (listed on pp. vi and vii), experts in their fields, who contributed to the book. They provided the up-to-date clinical information needed in a teaching text. Thank-you is also extended to the reviewers, who very conscientiously made suggestions to improve the text.

Both Emily McKinney and Sharon Murray, who, along with us, were authors and editors of the recently published combined book, *Maternal-Child Nursing* (2nd edition), provided input that helped us focus on needed improvements for this edition. Their suggestions were invaluable. Catherine Jackson, nursing editor, worked with us to make our vision for an improved text a reality. Much appreciation goes to Michele Hayden, our Managing Editor. Her untiring work on our behalf has made this process go as smoothly as possible; it has been a pleasure working with one so skilled at problem-solving. Steve Ramay, project manager, saw to it that the production process proceeded in a timely fashion and responded quickly to our editing and production concerns.

Finally, as educators we both teach and learn from our students. Some of the new features in *Nursing Care of Children: Principles & Practice*, 3rd edition, have their origin in wonderful feedback given by our students about their learning needs. We hope that this edition supports and strengthens students' ability and desire to learn about this exciting and ever-changing specialty of ours.

Susan Rowen James, RN, PhD (c)
Jean Weiler Ashwill, RN, MSN

SPECIAL FEATURES

Chapter Openers
Chapter opening pages contain *Learning Objectives* and *Key Terms* and *Definitions* to help guide the student's understanding of material presented.

Using Research to Improve Practice
These special *boxes* assist students to use *research* and *evidence-based* guidelines to evaluate nursing interventions in relation to desired outcomes of nursing care.

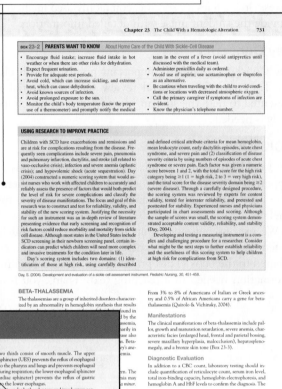

Electronic Resources
Electronic Resource boxes at the beginning of each chapter include a listing of associated activities on the *Companion CD* and *Evolve* website.

Clinical Reference
Special *Clinical Reference sections* open each alteration chapter, providing a review of basic anatomy and physiology, discussion of pediatric differences, and common diagnostic tests and medications.

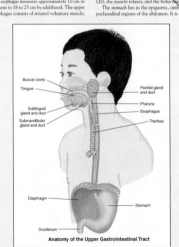

Marginal Notes
Handy *marginal notes* are placed throughout the text to highlight additional exercises and resources found on the *Companion CD* or *Evolve* website.

Procedures

Illustrated *Procedure boxes* provide clear, step-by-step instructions for common nursing tasks to assist students in clinical practice.

Pathophysiology

Pathophysiology boxes describe how disease conditions develop, presenting a scientific basis for understanding the therapeutic management and nursing care of an illness.

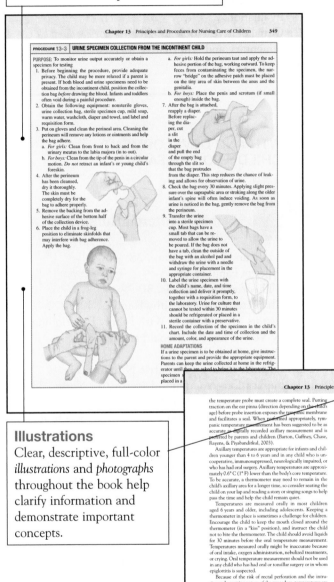

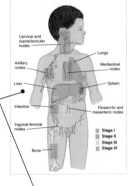

Illustrations

Clear, descriptive, full-color *illustrations* and *photographs* throughout the book help clarify information and demonstrate important concepts.

Critical To Remember

Critical To Remember boxes highlight vital information that is crucial to delivering safe nursing care.

Want to Know

Want to Know boxes guide the student in answering questions commonly asked and teaching the parents and child about self-care.

CONTENTS

22
The Child With a Cardiovascular Alteration, 664

26

The Child With a Musculoskeletal Alteration, 830

27
The Child With an Endocrine or Metabolic Alteration, 877

29
The Child With a Psychosocial Disorder, 963

30
The Child With a Cognitive Impairment, 997

31

The Child With a Sensory Alteration, 1019

APPENDIXES

CHAPTER 1

Introduction to Nursing Care of Children

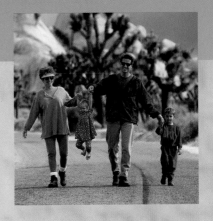

Learning Objectives

After studying this chapter, you should be able to:

- Describe the historic background of children's health care.
- Identify trends that led to the development of family-centered care of children.
- Describe issues that affect child health nursing, including cost containment, outcomes management, home care, and advances in technology.
- Discuss trends in infant and childhood mortality rates.
- Identify some of the effects of poverty and violence on children and families.
- Apply theories and principles of ethics to ethical dilemmas.
- Discuss ethical conflicts that the nurse may encounter in pediatric nursing practice.
- Relate how major social issues, such as poverty and access to health care, affect children's health.
- Describe the legal basis for nursing practice.
- Identify measures used to defend malpractice claims.
- Explain roles the nurse may assume in pediatric nursing practice.
- Explain the roles of nurses with advanced preparation for pediatric nursing practice.
- Explain the incorporation of critical thinking into nursing practice.
- Describe the steps of the nursing process and relate them to nursing care of children.
- Explain issues surrounding the use of complementary and alternative therapies.
- Discuss the importance of nursing research in clinical practice.

Definitions

advocacy   Speaking or arguing in support of a policy or a person's rights.

bioethics   Rules or principles that govern right conduct, specifically those that relate to health care.

case management   A practice model that uses a systematic approach to identify specific client needs and to manage client care to ensure optimal outcomes.

deontologic theory   Ethical theory that holds that the right course of action is the one dictated by ethical principles and moral rules.

ethical dilemma   A situation in which no solution seems completely satisfactory.

ethics   Rules or principles that govern right conduct and distinctions between right and wrong.

infant mortality rate   Number of deaths per 1000 live births that occur within the first 12 months of life.

malpractice   Negligence by a professional person.

morbidity   Ratio of sick to well persons in a defined population.

negligence   Failure to act in the way a reasonable, prudent person of similar background would act in similar circumstances.

neonatal mortality rate   Number of deaths per 1000 live births that occur before 28 days of life.

nurse practice acts   Laws that determine the scope of nursing practice in each state.

standard of care   Level of care that can be expected of a professional. This level is determined by laws, professional organizations, and health care agencies.

standardized procedures   Procedures determined by nurses, physicians, and administrators that allow nurses to perform duties usually part of the medical practice.

utilitarian theory   Ethical theory that holds that the right course of action is the one that produces the greatest good.

WIC   A Special Supplemental Food Program for Women, Infants, and Children that provides nutritious food and nutrition education to low-income pregnant and postpartum women and their children.

Audio Glossary

Electronic Resources

Additional information related to the content in Chapter 1 can be found on:

the interactive companion CD-ROM

- Audio Glossary
- NCLEX Review Questions

or the companion website at *evolve*
http://evolve.elsevier.com/james/ncoc

- NANDA-Approved Nursing Diagnoses
- NCLEX Review Questions
- Resources for Health Care Providers and Families
- WebLinks

PRINCIPLES OF CARING FOR CHILDREN

To better understand contemporary child health nursing, the nurse needs to understand the history of this field, trends and issues affecting contemporary practice, and the ethical and legal frameworks within which pediatric nursing care is provided.

HISTORIC PERSPECTIVES
Nursing of Children

The nursing care of children has been influenced by multiple historic and social factors. Children have not always enjoyed the valued position that they hold in most families today. Historically, in times of economic or social instability, children have been viewed as expendable. In societies in which the struggle for survival is the central issue and only the strongest survive, the needs of children are secondary. The well-being of children in the past depended on the economic and cultural conditions of the society. At times, parents have viewed their children as property and children have been bought and sold, beaten and, in some cultures, sacrificed in religious ceremonies. At times, infanticide has been a routine practice. Conversely, in other instances, children have been highly valued and their birth considered a blessing. Viewed by society as miniature adults, children in the past received the same remedies as adults and, during illness, were cared for at home by family members, just as adults were.

Societal Changes

On the North American continent, as European settlements expanded during the seventeenth and eighteenth centuries, children were valued as assets to the community because of the desire to increase the population and share the work. Public schools were established, and the courts began to view children as minors and protect them accordingly. Devastating epidemics of smallpox, diphtheria, scarlet fever, and measles took their toll on children in the eighteenth century. Children often died of these virulent diseases within 1 day.

The high mortality rate in children led some physicians to examine common child-care practices. In 1748 William Cadogan's "Essay Upon Nursing" discouraged unhealthy child-care practices, such as swaddling infants in three or four layers of clothing and feeding them thin gruel within hours after birth. Instead, Cadogan urged mothers to breast-feed their infants and identified certain practices that were thought to contribute to childhood illness. Unfortunately, despite the efforts of Cadogan and others, child-care practices were slow to change. Later in the eighteenth century, the health of children improved with certain advances such as inoculation against smallpox.

In the nineteenth century, with the flood of immigrants to eastern American cities, infectious diseases flourished as a result of crowded living conditions; inadequate and unsanitary food; and harsh working conditions for men, women, and children. Twelve- and 14-hour workdays were common for children working in factories, whose earnings were essential to the survival of the family. The most serious child health problems during the nineteenth century were caused by poverty and overcrowding. Infants were fed contaminated milk, sometimes from tuberculosis-infected cows. Milk was carried to the cities and purchased by mothers with no means to refrigerate it. Infectious diarrhea was a common cause of infant death.

During the late nineteenth century, conditions began to improve for children and families. Lillian Wald initiated public health nursing at Henry Street Settlement House in New York City, where nurses taught mothers in their homes. In 1889 a milk distribution center opened in New York City to provide uncontaminated milk to sick infants.

Hygiene and Hospitalization

The discoveries of scientists such as Pasteur, Lister, and Koch, who established that bacteria caused many diseases, supported the use of hygienic practices in hospitals and foundling homes. Hospitals began to require personnel to wear uniforms and limit contact among children in the wards. In an effort to prevent infection, hospital wards were closed to visitors. Because parental visits were noted to cause distress, particularly when parents had to leave, parental visitation was considered emotionally stressful to hospitalized children. In an effort to prevent such emotional distress and the spread of infection, parents were prohibited from visiting children in the hospital. As hospital care focused on preventing disease transmission and curing physical diseases, the emotional health of hospitalized children received little attention.

During the twentieth century, as knowledge about nutrition, sanitation, bacteriology, pharmacology, medication, and psychology increased, dramatic changes in child health occurred. In the 1940s and 1950s, medications such as penicillin and corticosteroids and vaccines against many communicable diseases saved the lives of tens of thousands of children. Technologic advances in the 1970s and 1980s, which led to

TABLE 1-1 Federal Projects for Maternal-Child Care	
Program	**Purpose**
Title V of Social Security Act	Provides funds for maternal-child health programs
National Institute of Health and Human Development	Supports research and education of personnel needed for maternal and child health programs
Title V Amendment of Public Health Service Act	Established the Maternal and Infant Care (MIC) projects to provide comprehensive prenatal and infant care in public clinics
Title XIX of Medicaid program	Provides funds to facilitate access to care by pregnant women and young children
Head Start	Provides educational opportunities for low-income children of preschool age
WIC Program	Provides supplemental food and nutrition information
Healthy Start	Enhances community development of culturally appropriate strategies designed to decrease infant mortality rate and causes of low birth weights
Individuals with Disabilities Education Act (PL 94-142)	Provides free and appropriate education for all disabled children
National School Lunch/Breakfast Program	Provides nutritionally appropriate free or reduced-price meals to students from low-income families

more children surviving conditions that had previously been fatal (e.g., cystic fibrosis), resulted in an increasing number of children living with chronic disabilities. An increase in societal concern for children brought about the development of federally supported programs designed to meet their needs, such as school lunch programs, the Special Supplemental Program for Women, Infants and Children (WIC), and Medicaid, under which the Early Periodic Screening, Diagnosis, and Treatment program was implemented (Table 1-1).

Development of Family-Centered Child Care

Family-centered child health care developed from the recognition that the emotional needs of hospitalized children usually were unmet. Parents were not involved in the direct care of their children. Children were often unprepared for procedures and tests, and visiting was severely controlled and even discouraged.

Family-centered care is based on a philosophy that recognizes and respects the pivotal role of the family in the lives of both well and ill children. It strives to support families in their natural caregiving roles and promotes healthy patterns of living at home and in the community. Finally, parents and professionals are viewed as equals in a partnership committed to excellence at all levels of health care.

Most health care settings have a family-centered philosophy in which families are given choices, provide input, and are given information that is understandable by them. The family is respected, and its strengths are recognized.

The Association for the Care of Children's Health (ACCH), an interdisciplinary organization, was founded in 1965 to provide a forum for sharing experiences and common problems and to foster growth in children who must undergo hospitalization. Today the organization has broadened its focus on child health care to include the community and the home.

Through the efforts of ACCH and other organizations, increasing attention has been paid to the psychologic and emotional effects of hospitalization during childhood. In response to greater knowledge about the emotional effects of illness and hospitalization, hospital policies and health care services for children have changed. Twenty-four-hour parental and sibling visitation policies and home care services have become common. The psychologic preparation of children for hospitalization and surgery has become standard nursing practice. Many hospitals have established child life programs to help children and their families cope with the stress of illness. Shorter hospital stays, home care, and day surgery have also helped minimize the emotional impact of hospitalization and illness on children.

CURRENT TRENDS IN CHILD HEALTH CARE

In 2000, the Department of Health and Human Services launched *Healthy People 2010* (USDHHS, 2000), a comprehensive, nationwide health promotion and disease prevention agenda. *Healthy People 2010* serves as a road map for improving the health of all people in the United States. Box 1-1 lists some of the national health objectives that are applicable to children and families. The National Center for Health Statistics monitors the nation's progress toward meeting the objectives of *Healthy People 2010*. National data measuring the objectives are gathered from federal and state departments and from voluntary private, nongovernmental organizations.

Nursing care of children has changed in focus as national attention to health promotion and disease prevention has increased. Even acutely ill children have only brief hospital stays because increased technology has facilitated parents' ability to care for children in the home or community setting. For example, children who formerly might have been hospitalized for repeated episodes of acute asthma can now

BOX 1-1	**Selected *Healthy People 2010* Objectives**
1-1	Increase the proportion of persons with health insurance.
1-2	Increase the proportion of insured persons with clinical preventive services.
1-3	Increase the proportion of persons appropriately counseled about health behaviors.
1-6	Reduce the proportion of families that experience difficulties or delays in obtaining health care or who do not receive needed care for one or more family members.
1-14	Increase the number of states and the District of Columbia that have implemented guidelines for prehospital and hospital pediatric care.
7-7	Increase the proportion of health care organizations that provide patient and family education.
7-11	Increase the proportion of local health departments that have established culturally appropriate and linguistically competent community health promotion and disease prevention programs for racial and ethnic minority populations.
21-12	Increase the proportion of children and adolescents under age 19 years at or below 200% of the federal poverty level who received any preventive dental service during the past year.
21-13	Increase the proportion of school-based health centers with an oral health component.

be managed in the home setting by using peak flow readings for assessing respiratory status and nebulized medication to manage some exacerbations. Most acute illnesses are managed in ambulatory settings, leaving hospital admission for the extremely acutely ill or children with complex medical needs. Nursing care for hospitalized children has become more specialized, and much nursing care is provided in community settings such as schools and outpatient clinics.

The current practice of child health nursing requires nurses to understand the importance of adapting procedures to the specific needs of children and families and to think critically about children's developmental differences. For example, why do infants and children become so acutely ill so quickly? Is there a smaller margin of safety when administering fluids or medications to children? Other adaptations are directed toward issues such as protecting children, providing for their activity, assessing nonverbal behaviors, planning and carrying out nursing care, and teaching home care to children and families. Table 1-2 presents principles of caring for children.

Cost Containment

In the past few years the government, insurance companies, hospitals, and health care providers have made a concerted effort to reform health care delivery in the United States and control rising costs. This trend has involved a change in where and how money is spent.

One way in which those paying for health care have attempted to control costs is by shifting to a *prospective* form of payment. In this arrangement, clients no longer pay whatever charges the hospital determines for service provided. Instead, a fixed amount of money is agreed on in advance for necessary services for specifically diagnosed conditions. Any of several strategies may be used to contain the cost of services.

Diagnosis-Related Groups

Diagnosis-related groups (DRGs) are a method of classifying related medical diagnoses based on the amount of resources that are generally required by the patient. This method became a standard in 1987, when the federal government set the amount of money that would be paid by Medicare for each DRG. If the facility delivers more services or has greater costs than what it will be reimbursed for by Medicare, the facility must absorb the excess costs. Conversely, if the facility delivers the care at less cost than the payment for that DRG, the facility keeps the remaining money. Health care facilities working under this arrangement benefit financially if they can reduce the client's length of stay and thereby reduce the costs for service. Although the DRG system originally applied only to Medicare clients, most states have adopted the system for Medicaid payments, and many insurance companies use a similar system.

Managed Care

Health insurance companies also examined the cost of health care and instituted a health care delivery system that has been called *managed care*. Examples of managed care organizations are health maintenance organizations (HMOs), point of service plans (POSs), and preferred provider organizations (PPOs). HMOs provide relatively comprehensive health services for persons enrolled in the organization for a set fee or premium. Similarly, PPOs are groups of health care providers that agree to provide health services to a specific group of clients at a discounted cost. When the client needs medical treatment, managed care includes strategies such as payment arrangements and preadmission or pretreatment authorization to control costs.

Capitated Care

Capitation may be incorporated into any type of managed care plan. In a pure capitated care plan, the employer (or government) pays a set amount of money each year to a network of primary care providers. This amount might be adjusted for age and sex of the client group. In exchange for access to a guaranteed client base, the primary care providers agree to provide general health care and pay for all aspects of the clients' care, including laboratory work, specialist visits, and hospital care.

Capitated plans allow a predictable amount of money to be budgeted for health care, thereby ensuring that clients do not have unexpected financial burdens from illness. However, clients lose most of their freedom of choice regarding who will provide their care. Providers can lose money (1) if

TABLE 1-2   Nursing of Children: Principles of Care

Principle	Description
Growth and Development	The nurse applies growth and development principles to meet the child's physical and emotional needs. Involves understanding the principles of maturation, physiologic immaturity, and response to illness. Nursing care is tailored to the child's chronologic age and developmental level.
Health Promotion	Guides the child and family toward independent responsibility for health. Anticipatory guidance is education that facilitates health promotion by providing developmentally appropriate information about nutrition, exercise, safety, play, and wellness issues such as immunizations and injury prevention.
Family Focus	Family-centered care is at the core of nursing of children because of the intimate relationship between the child and family in areas of support, love, security, values, beliefs, attitudes, and health practices. Because the family is a partner in the child's care, the nurse provides information for appropriate decision-making, assesses family needs, and refers the family to appropriate resources within the community.
Child Advocacy	Includes specific responsibilities as child advocates in the areas of health promotion, violence, abuse, neglect, drug abuse, infant morbidity and mortality, and access to care. Nurses exercise legal and ethical responsibilities cautiously, being aware of their accountability.
Communication	Nurses use a variety of techniques to communicate with children and families in a developmentally appropriate manner. Includes use of play and other developmentally appropriate verbal and non-verbal communication techniques for effective communication.
Concepts Applied Across Age Groups	Integration of the principles of pediatric nursing care across many disorders and with all age-groups. Recognizes that with any health encounter, children may have needs related to play and activity, chronicity, nutrition, safety, illness, and family. Knowing pathophysiologic human development, family theory, and evidence-based principles enhances nursing care.

they refer too many clients to specialists, who may have no restrictions on their fees; (2) if they order too many diagnostic tests; or (3) if their administrative costs are too high. Some health care providers and consumers fear that cost constraints might affect treatment decisions.

Effects of Cost Containment

Prospective payment plans have had major effects on infant care, primarily in relation to the length of stay. Mothers who have a normal vaginal birth are typically discharged from the hospital at 48 hours, and mothers who give birth by cesarean section leave at 96 hours. Many mothers and infants developed problems with shorter lengths of stay, sometimes called "drive-through deliveries," that were mandated under early prospective pay arrangements. The problems often required disruptive readmission and more expensive treatment than might have been needed if the problem had been identified early. As a result, many states passed legislation requiring a minimum 48-hour length of stay for vaginal births and 4 days for cesarean births, unless the woman and her health care provider choose an earlier discharge time. Some insurance plans use a compromise, in which the woman who elects to leave 24 hours after vaginal birth is provided one or more home visits by a nurse to check on her status and that of her baby.

Reduced lengths of stay have also affected caregivers, particularly nurses. Since the mid-1990s, nurses have become increasingly concerned with meeting the needs of families who leave the hospital shortly after the birth of an infant or during an acute health episode. Nurses find providing adequate information about self-care and infant care especially difficult when the mother is still recovering from childbirth.

A concern exists that children with chronic health care conditions may receive a higher degree of denial of care. Denial of care can result in negative sequelae, leading to the need for additional care, missed school or work, pain, or worsening of the child's condition (Valet, Kutney, Hickson, & Cooper, 2004).

Managed care, provided appropriately, can increase access to a full range of health care providers and services, but it must be closely monitored. Child health nurses serve as child advocates in the areas of preventive, acute, and long-term care. The teaching timelines for preventive and home care have been shortened drastically, and the call to "begin teaching the moment the child enters the health care system" has taken on a new meaning. Parents and other caregivers are being asked to perform procedures at home that were once done by professionals in a hospital setting. Systems must be in place to monitor adherence, understanding, and the total care of the child. Assessment and communication skills need to be keen, and the nurse must be able to work with specialists in other disciplines.

Case Management

Case management is a practice model that uses a systematic approach to identify specific clients and manage care collaboratively to ensure optimal outcomes through access to the best available resources (Alfaro-LeFevre, 2004). In this model, a case manager or case coordinator, who focuses on both quality and cost outcomes, coordinates the services needed by the client and family. Inherent to case management is the coordination of care by all members of the health care team. The guidelines established in 1995 by the Joint

Commission on the Accreditation of Healthcare Organizations require an interdisciplinary, collaborative approach to client care. This concept is at the core of case management. Nurses who provide case management evaluate client needs, establish needs documentation to support reimbursement, and may be part of long-term care planning in the home or a rehabilitation facility.

Clinical Practice Guidelines

The Agency for Healthcare Research and Quality (AHRQ), a branch of the United States Public Health Service, actively sponsors research in health issues facing children. From research generated through this agency as well as others, evidence can be accumulated to guide the best clinical practices. Priority children's health issues for the AHRQ include acute care/injuries; adolescent health; asthma; attention deficit–hyperactivity disorder; chronic illness; and cost, use, and access to care. Other major areas for ongoing research include emergency care/hospitalization, mental health, newborns and infants, oral health, otitis media, preventive services, and quality of care/patient safety (AHRQ, 2002). For detailed information, see the organizations website at *www.ahcpr.gov.*

Clinical practice guidelines are an important tool in developing guidelines for safe, effective care. The AHRQ has developed several guidelines related to child care (AHRQ National Guideline Clearinghouse, 2005): lead exposure, sudden infant death syndrome prevention, car safety seats, management of gastroesophageal reflux disease, poisonings, and asthma control, among others. Continued research and sharing of information in this area are needed to ensure quality case management.

Outcomes Management

The determination to lower health care costs while maintaining the quality of care has led to a clinical practice model called *outcomes management.* This is a systematic method to identify client outcomes and focus care on interventions that will accomplish the stated outcomes for specific case types, such as the child with asthma. The planning tools used by the health care team to identify and meet stated outcomes are known as *clinical pathways.* Other names for clinical pathways include *critical paths, clinical paths, care paths, care maps, collaborative plans of care, anticipated recovery paths,* and *multidisciplinary action plans.*

Clinical Pathways

Clinical pathways are standardized, interdisciplinary plans of care devised for clients with a particular health problem. Clinical pathways identify client outcomes, specify timelines to achieve those outcomes, direct appropriate interventions and sequencing of interventions, include interventions from a variety of disciplines, promote collaboration, and involve a comprehensive approach to care. Although the concept of clinical pathways is not new, it has only recently been widely accepted as the use of case management has become widespread in various health care settings. The purpose, as in managed care and case management, is to provide quality care while controlling costs.

Clinical pathways can be used in settings other than the hospital. Home health agencies use clinical pathways, which may be developed in collaboration with hospital staff.

Facilities differ in how they use clinical pathways. For instance, they may be used for change-of-shift reports to indicate information about length of stay, individual needs, and priorities of the shift for each child. They may also be used for documentation of the child's nursing care plan and his or her progress in meeting the desired outcomes. Many pathways are particularly helpful in identifying families that need follow-up care (see p. 626 for an example of a clinical pathway).

Variances. Deviations, often called *variances,* may occur, either in the timeline or the expected outcomes. A variance is the difference between what was expected and what actually happened. A variance may be positive or negative. A positive variance occurs when a client progresses faster than expected and is discharged sooner than planned. A negative variance occurs when progress is slower than expected, outcomes are not met within the designated time frame, and the length of stay is prolonged.

Students' Use of Clinical Pathways. Clinical pathways are guidelines for care. Although a pathway provides insight into the scheduling of assessments and care, it is not meant to teach nursing skills and procedures. One purpose of this text is to provide ample information so that students can *use* clinical pathways in a clinical setting. This involves teaching *why and how to perform assessments* and interpreting the significance of the data obtained. Moreover, the text emphasizes ways of providing information, care, and comfort for children and their families as they progress along a clinical pathway.

Home Care

Home nursing care for children has experienced dramatic growth since 1990. Advances in portable technology, such as infusion pumps for the administration of intravenous fluids and various monitoring devices, allow nurses to perform complicated procedures in the home. In addition, consumers often prefer home care because of decreased stress on the family when the child is able to remain at home rather than be separated from the family support system because of the need for hospitalization.

Home care services may be provided in the form of telephone calls, home visits, information lines, and lactation consultations, among others. Infants with congenital anomalies, such as cleft palate, may need care that is adapted to their condition. Moreover, increasing numbers of technology-dependent infants and children are now cared for at home. The numbers include those needing ventilator assistance, total parenteral nutrition, intravenous medications, apnea monitoring, and other device-associated nursing care.

Nurses must be able to function independently within established protocols and must be confident of their clinical skills when providing home care. They should be proficient at interviewing, counseling, and teaching. They often assume a leadership role in coordinating all the services a child and family may require, and they frequently supervise the work of other care providers.

A model for community care of children is the school-based health center. School-based health centers provide comprehensive primary health care services in the most accessible environment. Students can be evaluated, diagnosed, and treated on site. Services offered include primary preventive care, including health assessments, anticipatory guidance, vision and hearing screenings, and immunizations; acute care; prescription services; and mental health and counseling services. Some school-based health centers are sponsored by hospitals, local health departments, and community health centers. A shift from inner city to rural areas has also occurred (Brindis et al, 2003). Many are used in off hours to provide health care to uninsured adults and adolescents.

Health Insurance

Access to care is an important component when evaluating preventive care and prompt treatment of illness and injuries.

Access to health care is strongly associated with having health insurance. Having health insurance coverage, usually employer sponsored, often determines whether a person will seek care early in the course of an illness. The number of uninsured children in the United States between 2003 and 2004 remained unchanged at 11.2% (Fig. 1-1). Health insurance coverage varied among children by poverty, age, race, and ethnic (Hispanic) origin (National Center for Health Statistics, 2004; DeNavas-Walt, Proctor, & Lee, 2005). Children in poor and near-poor families are more likely to be uninsured, have unmet medical needs, receive delayed medical care, have no usual provider of health care, and have higher

rates of emergency room service than children in families that are not poor. Five percent of all children have no usual place of health care (Dey & Bloom, 2005).

Public health insurance for children is provided primarily through Medicaid or the State Children's Health Insurance Program (SCHIP), a program that provides access for children not poor enough to be eligible for Medicaid but whose household income is less than 200% of poverty level. Medicaid-covered medical payments increased by 10.3% from 2001 to 2002. In 2002, 24.5% of children younger than 18 years were covered by Medicaid, a 3.3% increase over the previous year (National Center for Health Statistics, 2004). Medicaid provides health care for the poor, aged, and disabled, with pregnant women and young children especially targeted. Medicaid is funded by both the federal government and individual state governments. The states administer the program and determine which services are offered.

Medicaid can be frustrating for a family. The application process often takes weeks. The family must fill out lengthy, complicated forms, provide documentation of income, and then wait for determination of eligibility. Medicaid criteria may deny payment for some services that are routinely provided to those who hold private insurance. Welfare reforms instituted in 1996 made the eligibility process more difficult for legal immigrants. The Balanced Budget Act of 1997 resolved some of these issues, but foreign-born, non-English-speaking people find navigating the system of application excessively difficult (Truong & Ferguson, 2003).

Some physicians and dentists are unwilling to care for Medicaid clients who are likely to be at high risk. Many are especially unwilling if reimbursement is slow and less than that paid by other insurers. With their continual concern about malpractice suits, physicians may be less inclined to accept high-risk, lower-paying clients.

Oral health of children in the United States has become a topic of increasing focus. Services available through Medicaid are limited, and as many as 48% of national dental expenditures are out of pocket compared with only 18% for physician services (Gorbova & John, 2004). In addition, maternal periodontal disease is emerging as a contributing factor to prematurity, with its adverse effects on the child's long-term health.

During the late 1990s, insurance coverage among children increased because of the state insurance expansion for low-income children and SCHIP. The proportion of children with health insurance is lower among American Indian/Alaska Native and Hispanic children compared with white children and among poor, near-poor, and middle-income children compared with high-income children (AHRQ, 2004b). Besides the obvious implication of not having health insurance—the inability to pay for health care during illness—another important effect on children who are not insured exists: they are less likely to receive preventive care such as immunizations and dental care. This places them at increased risk for preventable illnesses and, because preventive health care is a learned behavior, these children are more likely to become adults who are less healthy.

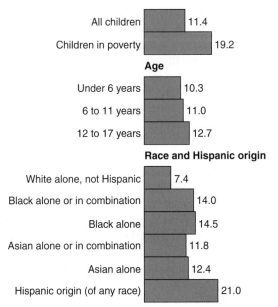

FIG 1-1 **Uninsured children by race, Hispanic origin, and age: 2003.** *(From DeNavas-Walt, C., Proctor, B. D., & Mills, R. J. (2003). Income, poverty, and health insurance coverage in the United States: 2003. U.S. Census Bureau, Current Population Reports. Washington, DC: U.S. Government Printing Office.)*

Health Care Assistance Programs

Many programs, some funded privately and others by the government, assist in the care of infants and children. The supplemental food program known as the WIC program, which was established in 1972, provides supplemental food supplies to low-income women who are pregnant or breast-feeding and their children up to the age of 5 years. The WIC program has long been heralded as a cost-effective program that provides nutritional support and links families with other services, such as prenatal care and immunizations.

Medicaid's Early and Periodic Screening, Diagnosis, and Treatment Program was developed to provide comprehensive health care to Medicaid recipients from birth to 21 years of age. The goal of the program is to prevent health problems before they become severe. This program pays for well-child examinations and for the treatment of any medical problems diagnosed during such checkups.

Public Law 99-457 is the part of the Individuals with Disabilities Act that provides financial incentives to states to establish comprehensive early intervention services for infants and toddlers with, or at risk for developmental disabilities. Services include screening, identification, referral, and treatment. Although this is a federal law and entitlement, each state bases coverage on its own definition of developmental delay. Thus coverage may vary from state to state. Some states provide care for at-risk children.

The Healthy Start Program, begun in 1991, is a major initiative to reduce infant deaths in communities with disproportionately high infant mortality rates. Strategies used include reducing the number of high-risk pregnancies, reducing the number of low-birth-weight and preterm births, improving birth weight–specific survival, and ameliorating specific causes of postneonatal death.

The March of Dimes, long an advocate for improving the health of infants and children, launched a campaign in 2003 to reduce the devastating toll that prematurity takes on the population. Between 1981 and 2003, the incidence of prematurity increased nearly 31%, often resulting in permanent health or developmental problems for survivors (March of Dimes, 2005). In 2004 a campaign was launched by the March of Dimes to expand funding for research into the causes of and potential interventions for preventing preterm births (see *www.modimes.org/prematurity* for information about this campaign).

STATISTICS ON INFANT AND CHILD HEALTH

Statistics are important sources of information about the health of groups of people. They may also be an indication of the value a society places on health care and the kind of health care available to the people. The newest statistics about infant and child health for the United States can be obtained from the National Center for Health Statistics (*www.cdc.gov/nchs*).

Death

Throughout history, infants have had high mortality rates, especially shortly after birth. Infant mortality rates began to fall when the health of the general population improved, basic principles of sanitation were put into practice, and medical knowledge increased. A further large decrease was a result of the widespread availability of antibiotics, improvements in public health, and better prenatal care in the 1940s and 1950s.

Infant Mortality

The infant mortality rate (death before the age of 1 year) increased from 6.8 infant deaths per 1000 live births in 2001 to 7.0 in 2002. This information was first reported in 2004. The rate in 2001 was the lowest rate ever recorded in the United States, and the 2002 rate was the first increase in the United States since 1958. Preliminary data for 2003 indicate that the increase may not continue. The upward move was primarily caused by an increase in the number of infants born weighing less than 750 g. The majority of infants born weighing less than 750 g die within the first year of life, contributing disproportionately to the overall infant mortality rate. This increase was not concentrated in any particular maternal age or race/ethnic group (Matthews, Menacker, & MacDorman, 2004).

Racial Disparity for Infant Mortality. Although infant mortality rates have declined for all racial and ethnic groups, large disparities remain (National Center for Health Statistics, 2004). Figure 1-2 compares the rates of infant mortality for all races from 2001 to 2002. The racial differences in both maternal and infant mortality rates are obvious when rates for African Americans are compared with those for other races. Much of the racial disparity for infant mortality is attributable to premature (born before 37 weeks' gestation) and low-birth-weight infants (less than 2500 g), both more common among African-American infants. Premature and low-birth-weight infants have a greater risk for short-term and long-term health problems as well as death (Anderson & Smith, 2003).

Poverty is an important factor in infant mortality. More nonwhites than whites are poor in the United States. Poor people are less likely to be in good health, be well nourished, or get the health care they need. Obtaining care becomes vital during pregnancy and infancy, and lack of care is reflected in the high mortality rates in all categories.

International Infant Mortality. A nation such as the United States would likely be expected to have one of the lowest infant mortality rates when compared with other developed countries. The most recent year for which comparative international data on infant mortality are available is 2000, slightly older than data for the United States only. These data show that the infant mortality rate in the United States is twenty-seventh compared with other countries in the world (Table 1-3). International rankings are difficult to compare because countries differ in how and when they compute statistics, but the numbers show the need for improvement in the United States.

The major reasons for the poor U.S. showing are (1) unequal access to health care for women of different socioeconomic levels and (2) excess of low-birth-weight and premature infants. Disorders related to short gestation, low birth weight, and congenital anomalies are the leading causes of

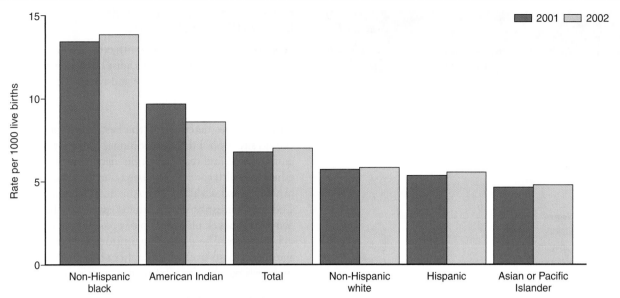

FIG 1-2 **Infant mortality rates by race and ethnicity, 2001 and 2002.** *(From Mathews, T. J., Menacker, F., & MacDorman, F. (2004).* Infant mortality statistics from the 2002 period linked birth/infant death data set, 53(10). *Hyattsville, MD: National Center for Health Statistics.)*

neonatal death. Sudden infant death syndrome and congenital anomalies are the leading causes of infant deaths after the first month of life.

Adolescent Pregnancy

U.S. adolescent birth rates have declined by one third since 1991. The rate for teens aged 15 to 19 years decreased 3% to a record low in 2003 of 41.7 per 1000 births (Martin et al, 2003; Martin et al, 2005).

The birth rate for younger teens, aged 10 to 14 years, declined to 0.6 per 1000, with the fewest reported in nearly 60 years. This decline was seen among all racial and ethnic subgroups as well as in almost all states. Teen mothers have the lowest level of prenatal care initiated during the first trimester and experience almost twice the rates of preterm delivery; the infant mortality rate in this group is two to three times higher than that for infants of mothers aged 20 to 44 years (Menacker, Martin, MacDorman, & Ventura, 2004).

Childhood Mortality Rates

Death rates for children have significantly declined over the past 20 years. Table 1-4 shows the leading causes of death in children aged 1 to 14 years. Although death rates attributed to unintentional injury have also dropped, they are still the leading cause of death in children aged 1 to 19 years. Homicide is the second leading cause of death for children older than 14 years. Other common causes of death in children include congenital malformations, malignant neoplasms, and cardiac and respiratory diseases. Self-inflicted injury is a leading cause of death in the adolescent population (National Center for Health Statistics, 2004).

Morbidity

Morbidity refers to illness. The morbidity rate is the ratio of sick to well persons in a population and is presented as the number of ill persons per 1000 population. This term is used

TABLE 1-3 Infant Mortality Rates for Selected Countries	
Country	**Infant Mortality (per 1000 Live Births)**
Singapore	2.5
Hong Kong	3.0
Japan	3.2
Sweden	3.4
Finland	3.8
Norway	3.8
Spain	3.9
Czech Republic	4.1
Germany	4.4
Italy	4.5
France	4.6
Austria	4.8
Belgium	4.8
Switzerland	4.9
Netherlands	5.1
Northern Ireland	5.1
Australia	5.2
Canada	5.3
Denmark	5.3
Israel	5.4
Portugal	5.5
England and Wales	5.6
Scotland	5.7
Greece	6.1
Ireland	6.2
New Zealand	6.3
United States	6.9

Based on 2000 data.
Reprinted from National Center for Health Statistics (2004). Health, United States, 2004 with chartbook on trends in the health of Americans. Hyattsville, MD: U.S. Government Printing Office.

TABLE **1-4**	Death Rates (per 100,000): Leading Causes of Death Among Children Ages 1 to 14 Years

Ages 1-4 Years

Unintentional injury	11.1
Congenital malformations	3.6
Malignant neoplasms	2.7
Homicide	2.6
Diseases of the heart	1-4
Pneumonia and influenza	0.7
Septicemia	0.7

Ages 5-14 Years

Unintentional injury	6.8
Malignant neoplasms	2.4
Congenital malformations	0.9
Homicide	0.8
Suicide	0.7
Diseases of the heart	0.6
In situ neoplasm/benign neoplasm	0.3

Reprinted from United States Department of Health and Human Services, Health Resources and Services Administration, Maternal and Child Health Bureau. (2003). *Child Health USA 2003.* Rockville, MA: Author.

in reference to acute and chronic illness as well as disability. Because morbidity statistics are collected and updated less frequently than mortality statistics, the presentation of current data in all areas of child health is difficult.

Diseases of the respiratory system are a major cause of hospitalization for children aged 1 to 9 years. Twelve percent of children younger than 18 years have been diagnosed with asthma and 13% have respiratory allergies, of which 9% are from hay fever and 13% are from other allergies. Seven percent of children have unmet dental needs, and dental decay is the second most common chronic disease among children (Dey & Bloom, 2005; USDHHS, 2005). Statistics regarding morbidity related to particular disorders are presented throughout this text as the disorders are discussed.

The Youth Risk Behavior Surveillance System has identified categories of health risk behaviors among youth that contribute to increased morbidity rates: tobacco use; unhealthy dietary behaviors; inadequate physical activity; alcohol and other drug use; sexual behaviors that may result in HIV infection, other sexually transmissible diseases, and unintended pregnancies; and behaviors that result in intentional injuries (violence, suicide) and unintentional injuries (motor vehicle crashes) (National Center for Health Statistics, 2004).

A link exists between children living in poverty and poorer health outcomes. Children who live in families of higher income and higher education have a better chance of being born healthy and remaining healthy. Access to health care, the health behaviors of parents and siblings, and exposure to environmental risks are among the factors contributing to the disparity in children's health (Velsor-Friedrich, 2003; National Center for Health Statistics, 2004).

ETHICAL PERSPECTIVES IN CHILD HEALTH NURSING

Pediatric nurses often struggle with ethical and social dilemmas that affect families. Nurses must know how to approach these issues in a knowledgeable and systematic way.

Ethics and Bioethics

Ethics involves determining the best course of action in a certain situation. Ethical reasoning is the analysis of what is morally right and reasonable. *Bioethics* is the application of ethics to health care. Ethical behavior for nurses is described in various codes, such as the American Nurses Association Code for Nurses (Box 1-2). Ethical issues have become more complex as developing technology has allowed more options in health care. These issues are controversial because a lack of agreement exists over what is right or best and because moral support is possible for more than one course of action.

Ethical Dilemmas

An ethical dilemma is a situation in which no solution seems completely satisfactory. Opposing courses of action may seem equally desirable, or all possible solutions may seem undesirable. Ethical dilemmas are among the most difficult situations in nursing practice. Finding solutions involves applying ethical theories and principles and determining the burdens and benefits of any course of action.

Ethical Principles

Ethical principles are also important in solving ethical dilemmas. Four of the most important principles are beneficence, nonmaleficence, autonomy, and justice (Box 1-3). Although principles guide decision making, in some situations the application of one principle may be impossible without encountering conflict with another. In such cases, one principle may outweigh another in importance.

For example, treatments designed to do good may also cause some harm. A child who undergoes chemotherapy may see improvement or disappearance of the cancer. However, the chemotherapy that cures the cancer can harm other body organs. In this instance the caregiver and parent need to weigh the principle of beneficence against the principle of nonmaleficence.

Solving Ethical Dilemmas

Although using a specific approach does not guarantee a right decision, it provides a logical, systematic method for going through the steps of decision making.

Decision making in ethical dilemmas may seem straightforward, but it may not result in answers agreeable to everyone. Many agencies, therefore, have bioethics committees to formulate policies for ethical situations, provide education, and help make decisions in specific cases. These committees include a variety of professionals such as nurses, physicians, social workers, ethicists, and clergy members. The child and family also participate, if possible. A satisfactory solution to ethical dilemmas is more likely to occur when a variety of people work together. At times, solutions to ethical dilemmas

---

BOX 1-2 | **ANA Code for Nurses**

1. The nurse provides services with respect for human dignity and the uniqueness of the client unrestricted by considerations of social or economic status, personal attributes, or the nature of health problems.
2. The nurse safeguards the client's right to privacy by judiciously protecting information of a confidential nature.
3. The nurse acts to safeguard the client and the public when health care and safety are affected by the incompetent, unethical, or illegal practice of any person.
4. The nurse assumes responsibility and accountability for individual nursing judgments and actions.
5. The nurse maintains competence in nursing.
6. The nurse exercises informed judgment and uses individual competence and qualifications as criteria in seeking consultation, accepting responsibilities, and delegating nursing activities to others.
7. The nurse participates in activities that contribute to the ongoing development of the profession's body of knowledge.
8. The nurse participates in the profession's efforts to implement and improve standards of nursing.
9. The nurse participates in the profession's efforts to establish and maintain conditions of employment conducive to high-quality nursing care.
10. The nurse participates in the profession's effort to protect the public from misinformation and misrepresentation and to maintain the integrity of nursing.
11. The nurse collaborates with members of the health professions and other citizens in promoting community and national efforts to meet the health needs of the public.

Reprinted from American Nurses Association. (1985). *Code for nurses with interpretive statements.* Washington, DC: Author.

BOX 1-3 | **Ethical Principles**

Beneficence: Doing or promoting good for others.
Nonmaleficence: Not risking or causing harm to others.
Autonomy: People have the right to self-determination. This includes the right to respect, privacy, and the information necessary to make decisions.
Justice: All people should be treated equally and fairly regardless of disease or social or economic status.

---

may be in conflict with what is legal, so nurses must consider both ethical principles and what is legal in their field and place of practice.

Ethical Concerns in Child Health Nursing

Cessation of Treatment

The decision to cease treatment is an ethical situation that is always difficult and seems to be compounded when the client is an infant or child. Children who would have died in the past can now have their lives extended through the use of life support. Parents must be involved in the decision-making process immediately and informed about available options. Laws in some states permit parents to provide advance directives for their minor children. When older children are involved, their views are considered.

In this age of resource allocation, debate centers on how to manage critical care resources. Many believe that these decisions should not be made at the bedside. The American Academy of Pediatrics (AAP), in its statement entitled *Ethics and the Care of Critically Ill Infants and Children* (1996), encourages society to engage in a thorough debate about the economic, cultural, religious, social, and moral consequences of imposing limits on which patients should receive intensive care.

Terminating Life Support

Decisions to terminate life support systems continue to present gut-wrenching ethical and legal situations to nurses, especially when an infant or child is involved. Contrary to the common belief that such decisions should be determined by what is termed *quality of life*, the legal system plays a major role in this area of health care.

Parents frequently become attached to a primary care nurse and request that the nurse participate in the decision regarding whether to terminate life support for their child. A nurse might be faced with such a situation in the neonatal intensive care unit (NICU) with a teenage parent of a premature infant with a congenital defect or in a chronic care oncology unit with a terminally ill child.

In such instances a team conference should be arranged with the parents, primary nurse, physician, and a hospital staff attorney who is knowledgeable about applicable laws in that particular state. Problems may arise when families, physicians, and nurses differ in their opinion of what is best.

The issue of when first to discuss with adolescents the idea of cardiopulmonary resuscitation, mechanical ventilation, and do-not-resuscitate (DNR) orders is always sensitive. Adolescents who have reached majority age must give consent if they are of sound mind. In most states, minority status ends at the age of 18 years.

LEGAL ISSUES

The legal foundation for the practice of nursing provides safeguards for health care and sets standards by which nurses can be evaluated. Nurses need to understand how the law applies specifically to them. When nurses do not meet the standards expected, they may be held legally accountable.

Safeguards for Health Care

Three categories of safeguards determine how the law views nursing practice: (1) state nurse practice acts, (2) standards of care set by professional organizations, and (3) rules and policies set by the institution employing the nurse. Additional information about nursing responsibilities is presented later in this chapter.

Nurse Practice Acts

Every state has a nurse practice act that determines the scope of practice for registered nurses in that state. Nurse practice acts define what the nurse is and is not allowed to do in caring for clients. Some parts of the law may be quite specific. Others are stated broadly enough to permit flexibility in the role of nurses. Nurse practice acts vary from state to state, and nurses must be knowledgeable about these laws wherever they practice.

In 1998 the National Council of State Boards of Nursing initiated a nurse licensure compact program. A nurse licensure compact allows a nurse who is licensed in one state to practice nursing in another participating state without having to be licensed in that state. Nurses must comply with the practice regulations in the state in which they practice. Since 1998, eighteen states have become participants in the nurse licensure compact program (National Council of State Boards of Nursing, 2005).

Laws relating to nursing practice also delineate methods, called *standard procedures* or *protocols*, by which nurses may assume certain duties commonly considered part of medical practice. The procedures are written by committees of nurses, physicians, and administrators. They specify the nursing qualifications required for practicing the procedures, define the appropriate situations, and list the education required. Standard procedures allow for changing the role of the nurse to meet the needs of the community and reflect expanding knowledge.

Standards of Care

Courts have generally held that nurses must practice according to established standards and health agency policies, although these standards and policies do not have the force of law. Standards of care are set by professional associations and describe the level of care that can be expected from practitioners. The Society of Pediatric Nurses is the primary specialty organization that sets standards for pediatric nurses (Box 1-4).

Other regulatory bodies, such as the Occupational Safety and Health Administration (OSHA), the Food and Drug Administration (FDA), and the Centers for Disease Control and Prevention (CDC), also provide guidelines for practice. Accrediting agencies, such as the Joint Commission on Accreditation of Healthcare Organizations and the Community Health Accreditation Program, give their approval after visiting facilities and observing whether standards are being met in practice. Governmental programs such as Medicare, Medicaid, and state health departments require that their standards be met for the facility to receive reimbursement for services.

BOX 1-4	ANA/SPN Standards of Care and Standards of Professional Performance for Pediatric Nurses

Standards of Care*

Comprehensive pediatric nursing care focuses on helping children and their families and communities achieve their optimum health potentials. This is best achieved within the framework of family-centered care and the pediatric nursing process, including primary, secondary, and tertiary care coordinated across health care and community settings.

Standard I. Assessment
The pediatric nurse collects health data.

Standard II. Diagnosis
The pediatric nurse analyzes the assessment data in determining diagnoses.

Standard III. Outcome Identification
The pediatric nurse identifies expected outcomes individualized to the client.

Standard IV. Planning
The pediatric nurse develops a plan of care that prescribes interventions to attain expected outcomes.

Standard V. Implementation
The pediatric nurse implements the interventions identified in the plan of care.

Standard VI. Evaluation
The pediatric nurse evaluates the child's and family's progress toward attainment of outcomes.

Standards of Professional Performance*

Standard I. Quality of Care
The pediatric nurse systematically evaluates the quality and effectiveness of pediatric nursing practice.

Standard II. Performance Appraisal
The pediatric nurse evaluates his or her own nursing practice in relation to professional practice standards and relevant statutes and regulations.

Standard III. Education
The pediatric nurse acquires and maintains current knowledge in pediatric nursing practice.

Standard IV. Collegiality
The pediatric nurse contributes to the professional development of peers, colleagues, and others.

Standard V. Ethics
The pediatric nurse's decisions and actions on behalf of children and their families are determined in an ethical manner.

Standard VI. Collaboration
The pediatric nurse collaborates with the child, family, and health care providers in providing client care.

Standard VII. Research
The pediatric nurse uses research findings in practice.

Standard VIII. Resource Utilization
The pediatric nurse considers factors related to safety, effectiveness, and cost in planning and delivering care.

*See the original source for measurement criteria.
Reprinted from the American Nurses' Association and the Society of Pediatric Nurses. (1996). *Statement on the scope and standards of pediatric clinical practice* (pp. 25-35). Washington, DC: American Nurses Publishing.

Agency Policies

Each health care facility sets specific policies, procedures, and protocols that govern nursing care. All nurses should be familiar with those that apply in the facilities in which they work. Nurses are involved in writing nursing policies and procedures that apply to their practice and as well as reviewing or revising them regularly.

Accountability

Nursing accountability involves knowledge of current laws. Accountability in child health nursing requires special consideration because the nurse must be accountable to the family as well as the child. For example, the Individuals with Disabilities Education Act (PL 94-142), which mandates free and appropriate education for all children with disabilities, provides for school nurses to be part of a team that develops an individual education plan for each child who is eligible for services. In school districts that are reluctant to involve the school nurse as part of the team, nurses may need to advocate for services for the child and family.

Both federal and state legislative bodies have addressed the issue of child abuse. Considerable variation exists among state laws in the investigative authority and procedures granted to child protective workers. When child abuse is suspected, issues often arise regarding whether a health care provider may investigate the home situation and obtain relevant records.

A recent issue pertaining to nursing accountability is inadequate hospital staffing as a result of budget cuts. Nurses have a duty to communicate concerns about staffing levels immediately through established channels. A nurse will not be excused from responsibility (e.g., late medication administration or injury resulting from inadequate supervision of a client) just as a hospital will not be excused for insufficient staffing because of budget cuts.

Accountability also involves competency. If a nurse is not competent to perform a nursing task (e.g., to administer a new chemotherapeutic drug), or if a child's status worsens to the point at which the care needs are beyond the nurse's competency level (e.g., a child requiring hemodynamic monitoring), the nurse must immediately communicate this fact to the nursing supervisor or physician. The fact that a child's transfer to the intensive care unit (ICU) was requested but denied because the ICU was at full capacity is an insufficient defense in a charge of nursing negligence. In addition, the fact that a call was placed to a physician but not returned is no excuse for harm caused to a child because of delayed treatment. The nurse has an obligation to pursue needed care through the established chain of command at the facility.

Malpractice

Negligence is failure to perform the way a reasonable, prudent person of similar background would act in a similar situation. Negligence may consist of doing something that should not be done or failing to do something that should be done.

Malpractice is negligence by professionals, such as nurses or physicians, in the performance of their duties. Nurses may

---

> ### CRITICAL TO REMEMBER
> **Elements of Negligence**
>
> *Duty.* The nurse must have a duty to act or give care to the client. It must be part of the nurse's responsibility.
> *Breach of duty.* A violation of that duty must occur. The nurse fails to conform to established standards for performing that duty.
> *Damage.* Actual injury or harm to the client must occur as a result of the nurse's breach of duty.
> *Proximate cause.* The nurse's breach of duty must be proved to be the cause of harm to the client.

be accused of malpractice if they do not perform according to established standards of care and in the manner of a reasonable, prudent nurse with similar education and experience. Four elements must be present to prove negligence: duty, breach of duty, damage, and proximate cause.

Prevention of Malpractice Claims

Malpractice awards have escalated in both number and amounts awarded to plaintiffs, resulting in high malpractice insurance for all health care providers. In addition, more health care workers practice defensively, accumulating evidence that they are acting in the client's best interest. For example, nurses must be careful to include detailed data when they chart.

Prevention of claims is sometimes referred to as *risk management* or *quality assurance*. Although prevention of all malpractice lawsuits is not possible, nurses can help defend themselves against malpractice judgments by following guidelines for informed consent, refusal of care, and documentation; acting as a client advocate; working within accepted standards and the policies and procedures of the facility; and maintaining their level of expertise.

Informed Consent

When clients receive adequate information, they are less likely to file malpractice suits. Informed consent is an ethical concept that has been enacted into law. Clients have the right to decide whether to accept or reject treatment options as part of their right to function autonomously. To make wise decisions, they need full information about treatments offered. Without proper informed consent, assault and battery charges can result.

The law mandates what procedures require informed consent. The law mandates what to inform about as "risks" specific to each procedure. Nurses must be familiar with those procedures requiring consent.

> ### CRITICAL TO REMEMBER
> **Requirements of Informed Consent**
>
> - Child's or family's competence to consent
> - Full disclosure of information
> - Child's or family's understanding of information
> - Child's or family's voluntary consent

Competence. Certain requirements must be met before consent can be considered informed. The first requirement is that the person giving consent be competent, or able to think through a situation and make rational decisions. A person who is comatose or severely cognitively disabled is incapable of making such decisions. Minors are not allowed to give consent; however, children should have procedures explained to them in terms appropriate for their age. In most states, minority status for informed consent ends at the age of 18 years.

Most states allow some exceptions for parental consent in cases involving emancipated minors. An *emancipated minor* is a minor child who has the legal competency of an adult because of circumstances involving marriage, divorce, parenting of a child, living independently without parents, or enlistment in the armed services. Legal counsel may be consulted to verify the status of the emancipated minor for consent purposes.

Most states allow minors to obtain treatment for drug or alcohol abuse or sexually transmissible diseases and to have access to birth control without parental consent. At present, laws governing adolescent abortion vary widely from state to state.

Full Disclosure. The second requirement is that of full disclosure of information, including the treatment's purpose and the expected results. The risks, side effects, and benefits as well as other treatment options must be explained to parents and children. They must also be informed regarding what would happen if no treatment were chosen.

For example, the National Childhood Vaccine Injury Act mandates that explanations about the risks of communicable diseases and the risks and benefits associated with immunizations should be given to all parents to enable them to make informed decisions about their child's health care. Parents need to know the common side effects and what to do in an emergency if any occur. The law stipulates that children injured by the vaccine must go through the administrative compensation system (funds from an excise tax levied on the vaccines) and reject an award before attempting to sue either the manufacturer or the person who gave the vaccine in a civil suit. Furthermore, the law mandates certain record-keeping and reporting requirements for nurses.

Understanding of Information. The parent must comprehend information about proposed treatment. Health professionals must explain the facts in terms the person can understand. Nurses must be advocates when they find that a parent does not fully understand a treatment or has questions about it. The nurse may be able to assist the parent in understanding the information. Otherwise, the nurse must inform the physician so that the parent's misunderstandings can be clarified.

Throughout hospitalization and discharge preparations, considerations should be given to those who do not understand the prevailing language and to the vision or hearing impaired. Foreign language and sign language interpreters must be obtained when indicated. Provision for those who cannot read any language or adults with a low education level must be considered as well.

Voluntary Consent. Parents and children must be allowed to make choices voluntarily without undue influence or coercion from others. Although others can give information, the parent or child alone makes the decision. Families should not feel pressured to choose in a certain way or feel that their future care depends on their decision.

Children cannot legally consent for treatment or participation in research. However, children should give voluntary assent for research participation. Assent involves the principles of competence and full disclosure. Children should be given information in a developmentally appropriate format. Clients 18 years and older must provide full consent. Dissent in children aged 13 to 17 years is considered binding in some states. Assent should be obtained for children aged 7 to 12 years, and dissent should be considered binding (Woodring, 2004).

The AAP Committee on Pediatric Emergency Medicine (2003) issued a policy regarding consent for emergency medical services for children and adolescents. The policy recommends that every effort be made to secure consent from a parent or legal guardian, but emergency treatment should not be denied if problems obtaining the consent occur.

Refusal of Care

Sometimes parents or children decline treatment, including hospitalization, offered by health professionals. They may refuse treatment when they believe that the benefits of treatment do not outweigh the burdens of the treatment or the quality of life they can expect after that treatment. Parents have the right to refuse care, and they can withdraw agreement to treatment at any time. When a person makes this decision, a number of steps should be taken.

First, the physician or nurse should establish that the parent and child understand the treatment and the results of refusal. The physician, if unaware of the decision, should be notified by the nurse. The nurse documents on the chart the refusal, explanations given to the parent, and notification of the physician. If the treatment is considered vital to the child's well-being, the physician discusses the need with the parent and documents the discussion. Opinions by other physicians may be offered as well.

Parents may be asked to sign a form indicating that they understand the possible results of rejecting treatment. This measure is to prevent a later lawsuit in which a parent claims lack of knowledge of the possible results of a decision. If no ethical dilemma exists, the parent's decision stands.

When parents refuse to give consent for what is deemed necessary treatment of a child, the state may be petitioned to intervene. The court may place the child in the temporary custody of the state or a private agency. The nurse may be asked to witness such a transaction when physicians act in cases of emergencies, such as a life-saving blood transfusion for a child despite parental objections based on religious beliefs.

Adoption

Nurses may care for infants involved in adoptions. The nurse may need to consult the birth parents, adoptive parents, social workers, obstetrician, or pediatrician to determine the various rights of the child, birth parents, and adoptive parents (e.g., in matters concerning visitation rights, informed consent, or discharge planning).

In open adoptions, the birth mother may opt to room in with the baby during hospitalization. The birth mother and adoptive parents typically have had contact before the delivery and have an informal agreement regarding shared responsibility for the baby. The birth mother may even participate in discharge planning because she may have extended rights to visit the child after adoption.

Issues may develop regarding the state of mind of the birth mother at the time of relinquishing parental rights (which cannot occur until after birth, unlike the relinquishment of the birth father's rights). State laws vary regarding the legal period necessary (1 day to several weeks after the birth of the child) before a birth mother can lawfully relinquish her rights to the child.

Some state laws allow the birth mother to relinquish her rights immediately after birth. In such cases, the nurse has the responsibility of protecting the birth mother and child to ensure that the birth mother is not coerced into making a decision while under the effects of medication. Factual documentation of such circumstances may be requested if the birth mother later asserts her rights to the child, claiming "undue influence" or "coercion."

Birth fathers have the same rights as the birth mother. Unless the birth father relinquishes his legal rights to the child, he may later assert his rights to the child after attachment has occurred with the adoptive parents. This situation may occur if the birth mother denies knowledge of the father's identity.

Documentation

Documentation, whether on paper or electronic media, is the best evidence that a standard of care has been maintained. All information recorded about a child should reflect that standard of care. This information includes both electronic and written nurses' notes, flow sheets, and any other data in the child's record. In many instances, notations on hospital records are the only proof that care has been given. When documentation is not present, juries tend to assume that care was not given. Although documentation is not listed as a step in the nursing process, it is an integral part of the process.

Documentation must be specific and complete. Nurses are unlikely to be able to recall situations that happened years in the past and, if sued, must rely on their documentation to explain their care. Documentation must show that the standards of care and facility policies and procedures in effect at the time of the incident were met. Documentation must demonstrate that the child was appropriately assessed, that continuing monitoring of problems was provided, that problems were identified and correct interventions were instituted, and that changes in the child's condition were reported to the primary care provider. If the nurse believes that the primary care provider has responded inappropriately, the nurse must refer the provider response through the appropriate chain of command for the facility and document the notification.

Documenting Discharge Teaching. Because of brief hospital stays, discharge teaching is essential to ensure that parents know how to care for their child. Nurses must document the teaching they perform as well as the parents' and child's understanding, if appropriate, of that teaching. Documenting information about the parents' degree of understanding of the teaching is important. The nurse should also note the need for reinforcement and how that reinforcement was provided. If follow-up home care is planned, teaching can be continued at home and documented on forms by the home care nurse.

Documenting Incidents. A type of documentation used in risk management is the *incident report*, often called a *quality assurance report*, *occurrence report*, or *variance report*. The nurse completes a report when something occurs that might result in legal action, such as an injury to a child or a departure from the expectations of the situation. The report warns the agency's legal department that a problem may have occurred. It also helps identify whether changing processes within the system might reduce the risk for similar incidents in the future. They are not intended to be punitive if an error was made. Incident reports are not a part of the child's chart and should not be referred to on the chart. Documentation of the incident on the chart should be restricted to the same type of factual information about the child's condition that would be recorded in any other situation.

The Nurse as Child and Family Advocate

Malpractice suits may be brought if nurses fail in their role of child advocate. Nurses are ethically and legally bound to act as the child's advocate. This means that the nurse must act in the child's best interests at all times. When nurses believe that the child's best interests are not being served, they are obligated to seek help for the child from appropriate sources. This usually involves taking the problem through the chain of command established at the facility. The nurse consults a supervisor and the child's physician. If the results are not satisfactory, the nurse continues through administrative channels to the director of nurses, hospital administrator, and chief of the medical staff, if necessary. All nurses should know the chain of command for their workplaces.

Nurses must be advocates for health promotion and prevention for vulnerable groups such as children. Nurses can participate in groups dedicated to the welfare of children and families, such as professional nursing societies, parent support groups, religious organizations, and voluntary organizations. Through involvement with health care planning on a political or legislative level and by working as consumer advocates, nurses can initiate changes for better quality health care.

Maintaining Expertise

Maintaining expertise is another way for nurses to prevent malpractice liability. To ensure that nurses maintain their expertise to provide safe care, most states require proof of continuing education for renewal of nursing licenses. Nursing knowledge changes rapidly, and all nurses must keep current.

Incorporating new information learned by attending classes or conferences and reading nursing journals can help nurses perform the way a reasonably prudent peer would perform. Journals provide information from nursing research that may be important in updating nursing practice. All nurses should analyze research articles to determine whether changes in pediatric care are indicated.

Employers often provide continuing education classes for their nurses. Many workshops and seminars are available on a wide variety of nursing subjects. Membership in professional organizations, such as state branches of the American Nurses Association or specialty organizations such as the Society of Pediatric Nurses, gives nurses access to new information through publications as well as nursing conferences and other educational offerings.

Maintaining expertise may be a concern when nurses "float" or are required to work with children who have needs different from those of their usual clients. In these situations, the employer must provide orientation and education so that the nurse can perform care safely in new areas. Nurses who work outside their usual areas of expertise must assess their own skills and avoid performing tasks or taking on responsibilities in areas in which they are not competent. Many nurses learn to provide care in two or three different areas and are floated only to those areas. This system meets the need for flexible staffing while providing safe care for children.

SOCIAL ISSUES

Nurses are exposed to many social issues that influence health care and often have legal or ethical implications. Some of the issues that affect child health care include poverty, homelessness, access to care, and allocation of funds.

Poverty

Children living in poverty are more likely to be in poor health and less likely to have used many types of health care (National Center for Health Statistics, 2004). The number of children living in households with cash incomes below the Federal poverty level is approximately 13 million, or 17.3% of all related children living in families, with children younger than 6 years more likely (19.9%) to live in poverty (DeNavas-Walt, Proctor, & Lee, 2005). Children living in single-parent, female-headed households are five times as likely to be poor as are children living in couple families (DeNavas-Walt, Proctor, & Lee, 2005).

Poverty becomes a health issue because it affects access to health care and decreases opportunities linked with health promotion. Poverty rates in the United States are geographic. The southern and western portions of the country have disproportionately more of the nation's poor population. Higher proportions of children in the West (13%) and South (12%) are uninsured than of children in the Midwest (7%) or Northeast (5%). Children in the West are also less likely to have a usual place of health care than children in other regions (Dey & Bloom, 2005).

Nurses can play a role in meeting the health care needs of infants and children by recognizing the adverse effect of poverty on health and identifying poverty as a practice concern. Several goals in the *Healthy People 2010* goals (USDHHS, 2000) have implications for pediatric nurses:

- To reduce the infant mortality rate to no more than 4.5 per 1000 live births and the childhood mortality rate to 18.6 per 100,000 for children 1 to 4 years old and 12.3 per 100,000 for children 5 to 9 years old; to similarly reduce the rate of adolescent deaths.
- To reduce the incidence of low birth weight to no more than 5% of live births and the incidence of very low birth weight to 0.9% of live births.
- To achieve and maintain effective vaccination coverage levels for universally recommended vaccines to 90% of children from 19 to 35 months of age and increase routine vaccination coverage for adolescents.
- To reduce vaccine-preventable diseases as follows: (1) measles, mumps, and rubella to zero cases and (2) pertussis in children younger than 7 years to no more than 2000 cases per year.
- To increase to 100% the proportion of persons with health insurance.

Poverty tends to breed poverty. In poor families, children may leave the educational system early, making them less likely to learn skills necessary to obtain good jobs. Childbearing at an early age is common and interferes with education and the ability to work. The cycle of poverty (Fig. 1-3) may continue from one generation to another as a result of hopelessness and apathy.

Homelessness

Families, 84% of which are composed of single women and their children, are the fastest-growing group of homeless people in the United States (National Resource Center on Homelessness and Mental Illness, 2003). In addition to poverty as a contributing factor to homelessness among women and their children, other factors include violence, substance abuse, and mental illness. Homeless children are poorly nourished and are exposed to violence, experience school absences with subsequent learning difficulties, and are at risk for depression and other emotional consequences (National Resource Center on Homelessness and Mental Illness, 2003).

Pregnancy and birth, especially among teenagers, are important causes contributing to homelessness. Adolescent mothers are more likely to be single and poor (Klein, 2005). Pregnancy interferes with a woman's ability to work and may decrease her income to the point at which she loses her housing. Without child care or a home address, she may have less chance of obtaining and keeping employment. In addition, her children are more likely to be sick because of inadequate food and shelter. Without money to pay for insurance or early health care, the chance that their children will need hospitalization is increased.

Federal funding has provided assistance with shelter and health care for homeless people. The homeless, however, have the same difficulties in obtaining health care as other poor people because of a lack of transportation, inconvenient hours of service, and lack of continuity of care.

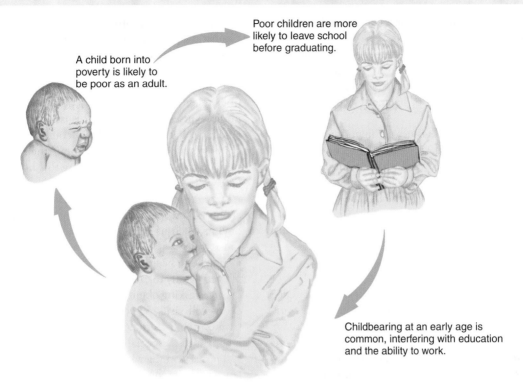

Poor children are more likely to leave school before graduating.

A child born into poverty is likely to be poor as an adult.

Childbearing at an early age is common, interfering with education and the ability to work.

FIG 1-3   **The cycle of poverty.**

Access to Health Care

Even people with incomes above the poverty level may not be able to pay for health care. The working poor have jobs but receive wages that barely meet their day-to-day needs. They have little opportunity to save for emergencies such as serious illness. In 2004, 11.2% of children younger than 18 years in the United States had no health insurance (DeNavas-Walt, Proctor, & Lee, 2005). Millions of others have limited insurance and would not be able to survive financially should serious illness occur. People without insurance seek care only when absolutely necessary. Health maintenance and illness prevention may seem costly and unnecessary to them. Some women receive no health care during pregnancy until they arrive at the hospital for birth, a situation that has potentially adverse consequences for newborns.

A decline in private, employer-paid insurance coverage has decreased the number of privately insured American children. This decline has had a tremendous impact on the low-income worker who does not have employer-paid coverage and cannot afford individually purchased insurance. Although Medicaid has expanded its coverage and SCHIP has enrolled many children of marginal income, some children still live in households whose families cannot afford to purchase private insurance and have not accessed public insurance programs. This issue is being addressed through a federal initiative called Insure Kids Now that publicizes the Medicaid and SCHIP benefits through community-wide publication and intense efforts to enroll children at schools and pediatricians' offices (USDHHS, 2005).

Greater restrictions on private insurance are blurring the distinction between private and public health coverage.

Many private health plans have restrictions such as prequalification for procedures, drugs the plan covers, and services that are covered. Persons with employer-sponsored health insurance often find that they must change providers each year because the available plans change, a situation that may negatively affect the provider-client relationship.

Allocation of Health Care Resources

In 2002 the United States spent $1.6 trillion on health care, a 9.3% increase from 2001 (National Center for Health Statistics, 2004). Expenditures climb every year, although the rate of growth slowed somewhat during the 1990s. However, the large population of "baby boomers," born from 1946 through 1964, is expected to need more health care dollars as they age.

Reforming health care delivery and financing is a complex area of national concern. How to provide care for the poor, the uninsured or underinsured, and those with long-term care needs is an area that must be addressed. In addition, major acute care facilities often deal with greater financial burdens because of the growing numbers of uninsured clients presenting for treatment who are often quite ill or severely injured. Escalating liability costs are another drain on health care dollars, leading some states to enact legislation that places a cap on awards for damages in malpractice cases.

Care Versus Cure

One problem to be addressed is whether the focus of health care should be on preventive and caring measures or on the cure of disease. Medicine has traditionally centered more on treatment and cure than on prevention and care. Yet prevention avoids suffering and is less expensive than treating diseases once they are diagnosed.

The focus on cure has resulted in technologic advances that have enabled some children to live longer, healthier lives. Financial resources are limited, however, and the costs of expensive technology must be balanced against the benefits obtained.

In addition, quality-of-life issues are important in regard to technology. For example, as a result of technologic advances, some very-low-birth-weight infants survive and go on to lead normal or near-normal lives. Others gain time but not quality of life. Families and health care professionals face difficult decisions about when to treat, when to terminate treatment, and when to acknowledge that suffering outweighs the benefits of treatment.

Health Care Rationing

Modern technology has had a great impact on health care rationing. Some might argue that such rationing does not exist, but it occurs when some people have no access to care and not enough money is available for all people to share equally in the technology available. Health care is also rationed when it is more freely given to those who have money to pay for it than to those who do not.

Many questions will need answers as the costs of health care increase faster than the funds available to pay for it. Is health care a fundamental right? Should a certain level of care be guaranteed to all citizens? What is that basic level of care? Should the cost of treatment and its effectiveness be considered when deciding how much government or third-party payers will cover? Nurses will be instrumental in finding solutions to these vital questions.

Violence

Women and children are the victims and sometimes the perpetrators of violence. Violence is a social problem as well as a health problem. Acts of violence can include child abuse, domestic abuse, and murder. Children who live in an environment of violence feel helpless and ineffective. These children have difficulty sleeping and show increased anxiety and fearfulness. They may perpetuate the violence they see in their homes when they are adults because they have known nothing else in family relationships.

Although victimization of children through violent crimes has decreased over the past decade, violence in schools continues to rise, and for many children violence or fear of violence is a daily stressor.

Experts in the field of education have cited socioeconomic disparity, language barriers, diverse cultural upbringing, lack of supervision and behavioral feedback, domestic violence, and changes within the family as possible causes for the increased violence. Traditional approaches to aggressive behavior in the school, such as suspension, detention, and being sent to the principal's office, have been ineffective in changing behavior and serve only to exclude the student from education, leading to an increased dropout rate (AAP, 2003). Nurses must educate themselves on the issue

of violence and, in turn, work with schools and parents to combat the problem. In addition, they should not ignore the child who is afraid to go to school or is having other school-related problems.

Children and adolescents are also exposed to violence from television, movies, video games, and youth-oriented music. Nurses need to make this issue a part of anticipatory guidance. Parents should be encouraged to monitor their children's media exposure and limit their children's television, computer, and video viewing to 2 hours or less per day (AAP, 2001).

The AAP (1999) encouraged clinicians to be concerned about adolescents who display aggressive or acting-out behaviors, such as lying, stealing, temper outbursts, vandalism, excessive fighting, and destructiveness. It further recommended that health care providers promote the responsibility of every family to create a gun-safe home environment. This includes asking about the presence of guns in the home at every well visit and counseling children, parents, and relatives on the importance of firearm safety and the dangers of having a gun, especially a handgun.

Nurses working with children should ask them about violence in their schools, homes, or neighborhoods and whether they have had any personal experience with violent behavior. In some cases contact with parents, human resource departments, police, or other authorities may be necessary to protect children and adolescents who are either in violent situations or at risk for violence.

THE PROFESSIONAL NURSE

As nursing care changed from the category-specific care of the infant or child to family-centered care, pediatric nursing entered a new era of autonomy and independence. Nurses today must be able to communicate with and teach children of many ages and levels of development and education. They must be able to think critically and use the nursing process to develop a plan of care that meets the unique needs of each child and family. They are expected to use current research to solve problems and collaborate with other health care providers.

The Role of the Nurse

The professional nurse has a responsibility to provide the highest quality care to every child and family. The American Nurses Association (ANA) Code for Nurses (see Box 1-2) provides guidelines for professional behavior. The code emphasizes the nurse's accountability to the client, the community, and the profession. The nurse should understand the implications of this code and strive to practice accordingly. Professional nurses have a legal obligation to know and understand the standard of care required of them. Nurses must maintain competence and a current knowledge base in their areas of practice. Standards of practice describe the level of performance expected of a professional nurse as determined by an authority in the practice.

Nurses who care for children in all clinical settings can use the ANA/Society of Pediatric Nurses (SPN) Standards of

Care and Standards of Professional Performance for Pediatric Nurses (see Box 1-4) and the SPN/ANA Guide to Family Centered Care as guides for practice. Other standards of practice for specific clinical areas, such as pediatric oncology nursing or emergency nursing, are available from nursing specialty groups.

As health care continues to move to family-centered and community-based health services, all nurses should expect to care for children, adolescents, and their families. Under the leadership of the Child and Family Expert Panel of the American Academy of Nursing, representatives from 10 pediatric and subspecialty organizations met to identify the commonalties of practice across all areas of pediatric practice and produced the document *Health Care Quality and Outcome Guidelines for Nursing of Children and Families*. The guidelines set forth in the document can serve as a framework for practice when caring for children and their families. Educators and administrators in health care should find them useful when planning programs (Betz, Muennich Cowell, Lobo, & Craft-Rosenberg, 2004; Betz, 2005).

Pediatric nurses function in a variety of roles, including those of care provider, teacher, collaborator, researcher, advocate, and manager.

Care Provider

The nurse provides direct nursing care to infants, children, and their families in times of illness, injury, recovery, and wellness. Nursing care is based on the nursing process. The nurse obtains health histories, assesses client needs, monitors growth and development, performs health-screening procedures, develops comprehensive plans of care, provides treatment and care, makes referrals, and evaluates the effects of care. Nursing of children is especially based on an understanding of the child's developmental stage and is aimed at meeting the child's physical and emotional needs at that level. Developing a therapeutic relationship with and providing support to children and their families are essential components of nursing care. Pediatric nurses practice family-centered care, embracing diversity in family structures and cultural backgrounds. These nurses strive to empower families, encouraging them to participate in their care and the care of their child.

Teacher

Education is an essential role of today's nurse. Nurses who care for children prepare them for procedures, hospitalization, or surgery, using knowledge of growth and development to teach children at various levels of understanding. Families need information as well as emotional support so they can cope with the anxiety and uncertainty of a child's illness. Nurses teach family members how to provide care, watch for important signs, and increase the child's comfort. They also work with new parents and parents of ill children so that the parents are prepared to assume responsibility for care at home after the child has been discharged from the hospital.

Education is essential for the promotion of health. The nurse applies principles of teaching and learning to change the behavior of family members. Nurses motivate children and families to take charge of and make responsible decisions about their own health. For teaching to be effective, it must incorporate the family's values and health beliefs.

Nurses caring for children and families play an important role in the prevention of illness and injury through education and anticipatory guidance. Teaching about immunizations, safety, dental care, socialization, and discipline is a necessary component of care. Nurses offer guidance to parents regarding child-rearing practices and the prevention of potential problems. They also answer questions about growth and development and assist families in understanding their children. Teaching often involves providing emotional support and counseling to children and families.

Factors Influencing Learning

A number of factors influence learning at any age, including the following:

- *Developmental level.* Developmental level influences whether a person learns best by reading printed material, using computer-based materials, watching videos, participating in group discussions, or playing. Teaching must be adapted to the child's developmental level rather than the child's chronologic age.
- *Language.* The ability to understand the language in which teaching is done determines how much the child and family learn. Families for whom English is not the primary language may not understand idioms, nuances, slang terms, informal use of words, or medical terms. An interpreter for the deaf may be necessary for the child or parent who is hearing impaired.
- *Culture.* People tend to forget or disregard content with which they disagree. The nurse's teaching can be most effective if cultural considerations are weighed and incorporated into the education.
- *Previous experiences.* Parents who have other children may need less education about infant and child care. They may, however, have additional concerns about meeting the needs of several children and about sibling rivalry.
- *Physical environment.* The nurse must consider privacy when discussing sensitive issues such as adolescent sexuality or domestic violence. A group discussion, on the other hand, may prompt participants to ask questions of concern to all members of the group, such as the experiences they can expect in labor.
- *Organization and skill of the teacher.* The teacher must determine the objectives of the teaching, develop a plan to meet the objectives, and gather all materials before teaching. The nurse must determine the best way to present the material for the intended audience. A summary of the information is helpful when concluding a teaching session.

Collaborator

Nurses collaborate with other members of the health care team, often coordinating and managing the child's care. Care is improved by an interdisciplinary approach as nurses work together with dietitians, social workers, physicians, and others.

Managing the transition from a hospital or any other acute care setting to the child's home or another facility involves discharge planning and collaboration with other health care professionals. The frequent use of home care makes collaboration increasingly important. The nurse must be knowledgeable about community resources, appropriate home care agencies for the type of child or problem, and financial resources. Cooperation and communication are essential as clients, including parents of children, are encouraged to participate in their care.

Researcher

Nurses contribute to their profession's knowledge base by systematically investigating theoretical or practice issues in nursing. Nursing does much more than simply "borrow" scientific knowledge from medicine and basic sciences. Nursing generates and answers its own questions based on research of its unique subject matter. The responsibility for research within nursing is not limited to nurses with graduate degrees. All nurses should apply research findings to their practice rather than base care decisions merely on intuition or tradition. Evidence-based practice is no longer an ideal but an expectation of nursing practice. Nurses can contribute to the body of professional knowledge by demonstrating an awareness of the value of nursing research and assisting in problem identification and data collection. Nurses should keep their knowledge current by networking and sharing research findings at conferences, by publishing, and by evaluating research journal articles.

Advocate

An advocate is a person who speaks on behalf of another. As the health care environment becomes increasingly complex, care can become impersonal. The wishes and needs of children and families are sometimes discounted or ignored in the effort to treat and cure. As the health professional who is closest to the child, the nurse is in an ideal position to humanize care and intercede on the child's behalf. As an advocate, the nurse considers the family's wishes in planning and implementing care. The nurse informs families of treatments and procedures, ensuring that the families are involved directly in decisions and activities related to their child's care. The nurse must be sensitive to the values, beliefs, and customs of families.

Nurses must be advocates for health promotion for vulnerable groups, such as children. Nurses can promote the rights of children and families by participating in groups dedicated to the welfare of children and families, such as professional nursing societies, parent support groups, religious organizations, and volunteer organizations. Through involvement with health care planning on a political or legislative level and by working as consumer advocates, nurses can initiate changes for better quality health care. Nurses possess unique knowledge and skills and can make valuable contributions in developing health care strategies to ensure that all clients receive optimal care.

Manager of Care

As a result of the decreased length of stay in acute care facilities, nurses often are not able to provide total direct client care. Instead, they delegate concrete tasks, such as giving a bath or taking vital signs, to others. As a result, nurses spend more time teaching and supervising unlicensed personnel, planning and coordinating care, and collaborating with other professionals and agencies. Moreover, nurses are expected to understand the financial squeeze resulting from cost-containment strategies and contribute to their institutions' economic viability. At the same time, they must continue to act as child advocates and maintain a standard of care.

Advanced Preparation for Pediatric Nurses

The increasing complexity of care and a focus on cost containment have led to a greater need for nurses with advanced preparation. Advanced practice nurses may practice as nurse practitioners or clinical nurse specialists, among other possibilities. Advanced practice nurses may also work as nurse administrators, nurse educators, and nurse researchers. Preparation for advanced practice involves obtaining a master's or doctoral degree.

Nurse Practitioners

Nurse practitioners are advanced practice nurses who work according to protocols and provide many primary care services that were once provided only by physicians. Most nurse practitioners collaborate with a physician but, depending on their scope of practice and their individual state's board of nursing mandates, they may work independently and prescribe medications. Nurse practitioners provide care for specific groups of clients in a variety of settings (primary care facilities, schools, acute care facilities, rehabilitation centers). They may address occupational health, women's health, family health, and the health of the elderly or the very young.

Pediatric nurse practitioners use advanced skills to assess and treat well and ill children according to established protocols. The health care services they provide range from physical examinations and anticipatory guidance to the treatment of common illnesses and injuries. Newborn nurseries and some children's hospital specialty units may be staffed by pediatric or neonatal nurse practitioners.

Family nurse practitioners are prepared to provide care for all family members, including children. They diagnose and treat clients holistically, with a strong emphasis on prevention.

School nurse practitioners receive education and training that is similar to that of pediatric nurse practitioners. However, because of the setting in which they practice, the school nurse practitioner receives advanced education in managing chronic illness, disability, and mental health problems in a school setting, as well as developing skills required to communicate effectively with students, teachers, school administrators, and community health care providers. School nurse practitioners expand the traditional role of the school nurse by providing on-site treatment of acute care problems and providing extensive well-child examinations and services.

Clinical Nurse Specialists

Clinical specialists are registered nurses who, through study and supervised practice at the graduate level (master's or doctorate), have become expert in the care of children and families. Four major roles have been identified for clinical nurse specialists: expert practitioner, educator, researcher, and consultant. These professionals often function as clinical leaders, role models, client advocates, and change agents. Unlike nurse practitioners, clinical nurse specialists are not prepared to provide primary care.

Implications of Changing Roles for Nurses

As nursing care has changed, so also have the roles of pediatric nurses with both basic and advanced preparation. Nurses now work in a variety of areas. Although they previously worked almost exclusively in the hospital setting, many now provide home care and community-based care. Some of the settings for children include the following:

- Acute care settings: in general hospital units, intensive care units, surgical units, postanesthesia care units, and emergency care facilities as well as on board emergency transport craft
- Clinics and physicians' offices
- Home health agencies
- Schools
- Rehabilitation centers and long-term care facilities
- Summer camps and day care centers
- Hospice programs and respite care programs
- Psychiatric centers

BOX 1-5	**Elements of Critical Thinking**

Characteristics of the Critical Thinker

Ability to recognize, examine, and reflect on one's own assumptions and biases

Open-mindedness, willingness to look at others' perspectives

Self-confidence

Ability to reason well by basing judgments on evidence and inclusive data and avoiding jumping to conclusions

Ability to recognize emotions and acknowledge mistakes

Inquisitiveness and curiosity

Creativity

Skills Required for Critical Thinking

Interpreting: collecting and organizing data and identifying patterns and meaning in the data collected

Analyzing: validating data, collecting additional information if needed, comparing to norms, proposing arguments or courses of action

Evaluating: assessing goals reached and outcomes achieved

Inferring: deriving conclusions after questioning evidence and considering alternatives

Explaining: stating and describing results based on evidence, providing rationales for courses of action or arguments

Self-regulating: continuing reflection on one's own thinking and making corrections when needed

---

Critical Thinking

In recent years critical thinking has received widespread attention in nursing. Clearly nurses must be concerned with the development of critical thinking skills, which are needed to pass the National Council Licensure Examination (NCLEX) as well as function clinically. Critical thinking skills underlie the steps of the nursing process.

Unlike undirected thinking, which is random and unfocused, critical thinking is controlled, purposeful, directed toward solving problems or developing opinions, based on evidence, and involves a thorough reflection and analysis of one's own thought processes. The critical thinker examines and questions assumptions (Lipe & Beasley, 2004). Critical thinking can improve clinical judgment by reducing habits that result in poor decision making and increase the ability to apply knowledge to clinical situations. It reduces the risk of decision making based on emotion, fatigue, or anxiety. Box 1-5 presents the elements of critical thinking.

NURSING OF CHILDREN: THE NURSING PROCESS

The nursing process is the foundation for all nursing. The nursing process consists of five distinct steps: (1) assessment, (2) nursing diagnosis, (3) planning, (4) implementation of the plan (interventions), and (5) evaluation. Despite the apparent complexity of the process, the nurse soon learns to use the steps of the nursing process in order when caring for clients.

Nursing of children, including care of a newborn, can present a challenge for many nursing students. Whereas use of the nursing process when caring for adults may involve only the client, in caring for infants and children it must involve the family as well. Therefore planning and interventions commonly state what the parent is expected to do or specify interventions such as teaching a parent. The involvement of a third party (the family) may be different to the nursing student who has applied the nursing process only to care of adults in the past.

Assessment

Nursing assessment is the systematic collection of relevant data to determine the client's and family's current health status, coping patterns, needs, and problems. The data collected include not only physiologic data but also psychologic, social, and cultural data relevant to life processes. Nurses must assess the belief systems, available support, perceptions, and plans of other family members in an effort to provide the best nursing care.

During the assessment phase, three activities take place: collecting data, grouping findings, and writing the nursing diagnoses. Data can be collected through interview, physical examination, observation, review of records, and diagnostic reports as well as through collaboration with other health care workers and the family. Two levels of nursing assessment are used to collect comprehensive data: (1) screening, or database, assessment and (2) focused assessments.

Screening Assessment

The screening, or database, assessment is usually performed during the initial contact with the child. Its purpose is to gather information about all aspects of the child's health. This information, called *baseline data*, describes the child's health status before interventions begin. It forms the basis for identifying both strengths and problems. An example of baseline data is the child's developmental and immunization history.

A variety of methods may be used to organize the assessment. For example, information may be grouped according to body systems. Assessment can also be organized around nursing models based on nursing theory, such as Roy's adaptation model, Gordon's functional health patterns, the North American Nursing Diagnosis Association's Human Response Patterns, or Orem's self-care deficit theory.

Focused Assessment

A focused assessment is used to gather information that is specifically related to an actual health problem or a problem that the child is at risk of acquiring. A focused assessment in an acute care setting is often performed at the beginning of a shift and centers on areas relevant to the child's diagnosis and current status. For example, the nurse would perform a focused assessment of the respiratory system several times during hospitalization for the child with acute asthma. In the outpatient setting, the nurse might perform a focused assessment to elicit information about a problem that brings the child to the facility.

Nursing Diagnosis

The data gathered during assessment must be analyzed to identify problems or potential problems. Data are validated and grouped in a process of critical thinking so that cues and inferences can be determined. The nurse identifies the child's response to actual or potential health problems and to normal life processes. The nursing diagnosis provides a basis for nursing accountability for interventions and outcomes.

Nursing diagnoses fall into three categories. An *actual nursing diagnosis* describes a human response to a health condition or life process affecting an individual, family, or community. It is supported by defining characteristics (manifestations, signs, and symptoms) that can be clustered in patterns of related cues or inferences. *Risk nursing diagnoses* describe human responses to health conditions or life processes that may develop in a vulnerable individual, family, or community. They are supported by risk factors that contribute to increased vulnerability. *Wellness nursing diagnoses* describe human responses to levels of wellness in an individual, family, or community that have a potential for enhancement to a higher state.

Each nursing diagnosis is a concise term or phrase that represents a pattern of related cues or signs and symptoms. One problem that nurses often encounter is writing nursing diagnoses that nursing actions cannot address. For example, a medical diagnosis, such as pyloric stenosis, cannot be treated by a nurse. However, saying that some nursing actions can

decrease the fluid volume deficit associated with pyloric stenosis is appropriate.

A nursing diagnosis consists of two sections joined by the phrase "related to." The statement begins with the child's response to the current problem and then describes the causative factor or factors. An example is *Interrupted Family Processes* related to *caring for a child with cancer*. The causative factors can be physiologic, psychologic, sociocultural, environmental, or spiritual. They assist the nurse in identifying nursing interventions as planning takes place.

Planning

The nurse next plans care for problems that were identified during assessment and are reflected in the nursing diagnoses. During this step, nurses set priorities, develop goals or outcomes that state what is to be accomplished by a certain time, and plan interventions to accomplish those goals.

Setting Priorities

Setting priorities includes (1) determining what problems need immediate attention (i.e., life-threatening problems) and taking immediate action; (2) determining whether problems exist that call for a physician's orders for diagnosis, monitoring, or treatment; and (3) identifying actual nursing diagnoses, which take precedence over at-risk diagnoses. For children with many health and psychosocial problems, a realistic number of nursing diagnoses must be chosen.

Establishing Goals and Expected Outcomes

Although the terms *goals* and *outcome criteria* are sometimes used interchangeably, they are different. Generally, broad goals do not state the specific outcome criteria and are less measurable than outcome statements. If broad goals are developed, they should be linked to more specific and measurable outcome criteria. For example, if the goal is that the child will maintain fluid balance, outcome criteria that serve as evidence might be urinary output appropriate for age, good skin turgor, and stable weight.

The following rules should be used when writing outcomes:

- Outcomes should be stated in client terms. This wording identifies who is expected to achieve the goal (the infant or child or the family).
- Measurable verbs must be used. For example, "identify," "demonstrate," "express," "walk," "relate," and "list" are verbs that are observable and measurable. Examples of verbs that are difficult to measure are "understand," "appreciate," "feel," "accept," "know," and "experience."
- A time frame is necessary. When is the child expected to perform the action? After teaching? By 1 day after hospitalization? Before discharge?
- Goals and outcomes must be realistic and attainable by nursing interventions only.
- Goals and outcomes are worked out in collaboration with the child and family to ensure their participation in the plan of care.

Implementation

Implementation is the action phase of the nursing process. Once the goals and desired outcomes are developed, nursing interventions that will help the child meet the established outcomes should be selected. During this phase, the nurse is constantly evaluating and reassessing to determine that the interventions remain appropriate. As the child's condition changes, so does the plan of care.

The type of nursing interventions implemented depends on whether the nursing diagnosis was an actual, risk, or wellness diagnosis. Nursing interventions for actual nursing diagnoses are aimed at reducing or eliminating the causes or related factors. Interventions for risk nursing diagnoses are aimed at (1) monitoring for onset of the problem, (2) reducing or eliminating risk factors, and (3) preventing the problem. For a wellness nursing diagnosis, interventions focus on supporting the child's or family's coping mechanisms and promoting a higher level of wellness.

Nursing interventions in care plans or protocols are most easily implemented if they are specific and spell out exactly what should be done. A well-written nursing intervention is specific: "Provide 30 mL of fluid (water or juice of choice) every 10 minutes while the child is awake." Vague interventions, such as "keep the child hydrated," do not provide specific steps to follow.

Evaluation

The evaluation determines how well the plan worked or how well the goals or outcomes were met. To evaluate, the nurse must assess the status of the child and compare the current status with the goals or outcome criteria that were developed during the planning step. The nurse then judges how well the child is progressing toward goal achievement and makes a decision. Should the plan be continued? Modified? Abandoned? Are the problems resolved or the causes diminished? Is another nursing diagnosis more relevant?

The nursing process is dynamic, and evaluation frequently results in expanded assessment and additional or modified nursing diagnoses and interventions. Nurses are cautioned not to view lack of goal achievement as a failure. Instead, it may be a sign to reassess and begin the process anew.

Collaborative Problems

In addition to nursing diagnoses, which describe problems that respond to independent nursing functions, nurses must also deal with problems that are beyond the scope of independent nursing practice. These are sometimes termed *collaborative problems*—physiologic complications that usually occur in association with a specific pathologic condition or treatment.

Nurses monitor to detect the onset of the complication and collaborate with physicians to manage changes in client status. Both physician-prescribed and nursing-prescribed interventions are necessary to minimize complications (Carpenito-Moyet, 2004b).

Planning

The identification of client-centered goals is important for a collaborative problem because the goals cannot be achieved by independent nursing action. Collaborative problems should reflect the nurse's responsibility in situations requiring physician-prescribed interventions. The nurse's responsibility includes monitoring for signs of complications and managing the complications with nursing-prescribed and physician-prescribed interventions (Carpenito-Moyet, 2004a).

Interventions

Nursing interventions for collaborative problems include (1) performing frequent assessments to monitor the status of the client and detect signs and symptoms of complications; (2) communicating with the physician when signs and symptoms of complications are noted; (3) performing physician-prescribed interventions, including standing orders and protocols, to prevent or correct the complication; and (4) performing nursing interventions described in the standards of care or policy and procedures manual.

Evaluation

Although client-centered goals or outcomes are not developed for collaborative problems, the nurse collects data, compares the data with established norms, and judges whether the data are within normal limits. If the data are not within normal limits, the nurse consults the physician for additional direction and implements physician-prescribed interventions and nursing interventions.

COMPLEMENTARY AND ALTERNATIVE MEDICINE

Today's nurse will likely encounter clients who use complementary and alternative medicine (CAM). CAM can be defined as a group of diverse medical and health care systems, practices, and products that are not presently considered part of conventional medicine (National Center for Complementary and Alternative Medicine, 2005). The therapies may be used instead of conventional medical therapy (alternative therapy) or in addition to conventional medical therapy (complementary therapy). Integrative medicine combines conventional medical therapies with CAM therapies that have substantial evidence regarding their safety and effectiveness.

A major concern in the use of CAM is safety. Those who use these techniques may delay needed care by a conventional health care provider, or they may take herbal remedies or other substances that are toxic when combined with conventional medications or when taken in excess. Adverse effects of CAM therapies may be unknown for children. Safety and effectiveness of botanical or vitamin therapies are often unregulated. Thus variable amounts of active ingredients from these substances may be taken. Some may not consider these therapies to be medicine and may not report them to their conventional health care provider, setting the stage for interactions between conventional medications and CAM therapies that have pharmacologic properties. Many people may not consider some of these therapies "alternative" because the therapy is mainstream in their culture.

Nurses may find that their professional values do not conflict with many of the CAM therapies. Nursing as a profession supports a self-care and a preventive approach to health care in which the individual bears much of the responsibility for his or her health. Nursing practice has traditionally emphasized a holistic, or body-mind-spirit, model of health that fits with CAM. Nurses already practice CAM therapies such as therapeutic touch fairly often. The rising interest in CAM provides an opportunity for nurses to participate in research related to the legitimacy of these treatment modalities.

The National Center for Complementary and Alternative Medicine, a division of the National Institutes of Health, has a website (*nccam.nih.gov*) to provide a source of information and classification of the therapies.

NURSING RESEARCH

As nursing and the health care system change, nurses will be challenged to demonstrate that what they do improves client outcomes and is cost effective. To meet this challenge, nurses must participate in research and encourage the use of research. With the establishment of the National Institute of Nursing Research as a member of the National Institutes of Health (*www.nih.gov/ninr*), nurses now have an infrastructure in place to ensure that nursing research is supported and that a group of well-prepared nurse researchers will be educated.

The amount of clinically based nursing research conducted is increasing rapidly as nurse researchers strive to develop an independent body of knowledge that demonstrates the value of nursing interventions. The challenge is to move the knowledge acquired by researchers into the clinical area.

Although students and inexperienced nurses may not participate in research projects, they must take advantage of the knowledge obtained by the research team. Professional journals are the best sources of new information that can help nurses provide improved care and demonstrate that what they do makes a difference in client outcomes.

KEY CONCEPTS

- Child health care in the United States has changed because of technologic advances, increasing knowledge, government involvement, and consumer demands.
- Family-centered child health care, based on the principle that families can make decisions about health care if they have adequate information, has greatly increased the autonomy of families and the responsibility of nurses.
- Prospective payment plans such as PPOs or HMOs control health care costs by negotiating reduced charges with providers such as facilities and physicians and by restricting client access to any provider of choice.
- Capitated plans are those in which a group of providers agrees to provide all services for clients for a set annual fee. If a client requires more costly care, the provider

network pays those added charges. If the client requires less care than the annual fee, the network keeps the remaining money.

- Case management and outcomes management have resulted in new tools to reduce the length of stay for infants and children in the health care setting. Preparation for continuation of care at home begins as soon as the child enters the health care system.
- Clinical pathways are interdisciplinary guidelines for assessments and interventions designed to accomplish the identified outcomes in the shortest time.
- Home care of children has increased because of the need to control costs and because of the availability of portable technology.
- The number of uninsured children continues to be excessive, reducing their chances of receiving preventive health care and increasing the costs of the late care they often seek.
- Infant mortality rates have declined dramatically in the past 50 years; however, the United States continues to rank well below other developed nations, and infant mortality rates still vary widely across ethnic groups.
- Unintentional injuries are the leading cause of death in children.
- Punitive approaches to ethical and social problems may prevent families from seeking care, particularly preventive care.
- Poverty is a major social issue that leads to questions about allocation of health care resources, access to care, government programs to increase health care to children, and health care rationing.
- The parents usually give consent for a minor child, although adolescents may be able to consent to their own treatment related to sexually transmitted diseases, contraception, and alcohol and drug abuse.
- Nurses are accountable for their practice and must be acquainted with laws, standards of care, and agency policies and procedures that affect their practice.
- Nurses can help defend malpractice claims by following guidelines for informed consent, refusal of care, and documentation and by maintaining their level of expertise.
- Documentation is the best evidence that the standard of care was met in care. Therefore nurses must ensure that their documentation accurately reflects the care given.
- Pediatric nurses function in a variety of roles, including care provider, teacher, collaborator, researcher, advocate, and manager.
- The care settings in which pediatric nurses may practice include acute care settings, clinics, physicians' offices, home health agencies, schools, rehabilitation centers, summer camps, day care centers, and hospices.
- Registered nurses with advanced education are prepared to provide primary care for children as certified nurse practitioners.
- Clinical nurse specialists function as educators, researchers, and consultants to provide in-depth interventions for many problems encountered in pediatric care.

- A primary responsibility of nurses is to provide information to children and their families; nurses must know the principles of teaching and learning to fulfill the role of educator.
- Nurses must learn to think critically by examining their own thought processes for flaws that can lead to inaccurate conclusions or poor clinical judgments.
- The nursing process begins with assessment and includes analysis of data that may result in nursing diagnoses. Nursing diagnoses are problems that nurses are legally accountable for identifying and managing independently.
- Collaborative problems are usually physiologic complications that require both physician-prescribed and nurse-prescribed interventions.
- Nurses must consider the impact of CAM when assessing the child and planning care.
- Professional journals are the best sources of information about scientifically sound research projects that demonstrate the effectiveness of nursing interventions.

REFERENCES AND READINGS

Ackley, B. J. & Ladwig, G. B. (2006). *Nursing diagnosis handbook: A guide to planning care* (7th ed.). St. Louis: Mosby.

Agency for Healthcare Research and Quality. (1996). *Clinical practice guidelines.* Retrieved May 21, 2005, from *www.ahrq.gov.*

Agency for Healthcare Research and Quality. (2002). AHRQ Publication No. 03-P008: *Program brief: Children's health highlights.* Rockville, MD: Author. Retrieved May 21, 2005, from *www.ahrq .gov/child/highlts/chhigh1.htm.*

Agency for Healthcare Research and Quality. (2004a). AHRQ Publication No. 05-0014: *2004 National healthcare disparities report.* Rockville, MD: Author.

Agency for Healthcare Research and Quality. (2004b) AHRZ Publication No. 05-0013: *2004 National healthcare quality report.* Rockville, MD: Author.

Agency for Healthcare Research and Quality. (2005). AHRQ Publication No. 05-PO11: *Fact sheet: Selected findings on child and adolescent health care from the 2004 national healthcare quality/disparities report.* Rockville, MD: Author.

Agency for Healthcare Research and Quality, National Guideline Clearinghouse. (2005). *Clinical practice guidelines.* Retrieved December 21, 2005, from *www.guideline.gov.*

Alfaro-LeFevre, R. (2004). *Critical thinking in nursing: A practical approach* (3rd ed.). Philadelphia: Saunders.

American Academy of Pediatrics Committee on Bioethics. (1996). *Ethics and the care of critically ill infants and children.* Elk Grove Village, IL: Author.

American Academy of Pediatrics Committee on Community Health Services. (2005). *Providing care for immigrant homeless, and migrant children.* Elk Grove Village, IL: Author.

American Academy of Pediatrics Committee on Emergency Medicine. (2003). Consent for emergency medical services for children and adolescents. *Pediatrics, 111*(3), 703-706.

American Academy of Pediatrics Committee on Public Education. (2001). Policy statement: Media violence. *Pediatrics, 108*(5), 1222-1226.

American Academy of Pediatrics Committee on School Health. (2003). Policy statement: Out-of-school suspension and expulsion. *Pediatrics, 112*(5), 1206-1209.

American Academy of Pediatrics Taskforce on Violence. (1999). Policy statement: The role of the pediatrician in youth violence prevention in clinical practice and at the community level. *Pediatrics, 103*(1), 173-181.

American Nurses Association. (2001). *The code of ethics.* Retrieved June 12, 2005, from *www.nursingworld.org/ethics/ecode.htm.*

American Nurses Association and Society of Pediatric Nurses. (2003). *The scope and standards of pediatric nursing practice.* Washington, DC: American Nurses Publishing.

Anderson, R. N., & Smith, B. L. (2003). Deaths: Leading causes for 2001. *National Vital Statistic Reports, 52*(10), Hyattsville, MD: National Center for Health Statistics. Retrieved February 5, 2004, from *www.cdc.gov/nchs/nvsr/nvsr52/nvsr52/_09.*

Betz, C. L. (2005). Health care quality and outcome guidelines for nursing of children and families. *Journal of Pediatric Nursing, 20*(3), 149-152.

Betz, C. L., Muennich Cowell, J., Lobo, M. L., Craft-Rosenberg, M. (2004). American Academy of Nursing child and family expert panel health care quality and outcomes guidelines for nursing of children and families: Phase II. *Nursing Outlook, 52*(6), 311-316.

Brindis, C. D., Klein, J., Schlitt, J., Santelli, J., Juszczak, L., & Nystrom, R. J. (2003). School-based health centers: Accessibility and accountability. *Journal of Adolescent Health, 32S*(65), 98-107.

Blumberg, S. J., Halfon, N., & Olson, L. (2004). The national survey of early childhood health. *Pediatrics, 113*(6), 1899-1906.

Carpenito-Moyet, L. J. (2004a). *Handbook of nursing diagnosis* (10th ed.). Philadelphia: Lippincott Williams & Wilkins.

Carpenito-Moyet, L. J. (2004b). *Nursing diagnosis: Application to clinical practice (10th ed.).* Philadelphia: Lippincott Williams & Wilkins.

Centers for Disease Control and Prevention. (2004a). *Infant mortality statistics from the 2002 period linked birth/infant death data set, 53*(10). Hyattsville, MD: Author.

Centers for Disease Control and Prevention. (2004b). Surveillance summaries. *MMWR, 53*(SS-2).

Cohen, R. A., Martinez, M. E., & Hao, C. (2005). *Health insurance coverage: Estimates from the national health interview survey, January-September 2004.* Hyattsville, MD: National Center for Health Statistics.

DeNavas-Walt, C., Proctor, B. D., & Lee, C. (2005). *Income, poverty, and health insurance coverage in the United States: 2004.* U.S. Census Bureau, Current Population Reports. P60-229. Washington, DC: U.S. Government Printing Office.

Dey, A. N., & Bloom, B. (2005). *Summary health statistics for U.S. children: National health interview survey, 2004. Vital and Health Statistics, 10*(227). Hyattsville, MD: National Center for Health Statistics.

Doenges, M. E., Moorhouse, M. F., Geissler-Murr, A. C. (2005). *Nursing diagnosis manual: Planning, individualizing, and documenting care.* Philadelphia: F.A. Davis.

Dowdell, E. B. (2004). Grandmother caregivers and caregiver burden. *American Journal of Maternal Child Nursing, 29*(5), 299-304.

Freid, V. M., Prager, K., MacKay, A. P., & Xia, H. (2003). *Chartbook on trends in the health of Americans. Health, United States, 2003.* Hyattsville, MD: National Center for Health Statistics.

Gorbova, M., & John, T. M. (2004). Taking a bite out of policies: A look at the policies affecting our nation's dental health. *Journal of Pediatric Nursing, 19*(1), 51-57.

Halfon, N., & Olson, L. (2004). Introduction: Results from a new national survey of children's health. *Pediatrics, 113*(6), 1895-1898.

Hamilton, B. E., Martin, J. A., & Sutton, P. D. (2003). *Births: Preliminary data for 2002, 51*(11). Hyattsville, MD: National Center for Health Statistics.

Honberg, L., McPherson, M., Strickland, B., Gage, J. C., & Newacheck, P. W. (2005). Assuring adequate health insurance: Results of the national survey of children with special health care needs. *Pediatrics, 115*(5), 1233-1239.

Ignatavicius, D. (2001). Six critical thinking skills for at-the-bedside success. *Dimensions of Critical Care Nursing, 20*(2), 30-33.

Klein, J. (2005). Adolescent pregnancy: Current trends and issues. *Pediatrics, 116*(1), 281-286.

Kogan, M. D., Schuster, M. D., Yu, S. M., Park, C. H., Olson, L. M., Inkelas, M., Bethell, C., Chung, P. J., Halfon, N. (2004). Routine assessment of family and community health risks: Parent views and what they receive. *Pediatrics, 113*(6), 1934-1943.

Lassetter, J. H., & Baldwin, J. H. (2004). Health care barriers for Latino children and provision of culturally competent care. *Journal of Pediatric Nursing, 19*(3), 184-192.

Lipe, S., & Beasley, S. (2004). *Critical thinking in nursing*. Philadelphia: Lippincott Williams & Wilkins.

March of Dimes. (2005). March of Dimes prematurity campaign. Retrieved December 21, 2005, from *www.modimes.org/prematurity*.

Markel, H., & Golden, J. (2005). Successes and missed opportunities in protecting our children's health: Critical junctures in the history of children's health policy in the United States. *Pediatrics, 115*(4), 1129-1133.

Martin, J. A., Kochanek, K. D., Strobino, D. M., Guyer, B., & MacDorman, M. F. (2005). Annual summary of vital statistics, 2003. *Pediatrics, 115*(3), 619-634.

Martin, J. A., Hamilton, B. E., Sutton, P. D., Ventura, S. J., Menacker, F., & Munson, M. L. (2003). *Births: Final data for 2002. National vital statistics reports, 52*(10). Hyattsville, MD: National Center for Health Statistics.

Matthews, T., Menacker, F., & MacDorman, M. (2004). *Explaining the 2001-02 infant mortality increase: Data from the linked birth/infant death data set. National Vital Statistics Reports, 53(12)*. Hyattsville, MD: National Center for Health Statistics.

Mayer, M. L., Cockrell Skinner, A., & Slifkin, R. T. (2004). Unmet need for routine and specialty care: Data from the national survey of children with special health care needs. *Pediatrics, 113*(2), e109-e115.

Menacker, F., Martin, J., MacDorman, M. F., & Ventura, S. J. (2004). *Births to 10-14 year-old mothers, 1990-2002: Trends and health outcomes. National Vital Statistics Reports, 53(7)*. Hyattsville, MD: National Center for Health Statistics.

Miller, V. A., Drotar, D., & Kodish, E. (2004). Children's competence for assent and consent: A review of empirical findings. *Journal of Ethics and Behavior, 14*(3), 255-295.

Nabors, L., Weist, M., Shugarman, R., Woeste, M., Mullet, E., & Rosner, L. (2004). Assessment, prevention, and intervention activities in a school-based program for children experiencing homelessness. *Behavior Modification, 28*(4), 565-578.

National Association of Pediatric Nurse Practitioners. (2004). *School-based and school-linked centers (position statement)*. Retrieved July 16, 2005, from *napnap.org/index.cfm?page=10&ssec=74*.

National Center for Complementary and Alternative Medicine. (2005). *What is complementary and alternative medicine (CAM)?* Retrieved July 16, 2005, from *nccam.nih.gov/health/whatiscam/*.

National Center for Health Statistics. (2005). *Health insurance coverage: Estimates from the national health interview survey, January-September 2004*. Hyattsville, MD: Author.

National Center for Health Statistics. (2004). *Health, United States, 2004, with chartbook on trends in the health of Americans*. Hyattsville, MD: Author.

National Council of State Boards of Nursing. (2005). *Just the facts: Nurse licensure compact*. Retrieved June 17, 2005, from *www.ncsbn.org*.

National Resource Center on Homelessness and Mental Illness. (2003). *What about the needs of children who are homeless?* Retrieved June 23, 2005, from *www.nrchmi.samhsa.gov*.

Neill, S. J. (2005). Research with children: A critical review of the guidelines. *Journal of Child Health Care, 9*(1), 46-58.

Nelson, R. (2005). Is there a doctor nurse in the house? A new vision for advanced practice nursing. *American Journal of Nursing, 105*(5), 28-29.

Paulsell, D., & Nogales, R. (2003). Quality child care for infants and toddlers from families with low incomes: Lessons learned from three communities. *Zero to Three, 23*(4), 4-10.

Rew, L., & Horner, S. D. (2003). Youth resilience framework for reducing health-risk behaviors in adolescents. *Pediatric Nursing, 18*(6), 379-388.

Rew, L., & Horner, S. D. (2003). Personal strengths of homeless adolescents living in a high-risk environment. *Advances in Nursing Science, 26*(2), 90-101.

Savage, M. F., Lee, J. Y., Kotch, J. B., & Vann, W. F. (2004). Early preventive dental visits: Effects on subsequent utilization and costs. *Pediatrics, 114*(4), e418-e423.

Shone, L. P., Dick, A. W., Klein, J. D., Zwanziger, J., & Szilagyi, P. G. (2005). Reduction in racial and ethnic disparities after enrollment in the state children's health insurance program. *Pediatrics, 115*(6). e697-e705.

Smith, P. J., Chu, S. Y., & Barker, L. E. (2004). Children who have received no vaccines: Who are they and where do they live? *Pediatrics, 114*(1), 187-195.

Society of Pediatric Nurses. (2005). *Protecting children and families involved in research (position statement)*. Retrieved June 24, 2005 from *www.pedsnurses.org/all.php?l=positions&x=3*.

Society of Pediatric Nurses. (2005). Safe staffing for pediatric nurses (position statement). Retrieved July 16, 2005, from *www.pedsnurses.org/home.php*.

Strickland, B., McPherson, M., Weissman, G., van Kyck, P., Huang, Z. J., & Newacheck, P. (2004). Access to the medical home: Results of the national survey of children with special health care needs. *Pediatrics. 113*(5), 1485-1492.

Truong, E., & Ferguson, S. (2003). Welfare reform at the crossroads: Pediatric nurses bridging the gap between self-sufficiency and health. *Journal of Pediatric Nursing, 18*(1), 60-63.

United States Department of Health and Human Services. (2000). *Healthy People 2010 online documents*. Retrieved June 17, 2005, from *www.healthypeople.gov/document/html/objectives/09-07.htm*.

United States Department of Health and Human Services, Health Resources and Services Administration, Maternal and Child Health Bureau. (2003). *Child health USA 2003*. Rockville, MD: Author.

United States Department of Health and Human Services, National Center for Vital Statistics. (2005). *Summary of health statistics for U.S. children. National health interview survey, 2004. Vital and health statistics, 10(227)*. Hyattsville, MD: Author.

United States Department of Health and Human Services Health Resources and Services Administration. (2005). *About insure kids now*. Retrieved December 27, 2005, from *www.insurekidsnow.gov*.

University of New Mexico College of Nursing. (2005). *What is critical thinking?* Retrieved December 27, 2005, from *hsc.unm.edu*.

Valet, R. S., Kutny, D. F., Hickson, G. B., & Cooper, W. O. (2004). Family reports of care denials for children enrolled in TennCare. *Pediatrics, 114*(1), e37-e42.

Velsor-Friedrich, B. (2003). Federally sponsored insurance programs for children: The State Children's Health Insurance Program. *Journal of Pediatric Nursing, 18*(2), 134-136.

Velsor-Friedrich, B., Pigott, T. D., & Louloudes, A. (2004). The effects of a school-based intervention on the self-care and health of African-American inner-city children with asthma. *Journal of Pediatric Nursing, 19*(4), 247-256.

Wilkinson, J. M. (2005). *Nursing diagnosis handbook with NIC interventions and NOC outcomes* (8th ed). Upper Saddle River, NJ: Pearson Prentice Hall.

Woodring, B. C. (2004). The role of the staff nurse in protecting children and families involved in research. *Pediatric Nursing, 19*(4), 311-313.

CHAPTER 2

Family-Centered Nursing Care

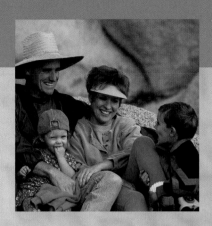

Learning Objectives

After studying this chapter, you should be able to:

- Explain the importance of family when caring for children.
- Describe different family structures and their impact on family functioning.
- Differentiate between healthy and dysfunctional families.
- List internal and external coping behaviors used by families when they face a crisis.
- Compare Western cultural values with those of other cultural groups.
- Describe the effect of cultural diversity on nursing practice.
- Describe common styles of parenting that nurses may encounter.
- Explain how variables in parents and children may affect their relationship.
- Discuss the use of discipline in a child's socialization.
- Evaluate the effects of an ill child on the family.

Definitions

anticipatory guidance Providing the family with information on what to expect regarding a future event, a potential problem or issue, or a child's next developmental phase.

coping Efforts directed toward managing and solving various problems, events, and stressors.

culture The sum of values, beliefs, and practices of a group of people that are transmitted from one generation to the next.

discipline The structure an adult sets for a child's life, designed to allow the child to interact socially in the real world in an appropriate manner; the training expected to produce a specific type or pattern of behavior.

egocentric Preoccupied with one's own interests and needs.

ethnic Pertaining to religious, racial, national, or cultural group characteristics, especially speech patterns, social customs, and physical characteristics.

ethnicity Condition of belonging to a particular ethnic group; also refers to ethnic pride.

ethnocentrism The opinion that the beliefs and customs of one's own ethnic group are superior to those of others.

family Two or more persons who are joined together by bonds of sharing and emotional closeness and who identify themselves as being part of the family (Friedman, 2003).

fatalism The belief that events are predestined.

nuclear family A family consisting of a two-generation relationship of parents and children, living together and more or less isolated from other close relatives.

stress Any situation or condition, positive or negative, requiring adjustment on the part of the individual, family, or group.

Audio Glossary

Electronic Resources

Additional information related to the content in Chapter 2 can be found on:

the interactive companion CD-ROM

- Audio Glossary
- NCLEX Review Questions
- Skill-Providing Culturally Sensitive Care

or the companion website at *evolve*
http://evolve.elsevier.com/james/ncoc

- NANDA-Approved Nursing Diagnoses
- NCLEX Review Questions
- Resources for Health Care Providers and Families
- WebLinks

No factor influences a person as profoundly as the family. Families protect and promote children's growth, development, health, and well-being until the children reach maturity. A healthy family provides children with love, affection, and a sense of belonging and nurtures feelings of self-esteem and self-worth. Children need stable families to grow into happy, functioning adults. Family relationships continue to be important during adulthood. Family relationships influence, positively or negatively, people's relationships with others. Family influence continues into the next generation as a person selects a mate, forms a new family, and often rears children.

For nurses caring for children, the whole family is the client. The nurse cares for the child in the context of a dynamic family system rather than caring for just an infant, or a child. The nurse is responsible for supporting families and encouraging healthy coping patterns during periods of normal growth and development or illness.

THE FAMILY AND NURSING CARE

Family structures in the United States are changing. The number of families with children that are headed by a married couple has declined, and the number of single-parent families has increased. In addition, roles have changed within the family. Whereas the role of the provider was once almost exclusively assigned to the father, both parents now may be providers, and many fathers are active in nurturing and disciplining their children.

Types of Families

Family types are sometimes categorized into three groups: traditional, nontraditional, and high risk. Nontraditional and high-risk families often need care that differs from the care needed by traditional families. Different family structures can produce varying stressors. For example, the single-parent family has as many demands placed on it for resources, such as time and money, as the two-parent family. Only one parent, however, is able to meet these demands.

Traditional Families

Traditional families (also called nuclear families) are headed by two parents who view parenting as the major priority in their lives and whose energies are not depleted by stressful conditions such as poverty, illness, or substance abuse. Traditional families can be single-income or dual-income families. Today, the family structure composed of two married parents and their children represents only 68% of families with children, down from 77% in 1980 (Federal Interagency Forum on Child and Family Statistics, 2005).

Single-income families in which one parent, usually the father, is the sole provider are a minority among households in the United States. Most two-parent families depend on two incomes, either to make ends meet or to provide nonessentials that they could not afford on one income. One or both parents must often travel as a work responsibility. Dependence on two incomes has created a great deal of stress on parents, subjecting them to many of the same problems that single-parent families face. For instance, reliable, competent child care is a major issue and has increased the stress traditional families experience. A high consumer debt load gives them less cushion for financial setbacks such as job loss. Having the time and flexibility to attend to the requirements of both their careers and their children may be difficult for parents in these families.

Nontraditional Families

The growing number of nontraditional families, designated as "complex households" by the U.S. Census Bureau (Simmons & Dye, 2003), includes single-parent families, blended families, adoptive families, unmarried couples with children, multigenerational families, and homosexual parent families (Fig. 2-1).

Single-Parent Families. Millions of families are now headed by a single parent, most often the mother, who must function as homemaker and caregiver and also is often the major provider for the family's financial needs. Divorce is the most common cause of single-parent families, although childbirth among unmarried women is also a major contributor. Widowhood of the parent sometimes occurs as well. The proportion of families with children that are headed by a single mother is now 23%, whereas single-father families, once rare, now comprise 5% of this group. Four percent of children live with neither parent (Federal Interagency Forum on Child and Family Statistics, 2005).

Slightly more than 50% of the 11 million children who live in poverty live in homes headed by a single mother, 40.5% live in homes headed by married parents, and 8.6% live in families headed by a single father (United States Department of Health and Human Services, 2003). Single parents may feel overwhelmed by the prospect of assuming all child-rearing responsibilities and may be less prepared for illness or loss of a job than two-parent families.

Blended Families. Blended families are formed when single, divorced, or widowed parents bring children from a previous union into their new relationship. Many times the couple desires children with each other, creating a contemporary family structure commonly described as "yours, mine, and ours." These families must overcome differences in parenting styles and values to form a cohesive blended family. Differing expectations of children's behavior and development as well as differing beliefs about discipline often cause family conflict. Financial difficulties can result if one parent is obligated to pay child support from a previous relationship. Older children may resent the introduction of a stepmother or stepfather into the family system. This can cause tension between the biologic parent, the children, and the stepmother or stepfather.

Adoptive Families. People who adopt a child may have problems that biologic parents do not face. Biologic parents have the long period of gestation and the gradual changes of pregnancy to help them adjust emotionally and socially to the birth of a child. An adoptive family, both parents and siblings, is expected to make these same adjustments suddenly when the adopted child arrives. Adoptive parents may add pressure to themselves by having an unrealistically high

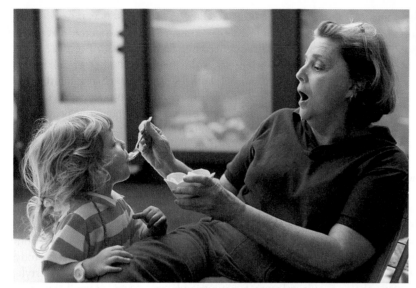

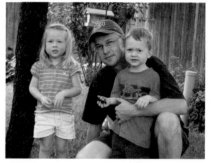

Busy parents may rely on grandparents for childcare or for an additional measure of love and attention for their children. Some grandparents raise grandchildren because of their own children's inability to do so.

Fathers are the primary childcare providers in a growing number of families. Fathers who are not the primary caregivers often participate more actively in caring for their children than the fathers of previous generations.

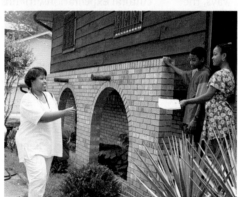

A single parent often experiences financial and time constraints. Children in single-parent families are often given more responsibility to care for themselves and younger siblings.

FIG 2-1   **The nurse caring for a child needs to know the child's family structure and the identity of the child's primary caregiver. This background becomes the context in which the nurse provides care. If family support is a concern, the nurse can provide information about local community resources. For example, in some communities, after-school programs and "warm lines" can help children with schoolwork and alleviate loneliness and fear.**

standard for themselves as parents. Additional issues with adoptive families may include possible lack of knowledge of the child's health history, the difficulty assimilating if the child is adopted from another country, and the question of when and how to tell the child about being adopted. Adoptive parents and biologic parents need information, support, and guidance to prepare them to care for the infant or child and maintain their own relationships.

Multigenerational Families. The multigenerational or extended family includes members from three or more generations living under one roof. This family structure is becoming increasingly common in the United States (Schwede, 2003). Elderly parents may live with their adult children, or in some cases adult children return to their parents' home, either because they are unable to support themselves or because they want the additional support that the grandparents provide for the grandchildren. The latter arrangement has given rise to the term *boomerang* families. Extended families are vulnerable to generational conflicts and may need education and referral to counselors to prevent disintegration of the family unit.

Grandparents or other older family members, because of the inability of the parents to care for their children, now head a growing number of households with children (Simmons & Dye, 2003). Approximately 3.6% of older people living with families in the United States are grandparents; of these, 42% are the primary caregivers for their grandchildren (Simmons & Dye, 2003). The strain of raising children a second time may cause tremendous physical, financial, and emotional stress.

Same-Sex Parent Families. Although families headed by same-sex parents are proportionately uncommon, they are increasingly recognized in the United States (Schwede, 2003). The children in such families may be the offspring of previous heterosexual unions, or they may be adopted children or children conceived by an artificial reproductive technique such as in vitro fertilization. This couple may face many challenges from a community that is unaccustomed to alternative lifestyles. The children's adaptation depends on the parents' psychologic adjustment, the degree of participation and support from the absent biologic parent, and the degree of community support.

Communal Family. Communal families include groups of people who have chosen to live together as an extended family group. Their relationship to each other is motivated by social value or financial necessity rather than by kinship. Their values are often spiritually based and may be more liberal than the traditional family. Traditional family roles may not exist.

FAMILY THEORIES AND MODELS

A theory helps organize facts in some sort of pattern. Scholars use different theories or models to explain the dynamics of family relations. These models provide a basis for family assessment and intervention by the nurse and other health professionals. Theories come from the social sciences, from therapists who work with families, and from nurses. Regardless of the underlying theory, most scholars agree that although the family is composed of individuals who interact with each other and their environment in unique ways, the family is also a whole unit. What affects an individual family member affects the family as a whole. Table 2-1 summarizes some pertinent family theories.

Characteristics of Healthy Families

In general, healthy families are able to adapt to changes that occur in the family unit. Pregnancy and parenthood create some of the most powerful changes that a family experiences.

Healthy families exhibit some common characteristics that provide a framework for assessing how all families function (Cooley, 2005):

- Members of healthy families communicate openly with one another to express their concerns and needs.
- Healthy family members remain flexible in their roles, with roles changing to meet changing family needs.
- Adults in healthy families agree on the basic principles of parenting so that minimal discord exists about concepts such as discipline and sleep schedules.
- Healthy families are adaptable and are not overwhelmed by life changes.
- Members of healthy families volunteer assistance without waiting to be asked.
- Family members spend time together regularly but facilitate autonomy.
- Healthy families seek appropriate resources for support when needed.
- Healthy families transmit cultural values and expectations to children.

Factors That Interfere With Family Functioning

Factors that interfere with the family's ability to provide for the needs of its members include lack of financial resources, absence of adequate family support, birth of an infant who needs specialized care, an ill child, unhealthy habits such as smoking or abuse of other substances, and inability to make mature decisions that are necessary to provide care for the children.

High-Risk Families

All families encounter stressors, but some factors add to the usual stress experienced by a family. The nurse must consider the additional needs of the family with a higher risk for being dysfunctional. Examples of these high-risk families are those experiencing marital conflict and divorce, those with adolescent parents, those affected by violence against one or more of the family members, those involved with substance abuse, and those with an ill child.

Marital Conflict and Divorce

Although divorce is traumatic to children, research has shown that living in a home filled with conflict is also detrimental to children (Grych, Harold, & Miles, 2003). Divorce can be the outcome of many years of unresolved family conflict. It can result in continuing conflict over child custody, visitation, and child support; changes in housing, lifestyle, cultural expectations, friends, and extended family relationships; diminished self-esteem; and changes in the physical, emotional, or spiritual health of the child and other family members.

Divorce is loss that needs to be grieved. The conflict and divorce may affect children, and young children may be unable to verbalize their distress. Nurses can help children through the grieving process with age-appropriate activities such as therapeutic play (see Chapter 11). Principles of active listening (see Chapter 3) are valuable for both adults and children to help them express their feelings. Nurses can also help newly divorced or separated parents through listening, encouragement, and referrals to support groups or counselors.

Adolescent Parenting

The pregnancy rate for teenagers in the United States remains among the highest among developed countries, although it has been declining since the early 1990s. In 2003 in the United States, 41.7 per 1000 live babies were born to teenagers between the ages of 15 and 19 years. Adolescent birth rates vary by race. During this same period, teenage birth rates fell for all race and ethnic groups, with the largest decline in non-Hispanic black teenagers. This group showed a 5% decline between 2002 and 2003 (Martin et al, 2003).

Teenage parenting often has a negative impact on the health and social outcomes of the entire family. Adolescent girls are at increased risk for a number of pregnancy complications such as hypertension or fetal growth restriction, and their infants are at increased risk for low birth weight, early death, and sudden infant death syndrome (Menacker, Martin, MacDorman, & Ventura, 2004). Those who become parents during adolescence are unlikely to attain a high level of education and, as a result, are more likely to be poor and often homeless. The father of the child often does not contribute to the economic or psychologic support of his children. Moreover, the cycle of teen parenting and economic hardship is more likely to be continued because children of adolescent parents are themselves more likely to become teenage parents.

TABLE 2-1	Summary of Family Theories	
Theory	**Overview**	**Applicable Terminology**
Systems theory	Originally developed by von Bertalanffy (1968) for use in physics and biology, systems theory views the family as being similar to the human body: a whole system that comprises interacting but distinct subsystems. The system, or family, changes and adapts over time under both internal and external influences, becomes more complex as it develops, and interacts with the external environment (suprasystem) through boundaries.	Wholeness: The family is an organized whole (more than just the sum of its parts), with family members being autonomous, interdependent, and interactive. Hierarchies and relationships exist within the family (e.g., parent-child). A change in one family member will affect every other member of the family as well as the family structure itself. Feedback: The process and patterns by which family members relate to each other and their community while maintaining homeostasis (internal balance) within the family system. These balancing features can be adaptive or maladaptive. Boundaries: Invisible lines of demarcation between family members and between the family and the environment. Boundaries can be open or closed and determine the relative isolation of family members from each other and the family from the community.
Bowen's family systems theory	Bowen (1976) described anxiety as a constant emotion in life and an emotion that can cause dysfunction in individuals and families. His theory describes adapting to stress by separating the emotion engendered by anxiety from the intellectual means of dealing with anxiety-producing stressors. This process of separating emotions from the intellect is accomplished by differentiating the self from the family. By looking at the emotional interactions within the family in an intellectual way, the family can understand past behaviors and choose to change.	Differentiation of self: The degree to which family members are emotionally separate from each other and able to distinguish thoughts from feelings. Multigenerational transmission process: The handing down of emotions from one generation to the next through the socialization of children. Dysfunctional adults tend to socialize their own children with the same dysfunctional coping styles and emotions that their own parents used. Family projection process: A process in which an anxious, undifferentiated parent becomes overly involved with one child as a way of decreasing anxiety. Unable to see the child's true character, the parent projects anxiety and inappropriate attributes onto the child. Eventually, the child might become what the parent has projected and unable to establish an individual identity separate from what the parent believes. Triangulation: The process by which tension between two family members is decreased by involving a third person in the relationship. Triangles can inhibit family members' creativity and flexibility to solve problems.
Duvall's family development model	Based on developmental theories applied to individuals (e.g., Erikson), Duvall and Miller (1995) described eight specific stages a family encounters during its development. These stages are defined by the age of the oldest child in the family. Goals, or developmental tasks, change as the family grows and matures. The goals of maintaining the marital relationship and kinship relationships with extended family appear in all stages. As with the developmental theorists, unsuccessful achievement of these goals or tasks can lead to family dysfunction. When the family transitions from one stage to the next, the resulting associated stress can cause a maturational family crisis. The major problem with this theory is that it is based primarily on the traditional nuclear family structure.	Stage I: beginning families. Major goal: establish a mutually satisfying relationship and connection with original families. Stage II: childbearing families (oldest child >30 months). Major goal: integration of the child into the family while maintaining marital and family relationships. Stage III: families with preschoolers (oldest child >6 years). Major goal: socialize children and meet family members' needs for space, safety, and privacy. Stage IV: families with schoolchildren (oldest child >13 years). Major goal: promote school and social achievement and healthy relationships with peers. Stage V: families with teenagers (oldest child >20 years). Major goal: facilitate teen's autonomy and sense of identity through open communication and maintaining the family's ethical and moral standards. Stage VI: launching young adults (the last child leaves home). Major goal: renewing and readjusting the marital relationship and caring for aging grandparents. Stage VII: families in middle-aged years (empty nest through retirement). Major goal: promote a healthy environment and sustain communication with grandparents and children; appropriately adapt to changes in financial resources. Stage VIII: families in retirement (retirement through the death of both spouses). Major goal: adjust to losses, maintain intergenerational connections, make sense of one's existence (Duvall & Miller, 1995).

Violence

Violence is a constant stressor in some families. Violence can occur in any family of any socioeconomic or educational status. Children endure the psychologic pain of seeing their mother victimized by the man who is supposed to love and care for her. In addition, because of the role models they see in the adults, these children may repeat the cycle of violence when they are adults and become abusers or victims of violence themselves.

Abuse of the child may be physical, sexual, emotional, or the abuse may be in the form of neglect (see Chapter 29). Often one child in the family is the target of abuse or neglect, whereas others are given proper care. As in adult abuse, children who witness abuse are more likely to repeat that behavior when they are parents themselves because they have not learned constructive ways to deal with their stress or discipline children.

Substance Abuse

Parents who abuse drugs or alcohol may neglect their children because obtaining and using the substance(s) may have a stronger pull on the parents than does care of their children. Children whose parents abuse substances are at risk for becoming a victim of violence (or witnessing violence), emotional effects of inconsistent parenting, social isolation, developmental delays, and other emotional and social consequences. In addition, these children are more likely to live in poverty and be homeless because so much money is spent maintaining the parent's substance habit (Children of Alcoholics Foundation, 2005; Sullivan, Chaliman, & Mooney, 2005).

The child may be the substance abuser in the home. The drug habit can lead a child into unhealthy friendships and may result in criminal activity to maintain the habit. School achievement is likely to plummet, and the older adolescent may drop out of school. Both children and adults can die as a result of their drug activity, either as a direct effect of the drugs or from associated criminal activity or risk-taking behaviors.

Child with Special Needs

When a child is born with a birth defect or has an illness that requires special care, the family is under additional stress (see Chapters 12 and 30). In most cases, their initial reactions of shock and disbelief gradually resolve into acceptance of the child's limitations. However, the parents' grieving may be long term as they repeatedly see other children doing things that their child cannot and perhaps will not ever do.

These families often suffer financial hardship. Health insurance benefits may quickly reach their maximum. Even if the child has public assistance for health care costs, the family often experiences a fall in income because one parent must remain home with the sick child rather than work outside the home.

Strains on the marriage and the parents' relationships with their other children are inevitable under these circumstances. Parents have little time or energy left to nurture their relationship with each other, and divorce may add yet another strain to the family. Siblings may resent the parental time and attention required for care of the ill child yet feel guilty if they express their resentment.

The outlook is not always pessimistic in these families, however. If the family learns skills to cope with the added demands imposed on it by this situation, the potential exists for growth in maturity, compassion, and strength of character.

HEALTHY VERSUS DYSFUNCTIONAL FAMILIES

Family conflict is unavoidable. It is a natural result of a perceived unequal exchange or an imbalance in the use of resources by individual members. Conflict should not be viewed as bad or disruptive; the management of the conflict, not the conflict itself, may be problematic. Conflict can produce growth and improved family functioning if the outcome is resolution as opposed to dissolution or continued conflict. The following three ingredients are required to resolve conflict:

1. Open communication
2. Accurate perceptions about the nature and degree of conflict
3. Constructive efforts to resolve the conflict, such as willingness to consider the view of the other, consider alternate solutions, and compromise

Dysfunctional families have problems in any one or a combination of these areas. They tend to become trapped in patterns in which they maintain conflicts rather than resolve them. The conflicts create stress, and the family must cope with the resultant stress.

Coping with Stress

When viewing the family as a balanced system that has interrelationships both internally and externally, stressors are viewed as forces that change the balance in the system. Stressful events are neither positive nor negative, but rather neutral until they are interpreted by the individual. Both positive and negative events can cause stress (Ingoldsby, Smith, & Miller, 2003). For example, the birth of a child is usually a joyful event, but it can also be stressful.

Some families are able to mobilize their strengths and resources, thus effectively adapting to the stressors. Other families fall apart. A family crisis is a state or period of disorganization that affects the foundation of the family (Ingoldsby et al., 2003).

Coping Strategies

Nurses can help families cope with stress by helping each family identify its strengths and resources. Friedman, Bowden, and Jones (2003) identified family coping strategies as internal and external. Box 2-1 identifies family coping strategies and further defines internal strategies as family relationship strategies, cognitive strategies, and communication strategies. External strategies focus on maintaining active community linkages and using social support systems and spiritual strategies. Some families adjust quickly to extreme crises, whereas other families become chaotic with relatively minor crises.

BOX 2-1	Coping Strategies of Families

Internal Coping Strategies

Relationship Strategies
- Family group reliance
- Greater sharing together
- Role flexibility

Cognitive Strategies
- Normalizing
- Controlling the meaning of the problem by reframing and passive appraisal
- Joint problem solving
- Gaining of information and knowledge

Communication Strategies
- Being open and honest
- Use of humor and laughter

External Coping Strategies

Community Strategy: Maintaining Active Linkages With the Community

Social Support Strategies
- Extended family
- Friends
- Neighbors
- Self-help groups
- Formal social supports

Spiritual Strategies
- Seeking advice of clergy
- Becoming more involved in religious activities
- Having faith in God
- Prayer
- Seeking renewal and connectedness in communion with nature

Reprinted from Friedman, M., Bowden, V., & Jones, E. (2003). *Family nursing* (5th ed.). Upper Saddle River, NJ: Prentice Hall.

Family functional patterns that existed before the crisis are probably the best indicators of how the family will respond to a crisis.

CULTURAL INFLUENCES ON PEDIATRIC NURSING

Culture is the sum of the beliefs and values that are learned, shared, and transmitted from generation to generation by a particular group. Cultural values guide the thinking, decisions, and actions of the group, particularly regarding pivotal events such as birth, sexual maturity, and death. *Ethnicity* is the condition of belonging to a particular group that shares race, language and dialect, religious faiths, traditions, values, and symbols as well as food preferences, literature, and folklore. Cultural beliefs and values vary among different groups, and nurses must be aware that individuals often believe their cultural values and patterns of behavior are superior to those of other groups. This belief, termed *ethnocentrism*, forms the basis for many conflicts that occur when people from different cultural groups have frequent contact.

Nurses must be aware that culture is composed of visible and invisible layers that could be said to resemble an iceberg (Fig. 2-2). The observable behaviors can be compared with the visible tip of the iceberg. The history, beliefs, values, and religion are not observed but are the hidden foundation on which behaviors are based and can be likened to the large, submerged part of the iceberg. To comprehend cultural behavior fully, one must seek knowledge of the hidden beliefs that behaviors express. One must also have the desire or motivation to engage in the process of becoming culturally competent to be effective in caring for diverse populations. Inherent in this process is the ability to be open and flexible with others, respect differences, build on similarities, and posses a willingness to learn from other cultures (Campinha-Bacote, 2003).

Religious beliefs often have a strong influence on families as they face the crisis of illness. Specific beliefs about the causes, treatment, and cure of illness are important for the nurse to know to empower the family to deal with the immediate crisis. Table 2-2 describes how some religious beliefs affect health care.

Implications of Cultural Diversity for Nurses

Many immigrants and refugees are relatively young, which means that nurses in most localities will provide care for families rearing children in culturally diverse circumstances. To provide effective care, nurses must be aware that culture is among the most significant factors that influence parenthood, health, and illness. Many health care workers' knowledge of other cultures and how to care for children and families in a culturally sensitive manner is limited. In addition to increasing the numbers of nurses from diverse populations, nurses in practice must be reached through innovative strategies to increase competence when caring for diverse populations (Jones, Cason, & Bond, 2004). Table 2-3 summarizes the characteristics of family roles, health care beliefs and practices, and communication styles of some cultural groups. These descriptions are merely generalizations. Each family is unique and needs to be assessed and evaluated individually.

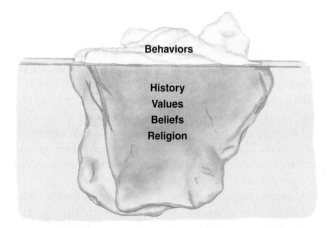

Behaviors

History
Values
Beliefs
Religion

FIG 2-2   **Visible and hidden layers of culture are like the visible and submerged parts of an iceberg. Many cultural differences are hidden below the surface.**

| TABLE 2-2 | Religious Beliefs Affecting Health Care |

Religion and Basic Beliefs

Practices

Christian Science

Based on scientific system of healing.
Beliefs based on Bible, science, and health with key to scriptures.
Seek to overcome evil through prayer, belief, and Christian acts.
Healing is divinely natural, not miraculous.

Birth: Use physician or midwife during childbirth. No baptism ceremony.
Dietary practices: Alcohol and tobacco are considered drugs and are not used. Coffee and tea may also be declined.
Death: Autopsy and donation of organs are usually declined.
Health care: May refuse medical treatment. View health in a spiritual framework.
Seek exemption from immunizations but obey legal requirements.
When Christian Science believer is hospitalized, parent or client may request that a Christian Science practitioner be notified.

Jehovah's Witness

Believe in God and Son Jesus Christ.
Expected to follow the example of Jesus Christ in daily living.
Expected to preach house to house about the good news of God.
Bible is doctrinal authority.
No distinction is made between clergy and laity.

Baptism: No infant baptism. Baptism by immersion of adults.
Dietary practices: Use of tobacco and alcohol discouraged.
Death: Autopsy decided by persons involved. Burial and cremation acceptable.
Birth control and abortion: Use of birth control is a personal decision. Abortion opposed based on Exodus 21:22-23.
Health care: Blood transfusions not allowed. May accept alternatives to transfusions, such as use of nonblood plasma expanders, careful surgical technique to minimize blood loss, and use of autologous transfusions.
Nurses should check unconscious clients for identification that states that the person does not want a transfusion.
Jehovah's Witnesses are prepared to die rather than break God's law.
Respect the health care given by physicians, but look to God and His laws as the final authority for their decisions.

The Church of Jesus Christ of Latter-Day Saints (Mormon)

Restorationism: True church of Christ ended with the first generation of apostles but was restored with the founding of Mormon Church.
Articles of faith: Mormon doctrine states that individuals are saved if they are obedient to God's divine ordinances (faith, repentance, baptism by immersion and laying on of hands, observance of Lord's Supper on Sunday).
Word of God can be found in the Bible, Book of Mormon, Doctrine, and Covenants, Pearl of Great Price, and current revelations.

Baptism: By immersion. Considered essential for the living and the dead. If a child older than 8 years is very ill, whether baptized or unbaptized, a member of the church's clergy should be called.
Holy Communion: Hospitalized client may desire to have a member of the church's clergy administer the sacrament.
Anointing of the sick: Mormons frequently are anointed and given a blessing before going to the hospital and after admission by laying on of hands.
Dietary practices: Tobacco and caffeine are not used. Mormons eat meat (limited) but encourage the intake of fruits, grains, and herbs.
Death: Prefer burial of the body. A church elder should be notified to assist the family.
Birth control and abortion: Abortion is opposed unless the life of the mother is in danger. Only natural methods of birth control are recommended. Other means are used only when the physical or emotional health of the mother is at stake.
Other practices: Believe in the healing power of "laying on of hands."
Cleanliness is important. Believe in healthy living and adhere to health care requirements.

Adapted from Carson, V. B. (1989). *Spiritual dimensions of nursing practice* (pp. 100-102). Philadelphia: Saunders; Betz, C. L., Hunsberger, M., & Wright, S. (1994). *Family-centered nursing care of children* (2nd ed., pp. 2230-2236). Philadelphia: Saunders; Taylor, E. J. (2002). *Spiritual care: Nursing theory, research, and practice.* Upper Saddle River, NJ: Prentice Hall; Spector, R. E. (2004). *Cultural diversity in health and illness* (6th ed). Upper Saddle River, NJ: Prentice Hall.

Western Cultural Beliefs

Nursing practice in the United States is based largely on Western beliefs. Nurses must recognize that these beliefs may differ significantly from those of other societies and that the differences may cause a great deal of conflict.

Leininger (1978) identified seven dominant Western cultural values. These values greatly influence the thinking and action of nurses in the United States but may not be shared by their clients:

1. *Democracy* is a cultural value not shared by families who believe that elders or other higher authorities in the group make decisions. Fatalism, or a belief that events and results are predestined, may also affect health care decisions.

2. *Individualism* conflicts with the values of many cultural groups in which individual goals are subordinated to the greater good of the group.

3. *Cleanliness* is an American "obsession" viewed with amazement by many.

4. *Preoccupation with time,* which is measured by health care professionals in minutes and hours, is a major source of conflict with those who mark time by different standards, such as seasons or body needs.

5. *Reliance on machines and equipment* may intimidate families who are not comfortable with technology.

6. *The belief that optimal health is a right* is in direct conflict with beliefs in many cultures in the world in which health is not a major emphasis or even an expectation.

TABLE 2-2   Religious Beliefs Affecting Health Care—cont'd

Religion and Basic Beliefs	Practices
The Church of Jesus Christ of Latter-Day Saints (Mormon)—cont'd	
Christ will return to rule in Zion, located in America.	Families are of great importance, so visiting should be encouraged. The church maintains a welfare system to assist those in need.
Roman Catholic	
Beliefs based on Bible, apostolic tradition, and contemporary revelation.	*Baptism:* Infant baptism by affusion (sprinkling of water on head). Original sin is believed to be "washed away." If death is imminent or a fetus is aborted, anyone can perform the baptism by sprinkling water on the forehead, saying "I baptize thee in the name of the Father, Son, and Holy Spirit." *Anointing of the sick:* Encouraged for anyone who is ill or injured. Always done if prognosis is poor. *Dietary practices:* Fasting and abstinence from meat optional during Lent. Fasting required for all, except children, elders, and those who are ill, on Ash Wednesday and Good Friday. No meat on Ash Wednesday and on Fridays during Lent strongly encouraged. *Death:* Organ donation permitted.
Hinduism	
Belief in reincarnation and that the soul persists even though the body changes, dies, and is reborn. Nonviolent approach to living. Congregation worship is not customary.	*Dietary practices:* Dietary restrictions vary according to sect. *Death:* Death rituals specify practices and who can touch corpse. Circumcision is observed by ritual.
Islam	
Belief in one God that humans can approach directly in prayer. Based on the teachings of Muhammad. Five Pillars of Islam. Compulsory prayers are said at dawn, noon, afternoon, after sunset, and after nightfall.	*Dietary practices:* Prohibit eating pork and using alcohol. Fast during Ramadan (ninth month of Muslim year). *Death:* Oppose autopsy and organ donation. Death ritual prescribes the handling of corpse by only family and friends. Burial occurs as soon as possible.
Judaism	
Beliefs are based on the Old Testament, the Torah, and the Talmud, the oral and written laws of faith. Belief in one God who is approached directly. Believe Messiah is still to come. Believe Jews are God's chosen people.	*Circumcision:* A symbol of God's covenant with Israel. Done on eighth day after birth. *Bar Mitzvah:* Ceremonial rite of passage for boys (approximately 13 years of age) into manhood. *Death:* Remains are washed according to rite by members of the Ritual Burial Society. Burial occurs as soon as possible.

7. *Admiration of self-sufficiency and financial success* may conflict with the beliefs of other societies that place less value on wealth and more value on less-tangible things such as spirituality.

Cultural Influences on the Care of People from Specific Groups

To provide the best care for all clients, the nurse should know common cultural beliefs and practices that influence nursing care. Because communication is an essential component of nursing assessment and teaching, the nurse must understand cultural influences that may form barriers to communicating with people from another culture.

Asian and Pacific Islander
"Asian" refers to populations with origins in many areas, such as the Far East, Southeast Asia, or the Indian subcontinent, including Vietnam, China, Japan, and The Philippines. "Pacific Islander" refers to the original peoples of Hawaii, Guam, Samoa, and other Pacific Islands. Their roots are in their ethnic viewpoint as well as their country of origin. They are not a homogeneous group, but differ in language, culture, and length of residence in the United States. Asians and Pacific Islanders comprise 4.4% of the U.S. population (Reeves & Bennett, 2003).

In the Asian culture, the family is highly valued and often consists of many generations that remain close to each other. The elders of the family are highly respected. Self-sufficiency and self-control are highly valued. Asian-Americans place a high value on "face," or honor, and may be unwilling to do anything that causes another to "lose face." When medication or therapy is recommended, they seldom say no. They may accept the prescription or medication sample but not take the medicine, or they may agree to undergo a procedure

TABLE 2-3 Cultural Differences in Families			
Cultural Group	**Family Roles**	**Health Care Practices**	**Communication**
African American	Children are important and valued Respectfulness, obedience, conformity to parent-defined rules, and good behavior are stressed The belief is that parents need to protect children from dangers outside the home through their parenting style Children are encouraged to engage in productive activities Some families have a patriarchal system, but a high percentage of families have a matriarchal system Growing number of grandparents are functioning as the primary parent Strong work and achievement orientation Self-reliance and education valued Strong church affiliations Deep respect for elders, especially grandmothers	Proper diet, rest, and a clean environment Prayer Sickness is viewed as a separation between God and man Home remedies Folk medicine Power of some people to heal (healers) May be suspicious of health-care providers Access to health care may be impeded either by intentional or unintentional insults such as an action or tone of voice	Speech is dynamic and expressive Facial expressions can be quite demonstrative Touch is important when interacting with family and those close to them What transpires in the family is considered private
Chinese	Children are highly valued Parents are permissive with young children, but when they are old enough to understand authority, they are required to obey Family members identify themselves in relation to others in the family The extended family is extremely important Each family maintains a recognized head Fathers, sons, and uncles are important in matters of politics and business Elder members of the family are venerated Children are expected to care for their parents Chinese who adopt Western ideas may find the ways of their elders to be too demanding; however, they respect and visit them frequently Maintaining reputation is important	Holistic health (health promotion and illness prevention): a state of spiritual and physical harmony Use a combination of traditional Chinese medicine and Western medicine Traditional Chinese medicine includes *acupuncture* (goal is to restore the yin and yang through the insertion of needles through specific points in the body known as meridians), *moxibustion* (goal is to restore the yin and yang through the application of heat to various meridians), *and herbal remedies* (reluctant to have blood drawn because blood is considered the source of life)	More than 30 different languages are spoken Rarely complain but silently withdraw May smile when they do not understand
Filipino	The family is the basic social and economic unit Emphasis on religious obligations Authority in the family is considered egalitarian Predominately two-income families Grandmothers often immigrate to United States to care for grandchildren while parents work	Seek out family for help when ill May use a combination of traditional medical care and alternative care suggested by family and friends Cleanliness is important Emphasis is on obtaining adequate rest, sleep, nutrition, and exercise May not seek out health care until illness is advanced	Interpersonal relationships are important and clear communication may be sacrificed to avoid conflict Often puzzled or offended by the precision and exactness of American communication Allowing time to respond communicates respect

Adapted from Purnell, L. D., & Paulanka, B. J. (2003). *Transcultural health care (2nd ed)*. Philadelphia: F.A. Davis; D'Avanzo, C. E., & Geissler, E. M. (2003). *Cultural health assessment (3rd ed)*. St. Louis: Mosby; Spector, R. E. (2000). *Cultural diversity in health & illness (5th ed)*. Upper Saddle River, NJ: Prentice Hall Health.

TABLE 2-3	Cultural Differences in Families—cont'd		
Cultural Group	**Family Roles**	**Health Care Practices**	**Communication**
Filipino—cont'd	Children are expected to attend college Children are taught to be respectful and heed the authority of older relatives Full disclosure of personal information may be withheld if the information is perceived as putting the family at risk for shame Family provides primary support during illness Strong value of reciprocal obligation	Pain is viewed as part of living an honorable life; may appear stoic and tolerate high levels of pain Self-sacrifice is believed to be virtuous, thus caretakers may not seek help until overwhelmed	Some individuals may avoid prolonged eye contact with authority figures as a form of respect Comfortable with silence, may wait for the other person to initiate conversation Touch is common with co-ethnics and insiders
Arabic	Women are subordinate to men and young people subordinate to older people Men are the breadwinners, decision makers, and protectors Women are responsible for the care and education of children Women attain power and status in advancing years Father is the disciplinarian and the mother the ally and mediator Family relationships are characterized by affection and sentimentality Children are dearly loved, indulged, and included in all family activities Family reputation is important and children are expected to behave in an honorable manner Methods of punishment include physical punishment and shaming	May be reluctant to share personal and family health information Women may prefer a female health care provider The authority of the physician is seldom questioned or challenged If a child is hospitalized family members are likely to remain with them Bad news may be kept from the ill person Associate good health with eating properly, consuming nutritious foods, and fasting to cure disease	Serious communication: may be passionate, loud, and gesturing Family may rely more on nonverbal cues and unspoken expectations Need to develop personal relationships with the health provider before sharing personal information Sensitive to the courtesy shown them
Japanese	Primary relationship is the mother-child relationship The mother-son relationship is particularly strong Infants are not allowed to cry Children may sleep with parents Education is valued Self-expression is not valued Corporal punishment is acceptable High respect for elders	Use Western medicine, herbs, and acupuncture May not voice discomfort May mail order traditional medications from Japan Seek both preventive and acute care	Relationship building and respect for privacy are important Saying "no" is impolite; better to drop the subject A high value is placed on "face" and "saving face" Smiling and laughter may be used to cover distress or embarrassment Prolonged eye contact is not polite Body space is respected and touching is limited to close acquaintances
Hispanic	Family takes precedence over work, school, and other aspects of life Patriarchal, with more of an egalitarian decision-making model in more educated and higher socioeconomic families	Use of both scientific and folk medicine May use folk medicine as an adjunct to traditional medical care Prayers, relics, faith, herbs, and spices may be used to ward off disease	Multiple indigenous languages and dialects Value touching, embracing approach with respect, and direction of questions to the dominant member of the group (usually the man)

Continued

TABLE 2-3 **Cultural Differences in Families—cont'd**

Cultural Group	Family Roles	Health Care Practices	Communication
Hispanic—cont'd	Machismo sees men as having strength, wisdom, more knowledge about sexual matters, and bravery Women are more maternal and are to be respected by their families Children are highly valued, protected, and not encouraged to leave home Physical punishment is often used as a means of discipline Show a great respect for traditions More flexible view of time, enjoy the present Religion is highly valued Education is valued, but access has often been difficult	Important to maintain a balance between "hot" and "cold" foods May seek the help of a *curandero* (folk healer), especially more traditionally oriented people May not seek health care until quite ill because they do not want to miss work May bring medications that require a prescription in the United States from their native country and share with family Pain is considered part of life and the will of God and may be endured quietly	Like to express their feelings and beliefs Sustained eye contact when speaking with an older person is considered rude Because of flexible view of time, may be late for appointments
Native American	Most tribes are matrilineal Children are valued and welcomed into the family Grandmothers are heavily involved in child care Family goals and bonds are important High respect for elders Emphasis is placed on learning the tribal culture Group activities are seen as more important than individual accomplishments Many remain traditional in their practice of religious activities	Wellness is a state of harmony with nature and others May combine native traditional medicine with Western medicine Asking questions to make a diagnosis may lead to mistrust May not express pain or request pain medication Care may be provided by a medicine man or healer	Language varies with each tribe Voice tones are quiet but not monotone May be comfortable with long periods of silence Direct eye contact is considered rude Children are usually bilingual and speak their native tongue mainly at home Dialects differ among tribes Talking loudly may be considered rude
Vietnamese	Patriarchal and extended family structure Children are expected to be obedient and devoted to their parents Children are valued Children usually are not disciplined at a young age, and corporal punishment is usually not used Young people may seek their own living conditions away from control of their elders High value placed on chastity in adolescents	Good health is achieved by attaining a balance between two opposing forces *am* (cold) and *duong* (hot); an excess of either force may cause illness May distrust Western methods of health care May try home remedies before seeking medical care Once in the health care system usually compliant May use skin pinching, cup suction, herbs, moxibustion, acupuncture, balms and oils, acupressure, massage	Some immigrants, even if they have been in the United States for some years, do not feel competent when speaking English Behavioral clues are important Approach in a quiet, unhurried manner Direct communication to the oldest member of the group May not give a direct answer to a question in order to avoid disharmony Expressions of emotion are considered a weakness Looking someone directly in the eyes may be considered disrespectful Negative emotions may be conveyed by silence or a smile

but not keep the appointment. Stoicism may make pain assessment difficult. Herbal medicines and practices such as acupressure may play an important part in healing for this culture.

Besides the national languages of Vietnam, Cambodia, and Laos, numerous languages are spoken within subgroups in each country. People from Southeast Asia speak softly and avoid prolonged eye contact, which they consider rude. Even people who have been in the United States for many years often do not feel competent in English. The nurse should watch for nonverbal cues, use simple sentences, avoid metaphors, ask for correction of understanding, and explain all points carefully (Purnell & Paulanka, 2003).

Families of some hospitalized Pacific Islander clients are involved in their direct care, which may include direct provision of food. Some individuals consult traditional healers. Education related to obesity, diabetes, and hypertension is more often needed (D'Avanzo & Geissler, 2003).

Hispanics

Hispanics, also called *Latinos,* include those whose origin is Mexico, Central and South America, Cuba, or Puerto Rico. They are a very diverse group. This group is now the fastest growing population in the United States. More than one in eight people in the United States are of Hispanic origin (Ramirez & de la Cruz, 2003).

Men are usually the head of household and considered strong (macho). Women are the homemakers. Hispanics usually have a close extended family and place a high value on children. Family is placed above work and other aspects of life.

Hispanics tend to be polite and gracious in conversation. Preliminary social interaction is particularly important, and Hispanics may be insulted if a problem is addressed directly without taking time for "small talk." This is counter to the value of "getting to the point" for many whites in the United States and may cause frustration for the client as well as the health care worker.

Religion and health are strongly associated. The *curandero,* a folk healer, may be consulted for health care before an American health care worker is consulted. Hispanics have great respect for health-care providers but may distrust them out of fear that they will disclose their undocumented status (Purnell & Paulanka, 2003).

African Americans

African Americans comprise 13% of the U.S. population (McKinnon, 2003). African Americans are often part of a close extended family, although many heads of household are single women. They have a sense of loyalty to their people and community, but they sometimes distrust the majority group.

The black minister is highly influential, and religious rituals such as prayer are frequently used. Illness may be seen as the will of God. Because of the close family and spiritual ties found within the culture, ill members are usually willingly cared for by the extended and nuclear family (Purnell & Paulanka, 2003).

American Indian and Alaska Native

The term American Indian and Alaska Native refers to people with origins in any of the original peoples of North and South America and who maintain tribal affiliation or community attachment. This group makes up 1.5% of the total U.S. population (Ogunwole, 2002). Many who consider themselves Native Americans are of mixed race. The largest American Indian tribal groups include Cherokee, Navajo, Latin American Indian, Choctaw, Sioux, and Chippewa. The largest tribe among Alaska Natives are the Eskimos (Ogunwole, 2002).

Native Americans may consider a willful child to be strong and a docile child to be weak. They have close family relationships, and respect for their elders is the norm. Native Americans may consider health to be a state of harmony with nature and may believe that supernatural influences have a great impact on health and illness. Native Americans may

highly respect a medicine man, whom they believe to be given power by supernatural forces. The use of herbs and rituals is part of the medicine man's curative practice.

Middle Easterners

Middle Eastern immigrants come from several countries, including Lebanon, Syria, Saudi Arabia, Egypt, Turkey, Iran, and Palestine. Islam is the dominant, and often the official, religion in these countries; its followers are known as *Muslims.* The man is typically the head of the household in Muslim families. Muslim women often prefer a female health care provider because of laws of modesty. Many Muslim women keep their head, arms to the wrists, and legs to the ankles covered. Islam requires believers to kneel and pray five times a day, at dawn, noon, afternoon, after sunset, and after nightfall. Muslims do not eat pork and do not use alcohol. Many are vegetarians.

Communication in these countries is elaborate, and obtaining health information may be difficult because Islam dictates that family affairs should be kept within the family. Personal information is shared only with friends, and the health assessment must be done gradually. When interpreters are used, they should be of the same country and religion, if possible, because of regional differences and hostilities. Because Islamic society tends to be paternalistic, asking the husband's permission or opinion when family members need health care is helpful.

Cross-Cultural Health Beliefs

More than 100 different ethnocultural groups reside in the United States, and numerous traditional health beliefs are observed among these groups. For example, definitions of health are often culturally based. People of Asian origin may view health as the balance of yin and yang. Those of African or Haitian origin may define health as harmony with nature. Those from Mexico, Central and South America, and Puerto Rico often see health as a balance of hot and cold.

Traditional Methods of Preventing Illness

The traditional methods of preventing illness rest in the person's ability to understand the cause of a given illness in their culture. These causes may include the following:

- Agents such as hexes, spells, or the evil eye, which may strike a person (often a child) and cause injury, illness, or misfortune
- Phenomena such as soul loss or accidental provocation of envy, jealousy, or hate of a friend or acquaintance
- Environmental factors such as bad air, and natural events such as solar eclipses

Practices to prevent illness developed from beliefs about the cause of illness. People must avoid those known to transmit hexes and spells. Elaborate methods are used to prevent inciting envy or jealousy of others and avoid the evil eye. Protective or religious objects, such as amulets with magic powers or consecrated religious objects (talismans), are frequently worn or carried to prevent illness. Numerous food taboos and traditional combinations are prescribed in traditional belief systems to prevent illness. For instance, people from many ethnic backgrounds eat raw garlic to prevent illness.

Traditional Practices to Maintain Health

A variety of traditional practices are used to maintain health. Mental and spiritual health are maintained by activities such as silence, meditation, and prayer. Many people view illness as punishment for breaking a religious code and adhere strictly to religious morals and practices to maintain health.

Traditional Practices to Restore Health

Traditional practices to restore health often conflict with Western medical practice. Some of the most common practices include the use of natural substances, such as herbs and plants, to treat illness. Religious charms, holy words, or traditional healers may be tried before an individual seeks a medical opinion. Wearing religious medals, carrying prayer cards, and performing sacrifices are other practices used to treat illness.

A variety of substances may be ingested for the treatment of illnesses. The nurse should try to identify what the child is taking and determine whether the active ingredient may alter the effects of prescribed medication.

Practices such as *dermabrasion,* the rubbing or irritation of the skin to relieve discomfort, are common among people of some cultures. The most popular form is *coining,* in which an area is covered with an ointment and the edge of a coin is rubbed over the area. All dermabrasion methods leave marks resembling bruises or burns on the skin and may be mistaken for signs of physical abuse.

Cultural Assessment

All health care professionals must develop skill in performing a cultural assessment so they can understand the meaning of health and illness in the cultural groups they encounter. When assessing the child and family from a cultural perspective, the nurse should consider the following:
* Ethnic affiliation
* Major values and beliefs
* Language barriers and communication styles
* Family and child-rearing practices
* Religious and spiritual beliefs
* Nutrition and food patterns
* Ethnic health care practices
* Health-promotion practices

After such an assessment, plans for care should show respect for cultural differences and traditional healing practices. A guiding principle for nurses should be one of acceptance of nontraditional methods of health care as long as the practice does not cause harm. In some instances, cultural practices may actually cause unintentional harm to children; in these circumstances the nurse may need to consult other professionals familiar with the particular cultural practice to provide appropriate care for the child and information for the family. Additional cultural information is presented throughout this text relating to specific areas in child health care.

PARENTING

Parenting implies the commitment of an individual or individuals to provide for the physical and psychosocial needs of a child. Many believe that parenting is the most difficult and yet rewarding experience an individual can have. Many parents assume this important job with little education in parenting or child rearing. If the parents themselves have had good parents as role models and seek resources, the transition to parenting is easier. Nurses are in a good position to provide parents with information on effective parenting skills through many venues, such as formal classes, anticipatory guidance at well-child checkups, and role modeling.

Parenting Styles

Three major parenting styles have been identified in the literature. Parenting style, which is the general climate in which a parent socializes a child, differs from parenting practices, the specific behavioral guidance parents offer children across the age span. Although the characteristics of parenting style are described below in their general categories, many specialists in child development acknowledge that some of the characteristics of several styles may be present in parents. In addition, researchers recognize that parenting styles may work in different ways in different cultures (Cardona, Nicholson, & Fox, 2000).

Authoritarian parents have rules. They expect obedience from the child without any questioning about the reasons behind the rule. They also expect the child to accept the family beliefs and principles without question. Give and take is discouraged.

Children raised with this style of parenting can be shy and withdrawn because of a lack of self-confidence. If the parents are somewhat affectionate, the child may be sensitive, submissive, honest, and dependable. If affection has been withheld, however, the child may exhibit rebellious, antisocial behavior.

Authoritative parents tend to show respect for the opinions of each of their children by allowing them to be different. Although the household has rules, the parents permit discussion if the children do not understand or agree with the rules. The parents emphasize that although they (the parents) are the ultimate authority, some negotiation and compromise may take place. This style of parenting tends to result in children who have high self-esteem and are independent, inquisitive, happy, assertive, and highly interactive.

Permissive parents have little or no control over the behavior of their children. If any rules exist in the home, they are inconsistent and unclear. Underlying reasons for rules may be given, but the children are generally allowed to decide whether they will follow the rule and to what extent. Limits are not set, and discipline is inconsistent. The children learn that they can get away with any behavior. Role reversal occurs: the children are more like the parents, and the parents are like the children.

Children who come from this type of home are typically disrespectful, disobedient, aggressive, irresponsible, and defiant. They tend to be insecure because of a lack of guidelines to direct their behavior. These children tend to be creative and spontaneous.

Regardless of the primary parenting style, parenting is more effective when parents are able to adjust their parenting techniques according to the child's developmental level and when parents are involved and interested in their children's activities and friends.

Parent-Child Relationship Factors

Relationships between parents and children are bidirectional, with the parents' behavior affecting the child and the child's behavior affecting the parenting. The parents' age, experience, and self-confidence affect the quality of the parent-child relationship, the stability of the marital relationship, and the interplay between the child's individualism and the parents' expectations of the child.

Parental Characteristics

Parenting is multidimensional. Sclafani (2004) noted that providing consistent discipline, meeting the child's needs for love and nurturance, and providing appropriate control and guidance are foundational parenting skills. Parent personality type, personal history of parenting as a child, abilities and competencies, parental skills and expectations, personal health, quality of marital relationship, and relationship quality with others all play a part in determining how a person parents.

In addition, parents who have had previous experience with children, whether through younger siblings, a career, or raising previous children, bring an element of experience to the art of parenting. Self-confidence and age can also be factors in a person's ability to parent. How an individual was parented has a major impact on how he or she will assume the role. The strength of the parents' relationship also affects their parenting skills, as does the presence or absence of support systems. Support can come from the family or community. Peer groups can provide an arena for parents to share experiences and solve problems. Parents with more experience are often an important resource for new parents.

Busy parents may rely on grandparents for child care or for an additional measure of love and attention for their children. Some grandparents raise grandchildren because of their own children's inability to do so.

Fathers are the primary child care providers in a growing number of families. Fathers who are not the primary caregivers often participate more actively in caring for their children than the fathers of previous generations.

A single parent often experiences financial and time constraints. Children in single-parent families are often given more responsibility to care for themselves and younger siblings.

Characteristics of the Child

Characteristics that may affect the parent-child relationship include the child's physical appearance, sex, and temperament. At birth, the infant's physical appearance may not meet the parents' expectations, or the infant may resemble a disliked relative. As a result, the parent may subconsciously reject the child. If the parents desired a baby of a particular sex, they may be disappointed. If parents are not given the opportunity to talk about this disappointment, they may reject the infant.

Temperament and Parental Expectations

Temperament can be described as the way individuals behave or their behavioral style. Several researchers have studied temperament. Chess and Thomas (1996) developed three temperament categories based on nine characteristics of temperament they identified in children (Box 2-2).

1. *Easy:* These children are even tempered, predictable, and regular in their habits. They react positively to new stimuli.
2. *Difficult:* These children are highly active, irritable, moody, and irregular in their habits. They adapt slowly to new stimuli and often express intense negative emotions.
3. *Slow to warm up:* These children are inactive, moody, and moderately irregular in their habits. They adapt slowly to new stimuli and express mildly intense negative emotions.

Some objection to the term *difficult* has been raised because it tends to have a negative connotation. That is the term established in temperament research, however, and parents should recognize that a "difficult" child is quite normal. As is true for other characteristics such as appearance, the parent-child relationship is likely to have less conflict if the child's temperament meets the parents' expectations.

BOX 2-2   Characteristics of Temperament in Children

1. Level of activity: the intensity and frequency of motion during playing, eating, bathing, dressing, or sleeping
2. Rhythmicity: regularity of biologic functions (e.g., sleep patterns, eating patterns, elimination patterns)
3. Approach/withdrawal: the initial response of a child to a new stimulus, such as an unfamiliar person, unfamiliar food, or new toys
4. Adaptability: ease or difficulty in adjustment to a new stimulus
5. Intensity of response: the amount of energy with which the child responds to a new stimulus
6. Threshold of responsiveness: the amount or intensity of stimulation necessary to evoke a response
7. Mood: frequency of cheerfulness, pleasantness, and friendly behavior versus unhappiness, unpleasantness, and unfriendly behavior
8. Distractibility: how easily the child's attention can be diverted from an activity by external stimuli
9. Attention span/persistence: how long the child pursues an activity and continues despite frustration and obstacles

Adapted from Chess, S., & Thomas, A. (1996). *Temperament: Theory and practice.* New York: Brunner-Mazel.

DISCIPLINE

Children's behavior challenges most parents. The manner in which parents respond to a child's behavior has a profound effect on the child's self-esteem and future interactions with others. Children learn to view themselves in the same way that the parent views them. Thus if parents view their children as wild, the children begin to view themselves as wild, and soon their actions consistently reinforce their self-image. In this way, the children will not disappoint the parents. This pattern is called a *self-fulfilling prophecy* and is a cyclic process.

Effective discipline requires knowledge of the target behavior, awareness of the principles that are related to behavioral change, and effective and consistent implementation of consequences (Larsen & Tentis, 2003). Discipline is designed to teach a child how to function effectively within society. It is the foundation for self-discipline. A parent's primary goal should be to help the child feel lovable and capable. This goal is best accomplished by the parent setting limits to enhance a sense of security until the child can incorporate the family's values and is capable of self-discipline.

When a child is in the health care system, the nurse has the opportunity to aid in the socialization of the child to some degree. Through both formal instruction and informal role modeling, the nurse can help the parent learn how to discipline a child effectively. Box 2-3 lists ways in which a parent or nurse can facilitate children's socialization and increase their self-esteem.

Dealing with Misbehavior

A child's misbehavior may be defined as behavior outside the norms of acceptance within the family. Misbehavior stretches the limits of tolerance in all parents, even the most patient. A parent's response to the child's misbehavior can have minor consequences such as short-term frustration or major consequences such as child abuse. To prevent these negative consequences, the nurse can help teach parents various strategies for effective discipline. The following are three essential

---

BOX 2-3	**Effective Discipline for Positive Socialization and Self-Esteem**

- Attend promptly to an infant's and young child's needs
- Provide structure and consistency for young children
- Give positive attention for positive behavior; use praise when deserved
- Listen
- Set aside time every day for one-on-one attention
- Demonstrate appreciation of the child's unique characteristics
- Encourage choices and decision making and allow the child to experience consequences of mistakes
- Model respect for others
- Provide unconditional love

---

components of effective discipline (American Academy of Pediatrics, 2004):

1. Maintaining a positive, supportive, loving relationship with the child
2. Using positive reinforcement and encouragement to promote cooperation and desired behaviors
3. Using "time out" or other alternatives that restrict activity instead of spanking or other forms of physical punishment

Punishment is used to eliminate a behavior and can be in the form of a verbal reprimand or physical action to emphasize a point. The American Academy of Pediatrics discourages the use of spanking or other forms of physical punishment (American Academy of Pediatrics, 2004).

Redirection

Redirection is a simple and effective method in which the parent removes the problem and distracts the child with an alternative activity or object. This method is helpful with infants through preadolescents.

Reasoning

Reasoning involves explaining why a behavior is not permitted. Younger children lack the cognitive skills and developmental abilities to comprehend reasoning fully. For example, a 4 year old may better understand that he will have to spend time in his room if he breaks his brother's toy rather than understanding the concept of respecting the property of others.

When this technique is used with older children, the behavior should be the object of focus, not the child. The child should not be made to feel guilt and shame because these feelings are counterproductive and can damage the child's self-esteem. The parent can focus on the behavior most effectively by using "I" rather than "you" messages.

A "you" message criticizes children and uses guilt in an attempt to get them to change their behavior. An example of a "you" message is "Don't take your little sister's toys away and make her cry. You're being a bad boy!" By contrast, an "I" message focuses on the misbehavior by explaining its effect on others. An example of an "I" message is "Your little sister cries when you take her toys away because she doesn't know that you will give them back to her."

Time Out

"Time out" is a method to remove the attention given to a child who is misbehaving. Time out involves placing the child in a nonstimulating environment where the parent can observe unobtrusively. For example, a chair could be placed facing a wall in a hall or bathroom. The child is told to sit on the chair for a predetermined time, usually 1 minute per year of age. If the child cries or fights, the timing is not begun until the child is quiet. The use of a kitchen timer with a bell is effective because the child knows when the time begins and when it has elapsed. At that time, the child is permitted to get up. After the child has calmed and the time is completed, discussion of the behavior that prompted the time out at a level appropriate to the child's age may be helpful.

Consequences

The consequences technique helps children learn the direct result of their misbehavior and can be used with toddlers through adolescents. If children must deal with the consequences of their behavior and the consequences are meaningful to them, they are less likely to repeat the behavior. Consequences fall into the following three categories:

1. *Natural:* Consequences that occur spontaneously. For example, a child loses a favorite toy after leaving it outside and the parent does not replace it.
2. *Logical:* Consequences that are directly related to the misbehavior. For example, when two children are fighting over a toy, the parent removes the toy from both of them for a day.
3. *Unrelated:* Consequences that are purposely imposed. For example, a child comes in late for dinner and, as a consequence, is not allowed to watch TV that evening.

Some parents have difficulty allowing their children to face the consequences of their actions. When parents choose to deny their children this experience, they lose an important opportunity to teach responsibility for one's actions.

Behavior Modification

The behavior modification technique of discipline rewards positive behavior and ignores negative behavior. This technique requires parents to choose selected behaviors, preferably only one at a time, that they desire to stop. They choose others that they want to encourage. The basic technique is useful for any age from toddlerhood through adolescence. For a young child, the selected positive behaviors are marked on a chart and explained to the child. For an older child, a contract can be written. The negative behaviors are kept in mind by the parents but are not recorded where the child can see them. A system of rewards is established. Stickers or stars on a chart for young children and tokens for older children are effective ways to record the behaviors. Children should receive a predetermined reward (e.g., a movie, book, or outing) after they successfully perform the behavior a set number of times. This system should continue for several months until the behavior becomes a habit for the child. Then the external reward should be gradually withdrawn. The child develops internal gratification for successful behavior rather than relies on external reinforcement. Children gain a sense of mastery and actually enjoy the process, often viewing it as a game.

Negative behaviors are simply ignored. If the parent refuses to give the child attention for the behavior, the child soon gives up that strategy. Consistency is the key to success for this technique, and many parents find this method difficult to enforce. Parents need to be warned that children frequently test the seriousness of this attempt by increasing their negative behavior soon after the parents begin ignoring it. If this technique is to be successful, the parents need to ignore the negative behavior every time.

Corporal Punishment

Corporal punishment usually takes the form of spanking. It is highly controversial and should be discouraged. The problems cited when corporal punishment is used include the following (American Academy of Pediatrics, 2004):

* The decrease in misbehavior is short term.
* Children learn that violence is acceptable.
* Children become accustomed to the pain, so some parents may feel that more severe pain is needed.
* Parents may experience rage and lose control, causing harm to the child.

Because of the negative consequences of spanking and because it is no more effective than other methods of discipline, the American Academy of Pediatrics (2004) recommends that parents be encouraged and assisted in developing methods of discipline other than spanking.

CRITICAL TO REMEMBER
Corporal Punishment as Discipline

Corporal punishment can lead to child abuse if the disciplinarian loses control. It can also lead to false accusations of child abuse by either the child or other adults. Because of the high cost and low benefit of this form of punishment, parents should think seriously before using it.

NURSING PROCESS AND THE FAMILY
Family Assessment

When assessing family health, the nurse first must determine the structure of the family. The structure is the actual physical composition of the family, the family's environment, and the occupations and education of its members. Diagrams can assist with this process. A *genogram*, which illustrates family relationships and health issues, looks like a family tree with three generations of family members represented. An *ecomap* is a pictorial representation of the family structure and relationships with factors in the external environment.

Next, the nurse needs to determine how well the family is fulfilling its five major functions as described by Friedman (2003):

1. *Affective function (personality maintenance function):* to meet the psychologic needs of family members—trust, nurturing, intimacy, belonging, bonding, identity, separateness and connectedness, need-response patterns, and the therapeutic role of the individuals in the family.
2. *Socialization function (social placement):* to guide children to be productive members of society and transmit cultural beliefs to the next generation.
3. *Reproductive function:* to ensure family continuity and societal survival.
4. *Economic function:* to provide and effectively allocate economic resources.
5. *Health care function:* to provide the physical necessities of life (e.g., food, clothing, shelter, health care), to recognize

illness in family members and provide care, and to foster a health lifestyle or environment based on preventive medical and dental health practices.

Health problems can arise from structural problems, such as too few or too many people sharing the same living quarters. If too few people are present, children may be left unattended; too many people may lead to overcrowding, stress, and the spread of communicable diseases. Environmental problems include impure drinking water, inadequate sewage facilities, damaged electric wiring and outlets, and inadequate sleeping conditions. Other environmental factors, such as rodents, crime, and noise, can affect health. Occupation and education can affect health through lack of adequate supervision of children; inability to purchase physical necessities, such as food; inability to purchase health insurance; and stress from employment dissatisfaction.

The Friedman Family Assessment Model consists of six broad categories (Box 2-4). Each category contains numerous subcategories. A nurse assessing a family should decide which subcategories are relevant on the basis of the family's goals, problems, and resources. Not all the subcategory assessment areas may need to be assessed. Other family assessment models that nurses can use are also available.

CRITICAL THINKING EXERCISE 2-1

Create a genogram of your family. Can you identify health issues and trends from looking at the genogram? What are the implications for nursing care?

Nursing Diagnosis and Planning

After using the various tools to assess the child's family completely, the appropriate nursing diagnoses are identified. These will differ according to the specific family assessment data. The following general nursing diagnoses can be used for families:

- Risk for caregiver role strain
- Compromised family coping
- Interrupted family processes
- Impaired parenting
- Ineffective family therapeutic regimen management
- Social isolation

Other diagnoses may also be appropriate. The expected outcomes for each diagnosis would be specifically tailored to the family's needs.

Intervention and Evaluation

Interventions also are specific for the child and family, but most family interventions are directed toward enhancing positive coping strategies and directing the family to appropriate resources. The nurse adapts general family interventions to each family's unique needs but in particular helps the family to do the following:

- Identify and mobilize internal and external strengths
- Access appropriate resources in the extended family and community

---

| BOX 2-4 | **Friedman Family Assessment Model (Short Form)** |

I. Identifying data
 1. Family name
 2. Address and phone
 3. Family composition
 4. Type of family form
 5. Cultural background
 6. Religious identification
 7. Social class status
 8. Family's recreational or leisure time activities
II. Developmental stage and history
 1. Family's present developmental stage
 2. Extent of family's fulfillment of developmental tasks
 3. Nuclear family history
 4. History of family of origin of both parents
III. Environmental data
 1. Characteristics of home
 2. Characteristics of neighborhood and larger community
 3. Family's geographic mobility
 4. Family's associations and transactions with community
 5. Family's social support system or network
IV. Family structure
 1. Communication patterns
 2. Power structure
 3. Role structure
 4. Family values
V. Family functions
 1. Affective function
 2. Socialization function
 3. Health care function
VI. Family stress, coping, and adaptation
 1. Family stressors, strengths, and perception
 2. Family coping strategies
 3. Family adaptation
 4. Tracking stressors, coping, and adaptation over time

Reprinted from Friedman, M. (2003). *Family nursing: Theory, research and practice* (pp. 593-594). Upper Saddle River, NJ: Prentice Hall.

- Recognize and enhance positive communication patterns
- Decide on a consistent discipline approach and access parenting programs if needed
- Maintain comforting cultural and religious traditions and sources of healing
- Engage in joint problem solving
- Acquire new knowledge by providing information about a specific health problem or issue
- Become empowered
- Allocate sufficient privacy, space, and time for leisure activities
- Promote health for all family members during times of crisis

Once families have participated in needed intervention, evaluation criteria are tailored to the specific intervention and individualized for the family.

KEY CONCEPTS

- Traditional families may be single-income or dual-income families. Two-income families are much more common at present.
- Nontraditional family structures may require nursing care that is different from that required by traditional families. These families may include single-parent, blended, adoptive, multigenerational (extended), and homosexual parent families.
- High-risk families have additional stressors that affect their functioning. Some high-risk families include families headed by adolescents; families affected by marital discord or divorce, violence, or substance abuse; or families with a severely or chronically ill member.
- All families experience stress; how the family deals with stress is the important factor.
- Identifying healthy versus dysfunctional family patterns can help the nurse implement effective strategies to care for the child and the family.
- Clients during health and illness are cared for within the framework of their families and their cultures.
- Traditional cultural beliefs may be used to prevent illness, maintain health, and restore health.
- Differing cultural beliefs and expectations between the health care provider and the family can create conflict.
- A knowledge of generally effective, healthy internal and external coping strategies can help the nurse offer the family specific suggestions for coping.
- The nurse can help parents learn effective discipline methods by teaching and role modeling.
- Assessing the structure and function of the family is a basic part of caring for any child.

REFERENCES AND READINGS

American Academy of Pediatrics Committee on Psychosocial Aspects of Child and Family Health. (1998). Guidance for effective discipline. *Pediatrics, 101*(4), 723-728.

American Academy of Pediatrics Committee on School Health. (2000). Corporal punishment in schools. *Pediatrics, 106*(2), 343.

American Academy of Pediatrics Committee on Pediatric Workforce. (2004). Ensuring culturally effective pediatric care: Implications for education and health policy. *Pediatrics, 114*(6), 1677-1685.

Ateah, C. (2003). Disciplinary practices with children: Parental sources of information, attitudes, and educational needs. *Issues in Comprehensive Pediatric Nursing, 26*(2), 89-101.

Bornstein, M. H., & Bradley, R. H. (2003). *Socioeconomic status, parenting, and child development.* Mahwah, NJ: Lawrence Erlbaum Associates.

Bowen, M. (1976). Theory in the practice of psychotherapy. In P. J. Guerin (Ed.). *Family therapy theory and practice* (pp. 42-89). New York: Gardner Press.

Bullock, B. M. (2003). Parenting together after divorce: Navigating the winds of change. *Journal of Zero to Three, 23*(3), 38-43.

Burr, W., Klein, S., Burr, R., Doxey, C., Harker, B., Holman, T., et al. (1994). *Reexamining family stress: New theory and research.* Thousand Oaks, CA: Sage.

Campinha-Bacote, J. (2003). *The process of cultural competence in the delivery of healthcare services.* Cincinnati, OH: Transcultural C.A.R.E. Associates.

Cardona, P., Nicholson, B., & Fox, R. (2000). Parenting among Hispanic and Anglo-American mothers with young children. *The Journal of Social Psychology, 140*(3), 357-365.

Casper, V. (2003). Very young children in lesbian and gay headed families: Moving beyond acceptance. *Journal of Zero to Three, 23*(3), 18-26.

Chess, S., & Thomas, A. (1996). *Temperament theory and practice.* New York: Brunner-Mazel.

Children of Alcoholics Foundation. (2005). *Effects of parental substance abuse on children and families.* Retrieved January 3, 2006, from *www.coaf.org.*

Cohen, F. (1984). Coping. In J. D. Matarazzo, S. Weiss, J. Herd, & S. Weiss (Eds.). *Behavioral health: A handbook of health enhancement and disease prevention* (pp. 261-274). New York: Wiley.

Coleman, M., & Ganong, L. H. (2004). *Handbook of contemporary families: Considering the past, contemplating the future.* Thousand Oaks, CA: Sage Publications.

Coleman, W. L., & Garfield, C. (2004). Fathers and pediatricians: Enhancing men's roles in the care and development of their children. *Pediatrics, 113*(5), 1406-1411.

Cooley, M. (2005). A family perspective in community/public health nursing. In F. Maurer & C. Smith (Eds.). *Community/public health nursing* (3rd ed., p. 285). St. Louis: Elsevier.

D'Avanzo, C. E., & Geissler, E. M. (2003). *Cultural health assessment* (3rd ed.). St. Louis: Mosby.

Duvall, E. M., & Miller, B. L. (1995). *Marriage and family development* (6th ed.). New York: Harper & Row.

Federal Interagency Forum on Child and Family Statistics. (2005). *America's children: Key national indicators of well-being 2005.* Retrieved July 2005 from *www.childstats.gov/americaschildren.*

Friedman, M. (2003). *Family nursing: Theory, research and practice* (pp. 593-594). Upper Saddle River, NJ: Prentice Hall.

Friedman, M. M., Bowden, V. R., & Jones, E. G. (2003). *Family nursing: Research, theory and practice* (5th ed). Upper Saddle River, NJ: Prentice Hall.

Giger, J. N., & Davidhizar, R. E. (2004). *Transcultural nursing: Assessment & intervention.* St. Louis: Mosby.

Graham, R. E., Ahn, A. C., Davis, R. B., O'Connor, B. B., Eisenberg, D. M., & Phillips, R. S. (2005). Use of complementary and alternative medical therapies among racial and ethnic minority adults: Results from the 2002 National Health Interview Survey. *Journal of the National Medical Association, 97*(4), 535-545.

Grych, J., Harold, G., & Miles, C. (2003). A prospective investigation of appraisals as mediators of the link between interparental conflict and child adjustment. *Child Development, 74*(4), 1176-1193.

Horn, I. B., Cheng, T. L., & Joseph, J. (2004). Discipline in the African American community: The impact of socioeconomic status on beliefs and practices. *Pediatrics, 113*(5), 1236-1241.

Ingoldsby, B. B., Smith, S. R., & Miller, J. E. (2003). *Exploring family theories.* Los Angeles: Roxbury.

Jones M. E., Cason, C. L., & Bond, M. L. (2004). Cultural attitudes, knowledge, and skills of a health workforce. *Journal of Transcultural Nursing, 15*(4), 283-290.

Kataoka-Yahiro, M, Ceria, C., & Caulfield, R. (2004). Grandparent caregiving role in ethnically diverse families. *Journal of Pediatric Nursing, 19*(5), 315-328.

Larson, M. A., & Tentis, E. (2003). The art and science of disciplining children. *Pediatric Clinics of North America, 50*(4), 817-840.

Leininger, M. (1978). *Transcultural nursing: Concepts, theories, practices.* New York: Wiley.

Linnard-Palmer, L., & Kools, S. (2004). Parents' refusal of medical treatment based on religious and/or cultural beliefs: The law, ethical principles, and clinical implications. *Journal of Pediatric Nursing,* *19*(5), 351-356.

Kalb, L. M., & Loeber, R. (2003). Child disobedience and noncompliance: A review. *Pediatrics, 11*(3), 641-652.

Martin, J. A., Hamilton, B. E., Sutton, P. D., Ventura, S. J., Menacker, F., & Munson, M. L. (2003). *Births: Final data for 2002. National vital statistics reports, 52*(10). Hyattsville, MD: National Center for Health Statistics.

Martin, J. A., Kochanek, K. D., Strobino, D. M., Guyer, B., & MacDorman, M. F. (2005). Annual summary of vital statistics-2003. *Pediatrics, 115*(3), 619-634.

McKinnon, J. (2003). *The Black population in the United States: March 2002.* Washington, DC: U.S. Census Bureau. Retrieved August 2005 from *www.census.gov/prod/2003pubs/p20-541.pdf.*

Menacker, F., Martin, J., MacDorman, M., & Ventura, S. (2004). *Births to 10-14 year-old mothers, 1990-2002: Trends and health outcomes. National vital statistics reports, 53*(7). Hyattsville, MD: National Center for Health Statistics.

Ogunwole, S. (2002). *The American Indian and Alaska Native population: 2002.* Washington, DC: U.S. Census Bureau. Retrieved August 2005 from *www.census.gov/prod/2002pubs/c2kb01-15.pdf.*

Purnell. L. D., & Paulanka, B. J. (2003). *Transcultural health care: A culturally competent approach* (2nd ed.). Philadelphia: F.A. Davis.

Ramirez, R. R., & de la Cruz, G. P. (2003). *The Hispanic population in the United States: March 2002.* Washington, DC: U.S. Census Bureau. Retrieved August 2005 from *www.census.gov/prod/2003pubs/p20-545.pdf.*

Reeves, T., & Bennett, C. (2003). *The Asian and Pacific Islander population in the United States: March 2002.* Washington, DC: U.S. Census Bureau. Retrieved August 2005 from *www.census.gov/prod/2003pubs/p20-540.pdf.*

Regalado, M., Sareen, H., Inkelas, M., Wissow, L. S., & Halfon, N. (2004). Parents' discipline of young children: Results from the National Survey of Early Childhood Health. *Pediatrics, 113*(6), 1952-1958.

Roy, K., & Burton, L. (2003). Kinscription: Mothers keeping fathers connected to children. *Journal of Zero to Three, 23*(3), 27-32.

Schneider, B., & Waite, L. J. (2005). *Being together, working apart: Dual-career families and the work-life balance.* Cambridge: Cambridge Press.

Schwede, L. (2003). *Complex households and relationships in the decennial census and in ethnographic studies of six race/ethnic groups.*

Census 2000 testing and experimentation program. Retrieved December 30, 2005, from *www.census.gov/pred/www/rpts/Complex%20Households%20Final%20Report.pdf*

Sclafani, J. D. (2004). *The educated parent.* Westport, CT: Praeger Publishers.

Shen, Z. (2004). Cultural competence models in nursing: A selected annotated bibliography. *Journal of Transcultural Nursing, 15*(4), 317-322.

Simmons, T., & Dye, J. (2003). *Grandparents living with grandchildren.* Retrieved December 30, 2005, from *www.census.gov/prod/2003pubs/c2kbr-31.pdf.*

Skidmore-Roth, L. (2004). *Mosby's handbook of herbs & natural supplements.* (2nd ed). St. Louis: Mosby.

Smitherman, L. C., Janisse, J., & Mathur, A. (2005). The use of folk remedies among children in an urban black community: Remedies for fever, colic, and teething. *Pediatrics, 115*(3), e297-e304.

Solomon, J. (2003). The caregiving system in separated and divorcing parents. *Journal of Zero to Three, 23*(3), 33-37.

Spector, R. E. (2004). *Cultural diversity in health and illness* (6th ed). Upper Saddle River, NJ: Prentice Hall.

Stevens Barnum, B. (2003). *Spirituality in nursing: From traditional to new age.* New York: Springer.

Sullivan, J., Chaliman, M., & Mooney, K. (2005). *Child welfare and substance abuse: Current issues and in-depth TA.* Presented at the NGA Center for Best Practices Institute on Child Welfare, Miami, FL.

Susman-Stillman, A. & Siebenbruner, J. (2003). For better or worse: An ecological perspective on parents' relationships and parent-infant interaction. *Journal of Zero to Three, 23*(3), 4-12.

Taylor, E. J. (2002). *Spiritual Care: Nursing theory, research, and practice.* Upper Saddle River, NJ: Prentice Hall.

United States Department of Health and Human Services, Health Resources and Services Administration, Maternal and Child Health Bureau. (2003). *Child Health USA 2003.* Rockville, MA: U.S. Government Printing Office.

Von Bertalanffy, L. (1968). *General systems theory.* New York: Braziller.

Wertlieb, D. (2003). Converging trends in family research and pediatrics: Recent findings for the American Academy of Pediatrics Task Force on the Family. *Pediatrics, 111*(6), 1572-1587.

Wright, L. M., & Leahey, M. (2005). *Nurses and families: A guide to family assessment and intervention* (4th ed). Philadelphia: F.A. Davis.

CHAPTER 3

Communicating With Children and Families

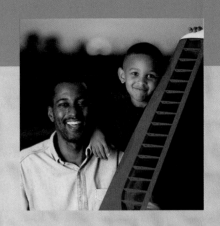

Learning Objectives

After studying this chapter, you should be able to:
- Describe six components of effective communication with children.
- Describe communication strategies that assist nurses in working effectively with children.
- Explain the importance of avoiding communication pitfalls in working with children.
- Describe effective family-centered communication strategies.
- Describe effective strategies for communicating with children with special needs.
- Describe warning signs of overinvolvement and underinvolvement in child/family relationships.

Definitions

active listening   Listening empathically to gain a better understanding of both the actual and the implied message.

empathy   Seeing from another's perspective while remaining objective.

empowerment   Provision of appropriate tools (education, information, support) to individuals that enable them to participate fully in decision making.

preparation   Provision of information before procedures, treatments, or events; facilitates coping.

self-esteem   Personal value that individuals place on themselves.

sensory information   Information gained from sight, taste, touch, smell, and hearing.

therapeutic relationship   A balance between appropriate involvement and professional separation in relating to child/family interactions.

win-win solution   Solution to a problem, such as the resolution of a conflict, which both parties can support as a common goal.

Audio Glossary

Electronic Resources

Additional information related to the content in Chapter 3 can be found on:

the interactive companion CD-ROM
- Audio Glossary
- NCLEX Review Questions
- Skill: Communicating With Children

or the companion website at *evolve*
http://evolve.elsevier.com/james/ncoc
- NCLEX Review Questions
- Resources for Health Care Providers and Families
- WebLinks

To effectively work with children and their families, nurses must develop keen communication skills. Parents and other family members play a crucial role in the lives of pediatric clients. To identify mutual goals and facilitate positive outcomes, nurses need to establish rapport with the family. An awareness of body language, eye contact, and tone of voice must accompany good verbal communication skills when listening to children and their families. The same awareness helps nurses assess their own communication styles.

COMPONENTS OF EFFECTIVE COMMUNICATION

Communication is much more than words going from one person's mouth to another person's ears. In addition to the words themselves, the tone and quality of voice, eye contact, physical proximity, visual cues, and overall body language convey messages. These nonverbals are often undervalued. Research has shown that verbal content makes up 7% of a message, whereas body language accounts for 55% and paralanguage (intonation, pauses, sighs) represents the remaining 38% (Topper, 2004). In choosing communication techniques to be used with children and families, the nurse considers cultural differences, particularly with regard to touch and personal space (see Chapter 2).

Touch

Touch can be a positive, supportive technique that is effective from birth through adulthood. Touch can convey warmth, comfort, reassurance, security, trust, caring, and support.

In infancy, messages of love, security, and comfort are conveyed through holding, cuddling, gentle stroking, and patting. Infants do not have cognitive understanding of the words they hear, but they sense the emotional support and they can feel, interpret, and respond to gentle, loving, supportive hands caring for them. Toddlers and preschoolers find it soothing and comforting to be held and rocked, as well as stroked gently on the head, back, arms, and legs (Fig. 3-1).

School-age children and adolescents appreciate giving and receiving hugs and getting a reassuring pat on the back or a gentle hand on their hand. The nurse, however, needs to request permission for any contact beyond a casual touch.

Physical Proximity and Environment

Children's familiarity and comfort with their physical surroundings affect communication. Normally, children are most at ease in their home environments. Once they enter a clinic, emergency department, or patient care unit, they are in an unfamiliar environment and they experience heightened anxiety. Hospital and clinic staff members have a tremendous advantage in knowing their clinic or unit as a familiar workplace. Nurses can gain a better picture of what a child is experiencing by trying to place themselves in the child's position and imagining the child's first impression of the triage desk, the reception desk, the admitting office, the treatment room, and the hospital room. The child's perspective is probably very different from an adult's. Creating a supportive, inviting environment for children includes the use of child-size furniture, colorful banners and posters, developmentally appropriate toys, and art displayed at a child's eye level.

Individuals have different comfort zones for physical distance. The nurse should be aware of differences and move cautiously when meeting new children and families, respecting each individual's personal space. For example, standing over the child and family can be intimidating. Instead, the nurse should bring a chair and sit near the child and family. This action puts the nurse at eye level. If a chair is not accessible, the nurse may also stoop or squat. The important part is to be at eye level while remaining at a comfortable distance for the child and family (Fig. 3-2).

The nurse should not overlook privacy or underestimate its importance. A room should be available for conducting private conversations away from roommates or family members and visitors. Privacy is particularly critical when working with adolescents, who typically will not discuss sensitive topics with parents present. The nurse's skill and ease with parents of adolescents will increase the adolescents' trust in the nurse. Hallway conversations, particularly outside a child's room, should be avoided because children and parents may overhear only some words or phrases and misinterpret the meaning. Overhearing may lead to unnecessary stress and mistrust between the health care providers and the child or family.

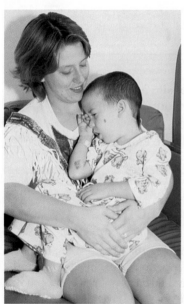

Touch is a powerful means of communicating. Toddlers and preschoolers often find touch in the form of cuddling and stroking to be soothing. Even older children who prize their independence find that a parent's hug or pat on the back helps them feel more secure.

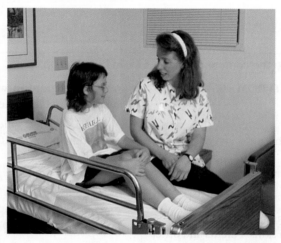

A child can communicate more easily with a nurse who is at eye level and at a comfortable conversational distance. The nurse may need to squat or even sit on the floor to talk with very young children.

FIG 3-1 **Communication with children is enhanced by direct eye contact and by body language that conveys attentiveness and openness.**

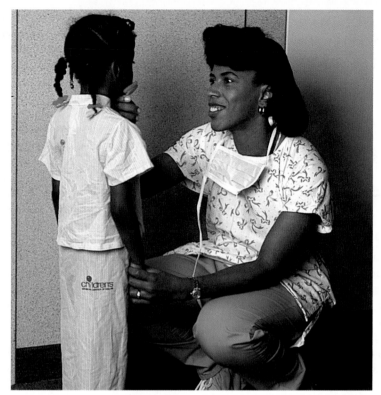

FIG 3-2   **For effective communication, the nurse needs to be at the child's eye level.**

Listening

Messages given must be received for communication to be complete. Therefore, listening is an essential component of the communication process. By practicing active listening skills, nurses can be effective listeners. *Active listening* skills include the following.

Attentiveness

The nurse should be intentional about giving the speaker undivided attention. Eliminating distractions is important, whenever possible. For example, the nurse should maintain eye contact, close the door, and eliminate potential distractions (e.g., TV, computer, video games).

Clarification Through Reflection

Using similar words, the nurse expresses to the speaker what was heard and understood about the content of the message. For example, when the child or family member says, "I hate the food that comes on my tray," a reflective response would be, "You are unhappy with the food you've been given?"

Empathy

The nurse identifies and acknowledges feelings expressed in the message. For example, if a child is crying after a procedure, the nurse might say, "I know it is uncomfortable to have this procedure. It is okay to cry. You did a great job holding still."

Impartiality

To understand and avoid prejudicing what is heard with personal bias, the nurse listens with an open mind. For example, if an adolescent expresses concern that she is having difficulty with relationships at school and that she feels disconnected socially because she is a lesbian, the nurse remains a supportive listener. The nurse can then help her identify ways to connect with peers and community resources and interact with her as with all children, regardless of the nurse's personal values and beliefs.

During shift report, descriptions of family must be shared objectively and impartially. Otherwise, perceptions of families may negatively affect how colleagues approach and interact with families.

To enhance the effectiveness of communication and maximize normal language patterns that contribute to language development, the nurse focuses on talking *with* children rather than *to* them and develops conversations with children.

The nurse must be prepared to listen with the eyes as well as the ears. Information will not always be audible, so the nurse must be alert to subtle cues in body language and physical closeness. Only then can one fully understand the messages of children. For example, when the nurse enters the room to complete an initial assessment of a 4-year-old child and observes the child turning away and beginning to suck her thumb, the child is communicating about her basic security and comfort level, although she has not said a word.

CRITICAL TO REMEMBER

Tips to Enhance Listening and Communication Skills

• Children understand better than they can talk.
• To develop conversations with children, ask open-ended questions rather than questions requiring *yes* or *no* responses.
• Comprehension is increased when the nurse uses different methods to present and share information.
• Use "people-first" language (e.g., "Sally in 428 has cystic fibrosis" instead of "The CF patient in 428 is Sally.")

Visual Communication

Eye contact is a communication connector. Making eye contact helps confirm attention and interest between the individuals communicating. Direct eye contact may be uncomfortable, however, for people in some cultures, so be sensitive to responses when making eye contact.

Clothing, physical appearance, and objects being held are visual communicators. Children may react to an individual's presence on the basis of a white lab coat, a bushy beard, a syringe, or a video game in hand. The nurse needs to think ahead and anticipate visual stimuli a child may find startling and those that may be pleasing and to make appropriate adjustments when possible. For example, it is a routine practice for nurses to bring a medication in a syringe for insertion into an intravenous (IV) line. Unless the purpose of the syringe is immediately explained, children might immediately assume they are about to receive an injection.

Some children, and some adults, are visual learners. They learn best when they can see or read instructions, demonstrations, diagrams, or information. Using various methods of presenting and sharing information will increase comprehension.

Concepts can be presented more vividly by using photographs, videotapes, dolls, computer programs, charts, or graphs than by using written or spoken words alone. The nurse needs to select teaching tools and materials that appropriately match the child's growth and developmental level.

Tone of Voice

The spoken word comes to mind most often when communication is the topic. Communication, however, consists of not only what is said but also the way it is said. The tone and quality of voice often communicate more than the words themselves.

Because infants' cognitive understanding of words is limited, their understanding is based on tone and quality of voice. A soft, smooth voice is more comforting and soothing to infants than a loud, startling, harsh voice. Infants can sense from the tone of voice whether the caregiver is angry or happy, frustrated or calm. The nurse can assess how aware of and sensitive to these messages infants are by observing their body language. Infants are relaxed when they hear a calm, happy caregiver and tense and rigid when they hear an angry, frustrated caregiver.

Children can detect anger, frustration, joy, and other feelings that voices convey, even when the accompanying words are incongruent. This incongruity can be very confusing for children. The nurse should strive to make words and their intended meanings match.

Verbal communication extends beyond actual words. All audible sounds convey meaning. An infant's primary mode of audible communication is crying. Crying is a cue to check basic needs, including hunger, pain, discomfort (e.g., wet diaper), or temperature. Cooing and babbling, also heard during the first year of life, generally convey messages of comfort and contentment. As children develop and mature, they will have increasing vocabularies to express their ideas, thoughts, and feelings.

The choice of words is critical in verbal communication. The nurse needs to avoid talking down to children but should not expect them to understand adult words and phrases. Technical health care terms should be used selectively, and jargon should be avoided (see Table 3-4).

Body Language

From the gentle caress of holding an infant to sitting and listening intently to an adolescent's story, body language is a factor in communication. An open body stance and positioning invite communication and interaction, whereas a closed body stance and positioning impede communication and interaction.

Using an open body posture improves the nurse's understanding of children and the children's understanding of the nurse. Nurses need to learn to read children's body language and should become more aware of their own body language. Table 3-1 compares open and closed body postures.

Timing

Recognizing the appropriate time to communicate information is a developed skill. A distraught child whose parents have just left for work is not ready for a diabetic teaching session. The session will be much more productive and the information better understood if the child has a chance to make the transition. The convenience of a schedule should be secondary to meeting a child's needs.

TABLE 3-1	**Open and Closed Body Postures**
Open	**Closed**
Leaning toward other person	Leaning away from other person
Arms loose at sides	Arms folded across chest
Frequent eye contact	No eye contact
Hands moving freely	Hands on hips
Soft stance, body swaying slightly	Rigid stance
Head up	Head bowed
Calm, slow movements	Constant motion, squirming
Smiling, friendly facial cues	Frowning, negative facial cues
Conversing at eye level	Conversing at diagonal eye level

FAMILY-CENTERED COMMUNICATION

Any discussion about effective ways to communicate with children must also include a discussion of effective communication with families. *Family-centered care* emphasizes that the family is intricately involved in the care of the child. Family-centered care is achieved when health care professionals can create partnerships with families, recognizing that the family is essential to the child and that the family has the right to participate fully in planning, implementing, and evaluating the child's plan of care.

Commitment to family-centered care means that the nurse respects the family's diversity. Children and parents live in a variety of family structures. An expanded definition of family is required in the twenty-first century, because *family* no longer refers to only the intact, nuclear family in which parents raise their biologic children. Therefore adolescent parents; extended families with aunts, uncles, or cousins parenting; intergenerational families with grandparents parenting; blended families with stepparents and stepsiblings; gay or lesbian parents; foster parents; group homes; and homeless children all qualify as contemporary family structures. The nurse should be prepared to identify the foundational strengths in all family structures (see Chapter 2). Family-centered care also means that the nurse truly believes that the child's care and recovery are greatly enhanced when the family fully participates in the child's care (Fig. 3-3).

Establishing Rapport

Critical to establishing rapport with families is the nurse's ability to convey genuine respect and concern during the first encounter. A nonjudgmental approach and a willingness to assist family members in effectively caring for their child demonstrate the nurse's interest in their well-being.

Availability and Openness to Questions

A nurse who does not take time to see how a child and family are doing—such as a nurse who leaves a room immediately after a treatment or administration of a medication—will not encourage or invite families to ask questions. Families want and need unrushed and uninterrupted time with the nurse. Sometimes this time can be made available only by purposefully scheduling it into the day. Encouraging families to write down their questions will enable them to take full advantage of their time with the nurse.

CRITICAL TO REMEMBER

Communicating With Families

- Include all involved family members. One essential step toward achieving a family-centered care environment is to develop open lines of communication with the family.
- Encourage families to write down their questions.
- Remain nonjudgmental.
- Give families both verbal and nonverbal signals that send a message of availability and openness.
- Respect and encourage feedback from families.
- Families come in various shapes, sizes, colors, and generations.
- Avoid assumptions about core family beliefs and values.
- Respect family diversity.

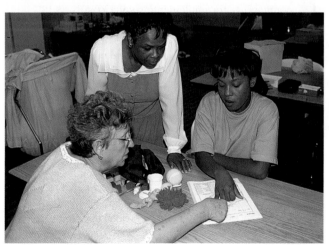

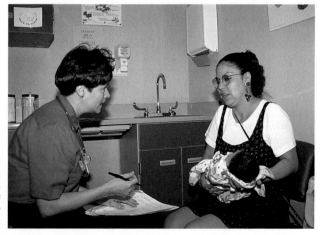

The nurse explains a child's test results to his mother and grandmother. Including all important family members in the child's health care reflects a commitment to family-centered care. *(Courtesy University of Texas at Arlington School of Nursing.)*

This nurse practitioner has learned Spanish to communicate better with her many Spanish-speaking clients. Speaking with family members in their own language encourages the family to remain in the health care system. The nurse is also using eye contact and has positioned herself at the mother's eye level. *(Courtesy Parkland Health and Hospital System Community Oriented Primary Care Clinic, Dallas.)*

FIG 3-3 **The child's continuing health care, both preventive and during illness, is enhanced by participation of the family.**

The nurse might encourage use of time by saying, "I know you have a lot of questions and are very anxious to learn more about your son's condition. I have another patient who has an immediate need, but I will be available in 10 minutes to meet with you. In the meantime, here is a parent handbook that gives general information about seizures. Please feel free to review it and write down any questions that we can discuss when I return."

Family Education and Empowerment

Educating parents about their child's condition, ensuring their continued involvement in planning and evaluating the plan of care, and teaching them the skills to participate empower the family. Families need support as they gain confidence in their skills, and they need guidance to assist them as they navigate through the health care experience. Communication is enhanced when families feel competent and confident in their abilities.

Effective Management of Conflict

When conflict occurs, it should be addressed in an expedient manner to prevent further breakdown in communication. Box 3-1 provides strategies for managing conflict, and Table 3-2 discusses the importance of choosing words carefully to make families feel welcome and to further facilitate family-centered care.

Feedback From Children and Families

The nurse must be alert for verbal as well as nonverbal cues. Routinely checking with family members about their experiences, satisfaction with communications, teaching sessions, and health care goals is an effective way to ensure that health care providers obtain appropriate feedback. To enhance the delivery of care, the nurse should explain how this feedback will be used. The nurse should listen and observe carefully to make sure that what family members are saying is truly what they are feeling.

BOX 3-1 | Strategies for Managing Conflict

- *Understand the parents' perspective (walk in their shoes)*. Imagine yourself as the parent of a child in a hospital where your values and beliefs are exposed and scrutinized. Try to understand their perspective better by encouraging them to share it.
- *Determine a common goal and stay focused on it*. Determine the agreed-on result, and work toward it. By staying focused on a common goal, the parties involved are more likely to find workable strategies to achieve the identified goal.
- *Seek win-win solutions*. Conflict should not be about who is right and who is wrong. Effective conflict management focuses on finding a solution whereby both people "win." By establishing a common goal, both parties win when this goal is achieved.
- *Listen actively*. Critical to resolving situations of conflict is the ability to listen and understand what the other person is saying and feeling. In active listening, the receiver actively and empathically listens to gain a better understanding of the actual and the implied message.
- *Openly express your feelings*. Talking about feelings is much more constructive than acting them out.

  The nurse might say, "I am very concerned about Jamie's safety when you leave his side rails down." *Avoid blaming*. Each party owns part of the problem. Pointing fingers and blaming others will not solve the problem. Instead, identify the part of the problem that each party owns and work together to resolve it. Seek win-win solutions.

- *Summarize the decision*. At the end of any discussion, summarize what has been decided and identify who is responsible for follow-up. This process ensures that everyone is clear about the decision and facilitates accountability for implementing solutions.

TABLE 3-2 Choosing Words Carefully

Poor Words	Rationale	Better Words	Rationale
Policies allowed or not permitted	Convey attitude that hospital personnel have authority over parents in matters concerning their children	*Guidelines, working together, welcome*	Convey openness and appreciation for position and importance of families
Noncompliant, uncooperative, difficult (when referring to parents and other family members)	Imply that health care providers make decisions and give instructions that families must follow without input	*Partners, colleagues, joint decision makers, experts about their child*	Acknowledge that families bring important information and insight and that families and professionals form a team
Dysfunctional, in denial, overprotective, uninvolved, uncaring (labeling families)	Pronounce judgment that may not incorporate full understanding of family's situation, reactions, or perspective	*Coping* (describing family's reactions with care and respect)	Leave room to build more complete and appreciative understanding of families over time

For example, while one nurse was teaching the mother of a 2-year-old child who was recently diagnosed with diabetes mellitus, the mother reported that, although she was the primary caregiver of her child, the child's grandmother frequently cared for the child while the mother was at work. The nurse therefore notified the other team members and altered the teaching plan for diabetes care to include the child's grandmother.

Spirituality

Children have rich spiritual lives although they do not use the same vocabulary as adults to describe them. Spiritual care is a vital coping resource for many children. Supporting children's existing faith and spiritual practices is recommended. Children can be assisted in maintaining their rituals, whether they are bedtime prayers, songs, or blessings at meals. Nurses can provide spiritual care in ways that offer hope, encouragement, comfort, and respect. Tapping into spiritual strength can improve the outcome of overall care (Rollins, Bolig, & Mahan, 2005). A resource to pursue in many hospital or health care settings is the pastoral care or chaplain's department.

TRANSCULTURAL COMMUNICATION: BRIDGING THE GAP

Conflict can arise when the nurse comes from a cultural background different from that of the child and family. Such differences could influence the approach to care. As the demographics in the United States continue to change, health care professionals will be challenged to become more transcultural in their approach to clients if they want to continue to be effective in their relationships with children and families. Health care professionals need to be aware of their own values and beliefs and need to recognize how these influence their interactions with others. They also need to be aware of and respect the child's and family's values and beliefs. In working with children and families, the initial assessment should address values, beliefs, and traditions. The nurse can then consider ways in which culture might affect communication style, methods of decision making, and other behaviors related to health care practices.

During the initial interview, the nurse should ascertain the following information related to the child and family:
- *Decision-making practices:* Are decisions made by individuals or collectively as a group?
- *Child-rearing practices:* Who are the primary caregivers? What are their disciplinary practices?
- *Family support:* What is the family structure? To whom do the patient and family turn for support?
- *Communication practices:* How is the information communicated to the rest of the family?
- *Health and illness practices:* Do family members seek professional help or rely on other resources for treatment and advice?

Once this information is obtained, the nurse can use this knowledge to individualize the treatment plan and approach for the child's and family's needs. For example, if the parents of a child with an Orthodox Jewish religious background request a kosher diet, the nurse facilitates the routine delivery of kosher meals and communicates the family's wishes to the rest of the team members so that they can also respect the family's customs. If the family of a child who has a severe brain injury requests the services of a healer, the nurse enables the family to arrange the visit. Coordinating the child's daily schedule to provide an uninterrupted visit with the healer is one aspect of family-centered care. When the nurse communicates the family's cultural preferences to other members of the health care team, communication and holistic care are enhanced.

THERAPEUTIC RELATIONSHIPS: DEVELOPING AND MAINTAINING TRUST

Trust is important in establishing and maintaining therapeutic relationships with families. Trust promotes a sense of partnership between nurses and families. Becoming overly involved with the child or family can inhibit a healthy relationship. Because nurses are caring, nurturing people and the profession demands that nurses sometimes become intimately involved in other people's lives, maintaining the balance between appropriate involvement and professional separation is quite challenging. Box 3-2 delineates behaviors that may indicate overinvolvement. Box 3-3 identifies behaviors that may indicate professional separation or underinvolvement. Whether nurses become too emotionally involved or find themselves at the other end of the spectrum being underinvolved, there is a loss of effectiveness in being an objective professional resource.

BOX 3-2	**Warning Signs of Overinvolvement**

- Buying gifts for individual children or families
- Giving out a home phone number
- Competing with other staff for the child's or family's affection
- Inviting the child or family to social gatherings
- Accepting invitations to family gatherings (e.g., birthday parties, weddings)
- Visiting or spending time with the child or family during off-duty time
- Revealing personal information
- Lending or borrowing money
- Making decisions for the family about the child's care

BOX 3-3	**Warning Signs of Underinvolvement**

- Avoiding child or family
- Calling in sick to not take assignment of a specific child
- Asking to trade assignments for a specific child
- Spending less time with a particular child

Family members may display feelings of incompetence, fear, and loss of control by expressing anger, withdrawal, or dissatisfaction. Most important in working with these families is to promote the parents' feelings of competence through education and empowerment. The nurse should keep parents well informed of the child's care through frequent phone calls and involvement in decision making. The nurse should promote their confidence, enhance their self-esteem, and foster their independence by teaching them the skills necessary to care for their child.

Nurses must be able to recognize their own personal and professional needs. Awareness of the motives for one's own actions will greatly enhance the nurse's ability to understand the needs of children and families and to give families the tools to manage care effectively.

CRITICAL TO REMEMBER
Maintaining a Therapeutic Relationship

Maintaining professional boundaries requires that the nurse constantly be aware of the fine line between empathy and overinvolvement.

NURSING CARE

Communicating With Children and Families

Assessment

A comprehensive needs assessment of the child and family elicits information about problem-solving skills, cultural needs, coping behaviors, and the child's routines. Any assessment requires the nurse to obtain information from the child and the family.

The nurse might say, "Mrs. Brown, I value your input as well as your child's. Hearing Michael explain his understanding of his diabetic dietary restrictions in his own words will help us gain better insight into how best to manage his care. Let's take a few minutes to hear from Michael, and then we can talk about your perspective."

Assessment enables the nurse to develop better insight by gathering information from multiple perspectives and facilitates the development of a more comprehensive plan of care. A thorough assessment of the child's communication skills presumes the nurse understands developmental milestones and can relate comprehension and communication skills to the child's cognitive and emotional development and language abilities. During the initial assessment of the child and family, the nurse should also describe routines and provide information about what the child and family can expect during their visit.

Nursing Diagnosis and Planning

The nursing assessment may suggest diagnoses that affect communication but that arise from the child's encounter with the health care system. Other diagnoses are related to the child's and family's communication abilities.

- Anxiety related to potential or actual separation from parents (e.g., a 4-year-old girl who becomes withdrawn and unable to cooperate with an office hearing test when separated from her mother).

  Expected Outcomes: The child verbalizes the cause of the anxiety and more readily communicates with the health care professional. The child exhibits posture, facial expressions, and gestures that reflect decreased distress.

- Fear related to a perceived threat to the child's well-being and inadequate understanding of procedures or treatments (e.g., a 7-year-old boy scheduled for tonsillectomy who wonders where his throat will be cut to remove his tonsils).

  Expected Outcomes: The child talks about fears and accurately describes the procedure or treatment.

- Hopelessness related to a deteriorating health status (e.g., an 11-year-old child in isolation with prolonged illness and uncertain prognosis).

  Expected Outcomes: The child verbalizes feelings and participates in care. The child makes positive statements, maintains eye contact during interactions, and has appetite and sleep patterns that are appropriate for age and physical health.

- Powerlessness related to limits to autonomy (e.g., a 3-year-old child with a C6 spinal fracture as a result of a motor vehicle trauma).

  Expected Outcomes: The child expresses frustrations and anger and begins to make choices in areas that are controllable. The child asks appropriate questions about care and treatment.

- Impaired Verbal Communication related to physiologic barriers or cultural and language differences (e.g., a 17-year-old adolescent who has had her jaw wired subsequent to orthodontic surgery).

  Expected Outcomes: The child with a physiologic barrier to communication effectively uses alternative communication methods. The child and family who speak and understand a different language appropriately communicate through an interpreter.

CRITICAL THINKING EXERCISE 3-1

The nurse caring for 8-year-old Jermaine observes him lying in his bed with his back facing the door. He is crying, although he quickly wipes his eyes when he sees the nurse at the door. Jermaine has been hospitalized because of leukemia. He lives in a small community 350 miles from the hospital. His parents visit on the weekends.

1. Identify two things that might be upsetting Jermaine.
2. What strategies could you use to encourage Jermaine to talk about his feelings related to the problems you have identified?

Interventions

Nurses working with children should determine the best communication approach for each child individually on the basis of the child's age and developmental abilities. Table 3-3

TABLE 3-3 Developmental Milestones and Their Relationship to Communication Approaches

Development	Language Development	Emotional Development	Cognitive Development	Suggested Communication Approach
INFANTS (0-12 mo) Infants experience world through senses of hearing, seeing, smelling, tasting, and touching.	Crying, babbling, cooing. Single-word production. Able to name some simple objects.	Dependent on others; high need for cuddling and security. Responsive to environment (e.g., sounds, visual stimuli). Distinguish between happy and angry voices and between familiar and strange voices. Beginning to experience separation anxiety.	Interactions largely reflexive. Beginning to see repetition of activities and movements. Beginning to initiate interactions intentionally. Short attention span (1-2 min).	Use calm, soft, soothing voice. Be responsive to cries. Engage in turn-taking vocalizations (adult imitates baby sounds). Talk and read regularly to infants. Prepare infant as you are about to perform care; talk to infant about what you are about to do. Use slow approach and allow child time to get to know you.
TODDLERS (1-2 yr) Toddlers experience world through senses of hearing, seeing, smelling, tasting, and touching.	Two-word combinations emerge. Participate in turn taking in communication (speaker/listener). "No" becomes favorite word. Able to use gestures and verbalize simple wants and needs.	Strong need for security objects. Separation/stranger anxiety heightened. Participate in parallel play. Thrive on routines. Beginning development of independence: "Want to do by self." Still very dependent on significant adults.	Experiment with objects. Participate in active exploration. Begin to experiment with variations on activities. Begin to identify cause-and-effect relationships. Short attention span (3-5 min).	Learn toddler's words for common items, and use them in conversations. Describe activities and procedures as they are about to be done. Use picture books. Use play for demonstrations. Be responsive to child's receptivity toward you and approach cautiously. Preparation should occur immediately before event.
PRESCHOOL CHILDREN (3-5 yr) Preschool children use words they do not fully understand, nor do they accurately understand many words used by others.	Further development and expansion of word combination (able to speak in full sentences). Growth in correct grammatical usage. Use pronouns. Clearer articulation of sounds. Vocabulary rapidly expanding; may know words without understanding meaning.	Like to imitate activities and make choices. Strive for independence but need adult support and encouragement. Demonstrate purposeful attention-seeking behaviors. Learn cooperation and turn taking in game playing. Need clearly set limits and boundaries.	Begin developing concepts of time, space, and quantity. Magical thinking prominent. World seen only from child's perspective. Short attention span (5-10 min).	Seek opportunities to offer choices. Use play to explain procedures and activities. Speak in simple sentences, and explore relative concepts. Use picture and story books, puppets. Describe activities and procedures as they are about to be done. Be concise; limit length of explanations (5 min). Engage in preparatory activities 1-3 hr before the event.

Continued

TABLE 3-3   Developmental Milestones and Their Relationship to Communication Approaches—cont'd

Development	Language Development	Emotional Development	Cognitive Development	Suggested Communication Approach
SCHOOL AGE CHILDREN (6-11 yr)				
School-age children communicate thoughts and appreciate viewpoints of others. Words with multiple meanings and words describing things they have not experienced are not thoroughly understood.	Expanding vocabulary enables child to describe concepts, thoughts, and feelings. Development of conversational skills.	Interact well with others. Understand rules to games. Very interested in learning. Build close friendships. Beginning to accept responsibility for own actions. Competition emerges. Still dependent on adults to meet needs.	Able to grasp concepts of classification, conversation. Concrete thinking emerges. Become very oriented to "rules." Able to process information in serial format. Lengthened attention span (10-30 min).	Use photographs, books, diagrams, charts, videos to explain. Make explanations sequential. Engage in conversations that encourage critical thinking. Establish limits and set consequences. Use medical play techniques. Introduce preparatory materials 1-5 days in advance of the event.
ADOLESCENTS (12 yr and older)				
Adolescents are able to create theories and generate many explanations for situations. They are beginning to communicate like adults.	Able to verbalize and comprehend most adult concepts.	Beginning to accept responsibility for own actions. Perception of "imaginary audiences." Need independence. Competitive drive. Strong need for group identification. Frequently have small group of very close friends. Question authority. Strong need for privacy.	Able to think logically and abstractly. Attention span up to 60 min.	Engage in conversations about adolescent's interests. Use photographs, books, diagrams, charts, and videos to explain. Use collaborative approach and foster and support independence. Introduce preparatory materials up to 1 wk in advance of the event. Respect privacy needs.

presents an overview of developmental milestones related to communication skills in children and some approaches to facilitate successful interactions.

Play. Play can greatly facilitate communicating with children. Approaching children at their developmental level with familiar forms of play increases their comfort and allows the nurse to be seen in a more positive, less threatening role.

Because play is an everyday part of children's lives and a method they use to communicate, they are less likely to be inhibited when participating in play interactions. Through play, children may express thoughts and feelings they may be unable to verbalize (see Chapters 5 through 8 for normal play activities and Chapter 11 for therapeutic play).

Storytelling. Storytelling is an innovative and creative communication strategy. It is also a skill that can be acquired and refined through practice. Familiarity with stories and frequent practice in storytelling increase a nurse's confidence and competence as storyteller. Storytelling can be a routine part of a nurse's day. Its purposes range from establishing rapport to approaching uncomfortable topics, such as loss, death, fear, grief, and anger. In storytelling, there is a teller and a listener. In individual situations, the child may be the teller or the listener, although in a shared story, adult and child may each take a turn in both roles (Box 3-4).

Explaining Procedures and Treatments. Preparation before a procedure, which includes explaining the reasons

---

BOX 3-4   Storytelling Strategies

- Capture a story on paper or on videotape as told by a child or group of children.
- Tell a "yarn story" with two or more people. A long piece of yarn with knots tied at varied intervals is slid loosely through the hands of the teller until a knot is felt, at which time the yarn is passed to the next person, who continues the story.
- Initiate a game of sentence completion, either oral or written, with sentences beginning "If I were in charge of the hospital …," "I wish …," "When I get home I will …," or "My family…."
- Read stories with themes related to issues a child is facing. The children's section of the local public library is an excellent resource.

for the procedure and the expected sequence of events and outcomes, can greatly reduce a child's fears and anxieties. Preparation enables the child to experience some mastery over events, gives the child time to develop effective coping behaviors, and fosters trust in those caring for the child. Adequate preparation is the key to helping a child have a successful, positive health care experience.

In general, the younger the child, the closer in time to the event should the child be prepared for it. For example, a 3-year-old child will generally be very anxious and therefore should be prepared immediately before, whereas teenagers would benefit from a longer preparation time so that they can develop strategies for dealing with the situation. Table 3-3 gives age-related attention span guidelines.

Key elements for communicating complete and accurate information are as follows (Gaynard et al., 1998):
- *Learn the procedure.* To explain a procedure adequately, the nurse must understand what is involved. What pieces of equipment will be used? Where will the procedure take place? Essentially, the nurse needs to learn what the child can expect to happen during the procedure.
- *Determine what information to share with the child and family.* The preparation should include information only about what the child will experience or perceive directly. Consultation with the family will allow the nurse to learn words and terminology used by the child. Table 3-4 offers other concrete suggestions of appropriate language for nurses to use in working with children.

TABLE 3-4 Considerations in Choosing Language

Potentially Ambiguous	Concrete Explanation
"The doctor will give you some dye." *To make me die?*	"The doctor will put some medicine in the tube that will help her see your _____ more clearly."
Dressing, dressing change. *Why are they going to undress me?* *Do I have to change my clothes?*	Bandages; clean, new bandages.
Stool collection. *Why do they want to collect little chairs?*	Use child's familiar term, such as "poop," "BM," or "doody."
Urine. *You're in?*	Use child's familiar term, such as "pee."
Shot. *When people get shot, they're really badly hurt.*	Describe giving medicine through a (small, tiny) needle.
CAT scan. *Will there be cats?*	Describe in simple terms, and explain what the letters of the common name stand for.
PICU. *Pick you?*	Explain as above.
ICU. *I see you?*	Explain as above.
IV. *Ivy?*	Explain as above.
Stretcher. *Stretch her? Stretch whom?*	Bed on wheels.
Special; funny (words that are usually positive descriptors). *It doesn't look/feel special to me.*	Odd, different, unusual, strange.
Gas, sleeping gas. *Is someone going to pour gasoline into the mask?*	"A medicine, called an anesthetic, is a kind of air you will breathe through a mask like this to help you sleep during your operation so you won't feel anything. It is a different kind of sleep." (Explain differences.)
"The doctor will put you to sleep." *Like my cat was put to sleep? It never came back.*	"The doctor will give you medicine that will help you go into a very deep sleep. You won't feel anything until the operation is over. Then the doctor will stop giving you the medicine, so you can wake up."
"Move you to the floor." *Why are they going to put me on the ground?*	Unit, ward. (Explain why the child is being transferred, and where.)
OR (or treatment room) table. *People aren't supposed to get up on tables.*	A narrow bed.

NOTE: Words or phrases that are helpful to one child may be threatening for another. Health care providers must listen carefully and be sensitive to the child's use of and response to language.

Modified with permission of the Child Life Council, Inc., 11820 Parklawn Dr., Rockville, MD 20852-2529, from Gaynard, L., Wolfer, J., Goldberger, J., Thompson, R., Redburn, L., & Laidley, L. (1998). *Psychosocial care of children in hospitals: A clinical practice manual from ACCH Child Life Research Project.* Rockville, MD: The Child Life Council, Inc.

Continued

TABLE 3-4 Considerations in Choosing Language—cont'd

Potentially Ambiguous	Concrete Explanation
"Take a picture." (X-ray, CT, and MRI machines are far larger than a familiar camera, move differently, and do not yield a familiar end product.)	"A picture of your insides." (Describe appearance, sounds, and movement of the equipment.)
"Flush your IV." *Flush it down the toilet?*	Explain.

Words can be experienced as "hard" or "soft" according to how much they increase the perceived threat of a situation. For example, consider the following word choices:

Harder	Softer
"This part will hurt."	"It (you) may feel (or feel very) sore, achy, scratchy, tight, snug, full, or _____ (other manageable, descriptive term)."
"The medicine will burn."	(Words such as scratch, poke, or sting might be familiar for some children and frightening to others.)
"The room will be very cold."	"Some children say they feel very warm." "Some children say they feel very cold."
"The medicine will taste (or smell) bad."	"The medicine may taste (or smell) different from anything you have tasted before. After you take it, will you tell me how it was for you?"
"Cut," "open you up," "slice," "make a hole."	"The doctor will make an opening."
"As big as _____" (e.g., size of an incision or of a catheter).	(Use concrete comparisons, such as "your little finger" or "a paper clip" *if* the opening will indeed be small.) "Smaller than _____."
As long as _____" (e.g., for duration of a procedure).	"For less time than it takes you to _____."
"As much as _____."	"Less than _____."
(These are open-ended and "extending" expressions.)	(These expressions help confine, familiarize, and imply the manageability of an event or of equipment.)

The unfamiliar usage or complexity of some common medical words or expressions can be confusing and frightening.

Potentially Ambiguous	Concrete Explanation
"Take your vitals" (or "your vital signs").	"Measure your temperature," "see how warm your body is," "see how fast and strongly your heart is working." (Nothing is "taken" from the child.)
Electrodes, leads.	"Sticky like a Band-Aid, with a small wet spot in the center, and small strings that attach to the snap (monitor electrodes); paste like wet sand, with strings with tiny metal cups that stick to the paste (EEG electrodes). The paste washes off easily afterward; the strings go into a box that will make a picture of how your heart (or brain) is working." (Show child electrodes and leads before using. Let child handle them and apply them to a doll or to self.)
"Hang your (IV) medication."	"We will bring in a new medicine in a bag and attach it to the little tube already in your arm. The needle goes into the tube, not into your arm, so you won't feel it."
N.P.O.	"Nothing to eat. Your stomach needs to be empty." (Explain why.) "You can eat and drink again as soon as _____." (Explain with concrete descriptions.)
Anesthesia.	"The doctor will give you medicine—you may hear it called 'anesthesia.' It will help you go into a very deep sleep. You will not feel anything at all. The doctor knows just the right amount of medicine to give you so you will stay asleep through your operation. When the operation is over, the doctor stops giving you that medicine and helps you wake up."

TABLE 3-5 Self-Esteem in Children: Communication Practices

Techniques to Enhance Self-Esteem	Practices That Harm Self-Esteem
Praise efforts and accomplishments.	Criticize efforts and accomplishments.
Use active listening skills.	Be too busy to listen.
Encourage expression of feelings.	Tell children how they should feel.
Acknowledge feelings.	Give no support for dealing with feelings.
Use developmentally based discipline.	Use physical punishment.
Use "I" statements.	Use "you" statements.
Be nonjudgmental.	Judge the child.
Set clearly defined limits, and reinforce them.	Set no known limits or boundaries.
Share quality time together.	Give time grudgingly.
Be honest.	Be dishonest.
Describe behaviors observed when praising and disciplining.	Use coercion and power as discipline.
Compliment the child.	Belittle, blame, or shame the child.
Smile.	Use sarcastic, caustic, or cruel "humor."
Touch and hug the child.	Avoid coming near the child, even when the child is open to touching, holding, or hugging. Touch and hold only when performing a task.
Rock the child.	Avoid comforting through rocking.

- *Provide sensory information.* Inviting children to see, hear, feel, taste, smell, and experience similar sensations during the preparation will greatly enhance their preparedness and diminish their anxieties. For example, in preparing a child for an IV line insertion, the nurse can show the child the catheter or explain the purpose of the tourniquet and allow the child to put it on or to put it on the arm of a doll, if the child so desires. The nurse should let the child smell an alcohol swab and feel its coolness when applied to the skin. Showing the child the treatment room and inviting the child to sit on the treatment table where the procedure will be performed are effective ways to convey information.

- *Explain the sequence of events.* Preparation includes a description of the sequence in which events will occur. Recognizing the procedure as a series of sequential steps allows children to anticipate appropriately and gives them a sense of control and a better understanding of the number of steps to expect before the procedure is over.

- *Explain how long the procedure will last.* Whenever possible, the nurse should invite the child to have simulated play experiences. Inviting the child to perform the procedure on a doll or stuffed animal is often effective and gives the child a real sense of time and firsthand experience with the sequence of events. If a concrete demonstration is not possible, the nurse should explain the timing in terms that the child can understand; for example, the nurse might say, "The procedure will last as long as it takes to sing your favorite song."

- *Monitor accuracy of information (feedback).* Feedback can be used to modify or reinforce future preparation sessions. Feedback also allows the nurse to correct any misunderstandings the child may have and provides an opportunity for the child to process verbally and express feelings about the experience.

Open, honest communication about treatments and procedures and attentiveness to the learning needs of the child will greatly facilitate achievement of the treatment goals.

Strategies for Enhancing Self-Esteem. Coopersmith (1967) defined self-esteem as a "personal judgment of worthiness that is expressed in the attitudes the individual holds toward himself or herself." Communication practices play an important role in the development of children's self-esteem. Nurses are in an excellent position to model communication practices that enhance self-esteem. Table 3-5 compares helpful and harmful communication practices.

The words adults choose, their tone of voice, and the place and timing of message delivery all influence the child's interpretation of the message. The interpretation may be positive, negative, or neutral. To enhance the child's self-esteem, adults should strive for positive language. Being attentive, engendering trust, demonstrating affection, and affirming goodness and talents are communication practices that contribute to building self-esteem (McClowry, 2003).

Evaluation

Although evaluation is traditionally thought of as a closure activity, evaluation should be a continuous activity throughout the nursing process. Keep expected outcomes visible, and assess whether they are being realized. Are the outcomes attainable? Could the wrong nursing diagnosis have been made? Adjust the plan of care as needed.

COMMUNICATING WITH CHILDREN WITH SPECIAL NEEDS

The opportunity to interact with children who have special communication needs presents an exciting challenge for nurses. To identify successful alternative methods of communication, the nurse needs to learn particular techniques for working with children and families. Alternative methods of communicating are critical. Children need to express their wants and needs accurately. Through adequate preparation and reassurance, the nurse can offer the child comfort and understanding. Successfully meeting this challenge is a rewarding experience for the nurse and a positive, supportive experience for the child and family.

CRITICAL TO REMEMBER
Communicating With Children With Special Needs

In working with children with special needs, the nurse must carefully assess each child's physical, mental, and developmental abilities and determine the most effective methods of communication.

The Child With a Visual Impairment

For the child with a visual impairment, the nurse can:
- Obtain a thorough assessment of the child's self-help skills and abilities (i.e., toileting, bathing, dressing, feeding, mobility).
- Orient the child to the surroundings. Walk the child around the room and unit several times, indicating landmarks (e.g., doors, closets, bedside tables, windows) while guiding the child by the hand or by the way the child prefers. Explain sounds that the child may frequently hear (e.g., monitors, alarms, nurse call bells).
- Encourage the parents to stay with the child. They can facilitate communication and greatly enhance the child's comfort in this unfamiliar environment.
- Keep furniture and other items in the same consistent place. Consistency aids in the child's orientation to the room, fosters independence, and promotes safety.
- Keep the nurse call bell in the same place and within the child's reach.
- Identify yourself when entering the room, and tell the child when you are departing.
- Carefully and fully explain all procedures.
- Allow the child to handle equipment as the procedure is explained.

The Child With a Hearing Impairment

For the child with a hearing impairment, the nurse can:
- Thoroughly assess the child's self-help skills and abilities.
- Identify the family's method of communication, and if possible, adopt it.
- Encourage a family member to stay with the child at all times to decrease the stress of hospitalization and facilitate communication.
- If sign language is used, learn the most frequently used signs and use them whenever able. Keep a chart of signs near the child's bed.
- Develop a communication board with pictures of most commonly used items or needs (e.g., television, cup, toothbrush, toilet, shower).
- Determine whether the child uses a hearing aid. If so, make sure that the batteries are working and that the hearing aid is clean and intact.
- When entering the room, do so cautiously and gently touch the child before speaking.
- Always face the child when speaking. If the child is a lip reader, face-to-face visibility will greatly enhance the child's ability to understand.
- Do not shout or exaggerate speech. This behavior distorts the face and can be very confusing. Rather, speak in a normal tone and at a regular pace.
- Remember that nonverbal communication can speak as loud as, if not louder than, speech (e.g., a frown or worried face can say more than words).
- When performing a procedure that requires standing behind the child, such as when giving an enema or assisting with a spinal tap, have another person stand in front of the child and explain the procedure as it is being performed.
- Whenever possible, use play strategies to help communicate and demonstrate procedures (see Table 3-3).

The Child Who Speaks Another Language

For the child who speaks another language, the nurse can:
- Thoroughly assess the child's abilities in speaking and understanding both languages.
- Ask family members if they would like an interpreter and involve them in the selection.
- Identify an interpreter, perhaps another adult family member, friend of the family, or other individual with proficiency in both languages. Other children should not be used as interpreters.
- Use an interpreter whenever possible but especially when explaining procedures, determining understanding, teaching new skills, and assessing needs.
- Use a communication board with the names of items printed in both languages.
- Learn the words and names of commonly used items in the child's language, and use them whenever possible. Using the familiar language not only aids in communication but also demonstrates sincere interest in learning the language and respect for the culture.
- Learn as much about the child's culture as possible and develop plans of care that demonstrate respect for the culture. Sincere attempts to learn to communicate with the child and family demonstrate your concern for their well-being.
- Use play strategies whenever possible. Play seems to be a universal language.

The Child Who Is Aphonic

For the child who is aphonic, the nurse can:

- Thoroughly assess the child's self-help skills and abilities. Determine the child's and family's methods of communicating and adopt these as much as possible.
- Encourage parents to stay with the child to decrease anxiety and foster communication.
- Determine whether the child uses sign language or augmented communication devices. Use a communication board if appropriate.
- Be attentive to and maximize the child's nonverbal communication. Facial grimaces, frowns, smiles, and nods are effective means of communicating responses and expressing likes and dislikes.
- If appropriate, encourage the child to use writing boards (dry erase, chalk, pads of paper) to write needs, wants, questions, and concerns.

The Child With a Profound Neurologic Impairment

Because hearing, vision, and language abilities are often hard to determine in the child who is profoundly neurologically impaired, assume the child can hear, see, and comprehend something of what is said. Use a friendly tone of voice that conveys warmth and respect. For the child with a profound neurologic impairment, the nurse can:

- Address the child when entering and exiting the room. Gently touch the child while saying the child's name.
- Speak softly, calmly, and slowly to allow the child time to process what you are saying.
- While in the room with the child, talk to the child. Do not talk as if the child were not there.

The nurse might say, "Jenny, I am going to wash your arm now," or "Jenny, now I am going to take your temperature by putting the thermometer under your arm." Identifying an assistant, the nurse might say, "Jenny, Kristi, another nurse, is here to help me lift you into your chair."

- Talk to the child about activities and objects in the room, things that the child might see, hear, smell, touch, taste, or sense.

For example, the nurse might say, "It is a sunny day today; can you feel the warm sun shining on you through the window?"

- When asking the child questions, allow the child adequate time to respond. Be careful to ask questions only of children who are capable of responding.
- Ascertain the child's ability to respond to simple questions. Some children can respond to *yes* or *no* questions by squeezing a hand or blinking their eyes (once for *yes* and twice for *no*).
- Be extremely attentive to any signs or gestures (e.g., facial grimaces, smiling, eye movements) that may convey responses to likes or dislikes. Signs or gestures may be the child's only means of communicating.

As with all children with special communication needs, thoroughly document and communicate to others who interact with the child any special techniques that work.

Providing information will greatly enhance continuity and more fully facilitate the child's ability to communicate.

KEY CONCEPTS

- Components of effective communication with children involve verbal and nonverbal interactions. Essential components include touch, physical proximity, environment, listening, eye contact, visual cues, pace of speech and tone of voice, and overall body language.
- Nurses should determine the best communication approach for an individual child on the basis of the child's age, developmental abilities, and cultural preferences. Strategies include play and storytelling, explaining procedures and treatments, and modeling communication practices that enhance self-esteem.
- Communication pitfalls, such as using jargon, talking down to children or beyond their developmental level, and avoiding or denying a problem, can lead to a breakdown in the relationship between the nurse and the child and family.
- Family-centered communication strategies include establishing rapport, identifying needs, establishing expectations, being available and open to questions, family education, empowerment, obtaining feedback from children and families, promoting effective conflict management, learning techniques for transcultural communication, and maintaining professional boundaries.
- In working with children with special needs, the nurse should carefully assess each child's physical, mental, and developmental abilities and determine the most effective methods of communication.

ANSWERS TO CRITICAL THINKING EXERCISE 3-1

1. Two areas that the nurse should explore are Jermaine's feelings about separation from his family and issues related to having leukemia, including the discomfort, treatment, and prognosis.

2. School-age children often do not readily discuss their feelings. The nurse needs to build trust with the child. Involving the child in a board game can be a useful strategy to help the child relax. As the game progresses, the nurse can begin to talk with the child, using a lead in such as, "You seem very quiet today" or "You seemed upset when I came into your room." The child can choose to validate or deny the nurse's observation.

   Another approach would be to say, "If you could have one wish today, what would it be?" Some children will use this as an opportunity to describe what they would like to change. The nurse can cue into this disclosure. It is important to remember that all children are different and what works for one child may not work for another. Every nurse caring for children needs to understand growth and development and learn related communication techniques.

REFERENCES AND READINGS

Allenbach, A., & Steinmiller, E. (2004). Waiting together: Translating the principles of therapeutic relationships one step further. *Journal for Specialists in Pediatric Nursing, 9,* 24-31.

Clarke, J. N., & Fletcher, P. (2003). Communication issues faced by parents who have a child diagnosed with cancer. *Journal of Pediatric Oncology Nursing, 20,* 175-191.

Coopersmith, S. (1967). *The antecedents of self-esteem.* San Francisco: Freeman.

Darley, M. (Ed.). (2002). *Managing communication in health care.* London: Harcourt.

Deering, C. G., & Jennings, D. (2002). Communicating with children and adolescents. *American Journal of Nursing, 102,* 34-42.

DiMatteo, M. R. (2004). The role of effective communication with children and their families in fostering adherence to pediatric regimes. *Patient Education and Counseling, 55,* 339-344.

Feudtner, C., Haney, J., & Dimmers, M. A. (2003). Spiritual care needs of hospitalized children and their families: A national survey of pastoral care providers' perceptions. *Pediatrics, 111* (Supplement), e67-e72.

Gaynard, L., Wolfer, J., Goldberger, J., Thompson, R., Redburn, L., & Laidley, L. (1998). *Psychosocial care of children in hospitals: A clinical practice manual from ACCH Child Life Research Project.* Rockville: Child Life Council.

Hallström, I., & Elander, G. (2004). Decision making during hospitalization: Parents' and children's involvement. *Journal of Clinical Nursing, 13,* 367-375.

Heck, K., & Parker, J. (2002). Family structure, socioeconomic status, and access to healthcare for children. *Health Service Research, 37,* 173-186.

Killam, P. (2003). Maintain relationships with challenging families. *Nurse Practitioner, 28,* 15.

Kloosterhouse, V., & Anes, B. D. (2002). Families' use of religion/spirituality as a psychosocial resource. *Holistic Nursing Practice, 17,* 61-76.

Leavitt, L.A. (2002). When terrible things happen: A parents' guide to talking with their children. *Journal of Pediatric Health Care, 16,* 272-274.

McClowry, S. G. (2003). *Your child's unique temperament: Insights and strategies for responsive parenting.* Champaign: Research Press.

Melnyk, B. M., Feinstein, N. F., Tuttle, J., Moldenhauer, Z., Herendeen, P., Veenema, T. G., Brown, H., Gullo, S., McMurtrie, M., & Small, L. (2002). Mental health worries, communication, and needs in the year of the U.S. terrorist attack: National KySS survey findings. *Journal of Pediatric Health Care, 16,* 222-234.

Narayanasamy, A. (2003). Transcultural nursing. How do nurses respond to cultural needs? *British Journal of Nursing, 12,* 185-194.

O'Neill, K. (2002). Kids speak: Effective communication with school-aged/adolescent patient. *Pediatric Emergency Care, 18,* 137-140.

Rollins, J. A., Bolig, R., & Mahan, C. C. (2005). *Meeting children's psychosocial needs across the health-care continuum.* Austin: Pro-Ed, Inc.

Ryan, E., & Steinmiller, E. (2004). Modeling family-centered pediatric nursing care: Strategies for shift report. *Journal of Specialists in Pediatric Nursing, 9,* 123-128.

Simons, J., & Roberson, E. (2002). Poor communication and knowledge deficits: Obstacles to effective management of children's post operative pain. *Journal of Advanced Nursing, 40,* 78-86.

Snyder, B. S. (2004). Preventing treatment interference: Nurses' and parents' intervention strategies. *Pediatric Nursing, 30,* 31-40.

Tates, K., Meeuwesen, L., Elbers, E., & Bensing, J. (2002). "I've come for his throat": Roles and identities in doctor-parent-child communication. *Child: Care, Health, & Development, 28,* 109-116.

Topper, E. F. (2004). Working knowledge: It's not what you say, but how you say it. *American Libraries, 35,* 76.

Walker, C. L., Wells, L. M., Heiny, S. P., & Hymovich, D. P. (2002). Family-centered psychosocial care. In C. R. Baggott, K. P. Kelly, D. Fochtman, & G. V. Foley (Eds.), *Nursing care of children and adolescents with cancer.* Philadelphia: Saunders.

Wanzer, M. B., Booth-Butterfield, M., & Gruber, K. (2004). Perceptions of health care providers' communication: Relationships between patient centered communication and satisfaction. *Health Communication, 16,* 363-384.

Wissow, L. S., & Kimel, M. B. (2002). Assessing provider-patient-parent communication in the pediatric emergency department. *Ambulatory Pediatrics, 2,* 323-329.

Young, B., Dixon-Woods, M., Windridge, K., & Henry, D. (2003). Managing communication with young people who have a potentially life threatening chronic illness: Qualitative study of patients and parents. *British Medical Journal, 326,* 305-310.

CHAPTER 4

Health Promotion for the Developing Child

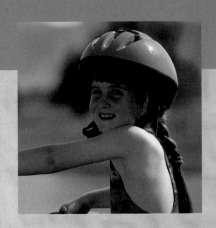

Learning Objectives

After studying this chapter, you should be able to:
- Define terms related to growth and development.
- Discuss principles of growth and development.
- Describe various factors, including genetics, that affect growth and development.
- Discuss the following theorists' ideas about growth and development: Piaget, Freud, Erikson, and Kohlberg.
- Discuss theories of language development.
- Identify methods used to assess growth and development.
- Describe the classifications and social aspects of play.
- Explain how play enhances growth and development.
- Identify health-promoting activities that are essential for the normal growth and development of infants and children.
- Discuss recommendations for scheduled vaccines.
- Discuss the components of a nutritional assessment.
- Discuss the etiology and prevention of childhood injuries.

Definitions

cephalocaudal   Progression from head to toe.
chronologic age   Age in years.
developmental age   Age based on functional behavior and ability to adapt to the environment; does not necessarily correspond to chronologic age.
dramatic play   Play in which children act out roles and experiences that may have happened to them, that they fear will happen to them, or that they have observed happening to someone else.
familiarization play   Use of materials that are commonly associated with health care situations in creative and playful activities.
growth spurts   Brief periods of a rapid increase in growth rate.
heredity   Transmission of genetic characteristics from parent to offspring.

learning   Behavior changes that occur as a result of both maturation and experience with the environment.
nutrients   Foods that supply the body with elements necessary for metabolism.
proximodistal   Progression from the center outward or from the midline to the periphery.
recommended dietary allowance (RDA)   Recommendations for the average amounts of nutrients that should be consumed daily by healthy people in the United States.
regression   Appearance of behavior more appropriate to an earlier stage of development; often used to cope with stress or anxiety.
symbolic play   Use of games and interactions that represent an issue or concern to be addressed.

Audio Glossary

Electronic Resources

Additional information related to the content in Chapter 4 can be found on:

the interactive companion CD-ROM
- Audio Glossary
- NCLEX Review Questions

or the companion website at *evolve*
http://evolve.elsevier.com/james/ncoc
- Denver Developmental Screening Test II
- NCLEX Review Questions
- WebLinks

Humans grow and change dramatically during childhood and adolescence. Normal growth and development proceed in an orderly, predictable pattern that establishes a basis for assessing an individual's abilities and potential. Nurses provide health care teaching and anticipatory guidance about the growth and development of children in many settings, such as newborn nurseries, emergency departments, community clinics and health centers, and pediatric inpatient units.

OVERVIEW OF GROWTH AND DEVELOPMENT

Nurses are frequently the members of the health care team whom parents approach. Parents are often concerned that their children are not progressing normally. Nurses can reassure parents about normal variations in development and can also identify problems early so that developmental delays can be addressed as soon as possible. Nurses who work with ill children must have a clear understanding of how children differ from adults and from each other at various stages. This awareness is essential to allow nurses to create developmentally appropriate plans of care to meet the needs of their young clients.

Definition of Terms

Although the terms *growth* and *development* often are used together and interchangeably, they have distinct definitions and meanings. Growth generally refers to an increase in the physical size of a whole or any of its parts or an increase in the number and size of cells. Growth can be measured easily and accurately. For example, any observer can see that an infant grows rapidly during the first year of life. This growth can be measured readily by determining changes in weight and length. The difference in size between a newborn and a 12-month-old infant is an obvious sign of the remarkable growth that occurs during the first year of life.

Development is a more complex and subtle concept. Development is generally considered to be a continuous, orderly series of conditions leading to activities, new motives for activities, and patterns of behavior.

Another definition of development is an increase in function and complexity that occurs through growth, maturation, and learning—in other words, an increase in capabilities. The process of language acquisition provides an example of development. The use of language becomes increasingly complex as the child matures. At 10 to 12 months of age, a child uses single words to communicate simple desires and needs. By age 4 to 5 years, complete and complex sentences are used to relate elaborate tales. Language development can be measured by determining vocabulary, articulation skill, and word use.

Maturity and learning also affect development. *Maturation* is the physical change in the complexity of body structures that enables a child to function at increasingly higher levels. Maturity is programmed genetically and may occur as a result of several changes. For example, maturation of the central nervous system depends on changes that occur throughout the body, such as an increase in the number of neurons,

myelinization of nerve fibers, lengthening of muscles, and overall weight gain.

Learning involves changes in behavior that occur as a result of both maturation and experience with the environment. Predictable patterns are observed in learning, and these patterns are sequential, orderly, and progressive. For example, when learning to walk, babies first learn to control their heads, then to roll over, next to sit, then to crawl, and finally to walk. The child's muscle mass and nervous system must grow and mature as well.

These examples show how complex and interrelated the processes of growth, development, maturation, and learning are. Children must be monitored carefully to ensure that these complicated events and activities unfold normally. Wide variations occur as children grow and develop. Each child has a unique rate and pattern of development, although parameters are used to identify abnormalities. Nurses must be familiar with normal parameters so that delays can be detected early. The earlier that delays are discovered and intervention initiated, the less dramatic their effect will be.

Stages of Growth and Development

To simplify analysis and discussion of the complex processes and theories related to growth and development, researchers and theorists have identified stages or age groupings. These stages serve as reference points in describing various features of growth and development (Box 4-1). Chapters 5 through 8 discuss the physical growth and cognitive, emotional, language, and motor development specific to each stage.

Parameters of Growth

Statistical data derived from research studies of large groups of children provide health care professionals with information about how children normally grow. Throughout infancy, childhood, and adolescence, growth occurs in bursts separated by periods when growth is stable or consistent.

Weight, height, and head circumference are parameters that are used to monitor growth. They should be measured at regular intervals during childhood. The weight of the average term newborn infant is approximately 7½ to 8 pounds (3.4 to 3.6 kg). Male infants are usually slightly heavier than female infants. Usually, the birth weight doubles by 6 months of age and triples by 1 year of age. Between 2 and 3 years of age, the weight quadruples. Slow, steady weight gain during childhood is followed by a growth spurt during adolescence.

BOX 4-1	**Stages of Growth and Development**

The following stages and age groupings refer to stages of childhood growth and development:

Newborn	Birth to 1 month
Infancy	1 month to 1 year
Toddlerhood	1 to 3 years
Preschool age	3 to 6 years
School age	6 to 11 or 12 years
Adolescence	11 or 12 to 21 years

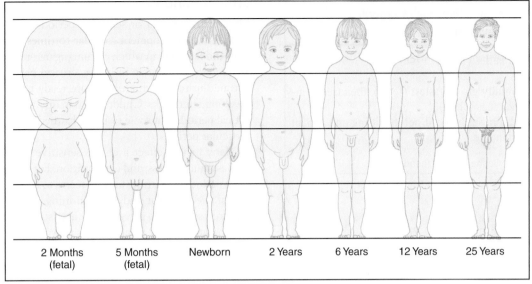

FIG 4-1 **Changes in body proportions with growth.**

The average newborn infant is approximately 20 inches (50 cm) long, with an average increase of approximately 1 inch (2.54 cm) per month for the first 6 months, followed by an increase of approximately ½ inch (1.27 cm) per month for the remainder of the first year. The child gains 3 inches (7.6 cm) per year from age 1 through 7 years and then 2 inches (5 cm) per year from age 8 through 15 years. Boys generally add more height during adolescence than do girls. Body proportion changes are shown in Figure 4-1.

Head circumference indicates brain growth. The normal occipital-frontal circumference of the term newborn head is 13 to 14 inches (33 to 35.5 cm). Average head growth occurs according to the following pattern: 4.8 inches (12 cm) during the first year, 1 inch (2.5 cm) during the second year; ½ inch (1.2 cm) per year from 3 to 5 years, and ½ inch (1.2 cm) per year from 5 years until puberty. The average adult head circumference is approximately 21 inches (53 cm).

Dentition, the eruption of teeth, also follows a sequential pattern. Primary dentition usually begins to emerge at approximately 6 to 8 months. Most children have 20 teeth by age 2½ years. Permanent teeth, 32 in all, erupt beginning at approximately age 6 years, accompanied by the loss of primary teeth (see Chapter 9). Although some parents place importance on eruption of the teeth as a sign of maturation, dentition is not related to the level or rate of development.

CRITICAL TO REMEMBER
Patterns of Growth and Development

Although heredity determines each individual's growth rate, the normal pace of growth of all children falls into four distinct patterns:
1. A rapid pace from birth to 2 years
2. A slower pace from 2 years to puberty
3. A rapid pace from puberty to approximately 15 years
4. A sharp decline from 16 years to approximately 24 years, when full adult size is reached

---

PRINCIPLES OF GROWTH AND DEVELOPMENT
Patterns of Growth and Development

Growth and development are directional and follow predictable patterns. The first direction of growth is *cephalocaudal*, or proceeding from head to tail (or toe). This means that structures and functions originating in the head develop before those in the lower parts of the body. At birth the head is large, a full one fourth of the entire body length, the trunk is long, and the arms are longer than the legs. As the child matures, the body proportions gradually change; by adulthood the legs have increased in size from approximately 38% to 50% of the total body length (see Fig. 4-1).

Directional growth and development are illustrated further by myelinization of the nerves, which begins in the brain and spreads downward as the child matures (Box 4-2). Growth of the myelin sheath and other nerve structures contributes to cephalocaudal development, which is illustrated by an infant's ability to raise the head before being able to sit and to sit before being able to stand.

A second directional aspect of growth and development is *proximodistal*, which means progression from the center outward, or from the midline to the periphery. The growth and branching pattern of the respiratory tract illustrates this concept. The trachea, which is the central structure of the respiratory tree, forms in the embryo by 24 days of gestation. Branching and growth outward occur in the bronchi, bronchioles, and alveoli throughout fetal life and infancy. Alveoli, which are the most distal structures of the system, continue to grow and develop in number and function until middle childhood.

Growth and development follow patterns, one of which is general to specific. As a child matures, activities become less generalized and more focused. For example, a neonate's response to pain is usually a whole-body response, with flailing of the arms and legs even if the pain is in the abdomen. As the child matures, the pain response becomes more localized

BOX 4-2 | **Directional Patterns of Growth and Development**

Cephalocaudal Pattern (Head to Toe)
Examples
- Head initially grows fastest (fetus), then trunk (infant), then legs (child).
- Infant can raise the head before sitting and can sit before standing.

Cephalocaudal (head to toe)

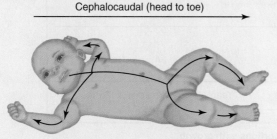

Proximodistal (from the center outward)

Proximodistal Pattern (From the Center Outward)
Examples
- In the respiratory system, the trachea develops first in the embryo, followed by branching and growth outward of the bronchi, bronchioles, and alveoli in the fetus and infant.
- Motor control of the arms comes before control of the hands, and hand control comes before finger control.

to the stimulus. An older child with abdominal pain guards the abdomen.

Another pattern is the progression of functions from simple to complex. This pattern is easily observed in language development. A toddler's first sentences are formed simply, using only a noun and a verb. By age 5 years, the child constructs detailed stories using many complex modifiers.

The rate of growth is not constant as the child matures. *Growth spurts*, alternating with periods of slow or stagnant growth, are observed throughout childhood. Spurts are frequently seen as the child prepares to master a significant developmental task, such as walking. An increase in growth around a child's first birthday may promote the neuromuscular maturation needed for taking the first steps.

All facets of development (cognitive, motor, emotional, language) normally proceed according to these patterns. Knowledge of these concepts is useful when determining how a child's development is progressing and when comparing a child's development with normal patterns.

Mastery of developmental tasks is not static or permanent, and developmental stages do not always correlate with chronologic age. Children progress through developmental stages at varying rates within normal limits and may master developmental tasks only to regress to earlier levels when ill or stressed. Also, people can struggle repeatedly with particular developmental tasks throughout life, although they have achieved more advanced levels of development.

Critical Periods

After birth, critical or sensitive periods exist for optimal growth and development. Similar to times during embryologic and fetal life, in which certain organs are formed and are particularly vulnerable to injury, critical periods are blocks of time during which children are ready to master specific developmental tasks. Children can master tasks outside these critical periods, but some tasks are learned more easily during particular periods.

Many factors affect a child's sensitive learning periods, such as injury, illness, and malnutrition. For example, the sensitive period for learning to walk seems to be during the latter part of the first year and the beginning of the second year. Children seem to be driven by an irresistible urge to practice walking and display great pride as they succeed. If a child is immobilized, for instance, for the treatment of an orthopedic condition from age 10 months to 18 months, the child may have difficulty learning to walk. The child can learn to walk, but the task may be more difficult than for other children.

Factors Influencing Growth and Development
Genetics
One factor that greatly influences a child's growth and development is genetics. Genetic potential is affected by many factors. Environment influences how and to what extent particular genetic traits are manifested. Genetics will be discussed in greater depth later in this chapter.

Environment
The environment is a significant determinant of growth and developmental outcome, both before and after birth. Examples of prenatal environmental factors include maternal smoking, alcohol intake, and disease, such as diabetes. Socioeconomic status, interpersonal relationships, and environmental hazards are only a few factors that affect children both before and after birth. Environmental factors that affect children are discussed in each individual growth-and-development chapter.

Culture
Culture is the way of life of a people, including their habits, beliefs, language, and values. It is a significant factor influencing children as they grow toward adulthood.

When gathering data, nurses must recognize how the common family structures and traditional values of various groups affect children's performance on assessment tests. The child's cultural and ethnic background must be considered when assessing growth and development. Standard growth curves and developmental tests do not necessarily reflect the normal growth and development of children of various cultural groups. Growth curves for children of various racial and cultural backgrounds are increasingly available. Nurse researchers and others conduct studies to determine the effectiveness of measurement tools for culturally diverse populations. In addition, culturally sensitive instruments are being developed to gather data to determine appropriate nursing interventions. To provide quality care to all patients, nurses must consider the effect of culture on children and families (see Chapter 2).

Nutrition

Because children are growing constantly and need a continuous supply of nutrients, nutrition plays an important role throughout childhood. Children need more nutritious food in proportion to size than adults do. Children's food patterns have changed over the years: they currently drink more low-fat and nonfat milk, consume fewer eggs, eat more snacks, and are more likely to eat their meals outside the home (Lucas, 2004). Nutrition is discussed in more depth later in this chapter.

Health Status

Overall health status plays an important part in the growth and development of children. At the cellular level, inherited or acquired disease can affect the delivery of nutrients, hormones, or oxygen to organs and also can affect organ growth and function. Disease states that affect growth and development include digestive or malabsorptive disorders, heart defects, and metabolic diseases.

Family

A child is an inseparable part of a family. Family relationships and influences are major determinants of how children grow and progress. Because of the special bond and influence of the family on the child, there can be no separation of child from family in the health care setting. For example, to diminish anxiety in a child, nurses sometimes attempt to reduce parental anxiety, which may then reduce the stress on the child. Nursing care of children involves nursing care of the whole family and requires skill in dealing with both adults and children.

> Nurses might reduce parental anxiety about an ill child by saying, "Your child is in the best place possible here at the hospital. You brought him in at just the right time so that we can help him."

Family structures are in a constant state of change, and these dynamic states influence how children develop. Within the family, relationships change because of marriage, birth, divorce, death, and new roles and responsibilities. Societal forces outside the family, such as economics, population shifts, and migration, change how children are raised. These forces cause changes in family structures and the outcomes of child rearing, which must be considered when planning nursing care for children. The family is discussed in Chapter 2.

Parental Attitudes. Parental attitudes affect growth and development. Growth and development continue throughout life, and parents have stage-related needs and tasks that affect their children. Superimposed on these developmental issues are other factors influencing parental attitudes: educational level, childhood experiences, financial pressures, marital status, and available support systems. Parental attitudes are also affected by the child's temperament, the child's unique way of relating to the world. Different temperaments affect parenting practices and whether a child's unique personality traits develop into assets or problems.

Child-Rearing Philosophies. Child-rearing philosophies, shaped by myriad life events, have an effect on how children grow and develop. For example, well-educated, well-read parents often provide their children with extra stimulation and opportunities for learning beginning at a young age. This enrichment includes extra parental attention and interaction—not necessarily expensive toys. Generally, development progresses best when enriched opportunities for learning are provided.

Other parents may not recognize the need to provide a rich learning environment at home, may not have time, or may not value this type of parenting. Children of these parents may not progress at the same rate as those raised in a more enriching atmosphere.

A significant point for parents to remember is that children must be ready to learn. If motor and neurologic structures are not mature, no amount of added stimulation will produce new behavior. The result of an overzealous approach toward accomplishing a specific task is frustration for both child and parent. For example, a child who is 6 months old will not be able to walk alone no matter how much time and effort the parent expends. However, at 12 to 14 months, a child usually is ready to begin walking and will do so with ease if given opportunities to practice.

THEORIES OF GROWTH AND DEVELOPMENT

Many theorists have attempted to organize and classify the complex phenomena of growth and development. No single theory can adequately explain the wondrous journey from infancy to adulthood. However, each theorist contributes a piece of the puzzle. Theories are not facts but merely attempts to explain human behavior. Table 4-1 compares and contrasts theories discussed in the text. The chapters on each age group provide further discussion of these theories.

Piaget's Theory of Cognitive Development

Jean Piaget (1896-1980), a Swiss theorist, made major contributions to the study of how children learn. His complex theory provides a framework for understanding how thinking during childhood progresses and differs from adult thinking. Like other developmental theorists, Piaget postulated that, as children develop intellectually, they pass through progressive stages (Piaget, 1962, 1967). The ages assigned to these periods are only averages.

During the *sensorimotor* period of development, infant thinking seems to involve the entire body. Reflexive behavior is gradually replaced by more complex activities. The world becomes increasingly solid through the development of the concept of *object permanence*, which is the awareness that objects continue to exist even when they disappear from sight. By the end of this stage, the infant shows some evidence of reasoning.

During the *period of preoperational thought*, language becomes increasingly useful. Judgments are dominated by perception and are illogical, and thinking is characterized, especially during the early part of this stage, by egocentrism. In other words, children are unable to think about another

TABLE 4-1 Theories of Growth and Development				
	Piaget's Periods of Cognitive Development	**Freud's Stages of Psychosexual Development**	**Erikson's Stages of Psychosocial Development**	**Kohlberg's Stages of Moral Development**
Infancy	**Period 1 (birth-2 yr): Sensorimotor Period** Reflexive behavior is used to adapt to the environment; egocentric view of the world; development of object permanence.	**Oral Stage** Mouth is a sensory organ; infant takes in and explores during oral passive substage (first half of infancy); infant strikes out with teeth during oral aggressive substage (latter half of infancy).	**Trust vs. Mistrust** Development of a sense that the self is good and the world is good when consistent, predictable, reliable care is received; characterized by hope.	**Premorality or Preconventional Morality, Stage 0 (0-2 yr): Naivete and Egocentrism** No moral sensitivity; decisions are made on the basis of what pleases the child; infants like or love what helps them and dislike what hurts them; no awareness of the effect of their actions on others. "Good is what I like and want."
Toddlerhood	**Period 2 (2-7 yr): Preoperational Thought** Thinking remains egocentric, becomes magical, and is dominated by perception.	**Anal Stage** Major focus of sexual interest is anus; control of body functions is major feature.	**Autonomy vs. Shame and Doubt** Development of sense of control over the self and body functions; exerts self; characterized by will.	**Premorality or Preconventional Morality, Stage 1 (2-3 yr): Punishment-Obedience Orientation** Right or wrong is determined by physical consequences: "If I get caught and punished for doing it, it is wrong. If I am not caught or punished, then it must be right."
Preschool Age		**Phallic or Oedipal/ Electra Stage** Genitals become focus of sexual curiosity; superego (conscience) develops; feelings of guilt emerge.	**Initiative vs. Guilt** Development of a can-do attitude about the self; behavior becomes goal-directed, competitive, and imaginative; initiation into gender role; characterized by purpose.	**Premorality or Preconventional Morality, Stage 2 (4-7 yr): Instrumental Hedonism and Concrete Reciprocity** Child conforms to rules out of self-interest: "I'll do this for you if you do this for me"; behavior is guided by an "eye for an eye" orientation. "If you do something bad to me, then it's OK if I do something bad to you."
School Age	**Period 3 (7-11 yr): Concrete Operations** Thinking becomes more systematic and logical, but concrete objects and activities are needed.	**Latency Stage** Sexual feelings are firmly repressed by the superego; period of relative calm.	**Industry vs. Inferiority** Mastering of useful skills and tools of the culture; learning how to play and work with peers; characterized by competence.	**Morality of Conventional Role Conformity, Stage 3 (7-10 yr): Good-Boy or Good-Girl Orientation** Morality is based on avoiding disapproval or disturbing the conscience; child is becoming socially sensitive. Kohlberg's Stages of Moral Development
				Morality of Conventional Role Conformity, Stage 4 (begins at about 10-12 yr): Law and Order Orientation Right takes on a religious or metaphysical quality. Child

TABLE 4-1	Theories of Growth and Development—cont'd			
	Piaget's Periods of Cognitive Development	**Freud's Stages of Psychosexual Development**	**Erikson's Stages of Psychosocial Development**	**Kohlberg's Stages of Moral Development**
School Age—cont'd				wants to show respect for authority, and maintain social order; obeys rules for their own sake.
Adolescence	**Period 4 (11 yr-Adulthood): Formal Operations** New ideas can be created; situations can be analyzed; use of abstract and futuristic thinking; understands logical consequences of behavior.	**Puberty or Genital Stage** Stimulated by increasing hormone levels; sexual energy wells up in full force, resulting in personal and family turmoil.	**Identity vs. Role Confusion** Begins to develop a sense of "I"; this process is lifelong; peers become of paramount importance; child gains independence from parents; characterized by faith in self.	**Morality of Self-Accepted Moral Principles, Stage 5: Social Contract Orientation** Right is determined by what is best for the majority; exceptions to rules can be made if a person's welfare is violated; the end no longer justifies the means; laws are for mutual good and mutual cooperation.
Adulthood			**Intimacy vs. Isolation** Development of the ability to lose the self in genuine mutuality with another; characterized by love.	
			Generativity vs. Stagnation Production of ideas and materials through work; creation of children; characterized by care.	**Morality of Self-Accepted Moral Principles, Stage 6: Personal Principle Orientation** Achieved only by the morally mature individual; few people reach this level; these people do what they think is right, regardless of others' opinions, legal sanctions, or personal sacrifice; actions are guided by internal standards; integrity is of utmost importance; may be willing to die for their beliefs.
			Ego Integrity vs. Despair Realization that there is order and purpose to life; characterized by wisdom.	**Morality of Self-Accepted Moral Principles, Stage 7: Universal Principle Orientation** This stage is achieved by only a rare few; Mother Teresa, Gandhi, and Socrates are examples; these individuals transcend the teachings of organized religion and perceive themselves as part of the cosmic order, understand the reason for their existence, and live for their beliefs.

person's viewpoint and believe that everyone perceives situations as they do. *Magical thinking* (the belief that events occur because of wishing) and *animism* (the perception that all objects have life and feeling) characterize this period.

At the end of the preoperational stage, the child shifts from egocentric thinking and begins to be able to look at the world from another person's view. This shifting enables the child to move into the *period of concrete operations*, where the child is no longer bound by perceptions and can distinguish fact from fantasy. The concept of time becomes increasingly clear during this stage, although far past and far future events remain obscure. Although reasoning powers increase rapidly during this stage, the child cannot deal with abstractions or with socialized thinking.

Normally, adolescents progress to the *period of formal operations*. In this period the adolescent proceeds from concrete to abstract and symbolic and from self-centered to other centered. Adolescents can develop hypotheses and then systematically deduce the best strategies for solving a particular problem because they use a formal operations cognitive style (Culbertson, Newman, & Willis, 2003).

Nursing Implications of Piaget's Theory

Although other developmental theorists have disputed Piaget's theories, especially the ages at which cognitive changes occur, his work provides a basis for learning about and understanding cognitive development. Piaget's theory is especially significant to nurses as they develop teaching plans of care for children. Piaget believed that learning should be geared to the child's level of understanding and that the child should be an active participant in the learning process. For health teaching to be effective, nurses must understand the different cognitive abilities of children at various ages. Nurses also must know how to engage children in the learning process with developmentally appropriate activities. Because illness and hospitalization are often frightening to children, especially toddlers and preschoolers, nurses must understand the cognitive basis of fears related to treatment and be able to intervene appropriately (see Chapter 11).

Freud's Theory of Psychosexual Development

Sigmund Freud (1856-1939) developed theories to explain psychosexual development. His theories were in vogue for many years and provided a basis for other theories. Freud postulated that early childhood experiences provide unconscious motivation for actions later in life (Freud, 1960). According to Freudian theory, certain parts of the body assume psychologic significance as foci of sexual energy. These areas shift from one part of the body to another as the child moves through different stages of development. Freud's work may help to explain normal behavior that parents may confuse with abnormal behavior, and it also may provide a good foundation for sex education.

Freud believed that during infancy sexual behavior seems to focus around the mouth, the most erogenous area of the infant body (oral stage). Infants derive pleasure from sucking and exploring objects by placing them in their mouths.

During early childhood, when toilet training becomes a major developmental task, sensations seem to shift away from the mouth and toward the anus (anal stage). Psychoanalysts see this period as a time of holding on and letting go. A sense of control or autonomy develops as the child masters body functions.

During the preschool years, interest in the genitalia begins (phallic stage). Children are curious about anatomic differences, childbirth, and sexuality. Children at this age often ask many questions, freely exhibit their own sexual organs, and want to peek at those of others. Children often masturbate, sometimes causing parents great concern. Although it is not universal, a phenomenon described by Freud as the Oedipus complex in boys and the Electra complex in girls is seen in preschool children. This possessiveness of the child for the opposite-sex parent, marked by aggressiveness toward the same-sex parent, is considered normal behavior, as is a heightened interest in sex. To resolve these disturbing sexual feelings, the preschooler identifies with or becomes more like the same-sex parent. The superego (an inner voice that reprimands and evokes guilt) also develops. The superego is similar to a conscience (Freud, 1960).

Freud describes the school-age period as the latency stage, when sexuality plays a less prominent role in the everyday life of the child. Best friends and same-sex peer groups are influential in the school-age child's life. Younger school-age children often refuse to play with children of the opposite sex, whereas prepubertal children begin to desire the companionship of opposite-sex friends.

During adolescence, interest in sex again flourishes as children search for identity (genital stage). Under the influence of fluctuating hormone levels, dramatic physical changes, and shifting social relationships, the adolescent develops a more adult view of sexuality. Adolescents' cognitive skills are not fully developed, however, and they often make questionable judgments about sexual matters and may have questions and concerns about their behavior and feelings (A. Freud, 1974; Litt & Martin, 1999).

Nursing Implications of Freud's Theory

Both children and parents may have questions and concerns about normal sexual development and sex education. Nurses must understand normal sexual growth and development to help parents and children form healthy attitudes about sex.

Erikson's Psychosocial Theory

Erik H. Erikson (1902-1994), inspired by the work of Sigmund Freud, proposed a popular theory about child development. He viewed development as a lifelong series of conflicts affected by social and cultural factors. Each conflict must be resolved for the child and adult to progress emotionally. How individuals address the conflicts varies widely. According to Erikson, however, unsuccessful resolution leaves the individual emotionally disabled (Erikson, 1963).

Each of eight stages of development has a specific central conflict or developmental task. These eight tasks are described in terms of a positive or negative resolution.

The actual resolution of a specific conflict lies somewhere along a continuum between a perfect positive and a perfect negative.

The first developmental task is the establishment of trust. The basic quality of trust provides a foundation for the personality. If an infant's physical and emotional needs are met in a timely manner through warm and nurturing interactions with a consistent caregiver, the infant begins to sense that the world is trustworthy. The infant begins to develop trust in others and a sense of being worthy of love. Through successful achievement of a sense of trust, the infant can move on to subsequent developmental stages.

According to Erikson, unsuccessful resolution of this first developmental task results in a sense of mistrust. If needs are consistently unmet, acute tension begins to appear in children. During infancy, signs of unmet needs include restlessness, fretfulness, whining, crying, clinging, physical tenseness, and physical dysfunctions such as vomiting, diarrhea, and sleep disturbances. All children exhibit these signs at times. If these behaviors become personality characteristics, however, unsuccessful resolution of this stage is suspected.

The toddler's developmental task is to acquire a sense of autonomy rather than a sense of shame and doubt. A positive resolution of this task is accomplished by the ability to control the body and body functions, especially elimination. Success at this stage does not mean that the toddler, even as an adult, will exhibit autonomous behavior in all life situations. In certain circumstances, feelings of shame and self-doubt are normal and may be adaptive.

Erikson's theory describes each developmental stage, with crises related to individual stages emerging at specific times and in a particular order. Likewise, each stage is built on the resolution of previous developmental tasks. During each conflict, however, the child spends some energy and time resolving earlier conflicts (Erikson, 1963).

Nursing Implications of Erikson's Theory

In stressful situations, such as hospitalization, children, even those with healthy personalities, evoke defense mechanisms that protect them against undue anxiety. *Regression*, a behavior used frequently by children, is a reactivation of behavior more appropriate to an earlier stage of development. This defense mechanism is illustrated by a 6-year-old boy who reverts to sucking his thumb and wetting his pants under increased stress, such as illness or the birth of a sibling. Nurses can educate parents about regression and encourage them to offer their children support, not ridicule. They can provide constructive suggestions for stress management and reassure parents that regression normally subsides as anxiety decreases.

Erikson's main contribution to the study of human development lies in his outline of a universal sequence of phases of psychosocial development. His work is especially relevant to nursing because it provides a theoretic basis for much of the emotional care that is given to children. The stages are further discussed in the chapters on each age group.

Kohlberg's Theory of Moral Development

Lawrence Kohlberg (1927-1987), a psychologist and philosopher, described a stage theory of moral development that closely parallels Piaget's stages of cognitive development. He discussed moral development as a complicated process involving the acceptance of the values and rules of society in a way that shapes behavior. This cognitive-developmental theory postulates that, although knowing what behaviors are right and wrong is important, it is much less important than understanding and appreciating why the behaviors should or should not be exhibited (Bear, Richards, & Gibbs, 1997; Kohlberg, 1964).

Guilt, an internal expression of self-criticism and a feeling of remorse, is an emotion closely tied to moral reasoning. Most children 12 years old or older react to misbehavior with guilt. Guilt helps them realize when their moral judgment fails.

Building on Piaget's work, Kohlberg studied boys and girls from middle- and lower-class families in the United States and other countries. He interviewed them by presenting scenarios with moral dilemmas and asking them to make a judgment. His focus was not on the answer but on the reasoning behind the judgment (Kohlberg, 1964). He then classified the responses into a series of levels and stages.

During the *Premorality* (preconventional morality) level, which has three substages (see Table 4-1), the child demonstrates acceptable behavior because of fear of punishment from a superior force, such as a parent. At this stage of cognitive and moral development, children cannot reason as mature members of society. They view the world in a selfish, egocentric way, with no real understanding of right or wrong. They view morality as external to themselves, and their behavior reflects what others tell them to do, rather than an internal drive to do what is right. In other words, they have an external locus of control. A child who thinks, "I will not steal money from my sister because my mother will spank me" illustrates premorality.

During the *Morality of Conventional Role Conformity* (conventional morality) level, which is primarily during the school age years, the child conforms to rules to please others. The child still has an external locus of control, but a concern for social order begins to emerge and replace the more egocentric thinking of the earlier stage. The child has an increased awareness of others' feelings. In the child's view, good behavior is that which those in authority will approve. If behavior is not acceptable, the child feels guilty.

Two stages, stage 3 and stage 4, characterize this level (see Table 4-1). This level of moral reasoning develops as the child shifts the focus of living from the family to peer groups and society as a whole. As the child's cognitive capacities increase, an internal sense of right and wrong emerges and the individual is said to have developed an internal locus of control. Along with this internal locus of control comes the ability to consider circumstances when judging behavior.

Level 3, *Morality of Self-Accepted Moral Principles* (postconventional morality) begins in adolescence, when abstract thinking abilities develop. The person focuses on individual rights and principles of conscience during this stage. There is an internal locus of control. Concern about what is best for all is uppermost, and persons step back from their own viewpoint to consider what rights and values must be upheld for the good of all. Some individuals never reach this point. Within this level is stage 5, in which conformity occurs because individuals have basic rights and society needs to be improved. The adolescent in this stage gives as well as takes and does not expect to get something without paying for it. In stage 6, conformity is based on universal principles of justice and occurs to avoid self-condemnation (Colby, Kohlberg, & Kauffman, 1987; Feldman, 1998; Kohlberg, 1964).

Only a few morally mature individuals achieve stage 6. These people, committed to a moral ideal, live and die for their principles.

Kohlberg believes that children proceed from one stage to the next in a sequence that does not vary, although some people may never reach the highest levels. Even though children are raised in different cultures and with different experiences, he believes that all children progress according to his description.

Nursing Implications of Kohlberg's Theory

To provide anticipatory guidance to parents about expectations and discipline of their children, nurses must be aware of how moral development progresses. Parents are often distraught because their young children apparently do not understand right and wrong. For example, a 6-year-old girl who takes money from her mother's purse does not show remorse or seem to recognize that stealing is wrong. In fact, she is more concerned about her punishment than about her misdeed. With an understanding of normal moral development, the nurse can reassure the concerned parents that the child is showing age-appropriate behavior.

THEORIES OF LANGUAGE DEVELOPMENT

Human language has a number of characteristics that are not shared with other species of animals that communicate with each other. Human language has meaning, provides a mechanism for thought, and permits tremendous creativity.

Because language is such a complex process and involves such a vast number of neuromuscular structures, brain growth and differentiation must reach a certain level of maturity before a child can speak. Language development, which closely parallels cognitive development, is discussed by most cognitive theorists as they explain the maturation of thinking abilities. The process of how language develops remains a mystery, however.

Passive, or receptive, language is the ability to understand the spoken word. Expressive language is the ability to produce meaningful vocalizations. In most people, the areas in the brain responsible for expressive language are close to motor centers in the left cerebral area that control muscle movement of the mouth, tongue, and hands. Humans use a variety of facial and hand movements as well as words to convey ideas.

Crying is the infant's first method of communication. These vocalizations quickly become distinct and individual and accurately convey such states as hunger, diaper discomfort, pain, loneliness, and boredom. Vowel sounds appear first, as early as 2 weeks of age, followed by consonants at approximately 5 months of age.

By age 2 years, children have a vocabulary of roughly 300 words and can construct simple sentences. By age 4 years, children have gained a sense of correct grammar and articulation, but several consonants, including "l" and "r," remain difficult to pronounce. For example, the sentence "The red and blue bird flew up to the tree" might be pronounced by the preschooler as "The wed and boo bud fwew up to the twee!"

The language of school-age children is less concrete and much more articulate than that of the preschooler. Between the ages of 5 and 10 years, children begin to understand the structure of language. By 12 years, the child has many of the cognitive and linguistic skills of adults (Kelly & Sally, 1999).

Infants learn much of their language from their parents. Children who are raised in homes where verbalization is encouraged and modeled tend to display advanced language skills. Also, in infancy, receptive ability (the understanding of language) is more developed than expressive skill (the actual articulation of words). This tendency, which persists throughout life, is important to realize when caring for children. In clinical situations, nurses must communicate what is happening to their young clients by use of simple, age-appropriate words, although the child may not verbalize understanding. Language development is discussed in more depth in chapters on each age group.

INFLUENCES OF HEREDITY ON GROWTH AND DEVELOPMENT

Heredity, the transmission of genetic characteristics from parent to offspring, is one of the most significant determinants of growth and development. Because all humans are products of the biologic composition of their parents, heredity must be considered when a child's growth and developmental patterns are assessed and when children with inherited diseases are cared for. Genetic disorders are common and have a significant effect on the growth and development of children. Because genetic diseases are complex and permanent, children, families, and entire communities are affected.

Nurses need a working knowledge of how common genetic traits are transmitted, how common chromosomal abnormalities occur, and what effects these resulting conditions have on children and families. Alert and skilled nurses can provide early assessment, identification, and referral to appropriate professionals for evaluation and counseling.

A significant nursing role is offering families support in coping with genetic abnormalities. Nurses can act as child and family advocates, helping them maneuver through the complexities of the health care system. Finally, nurses are in an excellent position to educate families and communities about the causes of birth defects and the prevention of environmentally induced disorders.

Genetics

Genetics is the study of how inherited characteristics, or traits, are transmitted and how genetic material, deoxyribonucleic acid (DNA), affects the physiology of cells. The transmission of traits from parents to their children is a complex process involving basic structures called *genes* and *chromosomes*.

Structure of Genes and Chromosomes

A review of the structure of genes and chromosomes aids in understanding how disorders occur. Chromosomes are composed of genes that in turn are composed of DNA (Fig. 4-2).

DNA

DNA is the basic building block of genes and chromosomes. It has three units: (1) a sugar (deoxyribose), (2) a phosphate group, and (3) one of four nitrogen bases (adenine, thymine, guanine, and cytosine).

DNA resembles a spiral ladder, with a sugar and a phosphate group forming each side of the ladder and a pair of nitrogen bases forming each rung. The four bases of the DNA molecule pair with one another in a fixed way, allowing accurate duplication of the DNA during each cell division.

- Adenine pairs with thymine.
- Guanine pairs with cytosine.

The sequence of base pairs within the DNA determines which amino acids are assembled to form a protein and the order in which they are assembled. Some of these proteins form the structure of body cells; others are enzymes that control metabolic processes within the cell. If the sequence of nitrogen bases in the DNA is incorrect or if some bases are missing or added, a defect in body structure or function may result.

Genes

A gene is a segment of DNA that directs the production of a specific product needed for body structure or function. Humans probably have between 30,000 and 40,000 genes, fewer than previous estimates, which ranged from 50,000 to 140,000 (Guyton & Hall, 2006; National Human Genome Research Institute, 2003/2005).

Genes that code for the same trait often have two or more alternate forms (alleles). Many alleles are normal, such as those that code for a person's blood type. Normal alleles that are common in the population, or polymorphisms, provide genetic variation and sometimes a biologic advantage. However, mutations often involve a change that harms function, such as those that cause the production of abnormal hemoglobin in sickle cell disease or that cause cells to grow in an uncontrolled way, causing cancer.

Genes are too small to be seen under a microscope, but many can be studied by tissue analysis:

- By measuring the products that the genes direct cells to produce, such as an enzyme or other substance
- By studying the gene's DNA directly
- By analyzing the gene's close association (linkage) with another gene that can be studied in one of the previous two ways.

Chromosomes

Genes are organized into 46 paired chromosomes in the nucleus of most somatic cells. Twenty-two chromosome pairs are autosomes, and the twenty-third pair makes up the sex chromosomes. Added or missing chromosomes or structurally abnormal chromosomes are usually harmful.

Mature gametes have half the chromosomes (23) of other body cells. One chromosome from each pair is distributed randomly in the gametes, allowing variation of genetic traits among people. When the ovum and sperm unite at conception, the total is restored to 46 paired chromosomes.

Cells for chromosomal analysis must have a nucleus and must be living. Chromosomes can be studied by using any of several types of cells: white blood cells, skin fibroblasts, bone marrow cells, and fetal cells from the chorionic villi (future placenta) or those suspended in amniotic fluid.

Unlike genes, chromosomes can be seen under the microscope, but only during division of live cells. Specimens must be obtained and preserved carefully to provide enough living cells for chromosomal analysis. Temperature extremes, clotting of blood, or adding improper preservatives can kill the cells and render them useless for analysis.

Chromosomes look jumbled when viewed under a microscope (Fig. 4-3). Photographing or using computer imaging allows the chromosomes to be displayed from largest to smallest pairs into a karyotype. The karyotype is then analyzed.

Transmission of Traits by Single Genes

Inherited characteristics are passed from parent to child by the genes in each chromosome. These traits are classified according to whether they are dominant (strong) or recessive (weak) and whether the gene is located on one of the autosome pairs or on the sex chromosomes. Both normal and abnormal hereditary characteristics are transmitted by these mechanisms.

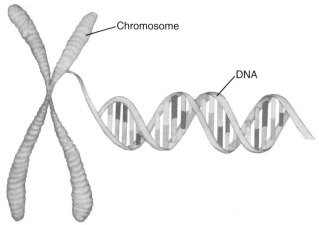

FIG 4-2 **Diagrammatic representation of the DNA helix, which is the building block of genes and chromosomes.**

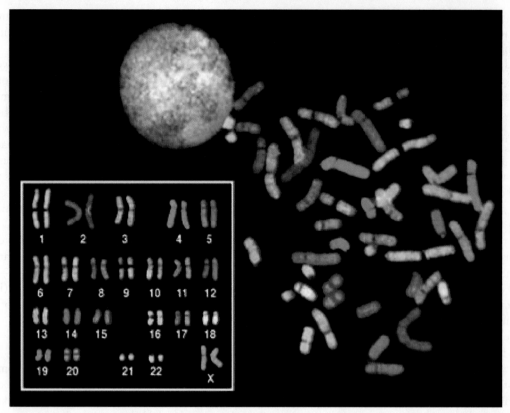

FIG 4-3   **When viewed before karyotyping, chromosomes appear jumbled. This photo is a spectral karyotype from a normal female.**   *(From National Human Genome Research Institute. [2002]. Retrieved October 22, 2005, from www.genome.gov/10000208.)*

Alleles

Because humans have a pair of matched chromosomes (except the sex chromosomes in the male), they have one allele for a gene at the same location on each member of the chromosome pair. The paired alleles may be identical (homozygous) or different (heterozygous).

Some alleles, both normal and abnormal, occur more frequently in certain groups than they do in the population as a whole. For example, the gene that causes Tay-Sachs disease is carried by about 1 of every 27 Ashkenazi Jews, whose families have their roots in Eastern Europe. Some non-Jewish French-Canadians and Cajun people from Louisiana also have a higher incidence of the disorder. However, an estimated 1 of every 250 people outside this group, including non-Ashkenazi Jews, carries the gene (National Tay-Sachs and Allied Diseases Association, Inc., 2003). Other disorders that are prevalent in certain ethnic groups are cystic fibrosis (primarily whites of northern European descent) and sickle cell disease (primarily people of African, Mediterranean, Indian, or Middle Eastern descent).

A new trait (harmful, neutral, or sometimes beneficial) may emerge because of a change in the gene within the gamete. The DNA in the gamete is then different from that in the person's somatic cells. The offspring who receives the new version of the gene will have it in all somatic cells and can transmit it to future generations.

Dominance

Dominance describes how a person's genetic composition is translated into the phenotype, or observable characteristics.

In the case of a dominant gene, one copy is enough to cause the trait to be expressed. For example, in the ABO blood system, genes for type A and type B are dominant. Therefore, a single copy of either of these genes is enough to be expressed in the person's blood type.

Two identical copies of a recessive gene are required for the trait to be expressed. The gene for blood group O is recessive. Only if a person receives a gene for blood group O from both parents will laboratory testing identify his or her blood group as O. If the person receives a gene for group O from one parent and a gene for group A from the other parent, group A will be expressed in laboratory blood typing.

Other alleles are equally dominant. The person who receives a gene for blood group A from one parent and group B from the other will have type AB blood because both alleles are equally dominant and both are expressed in blood typing.

Dominance and recessiveness are not absolute for all genes. Some people with a single copy of an abnormal recessive gene (carriers) may have a slightly abnormal level of the gene product (e.g., an enzyme) that can be detected by laboratory methods. These people usually do not have the disease because the normal copy of the gene directs production of enough of the required product to allow normal or near-normal function.

Chromosome Location

Genes located on autosomes are either autosomal dominant or autosomal recessive, depending on the number of identical copies of the gene needed to produce the trait. However, genes located on the X chromosome are paired only in females because males have one X and one Y chromosome.

A female with an abnormal recessive gene on one of her X chromosomes usually has a normal gene on the other X chromosome that compensates and maintains relatively normal function. However, the male is at a disadvantage if his only X chromosome has an abnormal gene. The male has no compensating normal gene because his other sex chromosome is a Y. The abnormal gene will be expressed in the male because it is unopposed by a normal gene.

Patterns of Single-Gene Inheritance

Three important patterns of single-gene inheritance are (1) autosomal dominant, (2) autosomal recessive, and (3) X-linked. Figure 4-4 summarizes characteristics and transmission of each pattern. Single-gene traits have mathematically predictable and fixed rates of occurrence. For example, if a couple has a child with an autosomal recessive disorder, the risk that future children from the same couple will have the disorder is 1:4 (25%) at every conception. The *risk* for the disorder is the same at every conception, regardless of how many of the couple's children are or are not affected.

Autosomal Dominant Traits

An autosomal dominant trait is produced by a dominant gene on a non-sex chromosome. The expression of abnormal autosomal dominant genes may result in multiple and seemingly unrelated effects in the person. The gene's effects may

Autosomal Dominant Inheritance Pattern

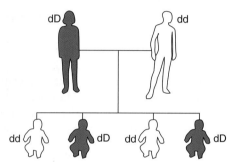

Each child has:
• 50% chance of having the disease
• 50% chance of being normal

No carrier state

No relationship to sex of the child

Example: Neurofibromatosis
Blood groups A and B

Key: d = normal gene; D = abnormal, *dominant* gene

Autosomal Recessive Inheritance Pattern

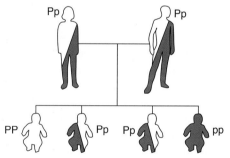

Each child has:
• 25% chance of having the disease
• 50% chance of being a carrier
• 25% chance of being normal

No relationship to sex of the child

Examples: Sickle cell disease
Cystic fibrosis

Key: P = normal gene; p = abnormal, *recessive* gene

X-Linked Recessive Inheritance Pattern

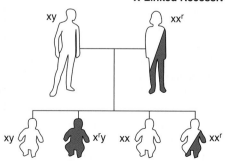

Each *female* child has:
• 50% chance of being a carrier
• 50% chance of being normal

Each *male* child has:
• 50% chance of having the disease
• 50% chance of being normal

Females do not usually have X-linked recessive disorders

Males are not usually carriers

Example: Hemophilia
Duchene muscular dystrophy

Key: xy = normal *male* sex chromosome pattern;
xx = normal *female* sex chromosome pattern;
r = sex-linked *recessive* gene

FIG 4-4 **Inheritance pattern and risk.**

CRITICAL TO REMEMBER
Single-Gene Abnormalities

- A person affected with an autosomal dominant disorder has a 50% risk of transmitting the disorder to each of his or her children.
- Two healthy parents who carry the same abnormal autosomal recessive gene have a 25% risk of having a child affected with the disorder caused by this gene.
- Parental consanguinity (blood relationship) increases the risk for having a child with an autosomal recessive disorder.
- One copy of an abnormal X-linked recessive gene is enough to produce the disorder in a boy.
- Abnormal genes can arise as new mutations that are then transmitted to future generations.

vary substantially in severity, leading a family to think that a trait skips a generation. A careful physical examination may reveal subtle evidence of the trait in each generation. Some people may carry the dominant gene but may have no apparent expression of it in their physical makeup.

In some autosomal dominant disorders, such as Huntington's disease, the person having the gene will always have the disease if he or she lives long enough. In other disorders, only a portion of those carrying the gene will ever exhibit the disease. New mutations often account for the introduction of autosomal dominant traits into a family that has no history of the disorder.

The person who is affected with an autosomal dominant disorder is usually heterozygous for the gene—that is, the person has a normal gene on one chromosome and an abnormal gene on the other chromosome of the pair, which overrides the influence of the normal gene. Occasionally, a person receives two copies of the same abnormal autosomal dominant gene. Such an individual is usually much more severely affected than someone with only one copy.

Autosomal Recessive Traits

An autosomal recessive trait occurs when a person receives two copies of a recessive gene carried on an autosome. Most people carry a few abnormal autosomal recessive genes without problems because a compensating normal gene produces enough of the gene's product for normal function. Because the probability that two unrelated people will share even one of the same abnormal genes is low, the incidence of autosomal recessive diseases is relatively low in the general population.

Situations that increase the likelihood that two parents will share the same abnormal autosomal recessive gene are as follows:

- Consanguinity (blood relationship of the parents)
- Membership in groups that are isolated by culture, geography, religion, or other factors

Many autosomal recessive disorders are severe, and affected persons may not live long enough to reproduce. Two exceptions are phenylketonuria and cystic fibrosis. Improved care of people with these disorders has allowed them to live into their reproductive years. If one member of a couple is affected by the autosomal recessive disorder, all their children will be carriers. Their risk for having similarly affected children is higher as well, depending on the prevalence of the abnormal gene in the general population.

X-Linked Traits

X-Linked Recessive Disorders. X-linked recessive traits are more common than X-linked dominant ones. Sex differences in the occurrence of X-linked recessive traits and the relationship of affected males to one another distinguish these disorders from autosomal dominant or recessive disorders. Males usually show the full effects of an X-linked recessive disorder because their only X chromosome has the abnormal gene on it. Females can show the full disorder in two uncommon circumstances:

- When a female has a single X chromosome (Turner syndrome, pp. 76-77)
- When a female child is born to an affected father and a carrier mother.

X-linked recessive disorders can be relatively mild, such as color blindness, or they may be severe, such as hemophilia. Also, those having the disorder may be affected with varying degrees of severity.

Chromosomal Abnormalities

Chromosomal abnormalities can be numerical or structural. They are quite common (50% or more) in the embryo or fetus that is spontaneously aborted. Chromosomal abnormalities often cause major defects because they involve many added or missing genes.

Numerical Abnormalities

Numerical chromosomal abnormalities are those involving added or missing single chromosomes and those with multiple sets of chromosomes. Trisomy and monosomy are numeric abnormalities of single chromosomes. *Polyploidy* describes abnormalities involving entire sets of chromosomes.

Trisomy. A trisomy exists when each body cell contains an extra copy of one chromosome, bringing the total number to 47. Each chromosome is normal, but there is an extra one in every cell. The most common trisomy is *Down syndrome*, or trisomy 21 (see Chapter 30). In Down syndrome, each body cell has three copies of chromosome 21. Trisomies of chromosomes 13 and 18 are less common and have more severe effects. The incidence of trisomies increases with maternal age, so most women who are 35 years old or older at conception are offered prenatal diagnosis to determine whether the fetus may have Down syndrome or another trisomy.

Monosomy. A monosomy occurs when each body cell has a missing chromosome, with a total number of 45. The only monosomy that is compatible with extended postnatal life is *Turner's syndrome,* or monosomy X. People with Turner's syndrome have a single X chromosome and they are female.

Live-born infants with Turner's syndrome have excess skin around the neck and edema that is most noticeable in the hands and feet. If Turner's syndrome is not identified and treated during infancy or childhood, an affected girl will remain very short and will not have menstrual periods nor will secondary sex characteristics develop. Heart and aortic defects are common. Severe defects are surgically repaired. Children with Turner's syndrome usually have normal intelligence, although they may have difficulty with spatial relationships or solving visual problems, such as reading a map.

Polyploidy. Polyploidy occurs when gametes do not halve their chromosome number during meiosis and retain both members of the pair or when two sperm fertilize an ovum simultaneously. The result is an embryo with one or more extra sets of chromosomes. The total number of chromosomes is a multiple of the haploid number of 23 (69 or 92 total chromosomes). Polyploidy usually results in an early spontaneous abortion but is occasionally seen in a live-born infant.

Structural Abnormalities

The structure of one or more chromosomes may be abnormal. Part of a chromosome may be missing or added, or DNA within the chromosome may be rearranged. Some of these rearrangements are harmless polymorphisms. Others are harmful, however, because important genetic material is lost or duplicated in the structural abnormality, or the position of the genes in relation to other genes is altered so that normal function is not possible.

Another structural abnormality occurs when all or part of a chromosome is attached to another (translocation). Many people with a translocation chromosomal abnormality are clinically normal because the total of their genetic material is normal, or balanced. If a parent has a balanced translocation, the offspring may have normal chromosomes or may have a balanced translocation like the parent. However, the offspring may receive too much or too little chromosomal material at conception and may be spontaneously aborted or may have birth defects. Either balanced or unbalanced chromosomal translocations may occur spontaneously in the child of parents who have no translocation.

Fragile X syndrome is a structural chromosome abnormality that often causes mental retardation among males. With this abnormality, a site on the X chromosome is more fragile than normal. Although females can also be affected with fragile X syndrome, males are more severely affected because the female has a second X chromosome that is usually normal. The fragile X syndrome is inherited in an X-linked dominant pattern, with males being most severely affected (Jorde, Carey, Bamshad, & White, 2003) (see Chapter 30).

Multifactorial Disorders

Multifactorial disorders result from an interaction of genetic and environmental factors. The genetic tendency toward the disorder is modified by the environment. These interactions may influence prenatal and postnatal development either positively or negatively. For example, two embryos may have an equal genetic susceptibility for the development of a disorder such as spina bifida (open spine) (see Chapter 28). However, the disorder will not occur unless an environment that favors its development, such as deficient maternal intake of folic acid, also exists.

Multifactorial disorders have two characteristics that distinguish them from other types of birth defects. They are typically (1) present and detectable at birth and (2) isolated defects rather than ones that occur with other unrelated abnormalities. A multifactorial defect may *cause* a secondary defect, however. For example, infants with spina bifida often have hydrocephalus because abnormal development of the spine and spinal cord disrupts spinal fluid circulation, allowing it to build up in the brain's ventricular system.

Multifactorial disorders represent some of the most common birth defects that a pediatric nurse encounters. Examples include many heart defects; neural tube defects, such as spina bifida; cleft lip and palate; and developmental dysplasia of the hip. Unlike single-gene traits, multifactorial disorders are not associated with a fixed risk of occurrence or recurrence in a family. The risks are an average rather than a constant

---

CRITICAL TO REMEMBER
Chromosomal Abnormalities

Numeric	Structural
Entire single chromosome added (trisomy)	Part of a chromosome missing or added
Entire single chromosome missing (monosomy)	Rearrangements of material within chromosome(s)
One or more added sets of chromosomes (polyploidy)	Two chromosomes that adhere to each other
	Fragility of a specific site on the X chromosome

CRITICAL TO REMEMBER
Multifactorial Birth Defects

- Multifactorial defects are some of the most common birth defects encountered in pediatric nursing practice. They result from interaction between genetic susceptibility and environmental factors during prenatal development.
- These are usually single, isolated defects, although the primary defect may cause secondary defects.
- Some occur more often in certain geographic areas.
- A greater risk for occurrence exists for any of the following:
  Several close relatives have the defect, whether mild or severe
  One close relative has a severe form of the defect
  The defect occurs in a child of the less frequently affected gender
- Infants who have several major or minor defects, or both, that are not directly related to each other, probably *do not* have a multifactorial defect but have another syndrome, such as a chromosomal abnormality.

percentage. Factors that may affect the degree of risk are number of affected close relatives, severity of the disorder in affected family members, sex of the affected child, geographic location, and seasonal variations.

Exposure to an Adverse Prenatal Environment

Avoiding exposure to harmful influences begins before conception because major organ systems develop early in pregnancy, often before a woman realizes that she is pregnant. Alcohol, substance, or cigarette use requires major lifestyle changes to avoid fetal or infant exposure. *Teratogens* are agents in the fetal environment that either cause or increase the likelihood that a birth defect will occur. Teratogens include certain medications, infectious agents, chemicals or pollutants, and ionizing radiation. Some maternal conditions, such as type I diabetes mellitus, can increase the risk of adverse effects on the fetus.

Genetic Counseling

Genetic counseling provides services to help people understand the disorder about which they are concerned and the risk that it will occur in their families. Genetic counseling is often available through facilities that provide maternal-fetal medicine services. State departments of mental health and mental retardation or rehabilitation services also may provide counseling services. Local chapters of the March of Dimes are an important source of information about birth defects and counseling sites. Fact sheets and other information about birth defects and their prevention are available on-line from the March of Dimes (www.modimes.org). Organizations that focus on specific birth defects provide valuable support and assistance in obtaining needed services for individuals and families affected by that disorder.

Focus on the Family

Genetic counseling focuses on the family rather than on an individual. One family member may have a birth defect, but study of the entire family is often needed for accurate counseling. This may involve obtaining medical records, including the mother's prenatal and perinatal history, or performing physical examinations or laboratory and other diagnostic studies on numerous family members. Examining photographs, particularly of deceased or unavailable family members, may be helpful, as would a genetic genogram. Counseling is impaired if family members are unwilling to provide their medical records or agree to examinations or laboratory studies. Moreover, those who seek counseling may be unwilling to request cooperation from other family members or to share the genetic information they acquire.

Genetic counseling is nondirective; that is, the counselor does not tell the individual or parents what decision to make but educates them about options for dealing with the disorder. Families often interpret the counseling subjectively, however. Some parents may regard a 50% risk of occurrence or recurrence as low, whereas others may think that a 1% risk is unacceptably high. The family's values and beliefs also influence whether they seek counseling and what they do with the information that is provided.

Process of Genetic Counseling

Genetic counseling is often a slow process that is not always straightforward. Several visits spread over months may be needed. In addition, some tests may be performed at only one or a few laboratories in the world, and several weeks may be needed to complete them. Despite a comprehensive evaluation, a diagnosis may never be established. An accurate diagnosis is crucial to provide families with the best information concerning what is known about the cause, the natural course of the disorder, options for caring for an affected child, the likelihood that the disorder will occur in others, the availability of treatment and services (including prenatal diagnosis for future pregnancies), and how to minimize future risk.

Comprehensive genetic counseling includes services of professionals from many disciplines, such as biology, medicine, nursing, social work, and education. These professionals provide added support for families; they may offer referral to parent support groups, grief counseling, and intervention for problems that accompany the birth of a child with a birth defect, such as socioeconomic or family dysfunction.

Nurses as Part of a Genetic Counseling Team

Nurses who participate on a genetic counseling team usually are educated in the specifics of genetic disorders and in specific counseling techniques. These nurses assist women or couples through the process of prenatal diagnosis, and support parents as they make decisions after receiving abnormal prenatal diagnostic results. They also help the family deal with the emotional impact of having a child with a birth defect and assist them to access needed services and support.

It is important for nurses to keep informed about advances in genetics and genetic counseling to provide accurate information to families. The Human Genome Project is an international effort begun in 1990 to identify all genes contained in the 46 human chromosomes. The full sequence of human genes was completed in April 2003 (National Human Genome Research Institute, 2003/2005). Information gained from this project may allow advances such as:

- Genetic testing to determine the risk for a disorder or the actual or probable presence of the disorder.
- Basing reproductive decisions on more accurate and specific information than has previously been available.
- Identifying genetic susceptibility to a disorder so that interventions to reduce risk can be instituted.
- Using gene therapy to modify a defective gene.
- Modifying therapy such as medication on the basis of an individual's genetic code or the genetic makeup of tumor cells.

The explosion of knowledge about the genetic basis for many diseases raises many legal and ethical issues for which we do not yet have answers. As our knowledge base grows, new issues are likely to emerge (National Human Genome Research Institute, 2003/2005):

- Genetic information has implications for others in the person's family, raising privacy issues.

- Identification of genetic problems could lead to poor self-esteem, guilt, and excessive caution, or, conversely, a reckless lifestyle.
- Presymptomatic identification of a genetically influenced illness could be a source of long-term anxiety.
- Genetic knowledge could affect one's choice of a partner.
- Discrimination may occur, such as the imposition of high insurance rates, the denial of insurance coverage, or an employer's decision not to hire a qualified person who has a greater chance of genetically influenced illness.

ASSESSMENT OF GROWTH

Because growth is an excellent indicator of physical well-being, accurate assessments must be made at regular intervals so that patterns of growth can be determined. Trained individuals using calibrated equipment and proper techniques should perform growth measurement. Methods of obtaining accurate measurements in children are described in Chapter 9. To minimize the chance of error, data should be collected on children under consistent conditions on a routine basis and values should be recorded and plotted on growth charts immediately.

Standardized growth charts allow an individual child's growth (height, weight, head circumference, body mass index [BMI]) to be compared with statistical norms. The most commonly used growth charts are those developed by the National Center for Health Statistics. Separate charts are available for boys and girls. One set of charts is used for children from birth to 36 months, and another set is used for children aged 2 years to 20 years (see Appendix B).

Because height and weight are the best indicators of growth, these parameters are measured, plotted on growth charts, and monitored over time at each well visit. Brain growth can also be monitored by measuring infant frontal-occipital circumference at intervals and plotting the values on growth charts. It is important to relate head size to weight because larger babies have bigger heads. These measurements are routinely performed during the first 2 years of life. Refer to Appendix A for recommendations for preventive health care.

BMI, which is a function of both height and weight, is an important measure of growth and overall nutritional status in children older than age 2 years. Child health professionals increasingly use the BMI when assessing growth (American Academy of Pediatrics [AAP] Committee on Nutrition, 2003), and BMI charts are included in the most recent versions of charts available from the National Center for Health Statistics.

Growth rate is measured in percentiles. The area between any two percentiles is referred to as a *growth channel*. Childhood growth normally progresses according to a pattern along a particular growth channel. Deviations from normal growth patterns may suggest problems. Any change of more than two growth channels indicates a need for more in-depth assessment.

Recognition of abnormal growth patterns is an important nursing function. The earlier that growth disorders are detected, diagnosed, and treated, the better the long-term prognosis.

ASSESSMENT OF DEVELOPMENT

Assessment of development is a more complex process than assessment of growth. To assess developmental progress accurately, nurses must gather data from many sources, including observations and interviews, physical examinations, interactions with the child and parents, and various standardized assessment tools. Refer to Appendix A for recommendations for preventive health care.

Observation is a valuable method most often used to obtain information about a child's developmental age (level of functioning). By watching a child during daily activities, such as eating, playing, toileting, and dressing, nurses gather a great deal of assessment data. Observation of the child's problem-solving abilities, communication patterns, interaction skills, and emotional responses can yield valuable information about the child's level of development. Similarly, interviews and physical examinations can provide much information about how the child functions.

In addition to these sources of data, many standardized assessment tools are available for nurses and other health care professionals to use for developmental assessment. Developmental assessment should be part of a newborn infant's assessment and of every well-child examination for several reasons. One reason is that parents want to know how their child compares with others and whether development is normal, especially if they had a difficult pregnancy or have developmentally delayed children. Developmental assessment tends to allay fears. Another reason is that abnormal development must be discovered early to facilitate optimal outcomes through early intervention.

Glascoe and Shapiro (2004) identified several pitfalls of screening:

- **Waiting until a problem is observable.** If the problem is obvious, refer the child immediately.
- **Ignoring screening results.** Good-quality screening is only 70% to 80% accurate and a wait-and-see attitude can delay valuable treatment.
- **Relying on informal methods.** Informal tools such as checklists often contain items sure to miss most children with problems.
- **Using a measure not suitable for primary care.** If a test is chosen that takes longer than the normal length of a well visit, it will only be used with children with observable problems (see above) or only key items on the test will be used. If the later is used, the screening tool becomes a checklist and losses its' validity.
- **Assuming Services are Limited or Nonexistent.** There are good services in every state, but health care providers must stay abreast of these resources. For information on programs, the National Early Childhood Technical Assistance Center has a website with contact information for every state and usually region for children 0 to 3 or 3 to 5 years (www.nectac.org). For children aged 5 years and older, a school psychologist in the child's school should be contacted. When parents have limited income, referrals may be made to Head Start, Early Head Start, or Migrant Worker Head Start.

Newborn Assessment

Two newborn screening tools are the Brazelton Neonatal Behavior Assessment Scale and the New Ballard Score. Refer to a maternity nursing text for more information related to these tools.

Prescreening Assessments

The AAP has issued a policy statement regarding developmental screening for all children, which emphasizes the importance of detecting early delays and referring for early intervention (AAP, 2001). Depending on the screening method used, developmental screening can take up to 30 minutes to administer—time not often available in a busy pediatric office or well clinic. Many providers have elected to do multilevel screening, first using a prescreening assessment tool and then administering (or referring for administration) a more comprehensive developmental assessment. Studies have suggested that parent concern is an important predictor of actual developmental delay in children (AAP, 2001; Glascoe, 2003; Glascoe & Shapiro, 2003). Some of the newer prescreening tools that are based on parent concerns, such as the Parents' Evaluation of Developmental Status and the Ages and Stages Questionnaires, have been found to be reliable and valid for detecting developmental delay (AAP, 2001; Glascoe & Shapiro, 2003). These screening tools are organized around major developmental areas (language, cognitive, social, behavioral, and motor). They are given to parents to complete in the office or clinic waiting room, take only 5 to 10 minutes to do, and are considered to be predictive for delay. The Prescreening Developmental Questionnaire is organized according to categories in the Denver Developmental Screening Test II (DDST-II). It is an objective measure of development and also is relatively easy and quick to administer (Frankenburg, 2002). Regardless of the screening method chosen, the AAP recommends periodic developmental screening for all young infants and children as part of well-child care (AAP, 2001). Despite the AAP policy related to improving developmental screening in the primary care setting, compliance in this area has been poor. Although many primary caregivers indicate that they assess children for developmental delays, they do not use an accompanying screening tool. The most common tool used is the Denver II (Sand et al., 2005).

Denver Developmental Screening Test II

The most widely used screening tool for infants and young children is the DDST-II (see the Evolve website). The DDST-II provides a clinical impression of a child's overall development and alerts the user to potential developmental difficulties.

The DDST-II, designed to be used with children between birth and 6 years of age, assesses development on the basis of performance of a series of age-appropriate tasks. There are 125 tasks or items arranged in four functional areas (Frankenburg & Dodds, 1992):

1. Personal-social (getting along with others, caring for personal needs)
2. Fine motor (eye-hand coordination, problem-solving skills)
3. Language (hearing, using, and understanding language)
4. Gross motor (sitting, jumping)

Items for rating the child's behavior are also included at the end of the test.

The test form is arranged with age scales across the top and bottom (see the Evolve website for a sample test form). After calculating the child's chronologic age (age in years), the test administrator draws an age line on the form. Each of the 125 tasks or items is arranged on a shaded bar depicting at which ages 25%, 50%, 75%, and 90% of the children in the research sample completed that particular item. The examiner assesses the child using the items clustered around the age line. The directions must be followed exactly during administration of the test. A score for performance on each item is recorded according to the following scale: pass (P), fail (F), no opportunity (NO), and refusal (R). At the completion of the test, the screener scores test behavior ratings (located at the bottom left of the form).

Interpretation of the test is based first on individual items and then on the test as a whole. Individual items are considered as "advanced, normal, caution, delayed, or no opportunity." Reliability and validity of the test can be altered if the child is not feeling well or is under the influence of medications. Parental presence and input as to whether the child is behaving as usual is desired (Frankenburg & Dodds, 1992).

The results of the test can be used to identify a child's developmental age and how a child compares with others of the same chronologic age. This information can be used to alert health care providers to potential problems. To ensure that the results are accurate, only individuals who are trained to administer the test in a standardized manner should perform testing. Training is obtained through study of the testing manual, review of the accompanying videotape, and supervised practice with children of various ages.

Although the DDST-II is widely used, it is a screening test only, not an intelligence quotient (IQ) test. It is not a definitive predictor of future abilities, and it should not be used to determine diagnostic labels. It is, however, a useful tool for noting problems, validating hunches, monitoring development, and providing referrals.

Implications for Nurses

To ensure the child's best performance, nurses must first establish rapport and create a comfortable screening environment. The test should be administered in a comfortably warm room with the child dressed but with restrictive clothing and shoes removed. Test materials should be located where the child can easily reach them. Only materials that are being used immediately for testing should be available to the child. All other materials should be out of sight. Young children may be held, but they should be able to rest their elbows on the testing table to manipulate objects.

Nurses should avoid making prejudgments about how a child will perform on the tests on the basis of the child's or the parents' physical appearance. It is important to avoid being

TeVonte ("T") is visiting the clinic for preventive health care shortly after his third birthday. The nurse will administer a DDST-II to evaluate his development in each of four areas: personal-social, fine motor-adaptive, language, and gross motor.

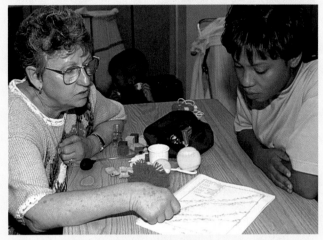

Before beginning T's DDST-II screening test, the nurse explains its purpose to his mother, Monifa Lee. The test assesses the child's performance of various age-appropriate tasks. The nurse emphasizes to the mother that the DDST-II is not an IQ test but rather compares her child's development with that of other children of the same age.

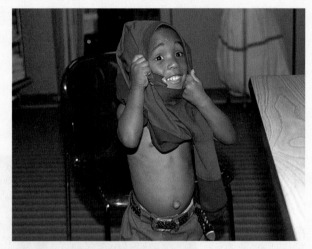

After verifying T's age, the nurse begins the test with personal-social items. After helping T remove his shirt, the nurse asks him to put it back on. T pulls the shirt over his head and then slips each arm into a sleeve.

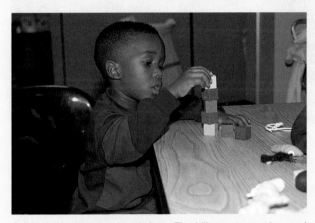

Colored cubes are used to evaluate T's ability to name colors and to build a tower. T is building a tower of eight blocks, which allows the tester to evaluate his fine motor-adaptive development.

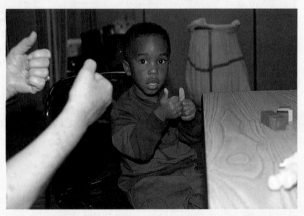

The nurse shows T how to wiggle his thumbs. T passes this part of the test because he keeps his fists closed and wiggles only his thumbs.

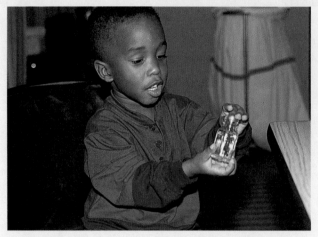

T plays with a raisin in a jar as part of the fine motor screening. The nurse observes to see whether T will pick up the raisin with his thumb and forefinger. T is really more interested in eating the raisin!

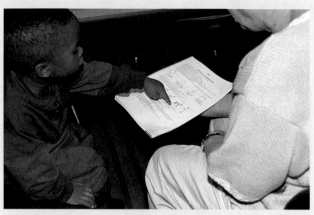

As she administers the DDST-II, the nurse evaluates T's speech, which is completely understandable, as it should be at his age. An additional part of the language test is to identify at least four of the pictures printed in the test manual. T correctly names the dog and other objects.

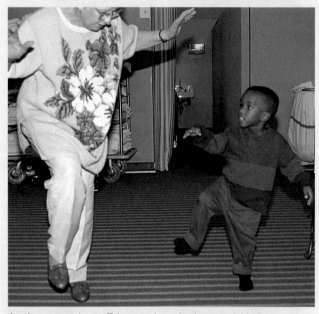

As the nurse shows T how to hop, he hops quickly in response. T's expression shows that he enjoys the gross motor part of the DDST-II.

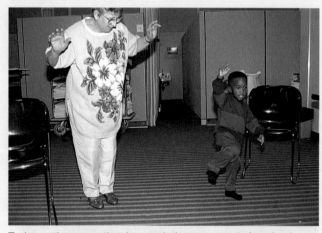

T shows the nurse that he can balance on each foot for 3 seconds. Note that he is effectively using his arms to help maintain his balance.

After completing the DDST-II, the nurse shares the results with T's mother. The screening indicates that T's development is appropriate for his age. The nurse recommends that TeVonte continue to have well-child screenings each year, including a DDST-II up to the age of 6 years.

misled by a child's charm, facial features, small or large size, handicap, or oddly shaped head. Children should be given every opportunity to perform to the best of their ability.

As the testing progresses, it is important to avoid causing unnecessary worry in parents. Doubts should not be expressed until the screener is certain that the child should be seen for further evaluation. The slightest suggestion of concern, which may be communicated by even a casual facial expression, can create unnecessary worry and diminished trust. The role of the nurse is to gather valid assessment data, determine deviations from normal, make appropriate referrals, and provide support. Diagnosing developmental delay is a function of other health care professionals.

At the completion of the DDST-II, the nurse should ask the parents whether the child acted in a normal and expected manner. If the parent responds negatively, the evaluation should be rescheduled. When explaining the results, emphasis should be placed on the items the child passed, those items the child failed but was not expected to pass, and finally those items the child failed and was expected to pass. Answer the parent's questions, and if indicated, refer for additional developmental testing.

NURSE'S ROLE IN PROMOTING OPTIMAL GROWTH AND DEVELOPMENT

Nurses are particularly concerned with preventing disease and promoting health. One aspect of preventive care is providing anticipatory guidance or basic information for parents about normal growth and development as their child approaches different age levels (see Appendix A).

Brazelton (1992) describes "touchpoints" as predictable times during which health care professionals can reach into a family system and, through supportive help, diminish or prevent problems. These points generally occur just before a growth or developmental spurt in which the child's behavior changes and the parents' normal modes of handling behavior do not work. During these periods the child becomes difficult to understand. The nurse can anticipate these predictable periods, which also provide a window of opportunity to offer information about normal growth and development and practical interventions to prevent problems characteristic of that age. Age-appropriate topics for anticipatory guidance are discussed in depth in the chapters on specific age groups

Developmental Assessment

Nursing care for children is not complete without addressing the developmental issues that are unique to each child. Because children grow and change rapidly, the nurse must use knowledge of theories of growth and development to create plans of care for both healthy and ill children. Assessment data are collected from a variety of sources, categorized, and analyzed with a theoretic knowledge base and clinical experience. A list of strengths and problems related to growth and development is generated. Nursing diagnoses are formulated with individualized goals, interventions, and evaluation to address specific problems that are related to, but differ from, physiologic and psychosocial needs.

Interview

During the initial interview, the nurse asks questions about the child's cognitive, language, motor, and emotional development. The parents' emotional state, level of education, and culture must be considered when information is gathered. The nurse might use the following questions and statements when interviewing the parents of a 4-year-old child:

- What does your child like to do at home?
- Does your child know the days of the week?
- Describe your child's typical day.
- Does your child attend preschool?
- Can your child throw a ball, ride a tricycle, climb?
- Can your child draw pictures, color them?
- How effective is your child's use of language?
- How did your child's development progress during infancy and toddlerhood?

The nurse also assesses the child's ability to think through situations and to communicate verbally. In addition, how the child interacts with other children and adults can be a measure of cognitive abilities. The number, type, length, appropriateness, and correct use of words and sentences are also noted. Careful observation of the child in a variety of situations, including play, provides valuable information about cognitive development.

A child's stage of emotional development can be assessed in a number of ways. From Erikson's theory, it is expected that the major conflict of a 4-year-old child would be developing a sense of initiative rather than a sense of guilt. If the child is hospitalized, however, regressive behaviors might be exhibited if the anxiety of hospitalization becomes overwhelming. Questions directed to the parents, such as those that follow, could help validate inferences about the child's psychosocial development:

- What types of play activities does your child like best?
- How does your child get along with other children? With adults?
- How does your child usually handle stressful situations?
- What do you do to help your child cope with problems?
- How does your child's ability to cope compare with that of your other children?
- Is the behavior exhibited your child's usual behavior?

The nurse can also obtain valuable information from careful observation of a child who is hospitalized. The nurse should note how the child deals with pain, intrusive procedures, and separation from parents.

Play

Although play is not work in the traditional sense, it is children's work. Play is those tasks, done to amuse oneself, that have behavioral, social, or psychomotor rewards. To adult observers, children's play may appear unorganized, meaningless, and even chaotic. Anyone who watches carefully, however, quickly discovers that play is a rich activity, intricately woven with meaning and purpose. In adulthood, work is any activity during which one uses time and energy to create a product or achieve a goal. Play in childhood is similar to adult work in that it is undertaken by the child to accomplish developmental tasks and master the environment.

Play is also an important part of the developmental process. Play is how children learn about shape, color, cause and effect, and themselves. In addition to cognitive thinking, play helps the child learn social interaction and psychomotor skills. It is a way of communicating joy, fear, sorrow, and anxiety.

Classifications of Play
Piaget (1962) described the following three types of play that relate to periods of sensorimotor, preoperational, and concrete operational functioning. These three types of play are overlapping and are linked to stages of cognitive development.

Sensorimotor, which is also known as *functional* or *practice play*, involves repetitive muscle movements and the introduction of a deliberate complication into the way of doing something. In this type of play the infant plays with objects, making use of their properties (falling, making noises) to produce pleasurable effects (Pellegrini & Smith, 2005).

Symbolic play, as its name suggests, uses games and interactions that represent an issue or concern to be addressed. Garvey (1979) identified three elements of symbolic play: one or more objects, a theme or plan, and roles. As children play, they incorporate some object (a toy syringe), use a theme (getting an injection), and then play the roles each player will have (child, nurse). Because there are no rules in symbolic play, the child can use this play not only to reinforce or learn the good things in life but also to alter those things that are painful.

Games include rules and usually are played by more than one person, although some games can be played by oneself. For example, the card game solitaire is played by one person, as are many video games. Games with rules rarely occur before age 4 years and are most common with the school-age child (Piaget, 1962). Games continue throughout life as adults play board games, cards, and sports.

Through games, children learn to play by the rules and to take turns. One common way children accomplish this is through board games. Young children often make up games with unique sets of rules, which may change each time the game is played. Older children have games with specific rules; younger children tend to change the rules.

Social Aspects of Play
As the child develops, more interaction with people occurs. Certain types of play are associated with, but not limited to, specific age groups.

Solitary Play. Solitary play is characterized by independent play (Fig. 4-5). The child plays alone with toys that are very different from those chosen by other children in the area. This type of play begins in infancy and is common in toddlers because of their limited social, cognitive, and physical skills. It is important for children in all age groups, however, to have some time to play by themselves.

Parallel Play. Parallel play is usually associated with toddlers, although it can be found in any age group. Children play side by side with similar toys, but there is a lack of interactive activity.

Associative Play. Associative play is characterized by group play without group goals. Children in this type of play do not set group rules, and although they may all be playing with the same types of toys and may even trade toys, there is a lack of formal organization. This type of play can begin during toddlerhood and continue into the preschool age.

Cooperative Play. Cooperative play begins in the late preschool years. This type of play is organized and has group goals. There is usually at least one leader, and children are definitely in or out of the group.

Onlooker Play. Onlooker play is present when the child observes others playing. Although the child may ask questions of the players, the child does not attempt to join the play (see Fig. 4-5). Onlooker play is usually during the toddler years but can be observed at any age.

Types of Play
Dramatic Play. Dramatic play allows children to act out roles and experiences that may have happened to them, that they fear will happen, or that they have observed in others. This type of play can be spontaneous or guided, and it often includes medical or nursing equipment. It is especially valuable for children who have had or will have multiple procedures or hospitalizations.

Hospitals and clinics with child life specialists on staff usually have a medical play area as part of the activity room. Nurses may provide opportunities for spontaneous and guided dramatic play. The nurse may choose to observe spontaneous play or be an active participant with the child. Occasionally nurses will want to structure the dramatic play to review a specific treatment or procedure. In guided play situations, the nurse directs the focus of the play. Specialized play kits may be developed for specific procedures, such as central line care, casting, bone marrow aspirations, lumbar punctures, and surgery, using supplies related to the hospital or clinic setting.

Familiarization Play. Familiarization play allows children to handle and explore health care materials in nonthreatening and fun ways (see Fig. 4-5). This type of play is especially helpful for but not limited to preparing children for procedures and the whole experience of hospitalization.

Examples of familiarization activities include using sponge mouth swabs as painting and gluing tools; making jewelry from bandages, tape, gauze, and lid tops; creating mobiles and collages with health care supplies; making finger puppets with plaster casting material; filling a basin with water and using tubing, syringes, medicine cups, and bulb syringes for water play; decorating beds, wheelchairs, and intravenous poles with health care supplies; and using syringes for painting activities.

Functions of Play
Play enhances the child's growth and development. Play contributes to physical, cognitive, emotional, and social development.

Physical Development and Play

Play aids in the development of both fine and gross motor activity. Children repeat certain body movements purely for pleasure, and these movements in turn aid in the development of body control. For example, an infant will first hit at a rattle, then will attempt to grasp it, and eventually will be able to pick up that same rattle. Next the infant will shake the rattle or perhaps bring it to the mouth.

The parent and child may make a game of repeating sounds such as "ma ma" or "da da," which increases the child's language ability. Repeating rhymes and songs can be a fun way for children to increase their vocabulary. Children love to color on a paper with a crayon and will scribble before being able to draw pictures and to color. This assists the child with eventually learning how to write letters and numerals.

Cognitive Development. Play is a key element in the cognitive development of children. Once a child has learned a general concept, further experiences with that concept expand from that beginning knowledge. Piaget gave the example of an infant learning to swing an object and then subsequently swinging other objects (Piaget, 1962). This could apply, for example, to things to be eaten, read, or ridden. Progression takes place as the child begins to have certain experiences, test beliefs, and understand the surrounding world.

Children can increase their problem-solving abilities through games and puzzles. Pretend play can stimulate several types of learning. Language abilities are strengthened as the child models significant others in role playing. The child must organize thoughts and be able to communicate with others involved in the play scenario. Children who play "house" create elaborate details of what the characters do and say.

Children also increase their understanding of size, shape, and texture through play. They begin to understand relationships as they attempt to put a square peg into a round hole, for example. Books and videos increase a child's vocabulary while increasing understanding of the world.

Emotional Development. Children in an anxiety-producing situation are often helped by role playing. Play can be a

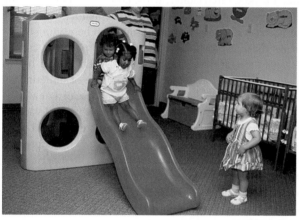

The little girl at right demonstrates onlooker play. She is interested in what is going on and observes another girl playing on the slide, but she makes no attempt to join the youngster on the slide.

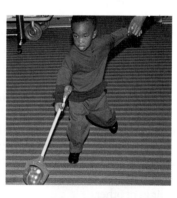

When engaging in solitary play, the child is playing apart from other children and with different types of toys. *(Courtesy University of Texas at Arlington School of Nursing.)*

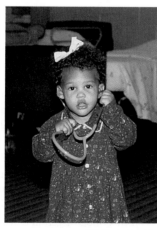

Playing safely with medical equipment (familiarization play) lessens its unfamiliarity to the child and can allay fears. A less fearful child is likely to be more cooperative and less traumatized by necessary care. *(Courtesy University of Texas at Arlington School of Nursing.)*

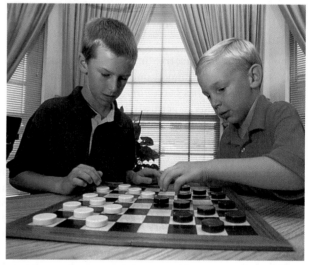

Games with rules, such as board games, help children learn boundaries, teamwork, taking turns, and competition. *(Courtesy Cook Children's Medical Center, Fort Worth, TX.)*

FIG 4-5 **Types of Play.**

way of coping with emotional conflict. Play can be a way to determine what is real and what is not. Children may escape through play into a world of fantasy and make-believe to make sense out of a sometimes senseless world. Play can also increase a child's self-awareness as an event or situation is explored through role playing or symbolic play.

As significant others in children's lives respond to their initiation of play, children begin to learn that they are important and cared for. Whether the child initiates the play or the adult does, when a significant person plays a board game with a child, shares a bike ride, plays baseball, or reads a story, the child gets the message, "You are more important than anything else at this time." This increases the child's self-esteem.

Social Development. The newborn infant cannot distinguish self from others and therefore is narcissistic. As the infant begins to play with others and things, a realization of self and others begins to develop. The infant begins to experience the joy of interacting with others and soon initiates behavior that involves others. Infants discover that when they coo, their mothers coo back. Children will soon expect this response and make a game of playing with their mothers.

Playing make-believe allows the child to try on different roles. When children play "restaurant" or "hospital," they experiment with rules that govern these settings.

Of course, most games, from board games to sports, involve interaction with others. The child learns boundaries, taking turns, teamwork, and competition. Children also learn how to negotiate with different personalities and the feelings associated with winning and losing. They learn to share and to take turns (see Fig. 4-5).

Moral Development. When children engage in play with their peers and their families, they begin to learn which behaviors are acceptable and which are not. Quickly they learn that taking turns is rewarded and cheating is not. Group play assists the child in recognizing the importance of teamwork, sharing, and being aware of the feelings of others.

HEALTH PROMOTION
Immunizations

Immunizations are effective in decreasing and, in some cases, eliminating childhood infectious diseases. Naturally occurring smallpox has been virtually eliminated, and the incidence of diphtheria, pertussis, tetanus, measles, mumps, rubella, and poliomyelitis has greatly declined in the United States. The incidence of diseases caused by *Haemophilus influenzae* type b (Hib) has been reduced by more than 95% since it was introduced to children in 1987 and infants in 1990. This pathogen was responsible for serious bacterial infections in infants and children with more than one half of Hib cases presenting as meningitis. In developing countries, Hib is still a leading cause of bacterial pneumonia deaths in children (Centers for Disease Control and Prevention [CDC], 2003). In 2000, the AAP issued a policy regarding the administration of pneumococcal conjugate vaccine to prevent pneumococcal infections in children younger than 2 years (AAP, 2000). Immunization since 2000 has

substantially reduced the number of cases of severe disease caused by the bacteria *Streptococcus pneumoniae*. Because the vaccine prevents spread of the bacteria between individuals, serious disease was less common even in people who were not targeted for vaccination (CDC, 2005a)

The threat of bioterrorism has generated interest in reintroducing smallpox vaccine. In 2002 the AAP issued a policy statement regarding routine administration of smallpox vaccine to children (AAP, 2002). Because children have a higher risk for adverse effects from the existing smallpox vaccine, the AAP supports the CDC recommendation for "ring" vaccination. This includes isolation of infected individuals and vaccinating contacts and contacts of contacts to contain the spread of disease (AAP, 2002).

The rubella virus, a major cause of birth defects, is no longer considered to be a major public health threat in the United States. Approximately 93% of the nation's children under age 2 years are vaccinated against measles, mumps, and rubella and more than 95% of the nation's children are vaccinated against rubella by the time they enter school (CDC, 2005c).

Pertussis (whooping cough) has been increasing in incidence in the United States, with most new cases occurring among adolescents (AAP, 2005a). The major contributing factor to this phenomenon is presumed to be waning of immunity during midadolescence. Because pertussis can be a serious problem resulting in school absences and health consequences, including possible exposure of underimmunized infants, the AAP recommends one dose of a new combined diphtheria-tetanus-acellular pertussis (Tdap) vaccine for children. The dose would be administered to 11- and 12-year-old children, so long as they have had the primary diphtheria-tetanus-acellular pertussis (DTaP) series and have not previously received the tetanus-diphtheria (Td) booster, and to older adolescents who have not received the Td booster or 5 years has elapsed since their last Td booster (AAP, 2005a).

Hepatitis A vaccine is recommended for all children at age 1 year (12-23 months). The 2 doses in the series should be administered at least 6 months apart. Children who are not vaccinated by age 2 years can be vaccinated at subsequent visits (CDC, 2006d).

Influenza vaccine is recommended annually for all healthy children age 6 months to 59 months and for older children who have conditions that can compromise respiratory function, or necessitate handling of respiratory secretions, or that increase the risk for aspiration. Household contacts of children in these groups, including siblings and caregivers, should also receive the vaccine. If not given previously, any child younger than 9 years needs to receive two doses initially, each dose being 1 month apart (AAP, 2004; AAP, 2006; CDC, 2006c).

Meningococcal conjugate vaccine (MCV4), should be administered to all children at age 11-12 years as well as to unvaccinated adolescents at high school entry (15 years). All college freshmen living in dormitories should also be vaccinated (AAP, 2006).

The U.S. Food and Drug Administration has licensed a rotavirus vaccine for use among infants. The Advisory Committee on Immunization Practices (ACIP) is recommending that all infants be immunized with 3 doses of the vaccine at 2, 4, and 6 months of age.

Obstacles to Immunizations

Major reasons identified for low immunization rates during health care visits are presented in Box 4-3. In the 1980s the safety of the pertussis portion of the diphtheria-tetanus-pertussis vaccine was questioned. Some parents elected not to immunize their children, which resulted in an increase in pertussis cases. Medical concern has led to the use in the United States of the acellular pertussis vaccine, which has fewer side effects.

The media play an important part in the immunization status of children. News programs that highlight the side effects of vaccines, rather than their individual and collective protective effect, create fear and misunderstanding in the public. Health care providers need to address this issue when recommending various immunizations to parents. It is important for nurses to be aware of vaccine controversies and know how to access appropriate, research-based information. The National Network for Immunization Information, an initiative of the Infectious Diseases Society of America, the Pediatric Infectious Diseases Society, the AAP, and the American Nurses Association, provides up-to-date information about immunization research. It can be accessed on-line at www.immunizationinfo.org.

Informed Consent

The National Childhood Vaccine Injury Act of 1986 requires that the benefits and risks associated with immunizations be discussed with parents before immunizations. The act also requires that families receive vaccine information statements (VISs) before immunization.

All health care providers who administer immunizations are required by federal law to provide general information about immunizations to the child and parents, preferably in the family's native language. This information describes why the vaccine is being given, the benefits and risks, and common side effects. Before providers administer a vaccine, parents should read the federally required information about that vaccine and have the opportunity to ask questions. The providers must use either VISs or a handout that provides all required information (AAP Committee on Infectious Diseases, 2003). It is necessary that the parents feel comfortable with the information and with the answers to any questions. It has been shown that VISs do increase the parents' knowledge level and are beneficial. Providing the information before scheduled vaccinations allows parents the time to read all the information. Providers are encouraged to obtain written informed consent for each vaccine administered. If signatures are not obtained, the client's medical record should document that the vaccine information was reviewed.

Immunization Schedule

Each January, recommendations regarding vaccinations in the United States are made by the Advisory Committee on Immunization Practices (ACIP) of the CDC, the AAP Committee on Infectious Diseases, and the American Academy of Family Physicians (AAFP). All states require immunizations for children enrolled in licensed child-care programs and school. Some states further require immunizations in the upper grades and at the time of college entrance. One group who may be overlooked includes children who receive home schooling. It is of utmost importance therefore that immunization records be traced and that vaccinations be given over the course of the fewest visits possible. State requirements can be obtained from each state health department. Refer to the Evolve website to access the current recommendations for immunization of healthy children in the United States.

Children With an Uncertain History of Immunization

When a lapse in immunization occurs, the entire series does not have to be restarted. Children's charts should be flagged to remind health care providers of these children's immunization status. For children of unknown or uncertain immunization status, appropriate immunization should be administered. Readministration of measles, mumps, and rubella (MMR) vaccine, Hib vaccine, inactivated poliovirus vaccine, or hepatitis B vaccine to someone who is immune has no harmful effects. For children older than 7 years, depending on age, the Td vaccine or Tdap vaccine, rather than the DTaP vaccine should be administered (CDC, 2006b).

International adoptees, refugees, and exchange students should be immunized according to recommended schedules for healthy infants and children. If written records of prior immunization are not available, the child begins the schedule

---

BOX 4-3	**Barriers to Immunization**

- *Complexity of the health care system,* which may lead to a delay in vaccinating children when parents become confused or frustrated with the health care system; special barriers include:
  —Appointment-only clinics
  —Excessively long waiting periods
  —Inconvenient scheduling
  —Inaccessible clinic sites
  —The need for formal referral from a primary health care provider
  —Language and cultural barriers
- *Expense* of immunization services
- *Parental misconceptions* about disease severity, vaccine efficiency and safety, complications, and contraindications
- *Inaccurate record keeping* by parents and health care workers
- *Reluctance of the health care worker* to give more than two vaccines during the same visit
- *Lack of public awareness* of the need for immunizations

TABLE 4-2   Recommended Immunization Schedule for Children and Adolescents Who Start Late or Who Are More Than 1 Month Behind

The tables below give catch-up schedules and minimum intervals between doses for children who have delayed immunizations. There is no need to restart a vaccine series regardless of the time that has elapsed between doses. Use the chart appropriate for the child's age.

Catch-Up Schedule for Children Aged 4 Months Through 6 Years

Vaccine	Minimum Age for Dose 1	Minimum Interval Between Doses			
		Dose 1 to Dose 2	Dose 2 to Dose 3	Dose 3 to Dose 4	Dose 4 to Dose 5
Diphtheria, Tetanus, Pertussis	6 wks	4 weeks	4 weeks	6 months	6 months[1]
Inactivated Poliovirus	6 wks	4 weeks	4 weeks	4 weeks[2]	
Hepatitis B[3]	Birth	4 weeks	8 weeks (and 16 weeks after first dose)		
Measles, Mumps, Rubella	12 mo	4 weeks[4]			
Varicella	12 mo				
Haemophilus influenzae type b[5]	6 wks	4 weeks if first dose given at age <12 months	4 weeks[6] if current age <12 months		
		8 weeks (as final dose) if first dose given at age 12-14 months	8 weeks (as final dose)[6] if current age ≥12 months and second dose given at age <15 months	8 weeks (as final dose) This dose only necessary for children aged 12 months-5 years who received 3 doses before age 12 months	
		No further doses needed if first dose given at age ≥15 months	No further doses needed if previous dose given at age ≥15 months		
Pneumococcal[7]	6 wks	4 weeks if first dose given at age <12 months and current age <24 months	4 weeks if current age <12 months	8 weeks (as final dose) This dose only necessary for children aged 12 months-5 years who received 3 doses before age 12 months	
		8 weeks (as final dose) if first dose given at age ≥12 months or current age 24-59 months	8 weeks (as final dose) if current age ≥12 months		
		No further doses needed for healthy children if first dose given at age ≥24 months	No further doses needed for healthy children if previous dose given at age ≥24 months		

1. **DTaP.** The fifth dose is not necessary if the fourth dose was administered after the fourth birthday.
2. **IPV.** For children who received an all-IPV or all-oral poliovirus (OPV) series, a fourth dose is not necessary if third dose was administered at age ≥4 years. If both OPV and IPV were administered as part of a series, a total of 4 doses should be given, regardless of the child's current age.
3. **HepB.** Admininster the 3-dose series to all children and adolescents <19 years of age if they were not previously vaccinated.
4. **MMR.** The second dose of MMR is recommended routinely at age 4-6 years but may be administered earlier if desired.
5. **Hib.** Vaccine is not generally recommended for children aged ≥5 years.
6. **Hib.** If current age <12 months and the first 2 doses were PRP-OMP (PedvaxHIB* or ComVax* [Merck]), the third (and final) dose should be administered at age 12-15 months and at least 8 weeks after the second dose.
7. **PCV.** Vaccine is not generally recommended for children aged ≥5 years.

TABLE 4-2 **Recommended Immunization Schedule for Children and Adolescents Who Start Late or Who Are More Than 1 Month Behind—cont'd**

Catch-Up Schedule for Children Aged 7 Years Through 18 Years

Vaccine	Minimum Interval Between Doses		
	Dose 1 to Dose 2	Dose 2 to Dose 3	Dose 3 to Booster Dose
Tetanus, Diphtheria[8]	4 weeks	6 months	6 months if first dose given at age <12 months and current age <11 years; otherwise 5 years
Inactivated Poliovirus[9]	4 weeks	4 weeks	IPV[2,9]
Hepatitis B	4 weeks	8 weeks (and 16 weeks after first dose)	
Measles, Mumps, Rubella	4 weeks		
Varicella[10]	4 weeks		

8. **Td.** Adolescent tetanus, diphtheria, and pertussis vaccine (Tdap) may be substituted for any dose in a primary catch-up series or as a booster if age appropriate for Tdap. A five-year interval from the last Td dose is encouraged when Tdap is used as a booster dose. See ACIP recommendations for further information.

9. **IPV.** Vaccine is not generally recommended for persons aged ≥18 years.

10. **Varicella.** Administer the 2-dose series to all susceptible adolescents aged ≥13 years.

Centers for Disease Control and Prevention (2006). *Recommended immunization schedule for children and adolescents who start late or who are more than 1 month behind.* Retrieved September 25, 2006 from http://www.cdc.gov/nip/recs/child-schedule-bw-print.pdf.

for children not immunized during infancy. Table 4-2 presents recommendations for immunizing children who were not immunized during infancy.

When taking an immunization history, the nurse should avoid asking the question, "Are your child's immunizations up to date?" This question will frequently be answered with "yes," but that does not give the nurse sufficient information. The nurse may gain more information by asking, "Can you tell me when and what was the last immunization your child had?"

Administration of Vaccines

The manufacturer's packaging insert for each vaccine includes recommendations for handling, storage, administration site, dosage, and route. Nurses responsible for handling vaccines should be familiar with storage requirements to minimize the risk of vaccine failures. When multidose vials are used, sterile technique should be used to prevent contamination. To ensure safe administration, the vaccines should be given by the recommended route. The deltoid muscle can be used in children aged 18 months and older. The ventrogluteal site may be used in older children (see Chapter 14). Vaccines given intramuscularly need to be injected deep into the muscle mass to avoid irritation and possible necrosis.

More than one immunization may be administered at the same age or time. Some vaccines are given as a combined vaccine. When more than one injection is to be given, vaccines should be administered with separate syringes, not mixed into one, unless provided for by the manufacturer.

They should be given at different sites (preferably in different thighs), and the site used for each vaccine should be recorded to identify possible reactions. The nurse should also record the lot number for each vaccine given. Box 4-4 lists nursing responsibilities associated with administering vaccines.

CRITICAL TO REMEMBER

Special Considerations Related to Immunizations

- The gluteal site is not recommended at any age for the administration of the hepatitis B vaccine. This is because there is diminished immunogenicity in the gluteal site. (AAP Committee on Infectious Diseases, 2003).

- When giving DTaP, Hib, and hepatitis B vaccines simultaneously, it is advisable to administer the most reactive vaccine (DTaP) in one leg and to inject the others, which cause less reaction, into the other leg.

- Siblings and household contacts of immunocompromised children should not receive the oral poliovirus vaccine but may be given the inactivated poliovirus vaccine.

- Live measles vaccine is produced by chick embryo cell culture, so there is a remote possibility of anaphylactic hypersensitivity in children with egg allergies. Most reactions from the MMR are reactions to other components of the vaccine, so MMR is not usually contraindicated for children with egg hypersensitivity (AAP Committee on Infectious Diseases, 2003).

- Any immunization may cause an anaphylactic reaction. All offices and clinics must have epinephrine 1:1000 available.

BOX 4-4	Nursing Responsibility in Administering Vaccines

- Know the recommended immunization schedule and the recommended alternative schedule for those with lapsed immunizations or unknown immunization history.
- Acquire up-to-date information because recommendations are revised frequently.
- Assess the family's beliefs and values to assist in the education of the family as to the rationale for immunizations, the risks and side effects, and the risks of nonimmunization.
- Take a careful history to determine possible contraindications or precautions and report any pertinent information to the practitioner. Educate the family as to the rationale for any contraindications.
- "Gloves are not required when administering vaccinations unless the persons who administer the vaccine will come in contact with potentially infectious body fluids or have open lesions" (AAP Committee on Infectious Diseases, 2003).
- Some vaccines come mixed in one syringe (e.g., DTaP-Hib). Other vaccines should not be mixed. Check manufacturer's recommendations.
- Administer vaccines according to the manufacturer's recommended sites.
- Aspirate to make sure that the needle has not been placed in a blood vessel.
- Wash hands before vaccine administration and between children.
- Review with the parents common side effects and the signs of potentially severe reactions that warrant contacting the practitioner.
- Instruct the parents that they may administer age-appropriate doses of acetaminophen every 4 to 6 hours for 24 hours if the child has discomfort related to vaccine administration.
- For painful or red injection sites, advise the parents to apply cold compresses for the first 24 hours; then use warm or cold compresses as long as needed.
- Give multiple administrations in different sites and record those sites in the medical record.
- Document parental consent in the medical record. Documentation should also include the type of vaccine, date of administration, manufacturer and lot number, expiration date, administration site, any data pertinent to risks and side effects, and the signature and title of the person administering the immunization.

Precautions and Contraindications

The main purpose of vaccination is to achieve immunity with the fewest possible side effects (Box 4-5). Most vaccines have no side effects; when side effects do occur, they are usually mild. Fever and local irritation are not uncommon after administration of DTaP vaccine, and fever and rash can occur 1 to 2 weeks after administration of live-virus measles vaccine.

BOX 4-5	Common Misconceptions About Administration and Safety of Vaccines

The following conditions or circumstances are *not* contraindications to the administration of vaccines:
- Mild acute illness with low-grade fever or mild diarrhea in an otherwise healthy child.
- A reaction to a previous dose of DTaP vaccine with only soreness, redness, or swelling in the immediate vicinity of the injection site.

Some severe side effects have been reported, however. These events are usually not predictable. Because cases have been reported of development of paralytic polio in healthy children after administration of oral polio vaccine, the AAP and the CDC now recommend a full schedule of inactivated polio vaccine. Reactions to the MMR vaccine have included anaphylactic reactions, both in children with and in those without a history of egg allergy. This has prompted consideration of other possible causative agents. For instance, the MMR vaccine contains neomycin, which may be the cause of the sensitivity.

Before a second dose of any vaccine is given, the nurse needs to ascertain and record whether any side effects or possible reactions occurred after the previous dose of that vaccine. The National Childhood Vaccine Injury Act of 1986 requires health care providers who administer vaccines to maintain permanent vaccination records and to report occurrences of certain adverse events stipulated in the act. Anaphylaxis or anaphylactic shock and encephalopathy are examples of two reportable events associated with the tetanus and pertussis vaccines. Providers administering immunizations must be aware of reportable events and comply with the provisions of the act.

Immunocompromised Children

In general, children who are immunologically compromised should not receive live bacterial or viral vaccines (e.g., MMR, varicella vaccine). There are some exceptions related to children with human immunodeficiency virus infection and in some specific instances of children in remission from cancer. Children with human immunodeficiency virus infection who are not severely compromised should receive MMR; varicella vaccine can be given, depending on the CD4 count (see Chapter 17).

Education

Immunization is a critical component of a child's health care. Knowledge of immunization schedules and an awareness of potential delays will aid the health care provider in identifying children who have not been fully immunized. Health care providers must provide parents with accurate information regarding immunizations because immunizations are the primary and safest means of managing preventable infectious diseases. All children in the United States should have access to appropriate immunization. The State Children's Health Insurance Program (see Chapter 1) and the Vaccines for Children program ensure that there are no financial barriers. Nevertheless, health providers need to be aware that, although immunization rates are increasing through efforts of the federal and state governments, disparities in immunization access for the poor and certain racial or ethnic minorities still exist (CDC, Office of Minority Health, 2004).

Nutrition and Activity

To provide care for infants and children, the nurse must understand the nutritional needs of the body. The body is nourished by food. Carbohydrates, fats, proteins, water, vitamins, and minerals (Box 4-6) are the basic *nutrients* in food. Carbohydrates, fats, and proteins provide energy, which is required by the cells of the body to transport all substances across the cell membrane, to synthesize substances within the cell, and to dispose of waste products.

Carbohydrates

Carbohydrates provide most of the energy needed to maintain a healthy body. They exist in two forms, simple and complex. Complex carbohydrates should make up the majority of calories consumed. Most complex carbohydrates are found in starch from cereal grains, roots, vegetables, and legumes. The more mature the vegetable, the higher the starch content. Foods that are good sources of complex carbohydrates are relatively inexpensive and easily obtained. Insufficient calorie intake causes the body to break down protein and fat for energy and glucose production. Carbohydrates are a food source for many of the essential nutrients, including fiber, vitamins C and E, the majority of B vitamins, potassium, and the majority of trace elements.

BOX 4-6	Common Sources of Nutrients
Carbohydrates	**Proteins**
Breads	Meat
Vegetables	Cheese
Cereals	Poultry
Rice	Eggs
Pasta	Fish
Fruits	Legumes
Dried peas and legumes	Milk
Fats	
Butter	
Cream	
Margarine	
Cheeses	
Shortening	
Nuts	
Oils	
Meats	

Fats

Fats serve as the secondary source of energy by providing 30% or less of daily calorie intake. The Food and Drug Administration recently required food manufacturers to list *trans* fat (i.e., *trans* fatty acids) on Nutrition Facts and some Supplement Facts panels. Trans fat, like saturated fat and dietary cholesterol, raises the low-density lipoprotein cholesterol. Trans fat can be found in processed foods made with partially hydrogenated vegetable oils such as vegetable shortenings, some margarines, crackers, candies, cookies, snack foods, fried foods, and baked goods. Dietary fat allows the absorption of the fat-soluble vitamins (A, D, E, K) and adds flavor to foods. The layer of fat beneath the skin plays a role in regulating body temperature. Fat is a component of cell membranes and acts as a protective padding for the internal organs. When excess calories are consumed, dietary fats are stored as excess body fat. The monounsaturated and polyunsaturated fats can raise high-density lipoproteins and decrease low-density lipoprotein cholesterol. For this reason, emphasis should be placed on replacing saturated fats with these fats whenever possible. Most whole grains, breads, pastas, and cereals are naturally low in fat. Families should be taught to choose lean meats, beans and low-fat dairy products and to limit their intake of processed foods such as crackers, cookies, cakes, and higher fat snacks.

Proteins

Dietary *protein* is necessary for building and maintaining body tissues. Proteins are involved in homeostasis by working with other elements in the blood to maintain fluid balance. Many vitamins and minerals are bound to protein carriers for transport. Proteins, as antibodies, aid in the regulation of the body's immune system.

Water

Water is essential for life. It transports nutrients to cells and waste products away from cells. It assists in the regulation of body temperature and in chemical reactions. Water lubricates joints and provides form and structure to the cells and the medium for body fluids. Water is found in most foods, including solids. Water requirements can be estimated by a variety of methods. The child's activity level and ambient temperature influence the amount of water needed.

Vitamins and Minerals

Vitamins and *minerals* are necessary in the regulation of metabolic processes. They are present in a wide variety of foods. Vitamins and minerals are added to processed formulas and to other foods such as cereals. It is generally not necessary for children to receive supplementation after infancy unless they are at nutritional risk (e.g., have anorexia or a chronic disease).

Dietary Guidelines

New guidelines for a healthful diet for Americans aged 2 years or older were published by the U.S. Department of Health and Human Services and the U.S. Department of Agriculture in 2005. This document, "2005 Dietary Guidelines for Americans" is the basis for a federal nutrition policy. The guidelines recommend that a variety of nutrient-dense foods and beverages within and among the basic food groups be consumed, but foods that contain saturated and trans fats, cholesterol, added sugars, salt, and alcohol should be limited. Special recommendations are given for children and adolescents (Box 4-7).

BOX 4-7	**Key Dietary Recommendations Specific to Children and Adolescents**

- Consume whole-grain products often; at least half the grains should be whole grains.
- Children 2 to 8 years should consume 2 cups per day of fat-free or low-fat milk or equivalent milk products.
- Children 9 years of age and older should consume 3 cups per day of fat-free or low-fat milk or equivalent milk products.
- Keep total fat intake between 30% to 35% of calories for children 2 to 3 years of age and between 25% to 35% of calories for children and adolescents 4 to 18 years of age, with most fats coming from sources of polyunsaturated and monounsaturated fatty acids, such as fish, nuts, and vegetable oils.

From United States Department of Agriculture. (2001). *Dietary guidelines for Americans, 2000* (5th ed.). Available on-line: www.usda.gov/cnpp.

The MyPyramid Food Guidance System was developed to provide food-based guidance to help implement the recommendations of the guidelines. The Dietary Reference Intakes nutrient-based recommendations are the starting point for all of the recommendations and tools shown. They were used as a major source of information by the Dietary Guidelines Advisory Committee in developing their science-based report. The Dietary Guidelines for Americans was then developed on the basis of the committee report. These all provide the basis for many consumer tools, such as the MyPyramid for Kids (Fig. 4-6). The MyPyramid illustrates the Food Guide Pyramid in a way that children younger than 6 years old can understand. The pyramid focuses on eating a variety of foods to get the required nutrients and adequate energy. The importance of grains, fruits, and vegetables is evident in the pyramid. Other web-based interactive tools and print materials can be accessed at http://www.nal.usda.gov/fnic/Fpyr/pyramid.html.

Energy, Calories, and Servings

Energy is measured in calories. Energy or calorie needs depend on the person's age, sex, height, weight, and level of physical activity. Calorie needs vary during childhood. Infants need sufficient calories to support rapid growth; therefore, fat is not restricted in children younger than 2 years. Fat intake should be between 30% to 35% of calories

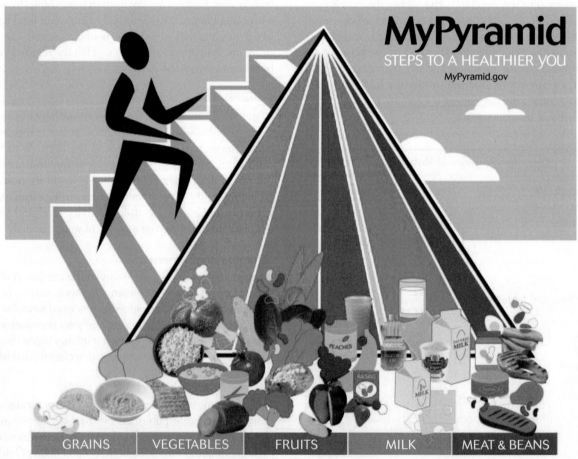

GRAINS   VEGETABLES   FRUITS   MILK   MEAT & BEANS

MyPyramid
STEPS TO A HEALTHIER YOU
MyPyramid.gov

FIG 4-6 **MyPyramid for Young Children.** *(Courtesy U.S. Department of Agriculture, 2005.)*

for children 2 to 3 years of age and between 25% to 35% of calories for children and adolescents 4 to 18 years of age, with most fats coming from sources of polyunsaturated and monounsaturated fatty acids, such as fish, nuts, and vegetable oils.

Physical Activity

Over the past several decades, children of all ages have become less active and more sedentary. The prevalence of overweight children aged 6 to 11 years has more than doubled in the past 20 years, going from 7% in 1980 to 16% in 2002. The rate among adolescents aged 12 to 19 years more than tripled, increasing from 5% to 16% (U.S. HHS National Center for Health Statistics, 2005). Physical activity, dietary behavior, and genetics affect weight across all age groups. American Indian, Hispanic, and African American children tend to be heavier than white children (Hardy, Harrell, & Bell, 2004). A person's BMI provides an indication of relative obesity, and this number (a function of weight and height) is being used more frequently to assess for obesity. Appendix B illustrates the BMI for children of various ages.

Any health promotion counseling during childhood and adolescence needs to include an emphasis on increasing the child's and parents' daily physical activity. Children particularly enjoy an activity if it is associated with fun and group involvement and they are more likely to participate in physical exercise if they see their parents exercising as well.

When counseling parents and children about increasing physical activity, the nurse can emphasize the following points (Calderon, Yucha, & Schaffer, 2005):

- Plan regular periods of exercise and engage in shared family activities
- Make exercise fun and a habitual activity
- Encourage students to participate fully in any physical education classes
- Encourage parents to investigate community physical activity programs in their community. City recreation centers, parks, and community YMCAs can provide fun places to engage in physical activities.

Cultural and Religious Influences on Diet

Dietary intake is profoundly affected by both cultural and religious beliefs. An understanding of these patterns will assist the nurse in both the assessment and implementation of nutrition-related behaviors. Hospitalized children who become stressed by being in a new and strange environment do not need the added stress of unfamiliar foods. Information regarding a child's food preferences can be obtained during a dietary history.

A child's religious beliefs may also have an affect on the types of foods eaten and the way in which they are served. Within religious groups there may be a variety of dietary observances. The nurse should assist and encourage the child and the child's family in communicating specific dietary needs.

Assessment of Nutritional Status

A nutritional assessment is an essential component of the health examination of infants and children. This assessment should include anthropometric data, biochemical data, clinical examination, and dietary history. From these data, a plan of care can be developed. In addition, children at risk can be identified and areas of prevention pursued through teaching and further evaluation and follow-up.

Anthropometric Data. Height and head circumference reflect past nutrition or chronic nutritional problems. Weight, skinfold thickness, midarm circumference, and BMI better reflect current nutritional status. The nurse should always be aware of the roles of birth weight and ethnic, familial, and environmental factors when evaluating anthropometric measurements. Infants and children should have anthropometric measurements done during each preventive health care visit.

Clinical Evaluation. The clinical evaluation includes a physical examination and complete history. Special attention is paid to the areas where signs of nutritional deficiencies appear: the skin, hair, teeth, gums, lips, tongue, and eyes. Clinical symptoms usually are not by themselves diagnostic but may suggest conditions, which are then confirmed by biochemical tests and diet histories. More than one deficiency may be present. (See also the section "Failure to Thrive" in Chapter 29.)

Dietary History. Obtaining an accurate history of dietary intake is difficult. The knowledge that what the child is eating is being recorded can influence what the parent feeds the child or what the child eats. Children often cannot remember what they have eaten. If the child or parent is not committed to the process, incomplete information may be obtained. It is still a useful assessment process, however, and should be used. Client teaching includes an understanding of the importance of recording the child's dietary intake and the need for accuracy. Common methods of assessing dietary intake include 24-hour recall, a food frequency questionnaire, or a food diary.

Twenty-Four-Hour Recall. With the 24-hour recall method, the child or parent is asked to recall everything the child has eaten in the past 24 hours. A questionnaire may be used, or the nurse may conduct an interview asking the pertinent questions.

The child or parent may have difficulty remembering the kinds and amounts of food eaten, or the family may have had an atypical day on the previous day or may not feel comfortable relating what was eaten the day being evaluated. How the child or parents see the nurse may influence the response; they may say what they think the interviewer wants to hear. Asking for information in relation to meals eaten as opposed to food groups may increase the accuracy of the assessment.

Food Frequency Questionnaire. The food frequency questionnaire elicits information on the intake of particular foods or food groups on a daily, weekly, or monthly basis. This tool can be used to validate the 24-hour recall data. As for all methods of assessment, this requires the interviewer to be nonjudgmental and objective. Putting the information into a questionnaire may be less threatening to the child and family and will save time.

Food Diary. When keeping a food diary, the child or parent records everything consumed during a specified period. Various sources recommend different lengths of time for keeping the diary; 3-day to 7-day records may be used. As in all nursing care, the nurse must evaluate what is a reasonable time to expect the family or child to keep the records. The time, place, and people present when the food was eaten may also be recorded. This provides the nurse with additional information, which may identify trends and other information related to the child's eating behaviors.

Safety

Unintentional injury is the most significant but under recognized public health threat facing children today. Unintentional injury is the leading cause of death in children. Across age groups, motor vehicle traffic injuries and firearm injuries are the two major causes of injury (CDC, 2005d). (See Chapter 10 for a more detailed discussion of the causes of injury in childhood.)

The number of childhood deaths is staggering, but it is only a fraction of the number of children who are hospitalized and require emergency treatment and who have a permanent disability as a result of injury. The economic burden to society is equally astounding, reaching billions of dollars yearly. What cannot be quantified is the emotional loss, suffering, and pain the child and family must endure once an injury has occurred.

All children are at risk for injury because of their normal curiosity, impulsiveness, and impatience. Everywhere they venture, they are exposed to potentially hazardous situations.

Injury Prevention

Injury prevention is a relatively new focus of health promotion. The term *accident*, with its implied meaning of random chance or lack of responsibility, has been replaced with *injury*, with its implication that injuries have causes that can be modified to prevent or lessen their frequency and severity. Safety education is a critical component of injury prevention. It increases awareness, it attempts to modify human behavior, and it reinforces changes implemented through legal mandates (e.g., seat belt laws) or product modification (e.g., crib design, air bags).

Nurses need to become proactive in childhood injury prevention by increasing children's and adults' awareness of safety issues (Box 4-8). Nurses who care for children are acutely aware of the devastating effects and complex problems injuries cause. From their experiences, they become well-informed advocates for childhood safety.

Anticipatory Guidance

To be most effective in providing anticipatory safety guidance, nurses must gear educational strategies to the child's level of growth and development. Knowledge of growth and development also helps the nurse understand the risks

---

BOX 4-8	What Nurses Can Do to Prevent Childhood Injuries

- Model safety practices in the home, work, and community.
- Educate parents and children through anticipatory safety guidance to help reduce needless injuries.
- Support legislative efforts that advocate prevention measures.
- Collaborate with other health care providers to promote safety and injury prevention.

CRITICAL TO REMEMBER
Relationship Between Safety and Childhood Development

Developmentally, children are vulnerable to injury for the following reasons:

- Children are naturally curious and enjoy exploring their surroundings.
- Children are driven to test and master new skills.
- Children frequently attempt activities before they have developed the cognitive and physical skills required to accomplish the task safely.
- Children often assert themselves and challenge rules.
- Children develop a strong desire for peer approval as they grow older.

---

associated with each age group and choose the educational strategy appropriate to a child's developmental level.

Early in their parenting experience, parents need to know how to provide a safe environment for their children and what behaviors they can expect at various developmental levels. Anticipatory guidance builds on the safety principles of the previous stage. Awareness of a child's changing capabilities allows the parent to be more alert and reactive to safety hazards that the child is likely to encounter. This awareness is especially important for first-time parents.

Simply telling parents to "watch your children" or to "child-proof" the home or telling a child to "be careful" has little educational impact. Educational efforts are much more likely to be effective if they focus on specific problems with specific solutions rather than providing broad or vague advice.

Teaching Strategies

Teaching can be formal or informal, simple or elaborate, as long as it provides relevant safety information and coincides with the child's or parents' cognitive abilities (Appendix A). For children younger than 5 or 6 years, it is advisable to incorporate the parents into the teaching process so that the parents can assist with reinforcement or questions the child later has about the safety issue. With younger children, who are easily distracted, the information should be presented in short sessions.

Many local and national organizations have safety information available for distribution. This information can be used to supplement the teaching process. Prepared materials range from pamphlets, booklets, posters, and audiovisual materials to entire teaching programs that can assist in providing injury prevention education to all age groups. Some programs offer the materials free of cost. Internet information, such as that obtained at www.kidsafe.com, can be extremely helpful to parents.

KEY CONCEPTS

- Growth, development, maturation, and learning are complex, interrelated processes that produce complicated series of changes in individuals from conception to death.
- Growth and development proceed from simple to complex, from proximal to distal, and from head to lower extremities.
- As children grow and develop, wide variations within normal limits occur.
- Weight, height, and head circumference, common parameters used to monitor growth should be measured and evaluated at regular intervals.
- The earlier that delays and deviations from normal are treated, the less severe the effect will be on growth and developmental outcomes.
- Numerous factors, including genetics, environment, culture, nutrition, health status, and family structure, affect how children grow and develop.
- Piaget's theory of cognitive development describes how children learn to deal with their environment through thinking and reasoning. Progress in learning during various periods is based on the child's ability to create patterns of understanding and behavior.
- Freud's psychosexual theory attempts to explain how humans struggle in both conscious and unconscious ways to become individual beings. During each stage of sexual development in children, a different area of the body is the focus of attention and pleasure.
- Erikson's theory of psychosocial development describes a series of crises emerging at specific times and in a particular order. These stages occur throughout life, and each must be resolved for an individual to progress emotionally.
- Kohlberg discusses moral development as a complex process involving progressive acceptance of the values and rules of society in a way that determines behavior. A maturing individual becomes less concerned with avoiding punishment and more interested in human rights and universal justice.
- Language development, a complex process involving extensive neuromuscular maturation, begins as undifferentiated crying at birth and proceeds throughout life to provide a vehicle for communication, thought, and creativity.
- The 46 human chromosomes are long strands of DNA, each containing up to several thousand individual genes.

- With the exception of those genes located on the X and Y chromosomes in males, genes are inherited in pairs that may be identical or different. Some genes are dominant, and some are recessive.
- Single-gene disorders are associated with a fixed risk of occurrence or recurrence. The type of single-gene abnormality (autosomal dominant, autosomal recessive, or X-linked) determines the level of risk.
- A variety of prescreening and screening tools, such as the DDST-II, are used by nurses to gain an overall picture of a child's developmental progress and to alert the nurse to potential developmental delays.
- To provide high-quality, developmentally appropriate care to children and parents, nurses must be aware of normal patterns of growth and development.
- Piaget described three types of play, related to periods of sensorimotor, preoperational, and concrete operational functioning: practice play, symbolic play, and games.
- Play enhances the child's growth and development through physical, cognitive, emotional, social, and moral development.
- Personnel who administer and handle vaccines must be aware of recommendations for handling, storing, and administering the vaccines. Special attention should be given to the site of administration, dosage, and route.
- When a lapse in immunization occurs, the entire series does not have to be restarted.
- Children who are immunologically compromised should not receive live bacterial or viral vaccines.
- The six basic nutrients are carbohydrates, protein, fat, vitamins, minerals, and water.
- Components of a nutritional assessment are anthropometric data, biochemical data, clinical examination, and dietary history.
- Many childhood injuries and deaths are predictable and preventable.
- Understanding the developmental milestones of each age group is important for promoting safety awareness for parents, caregivers, and children.

REFERENCES AND READINGS

American Academy of Pediatrics. (2001). Developmental surveillance and screening of infants and young children. *Pediatrics, 108,* 192-196.

American Academy of Pediatrics. (2002). Smallpox vaccine. (Electronic version). *Pediatrics, 110.*

American Academy of Pediatrics. (2005a). Pertussis in adolescents and adults: Should we vaccinate? *Pediatrics, 115,* 1675-1684.

American Academy of Pediatrics. (2005b). Responding to parental refusals of immunization of children. *Pediatrics, 115,* 1428-1431.

American Academy of Pediatrics Committee on Infectious Diseases. (2000). Technical report: Prevention of pneumococcal infections, including the use of pneumococcal conjugate and polysaccharide vaccines and antibiotic prophylaxis. *Pediatrics, 106,* 367-376.

American Academy of Pediatrics Committee on Infectious Diseases. (2003). *2003 Red book: Report of the Committee on Infectious Diseases* (26th ed.). Elk Grove Village, IL: The Academy.

American Academy of Pediatrics Committee on Infectious Diseases. (2004). *Pediatrics, 113,* 1441-1447.

American Academy of Pediatrics Committee on Infectious Diseases. (2005). *Pediatrics, 116,* 496-505.

American Academy of Pediatrics Committee on Infectious Diseases. (2006). *Pediatrics, 117,* 239-240.

American Academy of Pediatrics Committee on Nutrition. (2003). Prevention of pediatric overweight and obesity. *Pediatrics, 112,* 424-430.

American Heart Association. (2005). *Dietary guidelines for healthy children.* Retrieved October 11, 2005, from *www.americanheart .org/presenter.jhtml?identifier=4575.*

Bear, G. G., Richards, H. C., & Gibbs, J. C. (1997). Sociomoral reasoning and behavior. In G. C. Bear, K. M. Minke, & A. Thomas (Eds.), *Children's needs II: Development, problems and alternatives.* Bethesda, MD: National Association of School Psychologists.

Bornstein, M. H., & Bradley, R. H. (2003). *Socioeconomic status, parenting, and child development.* Rahway, NJ: Lawrence Erlbaum Associates.

Brazelton, T. B. (1992). *Touchpoints.* Menlo Park, CA: Addison-Wesley.

Bruce, B. S., Lake, J. P., Eden, V. A., & Denney, J. C. (2004). Children at risk of injury. *Journal of Pediatric Nursing, 19,* 121-127.

Calderon, K. S., Yucha, C. B., & Schaffer, S. D. (2005). Obesity-related cardiovascular risk factors: Intervention recommendations to decrease adolescent obesity, *Journal of Pediatric Nursing, 20,* 3-14.

Centers for Disease Control and Prevention. (2003). *Haemophilus influenzae serotype b (Hib) disease.* Retrieved October 29, 2005, from *www.cdc.gov/ncidod/dbmd/diseaseinfo/haeminfluserob_t.htm.*

Centers for Disease Control and Prevention. (2005a). *Direct and indirect effects of routine immunization with 7-valent pneumococcal conjugate vaccine on invasive pneumococcal disease—United States, 1998-2003.* Retrieved October 29, 2005, from *www.cdc.gov/od/oc/ media/mmwrnews/n050916.htm.*

Centers for Disease Control and Prevention. (2005b). *National, state, and urban area vaccination coverage among children aged 19-35 months—United States, 2004.* Retrieved October 29, 2005, from *www.cdc.gov/mmwr/preview/mmwrhtml/mm5429al.htm.*

Centers for Disease Control and Prevention. (2005c). *Rubella no longer major public health threat in the United States.* Retrieved October 2, 2005, from *www.cdc.gov/od/oc/media/pressure/r050321.htm.*

Centers for Disease Control and Prevention. (2005d). *Unintentional injury activities—2004.* National Center for Injury Prevention and Control. Atlanta, GA: Centers for Disease Control and Prevention and National Center for Injury Prevention and Control.

Centers for Disease Control and Prevention. (2006a). *Recommended childhood and adolescent immunization schedule—United States, 2006.* Retrieved January 7, 2006, from *www.cdc.gov.*

Centers for Disease Control and Prevention. (2006b). *Recommended immunization schedule for children and adolescents who start or who are more than 1 month behind.* Retrieved January 7, 2006, from *www.cdc.gov*

Centers for Disease Control and Prevention. (2006c). Prevention and control of influenza. *MMWR, 55*(Early Release), 1-41.

Centers for Disease Control and Prevention. (2006d). *Prevention of hepatitis A through active or passive immunization.* Retrieved June 28, 2006 from *www.cdc.gov.*

Centers for Disease Control and Prevention Office of Minority Health. (2004). *Highlights in minority health.* Retrieved October 9, 2005, from *www.cdc.gov/omh/Highlights/2004/HAug04.htm.*

Clements, R. L., & Fiorentino, L. (2004). *The child's right to play.* Westport, CT.: Praeger Publishers.

Colby, A., Kohlberg, L., & Kauffman, K. (1987). Theoretical introduction to the measurement of moral judgment. In A. Colby & L. Kohlberg (Eds.), *The measurement of moral judgment* (Vol. 1). Cambridge, England: Cambridge University Press.

Culbertson, J. L., Newman, J. E., & Willis, D. J. (2003). Childhood and adolescent psychologic development, *Pediatric Clinics of North America. 50,* 741-764.

Department of Health and Human Services & Department of Agriculture. (2005). *Dietary guidelines for Americans.* Retrieved October 2, 2005, from *http://www.healthierus.gov/dietaryguidelines.*

Dunkle, M. (2005). *Improving developmental screening through public policy.* Retrieved October 29, 2005, from *www.dbpeds.org.*

Elkind, D. (1970). *Children and adolescents: Interpretive essays on Jean Piaget.* New York: Oxford University Press.

Erikson, E. H. (1963). *Childhood and society* (2nd ed.). New York: Norton.

Feldman, R. S. (1998). *Child development.* Upper Saddle River, NJ: Prentice-Hall.

Flavell, J. (1963). *The developmental psychology of Jean Piaget.* Princeton, NJ: Van Nostrand.

Frankenburg, W. K. (2002). Developmental surveillance and screening of infants and young children, *Pediatrics, 109,* 144-145.

Frankenburg, W. K., & Dodds, J. B. (1992). *Denver II screening manual.* Denver: Developmental Materials.

Freud, A. (1974). *Introduction to psychoanalysis.* New York: International Universities Press.

Freud, S. (1960). *The ego and the id* (J. Riviere, Trans.). New York: Norton. (Original work published 1923.)

Garvey, C. (1979). What is play? In P. Chance (Ed.). *Learning through play.* New York: Gardner Press.

Glascoe, F. P. (2003). Parents' evaluation of developmental status: how well do parents' concerns identify children with behavioral and emotional problems? *Clinical Pediatrics, 42,* 133-138.

Glascoe, F. P. (2004). *Interpreting screening tests to families and encouraging follow through.* Retrieved October 29, 2005, from *www .dbpeds.org.*

Glascoe, F. P., & Shapiro, H. L. (2003). *Developmental screening.* Retrieved on August 12, 2003, from *www.dbpeds.org.*

Glascoe, F. P., & Shapiro, H. L. (2004). *Introduction to developmental and behavioral screening.* Retrieved October 29, 2005 from *www .dbpeds.org.*

Guyton, A. C., & Hall, J. E. (2006). *Textbook of medical physiology* (11th ed.). Philadelphia: WB Saunders.

Hardy, L. R., Harrell, J. S., & Bell, R. A. (2004). Overweight in children: Definitions, measurements, confounding factors, and health consequences. *Journal of Pediatric Nursing, 19,* 376-384.

Jorde, L. B., Carey, J. C., Bamshad, M. J., & White, R. L. (2003). *Medical genetics.* St. Louis: Mosby.

Kelly, D. P., & Sally, J. I. (1999). Disorders of speech and language. In M. D. Levine, W. B. Carey, & A. C. Crocker (Eds.). *Developmental behavioral pediatrics.* Philadelphia: WB Saunders.

Kohlberg, L. (1964). Development of moral character. In M. Hoffman & L. Hoffman (Eds.), *Review of child development research* (Vol. 1). New York: Russell Sage Foundation.

Kohlberg, L. (1984). *The psychology of moral development.* San Francisco: Harper & Row.

Litt, I. F., & Martin, J.A. (1999). Development of sexuality and its problems. In M. D. Levine, W. B. Carey, & A. C. Crocker (Eds.). *Developmental behavioral pediatrics.* Philadelphia: WB Saunders.

Lucas, B. L. (2004). Nutrition in childhood. In L. K. Mahan & S. Escott-Stump (Eds), *Food, nutrition & diet therapy.* Philadelphia: WB Saunders.

McDonald, E. K. (2003). Principles of behavioral assessment and management. *Pediatric Clinics of North America, 50,* 801-816.

National Human Genome Research Institute. (2003/2005). *About the human genome project.* Retrieved October 12, 2005, from *www .genome.gov/12011238.*

National Tay-Sachs and Allied Diseases Association, Inc. (2003). *Tay-Sachs disease: Classic infantile form.* Retrieved July 7, 2003, from *www.ntsad.org/pages/t-sachs.htm.*

Pellegrini, A. D., & Smith, P. K. (2005). *The nature of play.* New York: The Guilford Press.

Piaget, J. (1962). *Play, dreams and imitation childhood.* New York: Norton.

Piaget, J. (1967). *Six psychological studies.* New York: Random House.

Pinto-Martin, J. A., Souders, M. C., Giarelli, E., & Levy, S. E. (2005). The role of nurses in screening for autistic spectrum disorder in pediatric primary care. *Journal of Pediatric Nursing, 20,* 163-169.

Ploof, D., & Hamel, S. (2005). *Changing developmental screening practice in the real world.* Retrieved October 29, 2005, from *www.dbpeds.org.*

Richmond, P. G. (1971). *An introduction to Piaget.* New York: Basic Books.

Sand, N., Silverstein, M., Glascoe, F. P., Gupta, V. B., Tonniges, T. P., & O'Connor, K. G. (2005). Pediatricians' reported practices regarding developmental screening: Do guidelines work? Do they help? *Pediatrics, 116,* 174-179.

Schor, E. L. (2004). Rethinking well-child care. *Pediatrics, 114,* 210-216.

Sroufe, L. A., Egeland, B., Carlson, E. A., Carlson, E. A., & Collins, W. A. (2005). *The development of the person.* New York: Guilford Press.

Tschannen-Moran, B., Lewis, E., & Farrell, S. P. (2003). Childhood obesity: Policy issues in 2003. *Journal of Pediatric Nursing, 18,* 416-420.

United States Department of Agriculture, Food, and Nutrition Service. (2005). *MyPyramid for kids.* Retrieved October 29, 2005, from *teamnutrition.usda.gov/kids-pyramid.*

United States Department of Health and Human Services. (2000). *Healthy people 2010* (Conference edition, 2 vols). Washington, DC: U.S. HHS.

United States Department of Health and Human Services National Center for Health Statistics. (2005). *Prevalence of overweight among children and adolescents: United States 1999-2002.* Retrieved January 7, 2006 from *www.cdc.gov/nchs/.*

United States Food and Drug Administration. (2004). *Trans fat now listed with saturated fat and cholesterol on the nutrition facts label.* Retrieved October 15, 2005 from *www.cfsan.fda.gov/%7Edms/transfat.*

Wadsworth, B. J. (2004). *Piaget's theory of cognitive development* (5th ed.). Boston: Pearson Education.

Wake, M., Gerner, B., & Gallagher, S. (2005). Does parents' evaluation of developmental status at school entry predict language, achievement, and quality of life 2 years later? *Ambulatory Pediatrics, 5,* 143-149.

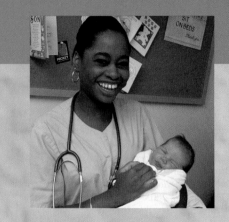

CHAPTER 5

Health Promotion for the Infant

Learning Objectives

After studying this chapter, you should be able to:

- Describe the physiologic changes that occur during infancy.
- Describe the infant's motor, psychosocial, language, and cognitive development.
- Discuss common problems of infancy, such as separation anxiety, sleep, irritability, and colic.
- Discuss the importance of immunizations and recommended immunization schedules for infants.
- Provide parents with anticipatory guidance for common concerns during infancy, such as immunizations, nutrition, elimination, dental care, sleep, hygiene, safety, and play.

Definitions

asphyxiation A state of suffocation that severely compromises oxygen delivery to the body.

café au lait spots Light brown birthmarks.

critical milestones Developmental milestones that, if not reached appropriately, would initiate a full developmental assessment. Critical milestones are based on the Denver Developmental Screening Test II milestones (see Chapter 4) and appear in the Growth and Development boxes throughout the health promotion chapters.

developmental milestones Benchmarks of development that indicate whether the infant is developing normally; not achieving milestones within a certain time frame might be cause for concern.

egocentrism Complete absorption with self; an inability to understand that others have a different point of view.

mistrust The negative resolution of the first developmental task, according to Erikson's theory; results in acute emotional tension and behavioral signs of unmet needs.

mongolian spots Bruiselike marks that occur mostly in newborn infants with dark skin tones.

object permanence The realization that objects continue to exist even though they are out of sight.

parent-infant attachment A sense of belonging to or connection between a parent and infant.

pincer grasp The use of index finger and thumb to grip objects.

sensorimotor stage Piaget's first stage of cognitive development, in which infants and young toddlers use mainly senses and movement to begin to understand and control their environment.

stranger anxiety The infant's ability to distinguish between caregivers and others, to prefer parents to other caregivers, and to become distressed when separation occurs.

trust The basic emotion established during infancy as a result of satisfying interactions between child and caregiver; provides the foundation on which a healthy personality is built.

Electronic Resources

Additional information related to the content in Chapter 5 can be found on:

the interactive companion CD-ROM

- Audio Glossary
- NCLEX Review Questions
- Pediatric Assessment & Video Clips

or the companion website at *evolve*
http://evolve.elsevier.com/james/ncoc

- NCLEX Review Questions
- Pediatric Assessment & Video Clips
- WebLinks

During no time after birth does a human being grow and change as dramatically as during infancy. Beginning with the newborn period and ending at 1 year, the infancy period, a child grows and develops from a tiny bundle of physiologic needs to a dynamo, capable of locomotion and language and ready to embark on the adventures of the toddler years.

GROWTH AND DEVELOPMENT OF THE INFANT

Although historically adults have considered infants unable to do much more than eat and sleep, it is now well documented that even young infants can organize their experiences in meaningful ways and adapt to changes in the environment. Evidence shows that infants form strong bonds with their caregivers, communicate their needs and wants, and interact socially. By the end of the first year of life, infants can move about on their own, elicit responses from adults, communicate through the use of rudimentary language, and solve simple problems.

Infancy is characterized by the need to establish harmony between the self and the world. To achieve this harmony, the infant needs food, warmth, comfort, oral satisfaction, environmental stimulation, and opportunities for self-exploration and self-expression. Competent caregivers satisfy the needs of helpless infants, providing a warm, nurturing relationship so that the children have a sense of trust in the world and in themselves. These challenges make infancy an exciting yet demanding period for both child and parents.

Nurses play an important role in promoting and maintaining health in infants. Although the infant mortality rate in the United States has declined markedly over the past 30 years (see Chapter 1), many infants still die before the first birthday. The leading cause of death in infants under 1 year of age is congenital anomalies, followed by complications related to short gestational age and sudden infant death syndrome (SIDS) (U.S. Department of Health and Human Services (DHHS) National Center for Health Statistics, 2005). Unintentional injuries rank sixth in this age group and contribute to mortality and morbidity rates in the infant population (Centers for Disease Control and Prevention National Center for Injury Prevention and Control, 2004). Nurses provide anticipatory guidance for families with infants to reduce morbidity and mortality rates. Providing parents with information about immunizations, feeding, sleep, hygiene, safety, and other common concerns is an important nursing responsibility. Appropriate anticipatory guidance can assist with achieving some of the goals and objectives determined by the U.S. government to be important in improving the overall health of infants (Box 5-1). Nurses are in a good position to offer anticipatory guidance on the basis of the infant's growth and achievement of developmental milestones. Table 5-1 summarizes growth and development during infancy.

Physical Growth and Development

Growth is an excellent indicator of overall health during infancy. Although growth rates are variable, infants usually double their birth weight by 6 months and triple it by

BOX 5-1	*Healthy People 2010* Objectives for Infants
1-12	Establish a single toll-free telephone number for access to poison control centers on a 24-hour basis throughout the United States.
8-11	Eliminate elevated blood lead levels in children.
14-1	Reduce or eliminate indigenous cases of vaccine-preventable disease.
14-5	Reduce invasive pneumococcal infections.
15-7, 8	Reduce nonfatal and fatal poisonings.
15-9	Reduce deaths caused by suffocation.
15-13	Reduce deaths caused by unintentional injuries.
15-20	Increase use of child restraints.
15-33	Reduce maltreatment, and maltreatment fatalities, of children.
28-11	Increase the proportion of newborn infants who are screened for hearing loss by age 1 month, who have audiologic evaluation by age 3 months, and who are enrolled in appropriate intervention services by age 6 months.

Modified from U.S. Department of Health and Human Services. (2000). *Healthy People 2010* (Conference edition, in 2 volumes). Washington, DC: U.S. Department of Health and Human Services.

1 year of age. From an average birth weight of 7½ to 8 pounds (3.4 to 3.6 kg), neonates lose 10% of their body weight shortly after birth but regain birth weight by 2 weeks. On average, they gain ½ to ⅔ ounce per day. During the first 5 to 6 months, the average weight gain is 1½ pounds (0.68 kg) per month. Throughout the next 6 months, the weight increase is approximately 1 pound (0.45 kg) per month. Weight gain in formula-fed infants is slightly greater than in breastfed infants.

During the first 6 months, infants increase their birth length by approximately 1 inch (2.54 cm) per month, slowing to ½ inch (1.27 cm) per month over the next 6 months. By 1 year of age, most infants have increased their birth length by 50%.

The head circumference growth rate during the first year is approximately ⁴⁄₁₀ inch (1 cm) per month. Usually the posterior fontanel closes by 2 to 3 months of age, whereas the larger anterior fontanel may remain open until 18 months. Head circumference and fontanel measurements indicate brain growth and are obtained, along with height and weight, at each well-baby visit. Chapter 9 discusses growth rate monitoring throughout infancy.

Maturation of Body Systems

In addition to height and weight, organ systems grow and mature rapidly in the infant. Although body systems are developing rapidly, the infant's organs differ from those of older children and adults in both structure and function. These differences place the infant at risk for problems that might not be expected in older individuals. Knowledge of these differences provides the nurse with important rationales on which to base anticipatory guidance and specific nursing interventions.

TABLE 5-1   Summary of Growth and Development: The Infant

Physical	Motor	Psychosocial	Sensory/Cognitive	Language/Communication
1-2 months Fast growth; weight gain of 1½ pounds (0.68 kg) per month and height gain of 1 inch (2.54 cm) per month during first 6 months. Upper limbs and head grow faster. Primitive reflexes present; strong suck and gag reflex. Obligate nose breather. Posterior fontanel closes by 2-3 months.	**Gross** May lift head when held against shoulder. Head lag. **Fine** Palmar grasp. *1 month:* Immediately drops object placed in hand. Fist usually clenched (grasp reflex). *2 months:* Holds objects momentarily. Hands often open (grasp reflex fading).	Erikson's stage of trust vs. mistrust. Infant learns that world is good and "I am good." This stage is the foundation for other stages. Child is entirely dependent on parents and other caregivers. Needs should be met in a timely fashion. Touch is important.	Piaget's sensorimotor phase. *1 month:* Notes bright objects if in line of vision. Vision 20/100. Reflexes dominate behavior. *2 months:* Begins to follow objects.	Strong cry. Throaty sounds. Responds to human faces. *6-8 weeks:* Begins to smile in response to stimuli.
3 months Primitive reflexes fading.	**Gross** Can get hand to mouth. Can lift head off bed when in prone position. Head lag still present but decreasing. **Fine** Holds objects placed in hands. Grasp reflex absent.	Smiles in response to others. Uses sucking to soothe self.	Follows an object with eyes. Plays with fingers.	Babbles, coos. Enjoys making sounds. Responds to voices, watches speaker.
4-5 months Can breathe when nose is obstructed. Growth rate declines. Drooling begins in preparation for teething. Moro, tonic neck, and rooting reflexes have disappeared.	**Gross** Plays with feet; puts foot in mouth. Bears weight when held in a standing position. Turns from abdomen to back. **Fine** Begins reaching and grasping with palm. Hits at object, misses.	Mouth is a sensory organ used to explore environment. Attachment is continuing process throughout infancy. Has increased interest in parent, shows trust, knows parent. Shows emotions of fear and anger.	*4 months:* Brings hands together at midline. Vision 20/80. Begins to play with objects. Recognizes familiar faces. Turns head to locate sounds. Shows anticipation and excitement. Memory span is 5-7 minutes. Plays with favorite toys.	Crying becomes differentiated. Babbling is common. Begins consonant sounds: *H, N, G, K, P, B* (4 months). Makes vowel sounds: *ee, ah, ooh* (5 months).

Neurologic System. Brain growth and differentiation occur rapidly during the first year of life and they depend on nutrition and the function of the other organ systems. At birth, the brain accounts for approximately 10% to 12% of body weight. By 1 year of age, the brain has doubled its weight, with a major growth spurt occurring between 15 and 20 weeks of age and another between 30 weeks and 1 year of age. Increases in the number of synapses and expanded myelination of nerves contribute to maturation of the neurologic system during infancy. Primitive reflexes disappear as the cerebral cortex thickens and motor areas of the brain continue to develop, proceeding in a cephalocaudal pattern: arms first, then legs (Box 5-2).

Respiratory System. In the first year of life, the lungs increase to three times their weight and six times their volume at birth. In the newborn infant, alveoli number approximately 20 million, increasing to the adult number of 300 million by age 8 years. During infancy, the trachea remains small, supported only by soft cartilage.

The diameter and length of the trachea, bronchi, and bronchioles increase with age. These tiny, collapsible air passages, however, leave infants vulnerable to respiratory

TABLE 5-1	Summary of Growth and Development: The Infant—cont'd

Physical	Motor	Psychosocial	Sensory/Cognitive	Language/ Communication
6-7 months Weight gain slows to 1 pound (0.45 kg) per month. Length gain of ½ inch (1.27 cm) per month. Birth weight doubles; tooth eruption begins; chewing and biting occur. Maternal iron stores are depleted.	**Gross** Sits, leaning forward on both hands; when supine, lifts head off table. Turns from back to abdomen. **Fine** Transfers objects from one hand to another. Picks up object well with the whole hand.	Smiles at self in mirror. Plays peek-a-boo. Begins to show stranger anxiety.	Can fixate on small objects. Adjusts posture to see. Responds to name. Exhibits beginning sense of object permanence. Recognizes parent in other clothes, places. Is alert for 1½-2 hours.	Produces vowel sounds and chained syllables. Begins to imitate sounds. Belly laughs. Babbles (one syllable) with pleasure. Calls for help. "Talks" to toys and image in mirror.
8-9 months Continues to gain weight, length. Patterns of bladder and bowel elimination begin to become more regular.	**Gross** Sits steadily unsupported. Can crawl and pull up. **Fine** Pincer grasp develops. Reaches for toys. Rakes for objects and releases objects.	Stranger anxiety is at its height. Separation anxiety is increasing. Follows parent around the house.	Beginning development of depth perception. Object permanence continues to develop. Uses hands to learn concepts of in and out.	Stringing together of vowels and consonants begins. First few words begin to have meaning (Mama, Daddy, bye-bye, baby). Begins to understand and obey simple commands, such as, "Wave bye-bye." Responds to "No!" Shouts for attention.
10-12 months Birth weight triples; birth length increases by 50% *(12 months)*. Head and chest circumference equal. Babinski reflex disappears.	**Gross** Can stand alone. Can walk with one hand held but crawls to get places quickly. **Fine** Releases hold on cup. Finger-feeds self *(10 months)*. Feeds self with spoon *(12 months)*. Holds crayon to mark on paper. Pincer grasp is complete *(12 months)*.	Has mood changes. Quiets self. Is quieted by music. Tenderly cuddles toy.	Vision 20/40. Searches for hidden toy. Explores boxes, inserts objects in container. Symbol recognition is developing (enjoys books).	Can say two or more words. Says "Mama" or "Dada" specifically. Waves bye-bye. Begins to differentiate between words. Enjoys jabbering. Vocalization decreases when walking. Knows own name.

difficulties caused by infection or foreign bodies. The eustachian tube is short and relatively horizontal, increasing the risk for middle ear infections.

Cardiovascular System. The cardiovascular system undergoes dramatic changes in the transition from fetal to extrauterine circulation. Fetal shunts close, and pulmonary circulation increases drastically (see Chapter 22). During infancy, the heart doubles in size and weight, the heart rate gradually slows, and blood pressure increases.

Immune System. Transplacental transfer of maternal antibodies supplements the infant's weak response to infection until approximately 3 to 4 months of age. Although the infant begins to produce immunoglobulins (Ig) soon after birth, by 1 year of age the infant has only approximately 60% of the adult IgG level, 75% of the adult IgM level, and 20% of the adult IgA level. Breast milk transmits additional IgA protection. The activity of T lymphocytes also increases after birth. Although the immune system matures during infancy, maximum protection against infection is not achieved until early childhood. This immaturity places the infant at risk for infection.

Gastrointestinal System. The stomach capacity of a neonate is approximately 10 to 20 mL, but with feedings the

---

BOX 5-2	**Infant Reflexes**

Rooting: Stroke or touch the infant's cheek or mouth; the infant should respond by searching for and attempting to suck the examiner's finger.

Sucking: If a nipple or finger is placed in the mouth so that it touches the hard palate, the infant should suck vigorously. This reflex is also indicative of functional gag and swallowing reflexes.

Ciliary: Stroking the eyelashes results in closure of one or both of the eyes.

Doll's eyes: If the infant is placed in a supine position and the head is turned from side to side, the eyes should move to the opposite side.

Moro: Holding the infant in a supine position then displacing the body downward a few centimeters causes the infant to extend, then abduct the extremities, with fingers spread in a symmetrical fashion. This may also elicit a cry.

Tonic neck: When the infant is placed in a supine position, the head is turned to one side with the opposite arm and leg extended and the arm and leg on the same side are flexed. If the head is turned to the other direction, the positioning of the extremities is reversed. This reflex may or may not be present at birth, and its absence is not considered abnormal. This is sometimes called the fencing reflex.

Palmar: If a finger is placed in the palm, the infant should respond by grasping the examiner's finger. The grasp should be symmetrical. If pressure is put on the balls of the feet, the infant should grasp with the toes.

Step: Being held upright with feet touching a flat surface causes the infant to make stepping motions.

Babinski: If the infant's foot is stroked on the outside (little toe) edge, the toes fan up and outward.

---

capacity increases rapidly to approximately 200 mL at 1 year of age. In the gastrointestinal system, enzymes needed for the digestion and absorption of proteins, fats, and carbohydrates mature and increase in concentration. Although the newborn infant's gastrointestinal system is capable of digesting protein and lactase, the ability to digest and absorb fat does not reach adult levels until approximately 6 to 9 months of age.

CRITICAL TO REMEMBER

Intake and Output in the Newborn Infant

First 2 days of life
- Intake: 65 mL/kg (30 mL/pound) a day
- Output: 2-6 voids

After the first 2 days
- Intake: 100-150 mL/kg (45-68 mL/pound) a day
- Output: 5-25 voids

Renal System. Kidney mass increases threefold during the first year of life. Although the glomeruli enlarge considerably during the first few months, the glomerular filtration rate remains low. Thus, the kidney is not effective as a filtration organ or efficient in concentrating urine until after the first year of life. Because of the functional immaturity of the renal system, the infant is at great risk for fluid and electrolyte imbalance.

CRITICAL TO REMEMBER

Risks Caused by the Infant's Immature Body Systems
- An immature respiratory system places the infant at risk for respiratory infection.
- An immature immune system places the infant at risk for infection.
- An immature renal system places the infant at risk for fluid and electrolyte imbalances.

Motor Development

During the first few months after birth, muscle growth and weight gain allow for increased control of reflexes and more purposeful movement. At 1 month, movement occurs in a random fashion, with the fists tightly clenched. Because the neck musculature is weak and the head is large, infants can lift their heads only briefly. By 2 to 3 months, infants can lift their heads 90 degrees from a prone position and can hold them steadily erect in a sitting position. During this time, active grasping gradually replaces reflexive grasping and increases in frequency as eye-hand coordination improves (see Table 5-1).

The Moro, tonic neck, and rooting reflexes disappear at approximately 3 to 4 months. These primitive reflexes, which are controlled by the midbrain, probably disappear because they are suppressed by growing cortical layers (Box 5-2). Head control steadily increases during the third month. By the fourth month, the head remains in a straight line with the body when the infant is pulled to a sitting position. Most infants play with their feet by 4 to 5 months, drawing them up to suck on their toes. Parents need anticipatory guidance about ways to prevent accidents by "baby-proofing" their homes before each motor development milestone is reached (Box 5-3).

The nurse might, for instance, explain, "Infants grow and mature very rapidly, and you will be very busy with a new baby. Now is the time to 'baby-proof' your home before Mary turns over and begins crawling and reaching for objects. By doing this now, you can prevent later injuries and worries."

During the fifth and sixth months, motor development accelerates rapidly. Infants of this age readily reach for and grasp objects. They can bear weight when held in a standing position and can turn from abdomen to back. By 5 months, some infants rock back and forth as a precursor to crawling.

| BOX 5-3 | **PARENTS WANT TO KNOW** How to "Baby Proof" the Home |

By the time babies reach 6 months of age, they begin to become much more active, curious, and mobile. Although your baby might not be creeping or crawling yet, it is difficult to predict when that will happen. For this reason, you need to be prepared by making sure your house and the toys with which the baby plays are safe. Babies learn through exploring and participating in many different types of experiences. By keeping the baby's environment safe, you can encourage these experiences for your baby.

Be sure to check the following:
- All small or sharp objects or dangerous substances should be out of the baby's reach. Get down to the baby's eye level to be sure. This includes plants and paint chips, which can be poisonous. Be sure to check that any bedside table near the baby's crib is kept clear of ointments, creams, pins, or any other small objects. Be sure to check that small pieces from older siblings' toys are put away. Keep money put away.
- Put plastic fillers in all plugs, and put cabinet and drawer locks on all cabinets and drawers. Doorknob covers are also available that prevent the infant from opening the door.
- Remove front knobs from the stove. Be sure to keep all pot and pan handles turned away from the edge of the stove.
- Remove from lower cabinets and lock away all dangerous or poisonous substances, including such items as

pet food, household cleaning agents, cosmetic aids, pesticides, plant fertilizers, paints, matches, medicines, and plastic bags. Be sure to store these products in their original containers. Never give a small child a latex balloon.
- Place a gate on the top and bottom of stairways. Be sure the gate does not have openings that can trap the baby's head, hands, or fingers.
- Remove heavy containers from table tops covered with a tablecloth. Do not hold the baby on your lap while drinking or eating any kind of hot foods.
- Pad furniture with sharp edges. Be sure all windows have screens.
- Keep household hot water temperature at less than 120° F; always test water temperature before bathing the baby. **Never leave a baby unattended near water** (toilet, bathtub, swimming pool). Keep water containers or tubs empty when not in use. Be sure there is no direct entrance to a back yard swimming pool through the house.
- Shorten all hanging cords (appliance, window cords, telephone) so they are out of the baby's reach. Be sure pull toy cords are shorter than 12 inches.
- Have your house tested for sources of lead.
- Never leave your baby unattended or in the care of a young sibling.

Six-month-old infants can sit alone, leaning forward on their hands. This ability provides them with a wider view of the world and creates new ways to play. Infants of this age can roll from back to abdomen and can raise their heads from the table when supine. At 6 to 7 months, they transfer objects from one hand to another. In addition, they can grab small objects with the whole hand and insert them into their mouths with lightning speed.

At 6 to 9 months, infants begin to explore the world by crawling. By 9 months, most infants have enough muscle strength and coordination to pull themselves up and cruise around furniture. These new methods of mobility enable the infant to follow a parent or caregiver around the house.

By 6 to 7 months, infants become increasingly adept at pointing to make their demands known. Six-month-old infants grasp objects with all their fingers in a raking motion, but 9-month-olds use their thumbs and forefingers in a fine motor skill called the *pincer grasp*. This grasp provides infants with a useful yet potentially dangerous ability to grab, hold, and insert tiny objects into their mouths.

Nine-month-old infants can wave bye-bye and clap their hands together. They can pick up objects but have difficulty releasing them on request. By 1 year of age, they can extend an object and release it into an offered hand. Most 1-year-old children can balance well enough to walk when holding

another person's hand. They often resort to crawling, however, as a more rapid and efficient way to move about.

An increased ability to move about, reach objects, and explore their world places infants at great risk for accidents and injury. Nurses provide information to parents about how quickly infant motor skills develop.

Cognitive Development

Many factors contribute to the way in which infants learn about their world. Besides innate intellectual aptitude and motivation, infants' sensory capabilities, neuromuscular control, and perceptual skills all affect how their cognitive processes unfold during infancy and throughout life. In addition, variables such as the quality and quantity of parental interaction and environmental stimulation contribute to cognitive development.

Cognitive development during the first 2 years of life begins with a profound state of egocentrism. Egocentrism is the child's complete self-absorption and the inability to view the world from anyone else's vantage point. As infants' cognitive capacities expand, they become increasingly aware of the outside world and their separateness from it. Gradually, with maturation and experience, they become capable of differentiating themselves from others and their surroundings.

Text continued on p. 108

The First Year: Growth and Development Milestones

During the first year after birth, the infant's development is dramatic as the child grows toward independence. Knowledge of developmental milestones helps caregivers determine whether the baby is growing and maturing as expected. The nurse should remember that these markers are averages and that healthy infants often vary. Some infants reach each milestone later than most. Knowledge of normal growth and development helps the nurse promote the safety of children. Parents should be taught to prepare for the child's safety before the child reaches each milestone.

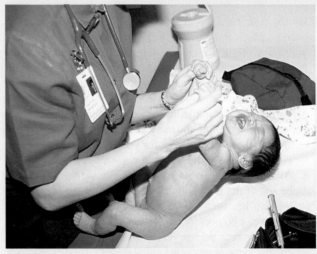

This 18-day-old infant demonstrates substantial head lag as the nurse lifts her trunk from the examining table. Weak neck muscles, combined with a large head, limit her ability to keep her head aligned with her spine as she is pulled toward a sitting position.

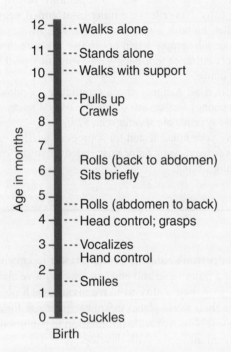

Age in months

12	Walks alone
11	Stands alone
10	Walks with support
9	Pulls up / Crawls
8	
7	
6	Rolls (back to abdomen) / Sits briefly
5	
4	Rolls (abdomen to back) / Head control; grasps
3	Vocalizes / Hand control
2	
1	Smiles
0	Suckles

Birth

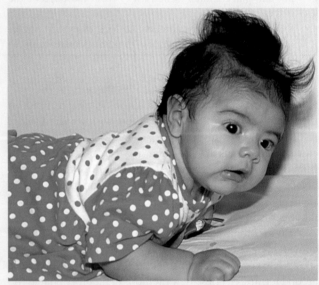

This 2-month-old infant can lift her head from the prone position and briefly hold it erect.

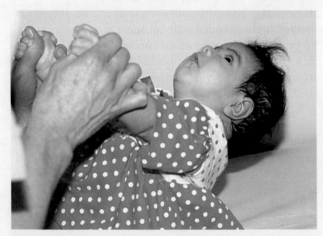

By 2 months, this infant has much less head lag as her neck muscles become stronger and better able to support her head.

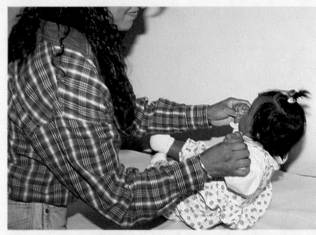

Head control steadily increases so that by 4 months this infant keeps her head in a straight line as her mother pulls her to a sitting position.

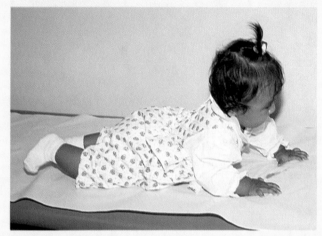

This 4-month-old infant can easily lift her head from a prone position and hold it steadily erect.

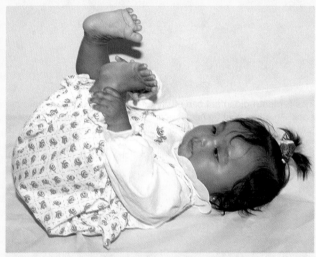

This 4-month-old infant takes pleasure in exploring her own body. She begins playing with her feet and often puts her toes in her mouth.

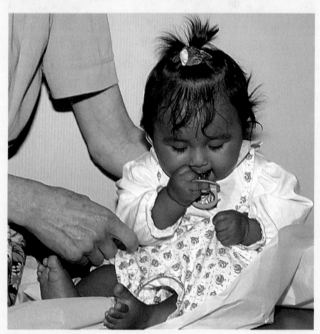

By 4 months, the infant can purposefully grasp objects with the palms of her hands.

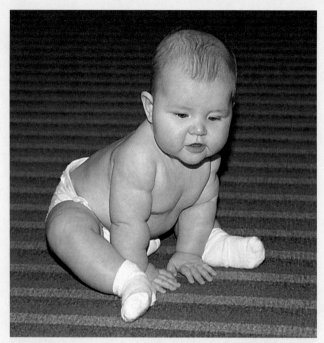

At 6 months, this infant can sit briefly if she leans forward on both hands for support. This position is called the *tripod sitting position*.

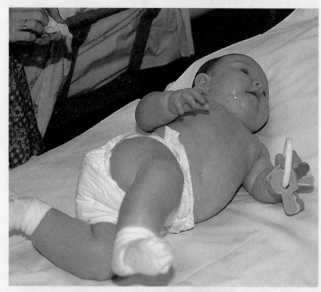

This 6-month-old infant can easily turn from her abdomen onto her back. An adult must be near if an infant of this age is on an elevated surface, such as an examining table or diaper-changing table. To reduce the risk of accidents, the nurse should teach parents about safety measures before the child reaches each developmental milestone.

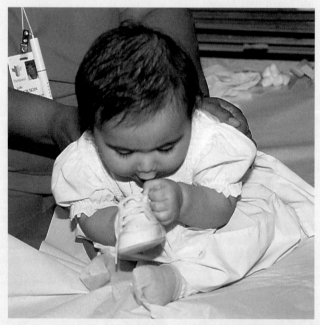

This 7-month-old infant can sit unsupported and hold her shoe. Note also that she explores it with her mouth. The nurse should teach parents that everything infants of this age can hold in their hands will go into their mouths. Parents must put dangerous materials, such as medications, cleaning solutions, and items small enough to swallow, well out of reach.

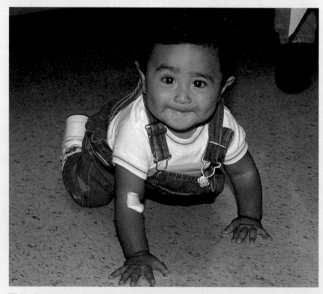

This 9-month-old infant crawls quickly, keeping his belly off the floor.

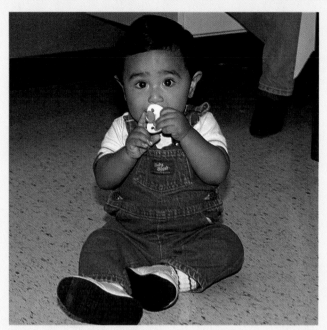

At 9 months, this infant can move easily from a crawling to a sitting position and can sit steadily with no support. He also begins grasping objects with the finer pincer grasp rather than the palmar grasp. If a parent tries to hide something, such as a pacifier, he will not forget the object and will search for it.

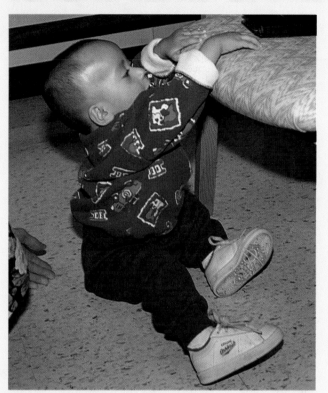

At 1 year, this infant can pull to a standing position. On a slick, hard floor such as this, an adult should be near to catch him if he slips backward while trying to pull up.

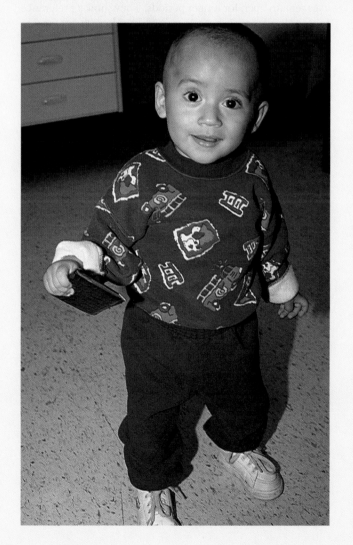

After pulling himself to a standing position, this 1-year-old child can stand alone.

After the first year, motor development is less dramatic. Nevertheless, to promote the child's safety and normal development, nurses must continue to prepare parents for new milestones.

Photos courtesy Parkland Health and Hospital Systems Community Oriented Primary Care Clinic, Dallas; and University of Texas at Arlington School of Nursing.

According to Piaget's theory (1952), cognitive development occurs in stages or periods (see Chapter 4). Infancy is included in the *sensorimotor stage* (birth to 2 years), during which infants experience the world through their senses and their attempts to control the environment. Learning activities progress from simple reflex behavior to trial-and-error experiments.

During the first month of life, infants are in the first substage, *reflex activity,* of the sensorimotor period. In this substage, behavior such as grasping, sucking, or looking is dominated by reflexes. Piaget believed that infants organize their activity, survive, and adapt to their world by the use of reflexes.

Primary circular reactions dominate the second substage, occurring from age 1 to 4 months. During this substage, reflexes become more organized and new schemata are acquired, usually centering on the infant's body. Sensual activities such as sucking and kicking become less reflexive and more controlled and are repeated because of the stimulation they provide. The baby also begins to recognize objects, especially those that bring pleasure, such as the breast or bottle.

During the third substage, or the stage of *secondary circular reactions,* infants perform actions that are more oriented toward the world outside their own bodies. The 4- to 8-month-old infant in this substage begins to play with objects in the external environment, such as a rattle or stuffed toy. The infant's actions are labeled *secondary* because they are intentional (repeated because of the response that is elicited). For example, a baby in this substage intentionally shakes a rattle to hear the sound.

By age 8 to 12 months, infants in the fourth substage, *coordination of secondary schemata,* begin to relate to objects as if they realize that the objects exist even when they are out of sight. This awareness is referred to as *object permanence* and is illustrated by a 9-month-old infant seeking a toy after it is hidden under a pillow. In contrast, 6-month-olds can follow the path of a toy that is dropped in front of them; however, they will not look for the dropped toy or protest its disappearance until they are older and have developed the concept of object permanence.

Infants in the fourth substage solve problems differently from how they solve problems in earlier substages. Rather than randomly selecting approaches to problems, they choose actions that were successful in the past. This tendency suggests that they remember and can perform some mental processing. They seem to be able to identify simple causal relationships, and they show definite intentionality. For example, when an 11-month-old child sees a toy that is beyond reach, the child uses the blanket that it is resting on to pull it closer (Flavell, 1964; Piaget, 1952).

Cognitive development in the infant parallels motor development. It appears that motor activity is necessary for cognitive development and that cognitive development is based on interaction with the environment, not simply maturation. Infancy is the period when the child lays the foundation for later cognitive functioning. Nurses can promote the cognitive development of infants by encouraging parents to interact with their infants and provide them with novel, interesting stimuli. At the same time, parents should maintain familiar, routine experiences through which their infants can develop a sense of security about the world. Within this type of environment, infants will thrive and learn.

CRITICAL TO REMEMBER
Possible Signs of Developmental Delays
- Lack of eye muscle control after 4 to 6 months suggests vision impairments and the need for further evaluation.
- Lack of a social smile by 8 to 12 weeks requires further evaluation and close follow-up

---

Sensory Development

Vision

The size of the eye at birth is approximately one half to three fourths the size of the adult eye. Growth of the eye, including its internal structures, is rapid during the first year. As infants grow and become more interested in the environment, their eyes remain open for longer periods. They show a preference for familiar faces and are increasingly able to fixate on objects. Visual acuity is estimated at approximately 20/100 to 20/150 at birth but improves rapidly during infancy and toddlerhood. Infants show a preference for high-contrast colors, such as black and white and primary colors. Pastel colors are not easily distinguished until about 6 months of age.

Young infants may lack coordination of eye movements and extraocular muscle alignment but should achieve proper coordination by age 4 to 6 months. A persistent lack of eye muscle control beyond the age of 4 to 6 months needs further evaluation. Depth perception appears to begin at approximately 7 to 9 months and contributes to the infant's new ability to move about independently.

Hearing

Hearing seems to be relatively acute, even at birth, as shown by reflexive generalized reactions to noise. With myelination of the auditory nerve tracts during the first year, responses to sound become increasingly more specialized. By 4 months, infants should turn their eyes and heads toward a sound coming from behind, and by 10 months infants should respond to the sound of their names. The National Institutes of Health and the American Academy of Pediatrics (AAP) have recommended that all newborn infants be screened for hearing impairment either as neonates or before 1 month of age and that infants who fail newborn screening have audiologic examination to verify hearing loss before age 3 months (AAP, 2000). Because some children manifest hearing loss later in infancy and childhood, periodic, objective, and age-appropriate hearing screening should be performed throughout childhood (Cunningham & Cox, 2003).

Language Development

The acquisition of language has its roots in infancy as the child becomes increasingly intrigued with sound, begins to realize that words have meaning, and eventually uses simple sounds to communicate (Box 5-4). Although young infants probably understand tones and inflections of voice rather than words themselves, it is not long before repetition and practice of sounds enable them to understand and communicate with words. Infants can understand more than they can express.

The social smile develops early in the infant, usually by 3 to 5 weeks of age (Fig. 5-1). This powerful communication tool helps to foster attachment and demonstrates that the infant can differentiate between people and objects within the environment. The infant who does not display a social smile by the age of 8 to 12 weeks needs further evaluation and close follow-up because of the possibility of developmental delay.

During infancy, connections form within the central nervous system, providing fine motor control of the numerous muscles required for speech. Maturation of the mouth, jaw, and larynx; bone growth; and development of the face help prepare the infant to speak.

Vocalization does not appear to be reflexive but rather is a relatively high-level activity similar to conversation. Parents usually elicit vocalization in infants better than other adults can. Infants' brains process speech and language in the environment, using cues, structure, and distributional patterns to construct their native tongue (Karmiloff-Smith, 1995).

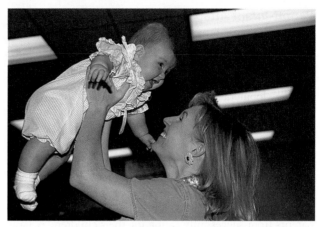

FIG 5-1 **This 6-month-old infant responds delightedly to her mother with a true social smile. Such interactive responses between parent and child promote communication and emotional development.**

Although there is great variability, most children begin to make nonmeaningful sounds, such as "ma," "da," or "ah," by 4 to 6 months. The sounds become more meaningful and specific by 9 to 15 months, and by age 1 year the child usually has a vocabulary of several words, such as "mama," "dada," and "bye-bye." Infants who have older siblings or who are raised in verbally rich environments sometimes meet these developmental milestones earlier than other infants.

Psychosocial Development

Most experts agree that infancy is a crucial period during which children develop the foundation of their personalities and their sense of self. According to Erikson's theory of psychosocial development (1963), infants struggle to establish a sense of basic *trust* rather than a sense of basic *mistrust* in their world, their caregivers, and themselves. If provided with consistent, satisfying experiences delivered in a timely manner, infants come to rely on the fact that their needs will be met and that, in turn, they will be able to tolerate some degree of frustration and discomfort until those needs are met. This sense of confidence is an early form of trust and provides the foundation for a healthy personality.

On the other hand, if infants' needs are ignored or met in a consistently haphazard, inadequate manner, they have no reason to believe that their needs will be met or that their environment is a safe, secure place. According to Erikson, without consistent satisfaction of needs, the individual develops a basic sense of suspicion or mistrust (Erikson, 1963).

Parallel to this viewpoint is Freudian theory, which regards infancy as the oral stage (Freud, 1974). The mouth is the major focus during this stage. Observation of infants for a few minutes shows that most of their behavior centers on their mouths. Sensory stimulation and pleasure as well as nourishment are experienced through their mouths. Sucking is an adaptive behavior that provides comfort and satisfaction while enabling infants to experience and explore their world. Later in infancy, as teething progresses, the mouth becomes an effective tool for aggressive behavior (see Chapter 6).

BOX 5-4	**Language and Development: Developmental Milestones in Infancy**

1 to 3 Months
Reflexive smile at first, and then smile becomes more voluntary; sets up a reciprocal smiling cycle with parent. Cooing.

3 to 4 Months
Crying becomes more differentiated. Babbling is common.

4 to 6 Months
Plays with sound, repeating sounds to self. Can identify mother's voice. May squeal in excitement.

6 to 8 Months
Single consonant babbling occurs. Increasing interest in sound.

8 to 9 Months
Stringing of vowels and consonants together begins. First few words begin to have meaning (Mama, Daddy, bye-bye, baby). Begins to understand and obey simple commands such as "Wave bye-bye."

9 to 12 Months
Vocabulary of two or three words. Gestures are used to communicate. Speech development may slow temporarily when walking begins.

Parent-Infant Attachment

One of the most important aspects of infant psychosocial development is parent-infant attachment. Attachment is a sense of belonging to or connection with each other. This significant bond between infant and parent is critical to normal development and even survival. Initiated immediately after birth, attachment is strengthened by many mutually satisfying interactions between the parents and the infant throughout the first months of life.

For example, noisy distress in infants signals a need, such as hunger. Parents respond by providing food. In turn, infants respond by quieting and accepting nourishment. The infants derive pleasure from having their hunger satiated and the parents from successfully caring for their children. A basic reciprocal cycle is set in motion in which parents learn to regulate infant feeding, sleep, and activity through a series of interactions. These interactions include rocking, touching, talking, smiling, and singing. The infants respond by quieting, eating, watching, smiling, or sleeping.

Conversely, continuing inability or unwillingness of parents to meet the dependency needs of their infants fosters insecurity and dissatisfaction in the infants. A cycle of dissatisfaction is established in which parents become frustrated as caregivers and have further difficulty providing for the infant's needs.

If parents can adapt to their infant, meet the infant's needs, and provide nurturance, attachment is secure. Psychosocial development can proceed on the basis of a strong foundation of attachment. On the other hand, if parents' personalities and abilities to cope with infant care do not match their infant's needs, the relationship is considered at risk.

Although the establishment of trust depends heavily on the quality of the parental interaction, the infant also needs consistent, satisfying social interactions within a family structure. Family routines can help to provide this consistency. Touch is an important tool that can be used by all family members to convey a sense of caring.

CRITICAL TO REMEMBER
Promotion of Parent-Infant Attachment

The establishment of a healthy parent-infant bond is an essential task in the newborn period. The nurse can aid the development of the bond by:
- Encouragement and support of breastfeeding
- Teaching about quiet/alert states and normal newborn appearance
- Providing positive feedback for learning new infant care-taking skills
- Attend to the mother's physical needs.

Stranger Anxiety

Another important aspect of psychosocial development is stranger anxiety or separation anxiety. By 6 to 7 months, expanding cognitive capacities and strong feelings of attachment enable infants to differentiate between caregivers and strangers and to be wary of the latter. Infants display an obvious preference for parents over other caregivers and other unfamiliar people. Anxiety, demonstrated by crying, clinging, and turning away from the stranger, is manifested when separation occurs. This behavior peaks at approximately 7 to 9 months and again during toddlerhood, when separation may be difficult (see Chapter 6).

Although stressful for parents, stranger anxiety is a normal sign of healthy attachment and occurs because of cognitive development (object permanence). Nurses can reassure parents that, although their infants seem distressed, leaving the infant for short periods does no harm. Separations should be accomplished swiftly, yet with care, love, and emphasis on the parents' return.

HEALTH PROMOTION FOR THE INFANT AND FAMILY

Parents, particularly new parents, often need guidance in caring for their infant. Nurses can provide valuable information about health promotion for the infant. Specific guidance about everyday concerns, such as sleep, crying, and feeding, can be offered, as well as anticipatory guidance about injury prevention. An important nursing responsibility is to provide parents with information about immunizations and dental care. Nurses can offer support to new parents by identifying strategies for coping with the first few months with an infant. The schedule of well visits corresponds with the schedule recommended by the AAP (see Appendix A). At each well visit the nurse assesses development, administers appropriate immunizations, and provides anticipatory guidance. The nurse asks the parent a series of general assessment questions (Box 5-5) and then focuses the assessment on the individual infant.

Immunization

The importance of childhood immunization against disease cannot be overemphasized. Infants are especially vulnerable to infectious disease because their immune systems are

---

BOX 5-5	**Continuing Assessment Questions**

- Nutrition—How much is your child eating, how often, what kind of foods?
- Elimination—How many wet diapers, stools? Consistency of stools?
- Safety—Use of car restraints? Gun violence?
- Hearing/vision—Any concerns?
- Can you tell me about the times you would feel it necessary to call your doctor?
- How is the family adjusting to the baby?
- Are you getting enough time alone and time together?
- Has there been any change in the household or family's lifestyle?
- Are there any financial concerns?
- Are there any other questions or concerns?

immature. Term neonates are protected from certain infections by transplacental passive immunity from their mothers. Breastfed infants receive additional Igs against many types of viruses and bacteria. Transplacental immunity is effective only for approximately 3 months, however, and for a variety of reasons many mothers choose not to breastfeed. In any case, this passive immunity does not cover all diseases, and infection in the infant can be devastating. Immunization offers protection that all infants need.

Nurses play an important role in health promotion and disease prevention related to immunization. Nursing responsibilities include assessing current immunization status, removing barriers to receiving immunizations, tracking immunization records, providing parent education, and recognizing contraindications to the receipt of vaccines. Chapter 4 provides detailed information regarding immunizations and their schedule.

CRITICAL THINKING EXERCISE 5-1

Mary Brown and her 4-week-old daughter, Tonja, are being seen for a well-baby checkup. Tonja is Mrs. Brown's first child. Mrs. Brown looks very tired and begins to cry when you ask her how she is doing.
1. What are some of the possible causes the nurse should explore?
2. How can you explore these possible causes?
3. What are some of the appropriate nursing measures?

Skin Care

Cord care should be performed after each bath and each diaper change. The umbilical stump and the area where it attaches to the abdomen are cleaned with rubbing or isopropyl alcohol. The umbilical cord usually falls off about 10 days after birth. Some slight bleeding may be noted. Parents should be taught to recognize the signs and symptoms of umbilical infection (Box 5-6).

Seborrheic dermatitis, or cradle cap, is seen in some infants. It appears as thick, yellow, scaly patches that are found on the scalp (most often over the anterior fontanel) but that may also appear on the eyebrows or eyelid. The scales may be removed by warming a small amount of baby oil, applying it to the patches, and allowing it to penetrate the crust. The crusts may then be washed away with baby shampoo. It is important to reassure parents that the condition is temporary and usually disappears by 12 months.

Some infants have *acne neonatorum*, an acne-like condition that is probably caused by hormonal changes. It generally appears when the infant is approximately 2 to 4 weeks old, and it is self-limiting, disappearing in several weeks to months.

The diaper area, including the gluteal folds, should be cleaned and thoroughly dried with each diaper change. Either warm water or baby wipes can be used. Parents should be cautioned not to use commercial baby wipes if any diaper rash is noted. It is important to teach parents to wipe females from front to back and to clean under the scrotum of males.

Feeding and Nutrition

Because infancy is a period of rapid growth, nutritional needs are of special significance. During infancy, eating progresses from a principally reflex activity to relatively sophisticated, yet messy, attempts at self-feeding. Because the infant's gastrointestinal system continues to mature throughout the first year, changes in diet, the introduction of new foods, and even upsets in routines can result in feeding problems.

Parents often have many questions and concerns about nutrition. They are influenced by a variety of sources, including relatives and friends who may not be aware of current scientific practices regarding infant feeding. To provide anticipatory guidance, the nurse must have a clear understanding of gastrointestinal maturation and knowledge about breastfeeding and various infant formulas and foods. Families and cultures vary widely in food preferences and infant feeding practices. The nurse must remain cognizant of these differences when providing anticipatory guidance related to infant nutrition.

CRITICAL TO REMEMBER
Essential Information for Infant Nutrition
- Breast milk or commercially prepared iron-fortified formula provides optimal nutrition throughout infancy.
- Formula must be prepared according to instructions, and leftover formula should be stored according to the manufacturer's directions.
- Some health care providers discourage the use of powdered formula until the infant is older than 6 weeks.

BOX 5-6	**PARENTS WANT TO KNOW** Care of the Umbilical Cord

Call your health provider if you observe:
- Bleeding
- Bad odor
- Redness
- Drainage
- The cord does not fall off after 2 weeks

Do:
- Dip a cotton swab in alcohol and clean around the base of the cord (including the folds of skin) with every diaper change.
- Fold the diaper back below the cord.

Don't:
- Give tub baths until the cord falls off.

HEALTH PROMOTION

NEWBORN TO 1-MONTH

FOCUSED ASSESSMENT

How have you been feeling? Have you made your post-partum checkup appointment?

How have you and your partner been adjusting to the baby? Do you have other children? How are they adjusting?

Have you discussed child-rearing philosophies?

Does anyone in your household smoke cigarettes?

Does anyone in your household use substances?

Have you recently been exposed to or had any sexually transmissible disease?

Have you experienced any periods of sadness or feeling "down"?

Do you have any concerns about the costs of the baby's care?

Do you feel that you and the baby are safe?

DEVELOPMENTAL MILESTONES

Personal/social: looks at parent's face; fixates, tracks, follows to midline; smiles responsively; prefers brightly colored objects

Fine motor: newborn reflexes present

Language/cognitive: prefers human female voice: responds to sounds; begins to vocalize

Gross motor: equal movements; lifts head; lifts head and chin (by 1 month)

HEALTH MAINTENANCE

Physical Measurements

Weight—7.5-8 pounds (3.4-3.6 kg) average. Loses 10% of body weight after birth but gains it back by 2 weeks. Gains ½ ounce a day on average.

Length—Average 20 inches (50 cm). Gains 1 inch (2.5 cm) a month for the first several months.

Head Circumference—13-14 inches (33-35.5 cm). Gains average of ½ inch (1.2 cm) per month until 6 months of age. Posterior fontanel closes by 2-3 months; anterior by 12-18 months.

Immunizations

Thimerosal-free hepatitis B #1 at birth and #2 at 1 month. Be sure to discuss side effects. Give the parent information about upcoming immunizations. If planning to use combination vaccine (diphtheria-tetanus-acellular pertussis, hepatitis B, polio) instead of hepatitis B #2, wait until 2 months for second hepatitis B.

Health Screening

Phenylketonuria and other metabolic diseases

Hearing screening

Visual inspection for congenital defects

ANTICIPATORY GUIDANCE

Nutrition

Breast milk on demand at least every 2-3 hours

Iron-fortified formula 2-3 ounces every 3-4 hours

Vitamin D supplement 200 IU/day for breastfed infants and for formula-fed babies consuming less than 16 ounces/day

Place on right side after feeding

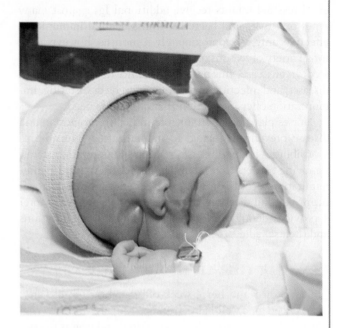

Elimination

6 wet diapers

Stools related to feeding method

Dental

Continue prenatal vitamins and calcium if breastfeeding

Sleep

Place on back to sleep in parent's room in a separate crib/cradle/bassinet. Keep loose or soft bedding and toys out of the crib, offer pacifier for nap and bedtime if not breastfeeding.

16 or more hours

Hygiene

Sponge bathe until cord falls off

Circumcision care

Safety

Be sure crib is safe: slats <2⅜ inches apart, firm mattress that fits the crib

Eliminate all environmental smoke

Rear-facing approved infant car seat

Fire prevention: smoke detectors, fire extinguishers

Water temperature <120 degrees

Cardiopulmonary resuscitation and first aid classes; emergency phone numbers

Violence: discuss shaking, guns in the home

Factors Influencing Choice of Feeding Method

The AAP strongly recommends breastfeeding for all infants, including premature and sick newborns, with rare exceptions (AAP Work Group on Breastfeeding, 1997; AAP, 2005a; Dobson & Murtaugh, 2001). Mothers who breastfeed need instruction and support as they begin. They are more likely to succeed if they are given practical information. Many facilities provide lactation consultants or home visits, or nursing staff may call to assess the mother's needs. Significant others are included in teaching to provide a support system for the mother.

A goal set by the U.S. DHHS for the year 2010 is for 75% of all new mothers to breastfeed at the time of birth facility discharge, for at least 50% to be breastfeeding at 6 months, and 25% at 1 year (U.S. DHHS, 2000). In 2000, 68.4% of mothers began to breastfeed their newborn infants. At 6 months, 31.4% of mothers were breastfeeding. At 12 months, the rate was 17.6% breastfeeding. These statistics show a gradual but steady increase since 1991 (Ross Products Division, 2003), but continued improvement is needed. Table 5-2 lists the benefits of breastfeeding.

In an effort to promote breastfeeding, the United Nations Children's Fund and the World Health Organization advocate that birth facilities become certified as "baby-friendly" hospitals, where policies are initiated to actively encourage breastfeeding. Guidelines to becoming certified as a baby-friendly hospital emphasize education of staff and parents about breastfeeding, early initiation of breastfeeding, demand feeding, avoidance of formula and pacifiers, and rooming-in.

Some parents prefer a combination of breastfeeding and bottle feeding. Giving breastfeeding infants formula leads to a decrease in breastfeeding frequency and milk production, making successful breastfeeding less likely (AAP & American College of Obstetricians and Gynecologists, 2002). Women who use a combination of breast milk and formula are likely to breastfeed for shorter durations than women who breastfeed exclusively (Chezem et al., 2003).

Unless medically indicated, it is best to delay giving formula until lactation has been well established. However, if the mother chooses to feed both breast milk and formula, the nurse should support her so that the infant receives the benefits of breast milk at least part of the time.

Some mothers choose to give a bottle daily or only occasionally, such as when a babysitter is with the infant. This allows the mother to be away from the infant for longer periods of time yet allows the closeness with the infant that many mothers enjoy and the physical advantages of breastfeeding to continue. Mothers may choose to use breast milk or formula for occasional bottle feedings.

Support from Others. The influence of family members is often an important determinant of whether mothers breastfeed. The mother with little support or with active discouragement from her family will probably have a difficult time nursing. Educating family members about the advantages of breastfeeding and how to deal with problems may lead to their encouragement of the breastfeeding mother. Some women choose not to breastfeed because their partner objects. However, one study of men from African American, Hispanic, and other cultures found that 81% wanted their infants to be breastfed (Pollock, Bustamante-Forest, & Giarratano, 2002).

Encouragement from the woman's health care provider may increase the chance that she will breastfeed. One study found that women were more likely to still be breastfeeding at 12 weeks if they had received encouragement from their provider (Taveras et al., 2003). The support the mother receives from the nurse plays a significant part in whether she feels comfortable with the feeding method she chooses. Those who do not feel confident in their ability to breastfeed are less likely to continue breastfeeding if they encounter difficulties at home.

If the mother has difficulty breastfeeding, the infant is exhibiting any problems related to diminished milk supply, or the infant has a medical problem (e.g., jaundice, cleft lip or palate) that would interfere with breastfeeding, the nurse can refer the mother to a lactation specialist or

---

TABLE 5-2	Benefits of Breastfeeding

For the Infant	**For the Mother**
Allergies are less likely to develop.	Oxytocin release enhances involution of uterus.
Immunologic properties help prevent infections. May have fewer respiratory, ear, and gastrointestinal infections and less risk for SIDS.	Mother loses less blood because of delayed return of menses.
Composition meets infant's specific nutritional needs.	Mother more likely to rest while feeding.
Nutritional and immunologic properties change according to infant's needs.	Mother likely to eat balanced diet that improves healing.
Breast milk easily digested.	Frequent, close contact may enhance bonding.
Protein, fat, and carbohydrate in most suitable proportions.	Convenient: always available, no bottles to prepare, no formula to buy or heat.
No possibility of improper (and potentially dangerous) dilution.	Economical: eliminates cost of formula and bottles.
Breast milk unlikely to be contaminated; not affected by water supply.	Traveling easier: no bottles to prepare, carry, refrigerate, or warm.
Less likely to result in overfeeding.	May reduce the risk of some cancers.
Infant unlikely to have constipation.	

organizations such as La Leche League. La Leche League chapters are available in most communities and are listed in the telephone book. Support groups may also be provided by the birth facility.

Culture. Cultural influences may dictate decisions about how a mother feeds her infant. For example, many Mormon women believe that breastfeeding is an important part of motherhood. Muslim women often breastfeed for the first 2 years. Immigrants from countries where breastfeeding is not the norm may breastfeed for shorter durations. In addition, formula feeding may be seen as a symbol of the new way of life.

Nurses should be particularly watchful for ways to help mothers from other cultures who might wish to breastfeed but fail to do so because of lack of support. Canadian Mohawk mothers were more likely to breastfeed when a woman from their community worked with them and the grandmother in promoting the value of breastfeeding (Banks, 2003).

Some Asian and Hispanic mothers give their infants formula while in the birth facility and do not begin to breastfeed until at home. This practice may be because of modesty about nursing in front of others in the birth facility and lack of understanding about the value of colostrum. Some Korean women believe they should not breastfeed for the first 3 days after birth (Windsor, 2003). Women in some cultures believe that colostrum may be "spoiled" because it has been in the breasts for a long time. They may express colostrum and discard it before they begin to breastfeed the infant.

Certain foods are used to increase milk production in some cultures. Examples include broth from blue cornmeal for Navajo Indians, chocolate for women from Guatemala, and anise or sesame seed for Hispanic women (Biancuzzo, 2003).

Employment. Returning to work or school is a major cause of discontinuation of breastfeeding by 10 to 12 weeks (Taveras et al., 2003). The mother may choose formula from the beginning, plan a short period of breastfeeding before weaning the infant to formula, or use a combination of breastfeeding and bottle feeding with breast milk or formula. Nurses who provide practical information about breastfeeding and working may help a mother continue breastfeeding for a longer period.

Women who will be using a breast pump at work should have a place to pump once or twice during breaks or lunch time. The place should be clean and private. If the woman pumps a couple of times a day for a week or two before returning to work, she will be adept at using the pump and will have a supply of breast milk for the caregiver to use while she is at work. Frequent breastfeeding during the evening and weekends will help her maintain her milk supply.

Other Factors. Other factors may also influence a woman's decision. Her knowledge and experience with infant feeding are important. Women who are most likely to breastfeed are older than 35 years, are white, have a college education, and live in the western part of the United States. Those with the lowest breastfeeding rates are African American, have a grade-school education, are employed full-time, are younger than 20 years, and live in the southern United States (Ross Products Division, 2003). Consistent with previous research, the National Immunization Survey breastfeeding data also revealed that non-Hispanic black and socioeconomically disadvantaged groups have lower breastfeeding rates (Centers for Disease Control and Prevention, 2004).

Normal Breastfeeding

The pediatric nurse may encounter mothers of newborn infants on the pediatric unit and therefore should have current knowledge of both advantages of breastfeeding and proper breastfeeding techniques.

Advantages. Breast milk contains a more complete protein than cow's milk–based formulas, is more easily digested, and results in more rapid gastric emptying time. For this reason, infants who breastfeed need to eat more frequently than do formula-fed infants. Breastfeeding is convenient, economical, and enhances mother-infant attachment and interaction.

Human milk changes to meet the changing nutrient needs of the infant. Human milk and colostrum contain immunologic and antibacterial components not available in formula. Human milk is higher in lactose, which is converted to monosaccharide galactose, essential for central nervous system development and growth.

The fat content of breast milk is higher in monounsaturated fat, which is more easily digested and absorbed than fat in formulas. The fat content varies during the feeding and the time of day. The milk produced at the end of a feeding (hindmilk) and in the middle of the day has a higher fat content. Because the milk at the beginning of a feeding (foremilk) has less fat content than at the end, it is important that the length of feeding time be sufficient for the infant to derive benefits from the higher-fat hindmilk.

Infants who are exclusively breastfed need vitamin D supplementation to prevent rickets. The AAP (Gartner & Greer, 2003) recommends vitamin D supplementation of 200 IU/day for all breastfed infants and for formula-fed infants who consume less than 16 ounces of vitamin D–fortified formula a day.

Breastfeeding Techniques. A breastfeeding mother can use one of several positions for feeding (Box 5-7). It is important for the infant's head and body to be directly facing the breast in a "tummy to tummy" position at a height that prevents pulling or tension on the nipple. Hand position for feeding is important. Either a "C" position (see Box 5-7) or a "V" position is acceptable. In the "V" position, the mother uses both forefinger and middle finger to lift and support the breast. Because suckling releases *prolactin* (the hormone responsible for milk production), the more frequently the infant feeds, the better the mother's milk supply.

Breastfeeding Concerns. Because they cannot visually observe the amount of milk the infant is receiving, many mothers become concerned that the baby is not receiving enough. The nurse assists the mother to observe the infant swallow

| BOX 5-7 | **PARENTS WANT TO KNOW** Guidelines for Breastfeeding |

1. Wash hands. Wash nipples with warm water, no soap.
2. There are three basic positions:
   a. Cradle position: Cradle your infant in one arm, with the head resting in the bend of your elbows. The infant's mouth is close to the breast. You can be sitting up straight in bed, with pillows supporting your back or sitting in a chair. Sometimes a pillow may be needed on your lap to elevate the infant to the nipple level.

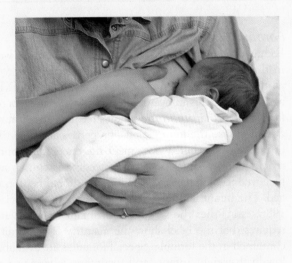

   b. Lying-down position: Lie on your side in bed with your infant lying on the side facing you.

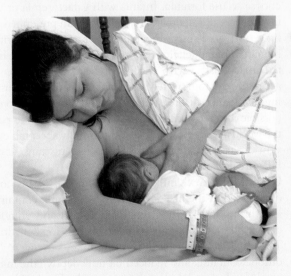

   c. Football hold: A pillow is needed to be successful with this position. Sit in a chair and place a pillow next to you on the nursing side. The pillow supports the elbow and your infant's buttocks and should bring your infant's head up to the level of your breast.

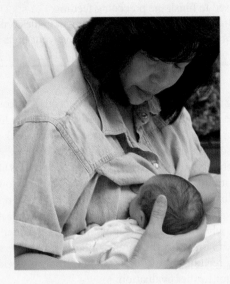

3. Hold the breast so the nipple brushes the center of the infant's lips and wait for the infant to open the mouth.
4. Your infant's mouth should be opened wide, as with a yawn, and should cover the entire areola, or a large amount of the areola. If necessary, apply pressure to your infant's chin with your index finger to open the infant's mouth wider. Your breast needs to be placed far back into the infant's mouth to drain the breast adequately. Your hand position is important: Hold your hand in a "C" position around your breast with the thumb on top behind the areola and the fingers against the chest wall and supporting the underside of the breast.

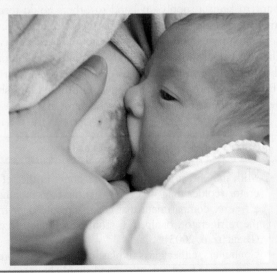

Continued

BOX 5-7 | **PARENTS WANT TO KNOW** Guidelines for Breastfeeding—cont'd

5. Both breasts are used in each feeding, usually 10 to 15 minutes on the first side, followed by burping before beginning the second side. The length of time on the second side is related to the quality of the infant's suckling. At the next feeding, your infant starts to feed on the breast used to finish the preceding feeding.
6. Break suction by placing your finger in the corner of your infant's mouth and quickly remove your breast.

7. The neonate is nursed shortly after birth and approximately every 2 to 3 hours thereafter for a total of 8 to 12 feedings a day.
8. Infants should be burped after each breast and at the end of the feeding.
9. Nipples often become tender during the first week of nursing but should not become sore. Soreness and prolonged feedings are most often the result of an infant who is not latched onto the breast properly.

---

during feeding. An infant who is receiving adequate milk will be gaining weight, appear satisfied after feedings, have at least six wet diapers a day (after the first week), and have loose, golden (mustard color and texture) stools.

Although infants are sleepier the few first days after birth, some infants continue this pattern and need some gentle stimulus to either wake for a feeding or to wake up during a feeding. It is best to completely remove the breast from an infant who has fallen asleep while nursing rather than jiggling the breast in the infant's mouth. Excessive sleepiness during feeding in an infant younger than 6 weeks may be cause for further evaluation.

Because movement of the tongue is different between bottle feeding and breastfeeding, it is best to avoid bottle feeding until the mother's milk supply is fully established. Some lactation specialists advise mothers to avoid pacifier use as well. The AAP (2005d), in its revised recommendations for preventing SIDS in infants, states that evidence suggests that giving an infant a pacifier for nap or night sleep may be protective against SIDS. It recommends that pacifiers be offered to all bottle-fed infants and to breastfed infants older than one month (AAP, 2005d).

Milk Storage. Many mothers choose to pump and store breast milk, either because they have returned to work or want to keep a supply on hand so others could feed the infant. Expressed breast milk is relatively free from bacterial contamination, but it can become contaminated when artificially collected and stored. Hands and collection equipment should be clean and the expressed milk stored appropriately (Box 5-8). Expressed milk not used within 24 hours should be frozen; thawed milk should not be refrozen.

BOX 5-8 | **Tips for Storing Breast Milk**

- Milk may be stored for 24 to 48 hours in the refrigerator (colder than 4° C [39° F]), up to 3 months in a freezer compartment that has a separate door from the refrigerator, or up to 6 months in a deep freezer (Biancuzzo, 2003).
- Containers, either glass or plastic, used to store breast milk should have a tight cap and should be sterile.
- To thaw breast milk, either thaw in the refrigerator or by holding under warm, running water.

Formula Feeding

Formula given by bottle is a choice selected by many women in the United States. This method is often easier for the mother who must return to work soon after her infant's birth, and it has the advantage of allowing other members of the family to participate in the infant's feeding. Infant formula does not have the immunologic properties and digestibility of human milk, but it does meet the energy and nutrient requirements of infants. If bottle feeding is chosen as the preferred feeding method, the formula should be iron fortified. The Infant Formula Act of 1980, which was revised in 1986, establishes the standards for infant formulas. It also requires that the label show the quantity of each nutrient contained in the formula. Special formulas are available for low-birth-weight infants and for infants allergic to cow's milk–based formulas.

There are some physiologic reasons why some mothers choose to use formula. Infants with galactosemia or whose mothers use illegal drugs, are taking certain prescribed drugs, have untreated active tuberculosis, or are infected with the human immunodeficiency virus (HIV) should not be breastfed. In countries with access to clean water and cultural acceptance of formula feeding as an alternative to breastfeeding, avoidance of breastfeeding by HIV-infected women is possible and recommended (CDC, 2005). In some parts of the world affordable, feasible and culturally acceptable interventions to decrease the risk of breastfeeding transmission of HIV are desperately needed (AAP, 2003a).

Cow's Milk. Cow's milk (whole, skim, 1%, 2%) is not recommended in the first 12 months. Cow's milk contains too little iron, and its high renal solute load and unmodified derivatives can put small infants at risk for dehydration. The tough, hard curd is difficult for infants to digest. In addition, skim milk and reduced-fat milk deprive the infant of needed calories and essential fatty acids. The incidences of allergy and iron deficiency anemia are higher in infants who are given cow's milk than in those who receive breast milk or formula.

Types of Formula. Formula can be purchased in three different forms.

Ready-to-Use Preparations. Ready-to-use formula can be poured directly into a bottle from a can, or it is available in bottles to which a nipple is added. Ready-to-use formula is the most expensive of the available formulas, but it is the most convenient. This formula would be the formula of choice if the water supply were unsafe. Ready-to-use formula should be refrigerated after opening and discarded after 24 hours or according to the manufacturer's recommendation.

Concentrated Liquid. Concentrated liquid is mixed with water according to instructions after the top of the can is washed before opening. It is important for the nurse to emphasize that the parent carefully check the formula can to avoid confusing concentrated formula with ready-to-use formula. Once opened, the can is refrigerated and discarded after 24 hours.

Powdered Formula. Powdered formula is mixed with warm water according to manufacturer directions, usually one scoop of powder for each 2 ounces of warm water in a bottle. It is important to emphasize that the powder should be uniformly dissolved before it is fed to the infant. Powdered formula is convenient and economical because it can be mixed one bottle at a time without waste.

Although commercially prepared formulas have many similarities, there are also differences. Some commonly used brands are Enfamil, SMA, Similac, Gerber, and Good Start. There are formulas specifically designed for infants older than 6 months, but it is not necessary to change to a different formula when a child reaches that age. Some formulas are designed for feeding low-birth-weight or ill infants. These include high-calorie formulas (24 cal.) and predigested formulas (e.g., Pregestimil, Neutramagen). All formulas given to infants should be iron fortified.

Formula can be fed at room temperature or warmed in hot water. Advise the parent not to warm the formula in the microwave because the formula will be warmer than the container and could burn the infant. Testing the temperature of the formula by sprinkling a few drops on the inside of the wrist can prevent giving formula that is too hot.

Newborn infants usually consume 2 to 3 ounces of formula per feeding in six to eight feedings a day. Intake increases as the infant grows.

Formula Preparation. Many different types of bottles and nipples are available. Mothers may use glass or plastic bottles or a plastic liner that fits into a rigid container. A variety of nipples is also available; the nipple choice usually is based on parent or infant preference.

Depending on the formula choice, the mother can prepare a single bottle or a 24-hour supply. Bottles and formula are not routinely sterilized where sanitary conditions are adequate, refrigeration is available, and the infant has a normal immune system. Clean technique, which consists of good handwashing and washing of all equipment is sufficient. Glass and plastic bottles can be washed in the dishwasher; nipples should be cleaned in hot, sudsy water and air dried. If safety of the water supply is questionable, sterilization, by aseptic or terminal method, is required. In the aseptic method, the bottles, nipples, and other supplies are sterilized separately from the formula by boiling for 5 minutes. Then the bottles are removed from the water with tongs, formula and water are added, and the bottles capped and refrigerated. In the terminal method, formula is poured in unsterilized bottles, loosely capped, and placed in a sterilizer or pan of water to be boiled for 25 minutes. The caps are tightened and the bottles are refrigerated.

Formula Feeding Techniques. It should not be assumed that parents know how to bottle feed an infant. The nurse may need to teach them how often and how much to feed, how to hold and cuddle while feeding, when and how to burp, and how to prepare formula. The nurse demonstrates to the mother how to position the infant in a semiupright position, preferably in a cradle hold (Fig. 5-2) to facilitate face-to-face contact. To minimize excessive intake of air during feeding, the bottle should be held so that the nipple is completely filled with formula. Advise the parent to burp the infant frequently, approximately every ½ to 1 ounce. To burp the infant, the parent holds the infant upright, either against the parent's shoulder or sitting on the parent's lap sideways with the child supported. Gentle rubbing of the back usually will elicit a burp.

Caution mothers not to prop the bottle. Propping increases the likelihood of choking if regurgitation occurs and eliminates the holding and cuddling that should accompany feeding. Infants who go to sleep with a bottle propped are at risk for aspiration. Pooled milk in the mouth leads to cavities once the teeth are in. Otitis media is more common in infants who sleep with a bottle or who have a propped bottle.

The mother should not try to coax the infant to finish the bottle at each feeding. This action could result in regurgitation and excessive weight gain. Discarding unused formula within an hour prevents feeding the infant formula contaminated by rapidly growing bacteria.

Weaning

Weaning is the replacement of breast or bottle feedings with drinking from a cup. Infants usually have a decreasing interest

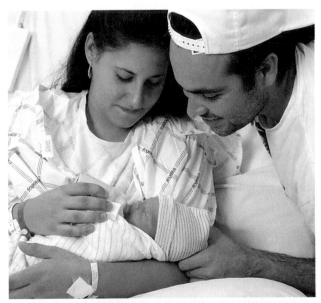

FIG 5-2 **This mother holds her infant close during bottle feeding. The bottle is positioned so the nipple is filled with milk at all times. The father offers encouragement.**

HEALTH PROMOTION

THE 2-MONTH-OLD INFANT

FOCUSED ASSESSMENT

How have things been going in the family?

Are you getting enough opportunities to continue relationships and activities away from the baby?

Will you describe the baby's personality?

Did the baby have any reaction to the last immunizations? If so, what happened?

Developmental Milestones

Personal/social: smiles spontaneously; enjoys interacting with others

Fine motor: follows past midline; reflexes disappear

Language/cognitive: vocalizes "ooh" and "ah" sounds; attends to voices

Gross motor: beginning head control when upright; lifts head 45 degrees onto forearms

Critical Milestones*

Personal/social: smiles responsively; looks at faces

Fine motor: follows to midline

Language/cognitive: vocalizes making cooing or short vowel sounds; responds to a bell

Gross motor: lifts head; equal movements

HEALTH MAINTENANCE

Physical Measurements

Measure length, weight, and head circumference and plot on growth charts

Immunizations

Diphtheria, tetanus, acellular pertussis (DTaP)#1; inactivated poliovirus (IPV) #1 (May substitute DTaP, hepatitis B, and polio combination vaccine); *Haemophilus influenzae* type b (HIB)#1; pneumococcal #1; rotavirus #1

Discuss potential effects

Health Screening

Hearing screen if not done at birth

Check eyes for strabismus

Assess ability to follow past midline

ANTICIPATORY GUIDANCE

Nutrition

Breastfeed on demand with increasing intervals

Formula, 4 to 6 ounces six times per day

Vitamin D supplementation 200 IU/day for breastfeeding infants

Elimination

Six wet diapers

Stools related to feeding method; may decrease in number

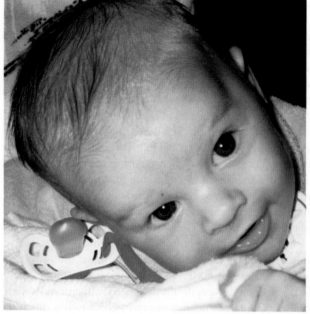

Photo courtesy Lisa Newton.

Dental

Continue prenatal vitamins and calcium if breastfeeding

Do not prop baby's bottle

Sleep

Place on back to sleep in parent's room in a separate crib/cradle/bassinet. Keep loose or soft bedding and toys out of the crib, offer pacifier for nap and bedtime.

Begin to establish nighttime routine

Play with baby when awake

Hygiene

Bathe several times per week

Watch for diaper rash and seborrheic dermatitis

Safety

Review house and environmental safety and conditions for calling the doctor; posting of emergency numbers near the telephone, car safety, and violence, avoidance of exposure to cigarette smoke

Discuss preventing falls; burns from hot liquids

Play

Imitate vocalizations and smile

Sing

Change infant's environment

Encourage rolling over

*Guided by Denver Developmental Screening Test II.

---

in the breast or bottle starting between ages 6 and 12 months. This varies from infant to infant, but if solids and a cup have been introduced, the infant will probably begin to indicate a readiness for the cup. Even young infants can be weaned to a regular plastic cup, although they will not be ready to hold the cup themselves until later. Some parents choose to use a sippy cup—a cup with a tight cover that prevents contents

from spilling when dropped. When weaning is begun after age 18 months, the infant may resist because of increased attachment to the breast or bottle.

Behaviors that might indicate a readiness to begin weaning include:

- Throwing the bottle down
- Chewing on the nipple

- Taking only a few ounces of formula
- Refusing the breast or dawdling

Weaning should not take place during times of change or stress (e.g., illness, starting child care, the arrival of a new baby). Weaning is a gradual process and should start with the replacement of one bottle or breastfeeding at a time. If breastfeeding must be terminated before age 6 months, it should be replaced with bottle feedings to meet the infant's sucking needs. The older infant who has learned to use a cup may not need to use a bottle.

The first bottle or breastfeeding eliminated should be the one in which the infant is least interested. Initially the infant may accept the cup only after drinking some formula from the bottle or milk from the breast. The infant is next offered the cup before the feeding. In approximately 1 week, another feeding can be eliminated if the infant is not resisting the change. The bedtime feeding is usually the last feeding to be eliminated.

During weaning, the child is giving up time that had been spent being held in the parent's arms. The parent needs to respond to the infant's continued need to be held and cuddled. Infants should not be allowed to carry bottles or sippy cups around as toys, to take them to bed, or to use them as pacifiers. Infants who indicate sucking needs should be given pacifiers.

Juices

Once the infant takes fluids from a cup, the parent can introduce small amounts (4-6 ounces/day) of fruit juice. A 6-ounce glass of fruit juice equals one fruit serving. Fruit juice lacks the fiber present in whole fruit. Nurses must be aware of the nutritional benefits and limitations of juice. The following are conclusions related to the intake of juice as determined by the AAP Committee on Nutrition (2001, p. 1212):

- Because fruit juice offers no nutritional benefits over breast milk or formula, it should not be given to infants younger than 6 months of age.
- Whole fruit is more nutritious for older infants and children, so excessive fruit juice should be avoided. However, 100% fresh or reconstituted fruit juice can be healthy when consumed as part of a well-balanced diet.
- Fruit drinks are not nutritionally equivalent to fruit juice.
- Other methods for treating diarrhea are more effective than fruit juice.
- Excessive fruit juice consumption can contribute to malnutrition because it either provides too many additional calories or it interferes with the consumption of more nutritious foods.
- Unpasteurized juice may contain pathogens that can cause serious illness.
- Calcium-fortified fruit juice provides a source of calcium but not other vital nutrients present in breast milk, formula, or cow's milk.

Because prolonged exposure of the teeth to sugars in juice can contribute to dental caries, parents should be encouraged to offer juices to their infant only by cup rather than the bottle. Certainly infants should not be given juice at bedtime.

In infants with a family history of allergies, orange and tomato juice should be delayed until age 1 year. Some prepared foods and dinners contain orange juice and tomato juice. Parents should be taught to read labels. Juice is not warmed because heating destroys vitamin C. Juices should be kept in a covered container in the refrigerator to prevent the loss of the vitamin. Juices should not be given in the bottle at night to avoid the development of nursing-bottle caries.

Water

Sufficient water is provided in breast milk and in prepared formula during the nursing period. When solid foods are introduced, it may be necessary to add water because some foods (e.g., strained meats, high-meat dinners) have a high renal solute load. Infants should be offered water as part of a feeding or during the day. Additional water is necessary when intake is low or the infant has fluid loss because of illness (fever, respiratory disease). Young infants do not need fluoridated water.

Solid Foods

The early introduction of solids may be detrimental to growth because the solids the infant eats cannot be adequately digested because of the immaturity of the gastrointestinal system. In addition, the nutrients in breast or formula milk will not be taken in because the infant's appetite has been satisfied with the less nutritious solids. In contrast, failure to offer solids by age 6 months may result in difficulty accepting solid feedings at a later time (AAP, 1998).

The feeding of semisolid foods should be delayed until the infant's consumption of foods is no longer a reflexive process and the infant has the fine and gross motor skills needed to consume them (usually between 4 and 6 months of age) (Story, Holt, & Sofka, 2002). The infant goes through a so-called *transitional period*, during which prepared foods are introduced and given together with human milk or formula. Each infant's growth and development vary, and milestones indicate the infant's readiness for solid foods (Box 5-9).

Solids should be introduced one at a time in small amounts (1 teaspoon to 2 tablespoons) for several days before introducing a new food. This is done to avoid confusion should a food intolerance be present. The order of introduction is

---

BOX 5-9	Readiness for Introduction of Solids

- Infant can sit.
- Birth weight has doubled and infant weighs at least 13 pounds.
- Infant can reach for an object and maintain balance.
- Infant indicates a desire for food by opening mouth and leaning forward.
- Extrusion reflex has disappeared (4 to 5 months).
- Infant moves food to back of mouth and swallows during spoon feedings.

HEALTH PROMOTION

THE 4-MONTH-OLD INFANT

FOCUSED ASSESSMENT

What new activities is the baby doing?

Is the baby able to settle down to sleep without needing to be consoled?

Are both parents included in the baby's care?

Is the mother considering going back to work in the near future?

DEVELOPMENTAL MILESTONES

Personal/social: loves moving faces; knows parents' voices

Fine motor: follows an object 180 degrees; binocular vision; bats objects; begins to hold own bottle

Language/cognitive: initiates conversation by cooing; turns head to locate sounds

Gross motor: supports weight on feet when standing; pulls to sit without head lag; begins to roll prone to supine

CRITICAL MILESTONES*

Personal/social: smiles responsively; smiles spontaneously; stares at own hand

Fine motor: grasps a rattle; follows past midline; brings hands to middle of body

Language/cognitive: laughs and squeals out loud; vocalizes; makes "ooh" sounds

Gross motor: lifts head and chest 45 and 90 degrees when prone; head steady when sitting

HEALTH MAINTENANCE

Physical Measurements

Continue to measure and plot length, weight, and head circumference

Posterior fontanel closed

Immunizations

Diphtheria-tetanus-acellular pertussis (DTaP)#2, inactivated poliovirus (IPV)#2 (combination diphtheria-tetanus-acellular pertussis, hepatitis B, polio vaccine as an alternative). *Haemophilus influenzae* type b (HIB)#2, pneumococcal #2; rotavirus #2

Review side effects and ask about previous reactions

Health Screening

Assess for strabismus

No additional screening required

ANTICIPATORY GUIDANCE

Nutrition

Maintain breastfeeding schedule

Formula, 5 to 6 ounces five or six times per day

Bottle supplement if breastfeeding mother has returned to work

Vitamin D supplementation 200 IU/day for breastfeeding infants

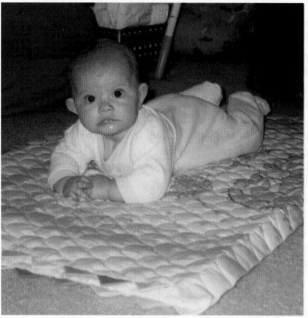

Photo courtesy Michele Hayden.

Elimination

Similar to 2-month-old

Dental

May begin drooling in preparation for tooth eruption

Sleep

Place on back to sleep in parent's room in a separate crib/cradle/bassinet. Keep loose or soft bedding and toys out of the crib; offer pacifier for nap and bedtime if not breastfeeding.

Total sleep: 15 to 16 hours

Encourage self-consoling techniques

Hygiene

Continue daily routine of cleanliness

Safety

Review car safety and violence, exposure to cigarette smoke

Discuss choking hazards and management of choking; avoidance of walkers; playpen and swing safety; begin child-proofing

Play

Talk with the baby frequently and from different locations

Respond verbally and smile as infant does; cuddle

Sing; expose to different environmental sounds

Supervised water play

Provide bright rattles, tactile toys, mirror

*Guided by Denver Developmental Screening Test II.

not critical, but iron-fortified rice cereal is most often recommended as a first food because it is high in iron, is easily digested, and has a low allergenic probability. Other commercially available infant cereals include oatmeal, barley, mixed grain, and cereals with added fruit. When foods are first being introduced, mixed grains and cereals with added fruit should be avoided. Foods should not be mixed with formula and fed through a nipple with a large hole. This deprives the child of the chewing experience and changes the texture and taste of the food.

Several commercially prepared fruits and vegetables are available. In addition, fruits and vegetables can easily be steamed or boiled and then pureed in a blender or food processor at home. It is usually necessary to add a small amount of water during the blending process. The parent should not give an infant home-prepared orange or dark leafy vegetables before age 4 to 6 months because of the elevated nitrate levels, which can cause methemoglobinemia. In addition, infants for whom formula is prepared with well water remain at high risk for nitrate poisoning (AAP Committee on Nutrition and Committee on Environmental Health, 2005). As with cereals, mixed fruits should be avoided until the infant is older and has tolerated individual foods.

Although most sources indicate that the order of introduction of foods is arbitrary, the introduction of meat usually follows cereal, fruit, and vegetables after age 6 months. The infant may be given ground liver, lean beef, or a variety of commercially prepared meats. The parent should avoid giving the infant mixed meats and vegetables; these baby foods may not contain enough meat.

Salt and sugar should not be added to commercial or home-prepared foods. Parents should avoid using canned foods or home-prepared foods that contain large amounts of sugar and salt. Feeding honey to infants under age 12 months has been associated with botulism and should therefore be avoided.

Finger Foods. Between age 8 and 10 months the infant can be introduced to finger foods. At this time the pincer grasp is developing and the infant can pick up foods. The infant will have a palmar grasp before this time and soft foods can be given, but the infant will mainly "play" with the food. This can be a positive experience that enables the infant to feel different textures and increase fine motor skills.

Finger foods should be bite-size pieces of soft food. Arrowroot biscuits, cheese sticks, slices of canned peaches or pears, cut pieces of bananas, and breads can be offered. As children's fine motor skills increase, they may enjoy eating some of the dry cereals, such as Cheerios. Be sure pieces of larger finger foods are not round and are small enough that they will not block the infant's airway, causing a choking hazard. Encourage parents to remain with an infant who is eating finger foods.

Snacks. When the infant is on a three-meals-a-day schedule, small snacks are an appropriate addition to the nutritional intake. Because infants have small stomachs, they may not be content to wait until the next meal before eating. Snacks should be nutritious, and parents should resist the urge to give infants a bottle to satisfy their hunger. Some of the finger foods just listed are nutritious snacks. If the infant is not hungry at mealtime, the snack should be given in a smaller portion or eliminated.

Food Allergies

The early introduction of solid foods may be associated with a higher incidence of food allergy, although recent evidence suggests that this may not be true in the development of eczema and asthma (Zutavern et al., 2004). Some of the more common suspected allergens include cow milk, egg, soy products, fish, peanuts, chocolate, corn, and wheat. Cow's milk protein intolerance is the most common food allergy during infancy, but this usually does not last past age 3 or 4 years.

Some of the common clinical manifestations of food allergies are abdominal pain, diarrhea, nasal congestion, cough, wheezing, vomiting, and rashes. Many children will outgrow their allergic response to certain foods; for example, 70% to 80% of infants with a milk allergy will tolerate milk by age 4 years. Children in whom food allergies develop after age 3 years tend not to outgrow them.

In addition to delaying the introduction of solid foods until the infant is 6 months old, other recommendations for minimizing the risk of food allergy include exclusive breastfeeding (or bottle feeding breast milk) for at least 4 to 6 months, prenatal avoidance of peanuts, and postnatal maternal avoidance of allergenic substances (Zeiger, 2003). In addition, AAP guidelines recommend delaying cow's milk for at least 1 year, egg white for 2 years, and peanuts, tree nuts, and fish until the child is 3 years old (Zeiger, 2003).

Dental Care

Eruption of the infant's first teeth is a developmental milestone that has great significance for many parents. Deciduous, or "baby," teeth usually erupt between 5 and 9 months of age. The first to appear are the lower central incisors, followed by the upper central incisors and then the upper lateral incisors. The next teeth to erupt are usually the lower lateral incisors, first primary molars, canines, and the second primary molars. The average child has six to eight teeth by the first birthday.

Teething

Although sometimes asymptomatic, teething is often signaled by behavior such as night wakening, daytime restlessness, an increase in nonnutritive sucking, excess drooling, and temporary loss of appetite. Some degree of discomfort is normal, but a health care professional should further investigate elevated temperature, irritability, ear tugging, or diarrhea.

To help parents cope with teething, nurses can suggest that they provide cool liquids and hard foods (e.g., dry toast, Popsicles, frozen bagels) for chewing. Hard, cold teethers and ice wrapped in cloth may also provide comfort for inflamed gums. Nurses should explain to parents that over-the-counter topical medications for gum pain relief should be used only as directed. Home remedies, such as rubbing the gums with whiskey or aspirin, should be discouraged, but acetaminophen administered as directed for the child's age can relieve discomfort. Although these interventions can be helpful, parents should understand that absolute relief comes only with tooth eruption.

Assessment of Dental Risk

The AAP and the American Dental Association have issued recommendations about prevention and treatment of dental caries in infants and young children (AAP, 2003b). The risk of tooth decay begins in infancy and is higher in families with a history of dental caries. Viewed as an infectious process, mothers with dental caries can transmit bacteria that cause caries to their infants through sharing of eating utensils, toothbrushes, or a pacifier given to an infant after having been in the mother's mouth (AAP, 2003b). Taking a dental history from a mother can provide information about an infant's risk, and this should occur as early as the infant's teeth begin to erupt. Infants with observable dental caries should be referred to a dentist as soon as these are observed by the health care provider (AAP, 2003b).

Cleaning Teeth

Because the primary teeth are used for chewing until the permanent teeth erupt and because decay of the primary teeth often results in decay of the permanent teeth, dental care must begin in infancy. The parent can use cotton swabs or a soft washcloth and water to clean the teeth with the infant positioned in the parent's lap or on a changing table. The teeth should be cleaned at least twice a day, and juice should be limited to no more than 1 cup a day given at meals (AAP, 2003b). Toothpaste should not be used until the child is older and can spit and will not swallow the toothpaste. This is recommended so the infant will not ingest excessive amounts of fluoride.

Appropriate amounts of fluoride, however, are necessary for the development of healthy teeth. Infants receive fluoride when formula and cereal are mixed with water from fluoridated water supplies. Fluoride supplementation is recommended only for children who do not live in areas where the water has sufficient amounts of fluoride.

Bottle-Mouth Caries

Bottle-mouth caries, or nursing-bottle caries, is a well-described form of tooth decay that can develop in infants and children. The decay pattern usually involves the incisors initially and then spreads to other teeth. Decay may be so serious that tooth loss occurs prematurely. When the infant is allowed to fall asleep with a bottle containing milk or juice, the carbohydrate-rich solution bathes the teeth for a long period and may cause dental caries.

Nurses should discourage parents from giving bedtime bottles of milk or juice to infants. If a nighttime bottle is necessary, plain water is an acceptable substitute for carbohydrate-rich liquids. A pacifier is an acceptable alternative to a nighttime bottle, although the practice of dipping the pacifier in corn syrup or honey to encourage acceptance poses the same problem. An additional danger of the use of honey in infancy is botulism.

Sleep, Rest, and Crying

Newborn infants may sleep as much as 17 to 20 hours per day. Sleep patterns vary widely, with some infants sleeping only 2 to 3 hours at a time. At approximately 3 to 4 months of age, most infants begin to sleep for longer periods during the night, although some children do not sleep through the night consistently until the second year.

Often one of the most difficult tasks for new parents is the regulation of their infant's sleep-wake cycles. Parents need anticipatory guidance about what to expect regarding sleep, rest, and crying. It is important to remember that rocking an infant to sleep provides warmth and security for the infant; however, to initiate good sleep habits, the parent should put the infant in the crib while the infant is drowsy and before the infant falls completely asleep.

For several years, the AAP has recommended placing all infants on their back to sleep (AAP, 2005d). In a recent revision of their policy about SIDS, the AAP has issued several other recommendations for preventing SIDS. These include (AAP, 2005d) the following recommendations:

- Putting the infant to sleep for nap or night in the parent's room in a place other than the parent's bed (e.g., cradle, bassinet, crib)
- Being sure that the mattress surface is firm and that there is no soft or loose bedding (e.g., sheets, blankets, quilts) or toys in the crib
- Avoiding exposing the infant to environmental smoke and avoiding overheating the infant
- Offering the infant a pacifier at nap and bedtime
- Not using commercially marketed monitors that purport to reduce the risk of SIDS
- Providing opportunities during awake time for "tummy play"

Additional information about SIDS is discussed in Chapter 21.

Safety

The rapidly growing infant becomes mobile seemingly overnight. With newfound mobility comes the potential for unintentional injury. As the infant's musculature strengthens and coordination improves, the infant has an insatiable desire to explore. Without the cognitive skills needed to differentiate danger from safety, the rolling, crawling, toddling infant is at great risk for accidents.

Infants are totally dependent on others for safety and protection. They are especially vulnerable to serious injury because of their relatively large head size. Motor development progresses to the point where infants quickly master new skills to learn more about their environment. They begin impulsively to reach out and move toward interesting objects around them.

HEALTH PROMOTION

THE 6-MONTH-OLD INFANT

FOCUSED ASSESSMENT
What kind of new activities is the baby doing?
Have you begun to give the baby solid foods?
How is any child care working out?
Have you done anything about child-proofing your home?

DEVELOPMENTAL MILESTONES
Personal/social: interacts readily and noisily with parents and familiar people; may be cautious with strangers
Fine motor: rakes objects with the whole hand; begins to transfer; mouths; can hold an object in each hand
Language/cognitive: begins to imitate sounds (raspberries, clucking, kissing); babbles; says single sounds; beginning object permanence; awareness of time sequence
Gross motor: tripod sitting unsupported; gets on hands and knees; bears full weight on legs; "swims" when prone

CRITICAL MILESTONES*
Personal/social: reaches for toy out of reach; looks at hand; smiles spontaneously
Fine motor: looks at raisin placed on contrasting surface; reaches out; follows completely side to side
Language/cognitive: turns to rattle sound made out of vision on each side; squeals; laughs
Gross motor: rolls over both directions; no head lag; lifts head and chest completely

HEALTH MAINTENANCE

Physical Measurements
Birth weight doubles
Continue to measure and plot length, weight, and head circumference

Immunizations
Diphtheria-tetanus-acellular pertussis (DTaP)#3 (combination diphtheria-tetanus-acellular pertussis, hepatitis B, and polio vaccine as an alternative); *Haemophilus influenzae* type b (HIB)#3; pneumococcal #3; rotavirus #3; monovalent inactivated poliovirus (IPV)#3 may be given between now and 18 months
Influenza vaccine annually until 59 months of age. Two doses initially, separated by at least 4 weeks.
Ask about previous reactions
Review side effects

Health Screening
Initial lead screening risk assessment (see Box 5-11)

ANTICIPATORY GUIDANCE

Nutrition
Begin introducing solid foods one at a time by spoon; use iron-fortified cereals
Avoid citrus and egg white; read labels
Hold or place in infant seat for feeding
Begin using a cup
Vitamin D supplementation 200 IU/day for breastfed infants and infants whose formula intake is less than 16 ounces/day

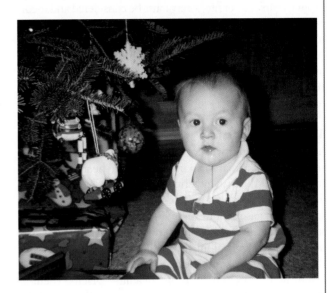

Elimination
Stools darken and become more formed as solids are increased

Dental
Tooth eruption begins with lower incisors
May have some pain and low-grade fever (<101° F)
May be fussy
Begin fluoride supplements as recommended
Clean teeth and gums with wet cloth
Do not put to sleep with a bottle

Sleep
Place on back to sleep (infant may roll over to prone position) **in a separate crib. Keep loose or soft bedding and toys out of the crib; offer pacifier for nap and bedtime if not breastfeeding.**
Can move to a separate room
12 to 16 hours each day
Sleeps all night; two or three naps
Maintain or establish sleep routine

Hygiene
Continue daily routine of cleanliness
Clean toys frequently

Safety
Review choking, walkers, violence, exposure to cigarette smoke
Discuss child-proofing, drowning prevention, poison prevention (see Chapter 10)

Play
Expose to different sounds and sights
Begin social games (pat-a-cake, peek-a-boo)
Provide bath toys, rattles, mirror, large ball, soft stuffed animals
Encourage to sit unsupported
Encourage to rock on hands and knees

*Guided by Denver Developmental Screening Test II.

Because of an infant's dependence, parents and caregivers are the primary recipients of anticipatory safety guidance. From the first day of life, safety must be considered and incorporated into the infant's world. Providing a safe environment for a rapidly growing infant is challenging. Potential safety hazards multiply as the baby learns to creep, crawl, climb, and explore. Some parents may not have a complete awareness of the safety issues that must be addressed to protect the infant from injury.

Motor Vehicle Safety

Injuries associated with automobile crashes constitute the single greatest threat to an infant's life and health. Restraining seats are the only practical means of reducing this risk. The crushing forces of a crash or sudden stop, even at low speed, can cause serious injury to the infant. Without a car safety seat, an infant involved in a collision or sudden stop becomes an unguided missile, colliding with the interior of the car or, worse, being ejected from the vehicle. In a collision, infants are usually thrust headfirst, placing them at greater risk for head, facial, or spinal injuries because of the weight of the head combined with poor neck muscle support (Kamerling, 2002).

Infant safety in motor vehicles depends entirely on adults. Parents must be informed that they cannot protect their child from injury in a crash by cradling or holding the infant on their laps. Adults are neither strong enough nor quick enough to prevent the sudden forward motions or to overcome the inertial forces (external forces of motion caused by impact) exerted in a crash. An unrestrained adult is propelled forward, trapping and crushing the infant between the adult's body and the hard surfaces inside the car on impact. The only way to prevent injuries and death to an infant in a car is to use a car safety seat for each trip, no matter how short.

A lifelong practice begins with the newborn infant's first ride home. Getting a child accustomed to using a safety seat at a young age establishes a safety habit and may reduce resistance later (Fig. 5-3). All car safety seats should be placed in the rear seat of the vehicle, preferably in the middle, away from the possibility of injury from a side crash. Newborns and infants should be in a rear-facing seat with a three- or five-point harness until they are 1 year of age and weigh 20 pounds (AAP, 2005b). Front-facing seats (Fig. 5-4) should be tethered to the tether anchor (available in cars made after 2000). LATCH (Lower Anchors and Tethers for Children) systems, which secure the seat without need for the seat belt, keep the seat tightly anchored to the car. Both car (those made after 2002) and seat must have the LATCH system for it to work without the seatbelt (AAP, 2005b). Children should remain in an approved car safety seat or booster seat until they are approximately 4 feet 9 inches tall (between 8 and 12 years) (AAP, 2005a).

Some injuries and deaths have been associated with the deployment of air bags. Infants and children younger than 12 years should not be restrained in the front seat of cars equipped with passenger-side air bags. When deployed, the air bag can severely jolt the car safety seat and harm the infant. The National Highway Traffic Safety Administration and the AAP recommend placing all children 12 years and younger in the rear seat with the appropriate restraint (Durbin, Chen, Smith, Elliott, & Winston, 2005). Placing the infant or young child in the middle of the rear seat avoids injury from side airbag deployment.

Providing a Safe Home Environment

During infancy and early childhood, when children are typically limited to the home environment, safety in and around the home is a top priority. With the exception of injuries and deaths related to motor vehicle crashes, most childhood injuries occur in the home. Parents must also consider safety as a factor when selecting day care facilities for their child.

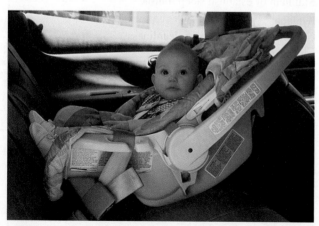

FIG 5-3 The infant rides facing the rear of the vehicle, ideally in the middle of the back seat. The infant seat is secured to the vehicle with the seat belt, and straps on the car seat adjust to accommodate the growing baby.

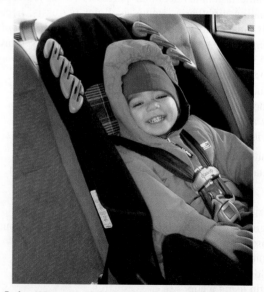

FIG 5-4 When the child reaches 1 year of age and weighs 20 pounds, the car safety seat can be adjusted to a forward-facing upright position. This seat is appropriate for the toddler until the child reaches about 40 pounds. The safety straps should be adjusted to provide a snug fit, and the seat should be placed in the back seat of the car, ideally in the middle.

Burn Safety. Infants are especially vulnerable to inflicted burns, particularly scald burns, and scald burns are a leading cause of emergency admissions in infants and young children (Titus, Baxter, & Starling, 2003). Infants' limited mobility makes it impossible for them to escape from immersion in hot water. Parents should be instructed to decrease the setting on hot water heaters to 120° F to prevent accidental scalds. Infant skin is thin, causing burns to occur faster at lower temperatures than in adults. With water temperature settings of 140° F, it takes only 3 seconds for the child to suffer serious burns. Lowering the temperature by 20° F causes the same degree of burn injury in 8 to 10 minutes of submersion. An adult should test the water temperature before the infant is submerged to decrease the risk of accidental scald injuries.

Burn injuries in infants can also be caused by a variety of other sources. Exposure to sunlight can result in serious sunburn to their delicate skin. Parents should be encouraged to apply sun blocks and sunscreens (minimum sun protection factor 15) liberally to older infants and to protect the face and head with a hat when exposing the infant or toddler to sunlight, even for brief periods and on cloudy days. Young infants should not be exposed to strong sunlight, and sunscreen should not be used on infants younger than 6 months old (AAP, 2003c).

Advise parents to avoid smoking, drinking hot liquids, or cooking while holding an infant. As infants begin to crawl around on the floor, open electrical sockets should be covered with appropriate socket protectors. Open stoves or fireplaces are especially intriguing to an exploring infant and should be outfitted with a guard or grid. Cool mist vaporizers should be used rather than steam vaporizers to prevent scald injuries to a curious infant.

Safe Baby Furnishings. Baby furniture, although seemingly benign, can present lethal hazards to a growing infant. Parents should be aware of safety considerations when planning or decorating the infant's room. Parents need to be aware that older furniture that has been handed down may not meet current safety regulations. In older cribs, the gaps between slats may be large enough that infants could entrap their heads, or the paint may contain lead.

Hanging toys or mobiles placed over the crib should be positioned well out of the infant's reach to prevent entanglement and strangulation. Encourage the parent to avoid placing large toys in the crib because an older infant may use them as steps to climb over the side, resulting in a serious fall. Cribs should be positioned away from curtains or blinds to prevent accidental entanglement in dangling cords (Box 5-10).

Preventing Falls. Infants are often placed on surfaces at heights that are convenient for the adult, such as on changing tables, counters, or furniture. These surfaces often have no restraining barriers. Infants begin to roll over as early as 2 months, and as they begin to scoot or crawl, fall injuries from these elevations are common. There must be constant adult supervision when infants are placed at such heights (Fig. 5-5). If the parent or nurse must move away from the infant, the adult should either take the infant or, if supplies are close, place a hand on the infant while reaching. At home, parents may choose to place their child on the floor for changing diapers or providing other care.

Falls from infant seats or out of high chairs are common, and falls from infant strollers have resulted in significant injury to young children improperly restrained in the stroller (Powell, Jovtis, & Tanz, 2002). Injuries can be prevented with supervision and the use of safety restraining straps to limit the mobility of the infant (see Fig. 5-5).

As infants begin to crawl, placing gates at the top and bottom of stairs can prevent falls. Infant walkers are dangerous and are not recommended. They allow infants mobility and the freedom to explore surroundings before they have developed the ability to interpret heights or protect themselves from falls.

Preventing Asphyxiation. Asphyxiation (suffocation) occurs when air cannot get into or out of the lungs and oxygen supplies are consequently depleted. Carbon dioxide levels then increase, causing life-threatening disruption of cardiac and cerebral functioning. Choking occurs when substances or objects are *aspirated* into the airway or into the branches of the lower airways, causing partial or complete obstruction of the lungs. Strangulation is typically thought of as a constriction of the neck, but it also includes blockage of the nose and mouth by airtight materials, such as plastic. This blockage prevents air exchange. Store all plastic bags or covers out of the infant's reach. Choking is a major concern in the first

---

BOX 5-10	**PARENTS WANT TO KNOW** Crib Safety

- The distance between slats must be no more than 2⅜ inches wide to prevent entrapment of the infant's head or body. Mesh-sided cribs should have mesh openings smaller than ¼ inch (6 mm).
- The interior of the crib must snugly accommodate a standard-size mattress so that the gap is minimal, less than the width of two adult fingers. Excessive space could allow the infant to become wedged, potentially suffocating.
- Decorative enhancements on the crib are not recommended because they can break apart and be aspirated

by the infant. Design cutouts can trap an infant's arm or neck, causing death or serious injury.
- Corner posts or finials that rise above the end panels can snag garments and inadvertently strangle infants.
- The drop side must be impossible for an infant to release. Activating the drop side must take either a strong force (at least 10 pounds) or a distinct action at each locking device. Never leave the drop side down when an infant is in the crib.
- Wood surfaces should be free of splinters, cracks, and lead-based paint.

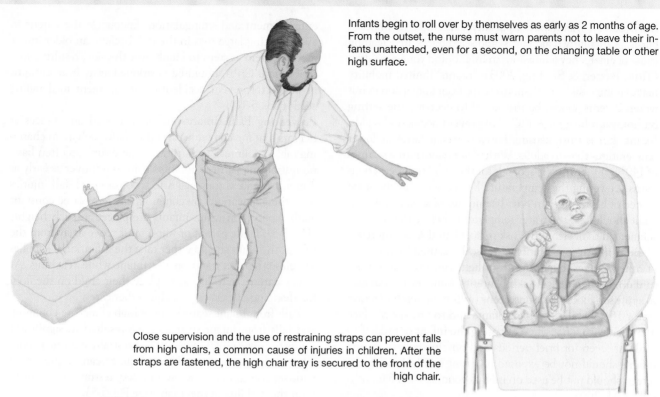

Infants begin to roll over by themselves as early as 2 months of age. From the outset, the nurse must warn parents not to leave their infants unattended, even for a second, on the changing table or other high surface.

Close supervision and the use of restraining straps can prevent falls from high chairs, a common cause of injuries in children. After the straps are fastened, the high chair tray is secured to the front of the high chair.

FIG 5-5   **Safety education for parents of infants should emphasize the need for constant supervision and the use of restraining devices to prevent falls.**

few months of an infant's life, when aspiration of feedings or vomit can occur easily because of the immature swallowing mechanism. Parents should be taught to position infants on their sides after feedings and to avoid placing small infants in bed with a bottle propped in their mouths.

As infants grow, they begin to explore the world around them by placing anything and everything in their mouths. Size, shape, and consistency are major determinants of whether a food or object is likely to be aspirated by an infant. Food that is round or similar to the size of the airway is especially dangerous. Dangerous foods include sliced hot dogs, hard candy, peanuts, grapes, raisins, and chewing gum. These foods should be avoided until the child is able to chew thoroughly before swallowing. Food should be cut into small pieces, and the child should be supervised while eating. Advise parents to strongly discourage infants and young children from playing, singing, or other activities while eating, to avoid choking. Infants are equally endangered by rattles, pieces of toys, ribbons from stuffed animals, and common household objects such as coins, buttons, pins, or beads found on the floor or within their reach. Balloons should not be given to infants or young children or used where an infant or young child plays.

Anticipatory guidance for parents includes performing a thorough inspection of the infant's surroundings to remove all potential items that infants could grasp, place in their mouths, and choke on. Parents can be encouraged to crawl through the home to gain a better perspective of the infant's environment. Parents can then substitute safe objects for exploration.

Ornaments or toys with detachable parts are not recommended for infants because of the aspiration risk. In 1979 the Consumer Product Safety Commission established a toy standard to prevent choking hazards in nonfood products targeted for children younger than 3 years. Parents should take extra care to note the presence of small detachable parts on toys before allowing the infant to play with the items. Although the government regulates the size of parts on infants' toys, older children's toys are not regulated by the same standard. As the infant explores an older sibling's or a playmate's territory, adult supervision is important.

To prevent strangulation injuries, parents should not place a pacifier on a string or cord around the infant's neck, not put an infant to sleep with a bib in place, and not position a crib near blinds or curtain cords. Crib slats should comply with the 2⅜-inch width requirement to prevent head entrapment.

In addition to inspecting and providing a safe environment for the infant, instruct parents in the appropriate action to take if the infant chokes (see Chapter 10 for a discussion of emergency procedures).

Preventing Lead Exposure. Although lead poisoning in the United States has decreased markedly since the elimination of lead paint and solder used in homes and leaded gasoline, lead poisoning remains a significant risk, especially in cities where old housing predominates. In addition, paint from old homes can enter the soil and get on children's hands when they are playing. Children inhale lead dust as homes are being renovated. The lead risk assessment begins as the infant begins to be mobile (6 months of age). Risk should

---

HEALTH PROMOTION

THE 9-MONTH-OLD INFANT

FOCUSED ASSESSMENT

What kind of new things is your baby doing?

How has the baby reacted to solid foods?

Do you live in a house built before 1978?

Do you live near sources of environmental lead?

Do you regularly come in contact with someone who uses lead?

Do you have a family member who has had lead poisoning?

DEVELOPMENTAL MILESTONES

Personal/social: stranger wariness; waves bye-bye; plays social games; begins to indicate wants

Fine motor: beginning pincer grasp; actively searches for out-of-sight objects; bangs toys together

Language/cognitive: uses consonant sounds and several vowel sounds; beginning to attach meaning to words; understands some symbolic language (blow a kiss); knows own name; says Mama and Dada specifically

Gross motor: gets to a sitting position; pulls up to stand; creeps and crawls; walks holding on to furniture; may briefly stand alone

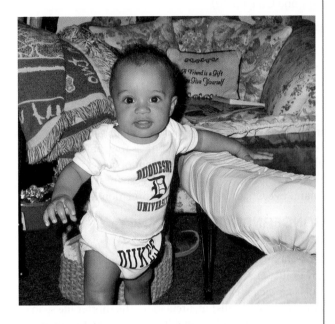

CRITICAL MILESTONES*

Personal/social: feeds self finger foods; tries to get toys; looks at hands

Fine motor: transfers; rakes a raisin or Cheerio; picks up and holds a small object in each hand

Language/cognitive: imitates sounds; says single syllables; begins to put syllables together

Gross motor: no head lag; sits without support; stands holding onto furniture

HEALTH MAINTENANCE

Physical Measurements

Continue to measure and plot length, weight, and head circumference

Immunizations

Hepatitis B #3 (can give between 6 and 12 months); omit if combination vaccine has been used previously

Influenza vaccine annually

Provide information about upcoming measles-mumps-rubella and varicella vaccines

Health Screening

Lead risk assessment (routine lead screen at 9 or 12 months, usually in conjunction with hemoglobin and hematocrit)

Hemoglobin or hematocrit (screen at 9 or 12 months)

ANTICIPATORY GUIDANCE

Nutrition

Continue to breastfeed on established schedule

Formula, 16 to 32 ounces/day

Vitamin D supplementation 200 IU/day if breastfed or taking less than 16 ounces/day of formula

Continue iron-fortified cereal

Begin to introduce soft, mashed table foods

Encourage cup, rather than bottle

Avoid giving large pieces of food

Elimination

Urinary and bowel patterns consistent

Appearance of undigested food in stools

Dental

Four teeth

Brush erupted teeth with soft toothbrush and water

Continue fluoride supplementation as recommended

Sleep

Night waking diminishes if managed appropriately

Hygiene

More vigilant cleanliness of diaper area as bladder volume increases

Wash infant's hands and face frequently

Keep toys clean

Safety

Review child-proofing, violence, exposure to cigarette smoke

Discuss lowering crib mattress, household and plant poisons, burn prevention, sunscreen use, avoiding sources of lead

Play

Social games

Provide cloth, cardboard, or plastic books

Cuddle, rock, hug

Ball rolling

Pots and pans with wooden spoons

Plastic stacking or nesting containers

Hide-and-seek games with toys

*Guided by Denver Developmental Screening Test II.

be assessed at every well visit beginning at the 6-month visit and education or treatment initiated as appropriate (Box 5-11 and Chapter 10).

Play

One sign of infants' cognitive development is the beginning evidence of play. Early signs of play are related to infants' motor and cognitive development. They mouth, shake, inspect, and reach for objects. Infants observe and engage other members of the family. In fact, human involvement is the most important component of play. A familiar game that we all have played is peek-a-boo. Not only is this game fun, but it is also associated with the development of object permanence. Box 5-12 outlines appropriate play activities and toys for the infant. See Chapter 4 for more information related to play.

CONCERNS DURING INFANCY
Jaundice

Most infants have some physiologic jaundice after the first day of life, characterized by a yellow gold color of the skin. This jaundice is caused by the increased number of erythrocytes (red blood cells) in circulation, the shorter life span of the erythrocytes, and the inability of the immature neonatal liver to conjugate (indirect) bilirubin out of the bloodstream. Because unconjugated bilirubin is bound to albumin, any medications that can interfere with these albumin-binding sites (e.g., phenobarbital) may also interfere with the excretion of bilirubin.

Indirect bilirubin levels usually peak at about 2 to 4 days of age. Their maximum level is usually 5 to 6 mg/dL. After this point, levels should continue to fall. Jaundice appears first on the face and progresses downward; jaundice of the

---

BOX 5-11	**Lead Exposure Risk Assessment**

- Do you live in, or is your child exposed to, housing that was built before 1950 that has peeling paint or plaster, or before 1978 that is being renovated?
- Do you live near any sources of environmental lead, such as smelters or places that use leaded gasoline?
- Does your child regularly come in contact with a household member who works with lead or lead solder (e.g., plumber, construction worker, stained glass artisan)?
- Does your child have a sibling who has or has had lead poisoning, or has any other household member had lead poisoning?
- In addition, has the infant or child been exposed to any other sources of lead: vinyl miniblinds, imported ceramics or toys, old baby furniture, leaded crystal? If the infant has any risk factors, a capillary test for lead should be performed. Otherwise, a routine capillary lead screening should be done at the 9-month or 1-year visit.

Modified from Rhode Island Department of Health. (2003). Lead screening and referral guidelines. Retrieved Feb. 27, 2004, from www.health.state.ri.us.

BOX 5-12	**Age-Related Activities and Toys for Infants**

General Activities

The infant enjoys watching other members of the family, being rocked, being taken for a walk in a stroller, time spent in a swing, supervised time on a blanket on the floor, crawling, walking, and being sung and read to.

Play is narcissistic; it is difficult, if not impossible, to direct play.

Human interaction is the most important component of play.

Toys and Specific Types of Play

Oral movements (playing with the nipple of the bottle, lip movements unrelated to sucking); peek-a-boo; playing with the caretaker's fingers, hair, and face and the infant's own body parts; and playing in water.

Soft stuffed animals, crib mobiles, squeeze toys, rattles, busy boxes, mirrors, musical toys, water toys during the bath, blocks, safe kitchen utensils, push toys (after infant begins to walk).

Contrasting colors for young infants (black-and-white mobiles).

Large picture books.

---

feet represents a markedly elevated bilirubin. For a serum bilirubin more than 15 mg/dL, phototherapy treatment may be considered.

Two types of jaundice have been identified in breastfed infants. The first type is early-onset jaundice, which seems to be related to insufficient intake of breast milk. As with formula-fed infants, this type of jaundice occurs 2 to 4 days after birth and usually resolves within 1 week. Early and frequent breastfeedings appear to decrease the incidence. The second type of jaundice is termed *breast milk jaundice*. This type of jaundice appears at 3 to 5 days of age and may last several weeks. This type of jaundice may be related to certain factors in the breast milk that alter the conjugation or absorption of bilirubin. Treatment approaches include phototherapy or temporarily discontinuing breastfeeding. See Chapter 23 for home care of the infant receiving phototherapy.

Circumcision

Circumcision, the removal of the prepuce (foreskin), a fold of skin that covers the glans penis, is a frequently performed surgical procedure during the newborn period. Although the foreskin can be retracted easily for cleaning in the older child, the prepuce is not usually fully retractable until age 3 years or older. The prepuce should never be forcibly retracted in any infant because trauma and adhesions can result. Circumcision is a controversial procedure, and parents may have questions about whether to choose to have it performed.

The (AAP states that, although there are potential benefits of the procedure, data are not sufficient to recommend routine neonatal circumcision (AAP & ACOG, 2002).

HEALTH PROMOTION

THE 12-MONTH-OLD INFANT

FOCUSED ASSESSMENT

Have parents discussed and agreed on approaches to discipline?

Is the baby able to follow directions and carry out requests?

Have the parents assessed the home and environment for sources of lead?

DEVELOPMENTAL MILESTONES

Personal/social: rolls or throws a ball with another person; explores; drinks from a cup; indicates wants without crying

Fine motor: actively looks for hidden objects; puts blocks in containers; uses simple toys appropriately

Language/cognitive: names the appropriate parent; begins to say one to three single words; understands simple requests

Gross motor: stands alone for increasing lengths of time; stoops and recovers; walks holding onto a hand; may begin to walk alone and climb stairs (on knees)

CRITICAL MILESTONES*

Personal/social: plays pat-a-cake; feeds self; works to get a toy

Fine motor: developed pincer grasp; bangs objects together; picks up two cubes

Language/cognitive: jabbers; combines syllables; mama/dada is nonspecific

Gross motor: stands briefly without support; gets to sitting position; pulls to stand

HEALTH MAINTENANCE

Physical Measurements

Continue to measure and plot length, weight, and head circumference

Weight is usually triple birth weight

Length is 50% more than birth length

Immunizations

Hepatitis B #3 (if not given previously); measles-mumps-rubella (MMR) #1; varicella vaccine; pneumococcal booster (if not scheduled to be given at 15 months)

Influenza vaccine annually

Hepatitis A #1

Health Screening

Hemoglobin/hematocrit if not done earlier

Lead screen if not done earlier

Tuberculosis if at risk

ANTICIPATORY GUIDANCE

Nutrition

May begin whole milk (2 or 3 cups daily)

Offer a variety of table foods from different food groups

Begins to use table utensils

Usually eats three meals and snacks

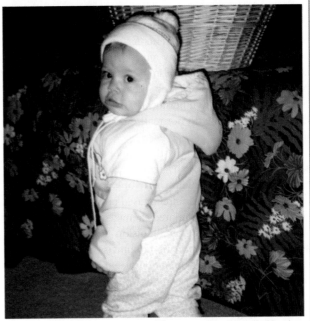

Photo courtesy Michele Hayden.

Avoid giving foods high in salt and sugar

Discuss high chair safety

Elimination

Remains dry for longer periods

Bowel movements decrease in number and become more regular

Dental

Eight teeth

Continue fluoride as recommended and brushing

Sleep

Sleeps through the night and has one or two naps

Hygiene

Continue as previously

Safety

Review poisons, burns, violence, exposure to cigarette smoke

Discuss changing to front-facing car seat (if infant weighs 20 pounds) placed in rear seat, falls, water safety, toy and toy box safety, bike passenger helmet

Play

Beginning parallel play

Push-pull toys

Various-size balls

Picture books

Dolls and stuffed animals

"Busy" box

Sandbox

*Guided by Denver Developmental Screening Test II.

Circumcision may reduce urinary tract infections, some sexually transmitted infections, inflammation of the glans or prepuce, and cancer of the penis. Other factors may be causative factors in these conditions as well.

Some parents choose circumcision for religious, cultural, or social reasons. Jewish parents may have their infants circumcised on the eighth day after birth as part of a special ceremony. Muslim culture also includes circumcision. Some parents want their son to look like his circumcised father or peers. Others feel circumcision is an expected part of newborn care, and some do not realize that they have a choice in the matter.

Lack of knowledge about the care of the prepuce leads to some circumcisions. Poor hygiene may increase the risk of infections and other problems. Teaching the parents and child the proper care of the uncircumcised penis can prevent surgery and complications related to inadequate cleanliness.

Many parents reject circumcision and the reasons are as varied as those supporting circumcision. Major reasons include (1) the benefits do not outweigh the risks, (2) belief that it is cosmetic surgery and not necessary, (3) unwillingness to subject the infant to pain, (4) culture, and (5) potential complications.

Only healthy newborn infants should undergo circumcision. Infants with blood dyscrasias may have excessive bleeding if circumcised. For the repair of anatomic abnormalities of the penis, such as hypospadias or epispadias, an intact prepuce may be needed for use in plastic surgery (see Chapter 20).

Circumcision may be performed in the hospital before the infant is discharged or in an outpatient setting during the first week. Circumcision is performed with a scalpel, Gomco clamp, or Hollister Plastibell. Pain control can be achieved through a dorsal penile nerve block, lidocaine infiltration on the prepuce, or topical anesthetic cream (EMLA cream). If a Gomco clamp was used, petrolatum gauze strips or petroleum jelly ointment are placed over the circumcision site and it is covered with gauze to prevent the diaper from sticking to it. Petroleum jelly should not be used with a Plastibell because it might make the Plastibell slip off too soon. The diaper is attached loosely to prevent pressure.

The wound is checked frequently for bleeding during the first few hours after the procedure. The nurse describes to the parents that spotting of blood can occur but emphasizes that the physician should be notified for more extensive bleeding. The normal yellowish exudate that forms over the site should be described and differentiated from purulent drainage. Signs of complications should be discussed fully.

Noting the first urination after circumcision is important because edema could cause an obstruction; the mother is instructed to call the physician if there is no urinary output within 6 to 8 hours. Box 5-13 describes the home care of the child who has been circumcised.

Although nurses usually teach parents of circumcised infants how to care for the penis, they may not think about providing teaching for parents who decide against circumcision. They should include care of the intact penis in the teaching plan for these parents.

The Infant with Colic

Colic usually refers to unexplained crying or fussing in infants, which may be characterized by infants pulling up their arms and legs. Periods of crying tend to occur at the same time of day, often in the late afternoon or evening. To be diagnosed with colic, an infant must have the symptoms several times daily for several days a week. It has also been defined as crying for more than 3 hours a day, more than 3 days per week, for more than 3 weeks (Wessel, Cobb, Jackson, Harris, & Detwiler, 1954). Most infants outgrow symptoms of colic by 3 to 4 months of age.

Etiology

The cause of colic is unknown, but several theories have been researched. The possibilities include but are not limited to allergy, cow's milk intolerance, maternal anxiety, familial stress, and too rapid feeding or overfeeding. It is highly likely that more than one factor may be involved. Colic is more common in infants with sensitive temperaments, who seem to need increased attention.

Management

The physician must determine whether, in fact, the infant is crying because of colic and not because of an acute condition such as intussusception, otitis media, or a fracture. Symptoms of milk allergy other than crying should be present before formula changes are made. Anticholinergics, motility-enhancing agents, barbiturates, and antiflatulents might be

---

BOX 5-13	**PARENTS WANT TO KNOW** Care for Circumcision

Call the health care provider if your infant:
- Does not urinate within 6 hours after circumcision
- Has swelling of the entire penis
- Bleeds more than tiny drops
- Shows drainage (clear or white)
- Has a fever—rectal temperature 100.4° F (38° C) or higher

Do the following:
- Apply the diaper loosely
- Give sponge baths until circumcision is healed

- Clean penis with clear water
- If Gomco clamp is used, put petroleum gauze dressing on the penis

Don't
- Clean the penis with alcohol wipes
- Remove the yellowish crusty material that forms on the penis during healing—this represents a normal healing process
- Place a dressing on a Plastibell

prescribed. Many practitioners avoid using these drugs because of their limited success, lack of scientific data, and possible side effects. Chamomile tea, which has been used for thousands of years, has a calming and sedating effect and is effective in some infants (Garrison & Christakis, 2000). It is readily available in most grocery stores, and allergic reactions are rare. If parents are using herbs such as chamomile, the nurse should be sure they know the appropriate dose, are aware of possible allergic reactions, and do not use so much as to interfere with adequate breast milk or formula intake.

Nursing Considerations

Because the etiology of colic and the care of an infant with colic are so individualized, it is very important that the nurse obtain a thorough history. The nurse should provide a concerned and caring atmosphere during the assessment and reassure the parents that colic is not related to bad parenting. It should be determined whether any other symptoms are associated with the crying. The infant's eating habits, including whether the infant is breastfed or bottle-fed, should be discussed. The nurse should ask the parents whether commonalities are associated with the crying (time of day, associated activities, family members present) and ask what has been tried, what works, and what does not work. If the parents are unsure, they should keep a diary for 48 to 72 hours to determine patterns. The nurse should assess the parents' stress level and support system.

The nurse should educate the parents regarding the normal growth and development needs of infants related to sleep and awake times, feeding, soothing, and holding and listen to the parents with an empathic ear. Parents should be encouraged to soothe their infant by rocking and cuddling. Some infants will quiet when given a massage, pacifier, or warm bath. If the parent is busy, a swing may provide a soothing, rhythmic effect. Some of the same strategies for soothing infants may also be effective in quieting infants with colic.

Some infants seem most distressed during high-activity times when the family may be busy preparing meals, doing chores, gathering at the end of the day, and so forth. By assisting parents to see such trends, the nurse can help them establish alternative routines to decrease the infant's stimuli. The parent may choose to feed the infant away from all the activity or to have a later dinner. Each family will be unique, and the nurse's role is to facilitate problem solving.

If, after 30 minutes, none of the interventions are effective, the infant should be placed in the crib. If crying continues for more than 15 to 20 minutes, pick the infant up again and try to soothe.

All families need extra support after the birth of an infant. If the infant has colic, the need increases. During the first few months after the addition of a new baby, demanding work schedules, lack of recovery time from childbirth, the needs of other family members, physical exhaustion, and sleep deprivation can combine with the presence of a fretful infant to create stressful situations for the entire family. Sometimes infant temperament and parental coping styles are not compatible.

The nurse might, for example, explain to new parents, "Parenting is very much a challenge even when parents care about their baby as much as you do. It is difficult at first even to discern what Avery is telling you when she cries. But you will feel more and more comfortable, even see that she has a different cry when she is hungry and when she is tired."

In validating the parents' feelings, the nurse recognizes that the infant's irritability or colic is real, not imagined, and that the infant is a challenge to handle. The nurse can reassure the parents that the infant is healthy, normal, and gaining weight and that the parents are competent in their nurturing role.

The emotional reserves of the parents can be restored through rest and pleasurable activities. Parents may need brief periods of relief from infant care responsibilities. Grandparents or other family members may be able to provide the parents with an evening out or a night of uninterrupted sleep. This direct support can help restore the parents' energy to cope with daily activities and feel more relaxed and confident in their parenting.

Patterns of Crying

Crying is a mode of communication for infants. It is especially challenging for new parents to learn and accurately interpret their individual infant's cry. Some infants respond readily to attempts to comfort them, sleep a great deal, and fit easily into their family's lifestyle. Other infants cry more readily and for longer periods and spend more time in a fretful, restless state than others. These infants often have more colic symptoms and sleep problems. This irritability may be caused by health problems, such as feeding difficulties, infection, or allergies, but often no clear cause emerges. In some cases, the temperament of the infant may be the cause.

Nurses can suggest that parents, after ruling out physiologic causes for crying (e.g., hungry, soiled, gassy) console their infants when they cry by holding them, talking softly, or humming. Gently stroking an infant's head, back, and arms may also be soothing. Infant massage techniques and simply "centering" are easily accomplished by positioning the infant's arms and legs toward the midline of the body. Swaddling a new infant is a consoling technique that assists the infant to center.

Specific strategies to diminish infant irritability include activities such as taking the baby for a car ride, carrying the infant in a front pack close to the parent's chest, or swinging the baby in an infant swing. Vertical positioning and constant motion, such as that obtained when walking with the baby carried over the shoulder, are sometimes helpful. The football-carry position, with gentle patting on the back, can also be tried. Sometimes irritable infants need to be left alone to cry for brief periods. If parents choose this strategy, they must be cautioned to limit the crying time and to check the baby frequently.

Few interventions are consistently successful because infant responses may vary. Providing parents with strategies, however, helps decrease their anxiety and increase their feelings of control and competence. As infants grow and develop, they are better able to regulate their sleep-wake cycles. Generally, during the third or fourth month of life, sleep problems and irritability improve.

KEY CONCEPTS

- During the first year of life, the infant's organs grow and mature at a rapid rate, yet organ systems of infants remain very different from those of older children and adults.
- Weight gain and muscle growth during infancy allow the infant to have increased control of reflexes and increasingly coordinated movement.
- Sensory capabilities, neuromuscular control, perceptual skills, the quality and quantity of parental interaction, and environmental stimulation all affect cognitive development during infancy.
- Infants develop language first by listening to sounds of caregivers, then by realizing that certain sounds have special meaning, and eventually by using simple words to communicate.
- Infancy is the period during which children develop the foundation of their personalities, struggling to establish a sense of basic trust rather than mistrust.
- One of the most important features of psychosocial development during infancy is parent-infant attachment, or the sense of belonging with one another.
- Common problems during infancy, such as separation anxiety, sleep disorders, and fretfulness, cause parents concern and distress. Nurses should be available with information and support to provide anticipatory guidance.
- Nurses play an important role in health promotion and disease prevention related to immunizations.
- Because infancy is a period of very rapid growth and development, nutritional needs are of special significance. Parents frequently have many questions and concerns about nutrition.
- Breast milk or commercially prepared formulas provide the foundation of nutrition throughout infancy.
- Solid foods are usually introduced between 4 and 6 months of age in small amounts, one food at a time, on the basis of the infant's growth and development.
- Weaning usually begins between ages 6 and 12 months. It should never take place during stress, and the infant should receive breast milk or formula in the cup until age 12 months.
- Teething usually begins between 5 and 9 months of age. Some degree of discomfort is normal, and parents often need suggestions for coping with teething.
- Bottle-mouth caries or nursing-bottle syndrome is a form of tooth decay that can develop in infants and children as a result of prolonged breastfeeding or bottle feeding, especially at night.

- Colic can be very stressful for parents. The cause of colic is unknown, and care of the infant must be individualized. Support of the parents is very important.
- Improved motor development coupled with a keen desire to explore the environment places the infant at great risk for unintentional injury.
- Play enhances the infant's growth and development.

ANSWERS TO CRITICAL THINKING EXERCISE 5-1

1. Because this is Mrs. Brown's first child, she might be insecure about caring for Tonja. She might not be aware of normal growth and developmental milestones for this age. Tonja may be awake for long periods at night or she may have colic, depriving Mrs. Brown of sleep. Mr. Brown may travel or need to be away from home with his job and may not be available to help with Tonja. Mrs. Brown may not have an extended family to help her with the care of the infant. Mrs. Brown may have postpartum depression.

2. Trust must be established, and this can be accomplished by supporting Mrs. Brown and encouraging her to verbalize her concerns. Mothers of newborn infants often need reassurance that they are doing a good job, and they need to be given permission to ask any question, no matter how insignificant they or the nurse might think the question is. The nurse can validate Mrs. Brown's feelings of being overwhelmed.

3. The nurse must determine whether Mrs. Brown has a support system and, if not, problem solve with her to provide the support she needs. If Tonja is colicky, Mrs. Brown will need added support and the various interventions will need to be discussed. The nurse ends the visit by giving Mrs. Brown permission to contact her as questions and problems arise. The nurse also makes a note to contact Mrs. Brown by phone in a couple of days to see how she is doing.

REFERENCES AND READINGS

Agran, P., Anderson, C., Winn, D., Trent, R., Walton-Haynes, L., & Thayer, S. (2003). Rates of pediatric injuries by 3-month intervals for children 0 to 3 years of age. *Pediatrics, 111,* e683-e692.

American Academy of Pediatrics. (1998). *Pediatric nutrition handbook.* Elk Grove Village, IL: American Academy of Pediatrics.

American Academy of Pediatrics. (2000). Year 2000 position statement: Principles and guidelines for early hearing detection and intervention programs. *Pediatrics, 106,* 798-817.

American Academy of Pediatrics. (2003a). Human milk, breastfeeding, and transmission of human immunodeficiency virus type I in the United States. *Pediatrics, 112,* 1196-1205.

American Academy of Pediatrics. (2003b). Oral health risk assessment timing and establishment of the dental home. *Pediatrics, 111,* 1113-1116.

American Academy of Pediatrics. (2003c). *Summer safety tips.* Retrieved June 10, 2003, from *www.aap.org.*

American Academy of Pediatrics (2005a). Breastfeeding and the use of human milk. *Pediatrics, 115,* 496-506.

American Academy of Pediatrics (2005b). *Car safety seats: A guide for families 2005.* Retrieved December 10, 2005, from *www.aap .org/family/carseatguide.htm.*

American Academy of Pediatrics (2005c). Effects of child age and body size on serious injury from passenger air-bag presence in motor vehicle crashes. *Pediatrics, 115,* 1579-1585.

American Academy of Pediatrics. (2005d). The changing concept of sudden infant death syndrome: Diagnostic coding shifts, controversies regarding the sleeping environment, and new variables to consider in reducing risk. *Pediatrics, 116,* 1245-1255.

American Academy of Pediatrics, Committee on Environmental Health. (2005). Lead exposure in children: Prevention, detection, and management. *Pediatrics, 116,* 1036-1046.

American Academy of Pediatrics, Committee on Nutrition. (2001). The use and misuse of fruit juice in pediatrics. *Pediatrics, 107,* 1210-1213.

American Academy of Pediatrics Committee on Nutrition. (2003). *Pediatric nutrition handbook* (5th ed.). Elk Grove Village, IL: American Academy of Pediatrics.

American Academy of Pediatrics, Committee on Nutrition and the Committee on Environmental Health. (2005). Infant methemoglobinemia: The role of dietary nitrate in food and water. *Pediatrics, 116,* 784-786.

American Academy of Pediatrics Work Group on Breastfeeding. (1997). Breastfeeding and the use of human milk. *Pediatrics, 100,* 1035-1039.

American Academy of Pediatrics, & American College of Obstetricians and Gynecologists. (2002). *Guidelines for perinatal care* (5th ed.). Elk Grove Village, IL, and Washington, DC: American Academy of Pediatrics and American College of Obstetricians and Gynecologists.

Banks, J. W. (2003). Ka'nistenhsera Teiakotihsnie's: A Native community rekindles the tradition of breastfeeding. *AWHONN Lifelines, 7,* 340-347.

Biancuzzo, M. (2003). *Breastfeeding the newborn: Clinical strategies for nurses* (2nd ed.). St. Louis: Mosby.

Centers for Disease Control and Prevention. (2004). *Breastfeeding: Data and statistics: Breastfeeding practices—Results from the 2004 National Immunization Survey.* Retrieved December 9, 2005, from *www.cdc.gov/breastfeeding/data/NIS_data/data_2004.htm.*

Centers for Disease Control and Prevention. (2005). *Infant feeding in the context of HIV infection.* Retrieved January 8, 2006, from *www .cdc.gov/nchstp/.*

Centers for Disease Control and Prevention, National Center for Injury Prevention and Control. (2004). *CDC's unintentional injury activities—2004.* Atlanta: Centers for Disease Control and Prevention.

Chezem, J., Friesen, C., & Boettcher, J. (2003). Breastfeeding knowledge, breastfeeding confidence, and infant feeding plans: Effects on actual feeding practices. *Journal of Obstetric, Gynecologic, and Neonatal Nursing, 32,* 40-47.

Cobb, M. A. B. (2003). Promoting breastfeeding. *AWHONN Lifelines, 5,* 418-423.

Cohen, M. H., Kemper, K. J., Stephens, L., Hashimoto, D., & Gilmour, J. (2005). Pediatric use of complementary therapies: Ethical and policy choices. *Pediatrics, 116,* e568-e575.

Cunningham, M., & Cox, E. (2003). Hearing assessment in infants and children: Recommendations beyond neonatal screening. *Pediatrics, 111,* 436-441.

Dobson, B., & Murtaugh, M. A. (2001). Position of the American Dietetic Association: Breaking the barriers to breastfeeding. *Journal of the American Dietetic Association, 101,* 1213-1220.

Durbin, D. R., Chen, I., Smith, R., Elliott, M., & Winston, F. (2005). Effects of seating position and appropriate restraint use on the risk of injury to children in motor vehicle crashes. *Pediatrics, 115,* e305-e309.

Erikson, E. H. (1963). *Childhood and society* (2nd ed.). New York: Norton.

Flavell, J. H. (1964). *The developmental psychology of Jean Piaget.* New York: Van Nostrand.

Freud, A. (1974). *Introduction to psychoanalysis.* New York: International Universities Press.

Garrison, M., & Christakis, D. (2000). A systematic review of treatments for infant colic. *Pediatrics, 106,* 184-190.

Gartner, L., & Greer, F. (2003). Prevention of rickets and vitamin D deficiency: New guidelines for vitamin D intake. *Pediatrics, 111* 908-910.

Hill, D. J., Heine, R. G., Hosking, C. S., Francis, D. E., Brown, J., Speirs, B., Sadowsky, J., & Carlin, J. B. (2005). Effect of a low-allergen maternal diet on colic among breastfed infants: A randomized, controlled trial. *Pediatrics, 116,* e709-e715.

Hong, T. M., Callister, L. C., & Schwartz, R. (2003). First-time mothers' views of breastfeeding support from nurses. *MCN: The American Journal of Maternal/Child Nursing, 28,* 10-15.

Iglowstien, I., Jenni, O., Molinari, L., & Largo, R. (2003). Sleep duration from infancy to adolescence: Reference values and generational trends. *Pediatrics, 111,* 302-307.

Kamerling, S. N. (2002). Airbags & children: Making correct choices in child passenger restraints. *MCN, The American Journal of Maternal/Child Nursing, 27,* 264-273.

Karmiloff-Smith, A. (1995). The extraordinary cognitive journey from foetus through infancy. *Journal of Child Psychology and Psychiatry, 36,* 1293-1313.

Khakoo, G. A., & Lack. G. (2004). Introduction of solids to the infant diet. *Archives of Diseases in Childhood, 89,* 295.

Labarere, J., Gelbert-Baudino, N., Ayral, A. S., Duc, C., Berchotteau, M., Bouchon, N., Schelstraete, C., Vittoz, J. P., Francoies, P., & Pons, J. C. (2005). Efficacy of breastfeeding support provided by trained clinicians during an early, routine, preventive visit: A prospective, randomized, open trial of 226 mother-infant pairs. *Pediatrics, 115,* e139-e146.

Malnory, M., Johnson, T. S., & Kirby, R. S. (2003). Newborn behavioral and physiological responses to circumcision. *MCN: The American Journal of Maternal/Child Nursing, 28,* 313-317.

Miller-Loncar, C., Bigsby, R., High, P., Wallach, M., & Lester, B. (2004). Infant colic and feeding difficulties. *Archives of Disease in Childhood, 89,* 908-912.

Mofidi, S. (2003). Nutritional management of pediatric food hypersensitivity. *Pediatrics, 111,* 1645-1653.

Nagaraja, J., Menkedick, J., Phelan, K. J., Ashley, P., Zhang, X., & Lanphear, B. P. (2005). Deaths from residential injuries in US children and adolescents, 1985-1997. *Pediatrics, 116,* 454-461.

Neu, M., & Robinson, J. (2003). Infants with colic: Their childhood characteristics. *Journal of Pediatric Nursing, 18*(1), 12-20.

Piaget, J. (1952). *The origins of intelligence in children.* New York: International Universities Press.

Pollock, C., Bustamante-Forest, R., & Giarratano, G. (2002). Men of diverse cultures: Knowledge and attitudes about breastfeeding. *Journal of Obstetric, Gynecologic, and Neonatal Nursing, 31,* 673-679.

Powell, E., Jovtis, E., & Tanz, R. (2002). Incidence and description of stroller-related injuries to children. *Pediatrics, 110,* e62.

Ross Products Division. (2003). *Breastfeeding trends through 2000. Mothers' survey.* Columbus, OH: Ross Products Division, Abbott Laboratories, Inc. Retrieved Oct. 27, 2003, from *www.ross .com/aboutross/survey.*

Savage, M. F., Lee, J. Y., Kotch, J. B., & Vann, W. F. (2004). Early preventive dental visits: Effects on subsequent utilization and costs. *Pediatrics, 114,* e418-e423.

Skidmore-Roth, L. (2004). *Mosby's handbook of herbs & natural supplements* (2nd ed.). St. Louis: Mosby.

Smitherman, L. C., Janisse, J., & Mathur, A. (2005). The use of folk remedies among children in an urban black community: Remedies for fever, colic, and teething. *Pediatrics, 115,* e297-e304.

Story, M., Holt, K., & Sofka, D. (2002). *Bright futures in practice: Nutrition* (2nd ed.). Arlington, VA: National Center for Education in Maternal and Child Health.

Taveras, E. M., Capra, A. M., Braveman, P. A., Jensvold, N. G., Escobar, G. J., & Lieu, T. A. (2003). Clinician support and psychosocial risk factors associated with breastfeeding discontinuation. *Pediatrics, 112,* 108-115.

Titus, M. O., Baxter, A., & Starling, S. (2003). Accidental scald burns in sinks. *Pediatrics, 111,* e191-e194.

U.S. Department of Health and Human Services. (2000). *Healthy People 2010* (Conference edition, in 2 volumes). Washington, DC: U.S. Department of Health and Human Services.

U.S. Department of Health and Human Services National Center for Health Statistics. (2005). *NVSS linked birth and infant death data.* Retrieved January 9, 2006, from *www.cdc.gov/nchs/.*

Velsor-Friedrich, B. (2002). The silent epidemic: Lead poisoning. *Journal of Pediatric Nursing, 17,* 59-61.

Wessel, M. A., Cobb, J. C., Jackson, E. B., Harris, G. S., & Detwiler, A. C. (1954). Paroxysmal fussing in infancy, sometimes called "colic". *Pediatrics, 14,* 421-435.

White, B. L. (1975). *The first three years of life.* Englewood Cliffs, NJ: Prentice-Hall.

Windsor, J. (2003). Korean women and breastfeeding. *AWHONN Lifelines, 7,* 61-64.

Woolf, A. D. (2003). Herbal remedies and children: Do they work? Are they harmful? *Pediatrics, 112,* 240-246.

Zeiger, R. S. (2003). Food allergen avoidance in the prevention of food allergy in infants and children. *Pediatrics, 111,* 1662-1671.

Zutavern, A., von Mutius, E., Harris, J., Mills, P., Moffatt, S., White, C., et al. (2004). The introduction of solids in relation to asthma and eczema. *Archives of Disease in Childhood, 89,* 303-308.

CHAPTER 6

Health Promotion During Early Childhood

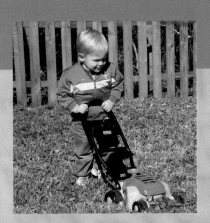

Learning Objectives

After studying this chapter, you should be able to:
- Describe the physiologic changes and the motor, cognitive, language, and psychosocial development of the toddler and preschooler.
- Provide parents with anticipatory guidance related to the toddler and preschooler.
- Discuss the causes of and identify interventions for common toddler behaviors: temper tantrums, negativism, and ritualism.
- Identify strategies to alleviate a preschool child's fears and sleep problems.
- Discuss strategies for disciplining a toddler and a preschooler.
- Describe signs of a toddler's readiness for toilet training, and offer guidelines to parents.
- Offer parents suggestions for promoting school readiness in the preschool child.

Definitions

associative play Group play without group goals.
autonomy The ability to function independently without the control of others.
caries Tooth decay.
cooperative play Organized play with group goals.
dysfluency Disorders in the rhythm of speech in which individuals know precisely what they wish to say but are unable to do so because of an involuntary, repetitive prolongation or cessation of sound.
irreversibility The inability to understand a process in reverse or mentally undo an action that has been performed.
negativism The attitude of opposing or resisting the directions of others.

parallel play Playing alongside but not with other children.
physiologic anorexia Decreased appetite because of relatively decreased caloric need.
regression The return to a behavior characteristic of an earlier stage of development.
ritualism The need to maintain sameness and reliability.
symbolic play The use of games and interactions that represent an issue or concern to be addressed.
symbolic thought The ability to allow a mental image (word or object) to represent something that is not present.
transductive reasoning Reasoning from the particular to the particular rather than from the general to the particular.

Audio Glossary

Electronic Resources

Additional information related to the content in Chapter 6 can be found on:

the interactive companion CD-ROM
- Audio Glossary
- NCLEX Review Questions
- Pediatric Assessment & Video Clips
- Skills: Car Seat Safety
  Fostering Healthy Sleep Patterns in Children
  Instructing Families in Child Safety

or the companion website at evolve
http://evolve.elsevier.com/james/ncoc
- NCLEX Review Questions
- Pediatric Assessment & Video Clips
- Resources for Health Care Providers and Families
- WebLinks

The developmental changes that mark the transition from infancy to early childhood are dramatic. During the toddler years, ages 12 through 36 months, the child begins to venture out independently from a secure base of trust established during the first year. The preschool period, ages 3 through 5 years, is a time of relative tranquility after the tumultuous toddler period.

GROWTH AND DEVELOPMENT DURING EARLY CHILDHOOD

The toddler years are characterized by a struggle for autonomy as the child develops a sense of self separate from the parent. Boundless energy and insatiable curiosity drive the toddler to explore the environment and master new skills (Fig. 6-1).

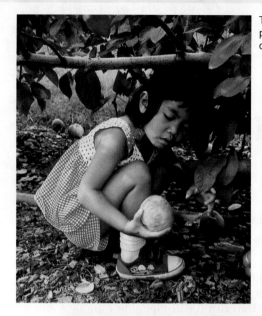

The toddler is enchanted by a world filled with discovery. Curiosity provides resources for the tremendous cognitive growth that occurs during this period.

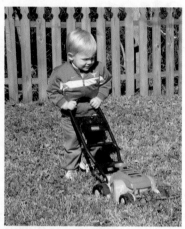

Toddlers enjoy push-pull toys. Toys should be strong and sturdy; wheeled toys should not tip over easily.

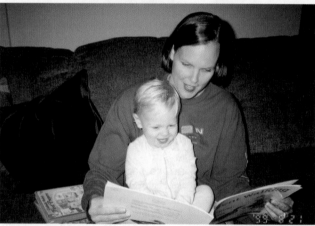

Reading simple stories provides quiet, enjoyable times for toddlers and parents and enhances speech and language development.

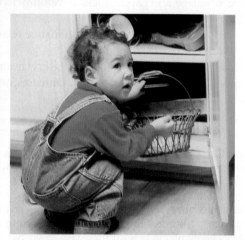

Pots and pans are popular toys for inquisitive toddlers. However, exploring cupboards can be a dangerous activity for toddlers. Toxic cleaning substances and other dangerous objects must be kept behind locked doors or otherwise out of reach.

FIG 6-1 **Growth and development of the toddler.**

The combination of increased motor skills, immaturity, and lack of experience places the toddler at risk for unintentional injury. Toddlers' egocentric and demanding behaviors, often marked by temper tantrums and negativism, have given this age the label "the terrible twos."

The preschooler becomes increasingly independent, mastering many self-care and motor skills and developing greater social and emotional maturity (Fig. 6-2). The preschooler is imaginative, creative, and curious. Many parents describe this period as their favorite age as they watch the dramatic transformation of a chubby toddler into an agile, articulate child who is ready to enter the world of peers and school.

The nurse's roles as health care provider, family counselor, and child advocate continue during the toddler and preschool years. Well-child checkups provide the nurse with opportunities for anticipatory guidance related to growth and development, safety, nutrition, and some of the common age-related concerns of parents (Box 6-1).

Physical Growth and Development

The Toddler

Physical growth slows during the toddler years. The average weight gain is 2.25 kg (5 pounds) per year. A child's birth weight has quadrupled by age 2 to 3 years. The rate of increase in height also slows, with the average toddler growing approximately 7.5 cm (3 inches) per year.

The brain grows at a slower rate during this period than during infancy. Head circumference reflects this growth, increasing approximately 3.7 cm (1½ inches) during the toddler years compared with the growth of 12 cm (4⅘ inches) in the first 12 months. By the age of 2 years, the head circumference has reached 90% of its adult size.

Immature abdominal musculature gives the toddler a potbellied appearance, with an exaggerated lumbar curve. The child's short legs may appear slightly bowed, and the feet seem flat because of a plantar fat pad that disappears around the age of 2 years. During the toddler years, muscle

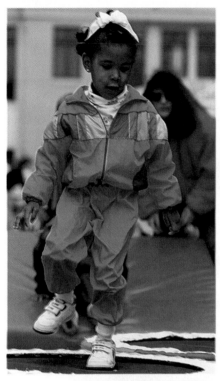

As the brain matures, the preschool child's motor development matures. Opportunities for practice contribute to the development of motor skills. *(Courtesy Cook Children's Medical Center, Fort Worth, TX.)*

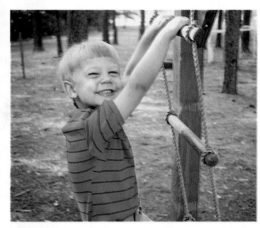

This 4-year-old's motor development has increased to the point that he can jump and climb well. A 4-year-old can also throw a ball overhand and cut on a curved line with scissors.

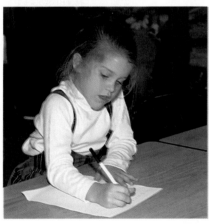

This 5-year-old is printing her name in readable letters. Children of this age can usually skip and can both throw and catch a ball. *(Courtesy University of Texas at Arlington School of Nursing.)*

FIG 6-2 **Growth and development of the preschooler.**

BOX 6-1	*Healthy People 2010* Objectives for Toddlers and Preschoolers
14-4	Reduce bacterial meningitis in young children.
14-24	Increase the proportion of young children who receive all vaccines that have been recommended for universal administration for at least 5 years.
15-3	Reduce firearm-related deaths. Reduce deaths caused by unintentional injuries.
15-29	Reduce drownings.
19-4	Reduce growth retardation among low-income children younger than 5 years.
21-2	Reduce the proportion of children, adolescents, and adults with untreated dental decay.
27-9	Reduce the proportion of children who are regularly exposed to tobacco smoke at home.

Modified from U.S. Department of Health and Human Services. (2000). *Healthy People 2010.* Washington, DC: Author.

tissue gradually replaces much of the adipose tissue (baby fat) present during infancy. As the musculoskeletal system matures and the child walks and runs more, the cherubic toddler disappears and the child grows into a taller, leaner preschooler.

The Preschooler

The growth of the preschool child is slow and steady. Height and weight gains are minimal during this period. The average weight gain is approximately 2.25 kg (5 pounds) per year, and the height gain averages 5 to 7.5 cm (2 to 3 inches) per year. Children attain half their adult height between the ages of 2 and 3 years. During this time, growth occurs more rapidly in the legs than in the trunk, accumulation of adipose tissue declines, and the child's appetite decreases. As a result, the preschooler loses the potbellied appearance of the toddler, becoming

---

THE 15- TO 18-MONTH-OLD CHILD

FOCUSED ASSESSMENT

What new activities is your child doing?

Can the child say single words? Put words together? Understand most of what you say? Communicate needs and wants?

What kinds of foods does your child eat and how often? Does the child have a problem with eating nonfood items? Is your child able to eat independently?

How does your child move from one area in the house to another?

How does your child behave when frustrated? How do you and your partner handle this?

What kinds of activities do you enjoy doing with your child?

DEVELOPMENTAL MILESTONES

Personal/social: may exhibit negativism, ritualism, and increasing tolerance of separation from parents; undresses; begins temper tantrums when frustrated; may have a transition object; begins to understand gender differences

Fine motor: turns book pages; begins to imitate vertical and circular strokes; vision 20/50 by 18 months; drinks from a cup by holding it with two hands

Language/cognitive: increasing receptive language; begins to understand and say "no"; may begin to put two words together; can point to familiar objects; begins to use memory; understands spatial and temporal relations and increased object permanence; has a basic moral understanding (reward and punishment); understands simple directions; by 18 months has a vocabulary of approximately 30 words; holographic speech (uses single words with gestures to express whole ideas)

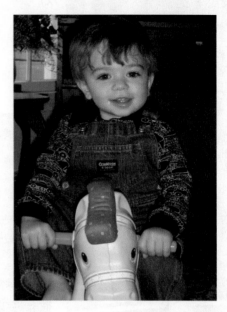

Gross motor: walks with increasing confidence and begins to run; climbs stairs first by creeping, then walking with hand held; jumps in place; begins to throw a ball overhand without falling

CRITICAL MILESTONES*

Personal/social: begins to imitate; helps in the house; feeds self with increasing skill (still rotates the spoon, if used) and holds a cup

Fine motor: builds a tower with increasing number of blocks; scribbles; able to put a block in a cup

* Guided by DDST II.

---

slimmer and more agile. Muscles grow faster than bones during the preschool period. Muscle strength is influenced by nutrition, genetic makeup, and the opportunity to exercise and use the muscles. "Knock knees" (see Chapter 26) are common in 3-year-olds and are often associated with occasional stumbling and falling. Maturation of the knee and hip joints usually corrects this problem by age 4 or 5 years.

As the lungs grow, the vital capacity increases and the respiratory rate slows. Respirations remain primarily diaphragmatic until age 5 or 6 years. The heart rate decreases and the blood pressure increases as the heart increases in size (see Chapter 9 for vital sign ranges). Cardiovascular maturation enables the preschooler to engage in more sustained and strenuous activity.

All 20 deciduous teeth are present by age 3 years. Deciduous teeth may begin to fall out at the end of the preschool period. The first permanent teeth to erupt, the back molars, usually appear in the early school-age years.

Motor Development

The Toddler

Learning to walk well is the crowning achievement of the toddler period. The child is in perpetual motion, seemingly compelled to pull up, take a few steps, fall, and repeat the process over and over, oblivious to bumps and bruises. The toddler will repeat this performance hundreds of times until the skill of walking has been perfected.

The age at which children learn to walk varies widely. Most children can walk alone by 15 months. By 18 months of age, toddlers walk well and try to run but fall often. At approximately 15 months of age, many toddlers become avid climbers. Chairs, tables, and bookcases all present irresistible challenges and risks for injury. Parents may have difficulty keeping the toddler in a crib and may decide to move the child to a regular bed.

Toddlers are also engaged in perfecting fine motor skills. Hand-eye coordination improves with maturity and practice. Mealtimes are still messy. Although most 18-month-olds

HEALTH PROMOTION

THE 15- TO 18-MONTH-OLD CHILD—cont'd

CRITICAL MILESTONES—cont'd

Language/cognitive: says three to 10 single words; can point to several body parts

Gross motor: walks well forward and backward; stoops and recovers

HEALTH MAINTENANCE

Physical Measurements

Continue to measure and plot length, weight, and head circumference

Anterior fontanel closed by 18 months

Immunizations

15 months: *Haemophilus influenzae* type b (Hib) #4; measles, mumps, rubella (MMR) #1 (if not given at 1 year); varicella (if not given at 1 year); pneumococcal (if not given at 1 year); hepatitis B #3 (if not given earlier)

18 months: diphtheria, tetanus, acellular pertussis (DTaP) #4; inactivated poliovirus (IPV) #3 (if not given earlier); hepatitis B #3 (if not given earlier); varicella (if not given earlier)

Influenza vaccine annually

Hepatitis A #2 (6 months after first dose)

ANTICIPATORY GUIDANCE

Nutrition

Calorie, protein, and fluid requirements decrease slightly; offer a variety of foods every 2 to 3 hours

Give 2 or 3 cups of whole milk daily for calcium

Vitamin D supplementation 200 IU per day if drinking less than 16 ounces/day of milk

Make mealtimes pleasant: use appropriate-size utensils, colorful dinnerware

Child may have fussy eating habits (physiologic anorexia)

Resist giving food as a comfort measure

Do not allow child to walk or play with food in the mouth

Elimination

Sphincters become physiologically under voluntary control, but child is usually not ready for toilet training; advise parents to wait but discuss signs of readiness

Dental

Continue to brush with a soft toothbrush twice daily

Give fluoride if water is not fluoridated

Maintain a diet low in sugar

Do not put the child to sleep with a bottle

Sleep

Sleep cycles decrease and the child has longer awake periods

Still naps one or two times per day

May resist going to bed; likes a bedtime routine

Hygiene

Begins to participate in self-care (washes face and hands with assistance)

Safety

Review car safety, violence, falls, water safety, toy and toy box safety, bike passenger helmet, poisons

Discuss choking, toy safety, firearm access, burn prevention, sun protection

Play

Provide push-pull toys with short strings

Noise-making toys

Dolls and stuffed animals (watch for small parts)

Musical toys

Art supplies: large crayons, finger paints, clay

Large blocks and balls

---

can hold a cup with both hands and drink from it without much spilling, eating with a spoon is difficult. Most of the food conveyed in a spoon is spilled. Children need a great deal of practice with a spoon before they can feed themselves without spilling. Most toddlers can feed themselves with a spoon by their second birthday if they have been allowed to practice.

At 18 months of age, the toddler enjoys removing clothing. By 24 months, the toddler can put on simple items of clothing but cannot differentiate front from back. Children at this age also can zip large zippers, put on shoes, and wash and dry their hands. Two-year-olds brush their teeth but need help in adequately removing plaque.

The toddler's increasing motor skills allow more independence in all areas of daily life. Feeding, dressing, and play provide opportunities for the child to develop autonomy. Motor development in this age group is far ahead of development of judgment and perception. This difference in timing of the development of different skills increases the risk for injury.

The Preschooler

Coordination and muscle strength increase rapidly between the ages of 3 and 5 years. Increases in brain size and nerve myelinization enable the child to perfect fine and gross motor skills.

Motor abilities vary widely among children. Although motor skill is less influenced by environment than other areas of development, such as language, opportunities to practice may contribute to better motor skills. For example, a 4-year-old who often plays catch with a sibling or parent generally finds playing Little League baseball as a 7-year-old easier than a child without a similar experience.

Handedness begins to emerge at approximately 3 years and is usually clearly established by 4 years. The nurse should encourage parents to provide left-handed children with appropriate tools, particularly left-handed scissors. Left-handed children should not be forced to use their right hand because coordination is usually better when they use the dominant side. Eye-hand coordination is usually good enough by age

5 years for a child to hit a nail on the head with a hammer. Increased coordination allows the child to perform many self-care skills and become more independent.

By age 4 or 5 years, the child is independent and can dress, eat, and go to the bathroom without help. Unlike the toddler, who must be restrained to avoid injury, the older preschooler can usually be trusted to heed verbal warnings of danger.

Cognitive and Sensory Development

The Toddler

Toddlers are consumed with curiosity. Their boundless energy and insatiable inquisitiveness provide them with resources for the tremendous cognitive growth that occurs during this period.

Toddlers between the ages of 12 and 18 months are in Piaget's sensorimotor period (Piaget, 1952) (see Chapter 4). Learning in this stage occurs mainly by trial and error. Toddlers spend most of a busy day experimenting to see what will happen as they dump, fill, empty, and explore every accessible area of their environment. Between 19 and 24 months, the child enters the final stage of the sensorimotor period. Object permanence is firmly established by this age. The child has a beginning ability to use symbols and words when referring to absent people or objects and begins to solve problems mentally rather than by repeating an action over and over. A toddler at this stage is often seen imitating the parent of the same sex performing household tasks (termed *domestic mimicry*). Late in this stage, the child displays *deferred imitation* (e.g., imitating the parent putting on makeup or shaving hours after that parent has left for work). The 18-month-old has a beginning ability to wait, as evidenced by the toddler appropriately responding to a parent or caregiver who says "just a minute." The child's concept of time is still immature, however, and "a minute" may seem like an hour to the toddler.

Toddlers think in terms of the predictable routines of their daily schedule. When talking with the toddler, the nurse should use time orientation in relation to familiar activities. For example, a toddler understands "Your mother will be here after your nap" better than "Your mother will be here at 2 o'clock."

Many hours each day are spent putting objects into holes and smaller objects into each other as the child experiments with sizes, shapes, and spatial relations. Toddlers enjoy opening drawers and doors, exploring the contents of cabinets and closets, and generally wreaking havoc throughout the house as well as exposing themselves to potential danger.

According to Piaget (1952) the preoperational stage of cognitive development characterizes the second half of early childhood (see Chapter 4). This stage is divided into two phases: the preconceptual phase (2 to 4 years) and the intuitive phase (4 to 7 years). During the preconceptual phase, the child is beginning to use symbolic thought—the ability to allow a mental image (words or ideas) to represent objects or ideas. Mental symbols allow the child to remember the past and describe events that happened in the past. At

approximately 24 months, children enter the preconceptual phase, which ends at age 4 years. Children begin to think and reason at a primitive level. Two-year-olds have a beginning ability to retain mental images. This ability allows them to internalize what they see and experience. Symbols in the form of words can be used to represent ideas. Increasing amounts of play time are spent pretending. A box may become a spaceship or a hat; pebbles may be money or popcorn. The child's rapidly increasing vocabulary enhances symbolic play. The toddler begins to think about alternative solutions to a problem and can even consider the consequences of an action without carrying it out (touching a hot stove, running too fast on a slippery sidewalk).

The toddler's thinking is immature, limited in its logic, and bound to the present. Egocentrism, animism, irreversibility, magical thinking, and centration characterize the preoperational thought of the toddler (Table 6-1). The predominant words in the toddler's language repertoire are "me," "I," and "mine."

The Preschooler

By age 3 years, the brain has reached two thirds of its adult size. Maturation of the central nervous system contributes to the child's increasing cognitive abilities.

The 3-year-old can retain a mental image of a loved one and can periodically "refuel" by thinking about that person. A photograph can help some children cope with separation by bridging the gap between physical presence and mental image. Preschoolers' ability to remember their parents and recognize that their needs can be met even though their parents are not present increases their ability to tolerate separation.

Because preschoolers still engage in animism, they often endow inanimate objects with lifelike qualities during play. A doll may become a crying baby, or a teddy bear may become a friend who listens sympathetically. Symbolic play is important for emotional development because it allows the child to work through distressing feelings. For this reason, allowing a child to play with medical equipment after a painful procedure can be therapeutic. Four-year-olds who have received injections may be found working out their feelings by giving their dolls "lots of shots."

During the preconceptual phase, reality may be distorted by transductive reasoning. The preschool child reasons from particular to particular rather than from particular to general, and vice versa, as adults do. The child cannot understand that relationships exist and cannot view the whole in relation to its parts. The preschool child has difficulty focusing on the important aspects of a situation. To a child, everything is important and interdependent. This type of thinking is called *field dependency*. For example, the preschooler may have difficulty falling asleep at night because the parent did not follow the usual bedtime routine. Objects, routine, and sameness are important to the preschool child. Rituals provide the preschool child with a feeling of control.

The second phase of Piaget's preoperational stage, the intuitive phase, is characterized by centration and lack of reversibility. *Centration* is the tendency to center or focus

TABLE 6-1 Characteristics of Preoperational Thinking	
Characteristic	**Example**
Egocentrism: Views everything in relation to self; is unable to consider another's point of view.	Toddler takes a toy away from another child and cannot understand that the other child wants (or has a right to) the toy, too.
Animism: Believes that inert objects are alive and have wills of their own.	Toddler trips over a toy and scolds the toy for hurting her. She believes that the toy hurt her on purpose.
Irreversibility: Cannot see a process in reverse order. Cannot follow a line of reasoning back to its beginning. Cannot hold onto two or more sequential thoughts simultaneously.	If the child takes a toy apart, the child cannot remember the sequence for putting it back together.
	If a child is taken on a walk, the child cannot retrace steps and find the way home.
Magical thought: Believes that magical thought is the cause of events and that wishing something will make it so.	Toddlers often feel extremely powerful and believe that their thoughts cause events to happen.
	May believe that parents are all-powerful and can read minds or have magical powers.
Centration: Tends to focus on only one aspect of an experience, ignoring other possible alternatives. Focuses on the dominant characteristic of an object, excluding other characteristics.	May have difficulty putting together a puzzle, concentrating on only one detail of a piece (e.g., shape) and ignoring other qualities (e.g., color, detail).
	Cannot follow more than one direction at a time.

on one part of a situation and ignore the other parts. The child cannot understand logical relationships and is unable to focus on more than one aspect of a situation at a time. For example, the child may not be able to follow a sequence of directions but will perform well if the directions are given one at a time.

The 4- or 5-year-old shows *irreversibility* in thought. Children this age cannot reverse a process or the order of events. They may be able to take a complex puzzle apart but have difficulty putting it back together. The 4- or 5-year old also lacks reversibility for mathematical processes. The child may be able to add 3 and 1 and get 4, but reversing the problem (4 − 1 = 3) would be too difficult.

The preschool years are a period of rapid learning. The preschool child is curious and wants to know how things work. Preschoolers' thinking is still magical and egocentric (self-centered). Children at this age tend to understand events only as these events affect them, believing that everyone else has had the same experience. Children seeing their mother in distress may bring her a doll, assuming that it would comfort the mother as it does the child.

Preschool children often think that their thoughts are powerful enough to cause things to happen. They may frighten themselves with some of their ideas, believing that they may become what they imagine they will be. Preschoolers may feel overwhelmed by guilt when a sibling is hospitalized because they believe that their hostile feelings caused the sibling's illness. Likewise, a child of this age may say, "I got sick because I was bad."

Language Development

The Toddler

The acquisition of language is one of the most dramatic developments of early childhood. Although the age at which children begin to talk varies widely, most can communicate verbally by their second birthday. The rate of language development depends on physical maturity and the amount of reinforcement that the child has received. Between 15 and 24 months of age, language ability develops rapidly. Toddlers understand many more words than they can say because receptive language (what the child understands) develops sooner and more quickly than speech. Sometime after 18 months, many children experience a sudden spurt in speech production and comprehension, resulting in a vocabulary of 300 or more words at 24 months. By 2 years of age, roughly 60% to 70% of toddlers' speech should be understandable. Because children of 24 to 30 months are less egocentric and better able to consider another's point of view, they engage in more conversation with others and less monologue.

If language development is not progressing normally, parents should be advised to pursue follow-up care. Children of bilingual families, children who are twins, and children other than firstborns may have slower language development. Because language development depends on adequate hearing, delayed language can be seen in children who have had repeated ear infections or who have undiagnosed hearing loss (see Chapter 31).

Parents can promote language development by talking to their children and incorporating teaching into daily routines. Feeding, bathing, dressing, and going on outings to both new and familiar places offer opportunities for verbal interaction and the practice of growing language skills. The child should be encouraged to express needs rather than have the parent anticipate and provide what the child wants before the child asks for it. Reading simple, entertaining stories with colorful pictures provides quiet, enjoyable times for toddlers and parents and enhances speech and language development.

The Preschooler

A dramatic increase in language skill in the preschool period promotes self-control and increases the child's ability to direct and be directed by others. Children at this age may be heard talking to themselves about things they have heard or been taught.

The preschooler's vocabulary increases rapidly, from 300 words at 2 years of age to more than 2100 words at 5 years. In less than 3 years, the child grows from a toddler who knows only a few words into a child who skillfully uses an extensive vocabulary to describe events, share feelings, and ask questions. Three-year-olds speak in short, telegraphic sentences. They may talk to themselves or to imaginary friends. A delightful characteristic of young preschoolers is the tendency to engage in lengthy monologues, regardless of whether anyone is listening or even present. Such self-talk provides the child with opportunities to practice speech and is often accompanied by symbolic play.

By 4 years old, children talk incessantly and tend to boast and exaggerate. They enjoy rhymes and silly ways to use similar words. Four-year-olds expect more detailed answers to their questions. They may use speech aggressively and may use profanity to gain attention. "Bad" language should be ignored, thus depriving the child of reinforcement of the behavior. When children feel that they gain power over their parents by using bad language, these verbalizations will continue.

Five-year-olds speak in sentences of adult length and use all parts of speech. They usually are proficient storytellers who produce elaborate tales for anyone who will listen. Their tendency to mix fantasy with reality may be perceived by adults as lying. The child of 5 years usually can recite the days of the week and can name the seasons.

Nurses can teach parents strategies to promote their child's language development. It is important for parents to talk with the child and respond to the child's attempts at communication. Reading to the child and making reading materials available can help build vocabulary and promote a lifelong love of reading. Watching educational television programs with their child may augment parents' communication skills with their child. Preschoolers spend a lot of time asking "how" and "why" questions, often taxing parents' patience. Short, simple, honest answers encourage vocabulary building and boost self-esteem.

Psychosocial Development

The Toddler

The toddler is developing a sense of autonomy, giving up the comfort of dependence enjoyed during infancy. If a basic sense of trust was established during the first year, the toddler can venture forward and separate from parents for short periods to explore and experience the world.

According to Erikson (1963), the toddler is struggling with the developmental task of acquiring a sense of autonomy while overcoming a sense of shame and doubt. Toddlers discover that they have a will of their own and that they can control others. Asserting their will and insisting on their own way, however, often lead to conflict with those they love, whereas submissive behavior is rewarded with affection and approval. Toddlers experience conflict because they want

to assert their own will but do not want to risk losing the approval of loved ones. If the child continues to practice dependent behavior, doubt related to abilities develops. Toddlers may feel shame for independent impulses, particularly if frequent punishment is associated with their actions.

The toddler learns which behaviors gain approval and which result in censure and punishment. Two-year-olds do not have a conscience but avoid punishment by controlling their behavior. Right and wrong are determined by the consequences of actions.

At approximately 15 months toddlers begin to demonstrate their developing autonomy with two almost universal behaviors: negativism and ritualism.

Negativism. Negativism, one of the most dramatic expressions of independence, is shown in a variety of ways. The toddler's favorite word seems to be "no." Unable to distinguish between requests and directives, the toddler seems to believe that saying "yes" would mean giving up free will. The child often seems to delight in this test of wills with the parent. Negativism may result in screaming, kicking, hitting, biting, or breath holding. Parents often interpret the child's negative behavior as being bad or stubborn. Nurses can help parents understand their toddler's behavior as an important sign of the child's progress from dependence to autonomy and independence. The nurse should give support and encourage the parent to deal with the toddler's trying behavior with patience and a sense of humor. Although general permissiveness is not recommended, too much pressure and forceful methods of control often lead to defiance, tantrums, and prolonged negative behavior.

Ritualism and the Importance of Routine. Ritualism helps the child venture out and away from the safety of the parents by ensuring uniformity and security. Ritualism allows the toddler to have a sense of control. The child feels more confident with a secure home base. The toddler insists on sameness. Milk may have to be poured into the same cup, parents may have to sit in the same chairs at dinnertime, and a specified routine may have to be followed countless times throughout the day. The child may be unable to go to sleep unless a bedtime ritual is followed exactly (e.g., a drink of water, two stories, prayers, and a teddy bear). The child may experience distress if this routine is not followed exactly the next night. Failure to recognize the importance of such rituals may increase stress and insecurity.

Events such as hospitalization, during which continuity of routine cannot be ensured, are difficult for the toddler. The nurse can decrease the stress of hospitalization by incorporating the child's usual rituals and routines from home into nursing care activities. Keeping hospital routines as similar to those of home as possible and recognizing ritualistic needs give the toddler some sense of control and security and decrease feelings of helplessness and fear. See Chapter 11 for further discussion of the hospitalized child.

Separation Anxiety. Separation anxiety peaks again in the toddler period. Although the concept of object permanence is fully developed in the toddler, children at this stage have

HEALTH PROMOTION

THE 2-YEAR-OLD CHILD

FOCUSED ASSESSMENT

How are you handling any discipline problems your child may be having?

Do you have any concerns about any daycare arrangements you have?

Does your child use a bottle or a cup?

How do you deal with temper tantrums?

How does your child communicate with others?

What, if anything, have you done to begin toilet training your child?

What activities do you enjoy doing together?

DEVELOPMENTAL MILESTONES

Personal/social: imitates household activities and begins to do helpful tasks; uses table utensils without much spilling; drinks from a lidless cup; removes a difficult article of clothing; begins developing sexual identity; is stubborn and negativistic: wants own way in everything; brushes teeth with help; is learning to walk; understands "soon"

Fine motor: puts blocks into a cup after demonstration; builds tower of four to six blocks; able to imitate a horizontal and circular stroke with a crayon; opens a doorknob; turns book pages one at a time; can unzip and unbutton

Language/cognition: has an approximately 300-word vocabulary, two-word sentences; points to six body parts and pictures of several familiar objects (e.g., bird, man, dog, horse); understands cause and effect, object permanence, sense of time; follows two-step directions; uses egocentric language (I, me, mine)

Gross motor: stoops and recovers well; walks forward and backward; climbs stairs holding the railing; runs, jumps, kicks a ball

CRITICAL MILESTONES*

Personal/social: removes one article of clothing; feeds a doll; uses a spoon or fork

Fine motor: holds a pencil and spontaneously scribbles; dumps a raisin out of a bottle on command after demonstration; builds a two-block tower

Language/cognitive: points to two pictures; says three to six words

Gross motor: runs; walks up steps; kicks a ball forward

HEALTH MAINTENANCE

Physical Measurements

Gains approximately 5 pounds/yr (2.25 kg)

Length is approximately half eventual adult height

Grows approximately 3 inches/yr (7.5 cm)

Immunizations

Influenza vaccine annually

*Guided by DDST II.

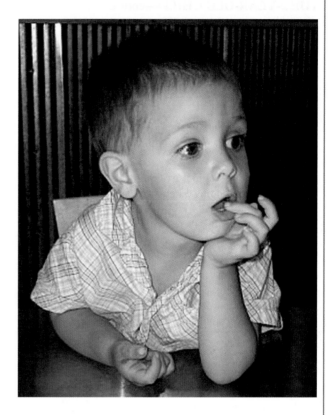

Health Screening

Hemoglobin and lead screen

Baseline cholesterol (if at risk)

Tuberculosis (TB) screening (if at risk)

ANTICIPATORY GUIDANCE

Nutrition

May begin low-fat milk

Daily diet: 2 or 3 cups milk, two servings of protein, three small servings of vegetables, two servings of fruit, and six servings of bread

Modify diet for children with elevated cholesterol (<300 mg/day, no more than 30% calories from fat and 10% from saturated fat): egg substitute, low-fat cheeses and meats

Decrease added fat and high-calorie, high-fat desserts; increase fruits, vegetables, and carbohydrates

Vitamin D supplementation 200 IU per day if drinking less than 16 oz/day of milk

Elimination

Bowel movements decrease in number and become more regular

Child remains dry for several hours

Begin to think about a positive approach to toilet training

Continued

HEALTH PROMOTION

THE 2-YEAR-OLD CHILD—cont'd

Dental

Sixteen teeth; may use pea-sized amount of fluoridated toothpaste, encourage not to swallow

Schedule first dental visit

Sleep

12 to 14 hr/day

Usually a long afternoon nap

Limit television viewing to no more than 1 hour daily

Hygiene

Girls are prone to vaginal irritation; advise to wipe from front to back; adding ¼ cup vinegar to bath water can relieve irritation

Boys' foreskin begins to retract; retract gently to clean; never force

Safety

Review toy safety, firearm safety, burn prevention, and other previously discussed subjects

Discuss choking on food, street safety, water safety, outside poisons, playground safety, sun protection

Self-Esteem and Competence

Model appropriate social behavior

Encourage your child to learn to make choices

Help your child to appropriately express emotions

Spend individual time with your child daily

Provide consistent and loving limits to help your child learn self-discipline

Begin toilet training only when your child is ready (dry for 2 hours, able to pull pants down, can use appropriate toileting words, can indicate the need to use the toilet)

Play

Parallel play; play begins to become imitative and imaginative

Choose toys that are safe and durable: balls, picture books, puzzles with large pieces, sandbox toys, trucks, riding toys, household toys (e.g., broom, mop, carpet sweeper)

---

difficulty differentiating their own feelings from those of their parents. Although the children experience a strong desire to be independent and leave their mothers, they fear that their mothers also want to leave them. A toddler may strike out independently across the room, only to rush back in tears to the mother, as if the child were frightened and angry with the mother for leaving. For a brief period, the parent may find talking on the telephone without interruption or even going into the bathroom without being followed virtually impossible. Leave taking and brief separations are acceptable to a toddler if they are the toddler's idea, but the parent's departure may cause desperate clinging and crying. Games such as hide-and-seek help the child master fears of separation. By repeating separation under conditions the child can control, the toddler is helped to overcome the anxiety associated with separation. The child learns from experience that loved ones will return after separation.

Being left with a stranger can be stressful. Toddlers should be told honestly and clearly about a separation shortly before it occurs. The parent or nurse should reassure the child that the parent is coming back. When a parent returns, the toddler often shows anger at being left by ignoring the parent or by pretending to be more interested in play than in going home. Parents of hospitalized toddlers are frequently distressed by such behavior when they visit their child (see Chapter 11).

Tolerating brief separations from parents is an important developmental task for the toddler. Transition objects, such as a favorite blanket or toy, provide comfort to the toddler in stressful situations, such as separation, illness, or even bedtime. Such objects help children make the transition from dependency to autonomy. Toddlers may become so attached to an object that they can hardly bear to part with it, even for a brief time while it is being laundered.

The nurse can offer support by explaining that the behavior is a normal growth and development milestone and telling the parents that plenty of affection and attention are needed to help the toddler cope with the stress of separation. The nurse counsels parents to leave a toddler only briefly at first and, if possible, to delay extended separations until the toddler can handle them better. The nurse who helps parents understand normal toddler behavior in response to separation helps parents cope with the frustrations of this transition.

Play. Toddlers spend most of their time at play. Play is serious business to the toddler—it is the child's work. Many hours are spent each day in play, perfecting fine and gross motor skills, learning to control inner urges, and gaining self-esteem. Play during this period reflects the egocentric toddler's developmental level. The toddler engages in parallel play, in which children play alongside but not with other children (Fig. 6-3). Little regard is given to the feelings of others. Children engaged in this type of play frequently grab toys away from other children or may hit or fight to obtain a wanted toy. Because toddlers are egocentric, they do not realize that they are hurting the other child and feel no shame for aggressive actions.

Imitation and acting out scenes of everyday life are common as the toddler begins to try out roles and identify with adults. Active, large-muscle play helps the toddler vent frustrations and dissipate excess energy. The nurse can help parents understand how play enhances the toddler's development. The nurse should encourage parents to play with their toddler and provide opportunities for the toddler to play with other children. The nurse teaches parents about

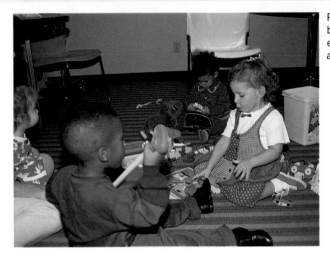

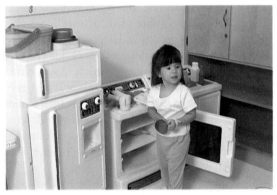

Parallel play occurs when children play side by side with similar toys but no organized group activity occurs. The children play *beside* each other but not *with* each other. *(Courtesy University of Texas at Arlington School of Nursing.)*

Symbolic play consists of activities that children use to express their perception of reality. This little girl is acting out a familiar adult scenario as she manipulates child-size toys that represent kitchen equipment.

FIG 6-3 **Types of play.**

child-proofing the house on a daily basis. Toys must be strong, safe, and too large to swallow or place in the ear or nose. Toddlers need supervision at all times. A variety of play materials, which need not be expensive, and a safe play environment enhance the toddler's development (Box 6-2).

Psychosexual Development. At approximately 18 months, toddlers enter Freud's anal stage. Freud (1960) theorized that as children focus on mastery of bowel and bladder functions, their attention is also directed to the genital area. Even

before the age of 2 years, children are aware of their own gender and begin to develop a sense of gender identity. By 2½ or 3 years, toddlers can correctly identify anatomic pictures of boys and girls. Gender identity is not fully established until age 5 years, when the child understands gender as permanent (i.e., that gender does not change with the addition of a wig or a dress) (Kohlberg, 1966).

Children begin to be aware of expected gender role behaviors at an early age. By age 3 years most toddlers show

---

BOX 6-2	**Age-Related Activities and Toys for Toddlers and Preschoolers**

General Activities

Toddler

The toddler fills and empties containers, begins dramatic play, has increased use of motor skills, enjoys feeling different textures, explores the home environment, imitates orders, likes to be read to and look at books and television that are age-appropriate.

Toys should meet the child's need for activity and inquisitiveness.

The child also enjoys manipulating small objects such as toy people, cars, and animals.

Preschooler

Dramatic play is prominent.

The child likes to run, jump, hop, and, in general, increase motor skills.

The child likes to build and create things (e.g., sand castles and mud pies).

Play is simple and imaginative.

Simple collections begin.

Toys and Specific Types of Play

Toddler

Continued exploring of the body parts of self and others; mechanical toys; objects of different textures such as clay, sand, finger paints, and bubbles; push-pull toys; large ball; sand and water play; blocks; painting; coloring with large crayons; nesting toys; large puzzles; trucks; dolls.

Therapeutic play can begin at this age.

Preschooler

Riding toys, building materials such as sand and blocks, dolls, drawing materials, crayons, cars, puzzles, books, appropriate television and videos, nonsense rhymes, singing games, pretend play as something or somebody, dress-up, finger paints, clay, cutting, pasting, simple board and card games.

an awareness of gender role stereotypes and tend to imitate the same-gender parent during play. Gender role identification continues throughout the toddler and preschool years as the child incorporates the attitudes, roles, and values of the same-gender parent. Although gender role stereotypes have relaxed somewhat in recent years, children behave according to adult expectations. Children learn behavior by reinforcement and punishment as well as by imitation. If a boy repeatedly hears that boys do not play with dolls, he will spurn such "girls' toys" and will play with toys that his parents consider masculine to gain their praise and approval. Nurses should be aware of their own biases about gender-typed behaviors and should support the parents in their choice of toys and activities for their child. The nurse can be most helpful by encouraging parents to make traditionally gender-typed toys available to both boys and girls if this approach is consistent with the parents' beliefs. Parents' expectations of appropriate gender role behavior differ according to their cultural backgrounds. In most cultures, boys and girls are treated differently and thus are taught "male" and "female" behaviors.

Parents are often concerned about their toddler's interest in and curiosity about gender differences. Sex play and masturbation are common among toddlers. Nurses can reassure parents that self-exploration or exploration of another toddler's body is normal behavior during early childhood. Parents should respect the child's curiosity as normal without judging the child as "bad." The child should be told that touching private parts is something that is done only in private. When parents discover children involved in sex play, casually telling them to dress and directing them to another activity can limit sex play without producing feelings of shame or anxiety. The nurse should explain to parents that positive attitudes toward sexuality are learned from parents who are comfortable with their own sexuality. As young children learn about their bodies and explore anatomic differences, they frequently ask questions about where babies come from or why "Brian looks different from Emily." Honest, straightforward answers that use the correct terminology satisfy the toddler's curiosity and lay the foundation for healthy sexual attitudes.

CRITICAL TO REMEMBER
Important Tasks of the Toddler Period
- Recognition of self as a separate person with own will
- Control of impulses and acquisition of socially acceptable ways to communicate wants and needs
- Control of elimination
- Toleration of separation from the parent

The Preschooler
The preschool years are a critical period for the development of socialization. Children need opportunities to play with others to learn communication and social skills. They also need appropriate guidance to learn acceptable behavior.

According to Erikson (1963), the preschooler's developmental task is to achieve a sense of initiative. The preschooler is busy learning how to do things and takes great pride in new accomplishments. If the child acts inappropriately or is repeatedly criticized or punished for attempts to explore and learn, feelings of guilt, anxiety, shame, and fear may result. For example, an adult's comment, "That's nice, but it would look better if you did it this way," may cause the child to feel inferior. Such subtle criticism can make the child reluctant to try new activities. A feeling of inferiority also may develop if adults are always doing things for the child rather than encouraging independence. The child who does not achieve a sense of initiative will feel defeated, angry, and afraid of people and new situations. Nurses can promote healthy psychosocial development in preschoolers and help them gain a sense of initiative by teaching parents the importance of providing the child with opportunities to explore in a safe, stimulating environment. Adults should encourage the preschooler's imagination and creativity and should praise appropriate behavior.

Play. Learning to relate to age mates is another developmental task that is significant during the preschool period. Preschoolers need experience playing with other children to learn how to relate to other people. Three-year-olds are capable of sharing and are more likely to do so than toddlers. Four-year-olds tend to be more argumentative and less generous with playmates. Although this behavior may appear to be a step backward to parents, it is actually a sign of growth because 4-year-olds feel more secure in a group and are testing their roles and communication skills. The 5-year-old enjoys playing with other children and generally can play with another child for longer periods before arguments develop.

Children between the ages of 3 and 5 years enjoy parallel and associative play. Children learn to share and cooperate as they play in small groups. During play, preschoolers learn simple games and rules, language concepts, and social roles. Play is often imitative, dramatic, and creative. Various roles are explored through play as children imitate significant adults. Preschoolers enjoy dress-up clothes, housekeeping toys, doll houses, and other toys that encourage pretending (see Fig. 6-3). Tricycles and climbing toys help develop muscles and coordination. Preschoolers also enjoy materials for cutting, pasting, and painting. Such manipulative and creative materials stimulate imagination and fine motor development (see Box 6-2).

Imaginary friends are common near the age of 3 years. Boundaries between reality and fantasy are blurred at this age, and "pretend" can seem real, especially during play. Imaginary friends serve many purposes. They may take the blame when the child misbehaves, allowing the child to save face when feeling guilty about a certain behavior. Imaginary friends may be companions during lonely times. They may accomplish a task with which the child is struggling or allow the child to practice roles. For example, the child may scold an imaginary friend and administer punishment, just as a parent would. Imaginary friends seem to be more common in highly imaginative and intelligent children.

Psychosexual Development. Sexual identity and body image are developing. Sexual curiosity and explorations are normal. Preschoolers are curious about anatomic differences and seek to investigate them. Preschoolers show interest in the differences between the sexes and often compare their bodies with those of others. Playing doctor and hiding with a friend to investigate anatomic differences are common activities during the preschool period. The nurse can reassure parents that the child is simply learning about his or her body and that the parents can direct the child to another activity. Preschoolers are interested in where they came from and how babies are made. Parents should be encouraged to assess what the child already knows about the subject and to determine why the child is asking the question. The parent should answer questions simply, honestly, and matter-of-factly. The child usually neither wants nor understands detailed explanations.

Parents greatly influence their children's sexual development. Positive signs of physical and emotional intimacy between parents send a positive signal to the child. A warm, accepting, matter-of-fact attitude toward sexual matters promotes a positive, healthy perspective in children. Parents can create an atmosphere of acceptance in the early preschool years when the first questions arise. A parental attitude of "You can ask me anything" can set the stage for healthy interaction from early childhood into adolescence, when parental guidance is so important.

Masturbation is common and may increase in frequency when the child is under stress. Parents often express concern about such behavior. The nurse can help parents handle these situations by explaining that such self-comforting behaviors are normal for this age. If the parent discovers the child masturbating, simple redirection of the child's attention without punishing, shaming, or reprimanding is best. Children should be taught that touching their genitals is not appropriate in public.

At this age, a sense of rivalry with the same-gender parent develops. Preschool boys commonly compete with their fathers for the attention of their mothers. A girl likewise may become "Daddy's girl," often cuddling and flirting with her father while excluding her mother from the relationship. This rivalry is usually resolved early in the school-age period as the child identifies strongly with the same-gender parent and same-gender peers. According to Freudian theory, the oedipal stage is resolved when the child strongly identifies with the parent of the same gender. By the end of the preschool period, the child identifies with and imitates the same-gender parent. In single-parent and nontraditional families the child should have a friendly, stable relationship with an adult relative or friend of the same sex who can serve as a role model. By age 3 years, children know gender differences. They imitate masculine and feminine behaviors in play, and gender identity is well established by 6 years.

Spiritual and Moral Development. Learning the difference between right and wrong (the development of a conscience) is another important task of the preschool period. According to Kohlberg (1964), children between the ages of 4 and 7 years are in the second stage of the preconventional level of moral development. In this stage, children obey rules out of self-interest. They tend to believe that if the consequences of an action are personally advantageous, the action is right. An "eye-for-an-eye" orientation guides their behavior.

The preschooler begins to use self-control to resist temptation and tries to "be good" to avoid feelings of guilt. Preschoolers determine right from wrong by the consequences of disobeying their parents' rules. At this age, children have little understanding of the reason for a rule. For example, when asked why hitting another child is wrong, the preschooler might reply, "Because my mother says so." Preschoolers adhere to parents' rules dogmatically, deciding whether to break a rule based on the resulting punishment.

Preschoolers often have difficulty applying rules in different situations. The child may know that hitting a sibling is wrong but may not understand that hitting another child at daycare is also wrong. Because the preschooler is egocentric, understanding another's viewpoint is difficult. The child begins to develop a conscience as a result of consistent rewards for good behavior and punishment for bad behavior.

The preschool child's concept of God is concrete. The family's religious beliefs and customs, such as bedtime prayers, mealtime grace, and Bible stories, are important to preschoolers. Such rituals, practiced in an atmosphere of love, can be deeply meaningful and comforting to children of this age.

HEALTH PROMOTION FOR THE TODDLER OR PRESCHOOLER AND FAMILY
Nutrition

The rate of growth slows during the toddler and preschool period, as does the child's appetite. This is sometimes referred to as *physiologic anorexia*. The child's food experiences during this period can have a lasting effect on how food and meals are viewed. The family is the primary influence at this time, although television plays an important role. Children should be discouraged from eating while watching television, and family mealtimes should be encouraged.

Nutritional Requirements

The U.S. Department of Agriculture (USDA) and the U.S. Department of Health and Human Services (USDHHS) published new nutritional guidelines in 2005 (see Box 4-7 and Fig. 4-6). Children 2 to 8 years should consume 2 cups per day of fat-free or low-fat milk or equivalent milk products. Yogurt and cheese are other milk-group sources. Total fat intake should remain between 30% and 35% of calories for children aged 2 to 3 years and between 25% and 35% of calories for children aged 4 years and older. Most fats should come from sources of polyunsaturated and monounsaturated fatty acids, such as fish, nuts, and vegetable oils (USDHHS & USDA, 2005). Poultry, fish, and lean meat are good sources of iron. Low-sugar breakfast cereals are sources of iron and vitamins. Snacks of fruits and vegetables assist in meeting the child's nutritional requirements (Box 6-3).

Many similarities exist in the nutritional needs of the toddler and the preschooler. Children this age who eat well-balanced diets should not experience iron deficiency. If milk

BOX 6-3	**Nutritious Snacks**

- Fresh fruit
- Celery sticks with cheese spread
- Yogurt
- Bagels
- Carrot sticks
- Graham crackers
- Pretzels
- Puddings

remains the primary food, however, it will replace foods rich in iron, vitamins, and minerals, such as dark-green leafy vegetables, meats, and legumes. The child who is healthy does not need vitamin supplementation. However, giving a daily children's multivitamin containing 100% of the recommended daily allowance (RDA) is not harmful.

Solid Foods

Children at this age are increasing their proficiency in using a spoon and cup. By age 2 years, children can hold a cup in one hand and use a spoon well (Fig. 6-4). By age 12 months, most children are eating the same foods as the rest of the family. The child should be offered three meals and two snacks each day.

By age 3 to 4 years, the child begins to use a fork. The child continues to develop fine motor skills and by the end of the preschool period should begin to use a rounded knife for cutting.

One method to determine serving size for children is 1 tablespoon of solid food per year of age. Children may

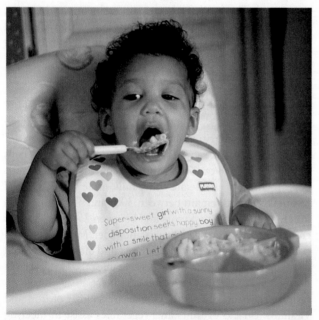

FIG 6-4 **By age 1 year, most children are eating the same foods as the rest of the family. Toddlers should be offered three meals and two healthy snacks each day. Most 2-year-olds can drink from a cup and use a spoon well if given the opportunity to practice.**

be more likely to try new foods and eat nutritious meals if smaller portions are served. Foods of different textures, colors, consistencies, tastes, and temperatures should be offered. The child should sit in a chair that allows easy access to the food; the dishes should be small, nonbreakable and, when possible, steady enough to prevent spilling. Thick, short-handled spoons and forks and shallow bowls increase the toddler's ability to eat successfully.

Foods that could be aspirated should continue to be avoided during the toddler period. Soft drinks and candy need to be discouraged. Sugar is a source of calories and is naturally present in breast milk as lactose, in fruits as fructose, and in grain products as maltose. A diet with too much sugar, however, can replace other more nutritious foods and increase tooth decay. Artificial sweeteners and foods that contain artificial sweeteners are not recommended for children younger than 2 years.

Age-Related Nutritional Challenges

Food Jags. The volume of food the child eats may vary from day to day. The child may want the same food at every meal for several days and then suddenly reject the food completely. Children this age may refuse foods because of odor and temperature. They may not like mixing foods and therefore may not eat casseroles. This dislike does not seem to apply to foods such as pizza, spaghetti, and macaroni and cheese. Many children prefer juices to milk and water. Too much milk is not good, but neither is too much juice, which can replace other foods and their nutrients. For toddlers and preschoolers, juices should be limited to no more than 4 to 6 ounces a day (American Academy of Pediatrics [AAP] Committee on Nutrition, 2001). Parents and older siblings can affect how a child views a food and should be careful about making negative comments about a certain food. Children should be assisted in developing tastes for new foods through role modeling and making the foods available.

Physiologic Anorexia. The nurse should teach parents appropriate ways to approach the child who is experiencing physiologic anorexia. Advise parents not to allow their child to fill up with snacks, milk, and juices. Small portions should be offered so that the child does not feel overwhelmed by the amount of food. Mealtimes should be pleasant and not times to discuss discipline problems or even the child's poor appetite. Children should not be made to sit at the table after the rest of the family has left. This will only create a negative association with mealtime. Parents need to maintain a balance between ignoring their child's nutritional intake and making it the focus of their parenting.

The nurse can encourage parents to focus more on their child's weekly nutritional intake, rather than on one day's intake. Frequently children are the best judges of what they need, and they may eat primarily fruit one day and peanut butter the next. Nutritional consumption tends to balance out over a week. Box 6-4 illustrates ways parents can increase their child's nutritional intake.

- Limit to two nutritious snacks per day, and give only at toddler's request.
- Limit to 4 to 6 oz of juice per day.
- Introduce to finger foods at age 8 to 10 months, and continue to make these types of food available.
- Limit to 16 to 24 oz of milk per day.
- Keep mealtimes pleasant.
- Do not force feed.
- Do not feed children who can feed themselves.

Dental Care

Most toddlers have a complete set of 20 deciduous teeth by the time they are 30 months old. Although the exact time of eruption of teeth varies, an approximate rule of thumb to assess the number of teeth is the age of the toddler in months minus six. One tooth usually erupts for each month of age past 6 months up to 30 months of age.

Permanent teeth are calcifying during the toddler period, long before they are visible. Proper care of the deciduous teeth is crucial for the toddler's general health and for the health and alignment of the permanent teeth. Deciduous teeth play an important role in the growth and development of the jaws and face and in speech development. Premature loss of the deciduous teeth complicates eruption of the permanent teeth, often leading to malocclusion. Nurses need to be aware that some parents do not understand the value of preserving primary teeth.

Because toddlers do not have the manual dexterity to remove plaque adequately, parents must be responsible for cleaning their teeth. Children can be encouraged to brush their teeth after the teeth have been thoroughly cleaned by a parent. Because toddlers like to imitate, watching parents brush their teeth can be motivating. A small, soft, nylon bristle brush works best. Optimal access and visibility are provided if the parent sits on the floor or bed with the child's head in the parent's lap and the child's body perpendicular to the parent's. This position also gives the parent some control of the child's head movement. Fluoride toothpaste is not recommended for young children because they often do not like the taste or, if they do, tend to swallow it. If the child receives fluoride from other sources, such as water or supplements, excess amounts of fluoride may be ingested if fluoride toothpaste is swallowed. Ingestion of excessive amounts of fluoride may lead to *fluorosis*, which produces white speckles or brown discoloration of the enamel. Ideally, teeth should be brushed after every meal and especially at bedtime. Flossing between teeth helps remove plaque and should be done daily by the parent after the toddler's teeth are brushed.

Fluoride makes tooth enamel resistant to acid attack, preventing decay. Fluoride supplementation (0.25 mg/day for age 6 months to 3 years, 0.5 mg/day for 3- to 6-year-olds) is recommended only for children who do not live in areas where the water has sufficient amounts of fluoride (United States Preventive Services Task Force, 2004).

A diet that is low in sweets and high in nutritious food promotes dental health. Sweets are most likely to cause caries if they are sticky or if they are eaten between meals rather than with meals. Encourage the parent to offer nutritious snacks, such as fresh fruit, yogurt, or cheese, instead of candy, soda, or cookies.

The child should first see the dentist 6 months after the first primary tooth erupts and no later than age 30 months. The first appointment should precede any needed dental work so that the visit is enjoyable and free from discomfort. This visit provides an opportunity for early assessment of the child's dental health as well as for teaching parents good preventive dental health practices.

Because the enamel on primary teeth is thinner than on permanent teeth, preschoolers' teeth are prone to destruction from decay. The distance from the tooth surface to the pulp is shorter also, so tooth abscesses from caries can occur rapidly. Untreated caries can lead to pain, abscess formation, and poor digestion because of ineffective chewing. Many parents do not realize that the deciduous teeth are important to protect the dental arch. If deciduous teeth are lost early (e.g., because of decay), the remaining teeth may drift out of position, block proper eruption of the permanent teeth, and lead to malocclusion.

Nurses play an important role in the promotion of dental health by teaching proper tooth cleaning, including the removal of plaque and the importance of adequate fluoride ingestion; encouraging a balanced diet limited in sweets; and recommending twice-yearly visits to the dentist. Preschoolers can usually brush their own teeth (Fig. 6-5). Short back-and-forth or up-and-down strokes are easiest for the child to manage. Parents should monitor the child's tooth brushing and

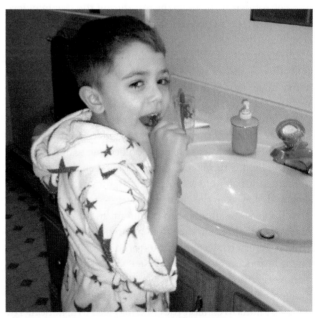

FIG 6-5 **Care of the deciduous teeth promotes healthy development of the permanent teeth. Some toddlers and preschoolers enjoy brushing their own teeth, but because toddlers and preschoolers lack the manual dexterity to remove plaque adequately, parents must assume this responsibility.**

inspect the child's teeth to be sure that all plaque has been removed. Parents must help with flossing because it requires more manual dexterity than preschoolers have.

Sleep and Rest

During the second year, children require approximately 12 to 14 hours of sleep each day. Most 2-year-olds take one nap each day until the end of the second or third year, when many children give up the habit. Toddlers often resist going to bed, using dawdling or even temper tantrums to postpone separation from loved ones and the exciting events of the day. Firm, consistent limits are needed when toddlers try stalling tactics, such as asking for one more drink of water.

Warning the child a few minutes before it is time for bed may reduce bedtime protests. Winding down with a quiet activity for 30 minutes before bedtime also helps toddlers prepare for sleep. Bedtime offers an opportunity for some snuggle time, when the parent and toddler can read a story and share the events of the day. Children of this age often have trouble relaxing and falling asleep. A warm bath before bedtime promotes relaxation. Bedtime rituals are important and should be followed consistently. Transition objects, such as a favorite blanket or stuffed animal, are often an important part of the child's bedtime routine.

Because preschoolers expend so much energy growing and learning, they need adequate rest. The preschooler needs an average of 10 to 12 hours of sleep in a 24-hour period. Some preschoolers do well without a nap during the day, but others still need a nap. Resistance to naps is common at this age. The child usually does not want to leave family or playmates, toys, and exciting activities to go into a darkened room to lie down and rest. A quiet time spent listening to music or looking at a favorite book may help the child relax and get some rest. Insufficient rest during the day may lead to irritability, decreased resistance to infection, and difficulty sleeping at night.

Sleep problems are more common during the preschool years than in any other period of childhood. Because of their active imaginations and immaturity, preschoolers often have nightmares and have trouble falling asleep at night. Because the boundaries between reality and fantasy are not well defined for children of this age, monsters and scary creatures that lurk in the preschooler's imagination become real to the child after the light is turned off. Patient and repeated reassurance from a caring parent may be needed. Nightmares—frightening dreams that awaken the child from sleep—are common among preschoolers. A familiar environment and comfort with a hug and verbal reassurance from a parent usually enable the child to return to sleep. Night terrors differ from nightmares. Night terrors occur during deep sleep, and the child remains asleep even though the eyes may be open. The child does not awaken but moans, screams, or cries and does not recognize parents. Efforts to comfort the child may lead to agitation. The child does not remember the episode in the morning, even if awakened during the night terror. Parents should be instructed not to attempt to comfort or awaken the child during a night terror but should allow the child to sleep.

The nurse should assess sleep patterns during well-child visits and address parental concerns. The nurse can reassure parents that resistance to going to bed, fears, and nightmares are normal for children of this age. The nurse should assess the frequency of sleep problems and parents' reactions to them. If sleep problems occur often and are disruptive to the family, further investigation and intervention may be indicated.

Ritualistic techniques and transition objects that help decrease bedtime resistance in the toddler continue during the preschool period. Avoiding high-carbohydrate snacks and excitement before bedtime promotes relaxation. Children should not be forced to face their fears alone by sleeping in a completely dark room or with the door shut. Parents can search the room to reassure the preschooler that the room is safe. Progressive head-to-toe relaxation is an effective technique for helping preschoolers fall asleep. A set bedtime promotes security and healthy sleep habits.

A child who has slept for a long time at the babysitter's or at daycare may not be ready to sleep again. Communication with the child's daytime caretaker is important to determine whether the child is maintaining a balance of activity, rest, and sleep.

CRITICAL THINKING EXERCISE 6-1

Mr. and Mrs. Thomas have brought 2-year-old Todd to the clinic for his annual physical examination. The parents report that bedtime is a major production almost every night. They state that he cries, comes out of his room, and displays various other behaviors that delay sleep. They wonder if he has a sleep disorder. They relate that, other than an occasional temper tantrum, they do not have any other concerns.

1. What information do you need from the parents to assess the problem?
2. After you have the above information, what advice should you give the Thomases?

Discipline

Effective discipline strategies should involve a comprehensive approach that includes consideration of the parent-child relationship, reinforcement of desired behaviors, and consequences for negative behaviors (AAP Committee on Psychosocial Aspects of Child and Family Health, 1998/2004). One goal of discipline and limit setting is to teach self-control. Eventually the child internalizes controls established by parental limits and begins to develop a conscience.

Toddlers need and want discipline to feel secure. They have little control over their behavior and need limits to learn how to behave and how to follow the rules and expectations of society. Toddlers' negativism, intense emotions, and curiosity place them at risk for injury. Because they are usually unaware of the consequences of their actions, vigilance and limits are needed for safety. Toddlers are frightened by a lack of limits and will deliberately test their parents until they are shown how far they can go. Firm discipline promotes

---

| BOX 6-5 | **PARENTS WANT TO KNOW**   Guidelines for Disciplining a Toddler |

- Discipline must be consistent. Inconsistency is confusing and counterproductive. Consistent follow through every time is important.
- Discipline must be immediate. Consequences of behavior should occur as soon as possible after the behavior occurs. Threats such as "Just wait until your father gets home!" are confusing and ineffective for a child of this age.
- Discipline must be realistic and age appropriate. Toddlers should not be expected to act like "little ladies" or "little gentlemen."
- Discipline must be related to the incident. Consequences that are logical results of a behavior are most effective.

- Limits must be clearly explained to the child.
- Toddlers must be given time to respond to instructions.
- Withdrawal of love should never be used as punishment. Comforting the child after discipline promotes positive feelings. Love is the key to effective discipline.
- Arguments and extensive explanations should be avoided.
- Praise for good behavior should be used to build self-confidence and self-esteem.
- The toddler must be separated from the behavior: "I love you very much. Hitting your sister needs to stop."

---

the development of autonomy by giving the child a feeling of freedom within bounds.

Toddlers often repeat parental prohibitions to themselves while engaging in a forbidden activity. For example, a toddler may walk over to an electrical outlet, knowing that it is out of bounds, and mumble, "No, no, hurt!" while playing with the outlet. Although remembering the prohibition, the toddler lacks sufficient self-control to prevent the behavior.

Effective discipline techniques for children of this age include a time-out (1 minute per year of age), diversion, and positive reinforcement. Teaching parents how to discipline their child helps avoid problems related to the incorrect use of discipline. Parents must be consistent. Physical punishment, such as spanking, is one of the least effective discipline techniques (see Chapter 2).

Preschoolers struggle to gain control over their strong inner impulses. To achieve this control, they need limits set on their behavior. When limits are set, the child feels more secure and can explore the environment and try new roles in an atmosphere of freedom and safety. Appropriate limit setting helps the child learn self-confidence, self-control, and moral values. The child must be consistently disciplined for acts that are destructive, socially unacceptable, or morally wrong. Limits must be clearly defined and consistently enforced to be effective. To prevent confusion and anxiety, the consequences of misbehavior should be spelled out in advance and carried out immediately after misbehavior occurs. When the child is disciplined for misbehavior, a simple, truthful explanation of why the behavior was unacceptable should be given.

> The focus of the explanation should be on the behavior rather than on the child. For example, "I don't like to see you throwing toys" is a better response than "I don't want to be around you when you act like that" or "You're a bad girl for doing that."

Discipline techniques that are effective with preschoolers include the following:
- Time-out (removing the child from a situation for a short period and offering an explanation for the punishment).

- Time-in (frequent, brief, nonverbal, physical contact when the child is acting appropriately). For example, the mother periodically strokes the child's hair or rubs his back when he is quietly playing on the floor near her while she talks on the telephone. The child who receives this type of reinforcement is more likely to continue what he is doing and much less likely to interrupt the mother.
- Offering restricted choices (e.g., "You may drink your juice in the kitchen or you may go into the living room without your juice.").
- Diversion (e.g., "You must stop marking on the wall with crayons. Here, mark on this paper instead.").

Consistent positive reinforcement for desired behavior is a powerful tool. If the parent does not care or is too busy to enforce rules consistently, the child will not internalize rules and will not feel guilty about breaking them. The child will be unruly and will be unable to follow the rules set by society.

Spending enjoyable time with their children is another way parents can model positive behaviors. Having good times with children increases their self-esteem and reinforces good behavior. Chapter 2 and Box 6-5 present additional discussions of discipline.

Toddler Safety

Understanding the developmental changes a toddler undergoes helps the nurse and parent appreciate why children are more injury prone in this stage of development than at any other time. Constant supervision is challenging for parents but is the most important factor in preventing injuries in this energetic age group.

Car Safety

Motor vehicle injuries are a significant threat to the toddler. Although toddlers begin to develop more independent behaviors, they are still wholly reliant on an adult for protection while traveling in a car. Toddlers should be secured in a forward-facing, upright, approved car safety seat, placed in the middle of the rear seat. Harness safety straps (for children weighing 40 pounds or less) should be adjusted to provide a snug fit (AAP, 2003a).

Skill: Car Seat Safety

Because children begin to imitate their parents at an early age, the nurse encourages parents to model safe behavior by consistently wearing their seatbelts. As the toddler's cognitive and fine motor skills develop, some children wiggle free of the restraining system despite releases that are designed to be difficult for a child to operate. Parents must insist on compliance in spite of temper tantrums.

Because of the toddler's short physical stature, adults should visually inspect the area surrounding the automobile before placing it in gear. A toddler near the car may not be visible and can sustain serious crushing injuries if run over by the car or trapped between the car and a stationary object. Toddlers may also dart out on foot into oncoming traffic. Parents need to closely supervise play activities and remain physically close to the toddler to prevent these types of injuries.

Toddlers and infants should never be left unattended in a car, even for a moment. Exposure to extreme heat or cold is dangerous in this age group. Injuries have occurred when parents have left cars running for various reasons and curious toddlers have disengaged the gears, causing the car to roll and collide with other objects.

CRITICAL TO REMEMBER
Car Safety

Toddlers should be restrained in an upright, forward-facing position in a car safety seat until they outgrow the manufacturer's weight or height recommendations (usually 40 lb [18.14 kg] and at 3 to 5 years of age).

Car doors should be locked while the car is in motion to prevent a curious toddler from opening the door.

Until passenger vehicles are equipped with air bags that are safe and effective for children, children younger than 13 years should not ride in a front passenger seat that is equipped with an air bag.

A booster seat with lap and shoulder belt is recommended for a preschooler who weighs more than 40 lb. It raises the child to a level that accommodates the car's seatbelt system. Children usually use a booster seat until they are tall enough to properly wear the seat/shoulder belt (height, 4 ft 9 in) (AAP, 2003a).

Airplane Safety

The lack of regulations to ensure that children younger than 2 years are properly restrained during airplane flights is an ongoing cause for concern. The AAP recommends a mandatory federal requirement for restraint use for children on aircraft. Children younger than 2 years should be restrained during takeoff and landing and during turbulence and as much as is feasible during flight. Children should be placed in properly secured rear-facing car safety seats until they are at least 1 year old and weight 9.07 kg (20 pounds). A forward-facing seat labeled for use on aircraft should be used for children at least 1 year old and 9.07 kg (20 pounds) to 18.14 kg (40 pounds) (AAP Committee on Injury and Poison Prevention, 2001/2005).

Fire and Burn Safety

Toddlers, with their increased mobility and developing fine motor skills, can reach hot water, open fires, or hot objects placed on counters and stoves above their eye level. This age child is at increased risk to reach up and pull a hot liquid off of a surface or grab or overturn a container of hot water onto himself or herself. One-year-old boys are at the highest risks for scalds and burns (Drago, 2005). They may pull objects off stoves, pull down cords attached to small appliances, open oven doors, and place electric cords or frayed wires into their mouths. They may drink liquids that are dangerously hot. The nurse should emphasize to parents to remain in the kitchen when preparing a meal, use the back burners on the stove, and turn pot handles inward and toward the middle of the stove to reduce the toddler's risk of burn injuries. Dangling cords from irons or other small appliances should not be accessible to toddlers. Open fires and heaters are also inviting. Sturdy guards fixed to the wall prevent young children from getting too close to these burn hazards. In addition, curious toddlers are fascinated with matches and lighters, which must be kept out of reach.

Toddlers depend on adults for their protection in the event of a house fire. Anticipatory guidance emphasizes the importance of smoke detectors and escape plans.

Preventing Falls

Toddlers move quickly and climb everywhere. Toddlers can fall from playground equipment, off tricycles, and out of windows. Falls from above the first floor of a building can result in serious injury. A chair next to a kitchen counter or table allows the toddler easy access to dangerously high places. Because climbing and exploration are normal aspects of the developmental process, safety education for the parent emphasizes constant supervision and some anticipatory planning, such as moving furniture, installing screen guards, and restricting access to potential climbing hazards.

Water Safety

Toddlers love to play in water. Most drownings occur when a child is left alone in a bathtub or falls into a residential pool. Even when a child survives a submersion injury, the risk of permanent brain and lung damage is great (see Chapter 10). Parents should not leave a child alone in or near a bathtub, pail of water, wading or swimming pool, or any other body of water, even for a moment. A toddler can drown in as little as 1 inch of water. Toilet lids need to remain closed. Toddlers can inadvertently fall headfirst into a toilet or bucket, and they lack the upper-body strength and coordination to remove themselves from submersion. Fencing on all four sides with a locked entry should surround in-ground swimming pools. Drowning prevention requires constant parental supervision of the toddler.

Preventing Poisoning

Children younger than 5 years are the most common victims of poisoning, and children ages 1 to 3 years are at the highest risk (CDC, 2004). The home is the site of exposure in most cases, with poisoning from medication ingestion being the major cause (Agran et al., 2003). With exploration, everything eventually finds its way to the child's mouth, even if it does not smell or taste good. Small children who are thirsty or hungry will ingest poisons that look or smell inviting.

The nurse can help parents poison proof the home and teach them the appropriate action to take if an ingestion occurs: immediately contact a poison control center or a physician (Box 6-6). The AAP no longer recommends keeping syrup of ipecac in the home (AAP, 2003b). In case of ingestion, the parent should immediately call the local poison control center. If the child is unconscious, having a seizure, or not breathing, the parent should immediately call 911 or the local emergency number (AAP Committee on Injury, Violence, and Poison Prevention, 2003).

Medicine should not be called candy and, because young children often mimic their parents, adults should be discouraged from taking medicine in the child's presence. The nurse needs to advise parents to take the same precautions when small children go to a grandparent's home to visit. Childproof caps slow the child but are not an absolute barrier. Labels with characteristic symbols, such as the skull and crossbones or "Mr. Yuk," help provide visual cues to young children; however, labels are not absolute deterrents for a determined child. The best way to prevent toxic ingestions is by carefully storing all potential poisons in a place that is inaccessible to children.

Preschooler Safety

Preschoolers are active and inquisitive. They have greater self-control, but their understanding of danger is not fully developed. Safety becomes even more challenging for the parent because preschoolers are no longer content with their own backyards. Preschoolers are mesmerized by cartoons that depict make-believe situations. They see cartoon characters engaging in daring endeavors and walking away unharmed. Because of their magical thinking, preschoolers may believe that these feats are possible and may attempt them.

Safety education can now be directed toward the child as well as the parent. Children of this age have a strong sense of rhythm, and songs and rhymes about safety can enhance the learning process. Instruction should be simple, with one concept introduced at a time. Short stories, puppet shows, songs, coloring activities, and role-playing games are all suitable learning activities that help preschoolers learn safety-conscious behaviors.

Car Safety

Preschoolers need to remain in an approved car safety seat until they weigh 18.14 kg (40 pounds) or are too tall for the safety seat according to manufacturer's recommendations. Once a child has outgrown the child car safety seat, an approved booster seat, positioned high enough to safely use the lap/shoulder belt, is strongly recommended (Fig. 6-6). Although preferable to no restraints at all, standard seatbelts alone can contribute to injury because they fit poorly over the small frame of the preschooler. The standard shoulder harness often crosses the child's face or neck, and the lap belt is positioned across the mid-abdomen rather than across the bony structure of the pelvis. Booster seats are designed to raise the child high enough so that the restraining straps are correctly positioned over the child's smaller body frame.

BOX 6-6	**PARENTS WANT TO KNOW** Childhood Poison Prevention

- Keep all poisons, medicines, cleaners, and toxic substances out of the reach of children. Never discard poisons in a wastebasket.
- Parents should be familiar with poisons commonly found in or near the home, including detergents, drain cleaner, dishwashing soap, furniture polish, cleaning agents, window cleaners, all medicines, vitamins, children's medications, sprays, powders, cosmetics, fingernail preparations, hair care products, sachets, mothballs, rodent poisons, fertilizers, gasoline, antifreeze, paints, glues, insecticides, cigarette butts, plants, and shrubs.
- Poisons should be stored in areas that are secured with locks or protected by child-resistant safety latches.
- Medicines and all harmful substances should be purchased in child-resistant packages.
- Alcoholic beverages should be kept out of the reach of children or locked in a separate cabinet. Parents should be discouraged from giving sips of alcohol to children because small amounts can be toxic to young children.
- Children should not be allowed to chew on plants or shrubs.
- Ashtrays should be kept empty and out of the reach of small children.

- Handbags and overnight luggage of guests in the home often contain medicines or other toxic substances and should be kept out of a child's reach.
- Poisons or harmful substances should always be stored in the original container. Parents should be discouraged from placing toxic substances in food or beverage containers for storage.
- Children should be taught to ask an adult before they touch a nonfood substance.
- Parents should poison-proof all areas of the home, especially the kitchen, bathroom, pantry, bedroom, garage, basement, and work areas. Grandparents and other caregivers should be encouraged to do the same.
- The telephone number of the local poison control center should be posted for immediate access in the event of a poisoning. The National Poison Help Line number (800-222-1222) will connect to the local poison control number, which is staffed 24 hours a day, 7 days a week. Parents should be instructed, when contacting the poison control center, to have on hand the substance with the label for prompt identification of toxic ingredients. Additionally, parents should not administer anything to the child without contacting the poison control center first.

HEALTH PROMOTION

THE 3-YEAR-OLD CHILD

FOCUSED ASSESSMENT

How are you handling any discipline problems your child may be having?

Have you been able to encourage your child to be independent and express ideas that may be different from yours?

Is your child in preschool or daycare? How many hours or days?

How does your child get along with other children the same age?

How well does your child communicate with others?

How well is your child doing with toilet training?

What activities do you enjoy doing together?

DEVELOPMENTAL MILESTONES

Personal/social: puts on articles of clothing; brushes teeth with help; washes and dries hands using soap and water; notices gender differences and identifies with children of own gender; exhibits sexual curiosity, may begin to masturbate; knows own name and names one or more friends; increasing independence, may start preschool; ritualistic; understands taking turns and sharing but may not be ready to do so; begins to show fears (dark, shadows, animals)

Fine motor: vision approaches 20/20; builds a tower of at least eight blocks; begins purposeful drawing, can imitate a circle and a cross and draw a person with three parts; feeds self well

Language/cognition: increasing vocabulary with intelligible speech, although stuttering is common (thinks faster than can talk); names four familiar objects and begins to describe qualities or actions of objects; knows meaning of common adjectives (sleepy, hungry, hot); begins color identification; uses symbolic language; still egocentric; increased concept of time, space, causality; constantly

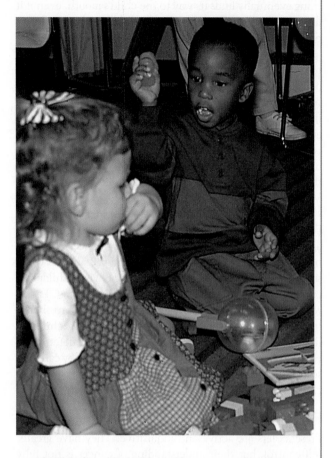

asks "how" and "why" questions; can count to three; can tell full name, age, and gender

Gross motor: jumps with both feet up and down and over a short distance; throws a ball overhand; catches a large ball with both hands; balances on each foot for at least 2 seconds; begins to ride a tricycle

---

Parents continue to have primary responsibility for ensuring that a child is safely restrained before the vehicle is started and in motion. Parents must insist that children remain restrained at all times and that seatbelts be used correctly. Although riding in the open bed of a pickup truck or in the cargo area of a van or station wagon may seem fun and relatively harmless, it can be deadly in the event of a crash. It is restricted in some states (AAP Committee on Injury and Poison Prevention, 2000/2004).

Fire and Burn Safety

Preschoolers imitate adults in all types of daily routines and activities. They may attempt household activities before they are able to manage an appliance safely (e.g., stove, iron, oven), increasing the risk of burn injuries. Matches and lighters continue to fascinate preschoolers. With their increased fine motor skills, preschoolers may be able to ignite

a flame. Preschoolers should be taught that lighters and matches are adult tools and instructed to tell an adult immediately if they find these items. These actions can prevent burn injuries.

Children younger than 5 years are at the greatest risk for burn deaths in a house fire. They often panic and hide in closets or under beds rather than escape safely. Parents need to practice fire drills with their children to teach them what to do in the event of a house fire. Preschoolers should become familiar with the sounds emitted by smoke alarms and be taught to crawl under smoke and to check doors for heat.

Preschoolers are at an ideal age to learn what to do if their clothing ignites in flames. Instruct preschoolers to stop immediately if their clothes catch on fire and to cover their face and mouth with their hands. They should then drop to the ground and roll to smother the flames. This simple

---

HEALTH PROMOTION

THE 3-YEAR-OLD CHILD—cont'd

CRITICAL MILESTONES*

Personal/social: brushes teeth with help, puts on clothing, feeds a doll

Fine motor: builds a tower of at least four to six cubes

Language/cognition: points to and names four familiar pictures (cat, horse, bird, dog, man); speech understandable 50% of the time

Gross motor: throws a ball overhand; jumps; kicks a ball forward

HEALTH MAINTENANCE

Physical Measurements

Continue to plot height and weight

Change to height growth chart if child able to stand while being measured

Growth rate is similar to that of a 2-year-old

Immunizations

Administer any immunizations not given previously according to the recommended schedule

Influenza vaccine annually

Health Screening

Objective vision screening using an appropriate chart (see Chapter 9)

Objective hearing screening with age-appropriate audiometry equipment

Blood pressure measurement

Hemoglobin, hematocrit, and lead screening

Tuberculosis (TB) screening if at risk

Cholesterol screening if at risk

ANTICIPATORY GUIDANCE

Nutrition

Similar to that of a 2-year-old

Elimination

Usually is toilet trained but not at night

Dental

Continue to have the child brush with toothpaste and take recommended fluoride (0.5 mg/day if water is not fluoridated)

Child should see the dentist every 6 months

Sleep

Similar to that of a 2-year-old

May relinquish the nap

Consider changing to a full bed if climbing out of the crib

May begin to experience night terrors

Hygiene

Similar to that of a 2-year-old

Remind the child about good handwashing, especially after toileting and before meals

Safety

Review choking on food, street safety, water safety, sun protection, outside poisons, playground safety

Discuss bike and tricycle safety, fire safety, car seats (change to a forward-facing approved booster seat when the child's weight exceeds 40 lb)

Self-Esteem and Competence

Model appropriate social behavior

Encourage your child to learn to make choices

Help your child to express emotions appropriately

Spend individual time with your child daily, and encourage your child to talk about the day's events

Provide consistent and loving limits to help your child learn self-discipline

Play

Similar to that of a 2-year-old

Likes imitative toys, large building blocks, musical toys, and riding toys such as large trucks

*Guided by DDST II.

---

command (stop, drop, roll) can help prevent severe burn injuries. Teaching specific behaviors educates children to remain calm and not panic.

Firearm Safety

Guns are often kept in the home loaded and readily accessible to young children. Parents should be encouraged to evaluate their need for a firearm in the home critically. Do the potentially devastating risks outweigh any benefits of keeping a weapon in the home? The nurse should talk to all parents about gun safety at every well visit because, even though parents may not keep a gun in the house, children may visit friends whose parents do. Parents who choose to keep a gun in the home should receive anticipatory guidance about injury prevention. Guns kept in the home should always be unloaded, stored with trigger guards in place, securely locked in metal vaults, and inaccessible to all children.

Personal Safety

Preschoolers have an interest in establishing relationships with others as they expand the boundaries of their world. With the child's increasing assertion of independence, parents are less able to provide the constant protection they once did.

Teaching children about personal safety encourages them to develop skills to detect danger and teaches appropriate ways to handle threatening situations. Strangers are often portrayed as evil characters, when in reality their appearance and approach may be nonthreatening and friendly. Distinguishing a stranger from a well-intentioned person is challenging and often difficult for the preschooler. Basic guidelines that a child needs to know about personal safety include saying no, getting away, and telling an adult.

Children need to know how to access emergency help if they need it. Parents should help their children learn to

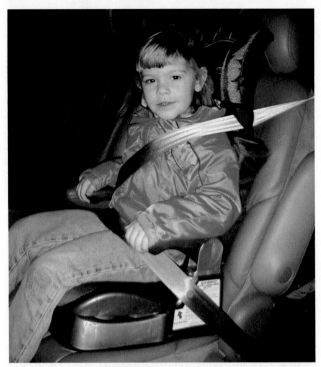

FIG 6-6   **A high-back booster seat designed to properly hold a car lap and shoulder belt is strongly recommended for children who have outgrown a child safety seat. Booster seats raise the young child high enough to allow the car seatbelts to be correctly positioned over the child's chest and pelvis.**   *(Photo courtesy M. Hayden.)*

identify safety officials and how to dial 911 or other locally appropriate emergency numbers. Children need to respond to emergency operators with their full name, address, parent's name, and other appropriate information and should remain on the phone until help arrives. Parents can practice this safety skill with their children to ensure proper reactions in an emergency and help the child understand what constitutes an emergency situation.

Sexual Abuse

Sexual abuse is another threat to personal safety. Preventing sexual abuse begins with teaching children the normal, healthy boundaries of their bodies and what constitutes inappropriate behavior. Often the perpetrators are known and trusted by the child. Abusers frequently intimidate the child into silence with threats of personal harm or suggestions that the child initiated the behavior. Children need to know that no matter how great the threat, if someone is touching their body in an inappropriate way, they should always tell an adult. If that adult cannot help them, they should tell as many adults as necessary until the inappropriate behavior is stopped (see Chapter 29).

Selected Issues Related to the Toddler

Toilet Training

Control of elimination is one of the major tasks of toddlerhood. Successful toilet training depends on both the child's and parent's readiness. The parent must be willing to spend

the necessary time and emotional energy to encourage the child on a daily basis.

Toilet training is one of the most frustrating and time-consuming tasks that parents face. It can be so frustrating for some that researchers have linked toilet training accidents with many cases of child abuse. Parents who do not understand normal growth and development patterns often have unrealistic expectations and can become frustrated to the point of rage.

The nurse can assist parents by explaining developmental milestones and encouraging parents not to begin training until the child shows signs of readiness. Toilet training proceeds at different times in different cultures. Helping the parent recognize signs of readiness and factors that interfere with toilet training, such as stress, can make the training easier (Box 6-7). The parent may not have the necessary reserves of patience and energy for toilet training during stressful times, such as near the birth of another child or while moving to a new house. Training may be easier if it is postponed until routines return to normal.

The nurse can assist parents in toilet training the toddler by explaining the importance of maturation to successful toilet training. Parents need to know that both physical readiness and psychologic readiness are necessary for toilet training to be successful. Myelinization of the spinal cord, which usually occurs between 12 and 18 months, must be complete before the child can voluntarily control bowel and bladder sphincters. The nurse can offer anticipatory guidance to parents by teaching them the signs that the toddler is ready for toilet training. The average toddler is not ready for toilet training to begin until 18 to 24 months of age. Waiting until the child is 24 to 30 months old makes the task considerably easier because toddlers of this age are less negative and usually are more willing to control their sphincters to please their parents.

There are no set rules or timetables for toilet training (Fig. 6-7). The age at which toilet training is usually begun varies from culture to culture. If the child resists, training may be stopped for 30 to 60 days before beginning again. Bowel control is usually achieved before bladder control.

BOX 6-7	Signs of Readiness for Toilet Training

Physical Readiness
Child can remove own clothing.
Child is willing to let go of a toy when asked.
Child is able to sit, squat, and walk well.
Child has been walking for 1 year.

Psychologic Readiness
Child notices if diaper is wet.
Child may indicate that diaper needs to be changed by pulling on diaper, squatting, or repeating a word or phrase.
Child communicates need to go to the bathroom or can get there by self.
Child wants to please parent by staying dry.

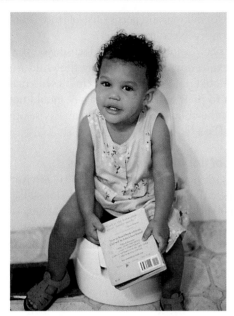

FIG 6-7 **No set rules exist for toilet training. The nurse can help parents understand that both physical readiness and psychologic readiness are necessary for success.**

Some children do achieve daytime bladder control before bowel control. This phenomenon is referred to as *toileting refusal,* and it can be distressful to parents. Daytime bladder control occurs before nighttime bladder control. Studies suggest that the earlier intensive toilet training begins, the longer it takes for the child to be trained. Optimal age for beginning toilet training is 27 months (Blum, Taubman, & Nemeth, 2003). Some studies suggest that children are completing toilet training much later than previous generations. Reasons cited for this include initiation of toilet training at an older age, presence of stool toileting refusal, and presence of frequent constipation (Blum et al., 2004).

A relaxed, child-centered approach is most successful, with plenty of praise for each success. Punishment and coercive techniques cause feelings of shame and lead to power struggles. The child should not be forced to sit on the toilet for long periods. Successful toilet training is a gradual process, and relapses must be expected. Toileting accidents often occur when children are too busy playing to notice a full bladder until too late. Many children cannot remain completely dry until the age of 3 years. Parents should respond to accidents with tolerance instead of scolding or shaming the child.

Temper Tantrums

Temper tantrums are a common toddler response to anger and frustration and often result from thwarted attempts at mastery and autonomy. Tantrums may also occur as an emotional release of tension after a long, tiring day. Unable to express anger in more productive ways because of limited language and reasoning abilities, toddlers may react by screaming, kicking, throwing things, or even biting themselves or banging their heads. Tantrums occur more often when toddlers are tired, hungry, bored, or excessively stimulated.

The nurse can help parents by identifying strategies to decrease the frequency of tantrums. Limiting situations that are too much for the child to handle is helpful. Anticipating periods of fatigue, having a snack ready before the child gets too hungry, and offering the toddler choices when possible can minimize temper tantrums. Parental practices such as inconsistency, permissiveness, excessive strictness, and overprotectiveness increase the probability of tantrums.

Toddlers need appropriate and consistent limits. Letting the child know that temper tantrums will not be tolerated gives the child a sense of security. The intensity of a toddler's outburst almost seems to be a plea for someone to stop the behavior. Probably the most effective method for handling tantrums is to isolate safely and ignore the child. The child should learn that nothing is gained from a tantrum, not even attention. Giving in to the child's demands or scolding the child only increases the behavior. Toddlers stop using tantrums when they do not achieve their goals and as their verbal skills increase. Once the tantrum has subsided and the toddler has regained some self-control, the parent should comfort and let the child know that limits are necessary and that the child is loved. Acknowledging the child's angry feelings and rewarding more mature ways of expressing them assist the child in gaining self-control.

Sibling Rivalry

Sharing parents' love and attention is difficult for most toddlers. Often toddlers have intense feelings of jealousy and envy toward a new infant sibling. Toddlers' egocentrism makes understanding that a parent can love more than one child at a time difficult.

Because the infant needs a great deal of time and attention, the toddler's routine is disrupted. The toddler has limited resources to cope with such stress and may react by treating the baby roughly, damaging property, or harming pets. The toddler may seem to regress by asking for a bottle or pacifier or by using baby talk.

Any changes, such as moving the toddler to a new bedroom or beginning daycare, should be made as far in advance as possible so that the toddler will not feel displaced by abrupt changes when the baby arrives. Many hospitals offer sibling preparation classes. When the mother and infant come home from the hospital, the mother's first concern should be greeting the older sibling. The father or another caregiver should carry the newborn, allowing the mother's arms to be free to hug the waiting toddler and express how the child was missed. A toddler's jealous feelings can become intense when visitors lavish gifts and praise on the baby. Giving an inexpensive gift to the toddler each time the baby receives one can minimize these feelings. Visitors should be encouraged to pay attention to the older child as well as the baby. Parents should anticipate behavior changes, even if the toddler has been prepared for the arrival of a new baby. The parents should be present when the toddler is with the infant to prevent the toddler from inadvertently harming the newborn sibling.

Toddlers should be helped to recognize and identify negative feelings toward a new sibling. Firm limits must be set, however, if the toddler tries to harm the baby. The child may be told "It's okay to feel like you don't like the baby right now, but it's not okay to hurt the baby." Praise should be given for affectionate, cooperative behavior.

Planned, uninterrupted private time is important to maintain feelings of closeness between parent and toddler. Even 10 or 15 minutes each day while the baby is sleeping is valuable. Allowing the toddler to choose an activity for this time with the parent makes it even more special. This special time should be given to the child each day, regardless of the child's behavior.

CRITICAL TO REMEMBER

Strategies to Decrease Sibling Rivalry

Including the toddler in preparations for the new baby
Explaining to the toddler what new babies are like
Letting the child feel the fetus move
Reading picture books about new siblings
Talking about changes that the newborn might create
Acknowledging the older child's feelings about these changes
Referring to the baby as "ours"

Selected Issues Related to the Preschooler

Stuttering

Stuttering, or stammering, is a disturbance in the flow and time patterning of speech. During the preschool years, children often have experiences they want to share but have difficulty putting the words together. Children this age commonly repeat whole words or phrases and interject "uh" and "um" in their speech. As the child's communication skills develop, most grow out of their normal dysfluency. Dysfluency tends to be more common during times of excitement, when formulating long and complex sentences, when trying to think of a particular word, and during times of stress.

Reactions to stuttering can increase the dysfluency. Indications for referral include whole-word or part-word repetitions, sound prolongations, word blockages, facial tension,

avoidance of talking, and persistence of stuttering for longer than 6 months (Needlman, 2004).

Parents can help their child by focusing on the ideas the child is expressing, not on the way the child is speaking. Parents should not complete their child's sentences or draw attention to their child's speech. They should not criticize or correct the child's speech and should advise others to do the same (Box 6-8).

Preschool and Daycare Programs

A quality daycare program provides an environment in which the child can expand social and play skills as well as manipulate play materials unavailable at home.

Working mothers often express guilt and concern about the effect of daycare on their child's emotional well-being and cognitive development. Some concerns about the effect of daycare on the child's development can be minimized by careful selection of the daycare facility.

The nurse is in an excellent position to advise parents about childcare. Parents need specific advice about options that are affordable but will not compromise the child's health and development. Parents must visit the daycare center to evaluate the quality of the program. They need to evaluate the attitude and qualifications of the caregivers as well as operating procedures, costs, childcare and disciplinary practices, meals, safety precautions, sanitary conditions, and the child/staff ratio.

The child needs preparation before beginning daycare and information about what to expect in simple, concrete terms. Emphasizing the exciting parts of the experience will help the child view the experience positively. The parent should also explain the reason for separation. Imaginative preschoolers may believe that they are being "sent away" because of some misdeed.

When parents must take their child to a baby-sitter or daycare center, they should give the child an explanation for the separation. A statement such as "I have to work so I can buy food and clothes for the family and toys for you" is not adequate. In response to this explanation, one 3-year-old boy wailed, "But I have enough toys!" More effective would be to explain the separation by saying, "We both have work to do. My work is at my office, and your work is at school."

BOX 6-8	**PARENTS WANT TO KNOW** How to Help the Child Who Stutters

- Listen closely when your child speaks.
- Speak slowly, and pause frequently. This provides a model for the child and gives the child more time to understand what is being said and formulate thoughts.
- Provide opportunities for your child to talk without distractions or competition from other family members.
- Reduce pressure to communicate by limiting the number of questions asked that require an immediate answer.
- Limit time pressure. Do not ask a second question before the first question is answered.

- Observe situations that increase or decrease fluent behavior. Increase those times when the child is more fluent.
- Recognize that certain environmental factors may have a negative effect on fluency: competition to speak, excitement, time pressure, arguments, fatigue, new situations, unfamiliar listeners.
- Repeat or rephrase what your child says to verify that it has been understood.

Modified from American Speech-Language-Hearing Association. (2001). Stuttering: do's & don'ts for parents. *Healthtouch On-line for Better Health*. Retrieved July 11, 2006 from http://www.healthtouch.com/bin/EContent_HT/showAllLfts.asp?lftname5ASLHA021&cid=HT.

HEALTH PROMOTION

THE 4- AND 5-YEAR-OLD CHILD

FOCUSED ASSESSMENT

Have you been able to encourage your child to be independent and express ideas that may differ from yours?

Is your child in preschool or daycare? How many hours or days?

How does your child get along with other children the same age?

How well does your child communicate with others?

Has your child's play become more imaginative? Does your child describe any fears?

Has your child become independent in feeding, cleanliness, toileting, and dressing?

Do you give your child small responsibilities or chores to do around the house?

What activities do you enjoy doing together?

DEVELOPMENTAL MILESTONES

Personal/social: develops a sense of initiative; learns new skills and games; begins problem solving; develops a positive self-concept; develops a conscience: begins to learn right from wrong and good from bad (based on reward and punishment); learns to understand rules; identifies with parent of same gender, often closely imitating characteristics; aware of gender differences; independence in self-care; sociable and outgoing (might be aggressive or bossy); has an attention span of approximately 20 minutes

Fine motor: proficient holding a crayon or pencil, draws purposefully; copies circle, cross, square, diamond, and triangle; draws a person with several body parts; drawings resemble familiar objects or people; may begin to write name or numbers; can tie shoelaces

Language/cognitive: vocabulary of 1500 words; begins to understand concepts of size and time (related to familiar events such as meals and bedtime); understands two opposites (e.g., same/different, hot/cold, big/little); can follow several directions consecutively; uses four-word sentences with prepositions (e.g., on, under, behind); defines five words, counts to five, names four colors; begins to see others' viewpoints; uses magical thinking; very imaginative; can complete an 8- to 10-piece puzzle

Gross motor: hops on one foot or alternate feet; walks heel to toe (front and back); balances on each foot for longer time; begins to ride bike with training wheels; throws and catches a ball; walks downstairs using alternate feet

CRITICAL MILESTONES*

Personal/social: puts on a T-shirt; washes and dries hands; names a friend

Fine motor: imitates a vertical line; wiggles thumbs; builds a tower of eight cubes

Language/cognitive: knows two adjectives (e.g., tired, hungry, cold); identifies one color; knows the use of two objects (e.g., cup, chair, pencil)

Gross motor: balances on each foot for 1 second; jumps forward; throws a ball overhand

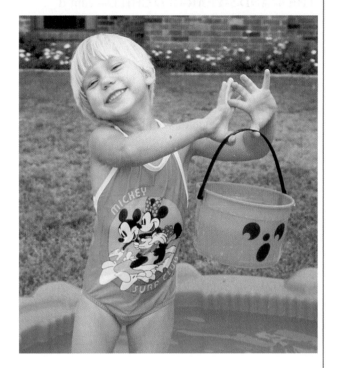

HEALTH MAINTENANCE

Physical Measurements

Weight increases 2.25 kg/yr (5 pounds)

Height increases approximately 7.5 cm/yr (3 inches)

Immunizations

Diphtheria, tetanus, acellular pertussis (DTaP) #5; inactivated poliovirus (IPV) #4; measles, mumps, rubella (MMR) #2

Influenza vaccine annually

Health Screening

Hemoglobin and lead screen

Vision

Audiometry

Blood pressure

Cholesterol if at risk

Tuberculosis (TB) if at risk

ANTICIPATORY GUIDANCE

Provide information and health teaching to the child as well as the parent

Nutrition

Continue as for a 3-year-old

Provide nutritious snacks (child too often in a hurry to eat at mealtime)

Begin to emphasize table manners

Elimination

Bowel movements once or twice daily

Urinary output 1000 mL/day

Nighttime control achieved

---

* Guided by DDST II.

Continued

HEALTH PROMOTION

THE 4- AND 5-YEAR-OLD CHILD—cont'd

Dental

Dental examinations every 6 months

Continue brushing and fluoride

Child might begin to lose deciduous teeth

Sleep

10 to 12 hours, no nap

May experience night terrors or nightmares

Safety

Review bicycle safety, playground safety, fire safety, poisoning (outside plants), pedestrian safety, automobile safety, sun protection

Discuss gun safety, stranger awareness, good touch versus bad touch

Self-Esteem and Competence

Model appropriate social behavior; begin to include participation in religious services

Encourage your child to learn to make choices

Help your child to express emotions appropriately

Spend individual time with your child daily and encourage your child to talk about the day's events

Provide consistent and loving limits to help your child learn self-discipline

Encourage curiosity, and provide formal learning experiences

Establish opportunities for your child to do small household chores

Assess your child's readiness for kindergarten entrance, and begin to prepare the child for the school experience

Play

Peak of imaginative play: misbehavior projected onto inanimate object or imaginary friend; participate in imaginary play; encourage curiosity and creativity

Teach songs and nursery rhymes

Read to the child frequently

Teach basic skills of sports and games

Provide playground equipment, household and garden tools, dress-up clothes, building and construction toys, art supplies, more sophisticated books and puzzles

---

The parent should reassure the child ("I'm really going to miss you today, and I wish you could be with me") and let the child know that separation is painful for the parent as well but is necessary. At the end of the day, when picking up the child, the child should be told how happy the parent is to see him or her. By responding to the child's feelings, parents can lessen the stress of separation.

Transition objects may help the child adjust to the new environment. Providing the staff with information about the child's interests, home routine, special terms, and names of pets and siblings helps the new caregiver make the child feel more comfortable. Parents should always assure the child that they will return to take the child home at the end of the day.

Preparing the Child for School

Preparation for school begins long before the preschool period. The earliest interactions between parent and infant lay the foundation for school readiness. Probably the most important factor in the development of academic competency is the relationship between parent and child. Parents who are attuned to their child and who structure the environment to provide challenges as well as security facilitate the child's cognitive growth. An interesting environment, combined with parental encouragement and support, maximizes the child's potential.

Parents are the child's first and most important teachers. They structure the child's environment and offer opportunities for learning. Visiting a zoo, fire station, or museum and talking about the experience increase the child's general knowledge and vocabulary. Cooking together, playing simple games, or putting together puzzles also fosters intellectual development. Playing with clay, paint, and scissors promotes fine motor skills and provides opportunity for self-expression. Reading to the child is one of the most valuable activities for promoting school readiness. Listening to stories and discussing them can promote reading readiness. Dramatic play encourages reading readiness by providing opportunities for symbolic thinking and problem solving.

Preschool and daycare programs can supplement the developmental opportunities provided by parents at home. Opportunities to play with other children and learn how to share the attention of an adult are some benefits of a good preschool program. Head Start programs offer low-income children and their families opportunities for remedial and supportive activities. Kindergarten provides a transition between home and first grade through a structured learning environment. In kindergarten, children prepare for school by learning to cooperate with other children, developing listening skills, and forming a positive attitude toward school.

Nurses can provide parents with strategies designed to promote safety as part of preparation for school. Teaching children about street safety and dealing with strangers and ensuring that children know their telephone numbers and addresses are important aspects of preparation for school.

Not every 5-year-old is ready for kindergarten. Both chronologic age and developmental maturity should be considered when assessing a child's readiness for school (Box 6-9). At this age, boys tend to lag behind girls developmentally by approximately 6 months.

BOX 6-9	**Checklist for School Readiness**

- Child is physically healthy and strong enough to enjoy the challenge of going to school and handle the increased stresses involved.
- Child attends to own toileting needs and washes hands independently.
- Child can separate from parent and spend several hours each day in an unfamiliar place with adults and children who are largely unknown at first.
- Child's attention span is long enough that child can sit for a fairly long period and concentrate on one thing at a time, gradually learning to enjoy the practicing and problem-solving activity involved.
- Child can listen to and follow two- or three-part instructions.
- Child can restrict talking to appropriate times.
- Child is able to tolerate the frustration of not receiving immediate attention from the teacher or others; can wait for and take turns.
- Child has some basic hand-eye skills necessary for learning to read and write.
- Child can hold a pencil properly and turn pages one at a time.
- Child knows the alphabet and can recognize some letters visually.
- Child counts to 10.
- Child recognizes the colors of the rainbow.

KEY CONCEPTS

- The slower physical growth rate of the toddler (compared with an infant) leads to a reduced demand for calories and decreased appetite (physiologic anorexia).
- The combination of increased motor skills, immaturity, and lack of experience places the toddler at risk for unintentional injury. Anticipatory guidance for the parents about childproofing the home is an essential nursing role.
- Children's coordination and muscle strength increase rapidly between the ages of 3 and 5 years. Increases in brain size and nerve myelinization enable the child to perfect fine and gross motor skills. The preschool child has the skills needed to engage in activities such as running, riding a tricycle, cutting with scissors, and drawing.
- Toddlers' behavior is characterized by negativism, ritualism, and egocentrism.
- The preschool years are a critical period for the development of socialization. Children need opportunities to play with others to learn communication skills and ways to get along with others. Preschool children learn to share and cooperate as they play in small groups. Their play is often imitative, dramatic, and creative.
- Preschoolers' thinking is still magical and egocentric. They tend to understand events only as those events affect them, believing that everyone else has the same experience. Preschool children may be overwhelmed by guilt

feelings if a loved one is injured or becomes ill because they believe their thoughts are powerful enough to cause events to happen.

- Toddlerhood is characterized by the struggle for autonomy as the child develops a sense of self as separate from the parent. Erikson defines the toddler's task as centered on autonomy versus shame and doubt.
- According to Erikson, the developmental task of the preschooler is to gain a sense of initiative. The preschooler is busy learning how to do things and takes great pride in new accomplishments.
- Gender identity and body image are developing in the preschool period. Sexual curiosity, anatomic explorations, and masturbation are common. The nurse should encourage parents to answer the preschooler's questions simply and honestly. Children should not be shamed or punished for self-comforting behaviors or for investigating gender differences.
- Food jags and physiologic anorexia are common occurrences in the young child.
- Toddlers need approximately 12 to 14 hours of sleep per day.
- The preschooler needs an average of 10 to 12 hours of sleep in a 24-hour period. Because of the preschooler's active imagination and immaturity, sleep problems are common.
- Firm, consistent discipline helps toddlers learn self-control. Effective discipline techniques include time-outs, diversion, and positive reinforcement.
- Preschool children need consistent discipline to learn acceptable behavior. Appropriate limit setting helps the child learn self-confidence, self-control, and moral values. Discipline techniques that are effective at this age include time-out, time-in, the use of restricted choices, and diversion.
- All 20 deciduous teeth are present by age 3 years. Proper care of deciduous teeth is crucial for the child's general health and for the health and alignment of permanent teeth. Nurses should teach parents the importance of good oral hygiene, adequate fluoride intake, good nutrition, and regular dental checkups.
- Nurses can help parents with toilet training by explaining the signs of physical and psychologic readiness. Readiness depends on myelinization of the nerve pathways that enable the child to control the bowel and bladder sphincters.
- Sibling rivalry can be minimized with techniques such as including the toddler in preparations for the new baby, acknowledging the toddler's negative feelings while setting appropriate limits, and affirming the toddler as special and loved.
- The nurse plays an important role in helping parents prepare their children for school and in assessing children's readiness for school. Parents can help their child succeed in school by providing a stimulating environment and encouragement and support.
- Health promotion for the toddler or preschool child includes ensuring adequate sleep, optimal nutrition, dental care, immunizations, and prevention of injuries.

ANSWERS TO
CRITICAL THINKING EXERCISE 6-1

1. The nurse needs to know if the child has a bedtime ritual. If a ritual exists, the nurse determines what it is and whether it is consistently implemented. Even though the parents volunteered that they did not have any other concerns, the nurse should ask about Todd's daily routine. Questions related to his play activities, eating habits, and daily routine might be helpful. The parents should be asked what discipline methods they use and if they are effective (i.e., what the parents do when Todd resists their instructions). This information will give the nurse a general idea of what the child's environment is like. The nurse is trying to determine whether the parents are supporting this child's need for structure while allowing him to venture out. The nurse is looking for balance and gathering information to determine whether consistent limits are set within the family.

2. Two-year-old children need limits set to feel secure. They do not have the maturity to control their behavior. They must be taught the rules. Toddlers often delay going to bed. The parents should be told that this behavior is part of normal growth and development. By providing a bedtime ritual, which may include quiet time, a snack, a story, and perhaps a prayer, parents help children find security in a routine that is repeated night after night. Children begin to know that their parents expect them to stay in bed and that they cannot manipulate their parents. Children who "wear their parents down" are confused and are not given the sense of control that they need to explore and become autonomous. Parents should be assured that by creating a consistent environment, they will help their child and save themselves a good deal of frustration.

REFERENCES AND READINGS

Agran, P., Anderson, C., Winn, D., Trent, R., Walton-Haynes, L., & Thayer, S. (2003). Rates of pediatric injuries by 3-month intervals for children 0 to 3 years of age. *Pediatrics, 111*(6), e683-e692.

American Academy of Pediatrics. (2003a). *Car safety seats: a guide for families 2003.* Retrieved November 6, 2005, from *www.aap .org/family/carseatguide.htm.*

American Academy of Pediatrics. (2003b). *Handling a poison emergency.* Retrieved December 30, 2005, from *www.aap.org.*

American Academy of Pediatrics, Committee on Injury, Violence, and Poison Prevention. (2003). Poison treatment in the home. *Pediatrics, 112*(5), 1182-1185.

American Academy of Pediatrics Committee on Injury and Poison Prevention. (2000, reaffirmed 2004). Children in pickup trucks. *Pediatrics, 106*(4), 857-859.

American Academy of Pediatrics Committee on Injury and Poison Prevention. (2001, reaffirmed 2005). Restraint use on aircraft. *Pediatrics, 108*(5), 1218-1222.

American Academy of Pediatrics Committee on Nutrition. (2001). The use and misuse of fruit juices in pediatrics. *Pediatrics, 107*(5), 1210-1213.

American Academy of Pediatrics Committee on Psychosocial Aspects of Child and Family Health. (1998, reaffirmed 2004). Guidance for effective discipline. *Pediatrics, 101*(4), 723-728.

Ateah, C. (2003). Disciplinary practices with children: parental sources of information, attitudes, and educational needs. *Issues in Comprehensive Pediatric Nursing, 26,* 89-101.

Banks, J. B. (2002). Childhood discipline: challenges for clinicians and parents. *American Family Physician, 66*(8), 1447-1452.

Blum, N., Taubman, B., & Nemeth, N. (2003). Relationship between age at initiation of toilet training and duration of training: a prospective study. *Pediatrics, 111*(4), 810-814.

Blum, N. J., Taubman, B., Nemeth, N. (2004). Why is toilet training occurring at older ages: a study of factors associated with later training. *The Journal of Pediatrics, 145*(1), 107-111.

Centers for Disease Control and Prevention. (2004). Surveillance for fatal and nonfatal injuries: United States, 2001. *MMWR, 53*(SS07), 1-57.

De la Cruz, G. G., Rozier, R. G., & Slade, G. (2004). Dental screening and referral of young children by pediatric primary care providers. *Pediatrics, 114*(5), e642-e652.

Drago, D. A. (2005). Kitchen scalds and thermal burns in children five years and younger. *Pediatrics, 115*(1), 10-16.

Duncan, P., Dixon, R., & Carlson, J. (2003). Childhood and adolescent sexuality. *Pediatric Clinics of North America, 50*(4), 741-764.

Durbin, D. R., Chen, I., Smith, R., Elliott, M. R., & Winston, F. K. (2005). Effects of seating position and appropriate restraint use on the risk of injury to children in motor vehicle crashes. *Pediatrics, 115*(3), e305-e309.

Erikson, E. H. (1963). *Childhood and society* (2nd ed.). New York: Norton.

Freud, S. (1960). *The ego and the id* (J. Riviere, Trans.). New York: Norton.

Gaylord, C. M. (2004). Picky eating: a toddler's continuing approach to mealtime. *Pediatric Nursing, 30*(2), 101-107.

Hardy, L. R., Harrell, J. S., & Bell, R. A. (2004). Overweight in children: definitions, measurements, confounding factors, and health consequences. *Journal of Pediatric Nursing, 19*(6), 376-384.

Jenni, O. G., & O'Connor, B. B. (2005). Children's sleep: an interplay between culture and biology. *Pediatrics, 115*(1), 204-216.

Kohlberg, L. (1964). Development of moral character. In M. Hoffman & L. Hoffman (Eds.), *Review of child development research, vol. 1.* New York: Russell Sage Foundation.

Kohlberg, L. (1966). A cognitive developmental analysis of children's sex-role concepts and attitudes. In E. E. Macoby (Ed.), *The development of sex differences.* Stanford, CA: Stanford University Press.

Lucas, B. L. (2004). Nutrition in childhood. In L. K. Mahan & S. Escott-Stump (Eds.), *Food, nutrition & diet therapy.* Philadelphia: Saunders.

Krol, D. M. (2004). Educating pediatricians on children's oral health: past, present, and future. *Pediatrics, 113*(5), e487-e492.

Lewis, C., Lynch, H., & Richardson, L. (2005). Fluoride varnish use in primary care: what do providers think? *Pediatrics, 115*(1), e69-e76.

Needlman, R. D. (2004). Growth and development. In Behrman, R. E., Kliegman, R. M., & Jenson, H. B. (Eds.), *Nelson textbook of pediatrics* (17th ed., p. 45). Philadelphia: Saunders.

Newgard, C. D., & Lewis, R. J. (2005). Effects of child age and body size on serious injury from passenger air-bag presence in motor vehicle crashes. *Pediatrics, 115*(6), 1579-1585.

Piaget, J. (1952). *The origins of intelligence in children.* New York: International Universities Press.

Schonwald, A., Sherritt, L., Stadtler, A., & Bridgemohan, C. (2004). Factors associated with difficult toilet training. *Pediatrics, 113*(6), 1753-1757.

Schum, T. R., Kolb, B. S., McAuliffe, T. L., Simms, M. D., Underhill, R. L., & Lewis, M. (2002). Sequential acquisition of toilet-training skills: a descriptive study of gender and age differences in normal children. *Pediatrics, 109*(3), e48.

Stevenson, M., Rimajova, M., Edgecombe, D., & Vickery, K. (2003). Childhood drowning: barriers surrounding private swimming pools. *Pediatrics, 111*(2), e115-e119.

United States Department of Health and Human Services. (2000). *Healthy People 2010.* Washington, DC: Author.

United States Department of Health and Human Services & United States Department of Agriculture. (2005). *Dietary guidelines for Americans 2005.* Retrieved December 30, 2005 from *www.healthierus .gov/dietaryguidelines.*

United States Department of Agriculture, Food and Nutrition Service. (2005). *MyPyramid for kids.* Retrieved October 29, 2005, from www.mypyramid.gov/Kids/index.html.

United States Preventive Services Task Force. (2004). *Prevention of dental caries in preschool children.* Retrieved January 29, 2006, from www.ahrq.gov/clinic/uspstf/uspsdnch.htm.

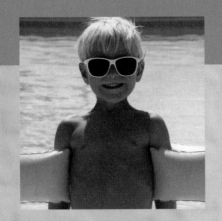

CHAPTER 7

Health Promotion for the School-Age Child

Learning Objectives

After studying this chapter, you should be able to:

- Describe the school-age child's normal growth and development and assess the child for normal developmental milestones.
- Describe the maturational changes that take place during the school-age period and discuss implications for health care.
- Identify the stages of moral development in the school-age child and discuss implications for effective parenting strategies.
- Discuss the effect school has on the child's development and implications for teachers and parents.
- Discuss anticipatory guidance related to various health and safety issues seen in the school-age child.
- Describe anticipatory guidance that the nurse can offer to decrease children's stress.

Definitions

caries   Decay of the teeth.
conservation   Ability to understand that certain properties of objects do not change simply because their order, form, or appearance has changed.
malocclusion   Misalignment of the teeth or dental arches; teeth may be crowded, crooked, or out of alignment.

menarche   Onset of menstruation.
self-care children   Children who care for themselves at home after school; formerly called latch-key children.

Electronic Resources

Additional information related to the content in Chapter 7 can be found on:

the interactive companion CD-ROM

- Audio Glossary
- NCLEX Review Questions
- Pediatric Assessment & Video Clips

or the companion website at *evolve*
http://evolve.elsevier.com/james/ncoc

- NCLEX Review Questions
- Pediatric Assessment & Video Clips
- WebLinks

Middle childhood, ages 6 to 12 years, is probably one of the healthiest periods of life. Slow, steady physical growth and rapid cognitive and social development characterize this time. During these 6 years, the child's world expands from the tight circle of the family to include children and adults at school, at a worship community, and in the community at large. The child becomes increasingly independent. Peers become important as the child starts school and gradually moves away from the security of home. This period is a time for best friends, sharing, and exploring.

The school years also are a time that can be stressful for a child, and this stress can impede the child's successful achievement of developmental tasks. The *Healthy People 2010* objectives (Box 7-1) that relate to school-age children include such goals as reducing stress and obesity, improving access to dental care, and preventing high-risk behaviors.

GROWTH AND DEVELOPMENT OF THE SCHOOL-AGE CHILD

The school-age child develops a sense of industry and learns the basic skills needed to function in society. The child develops an appreciation of rules and a conscience. Cognitively, the child grows from the egocentrism of early childhood to more mature thinking. The ability to solve problems and

BOX **7-1**	***Healthy People 2010* Objectives for School-Age Children**
6-2	Reduce the proportion of children and adolescents with disabilities who are reported to be sad, unhappy, or depressed.
6-9	Increase the proportion of children and youth with disabilities who spend at least 80% of their time in regular education programs.
15-23	Increase the use of helmets by bicyclists.
18-7	Increase the proportion of children with mental health problems who receive treatment.
19-3	Reduce the proportion of children and adolescents who are overweight or obese.
19-5, 6, 7	Increase the proportion of persons aged 2 years and older who consume at least two daily servings of fruit; three daily servings of vegetables, with at least one third being dark-green or deep-yellow vegetables; and six daily servings of grain products, with at least three being whole grain.
19-8, 9	Increase the proportion of persons aged 2 years and older who consume less than 10% of calories from saturated fat and who consume no more than 30% of calories from fat.
19-15	Increase the proportion of children and adolescents aged 6 to 19 years whose intake of meals and snacks at schools contributes proportionally to good overall dietary quality.
20-1	Reduce the proportion of children and adolescents who have dental caries in their primary or permanent teeth.
21-8	Increase the proportion of children who have received dental sealants to their molar teeth.
22-11	Increase the proportion of children and adolescents who view television 2 or fewer hours per day.
27-3	Reduce initiation of tobacco use among children and adolescents.

Modified from U.S. Department of Health and Human Services. (2000). *Healthy People 2010* (Conference edition, in 2 volumes). Washington, DC: U.S. Department of Health and Human Services.

make independent judgments that are based on reason characterizes this new maturity. The child is invested in the task of middle childhood: learning to do things and do them well. Competence and self-esteem increase with each academic, social, and athletic achievement. The relative stability and security of the school-age period prepare the child to enter the emotional and physical changes of adolescence.

Physical Growth and Development

The school-age years are characterized by slow and steady growth. The physical changes that occur during this period are gradual and subtle. Although growth rates vary among children (Fig. 7-1), the average weight gain is 2.5 kg (5½ lb) per year

and the average increase in height is approximately 5.5 cm (2 inches) per year. During the early school-age period, boys are approximately 1 inch taller and 2 lb heavier than girls. At around age 10 or 12 years, girls begin to catch up in size as they undergo the preadolescent growth spurt. By age 12 years, girls are 1 inch taller than boys and 2 lb heavier. This growth spurt, which signals the onset of puberty, occurs usually between ages 12 and 14 years and occurs 2 years later in boys than in girls.

Body Systems

School-age children appear thinner and more graceful than preschoolers do. Musculoskeletal growth leads to greater coordination and strength. The muscles are still immature, however, and can be injured from overuse. Growth of the facial bones changes facial proportions. As the facial bones grow, the eustachian tube assumes a more downward and inward position, resulting in fewer ear infections than in the preschool years. Lymphatic tissues continue to grow until about age 9 years; immunoglobulin A and G (IgA, IgG) levels reach adult values at approximately 10 years. Enlarged tonsils and adenoids are common during these years and are not always an indication of illness. Frontal sinuses develop at age 7 years. Growth in brain size is complete by 10 years. The respiratory system also continues to mature. During the school-age years, the lungs and alveoli develop fully and fewer respiratory infections occur.

Dentition

During the school-age years, all 20 primary (deciduous) teeth are lost and are replaced by 28 of the 32 permanent teeth. All permanent teeth, except the third molars, erupt during the school-age period. The order of eruption of permanent teeth and loss of primary teeth is shown in Figure 9-6. The first teeth to be lost are usually the lower central incisors, at around age 6 years. Most first-graders are characterized by a snaggle-tooth appearance (see Fig. 7-1), and visits from the "tooth fairy" are important signs of growing up.

Sexual Development

Puberty is a time of dramatic physical change. It includes the growth spurt, development of primary and secondary sexual characteristics, and maturation of the sexual organs. The age at onset of puberty varies widely, and puberty is occurring at an earlier age than previously thought. Onset of puberty is no longer unusual in girls who are 9 or 10 years old. On the average, African American girls begin puberty 1 year earlier than white girls (Herman-Giddens, Kaplowitz, & Wasserman, 2004). The reason for the earlier development among African American girls is not known. Puberty begins about 1½ to 2 years later in boys. Menarche, the onset of menstruation, occurs, on average, during the twelfth year. Females who are significantly overweight tend to have earlier onset of puberty and menarche. Because puberty is occurring increasingly earlier, many 10- and 11-year-old girls have already had menarche. Wide variations in maturity at this age are a common cause of embarrassment because the school-age child does not want to appear different from peers. Children

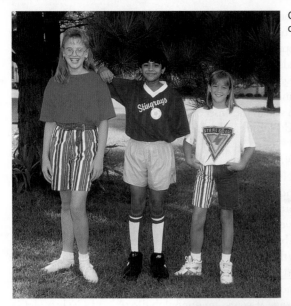

Children of the same age can vary significantly in height and physical development.

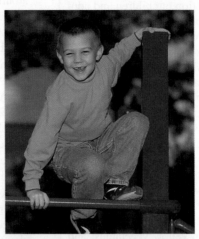

School-age children often have a snaggle-tooth appearance while they are losing their primary teeth.

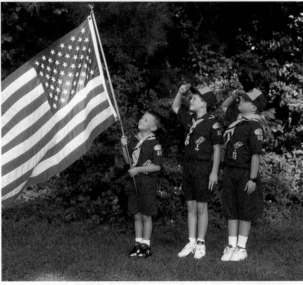

Organizations such as Boy Scouts help foster self-esteem and competence.

FIG 7-1   **Growth and development of the school-age child.**

who mature either early or late may struggle with feelings of self-consciousness and inferiority. Table 8-1 describes the usual sequence of appearance of secondary sex characteristics during the school-age and adolescent periods.

Because of the earlier onset of puberty, sex education programs should be introduced in elementary school. Nurses are in an excellent position to serve as resource persons for parents and teachers who are responsible for sex education. Children's questions about sexuality and related issues should be answered honestly and matter of factly. If sex education is presented within the context of learning about the human body, with its wonders and mysteries, children are less likely to feel embarrassed and anxious. Regardless of whether sex education is a part of a formal school curriculum, children need accurate information. Basic anatomy and physiology, information about body functions, and the expected changes of puberty should be introduced to children before the onset of puberty. Older school-age children need information about

menstruation, nocturnal emissions, and reproduction. Sex education programs must also include information about responsible sexuality and related issues, such as teenage pregnancy, human immunodeficiency virus (HIV), and sexually transmissible diseases.

CRITICAL TO REMEMBER
Components of Sex Education
- Basic anatomy and physiology
- Body functions
- Expected changes related to puberty
- Menstruation, nocturnal emissions
- Reproduction
- Teenage pregnancy
- Human immunodeficiency virus (HIV) infection prevention
- Sexually transmissible diseases

BOX 7-2	**Age-Related Activities and Toys for the School-Age Child**

General Activities

Play becomes organized with more direction.

Early school-age child continues dramatic play with increased creativity but loses some spontaneity.

Child is aware of rules when playing games.

Child begins to compete in sports.

Toys and Specific Types of Play

Collections, drawing, construction, dolls, pets, guessing games, complicated puzzles, board games, riddles, physical games, competitive play, reading, bike riding, hobbies, sewing, listening to the radio, watching television and videos, cooking.

Motor Development

Development of Gross Motor Skills

During the school years, coordination improves. A developed sense of balance and rhythm allows children to ride a two-wheeled bicycle, dance, skip, jump rope, and participate in a variety of sports. As puberty approaches in the late school-age period, children may become more awkward as their bodies grow faster than their ability to compensate.

Importance of Active Play

School-age children spend much of their time in active play, practicing and refining motor skills. They seem to be constantly in motion. Children of this age enjoy active sports and games as well as crafts and fine motor activities (Box 7-2). Activities requiring balance and strength, such as bicycle riding, tree climbing, and skating, are exciting and fun for the school-age child. Coordination and motor skills improve as the child is given an opportunity to practice.

Children should be encouraged to engage in physical activities. During the school-age years, children learn physical fitness skills that contribute to their health for the rest of their lives. Cardiovascular fitness, strength, and flexibility are improved by physical activity. Popular games such as tag, jump rope, and hide-and-seek provide a release of emotional tension and enhance the development of leader and follower skills.

Team sports, such as soccer and baseball, provide opportunities not only for exercise and refinement of motor skills but also for the development of sportsmanship and teamwork. Nurses should advise parents on ways to prevent sports injuries and how to assess a recreational sports program (Box 7-3). Sports activities should be well supervised, and protective gear (e.g., helmets for T-ball, shin guards for soccer) should be mandatory.

Obesity is has become a major problem in children in the United States, with 19% of children aged 6 to 11 years being overweight or obese (National Center for Health Statistics, 2005). Time spent watching television or playing computer games often diminishes a child's interest in active play outside. Nurses can help reverse this trend by advising parents to limit their children's television watching time to 2 hours or less per day and to encourage them to engage in more active play. Parents should provide adequate space for children to run, jump, and scuffle. Children should have enough free time to exercise and play. Parents need to role model both good nutrition and exercise.

Preventing Fatigue and Dehydration

Because children enjoy active play and are so full of energy, they often do not recognize fatigue. Six-year-olds in particular will not stop an activity to rest. Parents must learn to recognize signs of fatigue or irritability and enforce rest periods before the child becomes exhausted. Because the child's metabolic rate is higher than an adult's and sweating ability is limited, extremes in temperature while exercising can be dangerous. Dehydration and overheating can pose threats to the child's health. Frequent rest periods and adequate hydration are essential for the child during physical exercise.

BOX 7-3	**PARENTS WANT TO KNOW** About Assessing an Organized Recreational Sports Program

Whenever your child begins playing in an organized recreational sports program, you need to consider the following:

- *Coaches' training:* Coaches not only need to understand how to play a sport and to teach it to young children but also should have undergone a training program in injury prevention and first aid. Check to see that the training emphasizes preventing overuse injuries.
- *Coaches' attitude:* Coaches should have a positive, encouraging manner with children—not critical and demeaning. Check whether the coach emphasizes skill development and plays all the children, regardless of whether required to. Be sure the coach is a good role model on the field and is courteous to referees, other coaches, and the children. Avoid coaches who have a "win at all costs" philosophy.

- *Safety:* Check to see that protective and athletic equipment is used correctly by all children participating in the sport. Facilities and equipment should be well maintained and safe. Children should be divided into teams according to size and maturation level rather than by age. Many sports programs require a preseason physical examination.
- *Enjoyment:* Sports programs can do wonderful things for your child's skill development, confidence, sense of cooperation, and self-esteem. Remember that it is your child playing the sport and not you. Be encouraging and positive, help the child when asked, and cheer the team on in an appropriate manner.

Development of Fine Motor Skills

Increased myelinization of the central nervous system is shown by refinement of fine motor skills. Balance and hand-eye coordination improve with maturity and practice. School-age children take pride in activities that require dexterity and fine motor skill, such as model building, playing a musical instrument, and drawing.

Cognitive Development

Thought processes undergo dramatic changes as the child moves from the intuitive thinking of the preschool years to the logical thinking processes of the school-age years. The school-age child gains new knowledge and develops more efficient problem-solving ability and greater flexibility of thinking. The 6-year-old and the 7-year-old remain in the intuitive thought stage (Piaget, 1962) characteristic of the older preschool child. By age 8 years, the child moves into the stage of concrete operations, followed by the stage of formal operations at around 12 years. See Chapter 4 for a discussion of formal operations and Chapter 30 for a discussion of the child with cognitive deficits, including mental retardation and developmental disabilities.

Intuitive Thought Stage

In the intuitive thought stage (6 to 7 years), thinking is based on immediate perceptions of the environment and the child's own viewpoint. Thinking is still characterized by egocentrism, animism, and centration (see Chapter 6). At 6 and 7 years old, children cannot understand another's viewpoint, form hypotheses, or deal with abstract concepts. The child in the intuitive thought stage has difficulty forming categories and often solves problems by random guessing.

Concrete Operations Stage

By age 7 or 8 years, the child enters the stage of concrete operations. Children learn that their point of view is not the only one as they encounter different interpretations of reality and begin to differentiate their own viewpoints from those of peers and adults (Piaget, 1962). This newly developed freedom from egocentrism enables children to think more flexibly and to learn about the environment more accurately. Problem solving becomes more efficient and reliable as the child learns how to form hypotheses. The use of symbolism becomes more sophisticated, and children now can manipulate symbols for things in the way that they once manipulated the things themselves. The child learns the alphabet and how to read. Attention span increases as the child grows older, facilitating classroom learning.

Reversibility. Children in the concrete operations stage grasp the concept of *reversibility*. They can mentally retrace a process, a skill necessary for understanding mathematic problems (5 + 3 = 8 and 8 − 3 = 5). The child can take a toy apart and put it back together or walk to school and find the way back home without getting lost. Reversibility also enables a child to anticipate the results of actions—a valuable tool for problem solving.

The understanding of time gradually develops during the early school-age years. Children can understand and use clock time at around age 8 years. Although 8- or 9-year-old children understand calendar time and memorize dates, they do not master historic time until later.

Conservation. Gradually, the school-age child masters the concept of *conservation*. The child learns that certain properties of objects do not change simply because their order, form, or appearance has changed. For example, the child who has mastered conservation of mass recognizes that a lump of clay that has been pounded flat is still the same amount of clay as when it was rolled into a ball. The child understands conservation of weight when able to correctly answer the classic nonsense question, "Which weighs more, a pound of feathers or a pound of rocks?" The concept of conservation does not develop all at once. The simpler conservations, such as number and mass, are understood first, and more complex conservations are mastered later. An understanding of conservation of weight develops at 9 or 10 years old, and an understanding of volume is present at 11 or 12 years.

Classification and Logic. Older school-age children are able to classify objects according to characteristics they share, to place things in a logical order, and to recall similarities and differences. This ability is reflected in the school-age child's interest in collections. Children love to collect and classify stamps, stickers, sports cards, shells, dolls, rocks, or anything imaginable. School-age children understand relationships such as larger and smaller, lighter and darker. They can comprehend class inclusion—the concept that objects can belong to more than one classification. For example, a man can be a brother, a father, and a son at the same time.

School-age children move away from magical thinking as they discover that there are logical, physical explanations for most phenomena. The older school-age child is a skeptic, no longer believing in Santa Claus or the Easter Bunny.

Humor. Children in the concrete operations stage have a delightful sense of humor. Around the age of 8 years, increased mastery of language and the beginning of logic enable children to appreciate a play on words. They laugh at incongruities and love silly jokes, riddles, and puns ("How do you keep a mad elephant from charging? You take away its credit cards!"). Riddle and joke books make ideal gifts for young school-age children. Research suggests that children who have a good sense of humor use it as a positive coping mechanism for stress associated with maturational and situational life events (Taxis, Rew, Jackson, & Koozekanani, 2004).

Sensory Development

Vision

The eyes are fully developed by age 6 years. Visual acuity, ocular muscle control, peripheral vision, and color discrimination are fully developed by age 7 years. Just before puberty, some children's eyes undergo a growth spurt, resulting in myopia. Children with poor visual acuity usually do not complain of vision problems because the changes occur so gradually that they are difficult to notice. Usual behaviors that parents notice include squinting, moving closer to the television, or complaints of frequent headaches. The young child may never have had 20/20 vision and has nothing with which to compare the imperfect vision. For these reasons, yearly vision screening is important for school-age children.

Hearing

With maturation and growth of the eustachian tube, middle ear infections occur less frequently than in younger children. However, chronic middle ear infections are a problem for a few children, when they result in hearing loss. Annual audiometric screening tests are important to detect hearing loss before unrecognized deficits lead to learning problems (see Chapter 31).

Language Development

Language development continues at a rapid pace during the school-age years. Vocabulary expands, and sentence structure becomes more complex. By age 6 years, the child's vocabulary is approximately 8,000 to 14,000 words. There is an increase in the use of culturally specific words at this age. Bilingual children may speak English at school and a different language at home.

Reading effectively improves language skills. Regular trips to the library, where the child can check out books of special interest, can promote a love of reading and enhance school performance. School-age children enjoy being read to as well as reading on their own. Older children enjoy horror stories, mysteries, romances, and adventure stories.

School-age children often go through a period in which they experiment with profanity and "dirty" jokes. Children may imitate parents who use such words as part of their vocabulary.

Psychosocial Development

Development of a Sense of Industry

According to Erikson (1963), the central task of the school-age years is the development of a sense of industry. Ideally, the child is prepared for this task with a secure sense of self as separate from loved ones in the family. The child should have learned to trust others and should have developed a sense of autonomy and initiative during the preceding years. The school-age child replaces fantasy play with "work" at school, crafts, chores, hobbies, and athletics. The child is rewarded with a sense of satisfaction from achieving a skill as well as with external rewards, such as good grades, trophies, or an allowance. School-age children enjoy undertaking new tasks and carrying them through to completion. Whether it is baking a cake, hitting a home run, or scoring 100 on a math test, purposeful activity leads to a sense of worth and competence. Successful resolution of the task of industry depends on learning to do things and do them well. School-age children learn skills that they will need later to compete in the adult world. A person's fundamental attitude toward work is established during the school-age years.

Fostering Self-Esteem

The negative component of this developmental stage is a sense of inferiority. If a child cannot separate psychologically from the parent or if expectations are set too high for the child to achieve, feelings of inferiority develop. If a child believes that success is unattainable, confidence is lost and the child will not take pleasure in attempting new experiences. Children who have this experience will then have a pervasive feeling of inferiority and incompetence that will affect all aspects of their lives. The child who lacks a sense of industry has a poor foundation for mastering the tasks of adolescence. The reality is that no one can master everything. Every child will feel deficient or inferior at something. The task of the caring parent or teacher is to identify areas in which a child is competent and to build on successful experiences to foster feelings of mastery and success. Nurses can suggest ways in which parents and teachers can promote a sense of self-esteem and competence in school-age children (Box 7-4).

At this age, the approval and esteem of those outside the family, especially peers, become important. Children learn that their parents are not infallible. As they begin to test parents' authority and knowledge, the influence of teachers and other adults is felt more and more. The peer group

---

BOX 7-4 | **PARENTS WANT TO KNOW** About How to Promote Self-Esteem in School-Age Children

- Give your children household responsibilities according to their developmental level and capabilities. Set reasonable rules, and expect the child to follow them.
- Allow your child to solve problems and make responsible choices.
- Give praise for what is praiseworthy. Do not be afraid to encourage your child to do better. Refrain from being critical, but gently point out areas that could be improved.
- Allow your children to make mistakes and encourage them to take responsibility for the consequences of their mistakes.

- Emphasize your child's strengths and help improve weaknesses.
- Do not do your children's homework for them because this will make them think you do not trust them to do a good job; provide assistance and suggestions when asked and praise their best efforts.
- Model appropriate behavior toward others.
- Provide consistent and demonstrative love.

becomes the school-age child's major socializing influence. Although parents' love, praise, and support are needed, even craved during stressful times, the child begins to prefer activities with friends to activities with the family. As the child becomes more independent, increasing time is spent with friends and away from the family.

The concept of friendship changes as the child matures. At 6 and 7 years old, children form friendships merely on the basis of who lives nearby or who has toys that they enjoy. By the time children are 9 or 10 years old, friendships are based more on emotional bonds, warm feelings, and trust-building experiences. Children learn that friendship is more than just being together. Children at 11 and 12 years are loyal to their friends, often sharing problems and giving emotional support. School-age children tend to form friendships with peers of the same sex. Developing friendships and succeeding in social interactions lead to a sense of industry. Friendships are important for the emotional well-being of school-age children. Friends teach children skills they will use in future relationships.

Children learn a body of rules, sayings, and superstitions as they enter the culture of childhood. Rules are important to children because they provide predictability and offer security. Learning the sayings, jokes, and riddles is an important part of social interaction among peers. Sayings such as "Step on a crack and you'll break your mother's back" or "Finders, keepers; losers, weepers" have been part of the lore of childhood for generations.

Children become sensitive to the norms and values of the peer group because pressure to conform is great. Children often find that it is painful to be different. Peer approval is a strong motivating force and allows the child to risk disapproval from parents.

The school-age years are a time of formal and informal clubs. Informal clubs among 6-, 7-, and 8-year-olds are loosely organized, with fluid membership. Membership changes frequently and it is based on mutual interests, such as playing ball, riding bikes, or playing with dolls. Children learn interpersonal skills, such as sharing, cooperation, and tolerance, in these groups.

Clubs among older school-age children tend to be more structured, often characterized by secret codes, rituals, and rigid rules. A club may be formed for the purpose of exclusion, in which children snub another child for some reason.

Formal organizations, such as Boy Scouts, Girl Scouts, Campfire Boys and Girls, and 4-H, organized by adults, also foster self-esteem and competence as children earn ranks and merit badges. Transmission of societal values, such as service to others, duty to God, and good citizenship, is an important goal of these organizations.

Spiritual and Moral Development

Middle childhood years are pivotal in the development of a conscience and the internalization of values. Tremendous strides are made in moral development during these 6 years. Several theorists have described the dramatic growth that occurs during this stage.

Piaget

Piaget (1962) asserted that young school-age children obey rules because powerful, all-knowing adults hand them down. During this stage, children know the rules but not the reasons behind them. Rules are interpreted in a literal way, and the child is unable to adjust rules to fit differing circumstances. The perception of guilt changes as the child matures. Piaget stated that up to about age 8 years, children judge degrees of guilt by the amount of damage done. No distinction is made between accidental and intentional wrongdoing. For example, the child believes that a child who broke five china cups by accident is guiltier than a child who broke one cup on purpose. By age 10 years, children are able to consider the intent of the action. Older school-age children are more flexible in their decisions and can take into account extenuating circumstances.

Kohlberg

Kohlberg (1964) described moral development in terms of three levels containing six stages (see Chapter 4). According to Kohlberg's theory, children 4 to 7 years old are in stage 2 of the preconventional level, in which right and wrong are determined by physical consequences. The child obeys because of fear of punishment. If the child is not caught or punished for an act, the child does not consider the act wrong. At this stage, children conform to rules out of self-interest or in terms of what others can do in return ("I'll do this for you if you'll do that for me."). Behavior is guided by an eye-for-an-eye philosophy.

Kohlberg describes children between the ages of 7 and 12 years as being in stage 3 of the conventional level. A good-boy or good-girl orientation characterizes this stage, in which the child conforms to rules to please others and avoid disapproval. This stage parallels the concrete operations stage of cognitive development. Around the age of 12 years, children enter stage 4 of the conventional level. There is an orientation toward respecting authority, obeying rules, and maintaining social order. Most religions place the age of accountability at approximately 12 years.

Family Influence

Children manifest antisocial behaviors during middle childhood. Behaviors such as cheating, lying, and stealing are not uncommon. Often, children lie or cheat to get out of an embarrassing situation or to make themselves look more important to their peers. In most cases, these behaviors are minor; however, if they are severe or persistent, the child may need referral for counseling.

Parents and teachers profoundly influence moral development. Parents can teach children the difference between right and wrong most effectively by living according to their values. A father who lectures his child about the importance of honesty gives a mixed message when he brags about fooling his boss or cheating on his income tax return. The moral atmosphere in the home is a critical factor in the child's personality development.

Children learn self-discipline and internalization of values through obedience to external rules. School-age children are legalistic, and they feel loved and secure when they know that firm limits are set on their behavior. They want and expect discipline for wrongdoings. For moral teaching to be effective, parents must be consistent in their expectations of their children and in administering rewards and punishment.

Spirituality and Religion

Spiritually, school-age children become acquainted with the basic content of their faith. Children reared within a religious tradition feel a part of their religion. Although their thinking is still concrete, children begin to use abstract concepts to describe God and are able to comprehend God as a power greater than themselves or their parents. Because school-age children think literally, spiritual concepts take on materialistic and physical expression. Heaven and hell fascinate them. Concern for rules and a maturing conscience may cause a nagging sense of guilt and fear of going to hell. Younger school-age children still tend to associate accidents and illness with punishment for real or imagined wrongdoing. One 6-year-old child hospitalized for an appendectomy said, "God saw all the bad things I did, and He punished me." Reassurance that God does not punish children by making them sick reduces anxiety.

HEALTH PROMOTION FOR THE SCHOOL-AGE CHILD AND FAMILY

It is recommended that during middle childhood children should visit the health care provider every 2 years. Many school districts require documentation of a routine physical examination at least once during the elementary school years after the kindergarten visit. If children are participating in organized sports or attending camp, an annual physical examination might be required.

Nutrition During Middle Childhood

Nutritional Requirements

Growth continues at a slow, regular pace, but the school-age child begins to have an increased appetite. Energy needs increase during the later school-age years. Children in this age group tend to have few eating idiosyncrasies and generally enjoy eating to satisfy appetite and as a social function. Children who developed dislikes for certain foods during earlier periods may continue to refuse those foods. School-age children are influenced by family patterns and the limitations their activities put on them. They may rush through a meal to go out to play or watch a favorite program on television.

Children should choose a variety of culturally appropriate foods and snacks daily. Dietary recommendations for school age children include 6 ounces of grains; 2½ cups of vegetables; 1½ cups of fruit; 5 ounces of meat, fish, or beans; and 3 cups of nonfat milk or dairy products (U.S. Department of Agriculture, 2005). They need to limit saturated fat intake and processed sugars. Caloric and protein requirements begin to increase at about age 11 years because of the preadolescent growth spurt. The requirements for boys and girls also begin

to vary at this age. A gradual increase in food intake will also take place. The nurse should ask children to describe specifically what they eat at meals and for snacks to develop a more comprehensive picture of their eating habits.

When children's nutritional status is assessed, it is important to also assess any body image concerns; be sure to ask children how they feel about the way they look. Eating disorders, although thought to be a problem of adolescence, can begin in the late elementary school years.

Age-Related Nutritional Challenges

During the school years, the child's schedule changes and more time is spent away from home. Most children eat lunch at school, and they usually have a choice of foods. Even if the parent packs a lunch for the child to take to school, there are no guarantees that the child will eat the lunch. Children sometimes trade foods with other children or may not eat a particular item. It is also during this period that the child becomes more active in clubs, sports, and other activities that interrupt the normal meal schedule.

The federal government funds the School Lunch Program, which provides lunches free or at a reduced cost for low-income children. The School Lunch Program includes approximately one third of the recommended daily dietary allowances for a child. School lunch programs usually follow the dietary guidelines to meet recommended nutritional requirements; however, many school lunches are somewhat high in fat. Some schools also offer breakfast and milk programs. Many schools offer low-nutrient, high-calorie snacks as an add-on to the school lunch or in snack machines available in various locations throughout the school. In some cases, children use their lunch money to buy snacks. Advise parents to communicate with their children about appropriate lunch and snacks in school and to know what is being offered in the school cafeteria.

School-age children usually request a snack after school and in the evening. Encourage parents to provide their children with healthy choices for snacks. By not buying foods high in calories and low in nutrients the parent can remove the temptation for the child to choose the less healthy foods.

Unpredictable schedules, advertising, easy access to fast food, and peer pressure all have an effect on the foods a child chooses. The child may begin to prefer "junk foods," which do not have much nutritional value. Most of these foods are high in fat and sugar. In addition, school-age children often skip breakfast. The family plays an important role in modeling good eating habits for the child. Schools also have a responsibility to provide nutritious meals for children.

Dental Care

Although the incidence of dental caries (tooth decay) has declined in recent years, tooth decay remains a significant health problem among school-age children. Unfortunately, many parents and school-age children consider dental hygiene to be of minor importance. Many parents erroneously believe that dental care, even brushing, is not important for

THE 6- TO 8-YEAR-OLD CHILD

FOCUSED ASSESSMENT

Ask the child the following:

- Can you tell me how often and what foods you like to eat? How often do you eat at fast-food restaurants? How do you feel about how much you weigh? Do you think you need to gain or lose any weight?
- What types of physical activities do you like to do? How often do you do them? Do you have any quiet hobbies that interest you? How many hours each day do you watch television? What is your favorite television program?
- How often do you brush your teeth, floss, and see the dentist? Do you take fluoride?
- What time do you go to bed at night? What time do you get up in the morning? Do you have any trouble falling asleep, or do you wake up in the middle of the night?
- How often do you have a bowel movement? Are there any problems with urination? (Use the child's familiar terminology if known.) Do you wet the bed? If so, how often?
- What grade in school are you? Are you doing well in school or having any problems? Do you feel safe at school? Do you participate in any before-school or after-school programs?
- Tell me about your friends. Do they like to do the same things you like to do?
- How do you get along with other members of your family? Is there a special family member you could talk to if you are having a problem? If so, who?
- Do you do any or all of the following: use a seat belt every time you get in a car; wear a helmet every time you ride a bike; wear a helmet and protective pads every time you skate or use a scooter; use sunscreen; swim with a buddy and only when an adult is present; always look both ways before crossing the street; use the right equipment when you play sports; know to avoid strangers and how to call for help if needed?
- Has anyone ever physically harmed you or touched you in a way that made you uncomfortable?

Ask the parent the following:

- Are there any concerns related to the child's nutrition, body image, physical activity, oral health, sleep,

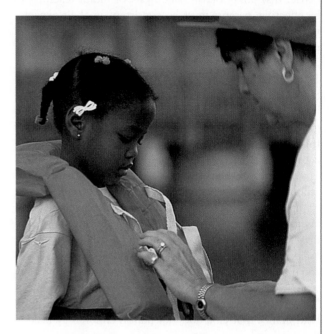

elimination, school, family interactions, self-esteem, and ability to practice safety precautions?
- Is there a gun in the home? If so, is it locked away and the ammunition stored in a separate place?
- Do you have a swimming pool? If so, is it fenced on all four sides and not directly accessible from the house?
- Do you have a fire escape plan that you practice regularly?

DEVELOPMENTAL MILESTONES

Personal/social: develops positive self-esteem through skill acquisition and task completion; peer group becoming the primary socializing force; outgoing and boisterous, "know-it-all," but becomes more reflective and quiet by age 8 years; loves new ideas and places; has a good sense of humor, may tell crude jokes; may be argumentative and use tension-releasing behaviors such as nail biting, hair twisting, wriggling; likes to make things but often does not finish projects; loves family members but worries about them; has a strong sense of fairness and justice—uses rules to define cooperative relationships with others (sees rules as being imposed by others)

---

primary teeth because they will all fall out anyway. However, premature loss of these deciduous teeth can complicate eruption of permanent teeth and lead to malocclusion.

School-age children are able to assume responsibility for their own dental hygiene. Good oral health habits tend to be carried into the adult years, reducing cavity formation for a lifetime. Thorough brushing with fluoride toothpaste followed by flossing between the teeth should be done after meals and especially before bedtime. Proper brushing and flossing and a well-balanced diet promote healthy gums and

prevent cavities. Sugary or sticky between-meal snacks should be limited. Candy that dissolves quickly, such as chocolate, is less cariogenic than sticky candy, which stays in contact with teeth longer. Information related to fluoride supplementation is given in Chapter 6.

Malocclusion

Good *occlusion*, or alignment, of the teeth is important for tooth formation, speech development, and physical appearance. Many school-age children need orthodontic braces

HEALTH PROMOTION

THE 6- TO 8-YEAR-OLD CHILD—cont'd

DEVELOPMENTAL MILESTONES—cont'd

Fine motor: ties shoelaces, buttons and zips clothes, dresses and undresses without help; can print, draw, color well, model clay, and cut with scissors; visual acuity is fully developed

Language/cognitive: vocabulary expands; understands the different properties of language: play on words, puns, mnemonics, jokes; adapts well to changing physical properties of objects (e.g., conservation, reversibility, identity); improved long-term memory; organizes concepts and classifies in several ways; uses various memory strategies to improve school work

Gross motor: improved muscle mass and coordination allow for participation in a variety of sports and games

HEALTH MAINTENANCE

Physical Measurements

Average weight gain is 2.5 kg (5½ lb) per year

Average increase in height is approximately 5.5 cm (2 inches) per year

Continue to plot height and weight

Plot body mass index (see Appendix B)

Note any breast budding or signs of other secondary sex characteristics

Immunizations

If not given earlier, administer measles, mumps, rubella (MMR) #2; diphtheria, tetanus, acellular pertussis (DTaP) #5 (if younger than 7 years); and inactivated poliovirus (IPV) #4

Administer other immunizations if not up to date

Health Screening

Objective hearing and vision screening

Speech assessment for fluency

Hemoglobin or hematocrit

Urine for sugar and protein

Blood pressure

Lipid screen if at risk

Tuberculosis screening if at risk (see Chapter 21)

ANTICIPATORY GUIDANCE

Provide health teaching to the child as well as to the parent

Nutrition

Follow recommended servings according to the dietary guidelines; teach the child how to keep track of servings and to give input into meal preparation

Advise to avoid fast foods and to eat a nutritious breakfast

Watch calcium and iron intake

Elimination

Regular bowel movements according to the child's pattern; treat constipation by increasing water intake and intake of fresh fruits and vegetables

Occasional bed-wetting is within the norm; refer for more serious problems (see Chapter 20)

Dental

Provide regular dental care every 6 months

Continue regular brushing with fluoride toothpaste and flossing (may need assistance with this)

Continue fluoride supplements if water is not fluoridated

May need dental sealants as permanent molars erupt

Sleep

Facilitate an individually appropriate sleep pattern; school-age children usually go to bed by 9 PM and are up by 7 AM

If the child is not tired, advise the parent to allow a quiet reading time in bed

Safety

Review gun safety; bicycle, skating, and scooter safety; playground safety; fire safety; automobile and pedestrian safety; water safety; sun protection; good touch versus bad touch, stranger awareness

Discuss exposure to contact allergens (poison ivy, oak, sumac), tick checks, sports safety, use of reflective clothing if out at night

Play

Encourage developing collections, playing complicated board and card games, crafts, electronic and science-related games

Advise limiting television watching to no more than 2 hours a day

Self-Esteem and Competence

See Box 7-4

---

to correct malocclusion, a condition in which the teeth are crowded, crooked, or out of alignment. Factors such as heredity, cleft palate, premature loss of primary teeth, and mouth breathing lead to malocclusion. Thumb sucking is not believed to cause malocclusion unless it persists past the age of 5 or 6 years. Malocclusion becomes particularly noticeable between the ages of 6 and 12 years, when the permanent teeth are erupting.

Children with braces are at increased risk for dental caries and must be scrupulous about their dental hygiene. School nurses can encourage children who wear braces to brush after every meal and snack, eat a nutritious diet, and visit the dentist at least once every 6 months. Use of a water pick keeps gums healthy and helps remove food particles from around wires and bands.

Braces cause many children to feel self-conscious and may be difficult for a school-age child to accept. However, for some children, orthodontic appliances may be a status symbol. Parental support and encouragement are important to help the child adjust to orthodontic treatment.

Preventing Dental Injuries

During the school-age years, injuries to the teeth can occur easily. Many injuries can be avoided by use of mouth protectors. These resilient shields protect against injuries by cushioning blows that might otherwise damage teeth or lead to jaw fractures (American Dental Association, 2005). Children should wear a mouth protector when participating in contact sports, bike riding, or in-line skating. Custom-made mouth protectors constructed by the dentist are more expensive than stock mouth protectors purchased in stores, but their better fit makes them more comfortable and less likely to interfere with speech and breathing.

Dental Health Education

Health education curricula need to be designed to foster attitudes and behaviors among children that promote good personal oral hygiene practices and awareness of the risks of dental disease. The school nurse is in an excellent position to educate children about dental health and to detect problems such as untreated caries, inflamed gums, or malocclusion. The nurse should look for signs of smokeless tobacco use (irritation of the gums at the tobacco placement site, gum recession, stained teeth) and should take this opportunity to explain to the child the risks of using tobacco. The use of snuff and chewing tobacco carries multiple dangers, including a greatly increased risk of oral cancer and heart disease.

Sleep and Rest

The number of hours spent sleeping decreases as the child grows older. Children aged 6 and 7 years need about 12 hours of sleep per night. Some children also continue to need an afternoon quiet time or nap to restore energy levels. The 12-year-old needs about 9 to 10 hours of sleep at night. More sleep is needed when the child enters the preadolescent growth spurt. Adequate sleep is important for school performance and physical growth. Inadequate sleep can cause irritability, inability to concentrate, and poor school performance.

To promote rest and sleep, a period of quiet activity just before bedtime is helpful. A leisurely bedtime routine, with adequate time for the child to read, listen to the radio or compact discs, or just daydream, promotes relaxation. Children who do not obtain adequate rest often have difficulty getting up in the morning, creating a family disturbance as they rush to get ready for school, perhaps skipping breakfast or leaving the house in the heat of frustration. A set bedtime and waking time, consistently enforced, promote security and healthful sleep habits. Bedtime offers an ideal opportunity for parent and child to share important events of the day or give a kiss and a hug, unthinkable in front of peers earlier in the day.

Occasionally, school-age children have sleep problems, most commonly sleepwalking and sleep terrors (night terrors). Both conditions occur during deep sleep. Children with night terrors scream and appear excessively frightened; they may be difficult to console during the episode, but the episode is self-limiting, usually lasting less than 30 minutes. Children who walk in their sleep do not respond to their environment and are in danger of injuring themselves. Episodes of both sleep terrors and sleepwalking are frightening to parents, but the child is unlikely to remember the episode on awakening. The nurse can advise a parent to quietly soothe the child during an episode and protect the child from harm. Episodes may increase when the child is under stress.

CRITICAL THINKING EXERCISE 7-1

Mrs. George states that Megan, 11 years old, has recently started to leave her belongings throughout the house and that her room is always a mess. Mrs. George states that she is frustrated and feels as if she is constantly asking Megan to pick her things up and clean her room.

1. What assumptions might a nurse make on the basis of Mrs. George's report about her daughter's behavior?
2. What other data does the nurse need to clarify to best help Mrs. George and Megan in this situation?
3. What are some possible approaches the nurse might suggest to Mrs. George?

Discipline

Because school-age children possess a strong sense of justice and believe in the importance of rules, they want and expect limits to be set on their behavior. Firm, consistent limits increase children's sense of security and reinforce the message that an adult cares about them. Realistic expectations, clearly defined rules, and logical consequences help children develop self-discipline and increased self-esteem. Some families have meetings where they discuss how responsibilities in the family will be shared. The child is made to feel more a part of the solution rather than the problem.

Responsibility can be developed in children through the use of natural and logical consequences related to actions. Children become accountable for their actions. If a child leaves a toy outside and it is damaged, the parent is empathetic but does not replace the toy. The parent does not get in a power struggle, nor does the parent verbally attack the child. The child begins to understand that there are consequences to actions. This type of discipline, correctly used, will allow the parent to separate the deed from the doer; not pass moral judgment; focus on the present, not the past; and show respect and firm kindness. In addition, the child will be given choices and the consequence will relate to the logic of the situation.

Teachers' disciplinary efforts are often thwarted when parents do not support them or when they show no concern about their children's misbehavior in school. Teamwork between parents and teachers is essential for effective discipline. Regular parent-teacher conferences help make discipline effective.

Safety

Unintentional injury is the leading cause of death in children of every age group. Although the death rate from unintentional injury is lower in children aged 5 to 9 years than it is during early childhood, with the exception of injury from falls, the annual incidence of nonfatal unintentional injury is higher (Rivara & Grossman, 2004).

Approaches to safety education vary as the child grows older. Physically, middle childhood is a period of great activity, with the child moving back and forth between the home environment and the community. The school-age child has less fear when playing and frequently imitates adults by using tools and household items. Children in this age group enjoy helping with adult routines and chores around the home. Anticipatory guidance related to safety is very important as children develop and try new projects that require use of more dangerous or sophisticated equipment.

Safety education is best accomplished by simply stating safety rules and providing reinforcement through short projects and immediate rewards. Role-playing activities and error-detection picture games are excellent ways to reinforce safety lessons. Children in this age group are inquisitive and will frequently ask questions. The answers to their questions should contain concrete rationales. Group projects with safety topics help foster independent thinking while promoting interactions with the child's peer group.

Car Safety

If the child has attained a height of 4 feet 9 inches and is between the ages of 8 and 12 years, the child may be large enough to use the vehicle's three-point restraining system. The child needs to be tall enough that the shoulder belt crosses the middle of the chest and the lap belt rides low onto the thighs (American Academy of Pediatrics [AAP], 2006a). Smaller and younger children can remain in an approved booster seat, which will position the belts properly in relation to the child (AAP, 2006a). Adherence often is determined by family values, with use or nonuse reflecting parental practices. Children should sit in a rear seat away from car passenger safety airbags.

Fire and Burn Safety

Parents should continue to reinforce safety procedures associated with fire safety. Routine fire drills should be practiced in the home. Repetition of family drills helps ensure that the child will respond correctly and automatically to smoke alarms. Children of this age can better comprehend cause-and-effect relationships, so they can understand why they should not play with potentially flammable substances.

School-age children are eager to help parents with daily chores such as cooking or ironing. Parents need to invest the time to teach their children how to use tools and appliances properly and must establish guidelines to avoid burn injuries as a result of the child's inexperience.

Fireworks create another burn hazard for children. Each summer, many children are seriously burned or permanently scarred by fireworks. To prevent serious burn injuries, the federal government, under the federal Hazardous Substance Act, prohibits the sale of the more dangerous fireworks to the general public. However, a degree of risk always is associated with any fireworks. There are no absolutely safe fireworks for children or adults. Fireworks are best left to the experts and viewed from a safe distance. Encourage families to enjoy the many community-sponsored fireworks displays.

CRITICAL TO REMEMBER
Fire Safety Rules

Know two specific escape routes from each area in the home.

Know how to dial 911.

Know how to crawl under the smoke to leave a burning house.

Have a predetermined meeting area outside the house.

Never return to a burning house.

Practice fire drills.

Bicycle, In-Line Skate, Scooter, and Skateboard Safety

Mastering the ability to ride a bicycle is a milestone in a child's life, leading to independence. The bicycle is typically considered a toy but is actually a vehicle that is capable of speedy transportation. Bicycle injuries are the fourth leading cause of nonfatal injury and the fifth leading cause of fatal injury in children 5 to 9 years of age (Centers for Disease Control and Prevention [CDC], 2005). For this reason, the public health community supports the mandatory use of bicycle helmets. Research has demonstrated that the use of a helmet can reduce the incidence of head injury by as much as 88% when it is fitted properly (AAP Committee on Injury and Poison Prevention, 2001).

Bicycle safety practices actually begin when the child is a passenger in a bicycle seat on the back of a parent's bike. They continue as the child learns to ride a tricycle and progressively build as the child becomes more skilled and begins to ride a bicycle. A helmet and other safety accessories are essential for protection, but they are only an adjunct to the child's skill level and knowledge of the rules of the road. A young cyclist is unpredictable and may be preoccupied with managing the bicycle itself. For this reason, parents should set limits on where, when, and how far the child may ride until the child can competently maneuver the bicycle. When parents on bicycles accompany children, it is essential that the parents wear helmets and follow the rules of the road to role model appropriate safety and emphasize the importance of the helmet and the rules. Khambalia and colleagues (2005) demonstrated a high correlation between adult helmet use and child helmet use, emphasizing the importance of modeling helmet behavior.

In-line skating and skateboarding are recreational activities that are popular with school-age children. Balancing, stopping, and turning are challenging and require motor skills similar to those required for bicycling. As the child begins to learn these skills, falls are frequent and protective gear is essential. Helmets and protective pads covering the knees and elbows help protect the most vulnerable areas of the child's body from serious injury. Key educational points and an overview of safety principles are described in Box 7-5.

Unpowered scooters are very lightweight, small versions of an older, more stable type of scooter used by children in the 1950s. They are propelled by one foot and have a very narrow base and small wheels. Because of their portability, both adults and children use them, many times on crowded city sidewalks. Since the introduction of unpowered scooters in the late 1990s, scooter-related injuries have markedly increased and approximately 90% of the visits to emergency rooms for scooter-related injuries were for children (AAP Committee on Injury and Poison Prevention, 2002/2005). Recommendations for safe operation of scooters are similar to those for in-line skating, with the exception of wrist pad use.

Pedestrian Safety

Children between the ages of 5 and 9 years are at the greatest risk for automobile-pedestrian injuries. The tremendous forces of impact and the lack of protection for the pedestrian can lead to severe injury. Children are commonly struck when they dart into traffic, especially where parked cars obscure the driver's view of the child (e.g., crossing the street in front of a school bus, playing near cars in driveways or yards).

Several factors predispose this age group to such injuries. Their smaller physical stature limits their visibility to drivers until too late. In addition, children in this age group have the misconception that if they can see the car, the driver must be able to see them and will be able to stop instantly. Focused on play activities, they often impulsively dart into the street, oblivious to boundaries and potential traffic dangers.

Children learn traffic safety by watching and doing. Exposure to traffic increases as the child begins to walk to and from school and friends' houses. Parents have the responsibility of practicing pedestrian safety hundreds of times before the child is allowed to venture across streets alone.

Water Safety

School-age children learn to swim well enough to keep their heads above water for a short time at about 8 years old. The length of time they can keep their heads above water and their swimming ability increase with age and experience. The incidence of drowning decreases in this age group; however, adult supervision is still needed to prevent a water-related injury. School-age children often overestimate their swimming capabilities and endurance. As their swimming abilities improve, anticipatory guidance can include general swimming safety. Children should be taught to stay away

---

BOX 7-5 | **PARENTS WANT TO KNOW** About Bicycle, In-Line Skating, Scooter, and Skateboard Safety

- Children should always wear a helmet when bike riding, in-line skating, or skateboarding. This safety practice should begin when the child begins to learn these activities.
- Helmets should fit properly and snugly on the head. Helmets need to be lightweight and ventilated and have reflective trim.
- Children should be taught not to ride at dusk or in the dark. They should always call home for a ride if it is after dark.
- Children should not ride two on a bicycle.
- Riding barefoot, in thongs, or in slippers is dangerous. Children need to avoid using audio headsets while riding a bicycle because headsets can diminish hearing capabilities.
- Encourage children to stay on sidewalks, paths, or driveways until they have mastered advanced biking skills and know the rules of the road.
- While riding or in-line skating, children should avoid uneven road surfaces, gravel, potholes, or bumps.
- Bicycles should be equipped with reflectors and lights. With their parents' help, encourage children to routinely inspect their own bicycles to ensure that they are functioning properly (e.g., brakes, tires, lights).
- Proper sizing is important when purchasing a bicycle for a child. Oversized bicycles are responsible for many injuries. The child should be able to place the balls of both feet on the ground when sitting on the seat with the hands on the handlebars.

- The child should be able to straddle the center bar with both feet flat on the ground. There should be about 1 inch of clearance between the crotch and the bar.
- The handlebars should be within easy reach for the child.

Rules of the Road

- Children younger than 8 years old should ride only with adult supervision and not in the street. Limit in-line skating or skateboarding to areas where there is no car traffic.
- Children should not ride bicycles on roads with heavy traffic.
- A bicycle should be ridden on the right side of the road, with the traffic. Bike riders must obey all traffic laws, traffic signs, and lights.
- Children need to learn the appropriate hand signals and use them every time before turning.
- Bicycles should be walked across busy intersections, not ridden.
- Children need to learn to stop, look left, look right, and look left again before entering a street or leaving a driveway, alley, or parking lot.
- Children should stop at all intersections, marked and unmarked.
- Children riding bicycles should obey all stop signs and red lights.
- Children should look back and yield to traffic coming from behind before turning left at intersections.
- Basic bicycle safety rules apply to scooters, in-line skates, and skateboards.

from canals and the fast-moving waters of creeks and rivers. Advise parents to teach children to wade into shallow water or to jump feet first into water of unknown depth to prevent neck injuries. Safety near the water includes never running, pushing, or jumping on others who are in the water.

Selected Issues Related to the School-Age Child

Adjustment to School

Most children are eager to start school, particularly if they have older siblings. They even look forward to bringing home their books and doing "real" homework. This enthusiasm usually fades quickly, however. Most children adjust well to first grade, enjoying the opportunities it provides for peer interaction and stimulating experiences. First grade may be the child's first experience of being away from home. For these children, starting school may be a frightening experience. Even children who have attended preschool have some anxiety about beginning first grade. Adjustment to school depends on a variety of factors, including the child's physical and emotional maturity, the child's experiences, and the parents' ability to support the child and accept the separation (see Chapter 6).

Peer Influence. School is often the first experience a child has with a large number of children of the same age. From peers children learn how to cooperate, compete, bargain, and follow rules. Peer approval is of major importance as children look to their friends for recognition and support. The influence of peers becomes stronger as the child grows older.

Influence of Teachers. Teachers have a significant influence on children's social and intellectual development. An effective teacher makes learning fun and capitalizes on the child's interests and talents. Teachers guide the child's learning by rewarding success and helping the child learn from and deal with failures. The teacher plays an important role in preventing feelings of inferiority in the child. By structuring the learning environment so that the child experiences success, the teacher bolsters feelings of industry.

The student-teacher relationship is a key factor in school success. Effective teachers motivate students by being warm and understanding, showing interest, and communicating at the child's level. Children value the opinion of such teachers and will work to gain their approval. Favorite teachers serve as role models and are often objects of hero worship by their students.

Even excellent teachers cannot do an effective job alone. They need the support of parents and school administrators to maximize children's learning potential.

Parents' Role. Parents play a key role in their children's academic success. By taking an active interest in children's progress and encouraging them to do their best, parents can foster learning. Positive reinforcement should be given for honest efforts, not just good grades. Parents should enforce rules that encourage self-discipline and good study habits (e.g., no television until homework is finished). The child must create and adhere to a schedule for completing large assignments to prevent last-minute panic. If the child does not have a desk or another private place for homework, the kitchen table or another quiet, well-lighted area should be made available during study time. The television should be turned off during study time and distractions kept to a minimum. Adequate sleep is important for school performance. Parents may need to enforce bedtime rules to meet the child's needs. Rewarding children for meeting deadlines and for being organized encourages them to take responsibility for their learning and fosters skills that are important for success in jobs as adults.

Parents need to communicate with teachers and stay informed about their children's progress. Visiting the classroom and attending parent-teacher conferences and school activities are important. Showing respect and support for the teacher facilitates learning.

School Refusal. *School refusal* is a descriptive term for behavior that may indicate the presence of a specific phobia, separation anxiety, truancy, or social phobia (Kearney & Bates, 2005). In the past, the term was used interchangeably with *school phobia* and *school avoidance*. There is much discussion over the diagnosis and treatment of children who refuse to attend school and the appropriate label for these children. School phobia can be distinguished from a separation anxiety disorder in that with school phobia the child does not have distressing symptoms anywhere else but in school. Children with separation anxiety disorder experience distress any time they are separated from their parents, including at school (Varley & Smith, 2003).

School refusal has been defined as frequent absences from school, academic disengagement or disruption, or dropping out (Kearney & Bates, 2005). Some school-refusing children show specific fears of school or school-related situations (tests, bullies, teacher reprimands, undressing for gym). Because some children with school refusal behaviors have intense emotional distress related to school attendance, they are labeled *phobic*. The confusion over the use of these terms can make assessment and treatment of these children difficult. For an additional discussion of separation anxiety, see Chapter 29.

Children may go to school unwillingly or may refuse and have temper tantrums if the parents insist on taking the child to school. Younger children may complain of stomachaches, headaches, nausea, and vomiting. Older children may complain of palpitations and feeling faint. These symptoms typically resolve when the child returns home.

Helping a Child Overcome School Refusal. In uncomplicated cases, the parent needs to return the child to school as soon as possible. If symptoms are severe, a limited period of part-time or modified school attendance may be necessary. For example, part of the day may be spent in the counselor's or school nurse's office, with assignments obtained from the teacher. The child should be gently questioned about factors at school that cause worry or fear. Specific causes, such as a bully or an overly critical teacher, should be dealt with immediately. Parents must support each other because the child may play one parent against the other to avoid school. Parents should be empathetic yet firm and consistent in their insistence that the child attend school. Parents should not pick the child up at school once the child is there. Positive reinforcement for school attendance is essential. Encouraging and maintaining peer contacts and emphasizing the positive aspects of school are helpful. The principal and teacher should be told about the situation so that they can cooperate with the treatment plan. More complicated cases require more in-depth evaluation and referral for the treatment of potential underlying issues.

Self-Care Children

The number of children who let themselves into their homes after school and are left alone continues to grow as the number of dual-income and single-parent families increases. These children are called *self-care children* or *home alone children*, previously referred to as *latch-key children*. Approximately 15% of all children aged 5 to 14 years in the United States care for themselves regularly (6.3 hours a week), and 1% are 5 and 6 years old (Johnson, 2005).

Parents often feel guilty about leaving children alone and may feel concern for their children's safety. Potential positive outcomes of this experience are learning to be independent and responsible. Because of time spent unsupervised at home, the risk of children engaging in problem behaviors (smoking, alcohol use, inappropriate eating) increases. The quality of the parent-child relationship and parents who are emotionally supportive and establish firm rules play a role in moderating adverse effects on the child in self-care.

Nurses can help families by offering support and education to parents and children to reduce the risks for self-care children. Parents need to know how to prepare their children for self-care, teaching them specific strategies for staying safe at home alone. Nurses can serve as child advocates by working to develop expanded after-school childcare programs in the community. A number of communities have established after-school telephone help lines to provide information, support, and assistance to self-care children. Nurses should also know the laws relating to self-care in their state of practice. Some state and local regulations prohibit self-care in young children (American Academy of Child and Adolescent Psychiatry, 2004).

Obesity

When intake of food exceeds expenditure, the excess is stored as fat. Obesity is an excessive accumulation of fat in the body. There is an increase of weight beyond that considered desirable with regard to age, height, and bone structure.

Obesity can be a precursor of hyperlipidemia, sleep apnea, cholelithiasis (gallstones), orthopedic problems, hypertension, and diabetes. In addition, children who are obese can have psychosocial difficulties, eating disorders, and inappropriate expectations because their greater growth makes them appear older than they are (Brown & Kahwati, 2004). Because the obese child develops increased numbers of fat cells, which are carried into adulthood, preventing obesity in childhood can reduce the risk of obesity in adulthood and plays a role in preventing disease.

Cultural, genetic, environmental, and socioeconomic factors have been linked to childhood obesity. Children with low metabolic rates and an increased number of fat cells tend to gain more weight. Children with one or both parents overweight are at increased risk for obesity (Kumanyika & Grier, 2006). It is often very difficult to isolate factors contributing to obesity in a family in which the parents are obese. When a parent lacks nutritional knowledge, it is reflected in the meals and snacks provided in the home. The child is at risk for development of the same habits. Obesity is more prevalent among children raised in urban communities and in smaller families. In addition, obesity varies among different ethnic groups, geographic regions, and socioeconomic classes (Kumanyika & Grier, 2006).

Unstructured meals, "meals on the run," and meals at fast-food restaurants can lack proper nutrition and be high in calories. Lack of exercise also contributes to obesity. Recent studies have shown that, as school-age children get older, they are less likely to be involved in regular physical exercise (CDC, 2005). The child who is given food for reward or punishment attaches more to eating than gaining nutrition. Some people still think that a fat baby is a healthy baby. This type of thinking leads to overfeeding.

Although the child may undergo an initial weight loss, the long-term success rate for the elimination of obesity is poor. Positive outcomes are increased when the child has a support system and understands the importance of diet and exercise.

Assessing the Scope of the Problem. There is no generally accepted definition of obesity. The child who is obese looks overweight. In addition, a body mass index (BMI) greater than the 95th percentile for age or a triceps skinfold measurement above the 95th percentile indicates overweight. Children with BMIs greater than the 85th percentile are at risk for being overweight (CDC, 2004b).

Generally, obesity is caused by increased calorie intake combined with decreased physical activity. The amount of time spent watching television, at a computer, and playing video games takes away from time the child could be participating in active exercise. The possibility of disease as a contributing factor must be evaluated. Increased weight gain has been associated with central nervous system tumors, hypothyroidism, Cushing syndrome, and Turner syndrome.

Prevention. Early identification of risk factors can target the child who needs special attention and support. All children should be taught healthy eating habits and the importance of regular exercise. School- and community-based interventions can, along with regular guidance from health providers, assist with obesity prevention (Brown & Kahwati, 2004).

Interventions and Anticipatory Guidance. Take a dietary history and evaluate the child's eating habits and patterns. The child or parents (or both) should keep a food diary for 1 week. The diary should include the time, place, and type and amount of food eaten and the reason for eating. The general dietary habits of the family should also be assessed.

One of the key elements of successful weight reduction in the child or adolescent is ownership by the child of whatever

BOX 7-6	**PARENTS WANT TO KNOW** About How to Prevent and Manage Obesity

You can help prevent and manage obesity in your child by doing the following:
- Do not use food as a reward.
- Establish consistent times for meals and snacks and do not allow in-between eating.
- Offer only healthy food options (ask the child to choose between an apple or popcorn, not an apple or a cookie). Avoid keeping unhealthy food in the house and minimize trips to fast-food restaurants.

- Be a role model by improving your own eating habits and levels of activity.
- Encourage the child to do fun, physical activities with the family.
- Praise the child for making appropriate food choices and for increasing physical activity levels.

plan is proposed. Care should be taken to avoid a power struggle between the parent and child. Obviously the young child will need more parental involvement than the older child or adolescent. The family should be willing to support the child but should not take on the role of watchdog (Box 7-6).

Caloric requirements vary depending on the age and gender of the child. By changing the obese child's lifestyle to include exercise and nutritional foods in smaller servings, the possibility of success is increased. Teach the family and child how to select and prepare foods that are tasteful and how to restrict serving size. The child's favorite foods should be identified and incorporated whenever possible. Because snacks are an important aspect in childhood nutrition, nutritious snacks should be identified. Involving the whole family will create family behaviors that support the child's new eating and activity behaviors.

The parent needs to limit television and computer game time. Children should be involved in regular physical exercise at school and at home. Children can be encouraged to ride their bicycles or to walk rather than ride in a car to a friend's house to play. Planned physical activities should be part of the child's after-school and weekend routine.

Some older children and adolescents may find success in a support group, such as Weight Watchers or Overeaters Anonymous. Some centers have a special group for children. Other support groups may be associated with schools, summer camps, and children's hospitals in the community.

A team approach is often necessary for successful weight reduction. Psychologic support may be essential for the child and family to be successful. A registered dietitian can provide expertise in the identification and planning of foods not only that are nutritional but also that the child likes.

Stress

Today's children are subjected to stress as no generation has been before. Alarming increases in drug abuse, childhood suicide, child abduction and murder, and school failure attest to the overwhelming stress that children experience. Rapid, bewildering social change and ever-increasing demands for achievement often pressure children to grow up too quickly.

Stressed children may not show serious symptoms during childhood but may develop patterns of emotional response that can lead to serious illness as adults (Box 7-7).

Sources of Stress in Children. Growing up is stressful, even for well-adjusted children with loving, supportive families. Children experience stress from societal change, school, competitive athletics, rushed schedules, and the media.

Middle-class children in particular are pressured to grow up quickly. Achievement-oriented parents, focused on success and financial gain, often view children as extensions of themselves and unwittingly expect too much of their children. Pressure on children to succeed, to win, and to be the best and brightest is great, especially when parents value academic achievement. Children are often pressured into a frenzied schedule of music, dance, sport, and art lessons and may have little time for family meals or playing with friends. Self-esteem and peer relationships often suffer. Ryan-Wenger and colleagues (2005) examined how stressors for children have changed over the past three decades. From 30 years ago, when the majority of stress in children was related to family issues, problems in school or with friends, or concerns about appearance, to the present, stressors have changed to include fear for safety (bullying, inappropriate touch), violence in the world and the child's environment, concerns about homework, worries about family fighting and "too many things to do" (Ryan-Wenger, Sharrer, & Campbell, 2005, p. 288).

BOX 7-7	**Manifestations of Stress in Children**

How children perceive stress influences its effects. It is not just the stress but how the child perceives and responds to the stress that determines whether the child has symptoms of stress.

Intervention is needed when a child shows the following signs of stress:
- Unhappiness, moodiness
- Irritability, increased aggressive behavior
- Fatigue, inability to concentrate
- Hyperactivity
- Changes in eating or sleeping habits
- Physical complaints (nausea, headaches, stomachaches)
- Bed-wetting
- Substance abuse
- Diminished school performance
- Suicidal behavior

HEALTH PROMOTION

THE 9- TO 11-YEAR-OLD CHILD

FOCUSED ASSESSMENT

Ask the child the following:

- Can you tell me how often and what foods you like to eat? How often do you eat at fast-food restaurants? How do you feel about how much you weigh? Do you think you need to gain or lose any weight?
- What types of physical activities do you like to do? How often do you do them? Do you have any quiet hobbies that interest you? How many hours each day do you watch television? What is your favorite television program?
- How often do you brush your teeth, floss, and see the dentist? Do you take fluoride?
- What time do you go to bed at night? What time do you get up in the morning? Do you have any trouble falling asleep or do you wake up in the middle of the night?
- How often do you have a bowel movement? Are there any problems with urination? (Use the child's familiar terminology if known.) Do you wet the bed? If so, how often?
- What grade in school are you? Are you doing well in school or having any problems? Do you feel safe at school? In what before- or after-school programs do you participate?
- Tell me about your friends. Do they like to do the same things you like to do? Do they pressure you to do things you would rather not do? Do you or your friends smoke or take any substances (alcohol, drugs)?
- How do you get along with other members of your family? Is there a special family member you could talk to if you are having a problem? If so, who?
- Do you do any or all of the following: use a seat belt every time you get in a car; wear a helmet every time you ride a bike; wear a helmet and protective pads every time you skate or use a scooter; use sunscreen; swim with a buddy and only when an adult is present; always look both ways before crossing the street; use the right equipment when you play sports; know to avoid strangers and how to call for help if needed?
- Has anyone ever physically harmed you or touched you in a way that made you uncomfortable? Have you ever thought about harming yourself?

Ask the parent the following:

- Are there any concerns related to the child's nutrition, body image, physical activity, oral health, sleep,

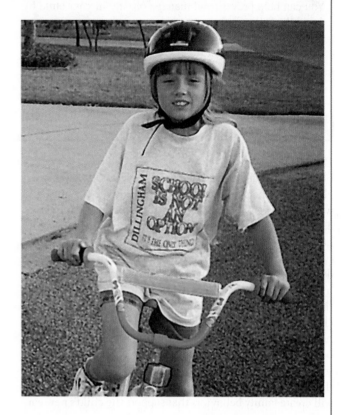

elimination, school, family interactions, self-esteem, and ability to practice safety precautions?
- Is there a gun in the home? If so, is it locked away and the ammunition stored in a separate place?
- Do you have a fire escape plan that you practice regularly?
- What types of information have you given to your child about puberty and sexual activity?
- Do you feel uncomfortable talking with your child about sensitive issues?

DEVELOPMENTAL MILESTONES

Personal/social: peers' opinions become more important than parents'; clubs, with secret codes and rituals, are at a peak; hero worship; fairly responsible, dependable, and polite to adults; boys tease girls, and girls may become "boy crazy"; may become angry but is learning to control it; critical of own work; rebelliousness may begin; ready for away-from-home experiences, such as camp

---

Economically deprived children must cope with an even greater burden of stress. Faced with the dangers of violence, drug and alcohol addiction, and gangs, these children must fight daily for survival. Children from lower-income families travel dangerous streets to and from school and suffer from the insecurity and uncertainty of poverty. Children who are homeless—as is increasingly common—have the added stress of living on the street or in shelters and having decreased access to appropriate nutritional, health, and educational resources. Both homeless and low-income children have significant adversity in their lives, with homeless children having increased stress (Culbertson, Newman, & Willis, 2003).

School Pressures. School can be a source of stress for children. Some children are unable to cope with the competitive, test-regulated curricula of school. They find it difficult to keep up with the unrelenting academic pressure. School

---

HEALTH PROMOTION

THE 9- TO 11-YEAR-OLD CHILD—cont'd

DEVELOPMENTAL MILESTONES—cont'd

Fine motor: hand-eye coordination fully developed; fine motor control approximates adults'

Language/cognitive: reads more and enjoys comics and newspapers; understands fractions, conservation of volume and weight; likes to talk on the telephone; interested in how things work

Gross motor: may begin to be more awkward as growth spurt begins; may drop out of team sports to avoid embarrassment

HEALTH MAINTENANCE

Physical Measurements

Girls are 2.54 cm (1 inch) taller and 0.9 kg (2 lb) heavier on average than boys

About 90% of facial growth has been attained

Boys have greater physical strength

Girls may have rapid growth spurt and menarche

Immunizations

Review immunization records

Administer immunizations if not up to date; some children may need measles, mumps, rubella (MMR) #2; varicella; hepatitis B series; tetanus and diphtheria (Td) if more than 5 years since last dose. Give tetanus, diphtheria, acellular pertussis (Tdap) if child is 11 years old and has had the primary diphtheria, tetanus, pertussis series

Health Screening

Objective hearing and vision screening (may become myopic as growth spurt begins)

Hemoglobin or hematocrit

Urine for sugar and protein

Blood pressure

Baseline lipid screen

Tuberculosis screening if at risk (see Chapter 21)

Scoliosis screening

ANTICIPATORY GUIDANCE

Provide health teaching to the child and the parent

Nutrition

Follow recommended servings according to the dietary guidelines; teach the child how to keep track of servings and to give input into meal preparation

Advise to avoid fast foods and to eat a nutritious breakfast

Watch calcium and iron intake

Assess adequacy of diet and snacks

Elimination

Regular bowel movements according to the child's pattern

Dental

Provide regular dental care every 6 months

Continue regular brushing with fluoride toothpaste and flossing

Continue fluoride supplements if water is not fluoridated

May need dental sealants as permanent molars erupt

May need referral to orthodontist for malocclusion

Sleep

Facilitate an individually appropriate sleep pattern; school-age children usually go to bed by 9 PM and are up by 7 AM

If the child is not tired, advise the parent to allow a quiet reading time in bed

Hygiene

May resist baths and showers, may wear the same clothes every day, bedroom is usually messy

Early reluctance to keep clean may be followed by a period of overcleanliness (multiple showers daily, new outfit after each shower)

Safety

Review gun safety; bicycle, skating, and scooter safety; playground safety; fire safety; automobile and pedestrian safety; water safety; sun protection; exposure to outside allergens and ticks; sports safety; use of reflective clothing if out at night

Continue to have child belted in the back seat of the car away from airbags

Discuss not allowing others into the home if parent is not there; how to contact emergency services; not to open doors to strangers; avoiding listening to loud music through earphones

Play

Encourage reading age-appropriate fiction, developing collections, playing complicated board and card games, crafts, electronic and science-related games

Advise limiting television watching to no more than 2 hours a day

Self-Esteem and Competence

See Box 7-4

---

imposes long-term stress on these children, and they tend to dislike school and stay home whenever they can. They are often tardy and may abuse alcohol and drugs. Eventually, they may drop out of school. These children rarely return to complete their education.

Other children, particularly those who are academically gifted, find school stressful because it is tedious. Boredom can be stressful. Meaningless, repetitive schoolwork can cause

bright, talented children to become chronically fatigued, inattentive, and careless.

Physical Threats. Children also face other types of stress at school. Violence and theft in schools are national problems. School-age children commonly voice fears of being beaten up or held up. The child who leaves a bike unlocked or a watch or jacket unattended quickly learns the hazards of such carelessness. Students who abuse drugs or participate in gang activity create a pervasive attitude of wariness and fear and are a real source of stress for children.

Competitive Sports. Participation in competitive sports is stressful for some children. Fear of failure, especially in front of a cheering crowd, can be overwhelming. Some parents contribute to competitive stress by overemphasizing the importance of winning. Because of their own needs or interests, some parents push their children to participate in organized sports at an early age (Fig. 7-2).

Tight Schedules and Adaptation Overload. As the number of single parents and working mothers increases, so does the stress on children who must adapt to parents' work schedules. Many children are rushed from home to school to carpool to day care or a babysitter. Children must draw on their energy reserves to exercise self-control in these varying situations and may not be able to cope. Fatigue and exhaustion from such demands often result in behavioral problems and regression.

Family Pressures. In today's mobile society it is not unusual for families to move and for children to have to leave other family members and friends. Attending a new school, making new friends, and losing former support systems can be very stressful for children. This happens at a time when one or both parents are also making major adjustments in their lives, and they may not have the time and energy to meet all of the child's needs.

Overhearing parents quarrel produces anxiety and fear in children and erodes a child's sense of security. Some parents, although physically present, may be emotionally unavailable to children because of their own stresses. Divorce and separation are especially painful. Changes frequently caused by divorce, such as moving to a new house, attending a new school, and, usually the most stressful of all, separation from one of the parents, can cause great stress for children.

Media Influence. The media are a common source of stress for today's children. Sexual and violent material portraying loss of control may frighten children because it suggests that they may not be able to master their own sexual and aggressive impulses. Television exposes children to vivid portrayals of the problems of today's society for many hours

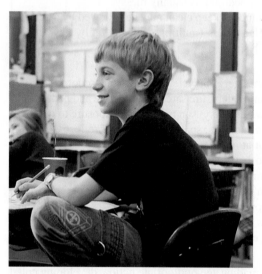

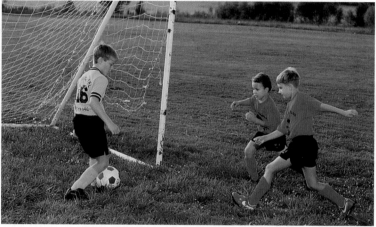

Attention span increases during the school-age years, facilitating classroom learning.

The nurse is in an excellent position to help parents and children identify factors that produce stress and to suggest ways to cope with its effects. Participation in competitive sports is stressful for some children, especially if parents push their child to play organized sports at an early age or overemphasize the importance of winning. Focusing on having fun and on the excitement of the game decrease competitive stress.

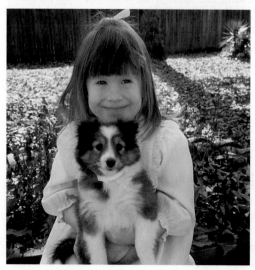

Spending time playing with and caring for pets can be fun and relaxing. Children who are given time and encouragement to play are better able to deal with the stresses of life.

FIG 7-2   **Health promotion for the school-age child and family.**

of their day. It also tends to isolate children from their parents and peers. Hours spent watching television can limit children's participation in more creative play and contact and interaction with others.

Interventions and Anticipatory Guidance. The nurse is in an ideal position to help parents and children identify factors that produce stress and to suggest ways to cope with its effects. Parents can meet basic psychologic needs, influence self-esteem, shape values, control exposure to stressful events, and provide support. Parents may need guidance about realistic expectations from their children. Parents should watch for behavior changes in their children that may indicate signs of stress and offer appropriate reassurance. If significant tension is in the home, parents can try to resolve conflicts by negotiating rather than continuing to build an emotionally charged atmosphere. Parents should examine the child's schedule to make sure the child is not overburdened with school and extracurricular activities.

CRITICAL TO REMEMBER
Sources of Stress for School-Age Children
- Societal change
- School
- Competitive sports
- Tight schedules
- Family pressures
- Influence of the media
- Fear of violence
- Chaotic living conditions

Close communication with teachers is important to prevent and deal with school-related stress. Becoming interested in and involved with the child's schoolwork conveys support and caring. Parents need to become active in parent-teacher associations and other community organizations to find solutions to the problems of violence and crime in the schools.

Children should be allowed to decide whether to participate in competitive athletics. It is important for parents to talk to coaches to determine what is expected of their children. Corrective instruction rather than punishment should be given for errors. Parents should serve as role models for good sportsmanship.

Limiting the number of hours that children watch television and helping them select appropriate programs can decrease its negative effects. Watching television with children and discussing the content of programs are also helpful.

Children need to have time just to play. Parents should recognize that play is the child's work. Whether it is shooting baskets in the driveway, working on a collection, or building a model, play reduces stress for children. Toys and games that provide the greatest opportunity to use imagination are the best stress relievers. Most children love animals. Spending time playing with and caring for pets can be relaxing and

fun. Children who are given the time and encouragement to play are better able to deal with the stresses of life (see Chapter 4).

One of the most effective antidotes for childhood stress is a loving, attentive parent who takes the time to listen. A sympathetic adult who understands the stresses of childhood can offer valuable support. Discussion and modeling of ways to deal with the inevitable stresses of life can teach the child valuable lessons for living in today's society.

KEY CONCEPTS

- Slow, steady physical growth and rapid social and cognitive development characterize the school-age period, from 6 to 12 years. Average weight gain in the school-age child is 2.5 kg (5½ lb) per year, and the increase in height is approximately 5.5 cm (2 inches) per year. During the early school-age period, boys are approximately 2.54 cm (1 inch) taller and 0.9 kg (2 lb) heavier than girls.
- During the school-age years, children gradually move away from home and parents as a primary source of support and they enter the wider world of peers and school.
- Physical changes include increased height and weight, increased muscle mass, maturation of body systems, and increased antibody production. During the school-age period, all 20 primary teeth are lost and are replaced by 28 of the 32 permanent teeth.
- The age at onset of puberty varies widely, but puberty is occurring at an earlier age than in the past. On average, African American girls enter puberty approximately 1 year earlier than white girls.
- School-age children enjoy a variety of activities. Cooperative play and team sports are typical of this age group.
- According to Erikson, the developmental task of this period is the development of a sense of industry.
- The child develops a conscience and internalizes cultural and social values. The child is able to understand and obey rules.
- Thinking becomes less egocentric as children learn to consider viewpoints different from their own. School-age children can solve problems, form hypotheses, and make judgments based on reason.
- School-age children experience an increase in appetite, and older school-age children have increased energy needs as they approach puberty.
- Sources of stress for school-age children include societal change, school, competitive athletics, rushed schedules, fear of violence from gangs or bullies, chaotic living conditions if homeless, and the media. Teaching children coping strategies can reduce the effects of stress.
- Dental care is increasingly important as the primary teeth are replaced by permanent teeth.
- Safety issues are related to the child moving more from the home environment to the community, less fear when playing, and the increased use of tools and household items.

1. The nurse might assume that Mrs. George is inconsistent in her expectations. Consequences may not be associated with Megan's behavior. Mrs. George is engaging in a power struggle with Megan. Mrs. George's expectations of a clean room may differ from Megan's.

2. The nurse can begin to gather data by asking Mrs. George to describe a typical day when she feels upset with Megan's behavior. The nurse can further ask, "What is your response to her behavior?" On the basis of Mrs. George's response, the nurse can determine how the mother is reacting to Megan's behavior and begin to develop strategies. The nurse can determine whether Mrs. George has an emotional response to the situation and reacts or whether she remains focused and has a plan of action.

3. Some children respond to family meetings where they are involved in the decision making related to the goals of the household. After the family agrees on a solution, there must be consequences to not following the plan. The family might discuss putting items left in a public area into a holding box for a time. Or, if Megan does not pick up her room and dirty clothes do not make it to the hamper, her clothes will not be washed. Consistency and consequences are the foundation for making such a plan work. This is one way to develop a responsible child.

REFERENCES AND READINGS

American Academy of Child and Adolescent Psychiatry. (2004). *Home alone children.* Retrieved April 5, 2006, from *www.aacap.org.*

American Academy of Nursing Child and Family Expert Panel. (2005). Health care quality and outcome guidelines for nursing of children and families: From the AAN Expert Panel on Children and Families. *Pediatric Nursing, 31,* 149-150.

American Academy of Pediatrics. (2006a). *Car safety seats: A guide for families 2006.* Retrieved April 14, 2006, from *www.aap.org/family/carseatguide.htm.*

American Academy of Pediatrics. (2006b). Dietary recommendations for children and adolescents: A guide for practitioners [Electronic version]. *Pediatrics, 117,* 544-559.

American Academy of Pediatrics Committee on Injury and Poison Prevention. (2001). Bicycle helmets. *Pediatrics, 108,* 1030-1032.

American Academy of Pediatrics Committee on Injury and Poison Prevention. (2002/2005). Skateboard and scooter injuries. *Pediatrics, 109,* 542-543.

American Dental Association. (2005). *Mouthguards.* Retrieved April 5, 2006, from *www.ada.org/public/topics/mpouthguards_faq.asp.*

American Heart Association. (2006). *Dietary guidelines for healthy children.* Retrieved March 30, 2006, from *www.americanheart.org.*

Brown, A., & Kahwati, C. (2004). Prevention of overweight in children and adolescents. *American Family Physician, 69,* 2591. Retrieved April 9, 2006, from Gale Group database.

Centers for Disease Control and Prevention. (2004a). Surveillance for fatal and nonfatal injuries—United States, 2001. *MMWR, 53,* 1-57.

Centers for Disease Control and Prevention. (2004b). Prevalence of overweight among children and adolescents: United States 2000. Retrieved April 5, 2006, from *www.cdc.gov.*

Centers for Disease Control and Prevention. (2005). *Physical activity and the health of young people.* Retrieved March 30, 2006, from *www.cdc.gov.*

Centers for Disease Control and Prevention. (2006). *2006 Childhood and adolescent immunization schedule.* Retrieved April 15, 2006, from *www.cdc.gov.*

Culbertson, J., Newman, J., & Willis, D. (2003). Childhood and adolescent psychologic development. *Pediatric Clinics of North America, 50,* 741-764.

Erikson, E. (1963). *Childhood and society* (2nd ed.). New York, NY: Norton.

Guilleminault, C., Palombini, L., & Chervin, R. (2003). Sleepwalking and sleep terrors in prepubertal children: What triggers them? *Pediatrics, 111,* e17-e25.

Herman-Giddens, M., Kaplowitz, P., & Wasserman, R. (2004). Navigating the recent articles on girls' puberty in pediatrics: What do we know and where do we go from here? *Pediatrics, 113,* 911-917.

Hodges, E. (2003). A primer on early childhood obesity and parental influence. *Pediatric Nursing, 29,* 13-17.

Johnson, J. (2005). *Who's minding the kids? Child care arrangements: Winter, 2002.* Retrieved April 5, 2006, from *www.sipp.census.gov/sipp/p.70s/p70-101pdf.*

Kearney, C., & Bates, M. (2005). Addressing school refusal behavior: Suggestions for frontline professionals. *Children and Schools, 27,* 207-216.

Khambalia, A., MacArthur, C., & Perkins, P. (2005). Peer and adult companion helmet use in association with bicycle helmet use by children. *Pediatrics, 116,* 939-942.

Kohlberg, L. (1964). Development of moral character. In M. Hoffman & L. Hoffman (Eds.). *Review of child development research* (Vol.1). New York: Russell Sage Foundation.

Kumanyika, S., & Grier, S. (2006). Targeting interventions for ethnic minority and low-income populations (rates of childhood obesity). *Future of Children, 16,* 18-39.

Larsen, M., & Tentis, E. (2003). The art and science of disciplining children. *Pediatric Clinics of North America, 50,* 817-840.

National Center for Health Statistics. (2005). Prevalence of overweight among children and adolescents: United States 2003-2004. Retrieved April 15, 2006, from *www.cdc.gov/nchs.*

National Mental Health Association. (2005). *Back to school. Bullying and what to do about it.* Retrieved December 29, 2005, from *www.nmha.org.*

Piaget, J. (1962). *Play, dreams, and imitation in childhood* (C. Gattegno & F. M. Hodgson, Trans.). New York, NY: Norton.

Pratt, H., Patel, D., & Greydanus, D. (2003). Behavioral aspects of children's sports. *Pediatric Clinics of North America, 50,* 879-899.

Rivara, F., & Grossman, D. (2004). Injury control. In R. Behrman, R. Kliegman, & H. Jenson (Eds.). *Nelson textbook of pediatrics* (17th ed., pp. 256-263). Philadelphia: WB Saunders.

Ryan-Wenger, N., Sharrer, V., & Campbell, K. (2005). Changes in children's stressors over the past 30 years. *Pediatric Nursing, 31,* 282-291.

Stevenson, M., Rimajova, M., Edgecombe, D., & Vickery, K. (2003). Childhood drowning: Barriers surrounding private swimming pools. *Pediatrics, 111,* e115-e119.

Taxis, J., Rew, L., Jackson, K., & Koozekanani, K. (2004). Protective resources and perceptions of stress in a multi-ethnic sample of school-age children. *Pediatric Nursing, 30,* 477-487.

U.S. Department of Agriculture. (2005). *Dietary guidelines for Americans, 2005.* Retrieved March 30, 2006, from *www.health.gov/dietaryguidelines/dga2005/document.html.*

Varley, C., & Smith, C. (2003). Anxiety disorders in the child and teen. *Pediatric Clinics of North America, 50,* 1107-1138.

Whitlock, E., Williams, S., Gold, R., Smith, R., & Shipman, S. (2005). Screening and interventions for childhood overweight: A summary of evidence for the U.S. Preventive Services Task Force. *Pediatrics, 116,* e125-e144.

CHAPTER 8

Health Promotion for the Adolescent

Learning Objectives

After studying this chapter, you should be able to:

- Describe the adolescent's normal growth and development.
- Identify the sexual maturity rating and Tanner stages and recognize deviations from normal.
- Describe the developmental tasks of adolescence.
- Describe the concept of identity formation in relation to adolescent psychosocial development.
- Describe appropriate health-promoting behaviors for adolescents and young adults.
- Provide anticipatory guidance for adolescents and their families regarding risk-taking behaviors, nutrition, and safety.
- Discuss the prevalence of adolescent violence and strategies to deal with aggressive behavior.
- Discuss adolescent sexuality and related health risks

Definitions

adolescence Period between the onset of puberty and the cessation of physical growth; the passage from childhood to adulthood.

autonomy Independent will and the capacity to be self-governing.

egocentrism Concern with oneself; the lack of differentiation between one's own views and those of others.

identity formation The acquisition of psychosocial, sexual, and vocational identity.

primary sexual characteristics Internal and external reproductive organs in males and females (i.e., uterus, fallopian tubes, ovaries, vagina, vulva, penis, testes, spermatic cord).

puberty Period of time during which adolescents experience a growth spurt, develop secondary sexual characteristics, and achieve reproductive maturity.

pubescence Period of time before sexual maturity, characterized by the development of breast tissue and pubic hair in girls and genital growth and pubic hair in boys.

reproductive maturity The establishment of menstruation and ovulation in females and the development of spermatogenesis in males.

risk-taking behaviors Behaviors that predispose the adolescent to physical or psychosocial harm.

secondary sexual characteristics Physical characteristics of males and females influenced by reproductive hormones but having no direct role in reproduction (i.e., voice, body shape, pubic hair distribution, breasts).

sexual maturity rating Stages of sexual maturation based on pubic hair and breast development in girls and pubic hair and genital development in boys.

Electronic Resources

Additional information related to the content in Chapter 8 can be found on:

the interactive companion CD-ROM

- Audio Glossary
- NCLEX Review Questions
- Pediatric Assessment Video Clips

or the companion website at **evolve**
http://evolve.elsevier.com/james/ncoc

- NCLEX Review Questions
- Pediatric Assessment Video Clips
- WebLinks

Adolescence spans ages 11 to 21 years although the developmental tasks of early adolescence, as well as the beginning stages of sexual maturation, may overlap with the school-age years. Adolescence is a time of change for teenagers and their families, a transition from childhood to adulthood. During this transition period, dramatic physical, cognitive, psychosocial, and psychosexual changes take place that are exciting and, at the same time, frightening.

Healthy People 2010 (U.S. Department of Health and Human Services [USDHHS], 2000) objectives address many areas of adolescent health (Box 8-1). These areas include access to comprehensive health care and education about, and practice of, appropriate reproductive health practices, violence reduction, and decrease in risk factors.

ADOLESCENT GROWTH AND DEVELOPMENT

The adolescent tries out many new roles during this time as part of the important developmental task of identity formation. The peer group is of the utmost importance as adolescents experiment with new roles outside the confines of the family unit. When identity formation is complete, the young adult is emancipated from the family and establishes independence.

The rapid rate of physical growth during adolescence is second only to that of infancy. Adolescents come in many shapes and sizes, and the changes that take place during the teen years are obvious and dramatic. With physical changes come the development of secondary sexual characteristics and an intense interest in romantic relationships. In general, adolescents move from the same-sex friendships of childhood to the capacity for intimate, long-lasting relationships

as young adults. Sexual orientation and gender identity are often recognized during adolescence as the teenager engages in exploration and self-discovery.

Both parents and adolescents need the nurse's support and guidance in understanding and facilitating health-promoting behaviors. Nurses can assist adolescents and their families in the areas of health promotion, disease prevention, and management of common problems by using effective communication strategies, knowledge of normal growth and development, anticipatory guidance, and early identification of potential problems.

Physical Growth and Development

Physical development during the adolescent years is characterized by dramatic changes in size and appearance. Girls experience budding of the breasts followed by the appearance of pubic hair. Approximately 1 year after breast development, height increases rapidly. Growth in height in girls typically ceases 2 to 2½ years after menarche.

Boys also experience physical changes, but those changes are not as obvious as in girls. Boys first experience testicular

---

BOX 8-1	*Healthy People 2010* Objectives for Adolescents

3-9a	Increase the proportion of adolescents in grades 9 through 12 who follow protective measures that may reduce the risk of skin cancer.	14-27	Increase routine vaccination coverage levels of adolescents.
7-1	Increase high school completion.	15-32	Reduce homicides.
7-2	Increase the proportion of middle, junior high, and senior high schools that provide comprehensive school health education to prevent health problems in the following areas: unintentional injury, violence, suicide, tobacco use and addiction, alcohol or other drug use, unintended pregnancy, human immunodeficiency virus/acquired immunodeficiency syndrome (HIV/AIDS) and STD infection, unhealthy dietary patterns, inadequate physical activity, and environmental health.	15-38	Reduce physical fighting among adolescents.
		15-39	Reduce weapon carrying by adolescents on school property.
		18-2	Reduce the rate of suicide attempts by adolescents.
		19-12	Reduce iron deficiency among young children and females of childbearing age.
		22-6, 7	Increase the proportion of adolescents who engage in moderate physical activity for at least 30 minutes on 5 or more of the previous 7 days and vigorous physical activity that promotes cardiorespiratory fitness 3 or more days per week for 20 or more minutes per occasion.
9-7	Reduce pregnancies among adolescent females.		
9-8	Increase the proportion of adolescents who have never engaged in sexual intercourse before age 15 years.	25-1	Reduce the proportion of adolescents and young adults with *Chlamydia trachomatis* infections.
9-9	Increase the proportion of adolescents who have never engaged in sexual intercourse.	26-6	Reduce the proportion of adolescents who report that they rode, during the previous 30 days, with a driver who had been drinking alcohol.
9-10	Increase the proportion of sexually active, unmarried adolescents age 15 to 17 years who use contraception that both effectively prevents pregnancy and provides barrier protection against disease.	26-9	Increase the age and proportion of adolescents who remain alcohol and drug free.
		26-14	Reduce steroid use among adolescents.
9-11	Increase the proportion of young adults who have received formal instruction before turning age 18 years on reproductive health issues, including all the following topics: birth control methods, safer sex to prevent HIV, prevention of STDs, and abstinence.	26-15	Reduce the proportion of adolescents who use inhalants.
		26-16	Increase the proportion of adolescents who disapprove of substance abuse.
		27-2	Reduce tobacco use by adolescents.
13-1, 5	Reduce AIDS and the number of HIV infections among adolescents and adults.	27-17	Increase adolescents' disapproval of smoking.

Modified from U.S. Department of Health and Human Services. (2000). *Healthy People 2010*. Washington, DC: Author.

enlargement, followed in approximately 1 year by penile enlargement. Pubic hair usually precedes the growth of the penis. The growth spurt in boys occurs later than it does in girls, beginning between ages 10½ and 16 years and ending between 13½ and 17½ years. Growth does continue at a much slower pace for several years after the spurt but usually ceases between 18 and 20 years of age.

Muscle mass increases in boys, and fat deposits increase in girls. Because of greater muscle mass, fully developed adolescent boys tend to be larger and stronger than adolescent girls.

Psychosexual Development, Hormonal Changes, and Sexual Maturation

The physical development, hormonal changes, and sexual maturation that occur during adolescence correspond to Freud's final stage of psychosexual development, the genital stage (see Chapter 4). The genital stage begins with the production of sex hormones and maturation of the reproductive system. Sexual tension and energy are manifested in the development of sexual relationships with others, and sexual gratification is sought. Freud's theory suggests that personality development is closely related to psychosexual development, with an emphasis on aggressive and sexual impulses as determining factors of personality. Freud's theories about male dominance, sexual repression, and the Oedipus and Electra complexes make the psychosexual theory of development highly controversial even today.

Girls generally reach physical maturation before boys with the onset and establishment of menstruation (menarche). Menarche usually occurs between the ages of 9 and 15 years (average, 12.43 years) (Chumlea et al, 2003) with some girls maturing normally as young as 8 years (Midyett, Moore, & Jacobson, 2003). Studies suggest that African-American girls experience menarche slightly earlier (approximately 1 year) than whites (Herman-Giddens, Kaplowitz, & Wasserman, 2004). Over the past 25 years in the United States, the age of menarche has decreased and general body mass index has increased; population weight gain appears to be related to timing of maturity in girls (Anderson, Dallal, & Must, 2003). Most young women achieve reproductive maturity 2 to 5 years after the start of menstruation. During the 2 to 5 years before reproductive maturity, the female sex hormones gradually increase, ovulation occurs more frequently, and menstrual periods become more regular.

Ultimately, diet, exercise, and hereditary factors influence adolescents' height, weight, and body build. The earlier onset of puberty has implications for the timing of sex education programs and anticipatory guidance.

The physical growth of boys and girls is directly related to sexual maturation and occurs in a relatively predictable sequence. The secretion of sex hormones—estrogen in girls and testosterone in boys—stimulates the development of breast tissue, pubic hair, and genitalia. Hormonal secretion at the time of puberty is the result of a complex regulatory process among the environment, the central nervous system, the hypothalamus, the pituitary gland, the gonads, and the

adrenal glands. Puberty is a biologic process that brings about the period of peak height velocity (PHV), or the "growth spurt," the changes in body composition, and the development of primary and secondary sexual characteristics in both sexes. Although variable in both sexes, the PHV occurs at approximately age 12 years in girls and age 13½ years in boys. Table 8-1 describes five distinct stages in a *sexual maturity rating* (SMR) based on breast and pubic hair development in girls and genital and pubic hair development in boys and includes approximate age ranges for early, middle, and late puberty (Tanner, 1962). The beginning Tanner stages frequently occur in the school-age child, and Tanner stages 3 to 5 occur in adolescence.

CRITICAL TO REMEMBER
Understanding Tanner Staging

Knowledge of Tanner staging is essential for nurses to assess normal growth and development and provide adolescents and their parents with anticipatory guidance regarding sexual development. Nurses must remember, however, that sexual maturation and physical development are *highly variable* and that Tanner stages may overlap one another. A description of the adolescent's SMR provides greater information about the child's physical development than does chronologic age (age in years).

In boys, puberty is considered delayed if testicular enlargement or pubic hair development has not occurred by the age of 14 years. Absence of breast budding or pubic hair development in girls by 13 years is reason for referral. Some of the more common causes of delayed puberty are chronic illnesses, malnutrition, extreme exercise, and hypothyroidism.

Female Sexual Maturation

Sexual maturation in girls begins with the appearance of breast buds (*thelarche*), which is the first sign of ovarian function. Thelarche occurs at approximately age 9 to 11 years and is followed by the growth of pubic hair. The PHV is reached during thelarche, usually in Tanner stage 2 or 3. Linear growth slows, and menarche begins approximately 1 year after the PHV. As pubic hair increases in amount and becomes dark, coarse, and curly, axillary hair develops and the apocrine sweat glands reach secretory capacity in Tanner stage 3 or 4. Frequent showers and deodorants become important to the adolescent. With increasing hormonal activity, girls develop a more adult body contour by age 14 to 15 years. As breasts mature, the nipples project more and the pubic hair extends to the medial thighs; the young female is estimated to be at Tanner stage 5. Ovulation may be established, and conception can occur.

Male Sexual Maturation

The first sign of pubertal changes in boys is testicular enlargement in response to testosterone secretion, which usually occurs in Tanner stage 2. Slight pubic hair is present and the smooth skin texture of the scrotum is somewhat altered. As

TABLE 8-1   SMR: Tanner Stages of Adolescent Sexual Development

Boys

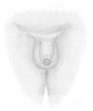 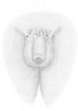 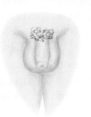 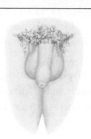 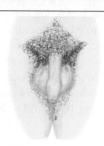

Stage 1	**Stage 2**	**Stage 3**	**Stage 4**	**Stage 5**
Pubic hair: none Penis: preadolescent Testes: preadolescent	Pubic hair: slight, long, straight, slightly pigmented at the base of the penis Penis: slight enlargement Testes: enlarged scrotum, pink, slight alteration in texture	Pubic hair: darker in color, starts to curl, small amount Penis: longer Testes: larger	Pubic hair: coarse, curly, similar to adult but less quantity Penis: larger, glans and breadth increase in size Testes: larger, scrotum darker	Pubic hair: adult distribution spread to inner thighs Penis: adult in size and shape Testes: adult

Early puberty: Testes, 9½-13½ yr; penis, 10½-14½ yr; pubic hair, 12-12½ yr

Middle puberty: Testes, 13½-14½ yr; penis, 13½-15 yr; pubic hair, 12½-14½ yr

Late puberty: Testes, 13½-17 yr; penis, 13½-16 yr; pubic hair, 13½-16½ yr

Breast Development In Girls*

 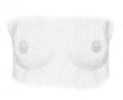 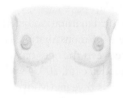 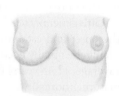

Stage 1	**Stage 2**	**Stage 3**	**Stage 4**	**Stage 5**
Preadolescent	Breast bud stage (thelarche): breast and papilla elevated as small mound, areolar diameter increased	Breast and areola enlarged, no contour separation	Areola and papilla form secondary mound	Mature, nipple projects, areola part of general breast contour

Early puberty: 9-13 yr

Middle puberty: 12-13 yr

Late puberty: 14-17 yr*

*Breast and pubic hair development may continue into late adolescence and increase with pregnancy.
Modified from Tanner, J. M. (1962). *Growth at adolescence* (2nd ed.). Oxford: Blackwell Scientific Publications; Marshall, W. A. & Tanner, J. (1969). Variations in pattern of pubertal changes in girls. *Archives of Disease in Childhood, 44*(235), 291-303. Modified with permission from Blackwell Scientific Publications and The BMJ Publishing Group.

TABLE 8-1	SMR: Tanner Stages of Adolescent Sexual Development—cont'd

Pubic Hair Development in Girls

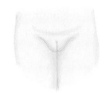 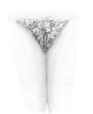 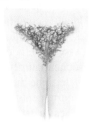

Stage 1	Stage 2	Stage 3	Stage 4	Stage 5
Preadolescent (none)	Sparse, lightly pigmented, straight medial border of labia	Darker, coarser, beginning to curl, increased over pubis	Coarse, curly, less in amount than adult, typical female triangle	Adult female triangle, adult quantity spread to medial surface of thighs

Early puberty: 10-11½ yr

Middle puberty: 11½-13 yr

Late puberty: 14½-16½ yr

testosterone secretion increases, the penis, testes, and scrotum enlarge. The PHV usually occurs during Tanner stages 3 and 4, and the voice deepens and "cracks" as the cartilage in the larynx enlarges. Axillary hair develops, and the eccrine and apocrine sweat glands respond to stressful or emotional stimuli. Skin surface bacteria metabolize secretions from the apocrine glands, and body odor develops. Gynecomastia (male breast enlargement) occurs in approximately two thirds of young males during early adolescence and may be unilateral or bilateral (Rapaport, 2004). This phenomenon is often disturbing to boys, and they need considerable reassurance that the breast tissue will decrease over time. During Tanner stages 4 and 5, increasing levels of testosterone cause sebaceous glands to enlarge and excessive sebum may result in acne. The voice continues to deepen, facial hair appears at the corners of the upper lip and chin, and ejaculation may occur. Nurses need to provide anticipatory guidance to adolescent boys regarding involuntary nocturnal emissions of seminal fluid ("wet dreams") and assure them that this occurrence is normal. By Tanner stage 5, genital maturation is complete, spermatogenesis is well established, facial hair is present on the sides of the face, and the male physique is adultlike in appearance. Gynecomastia significantly decreases or disappears, much to the adolescent male's relief.

Motor Development

Adolescents often engage in various forms of motor activity, from aerobic exercise to football. Motor activities such as sports and dancing provide an outlet for the adolescent's energy as well as an opportunity for competition, teamwork, and social relationships. Large muscle mass increases in adolescents, and coordination of gross and fine muscle groups improves. With practice, adolescents become more adept at athletics and also at art, music, sewing, and other activities that require fine motor skills. The bones are not completely

calcified until after puberty and are still fairly resistant to breaks in the young adolescent. Participants in sports activities should be grouped according to their size and their SMR rather than their chronologic age. A small, thin, late-maturing boy is less capable of competing with an early-maturing, muscular classmate, and injuries are more likely to occur.

Nurses, particularly school nurses, may be helpful in assessing adolescents' growth and development and counseling them about sports activities in which they can succeed rather than those in which they will meet with physical and psychologic failure. Adolescents should have a yearly physical examination if participating in high school athletics (Box 8-2); the school nurse keeps documentation of this. Because it is generally superficial, the school sports examination should not substitute for the recommended complete adolescent physical examination with counseling.

The development of the cardiovascular pump plays an essential role in the adolescent's participation in gross motor activities. Cardiopulmonary capacity increases during adolescence and is relatively mature in the late adolescent. The cardiovascular pump is not as efficient in young adolescents, whose lungs are smaller. Adolescents generally cannot run as fast or as long as young adults. The athlete's aerobic power, body composition, joint flexibility, and strength of skeletal muscles determine physical fitness.

CRITICAL TO REMEMBER
The Adolescent Who Is Involved in Athletics

Adolescents participating in athletics need the following:
- Adequate equipment
- Appropriate training schedules
- Frequent rest periods
- Adequate fluids to prevent injury, dehydration, and exhaustion

BOX 8-2	**Nursing Goals for Preparticipation Sports Physical Examination**

- Assess the adolescent athlete's general health.
- Identify conditions that could limit participation or predispose to injury.
- Assess the adolescent athlete's physical and psychosocial maturity.
- Determine the athlete's fitness relative to performance requirements.
- Assess legal insurance requirements for participation.
- Provide wellness counseling and anticipatory guidance.

Cognitive Development

Cognitive development influences every aspect of adolescent psychosocial development. Cognition moves from concrete to abstract thinking during the three phases of adolescent development. According to Piaget (1969), formal operations, or abstract thinking, characterize the last stage of cognitive development. Early abstract thinking encompasses inductive and deductive reasoning, the ability to connect separate events, and the ability to understand later consequences. Abstract thinking in late adolescence is increasingly logical, and young adults are capable of scientific reasoning, understanding complex concepts, and using analytic methods. Because of logical reasoning, adolescents are able to differentiate between others' perceptions and their own and to view social situations from a societal perspective.

In a review of adolescent cognitive development, Herrman (2005) cites research suggesting that the brain is still maturing during adolescence, and this maturational process affects cognitive and emotional processing. Areas of the brain that control coordination and physical skills and emotional intensity develop during early adolescence, with increased myelinization occurring in the cerebellum and amygdala. At this age, adolescents are physically capable of many skills and emotionally more likely to take physical risks. They have a heightened sensitivity to stress, demonstrated by an exacerbated stress response. During middle adolescence maturation in the mid-brain allows for increased organization and problem-solving skills and critical thinking. Finally, maturation in the frontal cortex assists the late adolescent to use rational thought to mediate intense emotion (Herrman, 2005).

The implications of this for nurses are especially apparent for health teaching. Adolescents think in different ways than adults. For example, sex education for ninth graders is quite different from that for college freshmen or adolescents with their first full-time jobs. The college freshman should be able to appreciate the later consequences of sexual behavior, whereas the young adolescent is focused on the here and now. Ask the ninth grader and the college freshman how an unwanted baby will affect their lives, and compare their answers.

For a variety of reasons (including poor comprehension ability, lack of education, and chronic substance abuse),

some older adolescents remain concrete thinkers. Nurses and educators must know their audiences and address them appropriately. Nurses may need to help parents learn how to communicate with their teens appropriately. Counseling a group of adolescent substance abusers may be ineffective if the consequence of their behavior is tied to the future when their thinking is in the present. A professional approach to communicating with teens includes the following:

- Enjoy them.
- Be patient and flexible.
- Know adolescent development; consider how the teen will look to peers.
- Be open to their ideas and opinions and willing to negotiate choices.
- Listen nonjudgmentally, keeping criticism to a minimum.
- Encourage problem solving and mutual decision making.
- Maintain confidentiality.
- Be an advocate, but do not take sides against a parent.
- Explore feelings about health care choices, and allow for questions and analysis of health care options.

Sensory Development

Adolescents' eyes and ears are fully developed, and with the exception of refractive errors and occasional minor infections of the eyes, ears, and sinuses, the sensory system remains quite healthy. Myopia occurs in early adolescence, between ages 11 and 13 years, often requiring frequent changes in corrective lenses.

Because of increased participation in competitive sports and outdoor activities, eye injuries are common in adolescence. Boys are more prone to eye injuries than are girls. Adolescents should always be required to wear safety or protective equipment when competing in sports or participating in any activity that may compromise eye safety.

Language Development

With the acquisition of formal operational thought and adequate intellectual capacity, adolescents are able to understand abstract concepts, process complex thoughts, and express themselves verbally. Adolescents who read extensively are generally more articulate and have a larger vocabulary than those who do not. Social development and self-confidence play a significant role in how well adolescents express themselves verbally to others. Shy, introverted adolescents may have difficulty speaking to a group or members of the opposite sex but may write expressively. Conversely, extroverted, social adolescents who have no trouble with verbal expression may lack the reading and writing skills for effective written communication.

Computer technology has added to the adolescent's avenues for creative expression. Adolescents are capable of expressing ideas in symbols and abstract concepts, and many enjoy interpreting or even developing complex computer programs. Computers have a symbolic language of their own that some adolescents find fascinating. Teens may become more proficient with computer technology than their parents. As well as teaching teens basic computer literacy, many high schools have computer clubs where students who excel in computer languages share ideas and knowledge of computer information systems. Because of safety concerns with young adolescents using the Internet, parents need to monitor computer use and investigate whether parental controls available through some Internet access companies are appropriate for their child.

Communicating with adolescents sometimes presents a challenge to parents and other adults. Although adolescents are capable of verbal expression, they are also intensely private and may not wish to divulge their thoughts and feelings to others. Developmentally, the verbally expressive 12-year-old may turn into a relatively uncommunicative 14-year-old. Conflict with parents increases tension in communication (Box 8-3).

Nurses who work with adolescents must develop communication skills that include assuring confidentiality, making no assumptions, remaining nonjudgmental, and posing open-ended questions. Questions such as "Tell me about your plans for the future" will glean more information than "Do you plan to go to college?" The question "Do you live with your parents?" makes an assumption about the living situation that could make the adolescent feel uncomfortable. "Describe where you live and who lives with you" gives the adolescent an opportunity to discuss the living situation.

Psychosocial Development

Identity formation is the major developmental task of adolescence; other tasks include the formation of a sexual and

---

BOX 8-3 | PARENTS WANT TO KNOW About Communicating with Adolescents

Parents need encouragement to maintain open communication with their teenager while not appearing too intrusive. Inundating adolescents with questions or going through their belongings causes feelings of invasion and a lack of trust. Adolescents get more out of discussions in which they participate than they do out of lectures and are more likely to respond positively to adults who listen and appear interested in what they have to say.

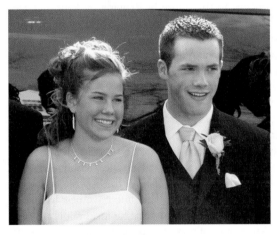

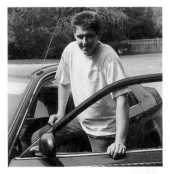

Relationships with the opposite sex are more mature by late adolescence. Late adolescents have more realistic expectations of both themselves and those who are important to them. They devote many hours and much anxious thought toward making events such as prom night memorable for a lifetime. Some adolescents may be left out because they are unpopular or shy or do not have the financial resources to participate in these special events.

With the freedom driving brings to the adolescent comes responsibility. The adolescent's inexperience and risk-taking behaviors can be a lethal combination.

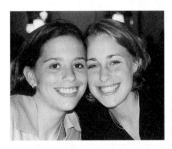

Although teens often have friends of both sexes, they are more comfortable sharing their hopes, dreams, secrets, and even embarrassing incidents with friends of the same sex.

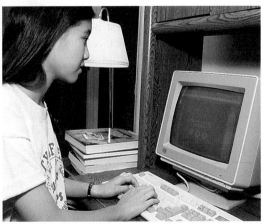

Computers in school and in many homes provide the adolescent with opportunities for learning, creative expression, communication, and entertainment. Adolescents often enjoy "surfing" the Internet, which can provide them with information not readily available locally. Parents must monitor their computer connections, however, for these networks sometimes allow access to people and activities that conflict with family values.

FIG 8-1 **Adolescent growth and development.**

vocational identity and the ability to emancipate oneself from the family or become independent (Fig. 8-1). Energy is focused within the self, and the adolescent is described as egocentric or self-absorbed. Frustrated parents often describe teenagers during this phase as self-centered, lazy, or irresponsible. In fact, they just need time to think, concentrate on themselves, and determine who they are going to be. Erikson (1968) described the conflict of this phase of psychosocial development as identity formation versus role confusion; this phase corresponds to Freud's genital stage of psychosexual development (see Chapter 4 for information on developmental theories).

In the transition period from childhood to adulthood, adolescents try new roles and experiment with the environment until they find a role that fits. The phase of experimentation has been termed the *moratorium*, meaning a period of delay granted to someone not yet ready to make more than a tentative commitment (Erikson, 1968). The adolescent's changing interests from year to year illustrate the lack of commitment. Parents may invest in expensive sports equipment or a musical instrument only to find it abandoned after a short time.

The peer group plays an essential role in adolescent identity formation. Teenagers take their cues on appearance, social behavior, and language from the peer group. The peer group serves as a safe haven as adolescents emotionally move away from the family and struggle to determine who they are. The peer group validates acceptable behavior, and teenagers feel secure in trying on new roles with peer group approval. Teens frequently spend all day with friends in school and all evening rehashing the day's events over the phone (Box 8-4). Changes in the adolescent's body image, psychosocial development, and peer group acceptance are closely related. Early and middle adolescents are particularly audience conscious and feel that they are the focus of everyone's attention. A bad hair day or a blemish may throw the adolescent into despair. Clothing, hairstyles, and material possessions that are accepted by the group become the most important. Nurses should counsel parents to negotiate choices with teens but always consider how peers will judge the child.

CRITICAL TO REMEMBER
The Adolescent and Erikson

- Identity formation and establishment of autonomy
- Acquisition of abstract reasoning leading to the following:
  Analytic thinking
  Problem solving
  Planning for the future

Early adolescence and middle adolescence are the periods when teens are prone to gang formation and activities. Peer modeling and peer acceptance, being of the utmost importance, lead some adolescents to form gangs that provide a collective identity and give them a sense of belonging. Peer pressure, companionship, and protection are the most

---

BOX 8-4	Age-Related Activities and Games for Adolescents

General Activities

Games and athletics are the most common forms of play.
Strict rules are in place.
Competition is important.

Games and Special Types of Play

Sports, videos, movies, reading, parties, hobbies, listening to favorite music, experimenting with makeup and hairstyles, talking on the telephone or cell phone, playing computer games.

---

frequently reported reasons for joining gangs, particularly those associated with violent or criminal acts.

Early and late adolescence have marked developmental differences. Each age group has unique reactions to the developmental tasks, which are influenced by the adolescent's cognitive thinking. According to Piaget (1969), adolescent cognition is characterized by the transition from concrete operational thought to formal operational thought, the ability to think logically and use deductive and abstract reasoning (see Chapters 4 through 7). The acquisition of formal operational thinking allows the adolescent to draw on past experience and apply knowledge to the future by drawing on logical consequences from a set of observations. Adolescents are capable of using abstract symbols such as those derived from higher-order mathematics, making and testing hypotheses, and considering and arguing philosophic issues. Problem-solving and decision-making skills become more highly developed, although adolescents may still be conflicted about idealism versus reality.

Early Adolescence

The early adolescent (11 to 14 years) has intense feelings about body image and the many physical changes taking place. Less confident with members of the opposite sex, early adolescents tend to group together and have best friends of the same sex. One has only to visit the local mall or movie theater to see groups of young teens of the same sex, observing but rarely speaking to groups of the opposite sex.

The early adolescent is quite egocentric and may move from obedience to rebellion regarding parental authority. Parents are often shocked by the sudden turn of events and are hurt by the teen's rejection. Providing parents with anticipatory guidance regarding age-specific developmental changes is a primary nursing function. For example, the happy-go-lucky 11-year-old may turn into the shy, self-absorbed 12-year-old who seems comfortable only in the presence of friends. Young teens, who are developmentally egocentric, fail to differentiate between how others see them and their own mental preoccupations, thinking everyone is as obsessed with them as they are with themselves. Elkind (1993) describes this phenomenon as a reaction to the imaginary audience. The belief in the imaginary audience is probably why young teens are so self-conscious; they believe everyone is critical of them, and indeed teens are quite critical of each other, especially those who are different. Self-conscious behavior may also be the result of the physical and emotional transition to middle adolescence. The early adolescent is losing the familiar role of the child but does not yet feel comfortable with the role of the adult. Ambivalence toward independence is common, and the teen who feels too grown up for a good-night kiss from a parent still falls asleep with a favorite teddy bear.

Elkind (1993) believes that because young teens are so audience conscious, they see themselves as unique and tell themselves a "personal fable" that supports feelings of invulnerability. They believe bad things will happen to others but not to them. Adolescent suicide attempts, for example, serve as a dramatic message to others, but young teens often do not realize the final consequences of their actions.

Middle Adolescence

Middle adolescence (15 to 17 years) is often described by parents as the most frustrating period of adolescent development. The real audience gradually replaces the imaginary audience, and teens become even more introspective and narcissistic. Conformity to peer group norms becomes even more important, and conflicts between teenagers and parents often escalate. Testing of limits, sulky withdrawal, and overt rebellion may occur over conflicts regarding curfews, friends, activities, appearance, cars, and money. The adolescent may feel more secure by associating with or becoming a member of a gang (Box 8-5). Nurses should counsel parents to

---

BOX 8-5	**Signs of Gang Involvement**

- Associating with new friends while ignoring old friends. The adolescent usually will not talk about the new friends or what they do together.
- A change in hairstyle or clothing and associating with other youths with the same style. Usually some of the clothing, such as a hat or jacket, has the gang's colors, initials, or "street" name on it. Parents may note tattoos on the body.
- Unexplained source of money or possessions (stereos, jewelry, cars).
- Indications of drug, alcohol, or inhalant abuse (e.g., paint or correction fluid on the clothes, the smell of chemicals on the breath or clothes).
- Change in attitude toward activities such as sports, Scouts, or church. Discipline problems at school, in public, or at home. Youth no longer accepts parents' authority and challenges it frequently.
- Problems at school, such as failing classes, skipping school, or causing problems in class.
- Fear of the police.
- Unexplained signs of fighting, such as bruises, cuts, or reports of pain.
- Graffiti on or around residence or possessions.
- Threats from rival gang members. Sometimes a family member is a victim of a drive-by shooting before the family realizes the youth is involved in a gang.

---

negotiate choices when possible and set limits that are perceived as reasonable by the adolescent. Consistent discipline and structure actually make adolescents feel more secure and assist them with decision making. With parental guidance, adolescents are able to make decisions that will result in desirable outcomes. Adults must keep in mind that middle adolescents are impulsive and impatient, however. Parental concern may be seen as interference rather than guidance and may be met with resistance and resentment.

Feelings about self-image and social relationships are intense. Middle adolescence is generally a time of transition from same-sex friendships to an extreme interest in the opposite sex; it is also a time when adolescents may acknowledge homosexual feelings. The proportion of teens who are sexually experienced and sexually active has declined slightly, as has the teen pregnancy rate (Centers for Disease Control and Prevention [CDC], 2004). Explanations for this slight decrease generally fall into two schools: one school points to abstinence education, and the other cites sex education that promotes more widespread and effective contraceptive use (Duncan, Dixon, & Carlson, 2003). Nurses and other health care providers cannot become complacent in response to this change in trends. The United States still has one of the highest adolescent pregnancy rates. In a recent survey by the CDC (2004) 7.4% of adolescents reported initiating sexual intercourse before age 13 years, and 46.7% of the ninth through twelfth graders surveyed had had sexual intercourse at least once. Of concern is the trend for early initiation of sexual intercourse.

Sexual activity is often related to peer pressure and self-esteem issues. Adolescents with low self-esteem are more vulnerable and are apt to engage in negative risk-taking activities associated with sexuality. Decisions about sexual activity are often impulsive and made with little regard to later consequences or prior preparation. In fact, according to the recent Youth Risk Behavior Surveillance (CDC, 2004), 37% of teenagers who are sexually active did not use a condom at last intercourse.

Another concerning trend among adolescents is the increasing participation in oral sex. Boekeloo and Howard (2002) reported a prevalence of oral sex in 14- and 15-year olds of 25%. Other studies have reported prevalence as high as 50% of teens engaging in oral sex (Halpern-Fisher, Cornell, Kropp, & Tschann, 2005). Questions about oral sexual activity are not currently included in the Youth Risk Behavior Surveillance. Halpern-Fisher et al (2005) state that adolescents intend to have oral sex for a variety of reasons, but primarily they believe it is more socially acceptable than vaginal intercourse and does not carry the same risks. Their research suggested that, although many adolescents know that HIV and other infectious diseases can be contracted from engaging in oral sex, an "important" percentage of adolescents see no risk from unprotected oral sex (Halpern-Fisher et al., p. 849).

Nurses and other health professionals who assess adolescent health status need to be more specific when interviewing adolescents about sexual activity. The question of whether an adolescent is sexually active is no longer sufficient; questions should be directed toward assessing participation in various specific types of sexual activity as well as the method of barrier protection used. Nurses may help by providing accurate information to assist adolescents in making appropriate sexual choices. Parents need encouragement to maintain open communication and guide teenagers in sexual decision making. Providing parental guidance about sexual behavior is not easy during middle adolescence, when privacy is of extreme importance and communication with parents tends to decrease. In addition, some parents may find sexual behavior a difficult topic to discuss and often avoid talking with teens regarding sexual issues altogether.

In the initial stages of establishing a vocational identity, adolescents are more likely to experience role confusion and have unrealistic expectations of themselves. Some adolescents will identify a role that holds their interest, whereas others will experiment with many roles, moving quickly from one role to another. Overidentification with glamorous roles takes precedence over reality and is enriched by daydreams and fantasy. A 15-year-old girl may spend time with her friends describing her future as a popular media star while failing to fold the laundry or do the dishes.

During middle adolescence, some teens acquire part-time jobs and identify various skills and interests. Part-time jobs are often a source of income for material possessions and activities not provided by parents. Such experiences help adolescents set realistic expectations about work, become more independent, and develop their self-esteem. Those who are successful in the working world demonstrate a sense of responsibility and tend to have more positive social interactions. However, some adolescents may allow work to interfere with educational activity and have difficulty setting priorities. School nurses, in collaboration with parents and teachers, are in an excellent position to identify working students and assist them in setting realistic guidelines for work and education.

Late Adolescence (18 to 21 Years)

Late adolescence is characterized by the ability to think abstractly, conceptualize verbally, and express thoughts and feelings about various aspects of life. Late adolescents tend to be idealistic about love, social issues, ethics, and lifestyles until their experiences modify their beliefs. Conformity becomes less important as teens progress through late adolescence. With the development of a unique identity, self-esteem increases and adolescents are able to resist group pressure if it is not in their best interest. Interactions with parents are less turbulent unless values clash, and relationships with both friends and family are maintained.

Emancipation (leaving home) is a major issue; late adolescents prepare themselves to meet this task through education or vocational training. Identifying realistic career goals is important, but many adolescents are not quite ready to make lifelong commitments. Changing career goals is not uncommon, but the nurse should watch for those adolescents who have set no career goals, who demonstrate apathy about the future, and who appear committed only to the present.

Boredom and apathy are often symptoms of a greater problem: depression.

Social relationships are more mature, although partner selection often continues to fluctuate. Friendships developed in late adolescence may last a lifetime, and expectations of friends and lovers become more realistic and less self-serving. The ability to consider others' needs increases, and recognition of societal needs is more apparent as the adolescent moves from adolescence to adulthood.

Failure to achieve identity formation may leave adolescents in role confusion and impede the successful mastery of the tasks of young adulthood. A positive ego identity depends on the adolescent's ability to accept the past, learn from experience, and become engaged in the future. Most adolescents move through the identity versus role confusion stage of development with minimal difficulty.

Moral and Spiritual Development

Children develop moral reasoning in a sequential manner, as described by American psychologist Lawrence Kohlberg (1984). As adolescents move from concrete to analytic thinking, they advance to Kohlberg's stage 4 conventional level or Kohlberg's stage 5 postconventional level of moral development. Adolescents who remain concrete thinkers may never advance beyond Kohlberg's stage 3 of moral reasoning: conformity to please others and avoid punishment. The teenager's sense of justice is developed through interpersonal relationships with peers, family, and other adult role models. Behaviors that are modeled and rewarded, such as helping the less fortunate and showing loyalty to friends, contribute to the development of a conscience, which operates as a moral guide for subsequent behavior. The middle to late teenager can appreciate that stealing from others is wrong regardless of whether one is caught and punished.

Adolescents and young adults develop a respect for law and order and a society-maintaining orientation (Kohlberg's stage 4). Young adults may even advance to the societal-perspective stage (Kohlberg's stage 5), which honors the moral rules of right and wrong, contractual agreements, majority opinion, and overall utility or the greatest good for the greatest number (see Chapter 4).

Older adolescents and young adults question the values of family and society and challenge existing moral codes before integrating their experiences and beliefs into a personal moral framework. Once the moral framework is developed, interpersonal relationships tend to be with those whose values and beliefs are similar.

Young adolescents in the stage of concrete operational thought are able to think logically. In this stage, children deal well with the observable but also begin to see other points of view and examine what they have learned. The young adolescent will accept religious teaching and examine how religious concepts relate to everyday life. Young adolescents are especially inclined to look to God for guidance when troubled.

Middle to late adolescents are capable of analytic thought and may begin to question the religious affiliation of the family, much as they question other family values. Older adolescents may explore different kinds of religion and share religious activities with the peer group.

Callaghan (2005) demonstrates a significant relationship between spiritual growth and assumption of responsibility for self-care in health promotion activities by adolescents. Nurses need to include an assessment of spiritual beliefs and values when working with adolescents and incorporate these values in nursing interventions, especially in the area of health promotion (Callaghan, 2005).

CRITICAL TO REMEMBER
Elements of Adolescent Care

Nurses working with middle adolescents must:
- Be approachable
- Maintain objectivity
- Encourage confidence
- Support parental authority
- Be a child advocate while not coming between adolescents and their parents
- Encourage the family to work as a mutually respectful unit

HEALTH PROMOTION FOR THE ADOLESCENT AND FAMILY

Adolescence is generally a period of wellness. Young people may seek health care for school or sports physicals, skin conditions (acne, contact dermatitis), acute minor illnesses (colds, flu), conditions related to sexuality (birth control, pregnancy, sexually transmissible diseases [STDs]), and the management of chronic illness (diabetes, epilepsy). Health promotion and disease prevention are achieved through adequate nutrition, rest, balanced exercise, and proper immunization against disease.

During well visits for health promotion, adolescents confer privately with the nurse and the health provider; separately, parents are asked about any concerns they might have. Confidentiality is often an issue when adolescents are seen in the health care setting. Nurses should encourage adolescents to involve their parents, but adolescents frequently ask that communication be kept confidential. The adolescent must understand that the nurse will respect this confidentiality unless the information shared suggests a potentially life-threatening danger either to the adolescent or to others.

CRITICAL THINKING EXERCISE 8-1

The nurse is caring for a 15-year-old girl, Heidi, who has been admitted to the hospital with dehydration. She is quiet and answers questions with a simple "yes" or "no." On the day Heidi is to be discharged, she says, "I'll tell you something, but you can't tell anyone else."
1. What factors must the nurse consider in this situation?
2. What would be the nurse's best response?

Screening tools are used in some settings to target areas of concern in an organized manner. Two of the more popular tools are HEADSS, which includes assessment of Home, Education/employment, Activities, Drugs, Sex, and Suicide (Cohen, MacKenzie, & Yates, 1991); and Guidelines for Adolescent Preventive Services (GAPS), which include parenting, development, drugs, sex, learning problems, depression, abuse, safety, and diet and fitness. GAPS is a comprehensive packet of services that includes screening and preventive services (American Medical Association, 1997). The home environment and relationships with peers also are important assessment areas. Health professionals must identify which tool best suits their philosophy of care. Ozer et al. (2005) suggest that using a screening instrument helps organize important areas of adolescent assessment and provides a basis for intervention and teaching; the instrument in their study encompassed areas previously mentioned and added a safety category particularly directed toward seatbelt and helmet use (Ozer et al., 2005).

Some clinics send a questionnaire before the visit so that the adolescent can complete it at home and return it during the visit. Some settings display their policy on confidentiality, always underlining the need to share information only if someone is in danger. Issues related to the time necessary for an adequate interview may arise in the present managed care environment. Nurses should be knowledgeable about communicating with adolescents and aware of when referral is warranted.

Nutrition During Adolescence

The accelerated growth (in linear height, weight, and muscle mass) and sexual maturation during adolescence increase teenagers' nutritional needs, including needs for protein, calories, zinc, calcium, and iron. Periods of intense growth require increased caloric intake, and the adolescent appears constantly hungry. Snacks and regular meals must contain adequate nutrients to meet the body's anabolic needs. Adolescents are generally interested in nutrition and the effect food has on their bodies. Teenagers tend to be concerned about their weight, complexion, sexual development, and acceptance by their peers. These issues, together with the adolescent's increasing independence, can have nutritional implications.

Age-Related Nutritional Challenges

The adolescent's food habits are influenced by many factors (Box 8-6). Unfortunately, this happens at a time when the body has increased nutritional needs. Boys tend to have

---

BOX 8-6	**Factors Influencing the Adolescent's Diet**

- Busy schedule (sports, activities, jobs)
- Body image concerns, which can lead to undereating
- Skipping breakfast
- Eating away from home
- Eating fast food frequently
- Beginning to buy and prepare own food
- Peer pressure
- Psychologic and emotional problems

fewer nutritional deficiencies than girls have because they take in more food and are less likely to be dieting. Soft drinks frequently replace milk. Fast foods and low nutrient "junk foods" sometimes become the mainstay of the adolescent's diet. The social aspect of food consumption gains importance, and adolescents may prefer to eat meals with peers at social gatherings and restaurants of their choice. Parental supervision of meals declines as the adolescent spends more time away from home and engages in extracurricular activities with peers.

Nutritional Guidance for the Adolescent

The nurse must understand growth and development to be successful in counseling adolescents and their parents about nutrition. Adolescents' increasing need to be independent and make their own choices should guide the nurse in teaching nutrition. The adolescent should always be involved in the planning.

The nurse needs to assess the adolescent's present diet and determine habits and eating patterns. The assessment should elicit how often the adolescent eats food from the different food groups and what foods the adolescent does not eat. Based on this information, nutritious foods for meals can be identified and a plan developed. In general, the United States Department of Agriculture (USDA) (2006) recommends 1800 calories/day for adolescent girls and 2200 calories/day for adolescent boys, with foods coming from a variety of groups, including whole grains, fruits and vegetables, dairy, and protein (plant and animal). Adolescents should drink at least three cups of milk a day and limit fats to 25% to 35% of total daily calories consumed. Adolescents need calcium to prevent future osteoporosis, and adolescent girls require adequate iron and folic acid (USDA, 2006).

The nurse can also assist the adolescent by pointing out nutritious fast foods and snacks. An awareness of nutritious fast foods can also aid the adolescent in meal selection. Many fast-food chains have salads with nonfat or low-fat dressings, grilled chicken sandwiches, pasta, and nonfat yogurt. Fat and salt contents have been reduced, and vegetable fats have replaced animal fats at some restaurants. Adolescents should be guided to mix an occasional hamburger and fries with a regular selection of more nutritious foods. Permission should be given to eat foods that may be untraditional at a particular meal, such as pizza for breakfast.

Many adolescents decide to follow a vegetarian diet during their teen years. The American Heart Association (AHA) (2006) confirms that a vegetarian diet, if correctly followed, is healthy for this population because the low-fat aspect of the diet can prevent future cardiovascular problems. If an adolescent wishes to follow a vegetarian diet, the nurse can assist with planning food choices that will provide sufficient calories and necessary nutrients. The focus is on obtaining sufficient calories for growth and energy through a variety of fruits and vegetables, whole grains, nuts, legumes, seeds, tofu, and soy milk; some vegetarians choose to eat eggs and dairy products as well (Mangels, 2003). As with any adolescent, nurses need to advise adolescents who follow a vegetarian

eating plan to avoid low-nutrient, high-fat foods (AHA, 2006).

Body image is of particular importance to adolescents. The media reinforce the belief that "thin is in." Adolescents hold themselves to standards set by the entertainment and advertising worlds, which emphasize fitness, glamour, and sexuality. Products that promise a quick weight loss or enhanced muscle mass with a lean physique are appealing to adolescents. Weight management techniques may include fasting, diet pills and laxatives, self-induced vomiting, and fad diets instead of low-fat, low-calorie, nutritionally sound diets and more aerobic exercise. Adolescents may not realize that unsound nutritional habits often follow them for a lifetime or that growth and development may be delayed or permanently impaired. School nurses are in an excellent position to identify adolescents who have nutritional problems or eating disorders and provide counseling or referral for adolescents and their families (see Chapter 29).

Hygiene

Adolescents in general are meticulous about personal hygiene. A major concern, however, is acne. Acne contributes to adolescent self-consciousness and, if severe, to decreased self-image. Nursing interventions to address acne are discussed in detail in Chapter 25.

Dental Care

The incidence of dental caries decreases in adolescence, but dental hygiene remains important. Most permanent teeth have erupted, with the possible exception of the third molars (wisdom teeth), which erupt by late adolescence or remain impacted and may be removed surgically. Several dental conditions are prevalent during the adolescent years: gingivitis, malocclusion, and dental trauma. Gingivitis is the inflammation and breakdown of the gingival epithelium; the gums appear pale and swollen and bleed easily. Increased hormonal activity at the time of puberty, diets high in sugar and simple carbohydrates, and the use of dental braces and appliances that make cleaning less effective are thought to contribute to the development of gingivitis.

Malocclusion (improper contact) occurs in approximately 50% of adolescents because of facial and mandibular bone growth and dental crowding. Treatment varies but generally entails dental devices such as braces to correct tooth position and redirect facial growth. Adolescents may be self-conscious if their peers are no longer in braces and may need reassurance that the condition is temporary. For economic reasons, some adolescents are unable to correct malocclusions and suffer the consequences indefinitely. Nurses can help by referring adolescents with no dental care to free clinics or agencies providing dental care at low cost. People with uncorrected malocclusions are at greater risk for dental trauma.

A tooth that has been completely knocked out of the mouth (avulsed) can sometimes be reimplanted. The sooner the reimplantation occurs, the greater is the likelihood of success. The prognosis is best if the injury is treated within 30 minutes. School and clinic nurses may be the first health

HEALTH PROMOTION

THE ADOLESCENT

FOCUSED ASSESSMENT

Ask the Adolescent the Following:

- Can you tell me how often and what foods you like to eat? How often do you eat at fast-food restaurants? How do you feel about how much you weigh? Do you think you need to gain or lose any weight? Do you ever make yourself vomit or take laxatives to control your weight?
- In what types of physical activities or organized sports do you participate? How often do you do them?
- How often do you brush your teeth, floss, and see the dentist? Do you take fluoride?
- What time do you go to bed at night? What time do you get up in the morning? Do you have any trouble falling asleep, or do you wake up in the middle of the night?
- How often do you have a bowel movement? Are there any problems with urination?
- What grade in school are you? How well do you think you are doing in school? Do any circumstances at school make you feel unsafe or threatened?
- Tell me about your friends. What types of activities do you do with them for fun? Do your friends pressure you to do things you would rather not do? Do you or your friends smoke cigarettes or take any substances (alcohol, drugs)?
- How do you get along with other members of your family? Do you have a special family member to talk to if you are having a problem? If so, whom?
- Do you do any or all of the following: use a seatbelt every time you get in a car; avoid getting into a car if the driver has been drinking; wear a helmet every time you ride a bike or motorcycle; wear a helmet and protective pads every time you skate; use sunscreen; swim with a buddy?
- Has anyone ever physically harmed you or touched you in a way that made you uncomfortable? Have you ever thought about harming yourself? Do you or does anyone you know own a gun?
- Have you begun dating? Have you been or are you sexually active? (If sexually active, ask about condom use and birth control methods and any incidence of STDs.) Do you have any questions or concerns about your sexual development (ask girls about the pattern and frequency of menstruation)?
- What kind of job do you have, if any? How many hours per week do you work?
- What kind of things do you do to stay healthy? Do you regularly take any medications or dietary supplements? Do you regularly perform breast or testicular self-examinations? Do you have any concerns about any aspect of your health?

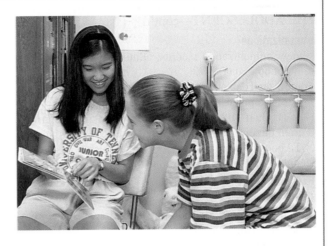

Ask the Parent the Following:

- Do you have any concerns related to the adolescent's nutrition, body image, physical activity, oral health, sleep, elimination, school, family interactions, self-esteem, or ability to practice safety precautions?
- Do you continue to stay involved in your child's life?
- What types of family rules do you consistently enforce?

DEVELOPMENTAL MILESTONES

Personal/social: experiences emotional and social turmoil associated with rapid changes in development and altered body image; is interested in opposite-sex relationships (some lead to a level of intimacy for which the adolescent is not ready); assumes varying roles to integrate social skills with new aspirations and to gain a sense of self; clarifies values and career directions; is more stable emotional control in later adolescence; may exhibit imaginary audience ("everyone is staring at me") or personal fable ("it will never happen to me")

Fine motor: adult fine motor control

Language/cognitive: becomes future oriented; views the world in broad perspective; hypothesizes several alternatives to a problem; thinks and reasons abstractly; develops moral reasoning

Gross motor: early growth-related awkwardness develops into coordinated muscle control

HEALTH MAINTENANCE

Physical Measurements

Girls achieve PHV approximately 2 years before boys

Average weight gain during growth spurt is 50% of adult weight, largely from body fat in girls and muscle mass in boys

Average height gain is 20% to 25% of adult height over a 2- to 3-year period (girls, 8.3 cm/yr; boys, 9.4 cm/yr)

Achieve Tanner stage 5 (see Table 8-1)

Continued

HEALTH PROMOTION

THE ADOLESCENT—cont'd

Immunizations

Review immunization records; administer immunizations if not up to date

Administer Tdap at age 11 to 12 years if primary DTaP series is complete and it has been 5 years since the last dose of DTaP. If Td booster has already been given, consider immunizing with Tdap if it has been 5 years since the Td booster dose.

Meningococcal vaccine (if available) at age 11 to 12 years or at entrance to high school, if not administered earlier.

Health Screening

Objective hearing and vision screening (may become myopic as growth spurt begins)

Hemoglobin or hematocrit

Urinalysis by dipstick

Blood pressure

Lipid screen if at risk

Tuberculosis screening if at risk (see Chapter 21)

Pap smear for sexually active girls

STD screening if applicable

Emotional and stress screening

ANTICIPATORY GUIDANCE

Nutrition

Follow recommended servings according to the Food Guide Pyramid; teach the adolescent how to keep track of servings and give input into meal preparation

Advise to avoid fast foods and eat a nutritious breakfast; watch calcium and iron intake; assess adequacy of diet and snacks; folic acid supplementation for adolescent girls

Teach principles of a vegetarian diet if applicable

Elimination

Regular bowel movements according to individual pattern

Dental

Provide regular dental care every 6 months

Continue regular flossing and brushing with fluoride toothpaste

Discuss emergency care for fractured or avulsed teeth (see Box 8-7)

Sleep

Facilitate an individually appropriate sleep pattern; usually needs 8 hours

Safety

Review gun safety; automobile and motorized vehicle driver and passenger safety; water safety; sun protection; fire safety; avoiding listening to loud music through earphones

Discuss techniques to combat violence, particularly dating violence; wear protective equipment in the workplace; no drinking and driving; learn cardiopulmonary resuscitation (CPR)

Emotional Health

Tell another if concerned about a friend

Take every threat of suicide as real

Learn stress-reduction techniques

Seek help if depressed or angry

---

professionals to see a child with a complete tooth avulsion and should be aware of the proper procedure (see Chapter 10). Parents should also know how to care for their child if such an incident occurs (Box 8-7).

Sleep and Rest

Along with increasingly independent activities, adolescents show a propensity for staying up late (particularly if working on a school project or attending a weekend party) and having difficulty waking up in the morning. Setting one's own bedtime and sleeping late on weekends are behaviors associated with gaining independence, although recent evidence suggests that sleeping late on weekends helps adolescents recover from sleep lost during the week (Hansen, Janssen, Schiff, Zee, & Dubocovich, 2005). Hours of sleep may vary from 6 to 8 hours during the week to 12 hours on the weekends, but an overall average of 8 hours per night is recommended for adolescents and young adults.

Rapid physical growth and increased activities contribute to the adolescent's fatigue, and frustrated parents may complain that their teenager has energy for everything but household and family chores. Nurses can educate teens and their parents to set realistic schedules that allow time for adequate rest and relaxation. Some teens may find themselves so overscheduled that they develop sleep disturbances from excess fatigue and anxiety. Adult sleep cycles are formed during adolescence, and sleep disturbances continue into the adult years. Persistent difficulty in falling asleep, wakefulness during the night, or early waking may be signs of emotional

---

| BOX 8-7 | **PARENTS WANT TO KNOW** About Caring for a Child with an Avulsed Tooth |

A tooth that has been completely knocked out of the mouth (avulsed) can sometimes be reimplanted. The sooner the reimplantation occurs, the greater is the likelihood of success. If the tooth can be recovered, it should be rinsed in lukewarm tap water and placed in saline, water, milk, or a commercial tooth preserving liquid. The tooth should not be scrubbed, and cleaning agents and disinfectants should be avoided. The child should be seen as soon as possible by a dentist or taken to the emergency room. The prognosis is best if the injury is treated within 30 minutes.

problems associated with tension, anxiety, or depression and may warrant referral.

Recently, several studies have suggested that adolescents' sleep patterns can interfere with their academic performance because the interaction between natural circadian sleep rhythm and social activities makes them less alert in the early morning (Hansen et al., 2005). These findings have implications for schools in terms of scheduling start times and planning tests for high school students. School districts in various sections of the country are beginning to address this issue by looking at later start times.

Exercise and Activity

Although adolescents are often involved in many activities, these activities do not always promote physical fitness. A recent national survey found that only 62.6% of adolescents regularly participate in vigorous physical exercise (20 minutes of exercise that causes sweating or breathing hard) 3 days a week (CDC, 2004). Regular exercise enhances physical and emotional development and promotes healthy sleep patterns. Healthy diet and exercise habits formed during adolescence can follow into adulthood and significantly reduce the risk of cardiovascular disease.

Adolescence is an ideal time to initiate an exercise program, either as a team sport or as an individual activity. Exercise need not always involve an athletic activity but should provide for a program that gradually increases exercise over a 1- to 3-week period with a goal of vigorous exercise of at least 20 minutes three or more times per week to enhance cardiovascular fitness (USDHHS, 2000). Nurses can assist adolescents in designing an exercise program that allows gradual fitness and provides warm-up and cool-down sessions. Exercise programs are highly personal and should be structured for enjoyment, with consideration of physical capabilities and limitations.

Safety

Injuries claim more lives during adolescence than all other causes of death combined. The predominance of injuries during adolescence results from a combination of factors: physical growth, psychomotor function, insufficient physical coordination for the task, energy, impulsivity, peer pressure, and inexperience. Impulsivity, inexperience, and peer pressure may place adolescents in unsafe situations. Feelings of invulnerability ("it can't happen to me") persist, and little thought may be given to the negative consequences of certain behaviors. Alcohol and other drugs that impair judgment are known to contribute to fatal injuries among adolescents, especially those involving firearms and motor vehicles (see Chapter 29 for a complete discussion of alcohol and substance abuse). The sad fact is that most serious or fatal injuries involving adolescents are preventable.

Nurses need to educate adolescents and their families about safety issues and injury prevention. Nurses in school and community action programs are increasingly focusing on preventing firearm and traumatic head injuries. Factual information with supportive explanations should be provided.

Expressing a genuine interest in adolescents as individuals and listening in a nonjudgmental way are also important steps to gain confidence and trust. Helping the adolescent recognize choices when faced with difficult or potentially dangerous situations is an important component of safety promotion with this age group.

The adolescent period is also a frightening time for parents because they are aware of the risks predisposing the adolescent to injury or death. Parents may request guidance from health care professionals in setting appropriate limits and establishing methods of effective enforcement. Parents should be encouraged to model the safe behaviors that they expect from the adolescent.

Car Safety

Obtaining a driver's license signifies a passage into adulthood and provides the adolescent with the means to explore and experience the world more freely. Driving is a complex activity, and proficiency requires skill, judgment, and experience. The adolescent's lack of judgment, opposition to authority, and need to express independence often result in a disregard for sound defensive driving practices. Risk-taking behaviors appear to play a major role in the high incidence of car-related injuries and deaths among teenagers. The young, inexperienced driver tends to drive faster and take more chances while operating a car than older drivers do. The Youth Risk Behavior Surveillance Survey of high school students found that 18.2% had rarely or never worn a seatbelt. In addition, during the 30 days preceding the survey, 30.2% had ridden with a driver who had been drinking alcohol (CDC, 2004).

The association between alcohol use and motor vehicle crashes by adolescents is alarming. Despite legal drinking age laws, alcohol is easily accessible to adolescents. The teenager's greater social activity, combined with the availability of alcohol, increases the incidence of impaired driving.

Nurses can promote car safety by supporting driver education programs for teenagers and the use of seatbelts. In addition, many schools and community organizations have developed prevention programs that are helpful in presenting the facts about drinking and driving to adolescents. Nurses should encourage teens and their parents to set up a ride-home agreement to discourage any driving after drinking alcohol. Adolescents need to know that they have an option available to them if they find themselves in a situation where the driver has been drinking. Dealing with the inconveniences of finding another ride home is much better than dealing with the injuries and damages of motor vehicle crashes.

Water Safety

Drowning is a needless cause of death in teenagers. Most drowning deaths occur in lakes, rivers, and ponds, with the rest occurring in public or private swimming pools. Risk-taking behaviors contribute greatly to deaths from drowning and to the incidence of spinal cord injuries. Adolescents are able to travel to areas that are free of adult supervision.

Frequently, alcohol and drugs are contributing factors. Given the combination of freedom and alcohol, adolescents may inadvertently place themselves at risk for injury by exceeding the limits for safe swimming and diving.

Safety promotion includes encouraging swimming lessons, water safety classes, and the completion of a course in cardiopulmonary resuscitation. Adolescents need to know how alcohol and drugs impair their ability to perform activities at which they are usually competent.

Suicide

Suicide is the third leading cause of death for teenagers 15 to 19 years (CDC, 2003). Between 1980 and 1990, suicide rates increased by 30% but have gradually decreased since. In 2001, the rate of suicide in the 15- to 19-year-old population was 7.9/100,000—a decrease of 7% from 1990 (National Center for Health Statistics, 2003). In a survey of adolescents, 16.9% seriously considered committing suicide during the previous 12 months (CDC, 2004). The identification of adolescents at risk for suicide is a priority. Depression is a common finding among suicidal youths; other risk factors include declining mental health, poor impulse control, poor school performance, family disorganization, conduct disorders, substance abuse, homosexuality, and recent stress. Nurses must be involved in identifying high-risk adolescents through the scientific study of these phenomena. Adolescents identified as at risk for suicide and their families should be targeted for supportive guidance and counseling before a crisis situation. Nurses should counsel parents that *all* adolescent suicidal gestures should be taken very seriously. Many adolescents do not know what type of drug ingestion or action will actually harm them. The suicidal gestures may appear minor to adults, but the actions may have serious intent (see Chapter 29).

Violence Toward Others

Violence continues to threaten the health and well-being of adolescents and society as a whole (see Chapter 1). Homicide is the fourth leading cause of death in children ages 10 to 14 years, and for teens ages 15 to 19 years it is the second leading cause of death after unintentional injury. The homicide rate increased dramatically during the 1990s but has decreased since then to 9.4/100,000 (National Center for Health Statistics, 2003). Factors contributing to violence are multiple and complex (Box 8-8). Contributing factors related to behavior provide the greatest opportunity for interventions initiated by health care professionals.

Nurses working with children, adolescents, and their families have the opportunity to include violence prevention as a component of anticipatory guidance. Ideally, prevention should begin when the child is young. Violence is a learned behavior. It is often reinforced by the actions of those closest to the child and by ever-increasing exposure to violence in the media. Assessing how a family deals with anger and resolves conflict provides insight into the way the child will likely react in similar situations. A family with violent tendencies should be referred to a counselor. Learning to react

---

BOX 8-8   **Factors Contributing to Adolescent Violence**

- Low socioeconomic status
- Crowded urban housing
- Single-parent family or limited parental supervision
- History of family violence or child abuse
- Access to guns
- Peer pressure or gang involvement
- Limited education
- Racism
- Drug or alcohol use or abuse
- Low self-esteem and hopelessness about the future
- Aggression

---

to anger or stress with nonviolent actions through conflict resolution is the goal for the youth. Unfortunately, intervention cannot be a one-time educational session. Efforts must be reinforced in multiple facets of the adolescent's life, such as in school, youth organizations, religious organizations, and home.

Parents need to be aware of the amount and type of violence to which their children are exposed in the media. Growing evidence suggests that exposure to media violence does lead to aggressive behavior by the children who watch the programs (Browne & Hamilton-Giachristis, 2005). Parents cannot isolate their children from all media violence, but they can be encouraged to monitor and limit their children's television viewing and to co-view and discuss with their children the implications of violence.

The availability of firearms is related to violent acts. In a survey of students in grades 9 through 12 conducted by the CDC, 17.1% reporting having carried a weapon within the 30 days preceding the survey (CDC, 2004). Carrying a weapon can establish a feeling of control or power, or it may be a response to fear of those with power. Regardless of the reasons, firearms in the hands of adolescents are impulsively used before the ramifications of such actions can be logically considered.

As society urgently seeks a solution to the growing problem of violence, health care professionals must become advocates of violence prevention. Opportunities for adolescents to discover and use less-violent means to express themselves or resolve day-to-day issues should be taught and promoted. Peer mediation programs in schools have been successful in preventing violent behavior among teens. Given the tragic effects of violence on the safety and health of American children, nurses should participate in efforts to resolve the complex issues of violence in society.

Selected Issues Related to the Adolescent

Body Piercing

Ear piercing has been popular with teens for many years. Today the tongue, lip, eyebrow, nose, navel, and nipple are also common sites. Generally, body piercing is harmless, but nurses should caution teens about performing these procedures under unsterile conditions and should educate teens about complications, such as bleeding, infection, keloid formation, and allergies to metal. Qualified personnel using sterile needles should perform piercing procedures. The area needs to be cleaned twice each day (more often for a tongue piercing).

Tattoos

Tattoos are increasingly popular among mainstream adolescents. Like clothing and hairstyles, tattoos serve to define one's identity. Unfortunately, tattoos are often the result of an impulsive decision by the adolescent and are performed by amateurs who are not qualified to do the procedure. Recent studies of a large sample of adolescents suggest a relationship between behavioral risk factors (multiple drug use, illegal activities, and school truancy) and adolescents who have body piercings or tattoos (Deschesnes, Fines, & Demers, 2005; Roberts & Ryan, 2002). Because of the invasiveness of the tattoo procedure, it should be considered a health-risk situation. Little regulation exists in the tattoo industry, and nurses should educate adolescents about the risks of blood-borne infections, skin infections, and allergic reactions to dyes used in the tattoo process. In addition, nurses need to be informed about tattoo removal to provide correct information to adolescents and their families (Box 8-9). Impulsive decisions to tattoo are often regretted, and teens or their parents may want the tattoo removed. Laser therapy is available for tattoo removal but is costly and not usually covered by insurance. Amateur tattoos are removed quite easily, but studio tattoos made with red and green dyes are quite difficult to remove. Tattoo removal requires several visits, and adolescents have to tolerate the tattoo's appearance during the removal process. Nurses need to caution adolescents with tattoos to notify health professionals of the tattoo if magnetic resonance imaging (MRI) is to be performed. The iron oxide in the tattooing dye can contribute to injury during MRI (Selekman, 2003).

Tanning

A "good" suntan does not exist. Convincing adolescents that tanning is harmful to their skin and is a risk factor for developing skin cancer later in life is difficult, however. The media (advertising, movies, television) promote the image of beach glamour: young, well built, and tanned. Although most companies that manufacture tanning products promote the sun protection factor (SPF) in their products, the advertised image remains a bronzed, attractive, young person. Most exposure to ultraviolet radiation occurs during childhood and adolescence, and skin cancers could be prevented with the appropriate and consistent use of sunscreens and sun blocks.

A recent study of the prevalence of indoor tanning salon use among white adolescents suggests that approximately 28% of adolescents in the United States, primarily girls, obtain a tan in a tanning salon relatively regularly (Demko, Borawski, Debanne, Cooper, & Stange, 2003). An area of concern is the fact that a percentage of the adolescents who use tanning salons do not use sun protection (either in the salon or when under natural sunlight) and are not aware of the dangers of exposure to this type of ultraviolet light. Adverse effects from tanning beds include eye injury, premature aging of the skin, and increased risk of skin cancer of all types (American Cancer Society, 2005). The American Dermatology Association (2004) has issued a policy stating that no one younger than 18 years should be permitted to use a tanning salon, that all equipment in tanning salons carry a warning of danger from the Surgeon General, and advertisements should not mislead clients into believing that salon tanning is safer than natural sunlight exposure. Nurses who are doing anticipatory guidance with teens must address these issues along with teaching about the risks of tanning in natural sunlight.

Nurses need to educate teens about the benefits and side effects of different sun protection products and encourage use for water sports and all activities that involve sun exposure. Teens involved in athletic activities are often exposed to the sun for long periods without protection. Teenagers may be cognizant of body exposure at a beach but may forget about the exposure of body parts during a long tennis match or a baseball game, especially on a cloudy day, when up to 80% of the sun's radiation reaches the ground. Nurses should caution teens receiving any type of medication about the side effects related to sun exposure. Some medications may potentiate the sun's ultraviolet rays, resulting in quicker burning. The side effects of sunscreen products include itching, burning, and redness immediately or up to 24 hours after the product is applied. Some people are allergic or sensitive to the sunscreen agent (e.g., para-aminobenzoic acid [PABA], PABA esters, cinnamates, anthranilates, benzophenones) or

---

BOX 8-9	**ADOLESCENTS WANT TO KNOW** About Tattooing

- Carefully consider tattooing by talking with others about the process.
- Avoid making an impulsive decision about obtaining the tattoo, the location of the tattoo, or what the tattoo will represent.
- Understand that tattooing carries a risk for complications such as infection, allergic reaction to the dye, scarring or keloid formation, and blood-borne diseases such as

hepatitis B or HIV; be sure you are immunized against hepatitis B. Tattoos are permanent and are expensive and painful to remove.
- Check the artist's technique; be sure that all equipment is sterile, the artist wears gloves, and the artist displays a certificate of inspection by the health department.
- Be sure to obtain written instructions about caring for your skin after tattooing.

Data from American Academy of Dermatology. (2006). *Tattoos, body piercing and other skin adornments.* Retrieved April 6, 2006, from *www.aad.org.*

other ingredients used, such as fragrances or preservatives. Sunscreen use should be discontinued if an allergic dermatitis is noted, and the teen should try another type of sunscreen. Numerous products are on the market with various ingredients that have protective capabilities. Sun damage can be prevented, and simple measures can minimize the effects of ultraviolet radiation on the skin. Many products are available over the counter or through professional salons that have the look of a tan when applied. Nurses can encourage adolescents to use these products rather than expose themselves to ultraviolet light.

Sexual Activity

Adolescent Sexuality. Adolescent sexuality refers to the thoughts, feelings, and behaviors related to the adolescent's sexual identity. Middle adolescence typically marks the initial period of dating and experimentation with heterosexual and homosexual behaviors, although in some cultures sexual experimentation occurs much earlier. Initially, group dating may be popular, but this is quickly replaced by dating in couples, who might be sexual partners. Intimate relationships in middle adolescence are usually short lived as adolescents experiment with their sexual identity. Of greatest concern to parents during the adolescent's stage of sexual experimentation are unwanted pregnancies, STDs, and the teen's feelings of despair over failed relationships. Adolescents themselves are often impervious to the possibility of negative consequences of their sexual experimentation and believe that "it can't happen to me."

Although homosexual behavior in adolescence does not necessarily indicate that the adolescent will maintain a homosexual orientation, gay and lesbian adolescents face many challenges growing up in a society that is often unaccepting. Those adolescents who self-identify their sexual preference as homosexual during high school are at increased risk for a variety of health risks and problem behaviors, including suicide, victimization, risky sexual behaviors, and multiple substance abuse (Duncan, Dixon, & Carlson, 2003).

Most very young teens have not had intercourse. The likelihood of teenagers having vaginal intercourse increases with age, however. The Youth Risk Behavior Surveillance System showed that more than 7.4% of the group had sexual intercourse before age 13 years and that 46.7% of all adolescents had been involved in sexual activity (CDC, 2004). Adolescence is a period of risk taking, and many adolescents choose to be sexually active and do so unprotected. In addition, sexual activity in adolescents is greatly correlated with other risk behaviors, especially alcohol and other substance use, so nurses must approach the issue from multiple perspectives.

Some underlying themes influence whether an adolescent delays engaging in sexual activity. Adolescents who demonstrate high levels of self-esteem are more likely to delay intercourse. A stable family environment, parental monitoring, regular church attendance, higher income level, and a positive parent-child relationship are factors that contribute to an adolescent's delaying intercourse (Klein, 2005).

The adolescent's limited cognitive abilities or lack of abstract thinking may influence contraceptive practices. Adolescents who feel invulnerable to pregnancy often cannot assimilate and apply to themselves information about sexual behavior, conception, and birth control. Lack of self-esteem and peer pressure also play a role in determining adolescents' sexual behavior. Teens may use sex to feel loved or desired, and they may fear abandonment by a partner if sex is refused. Some teens lack correct reproductive information and do not plan ahead for sexual encounters. Sexual activity is often impulsive, erratic, and unplanned because the relationships are relatively short term.

Nurses in schools and community clinics are in a position to identify teens at risk for pregnancy and provide guidance with appropriate information and referral in a confidential atmosphere. Nurses should strongly encourage adolescents to discuss sexuality, sexual behavior, and contraception with their parents whenever possible but must guarantee confidentiality of communication.

School sex education programs have had varying success. Many are either abstinence based or protection based. A combination of providing information about protection methods while emphasizing the benefits of abstinence may be more successful than either emphasis alone (Klein, 2005; USDHHS, 2000).

The nurse's professional role is to ensure that adolescents have the knowledge, skills, and opportunities that enable them to make responsible decisions regarding sexual behavior. Education regarding sexuality and contraception should be oriented to the developmental level of the individual or group. The nurse uses primary preventive intervention by assisting adolescents to develop coping strategies to meet their needs in ways other than through sexual behavior.

Contraception. Complete protection from pregnancy and STDs is achievable only through sexual abstinence. Because approximately half of adolescents between ages 15 and 19 years are sexually active, however, nurses need to feel comfortable with managing health concerns related to sexuality. Comprehensive health care includes providing services for sexually active adolescents. Health care providers should provide screening for and management of STDs, contraceptive services, and psychosocial counseling.

In the United States, nearly 1 million teens unintentionally become pregnant annually, and of these pregnancies, nearly 50% end in abortion (USDHHS, 2000). The average age for girls to initiate sexual activity is between 15 and 17 years; this age is slightly earlier in black girls (Klein, 2005). Most teens do not seek contraceptive information for 1 year after first intercourse, resulting in unintended pregnancy frequently occurring within the first several months after intercourse is initiated (Klein, 2005). When educating adolescents about birth control methods, consultation with both partners together is ideal. Open communication between partners is essential, and decisions about contraception should be mutual. Both male and female adolescents need to assume responsibility for sexual behavior. Regardless of the method of birth control selected (Table 8-2), all

TABLE 8-2	Methods of Contraception for Adolescents	
Method	**Advantages**	**Disadvantages**
Chance (no protection)	No cost; requires no preparation	High failure rate No disease prevention
Abstinence (no sex)	No cost; requires no preparation	May be difficult for sexually active teens
Withdrawal (withdrawal of penis from vagina before ejaculation)	No cost; requires no preparation	High failure rate Requires control and motivation by male No disease prevention
Periodic Abstinence (rhythm; no sex during fertile/ovulation period)	No cost; natural family planning	High failure rate Requires awareness of fertility times, motivation, and predictable menstrual cycle No disease prevention
Condom (male: latex, or non-latex, penile sheath to trap sperm; female: sheath inserted into the vagina)	Male condoms are inexpensive; allows for planning; effective with spermicide Disease prevention Male condoms readily available over the counter	Moderate failure rate; should be used in conjunction with other contraceptive method Requires planning Non-latex condoms may be used if allergic to latex Best used with spermicide Requires new condom with each successive intercourse Female condom more difficult to insert, not widely available
Diaphragm (rubber cup covers cervix to prevent sperm from entering; used with spermicide)	Allows for planning; may be inserted before sexual intercourse Once fitted, relatively inexpensive Disease prevention	Requires planning Messy creams and jelly Requires motivation and consistency of use Requires medical intervention and prescription Requires knowledge for insertion and use Must be left in for a minimum of 6 hours after sex; more spermicide must be applied for each successive intercourse Increases risk for toxic shock syndrome if left in more than 24 hours
Spermicides (creams, jelly, foam, suppositories placed in vagina to kill sperm before it enters cervix)	Available over the counter Effective if used with barrier method Disease prevention Relatively inexpensive Allows for planning Prescription not required	Requires planning High failure rate if used alone Messy Must reapply with each successive intercourse
Oral Contraceptives (combination products: suppress ovulation, increase thickness of cervical mucus, decrease thickness of uterine lining)	Not tied to sexual activity Highly effective; failure rate is <1% Allows for planning	Medical intervention and prescription needed Requires knowledge for use Expensive for teens Side effects include weight gain, breakthrough bleeding during cycles (varies with pill and patient); needs to be avoided if at risk for thrombolytic or embolic disorders Usually requires pelvic exam and regular follow-up No disease prevention

Modified from Hatcher, J., Trussell, J., & Stewart, F. (1994). The essentials of contraception: effectiveness, safety, and personal considerations. In *Contraceptive technology* (p. 113). New York: Irvington Publishers, Inc.; American Academy of Pediatrics Committee on Adolescence. (1999). Contraception and adolescents. *Pediatrics, 101*(5), 1161-1166; As-Sanie, S., Gantt, A., & Rosenthal, M. (2004). Pregnancy prevention in adolescents. *American Family Physician, 70*(8), 1517-1524.

Continued

TABLE 8-2   Methods of Contraception for Adolescents—cont'd

Method	Advantages	Disadvantages
Contraceptive Patch (thickens the cervical mucus and suppresses ovulation; applied to skin in upper torso (not breasts), upper outer arm, buttocks or abdominal area)	Not tied to sexual activity Patch is worn continuously, changed weekly for 3 weeks, then 1 week off; no need to remember to take medication daily Highly effective	Prescription required and periodic medical evaluation Side effects include skin irritation, nausea, vomiting, headache, breast tenderness; usually disappear after continued use Usually covered by Medicaid Requires back-up contraceptive method if schedule of patching is not closely followed or the patch comes off inadvertently Risk for thromboembolitic event is higher than that for oral contraceptives related to increased estrogen exposure
Injectable Contraceptive (Depo-Provera [DMPA], injectable progestin given every 3 months: suppresses ovulation for 12 weeks; combined hormone injections given monthly)	Highly effective Not tied to sexual activity No planning once injection has been received for 3 months Stops menses in 50% of users Can be used with lactating females, those with selected cardiac disease or chronic illnesses, and drug addicts	Requires medical intervention and intramuscular injection May have delay in fertility after use Side effects of progestin: irregular, heavy, or no bleeding; headaches; weight gain; depression Expensive Should not be used longer than 2 years because of increased risk for osteoporosis
Emergency Contraceptive Pills (combined estrogen and progestin taken within 72 hours and again 12 hours later; Plan B®-progestin only)	Approximately 70% to 85% effective in preventing pregnancy, depending on the medication used and the elapsed time since intercourse	Should not be used as routine contraception Requires medical intervention Contraindicated in teens who cannot use oral contraceptives or if longer than 72 hours after intercourse Nausea is the main side effect Pregnancy test required if no menses after 3 weeks of taking the medication Most physicians will require counseling for STD prevention and routine contraception

---

CRITICAL TO REMEMBER

Factors to Consider in Selecting Adolescent Contraception

- Cognitive development (concrete vs. abstract thinking)
- Understanding and acceptance of attitudes and values
- Sexual maturity rating
- Communication between partners
- Opportunity to counsel both partners
- Use of more than one method
- Frequency of intercourse
- Appropriate information (three messages per visit)
- Problem-solving abilities (appeal to logic and feelings of power over body)
- Communication with parents or other adults
- Physical and mental health
- Motivation of both partners
- Concrete, graphic instruction in all methods
- Number and gender of partners
- Encouragement that abstinence is all right

adolescents need frequent follow-up to maintain consistent contraception behaviors. Counseling teens about sexuality and contraception requires nurses who are open, forthright, and respectful of the decisions teens make about sexual activity. (See Chapter 16 for information about STDs.)

KEY CONCEPTS

- Adolescence is a period of transition from childhood to adulthood that is marked by important biologic and psychologic changes.
- Biologic development during adolescence is variable. Primary and secondary sexual characteristics are acquired through the influence of reproductive hormones in males and females.
- SMRs (Tanner stages) are somewhat variable but predictable stages of sexual maturation that are based on pubic hair and breast development in girls and pubic hair and genital development in boys.

- According to Erikson, the major developmental task in adolescence is the development of an identity and self-perception. Other developmental tasks include the development of a sexual identity, avocational/educational identity, and independence and autonomy.
- Early and middle adolescents are egocentric and concerned with themselves.
- Cognitive thinking during adolescence moves from concrete to abstract reasoning.
- According to Kohlberg, adolescents and young adults develop a respect for law and order and a society-maintaining orientation.
- Adolescents question the values of family and society before integrating their experiences and beliefs into a personal moral framework.
- Adolescents may be emotionally labile, with extreme highs and extreme lows.
- The pace of physical growth during adolescence is second only to the pace of growth during infancy.
- Poor eating habits and lack of aerobic exercise contribute to obesity and decreased overall physical fitness.
- Tanning, body piercing, and tattooing are behaviors associated with identity formation.
- Risk-taking behavior is considered part of normal growth and development.
- Safety issues related to sports activity, sexual activity, firearms, and the use of motor vehicles should be emphasized.
- Sexual maturation precipitates sexual activity; teen pregnancy and STDs are related issues.

ANSWERS TO CRITICAL THINKING EXERCISE 8-1

1. The main issues will be confidentiality and trust. To establish trust, the nurse must be honest with Heidi. The nurse must be clear about the boundaries before the conversation continues. Depending on what Heidi tells the nurse, she may want to encourage Heidi to share the information with her parents. Finally, if the information has the potential to cause harm to either Heidi or others, it *cannot* be kept confidential.
2. A therapeutic response would be, "Heidi, I want you to feel comfortable talking with me. I will keep what you tell me confidential unless it is something that might be harmful to you or others."

REFERENCES AND READINGS

Akinbami, L., Gandhi, H., & Cheng, T. (2003). Availability of adolescent health services and confidentiality in primary care practices. *Pediatrics, 111*(2), 394-401.

American Academy of Dermatology. (2004). *American Academy of Dermatology issues statement endorsing the World Health Organization's recommendation to restrict tanning bed use.* Retrieved April 6, 2006, from *www.aad.org.*

American Academy of Dermatology. (2004). *American Academy of Dermatology urges teens to heed warnings on dangers of tanning.* Retrieved April 6, 2006, from *www.aad.org.*

American Academy of Dermatology. (2006). *Tattoos, body piercings and other skin adornments.* Retrieved April 6, 2006, from *www.aad.org.*

American Academy of Pediatrics. (2006). Dietary recommendations for children and adolescents: a guide for practitioners. *Pediatrics, 117*(2), 544-559.

American Academy of Pediatrics Committee on Adolescence. (1999). Contraception and adolescents. *Pediatrics, 101*(5), 1161-1166.

American Cancer Society. (2005). *World Health Organization warns teens on tanning beds.* Retrieved April 6, 2006, from *www.cancer.org.*

American Heart Association. (2006). *Dietary guidelines for healthy children.* Retrieved March 30, 2006, from *www.americanheart.org.*

American Heart Association. (2006). *Vegetarian diets.* Retrieved March 30, 2006, from *www.americanheart.org.*

American Medical Association. (1997). *Guideline for adolescent preventive services (GAPS) recommendations monographs.* Retrieved April 6, 2006, from *www.ama-assn.org.*

Anderson, S., Dallal, G., & Must, A. (2003). Relative weight and race influence average at menarche: results from two nationally representative surveys of U.S. girls studied 25 years apart. *Pediatrics, 111*(4), 844-850.

As-Sanie, S. Gantt, A., & Rosenthal, M. (2004). Pregnancy prevention in adolescents. *American Family Physician, 70*(8), 1517-1524. Retrieved April 6, 2006, from *www.aafp.org/afp.*

Boekeloo, B., & Howard, D. (2002). Oral sexual experience among young adolescents receiving general health examinations. *American Journal of Health Behavior, 26*(4), 306-314.

Brooks, T., Woods, E., Knight, J., & Shrier, L. (2005). Body modification and substance use in adolescence: is there a link? *Journal of Adolescent Health, 32*(1), 44-49.

Browne, K., & Hamilton-Giachristis, C. (2005). Influence of violent media on children and adolescents: a public health approach. *Lancet, 365,* 702-710.

Callaghan, D. (2005). The influence of spiritual growth on adolescents' initiative and responsibility for self-care. *Pediatric Nursing, 31*(2), 91-96.

Carroll, R., Riffenburgh, R., Roberts, T., & Myhre, E. (2002). Tattoos and body piercings as indicators of adolescent risk-taking behaviors. *Pediatrics, 109*(6), 1021-1028.

Center for HIV Identification, Prevention, and Treatment Services: *HEADSS for adolescents.* (n.d.). Retrieved April 6, 2006, from *chipts.ucla.edu/assessment/Assessment_Instruments/Assessment_files_new/assess_headss.htm.*

Centers for Disease Control and Prevention. (2003). Deaths: leading causes for 2001. *National Vital Statistics Reports, 52*(9), 13.

Centers for Disease Control and Prevention. (2004). Youth risk behavior surveillance—United States, 2003. *MMWR: Morbidity and Mortality Weekly Report, 53*(SS02).

Centers for Disease Control and Prevention. (2005). *Physical activity and the health of young people.* Retrieved April 1, 2006, from *www.cdc.gov/HealthyYouth/PhysicalActivity.*

Centers for Disease Control and Prevention, National Center for Chronic Disease Prevention and Health Promotion, Division of Adolescent and School Health, Health Resources and Services Administration, Maternal and Child Health Bureau, Office of Adolescent Health, National Adolescent Health Information Center, University of California, San Francisco. (2004). *Executive summary—improving the health of adolescents and young adults: a goal for states and communities.* Atlanta, GA: Authors.

Chumlea, W. C., Schubert, C. M., Roche, A. F., Kulin, H. E., Lee, P. A., Himes, J. H., & Sun, S. S. (2003). Age at menarche and racial comparisons in U.S. girls. *Pediatrics, 111*(1), 110-113.

Cohen, E., MacKenzie, R., & Yates, G. (1991). HEADSS, a psychosocial risk assessment instrument: implications for designing effective intervention programs for runaway youths. *Journal of Adolescent Health, 12*(7), 539-544.

Demko, C., Borawski, E., Debanne, S., Cooper, K., & Stange, K. (2003). Use of indoor tanning facilities by white adolescents in the United States. *Archives of Pediatric and Adolescent Medicine, 157,* 854-860.

Deschesnes, M., Fines, P., & Demers, S. (2005). Are tattooing and body piercing indicators of risk-taking behaviors among high school students? *Journal of Adolescence, 29*(3), 379-393.

Duncan, P., Dixon, R., & Carlson, J. (2003). Childhood and adolescent sexuality. *Pediatric Clinics of North America, 50*(4), 765-780.

Elfenbein, D., & Felice, M. (2003). Adolescent pregnancy. *Pediatric Clinics of North America, 50*(4), 781-800.

Elkind, D. (1993). *Parenting your teenager.* New York: Ballantine Books.

Erikson, E. (1968). *Identity: youth and crisis.* New York: Norton.

Feroli, K. (2003). Adolescent sexually transmitted diseases: new recommendations for diagnosis, treatment, and prevention. *MCN: The American Journal of Maternal/Child Nursing, 28*(2), 113-118.

Halpern-Fisher, B., Cornell, J., Kropp, R., & Tschann, J. (2005). Oral versus vaginal sex among adolescents: perceptions, attitudes, and behavior. *Pediatrics, 115*(4), 845-851.

Hansen, M., Jannssen, I., Schiff, A., Zee, P., & Dubocovich, M. (2005). The impact of school daily schedule on adolescent sleep. *Pediatrics, 115*(6), 1555-1561.

Herman-Giddens, M., Kaplowitz, P., & Wasserman, R. (2004). Navigating the recent articles on girls' puberty in pediatrics: what do we know and where do we go from here? *Pediatrics, 113*(4), 911-917.

Herrman, J. (2005). The teen brain as a work in progress: implications for pediatric nurses. *Pediatric Nursing, 31*(2), 144-147.

Klein, J., & the Committee on Adolescence. (2005). Adolescent pregnancy: current trends and issues. *Pediatrics, 116*(1), 281-286.

Mangels, R. (2003). *Vegetarian nutrition for teenagers.* Retrieved March 30, 2006, from *www.vrg.org.*

Marshall, W. A., & Tanner, J. (1969). Variations in pattern of pubertal changes in girls. *Archives of Disease in Childhood, 44*(235), 291-303.

National Center for Health Statistics. (2003). *Health, United States, 2003.* Retrieved November 1, 2003, from *www.cdc.gov/nchs.*

Ozer, E., Adams, S. H., Lustig, J. L., Gee, S., Garber, A. K., Gardner, L. R., Rehbein, M., Addison, L., & Irwin, C. F., Jr. (2005). Increasing the screening and counseling of adolescents for risky health behaviors: a primary care intervention. *Pediatrics, 115*(4), 960-968.

Piaget, J. (1969). *The theory of stages in cognitive development.* New York: McGraw-Hill.

Prazer, G. E., & Friedman, S. B. (1997). An office-based approach to adolescent psychosocial issues. *Contemporary Pediatrics, 14*(5), 59-76.

Roberts, T., & Ryan, S. (2002). Tattooing and high-risk behavior in adolescents. *Pediatrics, 110*(6), 1058-1064.

Schneider, M. (2005). Limits to adolescents' indoor tanning access varies by state. *Family Practice News, 35*(20), 74.

Selekman, J. (2003). A new era of body decoration: what are kids doing to their bodies? *Pediatric Nursing, 29*(1), 77-80.

Tanner, J. (1962). *Growth at adolescence* (2nd ed.). Oxford: Blackwell Scientific Publications.

United States Department of Agriculture. (2005). *Dietary guidelines for Americans, 2005, Appendix A-1: the DASH eating plan at 1,600-, 2,000-, 2,600-, and 3,100- calorie levels.* Retrieved March 30, 2006, from *www.health.gov/dietaryguidelines/.*

U.S. Department of Health and Human Services. (2000). *Healthy People 2010.* Washington, DC: Author.

CHAPTER 9

Physical Assessment of Children

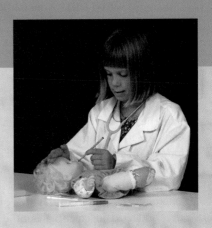

Learning Objectives

After studying this chapter, you should be able to:

- Apply principles of anatomy and physiology to the systematic physical assessment of the child.
- Describe the major components of a pediatric health history.
- Identify the principal techniques for doing a physical examination.
- Use a systematic and developmentally appropriate approach for examining a child.
- Describe the general sequence of the physical examination of the infant, the young child, the school-age child, and the adolescent.
- Describe normal physical examination findings.
- List common terms used to describe the findings on physical examination.
- Record physical examination findings in a systematic way.

Definitions

auscultation Elicitation and evaluation of sounds produced by the body, frequently by using a stethoscope to magnify body sounds.

circumduction Circular movement of a limb or an eye.

crepitation A dry, crackling sound or sensation.

development Changes that occur over time in function and psychosocial and cognitive behavior.

fasciculation A small, local, involuntary muscular contraction visible under the skin.

fremitus A vibration perceptible on palpation or auscultation.

growth Measurable physical and physiologic changes that occur over time.

history The aggregate of subjective data that describe past and present health status.

inspection Careful observation to identify physical findings.

obtund To render dull or blunt.

palpation The use of touch to determine factors such as texture, temperature, moisture, and organ size and location.

percussion Tapping of the body to determine the density, location, and size of organs.

systematic assessment Organized method of collecting data.

Audio Glossary

Electronic Resources

Additional information related to the content in Chapter 9 can be found on:

the interactive companion CD-ROM

- Animations: Abdominal Anatomy
  Cranial Nerves
  Organ Systems 3D Tour
- Audio Glossary
- NCLEX Review Questions
- Pediatric Assessment Video Clips
- Skills: Measuring Body Temperature
  Measuring Physical Growth

or the companion website at *evolve*
http://evolve.elsevier.com/james/ncoc

- NCLEX Review Questions
- Pediatric Assessment Video Clips
- WebLinks

Nurses perform physical assessments of infants and children in various settings—the clinic, the hospital, the school, and the home. The physical examination may be part of a well-child assessment, it may be the admission examination when a child enters the hospital, or it may be part of an initial assessment for home health care. The physical examination provides objective and subjective information about the child. The ability to perform a physical examination is fundamental to nursing care of the child and the nurse should not use short cuts or relinquish the physical examination. It allows health care providers to determine the child's health status, provide appropriate education, and make judgments about the need for nursing care.

GENERAL APPROACHES TO PHYSICAL ASSESSMENT

As when providing any nursing care for infants and children, the nurse applies knowledge of growth and development when preparing the child and performing the examination. Parents should be involved as much as possible, and the child should be encouraged to handle and play with instruments that are safe and clean, such as the stethoscope.

The physical examination is often the first direct contact between the nurse and the child. Establishing a trusting relationship between the child and the examiner is important. Throughout the examination the nurse should be sensitive to the cultural needs of and differences among children. Providing a quiet, private environment for the history and physical examination is important. The classic systematic approach to the physical examination is to begin at the head and proceed through the entire body to the toes. When examining a child, however, the examiner tailors the physical assessment to the child's age and developmental level.

> ### CRITICAL TO REMEMBER
> #### Adapting the Physical Examination to the Child
> The classic systematic approach to the physical examination is to begin at the head and proceed to the toes. For children, painful or frightening procedures should be left until last. Involving parents by asking them to hold or stand by the child can decrease children's anxiety and assist them in relaxing.

Infants Birth to 6 Months

Infants aged 1 to 6 months are responsive to human faces, are increasingly interested in their environment, and do not mind being undressed (see Chapter 5). Their examination should therefore be relatively easy. If the infant is nursing or asleep in the parent's arms, auscultate the heart, lungs, and abdomen without waking the baby. If the baby is awake, lay the baby on the examining table with the parent close by. As body parts are examined, incorporate evaluation of the primitive reflexes—palmar grasp, plantar grasp, placing, stepping, and tonic neck reflexes. Leave all uncomfortable procedures, such as abduction of the hips, speculum examination of the tympanic membranes, and eliciting the Moro reflex, until last. Before beginning the examination, undress the infant, leaving the diaper on a male child. Refocus an

unhappy infant by calmly talking in a soft voice, distracting with a rattle, or offering a pacifier.

Infants 6 to 12 Months

For an older infant, follow the same procedures used for the infant from birth to 6 months, but keep in mind that infants 6 months and older feel stranger anxiety and so are more difficult to examine. Distracting a child of this age with a toy or object may be useful. It is easier to do as much of the examination as possible with the child held on the parent's lap. Leave ear, oral, and other uncomfortable procedures until last.

Toddlers

Toddlers are the most challenging to examine because they are least likely to cooperate (see Chapter 6). To form a supportive relationship with the parent and toddler, the examiner begins by sitting or standing next to the parent. To facilitate relaxation, the examiner can provide a few toys and books and encourage the child to explore. Allowing the child to handle objects used during the examination can decrease fears. Communicating with the child, using age-appropriate words to describe what is about to be done, can also help decrease fear.

Portions of the examination can be done before the child is totally undressed. The order of the examination is flexible, and painful or frightening procedures should be left for last. Resistance and crying are common with toddlers. Assure the parent that the child's response to the examination is normal. The parent is the best assistant and can be asked, if willing, to hold the child's outstretched arms against the child's head or abdomen while the examiner's body immobilizes the lower half of the child's body.

Preschoolers

The preschool child is usually more cooperative, but these children still like to have their parents nearby (see Chapter 6). Preschool children are happy to show nurses that they can undress themselves. They can also be expected to cooperate. The nurse may proceed with the examination from the head to the toes but should still save the more invasive procedures, such as the speculum ear examination and the oral examination, until last. The examiner can reinforce the child's interest by allowing the child to participate in the examination and by praising the child for cooperating.

School-Age Children

To establish trust with the school-age child, the examiner asks the child questions the child can answer. Children in elementary school will talk about school, favorite friends, and activities (see Chapter 7). Older school-age children may have to be encouraged to talk about their school performance and activities. The examiner encourages the parent to support and reinforce the child's participation in the examination.

The examination proceeds from head to toe. Children of this age prefer a simple drape over their underpants or a colorful examination gown, and the examiner should be sensitive to the child's modesty. The examination is a wonderful opportunity to teach the child about the body and personal care. The nurse answers questions openly and in simple terms.

Community-based clinics promote optimal health in their clients. Children and their parents can develop a continuing relationship with a provider, which encourages them to return for needed care in both health and illness. This 2-year-old girl is having a routine checkup at the clinic today.

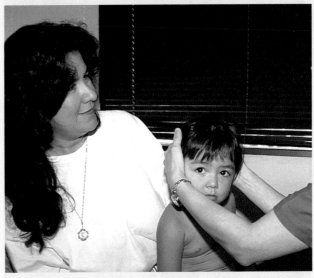

Communication and enlisting the trust of the child are vital elements in a successful physical examination. The girl remains in the security of her mother's arms as the nurse assesses her head. The little girl's anterior fontanel is not quite fully closed. The nurse reassures her mother that, although the fontanel is usually closed by 18 months of age, her child's open fontanel likely represents a normal variation. Note that the nurse is at the mother's eye level and makes eye contact with her, promoting effective communication.

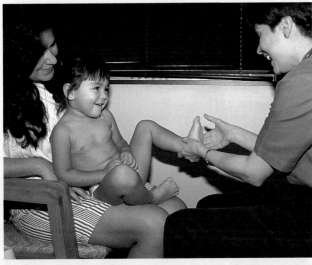

The nurse examines the child's feet for the presence of normal or abnormal reflexes and for straightness.

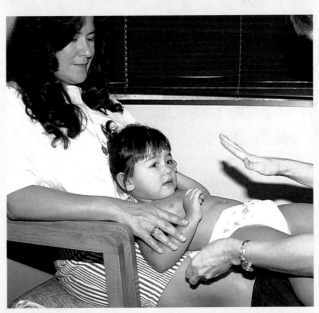

To limit the child's stress, the nurse creates an "examination table" by placing her knees next to the mother's knees. The child then lies across their laps as the nurse examines her thorax and abdomen.

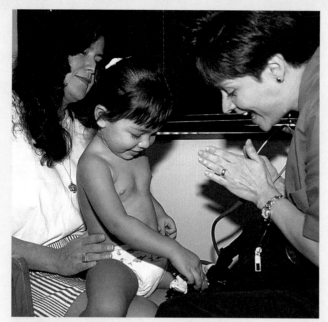

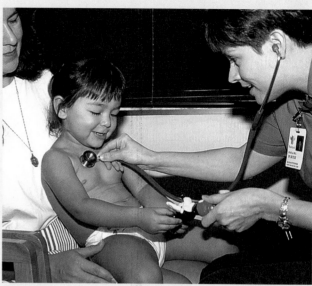

Allowing the child to check Mickey Mouse with a stethoscope before the nurse auscultates her chest enlists the child's cooperation and reduces her stress. This effort is especially important for assessments that are best done when the child is quiet. As the nurse auscultates her chest, the child is distracted by handling Mickey. Toddlers must be prepared for procedures immediately before they occur because a toddler's attention span is so short.

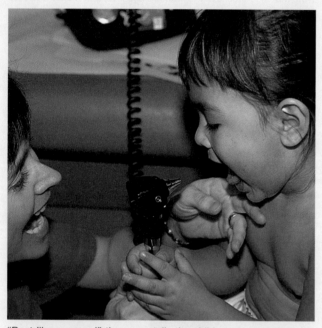

"Pant like a puppy!" the nurse tells the child as she examines her mouth and throat. Incorporating play and fun into examinations promotes the child's trust in the nurse and enlists her cooperation.

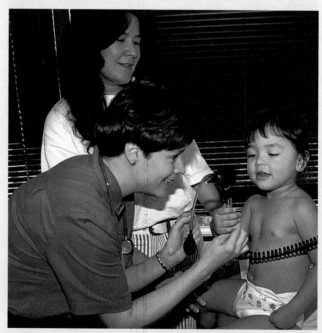

As in other examinations, the nurse helps the child examine the otoscope just before she uses it to examine her ears.

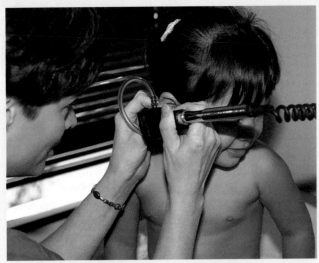

The nurse deftly examines the child's ears, pulling her pinna down and back. Ear examinations are especially important during the toddler years to identify fluid accumulation in the middle ear, which can interfere with hearing and speech development.

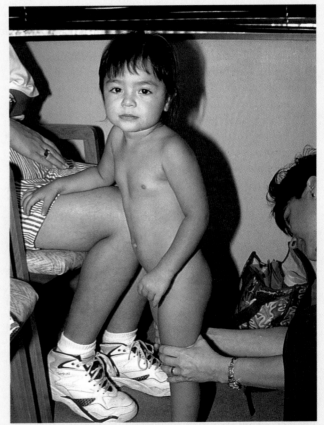

The nurse concludes the examination by checking the unclothed child for normal genital development, straightness of her spine and extremities, and evidence of previously undiagnosed hip dysplasia. To identify problems in motor development, the nurse observes the child's gait.

The nurse determines that this little girl's development is appropriate for her age. She is tall, like her mother, so the cherubic toddler appearance is less apparent than it might otherwise be. The nurse shares her findings as she does the examination and summarizes them for the mother at the end. Because the child is developing normally, she does not need to return to the clinic for a checkup until she is 3 years old.

(Photos courtesy Parkland Health and Hospital System Community Oriented Primary Care Clinic.)

Adolescents

Adolescents are most comfortable with a straightforward, uncondescending approach (see Chapter 8). Decisions about who should be present during the examination should be openly discussed with the adolescent. In most cases adolescents should be examined without the parent present. However, the parent should be given the opportunity to talk to the nurse about any concerns. The order of the examination is the same as for the school-age child.

It is best to incorporate the genital examination into the middle of the examination. If possible, proceed from the abdominal examination to the genital examination, to allow ample time for questions and discussions about this part of the examination. The physical examination provides the opportunity to assure the pubertal child about normal developmental stages and to answer concerns children this age frequently have about what is happening to their bodies. The adolescent is expected to undress and wear a gown. The adolescent is draped appropriately during the examination.

TECHNIQUES FOR PHYSICAL EXAMINATION

When performing the physical assessment, the nurse uses the four basic techniques of inspection, palpation, percussion, and auscultation, in that order. During the abdominal examination, the sequence is altered: inspection is performed first, and then auscultation, percussion, and palpation. The sequence of the abdominal examination is changed so as not to alter bowel sounds before determining their presence and characteristics. Percussion is performed to determine the size of abdominal organs before palpation.

Inspection

Most information is gathered during the physical examination by systematic and deliberate visual observations. The nurse first surveys an entire area of the body and then focuses on specifics, such as color, shape, size, or movement. Inspection can be both direct and indirect. Direct inspection relies on the examiner's senses of sight and hearing. Indirect inspection is accomplished with the use of special equipment, such as an otoscope, to examine a specific body area.

Palpation

During palpation, the nurse uses the sense of touch to make judgments about pulsations and vibrations and to locate structures and masses. Palpation allows the nurse to determine characteristics such as size, texture, warmth, mobility, and tenderness of various areas of the body.

Different parts of the hands are used to detect different characteristics. The fingertips are used to palpate the breast, lymph nodes, and pulses. The back of the hand is used to assess temperature. The palm of the hand is used to detect vibrations.

The type of palpation used is governed by the structure to be examined and the need to avoid any unnecessary discomfort to the child. Light palpation is accomplished by gently applying fingertip pressure to depress the skin surface approximately ½ to ¾ inch and then moving the fingertips in a circular motion.

CRITICAL TO REMEMBER

Using the Hands for Palpation

- Fingertips are used to palpate the breast, lymph nodes, and pulses.
- The back of the hand is used to assess temperature.
- The palm of the hand is used to identify vibrations.

Deep palpation identifies abdominal structures such as the liver, spleen, and kidneys and detects abdominal masses. Deep palpation follows light palpation. The surface is depressed approximately 1½ to 2 inches to identify underlying masses and abdominal structures. Bimanual palpation is performed with both hands. The examiner superimposes one hand over the other to increase pressure or places one hand near the other to capture and trap a mass or structure between them, such as the kidneys or spleen.

Percussion

To percuss, the nurse uses quick, sharp tapping of the fingers or hands to produce sounds. Percussion is performed to locate the position, size, and density of underlying structures. The three basic methods are:

- *Mediate*, or *indirect, percussion*, in which the finger of one hand is placed against the body surface and the finger of the other hand acts as the hammer
- *Immediate percussion*, performed by striking the finger of one hand directly against the body
- *Fist percussion*, in which the ulnar aspect of the fist is used to deliver a firm blow directly to the area

The method used depends on the area to be percussed. The nurse uses quick, light blows to create vibrations that penetrate approximately 2 inches below the surface. Sounds identified by percussion are classified as *flat, dull, resonant, hyperresonant,* or *tympanic* (Box 9-1).

Auscultation

Auscultation entails eliciting and listening to body sounds created in the lungs, heart, blood vessels, and abdominal viscera. The most common way to auscultate is to use a stethoscope. Most auscultated sounds result from air or fluid movement within the body. The diaphragm of the stethoscope is most effective in assessing high-pitched sounds, such

---

| BOX 9-1 | **Sounds Identified When Percussing** |

- *Flat:* high-pitched, soft-intensity sound elicited by percussing over solid masses, such as bone or muscle
- *Dull:* medium-pitched, medium-intensity sound elicited when percussing over high-density structures, such as the liver
- *Resonance:* low-pitched, loud-intensity sound elicited over a hollow organ, such as the lungs
- *Hyperresonance:* very low, very loud, with a booming quality heard over the lungs in young children
- *Tympany:* high-pitched, loud-intensity sound heard over air-filled body parts, such as the bowel or stomach

as heart and breath sounds. The bell of the stethoscope is most effective in hearing low-pitched sounds, such as blood pressure and vascular sounds. Auscultation requires a quiet environment. The nurse places the stethoscope on the skin in the appropriate area. Sounds heard are described according to pitch, intensity, duration, and quality.

Smell

While examining the child, the nurse uses the sense of smell to detect general body odors, common in children who are neglected or dirty. Odor may also indicate infection. Odors from the mouth, urine, or feces can be important. In particular, some diseases are characterized by odors coming from the mouth (Seidel, Ball, Dains, & Benedict, 2003).

SEQUENCE OF PHYSICAL EXAMINATION
General Appearance

During the first contact with the child and parent, the examiner forms an initial impression by making a general survey. The nurse determines the child's age, sex, and race and identifies clues concerning the child's behavior and health status. Because each child is a unique human, individual differences in behavior and health status related to growth and development will be evident. During the general survey, the examiner continually notes the parent-child interaction and the way the parent responds to the child's needs and behavior. Physical and emotional neglect as well as inadequate parental supervision for the child's age may be subtle or overt. These, together with other indicators of the child's health status, may provide clues to distress or abuse (Box 9-2).

History Taking

Taking an accurate history is the single most important component of the physical examination. Practitioners obtain three different types of health histories: the complete, or initial, history; the well, interim history; and the episodic, or problem-oriented, history.

In the *complete*, or *initial, history* (Box 9-3), data are gathered about the child from the time of conception to the

---

CRITICAL THINKING EXERCISE 9-1

Ann Maloney, a 17-year-old single mother, brings her 6-month-old daughter, Kerrie, to the clinic. This is Kerrie's first visit. Ms. Maloney had made several earlier appointments for Kerrie but was always unable to keep them. She states, "I am very busy trying to work and care for Kerrie. I have had to miss work because Kerrie has had lots of colds. I hate to take time off when she is well. My supervisor at work said that it was important for her to have her immunizations and a physical examination. I guess I messed up."

1. What assumptions could the nurse make about Ms. Maloney?
2. How should the nurse respond to Ms. Maloney's comment?
3. How can the nurse best act as an advocate for both Kerrie and her mother?

child's current status. The *well, interim history* includes data gathered about the child from the last well visit to the current visit. When doing a well, interim history, the examiner assumes that a database is in place. In a *problem-oriented*, or *episodic, history* (Box 9-4), information is gathered about a current problem. Information about the specific problem is then added to the existing database.

Recording Data

The information gathered during the history is documented concisely to provide all necessary information from pregnancy to the child's current status. Milestones in growth and development, immunizations, and family status are always included in the child's history.

Vital Signs

Vital signs are taken on every child at every visit in ambulatory settings and are monitored throughout the day in a hospitalized child. Assessment of vital signs (temperature, pulse, respirations, blood pressure) is an important way to measure and monitor vital body functions. Measuring vital signs provides the basis for decisions concerning the child's overall health and illness. In children, changes in vital signs are important signs of changes in health status. Table 9-1 describes normal vital signs by age, and Chapter 13 details the procedure for taking vital signs in children.

Temperature

The method for measuring children's temperature may vary from one setting to another. Some parents are comfortable taking a rectal or axillary temperature. Health care providers may use a tympanic membrane sensor or an electronic or digital thermometer. Currently, parents are encouraged to take axillary rather than rectal temperatures. Reasons for the recommendation are the invasive nature of rectal temperature measurements, the risk of injury, and their questionable accuracy with febrile children because feces retain body heat for hours after a fever has diminished. Axillary temperatures,

---

BOX 9-2	**Potential Indicators of Child Abuse**

- *Dress:* inappropriate for the weather; ragged or excessively dirty
- *Grooming and personal hygiene:* dirty teeth; broken and dirty fingernails; matted and dirty hair
- *Posture and movements:* crouching in a corner; slow, concentrated movements
- *Body image distortion:* being thin but describing self as fat
- *Speech and communication:* answering questions in words of one syllable; looking to others to respond first; seeking approval for answers
- *Facial characteristics and expressions:* fearful, anxious, tearful, sad, or angry expressions
- *Psychologic state:* labile, demanding, bizarre, overly dramatic, or condescending

BOX 9-3	The Complete History

The complete or initial history includes the following:

1. *Statistical information:* Name, age, address, telephone number, Social Security number, names of parents or guardians, and source of support.
2. *Client profile:* Times the child eats and sleeps, educational level, developmental level, race and nationality, religion, economic status, and health status perception. If an interpreter is used to gather the health history, the person's name is included in the record, usually in this section of the history. Also included is a statement about the reliability of an informant, such as an older sibling who answers questions concerning a younger sibling or an aunt or uncle who answers questions regarding a child visiting him or her.
3. *Health history:* Birth history, growth and development, common childhood illnesses, immunizations, previous hospitalizations, accidents or injuries, and allergies or allergic reactions and exact symptoms the allergy produced. The person taking the history should ask about medications taken daily or for an acute episode of an illness and should list all medications being taken, including dose and frequency. The parent should name both prescription and over-the-counter medications. The examiner also asks if the child has ever had a blood transfusion or has received any blood products. For any hospitalizations, serious illnesses, and injuries, the nurse should obtain the following information:
   a. Reason for admission
   b. Place of admission
   c. Length of stay
   d. Surgical procedures
   e. Outcomes
   f. Other
4. *Family history:* Information concerning the health status of the child's mother, father, siblings, and specific blood relatives such as aunts, uncles, and grandparents. If any are deceased, the history includes the age and cause of death. The purpose is to determine constitutional and hereditary factors that are likely to affect the child's health.
5. *Lifestyle and life patterns:* The child's interaction with the social, psychologic, physical, and cultural environment. Growth and development; use of street drugs, alcohol, and tobacco; roles and relationships; and family life information are all important.
6. *Review of systems:* A systematic review of the major anatomic and physiologic parts. A head-to-toe review focusing on the health function and maintenance of each body part should occur in this order:
   a. General appearance
   b. Head
   c. Hair
   d. Face
   e. Eyes
   f. Ears
   g. Nose and sinuses
   h. Mouth
   i. Throat
   j. Neck
   k. Lungs
   l. Heart
   m. Breasts
   n. Abdomen
   o. Kidneys and bladder
   p. Bowels, rectum, and anus
   q. Genitals
   r. Extremities

BOX 9-4	Problem-Oriented History

- *Chief complaint:* Use the child's own words.
- *Body location:* Place the problem somewhere on the body.
- *Quality:* Define what the problem is like for the child.
- *Quantity:* Describe the intensity of the problem for the child.
- *Chronology:* Determine when the problem began, the periodicity and frequency, and the course of symptoms.
- *Setting:* Identify where the problem occurs.
- *Aggravating and alleviating factors:* Find out what makes the problem better or worse.
- *Associated manifestations:* Document other related information.
- *Treatment:* Document what has been used to treat the problem. Be sure to ask about complementary therapies as well as traditional approaches.

when taken correctly, provide accurate information concerning changes in the child's health status.

Tympanic temperature measurements are frequently used in health care agencies because they can be performed quickly and involve less cross contamination; however, they may not be as accurate in detecting fever in infants and young children (Houlder, 2000). When recording a tympanic temperature, the nurse notes the side on which the temperature was elicited. Variation can occur from one ear to the other in the same child.

An oral thermometer may be used with older children, usually at 5 or 6 years old. For oral temperature measurements, an electronic thermometer is unbreakable and registers quickly but it may not be available (see Chapter 13 for a discussion of various methods of assessing temperature).

The TemporalScanner Thermometer (Exergin Corp., Watertown, Massachusetts) is a totally noninvasive system with advanced infrared technology. This new technology measures temperatures with a gentle stroke across the forehead. This thermometer can be used with neonates, infants, children, or adolescents. As the probe crosses over the temporal artery,

TABLE 9-1 Normal Vital Signs by Age					
	Temperature*		**Pulse Rate (beats/min)**	**Respiratory Rate (breaths/min)**	**Blood Pressure Range (mm Hg)**
Age	**Degrees Fahrenheit**	**Degrees Celsius**			
Newborn	96.8-99 (axillary)	36-37.2 (axillary)	120-160	30-60	Systolic: 60-99† Diastolic: 30-62†
4 yr	97.5-98.6 (axillary)	36.4-37 (axillary)	80-125	20-30	*Girls* Systolic: 91-104 Diastolic: 52-66 *Boys* Systolic: 93-107 Diastolic: 50-65
10 yr	97.5-98.6 (oral)	36.4-37 (oral)	70-110‡	16-22	*Girls* Systolic: 102-115 Diastolic: 60-74 *Boys* Systolic: 102-115 Diastolic: 61-75
16 yr	97.5-98.6 (oral)	36.4-37 (oral)	55-90	15-20	*Girls* Systolic: 111-124 Diastolic: 66-80 *Boys* Systolic: 116-130 Diastolic: 65-80

*The normal range of the child's temperature will depend on the method used. Temperatures exhibit circadian rhythms at all ages. Blood pressures represent values for the 50th and 90th percentiles at age and average height.
†Taken by Doppler measurement.
‡After age 12 yr, a boy's pulse is 5 beats/min slower than a girl's.

the sensor in its probe measures ambient temperatures, mathematically replaces the small temperature loss from cooling at the skin, and displays an accurate arterial temperature.

Pulse

Apical pulse rates are taken in children younger than 2 years old and in any child who has an irregular heart rate or known congenital heart disease. Radial pulse rates may be taken in children older than 2 years. To compensate for normal irregularities, the nurse counts the pulse for 1 full minute. Chapter 13 details the procedure for measuring pulse.

Arterial pulses are palpated to determine pulse rate and rhythm and to evaluate blood flow, arterial wall elasticity, and vessel patency. To determine the position of the heart in the anterior precordium, the nurse palpates the apical impulse in infants and children younger than 6 years old. In the acute care setting, an apical impulse is always palpated on every child and the location of the apical impulse is noted. Simultaneously, the examiner palpates and compares femoral, radial, and carotid pulses on children of any age. The nurse may also compare a carotid pulse with a femoral or radial pulse for equality of pulses. In infants, the nurse notes the pulsating anterior fontanel. The pulse may be increased significantly above normal in infants and children with anxiety, fever, exercise, inflammatory illnesses, shock, or heart disease. The resting heart rate changes with increasing age.

The rhythm of the heartbeat is assessed for equal spacing between consecutive beats. Irregular cardiac rhythms are not uncommon in children and are often related to changes in rhythm that occur in response to respiratory inspiration and expiration.

Respirations

The nurse observes the rate, depth, and ease of respiration in the child. Respirations vary with age. The respiratory rate, like the heart rate, is significantly influenced by emotion and exercise. In infants, the rate may be determined by observing abdominal excursion. In toddlers and older children, the nurse observes thoracic excursion. Because the movements are irregular, the rate should be assessed for 1 minute in infants and young children. Respirations are best counted when the child is not paying attention to the examiner. Respirations should be counted while the examiner continues to keep fingers on a pulse or the stethoscope on the chest, as though checking the pulses. This effort will ensure that the child is unaware that the examiner is counting respirations.

The depth and rhythm of respirations are determined subjectively and compared with norms for a particular age group. The ease or difficulty of respirations is a somewhat subjective observation. Respirations should be quiet and appear effortless. *Stridor*—a crowing noise heard on inspiration and heard louder over the neck—is worrisome in a child and may be a sign of croup or epiglottitis (see Chapter 21). Inspiratory stridor indicates a partial obstruction of the airway. Continuous inspiratory and expiratory stridor may be related to delayed development of the cartilage in the tracheal rings or to a relatively small larynx.

Blood Pressure

Blood pressure measurements are taken on all children at every ambulatory visit; in an acute-care setting, blood pressure is measured at least daily, and often more frequently, depending on the child's condition. The appropriate-size cuff must be used to auscultate the blood pressure. Blood pressure measurements in healthy ambulatory children are compared with standard norms (see Table 9-1 for the effects of age on vital signs). An auscultated blood pressure measurement that is equal to or exceeds the 90th percentile for the child's sex, height, and age (see Appendix C) must be confirmed before describing the child as being hypertensive. An average of at least three abnormal blood pressure measurements taken on separate occasions requires further evaluation. If an adolescent's blood pressure is greater than 120/80 mm Hg, the adolescent is considered to be prehypertensive even if this value is below the 90th percentile (AAP, 2004).

The size of the cuff is important. Cuffs that are too small will cause falsely elevated values; those that are too large will cause inaccurate low values (see Chapter 13 for determining appropriate cuff size). Several determinations may be needed to obtain values unaffected by anxiety. Instructing the child that the "balloon" will gently squeeze the arm or give the arm a "hug" will usually decrease anxiety. To alleviate anxiety, the child can also assist with taking a blood pressure on a doll, a stuffed animal, or the parent.

Anthropometric Measurement

Anthropometrics entails measuring the human body and assessing nutritional status as well as growth and development. Weight, height, and head circumference are always measured in children and are compared with averages for age group and sex. The amount of body fat should be measured on the basis of the body mass index (BMI), which is calculated according to a simple formula:

$$BMI = \frac{Weight \ (kg)}{Height \ (m)^2} \quad or \quad BMI = \frac{Weight \ (lb) \times 703}{Height \ (in)^2}$$

BMI tables can be accessed at *www.cdc.gov/nccdphp/dnpa/bmi/00binaries/bmi-tables.pdfhildren*. Midarm muscle circumference, skinfold thickness, and weight provide information about three body tissues (subcutaneous tissue, muscle, fat) altered by nutrition. Because children's body fat varies with age and sex, anthropometric measurements are most valuable when they are plotted on a growth curve and evaluated serially so that trends can be monitored.

Measuring height and weight are routine procedures that provide valuable information about a child's health. Children grow and develop rapidly, and this growth and development must be constantly evaluated. Physical measurements of a child reflect the rate of growth; a failure in growth, an acceleration in growth, or any change in growth pattern may be the first clue to serious problems. A child's falling off the child's own growth curve is the most significant indicator of changing health status. Measurements must be correct and accurate and are taken at every visit from birth to adulthood.

CRITICAL TO REMEMBER
Importance of Anthropometric Measurements

Anthropometric measurements reflect any change in the growth pattern and may be the first clue to a serious problem. Measurements must be taken at every health care visit from birth to adulthood. A child's falling off his or her own growth curve is a significant indicator of changing health status.

Height

The methods of measuring a child vary with the child's age. Infant and toddler length is best measured with the child lying down on a flat measuring board. This method is used until the child is able to stand independently. The child's head is held securely to the headboard, and the movable footboard is stretched to touch the child's heel. If a measuring board is not available for the infant and young child, it is possible to position the child's body on a flat surface, mark the point where the heel touches the surface, and then mark the point where the top of the head is lying on the surface, taking care to ensure that the child's legs and body are straight on the surface. The examiner then removes the child and measures the distance between the two points with a measuring tape. Measuring the length of the child in this manner is not as accurate as using a measuring board.

When a child is able to cooperate and stand without support, around age 2 years, the examiner stands the child in stocking feet next to a standard measuring tape that begins at the child's heel and is not displaced by room molding. A flat, hard surface is used to reach from the top of the child's head to the tape so that the examiner does not guess or add height because of the hair. If this is the first standing measurement, there may be a slight discrepancy from the lying measurement.

Once the measurement is taken, it must be plotted on a standardized growth chart appropriate for length or height measurement (see Appendix B). Height and weight are evaluated by determining whether the child is following a predictable percentile curve on a growth chart. Height and weight are related to hereditary factors and will vary from child to child.

Weight

The method and equipment for weighing vary with the child's age. All scales must be balanced first before weighing. Infants are placed in a lying position on a regular baby scale with all their clothing removed. Older children who are able to stand or walk without support may be weighed on the adult standing scale. On the older child, remove all clothing except underwear. Like height, weight is plotted on a standardized growth chart (see Appendix B).

Head Circumference

Head circumference is measured on all children from birth to age 36 months and plotted on a standard growth chart on all visits. Children older than 3 years with any questionable

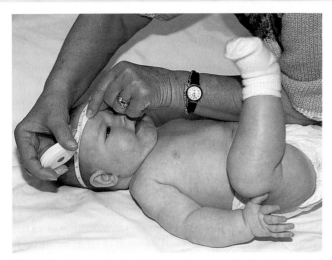

FIG 9-1 **Measuring head circumference.** The head circumference is measured from birth through age 36 months. The nurse uses a nonstretching tape and measures in a "hat band" position, just above the eyebrows and around the occipital prominence in the back. Chest circumference is also routinely measured in the newborn; it is usually smaller than the newborn's head circumference. *(Courtesy University of Texas at Arlington School of Nursing.)*

head size—megalocephaly or microcephaly—should have their head circumference measured at every visit. To measure the head circumference, a nonstretching measuring tape is wrapped above the supraorbital ridges and over the most prominent part of the occiput (Fig. 9-1).

The head circumference is plotted on a standardized growth chart. During the first year of life, the head circumference normally increases by 0.4 inch (1 cm) each month. Head circumference can reflect an abnormal rate of development, give some indication of nutritional status, and possibly indicate tumor growth.

Chest Circumference
Chest circumference is routinely measured only in the newborn infant. The newborn's head circumference is larger than the chest circumference. Chest circumference is almost equal to head circumference after age 1 year. To measure chest circumference, the measuring tape is wrapped around the chest at the nipple line. The measurement is taken between inspiration and expiration.

Midarm Circumference
Midarm circumference reflects muscle mass and fat. To measure midarm circumference, the midpoint on the arm between the acromial process and the olecranon process is determined. Then, with the arm hanging loosely at the side, the child's arm is measured at the midpoint with a tape measure. The measurement is recorded in centimeters. With a decrease in fat or muscle atrophy, the midarm circumference decreases. It will increase with weight gain.

Triceps Skinfold
Triceps skinfold thickness indicates total body fat because at least half of body fat is directly below the skin. Metal calipers

are used to obtain this measurement. On the nondominant arm, the midpoint of the arm is determined using the same method as is used for measuring midarm circumference. With the arm hanging loosely at the side, a fold of skin at the midpoint on the posterior aspect of the arm is grasped. To avoid error, the child is asked to flex the arm muscle after the examiner grasps the skin. If contraction is felt, muscle as well as fat has been grasped. The examiner applies the caliper and takes a reading after waiting 3 seconds. Fat stores decrease with long-term undernutrition and malnutrition.

Use of Growth Charts
An accurate record of an infant's or child's overall pattern of growth is best determined by serial measurements over months or years. The National Center for Health Statistics publishes growth charts (see Appendix B). The charts provide a single set of references to assess body size and monitor growth in infants, children, and adolescents in the United States. They are intended to serve as a reference rather than as growth standards or clinical ideals to be achieved.

National survey data for all racial and ethnic groups are combined to develop the growth charts. Racial and ethnic differences in growth appear to be attributable primarily to environmental influences. Special growth charts for premature infants, children with genetic alterations, such as Down syndrome, and cultural variations such as Asian children, are now available from the American Academy of Pediatrics (AAP). Special charts for premature infants are available.

The recently revised charts include these components:
- Infant charts for birth to age 3 years relate length, weight, and head circumference to age and relate weight to length. Special charts for premature infants are available.
- Charts for ages 2 through 19 years relate stature, weight, and BMI to age. BMI has been recommended for evaluating and tracking overweight children and adolescents. The 85th percentile line helps identify children at risk for overweight.

Separate charts exist for boys and girls.

To plot on a growth chart, the exact age of the child is determined on the chart's horizontal axis. The corresponding measurement is marked on the chart's vertical axis. The chart is marked where the two lines intersect. The percentile lines on these charts indicate the number of children expected to fall above and below the child's measurement.

Weight and height measurements above the 97th percentile or below the 3rd percentile on a standard growth chart may indicate a growth disturbance and need further investigation. BMIs between the 85th and less than the 95th percentile indicate a risk for being overweight; BMIs at or above the 95th percentile in children older than 2 years indicate overweight (Centers for Disease Control and Prevention, 2005).

Generally, African American children weigh less than white children during the first 2 years of life, but as they grow they tend to be taller and heavier than white children of the same age. Asian children are found to be shorter and lighter than their white counterparts.

Skin, Hair, and Nails

Skin

Skin assessment includes inspection and palpation. The entire skin surface is examined for color, texture, turgor, and presence of lesions. This examination may be combined with assessment of other areas of the body.

Inspection. The nurse observes the color and pigmentation of the skin. Skin color reflects the amount of melanin and can range from pink to black (Box 9-5). In dark-skinned infants and children, erythema will appear dusky red or violet, cyanosis will appear black, and jaundice will appear diffusely darker. In dark-skinned infants and children, it is best to determine the normal skin color and then compare any color change with the normal color. Increased pigmentation and thickening of the skin on the posterior neck, the armpits, and behind the knees and elbows (acanthosis nigricans) can be an indication of non–insulin-dependent diabetes mellitus in children (Gungor, Hannon, Libman, Bacha, & Arslanian, 2005). Color changes to the skin may be related to sun exposure or tattooing.

CRITICAL TO REMEMBER

Skin Inspection in Dark-Skinned Children

- Erythema: dusky red or violet
- Cyanosis: black or dusky
- Jaundice: diffusely darker than the child's normal color

Palpation. The examiner palpates the skin to assess moisture, temperature, texture, turgor, edema, and lesions.

Moisture is assessed by lightly stroking the skin surface and body creases. The external skin on exposed areas is normally drier than unexposed areas of the skin.

Temperature is assessed by using the back of the hand because it is more sensitive to skin changes. The two sides of the child's body are compared with each other.

Normal *texture* of the skin is described as being smooth and soft. Scars or excessive scar tissue should be noted.

Turgor is assessed by grasping the skin between the thumb and index finger and quickly releasing it (see p. 497). The skin normally returns to place without excessive skin markings.

BOX 9-5	**Skin Color Terminology**

- *Vitiligo:* areas of depigmentation
- *Nevi:* areas of increased pigmentation
- *Jaundice:* a yellow discoloration of the skin, best seen in the sclera of the eyes
- *Cyanosis:* a blue discoloration of the skin, best seen in all races in the mucous membranes of the mouth, particularly under the tongue
- *Carotenemia:* an orange color of the skin, best seen on the soles of the feet and palms of the hands
- *Pallor:* loss of skin color
- *Erythema:* diffusely red
- *Mottling:* discolored areas of the skin

Skin that "tents" when released indicates dehydration. The abdomen and upper arm are the best places to test for tissue turgor on a child.

Edema, the accumulation of excessive salt and water in the interstitial spaces, is identified by pressing the thumb into areas of the body that may appear puffy. The extremities and buttocks are classic areas to palpate for edema in the child. Periorbital edema is observed on the eyelids.

Lesions are identified, noting configuration, distribution, color, and size. Skin lesions are identified as primary lesions, arising from normal skin (e.g., freckle), or secondary lesions, resulting from an alteration of a primary lesion (e.g., scab). Configuration of a skin lesion refers to the arrangement or position of several lesions in relation to each other or to the arrangement of a single lesion. Distribution refers to the body location and the symmetry or asymmetry of lesions.

Hair

Hair normally covers the entire body except for the palms, soles, and parts of the genitalia. Hair is examined for texture, changes in color, unusual distribution, and cleanliness.

Scalp hair has a wide range of normal textures, including straight, curly, or kinky. The hair is usually shiny, silky, and strong. The examiner should keep in mind the age and development of the child. Fine, downy hair is normal for a newborn infant, whereas in an older child it would lead the examiner to consider nutrition and endocrine abnormalities. Brittle hair, identified when the hairs break off easily when bent between the fingers, also might indicate endocrine and nutrition abnormalities.

The color of the hair is genetically determined and may be anything from pale blond to black. Changes in color may be caused by depigmentation, hereditary factors, or chemicals applied to the hair. Hair texture varies widely with race.

The distribution of the hair over the head is identified. In most children, the hair begins in a whorl and then is distributed over the head. Some children may have more than one whorl. Scalp hair does not grow beyond the nape of the neck or down to the eyebrows. *Hirsutism* is defined as excessive hair growth; *alopecia* is unusual hair loss.

The hair is separated and examined for cleanliness, signs of trauma, lesions, or scaling. The scalp should be clean and free of any infestations. Most cases of head lice (*Pediculosis capitis*) are first detected when one or more children is seen scratching the head. Closer observation may reveal nits adhering to the hairs. Depending on their distance from the scalp, usually these are the whitish to sand-colored empty shells of eggs that have hatched (see Chapter 25 for further discussion of the integumentary system).

Nails

Nails are inspected and palpated for shape and contour. The nail surface is normally flat or slightly convex. The edges of the nails should be smooth, rounded, and clean. Clubbing of fingernails can be identified by looking at the index finger; the angle at the nail base and the fingertip should be less than 160 degrees. On palpation, the base of the fingernail should be firm. On touching the index fingernails back to back, a diamond of light below the knuckle and above where the fingernails touch will be present. In early clubbing, the diamond shape is decreased or not apparent (see Chapter 21).

Pressing and releasing on the nail edge assesses capillary refill; the nail will blanch, and then color will return to the nail within 1 to 2 seconds. A capillary refill time of more than 2 seconds may be caused by anemia, peripheral edema, vasoconstriction, or decreased cardiac output as a result of hypovolemia, shock, or congestive heart failure (Jarvis, 2004).

Lymph Nodes

Lymph nodes are inspected and palpated. Lymph tissue is found all over the body and must be evaluated as the examiner assesses body systems. Always assess for enlarged lymph nodes in the head and neck, the supraclavicular area, the axillary region, the arms, and the inguinal region (Fig. 9-2). At the time these areas are examined, the lymph nodes are assessed as well. When an enlarged lymph node or a mass is found during examination, its characteristics should be described (Box 9-6).

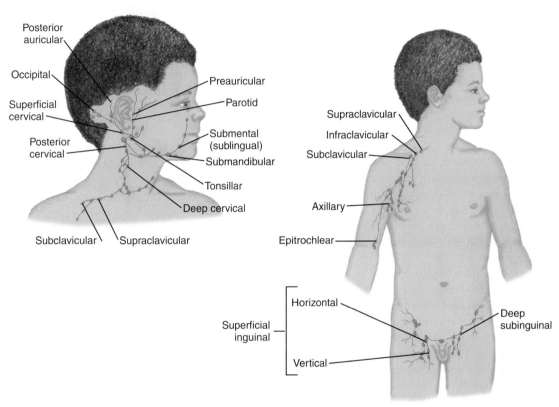

FIG 9-2 **Location of superficial lymph nodes.**

BOX 9-6	**Characteristics of Enlarged Lymph Nodes and Masses**

- *Location:* Identify the anatomic location of the enlarged lymph nodes or mass. Use imaginary body lines or body axes to assist in locating findings.
- *Size:* Describe in three dimensions: length, width, and thickness. Describe the shape: round or irregular.
- *Surface characteristics:* Describe the surface as smooth, nodular, or irregular on palpation.
- *Consistency:* Describe the nodes or masses as hard, soft, firm, resilient, spongy, or cystic on palpation.
- *Symmetry:* Evaluate paired anatomic structures for symmetry.
- *Fixed or mobile:* If a fixed mass is found, note whether it is fixed to underlying or overlying tissue. If a mobile mass is found, describe it in centimeters and describe its direction.

- *Tenderness and pain:* Describe whether the tenderness or pain is present on direct palpation or occurs without stimulation. Identify referred pain and rebound tenderness.
- *Erythema:* Describe the extent of any color change.
- *Heat:* Palpate with the back of the hand to identify any abnormal warmth.
- *Pulsatile nature:* Describe pulsations, if present, particularly when they are in an area where pulsations are not expected. All pulsating masses are auscultated for bruits.
- *Increased vascularity:* Describe the prominence of overlying veins or the presence of cyanosis of the area.
- *Transillumination:* If the mass is in an anatomic structure that can be transilluminated, record the results of the procedure.

To palpate for most lymph nodes, the examiner uses the distal portion of the fingers and gently but firmly moves the fingers in a circular motion to determine the node's characteristics and mobility.

Lymph nodes that are enlarged, warm, and firm and fluctuant are a sign of infection. Lymph nodes that are small, firm, and shotty (freely palpable and very small) are often palpable in healthy infants and children, up to the age of 12 years, in the cervical, axillary, inguinal, and occipital areas (Fox, 2002). An enlarged supraclavicular lymph node on the left in young children is called the *sentinel node* because it may suggest a Wilms tumor or other neoplastic disease.

Head, Neck, and Face

Head

The head is inspected and palpated. To examine the head, the examiner must see and feel. The head is evaluated from the front, the back, and the sides. The head is examined for symmetry, paralysis, weakness, and movement (Box 9-7).

Symmetry is assessed by looking at and feeling the entire head. If any lumps or bumps are seen or felt, the examiner notes their exact location, size, and density. The suture lines in infants should be palpated. Sutures are felt as prominent ridges in the neonate but usually flatten by 6 months.

Paralysis and weakness of the head are directly related to the condition of the neck muscles. That is, paralysis and weakness of the head will occur with paralysis or weakness of the neck muscles.

Head movement is evaluated by observing the child move the head. Head control is observed with the child in a lying position and while the examiner grasps the child's hands and pulls the infant into a sitting position. An infant younger than 4 months may show some head lag, but the infant in an upright position should be able to maintain the head upright for several seconds. Head lag after age 6 months may indicate poor muscle development. The head should be put through a full range of motion by asking the older child to look up, down, and sideways. After age 4 months, inability to move the head or to hold the head in an upright position may be related to paralysis or weakness of the neck muscles.

The fontanels are inspected and palpated for size, tenseness, and pulsation (Fig. 9-3). The posterior fontanel is closed by age 2 to 3 months. The anterior fontanel should be soft and flat when the child is sitting. Measure the width and length of an open anterior fontanel. The anterior fontanel should be less than 5 cm in length and width after age 12 months and should be completely closed by age 12 to 18 months. A sunken fontanel is associated with dehydration,

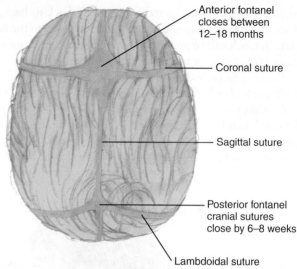

FIG 9-3   **Fontanels are inspected and palpated for size, tenseness, and pulsation.**

Anterior fontanel closes between 12–18 months

Coronal suture

Sagittal suture

Posterior fontanel cranial sutures close by 6–8 weeks

Lambdoidal suture

and a bulging fontanel can be associated with increased intracranial pressure. A bulging fontanel is normally seen when an infant cries, coughs, or vomits.

Neck

In the child, the neck is inspected and palpated for symmetry, size, and shape, which is directly related to use or disuse of the neck muscles. The infant's neck is relatively short and lengthens as the child grows. View the neck from the front, back, and both sides. Webbing of the neck—the presence of an extra fold of skin posteriorly—is associated with some chromosomal abnormalities such as trisomy 21, or Down syndrome.

The neck is mobile and supple. While palpating the child's neck, the thyroid gland is palpated by identifying the isthmus of the thyroid across the trachea. To identify an enlarged thyroid in a child, the examiner gently displaces the thyroid gland laterally and palpates thyroid tissue with the opposite thumb and fingers. The lobe may be more palpable when the child swallows.

Face

The child's face is inspected and palpated for dysmorphic features. Spacing and symmetry of facial features are noted. The face is observed for any changes in color or the presence of edema, such as cellulitis. The eyes are examined for size, position, and configuration. *Hypertelorism* is a condition in which the eyes are unusually widely spaced; in *hypotelorism*, the eyes are unusually close together. The child's nostrils should be oval in shape and equal in size, with no evidence of a hypoplastic philtrum (shallow crease or absence of a crease below the nose). The lips should be equal on either side of the midline. The child's ears are inspected for alignment. Low-set ears are identified when the auricle of the ear does not cross or touch the eye-occiput line. The position of the auricle should be almost vertical, with no more than a 10-degree lateral posterior angle (Fig. 9-4).

BOX 9-7	**Head Shape Terminology**

- *Normocephalic:* normal-size head
- *Microcephalic:* head small for body size and age
- *Macrocephalic:* abnormally large head
- *Bossing:* frontal enlargement

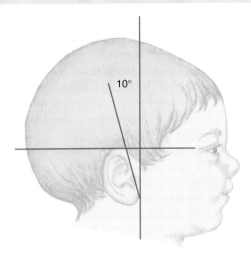

Normal alignment

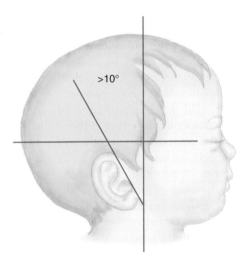

Low-set ears and
deviation in alignment

FIG 9-4 **The child's ears are inspected for alignment. Low-set ears could indicate mental retardation or renal anomalies.**

The functions of cranial nerve V (trigeminal nerve) and cranial nerve VII (facial nerve) are evaluated while assessing the face. Cranial nerve V is evaluated by observing chewing or sucking, which demonstrates the strength of the temporomandibular joint, and by touching the child's forehead and cheeks with a piece of cotton. The child should move the head or bat the object away. Cranial nerve VII is evaluated by having the child frown, smile, or make a face while the examiner observes for symmetry of movement. Having the child puff out the cheeks or whistle also allows the examiner to evaluate cranial nerve VII (Jarvis, 2004).

Nose, Mouth, and Throat

Nose

The examiner should wear gloves when doing the nasal examination, noting any drainage coming from the nose and describing the amount, color, and consistency.

The external nose is inspected and palpated. Patency can be determined by occluding one nostril and having the child sniff, and then repeating on the other side. The external nose is observed for symmetry, deformity, inflammation, or skin lesions. The "allergic salute," frequent wiping of the nose because of drainage, produces a transverse crease on the child's nose and indicates that the child has allergies. Palpate the entire external nose for septal deviation or other deformities. The sense of smell is mediated by cranial nerve I. This function can be evaluated by having the child close the eyes, occlude one nostril, and identify familiar odors, such as cinnamon, peppermint, orange, or cherry.

The nasal cavity can be examined by using a short, wide-tipped speculum on the otoscope and inserting it into the nasal vestibule, with care not to put pressure on the nasal septum. The nasal mucosa is inspected for color and moisture. The nasal mucosa is normally smooth and moist, with a bright pink color. In children with allergies, the mucosa is pale and appears boggy. With infectious diseases, the mucosa is erythematous and swollen; the nasal drainage may be yellow or green. The nasal septum is examined for intactness and for any deviation.

The *frontal* and *maxillary sinuses* are inspected and palpated (Fig. 9-5). The areas over the sinuses are examined for color and swelling. Puffiness and redness over the sinuses and dark circles under the eyes may indicate an inflammatory process in children. The frontal sinuses are palpated by pressing over the sinuses below the eyebrow. The maxillary sinuses are palpated by pressing upward with the thumbs under the maxillary bones.

Mouth and Throat

Assessment of the mouth in a young child should be performed at the end of the physical examination because it may create anxiety. The examination should proceed from the anterior structures to the internal structures of the mouth.

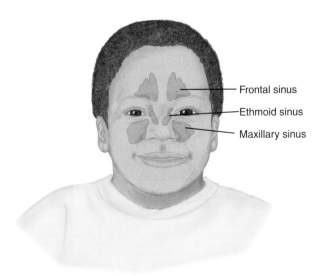

FIG 9-5 **The frontal, ethmoid, and maxillary sinuses.**

Frontal sinus
Ethmoid sinus
Maxillary sinus

The *philtrum*, the little notch between the nose and upper lip, should be intact. In children with dysmorphic features, the philtrum is absent or shallow.

The examiner should wear gloves when doing the oral examination. A tongue blade and a good penlight assist with visualization of the oral cavity. When the child opens his or her mouth, evaluate mouth odors. The mouth and internal structures are examined by inspection, palpation, and the sense of smell.

Lips are inspected for symmetry, color, moisture, cracking, or the presence of any lesions. The alveolar frenulum, which attaches the lips to the gums, should be intact. The lips are palpated to identify any masses.

The *buccal mucosa* is examined by holding the cheeks open with a tongue blade and examining for color, nodules, or lesions. Significant mouth odors should be noted. For many children, this part of the examination can be unpleasant. To facilitate the child's cooperation, the examiner may want to demonstrate on a doll or on the parent or allow the child to place the tongue blade in the parent's mouth. The buccal mucosa should be pink, smooth, and moist. Dark-skinned children may have patchy areas of hyperpigmentation. The opening of the *parotid gland* is found as a small dimple on the buccal mucosa opposite the upper second molar. The entire surface of the buccal mucosa is palpated for changes in consistency or masses.

Teeth are inspected for number, cavities, tooth formation, and occlusion. The number and characteristics of the teeth will change with growth and development (Fig. 9-6). The eruption of deciduous teeth begins around the sixth month of extrauterine life; all 20 deciduous teeth are present by age 30 months. Have the child bite down and gently part the lips and note the position of the teeth. The upper teeth slightly override the lower teeth. The color and shape of each tooth should be noted. The crown is white, with some

variation from person to person. Permanent teeth are larger and have a darker color than deciduous teeth. Brown or black discoloration of the teeth is usually caused by dental caries. Long-term use of certain medications (i.e., tetracycline, iron) may stain teeth. With excessive fluoride ingestion, the enamel of the permanent teeth may appear mottled. The shape of the tooth is determined by age, development, and the amount of wear.

The gums (*gingivae*) are inspected and palpated for color and swelling. The gum surface has a pink, stippled appearance and feels firm. Dark-skinned children may have a dark-pigmented line along the gingival margin.

The floor of the mouth can be inspected by asking the child to lift the tongue to the roof of the mouth. Observe the frenulum, the sublingual ridge, and Wharton's ducts, which lie on either side of the frenulum. The color of the floor of the mouth is pink.

The tongue is inspected and palpated. The dorsum of the tongue should appear dull red, moist, and glistening, with a white coat. The anterior portion of the tongue should have a slightly roughened appearance with papillae and small fissures. The tongue is palpated for indurations or ulcerations. While palpating the mouth of a young child, biting can be prevented by holding the child's cheeks.

Cranial nerve XII (*hypoglossal nerve*) is examined by asking the child to stick out the tongue as though licking a lollipop and observe for any deviation of the tongue to one side. The examiner can determine the strength of the tongue by placing a finger to the side of the child's cheek and asking the child to press the tongue against the examiner's finger. The tongue should feel equally strong on each side.

The hard palate, soft palate, and uvula are examined by asking the child to tilt the head back. The examiner inspects the hard palate for shape and color. The hard palate is whitish and convex, with transverse rugae. The examiner palpates

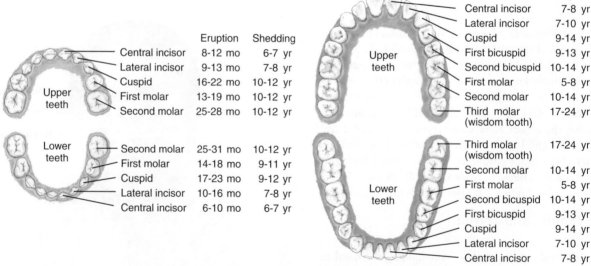

FIG 9-6   **Sequence of eruption of primary and secondary teeth.**

the hard palate for the height of the arch and intactness. The examiner can allow the infant to suck on a gloved finger while palpating the hard palate to determine the strength of the sucking reflex. The soft palate is continuous with the hard palate and is concave and pinker in color. The uvula varies in length and thickness and is located in midline as a continuation of the soft palate. Cranial nerves IX (*glossopharyngeal nerve*) and X (*vagus nerve*) are evaluated at this time. The child is asked to say "ah"; normally, the soft palate and the uvula rise symmetrically and phonation of "ah" is understood.

A tongue blade is used to depress the tongue and observe the oropharynx. This action can be unpleasant for the child. To minimize discomfort, the examiner slides the tongue blade along the side of the tongue until reaching the soft palate and then compresses the tongue to elicit the gag reflex (cranial nerve X) and observes the back of the throat. The tonsillar pillars are inspected with particular notation of size and color of tonsils. The tonsils are pink in color.

The size of tonsils varies; large tonsils are common in young children. Tonsils may have crypts where food particles collect. With inflammatory processes, the crypts may contain exudate. A child whose parents comment on the child's snoring or waking up by snoring may have grossly enlarged tonsils. The posterior wall of the pharynx should be smooth and glistening pink; the wall may have small, irregular spots of lymphatic tissue and small blood vessels (Seidel et al., 2003).

Eyes

The eyes are inspected, palpated, and evaluated for visual acuity and extraocular muscle function.

Visual Acuity

Visual acuity can be difficult to evaluate in a young child. Acuity develops over time, and evaluation requires the child's cooperation. Items needed for evaluating visual acuity in a child are an eye cover and vision charts (Box 9-8). The chart chosen will be determined by the child's age and development. The infant from birth to age 1 or 2 months gazes at black-and-white contrasting figures and faces. At age 4 weeks or older, an infant fixes on a brightly colored object and follows it.

The AAP recommends visual acuity testing for all children beginning no later than age 3 years (AAP, American Association of Certified Orthoptists, American Association

---

BOX 9-8	**Types of Eye Charts**

- *Snellen chart:* A standardized chart with graduated letters for testing far vision of children at 20 feet. Used with children older than 6 years.
- *Tumbling E (Snellen E):* A standardized chart using the letter *E* in various directions that is used with preschoolers aged 3 to 6 years to test far vision at 20 feet. Also available for a distance of 10 feet.
- *Lea chart:* A chart with four different symbols. Used for preschool-aged children. Designed for use at 10 feet.

- *HOTV chart:* A standardized chart with letters *H, O, T,* and *V* in graduated sizes. Designed for use at 10 feet with children aged 3 to 6 years.

- *Jaeger chart:* Standardized chart with graduated letters for testing near vision at 12 to 14 inches from the eyes. Used with children older than 6 years.
- *Ishihara chart:* A series of polychromatic cards with a pattern of dots printed against a background of many colored dots. Designed to test for color vision between ages 4 and 6 years.

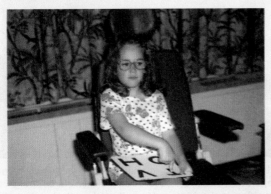

HOTV chart for children ages 3 to 6 years. The letters *H, O, T,* and *V* are presented at a distance, and the child points to the corresponding letter on the card resting on her lap. (From Goldbloom, R. B. [2003]. *Pediatric clinical skills* [3rd ed., p. 138]. Philadelphia: WB Saunders.)

for Pediatric Ophthalmology and Strabismus, & American Academy of Ophthalmology, 2003). Several groups have been researching the reliability and validity of vision screening methods for preschool age children (National Eye Institute, 2003; U.S. Preventive Services Task Force, 2004). Visual acuity tests that have evidence to support reliability and validity for preschool children include Lea cards, tumbling Es, and HOTV (Hartmann et al., 2000/2005).

Preschool children can be tested using the HOTV chart at 10 feet. A card with *H*, *O*, *T*, and *V* is given to the child to hold. One eye is covered, and the child is instructed to match the letters on the held card with the chart at 10 feet with the uncovered eye. The child holds the letters, or they are placed on a table directly in front of the child. Screening is begun at the 20/40 line for children younger than 4 years and at the 20/30 line for older children. The child passes the screening if the child correctly identifies four of the five symbols.

Older children's visual acuity can be tested by use of the Snellen chart, placed on a wall 20 feet away from the child. The chart should have no glare and should be well illuminated. No other materials should be around or near the chart. Test both eyes together first, and then test each eye separately. If the child has corrective lenses, the procedure should be repeated with the corrective lenses on. Unless the child is known to have very poor vision, testing is begun at the line on the chart for 40 feet. To determine at what level the child cannot see, the examiner finds the distance at which the child misses half plus one of the symbols on a line of the chart. The visual acuity is then designated as the smallest line at which the child is able to identify more than half the symbols on the line. For corrective lenses, the examiner notes the last date the child was examined for a prescription. Findings are recorded by noting the distance of the line correctly read for both eyes (i.e., right eye 20/20, left eye 20/20). This annotation means that the child has correctly interpreted the letters on the chart for 20 feet at a distance of 20 feet, which matches what the average child can see at that distance. If the child correctly identifies the letters on the line labeled *40 feet,* that child can see at 20 feet what the average child can see at 40 feet. Visual acuity changes with age and varies according to the test used. Normal ranges are as follows:

- *Birth:* fixates on objects (8 to 12 inches), 20/100 to 20/150
- *4 months:* 20/50 to 20/80
- *1 year:* 20/40 to 20/70
- *4 years:* 20/30 to 20/40
- *5 years:* 20/20 to 20/30

Color Vision

Color vision deficit, less correctly termed *color blindness,* is an inherited recessive X-linked trait that, in varying degrees, may affect the child's ability to discern traffic lights, brake lights, and color-coordinated clothing. Color discrimination occurs through integration of information from the cone pigments in the retinal layers of the eye. The genes for some colors are located on the X chromosome and, because boys have only one X chromosome, they are more likely to have color vision deficit. Color vision deficit may affect learning if the learning is color related. The condition is very rare in females but affects 8% to 10% of males.

Color vision is evaluated by Ishihara charts—a series of polychromatic cards. These cards have a pattern of colored pictures embedded in the charts. Children between ages 4 and 8 years are tested once and are asked to touch or identify the embedded patterns. A child with this deficit cannot see the patterns against the field of color.

Peripheral Vision

Visual fields are evaluated in older children to identify peripheral vision. The examiner's face is positioned directly in front and on the level of the child, about 2 feet away. The visual fields should roughly mirror the examiner's. The examiner covers one eye and has the child mimic by covering the opposite eye. Slowly a puppet or some other test object is brought from the periphery into the child's field of vision. The object should come from a position slightly behind the child's head, and the child is asked to say "now" when the object is in view (Fig. 9-7). Testing for visual acuity and visual fields evaluates cranial nerve II, the optic nerve, which mediates vision.

Binocular Vision and Strabismus

Extraocular muscle function is evaluated to test binocular vision and the presence of strabismus. Strabismus, or "crossed eyes," is the abnormal or incomplete development of binocular visual alignment. Three tests are performed: the corneal light reflex (Hirschberg) test, field-of-vision test, and cover/uncover (alternate cover) test.

Corneal Light Reflex Test. The corneal light reflex is assessed by shining a light directly onto the irises from a distance of about 40.5 cm (16 in). The reflection of the light should appear in exactly the same spot on both eyes. If the light falls off center in one eye, the eyes are malaligned. Children with *epicanthal folds*—vertical folds that partially or completely cover the inner canthi (Fig. 9-8)—may give a false impression of malalignment (pseudostrabismus).

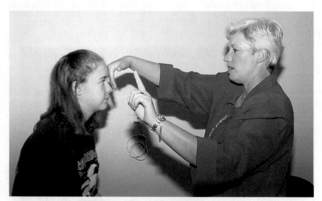

FIG 9-7 Visual fields (cranial nerve II) are tested in each eye separately. One eye is covered as the child stares straight ahead. An object is slowly moved from the side of the head into the field of vision. The child says "now" when first seeing the object.

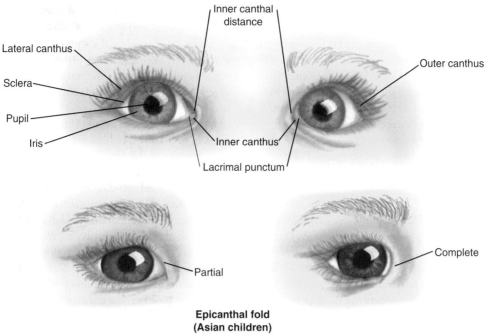

FIG 9-8 **External structures of the eye.**

Field-of-Vision Test. The six cardinal fields of vision are tested by holding the child's chin so that the head does not move and asking the child to follow a puppet or a familiar object held approximately 12 inches away from the face as the object is moved to each of the six cardinal positions. As the object is moved to the margins of each cardinal position, the examiner holds it momentarily in that position before proceeding back to the center. The eyes will track in a parallel fashion to each position. As the eyes are in the margins of each position, the examiner can note *end-stage nystagmus*, a gentle oscillation of the eye, which is considered normal. Children younger than 2 to 3 years may not be able to cooperate with this test.

Cover/Uncover Test. The cover/uncover test is used to detect deficits in binocular vision by interrupting fusion of the eyes as they gaze at a fixed object. One eye is covered with an opaque card while the child stares straight ahead, at which time the examiner observes the uncovered eye. A steady, fixed gaze is maintained by the uncovered eye. Next the covered eye is uncovered and observed for any movement; it should continue to stare straight ahead (Fig. 9-9).

The procedure is repeated with the opposite eye. Any movement in either eye in the process of covering or uncovering may indicate muscle weakness.

Testing for extraocular muscle function in children younger than 5 years is critical to identifying any muscle imbalance so that it can be corrected at an early age to preserve vision. Extraocular muscle function evaluates three cranial nerves: cranial nerve VI, the *abducent* nerve, which innervates the lateral rectus muscle (responsible for abducting the eye); cranial nerve IV, the *trochlear* nerve, which innervates the superior oblique muscle (responsible for down and inward movement of the eye); and cranial nerve III, the

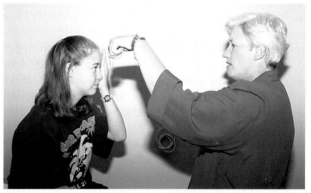

FIG 9-9 **The cover/uncover test detects small degrees of deviated eye alignment. With one eye covered, the child gazes straight ahead with the uncovered eye. The cover is then removed, and the eye should continue to stare straight ahead. Movement in either eye suggests muscle weakness. Extraocular muscle function is controlled by cranial nerves III, IV, and VI.**

oculomotor nerve, which innervates the superior, inferior, and medial rectus and the inferior oblique muscles (Seidel et al., 2003).

The random dot E stereo test, in which the child looks through special glasses to identify an E on a card, is now recommended as part of comprehensive vision testing for preschoolers and young school age children (Hartmann et al., 2000/2005).

External Eye

The external eye is evaluated for position and placement (see Fig. 9-8). The examiner notes whether the eyes are set wide apart or close together. Epicanthal folds are seen in Asian children and in some non-Asian children as well. The slant of the eyes is determined by drawing an imaginary line across the inner canthi (see Fig. 9-8).

The eyebrows are inspected for symmetry and hair growth and eyelashes for even distribution. The *lacrimal apparatus* is assessed by asking the child to look down. The outer part of the upper lid is palpated along the bony orbit for any discomfort, swelling, or redness. The *punctum* (tear duct) on the inner canthus is palpated for obstruction in the infant.

The eye globe is palpated for firmness and can be gently pushed into the orbit without causing discomfort. Palpation of the eye may cause anxiety in small children and should not be done unless there is a serious concern about the size of the eye.

Eyelids are inspected for color, swelling, discharge, and lesions. Note the position of the eyelids on the globe. With the eyelids open, the upper lid normally falls below the superior limbus but does not cover any of the pupil. The lower lids normally fall just at the inferior limbus. The limbus is the point where the sclera of the eye meets the color portion of the iris. When closed, the eyelids approximate each other completely, without tremor, fasciculations, or tics.

The *conjunctiva* has two portions to evaluate. The palpebral portion of the conjunctiva lines the lids. The palpebral conjunctiva is examined by pulling down as the child looks up. It is normally clear, with a pink color, and may have several small blood vessels visible. The upper lid can be inspected by everting the upper eyelid over a cotton-tipped applicator. Eversion of the upper eyelid is not normally done because eye manipulation may cause apprehension in a child. The bulbar portion of the conjunctiva is transparent and lies over the sclera, allowing the white of the sclera to be clearly visible.

The following anterior structures of the eye are inspected: sclerae, cornea and lens, anterior chamber, and irises. The sclerae are white. The sclera of dark-skinned children may have gray-blue or "muddy" color variations. Dark-skinned children may have small brown macules around the limbus (where the iris meets the sclera). These variations are normal. The corneas are clear, transparent, and very sensitive. Shining a light obliquely across the cornea highlights any abnormal irregularities on the corneal surface. The examiner illuminates the anterior chamber by shining a light across the eye from the temporal side to illuminate the entire iris without producing a shadow. The irises are round and contain muscle fibers that contract or expand in response to light. The pigmentation of the irises is uniquely different for each individual. The irises are similar in color but may exhibit some variation between them.

Pupils appear round, regular, and of equal size in both eyes. The *pupillary light reflex* is tested by darkening the room and asking the child to gaze into the distance. A light is brought from the side (temporally), and the examiner notes the change in the size of the pupil. Shining a light directly into a pupil causes the pupil to constrict (direct light reflex). The procedure is repeated while the opposite eye is observed. The opposite eye constricts (consensual light reflex) in response

to the light shone in the other eye. Pupils should constrict at equal speeds and to the same degree.

Pupil size should be the same in both eyes. In some children, pupils of unequal size are normal, but in general, unequal pupils call for a consideration of central nervous system injury. Asking the child to focus on a distant object can test accommodation. The pupils normally dilate. An object such as a puppet or a finger brought into the line of vision about 7 to 8 cm from the nose should cause pupillary constriction and convergence of the axes of the eyes (Seidel et al., 2003).

Ophthalmoscopic Examination

The ophthalmoscopic examination requires a cooperative child, practice, and patience. Lights in the room should be dim. Most children enjoy playing with the light of the "flashlight," and watching the light as you move it around the room facilitates cooperation. Minimally, all practitioners view the red reflex, but the procedure requires demonstration and practice. When the ophthalmoscope is placed in front of the pupil and the light hits the lens, a red color is reflected from the retina to the examiner. The retina, choroid, optic disc, macula, fovea centralis, and retinal vessels are also visible with the ophthalmoscope.

Ears

Assessment of the ears includes testing for hearing acuity, inspection and palpation of the external ear, and examination of the internal ear with the otoscope.

Hearing Acuity

Infant Assessment. Infants born in a hospital are tested for response of the acoustic nerve at the time of birth. In an infant, hearing is assessed by asking the parent to speak to the infant from behind and observing the infant's response to the parent's voice. The examiner can stand behind the infant and ring a bell or make a sound the infant is familiar with and observe the infant turning to locate the sound. A very young infant, younger than 4 months, may demonstrate a startle reflex to loud sounds.

Preschool and School-Age Assessment by Audiometry. In preschool and school-age children, the audiometer gives a precise (quantitative) assessment of the child's ability to hear. The child is placed in a soundproof room and is asked to identify tones played at a level the child can hear. With the audiometer, two tests are used to evaluate hearing: the sweep test and the pure tone hearing test. The *sweep test* is used to screen for hearing losses. The *pure tone test* is used to determine the exact extent of the hearing loss.

Preschool and School-Age and Adolescent Assessment: The Whisper Test. A whisper is heard as the examiner stands about 0.3 m (1 foot) behind or to the side of the child.

For a preschool child, the examiner stands in front of the child approximately 0.6 to 0.9 m (2-3 foot and gives the child a command such as, "Please put the toy on the floor."

Conduction Tests (Tuning Fork Hearing Tests). Tuning fork tests are qualitative tests done to determine the ability to

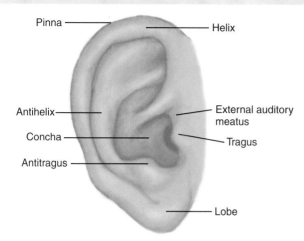

FIG 9-10   **Landmarks of the external ear.**

hear by air conduction and by bone conduction. In the normal child, air conduction of sound is greater than bone conduction. The *Rinne hearing test* is used to determine whether air conduction is greater than bone conduction. The *Weber hearing test* determines the child's ability to hear by bone conduction. Testing the child's hearing evaluates cranial nerve VIII *(acoustic nerve)*.

External Ear

The external ear is inspected and palpated. Ear placement and position are evaluated when assessing the face (see Fig. 9-4), but the external ear is also examined for any malformations or unusual markings (Fig. 9-10). Any discharge coming from the auditory meatus is noted, and its amount and characteristics are described. Soft, yellow-brown cerumen (ear wax) is normally seen in the external auditory meatus.

The bony prominence of the mastoid process behind the ear is palpated for tenderness. The auricles are gently pulled to determine whether discomfort is created.

Otoscopic Examination

The *tympanic membrane* is examined with the otoscope (Fig. 9-11). Many children may be apprehensive about this examination. If necessary, a small child is positioned on the parent's lap and the child's arms are secured. The examiner uses the largest speculum that will fit comfortably into the ear canal. In a child younger than 3 years, the ear canal is straightened by pulling the pinna of the ear down and back. If a child is 3 years old or older, the pinna is pulled up and back. As much of the canal as possible should be visible before inserting the speculum into the auditory meatus.

The canal is inspected for any lesions and for cerumen. The tympanic membrane is inspected for landmarks, color, and mobility. A puff of air is injected into the canal with an insufflation bulb, and the tympanic membrane is observed for movement. Normally, the tympanic membrane moves inward with a slight puff and outward with a slight release.

Thorax and Lungs

Assessment of the thorax and lungs consists of inspection, palpation, percussion, and auscultation, in that order. To assist with localizing findings on the thorax, anatomic landmarks such as the ribs and intercostal spaces are identified and imaginary lines are drawn on the surface (Fig. 9-12).

Location of lung tissue depends on the age and development of the child. In an infant, lung tissue on the anterior chest can be located from the apex, above the clavicle, to the level of the fifth rib in the midclavicular line. By age 6 years,

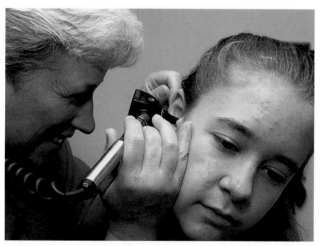

To straighten the ear canal of a child older than 3 years, the nurse pulls the child's pinna up and back.

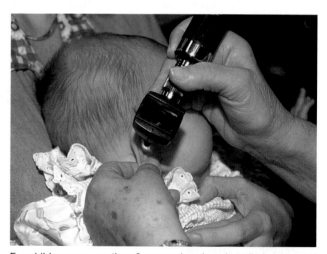

For children younger than 3 years, the pinna is pulled down and back.

FIG 9-11   **Inspection of the tympanic membrane with the otoscope. The auditory canal is inspected before the otoscope is inserted, to see the child's tympanic membrane.**

Continued

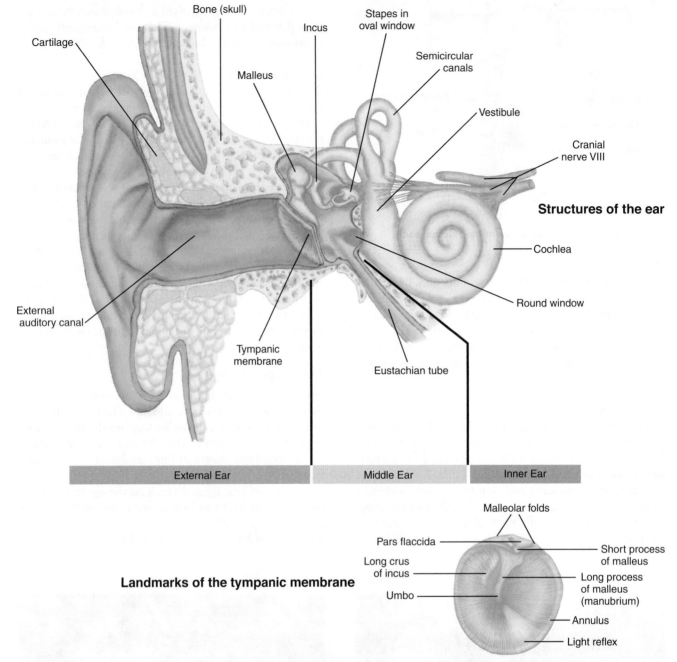

Structures of the ear

Landmarks of the tympanic membrane

FIG 9-11, cont'd   Inspection of the tympanic membrane with the otoscope. The auditory canal is inspected before the otoscope is inserted, to see the child's tympanic membrane.

lung tissue is assessed from the apex to the level of the sixth rib in the midclavicular line. Laterally, lung tissue is assessed from the axilla to the level of the eighth rib. Posteriorly, lungs are assessed from the level of the first thoracic vertebra to the tenth thoracic vertebra.

Inspection

Remove the child's shirt or clothing covering the chest. In adolescent females, the breasts should be kept covered and exposed only when necessary. Inspection of the chest includes observing the child for any cough, stridor, grunting,

hoarseness, snoring, wheezing, and type and amount of any sputum, if present. Respiratory rate and pattern are observed. In young children and infants, breathing is more diaphragmatic or abdominal (see Table 9-1 for the effect of age on vital signs). The chest wall should expand symmetrically during respiration. Respirations should be easy, regular, and without apparent distress. Rapid respirations, retractions, nasal flaring, and head bobbing may indicate respiratory difficulty.

Thoracic configuration is evaluated by determining the shape and symmetry of the chest from the front, sides, and

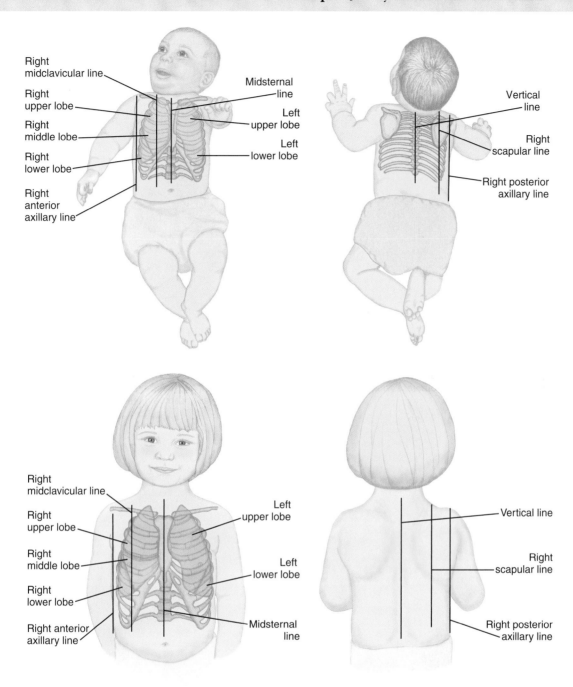

FIG 9-12 **Anatomic landmarks of the thorax in infants and children.**

back (Fig. 9-13). Two common alterations in structure in the anterior chest are *pectus carinatum* (pigeon chest) and *pectus excavatum* (funnel chest). *Scoliosis*, a lateral **S**-shaped curvature of the thoracic and lumbar vertebrae, is a common alteration of the posterior chest that may cause impaired pulmonary function.

Palpation
Palpation of the chest begins with the posterior chest. To alleviate fear in a young child, the examiner should stand in a position that allows the child visibility at all times. The posterior chest is palpated for areas of tenderness, tactile fremitus, and chest excursion.

To palpate for tenderness, the examiner touches the entire thorax with the palmar aspects of the fingers. This process elicits any points of discomfort or pain. The examiner notes any masses or edema (Fig. 9-14).

To evaluate for *tactile fremitus*, the examiner palpates the chest wall while the child says "ninety-nine." Vibrations felt on the chest wall are the result of vibrations produced in the vocal cords and transmitted to the chest wall through the respiratory tract.

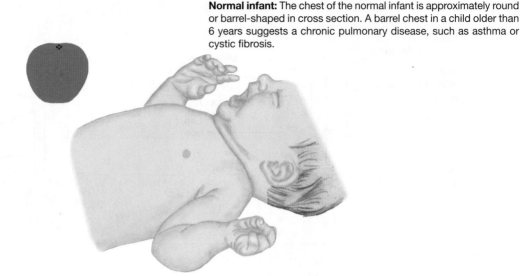

Normal infant: The chest of the normal infant is approximately round or barrel-shaped in cross section. A barrel chest in a child older than 6 years suggests a chronic pulmonary disease, such as asthma or cystic fibrosis.

Funnel chest (pectus excavatum): A funnel chest has a depression in the lower portion of the sternum. Compression of the heart and great vessels may cause murmurs.

Pigeon chest (pectus carinatum): In pigeon chest, the sternum is displaced anteriorly, increasing the anteroposterior diameter. Grooves in the chest wall accentuate the deformity.

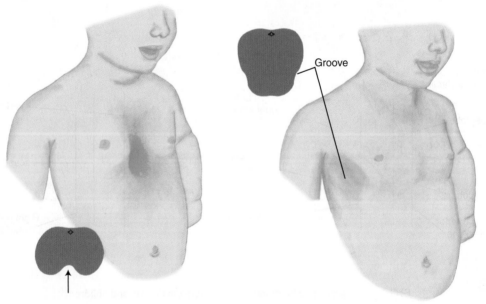

Groove

FIG 9-13 **Common alterations in chest configuration.**

Percussion of the chest is performed by advanced practitioners to determine changes in sound produced by the density of the underlying tissues.

Auscultation

Auscultating the chest with a stethoscope determines the characteristics of breath sounds. Breath sounds heard with the stethoscope are made by the flow of air through the respiratory tree and are characterized by intensity, pitch, quality, and duration.

It is best to listen to breath sounds with the child sitting upright if possible. Infants and toddlers can be held in the

parent's lap; have the parent assist with removal of clothing and positioning of the child. The examiner's position is on the side of the child, allowing the child to observe the examiner's movements. Before touching the chest, the examiner allows the young child to hold or play with the stethoscope and warms the stethoscope before placing it on the child's chest. The head of the stethoscope is cleaned with alcohol between patients.

An anxious or frightened child may cry during this part of the examination. Distracting the child or having the young child focus on another activity may facilitate listening. For the inconsolable child, the examiner listens to breath sounds

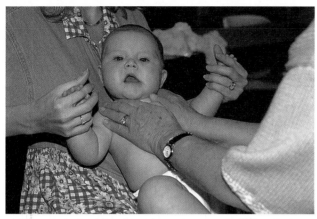

FIG 9-14   **To identify areas of fremitus, tenderness, symmetry, and depth and equality of expansion, the nurse palpates the child's posterior and anterior chest. When palpating any area, warm hands increase the child's comfort.**   *(Courtesy University of Texas at Arlington School of Nursing.)*

between each cry. If the young child is sleeping or comfortable in the parent's arms, the examiner listens to the chest first before proceeding to the rest of the examination.

For listening to the posterior thorax, the child is positioned with the head bent forward and hands folded in front. Having the child raise the arms overhead while sitting erect allows the examiner to listen laterally. To auscultate the anterior chest, have the child sit erect with the shoulders back (Fig. 9-15).

The examiner begins on the posterior thorax and has the child open the mouth and breathe in and out while the examiner listens with the diaphragm of the stethoscope. Having the young child blow bubbles, pretend to blow out

birthday candles, or blow a tissue increases breath sounds. Compressing the hand holding the stethoscope on the chest wall while placing the other hand on the opposite side of the chest accentuates expiration and makes end-expiratory sounds (e.g., wheezes) easier to hear. Having the child inhale deeply and then blow the breath out forcibly may assist with identification of adventitious breath sounds. The sequence for listening to breath sounds is posterior chest, right and left lateral chest, and anterior chest (Fig. 9-16).

Adventitious Breath Sounds

In addition to normal breath sounds, *adventitious sounds* may be audible with the stethoscope. Table 9-2 describes the origin and characteristics of adventitious sounds. Adventitious sounds are additional sounds heard in an abnormal clinical state. They are described by their quality. The examiner notes whether they are continuous or discontinuous and where they occur in the respiratory phase. The effects of coughing are also noted. When adventitious sounds are heard, they are described as to location, timing, and intensity.

Heart

The techniques for assessing the heart are inspection, palpation, and auscultation. The sequence of this examination depends on the age, growth, and development of the child being examined. For an infant or young child, the examiner may want to listen to the child's heart while the parent is holding the child, before doing other parts of the examination. Infants and children have varying degrees of dependence on parents and may be fearful of the examination. Percussion of the heart indicates primarily the size and shape of the heart and is not routinely done. The heart is

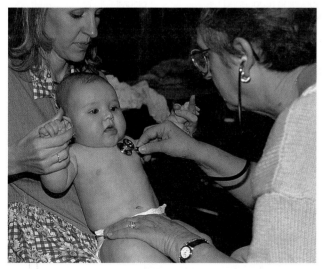

Infants and toddlers can be held sitting upright in the parent's lap while the nurse listens to breath sounds.

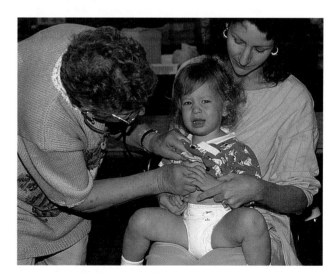

If the child is upset, the examiner may have to listen to breath sounds between cries. Keeping this child in the comfort of her mother's arms lessens her distress.

FIG 9-15   **To hear heart and breath sounds, the nurse auscultates the child's chest with a stethoscope in an orderly way. Auscultation is most easily done when the child is quiet, so this part of the examination is best performed first if the child is quiet or asleep. To allay fears and make the examination more comfortable, the child can play with the stethoscope first and warm the instrument. The child also can be distracted with a toy while the nurse is listening.**   *(Courtesy University of Texas at Arlington School of Nursing.)*

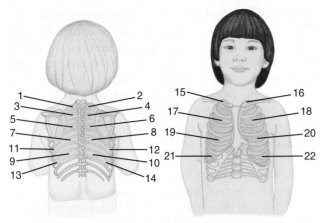

FIG 9-16   **Sequence for listening to breath sounds.**

assessed with the child in a supine position, in a left lateral recumbent position, and in a sitting position while leaning forward slightly.

Inspection

The anterior chest is systematically inspected, with special attention paid to the following five areas: second right intercostal space (aortic area), second left intercostal space (pulmonic area), left sternal border (right ventricular area), fifth left intercostal space in the midclavicular line (apex), and just below the xiphoid process (epigastric area). The areas will differ at different ages (Fig. 9-17). During infancy, the heart is more horizontal in the thorax, and the apex is one or two intercostal spaces above the fifth intercostal space

TABLE **9-2**	Origin and Characteristics of Adventitious Breath Sounds		
Sound	**Description**	**Mechanism**	**Clinical Example**
Discontinuous Sounds			
Crackles—fine (rales, crepitations); heard when fluid is in airways.	Discontinuous, high-pitched, short, crackling, popping sounds heard during inspiration and not cleared by coughing. You can simulate this sound by rolling a strand of hair between your fingers near your ear or by moistening your thumb and index finger and separating them near your ear. Described as discrete (short), discontinuous.	Inhaled air collides with previously deflated airways; airways suddenly pop open, creating crackling sound as gas pressures between the two compartments equalize.	*Late inspiratory* crackles occur with restrictive disease: pneumonia, congestive heart failure, and interstitial fibrosis. *Early inspiratory* crackles occur with obstructive disease: chronic bronchitis and asthma.
Pleural friction rub.	A very superficial sound that is coarse and low-pitched; it has a grating quality, as if two pieces of leather were being rubbed together. A pleural friction rub sounds just like crackles but close to the ear. It sounds louder if you push the stethoscope harder into the chest wall.	Caused when pleurae become inflamed and lose their normal lubricating fluid. Their opposing roughened pleural surfaces rub together during respiration. This sound is heard best in the anterolateral wall, where lung mobility is greatest.	Pleuritis, accompanied by pain with breathing. (Rub disappears after a few days if pleural fluid accumulates and separates pleurae.)
Continuous Sounds			
High-pitched wheeze heard with narrowing of the air passages from fluid, swelling, spasm, and tumors.	High-pitched, musical squeaking sounds that predominate in expiration but may occur in both expiration and inspiration. Coughing frequently will change the character of the sound.	Air squeezed or compressed through passageways narrowed almost to closure by collapsing, swelling, secretions, or tumors. The passageway walls oscillate in apposition between the closed and barely open positions. The resulting sound is similar to that produced by a vibrating reed.	Obstructive lung disease, such as asthma.
Low-pitched wheeze (sonorous rhonchi).	Low-pitched, musical snoring, moaning sounds. They are heard throughout the cycle, although they are more prominent on expiration and may clear somewhat by coughing.	Airflow obstruction as described by the vibrating reed mechanism. The pitch of the wheeze does not correlate with the size of the passageway that generates it.	Bronchitis.

NOTE: Although nothing in clinical practice seems to differ more than the nomenclature of adventitious sounds, most authorities concur on two categories: (1) discontinuous, discrete crackling sounds and (2) continuous, coarse, or wheezing sounds.

Cardiac Landmarks

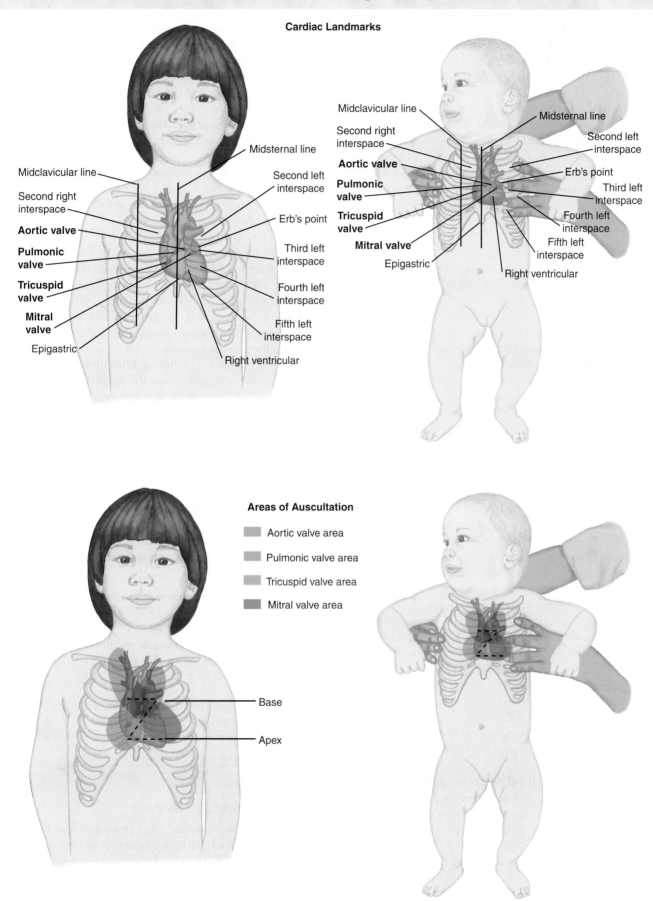

Areas of Auscultation

Aortic valve area

Pulmonic valve area

Tricuspid valve area

Mitral valve area

FIG 9-17   **Location of the heart within the thorax in the infant and the older child, showing landmarks and areas of auscultation.**

and lateral to the midclavicular line. The second intercostal space is located by identifying the sternal angle. The second rib is attached to the sternum just below or at the sternal angle. The second intercostal space is below the second rib. Other ribs and intercostal spaces are identified by their relationship to the second rib.

The precordium (anterior chest overlying the heart and great vessels) is inspected for *bulges, lifts, heaves,* and *apical impulse.* The apical impulse is the light tapping of the anterior chest wall every time the heart beats. The location of the apical impulse will change gradually as the child matures and by age 7 years can be seen at the fifth intercostal space in the midclavicular line.

Palpation

The examiner palpates the precordium with the fingertips for the presence of any pulsations at each individual area (see Fig. 9-17). The examiner locates the apical pulse, sometimes identified as the *point of maximal impulse (PMI),* or the point where the light tapping of the heart is felt the best and varies with age. In a child younger than 7 years, the PMI is located in the fourth intercostal space, lateral to the midclavicular line. The PMI in a child older than 7 years is located in the fifth intercostal space in the midclavicular line. Using the palmar aspect of the hand to feel for *thrills,* the examiner then palpates each individual area of the precordium. Thrills are palpable vibrations of the heart.

Auscultation

Auscultation of the heart is done by listening both with the bell and with the diaphragm of the stethoscope as the child is lying supine, in a left lateral recumbent position, and sitting up. To auscultate heart sounds, the examiner uses a systematic approach. Sounds heard with the stethoscope are predominantly produced with the closing of the heart valves. The four traditional areas for listening to heart sounds are the aortic valve area in the second right intercostal space, the pulmonic valve area in the second left intercostal space, the tricuspid valve area in the left lower sternal border, and the mitral valve area in the fifth intercostal space at the left midclavicular line (see Fig. 9-17). The position for listening to these areas depends on the age of the child. It is best to listen to heart sounds by inching the stethoscope across the precordium in a **Z**-shaped pattern, from the base of the heart across and down, or from the apex upward. All areas are auscultated with both the bell and the diaphragm of the stethoscope.

Sounds produced by the closing of the valves can be heard all over the precordium, so it will be necessary to concentrate on one heart sound at a time. The heart sounds are divided into two components—the first heart sound (S_1) and the second heart sound (S_2). S_1 is heard best at the apex of the heart, and S_2 is heard best at the base (see Fig. 9-17). S_1, phonetically described as *lub,* is produced by the closing of the mitral and tricuspid valves. S_2, phonetically described as *dub,* is produced by the closing of the aortic and pulmonic valves.

The physiologic splitting of S_2, an audible pause between the closing of the aortic and pulmonic valves, frequently heard in children of all ages, is considered normal. Splitting of S_2 can be heard best at the pulmonic area because ejection times on the right side of the heart are slightly longer than on the left side. Splitting of S_2 is greatest at the peak of inspiration and decreases or goes away during expiration.

The routine for assessing heart sounds is the following sequence:

1. Identify the rate and rhythm.
2. Identify S_1 and S_2.
3. Assess S_1 and S_2 separately to determine where they are best heard.
4. Listen for extra heart sounds.
5. Identify murmurs.

Normal Rate and Rhythm. The normal rate of a child's heart is different at different ages (see Table 9-1). Children's heart rates often increase with inspiration and slow down during expiration. To decrease the irregular rhythm associated with respirations, the examiner has the child hold the breath as the examiner continues to listen.

Extra Heart Sounds, Including Murmurs. Extra sounds (sounds heard over and above the normal heart sounds) may be described as opening snaps, ejection clicks, midsystolic to late systolic clicks, and murmurs. Snaps and clicks are short, high-pitched sounds heard with valve disorders and do not vary with respirations. *Murmurs* are blowing, swooshing sounds that occur because of some disruption in the blood flow into, through, or out of the heart. Innocent or functional heart murmurs are frequently heard in children. Innocent murmurs occur during systole, are heard best along the left sternal border, do not radiate, and change with position change. To describe and classify extra heart sounds, the nurse needs advanced training and practice.

CRITICAL TO REMEMBER
Normal Findings in Children

- Small, firm, nontender, and shotty (freely palpable and very small) lymph nodes may be palpable.
- Tonsils of varying sizes; often larger in young children.
- Pupils of equal size, round, and reactive to light and accommodation. (PERRLA)
- Pulses in upper and lower extremities; bilaterally symmetric.

Peripheral Vascular System

Arterial pulses are examined for decreased or absent pulses. Pulses are palpated, with the examiner noting the rate, rhythm, elasticity of the vessel wall, and equal force of bilateral pulses. The pulse force should be symmetric and should be the same for upper and lower extremities. Comparing opposite pulses is necessary in children. The examiner compares one femoral pulse with the opposite radial pulse for equality and compares one lower extremity pulse with an upper extremity pulse for equality. A diminished or absent femoral pulse, compared with the radial pulse, may be the only finding in coarctation of the aorta in infants and children.

Breast

The examiner inspects and palpates breast tissue. Developmental differences occur in response to circulating hormones and affect the appearance of breast tissue. In infants of both sexes, the breasts may appear engorged because of maternal estrogen crossing the placenta. *Thelarche,* or breast development, marks the beginning of puberty in preadolescent girls and can occur as early as age 7 years.

The examiner inspects the nipples for position and appearance. In infants, the nipple is flat and symmetric with darker areolar pigmentation. In preadolescent and adolescent girls, the Tanner sexual maturity rating is used to evaluate developmental levels (see Table 8-1). The nipples should be symmetric on the chest and should point in the same direction. Nipples may appear to be inverted or everted. An inverted nipple is significant if the inversion is of recent origin. The breast skin should be smooth and free of any dimpling. It is common to see some asymmetry during growth.

All adolescent girls should be taught how to do breast self-examination once they have reached menarche. Teaching self-examination to the adolescent and reinforcing its importance at every visit are important roles for the nurse. Many adolescents do not do breast self-examinations because of lack of knowledge or fear of finding something wrong. Once the adolescent is familiar with how her breasts look and feel, the natural and normal changes that occur in the breast as a result of hormonal fluctuations can be easily identified. Teach the adolescent girl to do breast self-examination 3 to 4 days after menses because the breasts are least tender and sensitive at that time (Fox, 2002).

The examiner uses the same technique to palpate the breast tissue and the axilla of the adolescent boy. In the male, the examiner expects to feel a thin layer of fatty tissue overlying the muscle. During puberty, some boys experience *gynecomastia*, an enlargement of breast tissue, felt as a smooth, firm, movable disk. It frequently affects only one breast and can be temporary.

Abdomen

The child's comfort should be considered during the abdominal examination. An empty bladder, warm hands, and positioning the child supine on the examining table with a pillow under the head and the knees flexed enhance abdominal relaxation. For an infant or young child, most of the abdominal examination can be done while the child is lying in the parent's lap. For an older child, the genitalia and breasts are draped. The child or parent should be questioned about urinary and bowel patterns.

The abdomen is divided into four quadrants that correlate with underlying anatomic structures (Fig. 9-18). Because bowel sounds are disturbed by percussion and palpation, the sequence of techniques differs in abdominal assessment. The abdomen is first inspected, then auscultated, then percussed, and last palpated.

Inspection

Abdominal inspection assesses contour, symmetry, characteristics of the umbilicus and skin, pulsations or movement, and hair distribution. *Contour* is the profile of the abdomen from the rib margin to the pubic bone and is best determined by looking tangentially across the abdomen. The contour is described as flat, scaphoid, rounded, or protuberant (Fig. 9-19). The abdominal contour provides an overall indicator of nutritional state. The abdomen should be symmetric bilaterally. The examiner looks for distention, bulging, visible mass, or asymmetric shape.

The umbilicus is normally midline and inverted. There should be no signs of discoloration, inflammation, or hernia. Throughout the neonatal period, the umbilical cord is inspected for signs of infection or bleeding.

The skin of the abdomen is inspected for color and the presence of scars, lesions, and striae. A fine venous network may be seen in infants and small children.

Inspect the abdomen for pulsations and movement. In thin children, the examiner may see the pulsations from the aorta beneath the skin in the epigastric area. Most children have abdominal movement with respirations. Peristalsis of the abdomen should not be visible.

Auscultation

Auscultation of the abdomen follows inspection. The diaphragm of the stethoscope is held lightly against the skin to note the character and frequency of bowel sounds. Bowel sounds are high-pitched, gurgling sounds heard in all four quadrants. They are irregular and can occur from 5 to 34 times per minute. The examiner begins in the lower right quadrant and listens in all four quadrants. To determine that there are no bowel sounds, the examiner must listen for up to 5 minutes in an area where no bowel sounds are heard.

The bell of the stethoscope is used to listen for bruits over the aortic, renal, iliac, and femoral arteries. The examiner also listens in the epigastric region and around the umbilicus for a venous hum—a soft, low-pitched, continuous sound.

Percussion

Advanced practitioners perform abdominal percussion. The technique reveals tympany, liver span, and splenic dullness.

Palpation

Abdominal palpation can identify any mass or tenderness and determine the size, consistency, and location of certain organs. The examiner should have warm hands before palpating the abdomen. Palpation of the infant or young child can be done in the parent's lap by laying the child's head and thorax across the parent's legs and extending the child's abdomen and legs across the examiner's legs. Flex the child's knees to prepare the child for palpation of the abdomen.

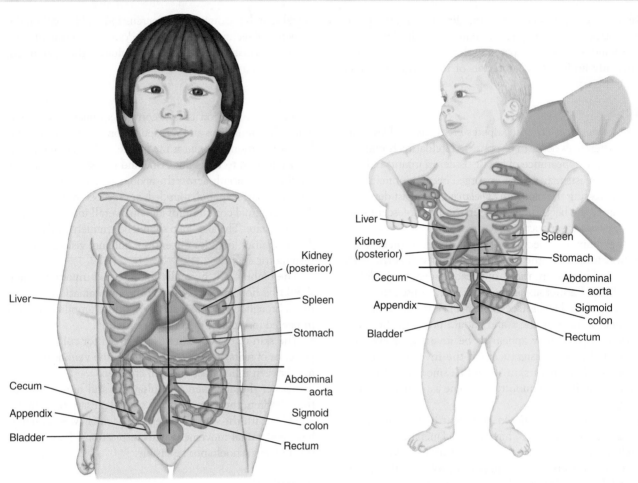

FIG 9-18   **Abdominal quadrants and structures.**

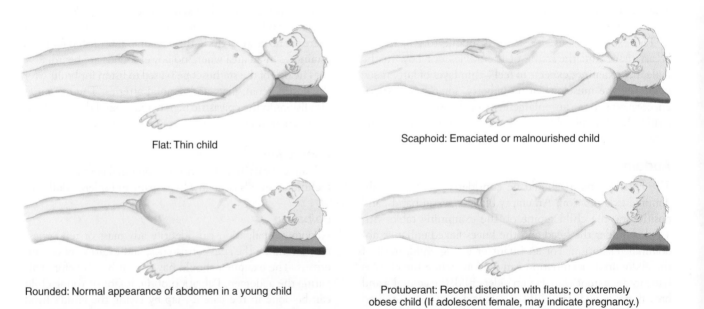

Flat: Thin child

Scaphoid: Emaciated or malnourished child

Rounded: Normal appearance of abdomen in a young child

Protuberant: Recent distention with flatus; or extremely obese child (If adolescent female, may indicate pregnancy.)

FIG 9-19   **Abdominal contours. The contour of the abdomen provides an indication of the child's overall nutritional state.**

Fear and anxiety may cause the child to resist when the examiner touches the abdomen. Distracting the young child with a toy or talking is helpful. Beginning with light palpation shows the child that palpation will not hurt.

Ask an older child who is anxious or ticklish to assist with this part of the examination. The child places a hand on the abdomen, and the examiner places a hand, with fingers touching the abdomen, on top of the child's hand and asks the child to push as the examiner pushes. This technique allows the child some control as the examination begins, and it reduces the sensation of tickling. To assist with relaxation of the abdominal muscles, the examiner can ask the child to take deep breaths.

The examiner begins with light palpation of all four quadrants using light, even pressure and pressing the palmar surface of the fingers no more than 1 cm into the abdomen. The hand is lifted while moving from area to area. Sudden jabs should be avoided. As the examiner circles around the abdomen, the abdomen should feel soft and smooth. Light palpation is useful in identifying areas of tenderness and muscular resistance. Guarding, resistance, or tenderness should alert the examiner to move cautiously with deeper palpation.

Tenseness can be either voluntary or involuntary. In a child, tenseness and rigidity may be caused by fear and anxiety. Distracting the child or waiting for the child to breathe will assist with determining whether the tenseness is voluntary or involuntary. The examiner gently indents the fingers into the abdominal wall during inspiration. With even pressure, the abdomen should feel soft. Rigidity, a constant, boardlike hardness, of the abdomen is usually associated with an acute inflammation of the peritoneum.

Using the same techniques, the examiner deeply palpates the abdomen. The examiner pushes down about 5 to 8 cm into the abdominal wall, beginning in the right lower quadrant. The entire abdomen is examined to identify palpable organs and masses.

To palpate the liver's edge, the examiner begins at the level of the umbilicus in the midclavicular line, using the side of the hand to indent the abdomen about 5 to 8 cm. With deep penetration of the abdominal wall, the hand is gently inverted toward the costal margin. Then the examiner progresses upward with the same maneuver until palpating the border of the liver. The edge of the liver is felt as soft and smooth. The firm border moves downward when the child takes a deep breath. In infants and young children, the examiner can begin at the costal margin and, using the palmar aspects of the fingers, indent the abdominal wall about 5 to 8 cm. The examiner should move down from the costal margin until the hand falls off the edge of the liver border. In infants and toddlers, the liver edge may be palpated 1 to 3 cm below the costal margin.

While palpating the abdomen, the examiner checks skin turgor and palpates the femoral pulses and inguinal lymph nodes. Advanced practitioners palpate the spleen and kidneys to determine the presence and size of masses or enlargement.

When areas of tenderness are elicited during palpation, a special procedure for identifying rebound tenderness is used. A site away from the identified tenderness is chosen. The examiner places a hand perpendicular to the abdomen, pushes down slowly and deeply into the abdomen, and then lifts the hand quickly. With peritoneal inflammation, the sudden release of the pressure will cause severe pain and muscle rigidity.

The child is turned over, and the buttocks are inspected. The buttocks in children are full, with symmetric folds. No evidence of scars or ecchymosis should appear on the buttocks. The sacrococcygeal area is examined for any dimples or tufts of hair.

Male Genitalia

The approach to examining the male genitals will depend on the child's growth and development. In an infant, toddler, or young child, the nurse tells the child what will occur and then the parent or guardian concurs that the nurse should proceed to examine the child's genitalia.

Objective signs of pubertal changes and the adolescent's perception of these changes have an impact on understanding physical signs experienced by this age group. Adolescent boys are normally apprehensive about the genital examination. Concerns arise from modesty, fear of pain, negative judgment, or a previous uncomfortable experience. A matter-of-fact approach and direct communication will facilitate this part of the physical examination. The genital examination is performed during or immediately after the abdominal examination. In the adolescent, the physical examination should not conclude with the genital examination so as to allow further opportunity for communication. A good practice is to conclude the physical examination with the musculoskeletal and neurologic examination after the genital examination has been completed.

Gloves should be worn during every genital examination. The examiner begins by inspecting the penis. The size of the penis is directly related to age and to growth and development. In infants and young boys, the penis is approximately 2 to 3 cm. Genital hair distribution is noted. The adolescent shows a wide variation in normal development of the genitals. Tanner stages are used for determining the level of development in the adolescent (see Chapter 8).

The skin on the penis normally appears wrinkled, hairless, and without lesions. In the adolescent, a dorsal vein may be prominent. Any indurations on the penile shaft should be noted. In the circumcised male, the glans looks smooth and without lesions. In an uncircumcised infant, the glans may not be visible. By the time the male is age 5 to 6 years, the foreskin may be easily retractable behind the corona of the glans. The adolescent is asked to retract the foreskin himself.

The meatus is evaluated by compressing the glans between the thumb and forefinger anteroposteriorly. The adolescent may be requested to compress the glans so that the examiner can see the meatus. The meatus in the male has a slitlike or

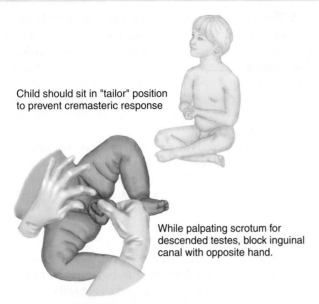

Child should sit in "tailor" position to prevent cremasteric response

While palpating scrotum for descended testes, block inguinal canal with opposite hand.

FIG 9-20   **When a boy's scrotum is examined, the cremasteric reflex may cause the testes to withdraw into the inguinal canals. To prevent this reflex, the examiner can have the boy sit in a tailor position. The examiner uses one hand to block the inguinal canal and the other to palpate.**

tear-shaped configuration and is located on the ventral surface, just millimeters from the tip of the glans. The meatus opening is pink, smooth, and without discharge.

The scrotum is inspected for size and configuration, which changes with growth and development. In the infant or young boy, the proximal portion of the scrotum is wider and the distal portion narrower. In the adolescent boy, the proximal portion is narrower and the distal portion wider. Asymmetry of the scrotum is normal, with the left half slightly lower than the right. The scrotum is movable and, to maintain optimal temperature of the testes, will move closer to or away from the body in response to environmental temperature.

The contents of the scrotum are palpated. The *cremasteric reflex* in young boys may cause the testes to withdraw into the inguinal canal, making palpation more difficult. If the boy is old enough, have him sit in a cross-legged, or "tailor," position, which will help prevent the cremasteric reflex by stretching the muscle, thereby preventing its contraction. In infants and young boys, before beginning the abdominal examination, the examiner warms the hands, blocks the inguinal canal with one hand, and palpates for the scrotal contents (Fig. 9-20). The examiner uses the thumb and first two fingers to palpate each testis and epididymis. The testes should be smooth, rubbery, and free of nodules. The size of the testes changes with growth and development. Tanner growth and development stages are used for appropriate interpretation. Because of the high incidence of testicular tumors in young men, adolescents should be taught to do testicular self-examination.

Female Genitalia

In general, the anogenital examination in prepubescent girls is limited to visual inspection and gentle palpation of the external area. Internal speculum examinations are not routine in prepubescent children. The appearance of the external genitalia in females varies from child to child and with growth and development. A relaxed, caring attitude will reassure both child and parent.

To safeguard privacy, reinforce modesty, and decrease anxiety, the child is draped appropriately. The examiner should communicate with the child what will be done and the parent or guardian concurs that it is appropriate to examine the genitalia. With the child in different positions, the genitals will differ in tone, relaxation, and appearance. Generally, the genitalia in young girls are examined with the child supine; the legs are gently drawn up onto the abdomen to expose the genitalia.

The examiner dons gloves and begins by inspecting the *mons pubis* and *labia majora*. The skin should be smooth and clean. The examiner notes the distribution of pubic hair. Tanner stages are used to determine appropriate growth and development (see Chapter 8).

In the newborn infant, the labia majora and minora may be edematous, with the *labia minora* often more prominent. In the infant, the *hymen* may protrude and may appear thick and vascular. The clitoris may appear relatively large. The hymen is centrally located and is about 0.5 cm in diameter. The examiner determines whether the hymen has an opening.

In the young girl or adolescent, the labia majora may be gaping or closed, shriveled or full, dry or moist, depending on the age and development of the child. The labia majora are usually symmetric (Fig. 9-21).

The examiner uses the fingers to gently spread the labia majora and then inspects and palpates the labia minora, the *clitoris*, the urethral orifice, and the *vaginal introitus*. The labia

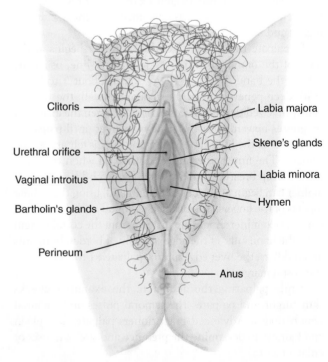

Clitoris

Urethral orifice

Vaginal introitus

Bartholin's glands

Perineum

Labia majora

Skene's glands

Labia minora

Hymen

Anus

FIG 9-21   **Postpubertal female genitalia.**

minora should appear symmetric, dark pink, and moist. On palpation, the tissue should be soft and homogeneous with no tenderness.

With the labia majora spread, the examiner can look superiorly and inspect the clitoris for size and length. The clitoris varies with growth and development. Progressing inferiorly, the examiner locates the urethral meatus, which may be close to or inside the vaginal introitus. The urethral meatus is usually in the midline and appears as a dimple posterior to the clitoris.

The vaginal introitus may be a thin, vertical slit or a large orifice with irregular edges, depending on the characteristics of the hymen. The hymen may or may not be stretched across the vaginal opening. By menarche, the opening should be at least 1 cm wide. The tissue is usually moist. The amount and characteristics of any vaginal discharge depend on the circulating hormones in the child. A normal vaginal discharge is odorless and may be cloudy or clear, thick or thin, and there may be a slippery sensation around the time of ovulation.

Normally, *Skene's glands,* located just inferior to the urethral meatus, are not seen or felt and have no discharge. Any discharge from Skene's glands indicates an infection. The examiner inspects and palpates *Bartholin's glands,* located in the posterolateral portion of the labia majora. Bartholin's glands should not be swollen or tender.

A speculum examination of the internal reproductive organs is not indicated for young girls. The adolescent girl has special needs during the genital examination, which is performed by advanced practitioners.

Musculoskeletal System

The musculoskeletal system is composed of the bones, joints, cartilage, ligaments, and muscles. Joint motions are defined as flexion, extension, abduction, adduction, internal rotation, external rotation, and circumduction. The musculoskeletal examination focuses principally on the upper and lower extremities and the spinal column. Musculoskeletal evaluation begins with observing the child during play or history taking. Observation of the child climbing, jumping, hopping, rising from a sitting position, and manipulating toys and other objects provides evidence of joint function, range of motion, bone stability, and muscle strength. Assessment of fine motor and gross motor ability is accomplished during the Denver II test for the child younger than 5 years old (see Chapter 4 and Evolve website).

General inspection begins with visual scanning of the body with use of a *cephalocaudal* (head-to-toe) organization. The child can be dressed in shorts or underwear during the examination. The examiner compares the two sides of the body for symmetry, contour, size, and involuntary movement. The examiner then inspects the two sides for areas of swelling or edema and for ecchymoses or other discolorations. The structural relationship of the feet to the legs and the hips to the pelvis, the upper extremities, the shoulder girdle, and the upper trunk are evaluated.

Common deformities of the extremities are *varus* and *valgus* deformities. With the reference point of the midline of the body, a varus deformity is a medial adduction or turning inward. A valgus deformity is a medial abduction or turning outward (see Chapter 26).

Injuries to the extremities caused by overexertion and strenuous movements are common in children. Sprains are the most common injury, followed by fractures, dislocations, and lacerations.

Deformities of the spine are *scoliosis, kyphosis,* and *lordosis,* which are discussed in Chapter 26.

Palpation of the skull, extremities and ribs for tenderness, swelling, deformity, or crepitus is performed on any child who is suspected of having injuries or circumstances that warrant suspicion of abuse.

Infants

During infancy, symmetric flexion of the arms and legs is noted. Limbs should be freely movable, with symmetry of the axillary, gluteal, femoral, and popliteal creases. The examiner inspects the hands, noting the shape, number, and position of the fingers and palmar creases. The clavicle should feel smooth, regular, and without crepitus. By age 2 months, the infant can lift the head while prone.

The examiner observes range of motion as the infant spontaneously moves the extremities. When the infant is lifted with the examiner's hands under the axillae, the infant with normal muscle strength wedges securely between the hands. The examiner checks the hips for congenital dislocation by comparing leg lengths. Place the baby's feet flat on the table, and flex the knees up. Look for the top of the knees to be the same height (Allis test). Posterior gluteal folds should be equal on both sides. The *Ortolani* and *Barlow maneuvers* are performed by a trained examiner on every visit until the infant is 1 year old (see Chapter 26).

Toddlers, Preschoolers, and School-Age Children

The examiner may want to start with the child's hands and arms by checking for range of motion and the presence of pain while the child is sitting. Children are willing to show their hands, so this is an excellent way to make contact with the child.

The child should stand so that the examiner can observe the posture from behind. The shoulders should be level and the scapulae symmetric. Lordosis is common in young children. Anteriorly, the examiner begins with the feet and observes for adduction and pronation of the foot. Pronation is common between ages 12 and 30 months because of the young child's broad-based stance. Adduction, or toeing in, is demonstrated when the child walks on the lateral side of the foot. Adduction tends to correct itself by age 3 years as long as the foot is flexible. *Genu varum* (bowleg) is present when a space of more than 2.5 cm is measured between the knees as the medial malleoli are held together. Genu varum is normal after the child has begun to walk and may persist until the child is 3 years old. *Genu valgum* means that more than 2.5 cm remains between the medial malleoli when the knees are held together. Genu valgum is present between ages 2 and 3½ years (see Chapter 26).

The child is instructed to stand on one leg and then the other while the examiner watches from behind. The iliac crest should stay level when the weight is shifted.

Adolescents

For adolescents, the examiner follows the sequence described for school-age children but with special attention to the spine. Adolescents frequently have kyphosis (see Fig. 26-10) caused by poor posture. Children aged 9 through 15 years should be screened for scoliosis (Box 9-9).

Range of Motion

The examiner notes the child's ability to perform active range-of-motion movements when the child is sitting, standing, and moving about the examination room. The equality of movement for each joint and for contralateral joints should be noted. There should be no pain, limitation of movement, spastic movement, joint instability, deformity, or crepitation during movement. Passive range-of-motion movements are performed on joints where limitations are noted. Passive range-of-motion movement is accomplished by the examiner anchoring the joint with one hand while the other hand slowly moves the joint to its limit. Active and passive ranges of motion should be the same.

Muscle Strength and Mass

The examiner assesses the strength of each muscle group. The child is asked to flex the muscle and then resist as opposing force is applied against flexion. Muscle tone should be firm on palpation. When appropriate, the evaluation of

---

| BOX 9-9 | **Screening Procedure for Scoliosis** |

To ensure early detection and treatment, children aged 9 through 15 years should be screened for scoliosis. At greatest risk are girls from 10 years old through adolescence.

The child should be unclothed or wearing only underpants so that the chest, back, and hips can be clearly seen. Have the child stand with his or her weight distributed equally on both feet, with legs straight and arms hanging loosely at the sides. Observe for the following signs of scoliosis:

- Nonpainful lateral curvature of the spine
- A curve with one turn (C curve) or two compensating curves (S curve)
- Lateral deviation and rotation of each vertebra, observed better by looking at the ribs as well as the spinal column itself
- Unequal shoulder heights
- Congenital scoliosis visible in the infant lying prone; the condition is sometimes more prominent if the infant is suspended prone
- Unequal scapular prominences and heights. (Note that the muscle masses may be somewhat unequal, especially if the child uses one shoulder more than the other, as in carrying books. Look for bony, not muscular, prominence.)
- Unequal waist angles
- Unequal rib prominences and chest asymmetry
- Unequal rib heights when the child stands in Adam's position (see photograph)

The physical examination should also include the following:

- Observation for equal leg lengths
- Examination of the skin for hairy patches, nevi, café au lait spots, lipomas, dimples
- Neurologic examination
- Cardiac examination for Marfan syndrome

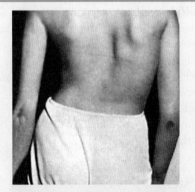

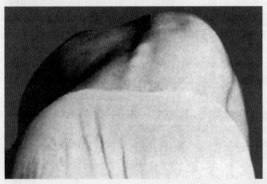

Adam's position with rib hump of structural scoliosis. Lateral curvature of thoracic and lumbar segments of the spine, usually with some rotation of involved vertebral bodies.

Functional scoliosis is flexible; it is apparent with standing and disappears with forward bending. It may be compensatory for other abnormalities such as leg-length discrepancy.

Structural scoliosis is fixed; the curvature is evident both when the individual stands and when the individual bends forward. Note the rib hump with forward flexion. When the child is standing, note unequal shoulder elevation, unequal scapulae, obvious curvature, unequal elbow level, and unequal hip level.

Data from Burns, C. E. (2000). Musculoskeletal disorders. In C. E. Burns, N. Barber, M. A. Brady, & A. M. Dunn (Eds.), *Pediatric primary care: A handbook for nurse practitioners* (p. 1147). Philadelphia: WB Saunders. Photographs from Delp, M. H., & Manning, R. T. (1981). *Major's physical diagnosis: An introduction to the clinical process* (9th ed., p. 450). Philadelphia: WB Saunders.

muscle strength is integrated with examination of the associated joint for range of motion. Evaluate the motor segment of cranial nerve V (*trigeminal nerve*) by applying opposing force to the temporalis muscle while the child clenches the teeth. Cranial nerve XI (*spinal accessory nerve*) is tested by assessing the strength of the sternocleidomastoid and trapezius muscles with rotation of the head from side to side and chin to shoulder.

When atrophy or hypertrophy is suspected, the examiner measures muscle mass. Muscles are best measured at their greatest circumference. With the joint used as a landmark, the distance from the joint to a point on the extremity is measured and compared with the opposite muscle. One measurement is not as significant as a series of measurements to determine changes in size of muscles.

Joints

The examiner palpates each joint for temperature, tenderness, swelling, crepitation, and masses. In children, fatigue, stiffness, or weakness, along with heat and redness, is frequently associated with disorders of the joints. Children will usually not move a joint if the joint is painful.

Gait

Assessment of the child's gait and the ability to ambulate is an essential part of both the musculoskeletal and the neurologic assessments. The developmental acquisition of the ability to walk follows a prescribed sequence in infants and toddlers (Table 9-3 and see Chapter 5).

Gait is assessed in two phases—stance and swing. The stance phase begins when the heel strikes the floor; then the weight is transferred to the ball of the foot, and the toes push off the floor. The swing phase consists of acceleration, swing through, and deceleration.

Neurologic System

The purpose of the neurologic examination in the child and adolescent is to identify any nervous system malfunction and to ascertain the extent of nervous system development and functioning. In cases of neurologic deficit, the examiner needs to determine the degree, type, and location of nervous system lesions. In the child, the examiner determines the degree to which the nervous system is functioning so that the healthy portion of the nervous system can be used for habilitation or rehabilitation. For the child younger than 5 years, neurologic functioning is best evaluated with the Denver II test (see Chapter 4 and Evolve website). For the child older than 5 years, adapt the sequence of the neurologic examination to the child's ability to understand and cooperate.

Brain dysfunction in infants and young children may be manifested by apnea, loss of consciousness, and seizures. Very young children may have milder nonspecific clinical signs such as irritability, recurrent vomiting, fever, or loss of appetite.

Testing cerebral function, cranial nerves, and cerebellar function gives a picture of nervous system functioning above the spinal cord. The child's age and development determine the sequence of the neurologic examination. The infant and younger child are not able to cooperate with neurologic testing. A review of developmental milestones attained helps establish the rate and consistency of development in the infant and younger child. The 3- or 4-year-old child cooperates with testing when it is approached as a game.

Cerebral Function

The evaluation of cognitive function focuses on appearance, behavior, orientation, speech patterns, memory, logic, and affect. The examiner needs to obtain information

---

TABLE 9-3   Gross Motor Development in the Infant: Progression to Walking

Activity	Age
Raises head and holds position	2 wk to 2 mo
Moves all extremities, kicking arms and legs when prone	2 mo
Draws up knees and raises abdomen off table; rocks back and forth while up on hands and knees; rolls over	3-6 mo
Sits alone, using hands for support (tripod fashion)	By 7 mo
Lurches forward and pulls legs to chest in "inchworm" fashion, may move backward in same fashion; creeps and rolls	By 9 mo
Crawls in one-sided manner (moves arm and leg on same side of body, then other side)	6-9 mo
Crawls in regular fashion, alternating arm and opposite leg	6-9 mo
Begins to pull up	By 11 mo
Cruises: attempts to walk with support or holding on to something stable	By 12 mo
Momentarily lets go and maintains balance for a few seconds	Once comfortable standing and holding on
Takes first steps (a broad stance with arms flexed for balance)	Once standing balance accomplished
Sits from a standing posture	By 12 mo
Walks alone	By 15 mo

from the primary caregiver about changes in the child's behavior, personality, appearance, and age-appropriate school performance. Evaluation of cognitive function in the older child and adolescent is based on observation of level of consciousness, awareness, thought processes, and communication.

The degree of response to sensory stimuli provides information about the older child's or adolescent's level of consciousness. The child is described as alert, lethargic, obtunded, stuporous, or comatose.

The older child and the adolescent have the ability to understand, think, feel emotions, and appreciate sensory information about the self and surroundings. Awareness is evaluated by observing the older child's or adolescent's level of orientation in relation to person, place, and time. The normally functioning child is oriented to person, place, and time.

Thought processes include abstract thinking, problem solving (simple calculations and concentration), insight, memory (recent and remote), and judgment. The child's school performance may or may not be an accurate indicator of thought processes. Factors that may influence thought processes are attention span, communication, perceptual problems, and emotional withdrawal and depression.

Language ability is evaluated through speech patterns and comprehension. Question the child about reading and writing ability. Is the child's speech intelligible? Does the child answer questions appropriately for age and developmental level? The normally functioning child is able to speak fluently, name objects correctly, and write both name and address (Box 9-10).

Cranial Nerves

Assessment of the cranial nerves (Table 9-4) should be incorporated into the examination of the system each nerve affects. Games, such as making faces or performing tests on a parent or the examiner, will enhance cooperation.

Cerebellar Function

Proprioception, balance, and coordination are tested by having the child perform specific movements. The cerebellum controls balance and coordination. Proprioception evaluates laterality and orientation in space. The techniques used vary with the child's age and development. The child should attempt the technique and show continued improvement with maturation (Box 9-11).

Motor System

Muscle size, muscle tone, involuntary movements, and muscle strength are assessed during the musculoskeletal examination.

While the child is at rest, the muscles are inspected and palpated for size, consistency, and possible atrophy. The examiner notes symmetry of posture and of muscle contours and outlines.

BOX 9-10	**Specific Cerebral Function Tests**

- *Sound recognition:* Can the child identify familiar sounds with the eyes closed?
- *Auditory and verbal comprehension:* Does the child answer questions and carry out instructions appropriate for age?
- *Recognition of body parts and sidedness:* Does the child recognize the parts of the body? Does the child know right from left?
- *Performance of skilled motor acts:* Can the child drink from a cup, button clothes, use a common tool?
- *Visual object recognition:* Can the child identify a familiar toy or object (e.g., wristwatch)?
- *Visual and verbal comprehension:* Can the child read appropriately and explain the meaning?
- *Motor speech:* Does the child imitate different sounds and phrases?
- *Automatic speech:* Can the child repeat series learned (e.g., nursery rhymes, days of the week)?
- *Volitional speech:* Does the child answer questions relevantly?
- *Writing:* Can the child write his or her name or the name of an object?

Muscle tone is evaluated by palpating the muscles at rest and noting resistance to passive movement. The examiner inspects the muscles for involuntary movements. Muscle strength is tested first without resistance and then against resistance. Corresponding muscles are compared on each side. The examiner then tests the major joints for flexion, extension, and other movements.

Sensory System

Sensory testing depends on the child's perception and interpretation of the stimuli and on the child's age and development. Sensory tests should first be done in an educational practice session before being done in a testing situation. Sensory testing compares both sides of the body, corresponding extremities, and the sensitivity of the distal and proximal parts of each extremity for each form of sensation. Sensory testing is performed to determine whether sensory changes involve one entire side of the body, are *dermatomal* (along nerve pathways in the skin) in distribution, or are confined to the peripheral nerves (Box 9-12). In an older child, primary forms of sensation, such as superficial tactile, superficial pain, sensitivity to temperature, sensitivity to vibration, deep pressure pain, and motion and position, can be tested. Cortical and discriminatory forms of sensation require interpretation by the cerebral cortex. They are evaluated by two-point discrimination, point localization, texture discrimination, *stereognostic* (touch recognition of objects) function, *graphesthesia* (identification of figures traced on the skin), and extinction phenomenon.

TABLE 9-4   Assessing Cranial Nerves

Cranial Nerve	Procedure
I (olfactory nerve)	The child is asked to identify familiar odors with the eyes closed. Each side of the nose is tested separately.
II (optic nerve)	Visual acuity is tested using the Snellen chart, HOTV chart for young children, or the tumbling E chart for very young children. Each eye is tested separately and then both eyes together. If corrective lenses are worn, the eyes are tested both with and without correction.
III, IV, VI (oculomotor, trochlear, abducens nerves)	The child is asked to follow a toy or the examiner's finger as the object moves in all directions of gaze (six cardinal fields of gaze).
V (trigeminal nerve)	The child is asked to identify a wisp of cotton on the face. Corneal reflex is tested by observing for blinking when the examiner approaches the face closely. The masseter and temporal muscles' strength can be evaluated by having the child bite down on a tongue blade as the examiner tries to remove it.
VII (facial nerve)	The child is asked to imitate the examiner's frown, wrinkled forehead, smile, and raised eyebrow. The child tries to keep the eyes closed while the examiner attempts to open them, to test the strength of the eyelid muscles. The sensory portion of the facial nerve can be evaluated by having the child identify the taste of sugar and salt placed on the anterior part of the tongue on each side.
VIII (acoustic nerve)	Cochlear nerve tests are tests for hearing. Audiometric testing is a quantitative evaluation of hearing. The Weber (lateralization) and Rinne (air and bone conduction) tests are qualitative evaluations of hearing.
IX, X (glossopharyngeal nerve, vagus nerve)	The glossopharyngeal and vagus nerves are tested together. With a tongue depressor, the gag reflex is tested by touching the posterior pharyngeal wall. The palatal reflex is tested by stroking each side of the mucous membrane of the uvula. The side touched should rise. Normal function of the vagus nerve is revealed by the child's ability to swallow and to speak clearly.
XI (accessory nerve)	The examiner palpates and notes the strength of the trapezius and sternocleidomastoid muscles against resistance, or the child shrugs the shoulders against resistance.
XII (hypoglossal nerve)	The child is asked to stick out the tongue, and the examiner notes any lateral deviation when it is protruded. The strength of the tongue is assessed by having the child push against the examiner's finger pressed against the cheek with the child's tongue.

Cranial nerves are tested when the system in which they occur is assessed.

Reflex Status

Most brain growth occurs in the first year of life. Primitive reflexes in the neonate are inhibited when more advanced cortical functions and voluntary control take over as the child matures and grows. Commonly elicited reflexes are illustrated in Table 9-5.

Motor maturation proceeds in a cephalocaudal direction. The ability to elicit a reflex requires an intact afferent nerve fiber, functional synapses in the spinal cord, intact motor nerve fibers, functional neuromuscular junctions, and competent muscle fibers. The examiner compares the responses on the right and left sides, which should be equal. Diminished or hyperreflexic responses are reported for further evaluation.

Neurologic "Soft" Signs

Neurologic soft signs are findings that indicate the child's inability to perform certain activities related to the child's age. They may provide subtle clues to an underlying central nervous system deficit or neurologic maturation delay.

Although these findings may fall in a gray area, they should be recorded and reported when they are observed. Children with multiple soft signs are often found to have learning problems (Seidel et al., 2003).

Children with soft neurologic signs need evaluation and monitoring because some children with medical, mental, or emotional problems may also demonstrate neurologic soft signs (Box 9-13).

CONCLUSION AND DOCUMENTATION

When the physical examination has been completed, the examiner should ask the parents and child, if age appropriate, whether they have any questions concerning the examination. Findings are documented in a complete and concise manner. Deviations from normal and risk factors should be identified and documented. Depending on the setting, referrals may be made.

TABLE 9-5 Evaluating Common Reflexes

Reflex	Evaluation
Deep Tendon Reflexes	Evaluation elicited by tapping briskly on a tendon or a bony prominence, evoking a sudden stretching of certain muscles and their resulting contraction. For an adequate response, the limb should be relaxed and the muscle partially stretched. The reflex is stimulated by directing a sharp blow of the reflex hammer onto the muscle's insertion tendon.
Biceps Reflex 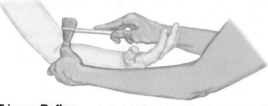	The child's arm should be flexed up to 45 degrees at the elbow. The biceps tendon in the antecubital fossa is palpated. The thumb is then placed on the biceps tendon, and a blow is struck on the thumb. The response is a visible or palpable flexion of the forearm.
Triceps Reflex 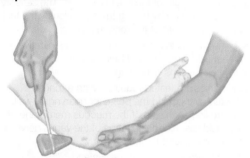	The arm is suspended by holding the upper arm and instructing the child to just let the arm "go limp." Alternatively, the forearm can be supported on the examiner's arm. The triceps tendon is struck directly just above the elbow. The response is extension of the forearm.
Brachioradialis Reflex 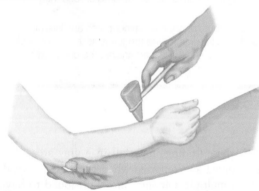	The child's arm is supported on the examiner's arm, and the elbow is flexed up to 45 degrees. The brachioradial tendon is struck with the reflex hammer 1-2 inches above the radial styloid process. The response is pronation and flexion of the elbow.
Patellar Reflex 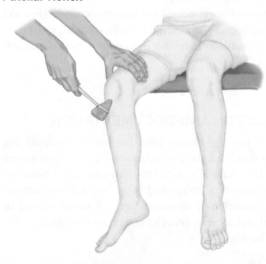	The lower leg is allowed to dangle freely by flexing the child's knee up to 90 degrees. The examiner supports the upper leg with the hand and strikes the patellar tendon just below the patella. The response is extension of the lower leg.

TABLE 9-5 Evaluating Common Reflexes—cont'd

Reflex	Evaluation
Achilles Reflex 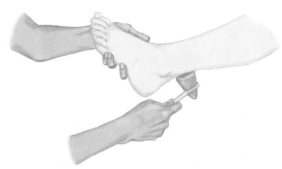	The hip is externally rotated, and the foot is held in dorsiflexion. The Achilles tendon is struck directly. The response is plantar flexion of the foot. An alternative way to elicit this reflex is to have the child kneel on a chair with the toes pointing toward the floor; the examiner then strikes the Achilles tendon directly.
Clonus Reflex	Eliciting a *clonus*—a continued, rapid flexion and extension of the foot and hand—is attempted in children. Clonus is elicited by suddenly and briskly dorsiflexing the foot or hand and applying sustained and moderate pressure. No rhythmic oscillating movements should be palpated.
Superficial Reflexes	Tested by stroking the skin with an object that is moderately sharp but not sharp enough to break the skin. The receptors are in the skin rather than the muscles.
Upper and Lower Abdominal Reflexes and Cremasteric Reflex 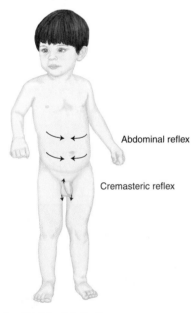 Abdominal reflex Cremasteric reflex	*Upper and lower abdominal reflexes:* While the child is in a supine position and with the abdomen exposed and knees slightly bent, the skin of the abdomen is stroked. Movement of stroking is from the side of the abdomen toward the midline at both the upper and lower abdominal levels. The response is ipsilateral contraction of the abdominal muscle with an observable movement of the umbilicus toward the side being stroked. *Cremasteric reflex:* In the male, light stroking of the inner aspect of the thigh causes the ipsilateral testicle to elevate. This reflex may cause withdrawal of the testicles into the inguinal canal when the abdomen is touched with very cold hands.
Plantar (Babinski) Reflex 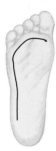	The lateral aspect of the sole of the foot, from the heel to the ball of the foot, is stroked in a movement curving medially across the ball. A fingernail or the wooden end of an applicator stick may be used. The response in an infant is dorsiflexion, fanning of the toes, and hyperextension of the great toe. Once a child is walking, the response is plantar flexion of the toes. Some children withdraw from this stimulus by flexing the hip and the knee.
Gluteal Reflex	When the buttocks are separated, the skin tenses at the gluteal area.

| BOX 9-11 | **Cerebellar Function: Tests of Balance and Coordination** |

Balance and coordination are tested by having the child perform the following movements:

- *Finger-to-nose test.* Child performs first with one hand, then with the other; first with the eyes open, then with the eyes closed. Ask child first to touch her finger to her nose and then to your finger as you change the position of your finger. Repeat this action with increasing rapidity. The tests are performed with each hand.

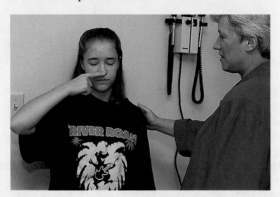

- *Rapid alternating movements.* Ask the child to rapidly pat his knee with the palms and backs of his hands by pronating and supinating the hands *(demonstrate first)*. Ask the child to touch his thumb to each of his fingers in rapid succession *(demonstrate first)*.

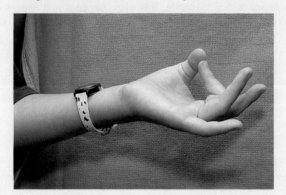

- Ask the child to stand erect, first with the eyes open and then with the eyes closed. Stand near the child to prevent injury if the child begins to fall.

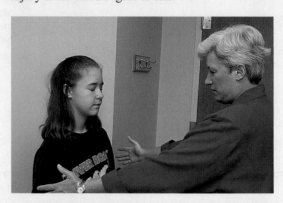

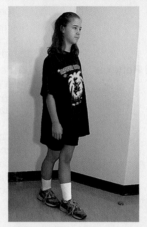

- Ask the child to walk in tandem fashion, placing her heel immediately in front of her opposite foot's toe and alternating while walking a straight line.

- Ask the sitting child to run each heel down the opposite shin. With the child lying down, ask the child to point to your hand with each big toe.

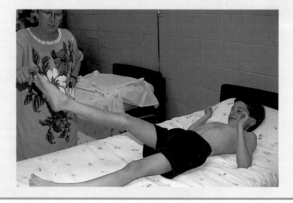

BOX 9-12	Tests for Evaluating Sensory Function

Primary Forms of Sensation

Check in sequence the hands, forearms, upper arms, trunk, thighs, lower legs, and feet for the following:

- *Superficial tactile sensation:* Touch the child with a wisp of cotton.
- *Superficial pain:* Touch the child with a pin or other sharp object. Be careful not to injure or frighten the child.
- *Sensitivity to temperature:* Touch the various parts of the child's body with test tubes containing warm and cold water. This test is infrequently done with children because of the difficulty of keeping water warm or cold enough for the child to distinguish the difference.
- *Sensitivity to vibration:* Hold a vibrating tuning fork to the bony prominences, noting the child's ability to perceive the vibration and tell you when the vibration stops.
- *Deep pressure pain:* Press the tip of your fingernail against the child's fingernail. The child will feel discomfort. You may also squeeze the Achilles tendon, calf, and forearm muscles, noting sensitivity.
- *Motion and position:* Hold the sides of the toes, thumbs, and fingers by grasping them between your index finger and thumb. Move the fingers and toes passively and ask the child to tell you the final position of the digit.

Cortical and Discriminatory Forms of Sensation

These forms of sensation are complex somatic sensory impressions that require interpretation by the cerebral cortex.

The following sensations can be evaluated, depending on the age and development of the child being tested:

- *Two-point discrimination:* Can the child differentiate between one and two points? With the child's eyes closed, various parts of the body are touched simultaneously with two sharp objects. Alternate touching the child with one point or two points. Different areas of the body differ in the distance by which the child can differentiate one from two points. This test is more appropriate for older children.
- *Point localization:* With the eyes closed, can the child locate the spot where the child was touched?
- *Texture discrimination:* Can the child recognize with the hands the difference in the feel of materials such as cotton, wool, and silk?
- *Stereognostic function:* Can the child identify familiar objects placed in each hand? Place several objects in a paper bag, and have the child identify them with each hand and show you the object.
- *Graphesthesia:* Can the child identify letters or numbers traced on the palm or back of the hand with a blunt point? Numbers are easier than letters for a young child to recognize.
- *Extinction phenomenon:* With the eyes closed, can the child identify touch on both sides? Touch opposite sides of the body in identical areas simultaneously. This test is used for older children only.

BOX 9-13	Examples of Neurologic "Soft" Signs

- Short attention span
- Poor motor coordination
- Clumsiness
- Frequent falling
- Hyperkinesis, voluntary or involuntary
- Uneven perceptual development
- Incomplete laterality, with no side clearly dominant
- Language disturbances: articulation disorders, dyslexia
- Motor outflow (movements involving more muscles than intended)
- Mirroring movements of the extremities (e.g., both hands in motion when only one is performing a function)

KEY CONCEPTS

- A systematic approach to the physical examination is to begin at the head and proceed through the entire body to the toes. The physical examination is tailored to the child's age and developmental level.
- The order of the examination should be flexible, and intrusive and frightening procedures should be done at the end of the examination. The examiner should develop creative approaches to complete the physical examination for children of different ages.
- An accurate history is the single most important component of the physical examination. The history and physical examination provide both subjective and objective data for identifying health and illness.

- Vital signs should be assessed on every visit in ambulatory settings and monitored on a routine basis in the hospitalized child.
- Assessment of vital signs is an important way to measure and monitor vital body functions.
- Examination findings are recorded completely and concisely. Deviations from normal and risk factors should be identified, recorded, and, when appropriate, reported for further evaluation.
- Anthropometrics measure the human body and assess nutritional status as well as growth and development. These measures are of most value when they are taken serially so that trends can be evaluated.
- The skin is observed for color and palpated to determine moisture, temperature, turgor, edema, and lesions.
- The general appearance of the child is observed for signs of abuse, both physical and psychologic.
- Examination of the lymph nodes is incorporated into the examination when that part of the anatomy is being assessed.
- The head is inspected for symmetry, movement, control, and shape.
- The fontanels are inspected and palpated for size, tenseness, and pulsation.
- The eyelids, eyebrows, palpebral fissures, nasolabial folds, mouth, and nose are inspected for spacing and symmetry.
- The nasal mucosa is inspected for color and moisture.
- Assessment of the mouth in a young child should be performed at the end of the examination because it may cause anxiety.
- The chart chosen to evaluate visual acuity is determined according to the age and development of the child and should be reliable and valid.
- Assessment of the thorax and lungs entails inspection, palpation, percussion, and auscultation.
- Auscultation of the heart is done by listening with both the bell and the diaphragm of the stethoscope with the child lying supine, in the left lateral recumbent position, and sitting up.
- An empty bladder, a warm room, and the child supine with a pillow under the head and the knees flexed will enhance abdominal relaxation.
- Examination of the genitalia may evoke concerns regarding modesty, fear of pain, negative judgment, or a previous uncomfortable experience. A matter-of-fact approach and direct communication will help create a positive experience.
- The musculoskeletal examination is predominantly directed toward the upper and lower extremities and the spinal column.
- The neurologic examination is done to identify any nervous system malfunction and to evaluate current nervous system development and functioning.
- When the physical examination has been completed, the examiner should ask the child and the parents if they have any questions concerning the examination.

ANSWERS TO CRITICAL THINKING EXERCISE 9-1

1. The nurse could assume that Ms. Maloney does not provide adequate care for her child. She might also assume that all teenage mothers lack the skills to be good parents. She might also assume that Kerrie has been neglected in other ways. In fact, however, Ms. Maloney may really be trying to meet all of Kerrie's needs but may not know what those needs are or how to meet them.

2. The nurse should display empathy and avoid displays of disapproval, perhaps by stating, "Children take a great deal of time and energy. You must be very busy trying to balance caring for Kerrie and working. Let's take some time today to look at how we can help you."

3. The nurse can take a thorough history and determine Kerrie's health status from conception to the present. A head-to-toe assessment will provide baseline data. Assuming that no abnormalities are present, the nurse will want to focus on anticipatory guidance related to nutrition, immunizations, safety, and any age-related growth and development issues. While doing the assessment, the nurse role models activities that increase Kerrie's language, motor, sensory, and psychologic skills. The nurse cannot provide care for Kerrie without meeting the needs of her mother. Support systems should be evaluated and, if weak, should be addressed. If Ms. Maloney understands that she needs to bring Kerrie to the clinic for preventive care, she is more likely to give clinic visits a higher priority. Teaching is therefore critical. Because of the history of this case, the nurse should assist Ms. Maloney in making the next appointment while in the clinic and should follow up with a call before the visit.

REFERENCES AND READINGS

Albert, D. M., & Jakobiec, F. A. (2000). *Principles and practice of ophthalmology* (2nd ed.). Philadelphia: WB Saunders.

Altman, C., Nihill, M., & Bricker, J. T. (2000). *Pediatric cardiac auscultation.* Philadelphia: Lippincott.

American Academy of Pediatrics, American Association of Certified Orthoptists, American Association for Pediatric Ophthalmology and Strabismus, & American Academy of Ophthalmology. (2003). Policy statement: Eye examination in infants, children, and young adults by pediatricians. *Pediatrics, 111,* 902-907.

American Academy of Pediatrics, National High Blood Pressure Education Program Working Group on High Blood Pressure in Children and Adolescents. (2004). The fourth report on the diagnosis, evaluation, and treatment of high blood pressure in children and adolescents. *Pediatrics, 114,* 555-576.

Angel, T., Nigro, J., & Levy, M. (2000). Infestations in the pediatric patient. *Pediatric Clinics of North America, 47,* 921-935.

Barkauskas, V. H., Stoltenberg-Allen, K., Baumann, L. C., & Darling-Fisher, C. (2002). *Health and physical assessment* (3rd ed.). St. Louis: Mosby.

Berkowitz, C. (2000). *Pediatrics: A primary care approach* (2nd ed.). Philadelphia: WB Saunders.

Block, S. L. (2005). The well-child checkup: Bright futures or dim economics? *Infectious Diseases in Children, 18,* 8-11.

Burns, C., Barber, N., Brady, M., & Dunn, A. (2000). *Pediatric primary care: A handbook for nurse practitioner* (2nd ed.). Philadelphia: WB Saunders.

Centers for Disease Control and Prevention: Body mass index formula (website). Retrieved June 21, 2005, from *http://www.cdc.gov/nccdphp/dnpa/bmi/bmi-adult/formula.htm.*

Centers for Disease Control and Prevention. (2005). *BMI—Body mass index: BMI for children and teens.* Retrieved January 14, 2006, from *www.cdc.gov.*

Cromwell, P., Munn, N., & Zolkowski-Wynne, J. (2005) Evaluation and management of hypertension in children and adolescents (part one): Diagnosis. *Journal of Pediatric Health Care, 19,* 172-175.

Eekhof, J., Neven, A. K., Verheij, T. J. (Eds). (2005). *Minor ailments in primary care—An evidence-based approach.* New York: Elsevier.

Erickson, B. (2003). *Heart sounds and murmurs across the lifespan* (3rd ed.). St. Louis: Mosby.

Flynn, J. (2003). Recognizing and managing the hypertensive child. *Contemporary Pediatrics, 20,* 38-60.

Fox, J. A. (2002). *Primary health care of infants, children, & adolescents* (2nd ed.). St. Louis: Mosby.

Goldbloom, R. (2003). *Pediatric clinical skills* (3rd ed.). Philadelphia: WB Saunders.

Greaser, J., & Whyte, J. J. (2004). Childhood obesity: Is there effective treatment? *Consultant for Pediatricians, 3,* 474-478.

Gungor, N., Hannon, T., Libman, I., Bacha, F., & Arslanian, S. (2005). Type 2 diabetes mellitus in youth: The complete picture to date. *Pediatric Clinics of North America. 52,* 1579-1609.

Hanson, E., & Neuhauser, T. (2003). *The complete history and physical exam guide.* Philadelphia: WB Saunders.

Hartmann, E. E., Dobson, V., Hainline, L., Marsh-Tootle, W., Quinn, G. E., Ruttum, M. S., Schmidt, P. P., & Simons, K. (2000/2005). Preschool vision screening: Summary of a task force report [Electronic version]. *Pediatrics, 106,* 1105-1112.

Houlder, L. (2000). The accuracy and reliability of tympanic thermometry compared to rectal and axillary sites in children. *Pediatric Nursing, 26,* 311-314.

Hymel, K. P., & Hall, C. A. (2005). Diagnosing pediatric head trauma. *Pediatric Annals, 34,* 358-370.

Jarvis, C. (2004). *Physical examination and health assessment* (4th ed.). St. Louis: Elsevier Saunders.

Jelinek, M., Patel, B. P., & Froehle, M. C. (Eds.). (2002) Bright futures in practice: Mental health (vol. 2). Toolkit. Arlington, VA: National Center for Education in Maternal and Child Health. Retrieved June 15, 2005, from *http://www.brightfutures.org/mental health.*

Krebs, N. F., Jacobson, M. S., for the American Academy of Pediatrics Committee on Nutrition. (2003). Prevention of pediatric overweight and obesity. *Pediatrics, 112,* 424-430.

Moran, R. (2003). Breaking the cycle of childhood obesity. *Clinical Advisor, February,* 62-67.

National Center for Health Statistics (2000). Pediatric growth charts. Retrieved July 12, 2006 from *www.cdc.gov/growthcharts.*

National Eye Institute (2004). Vision in preschoolers study (VIP study). Retrieved January 14, 2006, from *www.nei.nih.gov/.*

Rhee, H. (2005). Relationships between physical symptoms and pubertal development. *Journal of Pediatric Health Care, 19,* 95-103.

Schor, E. L. (2004). Rethinking well-child care. *Pediatrics, 114,* 210-216.

Seidel, H. B., Ball, J., Dains, J., & Benedict, G. W. (2003). *Mosby's guide to physical examination* (5th ed.). St. Louis: Mosby.

Story, M., Holt, K., & Sofka, D. (Eds.). (2002). *Bright futures in practice: Nutrition* (2nd ed.). Arlington, VA: National Center for Education in Maternal and Child Health.

Swartz, M. (2002). *Textbook of physical diagnosis history and examination* (4th ed.). Philadelphia: WB Saunders.

U.S. Preventive Services Task Force (2004). Screening for visual impairment in children younger than age 5 years. Retrieved January 14, 2006, from *www.ahrq.gov.*

Zitelli, B., & Davis, H. (2002). *Atlas of pediatric physical diagnosis* (4th ed.). St. Louis: Mosby.

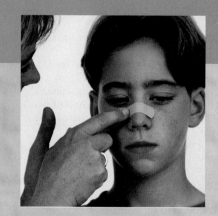

Emergency Care of the Child

Learning Objectives

After studying this chapter, you should be able to:

- Describe general principles that encourage cooperation and help make examination and treatment of children in emergency settings more comfortable for the child and family.
- List significant developmental issues when caring for infants, toddlers, preschool and school-age children, and adolescents.
- Compare the child's airway anatomy with that of an adult and explain the significance of the differences in managing the pediatric airway.
- Assess the early signs of shock in infants and children, recognizing that changes in heart rate and skin signs are more accurate signs of early shock than is decreased blood pressure.

- Define triage and list the most important factors to assess when obtaining an overall ("across the room") impression of an infant's or child's condition.
- Describe the general guidelines for cardiopulmonary resuscitation in infants and children and discuss what additional precautions and procedures are required for infants and children with traumatic injuries.
- List indications that suggest a child brought into the emergency care setting has been neglected or abused and discuss the nurse's responsibility for reporting possible neglect or abuse.
- Identify several possible roles for nurses in preventing traumatic injuries, poison ingestion, and environmental injuries.

Definitions

ABCDEs *Airway, breathing, circulation, disability, and exposure;* critical components of the primary assessment that require assessment and interventions in the stabilization of a critically ill or injured child.

airway management Correct positioning of the airway, appropriate interventions used to ensure patency of the airway, and adequate oxygenation and ventilation.

cardiopulmonary resuscitation Protocol performed when an individual's respiratory and cardiovascular systems require support to maintain vital functions; airway management, ventilation, and chest compressions are provided to improve tissue perfusion until definitive care is available.

dental emergency Injury or infection of a tooth or teeth occurring when the period of time to definitive care is critical for the survival of the tooth or to alleviate pain.

emergency Psychologic, medical, or traumatic condition that requires immediate care or care within 1 hour to prevent further deterioration.

envenomation Injection of venom by an animal (e.g., usually snakes, lizards, spiders, scorpions) into a human body.

environmental emergency Illness or injury occurring as a result of outside, or environmental, factors.

extracorporeal membrane oxygenation Temporary method of providing cardiovascular, pulmonary, and circulatory support for children for whom other methods of treatment are not effective.

hypothermia Cooling of body temperature to subnormal levels; temperature levels considered dangerous to infants and children are core body temperatures less than 35.6° C (96° F).

ingestion Swallowing of a potentially toxic substance, such as inappropriate amounts or types of medication, petroleum products, insecticides, or toxic plants.

shock Inadequate tissue perfusion, usually caused by illness or injury, that results in respiratory or cardiovascular compromise.

submersion injury Injury resulting from a near-drowning incident; may be immediately apparent or appear up to 48 hours after the submersion incident.

trauma Injury from an external cause, such as a motor vehicle collision, fall, gunshot wound, or stabbing; may be self-inflicted, may be deliberately inflicted or accidental, and may be psychologic in nature.

Continued

GENERAL GUIDELINES FOR EMERGENCY NURSING CARE

Many factors affect the psychologic impact of an emergency on both the child and family. In addition to the expected fears children have at various developmental stages (e.g., separation, pain, altered body image), an overriding concern expressed by both children and parents in emergency settings is fear of the unknown. The suddenness with which the child and family come in contact with emergency personnel, the necessity for rapid assessment and intervention, and the relative seriousness of the child's condition can intensify a fearful response and overwhelm normal coping mechanisms. In addition, children and families are unfamiliar with the setting, the staff of the health care facility, the equipment, and the procedures. Emergency nurses can use some simple interventions to make examination and treatment of children in the emergency setting more comfortable for the child and for the family and to decrease the adverse psychologic effects of the experience.

Communicate an attitude of calm confidence. This attitude can be difficult to maintain when the situation is critical, but families in crisis look to nurses for reassurance and expect to see competent, professional behavior. Speak quietly and calmly to the child and parents, and remain firmly in charge. Remember to talk to the family often throughout the visit; silence is a form of communication that is easily misinterpreted. Keep the parents informed of any untoward delays. Acknowledge the child's and family's fears (Eckle & MacLean, 2001).

Establish a trusting relationship with the child and family. Make eye contact with the child and family when you speak to them. Call the child by name to personalize care. Treat the child and family kindly and gently. To establish a trusting relationship, check back with the family and provide periodic updates if the child and family are separated. When parents are confident that they are being kept informed, they are less likely to make demands for additional attention and information. When speaking to the child and family, use simple, nonmedical terms and remember that children (and sometimes adults) can have inaccurate ideas of how their bodies function and the location of body parts. Providing comfort measures to the family members also builds a trusting relationship. Protect their privacy, direct them to a public telephone or cafeteria, and provide space where they can talk quietly.

Encourage caregivers to stay with the child. Family-centered care recognizes the partnership between health care workers and family in ensuring the well-being of the child. Nursing care is driven by the needs of the family and client rather than controlled by health care providers. According to comfort levels and ability, include the parents as partners in their child's treatment. Unless the child does not want a parent in the room (e.g., some adolescents), a parent can help calm the child, and many examinations and procedures can be performed with the child on a parent's lap. Although having

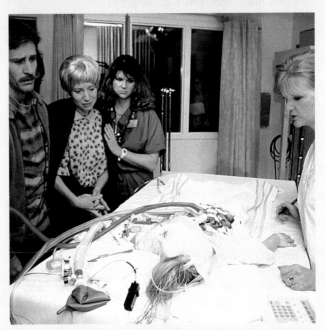

Encouraging parents to remain with their child in the emergency setting can bolster the family's coping. *(Courtesy Cook Children's Medical Center, Fort Worth, TX.)*

the family remain with the child can be calming and supportive, respect the family's right to leave if the child's condition or the painful nature of a procedure provokes more anxiety than the family member is able to handle.

> For parents who do not know exactly how to be of assistance in these situations, it can help to explain how a parent might help, such as "I think he might stay calmer if you hold his hand and tell him a story while I clean this burn" or "Try counting to 10 with her while I start this intravenous line."

Whenever possible, designate one staff member as the child's caretaker and liaison to the parents. In the unfamiliar emergency setting, the child and family find that having one contact person is less confusing. Consistency is helpful in a crisis because the child and family may feel overwhelmed in the busy and sometimes confusing emergency department environment.

Tell the truth. To establish a trusting relationship, be as honest as possible. If a procedure will be painful, tell the child (usually briefly beforehand). Only then can the child believe health care providers when they say that a procedure will *not* be painful. When a painful procedure is completed, tell the child you are finished and there will be no more pain. Keeping a child informed of what will occur by describing sensations (e.g., "This will feel cold and wet as I clean your arm.") is more helpful than describing the actual procedure.

Provide incentives and rewards. Provide positive feedback when either the child or the parents are being helpful. Children from 3 to 12 years of age especially appreciate verbal praise and concrete rewards for good behavior, such as stickers, fancy bandages, or inexpensive toys (Hawkins, 2004).

PEDIATRIC EMERGENCY EQUIPMENT

Airways:
    Oral: sizes 0-5
    Nasopharyngeal: sizes 12F-30F
Endotracheal tubes:
    Cuffed: sizes 3.5-9
    Uncuffed: sizes 2.5-6
Tracheostomy tubes: sizes 00-6
Stylet: sizes 6-14
Laryngoscope with blades:
    Straight: sizes 0-3
    Curved: sizes 2-3
Magill forceps
Oxygen equipment: infant, pediatric, and adult masks and cannulas
Bag-valve-mask: infant, pediatric, and adult sizes
Chest tubes: sizes 10F-40F
Flexible suction catheters: sizes 6F-12F
Pediatric peripheral IV equipment and solutions, including over-the-needle catheters: 18-24 gauge
Intraosseous device: 16-18 gauge
Nasogastric tubes: sizes 5F-18F
Urinary catheters: sizes 5-12
Length-based resuscitation tape
Defibrillator with adult and pediatric paddles
Monitors with pediatric-size electrodes and sensors
Blood pressure cuffs (neonatal, infant, child, and adult arm and thigh cuffs)
Heating source
    Fluid warmer
    Infrared lamp
    Overhead warmer

Adapted from Field, J. M., Hazinski, M. F., Gilmore, D. (2006). *Handbook of emergency cardiovascular care for healthcare providers.* American Heart Association.

Pediatric Emergency Medications

Medication	Use
Activated charcoal	Reduces drug absorption in toxic ingestions
Adenosine	Treats supraventricular tachycardia
Amidarone	Treats pulseless arrest, supraventricular and ventricular tachycardia
Atropine sulfate	Treats symptomatic bradycardia
Bretylium tosylate	Treats ventricular tachycardia; ventricular fibrillation prophylaxis
Calcium chloride	Treats hypocalcemia, hypomagnesemia, hyperkalemia, and calcium channel blocker overdose
Dextrose (25%, 50%)	Treats hypoglycemia, a common complication of dehydration, sepsis, and resuscitation
Inotropic agents	Treat hypotension or hypoperfusion, severe congestive heart failure, or cardiovascular shock
Epinephrine (1:1000 [endotracheal], 1:10,000 [intravenous/intraosseous])	Treats bradycardia or pulseless arrest (including ventricular fibrillatum, pulseless ventricular tachycardia, asystole, and pulseless electrical activity [PEA])
Lidocaine	Treats recurrent ventricular tachycardia, ventricular fibrillation, or ventricular ectopy
Magnesium	Treats torsades de pointes or hypomagnesemia
Naloxone hydrochloride	Reverses effects of some narcotics
Sodium bicarbonate (4.2%)	Treats severe acidosis associated with cardiac arrest, unstable hemodynamic status, hyperkalemia, or certain toxic ingestions

Adapted from Field, J. M., Hazinski, M. F., Gilmore, D. (2006). *Handbook of emergency cardiovascular care for healthcare providers.* American Heart Association.

Adults also appreciate being thanked for their patience and for their assistance in their child's care. All these techniques help create as positive an experience as possible.

Assess the child's unspoken thoughts and feelings. Try to determine what the child is thinking or feeling but not verbalizing. Encourage the child to express thoughts and feelings; sometimes the child might be misinterpreting a situation or need to express emotions.

In some cases, however, the child's and family's coping mechanisms break down, causing inappropriate behavior. If violence or abusive behavior is an issue, you might need to obtain assistance from law enforcement or hospital security officers. For an emotional crisis that does not involve abusive or aggressive behavior, the following simple rules apply:

- Encourage the person in crisis to move to a quiet place. Observers and stimuli from other sources tend to aggravate a crisis.
- Encourage the child or parent to talk about feelings as well as the "facts" of the situation. Use reflective statements.
- Avoid defensiveness, explanation, or justification of your own or others' behavior.

- Speak in simple sentences. Use sentences of no more than five words, with words no longer than five letters (e.g., "Let's sit down over here," "Let me help," "Please let go of that").
- Set limits. Avoid "yes" or "no" responses. Rather than saying, "Will you take this medicine?" (the small child will probably say "NO!"), ask "Would you rather take the pink or the yellow medicine first?"

When interacting with families in distress, a good general rule is to try to listen rather than talk. Simply being present for children and families and empathizing with them are useful interventions. Help families identify specific problems and their effective coping mechanisms and assist them to explore reasonable solutions.

When coping mechanisms break down entirely, however, some direction is necessary. Consulting social services, spiritual counselors (e.g., chaplain), or crisis intervention professionals can be helpful. Early intervention and support for appropriate coping mechanisms are far easier and less time consuming than intervening after a child's or parent's emotional decompensation.

Definitions

trauma score Numeric score assessed by health care providers to determine the extent of trauma; usually results from adding, subtracting, dividing, or multiplying numbers representing physiologic parameters or specific types of injuries; used for field triage and assessed serially to determine whether a person's condition is improving or deteriorating; also correlated with survivability.

traumatic brain injury One of the leading causes of death or permanent disability; severity of injury may range from mild to severe; can result in short-term and long-term disabilities.

triage Sorting process used to decide the urgency of an individual's illness or injury and allocate appropriate resources effectively; purpose is to ensure that the most seriously ill or injured people receive the appropriate level of care before those with less urgent or emergent conditions.

Electronic Resources

Additional information related to the content in Chapter 10 can be found on:

the interactive companion CD-ROM

- Animations: Bag Ventilation
  CPR, Pediatric
- Audio Glossary
- NCLEX Review Questions

or the companion website at **evolve**
http://evolve.elsevier.com/james/ncoc

- NCLEX Review Questions
- WebLinks

Very few experiences are as frightening to a family as a child's sudden illness or injury. Caring for children and families in the emergency setting therefore presents special challenges to the health care team. Nurses play an important role in emergency settings because they are most often responsible for the initial contact, triage, and continuing care throughout an emergency visit. The goals of emergency nursing care include addressing the child's physical problems, supporting the child's and family's coping mechanisms, and creating an atmosphere in which the family is valued and kept as intact as possible.

GROWTH AND DEVELOPMENT ISSUES IN EMERGENCY CARE

Emergency nursing care of children needs to address both the physiologic and psychologic differences in children in terms of age and development. Paying close attention to developmental issues assists in obtaining a more accurate assessment and can affect the course of care (see Chapters 5 through 8 for approaches to children of different ages). The nurse treats each child as an individual and avoids becoming judgmental when a child regresses to a "safer" developmental level. Although children of the same age group are similar, past experiences, cultural differences, and maturity levels may result in a range of behaviors. One toddler might be much more mature than another, and one adolescent might lean more toward school-age behaviors than another (Box 10-1).

The Infant

An infant experiences the world through the senses; hunger, satiation, cold, warmth, quiet, and noise affect the infant's comfort or discomfort. An infant has not learned patience and has little tolerance for physical or emotional discomfort,

including pain (see Chapter 15 for management of pain in infants and children).

Although infants are able to discriminate their parents from others, older infants (9 to 18 months of age) can exhibit signs of both separation and stranger anxiety. The nurse should allow the parent to hold the infant as much as possible for examination and treatment. This may not be possible in a critical situation, but nurses need to remember to reunite parent and child whenever feasible.

The Toddler

Toddlers are just beginning to explore the world and seem to have limitless energy and curiosity. They are also beginning to have a clearer image of themselves as autonomous and distinct beings. For this reason, they do not respond well to restrictions and tend to push any limits imposed. This tendency can be a problem in the emergency setting because some nursing care might involve securing and restraining the toddler, which makes the toddler feel vulnerable. The nurse should be sure to remove any restriction or restraint as soon as safety permits. Toddlers have little understanding of time, so procedures should be introduced just before they are initiated.

The Preschooler

The preschool child is talking and beginning to be more independent. This outward appearance of organization is somewhat misleading, however, because the preschool period is also the stage of fear and fantasy. Preschoolers are strong believers in cause-and-effect relations and tend to blame themselves for illnesses and injuries.

The preschool child may be more willing than the toddler to be separated from parents, but the nurse should keep this separation as brief as possible. The nurse can include the

BOX 10-1	**Working with Children in Emergencies: Developmental Guidelines**

Infants

Allow the use of a pacifier.

Use a quiet, soothing voice.

Touch, rock, or cuddle the infant. Holding the infant securely or swaddling a young infant can also be comforting.

Keep the infant warm; if the infant must be left undressed, use warming lights to ensure a comfortable temperature.

As much as possible, allay parents' fears so they will not be communicated to the infant.

Remember that infants feel pain (see Chapter 15 for pain interventions).

Toddlers

Give treatments and perform procedures with the toddler sitting up on the stretcher or examining table or on the parent's lap.

Perform the most distressing or intrusive parts of the examination last.

Reassure family members as much as possible; the child will benefit from their confidence.

Allow the child to have familiar objects (transitional objects) such as a blanket, doll, or toy to help feel safe.

Keep frightening objects out of the child's line of vision. Also try to keep machines that make loud noises away.

Praise (e.g., "You are so brave.") and distraction (e.g., bubbles, puzzles) will decrease anxiety and increase cooperation.

Preschoolers

Explain a procedure or treatment a few seconds rather than minutes beforehand, because allowing the child time to think about it may result in frightening fantasies or exaggerations.

Talk to preschool children throughout procedures, describing the sensations they are feeling or will feel and telling them how they can help.

Distract the child with noises or bright objects. Counting with some preschool children might help calm them during procedures.

Avoid criticizing the preschool child for crying, struggling, or fighting during a procedure.

Reassuring a child that the child did try his or her best to cooperate will help to build a positive self-image.

Encourage the preschool child to talk about how the illness or injury occurred. If the child is inappropriately taking responsibility for the illness or injury, try to reassure that the child is not to blame for the situation.

Preschoolers—cont'd

Remember that preschool children can seem to understand more than they actually do. Health care providers often overestimate understanding in a child of this age, so be sure to explain things in words the child understands.

Use positive terms, such as "make better" and "help," and avoid more frightening terms, such as "shot" and "cut."

Use adhesive bandages over small wounds and injection sites. Preschool children might imagine their blood leaking out through puncture wounds.

School-Age Children

Offer simple choices whenever possible to help the child feel more in control. The school-age child is capable of deciding in which arm to have an injection or in which hand to hold a nebulizer. Talk directly to the child, explaining procedures in simple terms. When explaining treatments or care options to the parent, include the child.

Ask the child about the level of understanding and allow time for questions.

Address the child's fears or concerns directly rather than treating them as foolish or inconsequential.

Give rewards, such as a sticker or inexpensive toy, after a procedure regardless of the child's behavior. Think of this gesture as a reward for undergoing the procedure, not as a judgment of "good" or "bad" behavior.

Adolescents

Preserve the adolescent's modesty; offer adolescents a choice regarding whether they want their parents present when obtaining history and during the examination.

Consider the legal issues regarding the right to privacy for pregnant adolescents and adolescents with sexually transmissible diseases.

Provide an opportunity for questions.

Listen to the adolescent's concerns nonjudgmentally and without belittling the young person.

Developing a teasing relationship with an adolescent is often a temptation, but this has potential for harm; the adolescent is easily embarrassed.

Explain procedures or treatments carefully and allow choices. Adolescents are capable of complex abstract thinking and can make intelligent and reasoned decisions about their own care.

parents in treatments and provide them with instructions on calming the child if they seem unsure. The nurse should not ask a parent to restrain the child because this role may be confusing to the child and difficult for the parent.

The School-Age Child

School-age children are interested in learning and gradually acquire reasoning skills, including some abstract think-

ing. They are able to understand the cause of illness and injury and are much less likely to fantasize and exaggerate. School-age children have extensive vocabularies, and they can understand simple explanations of procedures. They are also able to make decisions about their own care. By this time, they have developed personal techniques to help them through painful times. The nurse helps them use coping techniques that work for them.

The Adolescent

Although adolescents are at varying stages of puberty, they begin to resemble adults in appearance. They are also beginning to explore the adult world and develop their own unique identities. The nurse needs to remember, however, that even though adolescents may appear physically mature, they might not be emotionally mature and they continue to require support. Coping with extraordinary changes in their physical appearance, they are often concerned with whether they are "normal" and whether others have similar thoughts and feelings.

Although this is an age of risk taking, which can make them prone to serious injury, adolescents can be quite fearful of death. Although they are aware of the possibility of their own death, they avoid thinking about its reality. Adolescents consider themselves invincible and many experience overwhelmingly emotions when a friend dies unexpectedly.

Adolescence is an age of extremes—teenagers might either exaggerate or underplay the seriousness of a condition. Sometimes assessing the full extent of an adolescent's illness or injury is difficult. Expert care of the adolescent requires sensitivity to both verbal and nonverbal cues. Adolescents' privacy should be respected; approach them as one would an adult, giving them full attention and respect for their thoughts and feelings.

THE FAMILY OF A CHILD IN EMERGENCY CARE

Stress on the family results directly and indirectly from the child's illness or injury. The way a child perceives an illness or injury often is related to the parents' attitude, so caring for the child requires assessment of and intervention with the family.

The most common emotions experienced by parents of children cared for in emergencies are fear and anxiety. Past experiences may lessen or increase these emotions. Parents are afraid of the following possibilities:

- Their child might die. This fear is the greatest source of anxiety and can be present even when death is highly unlikely, such as in the case of minor illnesses or injuries. This anxiety is often the underlying cause of parents' anger toward health care providers.
- Their child might experience pain. As a rule, parents try very hard to protect children from pain. Even when pain is necessary, it is difficult for parents to understand and accept.
- The child's body may be permanently altered. Parents often fear that their children will have permanent scars or body changes.

Parental guilt is another frequently seen emotion. Parents can feel guilty for the following reasons:

- They feel responsible for their child's illness or injury.
- They are submitting their child to a painful experience.
- They do not have enough knowledge to make educated decisions about their child's care.

In addition, parents may have had negative experiences with health care providers in the past or have other concerns about siblings, financial arrangements, and work schedules.

The particular causes of stress for families in emergencies are unique to the circumstances and to the family involved. The nurse needs to ascertain who is the family (e.g., single parent, two parents, grandparent, other caregiver) and who are the decision makers (e.g., family members, religious leaders) and communicate accordingly. All the stressors combined could stretch parents' coping mechanisms to the limit and result in anger, withdrawal, or tearfulness. Stress also can manifest itself in hyperactivity—making numerous phone calls, repeating questions, and involving a large number of people.

Including family members in their child's care can reduce feelings of helplessness and promote positive coping mechanisms. Early assessment and appropriate support before problems occur are advantageous for both health care workers and the family.

EMERGENCY ASSESSMENT OF INFANTS AND CHILDREN

In the emergency setting, assessment of the ill or injured child must be rapid and accurate to identify abnormal findings quickly. In children, initial evidence of life-threatening conditions can be subtle, with few signs of impending respiratory or cardiopulmonary arrest. Making as many initial observations as possible without touching the child is extremely important so that assessments can reflect the child's baseline, or resting condition. For an apparently stable infant or young child, most of the examination required for general triage can be performed with the child on the parent's lap. The nurse also observes the relationship between the parents and child during the examination process.

The triage nurse usually performs the initial observation in the emergency setting and decides the level of care needed for the child. Triaging is an important skill that improves with experience. The nurse bases much of the initial assessment on an overall sense of how the child looks—sick or well (an "across the room" assessment). Because children do not try to cover up either how they feel or how they look, the nurse immediately receives a fairly accurate impression of illness or wellness.

Three essential factors combine to form a first impression: respiratory rate and effort, skin color, and response to the environment. Abnormalities are compared with the caregiver's perception ("Is this his normal color?"). If results of this assessment appear to be normal, the nurse completes a more thorough and in-depth evaluation. If the general impression is that the child is seriously ill, the nurse must intervene immediately and combine any additional evaluation with intervention.

Primary Assessment

Primary assessment, which is part of the initial triage assessment, consists of assessing the *ABCDEs*—*a*irway, *b*reathing, *c*irculation, level of consciousness (*d*isability), and *e*xposure. Because the two most common pathways to death in children are respiratory failure and shock, interventions include providing respiratory and circulatory support.

Airway Assessment

Although determining the cause of respiratory distress or failure in an ill child ultimately will be important, more important is recognizing symptoms and signs of respiratory distress. In the emergency setting, initial treatment is the same regardless of the cause.

Because of some differences in airway anatomy and physiology, children are at greater risk of airway problems than are adults (Table 10-1). When assessing children's airways, the nurse pays particular attention to breath sounds (often audible to the naked ear) as well as snoring, stridor, wheezing, and grunting. Snoring is caused by obstruction in the upper airway (often the tongue relaxing against the posterior pharynx) and can be heard in a child with decreased mental status. Stridor is a high-pitched sound heard on inspiration (laryngeal obstruction) or on both inspiration and expiration (midtracheal obstruction). Wheezing, a high-pitched, musical sound heard primarily on expiration, signals obstruction of the lower airway. Crackles or rales are fine, popping noises heard on inspiration; they usually indicate fluid in the lungs, such as in pneumonia.

Breathing Assessment

Level of consciousness, rate and depth of breathing, breath sounds, and the child's respiratory effort are indicative of relative oxygenation. Anxiety or decreased responsiveness may denote hypoxia. A rapid respiratory rate with shallow breathing indicates respiratory distress. Very slow breathing in an ill child is an ominous sign, indicating respiratory failure. A slowly breathing child might no longer have the energy for adequate ventilation. Increased work of breathing with quiet breath sounds may indicate an absence of air entry into lung fields. Abdominal breathing is normal in the infant or young child, so the nurse observes the rise and fall of the abdomen instead of the chest.

The use of accessory muscles for breathing invariably indicates respiratory distress. The child's chest wall is relatively weak and unstable, so retractions occur with increased work of breathing. Assessment of breathing includes observing the child for intercostal, substernal, suprasternal, supraclavicular, and infraclavicular retractions. As a child becomes exhausted, retractions may diminish, usually indicating respiratory failure. Nasal flaring with inspiration is another form of accessory muscle use. Grunting, a sound made by expiration against partially closed vocal cords, is a sign of hypoxemia and represents the body's effort to improve oxygenation by generating positive end-expiratory pressure.

The nurse observes the child's preferred body posture. A child in respiratory distress is upright with the jaw thrust forward, leaning forward on outstretched arms—the tripod position. This position helps maximize airway opening and the use of accessory muscles of respiration.

Once the work of breathing has been carefully observed, listening to the chest provides some useful information. Children have small chests, and breath sounds can be transmitted throughout the chest. The nurse therefore auscultates a child's chest at both sides of the body at the midaxillary line and over the trachea to confirm equality of breath sounds and distinguish upper from lower airway noises.

Normal respiratory rates for children vary by age and are faster than for adults (see Table 9-1). A respiratory rate greater than 60 breaths/min, however, is abnormal for any age. Another important adjunct for respiratory assessment is the pulse oximetry reading (see Chapter 13).

Cardiovascular Assessment

Cardiovascular assessment includes observing the child's skin color and temperature, checking capillary refill, and assessing central and peripheral pulse rate and quality. A child can compensate more effectively for fluid loss, through increased heart rate and peripheral vasoconstriction, than an adult can. Tachycardia and decreased peripheral perfusion are early signs of cardiovascular compromise in a child and require immediate intervention to prevent decompensation. Loss of circulating volume of 20% to 25% may initiate shock compensatory mechanisms without the child showing overt signs, such as altered mental status or hypotension (Caldwell & Ziglar, 2001). Hypotension is a late finding and suggests compensatory mechanisms are no longer adequate to maintain cardiac output.

TABLE 10-1	Primary Assessment in Pediatric Emergencies	
Assessment	**Pediatric Differences**	**Nursing Implications**
A—Airway Patency, positioning for air entry, audible sounds, airway obstruction (blood, mucus, edema)	The child's airway is narrower than an adult's and more easily obstructed by foreign bodies, small amounts of mucus, or tissue edema. Infants are preferential nasal breathers for the first several months of life; therefore nasal secretions can cause respiratory compromise. Children are more susceptible to infectious respiratory diseases that contribute to risk of airway obstruction. Edema and mucus in a narrow airway cause incrementally more obstruction than in a wider one. The tongue is relatively large in relation to the oral cavity and can more easily fall into the airway in the unconscious child. Cartilage of the larynx is relatively soft, and the trachea is thinner and more flexible than an adult's. The larynx is higher and more anterior, increasing the risk of obstruction and aspiration. The submandibular area is softer and can be more easily compressed to occlude the airway. Deciduous teeth are poorly anchored and easily dislodged. Altered mental status is an early sign of hypoxia.	Allow the child to maintain a position of comfort or manually position the airway (jaw thrust or head-tilt/chin-lift); encourage the child to avoid flexing or hyperextending the neck; use spinal immobilization and airway adjuncts as required.
B—Breathing Decreased level of consciousness, increased or decreased work of breathing, nasal flaring, use of accessory muscles of respiration (retractions), rate, pattern, quality, oxygen saturation	The chest wall is thin, softer, and more compliant. Rib alignment is more horizontal. The younger child is more susceptible to respiratory distress and failure. Retractions commonly occur with respiratory distress and can compromise the ability to increase tidal volume. The diaphragm is the predominant muscle of respiration. Pressure above or below the diaphragm can impede respiratory effort. Infants and children have a higher metabolic rate and increased oxygen demand. Hypoxia occurs more rapidly.	Provide supplemental oxygen; initiate assisted ventilation with bag-valve-mask, and prepare for intubation as indicated; provide gastric decompression with orogastric or nasogastric tube; provide comfort measures; encourage family presence to decrease anxiety.
C—Circulation Skin color, temperature, and capillary refill (<2 sec); rate and strength of peripheral and central pulses	The child's circulating blood volume per body weight is much larger than an adult's, even though actual blood volume is much smaller. Therefore small volume losses have more severe circulatory consequences. A higher percentage of fluid is located in the extracellular compartment, causing more rapid fluid shifts. A higher metabolic rate and oxygen demand require an increased heart rate; tachycardia is the first compensatory mechanism for decreased oxygenation—*not* hypotension.	Control bleeding through application of direct pressure; obtain vascular access; initiate volume replacement; perform chest compressions; defibrillate or provide synchronized cardioversion; initiate drug therapy.
D—Disability Level of consciousness or activity level; response to the environment (especially caregivers); pupillary response	A larger head/body ratio and weak neck muscles contribute to more serious head injury from shaking or impact. The anterior fontanel remains open until approximately age 18 mo. An open fontanel allows for expanded cranial volume, so signs of increased intracranial pressure, which indicate underlying brain injury, may be delayed. A thinner skull predisposes the child to more severe injury. Nerve myelinization is incomplete during infancy; unmyelinated tissue is more vulnerable to shearing injury.	Treat the underlying cause (e.g., signs of increased intracranial pressure; fluid or blood volume deficit; hypoglycemia; hypothermia; hypoxia); compare assessment with parent's perception (a deeply sleeping child may be difficult to arouse, which is "normal" to caregivers).
E—Exposure To identify underlying injuries or additional signs of illness	Bulging fontanel, periorbital edema, unusual rashes, and edema or exudate in the pharynx can indicate a variety of severe childhood communicable diseases. Bruising, unusual burns, vaginal tearing, rectal bleeding, and discharge suggest child abuse. Swelling, deformities can indicate underlying trauma to vital organs.	Remove all clothing, including diapers; save any clothing needed for evidence; maintain an appropriately warm environment.

Data from Bernardo, L. (1998). Multiple trauma. In M. Slota (Ed.), *Core curriculum for pediatric critical care nursing* (pp. 568-571). Philadelphia: Saunders; Emergency Nurses Association. (2004). *ENPC provider manual* (3rd ed., pp. 45-53). Park Ridge, IL: Author.

Disability: Neurologic Assessment

The infant's or child's level of consciousness is an essential component of the primary assessment. Alteration in level of consciousness (irritability or agitation, lethargy, or inability to recognize caregivers) can be the first sign of respiratory compromise or worsening condition.

A rapid neurologic assessment consists of two components: (1) pupillary reactivity and size; and (2) a brief mental status assessment (*AVPU*: *a*lert, responds to *v*oice, responds to *p*ain, *u*nresponsive). More thorough and sophisticated means of assessment are used later if needed (see Chapter 28). Serial assessment is imperative. Progressive loss of consciousness may be a result of hypoxemia, hypoglycemia, increased intracranial pressure, or another life-threatening condition.

Exposure

Primary assessment ends with exposure, or removing the child's clothing to identify additional injuries or indicators of illness. The nurse needs to preserve the child's clothing appropriately if it will be needed for evidence in any potential civil or criminal proceeding. Infants and children have a larger body surface area/weight ratio, making them at risk for hypothermia. Maintaining body temperature by shivering increases metabolic needs, such as oxygen and glucose, and the child has limited reserves. Methods to help the child maintain a normothermic state or help warming include over-bed warmers and heat lamps, warmed intravenous (IV) fluids and humidified oxygen, removal of wet clothes, and providing warmed blankets.

Secondary Assessment

After the primary assessment is complete and intervention (if necessary) has stabilized the child, the nurse begins the secondary assessment. Components of the secondary assessment include vital signs, assessing for pain, history and head-to-toe assessment, and inspection (Table 10-2).

Vital Signs

Vital signs are useful in the triage assessment of the child, but because age variations make their significance more difficult to interpret, they are not as reliable an indicator as in adult assessment. This variation is especially applicable to temperature. For example, an infant has an immature thermoregulatory system and may not have a fever or may even be hypothermic in the presence of infection, so the nurse needs to be alert for supporting signs. The nurse remembers that an alteration in one part of the vital signs may result in abnormal values in other parts. For example, an abnormally high heart rate and respiratory rate may be a result of hyperthermia, crying, pain, hypoxemia, or hypovolemia (see Chapter 13 for methods of obtaining a temperature).

When taking a child's vital signs, the nurse observes the respiratory rate first and then obtains the pulse; the nurse obtains the temperature and blood pressure last because these procedures can be the most upsetting for children. The nurse should be certain to use the correct size blood pressure cuff and take both the respiratory and heart rates

TABLE 10-2	Secondary Assessment in Pediatric Emergencies
Assessment	**Nursing Implications**
F—Full Set of Vital Signs; Family Presence	
Evaluate the child's vital signs, including temperature, for abnormal findings; obtain weight in kilograms. Family presence: assess the needs of the family for support and inclusion in care.	Continuously monitor the child's vital signs, including temperature; weigh child or obtain estimated weight if child's condition prohibits measured weight. Facilitate family presence and support in a culturally appropriate way.
G—Give Comfort Measures	
Discomfort is usually related to the underlying problem; use pain assessment scales for children.	Frequently monitor pain level and response to pain relief measures; include nonpharmacologic techniques for reducing pain.
H—Head-to-Toe Assessment; Obtain History	
Perform a complete head-to-toe assessment and obtain a history; during triage assessment, a focused assessment related to the chief complaint may be used.	Continuously monitor the child for changes in condition; assess for any unusual odors.
I—Inspect the Back; Isolate	
Observe the back for obvious or hidden injuries; assess for communicable illness or susceptibility to illness (immunocompromised clients).	Reinspect the back as indicated; provide isolation as indicated.

Modified from Emergency Nurses Association. (2004). *ENPC provider manual* (3rd ed., pp. 45-53). Park Ridge, IL: Author.

for one full minute because subtle differences are important in the child. Normal respiratory and heart rates are faster than an adult's, whereas the blood pressure is lower on average (see Table 9-1 and Appendix C for normal vital signs by age). An accurate weight, described below, should be obtained at this time, and monitors such as cardiac or pulse oximeter should be applied as indicated.

History and Head-to-Toe Assessment

A brief history provides information about prior illness or injury that might affect the emergency care of the child. One format often used for pediatric clients is the mnemonic *SAMPLE*:

S—signs and symptoms
A—allergies
M—medications taken (prescription, over-the-counter, and herbal or home remedies) and immunization history
P—prior illness or injury
L—last meal and eating habits
E—events surrounding this injury or illness (e.g., length of illness, mechanism of injury)

This mnemonic gives sufficient information to determine whether the child's medical history will play an important role in assessment and treatment of the current illness or injury. In emergency departments that care for children, a list of immunizations and the appropriate ages should be posted in a convenient location (see Evolve website).

After obtaining an appropriate history, the nurse begins to perform a head-to-toe assessment, documenting any findings that might affect the child's condition. Assessment findings are compared with the history to aid in diagnosis and look for inconsistencies. The nurse inspects all body surfaces, looking for fractures, lacerations, contusions, and penetrating injuries. The nurse also observes the skin for petechiae or rashes. The presence and pattern of any pain are described. The nurse pays particular attention to signs of pneumothorax or hemothorax (e.g., decreased breath sounds on the affected side, signs of hypoxemia, signs of shock). The nurse then palpates the child's abdomen and auscultates for the presence of bowel sounds. Any sign of hematuria suggests genitourinary injury or infection. Blood found at the urinary meatus suggests disruptive injury of the lower urinary tract, and a urinary catheter should not be inserted.

Diagnostic Tests

Once the child has arrived in the emergency setting and has undergone initial assessment and interventions, many diagnostic tests assist in the evaluation process. Standard protocols for laboratory tests usually include a complete blood count (CBC) with differential count, serum electrolytes, bedside glucose, and urinalysis. Additional studies may be necessary for the child who has multiple trauma. These include coagulation profiles, blood urea nitrogen (BUN), creatinine, glucose, amylase, lipase, SGOT (serum glutamic-oxaloacetic transaminase, also known as AST [*aspartate aminotransferase*]), SGPT (serum glutamic-pyruvate transaminase, also known as ALT [*alanine aminotransferase*]), and blood type and crossmatch.

Radiologic films may be obtained depending on the presenting problem and assessment data. Placement of a gastric tube, urinary catheter, or other device may be required.

Weight

Determining the child's weight is essential in emergency care because all medication dosages and fluid amounts are calculated according to the child's weight in kilograms. The nurse weighs the child on an appropriate scale if possible. If not possible, the nurse obtains a weight history from the parent.

Another way to determine the child's weight and medication dosages is through the use of a length-based resuscitation tape, such as the Broselow tape. A length-based resuscitation tape is placed on a gurney or stretcher next to the child, and the child's length is measured. The length is keyed to emergency medication dosages, usually listed on the tape. The tape also indicates fluid bolus volumes, defibrillation energy levels, and sizes of the pediatric airway, bag-valve-mask, laryngoscope, endotracheal tube, gastric tube, urinary catheter, chest tube, and IV catheter.

When all else fails or in preparation for the arrival of a seriously ill or injured child, three estimated average weights for children younger than 10 years (Brownstein & Rivara, 2000) can be used to estimate the child's weight:

1 year	10 kg
5 years	20 kg
10 years	30 kg

Parent-Child Relationship

Rapid triage assessment of the child also includes observation of the child in relation to the parents. If the relationship does not appear to be close, comfortable, and trusting, the nurse may want to explore further.

CARDIOPULMONARY RESUSCITATION OF THE CHILD
Airway and Breathing

Initial Assessment and Intervention

Whereas lethal arrhythmias related to heart disease are the most common causes of cardiopulmonary arrest in adults, factors leading to shock and respiratory failure are the most common causes of cardiopulmonary arrest in children. Early recognition of and intervention for respiratory distress and compensated shock can be lifesaving for the child. Assistance with ventilation and administration of fluids may prevent further deterioration in the child's condition. Once the child progresses to respiratory failure and shock, cardiopulmonary resuscitation (CPR) is necessary. Resuscitation of children requires attention to the differences between adults and children (see Table 10-1).

After appropriately opening and clearing the airway, the nurse looks for chest rise and listens and feels for exhaled breath against his or her cheek. When the child is not breathing or ventilation is not adequate after positioning the airway correctly, the nurse gives at least two, one second, breaths by a bag-valve-mask device, watching for the rise and fall of the chest. *The nurse should stop inflating the lungs when the chest just begins to rise and allow enough time for exhalation (longer than inhalation).* Endotracheal intubation by a provider skilled in the technique is necessary if the child cannot be ventilated adequately with these measures or if prolonged ventilation is anticipated. Ventilations should be given at a rate of 12 to 20/min, or approximately 1 breath every 3 to 5 seconds; each breath should be given over a 1-second period (American Heart Association, 2005a).

A pressure gauge attached to the bag-valve-mask device helps deliver breaths at the correct pressure, especially for infants and young children. Choosing the appropriate size mask and the correct volume bag is important. The mask should cover the child's mouth and nose but not place pressure on the eyes. A good fit ensures a seal around the face and under the chin. Gastric decompression by use of an orogastric or nasogastric tube is indicated during assisted ventilation.

Obstructed Airway Management

Inability to inflate the lungs suggests airway obstruction, a life-threatening emergency. When ventilation is not possible, the infant or child will die in a very short time.

Management of airway obstruction depends on the cause and on the child's age. Definitive treatment depends on diagnosis. Whereas adults more commonly choke while eating, children can choke while eating or playing. Foreign body aspiration, for example, is a problem frequently seen in young children, with a large number of aspirations attributed to coins, small toy parts, and certain foods, particularly candy, nuts, and grapes. More than 90% of pediatric deaths related to choking occur in children younger than 5 years of age (American Heart Association, 2005b). When a child is unable to ventilate adequately and aspiration of a foreign body is suspected as the cause, the nurse initiates maneuvers to remove the obstruction.

Although controversy remains about how to clear a foreign body from the airway, for children older than 1 year the American Heart Association recommends using the Heimlich maneuver for a conscious child. CPR should be initiated for all unresponsive infants and children with a foreign body aspiration. The rescuer tries to visualize the foreign body for removal prior to each ventilation sequence (American Heart Association, 2005b). Removal of a foreign body from an infant involves placing the infant in a downward-slant position and giving five back blows alternating with five chest thrusts. Blind finger sweeps to remove a foreign body are not recommended because of the risk of forcing the object farther down into the airway or cause injury to the supraglottic area. A finger sweep is used if the object is visible.

If obstruction continues after these maneuvers, subsequent actions may include direct laryngoscopy and use of a Magill forceps to remove the foreign body. Tracheostomy is used as a last resort. When the lower airway is obstructed because of a disease process, such as asthma, medication to open the airway may be necessary.

CRITICAL TO REMEMBER
Airway Obstruction in Children

When a child is in significant respiratory distress and the child is coughing or able to breathe adequately despite partial obstruction, the child should be allowed to maintain *whatever position is comfortable* until specialized care is available. In the smaller child, this position may be in the parent's or caregiver's arms. The nurse remains with the child and encourages the child to remain calm by reassuring in a soothing manner.

Circulation

The nurse feels for the pulse in the child older than 1 year by palpating the carotid artery and looking for signs of circulation such as movement. For an infant younger than 1 year, the nurse uses the brachial artery because the infant's relatively short, fat neck makes palpation of the carotid artery difficult. If no pulse is palpated after approximately 10 seconds, or if the infant's or child's heart rate is less than 60 beats/min and perfusion is poor after 30 seconds of assisted ventilation, the nurse begins chest compressions at a rate of at least 100 compressions per minute (American Heart Association, 2005b).

Rapid venous access for fluid resuscitation and medication administration is essential in the compromised child. During CPR or treatment of severe shock, an intraosseous line (IO; placed in the anteromedial tibia or distal femur) must be placed if venous access cannot be rapidly achieved. Immediate availability of fluid access site is more important than the route of administration. Children should be given IV fluid (usually lactated Ringer's or normal saline solution), 20 mL/kg, as a rapid bolus for symptoms of shock. The nurse administers additional boluses as needed after reassessing cardiovascular status and warms the solution before any rapid infusion. If more than 3 boluses are required for hemodynamic stability, administration of blood products may be required.

Epinephrine is the drug of choice for management of cardiac arrest, arrhythmias, and hemodynamic instability. It can be given through the endotracheal tube when necessary. Atropine diminishes vagally mediated bradycardia. Sodium bicarbonate is given on the basis of arterial blood gas results, and dextrose can be used on the basis of blood glucose results or for clients unresponsive to resuscitative efforts.

Although cardiac rhythm disturbances in children are rare, rapid heart rates can occur, including sinus tachycardia, supraventricular tachycardia, and ventricular tachycardia. Cardiac output is a function of stroke volume and heart rate. Because children are unable to increase stroke volume, they can increase cardiac output only by increasing their heart rate. As heart rates increase, cardiac filling time decreases and cardiac output falls.

Sinus tachycardia usually requires observation and determination of the cause (e.g., fever, shock, toxic ingestion). Vagal maneuvers (e.g., applying ice water to the face), cardioversion at 0.5 to 1.0 joules/kg, or adenosine may be necessary for symptomatic supraventricular tachycardia (heart rate >200 beats/min) (American Heart Association, 2005c). Ventricular tachycardia in a child is usually the result of congenital abnormalities, toxic ingestion, or chronic cardiac disease and requires complex interventions.

Resuscitation of the child requires a team effort. Training and rehearsal, such as mock codes, are helpful. Also helpful are national courses now available, such as the Pediatric Advanced Life Support (PALS) program provided by the American Heart Association and the Emergency Nursing Pediatric Course (ENPC) provided by the Emergency Nurses Association (Table 10-3).

Automatic external defibrillators (AEDs) are becoming increasingly more available in community settings. They

TABLE 10-3	Basic Life Support Maneuvers in Infants and Children	
Maneuver	**Infant (<1 yr)**	**Child (1 yr-onset of puberty)**
Airway	Head-tilt/chin-lift (if trauma is present, use jaw thrust)	Head-tilt/chin-lift (if trauma is present, use jaw thrust)
Breathing		
Initial	At least two effective breaths at 1 sec/breath	Two effective breaths at 1 sec/breath
Subsequent	12 to 20 breaths/min (approximate)	12 to 20 breaths/min (approximate)
Circulation: pulse check	Brachial, femoral	Carotid
Compression area	Just below nipple line	Center of chest between nipples
Compressed width	Two fingers; use two thumbs, encircling hands technique when there are two rescuers	Heel of one or two hands
Depth	Approximately one third to one half the depth of the chest	Approximately one third to one half the depth of the chest
Rate	100 breaths/min	100 breaths/min
Compression/ventilation ratio	30:2 for one rescuer; 15:2 for two rescuers	30:2 for one rescuer; 15:2 for two rescuers
Foreign body airway obstruction	Back blows, chest thrusts	Heimlich maneuver

Modified from American Heart Association. (2005). Highlights of the 2005 American Heart Association guidelines for cardiopulmonary resuscitation and emergency cardiovascular care. *Currents in Emergency Cardiovascular Care,16*(4), 1-27.

are effective for correcting serious rhythm disturbances in adults and are being used for children as well. The Pediatric Advanced Life Support Task Force, International Liaison Committee on Resuscitation has updated recommendations for use of AEDs in the pediatric population (American Heart Association, 2005a; Samson, Berg, & Bingham, 2002). These recommendations state that AEDs can be used safely in children ages 1 to 8 years whose circulation is absent, especially if equipped with child-sized external pads and a pediatric shock dose level. Additionally, AEDs should be able to identify shockable rhythms with a high degree of accuracy (Samson et al., 2002). In the community setting, CPR should be performed for at least 5 cycles before using an AED (American Heart Association, 2005a).

THE CHILD IN SHOCK

Shock is an acute, complex, unstable physiologic state of inadequate oxygen delivery to tissues. Decreased tissue perfusion (circulation of blood through the vascular bed of tissue) leads to tissue hypoxia and ischemia, metabolic acidosis and, if prolonged, irreversible tissue and organ damage (Caldwell & Ziglar, 2001). The causes of shock can be classified into three major categories: hypovolemic, cardiogenic, and distributive, with some overlaps (Sparrow & Willis, 2004). Regardless of the cause, the body will respond similarly to compensate for the alterations in perfusion and transport of oxygen and metabolic substrates that have occurred.

Etiology

Hypovolemic Shock

Hypovolemic shock is the most common cause of shock in children and is characterized by an overall decrease in circulating blood or fluid volumes. Hemorrhage, burns, and dehydration are the most common causes of hypovolemic shock. Blood loss can be caused by trauma or surgery; fluid and plasma losses can occur with vomiting and diarrhea, burns, and diabetic ketoacidosis.

Distributive Shock

Distributive shock is the result of an abnormality in the distribution of blood flow or inability of the body to maintain vascular tone through vasoconstriction.

Septic shock is the most common form of distributive shock and occurs when microbial toxins (from bacteria, viruses, fungi, or rickettsiae) are present in the blood. These toxins cause a cascade of metabolic, hemodynamic, and clinical changes, resulting in impaired organ perfusion and hypotension. Despite major advances in vaccines in the past 2 decades, septic shock continues to be a frequent reason for admission to pediatric intensive care units. Organisms responsible for septic shock vary with age and immunocompetence, but include group B beta-hemolytic streptococci, enteric gram-negative rods (*E. coli, Klebsiella,* Enterobacteriaceae), *Listeria monocytogenes,* and *Staphylococcus aureus* in neonates; *Streptococcus pneumoniae, S. aureus, Neisseria meningitides,* and *group A Streptococcus* in infants and children (Sparrow & Willis, 2004). Infants and children with debilitating illnesses, clients in the intensive care unit for prolonged periods with many invasive lines, and those who are immunosuppressed are at greatest risk for development of septic shock. Anaphylaxis, central nervous system or spinal injury, and drug intoxication are other forms of distributive shock.

Cardiogenic Shock

Cardiogenic shock occurs when myocardial function is impaired so that cardiac output is not sufficient to meet the body's metabolic demands. It is characterized by low cardiac output, cyanosis, respiratory distress differentiated extremity blood pressures, poor tissue perfusion, and poor response to fluid resuscitation (Koenig, Hijazi, & Zimmerman, 2004). The causes of cardiogenic shock include structural abnormalities related to congenital heart disease, infectious and noninfectious cardiomyopathies, intractable arrhythmias, trauma, ischemia, metabolic abnormalities, drug intoxication, and impaired cardiac function after intracardiac surgical repair.

Manifestations

Recognition of the clinical manifestations, with early intervention, is imperative for optimal treatment of shock (Box 10-2). In the early stages, the child is able to compensate with tachycardia, tachypnea, and vasoconstriction to maintain cardiac output. If the condition cannot be reversed, a decompensated state arises with altered perfusion (delayed capillary refill, weak pulses, cool extremities, hypotension) and profoundly altered mental status. Progression is cardiovascular collapse and death. Table 10-4 presents the general appearance of a child in shock.

CRITICAL TO REMEMBER
Hypotension in Children with Shock

Hypotension is a late sign of shock. The lower limits for systolic blood pressure in children are as follows:
- Infants younger than 1 month: 60 mm Hg
- Infants ages 1 to 12 months: 70 mm Hg
- Children older than 1 year: 70+ (twice the child's age in years) mm Hg

---

Diagnostic Evaluation

The diagnosis of shock in infants and children is established chiefly on the basis of clinical manifestations and medical history. A chest radiograph may help differentiate cardiogenic shock from hypovolemic and distributive shock. In cardiogenic shock, the heart is usually enlarged and may show signs of pulmonary edema. In hypovolemic or distributive shock, the chest radiograph is usually normal or shows signs of infiltrates (indicative of pneumonia) and the heart is smaller than normal (indicative of a decrease in circulating volume). An echocardiogram can identify underlying structural cardiac disease.

Laboratory studies used in a differential diagnosis include blood cultures and cultures of other sites that may be the source of infection (e.g., spinal fluid, urine, sputum, wound drainage, indwelling lines), arterial blood gas values, glucose levels, electrolytes, BUN, creatinine levels, CBC, and coagulation studies.

Therapeutic Management

The therapeutic management of the child in shock includes basic life support (maintaining airway, breathing, and circulation) and treating signs and symptoms.

Monitoring with pulse oximetry and increasing ambient oxygen are indicated in most cases. If vascular access cannot be obtained, an IO can be used until the child is resuscitated, at which time the temporary IO can be replaced with an IV line.

Hypovolemic Shock

Once the airway, breathing, and circulation are established, the next priority is adequate vascular access. A crystalloid infusion of warm normal saline or lactated Ringer's solution should be promptly initiated. If hypovolemic shock is caused by hemorrhage and symptoms persist after two or three crystalloid boluses, transfusions of typed and cross-matched packed red blood cells may be considered (Frankel & Mathers, 2004).

BOX 10-2	Manifestations of Shock in Children
Hypovolemic Shock Dry mucous membranes Depressed fontanel Cold, clammy skin Oliguria Poor skin turgor Delayed capillary refill **Distributive (Septic)** **Shock: Early** Vasodilation Extremities that are warm to the touch Tachycardia, tachypnea **Septic Shock: Late** Rapid, thready pulse Cyanosis Cold, clammy skin	**Septic Shock:** **Late—cont'd** Purpuric skin lesions Narrow pulse pressure Oliguria or anuria **Cardiogenic Shock** Hepatomegaly Cardiomegaly Increased central venous pressure Periorbital edema Crackles Diaphoresis Oliguria Reduced capillary refill Differences in proximal and distal pulses

---

TABLE 10-4	Assessing a Child's General Appearance: "Looks Good" Versus "Looks Bad"	
	"Looks Good"	**"Looks Bad"**
Color	Pink mucous membranes Consistent color over the trunk and extremities	Mottled color, "gray" or pale
Skin perfusion	Warm Brisk capillary refill (<2 sec)	Cold (peripheral to proximal cooling) Sluggish capillary refill (>2 sec)
Activity	Age appropriate (may be frightened, unhappy, unwilling to be separated from parents) Will engage in play	Fretful, then lethargic
Responsiveness	Age appropriate	Irritable (early), then lethargic Decreased response to painful stimulus is worrisome
Infant feeding	Eats well	Weak suck Tires during feeding May have respiratory distress during feedings

Modified from Hazinski, M. F. (1990). Shock in the pediatric patient. *Critical Care Nursing Clinics of North America, 2*(2), 313.

PATHOPHYSIOLOGY

SHOCK

Hypovolemic Shock

Hypovolemic shock results from an abnormal decrease in circulating volume. Water constitutes a much greater portion of an infant's or child's body weight than it does an adult's, and because the bulk of fluid volume in young children is located primarily in the extracellular tissue spaces, infants and young children are more susceptible to hypovolemic shock. Infants, with their large body surface area and increased metabolic rate, also experience increased insensible fluid loss, thus compounding hypovolemia. Because of their small body size, even relatively small blood losses can result in hypovolemia.

When intravascular volume is reduced, the body initially compensates by increasing the peripheral vascular resistance, stroke volume, and heart rate and redistributing the blood flow to the vital organs (brain, heart). If a fluid resuscitation is not initiated within an appropriate time frame, altered sensorium and oliguria will be noted and hypovolemic shock will eventually result in irreversible tissue organ damage (Caldwell & Ziglar, 2001).

Distributive Shock

Septic shock, the most common form of distributive shock, occurs when an invading organism infects a susceptible host, overwhelms the host's first and second lines of defense, and enters the bloodstream. The body's response to toxins or organisms in the blood, including endocrine, metabolic,

and immunologic reactions, can result in inflammatory and coagulation abnormalities. Endotoxins, produced by lysis of bacteria, cause maldistributed blood flow, cardiac dysfunction, oxygen supply and demand imbalance, and metabolic alterations. The end result can be organ ischemia, multiple organ dysfunction syndrome, and death (Burns, 2003).

Cardiogenic Shock

Cardiogenic shock is characterized by low cardiac output and hypotension, which result in inadequate oxygen delivery to the tissues. Unlike hypovolemic shock, the compensatory mechanisms that occur in a child with cardiogenic shock can cause further myocardial dysfunction. These compensatory mechanisms redistribute blood away from the peripheral, splenic, and mesenteric circulation to help maintain the circulation to the vital organs: the heart and brain. Initially, compensatory mechanisms increase the heart rate, myocardial contractility, and vasoconstriction. Subsequent events result in sodium and fluid retention, producing a greater workload on the left ventricle (afterload). The increased workload causes increased oxygen demands on the myocardium in response to a depleted oxygen supply. This process leads to myocardial ischemia, which further depresses cardiac function, thereby establishing a vicious cycle.

An alteration in contractility, as seen in an injury to the myocardium and myocarditis, results in a decreased stroke volume and the ventricle is unable to eject blood.

Colloids (albumin) are protein-containing fluids that may be used in volume resuscitation after the initial treatment with crystalloids. Colloids are used primarily for dehydration or body fluid losses other than blood.

Distributive Shock

The therapeutic management of distributive shock involves restoring hemodynamic status with fluid resuscitation and promptly treating the underlying cause. Inotropic medications and vasodilators are used to manage the cardiovascular instability. Vasoconstrictors may be used to increase vascular tone and counteract the effects of toxins. Steroids, medications to treat hypoglycemia and electrolyte imbalances, and administration of blood products may be required to combat complications of distributive shock (Maar, 2004). Maintaining a secure, patent airway may be necessary if significant respiratory distress occurs. Surgery also might be indicated to eliminate the source of infection (e.g., an abscess) or stabilize a central nervous system/spinal injury.

Cardiogenic Shock

Supplemental oxygen, vascular access, hemodynamic monitoring, and frequent assessments are imperative in shock management. The nurse uses assessment skills to recognize early signs of deterioration and response to therapeutic interventions. Invasive monitoring of central venous pressure,

arterial blood pressure, and pulmonary artery pressure helps identify hemodynamic changes and subtle clinical signs and symptoms of decreased cardiac output (e.g., cyanosis, decreased skin temperature, delayed capillary refill).

With an excess of intravascular fluid volume, diuretics may be prescribed. Usually furosemide (Lasix), 1 mg/kg, provides effective diuresis.

The heart rate must be in the normal range or higher than normal to improve the cardiac output. Children, especially infants younger than 6 months, have a decreased ability to increase stroke volume and thus depend much more on an increased heart rate to improve cardiac output. Pharmacologic therapy is the mainstay of medical treatment in children with cardiogenic shock. Frequently a combination of pharmacologic agents is necessary to stabilize the child. Enalaprilat, dopamine, and milrinone are the initial drugs of choice for treating cardiogenic shock (Koenig et al., 2004).

Extracorporeal membrane oxygenation (ECMO) is a means of providing short-term circulatory and respiratory support for infants and children in whom other methods of treatment are not effective. It has been successfully used in distributive and cardiogenic shock. Vital organ perfusion is maintained by ECMO to allow for recovery and stabilization required before definitive treatment such as antibiotic coverage or surgery can be implemented (Maar, 2004).

NURSING CARE

The Child in Shock

Assessment

Nursing assessment of a child in shock should be thorough, with attention focused on the cardiopulmonary system and neurologic status. A changing level of consciousness is one of the first indicators of a worsening condition, and early identification and treatment of shock in infants and children are crucial to decreasing morbidity and mortality rates. Initial concerns are ensuring a patent airway and monitoring the child's respiratory effort to confirm adequate air exchange with good chest expansion. Central circulation is assessed by checking a brachial, carotid, or femoral pulse. Assessment of level of consciousness is performed serially to detect early changes.

Hypovolemic Shock

A child in hypovolemic shock may have a history of trauma, vomiting and diarrhea, or anorexia. The parent may report a decrease in wet diapers or explain that the child has not voided recently. With trauma, the child may demonstrate obvious signs of injury or bleeding or covert symptoms suggestive of blunt trauma.

The child in hypovolemic shock requires frequent assessment of vital signs, including blood pressure (every 15 to 60 min). Skin color, turgor, and temperature should be closely monitored. The anterior fontanel (if present) should be assessed to determine whether it is depressed or full. A depressed fontanel may be a manifestation of dehydration, whereas a full or level fontanel usually suggests that fluid volume is adequate.

In addition, the nurse assesses and monitors the child's neurologic status closely. A depressed or deteriorating level of consciousness should be reported promptly. The nurse auscultates heart and lungs and palpates peripheral pulses. Capillary refill time, moistness of mucous membranes, and general muscle tone and strength should be assessed and urine output closely monitored. In very young children, weighing the diapers quantifies urine output. If the child has diarrhea, a urine bag or Foley catheter should be placed to monitor urinary output. The abdomen should be palpated and auscultated for the presence of bowel sounds. Abdominal injury must be ruled out, especially if the abdominal girth appears to be increasing, with evidence of abdominal distention. Any abnormal bruising or obvious trauma must be recognized quickly, because blunt abdominal trauma is a major cause of shock in children.

Distributive Shock

Early signs of distributive shock include hyperthermia or hypothermia. The temperature should be closely monitored. In early shock (the hyperdynamic phase), the skin is typically warm and flushed. In late shock (the hypodynamic phase), skin is ashen and cold. An exception is in the case of spinal injury, in which the body cannot maintain a normal temperature. Shock of any etiology may cause microcirculatory dysfunction leading to abnormal function of coagulation factors and platelets. Therefore the nurse observes the skin closely for signs of petechiae, oozing of blood from invasive lines, or purpuric lesions. The presence of petechiae that are spread diffusely over the body may indicate severe sepsis. In children, hypotension is a late sign of all types of shock.

Cardiogenic Shock

A child with cardiogenic shock requires close monitoring of the heart and lungs for adventitious sounds. The liver should be palpated and its size measured. The child's respiratory effort must also be assessed. Retractions, grunting, and nasal flaring may be apparent. Periorbital and peripheral edema or other signs of cardiac failure may be present. Close monitoring of the peripheral pulses and capillary refill is extremely important.

Nursing Diagnosis and Planning

The following nursing diagnoses and expected outcomes may be appropriate after assessment of the child with shock:

* Ineffective Tissue Perfusion (cardiopulmonary, cerebral, peripheral) related to decreased fluid volume (in hypovolemic shock); abnormal distribution of blood flow, metabolic acidosis, or both (in distributive shock); or decreased cardiac contractility (in cardiogenic shock).

  Expected Outcome: The child will maintain adequate tissue perfusion, as evidenced by strong peripheral pulses, appropriate skin turgor, normal capillary refill time, pink and warm mucous membranes and nail beds, vital signs within normal limits for age, and no evidence of dyspnea or altered mental status.

* Impaired Gas Exchange related to possible decreased pulmonary blood flow, increased interstitial fluid in alveoli, and inflammatory response of alveoli.

  Expected Outcome: The child will have adequate gas exchange, as evidenced by oxygen saturation level between 95% and 100% and normal arterial blood gas measurements.

* Risk for Infection related to invasive venous and arterial lines, indwelling catheters, presence of endotracheal tube, possible incisional wounds, and compromised state.

  Expected Outcome: The child will remain free from signs of infection, as evidenced by normal temperature, white blood cell count (WBC) within normal limits, no signs of redness or purulence from access sites, and negative blood cultures.

* Anxiety related to threat of a possible grave prognosis in a critically ill child.

  Expected Outcomes: The child, if verbal, and parents will verbalize symptoms of anxiety, seek information to ensure understanding of the condition, and demonstrate adequate coping skills.

Interventions

Interventions for the child in shock are directed toward maintaining tissue perfusion by improving cardiac output, ensuring adequate oxygenation, preventing infection, and enhancing child and family coping.

Maintaining Tissue Perfusion

Careful and frequent observation of the child's cardiovascular status is essential. Take vital signs and assess circulation every 1 to 2 hours. After establishing an adequate IV access, administer appropriate fluid replacement. Carefully document intake and output, and report urine output that is abnormal for age (see Chapter 18) or any major discrepancy between intake and output. Weigh the child daily on the same scale. Report any rapid weight gain to the physician.

Because infants have high glucose requirements and low glycogen stores, alterations in glucose metabolism are frequently seen in response to stress. Monitor blood glucose levels every 2 to 4 hours.

Administer ordered medications by IV pump to ensure appropriate delivery of medication. Because vasoactive drugs can cause tissue necrosis if infiltration occurs in peripheral tissues, these agents are administered preferably through a central line.

Ensuring Oxygenation

Observe and record respiratory rate and effort, skin color, chest expansion, and aeration. Note signs of respiratory distress and report them to the physician promptly. Administer oxygen as ordered, making sure the delivery mode is appropriate for the child's age. Monitor oxygen saturation, arterial blood gases, and hemoglobin levels. Maintain a patent airway, and have emergency endotracheal intubation and ventilation equipment available. Ensure normothermia and control pain and anxiety to decrease oxygen demands. Place gastric tube to decompress the stomach and allow full expansion of the thoracic cavity.

Preventing Infection

Because children in a compromised state are prone to infection, maintain strict aseptic technique when handling IV lines, invasive tubes, and incisional or puncture sites. Closely monitor the child's temperature and report any rectal temperature greater than 38° C (100.4° F) or less than 36° C (96.8° F). Observe secretions and body fluids, incisions, and puncture sites for erythema, edema, or purulence. Report positive culture results and elevated WBCs promptly. Administer ordered antipyretics and ensure adequate caloric intake. If the child is unable to tolerate oral or nasogastric feedings, discuss alternative methods of feeding with the physician.

Enhancing Coping

Provide concise, accurate information to parents. Determine the child's developmental level and level of comprehension. Provide simple explanations of procedures before initiating them. Provide information in a calm, relaxed, and concerned manner. Answer all questions honestly. Be empathetic.

Allow the child and parents to express their feelings, concerns, and anxieties. Encourage the parents to participate in the child's care as appropriate (e.g., bathing, combing hair, feeding). This assistance provides them with some control. Be nonjudgmental in response to parents' actions. Use available resources (e.g., social worker, chaplain, other family members) to help calm parents who are exhibiting uncontrolled feelings.

Elicit the parents' perceptions of the event and provide reassurance or clarify any misconceptions. Determine the availability of support systems and encourage their use. Help the parents identify coping mechanisms that have been effective in the past and encourage parents to determine whether these mechanisms may be effective during the current crisis.

Evaluation

* Does the child demonstrate pink mucous membranes, brisk capillary refill, alertness, responsiveness, and normal vital signs for age?
* Is the oxygen saturation at least 95% on room air, and are blood gas values within normal limits?
* Does the child demonstrate a normal breathing rate, pattern, and work of breathing?
* Is the child afebrile with negative culture results?
* Can the parents and child express their feelings to staff or significant others?
* Is the family demonstrating decreased anxiety by using available resources and effective coping mechanisms?

PEDIATRIC TRAUMA

Despite a 39% decline in unintentional injury deaths among children younger than 14 years from 1987 to 2000, injury is the leading cause of death for children (Wallis, Cody, & Mickalide, 2003). The Centers for Disease Control and Prevention (CDC) has consistently found that motor vehicle injuries are the leading cause of unintentional death in children younger than 18 years in the United States, followed by drowning and airway obstruction injury. Burns and poisoning are other major causes of unintentional death, whereas falls are the leading cause of nonfatal injuries requiring hospital emergency room treatment. The term *injury* is used in preference to accident when describing trauma because some trauma is not accidental and much of it is preventable.

Injury prevention and education have been credited with a decrease in unintentional deaths among children. Despite this, much more needs to be done. Successful prevention and education steps include motor vehicle safety restraints, firearm education, bicycle helmet programs, safety caps and locked medications, and eliminating potential hazards, such as old refrigerators and unfenced pools. Up-to-date educational resources can be obtained through organizations and websites such as those offered by the National SAFE KIDS Campaign, the CDC, and the U.S. Consumer Product Safety Commission. When child victims of trauma are discharged from the emergency department, the nurse provides injury prevention information to the families. Injury prevention is also discussed at every well-child visit through adolescence (see Chapters 5 through 8).

Mechanism of Injury

Injuries can be categorized as *blunt, penetrating,* and *multiple trauma.* Knowing the mechanism of injury and recognizing anatomic and physiologic differences in the pediatric population help identify common injury patterns and predict the child's needs and outcomes.

Blunt Trauma

Blunt or penetrating force causes tissue trauma. Blunt trauma occurs more frequently than all other injuries combined. Injuries sustained from blunt trauma are often less apparent but, nevertheless, can be extremely serious (Dayan & Klein, 2004).

Motor Vehicle Trauma. A common cause of blunt trauma is acceleration-deceleration force, often from motor vehicle collisions or falls. Just before a motor vehicle collision, both the occupant and the vehicle are traveling at the same speed. When the vehicle meets an opposing force, the speed of both the occupant and the vehicle rapidly decelerate. When this change occurs, four collisions take place: (1) the moving vehicle collides with the opposing object; (2) the occupant's body collides with the interior portion of the vehicle; (3) the occupant's internal organs and tissues collide with rigid internal structures; and (4) loose objects in the vehicle become projectile forces (Hawkins, 2004).

Unrestrained occupants in a motor vehicle collision have a higher incidence of injury than restrained occupants have because they are tossed around the interior of the vehicle or are ejected at the point of collision. This principle applies also to children riding unrestrained in the back of open pickup trucks; they become missiles ejected out of the vehicle into oncoming traffic or onto the road. Children who are held on an adult's lap during a motor vehicle collision can be instantly crushed between the rigid part of the automobile and the moving adult.

Child safety seats and safety belts, *when appropriately sized and correctly installed,* can prevent injury and save lives. Recently, childhood injuries and deaths have occurred as a result of airbag deployment. As of January 1, 2004, 141 children were killed by passenger airbags (National SAFE KIDS Campaign, 2005a). Twenty-three of these deaths were among infants in rear-facing child safety seats in front of a passenger airbag. Approximately 92% of all children killed by passenger airbags were either unrestrained or improperly restrained at the time of death. The National Highway and Traffic Safety Administration (www.nhtsa.com) advises that all children younger than 12 years be placed in rear seats in all cars, especially those with passenger airbags, and that infants younger than 1 year and weighing less than 20 lb must ride in a rear-facing infant safety seat.

Pedestrian Injury. Pedestrian injuries in children are also a significant problem, with the largest number of incidences occurring in children 5 to 14 years of age (Wallis et al., 2003). Most of these injuries occur during the daylight hours as the child darts out into the middle of the street between parked cars or stands unnoticed behind a vehicle backing out of a driveway.

When a child is hit by a motor vehicle, a triad of injuries, referred to as Waddell's triad, occurs (Fig. 10-1). This one traumatic event results in three different types of injuries:

1. After being struck by the bumper and hood of the car, the child sustains abdominal or thoracic injuries.
2. The child is then propelled into the air, lands on the ground, and sustains femur or other leg injury, as well as surface trauma.
3. As the child is propelled like a missile to the ground, the large size and weight of the child's head result in skull fracture or closed head injury to the contralateral side of the head.

Penetrating Trauma

Penetrating trauma includes stabbing, firearms, blasting, and impaling injuries. Damage to the body tissue can result from the penetrating object itself and secondarily from radiating energy forces along the pathway of the penetrating object. The severity of an injury depends on the location of impact and the type of object. For example, with gunshot wounds,

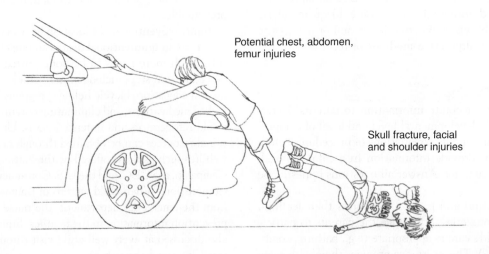

Potential chest, abdomen, femur injuries

Skull fracture, facial and shoulder injuries

what might seem like a fairly innocuous wound can actually be severe, depending on factors such as projectile, fragmentation, type of tissue struck, and striking velocity. Injuries from a stab wound depend on length of the instrument, applied velocity, and angle of entry.

Multiple Trauma

A child with multiple trauma incurs injuries to more than one body system. A positive outcome for a child who has sustained multiple trauma depends on rapid assessment and intervention, which begin at the scene of the accident and continue through the trauma center emergency department, the critical care and acute care units, and the rehabilitation phase. Ideally, a critically injured child should be rapidly transported to a trauma facility with the personnel, equipment, and commitment to provide specialized care to children.

At the trauma center, and even in the emergency department of the community hospital, the presence of qualified trauma team members to assess and treat the trauma patient is crucial. A trauma team consists of skilled surgeons, other physicians, nurses, social workers, and other health professionals, each with a specific role and duties during trauma resuscitation. The team assembles after notification of pending arrival by emergency personnel and readies the trauma room with personnel and equipment.

All clients with multiple trauma require a rapid, complete, and thorough assessment to determine the extent of injuries. As with the ill child, assessment of a child with multiple trauma includes primary and secondary surveys, with concurrent appropriate interventions.

Primary Survey

The goal of the primary survey is to assess and manage life-threatening injuries. The primary assessment (see "Primary Assessment," p. 255) proceeds with the following additions.

Airway Assessment and Management. The priority is to open and maintain the airway with the jaw-thrust maneuver to prevent movement of the cervical spine. The nurse inspects for loose teeth or other potential airway obstructions. Because the child's lower airway is narrow and easily obstructed by edema and mucus, oral suctioning may be required to keep the airway clear. A pediatric cervical collar and immobilization board secure a child when spinal cord injury is a concern (Fig. 10-2). To determine a correct fit, the cervical collar is measured for maximal stability: the chin must rest securely in the chin holder, with the collar below the ears and the lower end not extending below the upper part of the sternum. The cervical immobilization device and spinal immobilization device (long backboard) must remain in place until spinal injury has been ruled out.

When an alert child is brought to the emergency setting in the car seat, the nurse places rolled towels on either side of the child's head and secures these with tape to maintain cervical immobilization without removing the child from the seat. The child can then remain in the car seat until

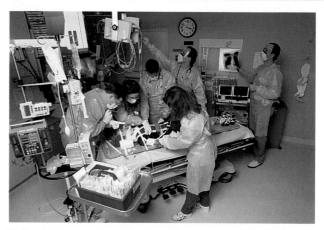

FIG 10-2 **The child with multiple trauma injuries must remain on an immobilization board (long backboard) with a cervical immobilization device in place until being evaluated for spinal injuries.** *(Courtesy Children's Medical Center, Dallas.)*

radiographs have shown no injury to the cervical spine or until a change in status is noted.

Breathing Assessment and Management. Pulse oximetry readings are an adjunct to evaluating ventilation and adequate oxygenation. Oxygen use in the child with multiple trauma is not contraindicated; therefore the nurse starts supplemental oxygen at a rate of 10 to 15 L/min by mask. If the child is alert and does not tolerate the mask, using blow-by oxygen with the tubing only or using a plastic cup attached to the end of the tubing might be less threatening to a child.

If ventilation is inadequate or absent, the nurse begins to ventilate the child (as described on p. 259) with a bag-valve-mask with a reservoir and high-flow oxygen. An oropharyngeal or nasopharyngeal airway maintains patency in a child with altered consciousness.

Endotracheal intubation may be needed for airway control and oxygenation in children with altered level of consciousness, lack of spontaneous respirations, or severe head injury. The nurse hyperventilates the child before this procedure and assists in evaluation of endotracheal tube placement after the procedure.

CRITICAL TO REMEMBER
Artificial Airways

- *Oropharyngeal airway:* Used in the unconscious child only. Determine the length of the airway by measuring the distance from the level of the teeth to the angle of the jaw. Use a tongue blade to depress and displace the tongue while inserting the airway curve down (in the anatomic position) and over the tongue.
- *Nasopharyngeal airway:* Select an airway with a diameter slightly less than the diameter of the child's nares, and determine the length of the airway by measuring the distance from the nares to the tragus of the ear.

While observing the child for respiratory difficulty, the nurse checks the neck for jugular vein distention or tracheal deviation (the cervical collar can be opened for this assessment and then closed, keeping the neck in alignment). Because respiratory difficulty can be caused by chest injury, the nurse observes the chest for contusions, penetrations, abrasions, and paradoxic movement. A chest tube insertion or intervention for cardiac tamponade may be indicated for a penetrating chest injury, or an occlusive dressing may be taped on three sides for an open pneumothorax.

Severe facial trauma, although rare in children younger than 5 years, can be life threatening, primarily because of the potential to obstruct ventilation—both fractures and soft tissue injury can cause narrowing of the airway. Facial trauma in children is treated as it is in adults. Nursing intervention includes ensuring an adequate airway and breathing, observing for possible progressive obstruction, and keeping the injured areas clean to prevent infection.

Circulation Assessment and Management. Cardiovascular assessment of the child focuses on early recognition and treatment of hypovolemia. Blood loss in children is usually caused by internal abdominal or chest injury, severe injuries to the extremities, or surface head trauma. As previously discussed, early indicators of shock in children are tachycardia, increased capillary refill time (>2 sec), mottled skin, agitation or apprehension, pallor, and cool extremities. Decreased level of consciousness, dusky skin color, clammy extremities, bradycardia, and hypotension are late signs, indicating that cardiac arrest is imminent.

Cardiac monitoring and frequent cardiovascular assessments are necessary during the acute stage. During this stage, any external hemorrhage is noted and controlled and IV or other access to the circulatory system is obtained.

The nurse assesses extremities for fractures and decreased peripheral circulation and splints any suspected fracture, assessing peripheral circulation after applying any splint. Assessment includes motor (Can the child move the extremity? Does the child feel pain?), circulatory (Does the child have good color, a strong pulse, and good capillary refill?); and neural function (Is sensation to the area intact? Does the child have any numbness or tingling in the extremity?). If neurovascular or circulatory compromise is present, immediate intervention is necessary.

Disability. During the primary survey phase, a brief neurologic examination is performed to establish level of consciousness along with pupil size and reactivity and muscle movement. AVPU can assess mental status. Sudden changes, such as agitation or somnolence, may indicate hypoxia or decreased cerebral perfusion.

Secondary Survey

After exposing the child by removing all the child's clothing and providing warming measures, the trauma staff assesses for pain, carefully inspects and documents all signs of injury by performing the head-to-toe assessment (including log rolling the child to inspect the back), and obtains a history of the injury.

Obtaining a History of the Injury. Determining the degree and severity of injuries is both an art and a science.

BOX 10-3	History of Injury Questions

For a Victim of a Motor Vehicle Collision
Was the child wearing a seatbelt or in a child's car seat?
What was the type of seatbelt (lap or lap and shoulder)?
What was the speed of the motor vehicle?
With what did the motor vehicle collide?
At what point on the motor vehicle was the location of impact?
Where was the victim seated in the motor vehicle?
How much damage was done to the motor vehicle?

For a Victim of a Fall
How far did the child fall?
How did the child land (on what part of the body)?
On what type of surface did the child land?
Was the child's fall broken by any objects?

For a Victim of a Penetrating Injury
How long and how wide was the blade of the knife?
How far away was the gun when it was fired?
What type of gun was used, and what was the caliber of the gun?

Diagnosis depends on knowing the mechanism of injury as well as the presenting signs and symptoms. Nurses can obtain a comprehensive history by asking specific questions (Box 10-3). Thorough assessment depends on a systematic trauma evaluation, which takes place along with life-saving intervention.

Trauma Scoring. Various kinds of scoring, performed and documented by on-site emergency medical personnel and nursing staff, are used as an objective measure of the severity of the injury caused by a traumatic event and sometimes to decide the facility most appropriate for treating the child. Most scoring systems are for the assessment of injury to adults and do not take into account the anatomic differences of children (Box 10-4).

BOX 10-4	Trauma Scoring Systems

Trauma Score (TS)
Adult scoring tool sometimes used with children
Assesses respiratory rate and effort, blood pressure, and capillary refill
Includes the Glasgow Coma Scale (GCS)

Revised Trauma Score (RTS)
Composed of the GCS, blood pressure, and respiratory rate

Pediatric Trauma Score (PTS)
Adapted for the pediatric client
Assesses size, airway, central nervous system response, systolic blood pressure, open wounds, and skeletal fractures

Assessing for Child Abuse. Child maltreatment can be a cause of injury (see Chapter 29 for an in-depth discussion of child abuse). Nurses working in emergency settings play an important role in both the assessment and reporting of child maltreatment. In acute care settings, time to assess parent-child interactions or observe at length the child's behavioral indicators is rare, although these actions may provide important information. The following important indicators raise the suspicion of child maltreatment in the emergency setting:

- A history inconsistent with physical findings
- Activity reportedly leading to the trauma that seems inconsistent with the age and condition of the child
- Delay in seeking treatment for the trauma
- A history of other emergency visits

The following physical findings should also raise the level of suspicion:

- Bruises or fractures in various stages of healing noted on radiography
- Injuries rarely found in children (e.g., long bone or rib fractures) when the history is not appropriate for the injury
- Patterns of injury indicating that a specific object caused injury (e.g., belt marks, cigarette burns)

The nurse carefully assesses these indicators in the context of the injury and in relation to the affect of the child and family. The nurse also observes the family's reaction to the child and staff, keeping in mind that people behave differently depending on culture, ethnicity, experience, and psychologic makeup. Above all, health care providers do not assume an investigative role—that is law enforcement's responsibility. Nurses are required to report suspicion of child maltreatment, however, and so must be careful to document any observations in detail. Remember that more than 90% of parents who have abused their children feel ashamed of doing so but are unable to control the impulse. When child maltreatment is suspected, the intervention of child protective services is essential to ensure the safety of the child (and that of other children in the home) and to prevent additional injury.

Nursing Considerations

The Child and Family

The most critical aspect of nursing care of the child with traumatic injury is continuous assessment of respiratory, circulatory, and neurologic status. The nurse observes injured children for the early signs of shock and intervenes immediately to prevent rapid and irreversible deterioration. Preparing for the many procedures and examinations required and observing the equipment used for monitoring should not interfere with close and continuous observation of the child's signs and symptoms.

Nursing care of the child also requires care of the family. When the family arrives at the hospital, one staff member should become the contact person and provide regular updates. Hospital staff supports family members when they visit their critically ill child. Information concerning their child's condition should be provided simply but completely, incorporating the family's educational and emotional status and readiness to learn. Family members are encouraged to touch and talk to their child if they so desire. Remember that informed consent must be obtained from the families of clients for all procedures unless the intervention is required to save the child's life.

The Child During Recovery

Regardless of the cause of the injury, most children with traumatic injury do well unless the injuries are extremely severe. Their cardiovascular systems are strong and their bodies are growing, allowing them to compensate for even the most serious injuries. Even children with severe traumatic brain injuries (TBI) have far more favorable chances of recovery than do adults; however, any TBI can result in short-term and long-term disabilities (CDC, 2003b). Children and their families require nursing support to recover from both the physical and psychologic effects of trauma; the need for rehabilitation must be considered from the moment the child arrives in the emergency setting.

CRITICAL THINKING EXERCISE 10-1

You are working in a small emergency department when a father brings in his 6-year-old daughter, who has been struck by a car while riding a bike. She is in her father's arms, her eyes are closed, and she is pale with mottled lower extremities. Blood is on the father's clothes.

1. What would your quick primary assessment consist of? What are you looking for?
2. What questions would you ask the father to obtain the history?
3. What do you think is wrong with her? Is this an emergency? Why or why not?
4. What interventions would you do? Which would you do first? Why?
5. What responses to your interventions would be expected? Why?

INGESTIONS AND POISONINGS

The term *poison exposure* is the ingestion of or contact with a substance that can produce toxic effects (CDC, 2003). The combination of small weight and size, curiosity, lack of fear, and evolving mobility place all children at risk of injury or death from toxic exposure and ingestion. Differences exist, however, in types of incident by age group. Younger children (1 through 5 years of age) are indiscriminately curious and can innocently ingest a toxic substance in a matter of seconds. As children grow, they gradually learn from parents to avoid dangerous substances, but accidental ingestions and exposures still can occur. In adolescence, the risk is higher for deliberate ingestion.

Incidence

More than half of all poison exposures occurred among children younger than 6 years. Mortality rate from poisonings is higher in the adolescent population as a result of adolescents using poisons to cause self-harm (CDC, 2004; *ED Nursing,* 2003). More than 90% of all poison exposures occur in homes. Most poisonings occur as a result of oral ingestion. Ocular or dermal exposure, inhalation, parenteral exposure, and envenomation account for the remainder of poisoning incidents. Children are poisoned by plants; household and personal care products such as cosmetics, cleaning substances, and medicines; lead; and carbon monoxide. Adolescent poisoning tends to occur as a result of alcohol and prescription and nonprescription ingestions.

Manifestations

Assessment and treatment of toxic exposure and ingestion go hand in hand. Although identification of the type and amount of the exposure is important, the child must initially be treated on the basis of physical signs and symptoms.

An accurate history of the ingestion is useful in planning for the child's care. History given by the child, parent, friend, or caretaker may not always be accurate or complete—areas of confusion are often present, especially in cases of unwitnessed ingestions. The information obtained in the history of the ingestion is combined with the child's presenting physical assessment to provide a complete picture of the event and plan treatment. Laboratory analysis in some cases may provide definitive diagnosis.

Most ingestions seen in emergency settings occur acutely, and the child is brought in immediately or when parents realize the event has occurred. An exception to this is lead poisoning. Although lead poisoning is relatively common, with an estimated 1 million children having elevated levels, it is rarely identified in the emergency setting. A child who has unusual neurologic signs or symptoms, neuropathy, or anemia that cannot be attributed to other causes may have lead poisoning. Elevated blood lead levels result primarily from exposure to lead-based paint or lead-contaminated dust and soil. Older miniblinds, improperly glazed pottery, folk remedies, imported toys, and cosmetics are also reported sources of lead poisoning (CDC, 2005). A careful history can assist in the diagnosis of lead poisoning, but testing serum lead levels provides the only accurate diagnosis. The child with a markedly elevated lead level usually is admitted to the hospital. Chelation therapy, if needed, is administered on an inpatient basis to remove lead from the blood and tissue. When a child is found to have elevated lead levels, other children in the home should be tested as well because of the environmental nature of the ingestion.

Diagnostic Evaluation

In cases of known or suspected ingestion, laboratory tests can be performed to assess serum levels of the substance and the effect of the toxin on body systems. Regional poison control centers and clinical pharmacists should be included as members of the treatment team. Measurements of serum glucose level and toxicologic analysis of urine, serum, and stomach contents are the most common laboratory tests ordered for possible toxic exposure or ingestion. Blood gases and chest radiographs are required if the child is hypoventilating, has other respiratory difficulties, or has been exposed to hydrocarbon (e.g., gasoline) or bleach. Baseline liver enzymes and kidney function tests may be drawn if the suspected substance is known to be toxic to these organs.

Therapeutic Management

The first step in treatment of a toxic exposure or ingestion is to assess ABCs and stabilize the child. Oxygen can be given and breathing supported with a bag-valve-mask device if necessary. If the child's level of consciousness is altered, endotracheal intubation may be necessary to protect the airway. When the child has ingested a sufficient amount of a substance to cause rapid deterioration in mental status, an intubation tray should be at the bedside even when the child is awake and alert. If the child is in shock or shows signs of compensated shock, IV fluid resuscitation is initiated. Cardiac rhythm disturbances can result from many ingested substances, so placement of a cardiac monitor and pulse oximeter is also indicated. Seizure precautions should be instituted in exposures to toxins with neurologic or metabolic side effects.

Care of the child who has been exposed to or ingested a toxic substance depends on the amount ingested and the toxicity of the ingested substance (Table 10-5). After initial stabilization, removing the poison, preventing its absorption, and limiting complications are primary goals. Several methods frequently used to treat toxic ingestions include removal of dermal and ocular toxins, dilution of the toxin, administration of activated charcoal, gastric lavage, and administration of an antidote.

Removal of Dermal and Ocular Toxins

Removing the child from a toxic environment, including removing contaminated clothes, brushing chemical powders from skin, and liberal washing, is mandatory with skin exposure. Copious irrigation of the eyes with water or normal saline is imperative with an ocular exposure. In cases of exposure to an alkaline substance, irrigation proceeds until eyes return to a normal pH (see Chapter 31).

Diluting the Ingested Toxin

Administering water or milk can dilute the toxic effects of acid or alkali ingestion. These substances, when ingested, can cause burning of tissue along the gastrointestinal tract. Because these caustic substances continue to cause damage until neutralized, inducing emesis is contraindicated.

Administration of syrup of ipecac in the home setting is no longer recommended by the American Academy of Pediatrics (AAP, 2003). Three rationales are given for the recommendation that ipecac not be kept in the home: (1) it does not completely remove the poison from the child's system, (2) vomiting is uncomfortable for the child and can lead to intolerance of other approaches to treating the ingestion

TABLE 10-5   **Common Poisonous Substances**

Substance	Pathophysiology	Clinical Manifestations	Treatment
Acetaminophen (Tylenol, many over-the-counter products)			
Toxic dose: uncertain, do not exceed recommended levels. Seriousness of ingestion determined by amount ingested and length of time before intervention and if toxicity is acute or cumulative. Other factors, such as decreased oral intake, have been linked with hepatotoxicity.	Metabolic byproducts deplete liver glutathione and cause damage to hepatic cells. Children younger than 6 yr seem to be more resistant to development of hepatotoxicity than older children and adults.	*First stage* (first 24 hr): malaise, nausea, vomiting, sweating, pallor, weakness. *Second stage* (24-48 hr): latent period with a rise in liver enzymes (aspartate and alanine aminotransferase) and bilirubin; right upper quadrant pain; prolonged prothrombin time. *Third stage* (3-7 days): jaundice, liver necrosis, signs of hepatic failure. *Fourth stage* (5-7 days): recovery or progression to death.	Institute gastric lavage within 1 hr of ingestion depending on amount ingested. Administer antidote: N-acetylcysteine (Mucomyst) as ordered. IV fluids. Sodium-restricted, high-calorie, high-protein diet.
Salicylates (aspirin, many over-the-counter products, oil of wintergreen)			
Toxic dose: single dose exceeding 200-280 mg/kg. Peak gastric absorption occurs within 2 hr of ingestion.	*First stage:* stimulation of respiratory center, leading to respiratory alkalosis. *Second stage:* loss of potassium; increase in metabolic rate; accumulation of ketones leading to metabolic acidosis, hypokalemia, and dehydration. Inhibition of prothrombin formation, decreased platelet levels and adhesiveness, capillary fragility (chronic poisoning).	Gastrointestinal effects: nausea, vomiting, thirst. Central nervous system effects: hyperventilation, tinnitus, confusion, seizures, coma, respiratory failure, circulatory collapse. Renal effect: oliguria. Hematopoietic effects: bleeding tendencies. Metabolic effects: sweating, dehydration, fever, hyponatremia, hypokalemia, dehydration, hypoglycemia.	Perform gastric lavage; administer activated charcoal to decrease absorption. IV fluids, sodium bicarbonate (enhances excretion), potassium replacement; volume expanders as needed to support circulation. Vitamin K for bleeding tendencies (chronic poisoning). Glucose for hypoglycemia. Hemodialysis in severe cases if child unresponsive to therapy.
Corrosives (toilet and drain cleaners, bleach, ammonia)			
Extent of damage depends on causticity of substance and amount ingested.	Severe chemical burns of mouth, throat, esophagus. "Splash" burns of eyes and skin. Alkali substances can continue to cause damage after initial contact. If damage is severe, long-term care is needed, including gastric button or tube, repeated esophageal dilations, and surgical repair of esophagus, sometimes with colon tissue transplant (done when child is older).	Whitish burns of mouth and pharynx, color darkens (red, swollen, oozing as ulcerations form and tissue erodes). Edema, difficulty swallowing, drooling. Respiratory distress, pain. Residual difficulty swallowing; subsequent healing of burns can produce esophageal strictures. Severe burns causing perforation can lead to vascular collapse and shock.	IV fluids while NPO. Analgesics, steroids, antibiotics, nasogastric tube feedings.
Hydrocarbons (gasoline, paint thinner, lighter fluid, turpentine, furniture polish)			
	Chemical pneumonitis from aspiration of hydrocarbon. Pneumonia and acute hemorrhagic necrotizing disease, usually in 24 hr.	Burning sensation in mouth and pharynx. Characteristic petroleum breath odor. Nausea, vomiting, anorexia, central nervous system depression, fever. Respiratory distress, wheezing.	Do not induce vomiting. Support ventilation; administer oxygen. IV fluids.

Continued

TABLE **10-5** Common Poisonous Substances—cont'd			
Substance	**Pathophysiology**	**Clinical Manifestations**	**Treatment**
Lead (paint chips from older homes, soil contaminated with lead, lead solder used in plumbing, vinyl miniblinds, improperly glazed pottery)			
Diet high in fat and low in iron and calcium increases lead absorption. Serum lead level >10 μg/dL: considered harmful; 10-15 μg/dL: more frequent screening indicated; 15-20 μg/dL: nutritional and educational interventions and environmental investigation; >20 μg/dL: possible removal and treatment.	Gastrointestinal tract is major route of absorption. Lead is deposited in blood, bone, and soft tissue. Major toxic effects occur in bone marrow, nervous system, and kidney. Amount of lead ingested, size of the particle, and repeated ingestion over time contribute to severity of lead poisoning.	Symptoms may be vague with insidious onset. Central nervous system effects: irritability, lethargy, hyperactivity, cognitive and perceptual-motor difficulties, clumsiness, seizures, coma, and death (associated with blood level of 100 mg/dL). Hematopoietic effect: anemia. Gastrointestinal effects: anorexia, nausea, vomiting, constipation, lead line along gums. Skeletal effects: increased density of long bones, lead line in long bones. Renal effects: glycosuria, proteinuria, possible acute or chronic renal failure. Kidney damage is reversible early in the disease, but with continued lead exposure, permanent kidney damage may occur.	Level >25 μg/dL: remove child from lead source, hospitalize if level is significantly higher. Administer chelating agents: succimer orally for lead level of 35-45 μg/dL; EDTA for level >70 μg/dL given IV over several hours for 5 days (causes lead to be deposited in bone and excreted by kidneys); bronchoalveolar lavage every 4 hr for six doses for level >70 μg/dL. Monitor kidney function because EDTA is nephrotoxic; monitor calcium levels because EDTA enhances excretion of calcium. Provide adequate hydration. Calcium, phosphorus, and vitamins C and D. Anticonvulsants. Oral or intramuscular iron for anemia. Follow-up lead levels to monitor progress (lead is excreted more slowly than it accumulates in the body).
Carbon monoxide			
Most often from improperly ventilated heaters; also from poorly ventilated vehicles. Cause of the exposure should be determined and eliminated.	An odorless, colorless gas that binds to receptors on hemoglobin more effectively than does oxygen, thereby causing hypoxia.	Headache, visual disturbances. Altered level of consciousness, cherry-red lips and cheeks, nausea, and vomiting.	100% oxygen by rebreathing mask. Serum carboxyhemoglobin levels, hyperbaric chamber treatment may be necessary for clients with high carboxyhemoglobin levels. Other interventions based on signs and symptoms.

(e.g., administration of activated charcoal), and (3) ipecac can be misused (e.g., by bulimic adolescents) (AAP, 2003). Parents are advised to call the poison control center immediately if they suspect their child has ingested a poisonous substance.

Gastric Lavage

Gastric lavage is used for gastric emptying in the first 1 to 2 hours after a poison ingestion. This method is selected when the toxic ingestion has potentially serious complications, such as seizures, decreased level of consciousness, respiratory or metabolic depression, and cardiac effects. Because of the danger of esophageal perforation, lavage should not be used after ingestion of corrosive substances. The nurse places the child on the left side, with the head lowered approximately 10 degrees in the Trendelenburg position. Depending on the size of the child, a 22F to 36F orogastric tube is inserted. In comatose children, endotracheal intubation is recommended

before beginning gastric lavage to protect the airway against aspiration of stomach contents. To prevent electrolyte disturbances, younger children are lavaged with normal saline or one-half normal saline. The nurse observes the returned fluid for any pill fragments or toxic substance and administers activated charcoal after completion of the lavage process if ordered. A specimen of lavage fluid may be sent to the laboratory for analysis in cases of an unknown substance.

Activated Charcoal

Activated charcoal is a charcoal substance with a porous surface that binds to the toxin and passes through the gastrointestinal system. Activated charcoal has become the recommended treatment for acute poisonings in the pediatric population, particularly for incidents in which identification of the poison is delayed. Activated charcoal can bind to the toxin at any point along the gastrointestinal tract. The longer the time between activated charcoal administration and the time the toxin was ingested, however, the less effective it will be. If the child has received ipecac, ongoing vomiting can delay administration and retention of activated charcoal.

Activated charcoal must have a stimulant, such as magnesium citrate, to counteract the side effect of constipation. Administering activated charcoal is a nursing challenge because the substance is unpalatable in both taste and appearance to young children. If gastric lavage has been performed, it is often easiest to administer the activated charcoal before removal of the gastric tube. In the toddler, having the child sit on a parent's lap and administering charcoal by oral syringe may be successful. Mixing the activated charcoal with chocolate milk or other flavoring sometimes makes it easier to drink. Placing the charcoal in a covered opaque or decorated container prevents the child from seeing the substance while drinking. Activated charcoal administration can be repeated to prevent reabsorption of the toxin from fluid secreted in the biliary tract. The dosage is usually 1g/kg in children.

Antidotes

Specific antidotes can be used to inhibit the absorption of the toxin at the receptor site or reduce the concentration. Examples of commonly used antidotes are acetylcysteine (Mucomyst) for significant acetaminophen ingestion and naloxone (Narcan) for narcotics (see Table 10-5).

NURSING CARE

The Child Who Has Ingested a Toxic Substance

Assessment

Accurate and rapid assessment of the poisoned child can mean the difference between life and death. Assess ABCs. Take frequent vital signs. Initiate respiratory or circulatory support as needed. Because shock is a result of ingestion of many toxic substances, blood pressure, tissue perfusion, and urine output are carefully monitored. Observe and document the child's mental status frequently to determine any changes in level of consciousness. Assess changes in pupil size or reactivity as well as occurrence of seizures.

The nurse needs to take the responsibility for assessing the cause of poisoning. A poison exposure is extremely distressing to parents. Defer detailed questioning until the child's condition is stabilized. If the ingestion was purposeful, psychologic consultation and referral should be provided. In some cases, child abuse must be ruled out.

CRITICAL TO REMEMBER
Assessment of Poison Ingestion

Obtain information about the following:
- Substance ingested if known
- Amount ingested (how many pills are missing?)
- Approximate time of ingestion
- Change in the child's condition
- Treatment administered at home

Nursing Diagnosis and Planning

The following diagnoses apply to the child and family:
- Risk for Injury related to insufficient parental knowledge about first aid for toxic ingestion and accidental poisonings.

  Expected Outcome: The parent will describe how to assess the child and access appropriate treatment if accidental poisoning occurs.
- Ineffective Breathing Pattern related to effects of toxic substances.

  Expected Outcome: The child will breathe in a way that maintains adequate oxygenation and ventilation, as evidenced by normal arterial blood gases and serum pH or pulse oximetry.
- Risk for Deficient Fluid Volume related to effects of ingested substances, treatment modalities, or decreased fluid intake.

  Expected Outcome: The child will maintain an hourly urine output appropriate for weight and age, with age-appropriate specific gravity.
- Compromised Family Coping related to sudden hospitalization and emergency aspects of illness.

  Expected Outcomes: The family will appropriately discuss the child's condition and treatment, verbalize feelings and concerns, and remain with the child as much as possible.
- Risk for Poisoning related to insufficient parental knowledge about poisoning prevention.

  Expected Outcome: The parent makes the necessary changes in the home environment to prevent future poisoning.

Interventions

Stabilizing the child is the nurse's priority in caring for the child who has ingested a poisonous substance. Nursing care also includes reducing the child's and the family's fear and anxiety, providing preventive teaching concerning the storage of poisons and supervision of children, and removal of the poison from the child's skin and mucous membranes to reduce further injury.

Parents usually are overwhelmed by feelings of guilt, fear, and anger when their child has ingested a poisonous substance. Providing an opportunity for them to express their feelings in a nonjudgmental atmosphere helps parents cope with this experience. Some aspects of treatment, such as placement of a gastric tube or support of ventilation, are disturbing and frightening to parents. Offer support by explaining treatment, including the parents in care (as appropriate), and informing them about the status of their child.

Ideally, nurses intervene with parents (and other caregivers such as grandparents, older siblings, and babysitters) before a poison exposure occurs. Knowledge of safety and "safe proofing" the environment is important before the child becomes mobile. Discussion of safe storage of medications and other potentially toxic substances as well as age-appropriate supervision of children are essential aspects of poison prevention. Advise the parent to post the poison control phone number clearly and to call the poison center before treating the child. This and other injury prevention information should be readily available in daycare, primary care, and emergency care settings and should be given to families proactively. Education through community programs to prevent poisoning and reduce drug abuse should be directed to young children as well as adolescents, parents, and caretakers. Simple ideas, such as not calling medication "candy," storing medication in the original containers, and labeling all cleaning products and containers should be encouraged.

Evaluation

* Do parents describe the appropriate actions to take in the event of a future poisoning?
* Are the child's oxygen saturation, blood gas measurements, and level of consciousness within normal limits?
* Is the child's hourly urine output appropriate for age and weight?
* Are family members remaining with the child and able to provide adequate support?
* Can parents and other caregivers describe poison prevention—common poisonous household hazards out of the child's reach, easily accessible poison control telephone number?

ENVIRONMENTAL EMERGENCIES

Active children are exposed to a variety of environmental hazards. Injuries from animal and snake bites, submersion injuries, and sun- and heat-related illnesses account for the majority of these hazards. This section focuses on animal, human, and snake bites; submersion injuries; and heat-related illnesses. Sunburn is discussed in Chapter 25.

Animal, Human, and Snake Bites

Etiology

Animal and Human Bites. Both animal and human bites involve soft tissue damage from crushing, lacerations, and puncture wounds. All animal bites have potential for infection. Although human bites are relatively rare, they carry the greatest risk of infection if they break the skin, particularly if they are on the scalp, face, hands, wrists, or feet. Serious injury can result from any type of bite, but most bites are not life threatening.

Snake Bites. Envenomation of children on land is usually from snakes, scorpions, and spiders. Envenomation can also result from marine animals, such as jellyfish, sea urchins, and stingrays. Fatalities from envenomation are rare; most fatalities occur from snake bites.

Incidence

Animal bites in the pediatric age group are most often from domestic animals and have the highest incidence in school-age boys. Most bites are from dogs, usually a dog familiar to the victim. Fatal dog attacks by certain aggressive breeds of dogs, such as pit bulls, have been reported (Melnick, 2005).

Cats are the most common family pets, and although a cat bite is less likely to cause serious injury initially, it is more likely to become infected than a dog bite (Daniels, Zook, & Lynch, 2004). Bites from pet birds, rats, ferrets, pigs, hamsters, turtles, fish, alligators, snakes, horses, and many other animals have been seen in emergency settings, as have bites from a variety of wild animals, such as raccoons, skunks, and coyotes.

In the United States, the two groups of poisonous snakes are pit vipers (Crotalidae), such as rattlesnakes, water moccasins, and copperheads, and coral snakes (Elapidae). Pit vipers are responsible for more than 95% of snake bites. Approximately 8,000 venomous snake bites occur in the United States annually—approximately half of them in children (Bowman, 2003).

Manifestations

Animal and Human Bites. Because of the risk of infection, human bites are more serious and can be differentiated from dog bites by the distance between the canine teeth; in human bites the distance is generally greater than 3 cm. A human bite is horseshoe shaped and rarely breaks the skin. Localized tissue damage and multibacterial infections are serious manifestations of animal and human bites. Dog bites run an additional risk because of the potential for serious structural damage (e.g., fractures, deep tissue injury) (Melnick, 2005).

Snake Bites. To determine the cause of envenomation, medical staff in emergency settings should have some knowledge of the venomous snakes likely to be encountered in the surrounding geographic area.

Smaller children are usually bitten on the hand or foot, whereas older children are more commonly bitten on lower extremities. More than half of snake bites occur when a person is purposely handling a known venomous snake (Bowman, 2003).

Regardless of whether the snake can be positively identified, treatment should be based on physical assessment and symptoms. The following local signs and symptoms most commonly suggest envenomation:
* Bite marks that look like fang marks
* Burning at the site
* Ecchymosis and erythema
* Pain or numbness
* Progressing edema

The following systemic signs and symptoms suggest severe envenomation:
* Nausea, vomiting
* Sweating, chills
* Numbness, paresthesia of the tongue and perioral region
* Hypotension
* Coagulopathies

Systemic signs and symptoms usually appear within 30 minutes or longer. When a substantial amount of venom has been injected and when treatment is delayed, envenomation can progress to coagulopathies, respiratory failure, renal failure, seizures, shock, and (rarely) death.

Therapeutic Management

Animal Bites. Emergency care for animal bites depends on the type of bite but usually includes thorough irrigation and debridement. Elevation and ice can be used to decrease pain and swelling (Daniels et al., 2004). Tetanus prophylaxis is given if the child's immunization is not up to date or if documentation is unavailable. Antibiotics are prescribed when a high probability of infection exists. Smaller bite wounds are often left open rather than sutured because puncture wounds and wounds closed with sutures have more potential for infection. A specialist should be consulted if tendon, bone, or compartment injury is suspected. Treatment of the child for rabies may be necessary, especially in cases of wild animal (e.g., raccoon, rat, skunk) bites.

Snake Bites. The following three factors influence the severity of bite from a venomous snake:

- The child's age, size, and general health
- Size of the snake (larger snakes produce more venom)
- Location of the injury (peripheral injuries account for 90% of the bites and are less severe)

When assessing the child with a snake bite, identification of the type of snake is helpful, but this is not always possible. In most cases, an expert in the treatment of snake bites should be consulted. Emergency treatments (e.g., use of a tourniquet, incision, and extraction of the venom; electric shock therapy; cryotherapy) are not recommended and can result in complications, including increased tissue loss and infection (Bowman, 2003). First aid (after assessment and maintenance of the ABCs) includes washing with soap and water, immobilization of the extremity in a position below the level of the heart; removal of clothes, rings, and other constricting items; and rapid transport to an emergency facility.

In the hospital setting, emergency management continues assessment and maintenance of the ABCs, insertion of an IV line if envenomation is suspected, laboratory studies including CBC, coagulation studies, electrolytes, creatinine phosphokinase, and urinalysis to assist in determination of need for antivenom therapy (Brown, 2005). Children with no progression of symptoms after 6 hours may be discharged. Children with any progression of symptoms should be admitted to the hospital. In cases of moderate to severe envenomation, the negative side effects of antivenin must be weighed against the positive effects. Antivenin therapy is the mainstay of treatment for snakebites. Indications for administration include worsening injury, coagulation abnormalities, or systemic effects.

Nursing Considerations

With severe bites, significant envenomation, or anaphylaxis, nursing interventions for bites and envenomation begin with attention to the ABCs and support of vital functions. With envenomation, nursing care includes keeping the child as calm as possible to help prevent spread of the toxin or venom. Hospitals may not have sufficient antivenin for severe envenomation, so nurses should make sure that available protocols include the location of centers to contact for additional antivenin.

Carefully clean the injury site of all bites, and give tetanus prophylaxis if immunizations are not up to date. When the bite or envenomation is located on an extremity, immobilize the extremity. Measuring the circumference of the affected extremity every 20 to 30 minutes will track progression of the injury as well as results of treatment.

If antivenin is to be administered, obtain a careful history of allergies because the most common antivenins are made from horse serum. Antivenin is most effective if given within 4 to 6 hours after injury, but it may be repeated if coagulopathies or bleeding is present. Document the type and location of the injury, the length of time since the injury, and the signs and symptoms resulting from the injury. All children who require antivenin should be monitored in an intensive care setting. To assess hypersensitivity, a small test dose of antivenin is given intradermally before the full dose.

Education concerning avoiding snake habitats, wearing protective clothing, and avoiding provocative behavior around snakes should be emphasized.

In most states, notification of the local animal control agency is required for animal bites. Document rabies immunization status of the animal, if available, in nursing notes. Quarantine of the animal responsible for the attack may be necessary if the animal can be found. Children who have been bitten by animals are at risk for developing posttraumatic stress syndrome (Melnick, 2005). Nurses should advise parents to observe the child closely for changes in behavior and refer for counseling, if needed.

Discharge instructions should include observation for signs and symptoms of infection and wound care. Provide injury prevention education to all families. Give parents information about how to teach their children to avoid animal bites, including avoiding strange animals and nonprovocative behavior in dealing with enraged animals.

Submersion Injuries (Near Drowning)

Known as the "silent event," submersion injury is the second leading cause of accidental death in children (National SAFE KIDS Campaign, 2005b). *Drowning* is submersion that results in asphyxia and death within 24 hours. If the child survives longer than 24 hours after submersion, the event is referred to as *near drowning*.

One of the most important nursing responsibilities related to drowning is prevention of injury, including water safety education and training, support of legislative efforts to pass drowning prevention measures, and teaching CPR. Nurses must emphasize the importance of adequate adult supervision when children are in or around water.

Etiology

Most drownings happen in residential swimming pools, although drownings can occur in any body of water, including hot tubs, spas, bathtubs, toilets, and even buckets. Open-water sites, such as lakes, rivers, and oceans, are more likely to be the site of accidents among teenagers. Alcohol is often a factor in teenage drownings because it alters judgment and increases risk-taking behaviors.

Incidence

According to the SAFE KIDS Campaign (2005b), although death by drowning in the child younger than 14 years has decreased 42% from 1987 to 2002, 838 children in this age group died in 2002 and, in 2003, nearly 4200 children required emergency room treatment. Nearly 60% of these children are 4 years old and younger. Boys are two to four times more likely than girls to die from drowning. Young children are most likely to drown in a home swimming pool, followed by the bathtub (Turner, 2004).

Manifestations

The child's condition after near drowning varies with the extent of injury. Five factors contribute to the child's eventual prognosis: (1) age, (2) submersion time and water temperature, (3) elapsed time before resuscitation efforts are instituted, (4) neurologic status, and (5) arterial blood gas measurements (especially pH). The child with the poorest prognosis is younger than 3 years, has been submerged longer than 5 minutes, is comatose, has an arterial pH less than 7.10, and has not had resuscitative efforts within the first 10 minutes of the incident (Modell, Idris, Pineda, & Silverstein, 2004; Orlowski & Szpilman, 2001).

The child who is conscious with adequate respirations might have mild hypothermia, show slight pulmonary

---

PATHOPHYSIOLOGY

SUBMERSION INJURY

Hypoxia causes the injury to organ systems when drowning occurs. Drowning progresses in a predictable sequence of events. Drowning victims panic, struggle, and attempt to hold their breath. In doing so, they begin to swallow water, which is then vomited and aspirated. This process can cause laryngospasm, which leads to hypoxia, seizures, and death (called *dry drowning* because laryngospasm prevents large amounts of water from entering the respiratory system). If the child becomes unconscious before laryngospasm, hypoxia causes loss of airway reflexes and subsequent aspiration of large amounts of water (leading to *wet drowning*). As hypoxia and acidosis progress, cardiopulmonary arrest occurs. Swallowing large amounts of fresh water also causes electrolyte shifts into the intracellular spaces, resulting in hyponatremia and cerebral edema.

Submerged children lose body heat quickly in cold water because of their relatively large body surface area. Severe hypothermia offers some protection to the brain through the diving reflex, which is stimulated when the face is submerged in cold water. This neurologic reflex shunts blood away from the periphery, increasing blood flow to the brain and heart. The diving reflex is stronger in young children. Irreversible brain damage usually occurs after 4 to 6 minutes of submersion, but some children have had a complete recovery after lengthy submersion (10-40 min) in very cold water.

---

changes on radiography, and demonstrate minor blood gas alterations. Children who are unconscious (stuporous or comatose) demonstrate consequences related to whether respirations are present or absent. If respirations are adequate, the child may have mild to moderate hypothermia and mild to moderate respiratory distress with abnormal chest radiography and arterial blood gas results. The child who has required resuscitative efforts is in markedly poorer condition, with altered mental status, metabolic acidosis and other arterial blood gas abnormalities, electrolyte disturbances, possible seizures, or shock, and may develop disseminated intravascular coagulation. Death is the result of complete cardiopulmonary arrest or cerebral anoxic-ischemic injury. Most long-term sequelae of near drowning are neurologic in origin (Orlowski & Szpilman, 2001).

Therapeutic Management

Prehospital Emergency Management. Treatment begins at the scene of the accident with rescue and removal from the water. The prehospital care the child receives can significantly affect the chances for a normal recovery. Prompt initiation of CPR and activation of the emergency medical system are imperative. The goal of prehospital care is to maintain adequate oxygenation and circulation, minimize secondary organ damage, and take proper precautions to stabilize possible cervical spine injuries.

Every child with submersion injury is considered hypoxic. When the brain is deprived of oxygen for even a short period, irreversible brain damage can occur. After the child's airway is opened, the nurse suctions the child's oropharynx to remove mucus and fluid and delivers 100% oxygen by mask or by bag-valve-mask in the child with inadequate respiratory rate or effort. Overinflation of the lungs must be avoided to prevent a pneumothorax. Pulse oximetry may not be available in prehospital management or may be inaccurate in the child with hypothermia. Assessment of breath sounds, chest symmetry and rise and fall, and central color are more reliable indicators of adequate respirations.

Elevating the head of the bed to 30 degrees may help lower intracranial pressure but should be done only if no spinal injury or shock is present. Intubation should be considered for unconscious and nonbreathing children.

A cardiac monitor is used for ongoing assessment of heart rate and rhythm. Ventricular fibrillation or asystole that is unresponsive to resuscitative efforts can occur in the severely hypothermic (28° C) child. Resuscitative efforts continue while aggressive warming measures are instituted. Children have been successfully resuscitated up to 40 minutes after a cold-water immersion. Because the presence of a cardiac rhythm does not ensure perfusion of the tissues, the prehospital team assesses the child's cardiovascular status at regular intervals in addition to observing the rhythm on the cardiac monitor.

The wet clothes are removed, and the child is covered with warm blankets. Increasing the ambient temperature of the transport vehicle may be indicated. Rapid transport to the local emergency department or tertiary center is critical in the severely hypothermic child.

Two IV lines should be started immediately in critically ill children with submersion injuries. Because of the electrolyte and fluid shift into the intracellular space, children can become hypovolemic and fluid resuscitation is required. Adequate circulation is necessary to maintain organ perfusion. The rescuer may obtain blood for laboratory analysis while inserting the IV lines. Standard blood studies for the submerged child include CBC, serum electrolytes, BUN, creatinine level, and serum amylase. If the child is in shock or has experienced significant trauma, typing and crossmatching of 2 to 4 units of blood should be included.

Both air and water can be swallowed during a submersion incident. Air may also be forced into the stomach with resuscitative efforts. Because gastric distention resulting from air and water in the stomach can prevent full expansion of the lungs, a gastric tube should be inserted to decompress the stomach, ensure full respiratory excursion, and prevent aspiration of stomach contents from vomiting.

Hospital Management. Emergency care, on reaching the emergency department, continues the prehospital goals of maintaining adequate oxygenation and circulation, and initiates other treatments on the basis of laboratory and radiologic findings. Arterial blood gases may indicate the need to correct acidosis with sodium bicarbonate. Continued hypothermia is addressed by initiation of warmed IV fluids and oxygen, overhead lights, and warmed blankets. Fluid and electrolyte corrections can be instituted.

The child is admitted to the hospital for observation, even if in stable condition after initial rescue and emergency treatment.

NURSING CARE

The Child With a Submersion Injury

Nursing care of the child with a submersion injury requires obtaining an accurate history, ensuring adequate oxygenation and tissue perfusion, and maintaining body temperature.

Assessment

Assessment of the child with a submersion injury focuses on the respiratory system. Airway and breathing are the priorities. Observe the child for rate and depth of respiration, work of breathing, and any change in mental status. Cardiovascular assessment includes assessment of capillary refill and heart rate. Take the child's temperature as soon as possible to determine any hypothermia.

An accurate history of the injury is important although often difficult to obtain. Whether the submersion incident occurred in salt or fresh water is irrelevant for early treatment, but subsequent intensive care may vary somewhat depending on the immersion fluid.

Nursing Diagnosis and Planning

The following diagnoses are applicable to the child with a submersion injury:

- Impaired Gas Exchange (actual or potential) related to bronchospasm, aspiration of fluid, surfactant elimination, or pulmonary edema.
  Expected Outcome: The child will demonstrate normal oxygen saturation, blood gas measurements, and clear breath sounds.
- Risk for Imbalanced Fluid Volume related to electrolyte imbalances that cause volume shifts from interstitial to intravascular space.
  Expected Outcomes: The child will maintain hourly urine output appropriate for weight and age and vital signs within normal limits; electrolytes will return to normal.
- Hypothermia related to prolonged exposure to cold water.
  Expected Outcome: The child will maintain body temperature between 36.5° C and 37.4° C.
- Compromised Family Coping related to the child's critical status.
  Expected Outcomes: The family will verbalize feelings (including feelings of guilt and anger) and concerns appropriately, exhibit an attitude of confidence in care, and provide support to the child.

Interventions

After the initial assessment and emergency management have been completed, the nurse monitors for changes from the baseline, anticipates the development of complications, and implements therapeutic management.

Providing Respiratory Support

Because hypoxia is the primary problem, with potential for damage to all major organ systems, attention to the pulmonary system is a priority. Assess level of consciousness and listen for adventitious breath sounds, which can signal the development of complications such as pulmonary edema, atelectasis, or pneumonia. Persistent hypoxemia, dyspnea, tachycardia, and respiratory alkalosis can also signal these pulmonary complications. If the child is intubated, maintain the airway and observe for signs of tube displacement or pneumothorax.

Restoring Appropriate Circulatory Status

Cardiovascular monitoring includes measuring vital signs, pulses, level of consciousness, skin temperature, color, and urine output. The well-perfused child is alert with age-appropriate behavior and has a capillary refill time of less than 2 seconds and urine output according to age (see Chapter 18). Maintain IV lines and administer fluid volume replacement as ordered.

Identifying and Preventing Neurologic Consequences

The neurologic system is monitored frequently. Common parameters include level of consciousness, pupillary response, movement of extremities, reflexes, and vital signs. Anticipate signs and symptoms of increased intracranial pressure up to 24 hours after the submersion event. Conventional measures to prevent increased intracranial pressure, such as positioning the head in the midline, elevating the head of the bed 20 to 30 degrees, preventing or managing elevated body temperature, and controlling pain and agitation, are instituted as ordered and as needed.

Restoring Fluid Balance

As a result of ingestion of large amounts of water during the near-drowning event, the child is at risk for development of alterations in fluid and electrolyte balance. Carefully monitor urine output, laboratory data, and physical signs and symptoms. Hyponatremia and water intoxication should be anticipated, particularly with a fresh-water submersion. Observe for changes in central nervous system functioning, especially seizures, as the serum sodium level drops.

Controlling Infection

The acutely ill child is at risk for local or systemic infection. Complications from organ damage, intubation and ventilation tubes, invasive monitoring lines, and urinary catheters are possible sources for infection. If infection is present, antibiotic therapy is started. Monitor the child's response to the therapy.

Maintaining Nutritional Status

In the gastrointestinal system, hypoxia leads to decreased blood supply to the bowel. Stress ulcers and gastrointestinal bleeding are not uncommon. Monitor gastrointestinal function in terms of what goes in (nothing by mouth [NPO], oral or enteral feedings), what goes on inside (bowel sounds, residual feedings), and what comes out (presence or absence of blood; amount, color, and consistency of stool).

The child's increased metabolic demands, along with disruption of gastrointestinal functioning, can result in a nutritional deficit. Implement nutritional therapy as ordered in the form of enteral feedings or total parenteral nutrition. If enteral feedings are ordered, monitor weight gain, residuals, amount and consistency of stools, and vomiting to ascertain tolerance of the feedings. If total parenteral nutrition is ordered, check the label with the order, administer the fluid as ordered, monitor laboratory values, and assess for any side effects.

Providing Emotional Care for the Family

Because children brought to the emergency department with CPR in progress rarely have a positive outcome, an important element of nursing care is psychologic intervention and support for the child's family. The most important nursing interventions with the family of any critically ill or injured child initially include attention to the family's physical needs and provision of information and hope.

Families should be encouraged to participate in the decision regarding their presence in the treatment area, especially if the child is likely to die and the family may not have an opportunity to see the child alive again. If the parents choose to be brought into the resuscitation room, one person should be their liaison, bringing them in, answering questions, and escorting them out at appropriate times. The American Heart Association Guidelines for CPR and emergency care (2005c) state that often families do not ask to be present during resuscitative efforts; nurses should be sensitive to this and offer the opportunity for family members to be present.

> Be honest with the family. If the child is in full arrest, a simple statement such as, "Your child (use the child's name if possible) is not breathing and has no heartbeat. We are supporting his breathing and helping his heart to beat right now." This statement is far better than "We're doing everything we can," which leaves much more room for doubt.

Parents react in many different ways, according to their cultures, religious beliefs, individual personalities, and past experiences. Remember that denial can initially be protective and allow the family to accept information gradually. Ask family members if they want other family members or clergy contacted. Religious rites, including baptism, may be quite important to families. A list of clergy from a variety of religions should be readily available for use by the nursing staff.

Providing hope for the family is always important. At times, the only hope may be that the child is not suffering, or did not suffer, and that the child is, or was, not alone. If the child survives the incident, the parents will have ample time to adjust to any adverse consequences, so insisting on their acceptance is not necessary at this point. Many miraculous recoveries have occurred after lengthy submersions, although these are usually in very cold water. In the emergency setting, however, predicting the ultimate outcome for a child is impossible. A realistically positive attitude, while acknowledging the strong possibility of long-term effects for the child, is the most reasonable approach.

Evaluation

- Does the child demonstrate adequate oxygenation and independent breathing? Are lung sounds clear?
- Is the child's urine output appropriate for weight and age? Have electrolyte levels returned to normal?
- Is the child's body temperature between 36.5° C and 37.4° C?
- Do the parents verbalize their feelings and concerns appropriately, and do they provide appropriate support for the child?

CRITICAL TO REMEMBER
Needs Expressed by Families of Critically Ill Children
The highest-ranked need identified for families in most research studies is the need for hope. Needs for privacy and comfort are also consistently identified as extremely important by the families of critically ill and injured children; these needs are usually ranked higher than the need for psychologic support from nursing staff. Another commonly cited need is to have a contact person to provide updates and answer questions.

HEAT-RELATED ILLNESSES

Heat-related illnesses include sunburn, heat cramps, heat rash, heat exhaustion, and heat stroke. The most serious types are heat exhaustion and heat stroke, both of which can ultimately result in death. Two important factors in evaluating the possibility of heat-related illnesses are environmental temperature and humidity. If the body is unable to maintain normal temperature through evaporation of sweat, as in the case of high humidity and exertion, thermoregulation systems can be overwhelmed, creating a cascade of potentially life-threatening events (Romanoff, 2005).

Incidence

Children's anatomic and physiologic differences make them more susceptible to sun- and heat-related illnesses. Approximately 80% of a person's sun and heat exposure occurs before 21 years of age. The majority of heat-related deaths involve very young or very old people. The majority of pediatric deaths are related to small children being left alone in closed vehicles. On average, 30 children die each year as a result of being trapped in hot vehicles. Most of these children are aged 3 years and younger (National SAFE KIDS Campaign, 2005a). Healthy habits such as use of sunscreen and adequate fluid intake should be taught early in life. This section focuses on heat-related illnesses; sunburn is discussed in Chapter 25.

Children involved in physical activity sweat less, create more heat in proportion to their body size, and adapt more slowly to warm environments than do adults (American Academy of Pediatrics, 2000). In addition, younger children have a greater body surface area/mass ratio, which causes their bodies to gain heat from the environment on a hot day.

Obese children are vulnerable because of increased insulation. Active children may continue playing without feeling the need to drink adequate amounts of fluids even in extremely hot environments.

Manifestations and Therapeutic Management

Symptoms of heat-related illness are wide ranging and, if left unrecognized or untreated, can quickly progress to heat exhaustion and the life-threatening state of heat stroke. Management of heat-related illness is dictated by the severity of symptoms. The first priority in all cases is to move the child to a cool place and start cooling measures such as loosening and removing wet clothes and applying cool cloths. Rehydration is instituted, either by oral fluids in cases of overexertion or by IV rehydration if the child is unable to tolerate the oral route. In cases of heat stroke, this is not sufficient. The child's temperature-controlling mechanisms are not working, the child is unable to sweat, and brain damage and death could result if the body is not cooled rapidly. Concurrent assessment and prompt stabilization of cardiopulmonary circulation are critical (Table 10-6).

Nursing Considerations

The nurse caring for a child with a heat-related emergency will assess and possibly intervene in stabilizing the ABCs, provide cooling measures aimed at progressively decreasing core temperature without causing shivering or increased metabolic demands, provide emotional support for the client and family, and provide education to promote healthy habits.

Depending on the severity of symptoms, the nurse will assess for respiratory compromise and intervene with the appropriate method of oxygen delivery. In the hospital setting, the child with heat exhaustion may benefit from cool oxygen

TABLE **10-6** Heat-Related Illness			
Type	**Pathophysiology**	**Clinical Manifestations**	**Treatment**
Overexertion	Muscles generate heat during strenuous exercise; body fluids are being lost through sweating; rapid breathing; increased metabolic demands	Dizziness; flushed skin; diffuse muscle cramps	Move to cool environment; offer oral fluids; loosen clothing
Heat exhaustion	Increased loss of body fluids; increased blood flow to the skin with resulting decreased oxygen and blood flow to vital organs	Heavy sweating; nausea; vomiting; dizziness or fainting; exhaustion; headache; cramps; cool, moist, or flushed skin; core body temperature may be slightly elevated	Move to cool environment; apply cool, moist cloths to skin; remove clothing or change to dry clothing; elevate legs; offer oral fluids if no altered mental status or vomiting
Heat stroke	Thermoregulation is ineffective; sweating has stopped; vascular collapse and severe central nervous system abnormalities are noted because of hyperthermia and insufficient circulating volume	Hot, dry, red skin; change in level of consciousness or coma; rapid, weak pulse; rapid, shallow breathing; elevated core body temperatures: $\geq 105°$ F ($40.6°$ C)	Emergency transport if not in an emergency setting; rapid cooling with moist, cool cloths and fans; administer oxygen by nonrebreather, or intubate for respiratory insufficiency; aggressive IV rehydration; intervene as needed to maintain vital functions

CRITICAL THINKING EXERCISE 10-2

You are at a seventh-grade baseball game when you are asked by a parent to look at her previously healthy child who is reporting nausea, leg and arm cramps, and dizziness. His baseball uniform is wet, and the child is sweating profusely. It is 92° F outside and it had rained earlier in the day.

1. a. What do you think is wrong with the child? Why?
   b. What are your interventions while on the baseball field?
   c. If he starts vomiting, what interventions may be anticipated?
2. What if this child has been playing in a baseball tournament all day, it is 95° F and muggy, and the child is found unconscious?
   a. What is wrong?
   b. What assessment would you perform? What would you expect to see if this child has heat stroke?
   c. What interventions could you do (at the baseball field)?
   d. What prehospital care would you tell the mother to anticipate?
   e. What hospital care would you tell the mother to anticipate?

blow-by or nasal cannula, whereas the child with heat stroke will require oxygen by nonrebreathing mask or even intubation in the case of an insufficient respiratory effort. The nurse performs serial assessments of circulation and disability to determine evaluation of IV fluid resuscitation.

As in other pediatric emergencies, the family should be involved early and to the extent they are comfortable. Family presence is encouraged, with the nurse or other member of the health care team available to provide clear explanations of procedures, answer questions, and provide support.

Involvement by the nurse in promoting healthy habits in the child and family is crucial. Young children should never be left alone in a vehicle, and they should be taught a car is not a toy. The danger of sun and heat exposure, along with adequate fluid intake, wearing light-colored, loose-fitting clothing, and adjustment of activity according to temperature and humidity levels are concepts the child, family, and community need to know and incorporate.

DENTAL EMERGENCIES
Incidence and Etiology

Injury to the teeth, particularly the anterior teeth, is common in children. Toddlers, because of their lack of coordination, receive dental injuries from falling from or onto furniture. School-age children are more likely to have their teeth injured on playgrounds and during sports activities. The first teeth begin to erupt at approximately 6 months of age. By approximately 2 years of age, a child has all 20 primary teeth. Permanent teeth come in at approximately 5 or 6 years of age. By adolescence, a child usually has the full complement

of 32 permanent teeth, although the eruption of wisdom teeth may be delayed. Injury to primary and permanent teeth is considered equally serious. Teeth are embedded in the bones of the maxilla and mandible. Injuries to teeth are usually divided into the following categories:

Concussion: the tooth is not displaced, but pressure may cause pain.

Subluxation: the tooth is moveable within the socket but is displaced less than 2 mm. The socket is not damaged.

Intrusion: the tooth is pushed into its socket with injury to the underlying structures.

Extrusion: an upper tooth is dislodged downward from the socket, or a lower tooth is dislodged upward.

Luxation: the tooth is moved laterally with tearing of the periodontal ligament.

Avulsion: the tooth is no longer in the socket, and the socket itself may be damaged.

Therapeutic Management

Dental emergencies require specialized care, which is often difficult to obtain immediately. Survival of the tooth depends on the periodontal ligament attachment, so concussion, subluxation, lateral luxation, and extrusion, in which the periodontal ligament is still attached, have a better prognosis than complete avulsion of a tooth. Intrusion of a tooth may damage underlying structures to a greater extent and diminish chances for tooth survival.

Time is of the essence in caring for dental injuries. With injury to a child's mouth, the nurse observes for missing teeth. If a missing tooth cannot be found in the oral cavity, possible aspiration should be considered in the presence of dyspnea. To determine whether other teeth are loose or malpositioned, the nurse gently palpates (using Standard Precautions) the teeth for movement or encourages the child to check with the fingers or tongue. A tooth that is loose in the socket should not be removed. If the position is not correct, repositioning may be necessary when a specialist is available.

In general, primary teeth are not replanted because damage to the developing tooth bud can occur. Complete avulsion of a permanent tooth requires care of the socket and the tooth itself. Survival of an avulsed tooth depends on prompt evaluation and replacement. Irreversible damage to the periodontal ligament because of dehydration of the open socket may occur after 60 minutes.

Emergency care by the dentist includes cleaning the tooth and socket, placing the tooth in the socket, and splinting the tooth. Tetanus immunization is given if needed, and an antibiotic may be prescribed.

Nursing Considerations

Parents should be instructed to keep the tooth moist. The tooth may be immersed in saline, water, milk, or a commercial tooth-preserving liquid. The tooth should not be cleaned or scrubbed. Although some recommend replacing the tooth in the socket immediately, a parent might replace the tooth backwards or the tooth or socket may not be clean or free of debris or clots, causing problems that would decrease the chances of tooth survival. The child should see a dentist, if possible, or should go to an emergency facility for care without delay.

Parents should be given careful discharge instructions and appropriate referrals for continuing care. When appropriate, reassure the family that first teeth are replaced by the second set of teeth and that a good cosmetic outcome can be provided in many ways, even with loss of a permanent tooth, with good follow-up care.

CRITICAL THINKING EXERCISE 10-3

Your friend's child is playing a soccer match at the local elementary school, and you have been invited to watch. During the match she trips and falls. She appears to have been accidentally kicked in the mouth by another player and her mouth is bleeding profusely.
1. What actions should you take if you are asked to help?
2. What actions will you take if you discover this child has lost one of her teeth?

┤ KEY CONCEPTS ├

- Because of children's smaller sizes, the different equipment and dosages needed for their care, and age-related psychologic differences, nursing care of ill and injured children may seem more complicated than care of adults.
- Familiarity with the issues related to the child's growth and development; continuing education in pediatric emergency care; and careful organization of pediatric equipment, supplies, referrals, and reference lists can help to decrease anxiety in health care providers and improve the care of children in emergency settings.
- Airway management is the most critical element in pediatric emergency care. Emergency assessment and triage should include airway assessment and intervention. Without adequate oxygenation and ventilation, clients have little hope of survival.
- Shock must be recognized early in the child and should always be considered a possibility when the heart rate increases, breathing increases, or changes occur in color, temperature, or moisture of the infant's or child's skin.
- Care of the family and the child's developmental stage should always be considered when providing nursing interventions in the emergency setting. The parents' reactions and the child's developmental factors affect adherence, cooperation, and anxiety levels.
- Trauma assessment of the child includes the standard primary and secondary survey and intervention but must also include assessment of skin signs, use of appropriate age-related tools for determining the level of consciousness, and prevention of or intervention for hypothermia.

- Injury prevention plays an important role in the nursing care of children. Motor vehicle injuries, ingestions, poisonings, and environmental injuries are largely preventable. Nurses can play an important role in offering anticipatory guidance and providing injury prevention materials and instruction to children and their families.

ANSWERS TO CRITICAL THINKING EXERCISE 10-1

Your primary assessment reveals: *airway:* clear, with small amount of vomitus noted in corner of mouth; *breathing:* rapid respirations, slightly shallow, no increased work of breathing; *circulation:* pulses rapid, peripheral pulses slightly weak, skin pale, mottled, and cool, capillary refill 3 seconds, active bleeding and deformity noted in left lower extremity; *disability:* eyes closed, responding to verbal stimuli.

The father states, "She was hit by a car going about 30 miles an hour. She flew up in the air about 20 feet. She was wearing her helmet. She cried immediately but is really sleepy now. This happened about 20 minutes ago. I just picked her up and ran. She had a snack about 2 hours ago. She has her shots, no allergies."
1. You would assess the ABCDs. *Airway:* Is the airway open? Any vomitus or other objects in the mouth? Is the child able to maintain her own airway? *Breathing:* Is she breathing? What is the rate and quality? Any increased work of breathing (e.g., retractions, grunting, head bobbing)? *Circulation:* What are the central and peripheral pulses (rate, quality), skin color and temperature, and capillary refill? Any active bleeding? *Disability:* What is her level of consciousness?
2. History: What happened? When? Was there loss of consciousness? Was she wearing safety equipment? Does she have her immunizations? Allergies? When was the last time she ate or drank?
3. Hypovolemic shock from blunt trauma. Yes, this is an emergency because of her increased heart rate and respiratory rate and decreased level of consciousness. You do not know the extent of injuries at this time. The child is attempting to compensate to increase cardiac output. If not treated, uncompensated shock can ensue, which causes metabolic disturbances, organ damage, and other sequelae of decreased oxygenation, leading to coma and death.
4. You would do the following (in this order): stabilize the cervical spine while applying oxygen, apply heart monitor and pulse oximetry, obtain vascular access, apply pressure to bleeding site, assess and treat pain, and provide support for the family. Next interventions include a fluid bolus of a crystalloid solution, 20 mL/kg; reassessment of effectiveness of interventions; assessment for extent of injuries; and stabilization of those injuries. You would expect laboratory

Continued

ANSWERS TO
CRITICAL THINKING EXERCISE 10-1—cont'd

studies (blood, urine); chest, cervical spine, and extremity radiographs; and cleaning and stabilizing of injuries. I&O is accurately measured and recorded. Treatment is aimed at stabilization and maintenance of ABCDs, so oxygen, monitoring, rehydration, and determination of the extent of injuries are priorities of care. The father needs to be supported, with coping strategies and support systems assessed to decrease anxiety and provide comfort during the stressful time of having a seriously ill child.

5. You would expect color to improve with oxygenation and rehydration and heart rate and respiratory rate to slowly return to normal. Injuries would be stabilized and bleeding stopped. The father will express understanding of treatment and will actively help comfort and distract the child.

ANSWERS TO
CRITICAL THINKING EXERCISE 10-2

1a. Heat exhaustion. The history of a hot, muggy day and outside activities. Physical symptoms: nausea, leg and arm cramps, dizziness, wet uniform, heavy sweating.

1b. Find shade or a car with air conditioning. Offer cool water or diluted sports drinks if not vomiting, have child change into dry clothes, caution child and family to avoid exertion, and check the other players for signs of overexertion.

1c. If unable to tolerate fluids, he needs to be taken to the hospital for IV hydration and observation.

2a. Possible heat stroke.

2b. Assess ABCDs. Expected findings would include the following: the child's breathing is shallow; he is not sweating, and his skin is red, dry, and hot to touch; his pulse is weak, rapid, and thready; he is tachypneic; and he is lethargic or comatose.

2c. Recognize that this is an emergency and **immediately call 911** or area emergency number. Move to a cool room or air-conditioned car while awaiting ambulance. Remove wet clothes, apply cool, wet cloths to body, and have a fan blowing on child. Monitor airway and breathing; assist if necessary. Maintain NPO status.

2d. Prehospital care will include high-flow oxygen, IV fluids, decreased ambient temperature in ambulance for continued cooling measures, ongoing assessment, and rapid transport to the emergency department. The mother needs to decide if she wants to go in the ambulance or follow in a friend's car.

2e. Hospital care will continue prehospital care with advanced monitoring and testing. Hospital personnel will provide more information and allow the mother to be with the child if she is comfortable.

ANSWERS TO
CRITICAL THINKING EXERCISE 10-3

1. First assess level of consciousness and ABCs. Initiate appropriate resuscitation if necessary. If the child is conscious and alert, observe her mouth carefully, being sure not to touch it without appropriate barrier protection.

2. If a tooth is missing, ask for help finding it. When it is found, your primary goal is to keep it moist to enhance eventual reimplantation. Milk, normal saline, or a commercially prepared tooth preservation solution is suggested. Do not try to replace the tooth in the socket. Alternatively, if a source of liquid is not readily available, wrapping the tooth in a wet handkerchief is an acceptable way of transporting it. Advise that the child be seen by dental personnel within 2 hours.

REFERENCES AND READINGS

American Academy of Pediatrics. (2003). Poison treatment in the home. *Pediatrics, 112*(5), 1182-1185.

American Academy of Pediatrics, Committee on Pediatric Emergency Medicine and American College of Emergency Physicians, Pediatric Committee. (2001). Care of Children in the Emergency Department: Guidelines for Preparedness. *Pediatrics, 107*(4), 777-781.

American Academy of Pediatrics, Committee on Sports Medicine and Fitness. (2000). Climatic heat stress and the exercising child and adolescent. *Pediatrics, 106*(1, Pt. 1), 158-159.

American Academy of Pediatrics: Committee on Drugs (2001). Acetaminophen toxicity in children. *Pediatrics, 108*(4), 1020-1024.

American College of Emergency Physicians, & American Academy of Pediatrics (2001). Care of children in the emergency department: guidelines for preparedness. *Annals of Emergency Medicine, 37*(4), 423-427.

American Heart Association. (2000). Guidelines 2000 for cardiopulmonary resuscitation and emergency cardiovascular care. *Currents in Emergency Cardiovascular Care, 11*(3), 1-30.

American Heart Association. (2005a). Highlights of the 2005 American Heart Association guidelines for cardiopulmonary resuscitation and emergency cardiovascular care. *Currents in Emergency Cardiovascular Care, 16*(4), 1-27.

American Heart Association. (2005b). 2005 American Heart Association guidelines for cardiopulmonary resuscitation and emergency cardiovascular care (Part 11 Pediatric Basic Life Support). *Circulation, 112*(24 suppl), IV-156-IV-166.

American Heart Association. (2005c). 2005 American Heart Association guidelines for cardiopulmonary resuscitation and emergency cardiovascular care (Part 12 Pediatric Advanced Life Support). *Circulation, 112*(24 suppl), IV-167-IV-187.

Bowman, M. J. (2003). From stingers to fangs: evaluating and managing bites and envenomations. *Trauma Reports, 4*(3), 1-9.

Brown, H. (2005). Venomous snakebite. *Nursing, 35*(5), 88.

Burns, J. P. (2003). Septic shock in the pediatric patient: pathogenesis and novel treatments. *Pediatric Emergency Care, 19*(2), 112-115.

Caldwell, J. & Ziglar, M. (2001). Hemorrhagic shock in children. *AJN. Emergency Nursing Update 2001, Sept,* 25-30.

Centers for Disease Control and Prevention. (n.d.). *Poisonings.* Retrieved August 20, 2005, from *www.cdc.gov/ncipc/factsheets/poisoning-overview.htm.*

Centers for Disease Control and Prevention. (2003a). Nonfatal dog bite-related injuries treated in hospital emergency departments—United States, 2001. *MMWR, 52*(26), 605-610.

Centers for Disease Control and Prevention. (2003b). *WISQARS™ (Web-based Injury Statistics Query and Reporting System).* webapp .cdc.gov/sasweb/ncipc/mortrate.html.

Centers for Disease Control and Prevention. (2004). Surveillance for fatal and nonfatal injuries—United States, 2001. *MMWR, 53*(SS07), 1-57.

Centers for Disease Control and Prevention. (2005). *Preventing lead poisoning in children.* Atlanta, GA: Author.

Daniels, J., Zook, E., & Lynch, J. (2004). Hand & wrist injuries: Part II, emergent evaluation. *American Family Physician, 69*(8), 949-956.

Dayan, P., & Klein, B. (2004). Acute care of the multiple trauma victim. In R. Behrman, R. Kliegman, & H. Jenson (Eds.). *Nelson textbook of pediatrics* (17th ed., pp. 312-316). Philadelphia: Elsevier Saunders.

Eckle, N., & MacLean, S. L. (2001). Assessment of family-centered care policies and practices for pediatric patients in nine US emergency departments. *Journal of Emergency Nursing, 27*(3), 238-245, 313-318.

Field, J. M., Hazinski, M. F., Gilmore, D. (2006). *Handbook of emergency cardiovascular care for healthcare providers.* American Heart Association.

Frankel, L., & Mathers, L. (2004). Shock. In R. Behrman, R. Kliegman, & H. Jenson (Eds.). *Nelson textbook of pediatrics* (17th ed., pp. 296-301). Philadelphia: Elsevier Saunders.

Hawkins, H. (Ed.). (2004). *Emergency nursing pediatric course provider manual* (3rd ed.). Park Ridge, IL: Emergency Nurses Association.

Hazinski, M. (Ed.). (2002). *Textbook of pediatric advanced life support.* Dallas: American Heart Association.

Ilardi, D. (2003). After mild traumatic brain injury: helping school staff meet the needs of students and families. *School Nurse News, May,* 31-35.

Is your care of pediatric poisonings outdated? (2003). *ED Nursing, 6*(8), 96-97.

Koschel, M. (2003). Is it child abuse? *American Journal of Nursing, 103*(4), 45-46.

Koenig, P., Hijazi, Z., & Zimmerman, F. (2004). *Essential pediatric cardiology.* New York: McGraw-Hill.

Lankster, M., & Brasfield, M. (2005). Update on PALS guidelines. *Critical Care Nursing Clinics of North America, 17*(1), 59-64.

Maar, S. (2004). Emergency care in pediatric septic shock. *Pediatric Emergency Care, 20*(9), 617-624.

Melnick, A. (2005). "Dog bites man" is news—how pediatricians can spread the word to parents and patients. *Contemporary Pediatrics, 22*(12), 55-60.

Modell, J., Idris, A., Pineda, J., & Silverstein, J. (2004). Survival after prolonged submersion in fresh water in Florida. *Chest, 125,* 1948-1951.

National Center for Injury Prevention and Control. (n.d.). *Traumatic brain injury.* Retrieved May 26, 2003, from *www.cdc.gov/ncipc/ factsheets/tbi.htm*

National Guideline Clearinghouse. (2005a). *Acetaminophen poisoning: an evidence-based consensus guideline for out-of-hospital management.* Retrieved January 22, 2006, from *www.guideline.gov.*

National Guideline Clearinghouse. (2005b). *Lead exposure in children: prevention, detection, and management.* Retrieved December 22, 2005, from *www.guideline.gov.*

National SAFE KIDS Campaign and General Motors. (2003). *Keep your kids safe: never leave your child alone.* Retrieved August 1, 2006 from www.gm.com/company/gmability.

National SAFE KIDS Campaign. (2005a.). *A car is not a child's toy: preventing heat injury and entrapment.* Retrieved August 19, 2005, from *www.hotelfun4kids.com/travelnews/safetynews/car_safety_heat.htm.*

National SAFE KIDS Campaign. (2005b.) *Injury fact sheets.* Retrieved August 18, 2005, from *www.usa.safekids.org.*

National SAFE KIDS Campaign. (2005c). *Sports/recreation: why kids are at risk.* Retrieved May 26, 2005, from *www.usa.safekids.org.*

Orlowski, J. P. & Szpilman, D. (2001). Drowning: rescue, resuscitation, and reanimation. *Pediatric Clinics of North America, 48*(3), 627-646.

Romanoff, B. (2005). Be cool about summer heat. *Nurseweek, 12*(17), 28.

Samson, R., Berg, R., & Bingham, R. (2003). Use of automated external defibrillators for children: an advisory statement from the Pediatric Advanced Life Support Task Force, International Liaison Committee On Resuscitation. *Pediatrics, 112*(1), 163-169.

Sparrow, A., & Willis, F. (2004). Management of septic shock in childhood. *Emergency Medicine Australia, 16,* 125-134.

Sztajnkrycer, M. J., & Bond, G. R. (2001). Chronic acetaminophen overdosing in children: risk assessment and management. *Current Opinion in Pediatrics, 13*(2), 177-182.

Taylor, S. (2003). Infections in children. *Topics in Emergency Medicine, 25*(2), 166-173.

Turner, J. (2004). Prevention of drowning in infants and children. *Dimensions of Critical Care Nursing, 23*(5), 191-193.

Wallis, A., Cody, B., & Mickalide, A. (2003). *Report to the nation: trends in unintentional childhood injury mortality, 1987-2000.* Washington, DC: National SAFE KIDS Campaign.

Wilkerson, R., Northington, L., & Fisher, W. (2005). Ingestion of toxic substances by infants and children. *Critical Care Nurse, 25*(4), 35-44.

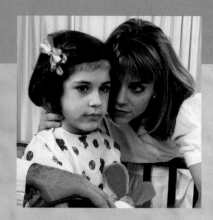

CHAPTER 11

The Ill Child in the Hospital and Other Care Settings

Learning Objectives

After studying this chapter, you should be able to:
- Discuss the nurse's role in various settings where care is given to ill children.
- List common stressors affecting hospitalized children.
- Describe the child's response to illness.
- Discuss the stages of separation anxiety.
- Describe the factors that affect children's response to hospitalization and treatment.
- Discuss the psychologic responses of families to the illness of a child in the family.

Definitions

denial A defense mechanism in which unpleasant realities are kept out of conscious awareness.
egocentric Preoccupied with one's own interests and needs.
regression Defense mechanism in which conflict or frustration is resolved by returning to a behavior that was successful in an earlier stage of development.

separation anxiety Distress and apprehension caused by being removed from parents, home, or familiar surroundings.
situational crisis Unanticipated event that poses a threat to an individual's psychosocial or psychologic well-being.
therapeutic play Guided play that promotes the child's psychophysiologic well-being.

Electronic Resources

Additional information related to the content in Chapter 11 can be found on:

the interactive companion CD-ROM
- Audio Glossary
- NCLEX Review Questions
- Skills: Admitting a Child to the Health Care System
        Preparing the Child for Surgery
        Therapeutic Play

or the companion website at *evolve*
http://evolve.elsevier.com/james/ncoc
- NCLEX Review Questions
- WebLinks

Because of current trends in health care management, the care of ill children continues to move from the traditional acute hospital setting to community-based settings and the home. Hospitalized children are more acutely ill than in the past, and their stays are shorter. In addition, the hospitalized child is more likely to have a chronic or terminal disease or to have special needs that require specialized care. These changes do not mean that the need for pediatric nurses has diminished; their role is ever changing and expanding. Pediatric nurses will continue to care for children in hospitals, schools, clinics, and homes.

All children experience some form of illness at some time. The ways in which stressors and developmental needs are addressed are important factors in resolving the immediate crisis and in dealing with future illnesses. The nurse is often the first person the child sees when the child enters the health care system, and the nurse spends more time with an ill child than does any other health care worker. The nurse therefore has a unique opportunity to influence that child's physical and emotional health.

SETTINGS OF CARE
The Hospital

Entering the hospital is somewhat like visiting a foreign country. The language, culture, activities, and expectations may be unfamiliar to the child and the family. The nurse acts as a "tour guide" and provides a safe environment, both physically and emotionally. Being the guide includes activities as diverse as explaining the jargon (e.g., NPO, IV, "vitals"), explaining procedures that are often painful, and facilitating the parents' access to hospital resources, such as social services, case managers, spiritual counselors, and ethics specialists. Above all, the nurse must educate the child and family about the disease process, its treatment, hospital procedures, and discharge issues.

Hospitalizations can be categorized according to length of stay, planned or unplanned admission, surgical or medical intervention, and outpatient (day) or inpatient status. Although they overlap, these categories provide a framework for examining the child's experience.

Another variable is the type of facility. Children may be hospitalized in a pediatric hospital, on a pediatric unit within a general hospital, or in a general hospital that occasionally admits children. Pediatric units within a general hospital or hospitals that do not have a specific pediatric unit may not have as many child-oriented services as a pediatric hospital has. Special play areas and child-size equipment and fixtures often are not available in general hospitals. Staff members who routinely do not care for children may be less comfortable in that role.

The nurse in this situation is aware of these challenges and can provide support for the child and the family, for example, by taking extra time when the child is admitted to explain routines and procedures or by placing the child close to the nurses' station. This support might include moving a cot into the room for the parent and ordering special foods for the child. Sometimes it means removing part of the food from a tray that is about to be served so that the child is not overwhelmed by the large servings intended for an adult. Ultimately, it means being sensitive to the needs of the child and the family.

24-Hour Observation

Children become ill quickly and recover quickly. For this reason, they may need acute care for a short time, such as when they are dehydrated or are having an acute asthma episode. At the end of 24 hours, the child is evaluated to determine whether further hospitalization is needed or whether discharge with home care instructions is appropriate.

The nurse must prepare the child and family for discharge and assess the parents' ability to care for the child at home. Instructions should be written, and the parent should be encouraged to ask questions. The nurse informs the parent about when to notify the primary health care provider in the event the child's condition worsens. An awareness of cultural differences enhances the nurse's assessment ability. For example, is the parent smiling because of contentment, or is the parent embarrassed to ask a question? Are parents nodding because they understand or because they are too embarrassed to say they cannot read? Many children's hospital units have a policy of contacting caregivers 1 to 2 days after the child is discharged, especially if the child left the facility at the end of 24 hours. Arrangements are made with the parent for a convenient time to be contacted. This policy allows the nurse to check on the child's condition and reinforce discharge teaching.

Emergency Hospitalization

Because of limited time for preparation, an emergency admission can be traumatic. The admission can be the result of trauma or acute sudden illness. The family may arrive at the hospital with little money, clothing, or other resources. Siblings may also be present, competing with the sick child for the parent's attention. In addition to caring for the sick child, the staff may be called on to help meet the family's basic needs for food, clothing, and a place to stay. A social service referral is appropriate in such situations.

Because of the intense level of activity in emergency departments, care of the family is often overlooked. The family may fear that the child will die or be permanently disabled. Although nurses may see many similar situations each day in which children do well, they must be sensitive to the family's fears, keep the family informed of the child's condition and care, and encourage a family member to stay with the child.

The time for preparing a child is usually limited in emergencies. Nurses must seize every opportunity to prepare children for the care they will receive. Holding and touching the child, talking softly, distracting the child, and involving the child in the procedure are methods of support used in emergencies. After the child is stable, the nurse returns and uses therapeutic communication to talk about the event. A child life specialist may also help the child express feelings. The use of dolls, puppets, and hospital equipment can aid children in communicating their feelings. (Chapter 10 provides more detailed information about caring for children and their families in an emergency setting.)

A 7-year-old boy was admitted to the medical-surgical unit after spending several hours in the emergency department because of acute asthma. Although his mother brought him to the hospital, she had his younger brother and sister with her and could not remain with him in the room. The boy remained quiet, but the nurse noticed that he watched every move she made. In such a case, the nurse might say, "Some kids say it's scary to come to the hospital and especially to be in the emergency room, with the bright lights and everyone rushing around. If you'd like, I can spend a little time with you and we can talk about being in the hospital."

Outpatient and Day Facilities

Outpatient facilities have evolved in an effort to keep children out of the hospital unless absolutely necessary. The outpatient facility may be part of a hospital, or it may be free standing. The child arrives in the morning; undergoes a procedure, test, or surgery; and goes home by the evening. Common procedures performed during such admissions include tympanostomy tube placement, hernia repair, tonsillectomy, cystoscopy, and bronchoscopy.

This mode of care has three main advantages: (1) it minimizes separation of the child from the family, (2) it decreases the risk of infection, and (3) it decreases cost. A disadvantage is that outpatient facilities that are not connected to a hospital may not be equipped for overnight stays. If complications develop that require continued observation and treatment, the child may have to be transferred to a hospital. This situation can be upsetting to the child and the family.

Although the procedure may be short, teaching the child and the parent is as important as in the acute-care setting. When possible, a tour of the facility before the procedure can decrease fear of the unknown. Parents have indicated that, although they like the idea of outpatient care, taking a child home afterward can be frightening.

Assessing the parent can assist the nurse in deciding whether the parent is capable of managing the child's care at home or whether home health care is needed. Written instructions specific to the child and procedure are helpful and reassuring. At the very least, a follow-up phone call to the home should be required. Parents should also be encouraged to call the facility if they have any concerns, and they should be given other resources to contact after the facility closes. Families who live far from the health care facility may want to spend the night at a nearby hotel or consider an overnight admission.

Rehabilitative Care

After a serious illness or trauma, the child's ability to function may change. After the acute situation has resolved, the child may be admitted to a rehabilitation hospital. Staff members from nursing, medicine, physical therapy, occupational therapy, and other areas collaborate to develop a treatment plan in which the child, family, and health professionals work to help the child regain previous abilities. Children with neurologic injuries, such as head injuries, or children with serious burns may thrive in this environment, which usually resembles a home environment with facilities available for the child to relearn the activities of daily living.

Nurses in rehabilitative settings must balance nurturing and firm discipline as they help children reclaim independence. Parents often need encouragement and support because they are torn between doing for their child and watching the child struggle to function independently. Overprotection is a common reaction, and parents can be assisted in identifying the child's developmental need to master the environment. The focus should be on what the child can do rather than on the child's limitations.

The Medical-Surgical Unit

Children admitted to the hospital are usually acutely ill or have a chronic disease or disability that requires frequent, often long-term hospitalizations. (Care of the child with a chronic disease is discussed in Chapter 12.) The average length of hospital stay for the acutely ill child has shortened significantly, and the need for teaching has increased in proportion.

Preparation for a planned hospitalization is essential. Some hospitals provide an opportunity for the child to visit the hospital before admission, and many pediatric hospitals host preoperative parties or classes to introduce children to the strange sights and sounds during a surgical experience.

Literature is available from public libraries and hospital sources. These types of literature may be presented in pamphlet, video, and book formats. Parents should make sure that these present a realistic picture of the hospital experience (Mansson & Dykes, 2004). Some children's hospitals also have libraries. Parents should answer questions honestly and encourage the child to talk about the hospitalization. Videos may also be available for family members to view together and then discuss.

The Intensive Care Unit

When a child is admitted to the intensive care unit, both the child and the parents experience increased stress because of the seriousness of the admitting diagnosis and the high-technology, unfamiliar environment. In addition, the child often is experiencing pain, uncomfortable procedures, noise, and constant lighting. In many instances, the child cannot eat or talk. Meanwhile, the parents are experiencing a parent's worst fear—the possible loss of a child.

The child and family need intense emotional support. All the normal responses to hospitalization are magnified and need to be assessed. When possible, planned admissions to the intensive care unit (e.g., for cardiac surgery) should be preceded by visits to the unit or special classes that provide information about special procedures and operations at a level the child can understand.

The parent should be encouraged to remain with the child and should be kept informed of the child's condition (Fig. 11-1). Procedures, equipment, and treatments should be explained, in appropriate language, to both the child and the parent. If the parent leaves and the child's condition changes or a new tube or piece of equipment has been added, the nurse should prepare the parent for the change before the parent sees the child. Nurses need to encourage parents to provide care and to touch their child as much as possible. The nurse's active listening is essential.

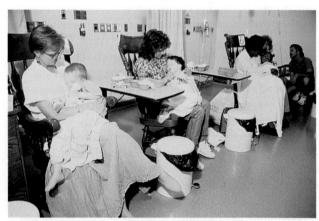

FIG 11-1   **When nursing care centers on the family, hospital rules must be altered. These parents are holding their children and rocking them in a postanesthesia care unit, normally a place off limits to those not on the staff.** (Courtesy Cook Children's Medical Center, Fort Worth, TX.)

Siblings of the seriously ill, hospitalized child can easily be overlooked. Siblings may need to talk, be comforted, or have the hospital experience explained to them. Parents may feel pulled between the ill child and the rest of the family. Often family members want to help but do not know what to do. Suggesting that a grandparent or other relative relieve a parent so that the parent has time with the ill child's sibling can help both the parent and the child. Helping parents by discussing options can relieve stress and may lead to solutions. Inclusion of family members in the provision of care, such as bathing and feeding, is important to both the family members and the child.

School-Based Clinics

The traditional areas of school health nursing that are still prevalent in many school systems include:

- *Health screening:* Vision, hearing, and growth checks can provide information about problems that may affect a child's ability to learn. When problems are identified, referral and follow-up services are provided.
- *Emergency care:* School nurses are the first to provide care for children involved in accidents, both on the playground and in the school building. Excellent assessment skills are necessary to determine the need for health care provider visits or emergency care.
- *Communicable disease management:* The nurse must assess children for illnesses that may be transmitted to other children, provide care and isolation until the parent can pick up the child from school and give advice concerning the safe time for re-entry into the school setting.
- *Health care advice:* The school nurse can be a source of referral for families in need of services.
- *Provision of specialized care for children with chronic health needs:* School attendance by children with many health care needs, including catheterization, gastric tube feedings, and suctioning, requires variation in the school nurse role to provide or supervise these specialized services.

School-based clinics have been part of health care for more than 25 years, but with the recent changes in health care delivery, this setting is now a site for expanding primary care. School-based clinics play an important role in providing care for children in remote rural communities and in underserved inner-city areas. School nurses, nurse practitioners, physicians, social workers, and other health care providers typically staff these clinics. This area of practice will continue to grow, and many believe that school-based clinics are the perfect setting for providing primary care for selected groups of children and adolescents because they are well situated to influence the health and well-being of underserved students (Selekman & Guilday, 2003).

Prevention remains the focus of school-based care as children learn health habits to prevent development of acute problems. Nurses identify children who need immunizations and provide immunizations when necessary. Screening that once required referral can often be handled on site. Through school-based clinics, children can receive medical services in a timely manner and avoid expensive emergency visits. For example, a child with an earache at school can be seen on site, treated, and sent home if warranted. The child's adherence to treatment can be monitored and a follow-up visit scheduled to determine whether treatment has been effective. Funding for school-based clinics is increasing, and they will continue to be a focus of health care delivery in the community.

Nurses in school-based clinics must be sensitive to parental concerns about certain topics in health care, especially areas related to sexuality (e.g., birth control, sexually transmissible diseases, abortion). Community involvement and support can dispel concerns and assist in setting guidelines for such clinics. School-based nurses must also be team members who act in collaboration with other health care workers and have a strong background in preventive health care and the ability to think critically.

The school-based clinic provides a setting for parental education in preventive health care, growth and development, anticipatory guidance, parenting skills, and care of acutely and chronically ill children. The nurse respects the rights and wishes of the parents, but respecting parents' wishes can be a challenge when the value systems of the health care provider and the parent differ. The pediatric nurse is a child advocate but must exercise caution unless the child is being harmed. (Child abuse is discussed in Chapter 29.)

The nurse is an integral part of children's health education in the school system. The American Academy of Pediatrics, along with other professional organizations, recommends that health education is a priority and should be a required subject for all school children in kindergarten through grade 12 (Taras et al., 2004). To be successful, health education programs should include active participation by the students in programs taught by qualified health educators and monitored by a school health committee. They should be taught separately from the regular curriculum and by qualified teachers who have had professional release time to develop an appropriate program of studies. Activities should be fun, be integrated with school services, and include family and community involvement (Taras et al., 2004).

Community Clinics

Community health clinics provide primary care for children and their families. In these settings, nurses, nurse practitioners, and physicians provide case management of illness and health promotion. Because most children enter this setting during illness, preventive health care is integrated into the child's acute care. Support services and groups (e.g., social services, a dental clinic, day care) may be available in the same center, and referrals to medical specialists and other health care providers are also available.

Although many children seen at community health clinics are ill, nurses must use the opportunity to take a health history to assess immunization, nutrition, anticipatory guidance, and growth and development. If the child is ill at the time of the visit, the nurse can set an appointment for the child to return for immunizations or other care that cannot be given when the child is ill (see Appendix A and the Evolve website).

In some urban areas, nurses are involved in primary prevention and offer information and education about childhood immunization, the signs and symptoms of childhood illnesses, injury prevention, and parenting skills (Fig. 11-2).

Home Care

Pediatric home care is the provision of skilled care within the child's home. Nurses in this setting are part of a multidisciplinary team that usually includes physicians, physical therapists, speech therapists, occupational therapists, and social workers. Children cared for at home include those receiving respiratory therapy, having dressing changes, receiving total parenteral nutrition, or needing skilled care because of a chronic illness or an injury.

Nurses who work in home care should have previous hospital experience in their practice area. The nurse must be able to make independent decisions and think critically and should have good clinical, documentation, communication, and teaching skills. To meet the needs of each child and family, the nurse must understand various cultures and socioeconomic backgrounds.

Although the separation of child from family is not a problem in home health care, the child may display many other effects of illness, such as fear of the unknown, loss of control, anger, guilt, and regression. In addition, care is taking place in the family's domain and the nurse is a guest in the home. Family members may have to adjust to unfamiliar noises and equipment, such as special beds, ventilators, or intravenous (IV) pumps, in their home. They may feel that they have lost their privacy and cannot "be themselves" because someone outside the family is frequently there. Awareness of siblings' needs is also a nursing goal in this setting.

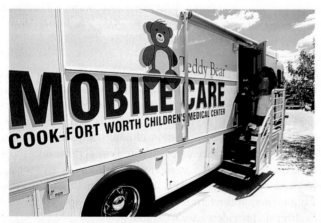

FIG 11-2   **Nurses today help take health care on the road to provide services to those who otherwise might not obtain them. This mobile van is stationed at a public school, where it offers health screenings and prevention services to children.** *(Courtesy Cook Children's Medical Center, Fort Worth, TX.)*

The nurse's role as a teacher is especially important because many tasks that the nurse might perform in the hospital are delegated to the family, with the nurse monitoring the care. Here the nurse acts as a case manager and coordinator of care.

CRITICAL TO REMEMBER
Children's Response to Illness

- Fear of the unknown
- Separation anxiety
- Fear of pain or mutilation
- Loss of control
- Anger
- Guilt
- Regression

STRESSORS ASSOCIATED WITH ILLNESS AND HOSPITALIZATION

Age, cognitive development, preparation, coping skills, and culture influence a child's reaction to illness. Previous experience with the health care system and the parent's reaction to the illness also affect the child.

Each child is unique, so predicting reactions to an illness is often difficult. Much of the research on the effects of hospitalization on children has been based on adult assumptions of the child's experience and on children's self-reports. Several categories have been identified: separation, physical harm or body injury, fear of the unknown, uncertainty about limits and outcomes, and loss of control (Melnyk, Feinstein, Moldenhouer, & Small, 2001; Visintainer & Wolfer, 1975). Previous experience with hospitalization may or may not help a child cope with the current experience. Including the parent in the child's care enhances coping (Tsuruta, Kusaba, Yamada, Murakata, & Nakatomi, 2005).

Although preschoolers and young school-age children experience separation anxiety, it is most significant in infants and toddlers, especially those aged 6 to 30 months. In times of stress, anxiety related to separation increases.

Each age group has its own fears related to pain and injury. The past decade has seen an expansion of knowledge about pain and its treatment, negating many erroneous beliefs about children and pain. Children quickly learn to associate health care activities and professionals with pain and injury. The fear is usually focused on "shots." (Chapter 15 discusses issues related to pain.)

A child's feeling of having control over a situation has been shown to affect the child's management of stressors (Ryan-Wenger, Sharrer, & Campbell, 2005). If children believe that they have personal control over a situation, they are more likely to feel confident and master a task, whether it is holding still while a needle is inserted or lying still while tomography is performed.

Although specific fears are related to the child's age, hospitalization puts all children at high risk for fears related to their unfamiliarity with the people, surroundings, and events.

The child has not developed trust in the health care provider and therefore does not know what to expect. The child may have real or imagined fears: Will the nurse know when I am hungry or hurting? Will the nurse hurt me?

The Infant and Toddler

Separation Anxiety

Infants and toddlers, especially those between 6 and 30 months, experience separation anxiety. Separation is this age group's major stressor, and it is traumatic to both the child and the parent. The child passes through several stages in reaction to the separation: *protest, despair,* and *detachment* (Bowlby, 1953) (Box 11-1).

In the initial phase, known as *protest,* the child demonstrates distress by crying and rejecting anyone other than the parents (Fig. 11-3). The child appears angry and upset. During the *despair* phase, the child feels hopeless and becomes quiet and withdrawn. Crying decreases, and the child becomes apathetic. If separation from the parent continues, the child enters the *detachment* phase. During this phase,

the child again becomes interested in the environment and begins to play. Nurses may misinterpret this phase as a positive sign that the child has adjusted to the hospitalization. In reality, the child has "given up." If the parents return during this stage, the child may ignore them and the parents may think that the child does not want to see them. The reaction, however, is a coping mechanism to protect the child from further emotional pain related to the separation.

Nurses in acute-care settings see the first two stages of separation—protest and despair—much more frequently than the final stage, detachment, which is more common in long-term separations. Parents may misunderstand their child's behavior. They may even perceive the child's reaction as a behavior problem. Nurses need to reassure parents that this reaction is a normal response to separation and that most children will not have any permanent effects from the event. As understanding of separation anxiety has evolved, visiting times have changed from structured hours to more flexible rooming-in situations (see Fig. 11-3).

Most practitioners believe that, if separation can be avoided, the child will be much more resilient during a hospitalization. Infants and toddlers go through the stages of separation. The older the child in this age group, the more elaborate the protest. The child not only cries but also may cling to the parent, kick, and generally create a scene. Parents need to understand that this behavior is a sign of healthy parent-child attachment. The toddler may resist bedtime and eating and may have temper tantrums more frequently than normal for this age. Regression may occur in toileting and eating. Nurses need to explain to parents that regression is normal and encourage parents to reinforce appropriate behavior while allowing the regressive behavior to occur.

BOX 11-1	**Stages of Separation**

- *Protest:* Child is agitated, resists caregivers, cries, and is inconsolable.
- *Despair:* Child feels hopeless and becomes quiet, withdrawn, and apathetic.
- *Detachment:* Child becomes interested in the environment, plays, and seems to form relationships with caregivers and other children. If parents reappear, the child may ignore them.

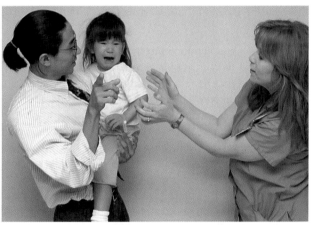

Hospitals try to reduce the stress of hospitalization for both parents and child by having rooming-in arrangements. Rooming in promotes parental attachment and provides many opportunities to teach parents how to care for their child's needs.

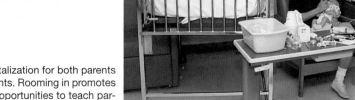

Between the ages of 6 and 30 months, a child is expected to have separation anxiety. The child initially reacts with protest, as this girl is doing. If separation continues, the child becomes quiet and withdrawn (despair phase). In the final phase (detachment), the child may ignore the parents.

FIG 11-3   **Separation is one of the stressors of hospitalization that affects both child and parent.** *(Courtesy T. C. Thompson Children's Hospital, Chattanooga, TN.)*

A parent might ask whether someone needs to be with a hospitalized toddler all the time and may be especially concerned because the parents work and have other children. The nurse may respond, "We encourage parents to stay with their children when they are in the hospital. If you have to leave, however, we will spend time with your child and check on your child frequently. You may call us at any time, day or night. When you return, perhaps you could bring a favorite toy or stuffed animal and something that reminds the child of you. A picture or a piece of clothing (transition object) will make your child feel more secure because it is familiar."

Fear of Injury and Pain

Previous experiences, separation from parents, restraint, and preparation affect the reaction of infants and toddlers to pain and body injury. The young child views injury and pain concretely. Nurses who have worked with toddlers know that most toddlers react to any intrusive procedure, whether it is painful or not. (See Chapter 15 for a more extensive discussion of pain in infants and toddlers.)

Loss of Control

According to Erikson, the major task of the toddler period is developing autonomy. Control is a major issue with this age group. The toddler experiences the environment through all the senses and loves to explore the environment. At the same time, toddlers need sameness (rituals, routines). Because of the changes in growth and development taking place in the toddler, familiar rituals and routines (e.g., those for eating, sleeping, playing) provide reassurance and stability.

Hospitalization, which has its own set of rituals and routines, can severely disrupt the toddler's life. The child may be confined to a crib, and the crib may have a cover over it. Because of safety issues, the child is not allowed to run in the halls. If the parents are unable to be with the child, the way the child is put to bed or bathed may be unfamiliar. Information obtained from parents about routines for feeding, going to bed, and playing can assist the nurse in maintaining usual and comforting routines. When children are unable to do things themselves, their sense of control and autonomy is weakened. They are frustrated and may have temper tantrums. Choices, even simple ones, can return some control to the child.

This lack of control is often exhibited in behaviors related to feeding, toileting, playing, and bedtime. The nurse should remember that each of these activities may have associated rituals and routines and that the child may also show some regression in these areas.

The Preschooler

Separation Anxiety

Separation anxiety occurs among preschoolers, but it is generally less obvious and less serious than in the toddler. Although the preschooler may already be spending some time away from parents at a day care center or preschool, illness adds a stressor that makes separation more difficult.

The preschooler expresses the same protest as the toddler but tends to be less direct. The nurse may find a preschooler quietly crying because the parents have told the child to "act like a big boy (girl)." Children of this age may refuse to eat or take medications, and they may be generally uncooperative. They may repeatedly ask when their parents will be coming for a visit; with access to a phone, the child may constantly call the parents. All these behaviors are signs that the child is having difficulty coping with the situation.

Fear of Injury and Pain

The preschooler fears mutilation. The child who must have surgery affecting a limb or other body part feels increased fear. The preschooler generally does not understand body integrity. Children of this age are also afraid of intrusive procedures, and, because of their literal interpretation of words, they often imagine treatments to be much worse than they are. Finally, the child's active imagination can go wild during illness. The preschooler may believe that the illness occurred because of some personal deed or thought or perhaps just because the child touched something or someone. (The preschooler's specific reactions to pain are discussed further in Chapter 15.)

Loss of Control

The preschooler has attained a good deal of independence in self-care and has been given more independence at home, preschool, or day care. Some children expect to maintain their independence in the hospital. For example, the preschooler may like to wander about the unit and may not be happy when restricted to the bed or room. Like the toddler, a preschooler likes familiar routines and rituals and may show some regression if not allowed to maintain some areas of control.

One 5-year-old boy refused to have his dressing changed by the nurse who cared for him during the previous day. She reported that he cried, pulled up the covers, and said that she was "mean." This behavior was unusual for him, and the nurse suspected that he had been told to do too many things and had not been given choices. In response, the nurse might say, "I know there have been many changes for you since you came to the hospital. Today, we are going to decide together what is going to happen. I see you have chosen a video to watch. Would you like me to change your dressing before you watch the video or after?" This approach gives the preschooler a choice and some control while maintaining boundaries.

Guilt and Shame

Because their thinking is egocentric and magical, preschoolers may believe that their illness is somehow related to a thought or deed. This belief can lead to feelings of guilt, shame, and increased stress at a time when the child has to cope with several other stressors. Because the child typically does not share these feelings with adults, parents and care-givers must be aware of the possibility of guilt and shame in this age group.

The nurse's role is to assess the child for this type of thinking and, through therapeutic communication, assist the child in identifying unfounded fears and beliefs. The child may be able to relate perceptions of what is happening. The use of puppets, dolls, and drawings can help children deal with their feelings. A tremendous decrease in anxiety can result when the nurse helps the child identify a perceived punishment and then reassures the child that nothing the child did could cause the illness.

The School-Age Child

Separation

The school-age child is accustomed to periods of separation from parents, but, as in the preschooler, as stressors are added the separation becomes more difficult. The younger school-age child may already have been feeling separation anxiety related to starting school.

Older children may be more concerned with missing school and the fear that their friends will forget them. The need to adjust to an unfamiliar environment and the regression seen in ill children, however, increase the likelihood that some separation anxiety will take place.

Fear of Injury and Pain

The school-age child is concerned with body disability and death. The child is more relaxed about having a physical examination or having the eyes or an ear examined but is uncomfortable with any type of genital examination. These children want to know the reasons for procedures and tests,

and they ask relevant questions about their illness. Because school-age children can understand cause and effect, they can relate actions to becoming ill. Their parents may tell them that if they do not get enough rest, wear warm clothes, or eat nutritious meals, they will get a cold. If they become ill, they associate their actions with the disease. (For further discussion of pain in the school-age child, see Chapter 15.)

Loss of Control

School-age children are "movers and shakers." They control their self-care and typically are highly social. They like being involved, and most fill their days with activities. Illness can change all these patterns. If children of this age have physical limitations, they can feel helpless and dependent (Fig. 11-4). Anxiety in response to loss of control, environmental changes, and the hospitalization experience can alter the way the school-age child appraises both the experience and the amount of resulting stress. School-age children who are highly anxious can view the hospital experience as uncertain and threatening (Board, 2005). Coping strategies used by these children include sleeping, talking with others, distraction (e.g., television, music, video games), and play; ineffective coping can occur if the child sees the strategies as unsuccessful for regaining control (Board, 2005).

Friends are important to children of this age group, and school-age children may think that their friends will forget them while they are ill. They are also accustomed to making choices about meals and activities. By capitalizing on the child's abilities and needs, the nurse can encourage children of this age to become involved in their own care. School-age children can select their own menus, assist with some treatments, keep their rooms neat, and visit with younger children

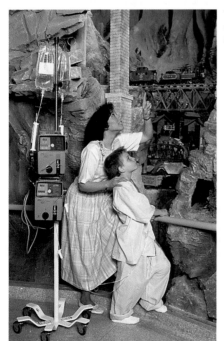

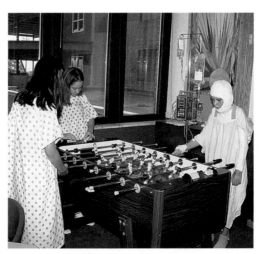

This multilevel "trainscape" in a children's hospital provides children and adults alike with a welcome respite from real-life stresses. *(Courtesy Children's Medical Center, Dallas, TX.)*

Hospitalized teens need to interact with their peers, as they do when they are well. A lounge area that is separate from the playroom used by younger children fulfills this need.

FIG 11-4   **Activities for the hospitalized child are important for growth and development, stress relief, socialization, and a sense of control.**

when it is appropriate for both. With these opportunities for independence, children retain a sense of control, enhance their self-esteem, and continue to work toward achieving a sense of industry.

The Adolescent

Separation

Adolescents often are unsure whether they want their parents with them when they are hospitalized. Some enjoy the freedom and the period of independence. Others, in response to the stress of illness, become more dependent and want their parents nearby. A third group cannot decide what they want, and this situation can be frustrating to parents. All these responses are consistent with the normal growth and development of adolescents.

Because of the importance of the peer group, separation from friends is a source of anxiety to the adolescent. Ideally, the peer group will support the ill friend. Some adolescents are reluctant to visit friends in the hospital, either because of their own health fears or because the reality of illness in someone their age is difficult for them to handle. Hospitalized adolescents may be upset if their friends simply go on with their lives, excluding them. Special activity areas and other opportunities for the adolescent to meet and interact with other hospitalized adolescents are important (see Fig. 11-4).

Fear of Injury and Pain

To the adolescent, appearance is crucial. Therefore an illness or injury that changes adolescents' perceptions of themselves can have a major impact. Even children who have seemingly adjusted to a chronic disease in their earlier years may have difficulty during adolescence simply because they do not want to be different. The adolescent who has diabetes may not want to eat different foods or take time out from an activity for injections. Adolescents do not want attention drawn to them, so they may eat the wrong foods and skip their medication.

Adolescents may also give the impression that they are not afraid, although they are terrified. Adolescents may think that being "cool" means being in control. They may question everything, or they may appear overly confident. Because of their concern with their bodies, they are guarded when any areas connected with sexual development are examined. Nurses need to be sensitive to adolescents' concerns and reassure them that they are normal, if in fact they are. Some adolescents also believe that they are invincible and that nothing can hurt them or cause death. This belief can cause them to take risks and to be nonadherent to treatment because they may not see the consequences of their behavior. (Pain management is discussed in Chapter 15.)

Loss of Control

Control is important to the adolescent. Some challenges in caring for an ill adolescent stem from control issues, and understanding this issue is key when caring for adolescents. Giving the adolescent some control avoids endless power struggles. Behaviors exhibited in response to loss of control may include anger, withdrawal, and general uncooperativeness.

Control issues can cause a major conflict between adolescents and parents. Parents often feel like ping-pong balls as they are bounced back and forth by a child who wants help 1 minute and rejects it the next. Parents who do not understand growth and development can become frustrated and angry over such behavior. Educating the parents increases understanding and facilitates parent-child communication (Melnyk et al., 2001).

Adolescents may also feel that they are losing control of their social lives as they sit on the sidelines of activities. Time to plan for the separation (e.g., scheduled surgery) allows a greater sense of control than an unplanned hospitalization (e.g., trauma).

Fear of the Unknown

The sights and sounds of the hospital can be frightening and confusing to the child. The child may have many questions: Why are the nurses wearing masks? Why does that alarm keep ringing? Am I dying? Why are they putting tubes in me?

The child's routines and rituals may have been disrupted, and the child may wonder what will happen next. Understanding these fears can assist the nurse in structuring care and teaching in a way that avoids unnecessary anxiety.

CRITICAL TO REMEMBER
Maintaining a Safe Place

A designated safe area can enhance the child's security. For example, intrusive procedures may cause discomfort or anxiety and might better be done in the treatment room rather than the child's room. The playroom should also be a place for playing, not treatments and administering medications. Nurses should consider the child's age, developmental level, coping skills, and parent/child preference when deciding where to perform procedures that may be painful or distressing.

Adapted from Fanurick, D., Schmitz, M., Martin, G., Koh, J., Wood, M., Sturgeon, L., & Long, N. (2000). Hospital room or treatment room: Where should inpatient pediatric procedures be performed? *Children's Health Care, 29,* 103-111.

Regression

Children may regress in toileting or may cry for a bottle although they have been weaned for several months. They may want more attention at bedtime or have temper tantrums. The older child may react to separation by clinging or crying or may have fears about shadows on the walls or noises in the halls.

Parents may be overly concerned about regression. They should be told that the child might continue the behavior at home. The child may need more emotional support while the parent slowly returns the child to normal routines. If the child has regressed in toileting, the parent should wait until the child has returned to a daily routine and then begin the toilet training again. Behavior that is appropriate for the child's age should be reinforced.

> The nurse might explain, "I know that you are concerned because David has been soiling his pants since he has been in the hospital. This soiling is a normal reaction to the stress of being ill and in the hospital. When he returns home and things return to normal for him, he will resume his previous schedule."

FACTORS AFFECTING A CHILD'S RESPONSE TO ILLNESS AND HOSPITALIZATION

Each child responds to illness or hospitalization differently. The expression "perception is everything" certainly applies to the ill child. How children perceive the incident will affect their responses before, during, and after the illness or hospitalization. How a child reacts is often related to the parents' response to the illness and the child's age, level of cognitive development, preparation, previous experiences, and coping skills.

If the child has had a previous illness or hospitalization, how that event unfolded and the child's response to it greatly affect the child's view of future occurrences. Children with chronic diseases who undergo multiple hospitalizations have a different perception of illness from those who have an occasional cold (see Chapter 12). A visit to a pediatrician's office will show the wide range of responses children have. Some older children have more negative responses as they begin to associate certain people, colors, and surroundings with what was for them an unpleasant experience.

In 2005 the American Academy of Nursing (AAN) released a document titled "Health Care Quality and Outcome Guidelines for Nursing of Children and Families" (AAN Expert Panel on Children and Families, 2005). These guidelines include 18 elements that guide nurses and other health professionals working with children and families both in the hospital and the community setting and include such important areas as family/provider collaboration, incorporation of cultural values in care, and accessibility of high-quality health care to prevent and manage physical and emotional illness (AAN Expert Panel on Children and Families, 2005). A second, and related, set of guidelines for consumers provides questions families can ask to assess whether their providers are meeting these guidelines. For the hospitalized child and family, nurses need to consider the following for all children and families, but especially hospitalized children: (1) Does the nurse adequately address questions and concerns? (2) Does the nurse provide opportunities for families to share and practice cultural values? (3) Does the nurse inform the family about and refer them to a range of health care services? (4) Does the nurse thoroughly educate the child and family about treatments and procedures? Is the care safe? Is the health care provided appropriate for the child's and family's needs and the child's level of development? (AAN Expert Panel on Children and Families, 2005).

Age and Cognitive Development

Children's developmental levels affect their reactions to illness. These differences should be considered when planning nursing care. Preparing a toddler for hospitalization or a procedure differs from preparing a school-age child. The content, the time frame, the setting, and the method of preparation are all based on the child's growth and development. Pediatric nurses must have a clear understanding of the cognitive abilities of children in each age group (Box 11-2).

Parental Response to Illness or Hospitalization

Children have sharp observation skills and know when their parents are anxious and upset. This anxiety is transferred to the child, and the child's anxiety then increases. If the parents talk outside their child's room or within hearing range but in whispers, the child begins to imagine what the parents are saying. All children, but especially preschoolers, who have such active imaginations, can invent elaborate stories to explain what is happening.

The parent who does not answer the child's questions or who does not tell the truth for fear it will frighten the child only confuses the child and weakens the child's trust in the parent. The child wants to believe that someone is in control and that that person can be trusted. Some parents cannot be honest with their children because of their own fears and insecurities. The nurse needs to assess all these issues.

Preparing the Child and Family

Stress has been defined as a nonspecific response of the body to any demand made on it. Perceived stressors, the conditioning factors brought to the situation, and the coping mechanisms used to adapt all affect each person's adaptation to a stress-producing situation (Selye, 1974). Preparing for an event (in this case, hospitalization) can decrease stress in several ways. During preparation, the child's and the parents' perceptions of the event can be explored. In addition, previous experiences that might affect the impending hospitalization and the use of previous coping strategies can be identified and discussed.

The depth and method of preparation vary among children and are based on an understanding of the child's individual needs. Variables that the nurse should consider include the child's age and developmental level, involvement of the family, timing, child's physiologic status and psychologic status, setting, sociocultural factors, and the child's experiences with illness and hospitalization.

Preparation sessions should be planned. Teaching is more effective if the nurse and family develop trust. Honesty and language appropriate for the child's age are imperative. When possible, all the child's senses should be involved. The child should be allowed to see the intensive care area before being admitted, to take the blood pressure of a stuffed animal, or to handle the mask that will be used in surgery. The nurse should avoid using medical terms that children and their parents may not understand. Literal interpretation of some words may be confusing and scary to some children, especially

| BOX 11-2 | **Developmental Approaches to the Hospitalized Child** |

Neonate
- Anticipate needs and fulfill them in a timely manner.
- Provide opportunities for nonnutritive (comfort) sucking and oral stimulation with a pacifier.
- Provide swaddling, with the infant's hands drawn to the midline and close to the face. Use soft talking to soothe.
- If the infant is very ill, provide a quiet, soothing environment. Pay close attention to light and sound stimulation.
- When stimulation is appropriate, provide stimulation for each sense (e.g., mobiles, music, smell, soft stuffed animals). Use contrasting colors and textures.
- Watch for cues of overstimulation, such as eye avoidance, extension of arms, splaying of fingers, and "zoning-out" behavior.
- Before painful procedures, provide comforting touch and nonnutritive sucking. Follow painful procedures with tucking, holding, and cuddling.
- Model and share appropriate behaviors with family members regarding stimulation, touch, verbalization, and feeding.
- Provide consistent caregivers when parents are not available.
- Collaborate with parents on ways to provide care to them.
- Involve the parents in the care of their infant as much as possible.
- Encourage parents to room in if possible.

Infant
- For the younger infant, provide the same care given for a neonate.
- The older infant will begin to anticipate painful procedures and fight. Use sheets and blankets to provide swaddling if necessary. Allow nonnutritive sucking for comfort.

- Expect regressive behavior and inform parents to expect it and why.
- Limit the number of caregivers to whom the infant must adjust.
- Request that parents bring the infant's security object (e.g., blanket, stuffed animal).
- Encourage parents to be present during procedures.

Toddler
- Expect regression and inform parents about behaviors.
- Follow home routines and rituals.
- Involve parents in the care of the toddler.
- Provide for rooming in if possible.
- Allow opportunities for mobility when it can be done safely.
- Use all possible methods of pain control when the child must have a painful procedure.
- Anticipate temper tantrums when the child's frustration level is high.
- Maintain a safe environment for the toddler's physical acting out and temper tantrums.
- Encourage the child to be independent (e.g., feed self, use potty chair, put on socks).
- Provide support when the toddler needs to be dependent (e.g., hold after a procedure, comfort if parents leave).
- Approach with a positive attitude ("I am going to give you your medicine.").

Preschooler
- Provide safe ways to act out aggression (e.g., with punching bags, painting, clay).
- Take time for communication. Answer questions with simple, concrete explanations. Explain all procedures honestly. Allow for choices whenever possible.

---

preschoolers (see Chapter 6). Some children assume that certain procedures include pain. Explanation and the opportunity to handle equipment, when possible, can help children master the fear of hospitalization and treatment.

Special attention should be given to prepare the family as well. Assuming that parents will understand complicated aspects of a child's care is a mistake. In fact, to thoroughly include families in the child's care, nurses must give information to family members that, like information given to the child, includes what the family will see, hear, and need to do (Daneman, Macaluso, & Guzzetta, 2003).

Coping Skills of the Child and Family

Coping is the process of contending with difficulties in an effort to overcome or work through them. How the child copes with illness or hospitalization is related to age, perception of the event, previous hospitalizations and encounters with the health care profession, support from significant others, and the child's and parents' coping skills.

Depending on age, children use words, behaviors, and physical actions to help them through stressful situations.

The child may also cope by ignoring or negating the event. The younger child is more likely to use emotional expression, whereas the older child and adolescent are more likely to withdraw or practice more self-control behaviors. For example, although the younger child might scream and kick during a procedure, the older child might remain stoic and say that it did not hurt, even though it did. Some children try to appear brave and meet self-imposed or parental expectations.

Breathing (e.g., blowing bubbles, pinwheels, party blowers) or singing helps with relaxation and offers a focus for the child. Teaching coping mechanisms and practicing them before a procedure can help a child feel more in control and successful. Distraction (e.g., water wheels, games, books) and imagery (e.g., tapes, scenarios) for older children are effective tools for coping. Parents, nurses, and child life specialists may all serve as facilitators for these techniques.

Psychologic Benefits of Hospitalization

Some think that hospitalization causes only negative psychologic effects. The stress of illness and hospitalization can actually be growth enhancing by promoting a child's coping

| BOX 11-2 | **Developmental Approaches to the Hospitalized Child—cont'd** |

Preschooler—cont'd

- Expect egocentric behavior.
- Provide for a safe and secure environment (e.g., with a night light, view of others, objects from home).
- Be consistent.
- Ask the parents how the child usually copes in new situations.
- Tell the child that he or she did not cause the illness.
- Involve parents in care and follow home routines.
- Place the child with other children of the same age if possible.
- Provide for play activities in the playroom and in the room.
- Accept regression if it occurs and explain it to parents.
- Encourage the child to be independent (e.g., feeding, dressing, toileting).

School-Age Child

- Inform the child of limits, and enforce them (e.g., no water fights, wheelchair races, leaving the unit).
- Involve the child in planning and implementing care (e.g., allow child to choose from menu and assist with some procedures).
- Explain all procedures and allow the child time for questions and answers. Use medical and scientific terminology and diagrams, body outlines, or anatomically correct dolls to explain the procedure.
- Accept regression but encourage independence.
- Provide privacy.
- Encourage the child to assist in keeping the room and belongings in order.
- Assist the child in contacting friends. Encourage parents to contact the teacher and have school friends send cards and letters.

- If the child's condition supports visits and calls from friends, encourage this contact.
- Provide for the child's educational needs by encouraging parents to bring in the child's homework and by scheduling study times. If the child will have a prolonged period of hospital or home care, arrange for a teacher to work with the child. Some hospitals have a hospital-based teacher.

Adolescent

- Provide privacy for care and visiting.
- Encourage the adolescent to wear street clothes and perform normal grooming.
- Encourage questions about appearance and the effects of illness on the adolescent's future.
- Use scientific and medical terminology to prepare the adolescent for procedures.
- Use body outlines and diagrams and give the rationale for the procedure.
- When possible, provide for a special activity area that is limited to adolescent use. Introduce the child to other adolescents on the unit.
- Encourage peers to call and visit if the adolescent's condition can tolerate this action.
- Assist parents in communicating, supporting, and guiding adolescents by providing them with information about growth and development.
- Allow favorite foods to be brought in if the adolescent does not need a special diet.
- Approach the adolescent with caring, understanding, and acceptance.
- Provide for educational needs, as for a school-age child.

skills and bolstering self-esteem. Children can increase their self-confidence as they overcome the anxiety related to hospitalization and perhaps master some self-care skills. They feel positive about their recovery or increased ability to cope with any disability they have. In addition, hospitalization offers an opportunity for children to ask questions and obtain new information. Some even become interested in a career in health care while observing professionals caring for them. Hospitalization can also be an opportunity to teach parents about children's growth and development, improve parenting skills, and assess the child's well care and immunizations.

PLAYROOMS IN HEALTH CARE SETTINGS

Hospitals and clinics often provide playrooms where children may go to play with toys, participate in age-appropriate arts and crafts, and socialize with other children. Children should always see this area as a safe place where procedures and treatments do not take place. Children, when their condition is stable, may be taken to the playroom in their beds and wheelchairs (Fig. 11-5). A separate activity area should be

provided, when possible, for adolescents to listen to music, play video games, and visit with their peers.

Play for hospitalized, or otherwise ill children, enables the child to gain control over stressful experiences. In a study of play patterns of children with leukemia, Gariepy and Howe (2003) suggested that play for ill children is somewhat different than for children who are well. Play was found to be less spontaneous, more repetitive, and more solitary. The authors suggested that ill children with high anxiety may not have the energy to play with others and may need to re-enact stressful experiences repetitively to cope and that a play routine might assist the child to manage stress (Gariepy & Howe, 2003). They recommended, however, that engaging ill children in play with others serves as an effective distraction from stress, so long as the type of play does not require excessive energy expenditure (Gariepy & Howe, 2003).

Therapeutic Play

When a child is hospitalized, one component of the child's plan of care is the use of *therapeutic play*. Therapeutic play differs from normal play in its design and intent. Members of

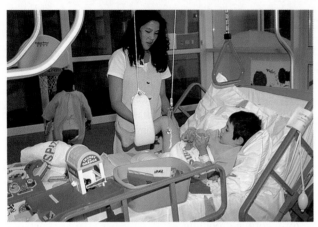

FIG 11-5   **Being in traction is no reason not to enjoy the hospital's play facilities. To give him a change of surroundings and allow him to interact with her and with other children, the play therapist wheels this child in his bed to the playroom. Because his mobility will be limited for a significant period, providing diversion is especially important.**   *(Courtesy Parkland Health and Hospital System, Dallas, TX.)*

the health team guide it, and activities are planned to meet the physical and psychologic needs of the child. Therapeutic play can provide an emotional outlet, instruct, and improve physiologic abilities (American Academy of Pediatrics Committee on Hospital Care, 2000). Supervised play with medical equipment helps reduce fear and separate reality from fantasy.

Child life specialists or play therapists are available in many hospitals to share their expertise in child growth and development and the use of play. Child life programs have as their goals maintaining normal living patterns, minimizing psychologic trauma, and promoting optimal development of the child and family. Nurses should also be involved in this type of activity, either in conjunction with the child life specialist or individually when a child life specialist is not available. Interpretations of the child's play behavior and some types of play therapy require guidance by a skilled health care worker.

Emotional Outlet Play

Emotional outlet play is often called *dramatic play*. During this type of play, the child acts out or dramatizes real-life stressors. These might include emotional stressors, such as abuse or neglect, or a painful physical stressor, such as a bone marrow aspiration. The hospitalized child who is separated from family and friends might use a wooden hammer and pegs to express anger over the separation. A child who has been sexually abused might not be able to communicate the experience verbally but may be able to use an anatomically correct doll to show what happened.

Many commercially crafted toys are available for dramatic play. Anatomically correct dolls and puppets are available. Some dolls have removable parts that enable the child to see the various organs of the body.

Children can express their inner beliefs and perceptions through drawing. A child may draw a very big bed with a tiny child on it surrounded by large, hovering adults or a huge syringe with a long needle. Children often express their thoughts and feelings through the use of paper and crayons or markers (Fig. 11-6) (Wikstrom, 2005).

Injection play is an appropriate intervention with the child who has to undergo frequent blood work, injections, IV therapy, or any other therapy involving syringes and needles. If a needle is used for this type of activity, safety is of the utmost importance and the nurse should assess the child's growth and development level before using this type of directed play. An adult is always present if a needle is used. The child can give a doll an injection and can thereby work through anger and anxiety. Wooden hammers and pegboards, Nerf balls, and boxing gloves are all avenues for release of stress or anger.

Teaching Through Play

Play can also be used to teach. It can be used in preoperative teaching and teaching before a new, painful, or extensive procedure (see Fig. 11-6). The nurse assesses the child's cognitive level before this type of teaching, and the play should be appropriate to the child's level.

Hospital equipment is often used in this type of play. The nurse might demonstrate taking a blood pressure on the child's stuffed animal before putting the cuff on the child. A breathing treatment might be "given" to the child's doll before the child is given the treatment. The nurse might use drawings and diagrams to explain procedures or surgery.

Some hospitals have preoperative visits during which children come to meet the people who will be taking care of them and see the physical surroundings. They may see the scrub gowns and masks worn by the surgical staff and visit a typical room. Children and parents can ask questions and meet other children and parents who are going through the same experience as they tour the area.

Enhancing Cooperation Through Play

Children with illnesses that require unpleasant or painful therapies often are uncooperative. Developing a plan that will stimulate and engage the child in the activity is a challenge. The nurse should include age-appropriate growth and development activities when planning care. The school-age child who loves competition and games is more likely to increase range of motion of an arm if points can be made each time the Nerf ball is thrown through the hoop.

Allowing the child to blow bubbles, a whistle, or a pinwheel or to simulate blowing out the nurse's penlight can enhance deep-breathing exercises. Range of motion can be accomplished by throwing Nerf balls, beanbags, and paper balls. The child who needs to increase intake can sometimes be motivated to drink more fluids if a graph shows the amount taken in and the child receives a reward when a selected goal is reached. Including the child in planning and identifying rewards and goals enhances motivation. Colorful stickers, baseball cards, small toys, and special pencils can be used as rewards.

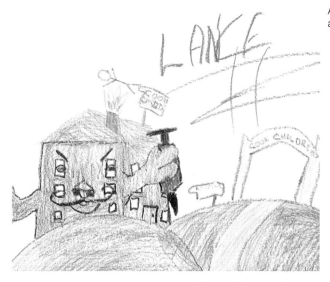

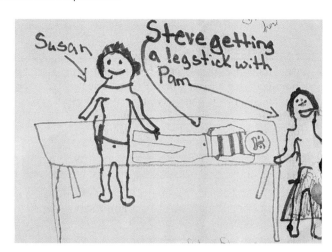

Art materials allow children to express their thoughts and feelings about health care problems.

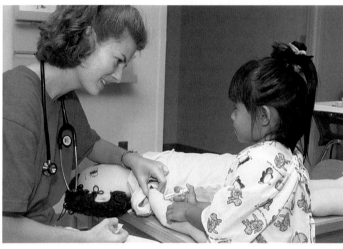

Giving a doll an injection can help a child work through anxiety and anger about injections she may be receiving.

FIG 11-6   **Therapeutic play can be used to teach children about medical procedures or help them work through their feelings about what has happened to them in the health care setting. Child life specialists or play therapists are often members of the team in children's hospitals to provide expert guidance for therapeutic play.**

Unstructured Play

In addition to therapeutic play, the nurse encourages unstructured play in the hospital setting. Through unstructured play, children can control events, ideas, and relationships.

Hospitals without a special room set aside for play should be encouraged to provide developmentally appropriate toys, games, and books. These items can be kept in a special box accessible to the nursing staff.

Evaluation of Play

Therapeutic play should be reflected in the child's nursing care plan. During the evaluation step of the nursing process, the nurse looks at the outcome criteria to determine whether the goals have been met. The nurse is asking whether play enhanced the care of the child. Is the child coughing and deep breathing every 2 hours? Is the child relating feelings of fear over the separation from parents? Is the child eating or sleeping? If the client goals have been achieved, the interventions have been appropriate and effective.

ADMITTING THE CHILD TO A HOSPITAL SETTING
Taking the History

The admission procedure sets the tone for the hospitalization. It should not be a series of questions but rather a time of collaboration between the nurse and the family. The time the family has spent in the emergency department, the seriousness of the illness, and other family needs (e.g., other children with grandparents or left with neighbors) may affect the interview process.

> The nurse can acknowledge the parent's concerns. For example, the nurse might say, "Mrs. Smith, I know you're concerned about your other children. Would you like to call your neighbor before I ask you some questions about Heidi and her illness?"

Most hospitals provide an admission interview form. Some of the information is essential for providing immediate care,

NURSING CARE PLAN

The Child in a Hospital Setting

Focused Assessment

Assess the child for any problems related to the hospital admission by identifying pertinent historical data on the admission data sheet and analyzing the results of the physical examination. Important assessment areas that can cause problems for hospitalized children include:

- *Nutrition:* Assess the child's calorie intake, and compare it with the requirements for age and weight. Note any abnormalities after plotting and recording height and weight percentiles. Determine the child's favorite foods and customary rituals around mealtimes, in addition to cultural or religious dietary practices that may restrict a child's food choices.
- *Elimination:* Assess any regression the child may be having in bowel or bladder control. Inquire about specific terms the child uses for elimination, and use these terms to provide comfort and assistance to the child. Although regression can be a normal response to the stress of hospitalization, it is distressing to the child and parent.

- *Sleep:* Understanding and communicating the child's usual sleep patterns and routines to others will assist in planning care. Determine usual bedtime, hygiene practices used before sleep, and bedtime rituals (e.g., rocking, prayers, stories, snacks). Note any alterations in the number of hours the child is sleeping, and compare with the norm for the child's age.
- *Self-Care:* Assess and note the child's usual self-care activities (e.g., eating, bathing, dressing, brushing teeth). Alterations may indicate increasing anxiety or loss of control.
- *Emotional/Social Status:* Assess for signs of anxiety or fear related to the hospital setting (e.g., crying, temper tantrums, withdrawal, decreased communication). Assess the child's ability to keep in touch with peers. Note whether the child readily participates in unit activities.

NURSING DIAGNOSIS   Imbalanced Nutrition: Less Than Body Requirements related to unfamiliar foods, separation from caregiver, strange environment, or disease process.

EXPECTED OUTCOMES   The child will:
- Eat the appropriate number of calories and variety of nutrients according to age.
- Maintain prehospital weight.

Intervention	*Rationale*
1. Identify the cause of the child's decreased intake.	1. Identifying the cause of any decreased appetite can assist in the elimination of the problem.
2. Encourage parents to bring foods from home and to be with the child during meals.	2. The parents' presence simulates the home environment and increases the likelihood that the child will eat.
3. Allow the child to select food from the menu. Communicate to other staff the types of foods the child particularly likes.	3. Allowing the child to select food gives the child control and provides an opportunity to select foods that the child likes and will eat.
4. Offer frequent, nutritious snacks and encourage parents to do the same.	4. Children may eat junk food and then refuse nutritious foods offered at mealtimes.
5. Offer small portions. Use small dishes, cups, and glasses.	5. Children may be overwhelmed by large portions and refuse to eat any of the food. Child-size tableware, especially if appropriately decorated, is more appealing to children.
6. If parents cannot be available during meals, allow the child to eat with other children.	6. Older children may distract the child and decrease separation anxiety.
7. Request a dietary consultation.	7. Registered dietitians can assist in planning age-appropriate nutritious meals.

Evaluation

- Is the child's nutritional intake appropriate for age?
- Did the child maintain baseline body weight during hospitalization?

NURSING DIAGNOSIS   Delayed Growth and Development, regression in toilet training or self-care skills, related to separation and hospitalization.

EXPECTED OUTCOME   The child will:
- Maintain usual self-care activities of feeding, toileting, dressing, and bathing. Any regression reverses quickly after discharge.

Intervention	*Rationale*
1. Follow home routines of elimination.	1. Cooperation will increase and anxiety will decrease if the child's normal routine and rituals are maintained.

NURSING CARE PLAN—cont'd

2. Do not scold the incontinent child.

3. Explain to parents that some regression in all self-care activities is normal in hospitalized children and that most children resume their normal routines soon after discharge.

4. Discourage parents from beginning toilet training during hospitalization.

5. Encourage the child to participate in self-care according to developmental abilities.

6. Assist the child when the ability to perform self-care is limited because of fatigue, discomfort, or other factors related to the disease process.

7. Provide the necessary equipment for self-care and place it within easy reach.

8. Offer choices and allow the child to make decisions when appropriate.

2. If the incontinence is caused by anxiety, scolding will only increase the anxiety.

3. Parents may be concerned about the child's regression and may increase the child's anxiety by focusing on the child's incontinence.

4. Toilet training can be an additional stressor at a difficult time.

5. Self-care increases the child's self-esteem and feeling of control.

6. The disease process may limit the child's ability, physically or mentally, to perform self-care.

7. Accessible equipment decreases the complexity of providing self-care by making the environment easier to manipulate.

8. Choice increases the child's sense of control.

Evaluation

- Is the child able to feed, toilet, dress, and bathe at the same level as before the illness?

- Does the child readily participate in self-care activities?

NURSING DIAGNOSIS   Disturbed Sleep Pattern related to unfamiliar environment, anxiety, or discomfort.

EXPECTED OUTCOME   The child will:
- Sleep the appropriate number of hours for age.

Intervention

1. Plan care to allow time for periods of sleep. Care can be organized so that vital signs can be measured and other procedures performed when medication is given.

2. Post a sign on the door when the child is asleep to prevent other staff and visitors from waking the child. Unplug the phone, turn off the television, close the door unless the child must be observed, and pull the blinds.

3. If the parents are not with the child, explain that you will be nearby and will check during the night. Provide a night light.

Rationale

1. Planning allows for uninterrupted sleep. Children who are awakened a short time after they have fallen asleep often have difficulty going back to sleep.

2. Environmental distractions can be major sleep interruptions.

3. Feelings of security are increased if the child understands that someone is watching.

Evaluation

- Does the child take naps and sleep an appropriate amount of time on the basis of age requirements?

NURSING DIAGNOSIS   Anxiety related to fear of the unknown and separation from significant others and familiar surroundings.

EXPECTED OUTCOMES   The child will:
- Display decreased indicators of distress (e.g., crying, withdrawal, irritability).
- Verbalize feelings of anxiety.
- Play appropriately and maintain contact with peers.

Intervention

1. Orient the child and parent to the hospital and the routines of the unit.

2. Prepare the child and parent for all procedures in an age-appropriate way.

3. Encourage parents to stay with the child when possible and to be involved in the child's care.

4. Hold, rock, and cuddle the infant or young child.

Rationale

1. Familiarity with the environment and its expectations will decrease anxiety caused by fear of the unknown.

2. Preparation for an event decreases anxiety and fear.

3. The presence of parents supports the parental role and decreases the child's separation anxiety.

4. Holding and cuddling children increase feelings of security and trust.

Continued

NURSING CARE PLAN—cont'd

5. If the parents cannot stay with the child, provide for a consistent caregiver.

6. Follow home routines and rituals when possible.

7. Encourage the parents to be honest with the child when they leave and to inform the nurse where they can be reached and when they will return. Encourage the parents to call while they are away. Older children can talk on the phone with their parents.

8. Encourage parents to bring transitional objects (e.g., blanket, teddy bear) and to provide reminders of themselves (e.g., pictures, scarf, handkerchief) if they cannot be with the child.

9. Take the child to the playroom and introduce to other children when appropriate or plan play activities (reading, board games, drawing) for a child unable to leave the room.

10. For the older child, arrange for peer contact through visits, phone calls, and letters.

11. Offer choices and allow the child to make decisions when appropriate.

12. Encourage the older child to wear street clothes and to decorate the room.

13. Provide opportunities for the older child to express feelings about the illness and hospitalization; communicate with a child life specialist about the child's identified needs (e.g., anxiety, anger, boredom, lack of information).

14. Provide information to the parents about diagnosis, treatment, and prognosis. Attend to their needs for sleep and nutrition.

5. Continuity of care provides the child with a consistent person with whom the child can develop a trusting relationship.

6. Familiar routines help the child predict events and reduce anxiety caused by the unfamiliar setting.

7. Trust is increased when parents and caregivers are honest with the child. If parents just disappear, the child will feel anger, abandonment, and acute anxiety. By keeping open lines of communication, the parent's anxiety is decreased.

8. Transitional objects give the child a feeling of security. Both transitional objects and reminders of the parents comfort the child and help decrease the anxiety related to separation.

9. Other children provide a form of distraction and assist the child in adapting to the environment.

10. The older child may fear being forgotten by peers. By maintaining contact and sharing information with peers, the child maintains a sense of importance and security.

11. Choice increases the child's sense of control.

12. Normal attire gives the child an opportunity for self-expression and makes the child feel more comfortable in the environment.

13. Fear and anxiety may decrease if the child has an opportunity to communicate feelings, have them validated, and participate in problem-solving techniques.

14. The child is affected by parents' anxiety. Helping the parents cope will help decrease their anxiety, which will in turn decrease the child's anxiety.

Evaluation

- Is the child playing and communicating with other children and staff and showing decreased signs of distress?

- Is the child able to express feelings of anxiety either verbally or through play?

and some can be collected later. By recognizing the family's needs, the nurse can structure each admission to fit that child and family. If the parent has entered the system through the emergency department, some of the questions may have previously been answered. By looking at the forms from other departments, repetition can be avoided, but data about allergies, medications taken at home, the history of the illness, and other relevant details must be repeated.

Although hospitals have policies and procedures for admission, the routine may need to be altered because of the child's condition. For example, a severely dehydrated child should have an IV infusion started and a child in pain should be medicated before any other interventions are performed. On the other hand, the primary needs of the child and family may be emotional. A parent who has just been told that

her child may have a terminal disease may have difficulty remembering the dates of the child's immunizations. In this situation, the nurse should provide the parent with support and assistance in mobilizing coping mechanisms and support systems rather than focusing on data gathering.

After the child and family are made comfortable (Fig. 11-7), the nurse obtains a thorough physical, health, and psychosocial history. This is followed by a detailed physical examination. For all types of admissions, the history is recorded on an admission data sheet which, depending on the facility, may be in electronic format. The format of the admission data sheet varies from hospital to hospital, but most admission forms ask for much of the same information: history; allergies; nutritional, sleep, elimination, and psychosocial information.

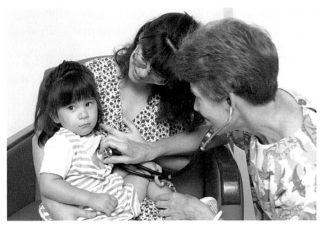

FIG 11-7 **To reduce the stress of unfamiliar surroundings and people, the nurse assesses this child while the girl remains in the security of her mother's arms.** *(Courtesy T.C. Thompson Children's Hospital, Chattanooga, TN.)*

Physical Examination

Initial Inspection

The initial inspection determines the need for any immediate or emergency care that must be provided before other information can be obtained.

Baseline Data

The physical examination should be thorough, and special attention should be given to the body system involved in the child's admission. Many admission forms have an outline of the child's body on which the nurse should indicate any bruises, scratches, or other skin markings that provide specific objective data. (The process of interviewing, taking a history, and physical assessment is explained in Chapter 9.)

Data collected at admission are used to formulate nursing diagnoses and the child's plan of care and should be placed in the body of the child's chart—not at the back of the chart, where this information can be forgotten.

THE ILL CHILD'S FAMILY

Through family-centered care, the nurse considers and treats the child in the context of the family and recognizes the family as the primary and continuing provider of care for the child. Although the nurse sometimes must plan care without involving the family, it is difficult to do so.

Parents

A child's illness may cause a situational crisis for the family. If the illness leads to hospitalization, either planned or unplanned, the family's anxiety increases. Ill children become the parents' central focus; parents can become very vigilant and committed to protecting the child and ensuring optimal care (Dudley & Carr, 2004; Stratton, 2004). Ensuring a positive parent/family/child/nurse collaboration is essential to a positive outcome from the hospital experience. The

literature describes several ways in which nurses can optimize care for hospitalized families:

- Establishing rapport, ensuring a consistent caregiver, providing compassion and being present for family members (Espezel & Canam, 2003; Stratton, 2004)
- Keeping family members informed about the child and what specifically they can do to collaborate in the child's care (Espezel & Canam, 2003; Griffin, 2003).
- Allowing the parents to decide how much time they wish to spend with their child and how involved they wish to be with the child's care; viewing families as partners in care (Griffin, 2003).
- Facilitating visitation policies that acknowledge cultural differences and different family configurations (Griffin, 2003) (Fig. 11-8).
- Addressing the health needs of family members as well as the health needs of the child (Hopia, 2005; Tsuruta et al., 2005).

Parents may wonder why their family is facing the crisis of a childhood illness or may believe that if they had sought treatment earlier the child would not be so ill. A parent may have delayed taking a child with a low-grade fever and vague symptoms to a physician. If the symptoms were a sign of serious illness, the parent may feel guilty for not having sought care earlier.

Parents have varied responses to a child's illness. They may initially deny that their child is ill, especially if the illness is serious. The period of denial may be followed by anger. The anger may be directed at the nurse, at another family member, or sometimes at God. When the immediate crisis is over, a period of depression may occur. At this point, the parents are usually exhausted, both physically and psychologically. Often, they have been spending long hours at the hospital while working and trying to care for the other children in the family.

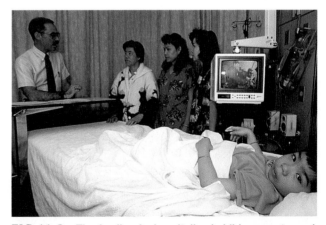

FIG 11-8 **The family of a hospitalized child may not speak the prevailing language. Interpreters on call at many hospitals help such parents communicate with hospital personnel and provide a familiar link to the parents' and child's culture and language.** *(Courtesy Cook Children's Medical Center, Fort Worth, TX.)*

The nurse needs to be aware of parents' feelings and to listen closely to what is said. The nurse can then assist the parents in working through their feelings.

The parental role often changes when the child is admitted to the hospital. The parent who had been in control before the admission is now in an unfamiliar environment. Parents may be confused as to what they can and cannot do. Can they bathe their child? Can they even hold their child, or will they disturb the tubes? When the parent is not given permission to perform some of the care, both the child and the parent suffer.

The needs of fathers are sometimes forgotten. The father may come to the hospital only after he has spent a day at work and then, after a short visit, may need to go home to be with other children. He may not be there when the primary care physician makes rounds and therefore receives most of his medical information from someone else. The father may think that he needs to be the strong one in the family and not show his fear and anxiety. In some families, the mother works outside the home while the father stays with the child. In either case, an awareness of each parent's role will assist the nurse in identifying the individual needs of the parents.

Because of dual roles, long separations, increased stress, and numerous other factors, the parents' marriage may be strained. This situation is especially likely in marriages that are already at risk. Even when both partners are at the hospital, they may not have any time alone.

Many children have stepmothers and stepfathers. In such cases, both sets of parents need recognition, support, and education. How the family copes with the child's illness depends on its coping strategies. A family that is already in crisis or one without support systems (e.g., family, friends, church) will have more difficulty adjusting to the change than a family that is organized and adjusted. A family that deals successfully with the crisis is strengthened by the experience. (For further discussion of the effects of illness on the family, see Chapter 2. For a discussion of the family with a child with a chronic illness, see Chapter 12.)

CRITICAL THINKING EXERCISE 11-1

Tommy, 4 years old, was admitted to the hospital with pneumonia. Tommy has cystic fibrosis. His family has recently moved to the area, and this is his first admission to your hospital. Tommy loves to play with his dinosaur collection and spends much of his day playing and watching his favorite videos. His mother visits for short periods during the lunch hour, and his father visits in the evening. Tommy cries when his parents leave. You mention to a colleague that you think Tommy's parents should spend more time with him. She responds, "We don't know what their other responsibilities are."
1. What other responsibilities might the family have?
2. What are some of the nursing interventions that would support a family with a child in the hospital?

BOX 11-3	**Caring for the Siblings of an Ill or Hospitalized Child**

Factors That Add to the Stress of Siblings
- Age younger than 10 years
- Emotional closeness to the hospitalized child
- Receiving only a limited explanation of the experience
- Fear of getting the illness themselves
- Being cared for outside their own home
- Perceiving that their parents are acting differently toward them
- Having a sibling who is progressively ill

Nursing Care Guidelines for Meeting the Needs of Siblings
- Encourage caregivers to have the ill child retell what happened. This experience may be uncomfortable for the adult, but it helps the sibling put the illness or accident in perspective.
- If the sibling has feelings of guilt, address the child's concerns directly. If the feelings of guilt continue, suggest a consultation with a counselor.
- Give parents educational materials, and show them how to use them with the sibling.
- Schedule a time for the sibling to visit. Prepare the sibling for the medical equipment and any changes in the ill child's appearance that may cause concern.
- If the sibling cannot visit, send photographs.
- Encourage the sibling to talk with the child on the telephone.

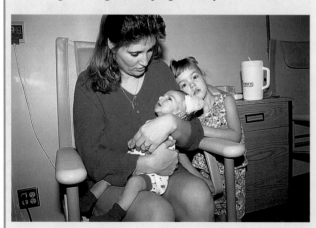

Her brother's repeated hospitalizations for problems associated with a diaphragmatic hernia have been difficult for this girl. Siblings of ill children may experience jealousy, insecurity, resentment, confusion, and anxiety. The nurse can help this child cope by paying attention to her when she is providing care to the infant. *(Courtesy Children's Medical Center, Dallas, TX.)*

Modified from Craft, M., Wyatt, N., & Sandell, B. (1985). Behavior and feeling changes in siblings of hospitalized children. *Clinical Pediatrics, 24,* 374-378.

Siblings

The illness or hospitalization of a brother or sister can be difficult for children. The ill child's siblings may experience jealousy, insecurity, resentment, confusion, and anxiety. Children often have difficulty understanding why their ill sibling is getting all the attention and why their parents seem so preoccupied and have so little time for them. They may worry that if their sibling could get sick, so could they. Preschool children, who engage in magical thinking, may worry that they somehow caused the illness. All these thoughts and feelings are compounded by children's difficulty expressing their feelings (Box 11-3). Although some are at greater risk than others, many children hold everything inside. The amount of stress the sibling experiences varies according to the well child's age and developmental level, closeness of the sibling relationship, who is caring for the sibling while the ill child is hospitalized, how often the well sibling can visit, and the type of perceived parental behavior changes.

NURSING CARE PLAN

The Family With a Hospitalized Child

Focused Assessment

Assess factors that affect a family's adjustment to illness and hospitalization; compare assessment with concerns expressed on the child's admission history. Was the admission an emergency? Were there previous admissions, and how did the parents perceive those hospitalizations? How serious is the illness or trauma? Are some factors unknown, such as the cause of the disease or the child's prognosis? Special attention should also be given to any information obtained in the admission interview.

Try to determine whether the parents and siblings are experiencing stress and how they are coping with hospitalization. Open-ended statements, such as "This must be difficult for you" may encourage communication in this crisis. Identify the parents' needs for sleep, nutrition, and information.

NURSING DIAGNOSIS Interrupted Family Processes related to the child's hospitalization and illness.

EXPECTED OUTCOMES The parents will:
- Participate in the child's care.
- Meet the needs of other family members.
- Use appropriate support systems.
- Identify ways to cope.
- Assist the child to move from a sick role to a well role.

Intervention

1. Orient the parents to the hospital and provide information related to their physical needs (e.g., food, sleep, bathing).
2. Encourage family members (parents, siblings) to express their feelings and to ask questions about the child's illness.
3. Provide the family with information about the child's condition, treatment, and support systems. Begin to prepare them for the child's discharge (Box 11-4).
4. Identify with the family the ways in which they are coping; support their parenting skills.

5. Refer the family to other professionals (e.g., social worker, clinical psychologist, clinical specialist, psychiatrist, clergy) when their problems are not within the scope of nursing.

Rationale

1. The parents' physical needs must be met for them to meet the child's needs and their own emotional needs. Meeting their needs indicates support by the caregiver.

2. Expression decreases anxiety and clarifies misconceptions.
3. Information gives parents a sense of control and decreases their anxiety.

4. Individuals are not always aware of their coping mechanisms, and the nurse should help the family evaluate the effectiveness of theirs.
5. Early identification of family problems can decrease the possibility of escalation of the problems. Collaboration with other health professionals can bring a holistic approach to the care of child and family.

Evaluation

- Are the parents able to participate in their child's care while meeting the needs of other family members?
- Do family members support each other and seek other resources when necessary?

- Are family members able to describe and use positive coping skills?
- Are the parents able to assist the child to move from a sick to a well role?

| BOX 11-4 | **PARENTS WANT TO KNOW** | Information for Discharge |

After assessing the family's knowledge, provide the information families need to know to help the child's transition from hospital to home:

- Information about the illness or trauma and expected outcomes. Tell the parents when they should consult the primary care physician or nurse.
- Medications or treatments to be given at home and information about times, route, side effects, and any special care to be taken when giving the medication. Providing written information is valuable.
- Information about any special nutritional needs.
- Specific activities the child may, may not, and sometimes should participate in.

- The date when the child may return to school.
- The date to bring the child back to the hospital, clinic, or office for follow-up care.
- Information about any referral agency needed for the child or family.
- The unit phone number and primary nurse's name.

Explain, demonstrate, and request a return demonstration of any treatments or procedures that will be done at home. This teaching should be a continuing process and not left until the time of discharge because learning takes place at different rates.

KEY CONCEPTS

- Pediatric nurses may care for children in the hospital, school, community, or home. Each setting requires special interventions.
- Common stressors affecting hospitalized children include fear of the unknown, separation anxiety, fear of pain or mutilation, and loss of control.
- Children may respond to illness with anger, guilt, and regression.
- The stages of separation anxiety are protest, despair, and detachment.
- The more stressed children become, the more difficult it is for them to separate from their parents.
- A child's reaction to pain and fear of injury are related to the child's developmental stage, previous experiences, separation from parents, restraint, and amount of preparation.
- Children who feel that they have control over their illness and hospitalization are more likely to feel confident and be cooperative.
- Regression is a common response to illness and hospitalization. The child returns to an earlier form of behavior.
- How children react to illness and hospitalization is affected by their perception of the event, age, cognitive ability, preparation, previous experiences, coping skills, and parent's response.
- Nursing care of the ill child is directed toward meeting the child's needs related to self-care, separation anxiety, growth and development, diversion, family, control, and pain.
- Parents may feel guilt, denial, anger, and depression when their child is hospitalized.
- Therapeutic play can provide an emotional outlet, instruct, or improve physiologic abilities.
- Play can be incorporated into nursing care when the nurse is teaching or providing a therapeutic intervention that the child finds unpleasant or painful. Adherence increases when deep-breathing and range-of-motion exercises, for example, are made fun activities.

ANSWERS TO CRITICAL THINKING EXERCISE 11-1

1. Families' two most common responsibilities are care of other children and work. A family with a child with cystic fibrosis has the added responsibility of caring for a child with a chronic disease who may or may not have frequent hospitalizations. In addition, family members have the expenses associated with the treatment of the child and, in most cases, cannot afford to miss work. They also risk losing their jobs because of missing work when the child is ill. Families often must balance work, caring for other children, and providing for the needs of the ill child.

2. In most cases, families of ill children are doing the best they can and may not know of available resources that might support them both emotionally and financially. The nurse should review the history obtained on admission to seek additional information about this family. In addition, the nurse should talk with the parents when they visit to determine whether they have a support system and whether a social service consultation is appropriate. Because the family is new to the area, their needs will probably be greater than the needs of a family surrounded by extended family and friends. If other family members and friends, such as grandparents or church members, are available, the nurse can guide them in identifying ways in which they might assist the family. The staff's awareness that Tommy is often alone can mobilize staff to spend extra time with him. The child life department, if one is available, should also be consulted.

REFERENCES AND READINGS

American Academy of Nursing Expert Panel on Children and Families. (2005). Health care quality and outcome guidelines for nursing of children and families: From the AAN Expert Panel on Children and Families. *Pediatric Nursing, 31,* 149-150.

American Academy of Pediatrics Committee on Hospital Care. (2000). Child life services. *Pediatrics, 106,* 1156-1160.

Board, R. (2005). School-age children's perceptions of their PICU hospitalization. *Pediatric Nursing, 31,* 166-175.

Bowlby, J. (1953). Some pathological processes set in train by early mother-child separation. *Journal of Mental Science, 99,* 265-272.

Bradley, S., & Connell, J. (2000). Visiting children in hospital: A vision from the past. *Paediatric Nursing, 12,* 32-35.

Bricher, G. (1999). Paediatric nurses, children, and the development of trust. *Journal of Clinical Nursing, 8,* 451-458.

Carlson, K., Broome, M., & Vessey, J. (2000). Using distraction to reduce reported pain, fear, and behavioral distress in children and adolescents: A multisite study. *Journal of the Society of Pediatric Nursing, 5,* 75-85.

Centers for Disease Control and Prevention. (1996). Guidelines for school health programs to promote lifelong healthy eating. *MMWR: Morbidity and Mortality Weekly Report, 45,* 1-33.

Craft, M., Wyatt, N., & Sandell, B. (1985). Behavior and feeling changes in siblings of hospitalized children. *Clinical Pediatrics, 24,* 374-378.

Daneman, S., Macaluso, J., & Guzzetta, C. (2003). Healthcare providers' attitudes toward parent participation in the care of the hospitalized child. *JSPN, 8,* 90-98.

Dokken, D. L., & Sydnor-Greenberg, N. (2001). Communication in healthcare: The parents' perspective. *Journal of Child and Family Nursing, 4,* 71-75.

Dowling, J. (2002). Humor: A coping strategy for pediatric patients. *Pediatric Nursing, 28,* 123-131.

Dudley, S., & Carr, J. (2004). Vigilance: The experience of parents staying at the bedside of hospitalized children. *Journal of Pediatric Nursing, Nursing Care of Children and Families, 19,* 267-275.

Elander, G., Hallstrom, I., & Runesson, I. (2002). Observed parental needs during their child's hospitalization. *Journal of Pediatric Nursing, 17,* 140-148.

English Long, E. (2003). Stress in families of children with sepsis. *Critical Care Nursing Clinics of North America, 15,* 47-53.

Erikson, E. (1963). *Childhood and society* (2nd ed.). New York: Norton.

Espezel, H., & Canam, C. (2003). Parent-nurse interactions: care of hospitalized children. *Journal of Advanced Nursing, 44,* 34-41.

Fanurick, D., Schmitz, M., Martin, G., Koh, J., Wood, M., Sturgeon, L., & Long, N. (2000). Hospital room or treatment room: Where should inpatient pediatric procedures be performed? *Children's Health Care, 29,* 103-111.

Gariepy, N., & Howe, N. (2003). The therapeutic power of play: Examining the play of young children with leukaemia. *Child: Care, Health, & Development, 29,* 523-537.

Godshall, M. (2003). Caring for families of chronically ill kids. *RN, 66,* 30-35.

Griffin, T. (2003). Facing challenges to family-centered care, I: Conflicts over visitation. *Pediatric Nursing, 29,* 135-137.

Hopia, H. (2005). Child in hospital: Family experiences and expectations of how nurses can promote family health. *Journal of Clinical Nursing, 14,* 212-222.

Instone, S. (2002). Developmental strategies for interviewing children. *Journal of Pediatric Health Care, 16,* 304-305.

Kristensson-Hallstrom, I., & Elander, G. (1997). Parents' experience of hospitalization: Different strategies for feeling secure. *Pediatric Nursing, 23,* 361-367.

Lau, B. (2002). Stress in children: Can nurses help? *Pediatric Nursing, 28,* 13-18.

Lynn-McHale, D., & Deatrick, J. (2000). Trust between family and health care provider. *Journal of Family Nursing, 6,* 210-231.

Mansson, E.W., & Dykes, A. K. (2004). Practice for preparing children for clinical examination and procedures in Swedish pediatric wards. *Pediatric Nursing, 30,* 182-229.

Melnyk, B. M., Feinstein, N. F., Moldenhouer, Z., & Small, L. (2001). Coping in parents of children who are chronically ill: Strategies for assessment and intervention. *Pediatric Nursing, 27,* 548-559.

Miles, M. S. (2003). Living with illness. Support for parents during a child's hospitalization. *American Journal of Nursing, 103,* 62-64.

Ryan-Wenger, N., Sharrer, V., & Campbell, K. (2005). Changes in children's stressors over the past 30 years. *Pediatric Nursing, 31,* 282-291.

Selekman, J., & Guilday, P. (2003). Identification of desired outcomes for school nursing practice. *Journal of School Nursing 19,* 344-350.

Selye, H. (1974). *Stress without distress.* New York: Lippincott.

Small, L. (2002). Early predictors of poor coping outcomes in children following intensive care hospitalization and stressful medical encounters. *Pediatric Nursing, 28,* 393-399.

Smit, E. M. (2000). Maternal stress during the hospitalization of the adopted child. *MCN: The American Journal of Maternal/Child Nursing, 25,* 37-42.

Stratton, K. (2004). Parents experiences of their child's care during hospitalization. *Journal of Cultural Diversity, 11,* 4-11.

Taras, H., Duncan, P., Luckenbill, D., Robinson, J., Wheeler, L., & Wooley, S. (2004). *Health, mental health and safety guidelines for schools.* Retrieved January 15, 2006, from www.schoolhealth.org.

Tsuruta, K., Kusaba, H., Yamada, M., Murakata, T., & Nakatomi, R. (2005). Health support program for family members with hospitalized child. *Pediatric Nursing, 31,* 297-304.

Visintainer, M., & Wolfer, J. (1975). Psychological preparation for surgical pediatric patient: The effect on children's and parents' stress response and adjustment. *Pediatrics, 56,* 187-202.

Webster, A. (2000). The facilitating role of the play specialist. *Paediatric Nursing, 12,* 24-27.

Wikstrom, B. (2005). Communicating via expressive arts: The natural medium of self-expression for hospitalized children. *Pediatric Nursing, 31,* 480-485.

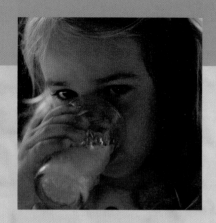

CHAPTER 12

The Child With a Chronic Condition or Terminal Illness

Learning Objectives

After studying this chapter, you should be able to:
- Define chronic illness.
- Analyze the effects of a chronic illness on the child and family.
- Discuss the concerns and needs of the child and family dealing with a chronic illness.
- Compare the stages of death and dying.
- Apply the concepts of death and dying as they relate to the pediatric client.

- Explain the concerns and needs of the child and family facing an impending death.
- Analyze the nurse's response to death and dying in the pediatric population.
- Use the nursing process to describe nursing care of the chronically ill and dying child.

Definitions

anticipatory grief The processes of mourning, coping, interacting, planning, and psychosocial reorganizing that occur as part of the response to the impending death of a loved one.
chronic illness or condition A condition or illness that is long term and either is without cure or has a residual effect that limits activities of daily living.
chronic grief Mourning after the death of an individual that is of excessive duration and interferes with the person's ability to return to normal living.
chronic sorrow Recurrent feelings of grief, loss, and fear related to the child's illness and the loss of the ideal, healthy child.
hospice care A system of comprehensive care that provides support and assistance to clients and families affected

by terminal illness; the purpose is to humanize the dying experience while providing the means for living as comfortably and as fully as possible; goals are accomplished by providing respectful, noninvasive care; pain and symptom control; and emotional, physical, psychological, and spiritual support.
illness trajectory The course of a chronic illness, including the work for and impact on the lives of all those involved.
normalization Responses used to counteract an illness or abnormal behavior to maintain appropriate and valued social roles.
palliative care Medical treatments or procedures that aim to promote comfort and quality of life rather than cure the underlying disease.

Electronic Resources

Additional information related to the content in Chapter 12 can be found on:

the interactive companion CD-ROM
- Audio Glossary
- NCLEX Review Questions

or the companion website at *evolve*
http://evolve.elsevier.com/james/ncoc
- NCLEX Review Questions
- Resources for Health Care Providers and Families
- WebLinks

Rapid advances in health care have changed the experience of chronic illness in childhood. Children with chronic illnesses are living longer, and an increasing number of children are living with illnesses previously considered fatal. Improvements in early diagnostic testing and treatment have enhanced quality of life as well as longevity.

CHRONIC ILLNESS DEFINED

A chronic illness or condition is one that is long term. It does not spontaneously resolve, is usually without complete cure, and frequently has residual characteristics that limit activities of daily living (ADLs) and require adaptation or special assistance. Box 12-1 lists some of the common chronic

BOX 12-1	**Common Chronic Conditions of Childhood**

Asthma (reactive airway disease)
Bleeding disorders (e.g., hemophilia)
Bronchopulmonary dysplasia
Cancer
Cardiac disorders
Cerebral palsy
Chronic renal failure
Congenital heart disease
Cystic fibrosis
Diabetes mellitus
Down syndrome
Hepatitis
Human immunodeficiency virus (HIV) infection and acquired immunodeficiency syndrome (AIDS)
Hydrocephalus
Inborn errors of metabolism
Juvenile rheumatoid arthritis
Lupus erythematosus
Muscular dystrophy
Neural tube defects
Phenylketonuria
Sickle cell disease
Seizure disorders

conditions of childhood. Severity varies among chronic conditions. Many, such as epilepsy, diabetes, or sickle cell disease, although not physically apparent may have a tremendous impact on the child and family. A chronic condition that is terminal but lasts only a short time may also have serious long-term effects on the surviving family. Although the first section of this chapter refers only to chronic conditions, this information also applies to terminal conditions. The federal Maternal and Child Health Bureau's Division of Services for Children with Special Health Care Needs (Health Resources and Services Administration, 2003) developed the following definition regarding the special needs of chronically and terminally ill children for planning and advocacy purposes:

Children with special health care needs are those who have or are at increased risk for a chronic physical, developmental, behavioral, or emotional condition and who also require health and related services of a type and amount beyond that required for children generally.

THE FAMILY OF THE CHILD WITH SPECIAL HEALTH CARE NEEDS
Impact on the Family

Improvements in technology, reimbursement provisions (insurance, state and federal funding), and allocation of health care resources have all affected the family's role in caring for the child with a chronic illness. Children with special needs can now be safely cared for in the home setting, with minimal periods of hospitalization. Such care, which includes psychosocial support, is the most desirable and cost-effective care for both child and family.

Although improved quality of life and longevity are positive developments, they do present certain difficulties. Despite health care advances, the child and family must live with a constant physical problem that requires consistent, ongoing attention and adaptation.

Chronic illness is stressful and can create situational crises for families. A situational crisis is an unexpected crisis for which the family's usual problem-solving abilities are not adequate. However, various studies show that some families reorganize and actually become stronger in response to a situational crisis. These families are considered resilient; that is, they are able to recover from adversities of a chronic illness. They do this through *normalization*, making necessary changes in their lives and adjusting to the presence of the chronic illness. They actively work on responses that will help counteract the illness and resulting abnormal behaviors to maintain social roles that are appropriate and valued.

Family resiliency implies present and future success at managing complex aspects of a crisis, such as having a child with a chronic condition (Patterson, 2002). Resilient families exhibit many important traits, but a predominant trait is family cohesiveness. This cohesion is achieved by active efforts to keep the family intact—by sharing the new responsibilities related to the chronic condition as well as the routine, enjoyable activities of family life. Although family life may be altered by the crisis, resilient families successfully manage the family tasks of equitable economic support, socialization, and protection of the vulnerable family members (Patterson, 2002). Families accomplish this by developing protective factors to counteract the risk inherent with caring for a child with a chronic illness. Patterson (2002) notes that processes that enhance resilience include the following:

- Reframing the situation to identify positive rather than negative aspects
- Successful coping that increases family self-efficacy, or the belief that the family can problem solve in new ways to meet the new challenges
- Maintaining high-quality communication patterns
- Being flexible
- Maintaining social integration
- Preserving family boundaries

Maintaining social integration involves balancing the needs of the family with the needs imposed by the child's condition as well as reciprocal interactions with the community relative to the child's needs. Resilient families are careful in allocating resources, including money, time, and energy, as they balance various needs. This balance ensures that no child in the family—ill or well—is neglected or overindulged. Additionally, it ensures that the condition-related needs of the ill child are balanced with normal growth and development needs and met without overprotection. In resilient families, the child's condition-related needs are incorporated into the family's daily life; they do not become the focus around which the activities of the entire family revolve. This integration helps achieve and maintain the family's new normality imposed by the illness. In such a family setting, baseball practices, school activities, ballet recitals, and other activities do not stop for either the ill child or the well sibling. Rather, care of the child, medical appointments, and treatments of the ill child are arranged around these activities to the degree possible. When conflicts do arise, parents (or other family members or friends) alternate responsibility for maintaining the activities of both the ill child and well siblings.

Equitable allocation of caregiving and encouragement of parental involvement with each other and well siblings help maintain appropriate family boundaries. When either of the two parents becomes primarily involved in meeting the needs of the ill child, the parental relationship suffers. To keep these boundaries intact, resilient families pay specific attention to maintaining a positive parental relationship. They also work to avoid showing favoritism toward the ill child.

Single-parent families may encounter additional difficulties that heighten the risks that the chronic condition will negatively affect resilience and impede normalization. Social support may not be inherent in the family structure, so these families are at increased risk for social isolation. Health care providers can refer single parents to support groups, put them in contact with other parents who have a child with a similar chronic condition, or organize group-sharing experiences between parents experienced in the care of the child with a particular chronic condition and parents of newly diagnosed children.

Boundary problems of a different sort can arise when the need for outside care and assistance increases, such as the presence of home health or hospice personnel. Whether they are in the home around the clock or for various shifts throughout the week, external family boundaries can be negatively affected. However, difficulties can be minimized if family members adopt an assertive role in managing the child's care and, along with the health care personnel, work to maintain professional relationships and boundaries with caregivers.

Resilient families consistently work to ensure appropriate communication, which may be more difficult because of new, condition-related language (medical or otherwise), an increased need for problem solving–based communication and, most importantly, the need to express emotions. Accepting the validity of all emotions and learning suitable means of expressing them may be difficult. However, many families report that the experience of living with a chronic illness brings about positive life changes, such as increased empathy, increased family unity, and new meanings to life.

Even when positive meaning is attached to a child's chronic condition, much flexibility is required of family members regarding family roles and expectations of family members. This flexibility is also required of the health care team, both for the benefit of the family and as a means of achieving a positive, collaborative relationship between the team and the family. The team becomes an integral part of family life. The quality of this relationship may affect how the entire family adapts to and copes with the child's condition.

For resilient families, coping is an active process that entails learning about their child's illness and available resources. These families do not sit idly by, letting others meet their child's needs. They are also the strongest advocates for their child. Subsequently, they have a tremendous need for any information concerning their child's condition. The nurse has an important role in helping families educate themselves and learn to meet their child's special health care needs.

At times of extreme stress, such as periods of unexpected physical setbacks, exacerbations, worsening, or relapse of the condition, as well as at the time of death, families may slip into less effective patterns of behavior and coping. Gentle reminders, support, and encouragement may be all the assistance that a resilient family needs to help members resume the behaviors that foster resiliency despite the many ongoing stressors and uncertainties of a chronic condition.

The Grieving Process

The most important aspect of a chronic illness is that it affects the entire family, not just the ill child. This scope of concern necessitates consistent family-centered nursing care (see Chapter 2). All family members respond to a chronic condition. However, responses vary according to their age and developmental level, their relationship and involvement with the ill child, and any previous experiences with a health care problem.

Chronic and terminal conditions involve the loss of health and result in grief. Grief is a normal psychophysiologic process that occurs in response to a specific loss. A normal and frequent response to such conditions includes the five stages of dying as defined by Elisabeth Kübler-Ross (1969). Her work identified the stages in relation to the anticipated death of an adult. However, they apply to children as well as adults and to the grief of a chronic condition as well as a terminal illness. The ill child, siblings, parents, and other family members may experience these stages.

The stages include denial, anger, bargaining, sadness or depression, and acceptance. During the first stage (*denial*), individuals react with disbelief and shock. Their feelings of "no, not me" and "no, not my loved one" occur whether they are explicitly told of the diagnosis or, in the case of the children, they figure it out on their own. *Anger* usually follows denial. This may include feelings of rage and resentment directed at themselves or at others. At this point, the questions of "why me?" and "why my loved one?" may also occur. Anger may recur at any time during the process of the illness. *Bargaining* then happens, whereby the individual attempts to postpone the inevitable. Although most bargaining is with a spiritual deity, bargaining with oneself or others may also take place.

Depression is the next stage. Such sadness may be for either past losses or those impending losses. Past losses may include physical losses, such as a change in appearance (e.g., hair loss), lifestyle changes, or changes in physical ability. Impending losses may include imminent loss of loved ones. It may also include preparing loved ones for the absence created by death.

The last stage is *acceptance*, whereby the individual is no longer depressed or angry. Although acceptance is not necessarily a happy stage, it is generally a time of comfort and peace.

Individuals need different periods of time to work through and resolve the feelings of one stage before proceeding to the next stage. The stages are not always experienced sequentially. Some fluctuation may recur across stages before acceptance and comfort are reached. Acceptance of a chronic illness can take place even in the presence of noticeable denial. Such denial might appear to be maintained throughout the course of the illness. Because children have less-predictable and variable protective mechanisms, they may use denial frequently—more so than adults will. An individual who has a positive, optimistic outlook and who focuses on concerns and tasks of the day rather than on fears about the condition may be using adaptive denial as a protective mechanism. This may assist in making decisions, lowering distress and anxiety, and supporting daily functioning (Lugton & Kindlen, 1999).

The period for the presence of denial is important. Short-term, true denial, although often considered maladaptive, may truly be adaptive. It is generally experienced as a normal stage of grieving after the onset of a chronic or terminal illness. Persistence of such denial over the course of the illness, however, is maladaptive (Walker, Wells, Heiney, Hymovich, & Weeks, 1993). Attempting to establish whether true, ongoing denial is present is important. Many times what appears to be denial is simply the individual's expression of the loss of their hopes for the ill child. This might be seen as a mother's talk of how beautiful her daughter will look as a bride. It might be a sibling's discussion as to how much fun he or she will have with the ill child next summer at camp. Family need to recognize and express the most difficult aspects of their impending loss to grieve fully and appropriately. Another aspect of what appears to be denial is the expression of the faith that a miracle will occur and that the child will not die after all.

As adjustment to the condition progresses, many parents experience *chronic sorrow*, or the recurrent feelings of loss and fear related to the child's disorder and the loss of the ideal, healthy child (Edwards, Hertzberg, Hays, & Youngblood, 1999). Chronic sorrow is a normal process and may never resolve. However, adaptation to the presence of the illness occurs. The family establishes a "new normal," and their life continues. Chronic sorrow, however, is not the same as chronic grief. Chronic grief refers to mourning after the death of an individual that is of excessive duration and interferes with the person's ability to return to normal living (Lugton & Kindlen, 1999).

The first step in supporting families and helping them deal with chronic sorrow is to listen, then recognize and acknowledge their emotions. The family can then be assisted to recognize the normality of such feelings and emotions themselves. Families should be gently encouraged to acknowledge and express feelings of chronic sorrow, to the degree with which they are comfortable. However, at the same time, they should be encouraged and assisted to verbalize and demonstrate realistic hopes and dreams.

Many organizations, both general and disease specific, offer a wealth of information, support, and assistance to families of a child with a chronic or terminal illness. They offer much beyond the information related to the child's condition. The nurse should introduce the family to such services and, as necessary, assist them to use these services fully. Conversely, a family's decision not to use such support services if that is their decision should be respected.

Such supportive services may be particularly important when observation and assessment of family behaviors indicate problems that may necessitate referral to a mental health professional. In caring for children with a chronic or terminal illness and their families, one issue that is frequently overlooked is that death may occur unexpectedly or earlier than anticipated. This is an important but difficult issue to address with families. It should be done in the early stage of the condition to prepare them if the death does happen in an unexpected manner. The nurse should support children and their families through all stages of the grief process. Supporting the family requires understanding the family's current knowledge base, coping skills, and personal beliefs as well as recognizing and attending to the grief-related problems that arise.

THE CHILD WITH SPECIAL HEALTH CARE NEEDS
Growth and Development Concerns

Children with chronic disorders have many different concerns and needs related to their conditions, not the least of which is successful navigation of the stages of growth and development. Children's responses to illness are influenced by their age at the onset of the disorder as well as growth and development considerations throughout the course of the illness. Nursing care is planned accordingly. (See Chapter 4 for a more complete discussion of the normal stages of growth and development.)

Chronic and terminal conditions often span a number of years and developmental stages. Regardless of the stage, concerns related to self-esteem, self-reliance, and autonomy are prevalent among children with chronic conditions. Many will experience altered body awareness and body image as a result of physical changes related to the illness or treatment. These changes frequently have a negative impact on children's self-esteem. Control and autonomy may be decreased because of hospitalizations and treatment regimens that offer few decision-making opportunities for the child. Socialization activities and adjustment may be limited as a result of hospitalization and the side effects of the illness or treatment. Side effects, including altered appearance, decreased physical ability, or increased susceptibility to infection, may interfere with age-appropriate socialization. At times a medical necessity (e.g., infection risk, bleeding risk) may not keep the child from participating; rather, the child declines because of fears regarding his or her appearance or physical abilities.

Such factors may profoundly affect a child's acquisition of age-appropriate growth and developmental skills, especially throughout adolescence. An important goal is to minimize the effects of illness and hospitalization and to maximize the child's potential to the optimal degree possible. This is true regardless of the age or developmental stage, and the nurse should understand issues concerning self-esteem and autonomy in relation to each stage of growth and development (Box 12-2).

Despite the understanding and interventions of family and staff, a variety of consequences may frequently occur

---

BOX 12-2	The Illness Experience: The Child and Adolescent

Infant
Developmental task: Achievement of awareness of being separate from significant other.

Impact of illness: Potential distortion of differentiation of self from parents or significant others.

Cognitive age/stage: Sensorimotor (birth to 2 years).

Major fears: Separation, strangers.

Interventions: Provide consistent caretakers. Minimize separation from parents and significant others. Decrease parental anxiety, which is projected to infant. Maintain crib and nursery as "safe place" where no invasive procedures are performed.

Toddler
Developmental task: Initiation of autonomy.

Impact of illness: Interference with or loss of developing sense of control, independence.

Cognitive age/stage: Preoperational (2 to 7 years): egocentric, magical, little concept of body integrity.

Major fears: Separation, loss of control.

Concept of illness: Phenomenism (2 to 7 years)—perceives external, unrelated, concrete phenomena as cause of illness (e.g., "being sick because you don't feel well"). Contagion—perceives cause of illness as proximity between two events that occurs by "magic" (e.g., "getting a cold because you are near someone who has a cold").

Interventions: Minimize separation from parents or significant others. Keep security objects at hand. Provide simple, brief explanations. Explain and maintain consistent limits. Encourage participation in daily care. Provide opportunities for play.

Preschooler
Developmental task: Creation of a sense of initiative.

Impact of illness: Interference with or loss of accomplishments, such as walking, talking, controlling basic body functions.

Cognitive age/stage: Preoperational thought—egocentric, magical, tendency to use and repeat words child does not understand, providing own explanations and definitions. Literal translation of words. Inability to abstract.

Major fears: Body injury and mutilation, loss of control, the unknown, the dark, being left alone.

Concept of illness: Phenomenism, contagion.

Interventions: Provide simple, concrete explanations. Advance preparation is important: days for major events, hours for minor events. Verbal explanations are usually insufficient, so use pictures, models, actual equipment, and medical play.

School-Age Child
Developmental task: Sense of industry.

Impact of illness: Potential feelings of inadequacy or inferiority if autonomy and independence are compromised.

Cognitive age/stage: Concrete operational thought (7 to 10 years).

Major fears: Loss of control, body injury and mutilation, failure to live up to expectations of important others, death.

Concept of illness: Contamination—perceives cause as a person, object, or action external to the child that is "bad" or "harmful" to the body (e.g., "getting a cold because you didn't wear a hat"). Internalization—perceives illness as having an external cause but being located inside the body (e.g., "getting a cold by breathing in air and bacteria").

Interventions: Provide choices whenever possible to increase the child's sense of control. Emphasize contact with peer group. Use diagrams, pictures, and models for explanations because thinking is concrete. Emphasize the "normal" things the child can do because the child does not want to be seen as different. Reassure children that they have done nothing wrong; hospitalization, for example, is not punishment.

Adolescent
Developmental task: Achieving a sense of identity.

Impact of illness: Potential alteration in or relinquishment of newly acquired roles and responsibilities.

Cognitive age/stage: Formal operational thought (11+ years): beginning of ability to think abstractly. Existence of some magical thinking (e.g., feeling guilty for illness) and egocentrism.

Major fears: Loss of control, altered body image, separation from peer group.

Concept of illness: Physiologic—perceives cause as malfunctioning or nonfunctioning organ or process; can explain illness in sequence of events. Psychophysiological—realizes that psychological actions and attitudes affect health and illness.

Interventions: Allow adolescent to be an integral part of decision making regarding care. Give information sensitively because adolescents react both to the content of information and to the manner in which it is delivered. Allow as many choices and as much control as possible. Be honest about treatment and its consequences. Stress the importance of cooperation and compliance. Additionally, emphasize decision making in which the adolescent can participate as well as the areas in life over which control can be maintained. Assist in maintaining contact with peer group.

From Gibbons, M. B. (1993). Psychosocial aspects of serious illness in childhood and adolescence. In A. Armstrong-Dailey & S. Goltzer (Eds.), *Hospice care for children*. New York: Oxford University Press. Based on Bibace, R., & Walsh, M. E. (1980). Development of children's concepts of illness. *Pediatrics, 66,* 912-918.

among children with a chronic condition or illness. Most are minimal, short lived, and expected as a part of the "normal" course of a chronic condition. For example, stranger anxiety may be heightened or may reappear months after previous resolution among infants and toddlers.

Temporary regression may be seen with children of all ages, including adolescents. However, it is more prevalent among older infants through the young school-age years. Toddlers use regression frequently as they attempt to cope with the stress of a serious illness. Despite the normalcy of regression, it may be unsettling to child and family because it involves the loss of recently acquired skills or the reappearance of behaviors seen when the child was younger. Common regressive behaviors include reverting back to a bottle, pacifier, or thumb sucking; a change in toileting skills; an increased incidence of bedwetting; and an increased use of "baby talk" or communication techniques more appropriate for younger ages.

Another possible difficulty is a fluctuation in the child's age-appropriate communication patterns between family and members of the health care team. Lack of communication or altered communication patterns with health care personnel may occur in the clinic or hospital setting, with regular patterns of communication resuming at home. Among older preschoolers, a lack of communication may be a form of withdrawal or an expression of stubbornness and a refusal to cooperate. This problem may also be seen in school-age children and adolescents and is usually related to issues involving independence and self-esteem. (Chapter 11 provides a more in-depth description of the impact of illness on the individual age groups.)

Parental Responses to Developmental Issues

Regardless of the developmental stage or the number of years that a chronic illness has existed, the basic guidelines for child rearing still apply to all children in the family. Boundaries, discipline, and consistency are equally important to both the ill child and the well sibling(s). A good example is the mother of a 3-year-old with cancer who would frequently remind both the ill child and her older sibling that cancer is no excuse for bad manners!

Experiencing a chronic illness is confusing, especially for children whose cognitive abilities are not sufficiently developed to allow understanding that could help them cope with the stress. When changes in a child's world begin to affect the only constant they know, their family, this is often reflected in the child's behavior. Negative behavior may result from the stress of the illness and changes in the family and environment. Previously existing negative behaviors may worsen, making treatment, a positive relationship, and cooperation with the health care team difficult. Future behavior and long-term development may be affected as well. At the time their child is diagnosed, parents should be reminded about the importance of maintaining previous rules and expectations. Chronically ill children have approximately twice as the frequency of behavioral or psychologic problems than healthy children. Despite this risk, most children with chronic health problems are psychologically healthy (Perrin, 2004).

> **CRITICAL TO REMEMBER**
> **Goals for Chronic Care**
> **Goals for the Child**
> - Achieve and maintain normalization
> - Obtain the highest level of health and function possible—physically, emotionally, and psychosocially
>
> **Goals for the Family**
> - Remain intact
> - Achieve and maintain normalization
> - Maximize function throughout the course of the illness

THE CHILD WITH A CHRONIC ILLNESS

The goal for any child with a chronic illness is to achieve and maintain the highest level of health and function possible—cognitively, emotionally, physically, and psychosocially. The aim is similar for the family system, including parents or guardians, siblings, and extended family members. Goals for the entire family are to remain intact, achieve and maintain normalization, and maximize function throughout the illness. This necessitates a family-centered approach to nursing care.

The nursing process for the child with a chronic illness is ongoing for the duration of the illness. It may be more complex because of goals that are both physical and psychosocial. The psychosocial environment is significant in that it greatly influences the manner in which the child relates to others and copes with stress. In addition, the entire family is involved as well as the ill child. Care is provided over a span of years and must often incorporate rapid changes in the child's growth and development. The nurse is prepared for a changing assessment, both physical and psychosocial, related to duration of care and fluctuations of the illness.

Planning and implementation of nursing care are based on several factors. The child's physical condition is the first consideration. Generalization across broad categories of illnesses, such as cancer, respiratory conditions, or cardiac problems, is not possible. Each illness includes specific implications, including subsequent disabilities. The child's growth and development across the span of the illness are also very important. Additionally, the needs, coping mechanisms, and available resources of child and family are also influencing factors. Nursing care includes assisting the child and family to accept, understand, and incorporate the illness appropriately into each stage of growth and development, regardless of the child's age at diagnosis.

Ongoing Care

Evaluations as well as subsequent modification of planning and implementation of care often take place on a daily basis because of the child's frequent physical changes. Unexpected setbacks, such as an exacerbation, relapse, critical infection, an undesirable response to medication, lack of physical progress, or the need to undergo a medical or surgical procedure unexpectedly or sooner than anticipated, may be a standard part of the illness. Goals may have to be repeatedly altered. All the changes may be stressful and difficult. This may be true even for the child and family who have been coping with an illness for a long period. Continuous support and reassurance are necessary throughout the illness.

Education

With an illness that continues for several years, numerous changes may occur because of the child's physical condition or the increasing age. Education involves the child and family, addressing both physical and psychosocial issues. This ensures that the family has an accurate knowledge base to provide care at home. It also serves to assist in psychosocial needs of the child and family.

One important consideration in relation to education and support for the ill child and siblings is use of a child life specialist (Fig. 12-1). The child life specialist uses methods that are educational, supportive, and therapeutic. These may include medical play, medical art, therapeutic play, and therapeutic art (see Chapter 11). All are similar in that they present the child with an opportunity for learning, increased expression of feelings, and coping methods for the difficult situations experienced as a result of the condition. The nurse may also use some of these techniques in daily care or when a child life specialist cannot be present. Child life services are used for siblings as well as the ill child.

Communication

Communication with the ill child may be more difficult than physical care (see Chapter 3). Communication is the most important factor in establishing a good relationship with the child and family. *Appropriate communication involves honesty as well as compassion. It is always based on the child's age and development.* Following these principles can help decrease the child's fears and misunderstandings. This may

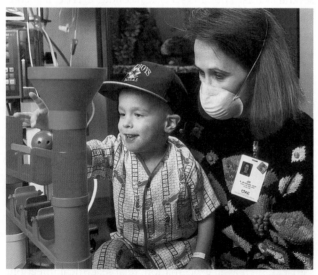

FIG 12-1 **The nurse or a child life specialist can use therapeutic play, medical play, and therapeutic art to enhance self-expression, education, and growth and development.** *(Courtesy Norm Tindell for Cook Children's Medical Center, Fort Worth, TX.)*

also help increase the child's confidence in nurses and other members of the health care team. Increased cooperation with the therapeutic regimen is an additional benefit. If fears and misunderstandings are not alleviated at the beginning and caregivers do not gain the child's trust, establishing trust at a later date can be difficult. This is particularly true when the nursing care involves unpleasant or painful medications and treatments.

To prevent misinterpretations and misunderstandings, the nurse can ask children to explain what they know and understand. The nurse should also strive to understand what the child is really asking. The classic example of miscommunication is the child who asks where she comes from and hears the entire story of reproduction, when all she really wanted to know was whether her family was from Texas or Oklahoma! Clarifying questions can help the nurse avoid providing more information than the child wants or can handle emotionally. Providing too much information may be overwhelming and frightening to the child. It may also inhibit future questions and interaction with the nurses.

Honesty and trust must be maintained at all times when caring for the child. These principles should be encouraged among the family and other members of the health care team. Complete honesty may cause problems for some individuals, family, or staff, especially when they face the difficult questions that often arise when caring for a chronically or terminally ill child. The most difficult and feared questions are usually centered on whether the child is going to die and why he or she became sick and is dying. These are followed closely by questions concerning the deaths of other children whom the child has known or with whom the child has developed a close relationship.

Children are often reluctant to question adults at all, much less ask questions whose answers they fear. Many times the child already knows the answer, so the question is really a test concerning honesty and a point of reference in the child's relationship with the adult (parent or staff). As with adults, children need honesty to establish trust. They may not understand the use of dishonesty as a means of protecting them against emotional pain or unpleasantness. Once a child has experienced dishonesty from an adult, she may feel that she cannot and will not trust the adults around her, parents or staff. Dishonesty may then have disastrous effects, particularly when trying to reassure the child and gain the child's cooperation. Often a chronic condition may progress to impending death, at which point the child's trust can be paramount to achieving comfort and peace.

For children with a chronic condition, honesty may increase their emotional pain to some degree. Conversely, it may help comfort them at the same time. Honest answers to a child's difficult questions are not always handled well by adults in the family. Realizing the importance of the child's trust, understanding and exploring feelings about providing honest answers to the child's questions and establishing and communicating guidelines up front is good practice for the nurse and family. The family may give instructions about communication that bring about conflict for the nurse, both professionally and personally. The family may ask that the nurse answer deceitfully concerning the serious nature of the illness or the fact that the child is expected to die. In many situations, a compromise is reached in that the nurse will not initiate conversations that may lead to the hard questions such as whether the child is expected to die. However, if the child initiates the conversation and asks such questions directly, the nurse will reply honestly, in terms approved by the family. This may not work with some families. In such instances, other members of the health care team can become involved to make communication decisions that best suit the needs of all involved. Such members might include physicians, a child life specialist, the social worker, and those who provide pastoral care.

Care of the Parents

Health care professionals can support parents in the following ways (Lindblad, Rasmussen, & Sandman, 2005):

- Increase the confidence of parents
- Acknowledge the parent as a person
- Acknowledge the parent as the child's caregiver
- Ease the parent's daily worries by providing information and easy access to the caregiver when questions and problems arise
- Acknowledge the child as valuable and unique
- Help the parents see the child's potential and abilities
- Help the parents understand the child's normal growth and development needs

Grief Education and Support

Nursing care should include education about the child's condition and treatment as well as education concerning the grief issues. The nurse helps all family members, including the child, to understand and express, in the manner most comfortable, their grief responses. Taking time to provide care and support in this area is as important as physical care. Many adults have not experienced illness or death before the child's diagnosis and are not accustomed to the idea of grief, much less grief as a normal, healthy process. In addition, some family members may have had a previous experience with dying, death, and grief that they perceive to have been negative and quite distressing. Both situations may increase support needs among the family.

The nurse educates the family about the importance of the grief process and provides opportunities for grieving. Such care may include conversations and time "being present" with family. Being present for all family members as the need arises entails the important aspect of listening and sitting in silence. Many times family members do not need or want conversation; they just want to be with someone who knows their child and is familiar with what they might be experiencing. This may be true even for siblings. Children who just want to be with an adult may require only that the person sit with them while they play. The expression of emotions is recognized to be more beneficial for most individuals than holding the emotions inside. However, for some, such expressions were not a normal or comfortable part of their life before their child's illness. Such patterns will likely not be altered. The nurse accepts this choice while letting the family know that a caring individual is available at any time if the need for talking and sharing arises.

Cultural and Religious Beliefs

Culture and religion influence the meaning of illness and death as well as customs observed by the family. The family's explanation of the child's disease can be revealing and may lead to more culturally sensitive interventions (Sterling, Peterson, & Weeks, 1997). When faced with an unfamiliar culture or religion, the nurse becomes familiar with beliefs and practices used and honored by the family. The nurse and the entire health care team should communicate acceptance of such beliefs and standards. Team members cannot assume that an individual or family belongs to a particular religion or denomination solely because of cultural background. In addition, they should not assume that the family adheres to all beliefs and practices of their chosen religion or denomination. If in doubt, the nurse should question the family, stressing that the questioning is an effort to provide the most comprehensive and appropriate care possible.

Health care professionals must deliver culturally sensitive care to families with chronically ill or disabled children. The meaning of chronic illness or disability to a family must be considered in light of that family's culture. Nurses must avoid cultural stereotyping and appropriately communicate with families to determine personal meaning of the illness or disability (Banks, 2003). Many excellent resources can provide the nurse with appropriate information regarding the impact of cultural and religious beliefs on illness and death, such as journals, research, textbooks, and the Internet. (See Chapter 2 for a more in-depth discussion about these issues.)

Referrals

To the degree possible, the nurse should endeavor to make sure that the physical, emotional, psychosocial, and intellectual needs of child and family are met. Additionally, nursing care includes assisting family members to provide for the child's physical and psychosocial needs themselves. Regardless of culture or religion, the nurse should not expect to be able to provide all the necessary support. This is related to a lack of both time and necessary expertise. At such times, the family should be referred to other personnel, such as members of the clergy, other spiritual counselors, and social workers. If these individuals cannot provide assistance, they are generally in a better position to refer the family to outside professionals or services. Members of the clergy generally have wider access to information on various religious beliefs as well as access to the necessary clergy from different religious sectors. The social work department will also be able to provide information concerning other helpful, necessary resources for the family. This information may include financial information, such as insurance and government assistance, housing and transportation assistance, and assistance with medical care and supplies.

Schooling

The face of public education and the child with special health care needs has changed dramatically. The Education for All Handicapped Children Act (PL 94-142) and subsequent amendments (most notably the Individuals with Disabilities Education Act, 1997) ensure a free public education for each child with a disability or other chronic condition. It also mandates that special education and support services be provided in the least restrictive environment for children aged 3 years and older. Consequently, children with a wide variety of physical needs are attending school with minimal difficulty or disruption. These needs range from the relatively simple needs (e.g., medication administration, respiratory treatments) to more extensive needs (e.g., gastrostomy tube feedings, tracheostomy tubes, ventilators). Facilitating the start of school or return to school for the child with special needs requires preparation and assistance for the child, the family, and school personnel. In addition to child and family, those involved should include a nurse from the hospital or clinic, school nurse, teacher, and counselor and director of special education.

A specific, structured plan of care is developed before the child's return to school. This is accomplished by the school system through a legally mandated process referred to as an *individualized educational program* (IEP) or *admission, review, and dismissal* (ARD). This plan is developed with input from the health care team, who are encouraged to attend the actual conference if possible. The plan includes cognitive and physical needs in relation to the child's school attendance. This plan includes those learning goals that might require alteration as a result of the special needs, as well as the specific task for achieving such goals. Both must be realistic in relation to the child's condition. The plan also addresses any special health care that is needed while the child is in school, such as medication, feedings, or other treatments. The planning conferences will be needed before the child is scheduled to start school for the first time after his or her condition is diagnosed. After the initial plan, the IEP or ARD must take place at least once a year or when changes in the child's condition occur that will necessitate changes at school. Most schools now offer children the opportunity to attend school full time as their condition allows and then change to homebound when necessary. Regardless of the type of school services the child is receiving, the hospital or clinic nurse may need to provide ongoing education and psychosocial support for the school nurse and other personnel, particularly if they are unfamiliar with the child's condition or the treatments it requires.

Special considerations are given in the school setting for a child who is immunosuppressed, whether related to the disease itself or treatment. Preventing the infection that can occur with immunosuppression is a challenge in the school setting regardless of the age of the child. Because of crowded conditions in school classrooms and the often inadequate infection control practices by children (e.g., good handwashing), preventing infection may be difficult. The school nurse should alert teachers to be particularly vigilant and notify the nurse if any infectious disease is present in the classroom. Families can also be reminded to notify the school if their child contracts certain serious illnesses such as chickenpox or strep throat. Such notification may or may not include information about the immunosuppressed child, as per the families' wishes. The school nurse can also use this as an opportunity to visit classrooms and present a health-teaching module on general infection-prevention practices. The school nurse should obtain information about the specific signs of infection that accompany specific conditions or treatments because they may differ from child to child. Information will also be required regarding how to contact the child's health care team directly and quickly if problems are suspected.

Ongoing psychosocial support may also be necessary for the child and family in relation to school. Parents may experience mixed emotions regarding their child's return to school. They are likely to be pleased and excited that the child is well enough to attend school. At the same time, they may be concerned about the child's well-being during school hours, particularly whether the special health care needs will be met appropriately. For children with a terminal condition, parents may also experience a degree of sorrow about being apart during what limited time they have with their child. The child's siblings may also experience similar feelings. The nurse can best provide support, or refer to those who can, by maintaining ongoing communication with the family, recognizing that problems and concerns with school may vary over time. Referral to others such as a spiritual counselor, social worker, or mental health professional may also be helpful for the psychosocial support families are seeking.

Regardless of whether the child is transitioning into or reentering school, all involved (child, family, health care and school personnel) must understand the impact of the condition or disability on the child's school day. They must also recognize when the child's participation in an activity must be altered and understand the need for adaptive tools or equipment (Edwards et al., 1999).

The Nurse as Liaison

The nurse is a liaison for the family in many different situations. The most important liaison work, however, is to link the family with other members of the health care team, particularly the physician. In this capacity, the nurse can help guarantee that family members receive accurate information and have an appropriate understanding of their child's condition as well as resulting psychosocial and physical needs. These efforts can facilitate the family's health care planning and help ensure a good relationship and appropriate communication with the health care team. Such efforts may also increase compliance with the treatment plan.

Care of the Siblings

Sibling concerns and needs in relation to the chronic illness vary according to age and development in a similar way as the child with the chronic illness. Fluctuations are common when the condition exists for several years. Siblings may have many of the same anxieties and fears as their parents.

Regardless of whether they are past the age of magical thinking, siblings often have feelings of guilt regarding their role in the ill child's condition. Many children with siblings have had thoughts of what life would be like without having to share material possessions and parental love with their sibling(s). When a sibling then becomes ill, the guilt and associated emotions may be overwhelming. The well sibling should be reassured about the normalcy of such feelings and that the illness is not the result of anything that was said or done by them or anyone else.

Nursing care of the sibling involves education regarding the ill child's condition, treatment, physical changes, disabilities, and expected disease progression. The sibling should always be kept up to date regarding changes in the ill child's condition. Ideally, from the standpoint of honesty, this means changes for good as well as bad. The same principles of honest communication apply to siblings as well as the child with the illness. However, what information is ultimately shared with siblings is at the parents' discretion. The hospital setting—rules, equipment, and personnel—must also be explained. If possible and suitable, the sibling may also be allowed to participate in physically caring for the ill child.

As with the ill child, siblings may also regress in developmental stage and activities. Parents frequently do not expect such behavioral changes from a well sibling and may need to be reminded that in the presence of a stressful event, regression is a normal coping mechanism for all children, both ill and well.

The nurse can help the sibling understand that illness creates stress, which may result in difficult or painful emotions, such as anger and jealousy. Children need to know that these emotions are a normal part of life, although they are often perceived as negative and harmful. Children must be allowed to have and express these feelings (Fig. 12-2). Whereas the physical and emotional needs of the ill child are generally well tended to, health care professionals and the family may too easily exclude siblings and neglect their psychosocial and emotional needs. Such oversight can lead to additional stress and problems that must be dealt with by the entire family. This, in turn, may negatively affect the ill child.

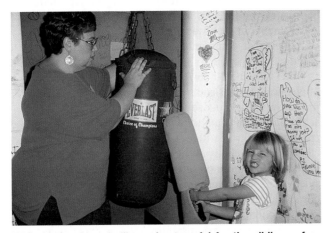

FIG 12-2 **Chronic illness is stressful for the siblings of an ill child. Siblings' emotional needs may be overlooked. Siblings should be given the opportunity to express negative feelings, such as anger and jealousy, through therapeutic art and play as well as through physical outlets such as striking a punching bag, as this little girl is doing.**

The nurse and family should include siblings as much as possible in the life and activities of the ill child, whether the child is hospitalized or receives outpatient care. The family will require education and input from the health care team regarding the pros and cons of sibling involvement. Spiritual or cultural beliefs may affect this type of decision. Many families choose to minimize siblings' time and involvement in the medical setting as a means of keeping their lives as normal and uninterrupted as possible. Other families try to maintain the existing degree of closeness between sibling and ill child and may choose the most complete involvement possible. This may include the presence of siblings during the day and for overnight visits if allowed by the institution. Regardless of the type of involvement selected and the reasons behind it, the family's decision should be honored and supported.

When more extensive involvement is chosen, the nurse should ensure that the sibling has received appropriate education to decrease misunderstanding and fear. Medical play, therapeutic play, and therapeutic art are excellent means of educating and providing support as well as alleviating fears and misunderstandings for the sibling. Such misunderstandings may be about the ill child's condition and medical treatment or the emotions and behavior they see in the adults around them. These interventions may also assist siblings to gain some understanding of their often intense and confusing emotional responses as well as how to express them in a healthy, appropriate manner.

Extensive sibling involvement may bring with it additional risks. The sibling may frequently be exposed to the ill child's intense physical and emotional experiences, which can certainly have emotional consequences for the sibling. Close attention from staff and family can help detect problems of this type if they occur. If problems become evident, appropriate team members, including nurses, physicians, child life specialists, clergy, and social workers, should provide support. As necessary, referrals can also be made to professional counseling services.

Nurses striving to teach, support, and include siblings in the hospital or clinic life of the ill child should collaborate with the child life specialist. This interaction can help the entire family discover, explore, and resolve feelings that may otherwise be problematic for both the ill child and the siblings.

The relationship between the ill child and siblings may be altered because of normal but unintentional feelings of resentment, jealousy, and competition as the ill child receives more attention. This change may be accentuated if the sibling spends extended time at the hospital, thus witnessing the extra attention given to the ill child. Siblings may experience guilt and shame about such feelings. The nursing staff, child life specialist, social worker, and chaplain can devote individual attention to the sibling separately from the ill child as a means of providing sibling support. The opportunity to verbalize emotions and interact with a caring, nonjudgmental individual may help siblings understand and accept the normality of their feelings. In addition, sibling support groups are a resource available at many hospitals.

The ill child often receives extra attention, including gifts, from family and friends during the course of the illness. Siblings may associate illness with such extra attention and gifts, subsequently experiencing real or imagined illnesses themselves as a bid for similar attention. An important aspect of sibling support is to encourage family and friends to remember the sibling when they give gifts to the ill child. It may also be helpful to remember siblings at their special times, such as birthdays or special times of accomplishment. Encouraging the parent to spend some time every day with each sibling is essential for the family to maintain emotionally positive relationships.

CRITICAL THINKING EXERCISE 12-1

How can the nurse apply the principles of family-centered nursing to the family with a chronically ill child?

Maintaining close contact with the sibling's school personnel and keeping them up to date regarding the current circumstances of the ill child are important. This can help personnel understand and support the sibling if behavioral issues are noted in school. This may also be helpful if increased absences are necessary because of problems with the ill child. Because the sibling's teacher and other personnel are generally not shared with the ill child, the sibling may turn more frequently to them for support than to members of the health care team. School personnel working with the sibling may need the same type of educational support as those working with the ill child. A school visit can be made and education provided to personnel as well as the sibling's peers and classmates. Family and members of the health care team determine the extent of information given to the children. As with school visits for the well child, education and support may best be provided by a nurse and child life specialist.

CRITICAL TO REMEMBER
Nursing Care for Children With Chronic Conditions and Their Families

- Caring for a child with a chronic condition means attending to the needs of the family system. Both parents and siblings may need additional support.
- The age and developmental level of the chronically ill child affect both the child's understanding and the family's needs. Goals may need to be frequently revised to meet the child's changing developmental needs.
- The nurse should listen carefully to the child's perception of the condition. A child's illness experience does not always match an adult's view of the physical limitations and emotional stress.

NURSING CARE PLAN

The Child With a Chronic Condition in the Community Setting

Focused Assessment

Assessment of the child involves the entire family system and its existing coping and adaptive mechanisms, regardless of whether the child is at home, attending school, or in the hospital. Note any inappropriate coping behaviors so suggestions and support for changing to healthy, beneficial mechanisms can be planned. Because coping is examined during the course of a chronic illness, the nurse needs to keep in mind the physiologic progression of the disease. As the condition progresses and the child's condition changes, so will the impact on the family and the coping mechanisms they use.

Explore the family's response to the child's illness and the family's recognition of the impact of illness on the entire family system. Discovering what each individual understands about the disease process and the treatment regimen can help determine whether misinformation or misinterpretation exists regarding information from the health care team. Explore and document the family's existing support system in the community. Such support helps with family coping and may influence the family's beliefs, responses, and methods of coping.

A collaborative assessment of the child's development as well as cognitive and physical abilities must be made. This assessment involves the child, family, school personnel, and interdisciplinary health care team. This baseline assessment of skills and abilities may be done within the context of developing a school IEP or a plan for a hospital admission. Ensure consistency of expectations and gauge the level of assistance that will be required. Assessment of psychosocial abilities should include family patterns of communication and behavior as well as emotional concerns.

The nurse should always assess the child's perception of physical changes and treatments, their effects, and their impact on the child's self-esteem. Issues of self-esteem, self-reliance, and autonomy are primary concerns for the child with a chronic illness. Even with apparently minor changes, altered body awareness and body image can lead to a negative impact on self-esteem. This assessment considers the special concerns of each developmental stage because these may change with the passing years. An 8-year-old child may be comfortable with and well adjusted to a physical change or disability yet may experience difficulties with the same circumstances on becoming an adolescent. The school nurse should communicate assessment findings when the child moves to a new school level.

NURSING CARE PLAN—cont'd

NURSING DIAGNOSIS	Risk for Delayed Growth and Development related to the effects of chronic illness or disability.
EXPECTED OUTCOMES	The child will:

- Experience minimal disturbance of normal growth and development (physical, cognitive, emotional, psychologic), as evidenced by minimal delays and documented by an age-appropriate developmental screening tool.
- Experience minimal disturbance of normal growth and development, as evidenced by ability to interact in an age-appropriate manner cognitively, emotionally, physically, and socially to the degree allowed by the existing disability.
- Experience minimal disturbance of normal growth and development, as evidenced by ability to perform usual, age-appropriate ADLs as allowed by the existing disability.

Intervention	*Rationale*
1. Educate the child and family about the physical conditions, expected physical changes or disabilities, and prescribed treatment. Education should be in a manner appropriate for the child's cognitive abilities rather than chronologic age.	1. Education encourages a sense of control and acceptance of the physical changes related to the condition as well as increased cooperation with the prescribed treatment. Many children with a chronic condition are wise beyond their years, with a cognitive ability that does not necessarily correspond to their chronologic age. These children—even those as young as 5 or 6 years—may be able to discuss medical matters knowledgeably, such as laboratory values or the results of a diagnostic procedure.
2. Set reasonable goals for improving and maximizing abilities in relation to any existing disability. Goal setting should be a group effort involving the child, family, school, and interdisciplinary team.	2. Goal setting assists children and families to increase their abilities and self-esteem through successful accomplishment of tasks. Goal setting may also increase a sense of situational control.
3. Assist the child to develop a sense of pride in existing abilities and to gain incentive to expand the range of physical abilities.	3. Focusing on activities or skills once enjoyed can provide incentive for achieving them again. For example, the child with prosthesis can strive toward becoming an accomplished skier again, but on one leg instead of two. Alternatively, the child can establish a goal of learning to drive an automatic-shift instead of a standard-shift automobile, receiving a driver's license along with peers.
4. Encourage and provide opportunities for autonomy and situational control by offering as many choices as possible. Include the child in age-appropriate decisions regarding treatment. Work with the school-age child to modify a school routine to better fit the child's educational and social schedule.	4. Autonomy and situational control are often lost as a result of limitations imposed by the condition or treatment. The child often cannot have a say in accepting a treatment or determining the type of treatment received. However, she can be made to feel a part of the decision-making process and planning. Situational control and autonomy are positively connected to self-esteem. Choices are not always possible, but when they are, no matter how small, they should be offered. Goal setting and the reasons for achieving the goal will be facilitated if the goal has meaning for the child—not just for the family or health care personnel.
5. Encourage and provide opportunities for the child to engage in normal, age-appropriate ADLs and self-care. Provide assistive devices and educate the child in their proper use. Keep equipment in a school health office for when the child needs it.	5. Self-care encourages independence and gives the child an opportunity to practice and improve abilities.
6. During hospital stays, provide regular street clothes (when possible) and items from home for grooming, eating, and recreation.	6. Personal items promote normalization despite an illness or disability and help minimize disturbances in the child's usual routines. Normalization also maintains and maximizes the child's sense of control.

Continued

NURSING CARE PLAN—cont'd

7. Provide age-appropriate activities both in and out of the hospital and encourage the child to continue regular peer interaction (e.g., sports, school clubs or activities, church, social groups) to the degree allowed by the child's physical condition or treatment. Advise the family to schedule clinic visits, treatments, and hospitalizations (if possible) so as not to interfere with social, school, or church events. During hospitalizations, support and encourage the completion of schoolwork as well as peer visits and activities (Fig. 12-3). Include well peers in special events during hospitalizations.

7. Ongoing social connections encourage development and maintenance of age-appropriate activities and developmental skills. Social involvement also positively contributes to the child's self-esteem and autonomy. Peers' misunderstandings and fear regarding the child's condition or the medical setting can be counteracted by the school nurse's or child life specialist's visits to the classroom.

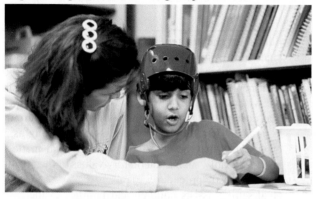

FIG 12-3   **Because more children with chronic conditions are living longer, more attend public school. However, these children are likely to be frequently hospitalized, so hospitals often provide an area where teachers can help them keep up with their studies.**   *(Courtesy Cook Children's Medical Center, Fort Worth, TX.)*

8. Encourage the child to participate in the general or disease-specific support groups found at most pediatric hospitals. Encourage participation in support groups, but accept the child's decision not to join if that is his or her choice. Disease-specific camps (e.g., for children with renal, endocrine, neurologic, pulmonary, hematologic, or oncologic conditions), at which all campers share the same problem, are also available.

8. Tremendous and valuable support can be derived from peers who have a similar medical situation. Support groups can provide acceptance and understanding not frequently found among those who are well. It may be appropriate to offer the strongest encouragement to access a support group when the child is initially diagnosed (i.e., when fears and concerns are likely to be increased). Because comfort levels and the type of support needed vary, however, such support groups may not be the best or only answer for every child.

Evaluation

- Does the child exhibit minimal developmental delays?
- Does the child exhibit age-appropriate cognitive, emotional, physical, and social interactions?

- Does the child perform age-appropriate ADLs as allowed by the existing disability?

NURSING DIAGNOSIS   Disturbed Body Image related to actual or perceived physical differences or disabilities resulting from a chronic illness.

EXPECTED OUTCOMES   The child will:
- Exhibit minimal disturbance of body image and adapt to physical changes or disabilities caused by the illness, as evidenced by stating or demonstrating acceptance of change or loss and an ability to adjust to lifestyle changes.
- Experience grief resolution regarding the loss or change, as evidenced by returning to previous social involvement.

Intervention

1. Encourage and provide opportunities for the child to verbalize all feelings, positive and negative, regarding the illness, physical change, or disability. Emphasize the normality of negative emotions.
2. Educate the child about physical changes or disability, expected limitations, or the progression of the disease, its duration, required assistive devices, and newly required self-care skills.

Rationale

1. Negative emotions will occur. To assist the child's progress to a positive, accepting attitude, these should be expressed and dealt with by the health care team and family in an accepting, nonjudgmental fashion.
2. Misperceptions concerning physical changes or disability may hamper acquisition of a positive, accepting attitude, compliance with treatment, and the acquisition of new skills.

NURSING CARE PLAN—cont'd

3. Encourage and assist the child to achieve as much independence as allowed by the physical change or disability. Provide specific suggestions to teachers and others in the community about how to facilitate the child's independence.
4. Provide constant reassurance about the child's self-worth and ability to be autonomous despite a physical change or disability. Teach the child and family the actual self-care skills necessitated by the physical change or disability.
5. Focus positively on the unchanged physical attributes of the child and the child's intact physical abilities. Teach and encourage the child, family, and others to do the same.
6. Assist the child to use aesthetic devices, such as wigs, special clothing, and makeup. Educate the child and family about more extensive measures, such as prosthetics and reconstructive surgery. Support any decision made about use of such measures.
7. Teach and encourage positive, accepting attitudes about physical differences. Foster new ideas regarding what constitutes physical attractiveness. Advocate for legislation to assist children with chronic illness.

8. Refer the child or family to appropriate professionals to manage coping or adjustment difficulties requiring therapeutic intervention.

3. Independence in self-care promotes self-esteem and a sense of control. Communicating concrete suggestions for facilitating independence contributes to a more coordinated approach.
4. An ongoing physical disability can cause poor self-esteem. It may also cause doubts regarding the child's ability to become and remain self-reliant and autonomous. These skills must be taught, encouraged, and supported.
5. Achieving and maintaining a positive body image (with resulting increased self-esteem) is often difficult when physical changes have resulted from a condition, treatment, or use of an assistive device.
6. Adults may consider physical changes, such as hair loss or scarring, to be minor when compared with limb loss or salvage, which results in disability. Children, however, often consider physical changes to be severe, resulting in negative emotions and poor self-esteem.
7. Minimizing or disguising physical changes is often necessary to foster a positive self-image. These adaptations may also be necessary to assist others to accept physical differences more easily. Many programs are available to help children adapt to physical changes. For instance, some offer advice about head coverings and makeup for the cancer patient (*Look Good, Feel Better,* a program of the American Cancer Society). Some provide fashion alternatives for those with braces or prosthetics. Disease-specific support groups provide information about available programs.
8. Some children experience serious problems such as depression. Early intervention may lead to acceptance, adjustment, and resolution of such problems.

Evaluation

- Does the child openly verbalize feelings, both negative and positive, regarding the condition, physical changes, or disability?
- Does the child verbalize acceptance of the condition, physical changes, or disability?

- Does the child return to his or her previous social involvement?

NURSING DIAGNOSIS Interrupted Family Processes related to intermittent situational crisis of chronic illness.

EXPECTED OUTCOMES The child and family will:
- Experience normal family functioning, as evidenced by maintaining usual family routines, meeting developmental needs of all family members, and maintaining usual expectations for the ill child.
- Experience appropriate psychosocial adjustment, as evidenced by expressing feelings, identifying ways to cope effectively, and using appropriate support systems.

Intervention

1. Assist the family achieve a positive, realistic view of the child in relation to the condition by providing appropriate information. Describe ways the family can continue appropriate behavioral expectations for the ill child within the limits of the child's condition.

Rationale

1. Education enables and encourages appropriate interaction with the health care team and compliance with treatment in addition to decreasing fears and misconceptions.

Continued

NURSING CARE PLAN—cont'd

2. Assist the family to identify fears and emotions pertaining to the child's illness. Emphasize that all feelings are normal and that appropriate verbalization is a positive and healthy part of coping.

3. Act as a role model for appropriate, accepting, positive attitudes and behaviors concerning the child.

4. Refer the family or child to additional resources (e.g., social worker, clergy, professional counselor) when necessary (i.e., if problems are beyond the nurse's scope or if the family requests referral).

5. Discuss with the family alternate approaches to maintaining usual routine.

2. Verbalization of feelings, with positive feedback, can help decrease stress and facilitate resolution of negative emotions.

3. Grief over the loss of a healthy child, discomfort with providing medical care, or a physical disability may hamper positive adjustment and acceptance. A positive role model may facilitate adjustment.

4. Situations requiring psychosocial assistance beyond the scope of nursing practice are not always indicators of family dysfunction requiring mental health intervention. When such intervention is indicated, however, early referral leads to a greater opportunity for positive outcomes.

5. By including some adaptations, families can maintain usual routines and meet the needs of all family members.

Evaluation

- Is the family able to maintain its usual routine and meet needs of all family members?
- Does the family treat the ill child as normally as possible to avoid overdependence?

- Do family members express their feelings? Has the family identified and utilized appropriate coping mechanisms, and are they using appropriate support systems?

THE TERMINALLY ILL OR DYING CHILD
The Child's Concept of Death

An understanding of death and dying in relation to childhood is necessary when caring for the child approaching death. The established and accepted guidelines concerning children's concepts of death are based on the stages of growth and development. As Wass (1985) explains, these concepts correlate with age and cognition (Table 12-1). In addition, a child's response to death is affected by culture, environment, and personal experiences with death (Gudas & Koocher, 2004).

Infants and Toddlers

Infants and toddlers view death in relation to the loss of a caretaker and the subsequent emptiness in their lives. They are also affected by the loss of comfort measures, such as when they experience pain or cold. Consequently, time with primary caregivers is quite important. As they approach death, they often sense the severity of their condition through their parents' nonverbal communication. Children of this age may react to the dying process based upon the sadness, anger, and anxiety conveyed by their parents. Reactions will be expressed through crying, attachment to the primary caregiver, and separation anxiety.

Preschoolers. Preschoolers view death as a separation or departure and believe it to be only temporary. Death is also seen as reversible. Magical thinking and egocentricity at this age often lead to guilt and shame because children may believe that their thoughts or actions caused the death. The child's first exposure to death frequently involves a dead animal, such as an insect, bird, or pet.

Preschoolers facing an impending death frequently view their condition as punishment for behaviors or thoughts. They respond with guilt, anger, sadness, and fear. Their

TABLE 12-1 The Child's Concept of Death

Age	Cognitive Stage	Concept
Infancy and toddlerhood (0-2 yr)	Sensorimotor	Death as loss of the caretaker
Early childhood (2-7 yr)	Preoperational	Death as a reversible and temporary separation
Middle childhood (school-age; 7-12 yr)	Concrete operations	Death as sad and irreversible but not necessarily inevitable
Adolescence (12+ yr)	Formal operations	Death as inevitable and irreversible but often a distant event

self-imposed guilt may cause them to believe that others, including parents, see them as "bad" and are angry with them. Feelings are kept inside, and children this age may withdraw from everyone, including those whom they love and on whom they depend. Their anger at those they care about and the intensity of that anger frightens them. Great patience and understanding are required of their parents and nurses, particularly when emotions are labile and subject to frequent, acute changes. Indeed, all children feel greater security when adults maintain discipline and suitable, customary limits, especially when dying children are experiencing multiple changes and discrepancies in their daily life.

School-Age Children

By the school-age years, death begins to be understood as a sad and irreversible event, yet it still may be considered inevitable only for adults. By the age of 10 years or so, children begin to understand that they too can die. Some associated feelings of guilt often persist for school-age children. They may continue to believe that thoughts or actions can cause death or that death serves as a punishment for wrongdoing.

The school-age child has increased cognition and other resources necessary to cope with the dying process. However, these same abilities may lead to additional questions and fears. School-age children may wonder why they are ill and must die so young. Fear about the process of dying and what follows may also arise. Even in children who have a foundation of faith and spiritual beliefs, this fear may persist because they do not have a concrete knowledge of what it is like after a person dies. They may also fear being without their parents' love and support, which they have always known. Moreover, school-age children may feel vulnerable and doubt their ability to cope with the knowledge of their impending death as well as the experience itself.

Adolescents

Most adolescents have a fully developed understanding of death as inevitable and irreversible. However, many adolescents view death as a distant event and may consider themselves invulnerable to death, related to their increasingly independent frame of reference. Although adolescents may understand death and dying, they do not necessarily have an emotional acceptance. Adolescents who are attempting to separate from their parents often test and break rules as they strive for independence. This process may cause guilt for the dying child, especially when contemplating the spiritual aspects of life and death.

As the result of their illness, adolescents may become isolated from their peers. The terminal illness or disability of a peer forces adolescents to face and question their own mortality and wholeness abruptly and unwillingly. Discomfort with this possibility is often the cause of infrequent visits or a total lack of visits, even from close friends. Adolescents may also become isolated from caring adults, family, and staff because of feeling that adults do not understand them. Consequently, many feel lonesome and fear that they will die without the love and support that they need and desire. Realizing that they face death when their lives are just beginning, many adolescents respond with anger and sadness, particularly when they consider the adult experiences that will be denied them. This may contribute to the onset of depression.

Responses to Death and Dying

The process of dying, as well as the actual death of a child, is a unique and complex situation. The responses of all persons involved—child, family, and staff—are affected by various factors, including personal and spiritual beliefs, previous experiences with illness and death, and experiences during the current illness and dying process. An individual's progression through the stages of grief and death is also important, as is the relationship with the dying child. At any given time, the child, parents, and siblings may all be experiencing a different stage of grief and expressing that grief in different ways.

The Child's Response

A child who is dying wants to feel safe and does not want to be alone or in pain. These concerns are frequently more intense and problematic with school-age children and adolescents. The child's responses to death and dying will be multiple and varied, not always fully correlating with the child's chronologic growth, development, and cognition. The frequently traumatizing experiences of a chronic condition and its treatment tend to make children more mature and wise beyond their years. In addition, children with a terminal illness may reach a point at which they consider their illness and treatment worse than death. Relief is frequently evident as the dying child works through the five stages of grief and dying. The responses and actions of the dying child may also be affected by the behaviors and feelings of those around them, particularly family and staff.

The child's response to dying and the resulting actions are often more precocious than would be expected, particularly among preschool children. Family or staff members often consider precocious actions and those of a spiritual nature to be inappropriate or unbelievable. They may possibly attribute these responses to physical alterations, such as a low hemoglobin level, altered neurologic status, or medications such as analgesics or sedatives.

Spiritual beliefs may influence the child and be reflected in conversation and actions. Children may speak of seeing or even interacting with angels or the Higher Being recognized by their specific faith. They may also speak of going to heaven to be with the angels or other spiritual beings. In addition, children may speak of going to play or be with another child or relative who has already died. This type of conversation may take place anywhere from several weeks to days or hours before death, with children actually giving specifics as to when they will see or be with deceased individuals. Such behaviors are commonly referred to as *nearing death awareness*.

Dying children often experience a heightened sense of understanding and awareness, particularly as death nears. Many know specifically when they will die. As seen with adults, death often occurs after children have successfully achieved closure of some type. Closure may be a special event in their life or that of a loved one, such as a graduation, holiday, or birthday. Frequently, closure also involves resolution of unfinished business, such as interacting with a loved one who has been absent or apologizing for things they have said or done.

One concept of pediatric death that families may have difficulty understanding and accepting is "allowing" their child to die. As noted by Kübler-Ross (1983), children are afraid not of death but of abandonment. Children who are enveloped by hope, joy, and love may sustain their grasp on life. For most children, allowing them to die means giving the child permission to die. A predominant issue of childhood is that children should obey their parents. This assumption is based on the knowledge that parents know best and provide guidance for their child to do what is safe and correct. A child's death may not occur as smoothly until parents tell the child it is all right to die.

Accordingly, most children, particularly those who are younger, need verbal "permission" to die, as well as reassurance that it is safe to do so. Such reassurance should include a description of what and whom to expect as they die and in the time afterward. Children may also need reassurance that the family, friends, and loved ones who are left behind will grieve yet will be all right and that they will take care of each other. Equally important to children of all ages is the knowledge that loved ones will remember them always.

The Parents' Response

When a child is initially diagnosed with any condition that is life threatening, every parent faces and begins to cope with the *possibility* of the child's death. When they are informed that nothing more can be done medically, parents face the *reality* of their child's death. The stages of grief associated with the child's illness must now be experienced in relation to the child's death. Acceptance does not always occur. Some parents may find it difficult or unacceptable to discontinue treatment. They may choose to continue treatment of a curative rather than a palliative nature. Such a choice, however, does not always indicate denial. It may simply represent a belief system based on spiritual or personal convictions. Legally, emotionally, and psychosocially, the family's decision must now be upheld and supported by members of the health care team. However, such treatment may prolong and worsen the child's dying experience by causing pain or other uncomfortable symptoms. The health care team should strive as diligently as possible to remain the child's advocate for a physically and emotionally comfortable death. This requires looking carefully at whether treatment is *doing for* the child as opposed to *doing to* the child. At such times, the team's experience with other children in similar situations may be useful in gently guiding the parents to move into the mindset of palliative care. This can enable child and family to make the most of the time left in an emotionally and physically comfortable manner.

> Parents will exhibit the need to talk about their child and the experience of their child's illness and death. They talk to assimilate the experience, but more importantly, they talk to remember their child.

When a chronic condition has extended over time, the parents' initial reaction to their child's death is often relief that the child is no longer suffering and that the uncertainty of their situation has ended. Many times, this relief and feeling of peace may begin before death, when it is known to be inevitable and imminent. Such relief may evoke feelings of guilt. Support and explanations regarding the normalcy of feeling relief may be necessary for parents. This may include a reminder that their feelings include relief that their child is no longer experiencing the illness along with the subsequent physical and emotional suffering. Relief at the death is followed by numbness, intense sadness, and a sense of profound loss and emptiness. The grief of a child's grandparent is similar to that of the parents yet, in a different manner, even greater. Grandparents grieve for themselves at the loss of their grandchild and also for *their own child,* the parent who has experienced the death of a child.

The Siblings' Response

As with their responses to the illness itself, siblings' responses to death and dying, as well as their progression through the stages of grief, vary according to age and development. Although children usually experience all five stages of grief and dying, these may not necessarily occur in the given sequence. Frequently, children move between the stages in a seemingly random fashion, often experiencing a stage several times. This process is an appropriate coping mechanism for children's cognitive and developmental needs and abilities. Issues dealt with successfully earlier in the illness, such as concern over having caused the illness or death, may resurface. Without appropriate guidance and assistance, these issues may persist. Siblings may experience other emotions, many of which are the same as those experienced by their parents. In relation to their level of cognition and development, however, they may not be as well equipped to understand, cope, and work their way through the grieving process as smoothly and successfully.

Unresolved grief may contribute to many problems in adult life. Because children work through the grieving process differently than adults do, they often need assistance to complete the process. Such assistance does not necessarily mean professional counseling. Many grief support centers are available to provide assistance for the child who has experienced the death of a loved one, including a sibling.

The most important aspect of providing support for the grieving child is to acknowledge that the loss of a sibling is *just as significant* as the parents' loss of their child. It is common practice for the health care team to send sympathy cards and other correspondence to parents after their child's death. This gesture can be taken an important step further by also addressing cards, phone calls, and other statements of sympathy to siblings individually. Such validation of their grief can be a first and important step in their successful navigation of the grieving process.

Caring for the Dying Child

Despite medical advances and current technology, many chronic disorders ultimately end in death. Providing nursing care to the child with a fatal illness who is nearing death as well as to family members requires a heightened level of understanding, compassion, and support. A family's coping abilities are often tested beyond measure. Nursing care includes assisting the family to withstand the tremendous pressures and meet the emotional demands of the situation (Fig. 12-4).

Professional Boundaries

Caring for dying children involves certain potential stressors for all involved, including the nurse. An important aspect of self-care is for nurses to recognize and acknowledge such stressors for themselves. Caring for the child who is approaching death can be rewarding, but it may also severely test the nurse's coping skills. Compassion is necessary, but also essential are awareness and maintenance of professional boundaries. These boundaries are necessary for the nurse to provide clinically sound, compassionate care while maintaining

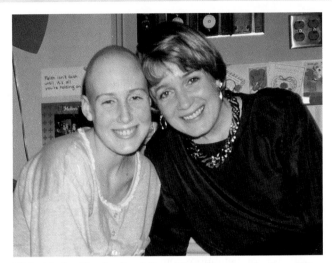

FIG 12-4 **The family of the child with a terminal condition needs compassion and support from the nurse. Nursing care includes physical care and support of the family's caregiving and assistance with the grieving process.** *(Courtesy Gwen T. Martin, Fort Worth, TX.)*

emotional, physical, and spiritual health. To provide professional care and support, nurses must understand and accept their own feelings and beliefs about death. Unresolved difficulties may interfere with appropriate nursing care. Methods to provide good self-care and resolve emotional or spiritual difficulties might include meeting with the hospital pastoral care team or a personal spiritual counselor. Nursing support groups mediated by a member of the clergy, social worker, or counselor may also be helpful. Taking part in patient care conferences or ethics committee meetings may be useful to understand patient care decisions that the nurse does not understand or possibly does not support. This could serve to reassure the nurse that the family has had appropriate education and support in making difficult decisions. It also provides nurses with education and support as they care for the child in the midst of the decision-making process.

Communication

Staff and family must be aware of the dying child's communication needs and patterns. Such awareness requires openness and acceptance on the part of all involved. Nurses and parents should assure the child that they will not abandon or leave the child alone and that loved ones will always be present. Children should consistently be reassured that the illness and approaching death are not the result of anything they have said or done or something they did not say or do.

Children must also be assured that none of their emotions and actions is wrong and that they are always loved and accepted. Children, parents, and siblings need assistance to understand their different, intense emotions, especially emotions such as anger and guilt, which are often perceived negatively. Parents, in particular, need opportunities away from the child to express their grief and anger. This opportunity helps minimize or prevent the child from feeling responsible for the parents' emotions. It also contributes to an environment that is as soothing, comfortable, and stress

free as possible in which parents can have uninterrupted time with their child and the opportunity to provide whatever level of physical care they wish to assume.

Regardless of age, most dying children will follow the rules and patterns of communication set by those closest to them. As death approaches, communication between child and family can decline in both extent and effectiveness. The nurse should take into account how communication was handled at previously stressful times, such as the time of diagnosis, relapse, or periods of disease exacerbation. Generally, what has been used in the past will continue to be effective during the dying process. The nurse should avoid blanket assumptions regarding the most appropriate or effective communication techniques for the family. Each circumstance should be carefully evaluated to assist the child and family experience the most effective, comfortable communication possible.

The most common issue that arises regarding a child's impending death is whether to inform the child of the prognosis. The needs of the child, parents, and staff frequently conflict, but all must be considered, with the ill child's needs taking precedence. The suggested approach is to adopt a policy that allows the child to maintain open awareness and communication with those who choose to do so and are comfortable doing so. Such open acknowledgment makes possible meeting the child's need for someone to know and acknowledge that the child is dying. Simultaneously, it allows mutual pretense and decreased communication with those who prefer that approach. This flexible system has been found to be effective and is prevalent among many dying children and their caregivers.

Despite such flexibility, nurses may be caught between children who wish to talk about their death and parents who forbid any such conversation. As the caregiver and primary advocate, the nurse should first meet the child's needs. Any skirting of the issues or dishonesty with the child may destroy the nurse-client relationship, possibly denying the child a much-needed source of comfort and support. The child is also likely to distrust the nurse as a result of such actions. This could be extremely detrimental in relation to the child's trust in the nurse's actions, especially giving medications for pain and symptom management. Nurses can inform the parents that they will not initiate any discussion with the child but that they need and intend to respond openly and honestly if and when the child initiates such a discussion. This policy allows nurses both to respect the wishes of the parents and provide assistance or support when needed by the child.

Words are not always necessary to provide assistance and support. Presence—simply sitting with the child—or a light touch, such as holding a hand, may be all the child needs. The silence itself may be a therapeutic intervention, or it may help open the door for desired verbal communication.

The Family's Beliefs and Practices

To support parents appropriately during the difficult time surrounding the death of their child, nursing care must impart consistent respect and acceptance. This effort must occur regardless of any differences between the spiritual or cultural beliefs and practices of the family and those of the nurse (Box 12-3) (see Chapter 2).

The nurse will encounter different beliefs and practices surrounding death and the grieving process. These practices may include wearing prayer cloths; the laying on of hands; holy water or oil; viewing religious pictures, icons, or other objects; extemporaneous prayer gatherings; or the preparation and serving of certain foods. Some practices may be troublesome to deal with because of concern over whether they are in the best interest of the child or emotionally or physically unsafe. Each situation should be dealt with individually, carefully weighing the potential emotional or spiritual benefits against proven safety issues.

Many parents have difficulty moving from active treatment with a goal of cure to palliative care only. Palliative care promotes comfort and quality of life as opposed to cure. Parents' last-ditch attempts at cure may include the use of unproven medications or treatments, such as those used in other countries. Although difficult to justify in our world of U.S. Food and Drug Administration (FDA)–approved

medical care, many of these attempts are not physically harmful to the child. Indeed, they may be emotionally beneficial to both parent and child because such efforts affirm that everything possible was tried, a notion that may be quite important to child and family. These efforts may also instill hope, which should not be taken from the child or parents under any circumstances. At times, however, such medication or treatment may be harmful to the child, as with painful intramuscular injections or treatments that may cause bleeding in a child with a low platelet count. In such instances, the staff may decide not to allow administration of the treatment. The decision and the rationale for it must be explained compassionately yet firmly, always noting that the decision was made in the best interest of the child.

Another area in which the family's beliefs and practices as well as strong emotions come into play is deciding about a do-not-resuscitate (DNR) order. A DNR order means cardiopulmonary resuscitation (CPR) or other interventions designed to initiate heartbeat and respiration after a cardiopulmonary arrest are not initiated. Even in the face of

---

BOX 12-3	**Resources on Death and Dying for Families and Health Professionals**

Internet Resources

Compassionate Friends (U.S.)—*www.compassionatefriends.org*—has brochures for parents and siblings in both English and Spanish. Discussion support groups and chat rooms are available for siblings.

Baby Steps (Canada)—*www.babysteps.com*—has an extensive book list, sharing rooms, and grieving rooms.

Book Selections for Children

Alley, R. W. (1998). *Sad isn't bad*. St. Meinrad, IN: Abbey Press.

Buscaglia, L. (2002). *The fall of Freddie the leaf: 20th anniversary edition*. Thorofare, NJ: Slack Incorporated. (all ages)

Fitzgerald, H. (2000). *A guide for teenagers and their friends*. New York: Simon & Schuster. (teens)

Peterkin, A. & Middendorf, F. (1992). *What about me? When brothers and sisters get sick*. Washington, DC: Magination Press.

Simon, J. (2001). *This book is for all kids, but especially my sister Libby. Libby died*. Kansas City, MO: Andrews McMeel. (preschool)

Book Selections for Adults—Parents and Nurses

Bluebond-Langner, M. (2000). *In the shadow of illness*. Princeton: Princeton University Press.

Coloroso, B. (2000). *Parenting through crisis: helping kids in times of loss, grief, and change*. New York: Harper Collins.

Grollman, E. A. (1990). *Talking about death*. Boston: Beacon Press.

Hilden, J. M., Tobin, D. R., & Lindsey, K. (2002). *Shelter from the storm: caring for a child with a life-threatening condition*. Cambridge: Perseus Press Group.

Ilse, S., & Leininger, L. (1985). *Grieving grandparents*. Maple Plain, MN: Wintergreen Press.

Power, P. W., & Dell Orto, A. E. (2003). The resilient family: living with your child's illness or disability. Notre Dame: Sorin Books.

Rothman, J. C. (1997). *The bereaved parent's survival guide*. New York: Continuum Publishing.

Schive, K., & Klein, S. D. (Eds.). (2001). *You will dream new dreams: inspiring personal stories by parents of children with disabilities*. New York: Kensington Publishing Corporation.

Seibeti, D., Drolet, J. C., & Fetro, J. V. (2003). *Helping children live with death and loss*. Carbondale, IL: Southern Illinois University Press.

Sourkes, B. M. (1996). *Armfuls of time: the psychological experience of the child with a life-threatening experience*. Philadelphia: University of Pittsburgh Press.

Book Selections for Nurses

D'Avanzo, C., & Geissler, E. (2002). *Pocket guide to cultural assessment* (3rd ed.). St. Louis: Mosby.

Field, M. J., & Behrman, R. (Eds.). (2003). *When children die: improving palliative and end-of-life care for children and their families*. Washington DC: National Academies Press.

Giger, J. N., & Davidhizar, R. E. (2004). *Transcultural nursing: assessment and intervention* (4th ed.). St. Louis: Mosby.

Lipson, J., Dibble, S., & Miniarik, P. (1996). *Culture and nursing care: a pocket guide*. San Francisco, CA: University of California San Francisco.

acknowledging their child's impending death, many families have a great deal of difficulty and uncertainty regarding not having their child resuscitated. They may also change their minds several times regarding the DNR. Assisting families at this time includes educating them regarding their choices, discussing their feelings about the matter, and exploring their wishes for their child. A reminder to parents that DNR does not mean withholding treatment *while the child is alive* may be helpful. Rather, it involves not initiating treatment *after the child has died*. Parents are reminded that if a DNR order is chosen, they may change their minds and revoke the order at any time. Most importantly, they are continually reassured that the child's comfort remains the top priority, regardless of the DNR status.

Parents often make treatment decisions that do not offer any hope of increased comfort and quality of life and are not based on cultural or spiritual beliefs. These decisions often do not seem to be in the best interest of the child. For instance, parents may refuse pain medication for their child because they feel the child will be more alert. They may request to continue treatments that are traumatic and offer no hope of long-term survival. The issue of pain medication may be more easily resolved than the question regarding whether treatments should be continued or extraordinary means should be used to keep the child alive. These situations may cause emotional, spiritual, and professional distress for the nurse. This may be particularly true if the action conflicts with the nurse's beliefs and seems useless for the child. To provide the necessary appropriate care, the nurse must cope with and resolve these situations. If unable to do so, the nurse should be given the option of not participating in the child's care. As mentioned, resolution of emotional, spiritual, or moral difficulties may include meeting with the hospital pastoral care team or a personal spiritual counselor. Nursing support groups mediated by a member of the clergy, social worker, or counselor may also be helpful. Taking part in patient care conferences or ethics committee meetings may be useful to understand patient care decisions that the nurse does not understand or possibly support. This could serve to reassure the nurse that the family has had appropriate education and support in making difficult decisions. It also provides the nurse with education and support when caring for the child in the midst of the decision-making process.

Pain Control

For all involved—child, family, and staff—the most troubling and emotional issue relating to the dying child is usually pain control. The nurse educates the child and family regarding pain control and then provides constant, consistent reassurance that everything possible and appropriate will be done to guarantee the child's continued comfort. Families and older children may express concerns about addiction in the same breath as concerns that pain relief will not be adequate. Without belittling the feelings of those involved, the nurse should reassure the family that their concerns regarding addiction are unfounded in the current situation.

The child and family are reminded that when a physical reason and need for pain medication exists, such as with a terminal condition, addiction does not and will not occur. Questions regarding increasing doses of narcotics and addiction may arise just as frequently in the care of children as they do in the care of adults. The child and family should be informed that the pain associated with terminal conditions may escalate acutely and frequently, with a corresponding decrease in the child's response to narcotics. The nurse should also emphasize that any necessary increase in medication dosage or change in regimen will always occur in response to escalating pain. The child and family must always know and believe that pain will be handled in a manner that provides comfort as well as the optimal environment for meeting their psychosocial and spiritual needs. (For further information and discussion of pain control for children, see Chapter 15.) Education regarding appropriate pain management, including myths and realities (see Chapter 15), should begin whenever pain medications are first used during the illness. Doing so can help ensure that education and information the family has already been given is simply being reinforced during the terminal phase of the illness.

Hospice Care

For many terminally ill children and their families, being outside the hospital environment, either in a home hospice program or at an inpatient hospice facility, may be the preferred choice for meeting their various needs during the dying process. *Hospice care* is a specialized, comprehensive system of care that provides support and assistance to the dying and their families in the last phase of a terminal illness. This phase is generally the last 6 months of a person's life. However, many hospice organizations also offer *palliative care*, for which they are a part of the patient's life before the last 6 months. This may be to assist with pain and symptom management, provide an extra system of support, or to develop a relationship with the family before the need for hospice services. Palliative care can occur while the child is still receiving treatment of a curative nature.

- The use of hospice care for children, either in a home setting or in an inpatient setting, is becoming increasingly common. In part, this increase is the result of the wide range of support services offered by hospice programs. Although specialized nursing and physician support is the primary reason hospice care is feasible, it is only one component of the array of services available through a comprehensive hospice program. These include other team members: social workers, chaplains, home health aides, and volunteers. The physical support services include pharmacy prescriptions, supplies, and medical equipment that are delivered for use in the home. The nurse can help families choose an appropriate hospice by asking the following questions (Kang et al., 2005): Has the agency had experience in caring for pediatric patients?
- If so, what was the experience like?

- Do they have staff who have been trained in end-of-life care for children?
- Are they available to come to the hospital to meet the family before discharge?
- Can they provide ongoing bereavement services after the child dies?

In general, death occurs peacefully for children, but home or an inpatient hospice facility may provide a more natural, comfortable, and relaxed backdrop than the traditional hospital setting. At home, children can have family, pets, friends, and the comfort of their own rooms and possessions nearby. Inpatient hospice care may be provided in a free-standing setting or as a separate unit within an acute care setting. Families may choose an inpatient hospice for the following reasons:

- Physical care requirements and emotional burdens are too great for family caregivers to manage.
- The physical symptoms may require aggressive management, or the child may have pain requiring intensive and complex medication control.
- The home may not be conducive to adaptations needed for the child's care (e.g., hospital bed, oxygen equipment, a private room).

Brief periods of inpatient hospice care may also be used to meet a family's respite care needs, providing an environment that is less threatening and more homelike than that available in a regular acute care setting.

Hospice care should always be offered to families along with the information necessary for making an educated choice. Some families may choose home-based hospice care but later admit the child to a hospital during the final hours or days of life. This choice, which always remains available to families, may be based on fears about pain control, adequate physical care of the child, or the emotional aspect of a death at home. Parents may be particularly anxious regarding how successfully they or siblings will cope with living in their home once a death has occurred there. This may lead to parents choosing hospitalization, even when their child prefers to die at home. Discussion of these fears early in the hospice experience is beneficial for the health care team and family. This will permit ample time to explore such fears and emotions, ideally leading to a choice that is acceptable and comfortable for child, siblings, and parents. In spite of such discussions, however, families may still elect hospitalization when death nears. The family's choices must be accepted and supported, regardless of the type or frequency of changes in decision making. Such changes may occur more frequently than anticipated depending on the changing physical and emotional status of child and family.

The Dying Process and the Time of Death

The care needs of the dying child are much like those of the chronically or seriously ill child. Much of the care is directed by the physical, emotional, and spiritual needs of the child and family. The goal of nursing care is to provide comfortable, peaceful time for the child and family with minimal disruptions. Whether the death is occurring at home, in the hospital, or on an inpatient hospice unit, the child's room should be secluded, comfortable, and quiet. This type of surroundings contributes significantly toward creating a meaningful time for the child and family.

Privacy for the Child and Family. Disruptions by staff and possibly even by friends or extended family should be discouraged and minimized to the extent desired by the child and family. Often, members of the immediate family will request private time with the dying child. Occasionally this request may cause others, such as grandparents, to become distraught or to insist on spending time with the child. In a hospital or inpatient hospice setting, this response is less difficult to handle. In such an environment, the nurse can more easily treat the matter as a request that the nurse is appropriately responsible to enforce. The nurse then saves the family the responsibility of being the "bad guy." In the home environment, the nurse has no such authority yet still remains an advocate for child and family. Therefore the nurse attempts to communicate the family's wishes to other family and friends. She also works to educate others about the importance of meeting the family's wishes and needs for privacy.

Regardless of whether privacy is requested for emotional or spiritual needs, it is important for physical reasons. The dying child's endurance will be greatly diminished, with increased needs for daytime napping and extended nighttime sleep. The child may also have difficulties with sleep, such as sleep deprivation, frequent wakefulness, or nightmares. Privacy and careful control of the number and frequency of visitors will help ensure as much normalcy and quality in sleep as possible. The knowledge that loved ones are present or close by is also helpful. In the home or inpatient hospice setting, where privacy may not be as great a problem, open doors or an intercom system (e.g., a baby monitor) can help reassure the child that loved ones are always available.

Changes in Family Routines. The availability of loved ones becomes more important to the dying child, who will experience increasingly frequent and prolonged periods of sleep. Regardless of the duration—moments, minutes, or hours—intervals spent with the child can become treasured memories. The nurse should therefore facilitate family contact as much as possible. Special care must be taken to explain to siblings the reasons for rearranging life around the ill child's wakeful times. Siblings must also be allowed to have their time with the ill child. Most important, their feelings should be explored and emotional support provided.

Family Concerns about Oral Intake. The entire family often needs heightened emotional support regarding nutrition and oral intake for the dying child. Disinterest in eating and drinking is a normal part of the dying process, yet diminishing nutritional needs can be one of the most difficult aspects of dying with which families must cope. Parents and siblings may worry that the child will starve to death and that hunger or thirst will add to other physical discomforts.

The nurse should remind the family that at a point before death—often days before or (rarely) weeks before—intake will cease as the child loses the ability to swallow. The family needs enhanced emotional support and reminders that lack of oral intake does not cause added discomfort for the dying child, even when it continues for an extended time. The family may also need to be educated that fluids may actually cause discomfort for the child by increasing lung secretions. Such secretions can necessitate suction, and the sounds of wet or rattling respirations can be emotionally distressing to the family. When kidney function is declining during the dying process, the child may also retain fluids. This can make the child uncomfortable and be visually distressing for the family.

Fluids and Oral Care. Although the lack of oral intake is normal and contributes to the child's comfort, some important nursing implications exist regarding care of the child. If the child has a dry mouth and is thirsty, small amounts of ice chips or fluids can be given when desired and requested by the child. Thirst is usually experienced only minimally, however. It is almost unheard of to have children experiencing a degree of thirst that cannot be satisfied by the amount of fluid they are able to swallow.

In light of decreased swallowing function and the possibility of aspiration, water would appear to be the best choice. Given the terminal situation, however, physical and emotional comfort can be enhanced by meeting the child's requests. Many children continue to drink their favorite fluid, such as milk or root beer, until the time of death. A lack of strength or coordination may make drinking from a glass or straw difficult. In such cases, fluids can be introduced into the child's mouth easily and without spilling, with a medicine dropper or small syringe. A catheter-tip syringe may be an even better choice because the child may find closing the mouth around the syringe's wide opening and long tip easier, although care must be taken with such a wide opening not to deliver too much fluid and cause choking. Many older children also find it easy to drink from the "sippy cups" used to assist toddlers as they first learn to drink. These cups usually have easy-to-grip handles, a secure lid, and a small spout that requires little strength for drinking. Drinking from a cup may also give the child a small sense of independence and control, which are often lost in the process of dying.

If oral discomfort occurs because of lack of fluids, several interventions may prove useful and appropriate. Good oral care will help minimize any discomfort. Sponge swabs can be used to clean the lips and mouth, but lemon and glycerin swabs should be avoided because of the drying effect from the alcohol content. Dryness can be further minimized by using artificial saliva preparations, which can be swished if the child is able and then swallowed or spit out. These preparations may also be applied with the sponge swabs along with agents to reduce inflammation or pain. Almost any type of lip balm or petroleum jelly products can be applied to dry, chapped lips. An important educational point will be to avoid lip products that have alcohol or fragrance because these might be irritating if the lips have areas that are irritated or open.

Good oral care will help minimize mouth odor and unsightliness, which may be distressing to the child and family. Providing oral care may also give the family a feeling of usefulness and an opportunity for much-needed physical contact with the child. Provision of physical care should therefore be encouraged in the amounts desired by family members and for as long as they wish, regardless of whether the child is alert enough to notice.

Responsiveness and Communication. A child's degree of awareness or wakefulness until the time of death is frequently an overwhelming concern for family members. This aspect of dying varies from person to person in both children and adults. Many children will experience a "good" period of time (either a few hours or an entire day) immediately before they die. This time may involve more strength than seen recently, more wakefulness, or more interest in family life around them. Such periods may cause family members to experience inappropriate hope for recovery. Preparing and educating families about the possibility of this occurrence are therefore important. The child may become unresponsive in the days or hours before death or may be intermittently responsive until the actual moment of death. The nurse should explain the possible variations to family members and remind them that hearing is the last sense to cease before death. For this reason, verbal communication and physical touch should be encouraged until death occurs, and even after as desired by the family.

Personal fears or beliefs occasionally make such actions difficult. This may simply reflect a different comfort level in relation to the dying process, a different need for personal space, or different expression of emotions. The absence of either verbal communication or physical touch may not necessarily be emotionally harmful to either child or family. The nurse, however, should investigate the cause and offer assistance only when lack of interaction indicates a negative effect. No matter what the type or level of touch and communication, family members should be reassured that a heightened awareness of the presence of loved ones is common for a dying individual, regardless of age. This information may impart an added sense of comfort and security.

Indicators of Imminent Death. Security and comfort may also come from knowing that reliable physical indicators usually signal the time when death is imminent. This phase may last a few hours or a few days. The heart rate increases, with a concomitant decrease in the strength and quality of peripheral pulses. Blood pressure also decreases. Pulses and blood pressure may become difficult or impossible to palpate, a state that can last for hours. Cardiac changes generally occur before respiratory changes but not always. Even if mild respiratory changes occur without significant cardiac changes, the nurse should remember how quickly and acutely a cardiac transition could occur. In some cases, apparently innocuous respiratory variations, with normal heart rate and blood pressure, have been followed by death in less than 30 minutes.

Family members more readily notice respiratory changes, which usually follow a typical pattern that is both visible and audible. The force of the respiratory effort may decline, as evidenced by rapid, shallow respirations. An increased work of breathing, along with apnea, may also be evident. The respiratory picture may fluctuate between the two states. Respirations may cease after rapid, increasingly shallow breaths. Cessation may occur after a period of Cheyne-Stokes respirations. This is a cyclic period of slowing respirations with apnea, followed by a speeding up to peak, and then slowing and becoming apneic again. Such respirations are often referred to as *agonal*. This description may impart the belief that they are painful, and thus the term should be avoided around family members.

Respirations may become more audible and may be accompanied by an expiratory sigh. This sigh often resembles moaning and may alarm family members because they interpret the sound to indicate pain. If the child is otherwise without verbal or physical indications of pain, the family should be reassured that the child's pain level is well controlled. The nurse can reinforce this information by educating the family as to the cause of the sounds and noting their correlation with each breath. If a strong belief continues that the child is in pain, then pain medications should be given.

All these variations in respiratory patterns will result in either hypoxia or hypercapnia. If hypoxic agitation occurs, it is treated with oxygen, morphine, or both. The morphine may be given IV if such access exists, or a concentrated liquid form may be given sublingually. Both measures provide physical comfort for the child and emotional comfort for the family. If the nurse is uncertain regarding whether the agitation results from hypoxia or pain, the child should be treated for pain as well. A rising carbon dioxide level may actually contribute to a peaceful and comfortable death through its sedative and analgesic qualities. Explaining this information may give the family an additional sense of comfort.

Continuing respiratory and cardiac changes may lead to cool extremities and cyanosis. These effects most often begin in the lower extremities and progress upward to the face. All these changes, although potentially distressing, are usually well handled by the family with adequate preparation and education.

Potentially most distressing is the noisy breathing caused by the rattling secretions in the upper airway. This rattling —often called the *death rattle*—occurs when the child has lost the strength and ability to clear airway secretions. Even with preparation, this sound can be extremely difficult for the family.

Pharyngeal suctioning can be helpful but may need to be done frequently and can be a source of discomfort for the child. Medications with a drying effect, such as diphenhydramine, atropine, or scopolamine, are used to decrease the secretions. Until a prescribed medication takes effect, the child can be positioned on the side to facilitate drainage of the secretions. A cloth should be placed appropriately and the family prepared to expect secretions draining from the mouth. The child is rarely aware of this respiratory occurrence, so the focus of care should be symptom management to ensure the emotional comfort of the family. When respirations have ceased, a short delay may occur before the heart stops beating. A final gasping noise may occur after the respirations and heartbeat have stopped. Reassure the family that this sound is normal and not painful.

The Family after Death. After death has occurred, family members should have the opportunity to spend as much time with the child as they desire. They might want to spend time with their child before the body is cleaned. This should not be a problem, although it might be preferable to finish body preparation and cleaning first because of the drainage, bleeding, and spontaneous elimination of body wastes that often occur at the time of death. Before the body is bathed, families often appreciate the opportunity to make hand and foot prints or cut a lock of hair as a remembrance of the child. Family members should be invited to assist in the bathing if they so desire. This final act of physical care may be a special means of closure.

Frequently siblings or other children are interested in this procedure. Adults may find such interest distressing, even if they themselves do not wish to participate. Encourage the family to allow the other children to participate, emphasizing that it may facilitate closure and correct or prevent fears and misconceptions about death or the deceased child. The nurse should respect whatever decisions are made and offer an explanation regarding what the care will involve, even if the family chooses not to participate. Rare occasions may occur when the family's time with the child or ability to participate in after-death care may be limited, such as if an autopsy is to be performed. This does occur even in the case of a terminal condition, perhaps to learn from the child's condition, such as when the body has been donated for medical research. When this is the case, families should be given the exact information before death regarding how much time they will have as well as how much involvement in after-death care will be possible.

The nurse should inform the family that the child can go to the funeral home either in a hospital gown or in personal

---

CRITICAL TO REMEMBER
Nursing Care for the Dying Child and the Child's Family

- The nurse should be available to assist both the dying child and the family but must not impose personal beliefs and expectations on either the child or the family members.
- The siblings of a dying child need time and attention. They, too, will experience grief and will need to resolve their feelings.
- Most family members need to talk about the experience of illness and death. Open communication helps support family resilience and helps family members remember the child after death.
- Caring for the dying child includes providing adequate pain control, oral care, privacy, and information on the signs of imminent death and what to expect in the immediate postmortem period.
- After death occurs, family members should have as much time as they desire with the child.

clothes and should reassure the family that the clothes will be returned after the child is dressed for burial. If the family will not be participating in postmortem care, the period just after death is a good time to choose clothing and a personal item, such as a blanket or toy. These items will also be returned. Sibling participation in this process is another good closure activity. As family members prepare to hold the deceased child, the nurse reminds them that physical change after death may occur very quickly. Changes include cooling of the body, cyanosis, or paleness, and stiffening. The nurse attempts to prevent further drainage of any body fluids, particularly if family members will be holding the child. The

---

NURSING CARE PLAN

The Terminally Ill or Dying Child

Focused Assessment

Nursing care of the dying child and the family is based on a complex set of issues. Circumstances affecting the child, parents, and siblings must be assessed and considered. Some of these circumstances include the family relationship and involvement with the child; the child's cognition, developmental stage, and previous experiences with illness and death; and the family's and child's experiences during the current illness. The nurse also explores the individual's progression through the stages of grief and dying. Children and their families may have experienced these stages in relation to the grief caused by a chronic illness; now they must experience them in relation to the impending death.

Anxiety can negatively affect the child physically, exacerbating pain or triggering other physical symptoms such as dyspnea. Negative psychosocial effects may also exist for both the child and the family. Anxiety and concerns exhibited during the current illness should be assessed, particularly during times of increased stress, such as at diagnosis or during disease exacerbations or relapses. The nurse also assesses the coping and adaptive mechanisms of both child and family.

NURSING DIAGNOSIS   Anticipatory Grieving related to the impending death of a child.

EXPECTED OUTCOMES   The child and family will:
- Experience appropriate progression through the five stages of grief, as evidenced by verbalization of an understanding of the five stages of grief, expression of all emotions in an appropriate manner, and expression of feelings by each family member in a communication style most comfortable for the individual.
- Exhibit behaviors indicating acceptance of the child's impending death and will provide care and support—emotional, physical, and psychosocial—in the manner desired by the child.

Intervention	Rationale
1. Explain the five stages of grief and their necessity for healthy grieving, including resolution to acceptance.	1. An understanding of the normal grieving process may be lacking. An explanation should facilitate grief progression and guide behaviors in each stage.
2. Identify the stage of grief being experienced and provide each family member with the opportunity to verbalize feelings corresponding to that stage. Provide positive feedback for appropriate progression.	2. Verbalization of feelings and receiving positive feedback guide behaviors and facilitate continuing progression.
3. Educate family about the stage of grief progression that are characteristic of children (the client and any siblings). Encourage patience with the extended period for a child's grief.	3. Understanding the ways in which children's coping mechanisms differ from those of adults facilitates acceptance and understanding by parents.
4. Offer all family members the opportunity to verbalize and act out, as necessary, all emotions in an appropriate manner.	4. Venting of emotions helps decrease stress and facilitate resolution of anger.
5. Exhibit a nonjudgmental attitude toward and acceptance of verbalization and behaviors.	5. An attitude of acceptance conveys care and support. It will also encourage appropriate, needed expression of all emotions, both negative and positive.
6. Encourage open, honest communication with the child to the degree requested. Demonstrate appropriate communication techniques.	6. Appropriate communication with the child will provide comfort and support. It will also ease closure and resolution of problems for the client.
7. Offer family members the opportunity to participate in the child's physical care, as desired by both parties. Demonstrate care in a gentle, supportive fashion.	7. Many individuals fear the atmosphere of dying and the provision of physical care. Learning by example will lessen fears and enhance provision of care.

Continued

NURSING CARE PLAN—cont'd

Evaluation

- Do the child (if cognitively able) and family verbalize an understanding of the five stages of grief and express all emotions in an appropriate manner and in a communication style most comfortable for each individual?
- Do the child and family exhibit behaviors that indicate acceptance of the impending death?

- Does the family provide physical, emotional, and psychosocial care and support in the manner and environment desired by the child?

NURSING DIAGNOSIS   Anxiety related to the threat of impending death.

EXPECTED OUTCOMES   The child and family will:
- Achieve anxiety control, as evidenced by open verbalization of all feelings and emotions and questions concerning the diagnosis and prognosis.
- Verbalize physical, emotional, and spiritual comfort.

Intervention

1. Educate the child and family about the terminal phase of illness, including what to expect physically, emotionally, and spiritually. Explain how needs will be met. Offer alternatives, such as hospice care.
2. Assure the child and family that the child will be safe and comfortable and will not be alone. Provide frequent reassurance as needed.
3. Provide as much privacy as possible for the child dying in the hospital setting. Allow and encourage parents and siblings to stay with the child if desired by the family. Regulate visitation by those outside the immediate family and friends as necessary.

4. Provide extensive opportunities for the family to care for the child. Teach family members the necessary physical skills. Allow the family to decline care when it is physically distressing or painful.

Rationale

1. Misconceptions may lead to increased fear and anxiety. Expression of feelings by family members may distress an otherwise comfortable child.

2. Fears about the child's comfort and security are the most common. Frequent reassurances are often necessary as the disease or symptoms worsen.
3. Families may need extended time for closure. Although visitors may be well meaning, their increased visits as death nears may interfere with time needed by the family. Because of concerns over hurt feelings, the family may have difficulty regulating visitors. If so, the staff must help by regulating visitors as a means of ensuring the family's privacy.
4. Children are usually most comfortable when cared for by family members. In some instances, however, the child and family may be more comfortable and less anxious if the staff provides certain care.

Evaluation

- Do the child and family openly and appropriately verbalize all feelings, emotions, and questions concerning the diagnosis and prognosis?

- Do the child and family exhibit physical, emotional, and spiritual comfort?

---

nurse prepares the family emotionally and provides towels if preventive measures are not possible or are ineffective.

The nurse should allow privacy for the family, promising to be close by and to return as needed or desired. The nurse always offers the support of clergy, even if no such involvement has previously occurred. If personal clergy has not been identified or is not available, the nurse reminds the family of the availability of hospital or hospice personnel. If a funeral home has not been chosen, clergy and social services personnel are good sources for assistance.

Some hospitals hold periodic memorials for children who have died. Attending these services or the funerals of children who have died supports the family through the bereavement period. Parents appreciate the efforts by staff both at the time of death and the period after (Macdonald et al., 2005).

The Nurse's Response to the Dying Child

Not all health care providers cope well with the reality of death. This limitation may hold serious implications for the nurse who chooses to work in an area where death is common. Caring for dying children and their families can be stressful and emotionally demanding. Even the nurse who works closely and frequently with dying children is not immune to the pressures and emotional responses experienced in such an environment. The demands of chronic or terminal illness may require increased emotional and psychosocial strength as well as clinical expertise.

The nurse's response to the dying process and death of a child correlates to a certain degree with the stages of grief and dying. The nurse who has become more accustomed to the reality and frequency of death may not experience each stage. Length of treatment and personal affinity often cause the nurse to become more involved with or closer to one child or another, a development that can lead to a more intense response or a delay in appropriate resolution of grief. In providing competent and caring nursing care, the nurse may have difficulty maintaining appropriate boundaries between personal involvement and professional care. A nurse who is compassionate yet can retain professionalism may be able to provide care more easily on a continuing basis in the area of terminal illness.

Regardless of the depth of involvement, level of professionalism, or the number of deaths encountered, however, every nurse who cares for dying children will experience loss and grief. Consequently, the nurse will need support through the difficult times. Both staff nurses and management must recognize this need. All must work together to provide mutual support through both active, organized support programs and simple acts of respect, concern, and care among colleagues. When a nurse begins working with dying children for the first time, having a more experienced nurse mentor may be helpful. This is true whether the nurse has many years experience or has experience working with dying adults. Parents caring for a dying child are frequently reminded that to provide such care they must care for themselves as well as they care for their child. This is equally true for the nurses who choose to care for children with chronic or terminal illnesses.

KEY CONCEPTS

- Children with chronic conditions are living longer, and more children are living with conditions that were once considered fatal. Despite improvements in quality of life and longevity, chronic illness remains stressful and is a situational crisis for families that requires ongoing attention and adaptation.
- The most important aspect of a chronic illness is that it affects the entire family, not just the child.
- Families dealing with chronic illness have many different concerns and needs. These including meeting the physical and emotional needs of the child, providing care for the rest of the family, and meeting financial burdens. The family must work together to meet the physical, emotional, psychosocial, and spiritual needs of each of its members.
- The stages of grief, as well as of death and dying, are applicable to pediatric clients but with special considerations for both child and family. The child's concepts of death and dying are based on the child's stage of growth and development. These concepts are further affected by age, cognition, and life experiences —intellectual, social, and psychological. Both ill children and their well siblings fluctuate in their understanding of death and dying as well as their response to the situation.
- The dying child, like the dying adult, desires the comfort, safety, and presence of loved ones.
- Parents must move from *fearing* the child's death to *acknowledging* the child's impending death. For parents caring for a dying child, pain is the greatest concern.

- The grief of parents is often more intense than that of the child's sibling. However, siblings' lesser cognitive abilities as well as their changing developmental needs and capabilities can make the grief of siblings more difficult to address.
- Grief is similar for all families (adults and children); grief must be processed and the loss integrated. Loved ones must understand that the person who has died is gone. They must also acknowledge and allow themselves to experience the resulting emotions. Family members must reinvest in life and go forward with their lives.
- Nursing care of the terminally ill or dying child can be extremely stressful and demanding. It requires strict attention to one's own physical, emotional, and spiritual health. Care of the caregiver is imperative if the nurse is to provide physical and psychosocial care for families at such a difficult time.

ANSWERS TO CRITICAL THINKING EXERCISE 12-1

The nurse can assist family members in problem solving and using their coping skills. The family is educated regarding the medical aspects of the disease and how to care for their child physically at home. Interpersonal communication among family members and the development of social supports should be encouraged. Siblings should be included in the assessment of the family and incorporated into the plan of care for the family. Community resources that support both child and family should be identified and the family helped to access such support systems as they see fit.

REFERENCES AND READINGS

American Academy of Pediatrics Committee on Children With Disabilities. (2000). Policy statement: provision of educationally-related services for children and adolescents with chronic diseases and disabling conditions. *Pediatrics, 105,* 448-451.

American Academy of Pediatrics Committee on Bioethics and Committee on Hospital Care. (2000). Policy statement: palliative care for children. *Pediatrics, 106,* 351-357.

American Academy of Pediatrics Council on Children With Disabilities. (2005). Policy statement: care coordination in the medical home: integrating health and related systems of care for children with special health care needs. *Pediatrics, 116,* 1238-1244.

Banks, M. (2003). Disability in the family: a life span perspective. *Cultural Diversity & Ethnic Minority Psychology, 9,* 367-384.

Carter, B. S., & Levetown, M. (2004). *Palliative care for infants, children and adolescents: a practical handbook.* Baltimore: The Johns Hopkins University Press.

Chernoff, R., Ireys, H., DeVet, K., & Young, K. (2002). A randomized controlled trial of a community-based support program for families of children with chronic illness: pediatric outcomes. *Archives of Pediatrics & Adolescent Medicine, 56,* 533-540.

Chesson, R. A., Chisholm, D., & Zaw, W. (2004). Counseling children with chronic physical illness. *Parent Education and Counseling, 55,* 331-338.

Contro, N. A., Larson, J., Scofield, S., Sources, B., & Cohen, H. J. (2004). Hospital staff and family perspectives regarding quality of pediatric palliative care. *Pediatrics, 115,* 1248-1252.

Cox, A. H., Marshall, E. S., Mandleco, B., & Olsen, S. F. (2003). Coping responses to daily life stressors of children who have a sibling with a disability. *Journal of Family Nursing, 9,* 397-413.

Edwards, P., Hertzberg, D., Hays, S., & Youngblood, N. (1999). *Pediatric rehabilitation nursing.* Philadelphia: Saunders.

Finnegan, A. (2004). Sexual health and chronic illness in childhood. *Paediatric Nursing, 16,* 32-36.

Freyer, D. R. (2004). Care of the dying adolescent: special considerations. *Pediatrics, 113,* 381-388.

Garro, A., Thurman, S. K., Kerwin, M. E., & Ducette, J. P. (2005). Parent/caregiver stress during pediatric hospitalization for chronic feeding problems. *Journal of Pediatric Nursing, 20,* 268-275.

Godshall, M. (2003). Caring for families of chronically ill kids. *RN, 66,* 30-35.

Gudas, L. S., & Koocher, G. P. (2004). In R. E. Behrman, R. M. Kliegman, & H. B. Jenson (Eds.). *Nelson textbook of pediatrics* (17th ed., p. 118). Philadelphia: Elsevier Saunders.

Guite, J., Lobato, D., Kao, B., & Plante, W. (2004). Discordance between sibling and parent reports of the impact of chronic illness and disability on siblings. *Children's Health Care, 33,* 77-92.

Hames, C. C. (2003). Helping infants and toddlers when a family member dies. *Journal of Hospice and Palliative Nursing, 5,* 103-110.

Health Resources and Services Administration, Maternal and Child Health Bureau. (2003). *Division of services for children with special health needs fact sheet.* Rockville, MD: U.S. Department of Health and Human Services.

Heller, K. S., & Solomon, M. Z. (2005). Continuity of care and caring: what matters to parents of children with life-threatening conditions. *Journal of Pediatric Nursing, 20,* 335-346.

Inkelas, M., & Garro, N. (2005). A picture of needs for children with special health-care needs: what we are learning from the national survey. *Journal of Pediatric Nursing, 20,* 207-210.

Institute of Medicine of the National Academies. (2003). *When children die: improving palliative and end-of-life care for children and their families.* Washington, DC: The National Academies Press.

Ipstein, I., Stinson, J., & Stevens, B. (2005). The effects of camp on health-related quality of life in children with chronic illnesses: a review of the literature. *Journal of Pediatric Oncology Nursing, 22,* 89-103.

Ireys, H., Chernoff, R., DeVet, K., & Kim, Y. (2001). Maternal outcomes of a randomized controlled trial of a community-based support program for families of children with chronic illness. *Archives of Pediatric and Adolescent Medicine, 155,* 771-777.

Jacobs, H. H. (2005). Ethics in pediatric end-of-life care: a nursing perspective. *Journal of Pediatric Nursing, 20,* 360-369.

Jennings, P. D. (2005). Providing pediatric palliative care through a pediatric supportive care team. *Pediatric Nursing, 31,* 195-200.

Johnson, C. P., & Kastner, T. A. (2005). Helping families raise children with special health care needs at home. *Pediatrics, 115,* 507-511.

Kang, T., Hoehn, K. S., Licht, D. J., Mayer, O. H., Santucci, G., Carroll, J. M., et al. (2005). Pediatric palliative, end-of-life, and bereavement care. *Pediatric Clinics of North America, 52,* 1029-1046.

Kastner, T. A. (2004). Managed care and children with special health care needs. *Pediatrics, 114,* 1693-1698.

Kübler-Ross, E. (1969). *On death and dying.* New York: Macmillan.

Kübler-Ross, E. (1983). *On children and death.* New York: Macmillan.

Kuebler, K. K., Davis, M. P., & Moore, C. D. (2005). *Palliative practices: an interdisciplinary approach.* St. Louis: Elsevier Mosby.

Langton, H. (2000). *The child with cancer: family centered care.* St. Louis: Saunders.

Lindblad, B. M., Rasmussen, B. H., & Sandman, P. O. (2005). Being invigorated in parenthood: parents' experiences of being supported by professionals when having a disabled child. *Journal of Pediatric Nursing, 20,* 288-297.

Lugton, J., & Kindlen, M. (Eds.). (1999). *Palliative care: the nursing role.* Philadelphia: Churchill Livingstone.

Lyon, M. E. (2004). What do adolescents want? An exploratory study regarding end-of-life decision-making. *Journal of Adolescent Health, 35,* 529-534.

Macdonald, M. E., Liben, S., Carnevale, F. A., Rennick, J. E., Wolf, S. L., Meloche, D., & Cohen, S. R. (2005). Parental perspectives on hospital staff members' acts of kindness and commemoration after a child's death. *Pediatrics, 116,* 884-890.

Patterson, J. M. (2002). Integrating family resilience and family stress theory. *Journal of Marriage and Family, 64,* 349-360.

Perrin, J. M. (2004). Developmental disabilities and chronic illness. In R. E. Behrman, R. M. Kliegman, & H. B. Jenson (Eds.). *Nelson textbook of pediatrics* (17th ed., p. 137). Philadelphia: Elsevier Saunders.

Rushton, C. H. (2005). A framework for integrated pediatric palliative care: being with dying. *Journal of Pediatric Nursing, 20,* 311-325.

Sterling, Y., Peterson, J., & Weekes, D. (1997). African-American families with chronically ill children: Oversights and insights. *Journal of Pediatric Nursing, 12*(5), 292-300.

Walker, C., Wells, L., Heiney, S., Hymovich, D., & Weeks, D. (1993). Nursing management of psychosocial care needs. In G. Foley, D. Fachman, & K. Mooney (Eds.). *Nursing care of the child with cancer.* Philadelphia: W. B. Saunders.

Wang, K. K. (2004). Technology-dependent children and their families: a review. *Journal of Advanced Nursing, 45,* 36-46.

Wass, H. (1985). Concepts of death: a developmental perspective. *Issues in Comprehensive Pediatric Nursing, 8*(1-6), 3-25.

Widger, K. A. (2004). What are the key components of quality perinatal and pediatric end-of-life care? A literature review. *Journal of Palliative Care, 20,* 105-112.

Williams, P., Williams, A., Graff, C., Hanson, S., Stanton, A., Hafeman, C., Liebergen, A., Leuenberg, K., Setter, R., Ridder, L., Curry, H., Barnard, M., & Sanders, S. (2003). A community-based intervention for siblings and parents of children with chronic illness or disability: the ISEE study. *The Journal of Pediatrics, 143,* 386-393.

CHAPTER 13

Principles and Procedures for Nursing Care of Children

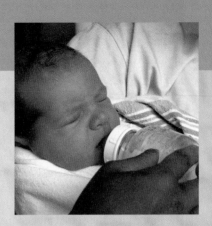

Learning Objectives

After studying this chapter, you should be able to:

- Describe how to prepare children and families for selected procedures frequently seen in an acute care setting and home care setting.
- Compare anatomic and physiologic differences in children and adults as they apply to selected procedures.
- Identify psychosocial considerations unique to children undergoing selected procedures.
- Describe techniques useful for eliciting cooperation from the child undergoing selected procedures.
- Describe step-by-step nursing actions and the rationales for performing selected procedures.

Definitions

antipyretic An agent that reduces or relieves fever.

apical pulse rate Heart rate determined by placing the stethoscope over the point of maximal intensity and counting for 1 minute.

auscultate To listen to body sounds (e.g., heart sounds, breath sounds).

enteral By way of the digestive system (e.g., enteral feeding).

epiglottitis Inflammation of the epiglottis.

hand hygiene Cleansing of the hands with soap and water, antiseptic handwash, alcohol-based hand rub, or surgical hand antisepsis (CDC, 2002; CDC, 2005a).

informed consent A requirement, both legal and ethical, that the child and the parent or guardian completely understand proposed procedures or treatments, including their benefits and risks.

lavage Wash.

pyrogens Substances that cause fever.

Standard Precautions Infection control guidelines developed by the National Center for Infectious Disease and the Hospital Control Practices Advisory Committee to prevent the spread of infectious organisms from blood, body fluids, secretions and excretions, mucous membranes, and nonintact skin.

Electronic Resources

Additional information related to the content in Chapter 13 can be found on:

the interactive companion CD-ROM

- Animations: Central Venous Access via Jugular Vein
        IV Line Placement
        PICC Line Placement
- Audio Glossary
- NCLEX Review Questions
- Skills: Infant Bathing
        Measuring Baby Temperature
        Measuring Oxygen Saturation
        Preparing the Child for Procedures
        Urine Specimen Collection

or the companion website at *evolve*
http://evolve.elsevier.com/james/ncoc

- NCLEX Review Questions
- Standard Precautions
- WebLinks

Children need preparation before and accurate information about any procedure that is performed. This information is essential to promote a sense of security, decrease fear, elicit cooperation, and improve coping skills. Parents also need preparation because their anxiety about a procedure may be transferred to the child.

Before preparing the child and family for any procedure, the nurse needs to plan how to carry out the procedure in the most effective manner. The nurse can implement strategies to help the child and parents through all phases of a procedure, including the anticipation and preparation for the procedure, the actual procedure, and the period after the procedure. Teaching before performing procedures also helps increase the child's and family's knowledge base.

CRITICAL TO REMEMBER
Standard Precautions

Always wash your hands and follow Standard Precautions before beginning any procedure. Wash your hands again when the procedure is finished.

PREPARING CHILDREN FOR PROCEDURES

Adequately preparing children and families for procedures, especially those that are painful, threatening, or invasive, necessitates a thorough, individualized assessment. This process should include an assessment of the child's age and developmental level, personality, existing level of knowledge, present level of understanding, past experience, coping skills, and family situation. The nurse can then match explanations and teaching to the specific needs of the child and family.

Explaining Procedures

Mentally reviewing the procedure before giving explanations is especially important if the procedure is seldom performed, new, or unfamiliar. Thinking about the procedure in advance provides an opportunity for the nurse to request sedation for the child, gather extra supplies, and obtain assistance as necessary. Gather all equipment to be used and check that it functions before beginning any procedure.

Explaining procedures includes demonstrating equipment and describing anything the child will feel, see, hear, and smell. Use words the child will understand, and use a developmentally appropriate approach. Relating the experience to an object or situation familiar to the child or one in which the child is interested helps.

Appropriately timing the explanation is critical. Many children respond better to procedures if the explanation is given either just before the procedure or step by step as the procedure unfolds. Some older children and adolescents like to be prepared well in advance in case they have questions that need answering. Advance preparation allows the child to express feelings about the procedure through role play. Often parents can inform the nurse about the best timing for their child, so the nurse needs to question the parents about the best approach for their child. If possible, time should be

allowed for questions and for the child to become familiar with the equipment (Box 13-1).

Also important for a child's successful coping with an invasive or painful procedure is the presence of someone the child trusts. Time spent establishing a trusting relationship with a child is time well spent. Trust in health care providers can enhance the child's unique coping strategies.

Before procedures, ensure the child's privacy by closing the door to the room and drawing a curtain around the bed or, optimally, by taking the child to a treatment room if

---

BOX 13-1 | **Tips for Preparing and Supporting Children Undergoing Procedures**

Before the Procedure
- Offer the child ways to cope with pain or discomfort. For example, some children can use coping strategies such as guided imagery. Others may listen to a radio, increasing the volume as the discomfort level increases. Give the child permission to cry or yell if necessary.
- Use developmentally appropriate words when discussing the procedure and expectations.
- Give the child as much choice as possible over what will happen. For example, when possible, the child could be allowed to choose an injection site or a site for intravenous catheter placement.
- Be sure the consent form has been signed, if applicable.
- Always wash your hands thoroughly before beginning any procedure and follow Standard Precautions.

During the Procedure
- Talk to the child during the procedure if the child desires. If the child is using a coping strategy such as guided imagery, however, talking will be a distraction and will decrease the child's ability to cope with what is happening.
- Keep the child informed of the procedure's progress.
- Tell the child when the procedure is nearly completed and the "worst is over."

After the Procedure
- *Praise* the child for *attempts* at cooperation even if the child did not do anything you asked. Trying counts! Specifically praise the child for accomplishing an expected task.
- Provide an opportunity for the child to vent feelings about the procedure. Remember that expressing feelings of anger is appropriate. Tell the child that you understand if the child does not want to talk with you right now and that you will return later.
- If parents were not present during the procedure, reunite the child with the parents and allow them to provide comfort and support.
- Reward the child by using age-appropriate methods such as stickers.
- Record the preparation process and procedure performance, who performed the procedure, the child's tolerance of the procedure, and its outcomes.

appropriate and comfortable for the child and parent. The treatment room contains suitable equipment for invasive procedures and is a private area away from the safe haven of a child's room or the playroom (Fig. 13-1). Visitors should be asked to leave, and parents might also choose to leave at this point, although parental participation is supported and encouraged.

Telling children or parents what they can do to help gives them control and decreases potential feelings of powerlessness. For example, if the child must hold an extremity still for the placement of an intravenous (IV) catheter or for blood work, the child must know about this need *before* the procedure is begun.

> You might say to the child, "We have talked about why you need to have blood taken from your arm, but you need to know how important it is for you to hold your arm very still while we are doing this. I will tell you everything that is going to happen so you can be prepared and know when to help. Do you think you can help us, or do we need to ask someone to help you remember?"

Offer children choices when feasible. For example, let a child choose the type of colorful bandage that will cover an injection site or whether to have a procedure done before or after the next television show. Do not threaten children with punishment for not cooperating. Nurses need to have realistic expectations that are based on the child's developmental level and knowledge of the child's capacity for cooperation.

Involve parents as much as they want according to what is possible during procedures. For example, a child might be much more cooperative in taking oral medications if the mother administers them. Often, by explaining what the parents will be seeing and what they can do, the nurse helps them feel comfortable staying with and supporting their child. The nurse should recognize, however, that parents might be uncomfortable remaining with their child during a painful or invasive procedure. Give parents permission to leave if they desire and assure them that they will be called if they are needed or as soon as the procedure is completed.

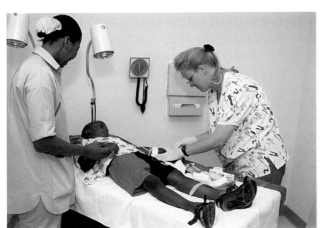

FIG 13-1   **Because a child should feel that the hospital room is a safe place, a treatment room is used for invasive or painful procedures. The parent is present, not to restrain the child, but to provide emotional support.**

CRITICAL TO REMEMBER
Preparation for Procedures

- A treatment room is the preferred location for performing painful procedures. It is a private area away from the safe haven of a child's hospital room, and it usually contains the necessary equipment for a variety of procedures (see Fig. 13-1).
- Ensure that a person the child trusts is there for support.
- Use terminology appropriate for the child's developmental level. Avoid using words or phrases that the child might misinterpret (e.g., dye, put to sleep, stick).
- Offer the child choices if appropriate.
- Tell the child and family how they can help with the procedure.
- Do not threaten punishment for lack of cooperation.
- Encourage parental participation in the procedure, but do not force an unwilling parent to stay.

Consent for Procedures

All surgical or diagnostic invasive procedures, particularly those that involve risk to the child, require *informed consent*. Some examples are lumbar puncture, chest tube insertion, and bone marrow aspiration. Both legal and ethical requirements exist to inform the child, if appropriate, and the child's parents of the benefits and risks of the proposed procedure or treatment. Informed consent must be obtained from the parent or legal guardian *before* the procedure is performed.

Other procedures, such as IV line insertions, specimen collection, and medication and oxygen administration, are covered under the general consent to treat that is signed at admission. It is now also customary to obtain *assent* from children 7 years old and older. Assent means that the child has been fully informed about the procedure and concurs with those giving the informed consent. Laws on informed consent vary from state to state, so nurses should become familiar with the laws and policies of their institution. (See Chapter 1 for specific information related to legal issues.)

The person performing the procedure should obtain the consent. Nurses need to check that the consent form is signed and witnessed, and they need to answer questions relating to the procedure. Occasionally an emergency or life-threatening situation arises in which contacting the parents or legal guardian for consent is not possible. In such cases administrative consent may be obtained to allow physicians to perform the indicated procedures. (See Chapter 1 for legal issues related to informed and emergency consent provisions.)

HOLDING AND TRANSPORTING INFANTS AND CHILDREN

Infants can be held in several positions (Fig. 13-2). Before the infant is discharged from the hospital, the nurse teaches new parents how to hold the infant, and nurses working on children's units should hold infants in similar ways. Hold the infant securely, anticipating sudden movement; because

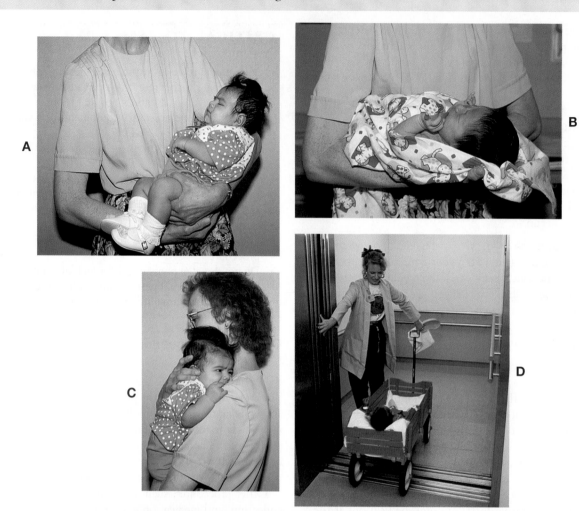

FIG 13-2 **Methods of transporting infants and children. The nurse carries the infant securely, anticipating sudden movement. A, Cradle carry. B, Football hold. C, Over-the-shoulder carry, which can be used until the infant is 6 to 7 months old. D, Transport can be fun for young children, especially when it is on wheels.** *(A, B, and C courtesy Parkland Health and Hospital System District Community Oriented Primary Care Clinic, Dallas; D courtesy Cook Children's Medical Center, Fort Worth, TX.)*

infants younger than 4 months do not have well-established head control, supporting the head is essential. Cradle infants up to 2 to 3 months of age by holding them in a horizontal position, supporting the back, and grasping the thigh (see Fig. 13-2, A). When using the football hold, tuck the infant between your body and elbow, with your arm carrying the infant's body and your hand supporting the head (see Fig. 13-2, B). When carrying the infant upright, hold the infant erect against your chest (see Fig. 13-2, C). Rest the infant's buttocks on your forearm, and support the infant's head and shoulders with your other arm. Even for infants with well-developed neck muscles and head control, this extra support prevents the infant from falling backward should the infant make a sudden move. Advise parents who use a backpack or front-facing baby carrier to be sure that the infant's head is supported in the carrier at all times.

Hospitalized infants and children sometimes must be transported to other areas within a hospital unit or even outside the unit. A change in location might be a response to changes in the child's condition or might be done to increase parental involvement in the child's care (e.g., rooming-in). Children may also be transported for specialized care (e.g., rehabilitation) or for diagnostic testing. In addition, children might be transported to different areas on the same unit (e.g., treatment room, playroom).

The method of transportation will depend on the child's age, developmental level, and physical condition; the destination; safety factors; and whether specialized equipment is needed to accompany the child. Any special accommodations should be arranged before the time of the planned transfer.

Infants and toddlers can also be transported in a bassinet or crib. The rails should always be up, and for older infants and toddlers the protective top should be in place. Strollers and wagons can be used to transfer older infants and toddlers to other areas on the unit (see Fig. 13-2, D). Use safety belts, and make sure the sides of the wagon are raised. Do not leave an infant or toddler unattended. In all methods of transfer, equipment (e.g., IV pump, enteral feeding pump, oxygen) can be pushed or pulled along with the transporting vehicle or, in some cases, stored on a lower shelf of the transport vehicle. Do not place equipment in the transporting unit with infants or young children.

Transport older children in the same manner as adults (e.g., in wheelchairs or on stretchers with the side rails raised). In some cases, such as for a child in traction, transporting the child in the bed is preferable. As for younger children, remember to use safety belts, raised sides, and constant supervision.

USING RESTRAINTS

Safety is of paramount concern for all children, particularly infants and toddlers. Nurses and parents need to be especially vigilant about raising side (crib) rails and keeping small objects away from young children. *Always place your hand on an infant's or young child's back or abdomen when the sides of the bed are down or when the child is in a high place; teach parents to do the same.* Keep small objects off bedside tables or any area within the child's reach.

Occasionally, to prevent trauma, temporarily restraining a child is necessary to suspend movement during certain procedures. In this instance, the restraint is removed as soon as the procedure is complete.

Some children are particularly active and prone to injury. Restraining the child might be the only option for maintaining the child's safety. All possible alternatives to restraint should be considered before applying the restraint. These alternatives might include using a sitter; behavior modification techniques, such as a time out; or diversional activities, such as reading. If restraint is considered for unruly or dangerous behavior, the cause of the behavior should also be examined. Causes can include hypoxia (decreased oxygenation), sedation, adverse drug reactions, and mental illness.

The Omnibus Budget Reconciliation Act of 1987 states that restraints should be used only as a last resort for the protection of the client and others. The legislation further specifies that restraints should not be applied merely for the staff's convenience.

Physical restraints include items such as mitts, elbow restraints, and ankle and wrist restraints. Jacket restraints (safety vests), which might be used primarily to keep children in bed after surgery, are used with caution on a general children's unit because extremely active children can get twisted and caught in the restraint. Most facilities require a physician's order stating why any restraint is needed and how long it will be in place. The restraint chosen should be the least restrictive device that will prevent injury. Less-restrictive protective restraints include such mechanisms as a plastic bubble top placed over a crib. Examples of restraints used for children are illustrated in Figure 13-3.

Elbow restraint

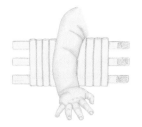

Prevents child from flexing and reaching face, head, IV and other tubes. Position so that it does not rub against the axilla.

Crib top bubble restraint

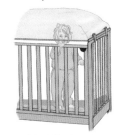

Prevents older infant and younger child from falling and climbing out of bed.

Mummy restraint (body restraint)

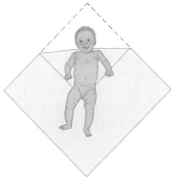 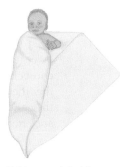 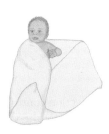 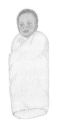

A restraint can be made from a sheet folded into a square of the appropriate size for the infant. Start by folding the top corner under the infant's shoulders and aligning the infant's head with the folded edge.

Fold one point of the sheet across the child and tuck it firmly behind the back.

Fold the bottom corner of the sheet up to cover and restrain the infant's feet.

Fold the remaining corner over the child and tuck firmly behind the back.

FIG 13-3 **Examples of pediatric restraints.**

Before placing the restraint, check the area to be restrained for any sign of compromised circulatory, integumentary, and neurologic systems. Also note any orthopedic alterations. If these conditions exist, extra monitoring of the restrained extremity will be needed.

Preparing the Child and Family

When restraints are applied, the child and family should be told why the restraint will be used, where it will be applied, what movement it will prevent, and how long it will be in place. Tell the child and family how often a nurse will check on the child. Have the call button readily available to older children so they can call the nurse as needed. If possible, consider and meet the child's developmental needs, such as thumb sucking. For example, an infant's or toddler's arm can be restrained so that the thumb can still be placed in the mouth.

Check the extremity distal to restraints for temperature, pulses, and capillary refill (circulation, sensation, motion) every 15 minutes for 1 hour after initial placement. After that, check and record findings at least every hour and more often if the child is aggressive or extremely active or if institution policy dictates more frequent assessment. Remove restraints every 2 hours to allow for range-of-motion movement and repositioning and to offer the child food or the opportunity to use the bathroom.

CRITICAL TO REMEMBER
Using Restraints

- Use the least restrictive restraint.
- Choose the proper device for the child's condition.
- Ensure proper fit of the device.
- Tie knots that can be easily untied for quick access.
- Secure ties to bed frames (not mattresses or side rails), to the frames of wheelchairs, or to another stable device.
- Frequently check and record the child's neurovascular status, behavior, and general condition.

Documentation

Record findings from hourly neurovascular checks and any other changes in the child's behavior or condition. Every 2 hours, record removal of restraints, range of motion, and position changes. Be particularly alert for skin irritation under the restraints.

INFECTION CONTROL
Hand Hygiene

Hand hygiene is the mainstay of infection control in health care settings and in the home. In 2002, the Centers for Disease Control and Prevention (CDC) published data regarding transmission of organisms by health care workers in hospital settings. By using evidence based on research that demonstrates that organisms are present both in hospitalized patients and on environmental surfaces, and that alcohol-based hand rubs are more effective for eliminating organisms,

the CDC (2002) issued the following new recommendations for hand hygiene:

1. If hands are contaminated with blood or body fluids, or visibly soiled, clean hands with soap and water.
2. If hands are clean, use an alcohol-based hand rub before and after patient contact, before putting on gloves for a procedure, and after removing gloves.
3. Put alcohol-based hand rub on the hands, rub over all surfaces of hands and fingers, and allow to thoroughly dry (total time, approximately 20 seconds).

Procedures described subsequently in this book assume that the nurse will use appropriate hand hygiene both before and after each procedure.

Standard Precautions

Standard Precautions, which are used in institutions and the workplace for infection prevention, apply to the following:

- Blood
- All body fluids, secretions, and excretions except sweat, regardless of whether they contain visible blood
- Nonintact skin
- Mucous membranes

Two tiers of precautions are under this system. *Standard Precautions,* precautions in the first tier, apply in the care of all hospitalized clients without regard for diagnosis or presumed infectious state. Second-tier precautions apply in the care of specific clients and are referred to as *Transmission-Based Precautions.* They are for clients known or suspected to be infected by pathogens that are transmitted through air or droplet or through contact with dry skin or contaminated surfaces.

The complete guidelines for applying Standard Precautions and Transmission-Based Precautions are quite detailed and extensive. Each facility is responsible for making these guidelines available and implementing the precautions.

Implementing Precautions

When Transmission-Based Precautions are in effect, the items with which the infected child comes in contact are also contaminated. These items include the bed, linens, IV pump, sink, and toys. Therefore the nurse who is going in the room to reset an IV pump, pick up soiled linens, and so forth must use whatever protective equipment is mandated by the type of precaution (gown, mask, gloves).

Children placed on Transmission-Based Precautions often need extra attention to avert boredom. They need more diversional activities, such as games or movies, and more psychosocial support. Young children, for example, may think that they are being punished. Visitors might hesitate to enter the child's room and may need additional support or reassurance from the nurse.

Family Teaching

Family education is crucial for effective infection control or prevention; emphasize to parents, other visitors, and other health care providers that infection control precautions are important and must be closely followed. Parents often state that they are there to visit only their child and do not understand the need to wear special clothing or equipment. The nurse needs to emphasize that some diseases, such as respiratory syncytial virus, can live on inanimate objects such as clothing for up to 48 hours and can spread throughout the hospital or to the home if infection control or prevention measures are not followed. Encourage family members to visit the child frequently because visits will decrease the child's sense of isolation. Advise the family that meticulous handwashing, both in the hospital setting and at home, is the best infection prevention.

BATHING INFANTS AND CHILDREN

The nurse can use bath time as a time to help parents interact with their infants. During the bath, the nurse assists the parent by demonstrating how to hold the infant securely and how to bathe the infant so that bath time is a positive time for parent and child. Encouraging the parent to observe the infant's physical and emotional characteristics during the bath can enhance attachment (Amy, 2001).

Strictly observing safety principles when bathing an infant or child can prevent falls, burns, or aspiration of water. When bathing an infant or a child in the hospital setting, take the opportunity to note any problems, such as altered skin integrity, surgical incisions, loss of sensation, abnormal skin color, bruising, paralysis, or any other condition that might warrant special consideration. Newborn infants can be immersed in water after the umbilical stump and circumcision sites (if applicable) have healed. The temperature of the bath water should not exceed 37.7° C (100° F)—that is, warm but not hot to the touch. If a bath thermometer is available, it should be used to check the temperature of the water. Otherwise, a temperature that is comfortable when tested on the inside of your wrist or elbow is appropriate.

Before bathing any child, assess the family's preferences and home practices. Factors to consider include the time of day usually set aside for the bath, bathing rituals, special equipment, any product allergies, and the type of bath preferred. You can also use this time to determine the amount of assistance needed and to address any learning needs related to hygiene. Because bathing is one of the few areas over which parents might be allowed to retain control when a child is hospitalized, it is important to allow them to make as many decisions as possible. Decision making also allows parents to maintain a part of the home routine with their child.

An infant who cannot sit unaided can be given either a sponge bath or a tub bath. Support the infant's body and head at all times during the bath (Fig. 13-4). Older infants and toddlers can be bathed in either a bedside tub or a regular bathtub. *Never leave an infant or small child unattended in the bath.* Older children can take showers if facilities are available. The nurse should use judgment in deciding how much supervision an older child needs while bathing. Privacy for the school-age child or adolescent is extremely important.

Special Considerations

Bed baths are frequently used for hospitalized infants and children. When bathing a newborn or young infant, soap is not necessary. In fact, soap can be too drying to the skin if used frequently. If soap is necessary or desired by the parent, use a gentle, nonalkaline soap.

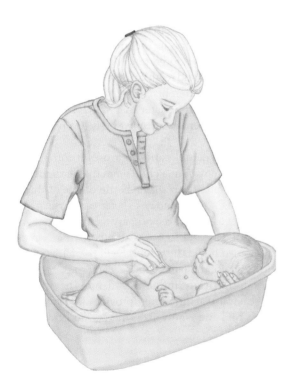

Using hand to support infant's neck and head

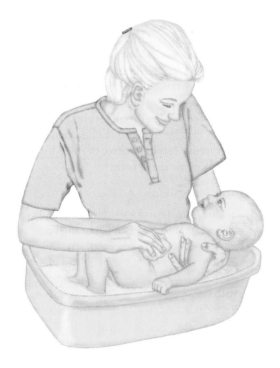

Using arm to support infant's neck and head

FIG 13-4 **When giving an infant a tub bath, the nurse supports the infant's body at all times.**

Skill: Infant Bathing

To prevent chilling when giving a sponge bath, be sure to keep the infant covered with a cotton blanket. Cover the entire body except for the body part being washed or rinsed. Begin the bath with the face, and clean the diaper area last. Clean any eye discharge with a wet cotton ball, and clean from the inner canthus outward. Use a clean cotton ball for each eye. Outer ears can be cleaned with a wet face cloth.

If bathing an infant in a bathtub, line a plastic infant tub with a towel to provide comfort as well as traction to prevent slipping. To prevent accidental drowning should the infant slip out of your grasp, fill the tub with no more than 3 inches of water.

When finished with the infant bath, wrap the infant in a dry towel or cotton blanket. Using the football hold and holding the infant over the tub, shampoo the infant's head with baby shampoo. Be sure to shampoo over the fontanel. Avoid using talcum powder or cornstarch in the infant's diaper area. When these substances get moist, they provide a medium for organism growth. Talcum powder and cornstarch, if accidentally inhaled, can result in respiratory complications.

The technique for bathing a child differs little from that used for bathing an adult. The nurse performs the same assessment as with any client and provides assistance as necessary.

Adjust the room temperature to a comfortable setting, and draw the curtain around the bed. As with any bed bath, the nurse begins with the face and proceeds in a head-to-toe progression. Obtain fresh water when it is time to rinse the child. As with the infant, drape the child adequately for privacy and warmth. To prevent chilling, dry each body section as it is rinsed. The bath can be followed with application of lotion or deodorant if desired.

Some bathing restrictions might apply to children with surgical incisions, skin traction, IV catheters, casts, urinary catheters, artificial airways, and feeding tubes. Some children are also restricted in position and mobility. For example, children who have undergone orthopedic or neurosurgical procedures often must remain supine. Other children may be intolerant of position changes because of underlying physiologic conditions or injury. It is imperative to assess for these special needs before beginning the bath.

Documentation

Documentation includes the type of bath, child or family participation, procedure tolerance, and any abnormal findings noted, such as bruising, rashes, or excoriation. Any lotions or other skin preparations used also should be recorded.

Parent Teaching

General principles of hygiene and safety might need to be reinforced with some parents. Instruction in the use of special bathing equipment, such as infant bathtubs, safety bars, or tub grips, should be included as part of discharge teaching and preparation. After approximately 1 year of age, a child can be bathed safely in a regular tub. To prevent injury or accidental drowning, appropriate supervision should be maintained at all times. Advise parents never to leave an older infant or young child alone in the bath; the risk of drowning, even in small amounts of water, is high. Infant bath seats, which adhere to the floor of a regular bathtub by suction cups, can also be dangerous. The older infant can slip out of the sides of the seat, especially when the seat is wet, or the suction cups can accidentally release, tipping the seat over.

ORAL HYGIENE

To remove excess food and bacteria, wipe infants' gums gently with a wet cloth after each feeding. After teeth erupt, a soft, damp cloth, a piece of gauze, or a child's soft toothbrush can be used after each feeding and before bed. Until the parent is assured that the child can manage correctly and independently, young children will need supervision when performing oral care. Even then, reminders to brush might be necessary.

Children should brush their teeth at least twice daily with a child's soft toothbrush and a *small* (pea-sized) amount of toothpaste. Children may ingest excessive amounts of fluoride if they are allowed to use large amounts of toothpaste or if they eat the toothpaste. Using the recommended amount of toothpaste and encouraging the child not to swallow the toothpaste will prevent *fluorosis* (brown spots on the teeth caused by too much fluoride).

Flossing is useful for cleaning between teeth and maintaining healthy gums. The child should begin to floss when all the primary teeth are in or when the child's molars begin to touch.

Immunosuppressed children, in particular, need excellent oral hygiene. Soft toothbrushes, sponge-covered toothettes, or moistened gauze sponges can be used for dental care in the child who is at risk for gingival bleeding (see Chapter 24).

Discharge teaching in the area of oral hygiene is quite important and often forgotten. Many parents do not realize that infants' gums and teeth can and should be cleaned. Children should have their first visit to a dentist by the time the first teeth erupt and no later than age 2½ years. Thereafter they should be seen on a regular basis (every 6 months) for checkups.

The risk of dental caries increases if formula, milk, or other liquids remain in a child's mouth overnight. Allowing an infant to fall asleep with a bottle of one of these liquids can cause a condition known as *bottle mouth syndrome*, which results in severely decayed primary teeth. Discourage parents from putting a child to bed with a bottle of formula, juice, or sweetened liquid. If the child will not fall asleep without a bottle, advise the parent to use water only.

Good nutrition influences dental health and vice versa. Dental teaching often provides a means for educating the child and family about proper nutrition and health maintenance.

FEEDING

Mealtimes can be difficult for the hospitalized child. Changes in routine, diet, and surroundings, as well as dietary restrictions and illness, affect the child's ability and desire to eat.

Refusing to eat might also be the only way the child can control the environment.

Assess the child's preferences and dislikes on admission and before ordering meals. Also note mealtime rituals and routines and cultural food variations. Serving favorite and preferred foods and offering nutritious snacks can ensure appropriate caloric intake.

The type and form of food chosen should be appropriate to the child's age and developmental status. (See Chapters 5 through 8 for a discussion of food types appropriate for each age group.) When planning meals, the nurse also considers whether the child has any special needs. For example, the child with an impaired gag reflex cannot tolerate the same foods as other children. Likewise, the child with nausea should not be offered favorite foods because these foods may become associated with the nausea when the child is feeling better.

Feeding a hospitalized infant seldom differs from feeding an infant at home. Types of foods, feeding schedules, and routines should mimic home schedules and routines when possible. If the infant's bottle or nipple brand is not available in the hospital, ask the parents to bring what the infant uses at home. Encourage parents to feed their children or be present at mealtimes. Feeding reinforces the special bond that develops between child and parent.

Facilitate feeding for the breastfeeding infant, providing a private, quiet, and relaxed location so mother and infant feel comfortable and not rushed. If the mother is pumping breast milk for use when she is absent, be sure to meticulously follow hospital policy for labeling, storing, and administering pumped breast milk.

Unless contraindicated by their medical condition, hold infants during feedings. Because of the risk of aspiration, *never prop a bottle* (i.e., do not leave it on a pillow or rolled blanket next to the infant's mouth). Frequent burping during and after feedings can reduce the incidence of regurgitation. Burp the infant by using the upright hold and gently patting or rubbing the infant's back. You can also seat the infant on your knees with your hand supporting the infant's chin. After feeding, position the infant on the right side to facilitate the flow of the feeding toward the lower end of the stomach and allow any swallowed air to rise into the esophagus. *Infants should not, however, be placed on their sides to sleep* (AAP, 2005).

Toddlers and preschoolers often use food as a source of control. They might exhibit "food jags," during which they will eat only one or two items for a period of several days. They enjoy finger foods but are beginning to use spoons or forks fairly competently. Use colorful plates and cups to encourage a reluctant child to eat. Also allow parents to bring the child's own cups or utensils from home to simulate the usual mealtime routines as closely as possible.

Cut foods into pieces appropriate in size and texture to decrease the risk of aspiration. Avoid foods such as hot dogs, popcorn, peanuts, and grapes, because if aspirated, these can occlude the airway. Do not allow young children to eat unsupervised. Secure them appropriately at a table, in a high chair, or in bed using an over-the-bed table during meals.

"Roaming" while eating should be discouraged. Allow children to feed themselves if possible, and restrict the feeding time to 15 to 20 minutes. Discontinue the meal if the child begins to play with the food.

Older children and adolescents seldom have difficulty expressing their dietary preferences. Difficulty may arise, however, when children this age are placed on a restricted or special diet. For example, the diabetic child often has difficulty staying on a restricted diet in the face of peer pressure. Support and clear limits are often needed to ensure cooperation. Referral to a dietitian may be necessary to help the child make appropriate food choices.

Special Considerations

Keeping accurate intake and output (I&O) measurements may be necessary for some children. Measure and record all intake, both oral and parenteral. All output, including output from urine and stool; drainage from tubes, stomas, or fistulas; and emesis, is also measured and recorded. To measure urinary output in an untrained child, weigh each wet diaper and compare the weight with the weight of a dry diaper of similar size. One gram of weight equals approximately one milliliter of output.

Documentation

Recording the child's nutritional intake assists in determining the child's overall health. Record food intake and preferences as well as observations about the child's appetite and eating patterns. Particularly note abnormal eating habits in an older child or adolescent—the age at which eating disorders are prevalent.

Parent Teaching

Parental education is extremely important, particularly if the hospital admission is related to eating disorders or accidents, such as food aspiration. Carefully instruct parents about any food or fluid restrictions or special diets. For example, a child with *phenylketonuria (PKU)* or type 1 diabetes mellitus (see Chapter 27) is at high risk for injury if the diet is not closely followed.

VITAL SIGNS

The principles of measuring vital signs in children are similar to those for adults, with some modifications. Obtain vital signs when the infant or child is quiet. If this timing is not possible, record any activity that affects accurate measurement (e.g., crying, playing).

Measuring Temperature

Temperature is an objective and reliable indicator of illness, and measuring temperature is an integral part of assessing children. A child's temperature can be measured in a variety of ways. Oral, rectal, axillary, and tympanic temperatures can be measured with electronic, digital, or tympanic membrane thermometers. The American Academy of Pediatrics no longer recommends the use of thermometers containing mercury for children in hospital or home settings (Goldman,

Shannon, & Committee on Environmental Health, 2001). Whatever temperature measurement method is chosen, the child's temperature should be measured at the same site and with the same device to maintain consistency and allow reliable comparison and tracking of temperatures over time. (See Table 9-1 for normal temperatures in children.)

Digital thermometers, which are electronic or run on a battery and measure the temperature quickly (usually in less than 30 seconds), can be used to measure temperatures orally, rectally, or in the axillary area. To prevent cross contamination, use disposable covers for obtaining temperatures.

Most hospital facilities use axillary or tympanic temperature measurement for infants and children too young to properly hold an oral thermometer (Fig. 13-5). Axillary or tympanic temperature measurement is less invasive than rectal temperature measurement but may be less accurate for measuring core temperatures in infants. For this reason, some institution policies require one rectal temperature measurement be done each shift on young infants.

The advantage to tympanic temperature measurement is that the measurements are obtained quickly, usually within a few seconds. For tympanic measurement to be accurate,

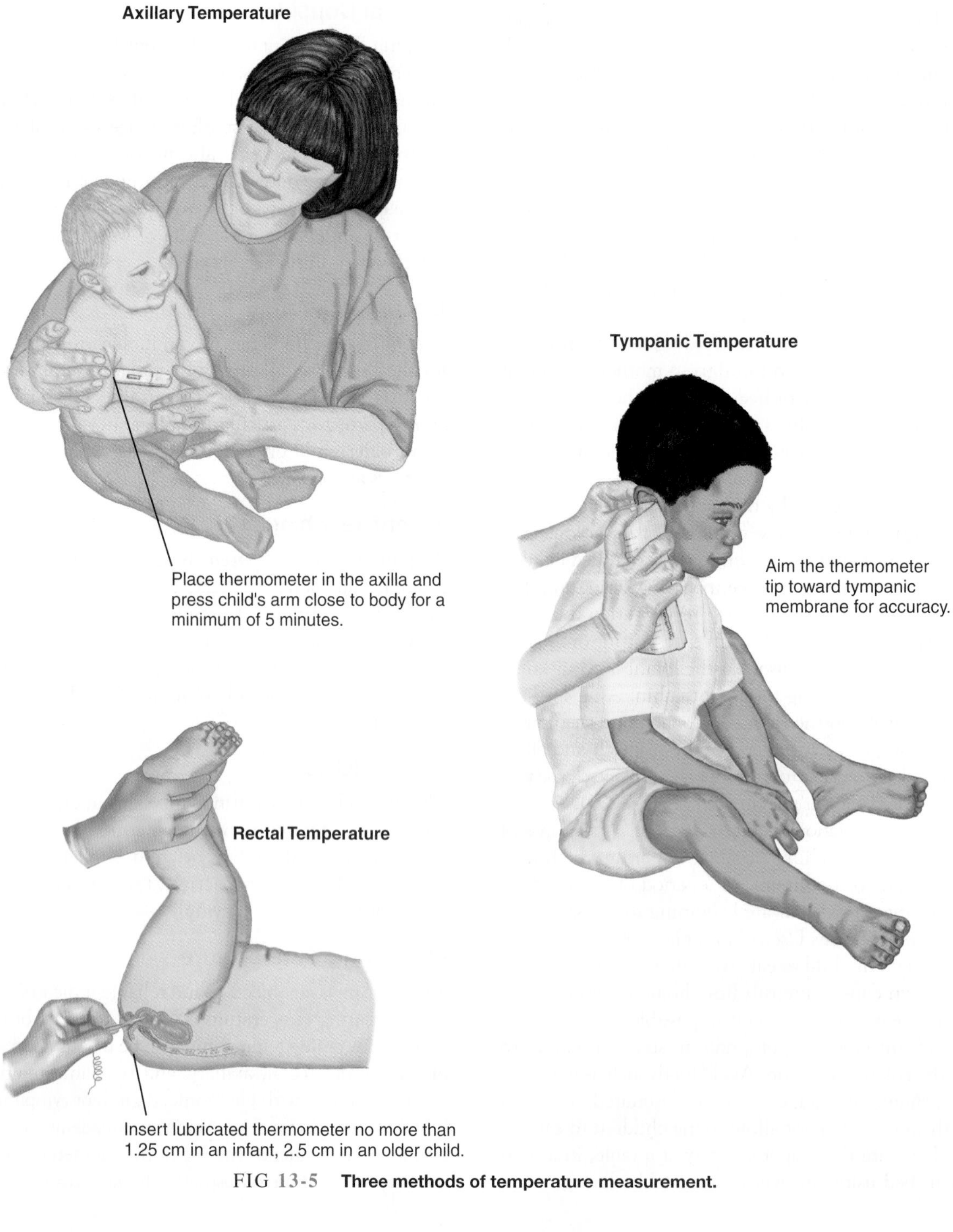

Axillary Temperature

Place thermometer in the axilla and press child's arm close to body for a minimum of 5 minutes.

Tympanic Temperature

Aim the thermometer tip toward tympanic membrane for accuracy.

Rectal Temperature

Insert lubricated thermometer no more than 1.25 cm in an infant, 2.5 cm in an older child.

FIG 13-5   **Three methods of temperature measurement.**

the temperature probe must create a complete seal. Putting traction on the ear pinna (direction depending on the child's age) before probe insertion exposes the tympanic membrane and facilitates a seal. When performed appropriately, tympanic temperature measurement has been suggested to be as accurate as digitally recorded axillary measurement and is preferred by parents and children (Barton, Gaffney, Chase, Rayens, & Piyabanditkul, 2003).

Axillary temperatures are appropriate for infants and children younger than 4 to 6 years and in any child who is uncooperative, immunosuppressed, neurologically impaired, or who has had oral surgery. Axillary temperatures are approximately 0.6° C (1° F) lower than the body's core temperature. To be accurate, a thermometer may need to remain in the child's axillary area for a longer time, so consider seating the child on your lap and reading a story or singing songs to help pass the time and help the child remain quiet.

Temperatures are measured orally in most children aged 6 years and older, including adolescents. Keeping a thermometer in place is sometimes a challenge for children. Encourage the child to keep the mouth closed around the thermometer (in a "kiss" position), and instruct the child not to bite the thermometer. The child should avoid liquids for 30 minutes before the oral temperature measurement. Temperatures measured orally might be inaccurate because of oral intake, oxygen administration, nebulized treatments, or crying. Oral temperature measurement should not be used in any child who has had oral or tonsillar surgery or in whom epiglottitis is suspected.

Because of the risk of rectal perforation and the intrusive and upsetting nature of the procedure, temperatures are measured rectally only when no other route can be used or when obtaining a core body temperature is necessary (see Fig. 13-5). Skin strips or dots to measure temperature are not as precise as other temperature measurements but can be used in the home setting to estimate whether a child has a fever (Box 13-2).

> ## CRITICAL TO REMEMBER
> **Measuring Temperature**
> - Follow an elevated tympanic or axillary temperature with a rectal core temperature measurement.
> - Report any core temperature measurement of less than 36° C (96.8° F) or more than 38° C (100.4° F), especially in an infant younger than 2 months.

Measuring Pulse

Apical pulse rate measurements (Fig. 13-6) are recommended for infants and children younger than 2 years and in any child who has an irregular heart rate or known congenital heart disease. Take the apical pulse when the child is quiet, and count for one full minute. Determine the apical heart rate before administering certain medications, such as digoxin.

Radial pulse measurements are appropriate for children older than 2 years (see Table 9-1 for normal pulse measurements). The procedure for taking a radial pulse is similar to that for an adult.

Evaluating Respirations

Infants often have irregular respiratory rates that change with stimulation, crying, and feeding. Some infants will initially exhibit a Cheyne-Stokes type of respiratory pattern, but this pattern should disappear by 4 weeks of age. Table 9-1 shows normal rates. When measuring respirations in an infant, observe the pattern of inspiration and expiration before auscultating; this helps determine any irregular rhythm. Measure the respiratory rate in an infant or young child by auscultating for one full minute. As with the apical pulse measurement, try to obtain the respiratory rate when an infant or young child is at rest. Either observe or auscultate respirations in the older child.

BOX 13-2 | PARENTS WANT TO KNOW   About Temperature Measurement

Accurately measuring your child's temperature, along with other symptoms, helps your physician determine whether your child needs to be seen for assessment and treatment. Feeling your child's forehead can give you a clue regarding whether the child's temperature should be measured but does not give accurate information about the child's body temperature. Temperature strips placed on the child's forehead also give only an approximate reading.

A variety of thermometer types are available at the drugstore. An inexpensive digital thermometer can be used to take oral, rectal, and axillary (under the arm) temperatures. Digital thermometers are easy to read because the numbers are displayed on a small screen. Pediatricians do not recommend using glass thermometers or other thermometers containing mercury for children.

The average body temperature, when measured orally, is 98.6° F (37° C). Mild increases can occur as a result of exercise, wearing excessive clothing, taking hot baths, hot weather, eating warm food, or drinking warm drinks. If you take your child's temperature and it is higher than you would expect it to be, encourage the child to sit quietly and retake the temperature in 30 minutes.

Your child has a fever if the temperature is greater than 100.4° F (38° C) when measured rectally, greater than 99.5° F (37.5° C) when taken orally, and greater than 99° F (37.2° C) when measured by the axillary method. If your infant is younger than 6 weeks, you should call your physician if the baby's rectal temperature is above 100° F (37.7° C).

In general, the height of the fever is not an indication of the seriousness of the illness. What is important is how your child is acting. If your child has a fever and is acting sick, notify your physician.

Measuring Blood Pressure

Blood pressure is assessed on hospital admission and may be assessed every shift, or more often if necessary. Unless a problem is suspected, however, blood pressure may not be assessed more than once per year during routine physical examinations. The National High Blood Pressure Education Program Working Group on High Blood Pressure in Children and Adolescents (2004) recommends auscultated blood pressure measurements as the standard for children.

Choosing the appropriate cuff size is extremely important because an inappropriate cuff size will yield a blood pressure reading that is higher or lower than the actual pressure. Recommendations for the method of choosing an appropriate cuff size vary, but the following is a suggested procedure (American Heart Association, 2005):

- Find the midpoint of the right upper arm between the shoulder (acromion) and the elbow (olecranon).
- Holding the bladder of the cuff *lengthwise,* the bladder width should cover approximately 40% of the upper arm circumference (UAC) at this point.
- If measured this way, when you wrap the cuff around the arm to take the blood pressure, the bladder should encircle 80% to 100% of the arm without overlap.

- Palpate the brachial artery, and place the stethoscope bell on the brachial artery below the cuff.
- Measure the blood pressure with the arm at heart level.

If using a different site than the arm for blood pressure measurement, use 40% of the circumference of the site used. Commercially designated blood pressure cuffs are standardized widths. Choose the closest standard width to the 40% circumference measure rather than the designated label on the cuff. Table 13-1 illustrates average bladder widths of commercial blood pressure cuffs. Blood pressure measurements will differ according to the measuring technique used and the site selected (see Appendix C for normal results).

Blood pressures can be measured in the upper arm, lower arm, thigh, calf, or ankle (Fig. 13-7). To ensure consistency, take measurements in the same limb, in the same place, and with the child in the same position. Remember that blood pressure measurements can differ depending on the site used.

When using electronic devices to measure blood pressure, follow the manufacturer's guidelines closely to ensure accuracy. For most devices, the first reading is considered a "priming" reading and the second reading is considered the true blood pressure measurement. If the blood pressure result

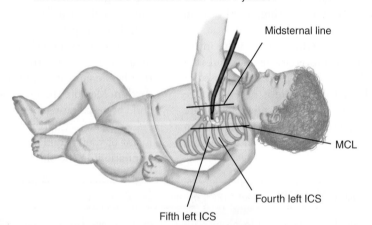

Apical pulse is lateral to the left midclavicular line (MCL) and fourth intercostal space (ICS) in children younger than 7 years and to the left MCL and fifth ICS in children older than 7 years.

Midsternal line

MCL

Fourth left ICS

Fifth left ICS

FIG 13-6   **Locating the apical pulse.**

TABLE 13-1	Recommended Dimensions for Blood Pressure Cuff Bladders		
Age Range	**Width, cm**	**Length, cm**	**Maximum Arm Circumference, cm***
Newborn	4	8	10
Infant	6	12	15
Child	9	18	22
Small adult	10	24	26
Adult	13	30	34
Large adult	16	38	44
Thigh	20	42	52

*Calculated so that the largest arm would still allow the bladder to encircle arm by at least 80%.
Reprinted from National High Blood Pressure Education Program Working Group on High Blood Pressure in Children and Adolescents. (2004). The fourth report on the diagnosis, evaluation, and treatment of high blood pressure in children and adolescents. *Pediatrics, 114*(2), 557. Reprinted with permission.

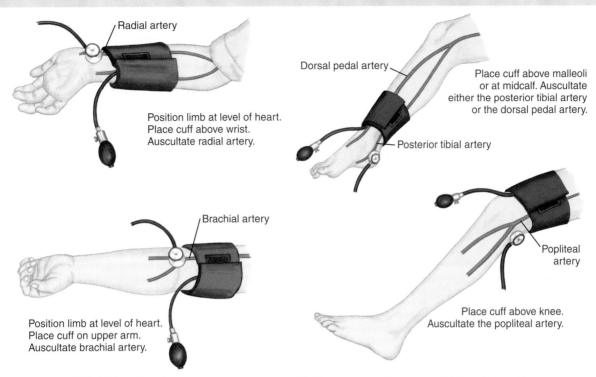

FIG 13-7 **Blood pressures can be measured in the upper arm, lower arm, thigh, calf, or ankle. An appropriate-size cuff must be used to obtain accurate results.**

is elevated when taken electronically, retake the blood pressure using auscultation.

The procedure for measuring blood pressure in children is similar to the procedure for adults. Recommendations state that the diastolic reading is the number at which sound is absent—not the number at which the sound quality changes (National High Blood Pressure Education Program Working Group on High Blood Pressure in Children and Adolescents, 2004). Auscultating the diastolic pressure in young children, however, may not be possible. The systolic blood pressure sometimes can be heard down to a measurement of zero. In this case, record the blood pressure as the systolic number over pulse (e.g., 90/P).

When auscultation of blood pressure in infants and toddlers is impossible, palpate the pulse to obtain a systolic reading. Find the location of the pulse below the cuff with your index and middle fingers and inflate the cuff, as for an auscultated pressure. As the cuff deflates, note the point at which the pulse is first felt. Record this systolic measurement as if you had heard the systolic beat down to zero.

Documentation of Vital Sign Measurement

Record all vital signs in the child's medical record. Include the method used to measure the vital signs, the measurement obtained, and any action taken. Record and report core temperatures of less than 36° C (96.8° F) or more than 38° C

CRITICAL TO REMEMBER
Measuring Vital Signs

- Temperatures should not be measured rectally in the immunosuppressed child or in any child who has had rectal surgery, diarrhea, or a bleeding disorder.
- Count respirations and measure the apical heart rate before taking other vital signs. Both signs are best measured on a sleeping child.
- Measure the apical heart rate for a full minute on any child younger than 2 years, on a child being assessed for the first time, on any child whose heartbeat is irregular, or on a child for whom treatment decisions are made on the basis of the heart rate.
- Observe the child's respiratory rate and effort for a full minute while the child is quiet. Abdominal movement

is normally observed in infants and young children, whereas thoracic movement can be noted in older children and adolescents.
- Evaluate the quality of respirations, symmetry of chest movement with each breath, and any noisy respirations (e.g., crackles, wheezes, friction rubs). Observe the child for any signs of respiratory distress, such as nasal flaring, grunting, stridor, retractions, increased work of breathing, cyanosis, or apneic periods.
- Always use a manual cuff to verify electronically measured blood pressures that indicate hypertension or hypotension.

(100.4° F). Record and report any other abnormal findings or findings that are significantly different for the individual child.

Preparing the Child and Family

Inform the child and family about the purpose of the procedure. Children who are fearful should be allowed to examine or handle the equipment while you explain how it is used.

> Tell young children that the blood pressure cuff feels like a "hug" or a "squeeze."

Many children have toy medical instruments at home and may be familiar with the concept of taking vital signs.

Parent Teaching

Some parents may need to learn how to take the child's temperature at home. Demonstrate how to take the child's temperature, and then observe the parent perform the procedure. Make sure the parent is comfortable with the procedure and is able to read the thermometer accurately.

Some parents may need to be taught how to determine their child's heart rate accurately as well as the acceptable range for their child. Special considerations relating to parents' notifying the physician may need to be made for children who are taking certain medications, such as digoxin.

If the child's condition requires home blood pressure monitoring, teach the procedure to the parent. You can provide helpful suggestions about the size of the cuff and methods to involve the child who might resist this procedure. For instance, parents might make a smaller cuff for the child's favorite doll or stuffed animal.

Special Considerations: Cardiorespiratory Monitors

Some children need cardiorespiratory monitoring so that heart rate, respiratory rate, blood pressure, and temperature can be continuously measured. Children who are acutely ill or who are undergoing procedures might be placed on a monitor to help health care providers detect subtle changes in the child's condition.

The procedure and indications for attaching a child to a cardiorespiratory monitor are no different from those for an adult. Monitors sound an alarm to warn of changes in the child's cardiorespiratory status. Remember that false alarms can occur. *Always look at the child and perform an assessment before intervening.* A flat line on the electrocardiogram (ECG) does not always signal a cardiac arrest. It may be nothing but a loose monitor lead. Check the manufacturer's recommendations for attaching leads and monitoring selected vital signs.

FEVER-REDUCING MEASURES

The body's internal thermostat, the hypothalamus, attempts to keep the body's temperature between 36° and 38° C (96.8° and 100.4° F). This regulation is done through a complex series of interactions that result in heat gain or loss. The body's mechanisms for conserving or producing heat are vasoconstriction and shivering. Heat is lost through radiation, conduction, convection, and evaporation.

Description of Fever

Fever is defined as a body temperature greater than 38° C (100.4° F) rectally or 37.5° C (99.5° F) orally that results from an insult or disease during which the body's set point temperature rises to a higher-than-normal level. After the cause of the fever is removed, the body resets its set point at the normal level.

The body's attempt to defend itself against illness is manifested by fever, which is triggered by endogenous *pyrogens* produced during the inflammatory response. Because research studies have not conclusively demonstrated whether fever is beneficial or detrimental, practitioners vary in their approach to managing fevers caused by infections. Mild degrees of fever may or may not require intervention, depending on the underlying cause and the child's response. Most fevers are brief and benign and resolve when the underlying infection resolves. Children with chronic cardiac or respiratory disease, those with neurologic disease, and those prone to febrile seizures should be treated for fever. Children with fevers of 40° C (104° F) or higher also should be treated.

Fever is uncomfortable, and children may become irritable. For every 1° C of temperature elevation, the body's metabolic rate increases 10% to 12%, resulting in increased insensible fluid loss, increased oxygen consumption, and increased stress on the cardiovascular system (Lorin, 2004). Regardless of the fever's cause, the child's comfort is the primary reason for treating a fever in a normally healthy child.

Medications and Environmental Management

Treatment can consist of environmental measures, antipyretics, or a combination of interventions. External cooling is one of the oldest and most common forms of fever management, particularly when the elevated temperature is caused by hyperthermia. Removing blankets and clothing and reducing the environmental temperature can reduce fever. Tepid sponge baths and the use of mechanical cooling blankets can reduce a moderate to high fever fairly quickly (Procedures 13-1 and 13-2). The challenge is to reduce the fever without causing shivering, which produces heat.

In febrile illnesses, the body attempts to resist external cooling, resulting in the need for antipyretics in addition to external cooling interventions. Fevers in children are treated with antipyretics such as acetaminophen and ibuprofen. Aspirin is avoided because of its association with Reye syndrome in children with viral illnesses such as influenza and varicella.

Children with elevated temperatures often have a loss of appetite. Dehydration can occur from decreased oral intake and increased insensible water loss through the lungs and the skin. Meet the need for adequate hydration by offering the child additional oral fluids. For those who refuse oral hydration or who are unable to take in adequate volume, consider the need for intravenous fluids.

PROCEDURE 13-1	**GIVING A COOLING BATH**

PURPOSE: To reduce fever

1. Explain the purpose and the reason for selecting the intervention with developmentally appropriate language. If possible, provide toys or some other distraction for the child. The parent can be present to help comfort or play with the child. The goal is to reduce the fever without causing the child to shiver.
2. Gather the following equipment: tepid water (water temperature between 29° and 32° C [approximately 85° and 90° F]), cotton blankets, washcloths, and toys. The use of rubbing alcohol is contraindicated because of skin irritation, the risk of neurologic depression from the fumes or absorption through the skin, and too-rapid cooling, which can result in shivering.
3. Assist the infant or child to sit or lie in a position of comfort in the bed. Place the infant or child on a cotton bath blanket.

WHEN BATHING THE CHILD OUTSIDE A TUB

4. Using tepid water, wet the washcloths or towels and place them on the child, exposing one area at a time. Tepid water, not ice water, is used because it allows the body temperature to drop gradually, thus avoiding heat-producing responses such as shivering, which are caused by too-rapid cooling. *If shivering occurs, the procedure should be terminated immediately.*

WHEN THE CHILD IS PLACED IN A TUB

5. Alternatively, the child can be placed in a tub of warm water, with cool water added until the desired temperature is reached. Gently pour or spray water over the child's back and chest. Continue this for 20 to 30 minutes. Use water toys to provide distraction during this nursing intervention. *Remember: an infant or young child should never be left unattended in the tub.*

6. After the bath, dry the child. Dress the child in lightweight clothing or pajamas and place in a dry bed.
7. Recheck the child's temperature approximately 30 minutes later to evaluate the effectiveness of the intervention.
8. Document in the nurses' notes the child's baseline vital signs, hydration status, general appearance, interventions used for fever reduction, the indications for the interventions, the duration, the child's response, and any problems identified. Also document any family teaching as well as the degree of understanding the information given.
9. Take the opportunity to teach the parent how to care for a child with an elevated temperature. Provide information about how to take a temperature, how to read a thermometer, normal temperature range, administration of antipyretics, the use of tepid baths, and when to seek professional help. Emphasize in your teaching that ice water and isopropyl alcohol should never be used for sponging or bathing the child with a fever.
10. Additional points to cover with parents include the importance of accuracy in dosing, the timing of doses, methods of administration, and appropriate medication choices when giving antipyretics. Parents need reassurance that fever is a common sign of illness and rarely poses a threat to the child's well-being.

HOME ADAPTATIONS

To manage a fever at home, advise the parent to dress the child in lightweight clothing. Consult the child's pediatrician before initiating tepid baths. If advised to use tepid baths, an infant tub or regular bathtub can be used. Advise the parent to keep the room at a comfortable temperature and discontinue the tepid bath if the child begins to shiver.

PROCEDURE 13-2	**USING A COOLING BLANKET**

PURPOSE: To reduce hyperthermia

1. Using developmentally appropriate language, explain the purpose and the reason for using a cooling blanket. Encourage the parent to be present to help comfort or distract the child.
2. You will need the following equipment: a commercial cooling blanket, sheets or small blankets as needed, and a temperature probe.
3. Place the cooling blanket on the bed and cover it with a sheet or thin blanket.
4. Connect the blanket to the cooling unit and set the control mode (manual or automatic) and the desired blanket or body temperature. Temperature parameters should be set according to the manufacturer's recommendations and physician's orders.
5. Check the child's skin condition before, during, and after use of the blanket, and record the findings.

6. Cover the child lightly to maintain privacy and reduce shivering.
7. To prevent too-rapid cooling or overcooling, monitor the child's vital signs frequently. A temperature probe can be used to monitor the child's temperature continually during this cooling method.
8. To reduce shivering, wrap the child's extremities with towels or baby blankets.
9. Keep the child completely dry to reduce the risk of frostbite from dampness.
10. Reposition the child who is on a cooling unit frequently and gently to reduce the risk of skin breakdown.
11. Record the type of unit used, the control mode and temperature settings selected, and the condition of the child's skin before, during, and after use.

DRUG GUIDE

ACETAMINOPHEN (TYLENOL, TEMPRA, PANADOL)
Classification: Nonnarcotic analgesic and antipyretic.
Action: Unknown; may act on hypothalamic heat-regulating center.
Indications: Mild fever and pain relief.
Dosage and route: Dosage is age and/or weight related; administered four or five times daily. Oral, rectal. Comes in a variety of oral preparations: infant drops (80 mg/0.8 mL), liquid or suspension (160 mg/5 mL), chewable tablets (80 mg/tab), caplets and chewables for older children (160 mg/tab), adult strength (325 mg/tab). Rectal suppositories in 80, 120, 125, 300, 325, and 650 mg.
Absorption: From the gastrointestinal tract; peak action in 1 to 3 hours.
Excretion: Duration approximately 4 to 5 hours.
Contraindications: Any previous sensitivity to the medication.
Precautions: Long-term use can cause liver damage. Other over-the-counter cold preparations can contain acetaminophen; if given concurrently they can increase the amount of acetaminophen above safe levels.
Adverse reactions: Blood dyscrasias, hypoglycemia, rashes or urticaria, liver damage with prolonged use.
Nursing considerations: Advise parents to be extremely careful not to confuse the liquid preparations; check the label carefully before giving the medication. Never refer to this or any other medication as "candy." Acetaminophen overdose must be treated immediately to prevent hepatic toxicity. In clients performing home glucose monitoring, acetaminophen can affect glucose readings. Parents should not continue to give their children this medication for fever that lasts longer than 2 days without checking with the health care provider.

Remember that infants who are being cared for in servo-controlled heating environments must be carefully monitored because of the potential for accidental dislodgment of the skin temperature probe. This problem can cause an increase in the heat production of the unit and a resulting increase in the infant's temperature. In addition, the insensible water loss in infants in these controlled units is greatly increased. These additional fluid losses must be considered when calculating fluid replacement.

Commercial Cooling Blankets

Commercial cooling blankets also can be used to control hyperthermia. These units, which can be controlled manually or automatically, lower the body temperature through cold transfer between the blanket and the child. Cooling unit operation varies among manufacturers. Read the operating manual before using this equipment. Some cooling blankets may be reusable, but blankets designed for single client use are preferred. Shivering, frostbite, and skin breakdown are concerns when using a cooling blanket.

SPECIMEN COLLECTION

Specimens are collected from children for the same reasons they are collected from adults, but children often need more of an explanation of the reasons and procedure for specimen collection. All explanations should be given in age-appropriate language, and children should be prepared for any sensations that they may experience.

Regardless of the type of specimen to be obtained, use Standard Precautions. The use of gloves, gowns, masks, eye protection, and handwashing provides protection for individuals coming in contact with potentially infectious materials. The use of equipment for Standard Precautions will vary according to the degree of "potential splash." *Any time a chance for contamination exists, use Standard Precautions.* Follow procedures for handling biologic hazards as directed by individual facilities on the basis of Standard Precautions.

Urine Specimens

Voided Specimens

Older children and adolescents often cooperate in the collection of urine specimens. Most can use a bedpan, urinal, or specimen cup with little difficulty. Younger children and preschoolers often have difficulty voiding on request. The nurse should take care to use familiar terms, such as "pee pee," "tinkle," or "potty," when telling the child what is needed. For younger children, have a potty chair or collection "hat" available that fits in the toilet. Parents can be helpful in obtaining a specimen from children this age. Parents may also be successful in obtaining specimens from older toddlers who are being toilet trained. Infants and young toddlers, however, are unable to void on request. Because they are not toilet trained, specimen collection devices are needed (Procedure 13-3).

If the specimen must be collected under special conditions (e.g., a midstream urine sample), the nurse carefully explains to the child what preparation is needed and verifies that the child understands all directions. An adult may need to accompany the child during the collection. A young child may be able to sit on the toilet but be unable to manipulate a specimen cup. The parent or nurse can hold the cup while the child voids. For a boy who wishes to stand while voiding, the cup can be held in the stream as he voids. If the specimen is to be carried to another room or down a hallway, provide a plastic bag or other container for transport.

If a midstream urine sample is needed and the child is at home, the nurse can describe the procedure to the parent over the telephone. The parent will need to boil a clean glass container and cover for 20 minutes in a covered pan. After letting the water cool, empty the water from the pan and carefully remove the container and the cover, being sure not to touch the inside of either. The urine is collected after the perineal area is cleaned (see Procedure 13-3). Advise the parent to place the specimen jar in a plastic bag and keep it refrigerated until bringing it to the laboratory for testing.

Although many methods have been used to collect nonsterile urine from incontinent children (e.g., placing plastic wrap in a diaper to catch urine), the most reliable

PROCEDURE 13-3	URINE SPECIMEN COLLECTION FROM THE INCONTINENT CHILD

PURPOSE: To monitor urine output accurately or obtain a specimen for testing

1. Before beginning the procedure, provide adequate privacy. The child may be more relaxed if a parent is present. If both blood and urine specimens need to be obtained from the incontinent child, position the collection bag *before* drawing the blood. Infants and toddlers often void during a painful procedure.
2. Obtain the following equipment: nonsterile gloves, urine collection bag, sterile specimen cup, mild soap, warm water, washcloth, diaper and towel, and label and requisition form.
3. Put on gloves and clean the perineal area. Cleaning the perineum will remove any lotions or ointments and help the bag adhere.
   a. *For girls:* Clean from front to back and from the urinary meatus to the labia majora (in to out).
   b. *For boys:* Clean from the tip of the penis in a circular motion. *Do not* retract an infant's or young child's foreskin.
4. After the perineum has been cleansed, dry it thoroughly. The skin must be completely dry for the bag to adhere properly.
5. Remove the backing from the adhesive surface of the bottom half of the collection device.
6. Place the child in a frog-leg position to eliminate skinfolds that may interfere with bag adherence. Apply the bag.

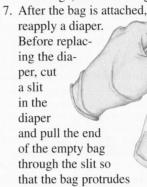

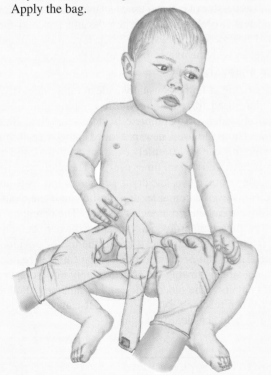

   a. *For girls:* Hold the perineum taut and apply the adhesive portion of the bag, working outward. To keep feces from contaminating the specimen, the narrow "bridge" on the adhesive patch must be placed on the tiny area of skin between the anus and the genitalia.
   b. *For boys:* Place the penis and scrotum (if small enough) inside the bag.
7. After the bag is attached, reapply a diaper. Before replacing the diaper, cut a slit in the diaper and pull the end of the empty bag through the slit so that the bag protrudes from the diaper. This step reduces the chance of leaking and allows for observation of urine.

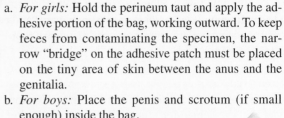

8. Check the bag every 30 minutes. Applying slight pressure over the suprapubic area or stroking along the older infant's spine will often induce voiding. As soon as urine is noticed in the bag, gently remove the bag from the perineum.
9. Transfer the urine into a sterile specimen cup. Most bags have a small tab that can be removed to allow the urine to be poured. If the bag does not have a tab, clean the outside of the bag with an alcohol pad and withdraw the urine with a needle and syringe for placement in the appropriate container.
10. Label the urine specimen with the child's name, date, and time collection and deliver it promptly, together with a requisition form, to the laboratory. Urine for culture that cannot be tested within 30 minutes should be refrigerated or placed in a sterile container with a preservative.
11. Record the collection of the specimen in the child's chart. Include the date and time of collection and the amount, color, and appearance of the urine.

HOME ADAPTATIONS

If a urine specimen is to be obtained at home, give instructions to the parent and provide the appropriate equipment. Parents can keep the urine collected at home in the refrigerator until they are asked to bring it to the laboratory. The specimen should be kept chilled during transport (i.e., placed in a cooler or plastic bag packed with ice).

noninvasive method is the pediatric urine collection bag or urine "wee bag." This collection device is a plastic bag with an opening lined with adhesive so that it can be attached to the perineum. It is available in two sizes, infant and pediatric, to accommodate almost any child. Twenty-four-hour collection bags are also available. These bags have a tube that extends from the end of the bag, allowing each void to be removed.

Although some facilities use sterile urine collection bags to obtain a specimen for urine culture, this method of collecting urine is considered inappropriate to rule out a urinary tract infection. Bags can become contaminated with organisms usually present in the perineal area. Most physicians choose to use straight catheterization or suprapubic aspiration (inserting a needle through the skin and directly into the bladder) to obtain urine for culture from an incontinent child.

Urinary Catheterization

Catheterizing a child is different from catheterizing an adult because of the child's unique psychologic and developmental needs (Procedure 13-4). Pediatric catheterization kits often contain a completely closed collection system (with the catheter end already enclosed in the collection tube). Choose a urinary catheter that is small enough so that it can be inserted easily into the urinary meatus but large enough to prevent leakage of urine. Avoid using feeding tubes as straight catheters because these could become coiled or knotted after insertion (Smith, 2003). Urinary catheters are available in sizes as small as 5F and can be matched to the child's age as follows:

- Infants up to 1 year old: 5F to 8F
- Children 1 to 5 years old: 8F
- School-age children: 8F to 12F
- Adolescents: 10F to 14F

PROCEDURE 13-4	**URINARY CATHETERIZATION**

PURPOSE: To obtain a sterile urine sample

1. Prepare the child for the procedure by using age-appropriate methods. Explain what the child will feel and what the child can do to "help." Demonstrating the procedure on a teaching doll may be helpful. Teach the child to take slow, deep breaths during the procedure, and have the child practice breathing before the procedure. Encouraging the child to sing also helps relax the appropriate muscles. The child might feel a need to urinate during the catheter insertion. Reassure the child that the feeling is normal. The assistance of another adult is often necessary with younger children.
2. Make sure the area is well lighted and gather all necessary equipment. If equipment is not contained in the catheterization kit, bring the appropriate-size catheter, sterile gloves (extra pairs in case of contamination), specimen cup, sterile topical anesthetic lubricant, label, and requisition form. If the child is to have an indwelling catheter, bring a closed drainage bag.
3. The procedure is the same as for an adult, with the following additions:
   a. Take extra care to be gentle when cleansing the meatus or glans penis.
   b. Choose the appropriate-size catheter (see text this page). Apply the lubricant according to manufacturer's directions.
   c. In girls, direct the catheter slightly upward and insert it gently through the meatus 1 to 2 inches (2.5 to 5 cm) or until urine appears. In boys, hold the penis at a 90-degree angle from the boy and gently insert the catheter 2 to 4 inches (5 to 10 cm) (longer in older boys) or until urine appears. Never force the catheter. The older child can assist in relaxing the external sphincter by bearing down.
4. When using an indwelling catheter, measure the distance from the catheter tip to the end of the balloon. Once urine

is observed, insert the catheter an additional amount at least equal to this distance before inflating the balloon, or follow institution policy regarding insertion length. Research-based recommendations on insertion suggest inserting an indwelling catheter until urine is visualized and then inserting it an additional amount before inflating the balloon: 2 inches (5 cm) for girls, 3 to 4 inches (7.5 to 10 cm) for boys newborn to preschool, and 5 inches (12.5 cm) for older boys.* These distances reduce the risk of the balloon inflating in the urethra. Before inserting a Foley catheter, inflate and deflate the balloon to check for function and leaks.

5. Record the date and time the procedure was performed as well as the size of catheter used and the amount, color, and appearance of the urine. Note how the infant or child tolerated the procedure. Deliver the labeled specimen promptly, together with the requisition form, to the laboratory.

HOME ADAPTATIONS

Catheterizing at home is usually a clean rather than sterile procedure used for children who have spina bifida, neurogenic bladder, or incomplete bladder emptying. Some families choose to use a new, packaged catheter each time; however, this can be extremely expensive when a child has to be catheterized several times per day. The alternative is to thoroughly rinse, clean, and dry the catheters and keep them in a clean, covered container or a plastic bag if the child is carrying the catheter in a pocket or pack. The parent needs to follow physician protocol for cleaning the perineum; this may include mild soap and water or the use of povidone-iodine. The infant or young child can be catheterized on a changing table, allowing the urine to empty into a diaper or small container; the older child can be catheterized on the toilet. When teaching a girl how to self-catheterize, use a mirror to help her identify landmarks.

---

*Smith, A., & Adams, L. (1998). Insertion of indwelling urethral catheters in infants and children: a survey of current nursing practice. *Pediatric Nursing, 24*(3), 229-234.

Some facilities recommend precatheterization topical application and instillation of an anesthetic lubricant, such as 2% lidocaine hydrochloride, to diminish discomfort associated with catheterization (Gerard, Cooper, Duethman, Gordley, & Kleiber, 2003). Some children, particularly those who undergo multiple urinary tract catheterizations (e.g., children with spina bifida), are at high risk for developing latex sensitivity. These children and other children with known or suspected latex allergy should be identified as early as possible, and latex-free catheters should be used.

Stool Specimens

Stool specimens are obtained to test for the presence of fat, blood, bacteria, parasites, or reducing substances in the stool. If a stool specimen from an incontinent child is needed, it often can be scraped from a diaper and placed in an appropriate container. If the stool is watery, a specimen may be collected by placing a piece of gauze in the diaper to absorb some of the stool or by applying a "wee bag" over the anus.

A bedpan or a specimen collector designed to be placed in the toilet can be used to obtain a specimen from an older child. Because older children may be embarrassed about providing a stool sample, the nurse should use a calm, matter-of-fact manner when explaining why the specimen is needed and the procedure for handling the specimen.

Blood Specimens

Nurses use a variety of techniques to collect blood samples from children. Because blood collection is an invasive procedure, it should be performed in a treatment room if one is available.

Regardless of the sampling procedure used, most children find blood collection distressing. Some are concerned about the pain involved, and others fear the perceived loss of body fluid. The use of a eutectic mixture of local anesthetics (EMLA), a topical anesthetic cream, can reduce the child's discomfort. To be effective, EMLA must remain on the site for at least 45 minutes before the needle is inserted (see Chapters 14 and 15). Other anesthetic systems that deliver lidocaine to a venipuncture site, such as iontophoresis or needle-free systems, have shown promise and act more rapidly than EMLA (Migdal, Chudzynska-Pomianowska, Vause, Henry, & Lazar, 2005).

In children who need long-term venous access for nutrition or medications and who have a central venous catheter or port in place, the nurse can obtain blood for laboratory studies from the central venous catheter or port. This procedure, however, may be performed *only* by specially trained, licensed personnel.

Venipuncture in children is often performed with a butterfly catheter (Procedure 13-5). The most commonly used sites are the veins of the hand and the antecubital area. Always follow Standard Precautions when collecting blood specimens or when assisting other personnel in collecting blood.

Jugular and Femoral Venipuncture

Jugular venipuncture and femoral venipuncture are performed by a physician, with the nurse assisting and monitoring the child. If obtaining blood from one of the large superficial

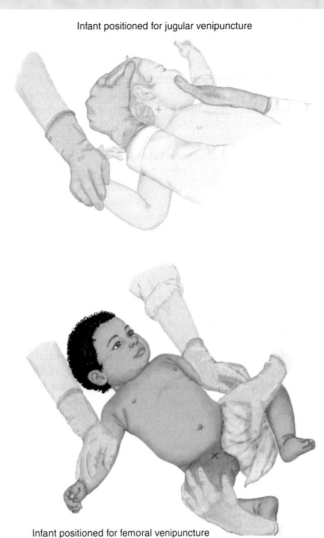

Infant positioned for jugular venipuncture

Infant positioned for femoral venipuncture

FIG 13-8 **Two additional sites for obtaining blood specimens from infants and young children are the large superficial external jugular veins and the femoral veins.**

external jugular veins, place the child in a mummy restraint (see Fig. 13-3), allowing enough area at the top edge of the restraint to permit access to the jugular vein. If a restraint is not used, the arms and legs can be held by a second nurse. The child's head is hyperextended to the side opposite the site, over the edge of a table or a small pillow (Fig. 13-8). After the venipuncture, apply pressure to the site for 3 to 5 minutes or until bleeding stops. Do not overextend the head to the point of causing airway problems.

If performing a femoral venipuncture, place the child supine in the frog-leg position to expose the groin area (see Fig. 13-8). One nurse stands above the child's head, holding the child's arms with the elbows and the legs with the hands. Place a cloth diaper over the infant's perineal area, tucked under the buttocks with the site exposed. The diaper protects the area in case the child urinates. Apply pressure to the site with a dry, sterile gauze square after the specimen is obtained.

Capillary Blood Sampling

When a small blood sample is needed, a disposable pediatric lancet (inserted 2.4 mm deep) can be used for a finger or

PROCEDURE 13-5	**VENIPUNCTURE**

PURPOSE: To obtain a blood sample for laboratory testing with minimal trauma to the child

1. As with any procedure, prepare the child using age-appropriate language. Be sure to include what the child will see and feel. Ask the parents whether it is better to prepare their young child in advance or to describe what you are doing as you are performing the procedure. Assistance is often necessary in restraining the child during the procedure. Parents may not wish to remain in the room. If EMLA is to be used, it must be applied at least 45 minutes in advance of the procedure; follow the timing directions for other topical anesthetics if used.

2. Take the child to the treatment room. Have the following equipment available: 23- or 25-gauge butterfly catheter, gloves, alcohol or povidone-iodine (Betadine) swabs or pads, syringe or syringes, labels, appropriate collection containers, requisition form, and tourniquet. (Note: Most tourniquets are composed of rubber tubing that is ½ to 1 inch wide. Although rubber bands have been used as tourniquets in infants, these are not preferred because they may abrade the skin.)

3. Restrain the child by having one nurse place one gloved hand under the child's arm (usually at the shoulder) and the other gloved hand on the child's hand. The sampling nurse is then able to draw the blood with less likelihood of missing the vein. The vein of the antecubital area is commonly used for venipuncture in children.

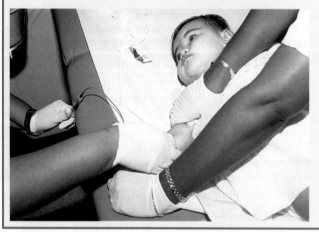

4. Put on gloves and apply a tourniquet tight enough to restrict blood flow toward the heart but not so tight as to cause pain or restrict arterial blood flow. Tourniquets are used to slow venous blood return to the heart and cause distention of the veins, thus making them more visible. To facilitate easy removal, the tourniquet should be looped when applied. To prevent hemoconcentration, a tourniquet should be left in place no longer than 2 minutes.

5. Lightly pat or rub the sample site to help the veins become more visible.

6. With a circular motion, clean the site with alcohol and allow to dry. If the child is immunocompromised, use povidone-iodine (Betadine) to cleanse the skin instead of alcohol. Do not use both together because they can damage the skin.

7. Insert the needle of the butterfly catheter into the vein, bevel side up.

8. When blood begins to flow into the catheter, avoid the temptation to place the syringe on the end of the catheter and attempt to speed up the blood flow by pulling back the plunger. Instead, to avoid venospasm, wait until the blood reaches the end of the catheter, attach the syringe, and slowly draw the appropriate amount of blood into the syringe. The tourniquet can be released when blood begins to flow into the syringe.

9. After obtaining the required amount of blood, withdraw the needle and apply pressure to the puncture site until the bleeding has stopped. Fill the appropriate specimen tubes or containers. Be sure to dispose of needles in the sharps container and contaminated gauze in the biohazard receptacle.

10. Comfort the child and offer praise for cooperation. Encourage the parent to provide comfort. Adhesive bandages are important because they help prevent bleeding from the puncture site. Specially colored or cartoon character bandages are available commercially and are appropriate for children's "boo boos." The nurse can also give the child a reward, such as a sticker.

11. Label the specimen with the child's name and record the date and time of collection, the amount of blood collected, the site used for puncture, and the reason blood was drawn (e.g., diagnostic test). Note the child's reaction to the procedure and the number of attempts made before a specimen was obtained.

(Courtesy Parkland Health and Hospital System Community Oriented Primary Care Clinic, Dallas, TX.)

heel puncture (Procedure 13-6). For finger punctures, the third (ring) finger of the nondominant hand should be used. Make the puncture just to the side of the finger pad rather than at the tip. Fewer nerve endings are in this location, and the area is highly vascular. The heel is used in infants; it is warmed first to increase blood flow. The heel is not used once the infant is walking because calluses make it more difficult to puncture.

Sputum Specimens

Sputum specimens are most frequently obtained to identify or rule out a respiratory infection. When obtaining any specimen, follow Standard Precautions. If splashing is anticipated, wear masks and goggles or protective eyewear in addition to gloves.

Obtaining sputum in the older child is relatively easy because most older children and adolescents can cough deeply

| PROCEDURE 13-6 | **CAPILLARY BLOOD SAMPLING** |

PURPOSE: To obtain a small sample of capillary blood

1. Prepare the child appropriately for the procedure by using developmentally appropriate explanations (finger poke, "owie"). You can warm the site before proceeding or have the older child wash the hands in warm water. If doing a heel stick on an infant, warm the heel for several minutes with a warm washcloth or a commercial warmer. To avoid a burn, the item used to warm the heel should not exceed 42° C (107.6° F).
2. Bring the child to the treatment room, where the following equipment should be available: disposable lancets or microlancets, alcohol or povidone-iodine (Betadine) swabs, sterile gauze pads, gloves, warm washcloth, specimen containers, and labels and requisition forms.
3. After putting on gloves and appropriately cleaning the site, make a puncture with the lancet across the fingerprint halfway between the center of the ball of the finger and its side. Use the third, or ring, finger of the nondominant hand. Do not use a bruised, edematous, or abraded finger, and avoid old puncture sites. If using the heel, use the lateral aspect of the heel and avoid any previously used site.
4. Wipe off the first drop of blood with a sterile gauze pad. To ensure adequate blood flow, gently massage the heel or the finger from its base to the tip.
5. Collect the blood in the appropriate container or containers. Apply pressure with sterile gauze until the bleeding stops. Apply a decorative adhesive bandage if the child desires. Do not apply an adhesive bandage on an infant.
6. Label the specimen with the child's name and record the date, time, amount of blood collected, site used for the puncture, and reason the blood was drawn. Note the child's reaction to the procedure and whether more than one puncture was necessary.

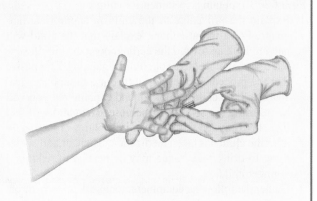

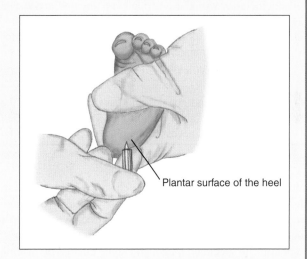

Plantar surface of the heel

| PROCEDURE 13-7 | **NASAL WASHING** |

PURPOSE: To obtain a nasopharyngeal secretion sample from an infant or young child

1. Prepare the child for the procedure by using developmentally appropriate language and describing any expected sensations (the procedure will make the child sneeze).
2. Gather the following equipment: butterfly catheter, syringe, sterile saline, gloves, goggles, sterile specimen container or pertussis kit, and labels and requisition form.
3. Ask for assistance restraining the child, or mummy wrap an infant to restrain the arms and legs.
4. Cut the "butterfly" (needle and wings) off the butterfly catheter and discard in a sharps container.
5. Attach a syringe (without needle) containing 1 to 3 mL sterile saline to the catheter and fill the catheter.
6. Put on gloves and goggles and place the child in a supine position; gently place the catheter into one nostril.
7. Instill the saline into the nostril and immediately withdraw into the syringe or aspirate secretions with a small sterile bulb syringe.
8. Place the saline or secretions into a sterile, labeled container.
9. Record the amount of saline instilled and the method of collection used. Note the date, time, amount, color, and consistency of secretions.

PROCEDURE 13-8	THROAT OR NASOPHARYNGEAL CULTURE

PURPOSE: To obtain a specimen for culture

1. Explain the procedure to the child in appropriate language. For a throat culture, explain that the child will need to look up toward the ceiling, open the mouth very wide, and may feel like coughing or gagging. Emphasize that the procedure does not hurt. For a nasopharyngeal swab, tell the child to look up and explain that you will be inserting the swab into the nose. The child will feel like sneezing. Do not do these procedures immediately after the child has taken medication, eaten, or had something to drink. Assistance may be needed to restrain a younger child.

2. Gather the following equipment: tongue depressor, throat or nasopharyngeal swab (cotton-tipped swab with a flexible wire extension), collection containers and labels (if not included with the swab), gloves, goggles, and sterile saline.

3. An older child can sit in a chair or sit upright in bed for the culture. A younger child should be placed supine on a bed or examining table.

THROAT CULTURE

4. Put on gloves and goggles and have the child open the mouth and say "ahhh." Eliciting a cry from an infant will give optimal access to the pharyngeal area. Insert a tongue depressor into the mouth with the nondominant hand so that it covers the anterior half of the tongue and depress the tongue to allow observation of the pharyngeal area. Swab the area quickly, avoiding the tongue, buccal mucosa, and palate. If the child opens the mouth wide enough for adequate visibility, a tongue depressor may not be needed. Only one swab should be used for each culture.

NASOPHARYNGEAL CULTURE

5. Ask the child to look up. Bend the wire so that, when the swab is inserted, the tip will go beyond the back of the nares and into the pharyngeal area. Dip the swab tip into saline and gently insert it into one nostril, down to the posterior nasopharynx. Leave it in place for several seconds and then remove.

6. After the specimen is obtained, place the swabs in the appropriate culture media and transport them to the laboratory.

7. If possible, offer the child cool fluids to drink after the procedure. Assist the parent to support and comfort the child during and after the procedure.

8. Record the date and time, the appearance of the specimen, and the child's response to the procedure.

---

and produce a sputum sample, which can then be placed in the appropriate container. Specimens are easily obtained from children with artificial airways by attaching a mucus or suction trap to a suction catheter and suctioning the airway to obtain the specimen. A cough can be elicited by placing a suction catheter into the back of the throat in an infant or young child.

Because younger children and infants can seldom produce a deep cough on demand and often swallow those secretions, obtaining sputum samples often requires a nasal washing, or *lavage* (Procedure 13-7). Nasal washing is particularly used to obtain a sample for identifying respiratory syncytial virus (RSV) and pertussis.

Throat and Nasopharyngeal Specimens

Throat cultures can identify the causative agent of sore throats or tonsillitis in children. Nasopharyngeal cultures are mainly used to identify pertussis (Procedure 13-8).

Cerebrospinal Fluid Specimens

Physicians perform lumbar punctures to examine the cerebrospinal fluid (CSF) for bacteria or abnormal cells, measure pressure within the cerebrospinal cavities, or inject certain medications (e.g., for pain control, to prevent or eradicate specific diseases, or as contrast agents for scans). A hollow spinal needle, inserted into the subarachnoid space between the third and fourth lumbar vertebrae, provides fluid exit and collection. An attached stopcock and manometer are used to measure spinal fluid pressure.

> **CRITICAL TO REMEMBER**
> **Throat Cultures**
> - Never attempt to obtain a throat specimen for culture in a child for whom a diagnosis of *epiglottitis* is suspected because the procedure could precipitate sudden airway obstruction.
> - Before obtaining a specimen for throat culture, assess for the presence of high fever of sudden onset, drooling, muffled voice, and erythema or exudate (signs of epiglottitis).

Because a lumbar puncture is frequently performed when a child is acutely ill, such as with meningitis or leukemia, this stressful procedure becomes even more stressful for the child and family. The nurse must provide a great deal of support and education for the child and family. The physician explains what is planned and obtains an informed consent from the parents or guardians. Only a physician or qualified nurse practitioner can perform a lumbar puncture. The nurse assists by positioning, restraining, and monitoring the child (see Chapter 28).

Bone Marrow Aspirates

Bone marrow aspiration is performed to obtain specimens of marrow for diagnostic testing, for evaluation of response to treatment, or for transplantation (see Chapter 24). The most common site of bone marrow aspiration in the child is the posterior iliac crest. Other sites include the anterior iliac crest and the tibia.

Because the reasons for a bone marrow aspiration include ruling out serious disease, such as leukemia, or assessing the progress of cancer treatment, the child and family need a tremendous amount of support and preparation before the procedure.

GAVAGE AND GASTROSTOMY

Because some infants and children are unable to tolerate adequate oral nutrition, the physician may select an alternative method of feeding. *Enteral feedings* are an option for infants and children who are premature, ill, or injured or who have congenital anomalies, respiratory distress, swallowing disorders, or neurologic impairment or have previously undergone surgery. Feedings are given through an orogastric, nasogastric, or transpyloric tube or through a gastrostomy tube or button.

Tube Route and Placement

Placement of a gastrostomy tube or gastrostomy button is a surgical procedure. The nurse usually places an orogastric (OG), nasogastric (NG), or nasointestinal tube (Procedures 13-9 and 13-10). Nasogastric tubes are used most frequently because the tube is easier to stabilize with nasal placement than with oral placement and has a decreased risk of inappropriate insertion into the respiratory tract. Because of increased mucus production caused by irritation from the tube, nasal placement can potentially interfere with respiratory function. Children with head or nasal anomalies or injuries and infants who are still preferential nose breathers (usually those 4 months old or younger) will need orogastric tube placement. A nasointestinal tube is more difficult to insert than an orogastric or nasogastric tube because it must exit the pyloric sphincter into the small intestine.

Controversy exists regarding measurement of the length of the tube to be inserted. The two most common methods of measurement are (1) from the nose to the ear and to the end of the xiphoid process and (2) from the nose to the ear and to a point midway between the xiphoid process and umbilicus. Studies have examined the role that height and, in low-birth-weight infants, weight play in gastric insertion distance. Additional research is needed in this area.

Tube Selection

Many types and sizes of tubes are commercially available. Factors influencing the selection of feeding tubes include the child's age and size, the viscosity of the formula, the reason for the enteral feeding, and whether an infusion device will be used. A feeding tube of size 5F to 10F is used in infants, and the size increases proportionately for older children. Selecting the smallest bore tube for the infusion and a tube of soft material will decrease the child's discomfort.

Safety Issues Related to Tube Placement

Tube placement must be verified at the time the tube is inserted, any time feeding is interrupted, before each bolus feeding or medication administration, and every 4 to 8 hours during continuous feeding (unless institution policy requires more frequent assessment). Although auscultation (listening for a distinctive "whooshing" or "gurgling" sound after insufflation of a small amount of air) is the most frequently used method for checking tube placement at the bedside, examination of aspirate and pH measurement of the aspirate are considered more reliable (Huffman, Jarczyk, O'Brien, Pieper, & Bayne, 2004; Metheny & Titler, 2001). Auscultation as a piece of confirmatory data relies on the nurse's experience because a similar sound can be heard if the tube is placed in the respiratory tract.

Aspiration of enteral fluid can indicate the probability of the tube being in the stomach (pH of 5 or lower), particularly when accompanied by grassy green, brown, or mucoid-flecked, clear aspirate. In children whose aspirate pH is greater than 5, the tube could be in the intestine beyond the pylorus or in the respiratory tract. Aspirate color can help distinguish the two, with intestinal aspirate being yellowish-green in appearance and respiratory aspirate looking more like gastric aspirate (Huffman et al., 2004). Respiratory tube placement is more of a risk in children who have decreased level of consciousness; who are uncooperative or restless; recently intubated or extubated; or who demonstrate decreased swallowing, cough, or gag reflexes (Metheny & Titler, 2001). Keep in mind that both formula and certain medications can alter pH of enteral secretions (Huffman et al., 2004). Most research done on tube placement in adults and children emphasizes that *radiographic confirmation of tube placement is the only definitive method of correct positioning* (Huffman et al., 2004).

Do not assume that a feeding tube has remained in proper position just because the external position has not changed. Tubes can become dislodged with suctioning, retching, or vomiting. Measuring, marking and documenting the external length of the tube immediately after insertion will assist in determining whether the tube has lost its original position.

Contraindications to Tube Placement

Determine any preexisting contraindications to the procedure, such as prior surgeries, trauma, or congenital anomalies (e.g., choanal atresia, tracheoesophageal fistula, esophageal strictures) that could interfere with passage of the tube. If any of these findings are present, the physician may use fluoroscopy to guide the insertion. *Do not reinsert a dislodged tube that was placed during or through a surgical repair. Notify the surgeon if the tube becomes dislodged.*

Gastrostomy Feedings

The procedure for gastrostomy feedings is similar to that for orogastric, nasogastric, or nasointestinal feedings. As with any tube feeding, hold the infant or young child, when possible, to associate the feeding with pleasant sensations and socialization and to promote normal development and bonding.

Special considerations for children with gastrostomy tubes or buttons include skin and stoma care. Assess the site for abnormal findings such as leakage, redness around

| PROCEDURE 13-9 | FEEDING TUBE INSERTIONS |

PURPOSE: To provide enteral nutrition

1. Using developmentally appropriate language, explain the procedure to the child and family and assess their needs and concerns (e.g., previous experience with tube insertion, ability to assist with the procedure, need for restraint). Therapeutic play can be used to allay the child's and parents' fears related to the procedure.

2. Gather the following equipment before starting the procedure: feeding tube of appropriate size and type, ¼- or ½-inch hypoallergenic tape, 20-mL syringe, sterile water for oral use, stethoscope, water-soluble lubricating jelly (for nasal insertion only), pH reagent strips, gloves, feeding pump and setup (enteral feeding bag or burette), and the enteral fluid to be administered.

3. Position the child on the back or right side with the head of the bed elevated. To facilitate cooperation and decrease fear, a small child can be held in a parent's arms, with the child's head on the parent's shoulder. An older child may sit up in the bed. Restrain if necessary.

4. Wash your hands and don gloves.

5. Measure the length of the catheter to be inserted, and mark with a waterproof marker or with tape:

   a. To place a nasogastric tube in a child, measure the distance from the tip of the nose to the earlobe and then down to the xiphoid process. Mark the total measurement on the tube.

   b. To place an orogastric tube in an infant, measure the tube from the tip of the nose to the earlobe and to the midpoint between the end of the xiphoid process and the umbilicus. The total measurement (nose-ear-xiphoid) should be marked on the tube with tape or indelible marker.

6. To facilitate passage through the nasopharynx, lubricate the tube with water or water-soluble lubricant. In neonates and for orogastric placement, use water only.

7. Insert the tube gently but firmly through the mouth or nose and down the throat. If you encounter obstruction or if the tube curls in the mouth, remove the tube and repeat this step. If the child gasps, coughs, gags, or turns cyanotic, withdraw the tube and wait for the response to subside before proceeding.

8. Continue to advance the tube gently to the predetermined mark. While advancing the tube, ask the cooperative child to swallow repeatedly when the tube reaches the pharynx, or give small sips of water through a straw if not contraindicated. Swallowing will ease insertion into the esophagus. Advance the tube 5 to 10 cm with each swallow. Giving an infant a pacifier will encourage swallowing. Direct the tube toward the back of the throat.

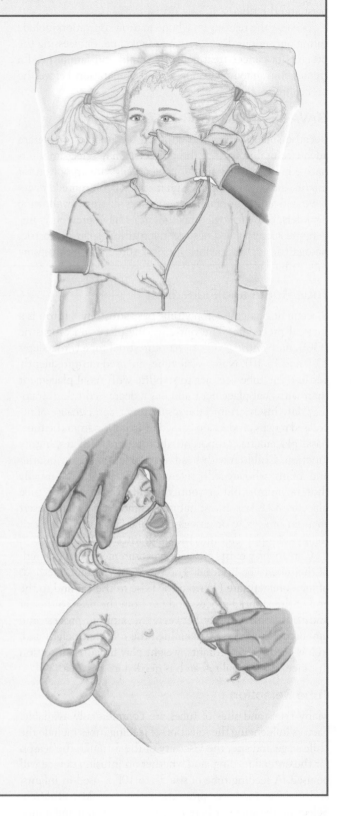

the site, drainage, bleeding, and skin breakdown. Clean the skin around the tube insertion site with soap and water once or twice daily, depending on the condition, and with each spillage. To facilitate complete cleansing, rotate gastrostomy buttons in a full circle during cleaning.

Capped gastrostomy tubes extend several inches from the insertion site. Check to ensure that no tension is on the external tube. If necessary, coil the tube and tape near the exit site. Gastrostomy buttons are placed close to the skin surface. They have a one-way valve that eliminates the

PROCEDURE 13-9 | **FEEDING TUBE INSERTIONS—cont'd**

9. Temporarily secure the tube with tape to stabilize it while you check the tube position.

10. Attach the syringe to the end of the tube, and insufflate 1 to 5 mL (more for an older child or adolescent) of air. Then, after withdrawing the air, attempt to aspirate the gastric contents for pH testing. Choking or soundless coughing may indicate placement in the trachea. Accidental placement of a small-diameter tube into the lungs may not be as apparent as with larger tubes, particularly if the child's cough or gag reflex is absent or suppressed; radiographic confirmation of small-bore tube placement usually is necessary.*

11. Check the pH of the aspirate to confirm gastric or intestinal placement. (Note: Administration of antacid and gastric acid inhibitors will alter the pH of the aspirate, thus affecting the reliability of the pH test.*)

12. If a nasointestinal tube with a guide wire has been used, remove the guide wire by holding the tube at the child's nostril or the corner of the mouth and slowly removing it. To allow gravity to assist in the advancement of the tube into the duodenum, keep the child on the right side. A plain abdominal film will be ordered by the physician to confirm tube placement in the duodenum.

13. Once tube placement is confirmed, tape the tube securely in place and label the tube with the date and time of insertion. Refer to your facility's policy and procedure manual for recommended frequency of tube change. With indelible marker, mark the tube just below the insertion site. This will assist with future assessments of tube placement.

14. Record in the nurses' notes the size and type of tube used, route, placement, pH testing results, measurement of visible length, date and time of insertion, child and family teaching, procedure tolerance, and any problems encountered.

HOME ADAPTATIONS

If the child is to receive enteral nutrition at home, teach the parent how to insert and check placement of the tube. Tube placement should be confirmed before each feeding or medication administration.† Describe comfort measures that may be helpful. Be sure to have the parent give a return demonstration before taking the child home. Make sure the parent has and knows how to read pH strips. Provide the parent with directions for reaching the health care provider if there is a question about tube placement.

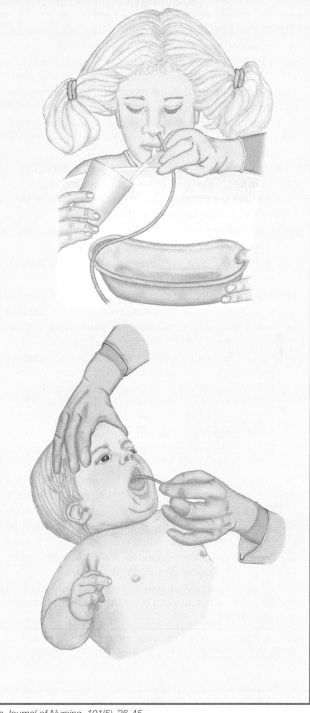

*Metheny, N., & Titler, M. (2001). Assessing placement of feeding tubes. *American Journal of Nursing, 101*(5), 36-45.
†Huffman, S., Jarczyk, K., O'Brien, E., Pieper, P., & Bayne, A. (2004). Methods to confirm feeding tube placement: application of research in practice. *Pediatric Nursing, 30*(1), 10-13.

need for clamping and offers the added advantage of allowing children to participate in regular childhood activities. When feeding a child with a gastrostomy button, you might need to place extension tubing between the button and the feeding pump.

Watch for signs that the tube or button may need to be replaced. These signs include leaking, tube occlusion, malfunction of the antireflux valve, or abnormal tube position. Report these findings to the physician.

Many children are discharged home with gastrostomy tubes in place. Parents must be able to provide all required care. Parent teaching is a major part of the nursing care of a child with a feeding tube. Parents must know how to check tube position, how to administer feedings, how to care for

PROCEDURE 13-10	ADMINISTERING ENTERAL FEEDINGS (VIA THE OROGASTRIC, NASOGASTRIC, OR NASOINTESTINAL ROUTE)

PURPOSE: To provide adequate nutrition in a child who cannot tolerate oral feedings

1. Using developmentally appropriate language, explain the procedure to the child and family. Assess their needs and concerns related to the procedure, such as previous experience with enteral feedings, ability to assist with the procedure, and need for restraint. Use therapeutic play to allay the child's and parent's fears related to the procedure.

2. The following equipment is needed: stethoscope, irrigation syringe, room-temperature formula and warm water, pacifier for neonates and infants, electronic feeding pump (for continuous tube feedings), and gloves.

INTERMITTENT FEEDINGS (BOLUS)

3. Technique:
   a. Position the child and remove the syringe or cap from the tube. Put on gloves.
   b. Check for proper tube placement (be sure the mark indicating insertion length is in its original place relative to the exit site), instill several milliliters of air, and aspirate for residual volume from the previous feed. Follow the facility's policy and procedure manual or physician's orders for disposition of residual volume. Follow institutional policy about flushing the tube with warm water before beginning the feeding. Flushing the tube before and after bolus feedings prevents build-up that can cause tube occlusion.*
   c. Remove the plunger from the syringe and attach the syringe to the tube.
   d. Pour room-temperature formula into the syringe and allow the feeding to flow slowly into the tube (usually over a period of 15 to 30 minutes). Raising or lowering the level of the syringe increases or decreases the flow of formula. Discontinue the feeding if signs of respiratory distress, cyanosis, abdominal distention, or vomiting occur. Notify the physician.
   e. After the prescribed volume has been infused, flush the tube with water and clear the tube by injecting 1 to 5 mL of air.
   f. Discard the used syringe and close or clamp the tube unless otherwise indicated.
   g. Leave the child lying on the right side with the head of the bed elevated for 30 to 60 minutes after the feeding.

CONTINUOUS FEEDINGS

4. Technique:
   a. Position the child and check tube placement. The aspirate will probably have the appearance of curdled milk if the tube is in the stomach or look bile stained if in the intestine. Because feeding can alter aspirate pH, the pH is a less reliable indicator of placement when a child is on continuous feeds.†
   b. Fill the feeding bag, volume-control set, or syringe and tubing with the prescribed formula.
   c. Attach infusion tubing to the feeding tube and begin the infusion at the prescribed rate.
   d. Check tube placement and residual volumes every 4 to 8 hours. Flush with water according to institution policy.
   e. To reduce the incidence of reflux and aspiration, keep the child positioned on the abdomen or right side.

5. If aspirate was present, record the amount, color, and consistency. Note whether it was re-fed or discarded. Note the type and amount of formula and the child's tolerance of the procedure. Note the position of the child after feeding and whether the tube is clamped or open (an open clamp allows venting of air).

HOME ADAPTATIONS

Assess the parents' ability to perform enteral feedings. Parents should be encouraged to make this as normal a procedure as possible (e.g., by holding the infant during feedings). Ask the parent to demonstrate the procedure before discharge. Assistance with home care can be provided by a home health agency. Advise the parent to follow manufacturer's recommendations about discarding opened unused formula left at room temperature.

*Reising, D., & Neal, R. (2005). Enteral tube flushing. *American Journal of Nursing, 105*(3), 58-63.
†Methany, N., & Titler, M. (2001). Assessing placement of feeding tubes. *American Journal of Nursing, 101*(5), 36-45.

CRITICAL TO REMEMBER
Enteral Feedings

- Begin the feeding *only* after tube placement in the stomach has been properly verified.
- Discontinue feedings and notify the physician if signs of respiratory distress, cyanosis, abdominal distention, or vomiting occur.
- Provide a pacifier to infants so that they can associate sucking with feeding. Encourage older children to sit at a table during meals to promote the normal socialization associated with eating.

- To avoid accidental overfeeding should the infusion pump malfunction, use only an amount of formula appropriate for a 4-hour feeding. Discard any formula that has been opened for more than 4 hours.
- Follow the facility's policy or procedure manual or physician's orders regarding disposing of residual volumes and the prescribed frequency for changing feeding equipment.

the tube, what symptoms should be reported, and what to do if the tube becomes dislodged. Booklets are available to assist the family in the care of the child with a gastrostomy tube or button.

ENEMAS

Enemas are given when stool needs to be removed from the bowel because of severe constipation or in preparation for a diagnostic procedure or surgery. Giving an enema to an infant or child differs little from the procedure for an adult. The differences are the type and amount of fluid administered and the distance that the enema tip is inserted into the rectum.

Enema Administration

Rectal damage and perforation can occur with improper insertion of the enema tip. Insert a lubricated tip gently 2.5 cm to 7.5 cm, depending on the age and size of the child. Commercially prepared single-use enemas come with a prelubricated tip of appropriate length.

Solutions and Volumes

The amount of the enema solution will vary with the age and size of the child. Unless the physician's orders specify a different amount, the values listed in Table 13-2 for volume of solution and depth of enema tip insertion into the rectum are recommended. Only isotonic solutions should be used with children. Plain tap water should never be used because it is hypotonic and can cause a rapid fluid shift and fluid overload.

After completing an enema, diaper the infant. Toddlers can use the bedpan or "potty" if possible. Older children

TABLE 13-2	Recommended Volume and Depth for Enema Tip Insertion, by Age	
	Volume (mL)	**Depth of Insertion**
Infants	120-240	1 in (2.5 cm)
2-4 yr	240-360	2 in (5 cm)
4-10 yr	360-480	3 in (7.5 cm)
11 yr and older	480-720	4 in (10 cm)

and adolescents can use the bedpan or bedside commode or be assisted to the bathroom. Record in the nurses' notes or I&O sheet the date and time the enema was given, the type and amount of solution, the amount and characteristics of stool, any unusual findings (e.g., blood, mucus, foreign bodies, worms), and the child's tolerance of the procedure.

OSTOMIES

Urinary and fecal diversion may be needed when normal methods of elimination are temporarily or permanently halted. Some conditions requiring the creation of a fecal stoma include imperforate anus, Hirschsprung disease, necrotizing enterocolitis, some cases of intestinal atresia, intussusception, Crohn disease, and ulcerative colitis (see Chapter 19). The anatomic location of the stoma will dictate the consistency of the stool. The higher the stoma, the more liquid is the stool.

Urinary diversion is usually the result of obstructive uropathy, congenital anomalies, or occasionally neurogenic bladder (see Chapter 28). The ureters can be brought out through the abdominal wall (ureterostomy) or connected to a segment of small bowel (ileal conduit).

Nursing care of the child with an ostomy focuses on minimizing the obstacles the child and family face in learning to care for the ostomy, maximizing skin integrity, encouraging the child and family to be actively involved in the treatment regimen, providing support and guidance, and making appropriate referrals to an enterostomal therapist or other support system. The actual management and care of pediatric ostomies differ little from that in adults with ostomies. The major difference is the need to use developmentally appropriate terminology to explain the procedure and care of the ostomy to the child and family. A teaching model, such as a doll with a stoma, can facilitate child and family education.

OXYGEN THERAPY

Hypoxemia, resulting from apnea or inadequate ventilation, occurs more rapidly in children than in adults because of children's higher metabolic rate and increased oxygen consumption. Because cardiopulmonary arrest in children can follow progressive respiratory distress, early recognition of subtle signs and symptoms of respiratory distress is a necessary skill for every nurse.

Oxygen is an essential body requirement for any energy-consuming activity or function. For infants and children who are unable to maintain a normal arterial oxygen pressure (PaO_2), supplemental oxygen may be needed. Because oxygen is a drug, a physician's order is needed for administration, except in an emergency situation. Follow your facility's policy for oxygen administration in emergencies.

Oxygen Delivery

Oxygen may be administered to children by nasal cannula, face mask (simple, nonrebreather, partial rebreather, Venturi, or aerosol), an oxygen hood, or an oxygen tent (Fig. 13-9). The method of delivery depends on the concentration needed and the child's ability to cooperate with the chosen method.

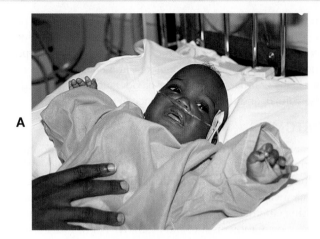

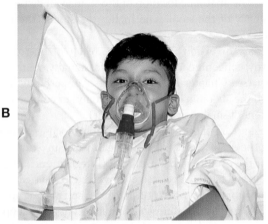

FIG 13-9 **Administering oxygen to children differs from the procedure in adults in the choice and size of equipment and in the greater need to educate and support the child and family. A, Nasal cannula. B, Simple face mask.** *(Courtesy Parkland Health and Hospital System, Dallas, TX.)*

In most facilities, a respiratory therapist is responsible for the setup, maintenance, and management of oxygen equipment. However, the nurse needs to have a working knowledge of the oxygen delivery system used.

The primary differences in oxygen delivery between children and adults are the size of the equipment and the teaching and emotional support needed for children receiving oxygen and their families. Usually an oxygen hood is used to provide maximal oxygenation for neonates and infants. Older infants and young toddlers may better tolerate a nasal cannula, blow-by oxygen, or face mask. Oxygen delivery by nasal cannula, the blow-by method, or a face mask works well for toddlers and preschoolers. School-age children and adolescents prefer nonrebreather masks to achieve maximal oxygenation.

Children experiencing difficulty breathing may be less than cooperative when an attempt is made to place a mask or cannula on the face. Explain to the child and family in developmentally appropriate language what will happen, why the mask is needed, and how it will feel. Provide assistance, if needed, to keep the oxygen delivery system in place. Check the physician's orders for the percentage of oxygen to be delivered and the method of delivery.

A nasal cannula is a low-flow delivery system indicated for infants and children who need modest amounts of supplemental oxygen (up to 40%). Flow rates should not exceed 6 L/min. The loop of the cannula can be enlarged to slip easily over the child's ears. Place the prongs in the nares and tighten the loop. If the child is active, tape the cannula to the sides of the child's face to maintain proper position. Be aware, however, that a flow rate exceeding 6 L/min can irritate the nasopharynx and cause gastric distention and regurgitation without appreciably improving the child's oxygenation.

The simple face mask and the Venturi mask are indicated for infants and children who need modest amounts of supplemental oxygen (35% to 60%, or a flow rate of 6 to 10 L/min). The Venturi mask can be adjusted to deliver specific concentrations of oxygen (e.g., 24%, 28%, 35%, 40%, or 50%). You must maintain a minimum flow rate of 6 L/min to prevent rebreathing of exhaled carbon dioxide.

Partial and full nonrebreathing masks are simple face masks with an attached reservoir that allows a portion of exhaled gas to remain in the bag and mix with oxygen. These masks supply oxygen concentrations of 50% to 60% at a rate of 10 to 12 L/min. A nonrebreather system can deliver almost 100% oxygen at a flow rate of 10 to 15 L/min.

Proper fit of an oxygen mask will ensure adequate oxygen delivery. When delivering oxygen by mask, select the correct size of mask to ensure a tight fit. Masks are available in preemie, newborn, infant, child, small adult, and adult sizes. To determine proper size, check to see that the mask extends from the bridge of the child's nose to the cleft of the chin. Attach the mask to the humidified oxygen source and adjust the flow rate to the prescribed level. Then place the mask over the child's face and adjust the nose clip and head strap.

In rare circumstances in which a child needs a humidified environment with oxygen, a cool mist tent may be indicated. In this instance, ensure the sides of the tent are completely tucked in to prevent escape of oxygen and that the child remains as dry as possible.

With the use of any oxygen administration system, safety is of great concern. Post "oxygen in use/no smoking" signs outside the child's door and over the bed. Although most health care facilities are nonsmoking facilities, remind parents and visitors that smoking is not allowed in the room. Toys that have the potential for producing a spark, including those that are battery powered, should not be permitted near the oxygen.

Documentation

Record in the nurse's notes the date and time; the type of oxygen administration system used; the percentage of oxygen delivered and the flow rate; the child's vital signs, skin color, respiratory effort, and lung sounds; the child's response to the procedure; and any teaching done with the child or family.

Parent Teaching

Infants and children often receive home oxygen therapy. Educate parents or caregivers about the operation of equipment to be used at home, equipment cleaning, safety factors, cardiopulmonary resuscitation, and available support services.

ASSESSING OXYGENATION

Pulse oximetry is a sensitive, reliable, noninvasive means of measuring oxygen saturation (SaO_2) in the blood. Oxygen saturation is the percentage of hemoglobin that is carrying the full complement of oxygen molecules (completely saturated). Pulse oximetry measures the absorption of light waves as they pass through highly perfused areas of the body, providing the nurse with valuable information and acting as an early warning of hypoxemia. Pulse oximetry is a valuable method of assessing oxygenation status in acutely ill infants and children. It accurately identifies children whose oxygenation status is marginal (Fig. 13-10; Procedure 13-11). The relation between oxygen saturation and actual oxygenation (as measured by PaO_2 [see Chapter 21]) is not 1:1. In general, a small decrease in oxygen saturation can represent a much larger decrease in PaO_2 (Popovich, Richiuso, & Danek, 2004). Because of this, nurses must quickly report any decreases in oxygen saturation.

Pulse oximetry has several advantages. It is noninvasive, requires no special site preparation, and in most cases yields an accurate measurement of oxygenation status in the neonate, infant, child, or adult. Also, values are available immediately. Despite some limitations, pulse oximetry has significant benefit in the assessment and care of the ill child. The immediate feedback it provides can alert the nurse to changes in oxygenation that require immediate intervention.

Pulse oximeter measurements reflect the child's oxygen saturation and the perfusion status. Potential sources of error in measurements include an abnormal hemoglobin value (e.g., in hyperbilirubinemia or carbon monoxide poisoning), decreased peripheral perfusion (e.g., in hypotension or hypothermia), ambient light interference, motion artifact, and

PROCEDURE 13-11	PULSE OXIMETRY

PURPOSE: To assess the child's oxygen saturation
1. Explain to the child and family the indication for the procedure and describe the appearance of the sensor (e.g., "E.T., the extraterrestrial") to enhance cooperation.
2. Bring the oximeter and sensor (finger probe, adhesive probe, or ear clip) to the child's room. The sensor will differ depending on whether the oximetry is intermittent or continuous.
3. Set the parameters for the alarm on continuous measuring oximeters.
4. Place the probe on the finger, toe, or foot. Avoid placing the probe on an extremity with an arterial line, blood pressure cuff, or intravenous (IV) line in place. Fingernail polish or artificial nails will need to be removed before placing the sensor. Do not wrap the sensor so tightly as to prevent venous flow and cause inaccurate readings.
5. Observe and record the pulse rate and oxygen saturation. The pulse rate on the oximeter should coincide with an apical pulse or pulse rate on a cardiac monitor. If no pulse is detected, reposition the sensor.
6. To check the skin condition, remove the sensor from the site at least every 2 hours. If using a portable oximeter, be sure to clean the sensor with alcohol or the manufacturer's recommended cleaning solution.
7. Record the child's response to the procedure and the pulse oximetry reading obtained, the percentage of oxygen (if in use), and the activity level of the child. Report any abnormal findings to the physician (<95%, except in children with chronic cardiac or respiratory disease who might have a lower "normal" pulse oximetry value).
8. Inform parents that an alarm will sound if the child's oxygen saturation falls below the set parameters. The alarm may also sound if the child is particularly active or the sensor becomes dislodged.

A

B

C

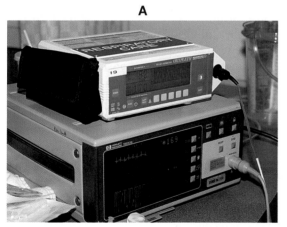
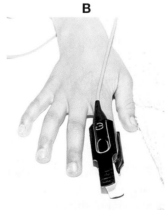
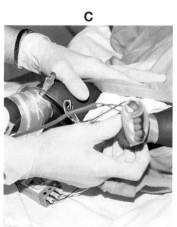

FIG 13-10 **A, The pulse oximeter is a reliable, noninvasive way to measure blood oxygen saturation, allowing rapid adjustments in oxygen delivery to meet the child's needs. The sensor is applied to a child's finger (B) or an infant's toe (C) to permit information to be sent to the pulse oximeter.** (*A courtesy Parkland Health and Hospital System, Dallas, TX.*)

skin breakdown from the adhesive used to secure the sensor. To eliminate the effects of ambient light, an opaque shield can be placed over the sensor site. Skin breakdown can be avoided by using a reusable sensor.

Under certain circumstances, capillary or arterial blood gases may need to be measured to establish correlation of oxygenation with pulse oximetry readings. Both capillary and arterial blood gas measurements are invasive. They measure the blood's oxygen content and the body's acid-base balance. Sampling can be done from indwelling arterial catheters or by arterial puncture.

The procedure for arterial blood sampling differs between the adult and pediatric populations. The differences include the sites used, the size of the equipment, the angle of entry, and the psychosocial interactions with the child and family. The preferred site in children is the radial artery, although alternatives (e.g., brachial artery) can be used. A capillary blood gas measurement provides similar information but is a less-painful and less-invasive procedure.

Because a respiratory therapist or trained nurse or other personnel must draw arterial blood for blood gas measurements, the novice nurse is primarily responsible for assisting with the procedure and restraining or comforting the child. Be sure to place the arterial blood gas specimen in ice for transport to the laboratory.

CRITICAL TO REMEMBER
Assisting with Arterial Blood Gas Sampling

- Position the child's wrist with the palm up but not hyperextended. Stabilize the extremity, allowing neither twisting of the wrist nor jerking of the shoulder.
- Do not hold the child's arm too tightly because a tight grip occludes arterial blood flow.
- The skin is punctured at an angle of 15 to 45 degrees. When the needle is withdrawn, it is withdrawn slowly to decrease the incidence of arterial spasm.
- After the needle is withdrawn, apply direct pressure to the site using a sterile 2 inch × 2 inch gauze pad for at least 5 minutes.
- If the analysis is not to be done immediately, place the sample on ice.
- Record the puncture site and the child's activity level at the time of the sampling.

CHEST PHYSIOTHERAPY

Chest physiotherapy (CPT) includes postural drainage, chest percussion and vibration, and coughing and deep-breathing exercises. These techniques can mobilize and eliminate secretions, reexpand the lungs, and promote efficient use of the respiratory muscles, particularly in children with cystic fibrosis. CPT also may be used prophylactically in postoperative clients. Contraindications to this therapy include head

injury, acute asthma, chest trauma with an unstable chest wall, osteogenesis imperfecta, and lung tumor.

In most health care facilities, CPT is the responsibility of the respiratory or physical therapist, but if respiratory therapy coverage is not available, the nurse performs this procedure (Procedure 13-12) when needed. Many children with chronic pulmonary disease receive this treatment at home, so the family must be educated in performing this aspect of the child's care. The goal of CPT is to prevent atelectasis and pneumonia.

Initiation of CPT requires a physician's order. The order should include the number of treatments per day, and it may specify the areas of the lungs to be treated. *Percussion* is rhythmic clapping with a cupped hand over the affected portion of the lung or the simulation of this movement with a percussion cup or mechanical percussor or vibrator. *Postural drainage* entails positioning the child to promote gravity-assisted drainage of the lungs. These two treatments are usually used in conjunction with each other and are carried out three or four times per day or more often if indicated. To decrease the risk of aspiration, treatments are performed before meals or 1½ hours after meals. Children receiving continuous feedings should have their feeding interrupted 1 hour before the treatment. The "lost volume" can then be replaced in the interval before the next treatment.

The length of the treatment depends on the child's ability to tolerate the procedure but is usually 20 to 30 minutes. Although several positions are possible for postural drainage, all of them may not be necessary at each session. Infants can be positioned on the lap with a pillow for the entire procedure. The pattern of postural drainage is similar to that for an older child.

TRACHEOSTOMY CARE

A *tracheostomy* is a surgically created opening (stoma) in the trachea. It is performed in children to bypass an upper airway obstruction, facilitate pulmonary toilet, or optimize mechanical ventilation. Tracheostomies can be either temporary or permanent. The use of tracheostomies for acute airway management has decreased because of the increased use of endotracheal intubation; tracheostomies continue to be used for long-term management of problem airways, with parents managing the tracheostomy care in the home setting (Montognino & Mauricio, 2004; Wilson, 2005).

Pediatric tracheostomy tubes vary in size and type. The tube most commonly used is made of Silastic, which is soft and flexible. It consists of two pieces: the outer cannula, which stays in the trachea to keep the stoma open, and an obturator, which guides the tube into place during tube changes. Some tubes have an inner cannula that can be removed for cleaning. Tracheostomy tubes with inner cannulas are often used for older children and for those who have increased mucus production.

Shiley single-lumen tracheostomy tubes are available in a variety of sizes (up to a No. 8 for an adult-size client). Tracheostomy tubes with inner cannulas are available in sizes No. 4 and larger.

PROCEDURE 13-12 | **CHEST PHYSIOTHERAPY**

PURPOSE: To mobilize secretions and facilitate effective airway clearance

1. If the child and family are not familiar with chest physiotherapy (CPT), explain the procedure to them using developmentally appropriate language. Show them the equipment and allow time for questions.
2. The following equipment is needed: a mechanical percussor, vibrator, or rubber cups (if being used instead of hands); stethoscope; towel or baby blanket; gloves; goggles; and tissues or collection container for sputum.
3. To provide a basis for determining response to the treatment, assess the child's baseline respiratory status before beginning the procedure. Before the treatment, ask the child to cough or suction the trachea to remove secretions that may have accumulated in the trachea. Wear gloves and goggles for suctioning or the collection of sputum.
4. Place the child in a postural drainage position.
5. Gently but firmly clap the chest wall with cupped hands. The sound should be hollow. Percussion cups and mechanical vibrators may be used instead of the hand. If the child is young, has sensitive skin, or is otherwise more comfortable, percussion can be done with a very light blanket or gown covering the chest.
6. Reposition the child as needed to complete the procedure, maintaining each position for approximately 5 to 10 minutes. Ask the child to cough between positions.
7. Encourage the child to take deep breaths during the treatment. Expiration after these deep breaths will often stimulate coughing. Use toys, such as pinwheel toys and non-latex balloons (with close supervision), or engage the child in blowing soap bubbles to optimize deep breathing and stimulate coughing. Assist with removal of secretions if needed.

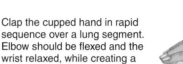

Correct hand position for percussion

Cup the hand to trap a pocket of air that will transmit vibrations through the chest wall to the secretions that need to be dislodged.

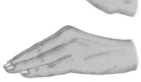

Clap the cupped hand in rapid sequence over a lung segment. Elbow should be flexed and the wrist relaxed, while creating a rapid, popping action.

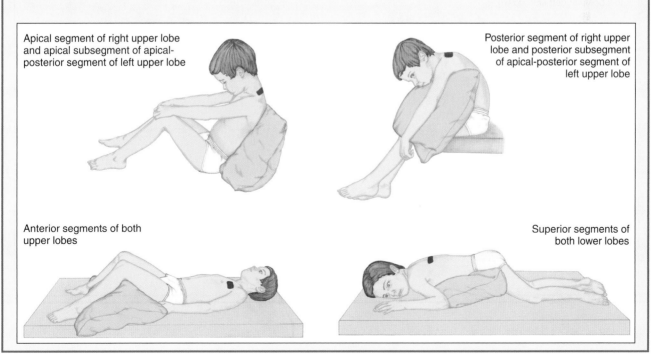

Apical segment of right upper lobe and apical subsegment of apical-posterior segment of left upper lobe

Posterior segment of right upper lobe and posterior subsegment of apical-posterior segment of left upper lobe

Anterior segments of both upper lobes

Superior segments of both lower lobes

Continued

PROCEDURE 13-12	CHEST PHYSIOTHERAPY—cont'd

8. Assess the child's vital signs and breath sounds after therapy is completed. Record the following in the nurses' notes: the date and time of CPT; positions used for drainage and length of time each is maintained; chest segments percussed or vibrated; color, amount, and tenacity of any secretions produced; any complications and nursing actions taken; the child's response to and tolerance of the procedure; and any teaching done with the child and family and their degree of understanding of the teaching.

HOME ADAPTATIONS

Determine the parent's ability to perform CPT at home. It can be done with the child on a regular bed, a couch, or the floor. A variety of devices (tilt tables, slant boards) are available to achieve the proper angle for the procedure. A piece of firm mattress foam purchased at an upholstery store, cut at an angle, and covered is an inexpensive alternative. Young children can achieve the appropriate positioning by lying over a large (3-foot size) ball or over a bean bag chair. Playing during the procedure makes the experience more pleasant for the child. Older children can perform some CPT techniques on themselves, particularly postural drainage and percussion of areas within reach. Observe the parents and child as they demonstrate the procedure. Provide written instructions for parents regarding the child's CPT needs. Teaching materials are available for families of children needing CPT performed at home. Assist the family in obtaining this literature and refer them to appropriate financial resources if needed.

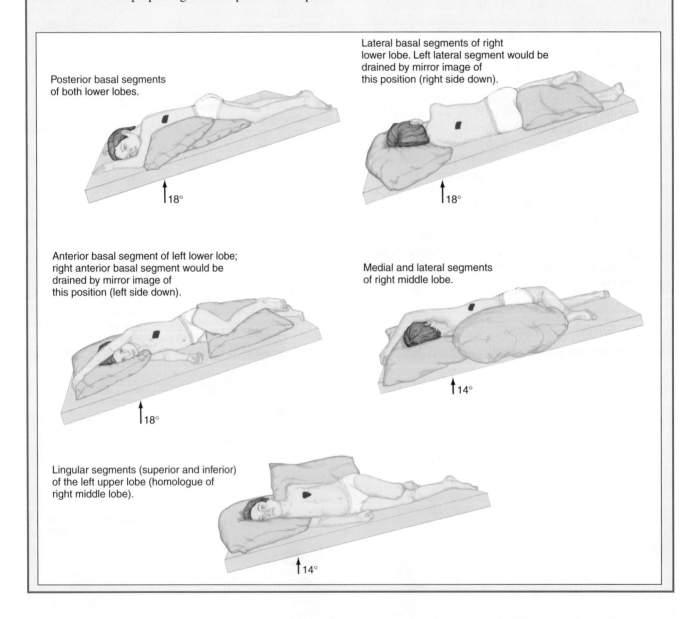

Posterior basal segments of both lower lobes. 18°

Lateral basal segments of right lower lobe. Left lateral segment would be drained by mirror image of this position (right side down). 18°

Anterior basal segment of left lower lobe; right anterior basal segment would be drained by mirror image of this position (left side down). 18°

Medial and lateral segments of right middle lobe. 14°

Lingular segments (superior and inferior) of the left upper lobe (homologue of right middle lobe). 14°

Suctioning

In children with tracheostomies, secretions are removed from the airway by a catheter inserted into the airway. Appropriate techniques and equipment for suctioning can prevent problems sometimes encountered during suctioning, such as hypoxia, tissue damage, and infection. Suctioning infants and children requires the use of a smaller suction catheter and lower suction settings than for the adult. Catheter sizes range from 5F to 14F, with smaller sizes used for smaller tubes. To avoid total airway occlusion, catheter size should be approximately half the inner diameter of the tracheostomy tube. The following suction settings for tracheostomy care vary by age:

* Neonates: 60 to 80 mm Hg
* Infants: 80 to 100 mm Hg
* Larger children: 100 to 120 mm Hg

Assess and record the child's breath sounds, respiratory rate, and character of respirations every 4 hours. Suction the tracheostomy every 2 to 4 hours or as needed. Always use Standard Precautions (Procedure 13-13). Providing a humidified environment keeps secretions more liquid and easier to suction.

Stoma Care

Routine tracheostomy care (Procedure 13-14) includes assessing the stoma area for signs of infection and skin breakdown, changing tracheostomy ties, cleaning the tracheostomy site and inner cannula, changing the tracheostomy tube, and suctioning. Clean the area around the tube at the time the tracheostomy ties are changed or more frequently if needed to keep the site clean and dry. Tracheostomy care can be given at various intervals but should be done at least every 8 hours. The tracheostomy tube is usually changed weekly. The tracheostomy tube is held in place with ties made of a durable, nonfraying material. These are changed daily or more frequently if they become soiled. *To prevent the tube*

| PROCEDURE 13-13 | **SUCTIONING A TRACHEOSTOMY TUBE** |

PURPOSE: To maintain patency of the tracheostomy tube

1. After using developmentally appropriate language to explain the procedure, its purpose, and other pertinent information to the child and parent, gather the following equipment: a sterile suction catheter of appropriate size, sterile gloves and goggles, normal saline, sterile cup, and equipment for ventilation.
2. Adjust the suction vacuum pressure to the prescribed level and put on the goggles. Pour normal saline into the sterile cup. Put on sterile gloves.
3. Lubricate the catheter with normal saline, then insert the catheter the length of the tracheostomy tube (measure another tracheostomy tube the same size) and an additional 0.5 cm *with suction off.* *
4. Apply intermittent suction according to facility policy (policies differ as to whether to suction while entering the tracheostomy tube).† Withdraw the catheter with a twisting or twirling motion. Limit insertion and suctioning time to less than 5 seconds to prevent hypoxia. Holding your own breath during suctioning is a good reminder. If you need a breath, then the child probably does too.
5. Reoxygenate between suction catheter passes and allow a sufficient recovery time after each pass. This time can include allowing the child to rest and take a few breaths, or it may involve "bagging" (giving oxygen by bag and mask). "Bagging" of children on ventilatory support is imperative.
6. Assess the child to determine whether secretions are still present. Auscultate to listen for air exchange. Repeat the procedure until the airway sounds clear, rinsing the suction catheter with normal saline between each insertion.

Normal saline lavage may be used if thick secretions are encountered. Refer to your facility's procedure or policy manual regarding this controversial issue.

7. Assess the child's breath sounds and respiratory rate after suctioning to evaluate the effectiveness of suctioning.
8. Discard the suction tube, other equipment, and gloves in an appropriate container. Record in the nurses' notes the date and time the procedure was performed, the amount and characteristics of the secretions obtained, the character of the breath sounds before and after suctioning, the child's response to the procedure, and any teaching done with the child and family, as well as their level of understanding and their response to the teaching.

HOME ADAPTATIONS

Tracheostomy suctioning at home is a clean rather than sterile procedure. The family will need a powered suction apparatus, catheters of appropriate size, normal saline, nonsterile gloves, boiled water, and the ordered catheter cleaning solution. The procedure for suctioning is as previously discussed, including presuctioning and postsuctioning assessments. Teach the parent to flush the catheter with boiled water, suction with air, and wipe the outer surface with alcohol or hydrogen peroxide.‡ Store the cleaned catheter in a clean, covered container.

The family will need much support and encouragement to feel comfortable with suctioning and tracheostomy care. The child can take baths, but care should be taken to prevent water from entering the trachea. Showers are not recommended. To avoid tracheal spasm, the tracheostomy can be covered loosely during cold or windy days.

*Wilson, M. (2005). Tracheostomy management. *Paediatric Nursing, 117*(3), 38-44.
†American Thoracic Society. (2000). Care of the child with a chronic tracheostomy. *American Journal of Respiratory and Critical Care Medicine, 161,* 297-308.
‡Suctioning of the patient in the home. (1999). *Respiratory Care, 44*(1), 91-98.

| PROCEDURE 13-14 | CLEANING AND CARE OF THE TRACHEOSTOMY SITE AND INNER CANNULA |

PURPOSE: To maintain a patent airway and prevent infection

1. Using developmentally appropriate language, explain the procedure, its purpose, and other pertinent information to the child and parent. Some hospital facilities use videotapes and stoma dolls to demonstrate the procedure.

2. If the facility does not have a preassembled tracheostomy care kit, assemble the following: a small tray to hold the cleaning solution, cotton-tipped applicators, pipe cleaners or a brush for cleaning the inner cannula, forceps, tracheostomy ties, sterile dressing (optional), gauze pad, gloves (sterile and nonsterile), towel or blanket roll, hydrogen peroxide, sterile normal saline, and goggles.

3. To hyperextend the head and neck to expose the site, position the child with a towel or blanket under the shoulders.

4. Wash your hands and open the tray, creating a sterile field.

5. Pour equal parts of normal saline and hydrogen peroxide in one small tray and normal saline in the other small tray. Use the large tray for holding cotton-tipped applicators, clean tracheostomy ties, and gauze pad.

6. Don nonsterile gloves and goggles and remove the dressing around the tracheostomy if present. Discard the dressing and gloves according to agency policy. A dressing placed between the skin and the tube can increase the risk for skin breakdown because it will absorb any secretions. For this reason, it may not be used in some facilities. Assess the stoma for redness, drainage or discharge, and skin breakdown.

7. Don sterile gloves and, using cotton-tipped applicators moistened in half-strength hydrogen peroxide solution, clean the child's neck under the tracheostomy tube flanges and tracheostomy tape and allow to dry. If the child has a tracheostomy without an inner cannula, skip to step 11.

8. Unlock the inner cannula (if using a three-piece tracheostomy system) by rotating it counterclockwise. Remove the inner cannula and, using pipe cleaners or a brush, quickly clean it in half-strength hydrogen peroxide solution. (Alternatively, it may be replaced with a new or extra inner cannula if available.) Rinse the cannula thoroughly in normal saline and inspect it for cleanliness. Repeat the cleaning procedure if necessary.

9. To remove excess moisture, tap the cleaned inner cannula on the edge of the sterile container. Do not dry the outside of the inner cannula because moisture will act as a lubricant during reinsertion.

10. Reinsert the inner cannula into the tracheostomy tube and lock it in place by rotating it clockwise.

    Note: Some facilities require two people to change ties, in which case the following procedure is used. While the assistant (wearing sterile gloves and goggles) gently holds the tube in place, remove the existing tape from the flanges. Clean the skin under the ties and inspect the skin for pressure sores from the ties.

11. Loop the new tracheostomy ties through the flange on one side of the tracheostomy (see p. 367). Bring the ties around the back of the child's neck and tie them securely to the opposite flange. Ties are tight enough if only one finger can be inserted between the ties and neck. Tie the ties on the side, not the back, of the neck to prevent confusing the tracheostomy ties with bib ties and to avoid putting pressure on the back of the neck. Use triple knots to prevent accidental untying and dislodging of the tracheostomy. Clean and assess the skin under the ties.

12. Carefully cut and remove the soiled tracheostomy ties and any excess clean tracheostomy tape. Make sure the tracheostomy tube is secure before leaving the bedside.

13. Discard used supplies in appropriate receptacles. Record in the nurses' notes the date, time and type of procedure, the condition of the stoma and skin, any abnormal findings or complications and the nursing action taken, the child's tolerance of the procedure, and any child and family teaching done, as well as their understanding of and involvement in the care.

HOME ADAPTATIONS

Assess the family's ability to perform the procedure. It may be necessary to engage the assistance of a home health agency if the family needs temporary assistance and support. Begin to teach tracheostomy care early in the child's hospitalization, and teach more than one family member how to do the care. All those caring for the child must also know cardiopulmonary resuscitation (CPR). Write clear instructions and observe all caregivers perform the procedures. Return demonstrations of the technique are imperative. Advise the caregiver that ½-inch width cotton seam binding, which can be found in fabric stores, makes acceptable tracheostomy ties.

from being accidentally dislodged while the ties are being changed, an assistant should be present to hold the tube in place.

Keep an extra tracheostomy tube of appropriate size at the bedside (or taped to the head of the bed) for easy access in an emergency. Because of the risk of aspiration and possible occlusion of the trachea, avoid giving the child small toys, toys with small parts, plastic bibs, and plastic bedding. In addition, do not use talcum powders and aerosol products near children with tracheostomies because of the risk of inhalation injury from breathing the particles.

Caring for an Infant with a Tracheostomy

Caring for the child with a tracheostomy can involve several steps, including respiratory therapy treatments, suctioning, and changing the ties that secure the tube. Because many children are discharged from the hospital with a tracheostomy, their parents and other home caregivers must be taught these procedures.

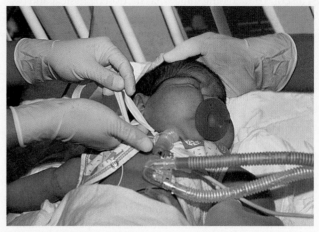

When changing the infant's tracheostomy ties, the nurse has an assistant hold the tube in place to reduce the chance that it will be displaced. The nurse makes sure the ties are snug but not too tight. When the new ties are in place, the nurse checks their snugness by inserting a finger beneath them.

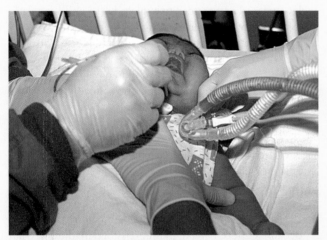

Secretions are removed from this infant's airway with a suction catheter. Appropriate techniques minimize problems with suctioning, such as hypoxia, tissue damage, or infection. The suction catheter is inserted into the tube with the suction turned off. After the appropriate length of tubing is inserted, suction is applied and the catheter is withdrawn using a twisting motion. Do not suction longer than 5 seconds at a time.

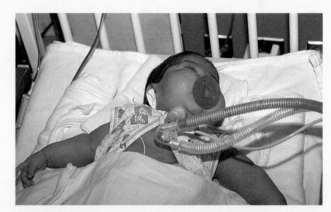

The infant who has a device such as a tracheostomy tube or a gastrostomy feeding tube still needs to suck. A pacifier fulfills this need. Because tracheostomy care is often tiring, the child should be allowed to rest afterward.

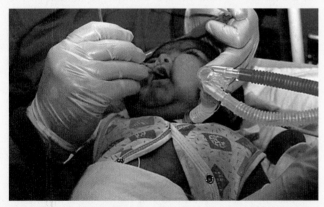

Often the oral cavity requires suctioning as well. The technique is similar to that for suctioning the tracheostomy: the catheter is inserted, and then suction is applied while the catheter is withdrawn.

Photos courtesy Parkland Health and Hospital System, Dallas.

SURGICAL PROCEDURES

The child undergoing surgery has increased physical and psychologic needs. Although each surgical procedure is unique, a general body of knowledge relates to all children experiencing surgery. Surgery can be an extremely traumatic event for a child.

With the rising cost of health care, managed care contracts, and the need for cost containment in health care, many surgeries are now performed on an outpatient basis. Ambulatory, or same-day, surgery uses the same standards of care that apply to all routine hospital admissions but with the added benefit of lower cost.

Preparation for Surgery

A multidisciplinary approach should be used when preparing a child for surgery. Include the following: parents, nursing staff, child life specialist, physician, and any other specialists involved in the child's care. Preparation for outpatient procedures depends on the type of procedure to be performed and the child's age and developmental level. Psychologic preparation for an outpatient experience is just as important as for an inpatient hospital experience. Indeed, much of the preparation is the same, regardless of whether the surgery will be performed on an outpatient or an inpatient basis, and a multidisciplinary approach to teaching is appropriate for both settings.

Assess the child's and family's physical and psychosocial needs. Both the child and the family will be anxious, so the nurse needs to be a calming influence. Being aware of the stressors of surgery will guide the nurse in providing family-centered care. These stressors include the following:

- Separation from significant others, unfamiliar surroundings, and care by strangers
- Preoperative testing
- Pain
- Fear of mutilation or disfigurement
- Disruption in routine
- Anesthesia
- Lack of privacy
- Disability

Fear of the unknown is another common fear that children have. By assessing the presence of these and other stressors, the nurse can develop a plan of care.

Preparing the child and family for surgery establishes a foundation of trust between the nurse and the family. Schedule formal sessions no more than 1 week before admission; younger children may need preparation closer to the operative day. Waiting too long to initiate preparation for surgery can give rise to fantasies and increase the child's fear. A preparation that is too close to surgery might not provide enough time to answer questions posed by the child or family so that they feel adequately prepared for the surgery.

Although preparation may vary from setting to setting, all teaching should be planned, use a developmental approach, and provide information that is simple and truthful. Many hospitals include a tour of the perioperative area. Conduct a review of the teaching on the day of the surgery. If a child life specialist participates in the preparation, that person should be present on the day of surgery.

The use of therapeutic play is an essential tool, both in preparation and perioperatively (see Chapter 11). Keeping the child busy is especially important if a waiting period is required before the scheduled surgery time. Provide age-appropriate toys in holding areas or in the child's room if that is where the child is waiting.

More and more often, parents are the primary educators for their child's surgical experience because of the increase in day surgery. Parents need to explain to the child as clearly as possible why the child is going to the hospital or surgery center and what will happen during the stay. Nurses can assist the parents in preparing their child. Books on hospitalization or surgery that are geared toward children help prepare them for the experience. Videotapes are also available.

Regardless of the procedure planned, some preoperative activities are routine. These include the following:

- No food or drink after a specified time
- A consent form for the procedure signed by the parent or guardian

In some instances, preoperative medication will be ordered. Reassure children that they will not be left alone and that they will not feel the procedure being done.

Because children are at greater risk for dehydration than adults, the period during which they can have nothing by mouth may be shorter. This period varies according to the protocol of the facility and the anesthesiologist (Box 13-3).

Some procedures require preoperative laboratory tests, such as a complete blood cell count, urinalysis, and chest radiograph. Most hospitals and surgical centers have preoperative checklists (similar to those used in adult care) that assist the nurse in documenting the child's preparation for the procedure. These lists usually include checking the child's identification, obtaining a signed consent form, obtaining laboratory results, administering preanesthetic medication, and obtaining other documentation. After the preanesthetic medication has been administered, the parent may hold the child or place the child on a stretcher with the side rails raised.

BOX 13-3	**Guidelines for Preoperative Fasting**

1. Fast from solid food and full liquids from the night before as directed. Some physicians allow a light breakfast early in the morning if surgery will be late in the afternoon (at least 6 hours after ingestion).
2. Stop breastfeeding at least 2 hours before the hospital arrival time. Unless otherwise instructed, stop formula feeding from the night before surgery.
3. Clear liquids, such as water, broth, ice pops, gelatin, and clear juices can be taken up to 2 hours before time of arrival to the hospital.

Preoperative Medication

Preoperative medication is primarily used to decrease anxiety in the child. In some settings, premedication is not used if the parents are present. Parents are increasingly present during the induction of anesthesia. Many safe and painless premedication methods are now available. If parents are to stay until anesthesia takes effect, nurses need to prepare parents properly for what they will see during anesthesia induction (e.g., sudden muscle relaxation, intubation) (Himes, Munyer, & Henly, 2005; Romino, Keatley, Secrest, & Good, 2005). After parents are asked to leave the child for surgery, the nurse keeps them informed of the anticipated length of the surgery and their child's status throughout the surgery.

Postanesthesia Care

After surgery, the child is taken to the postanesthesia care unit (PACU), or recovery room. There the nurse performs frequent assessments of the child's cardiorespiratory and circulatory systems until the child is fully awake. When the child awakens from surgery, the parent or parents should be present to comfort and calm the child. The child may also want a favorite toy or object. Providing warm blankets and a rocking chair as comfort measures can assist both the child and the parent. Pain medication should be provided as needed (see Chapter 15). Depending on the procedure performed, the child may be discharged from the hospital or admitted to an inpatient unit for the remainder of the hospital stay.

Postoperative Care

Most facilities have a specific protocol that is followed for postoperative care. After a surgical procedure, the child's vital signs are monitored frequently until they are stable. The surgical site is checked for drainage, and the child is assessed for pain. The use of patient-controlled analgesia (PCA) and the routine administration of analgesic afford effective pain control. See Chapter 15 for a more detailed discussion of pain management in children.

Atelectasis, a common complication of surgery, can result from the effects of anesthesia combined with other factors, such as inadequate respiratory inflation from pain or decreased respirations associated with pain medications. Auscultate the lungs to determine any abnormal breath sounds or areas of diminished or absent sounds. In addition, encourage early ambulation, deep breathing, and coughing. The use of incentive spirometers can increase respiratory movement. Games such as blowing cotton, a windmill, or bubbles can also facilitate air exchange for children unable or unwilling to use a spirometer.

Children generally recuperate more quickly in a familiar environment; as a result, they are discharged as soon as safely possible after surgery. Because of decreased lengths of stay, discharge planning begins at the time of admission. With an organized plan of care, the discharge planner works closely with the child and family to identify needs and resources and then develops an efficient, cost-effective plan for meeting those needs.

Some children need specialized care in the home after discharge from the hospital. The family's ability to provide some or all of the care will determine the extent of education provided before discharge and the need for involvement of a home health agency after discharge. The family and the nurse must identify the level of knowledge needed and any specific equipment or home modifications required to care for the child adequately at home. The home health agency is usually responsible for making the necessary arrangements for durable or disposable equipment. It is helpful, when possible, for equipment and supplies to be provided by the same agency that provides assistance with home nursing care. Some agencies also will provide education for the family before the child's discharge. To ensure the child and family the smoothest transition possible from hospital to home, these issues and delegation of responsibilities need to be addressed as soon as they are identified.

Nursing diagnoses frequently associated with the child undergoing surgery include the following:

- Anxiety and Fear related to separation from significant others, surgery, unfamiliar environment, and personnel
- Acute Pain related to the surgical incision
- Deficient Knowledge related to unfamiliarity with the procedure and expected outcomes
- Interrupted Family Processes related to the surgical procedure
- Risk for Deficient Fluid Volume related to nothing-by-mouth status before and after surgery, as well as to nausea and vomiting

ADDITIONAL INFORMATION

See Chapter 3 for assistance with communication challenges. Chapter 11 provides information on care related to hospitalization and separation, Chapter 15 discusses pain-related issues, and Chapter 18 presents nursing care as it relates to fluid balance. To deliver quality care, the nurse must identify the child's growth and developmental needs along with the care needs associated with the disorder for which the surgery is being performed.

KEY CONCEPTS

- Whenever possible, perform procedures in the treatment room, away from the child's room.
- Some procedures require informed consent. Children aged 7 years and older may need to give assent to some procedures. Because laws on informed consent vary from state to state, nurses must be familiar with the laws and policies of their institution.
- Use developmentally appropriate and descriptive words when preparing children for procedures.
- Praise children for attempts at cooperation during a procedure even if they did not follow instructions. Praise them for accomplishing an expected task.
- Documentation of a procedure includes recording the preparation, who performed the procedure, the child's tolerance, the actual procedure, and outcomes.

- Follow Standard Precautions when collecting all specimens. Standard Precautions are used with all hospitalized clients and are not based on diagnosis or presumed infectious state. Transmission-Based Precautions are used with clients known or suspected to be infected by pathogens that are conveyed by airborne or droplet transmission or by contact with dry skin or contaminated surfaces.
- Use restraints only as a last resort to protect the child and others.
- Because of children's developmental level and activity, be particularly conscious of safety measures when caring for children in a hospital setting.

ANSWERS TO CRITICAL THINKING EXERCISE 13-1

1. As a nurse, you are responsible to practice safely. This means checking the hospital policy and procedure manual before beginning any procedure and keeping current with evidence-based research. Because even experienced nurses disagree on the best approach to confirm feeding tube placement in children, using a combination of methods described in the literature increases the likelihood of an accurate assessment. Remember that the only truly accurate determination of placement is by radiography. In most institutions, nurses write procedures by committee. One way of ensuring that your institution's policy reflects evidence-based practice is to serve on the committee that periodically updates procedures.

2. If a question about tube placement arises (marginal pH measurements, questionable aspirate appearance), do not give an enteral feeding through the tube. Inform the physician about your findings. You can request that the physician order a radiographic confirmation. The tube may have to be removed and replaced.

REFERENCES AND READINGS

American Heart Association. (2005). Recommendations for blood pressure measurement in humans and experimental animals. Part 1: blood pressure measurement in humans: a statement for professionals from the Subcommittee of Professional and Public Education of the American Heart Association Council on High Blood Pressure Research. *Circulation, 111*, 697-716.

Amy, E. (2001). Reflections on the interactive newborn bath demonstration. *MCN: The American Journal of Maternal/Child Nursing, 26*(6), 320-322.

Attin, M., Cardin, S., Dee, V., Doering, L., Dunn, D., Ellstrom, K., Erickson, V., Etchepare, M., Gawlinski, A., Haley, T., Henneman, E., Keckeisen, M., Malmet, M., & Olson, L. (2002). An educational project to improve knowledge related to pulse oximetry. *American Journal of Critical Care, 11*(6), 529-534.

Barker, G. (2004). The baby bath: empowerment of the parents. *Creative Nursing, 4*, 11-12.

Barton, S., Gaffney, R., Chase, T., Rayens, M., & Piyabanditkul, L. (2003). Pediatric temperature measurement and child/parent/nurse preference using three temperature measurement instruments. *Journal of Pediatric Nursing, 18*(5).

Bowen, W. H. (2002). Fluorosis: is it really a problem? *Journal of the American Dental Association, 133*(10), 1405-1407.

Centers for Disease Control and Prevention. (2001). Recommendations for using fluoride to prevent and control dental caries in the United States. *Morbidity and Mortality Weekly Report, 50*(RR14), 1-42.

Centers for Disease Control and Prevention. (2002). Guideline for hand hygiene in health care settings. *Morbidity and Mortality Weekly Report, 51*(RR16), 1-44.

Centers for Disease Control and Prevention. (2005a). *Hand hygiene guidelines fact sheet.* Retrieved April 17, 2006, from *www.cdc.gov*

Centers for Disease Control and Prevention. (2005b). *Standard precautions.* Retrieved April 17, 2006, from *www.cdc.gov*

Clark, J., Lieh-Lai, M., Sarnaik, A., & Mattoo, T. (2002). Discrepancies between direct and indirect blood pressure measurements using various recommendations for arm cuff selection. *Pediatrics, 110*(5), 920-923.

Dunn, D. (2005). Preventing perioperative complications in special populations. *Nursing 2005, 35*(11), 36-45.

Gelmetti, C. (2002). Skin cleansing in children. *Journal of the European Academy of Dermatology and Venereology, 15*(Suppl 1), 12-15.

Gerard, L., Cooper, C., Duethman, K., Gordley, B., & Kleiber, C. (2003). Effectiveness of lidocaine lubricant for discomfort during pediatric urethral catheterization. *The Journal of Urology, 170*(2), 564-567.

Goldman, L., Shannon, M., & Committee on Environmental Health. (2001). Technical report: mercury in the environment: implications for pediatricians (RE 109907). *Pediatrics, 108*(1), 197-205.

Hanchett, M. (2002). Techniques for stabilizing urinary catheters. *American Journal of Nursing, 102*(3), 44-48.

Himes, M., Munyer, K., & Henly, S. (2005). Parental presence during pediatric anesthesia inductions. *AANA Journal, 71*(4), 293-298.

Huffman, S., Jarczyk, K., O'Brien, E., Pieper, P., & Bayne, A. (2004). Methods to confirm feeding tube placement: application of research in practice. *Pediatric Nursing, 30*(1), 10-13.

Jeffery, K. (2002). Therapeutic restraint of children: it must always be justified. *Paediatric Nursing, 14*(9), 20-22.

Lorin, M. (2004). Fever: pathogenesis and treatment. In R. Feigin, J. Cherry, G. Demmier, & S. Kaplan (Eds.), *Textbook of pediatric infectious diseases* (5th ed., pp. 100-106). Philadelphia: Saunders.

McConnell, E. (2002). Clinical do's and don'ts providing tracheostomy care. *Nursing 2002, 32*(1), 17.

Metheny, N., & Titler, M. (2001). Assessing placement of feeding tubes. *American Journal of Nursing, 101*(5), 36-45.

Metheny, N., Wehrle, A., Wiersema, L., & Clark, J. (1998). Testing feeding tube placement: auscultation vs. pH method. *American Journal of Nursing, 98*(5), 37-42.

Migdal, M., Chudzynska-Pomianowska, E., Vause, E., Henry, E., & Lazar, J. (2005). Rapid, needle-free delivery of lidocaine for reducing the pain of venipuncture among pediatric subjects. *Pediatrics, 115*(4), e393-e398.

Montagnino, B., & Mauricio, R. (2004). The child with a tracheostomy and gastrostomy: parental stress and coping in the home—a pilot study. *Pediatric Nursing, 30*(5), 373-401.

Mowery, B., & Suddaby, B. (2002). Tracheostomy troubles. *Pediatric Nursing, 28*(2), 162.

National High Blood Pressure Education Program Working Group on High Blood Pressure in Children and Adolescents. (2004). The fourth report on the diagnosis, evaluation, and treatment of high blood pressure in children and adolescents. *Pediatrics, 114*(2), 555-576.

Pagana K. D., & Pagana, T. (2006). *Mosby's manual of diagnostic and laboratory tests* (3rd ed.). St. Louis: Mosby.

Popovich, D., Richiuso, N., & Danek, G. (2004). Pediatric health care providers' knowledge of pulse oximetry. *Pediatric Nursing, 30*(1), 14-20.

Prinzhorn, J., & Churchwell, C. (2004). Fever management in children who are febrile is questionable. *Pediatric Nursing, 30*(4), 322-324.

Reising, D., & Neal, R. (2005). Enteral tube flushing. *American Journal of Nursing, 105*(3), 58-64.

Romino, S., Keatley, V., Secrest, J., & Good, K. (2005). Parental presence during anesthesia induction in children. *AORN Journal, 81*(4), 780-792.

Siberry, G., Diener-West, M., Schappell, E., & Karron, R. (2002). Comparison of temple temperatures with rectal temperatures in children under two years of age. *Clinical Pediatrics, 41,* 405-414.

Smith, A., & Adams, L. (1998). Insertion of indwelling urethral catheters in infants and children: a survey of current nursing practice. *Pediatric Nursing, 24*(3), 229-234.

Smith, L. (2003). Which catheter? Criteria for selection of urinary catheters for children. *Paediatric Nursing, 15*(3), 14-18.

Smith, L., & Callery, P. (2005). Children's accounts of their preoperative information needs. *Journal of Clinical Nursing, 14,* 230-238.

Sole, M., Byers, J., Ludy, J., Zhang, Y., Banta, C., & Brummell, K. (2003). A multisite survey of suctioning techniques and airway management practices. *American Journal of Critical Care, 12*(3), 220-230.

Wilson, M. (2005). Tracheostomy management. *Paediatric Nursing, 117*(3), 38-44.

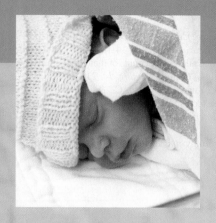

CHAPTER 14

Medicating Infants and Children

Learning Objectives

After studying this chapter, you should be able to:
- Describe different methods of administering medications to children.
- List the advantages and disadvantages of each route of administering medication to children.

- Describe the physiologic differences between children and adults that affect medicating a child.
- Describe psychosocial interventions for teaching and successful medication administration for each age group.

Definitions

blood-brain barrier Selective anatomic or physiologic capillary obstruction that prevents potentially harmful substances, such as certain medications, radioactive ions, and viruses, from entering the parenchyma of the brain.

central venous access device Venous access device in which the catheter is placed centrally rather than peripherally, usually in the superior vena cava or jugular vein; used for long-term intravenous therapy.

eutectic mixture of local anesthetics Cream used to numb the skin at a depth of 0.5 mm; used before needle punctures.

implanted venous access device Surgically implanted port or reservoir in which the catheter tip is placed in the superior vena cava; used for long-term intravenous therapy.

intermittent infusion port Intravenous catheter used to administer intermittent medications or fluids; remains clamped when not in use.

metered-dose inhaler Hand-held device that delivers "puffs" of medication for inhalation.

peripherally inserted central catheter Central line that is inserted peripherally (usually through an antecubital vein) into the superior vena cava.

pharmacodynamics Behavior of medications at the cellular level.

pharmacokinetics The time and movement relationships of medications.

sustained-release medication Medication taken in a single dose but designed to dissolve slowly, releasing medication into the bloodstream over a specified period of time (usually 12 to 24 hours).

tunneled central line A surgically placed central line that is held in place by a Dacron polyester cuff located in a subcutaneous tunnel; most commonly placed in the external jugular vein.

Electronic Resources

Additional information related to the content in Chapter 14 can be found on:

the interactive companion CD-ROM
- Animations: Central Venous Access via Jugular Vein
    IV Line Placement
    PICC Line Placement
- Audio Glossary
- NCLEX Review Questions
- Skills: Administering Oral Medications
    Calculating Safe Dosages for Children

or the companion website at *evolve*
http://evolve.elsevier.com/james/ncoc
- NCLEX Review Questions
- WebLinks

Medicating infants and children is one of the nurse's most important responsibilities. The nurse plays a key role in administering medications, supporting the child and family during the experience, and teaching the child and parents about pharmacologic aspects of the child's care. Although physicians or nurse practitioners prescribe medications, the nurse or caregiver is responsible for their administration. The nurse has a legal responsibility to administer medications safely and accurately. Safe administration of medications to children requires an understanding of the dosages of the medications used for children and the expected actions, possible side effects, and signs of adverse reactions or toxicity. Nurses should use reliable sources of information (e.g., pharmacists, drug handbooks, hospital formularies) when administering drugs that are unfamiliar or used infrequently and should question orders they do not understand before administering the medication.

Giving medications to children requires special skill. To gain the child's cooperation and to administer the medication in the least traumatic manner, the nurse needs to understand the physical characteristics and psychologic needs of children at each developmental level. The nurse should use developmentally appropriate strategies to handle children's fears, prevent injury, and enhance coping.

It is vitally important to provide parents with information about medications used in their child's treatment and to encourage parents to support their child during potentially uncomfortable experiences. Involving parents in the task of eliciting their child's cooperation not only makes the job easier but also gives the family a sense of self-management and control. If the parents will be asked to administer medications to their child at home, the nurse ensures that the parents are properly instructed before the child is discharged.

Adherence to properly taking the full course of a medication continues to be a problem for children and adolescents (Winnick, Lucas, Hartman, & Toll, 2005). Factors that improve medication adherence include allowing adequate time for the health provider to educate the parent and child, continuity of care, availability of the health provider to answer questions about the medication, a medication schedule that fits the family's and child's lifestyle, low cost, oral route, and low potential for side effects. Oral medications that taste good are more palatable to young children (Winnick et al., 2005). Any medication regimen should consider the child's or adolescent's developmental needs and should be presented to the child and family by a variety of educational and behavioral strategies. For example, strategies such as simple dosing schedules, personal interest expressed by the provider, and a variety of cues to help an older child remember to take the medication can be successful with increasing adherence (Staples & Bravender, 2002).

PHARMACOKINETICS IN CHILDREN

An understanding of pharmacokinetics and pharmacodynamics guides appropriate interventions in children. *Pharmacokinetics* refers to the actions of a drug (e.g., movement, biotransformation) within the human body over time, and *pharmacodynamics* is the behavior of a drug as it interacts with the biochemical and physiologic milieu of the body. The pharmacokinetic actions of absorption, distribution, metabolism, and excretion are influenced by the physiologic environment in which the drug moves, and this environment differs between adults and children (Fig. 14-1). The physiologic differences in body systems are most striking in the neonate.

Absorption

Oral Route

When a medication is given orally, several factors influence its absorption along the gastrointestinal (GI) tract. Because most medication absorption occurs in the small intestine, the drug must reach that location in a form suitable for maximum absorption. Four factors influence this process:

- Gastric acidity
- Gastric emptying time
- GI motility, or transit time through the GI tract
- Function of the pancreatic enzymes

Gastric Acidity. Infants' gastric secretions are less acidic than older children's or adults'. Secretions slowly increase in acidity during the first 2 years of life. Children, particularly infants, eat more frequently than adults and are more likely to have food and digestive enzymes present in their stomachs. Formula or milk can increase the alkalinity of gastric secretions, decreasing the absorption of medications that require a more acidic environment and enhancing the absorption of medications that require a more alkaline milieu. These factors can greatly affect serum drug levels.

Gastric Emptying. Gastric emptying is intermittent and unpredictable in infants but is usually slower than in older children. This slower pace can prolong the time it takes a medication to reach the intestinal absorption site.

Gastrointestinal Motility. Depending on whether the infant or young child has eaten recently, peristaltic activity in the intestine can be faster or slower than in the older child or adult. Infants up to 8 months of age tend to have prolonged motility. Certain adverse health conditions, such as diarrhea, can alter intestinal motility by increasing peristalsis. The longer the transit time in the intestine, the more medication is absorbed. Conversely, a shortened transit time decreases absorption.

Enzyme Activity. Pancreatic enzyme activity also is variable in infants for the first 3 months of life as the GI system matures. Medications that require specific enzymes for dissolution and absorption might not be digested to a form suitable for intestinal action.

Other Routes

Adequate absorption of medication administered intravenously (IV) depends on adequate peripheral perfusion. Medications given IV are immediately available for absorption into the child's bloodstream. The child's peripheral circulation is less reliable and more responsive to environmental changes than the adult's. As a result, vasoconstriction or vasodilation can occur and alter the absorption of a parenteral medication. Also, the cardiovascular system is less able to accommodate large or rapid changes in volume, and fluid overload can occur if volumes of IV infusions are not carefully monitored.

A child's muscle mass is less than an adult's. The infant's body weight is about 25% muscle, whereas the adult's is about 40%. Because of the smaller muscle mass in infants, fewer sites are available for intramuscular (IM) injections. Increased blood flow to muscle tissue is essential for adequate absorption. Blood flow to muscles in the young child is erratic and can affect the absorption of injected medications.

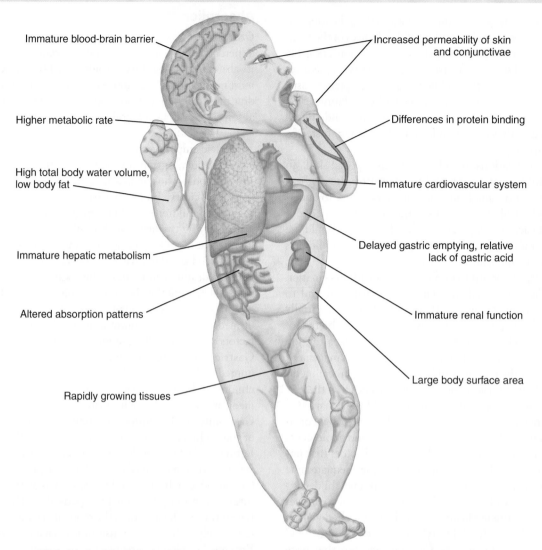

Immature blood-brain barrier

Increased permeability of skin and conjunctivae

Higher metabolic rate

Differences in protein binding

High total body water volume, low body fat

Immature cardiovascular system

Immature hepatic metabolism

Delayed gastric emptying, relative lack of gastric acid

Altered absorption patterns

Immature renal function

Rapidly growing tissues

Large body surface area

FIG 14-1   Physiologic differences between children and adults affect drug absorption, metabolism, distribution, and excretion. These differences are most extreme in the neonate.

Infants and young children have a thinner outer skin layer (stratum corneum) and a larger body surface area (BSA)/weight ratio. Because the ratio of BSA to weight varies inversely with length, the infant has more surface area relative to weight than the adult does. This difference affects the absorption of topical medications. Absorption of a similar dose of a topical medication in an infant and an adult is approximately three times greater in the infant because of the greater BSA and thinner skin layer (Reed & Gal, 2004).

Skin pH varies with age and can affect the absorption of topical medications. A child's skin is also more prone to irritation, making contact dermatitis and other allergic reactions more common. Irritated or open skin can enhance the absorption of topical medications.

Distribution

Distribution refers to the general and specific concentration of the medication in body fluids and tissues. The medication is distributed to body tissues through blood and body fluids.

Differences in Body Fluids

Fluid differences between children younger than 2 years and older children must be considered when the nurse determines dosages of medication. The body fluid content ranges from 75% of body weight in infants to 60% of body weight in children 2 years and older. Because of their greater fluid volume per weight, children need a higher dose per kilogram of a water-soluble medication to achieve the desired distribution effects (see Chapter 18).

A higher percentage of the young child's body fluid is located in the extracellular fluid compartment. During certain illnesses, this extracellular fluid can be lost rapidly, causing fluid depletion. It is important to adjust medication dosages accordingly in the ill infant or young child to avoid overdosing or underdosing.

Differences in Fat Percentages

Percentages of fat also change as the child grows. Fat makes up about 16% of an infant's weight, although total body fat varies from child to child. This percentage increases in a 1-year-old but decreases during the preschool years. The percentage of body fat affects the distribution of fat-soluble medications in children. Because the body fat must be saturated with a fat-soluble medication before the drug becomes detectable in the blood, dosages often must be varied to achieve the desired effects.

Differences in Proteins

Medications bind to plasma proteins, mainly albumin, for distribution. Only free, unbound medication can be absorbed by the body. Because infants have lower levels of plasma proteins than do older children, more unbound drug circulates and is available for absorption. This increased concentration of unbound drug alters the amount of medication needed to maintain a therapeutic drug level.

Blood-Brain Barrier

The blood-brain barrier does not fully mature until the child is about 2 years old. This immaturity causes the barrier to be less selective and allows for distribution of medication into the central nervous system. As a result, encephalopathy can occur with some medications.

The relative immaturity of the neurologic system also can lead to paradoxic effects from certain medications. For example, medications that normally cause sedation in adults may have the opposite effect in many children, causing hyperactivity.

Metabolism

Most medications are metabolized in the liver. Because the metabolic enzyme systems are less mature in newborn and premature infants, they might not be able to properly metabolize all the medication in a prescribed dosage. Toddlers and preschoolers can have a much greater metabolizing capacity than adults do for certain drugs. For this reason, larger dosages or more frequent administration of certain drugs (e.g., pain medications) might be needed for young children to achieve therapeutic results.

Excretion

Most medications are excreted through the renal system. The renal system also is immature at birth. The newborn infant's glomerular filtration rate is about 30% to 50% that of an adult's, and the renal tubules also function less efficiently. Adult rates are reached after approximately 1 year. Infants and young children cannot concentrate urine as well as older children or adults can.

Because of renal immaturity, medications might not be filtered out of the circulating blood volume and excreted in the urine (the primary method of medication excretion). As a result, medications can circulate longer and reach toxic blood levels. Likewise, loss of fluid may decrease the child's ability to excrete medications. Therefore dehydration has a serious effect on drug serum levels.

Concentration

To administer appropriately therapeutic medication doses to children, nurses need to be aware of the importance of knowing the concentration of certain medications in serum. Maintaining serum levels within a safe therapeutic range maximizes the effect of a medication while reducing the risk of toxicity. When certain medications are used, the physician will order peak and trough serum levels to be measured to monitor medication concentration. The peak concentration is not necessarily the highest concentration but the concentration of the medication after it has been distributed. The time at which a medication reaches peak concentration differs according to the specific medication but usually occurs a specified time after the medication has been administered.

The medication trough is the level at which the serum concentration is lowest. Trough levels usually are obtained just before the next medication dose. Knowing the usual therapeutic peak-and-trough range for a specific medication will assist the nurse in an accurate assessment of the child's response and the potential for toxic medication effects.

PSYCHOLOGIC AND DEVELOPMENTAL FACTORS

Growth and developmental principles and differences among age groups must always be considered when medicating a child. Eliciting support from the parent usually eases any concern the child may have (Box 14-1).

> Always approach children at their developmental level and provide developmentally appropriate explanations about a medication procedure. To decrease feelings of powerlessness, give the child as many choices as possible.

Honesty, reward, and praise are important for gaining trust and cooperation. The nurse should give honest explanations and tell the child when a procedure will be painful or uncomfortable. Also, tell the child approximately how long the pain will last and what the child can do to help during that time. Terms familiar to the child, such as "pinching" or "stinging," should be used.

> Praising the child after the procedure for attempts at cooperation is important and helps gain trust and cooperation for future procedures. Do not scold a child for failure to cooperate.

Restraints are seldom necessary for administration of medications. It is appropriate to ask a parent or other staff member to assist with holding a child during an injection if the child's movements appear to jeopardize safe administration of the medication. Approaches include taking the child to a procedure room where another staff member assists in helping the child remember to hold still. Physical restraint devices, such as arm boards and mummy restraints, are occasionally necessary. It is important to explain that the staff

BOX 14-1	PARENTS WANT TO KNOW	About Medication Administration

Parents want to know how they can help their children when a procedure for administering medication is expected to be uncomfortable. They also become concerned if the child refuses to take a medication that is intended to help the child recover from an illness. Nurses should do the following to empower parents:

- Obtain the following information before administering the medication:
  —Medication allergies or sensitivities
  —The child's ability to take medications (e.g., can the child swallow pills?)
  —What method the parent usually uses to administer the medication (e.g., mixing it with certain foods)
- Give the parent a thorough explanation about the medication before administration. Include information about why the child needs the medication, any possible side effects, and how and where you expect to administer the medication.

- Allow the parent to administer certain medications if the child is more comfortable (e.g., oral, otic, ophthalmic). Check the medication "rights" before you allow a parent to administer a medication. Show the parent the most acceptable position for administering the particular medication.
- Encourage the parent who is concerned that a medication might not be effective or might be making the child ill to express these concerns. Parents know their children and often are aware of subtle changes long before hospital personnel notice them.
- Help the parent determine the best way to administer the child's medication at home. Recommend the use of positive reinforcements such as rewards or stickers to increase cooperation. Encourage the parent to explain to the child why the medication is needed and to be firm that the child takes the medication.

person is helping the child remember to hold still. Do not threaten a child with restraint.

Rewards for good behavior often help the child feel better about the procedure. Rewards should always be safe and appropriate for the child's age. Stickers are a good choice for younger children. Older children might want a sticker or might choose a small toy or a privilege, such as watching a favorite video.

Infants

Infants are easier to medicate than toddlers but more difficult than children who can follow directions (see Chapter 5). Parents always need to know why the infant is receiving the medication. Because keeping a squirming infant still may be difficult, the nurse should get help in administering the medication if necessary. Maintaining a routine and cuddling and comforting the infant before and after the procedure are important interventions.

Toddlers and Preschoolers

Older toddlers (2 to 3 years) are prone to magical thinking and might view the administration of medication (especially if painful or intrusive) as punishment for "bad" thoughts (see Chapter 6). Give toddlers age-appropriate explanations, using play if possible. Allowing older toddlers to examine the equipment before the procedure might enhance cooperation. Because the toddler might react negatively to restraint, use as little restraint as possible and allow the toddler to sit on the parent's lap if the parent is willing. Praise and cuddling after the procedure are important. Rewards, such as stickers, are useful for this age group.

Preschoolers (3 to 5 years) continue to use magical thinking. They fear the unknown and they fear painful procedures (see Chapter 6). This age group benefits greatly from

therapeutic play and participation. The nurse should allow as much control over the procedure and offer as much choice as possible (e.g., "Do you want your medication with juice or milk?"). Ask preschoolers if they can hold still for a painful procedure; if they cannot, they usually will say so. Adhesive bandages are important to children in this age group after an invasive procedure, such as an injection. Preschoolers believe that these bandages "make it better"—an example of magical thinking.

School-Age Children

School-age children (6 to 12 years) fear loss of control, pain, and injury. At this age, a child can understand more complex explanations (see Chapter 7). Offer as much choice as possible. School-age children often cooperate fully, even with painful procedures, but might need a source of distraction (e.g., a radio to turn up as pain increases, counting out loud for the length of pain time) and support (see Chapter 15). School-age children still need praise, and rewards (e.g., stickers) are appreciated.

Adolescents

Adolescents (11 to 21 years) fear separation from peers and loss of control (see Chapter 8). Persons in this age group understand adult explanations and can assist in making decisions about their care. Often, however, adolescents exhibit a hyperresponse to procedures that can seem inconsistent with their age. It is important to praise their cooperation and find outlets for their frustration (e.g., drawing, writing).

CALCULATING DOSAGES

Medications for children usually do not have standard dosages. Instead, dosages are calculated on the basis of the child's weight (milligrams per kilogram [mg/kg]). This practice

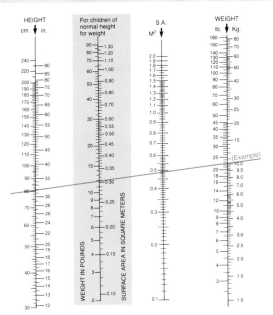

FIG 14-2 **Nomogram for calculating BSA, used for determining medication dosages for infants and children. *S.A.,* Surface area.** *(From Behrman, R. E., Kliegman, R. M., & Jenson, H. [2000]. Nelson textbook of pediatrics [16th ed., p. 2182]. Philadelphia: WB Saunders.)*

usually is the most reliable method for precisely determining doses. For example, for a child weighing 10 kg, the daily dose of amoxicillin is 20 to 40 mg/kg, or 200 to 400 mg/day.

Dosages can also be calculated based on body surface area (BSA) (milligrams per square meter [mg/m²]) or according to other standardized methods (Fig. 14-2). To calculate medications on the basis of surface area, the following formula is used:

$$\text{Approximate dose} = \text{BSA of child } (m^2)/1.7 \times \text{adult dose}$$

ADMINISTRATION PROCEDURES

Because the margin of safety is minimal in pediatric patients, accuracy is a prime consideration when administering medications. Inaccurate dosage calculations, the most common form of medication error in the pediatric setting (American Academy of Pediatrics [AAP], 2003; Hughes & Edgerton, 2005), can result in a tenfold or more dosage error if the decimal point is in the wrong place. Always verify medication doses for accuracy in the following areas: (1) recommended dosage in mg/kg/day, (2) number of divided doses recommended (e.g., every 4 hours, three times a day, every 12 hours), and (3) recommended route of administration. To further avoid errors, follow these procedures:

- Adhere to the "six rights" of medication administration: right child, right drug, right dose, right time, right route, and right documentation.
- Check the orders to be sure that all information is correctly transcribed. Note any allergies.
- Always double-check medication calculations before administration. Be sure the child's weight is accurately recorded.

- Double-check calculations of medications provided by the pharmacy in a unit dose form. Consult with the physician or pharmacist if there is any question about a dose.
- Ask another nurse to double-check the following medications:
  —Insulin
  —Narcotics
  —Chemotherapy
  —Digoxin or other inotropic drugs
  —Anticoagulants
  —K⁺ and Ca⁺⁺ salts

Many institutions also require two nurses to check any medication given by continuous infusion or by medication syringe pump. If the child is to receive a medication for off-label use, the nurse needs to verify the dose with the prescribing physician and the pharmacy, obtain written information about the potential adverse effects, and meticulously check any calculations, preferably with another nurse (Hughes & Edgerton, 2005). Providing accurate discharge instructions to parents is most important. The nurse should be sure to check the dosage conversion to lay terms (e.g., 1 teaspoon, not 5 mL) and be sure that it is accurately written so the parent can follow the instructions for administration.

Medication errors in the child population have been increasing. Most medication errors are system errors and result from breakdown in one part of the system of provider, pharmacist, unit clerk, and nurse (AAP, 2003). The AAP (2003) has made recommendations for reducing medication errors in the child population. These include the following:

- Reporting even minor errors (including disclosing an error to the child's family), so that system performance can be assessed and improved
- Ensuring that those who prescribe, fill, and administer medications to children are adequately educated and regularly updated
- Standardized equipment to be used for children, especially equipment used for parenteral delivery of medication, throughout a hospital setting
- Writing medication prescriptions clearly and without abbreviations; use a zero before a dose that is less than 1 and do not use a decimal point followed by a zero for doses that are whole numbers greater than 1

Although computer medication systems have the potential to reduce medication error, they are not foolproof and should not replace the nurse's responsibility for calculating and properly administering medications to children.

Administering Oral Medications

The oral route is the most widely used and economic method of administering medications. It is also one of the least reliable methods of administration because absorption is affected greatly by the presence or absence of food in the stomach, gastric emptying time, GI motility, and stomach acidity. The oral route can be less predictable also because of medication loss to spillage, leaking, or spitting out.

Oral medications are available in liquid (elixir or suspension), tablet or capsule, chewable tablet, or sprinkle (powder) forms. If the child cannot swallow tablets or capsules, the nurse determines whether the medication is available in a liquid form and, if it is not, determines whether it can be crushed.

Before administering oral medications, the nurse assesses the child's gag reflex and ability to swallow. The oral form used should be tailored to the child's developmental level and ability to successfully take the form prescribed. An assessment of the way the child takes medications at home also helps determine the proper form. Some older infants and toddlers can successfully take crushed tablets but refuse liquid forms.

CRITICAL THINKING EXERCISE 14-1

A father calls the office with questions for the triage nurse. The father explains that his 3-year-old son is refusing to take his medication because it tastes "yucky." The parent would like the physician to change the medication to something that tastes better. When asked, the father explains that the medication is penicillin liquid and that the child is taking it for treatment of a "strep throat." The father says the child is feeling much better now.

1. What information should the nurse give this father about the child's medication regimen?
2. How would the nurse approach encouraging the child to adhere to the medication regimen?

Medication Preparation

When preparing to administer an elixir or suspension, the nurse first ensures that the correct dose is drawn for administration. Physicians' orders often specify the dosage in milligrams, *not* milliliters, for liquid medications. It is important to calculate the milliliter dose properly on the basis of the number of milligrams per milliliter in the liquid medication on hand.

CRITICAL THINKING EXERCISE 14-2

You need to administer ibuprofen, 150 mg, to your 5-year-old patient. Ibuprofen comes in liquid form in a dose of 100 mg/5 mL.

1. How many milliliters will you give?
2. When the child is discharged, how many teaspoons will you instruct the parent to give?

Because tableware spoons vary in volume, use a calibrated spoon or dropper designed for medication administration. Calibrated syringes (preferably oral administration syringes) should be used for doses less than 5 mL or doses that are not in 5-mL increments. Pour larger volumes into calibrated plastic medicine cups. Avoid using paper measuring cups because their volumes tend to vary.

If a tablet is to be crushed and mixed with food or is available as a sprinkle or powder, mix it with a nonessential food,

such as applesauce or pudding, not orange juice or formula. Giving medication with a favorite food can alter the flavor of the food. Avoid using syrup or other high-sugar substances. Never give infants medication or foods mixed with honey because honey has been known to cause infantile botulism.

Determine a medication's compatibility with food before giving it to the child. Mix any medication with a small amount (5 to 10 mL) of food or liquid and give it to the child before a feeding, if not contraindicated.

Sustained-release tablets or capsules should never be crushed because their function is to release the medication slowly over a long period. Enteric-coated tablets (tablets covered with a substance that prevents the drug from dissolving until it reaches the intestine) can have an unpleasant taste or odor if crushed. Crushing also interferes with the function of the enteric coating.

Medication Administration

The method of administering oral medications differs according to the child's age and developmental level. Infants usually receive elixir or suspension forms of oral medications. Administer these with an empty nipple or oral syringe. First place the infant in an upright or semiupright position. The position used for feeding the infant can be used for administering medications. Open the infant's mouth by applying gentle pressure to the chin or both cheeks. If using a nipple, place the nipple in the infant's mouth and add the medication to the empty nipple when the baby begins to suck. Unpleasant-tasting medications should not be given through a nipple because the taste can cause a future aversion reaction to the nipple, thus interfering with feeding.

If using an oral syringe or medicine dropper to administer the medication, place the syringe or dropper gently in the infant's mouth along the side of the cheek and squirt the medication in slowly as the infant sucks (Fig. 14-3). Aiming

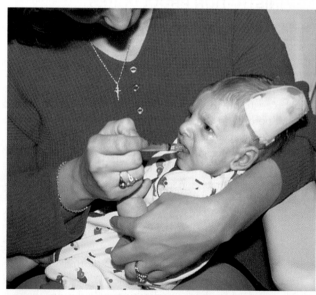

FIG 14-3 **Administering an oral medication with an oral syringe to an infant.** *(Courtesy Parkland Health and Hospital System, Dallas, TX.)*

the medication toward the back of the throat is dangerous because it can cause choking and aspiration.

Toddlers and preschoolers can easily take liquid medications from an oral syringe or medicine cup. If the liquid medication has an unpleasant taste, offer to let the child take it through a straw. If a straw is used, cut the straw in half to avoid a loss of medication. Allowing children to take their own medication, giving rewards as incentives, and providing choices that fit into the medication regimen enhance autonomy.

Preschoolers can usually manage chewable tablets without difficulty. Most older children can swallow tablets or capsules. The nurse, however, should determine whether the child can swallow pills. If not, the nurse should determine whether the medication can be crushed and mixed with food or a small amount of liquid. If the child cannot swallow tablets or capsules and the tablets or capsules cannot be crushed, the nurse needs to contact the pharmacy to identify another form for administration (elixir or suspension). If the child can swallow tablets and capsules, ask what the child prefers for the "chaser" (usually water or juice).

Administer oral medications with the child in an upright or slightly recumbent position. The nurse should always use the least amount of force or restraint possible to administer the medication safely and avoid choking and aspiration. The child who is reluctant to take a necessary medication can be positioned in the nurse's lap, as follows:

- Seat the child sideways on your lap, facing your dominant hand.
- Hug the child by bringing the arm closest to your body under your arm and around your waist or back.
- Bring your nondominant arm around behind the child's neck and hold the child's free arm or hand with yours. This position cradles the child's head between your arm and body (see Fig. 14-3).
- If the child is very resistant, secure the child's legs between yours as well.

If the child vomits or spits up after the administration of medication, notify the physician. Another dose may need to be reordered depending on how long it has been since administration, the type of medication, and the amount vomited.

Alternative Oral Routes

Oral medications can be administered directly into the GI tract through a feeding tube. If the medication is to be administered through a feeding tube, verify tube placement before administration (see Chapter 13) and, depending on the type of tube (e.g., transpyloric), determine whether the tube is the proper route for the medication. Before and after the medication is administered, flush the tube with water to ensure that the medication has reached the GI tract and to prevent blockage in the tube.

Administering Injections

Injected medications are rapidly absorbed by diffusing into either plasma or the lymphatic system. Although injection results in faster and more reliable absorption than the oral route, injections are stressful and threatening to children and are not preferred. Injections are used most often for one-time doses of antibiotics (e.g., ceftriaxone for the initial treatment of severe infection), immunizations, iron administration, purified protein derivative (PPD), and allergy skin testing. Injections are potentially more dangerous in infants than in older children because of the infant's decreased muscle mass and variable blood flow to muscles.

Appropriately preparing the child for injections can reduce emotional and anticipatory concerns. Depending on the child's developmental level, explain the reason for the injection, any sensations the child might experience, and the length of time they are anticipated to last. Tell the child that the injection is not a punishment but is needed to make the child better or keep the child healthy. Practice counting, singing, deep breathing, or other distraction techniques with the child in advance.

Offer parents the option to leave if they feel unable to cope with the procedure; inform them when the procedure is completed. Most parents prefer to remain. Some are willing to help reassure the child or hold the child during the procedure.

To reduce the risk of injury, it is sometimes necessary to restrain the child before administering an injected medication. Restraint can be accomplished by swaddling the child or obtaining the assistance of another health care professional. Toddlers and older children often respond better to injections if parents can hold and comfort them during the procedure (Fig. 14-4). The parent, however, must feel confident in the ability to keep the child still enough to prevent injury.

Children perceive injections to be very painful. Even with the best preparation, it is hard for a child to understand that the pain of an injection lasts only seconds. Ice applied to the anticipated injection site for several minutes before the injection can numb the pain sensation, but it can also reduce blood flow to the area, interfering with absorption. Topical anesthetic agents, such as eutectic mixture of local anesthetics (EMLA) cream or topical lidocaine, also have been shown to be effective in reducing injection pain (see p. 387).

Depending on age, children can be taught to deal with the pain of an injection using guided imagery, distraction, or other methods, such as taking a deep breath and blowing out the pain, singing, or counting. Sucrose solution given to very young infants can temporarily decrease pain (Ellis, Sharp, Newhook, & Cohen, 2004).

Careful documentation of the injection is also important. Documentation includes recording the amount of medication injected and the site used. If the child will receive several injections, it is important to rotate sites to prevent tissue irritation and possible muscle atrophy and wasting. Federal vaccine regulations now require nurses to record the vaccine manufacturer and lot number for each immunization given, as well as any prior vaccine reaction the child might have incurred.

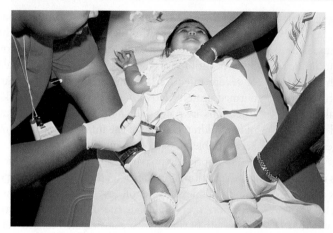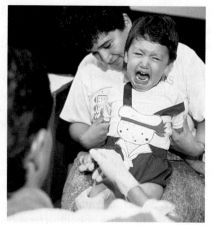

FIG 14-4 **Two methods of restraint for IM injection at the vastus lateralis site.** *(Left, Courtesy Parkland Health and Hospital System Community Oriented Primary Care Clinic, Dallas, TX. Right, Courtesy Cook Children's Medical Center, Fort Worth, TX.)*

Preparing and Administering Intramuscular Injections

When filling a syringe for an injection, it is important to remember that most syringes and needle hubs contain approximately 0.2 mL of dead space. Therefore, to keep the dose accurate, do not flush the needle and hub after injection. On the rare occasion that a Z-track method is used (a method in which a small air bubble locks in the medication), the dead space in the hub of the needle must be taken into account so as not to cause an overdose.

Select the site before the child is given an injection; the site should be soft, well vascularized, and healthy. It is important to avoid puncturing blood vessels, nerves, or bones and also to avoid injecting medications intended for IM administration into subcutaneous tissue. Inadvertent injection into any of these areas can result in accidental IV injection, pain, tissue sloughing, or nerve damage. The preferred IM injection sites in children are shown in Table 14-1.

Select an appropriate needle size (21 to 25 gauge) and length (½ to 1½ inches, depending on the child's size and the injection site) for the injection. Use the smallest size and length that will *safely and comfortably* administer the medication. For example, a viscous medication is less painful when injected through a larger-gauge needle. Also, consider the amount of body fat, the distance to the muscle, the size of the muscle, the volume of medication, and the properties of the medication.

Safe volumes for IM injection range from 0.5 to 2.5 mL, depending on the age and size of the child. Wipe the injection site with a skin cleanser and allow it to dry. Insert the needle at a 90-degree angle with a quick darting motion. Pull back gently on the plunger to aspirate for blood. If blood is noted, withdraw the needle to avoid giving the medication IV. Change the needle and the site. If no blood is noted, give the injection slowly. Unless contraindicated, massage the injection site afterward.

CRITICAL THINKING EXERCISE 14-3

You need to immunize an infant with hepatitis vaccine. The infant's dose is 2.5 μg. The type of vaccine you have on hand delivers 5 μg/mL. How many milliliters will you give the infant?

Administering Subcutaneous Injections

A subcutaneous injection is given into the tissue that lies just below the skin. This type of administration is used for medications that provide a sustained effect (e.g., heparin, insulin). A subcutaneous injection should be given only into healthy tissue. If circulation is impaired (e.g., because of edema, decreased temperature, shock), a subcutaneous injection should not be used because absorption will be altered.

Preferred subcutaneous injection sites are the fat pads located above the iliac crests, hips, lateral upper arms, and anterior thighs (Fig. 14-5). Children requiring frequent subcutaneous injections (e.g., children with type I diabetes mellitus) also use the abdomen, avoiding the 2-inch radius around the navel (Caffrey, 2003). Rotate sites to avoid the development of abscesses and to facilitate drug absorption.

CRITICAL TO REMEMBER
Guidelines for Maximum Safe Volumes for Intramuscular Injections

	Site			
Age	Deltoid	Ventro-gluteal	Dorso-gluteal	Vastus Lateralis
Premature	—	—	—	0.5 mL
Neonate	—	—	—	0.5 mL
Infant	—	—	—	1 mL
Young child (3-6 yr)	—	1.5 mL	1 mL	1.5 mL
Older child (6-14 yr)	0.5 mL	1.5-2 mL	1.5-2 mL	1.5 mL
Adolescent (15 yr to adult)	1 mL	2-2.5 mL	2-2.5 mL	1.5-2 mL

TABLE **14-1**	Preferred Intramuscular Injection Sites in Children		

Site	Key Points	Site	Key Points
Vastus lateralis	Located on anterior lateral thigh. Well developed at birth. Good choice for all age groups but usually used in children younger than 3 yr. Able to tolerate larger volumes and not located near vital structures, such as nerves and blood vessels. To locate appropriate site, divide leg into thirds; give the injection in middle outer third.	Dorsogluteal	Located by drawing diagonal line between posterior superior iliac spine and greater trochanter of femur. Dorsogluteal muscle is found above and lateral to this line. It develops with walking, so it should not be used until child has been walking for at least 1 yr. The child should be asked to "toe in" to avoid tensing muscle. Can hold 1 to 2.5 mL but has the slowest and poorest absorption of all sites.

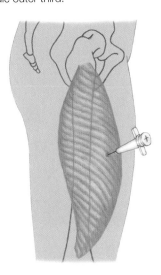

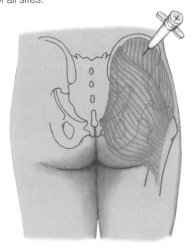

Site	Key Points	Site	Key Points
Ventrogluteal	Located by placing heel of hand on greater trochanter with fingers pointed toward child's head. Place index finger over anterior superior iliac spine and middle finger along iliac crest posteriorly as far as possible to form V. The injection is given in center of V. Site is safe for IM injection in children older than 18 mo because it is free of major blood vessels and nerves. Can generally hold larger volumes (up to 2.5 mL in adolescents). Care should be taken to avoid bone and joint.	Deltoid	Use part of muscle located about two fingerwidths below acromion process. This site is not used for injection in young children because small muscle mass cannot hold large volumes of medication or medications that must be injected deep into muscle mass. This is least painful site for injecting smaller volumes.

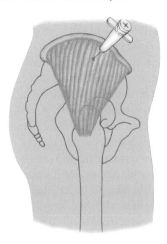

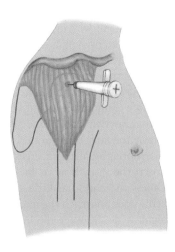

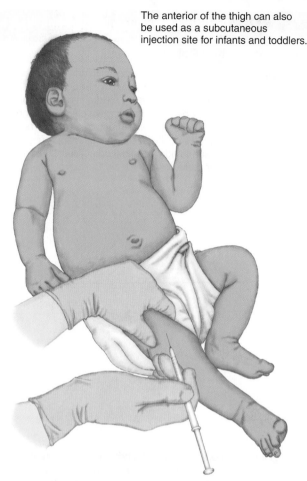

The anterior of the thigh can also be used as a subcutaneous injection site for infants and toddlers.

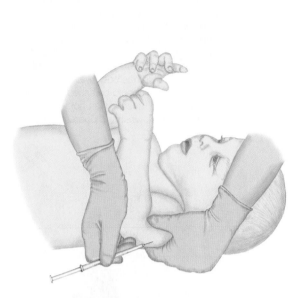

Use the dorsum of the upper arm of infants and toddlers for subcutaneous injections.

FIG 14-5   **Two of the preferred subcutaneous injection sites in children. The fat pads above the iliac crests and hips may also be used.**

Record the site of the subcutaneous injection to avoid using the same site again, which can cause tissue irritation.

Subcutaneous injections are usually given with a small (25- to 27-gauge), short (no more than ½- to ⅝-inch) needle to ensure that the medication is not inadvertently given IM. Insulin syringes come with even shorter, thinner needles (28- to 30-gauge, 5⁄16 inch). Volumes for subcutaneous injections are small, usually averaging 0.5 mL. Because the needle is so small and narrow, changing to a new needle after withdrawing medication through the stopper of a vial makes the injection more comfortable for the child.

Clean the site with alcohol and allow it to dry. Pinch the tissue to raise the fatty tissue from the muscle. The angle of needle insertion is usually 45 degrees, although some practitioners insert the ½-inch or 5⁄16-inch needle at a 90-degree angle. Unless the child has little subcutaneous tissue, the short needle does not reach the muscle, even if it is inserted at a straight angle. Massage the insertion site after administration unless massage is contraindicated for the injected medication, such as heparin.

If subcutaneous injections are to be done often (e.g., insulin administration), pay special attention to client education. Older children and adolescents can usually learn to perform this procedure without difficulty.

Intradermal Injections

Intradermal injections enter just below the outer layer of skin, the epidermis, and usually on the inner aspect of the forearm or on the upper back. They are most often used for testing (e.g., allergy, PPD). The needle is small (25- to 27-gauge) and short (½ to ⅝ inch). The volume is also small (usually 0.1 mL). After cleaning the site with alcohol and allowing it to dry, turn the bevel of the needle up and insert gently at a 15-degree angle. The needle will barely penetrate the skin. Inject the medication to form a wheal (similar in appearance to an insect bite) (Fig. 14-6). If the injection does not form a wheal or if bleeding is noted after the injection, administration was probably too deep and should be repeated. If several intradermal injections are made in the same area, each site should be marked with permanent ink for later identification.

The child who is to receive multiple injections might benefit significantly from carefully supervised needle play. In needle play, the child uses a syringe and needle to give shots to a doll. The nurse uses this play to prepare the child for injections and to help the child gain a sense of mastery over the experience of receiving an injection. The nurse offers a brief explanation of what will occur and why the child must receive an injection. Through therapeutic play, the child's anxiety is decreased.

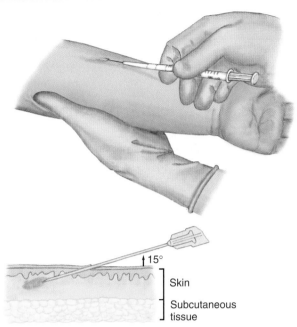

↑15°

Skin

Subcutaneous tissue

FIG 14-6   **Intradermal injection site and technique.**

Rectal Administration

The rectal route of administration is unreliable and is not used as often as other routes. It is most often reserved for times when a child cannot tolerate the oral route (e.g., because of nausea and vomiting). It has many possible complications, including the Valsalva response, rectal perforation, and other damage to the rectum or anus.

This route should not be used if the rectum is full of stool. Rectal administration is stressful for children because they fear intrusive procedures. Carefully prepare the child and give an explanation about the procedure. Tell the child the reason the medication is being given in this form and what the child can do to help. The child is also told whether the suppository must be retained or expelled.

Position the child on the left side with the right leg flexed, and expose the rectal area sufficiently for visibility. Adequate draping is essential for preschool and older children. Often the child needs help to relax. Distraction and deep-breathing exercises can help the child relax the external sphincter. Lubricate the suppository well with a water-soluble lubricant before insertion.

Advise the child to take a deep breath or bear down if possible to relax the sphincter further. Then gently insert the suppository past the internal sphincter. The child's rectal vault is not as long as an adult's, and the distance required to place medication is approximately 1 to 2 cm (½ to 1 inch). After insertion, hold the child's buttocks together until the urge to expel the suppository has passed.

Vaginal Administration

Although the vaginal route is not often used in infant, toddler, or preschool-age girls, it might be required for school-age or adolescent girls, most often to treat candidal infections or possibly for birth control. It is essential to explain the procedure, why it is indicated, and how the child can help.

Ask the child to void and then assist her into a supine position with the soles of her feet together and her knees resting on the bed (frog-leg position). Remember to drape the child and provide privacy. With a gloved hand, gently spread the labia so that the vaginal orifice is visible. If necessary, lubricate the tablet, suppository, or applicator with warm water or a water-soluble lubricant. Have the client take a deep breath and then gently insert the vaginal tablet, suppository, or applicator approximately 9 to 10 cm (3½ to 4 inches) along the posterior wall of the vagina. To reduce discomfort, the nurse should follow the natural angle of the vagina by pointing the finger or applicator toward the sacrum.

After the procedure is completed, the child might need to remain in a supine position for a time. Older school-age children and adolescents can be taught to instill their own vaginal medications. It is important that these girls receive good education and give a return demonstration of the procedure, especially if the instillations are contraceptives.

Ophthalmic Administration

Instillation of ophthalmic preparations is a clean rather than a sterile procedure (Procedure 14-1). Most pediatric ophthalmic solutions are available as either drops or ophthalmic ointment. If these preparations are refrigerated, allow them to warm to room temperature before instillation.

Before administering an ophthalmic preparation, note the expiration date and inspect the drops for color changes or cloudiness. Shake all suspensions well before instillation. Gently remove any exudate by wiping the child's eye with a sterile gauze pad from the inner to outer canthus. If exudates are dry or crusted, wipe with a warm, wet compress. Use a different pad for each eye.

Otic Administration

Otic procedures are clean rather than sterile procedures except in the case of a ruptured tympanic membrane (Procedure 14-2). Because cold ear drops can cause pain when they come in contact with the tympanic membrane, otic solutions should be allowed to warm to room temperature before administration.

Before administering ear drops, gently clean any exudate from the outer ear with sterile gauze. Because the risk of rupturing the tympanic membrane is high, never attempt to place anything inside the ear to clean the canal.

Nasal Administration

Although the mucous membrane route is generally used only for localized treatment, it has fairly rapid systemic absorption and, with a variety of novel administration devices, is being used more frequently for the administration of certain systemic medications (e.g., emergency medications, such as fentanyl and opioids, midazolam, antidiuretic hormone, steroids) (Wolfe & Bernstone, 2004).

When administering nose drops to an infant, the nurse or parent removes any excess mucus by gently suctioning with

| PROCEDURE 14-1 | ADMINISTERING AN OPHTHALMIC PREPARATION |

PURPOSE: To treat an eye infection, dilate pupils for diagnostic testing, or keep eyes moist.

1. Explain the purpose for the medication or lubricating drops. Tell the child how to help with the procedure. Explain that the child might have blurred vision for a short time afterward.
2. Gather needed equipment: eye drops or ointment, gauze pads, and tissues. Use appropriate hand hygiene before proceeding and after the procedure is complete. Wear gloves if contact with exudates is expected.
3. Assist the child into a supine position with the neck slightly hyperextended (e.g., by placing a rolled towel or small blanket under the shoulder blades).
4. If the drops are to be instilled into an infant's eyes, obtain assistance in restraining the child's arms and head or use a mummy wrap as necessary.
5. Instruct an older child to look upward and gently pull the lower lid down and away from the eye.
6. Place the drops or a ribbon of ointment into the space between the eye and lower lid, taking care not to contaminate the end of the dropper or tube.
7. If both drops and ointment are ordered, the drops should be administered first. If they are placed after the ointment, they will not be absorbed.
8. Have the child look down as the lower lid is released. Encourage the child to close both eyes and keep them closed for several seconds. Hand the child a tissue to gently blot any excess medication.
9. As with any procedure, praise the child for cooperation and assistance. Document the medication in the appropriate location.

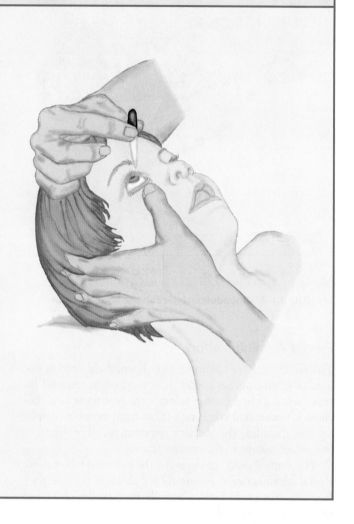

a bulb syringe before administration. To make eating more comfortable, saline nose drops followed by gentle suction should be given 20 to 30 minutes before feedings.

Receiving nose drops is stressful for young children, who might feel that they are drowning during the instillation. A thorough explanation of what the child will feel, why the medication has been ordered ("to help unstop your nose"), and what the child needs to do to help is necessary. Assistance with restraint may be necessary with the young child, or mummy restraint or swaddling may be used.

Assist the child into a supine position and hyperextend the neck slightly by placing a rolled towel or small blanket under the shoulder blades. Keeping the head in a midline position, instill the number of drops ordered into each naris. The head is kept in the same position to allow the drops to reach the ethmoid and sphenoid sinuses. Then briefly have the child turn the head slightly in each direction and back to midline to disburse the medication to the maxillary and frontal sinuses.

After the drops have been instilled, the child remains in the supine position for several minutes to allow the medication to be distributed to the sinuses. Instruct the child not to blow the medication out the nose. Praise all efforts at cooperation.

Topical Administration

Because skin is relatively impermeable when intact and has a large surface area, topical administration of drugs is generally limited to localized treatment. If the medication is applied to abraded skin, over a large area, or over a long period, however, systemic effects can result. Solvents added to the medication to break down skin oils and occlusive dressings also increase absorption. Monitor the child carefully for systemic absorption effects.

As with all other procedures, explain what will be done, why it will be done, and what sensations the child will experience. Clean the skin gently to remove any exudate, scales, or other residue and allow it to dry. To avoid contaminating the container, place the estimated amount of medication on a sterile pad. Wear gloves and apply the ointment or cream as ordered or as recommended by the manufacturer. Cover the site afterward with a sterile pad if ordered. Encourage the child to avoid touching or scratching the area and praise the child for cooperation.

PROCEDURE 14-2 | ADMINISTERING OTIC DROPS

PURPOSE: To treat inflammation or infection of the ear canal, relieve pain, or prevent otitis externa.

1. Explain any expected sensations to the child in developmentally appropriate terms (e.g., "It may sound like there is a butterfly flying inside your ear.") and describe how the child can help. Assistance in restraining a young child might be necessary.
2. Gather the following equipment: otic drops and cotton pieces. Use appropriate hand hygiene before and after the procedure.
3. Position the child lying down with the affected ear up or sitting with the head turned so the affected ear is up.
4. Brace the administering hand against the child's head above the ear.
5. If the child is 3 years or younger, pull the pinna of the ear back and down, holding near the lobe. If the child is older than 3 years, pull the pinna back and up.
6. Insert the required number of drops. Then gently massage the tragus (anterior portion) to ensure that the drops reach the tympanic membrane.
7. Pack cotton loosely into the canal, if ordered. Instruct the child not to remove the cotton or place anything inside the ear.
8. Keep the child on the unaffected side for several minutes after administration. If medication is to be administered in both ears, the procedure should be repeated in the other ear after a wait of at least 1 minute.
9. Document the medication in the appropriate place.

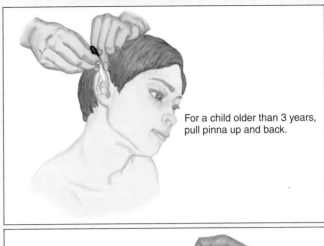

For a child older than 3 years, pull pinna up and back.

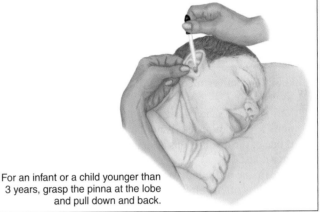

For an infant or a child younger than 3 years, grasp the pinna at the lobe and pull down and back.

Adolescents may be receiving medications by transdermal patch (e.g., nicotine patch, birth control). Transdermal patches deliver a steady dose of medication over a prescribed time period and are changed on a regular schedule. Nurses need to carefully explain how the patch is to be applied, proper disposal after use, and under what conditions medication absorption can be adversely affected (e.g., application of cold or heat). It is important to emphasize to the adolescent that a transdermal patch is a medication, like an oral medication, that, if used, should be reported to a health care provider (Paparella, 2005). In unconscious or unresponsive patients, nurses need to carefully search usual areas for patch placement (e.g., thorax, buttocks, upper arm, behind the ear) to avoid overdosing the patient (Paparella, 2005).

Inhalation Therapy

Respiratory medications, used frequently in children, are delivered either by nebulizer or a metered-dose inhaler—a hand-held device that delivers "puffs" of medication for inhalation. Although many inhaled medications have an unpleasant taste or smell, this route is a relatively nonthreatening form of medication delivery. Monitoring for desired therapeutic effects and systemic effects is essential because most medications used for inhalation have systemic side effects.

Nebulized medications are diluted in normal saline solution and administered with a hand-held small-volume nebulizer. The small-volume nebulizer aerosolizes the medication for the child to inhale. Medication can be delivered through a mask or through a plastic mouthpiece held between the lips or close to the face (Fig. 14-7). A mask is preferred for young children because they are seldom able to successfully hold a mouthpiece in place for the required length of time. Encourage the child to breathe deeply and slowly during the treatment.

Metered-dose inhalers offer an inexpensive, portable means of delivering inhaled medications. Many people, particularly children, have difficulty using a metered-dose inhaler correctly. The effectiveness of these medications is increased with the use of an inhalation aid, such as a spacer device. A spacer is a cylindric piece of hard or expandable plastic that attaches to the mouthpiece of the inhaler and is attached to a mouthpiece or mask. The child depresses the inhaler, and the medication enters the spacer, allowing the child time to deeply inhale the medication. For people who cannot afford a commercial spacer, a small plastic commercial water bottle can be used; an opening large enough for the inhaler mouthpiece can be cut into the large end, and the bottle opening at the other end is small enough to fit into the child's mouth. (See Procedure 14-3 for directions to use a metered-dose inhaler.)

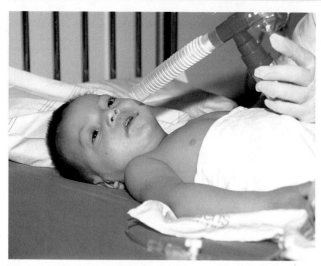

FIG 14-7 **Administration of nebulized medication to an infant.** *(Courtesy Children's Medical Center, Dallas, TX.)*

PROCEDURE 14-3	**USING A METERED-DOSE INHALER**

PURPOSE: To deliver medication directly to the respiratory system

1. Verify the physician's order for medication or medications to be administered and the number of puffs.
2. If one of the medications is an inhaled steroid, administer it last.
3. Explain the procedure to the child and parent or caregiver. It is often helpful to demonstrate the use of the inhaler and to explain specifically what the child is expected to do.
4. Place the inhaler in the spacer. Tell the child not to inhale too quickly or the spacer will whistle.
5. Tell the child to exhale ("big breath out") and place the spacer mouthpiece in the mouth or the spacer mask over the face. The child might be more comfortable holding the spacer and helping you.
6. Tell the child that you will squeeze the inhaler and release the medication into the spacer. Then direct the child to inhale ("big breath in") slowly. You may need to talk the child through this process.
7. Encourage the child to hold the breath for about 10 seconds or until you count slowly to 5.
8. Ask the child to exhale and then take another breath from the spacer and hold it for 10 seconds.
9. Repeat with another puff, if ordered. Praise the child for cooperation.
10. Rinse the inhaler adapter and spacer with cool water. Return the equipment to the medication room or designated area. Document.

Although both forms of delivering inhaled medications are effective, the nebulized medication offers the advantage of delivery with supplemental oxygen to children in an acute episode of respiratory distress. Nebulized medications can also be delivered to an unconscious or intubated child by inserting the aerosol administration device in-line between the child and a bag-valve-mask.

Educating the parent and child is important to ensure the effectiveness of this form of medication delivery. The technique must be demonstrated and a return demonstration given. Use of the metered-dose inhaler should be reviewed at each return visit.

INTRAVENOUS THERAPY

IV therapy is widely used for children. Fluids and electrolytes, nutrition, blood products, and medications can be delivered by the IV route. When used to administer medications, IV therapy produces a steadier and more therapeutic blood level and it is the only acceptable route of administration for some medications that might be irritating. The risks of IV therapy include possible fluid overload and possible complications from administration errors.

Intravenous Catheter Insertion

Typically, children's IV lines are infused through an over-the-needle catheter or a butterfly catheter. The type of catheter chosen often depends on hospital policy. Over-the-needle catheters are generally preferred because they are more flexible and stable, thus decreasing the risk of infiltration. Over-the-needle catheters come in even sizes (e.g., 22 and 24 gauge), and butterfly catheters are available in odd sizes (e.g., 23 and 25 gauge).

Venous access sites in children are shown in Figure 14-8. The rate and type of fluid to be infused, the projected length of time the IV line will be needed, and the availability of veins often determine site selection in children. The nurse also considers the child's developmental level. For example, placement of an IV line into a toddler's foot is often a poor choice because it inhibits walking, a newly learned skill. Avoid inserting an IV line into a dominant hand, if possible, because the site will interfere with activities of daily living. The hand, wrist, and antecubital sites are most frequently used in infants and children. Scalp veins are sometimes used in infants. Scalp veins have no valves and can be infused in either direction. IV catheters placed in this area can be adequately secured to allow the infant to move without dislodging the IV line.

Vein size and the kind of fluid to be infused also guide the choice of catheter. Generally, the smallest catheter through which fluids and medications can be safely infused should be used (often a 22- or 24-gauge catheter). For most children, a 20- to 24-gauge catheter provides adequate access.

Before an IV needle is inserted, explain the procedure to the child and parent. Include information about what will happen (what the child will see and feel) during each step of the procedure, why the catheter will be placed, where it will be placed (if possible), how long it will be in place (if known), and what function it will perform. Explain to the parent the purpose of both the IV therapy and any additional equipment (e.g., an infusion pump). Reassure the parent that once the IV catheter is in and stabilized, the child can

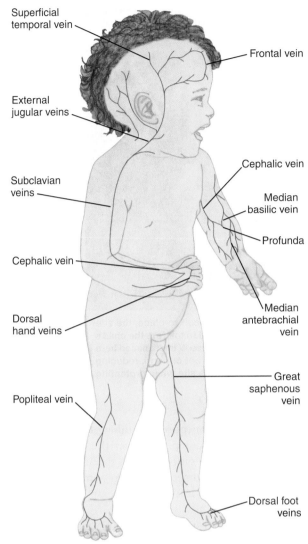

FIG 14-8   **Venous access sites in children.**

Labels on figure:
Superficial temporal vein
Frontal vein
External jugular veins
Cephalic vein
Subclavian veins
Median basilic vein
Profunda
Cephalic vein
Dorsal hand veins
Median antebrachial vein
Popliteal vein
Great saphenous vein
Dorsal foot veins

Have all the needed equipment ready in advance. Equipment includes an IV catheter of appropriate size, ordered IV solution, primed needleless infusion set, extension tubing with a T-connector, tape, sterile transparent occlusive dressing, a padded arm board, a tourniquet, alcohol pads, gloves, and blood-sampling tubes (if required). Povidone-iodine preparations might be necessary for immunosuppressed children or children with sensitivity to alcohol. Bacteriostatic normal saline solution, 3 mL, is used to flush the catheter after any required blood samples have been obtained.

Encourage parents to remain with the child if they desire. Parents should not, however, be expected to restrain the child during the procedure. Explain the procedure at each step. The nurse usually selects the IV site, beginning with the veins of the nondominant hand or forearm and moving proximally. As the catheter is inserted and the child experiences a "big sting" or "pinch," it might be helpful to advise the child to take a deep breath and blow out the pain.

Catheter placement is confirmed by a blood return, but a normal saline solution flush is needed to verify that there is no infiltration. After the catheter is placed, secure it in place with tape and a sterile, clear, occlusive dressing or tape. The clear dressing allows for adequate visibility of the insertion site. In addition, secure the catheter extension tubing to the extremity with tape. Be sure to leave the plastic clamp accessible.

After the IV catheter and tubing are fully stabilized, secure the extremity to a well-padded arm board if necessary to prevent injury. This is particularly important for active children. Secure the extremity in an anatomic position to prevent nerve damage. You can further protect the catheter by using a plastic shield. This can be a medicine cup that is cut in half

be held as usual. Bring the child to the treatment room for the procedure.

Assess the child's ability to hold the affected extremity still during the procedure. Give children suggestions for coping with the discomfort and have them practice coping techniques in advance if possible. Nonpharmacologic interventions include guided imagery (e.g., putting on an imaginary "magic glove" that keeps the hand from hurting) and distraction (e.g., music, novelty toys, seek-and-find books) (Ellis et al., 2004). Pharmacologic interventions include ice and topical numbing gels or pastes, such as EMLA cream or ELA-Max. Topical lidocaine can be used; however, it must remain on the skin almost as long as EMLA (45 to 60 minutes). Newer types of lidocaine administrations (e.g., by iontophoresis or helium gas actuator) can shorten the time to local anesthesia (Migdal, Chudzynska-Pomianowska, Vause, Henry, & Lazar, 2005). If the child is not able to hold still, obtain assistance before attempting to start the IV line. (See Chapter 15 for further discussion of pain management techniques.)

This boy's IV line is secured well enough so he can pretend that he is a famous basketball star as he shoots baskets in the playroom.

The foot is a useful site for the infant who is not walking or crawling.

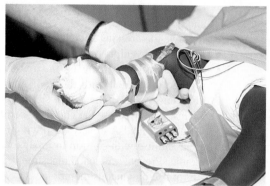

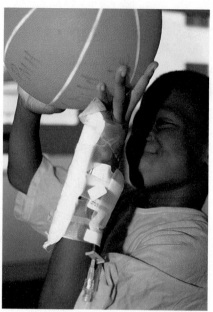

FIG 14-9   **Because children's veins are fragile and IV lines can be difficult to place, the site must be well protected to prevent the child from removing the catheter and to tolerate the child's activity. Hand veins may be good for preschoolers and older children because IV lines placed here do not limit walking. A padded arm board gently limits movement of the foot or hand, reducing the risk of infiltration of the IV fluid. A plastic shield allows visibility of the site while protecting it.** (*Courtesy Parkland Health and Hospital System, Dallas, TX.*)

and taped on the edges or a commercially available device (Fig. 14-9). Document in the child's record the location of the IV line, the location and condition of the site, the type of access device used (length and gauge of catheter or butterfly), and the date and time it was inserted.

Intravenous Monitoring and Maintenance

To prevent fluid overload in children receiving IV therapy, IV fluids or medications are administered through an infusion pump that delivers a preset volume at an hourly rate (Fig. 14-10). Most infusion pumps are easily programmable with dose limits to prevent accidental fluid overload. If available, a pump with a tamper-proof design should be used.

An additional safety feature used in many institutions is the in-line volume-control set and tubing (burette: Buretrol, Soluset, Metriset), which is used in place of regular IV tubing. A volume-control set usually has a 100- to 150-mL capacity (a 1- to 2-hour supply of fluid). The nurse programs the infusion pump to deliver only the amount in the volume-control set; the clamp between the burette and the IV container remains closed to prevent fluid from inadvertently dropping into the volume-control chamber. Medications can be mixed with an appropriate amount of fluid in the volume-control set by injecting the medication through the available port. The infusion pump is then set at a rate to infuse the amount in the burette over the correct time period.

To precisely administer very low volumes of fluid or medications, a volumetric infusion pump is used (Baxter, Bard). A syringe with the appropriate fluid volume or medication is attached to primed, low-volume tubing and placed in the pump. After connecting the tubing to the child, the nurse programs the pump to deliver the volume of fluid or medication in the syringe over a specified time period (see Fig. 14-10). Volumetric infusion pumps are used for both continuous and intermittent therapy and to deliver IV medications.

The nurse assesses and documents an IV site at least every hour (or according to institutional policy, if different) for signs and symptoms of infiltration or phlebitis. Use of a transparent dressing over the IV site facilitates assessment. Feel the temperature of the site and for any hardness of the vein, observe for any redness or swelling, and assess for pain. Depending on the facility, IV sites are charted "by exception," meaning that only adverse findings are documented in detail. One way to assess for infiltration is by observing for symmetry in the size and shape of limbs or scalp. Gently touch the site to determine whether it is soft or taut or whether the scalp site is boggy. If signs of complications (e.g., edema, erythema, pain, blanching, coolness, streaking of the skin above the vein) are noted, discontinue the infusion immediately and notify the physician. Elevating the extremity can decrease edema. Heat can be applied if the infused solution or medication is neither a vesicant nor a sclerosing agent.

Unlike adults' IV sites, because of the fragility of children's veins and the difficulty of finding a new site, children's IV sites are not changed every 72 hours. Change IV fluid containers every 24 hours and tubing according to hospital policy. Many facilities require tubing to be changed every 48 to 72 hours. Many institutions, however, change total parenteral nutrition tubing every 24 hours in an attempt to decrease infection rates.

Volumetric infusion pump.

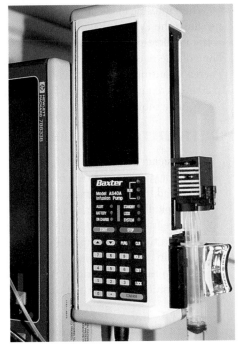 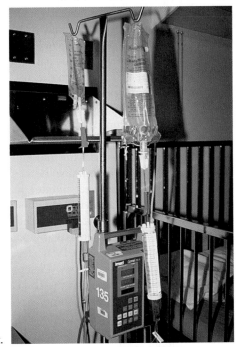

In-line volume-control set.

FIG 14-10   **Two types of infusion pumps.**   *(Courtesy Parkland Health and Hospital System, Dallas, TX.)*

Infusion Rates and Methods

In most instances the physician orders an hourly IV fluid infusion rate. The nurse verifies the rate with the physician's order and documents on the child's flow sheet the type of solution, the location of the site, and the ordered rate. The rate is based on normal fluid maintenance requirements and additional fluids to replace deficits as needed. At some facilities, nurses can adjust the child's IV rate to infuse fluids in the required time frame. In other facilities, a physician's order is needed to adjust the IV infusion rate. Before adjusting the rate, the nurse must know the maintenance rates appropriate for the child's weight, to avoid increasing the rate too much and causing fluid overload. Box 14-2 illustrates how the nurse can determine maintenance fluid rates according to the formula for daily fluid requirements.

It is most important to ensure that the appropriate amount of fluid is being absorbed. *Even if the child is receiving fluids through an infusion pump, the nurse checks the fluid absorption at least hourly.* Pumps can malfunction, risking fluid overload if they are not meticulously checked.

Administering Intravenous Medications

IV medications can be administered as a continuous infusion (e.g., potassium chloride) or intermittently (e.g., antibiotics). Methods of administering IV medications include piggyback, push, and retrograde methods. It is imperative that the appropriate method is chosen to meet the needs of the child and to fit any restrictions posed by the medication and fluid volume.

When administering IV solutions and medications to children, the nurse must consider the following:
- Type of IV solution
- Compatibility of the medication and the IV solution
- Dilution volume of the medication
- Amount of flush needed
- Administration rate

The administration method, type of IV tubing used, and hospital policies and procedures determine some factors, such as the amount of flush needed. Information about specific medications and their reconstitution, compatible fluids, and rates of infusion can be obtained from pharmacists, drug inserts, or texts.

BOX 14-2	**Calculating Daily Maintenance Fluid Rates**

≤10 kg	100 mL/kg
10-20 kg	1000 mL + 50 mL/kg for each additional kg between 10 and 20 kg
20 kg	1500 mL + 20 mL/kg for each additional kg over 20

The preceding formulas give the daily fluid requirements. To determine an hourly rate, take the total milliliters per day and divide by 24. For example:
1. A child weighing 15 kg should receive 1000 mL (1000 for the first 10 kg) + (50 × 5) (50 mL/kg for each 1 kg between 10 and 20) = 1250 mL/day.
2. The result is 1250 mL/24 hr = 52 mL/hr.

Intravenous Push Administration

Medications delivered by IV push are reconstituted, but not diluted in additional solution, and are pushed directly into the IV catheter through the port closest to the child. The volume of medication infused is small (usually 5 mL or less), and the effects (both desired and adverse) are immediate.

This method is used to give pain medications in the immediate postoperative period, administer sedatives, induce paralytic effects in ventilated patients, and administer other medications. To administer a medication by IV push, the nurse must first ensure that the medication can be administered safely in this way. Verify compatibility with the infusing solution (if there is a running IV line) and determine the administration rate (usually given in milligrams per minute). If hospital policy requires, check the medication with another nurse or physician before administering it. In explaining the procedure, reassure the child that the procedure is painless.

Before administering the medication, check the IV site for complications and the running IV line for patency. Clamp the IV tubing above the injection port closest to the child and clean the port with alcohol. Use povidone-iodine (Betadine) if the line is a central access catheter or the child is immunosuppressed. If the medication is not compatible with the infusing IV fluid or if the medication is going into an intermittent infusion port, flush the tubing with approximately 2 to 3 mL of normal saline solution before and after administering the medication. Be sure to wipe the access port with alcohol each time the port is entered and after the procedure is complete. Attach the medication syringe to the port and administer the medication at the prescribed rate. Medications given by IV push are usually administered slowly and should not be administered faster than the rate the manufacturer or the formulary suggests. Remove the medication syringe, wipe the port with alcohol, and cover the port if the IV administration system requires a port cover.

Monitor the child carefully for the effects of the medication, including undesired side effects. Evaluate by monitoring the child's vital signs (including blood pressure) and reassessing frequently.

Intravenous Piggyback Administration

Medications given by piggybacking an IV line frequently are diluted in at least 20 mL of IV solution and administered over at least 15 minutes. These medications might be diluted by the pharmacy and sent to the nursing unit in a separate IV bag, or they can be prepared on the unit with a needleless mixing system, which allows the powdered medication to enter the diluent bag. The nurse can dilute reconstituted medications by injecting them directly into a volume-control set containing a predetermined amount of IV solution. Medications given by IV piggyback to children should be administered through an infusion pump to avoid infusing the medication either too rapidly or too slowly. If the medications are to be diluted in the volume-control set, the nurse notes the total amount of fluid (volume of medication plus volume in the burette) when setting the pump for the correct infusion rate.

When infusing medications by piggyback, the nurse must also flush the IV tubing with fluid to complete the delivery of the medication out of the IV tubing and into the child. The volume needed for the flush varies and must be added when accounting for the total volume infused. Generally, 16 to 20 mL is required to flush the IV tubing adequately, unless low-volume tubing is used.

CRITICAL THINKING EXERCISE 14-4

The physician has ordered 1.4 g of IV ampicillin every 4 hours for your patient. You need to mix the ampicillin.
1. If you add 5 mL of normal saline solution to a 2-g vial of ampicillin, how many milliliters will you need to remove from the vial for the child?
2. You add the mixed ampicillin to 50 mL of the IV fluid to run in over the course of ½ hour. How fast will you need to run the IV line to deliver the medication in the appropriate amount of time?

The total volume to be infused should be within safe limits for the child. For example:
- Vancomycin, 150 mg, is ordered for a 15-kg child. The child's hourly maintenance rate is 52 mL.
- The recommended concentration for administering vancomycin is 5 mg/mL. To achieve that concentration, 30 mL of fluid would be needed ($150 \div 5$).
- Add a 20-mL flush, for a total volume of 50 mL to be administered over the course of 30 to 60 minutes.
- This amount is within the 52-mL hourly volume the child should be receiving.

Determine that the IV line is functioning and that the site is free of complications. Clean the injection port on the volume-control set with alcohol and add the medication to the required amount of diluent. Agitate the volume-control set gently to mix the medication and diluent. Set the pump to infuse the medication; the rate should be based on the volume actually in the volume-control set. It is important to set the pump to sound the alarm when the volume is infused so that the nurse can return and add the volume needed to complete the flush. Label the volume-control set with the name of the medication added. Document what has infused. All flush and medication volumes must be added to recorded intake and calculated into the total volume limits to avoid fluid overload.

If the child does not have a running IV line but is receiving medication intermittently by piggyback, be sure to flush the IV catheter with saline solution before attaching the piggyback set. This procedure ensures patency of the line. In some instances, depending on hospital equipment, the medication and the regular IV infusion can be run concurrently, so long as the medication is compatible with the running IV fluid.

Intravenous Retrograde Administration

The IV retrograde method uses smaller volumes (usually 1 mL) of both medication and flush solution and generally has a slightly shorter administration time than the piggyback method. The nurse clamps the IV tubing below the injection port nearest the child. After wiping the port with an appropriate cleansing solution, the nurse injects the medication into the port in a direction away from the child (retrograde), causing it to flow into the tubing above the injection port. The syringe is removed and the IV pump is then set to deliver the medication volume plus the amount of fluid needed to flush the IV tubing from the injection port to the child.

Some infusion pumps do not allow the pressure created by retrograde infusion. In this instance, an empty syringe is connected to the port closest to the IV pump. When the medication is inserted into the tubing at the port nearest the child, it displaces an equal volume of fluid into the empty syringe (Hadaway, 2005). It is important for the nurse to be familiar with the type of infusion pump used and the facility's policy and procedure for retrograde administration.

Venous Access Devices

Intermittent Infusion Ports
Intermittent infusion ports (saline or heparin locks) allow drugs to be administered IV without the need for a running IV line. The intermittent infusion port is an IV catheter that is placed, flushed with normal saline solution or heparin to maintain patency, and then locked with a male adapter. The port is accessed when needed for fluid or medication infusion. Site observation and site care are the same as for any IV catheter.

The frequency of flushing is controversial and is determined by hospital policy. Routine flushing with normal saline solution to maintain patency is performed every 6 to 12 hours. The device is flushed with saline solution before and after medication administration and with heparinized saline solution, if ordered, after blood is drawn or infused.

Central Venous Access Devices
Central venous access devices are venous access devices in which the catheter is centrally placed directly into a major blood vessel. These devices are most often used to administer medications, blood products, IV fluids, and parenteral nutrition over the long term to chronically ill children. These devices can be tunneled or nontunneled central catheters and implanted infusion ports. *Percutaneously implanted central catheters (PICCs)* are also used for children who need IV access for a period longer than peripheral IV catheters can be adequately maintained. All central venous access devices need routine care (dressing changes, flushing) according to facility protocol. Because these devices enter the central venous system, all procedures are done using aseptic technique.

Tunneled central lines are surgically placed lines that are held in place by a Dacron cuff located in a subcutaneous tunnel. They are most commonly placed in an external jugular vein but may also be placed in the cephalic, axillary subclavian, femoral, saphenous, or internal jugular veins. The tip of the tunneled catheter is threaded until it rests at the junction of the superior vena cava and right atrium. Tunneled central lines are usually flushed with heparin at least every 24 hours and after blood is infused or drawn.

Short-term or nontunneled central catheters are most frequently placed in the subclavian or femoral veins. These lines involve the placement of a large-gauge catheter that is then sutured in place.

An *implanted venous access device* (IVAD, Infusaport) consists of a catheter that is connected to a port or reservoir. Like the tunneled catheter, the catheter tip rests at the junction of the superior vena cava and right atrium. The port is under the skin and is accessed with a noncoring needle placed through the skin into the port. The needle is then covered with a bio-occlusive dressing, and an extension set is attached to the end. When the port is no longer needed for infusions or obtaining blood specimens, it is flushed with heparin and the needle withdrawn. The child with an implanted port can participate in all typical childhood activities except those with a potential for high-impact contact with the chest (e.g., competitive football).

PICC lines are long catheters made of polyurethane or silicone and threaded through an introducer placed in the antecubital vein. They are usually placed by specially trained nurses and are frequently used for home antibiotic therapy. After the catheter is threaded so that the tip is located in the superior vena cava, the introducer is removed. The catheter is then covered with a bio-occlusive dressing, and placement is verified by x-ray examination. These catheters are usually left in place for several weeks to months. The major complications of this type of line are phlebitis, infection, thrombosis, and catheter occlusion.

ADMINISTRATION OF BLOOD OR BLOOD PRODUCTS
Education of the child and parent is essential whenever a transfusion is administered. Children and parents must receive all necessary information honestly, consistently, and at a developmentally appropriate level. Information includes why the transfusion is necessary, how long it will take, what the child will feel and hear, and the types of blood products to be used. Ask the parent or caregiver about the child's transfusion history and whether the child has ever had a transfusion reaction. The nurse discusses the risks of receiving versus not receiving the blood product and explains each step as it is to be performed. It is important to use clear, concise, age-appropriate terminology.

Information about the types of blood products, the indications and procedures for their administration, and the identification and treatment of transfusion reactions is found in standard medical-surgical nursing texts. The key features of administration of blood products to children are as follows:

- To prevent circulatory hypervolemia, packed red blood cells are usually administered to infants and children.
- Identify the child and verify blood (type, Rh factor, donor number, expiration date) with another nurse or physician.
- Take vital signs, including blood pressure, before administering blood. Then take vital signs every 15 minutes for

the first 2 hours and every 30 minutes thereafter until the infusion is complete.

- Administer blood with normal saline solution (dextrose solutions cause hemolysis) on a piggyback setup through an appropriate filter.
- Use blood within 30 minutes of its arrival from the blood bank. Do not store blood in regular unit refrigeration. Return unused blood to the blood bank. Order only as much blood as can be used in 4 hours.
- The rate of infusion of packed red blood cells is approximately 2-3 mL/kg/hr over no more than 4 hours (Brunetti & Cohen, 2005). Run the infusion slowly for the first 15 minutes because many transfusion reactions are seen during this brief period. If the child has not displayed any signs of a reaction during this time, increase the rate to the ordered rate for the remainder of the dose.
- Cytomegalovirus-negative blood (blood that has tested negative for cytomegalovirus) is used for cytomegalovirus-negative, immunocompromised children; low-birth-weight neonates; bone marrow transplant recipients; and children younger than 2 years who are receiving chemotherapy.
- Blood that has been irradiated to prevent lymphocyte replication helps prevent graft-versus-host disease in immunocompromised children, such as bone marrow transplant recipients; it also is used in neonates.
- Although the type and crossmatch should be less than 48 hours old, infants younger than 4 months rarely form red blood cell antibodies and therefore usually undergo a type and crossmatch only once. These results can be used until the infant reaches 4 months of age or is discharged from the hospital.
- During the administration of blood or blood products, the child and parents should notify the nurse immediately if the child feels "bad" or has fever or chills, headache, nausea, pain at the needle site, or difficulty breathing. Children and parents often do not know how they are supposed to feel and will not notify the nurse of the signs and symptoms of a transfusion reaction. The child should not be left alone while receiving blood products.
- In neonates and small infants, auscultate the lungs before and frequently during a transfusion to detect signs of respiratory distress from fluid overload.
- If a reaction is suspected, stop the transfusion immediately and infuse normal saline solution through new tubing. Notify the physician. Continue to monitor vital signs. Monitor urine output hourly and send samples of the child's blood and urine to the laboratory.
- If the child's maintenance IV rate was decreased to avoid fluid overload, the blood sugar level must be monitored with reagent strips (Dextrostix) or another form of measurement because reducing the maintenance IV rate decreases the amount of IV glucose received by the child and may lead to hypoglycemia.
- After the transfusion, praise the child and family for their cooperation and help during the procedure.

CHILD AND FAMILY EDUCATION

Teaching children and their caregivers about medications is an essential part of therapy (Box 14-3). Statistics about adherence suggest that children taking medications for an acute or chronic condition do not adhere to their prescribed regimen (Winnick et al., 2005). In addition to factors such as forgetting to give a medication, refusal to take the medication because of unpleasant taste, and discontinuing a medication because symptoms have improved, lack of understanding about a medication and its effects is a major reason cited for nonadherence (Bartlett, Lukk, Butz, Lampros-Klein, & Rand, 2002; Staples & Bravender, 2002).

Teaching the family about medications begins with a thorough assessment that includes a list of all medications the child is currently taking, including over-the-counter medications. Any history of allergies to medications should be noted to prevent potential drug interactions.

Note as well any developmental needs or special learning needs, such as a hearing or speech disability, language

---

BOX 14-3 | PARENTS WANT TO KNOW About Medication Administration at Home

Address special medication problems before the child leaves the hospital or ambulatory care setting. Attention to this issue can help prevent medication errors or the child's and family's failure to follow the physician's order for home treatment. The parent and child (if old enough) will want to know:
- Name of the medication (trade, generic)
- Why it was prescribed
- What it is supposed to do
- How to take the medication (how much, how often, how long to take it, techniques for administering the medication)
- Acceptable measuring device for home administration of medications (oral syringe, small medicine spoon, small medicine cup)

- How to use calibrated droppers or syringes to measure and give the right amount of medication
- Expected or potential side effects and what to do if they occur
- When the nurse or physician should be notified of side effects
- Any dietary restrictions

If the child will need to take the medication during the school day, the health provider must give the parent a written order with the description of the medication, effects, side effects, and time of day the medication should be administered. This must be delivered to the school nurse, along with written permission from the parent for the medication to be administered and the medication in an original pharmacy container.

barrier, or illiteracy. The nurse must make provisions to accommodate the child's special needs. For example, information should be presented in a variety of ways (e.g., spoken, written, illustrated). Written instructions should accompany any oral instruction.

Problem solve with the family before discharge from the hospital, clinic, or physician's office. This process includes devising acceptable schedules for medication administration, suggesting alternative methods of administering oral medications (e.g., crushing and mixing with food), and identifying foods that might be mixed with the medications.

Emphasize taking the medication as ordered. Particularly highlight finishing the full course of a prescribed antibiotic, not changing dosages without consulting the physician, and returning for follow-up appointments.

Reinforce general safety information, such as keeping medications out of the reach of children and keeping all medications in their original containers. Evaluate your interventions by asking questions (scenarios work well), providing a demonstration, and asking for a return demonstration. Document all teaching and validation of understanding.

KEY CONCEPTS

- Standardized dosage ranges for many medications have not been established for children.
- Children's body proportions and composition differ from those of adults, and children's responses to medications differ accordingly.
- The nurse must incorporate principles of growth and development into medication administration.
- The margin of safety for medication administration is narrow for children.
- Oral medications should be administered with developmentally appropriate equipment.
- Injections are stressful to children and are not usually the first choice of administration route. Take care to choose the appropriate site for the child's size and age, and use the shortest and smallest-gauge needle possible to ensure safe administration of the medication.
- The rate and type of fluid to be infused and the availability and accessibility of veins often determine the site selected for venipuncture.
- Children receiving IV infusions should receive their fluids through a pump that can be set to deliver a predetermined amount of fluid safely. A volume-control set can be used as well to decrease the chance of fluid overload.
- A baseline assessment must be performed before a blood product is administered to a child. This assessment includes auscultating an infant's lungs so that signs of fluid overload during the transfusion are immediately recognized.
- As with any client, the infant or child receiving a transfusion needs to be carefully monitored throughout the procedure to assess effects and adverse reactions.

ANSWERS TO
CRITICAL THINKING EXERCISE 14-1

1. The nurse needs to emphasize the following to the father:
   a. Although symptoms have disappeared, it is important for the child to take the entire amount of medication.
   b. The medication prescribed is the one best able to treat the child.
   c. Some children do react adversely to certain tastes, but there are methods of disguising the taste.
   d. Children of this age will react positively to expectations for cooperation.
2. If, after a firm statement of expectation by the father for the child to take the medication, the child still refuses, suggest to the father that he try mixing the medication in a small (2 teaspoons) amount of a liquid (juice, soda) to disguise the taste. The nurse can also describe how to hold the child properly for administering an oral medication with control. If these methods do not work, the father should call back.

ANSWERS TO
CRITICAL THINKING EXERCISE 14-2

1. 100 mg/5 mL = 150 mg/x mL;
   100x = 750;
   x = 7.5 mL
2. 5 mL/1 tsp = 7.5 mL/x tsp;
   5x = 7.5;
   x = 1½ tsp

ANSWERS TO
CRITICAL THINKING EXERCISE 14-3

5 µg/1 mL = 2.5 µg/x mL;
5x = 2.5;
x = 0.5 mL

ANSWERS TO
CRITICAL THINKING EXERCISE 14-4

1. 2 g/5 mL = 1.4 g/x mL;
   2x = 7;
   x = 3.5 mL
2. 50 mL + 3.5 mL = 53.5 mL total fluid. Because you want to set the pump to deliver an hourly rate, you should do the following:
   53.5 mL/30 min = x mL/60 min;
   30x = 3210;
   x = 107 mL/hr
   _or_
   53.5 mL/0.5 hr = x mL/1 hr;
   0.5x = 53.5;
   x = 107 mL/hr

- Education of the child and parent is important to ensure that medications are administered to achieve therapeutic effects and avoid dangerous side effects.

REFERENCES AND READINGS

American Academy of Pediatrics. (2003). Prevention of medication errors in the pediatric inpatient setting. *Pediatrics, 112*, 431-436.

American Academy of Pediatrics Committee on Infectious Diseases. (2003). *2003 Red book: Report of the Committee on Infectious Diseases* (26th ed., pp. 17-33). Elk Grove Village, IL: American Academy of Pediatrics.

Bartlett, S., Lukk, P., Butz, A., Lampros-Klein, F., & Rand, C. (2002). Enhancing medication adherence among inner-city children with asthma: Results from pilot studies. *Journal of Asthma, 39*, 47-54.

Brunetti, M., & Cohen, J. (2005). Hematology. In J. Robertson & N. Shilkofski (Eds.). *The Johns Hopkins Hospital: The Harriet Lane handbook* (17th ed., pp. 335-361). St. Louis: Elsevier Mosby.

Caffrey, R. (2003). Diabetes under control. Are all syringes created equal? *American Journal of Nursing, 103*, 46-49.

Camara, D. (2001). Minimizing risks associated with peripherally inserted central catheters in the NICU. *MCN: The American Journal of Maternal/Child Nursing, 26*, 17-22.

Ellis, J., Sharp, D., Newhook, K., & Cohen, J. (2004). Selling comfort: a survey of interventions for needle procedures in a pediatric hospital. *Pain Management Nursing, 5*, 144-152.

Fortescue, E. B., Kaushal, R., Landrigan, C. P., McKenna, K. J., Clapp, M. D., Federico, F., Goldmann, D. A., & Bates, D. W. (2003). Prioritizing strategies for preventing medication errors and adverse drug events in pediatric inpatients. *Pediatrics, 111*, 722-730.

Hadaway, L. (2005). Giving medication by retrograde infusion. *Nursing 2005, 35*, 28.

Hodgson, B., & Kizior, R. (2004). *Saunders nursing drug handbook 2004*. Philadelphia: WB Saunders.

Hughes, R., & Edgerton, E. (2005). First, do no harm: reducing pediatric medication errors. *American Journal of Nursing, 105*, 79-84.

Klein, T. (2001). PICCs and midlines: Fine-tuning your care. *RN, 64*, 26-29.

McCloskey, D. (2002). Catheter-related thrombosis in pediatrics. *Pediatric Nursing, 28*, 97-106.

Medical Economics Data Production Co. (1999). *Physicians' desk reference* (53rd ed.). Montvale, NJ: Medical Economics.

Migdal, M., Chudzynska-Pomianowska, E., Vause, E., Henry, E., & Lazar, J. (2005). Rapid, needle-free delivery of lidocaine for reducing the pain of venipuncture among pediatric subjects. *Pediatrics, 115*, e393-e398.

Paparella, S. (2005). Transdermal patches: An unseen risk for harm. *Journal of Emergency Nursing, 31*, 278-281.

Pena, B., & Krauss, B. (2000). Pediatric sedation: Seeing patients safely through. *Contemporary Pediatrics, 17*, 42-52.

Reed, M., & Gal, P. (2004). Principles of drug therapy. In R. Behrman, R. Kliegman, & H. Jenson. (Eds.), *Nelson textbook of pediatrics* (17th ed., pp. 2427-2432). Philadelphia: WB Saunders.

Staples, B., & Bravender, T. (2002). Drug compliance in adolescents: Assessing and managing modifiable risk factors. *Pediatric Drugs, 4*, 503-513.

Strauss, R. (2004). Risks of blood component transfusion. In R. Behrman, R. Kliegman, & H. Jenson (Eds.). *Nelson textbook of pediatrics* (17th ed., pp. 1646-1650). Philadelphia: WB Saunders.

Walsh, K., Kaushal, R., & Chessare, J. (2005). How to avoid paediatric medication errors: A user's guide to the literature. *Archives of Diseases in Childhood, 90*, 698-702.

Winnick, S., Lucas, D., Hartman, A., & Toll, D. (2005). How do you improve compliance? *Pediatrics, 115*, 718-724.

CHAPTER 15

Pain Management for Children

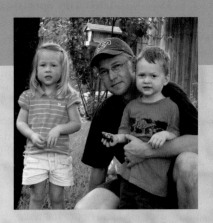

Learning Objectives

After studying this chapter, you should be able to:
- Define pain.
- Discuss the gate-control theory of pain.
- Discuss the myths and realities of pain and pain management.
- Discriminate between acute and chronic pain.
- Explain pain assessment in children according to developmental stages.

- Describe common pain assessment tools.
- Discuss nonpharmacologic and pharmacologic interventions that may be used for pediatric pain management
- Use the nursing process to describe nursing care of the child in pain.

Definitions

addiction A psychologic and neurobiologic state of need for and compulsive use of legal and illegal drugs.

adjuvant A pharmacologic or nonpharmacologic intervention with additive effects on pain management; designed to assist the primary pain management intervention.

epidural Situated within the spinal canal, on or outside the dura mater; synonyms are extradural and peridural.

neuropathic pain Pain resulting from trauma or malfunction in the peripheral or central nervous system.

nociceptive Impulse from a specific body area that gives rise to the sensation of pain.

opioid Natural and synthetic opium derivatives used for analgesia.

pain "An unpleasant sensory and emotional experience associated with actual or potential tissue damage or described in terms of such damage" (International Association for the Study of Pain, 1979).

pain threshold Level of intensity at which pain becomes appreciable or perceptible.

Electronic Resources

Additional information related to the content in Chapter 15 can be found on:

the interactive companion CD-ROM
- Audio Glossary
- NCLEX Review Questions
- Skill: Managing Pain

or the companion website at *evolve*
http://evolve.elsevier.com/james/ncoc
- NCLEX Review Questions
- Resources for Health Care Providers and Families
- WebLinks

Assessing and treating pain in children can be difficult. Infants and children are often unable or unwilling to communicate the presence, location, type, or intensity of pain. Parents may be reluctant to acknowledge or help validate their child's pain. They may also be hesitant to allow suitable pain management because of fears related to side effects from the use of opioids, including inaccurate fears regarding addiction. Additionally, some physicians and nurses continue to have inappropriate and outdated beliefs regarding pain and pain

management in infants and children. The American Academy of Pediatrics and the American Pain Society addressed the need for appropriate pain management in children in their joint statement presented in 2001. They noted that, despite comprehensive research, anecdotal experience, and ample knowledge from the past 10 to 15 years, the assessment and treatment of pain in children frequently remain inadequate (American Academy of Pediatrics [AAP], 2001). This remains true, even in the years since the statement was published. Despite the increasing knowledge regarding safe and effective pain management in children, as well as widespread anecdotal experience, this information has not been generally or effectively applied to routine clinical practice. It is well documented that the youngest children have the greatest probability of receiving insufficient pain medications, that pain medication administration varies by age and is underused for many children. It is also evident that overall pain medication administration for children lags behind that for adult patients (Pasero & McCaffery, 2005; Zempsky et al., 2004).

Increased and improved research in pediatric pain has led to more precise and improved pain assessment and better prescribing and administering of analgesics. The most current resources and strategies for pain management, however, are not always implemented, emphasizing the continuing need for educating all health providers. Nurses, having frequent interaction with physicians and other health care workers, can facilitate a significant improvement in the pain management for infants and children. They can also play a vital role in providing education to other health care personnel as well as parents and children with regard to appropriate pain management.

Individual nurses vary in their ability to assess pain. Some of these differences have been linked to lack of or inaccurate clinical knowledge regarding pain, lack of nursing experience, personal experiences with pain, personal assessment style, and practice setting (Franck, Greenberg, & Stevens, 2000). In addition, the behaviors of many health care professionals, including nurses, do not always correspond with the attitudes and beliefs they report concerning pain assessment and management (Simons & Roberson, 2002).

DEFINITIONS AND THEORIES OF PAIN

There are many definitions of pain. In a commonly accepted definition, pain is whatever the person experiencing the pain says it is, existing whenever the person says it does (McCaffery & Pasero, 1999). The International Association for the Study of Pain (1979, p. 249) defines pain as "an unpleasant sensory and emotional experience associated with actual or potential tissue damage, or described in terms of such damage." Both definitions underscore the fact that pain is complex, multidimensional, subjective, and personal.

Gate-Control Theory

Pain impulses travel between the initial site of injury and the brain, and certain mechanisms affect pain intensity. According to the gate-control theory, proposed by Melzack and Wall in 1965, a gating mechanism at the level of the dorsal horn in the spinal cord can facilitate or dampen the transmission of pain signals. Stimulation of the larger afferent nerves, which carry benign sensations, can blunt the transmission of pain signals. The gating mechanisms are influenced by the relative activity in the sensory fibers. Input from the large fibers closes the gate, whereas input from the small fibers opens it. For example, rubbing an injured part activates large-fiber activity, which decreases the ability of small-fiber activity to open the gate, thus decreasing the pain. The theory further

postulates that cognitive processes, such as attention, emotion, and memory, influence the gating mechanism and have an impact on the transmission of pain. The gate-control theory lends support for the use of both physiologic and psychologic interventions in pain management.

Acute and Chronic Pain

Children may have acute and chronic pain. Nursing assessment and the result of interventions will vary on the basis of the nature of the pain, acute or chronic. Acute pain usually has a sudden onset, is from an identifiable trauma, and continues for a limited time. Resolution generally occurs with healing of the trauma. Frequently, the acute pain experienced by children in the health care setting is procedural pain resulting from invasive procedures. This is particularly evident for children with cancer and other chronic illnesses that require frequent medical care. Acute pain is experienced with acute disease states, during and after invasive procedures, as well as after surgery, and trauma. Trauma can be physical, as with a motor vehicle collision or with purposeful inflicted injury (child abuse). Trauma can also be chemical as with tissue damage from the infiltration of a medication being given intravenously. Events that cause acute pain may persist, leading to the development of chronic pain.

Chronic pain continues for an unpredictable period beyond the expected recovery period, is unlikely to resolve quickly, and usually affects the child's ability to live a normal life. Children with conditions such as juvenile arthritis, sickle cell disease, and cancer have chronic pain. Improvements in pain management have enabled children with pain related to a chronic condition to live more comfortably, spending less time in the acute-care setting. They are also able to live their lives more normally in relation to school, play, and other activities of childhood (see Chapter 12). Nurses who work in the school, home health care, and hospice settings have added resources (e.g., knowledge, medication, equipment) to assist in the facilitation of more comfortable, normal lives for these children.

Nevertheless, Howard (2003) notes that chronic pain is much more prevalent that previously realized. This includes neuropathic pain, which is among the most difficult types of pain to treat. Accurate assessment and successful treatment of chronic pain is very difficult. It remains a significant, unsolved challenge in pediatric pain management, leading to concerns regarding the long-term functional consequences of chronic childhood pain.

RESEARCH ON PAIN IN CHILDREN

The past two decades have seen a tremendous increase in pediatric pain-related research, with information on acute and chronic pain being widely accessible in chapters of major texts and in entire texts devoted to pain. Articles appear frequently in various health care journals. There are also journals that focus exclusively on pain and pediatric pain. However, research on pain in neonates and infants is still limited.

In 1989 the Agency for Health Care Policy and Research, now renamed the Agency for Healthcare Research and Quality, was created to focus on the development of scientifically based practice guidelines for selected problems. Pain was a targeted area. The development of guidelines for the care of children with pain was based on retrieval and review of articles related to postoperative, procedural, and trauma pain. The research studies tested pain assessment tools and pharmacologic and nonpharmacologic pain relief. Other studies included the description of pain in children, the development of pain assessment tools, and other issues related to pain in children. This work produced a document titled *Acute Pain Management Guidelines in Infants, Children, and Adolescents: Operative and Medical Procedures* (Agency for Health Care Policy and Research, 1992a). This guide remains the starting reference point for pediatric pain management, for dosing and for choice of analgesics.

Other bodies of research and development have yielded additional standards of care for both acute and chronic pain. These include numerous publications from the World Health Organization, the American Pain Society (APS) (see Evolve website), the AAP, and the International Association for the Study of Pain. The World Health Organization three-step analgesic ladder was developed in the early 1980s to improve treatment for cancer pain. These guidelines are a basis of care for children and adults, particularly for the use of multidrug therapy. In 1999 the APS developed guidelines for acute pain, cancer pain, juvenile arthritis pain, and the acute and chronic pain associated with sickle-cell disease. In cooperation with the AAP, the APS issued recommendations for the assessment and management of acute pain in infants, children, and adolescents (AAP & APS, 2001). In addition, the Joint Commission on Accreditation of Healthcare Organizations added new standards that integrate pain assessment and management into their accreditation standards. The 2001 standards provide pain management education and guarantee all hospitalized patients the right to developmentally appropriate, comprehensive assessment and management of pain from admission until discharge (Joint Commission on Accreditation of Healthcare Organizations, 2001).

Academic literature, research, and standards of care regarding pediatric pain management have increased significantly. Despite these advances in research, knowledge, and clinical expertise, improvements in pediatric pain management are still required. Needs include research on nurse-physician collaboration for pediatric pain management, barriers to suitable pain management, continued education of health care providers about appropriate, effective pain management, increased information about pain management in neonates and infants, and, as new analgesics are introduced, their safety and efficacy for children should be tested, rather than depending on anecdotal experience to guide usage in the pediatric population.

One major area of specific concern is pain management for premature infants, neonates, and very young infants, particularly with regard to painful procedures (Halimaa, 2003; Lyon, 2005). Research is beginning, but much remains to be examined. Howard (2003) notes studies have discovered that pain experiences in early life may have long-term consequences. He cites evidence that there may be long-term behavioral changes that extend far beyond what is considered the normal recovery after the painful event. Important determinants of the long-term outcomes of infant pain

include timing, degree of injury, and the analgesic used. There are also concerns for older children in relation to their memories of painful experiences. Von Baeyer and colleagues (2004) note that the long-term consequences may include the child's' later reaction to painful events and acceptance of later health care interventions. In regard to use of adjuvants for infant pain management, beginning studies examining the use of oral sucrose with and without nonnutritive sucking of pacifiers are yielding exciting, positive results (Stevens et al., 2005; Thompson, 2005).

OBSTACLES TO PAIN MANAGEMENT IN CHILDREN

Obstacles to appropriate pain management in children include knowledge deficits, lack of confidence regarding pain management, accurate pain assessment, awareness of the adequacy of pain management interventions, lack of communication with patients and parents, and personal attitudes and beliefs about pain (Manworren, 2001; Simons & Roberson, 2002; Von Hulle & Denyes, 2004; Wang et al., 2003; Zisk, 2003). Nurses may also have the problem of working with a lack of knowledge concerning pain management on the part of parents and children. The two beliefs from parents and nurses that are most likely to interfere with the provision of adequate pain relief in infants and children are fear of addiction and fear of respiratory depression. Table 15-1 lists and refutes other prevalent myths about pain and pain management in children.

One strategy used by pediatric institutions to provide pain management education is a pain management team. The team may be composed of advanced practice nurses (APNs) as well as physicians. The team educates patients, families, nurses, physicians, and other health care disciplines. They also offer pain management recommendations to the health care team. The APNs maintain their expertise in pain management and thus can offer information and recommendations for pain management on the basis of the most current knowledge. Such personalization of education may provide the motivation for changes in beliefs and attitudes among staff as well as patients and families. The APNs can personalize pain education for the specific learning needs of staff. They can also reinforce education as frequently as is mandated or needed by health care team members.

Once nurses have overcome knowledge deficits and other barriers, for many there remains the problem of confidence regarding pain management. Despite knowledge regarding appropriate analgesic doses and accurate concerns as to side effects, many nurses still require day-to-day assistance in gaining autonomy in pain management. One solution seen at some medical centers is the use of pain resource nurses (PRNs). McCleary, Ellis, and Rowley (2004) detail the role of the PRNs in their 2004 study. PRNs are nurses for each unit who act as pain management coaches or mentors for their colleagues through provision of continuing support for best practice in pain management. Support is provided to nurses and other members of the multidisciplinary team. PRNs can be an important role in a comprehensive pain management program. They can provide invaluable assistance to the pain team by assuming a day-to-day support role for each unit.

| TABLE 15-1 | Pain and Pain Management in Children: Myths and Realities |

Myth	Reality
Neonates do not feel pain because of incomplete myelinization in peripheral nerves and CNS.	Myelinization is not necessary for pain perception. Central and peripheral structures required for nociception are present and functional early in gestation. Therefore infants have the neurological capacity for pain perception at the time of birth, even those born prematurely.[1]
Children have no memory of pain.	Feeding and sleeping differences have been reported in studies of infants who experienced pain, which suggests that the procedure had consequences extending beyond the event.[2]
There is a correct or given amount of pain for a specific injury or procedure-induced pain.	The amount of pain a child experiences varies and cannot be predicted because of cognitive, developmental, and emotional factors affecting the child.[3]
Children can easily become addicted to narcotic analgesics.	There is no identified characteristic of childhood physiology or development that indicates any increased risk of physiologic or psychologic dependence. The actual risk of addiction is very low.[4,5]
Narcotic administration can easily cause respiratory depression.	No data support the belief that children are at higher risk for respiratory depression than adults.[6] Respiratory depression is rare.[7]

[1]Franck, L. S., Greenberg, C. S., & Stevens, B. (2000). Pain assessment in infants and children. *Pediatric Clinics of North America, 47*, 487-512.
[2]Schechter, N. L. (1988). An approach to the child with pain. *Patient Care, 3*, 116-131.
[3]Chen, E., Joseph, M. H., & Zeltzer, L. K. (2000). Behavioral and cognitive interventions in the treatment of pain in children. *Pediatric Clinics of North America, 47*, 513-525.
[4]Agency for Health Care Policy and Research, Acute Pain Management Guideline Panel. (1992b). *Acute pain management: Operative or medical procedures and trauma. Clinical practice guideline* (AHCPR Publication No. 92-0032). Rockville, MD: Public Health Service, U.S. Department of Health and Human Services.
[5]Zeltzer, L., Bush, J., Chen, E., & Riveral, A. (1997). A psychobiologic approach to pediatric pain. Part II. Prevention and treatment. *Current Problems in Pediatrics, 27*, 264-284.
[6]Eland, J. (1990). Pain in children. *Nursing Clinics of North America, 25*, 871-884.
[7]Golianu, B., Krane, E. J., Galloway, K. S., & Yaster, M. (2000). Pediatric acute pain management. *Pediatric Clinics of North America, 47*, 559-587.

This allows the pain team nurse(s) more time to evaluate patients and provide recommendations for pain management.

Recognizing the necessity for and implementing appropriate pain management are accompanied by the continuing need to have access to the most current information. The World Wide Web or Internet can be a powerful tool for instant, up-to-date information. Nurses and families are cautioned to ensure that they obtain information from appropriate websites. Box 15-1 lists some suggested Internet resources. Given the rapidity with which Internet information changes, it is always prudent to ensure the appropriateness of the website and the accuracy of the information presented.

| BOX 15-1 | Pain Management Resources From the World Wide Web |

American Pain Society:
   www.ampainsoc.org
American Society for Pain Management Nursing:
   www.aspmm.org
National Institutes of Health Pain Consortium:
   www.painconsortium.nih.gov
National Foundation for the Treatment of Pain:
   www.paincare.org
Pain Foundation:
   www.painfoundation.org

ASSESSMENT OF PAIN IN CHILDREN

Pain in children is multidimensional and subjective (AAP, 2001; Bishop-Kurylo, 2002). It is affected by the type and duration of pain, developmental level, emotional status, previous pain experiences, culture and ethnicity, personality type, sex, genetic variations, and parental response to the child's pain. These factors should all be taken into consideration when assessing an infant or child in pain. Consequently, assessing pain in infants and children is more challenging than in adults. Infants and young children may not have the language or cognitive abilities to communicate their pain. Their crying and verbal responses occur for many other reasons including hunger, sleepiness, and anxiety. Accordingly, the nurse must use a combination of behavioral and physiologic signs together with an appropriate pain assessment tool to assess pain in infants and children (Spagrud, Piira, & Von Baeyer, 2003) (Box 15-2).

The role of vital signs in pain assessment is discussed below. However, there are changing views as to the accuracy and role of vital signs pain assessment. Some believe that there is actually very little evidence to support the use of vital signs to assess pain (Foster, Yucha, Zuk, & Vojir, 2003). Behavioral and physiologic signs can play an important role in instances where a child is giving a verbal report of pain that is different from nonverbal behaviors. An example might be a child who gives a verbal report of little or no pain out of concern that someone will be angry or that pain medication

| BOX 15-2 | **Pain Assessment According to Developmental Levels** |

Neonate and Infant
- Usually demonstrates changes in facial expression, including frowns, grimaces, wrinkled brow, expression of surprise, and facial flinching
- May demonstrate increases in blood pressure and heart rate and decrease in arterial saturation
- High-pitched, tense, harsh crying
- The neonate and young infant usually demonstrate a generalized or total body response that becomes more purposeful as the infant matures
- May thrash extremities; may exhibit tremors
- Older infants may localize the pain, rubbing the painful area or pull away, or guard the involved part

Toddler
- Likely to demonstrate loud crying
- Able to verbalizes words that indicate discomfort such as "ouch," "hurt," "boo-boo"
- May attempt to delay procedures perceived as painful
- May demonstrate generalized restlessness
- May guard the site
- May touch painful areas
- May run from the nurse

Preschooler
- May think the pain is punishment for something they have said or done
- Likely to cry and struggle

Preschooler—cont'd
- Able to describe the location and intensity of pain (e.g., "ear hurts bad")
- May demonstrate regression to earlier behaviors, such as loss of bladder and bowel control
- May demonstrate withdrawal
- May deny pain to avoid a possible injection
- May have been told to "be brave" and deny pain, even though it is present

School-Age Child
- Able to describe pain and quantify pain intensity
- Fears bodily injury
- Has an awareness of death
- May demonstrate stiff body posture
- May demonstrate withdrawal
- May procrastinate or bargain to delay procedure

Adolescent
- Perceives pain at a physical, emotional, and cognitive levels
- Understands cause and effect
- Able to describe pain and quantify pain intensity
- May have increased muscle tension
- May demonstrate withdrawal and decreased motor activity
- May use words such as "sore," "ache," or "pounding" to describe pain

might involve an injection. Visually, the nurse might see the child grimacing, perhaps with tears, laying rigidly in bed and not moving. Such nonverbal behaviors would lead the nurse to speak and interact gently with the child about level of pain to ensure appropriate pain management.

Although older children may be able to verbalize their discomfort, they are often afraid of treatment that includes a painful procedure such as an injection. They may have also been told to "be brave" and not verbalize or demonstrate the pain they are experiencing. Increasingly, it is also seen that even children as young as 5 or 6 years may be fearful of taking pain medication because of the emphasis on "saying no" to drugs. Such an emphasis is meant to focus on illegal substances or inappropriate use of prescription medications. Despite this fact, some children translate this to mean they must shy away from using even appropriate and necessary pain medications. The nurse can depend on the current bank of literature, research, and standards of care in providing the necessary education to parents and children to overcome such barriers to appropriate pain assessment and management.

Pain assessment is increasingly affected by the multicultural diversity of the pediatric population. Working to understand the impact of cultural differences on pain management is a crucial aspect of pediatric nursing care. Increasingly, studies and references detail pain management in different cultures (Gharaibeh & Abu-Saad, 2002; Jasaithong,

2002; Luffy & Grove, 2003; McCarthy, Chammas, Wilimas, Alaoui, & Harif, 2004; Wang et al., 2003). Such references can assist in understanding the diversity in words used for pain, descriptions of pain, and scaling of pain noted among different cultures. Studies detailing the validity of pain scales for different cultures are also discussed. The nurse is also encouraged to review the most current edition of a nursing text that deals with transcultural nursing care.

Assessment According to Developmental Level

Neonates and Infants

Neonates and young infants have immature central nervous systems lacking myelinization of pain fibers, therefore, clinicians believed these children to be incapable of perceiving pain. Research has challenged this assumption and demonstrated that neonates and infants do indeed feel pain (Bishop-Kurylo, 2002; McCaffery & Pasero, 1999; Stevens, Gibbins, & Franck, 2000). In addition, Franck, Greenberg, and Stevens (2000) note that research supports that the nociceptive processes between infants and adults differ in that in infants the primary transmission of pain impulses is along nonmyelinated C fibers, there is less precise pain signal transmission in the spinal cord, and there is a lack of descending inhibitory transmitters. For this reason, infants may actually have a lower pain threshold and perceive pain more intensely than adults or older children, as a result of the immature descending control mechanisms, which would thus limit their ability to modulate the pain experience.

Pain assessment for the neonate and infant is based on behavioral and physiological indicators. Behavioral indicators of infant pain are more easily assessed. These are detailed by multiple resources (Anand & Hickey, 1987; Craig, 1998; Franck et al., 2000; Grunau, Johnston, & Craig, 1990; McCaffery & Pasero, 1999) who note that such indicators include rapid changes of behavioral state, changes in sleep patterns, crying, fist clenching, grimacing, wrinkling of forehead, fussiness, and restlessness. Facial expression is considered the most reliable indicator of pain throughout populations of infants and children. Facial expression, in combination with short latency to onset of cry and a long duration of the first cry cycle, typifies infants' reactions to acute invasive procedures. Cries associated with pain may sound different from those associated with hunger, discomfort, and stress; these cries are higher pitched, tense, and harsh. Parents and nurses may therefore be able to differentiate between the usual cries of infants and the cries of pain.

Motor movements associated with pain in the neonate and infant progress from a generalized body response to more purposeful movements. For example, infants ages 9 to 12 months can use their hands to push the nurse away if they perceive a painful action about to begin. The responses of neonates to painful stimuli are sometimes described as total body responses (Fig. 15-1). The infant's extremities may thrash about, and some infants exhibit tremors. Older infants may rub the painful area, pull away, or guard the involved body part.

Franck, Greenberg, and Stevens (2000) note that an infant's behavioral state immediately before painful stimulation, such as sleep state, affects the vigorousness of the response. In addition, the responses of preterm infants are less vigorous than those of term infants, although they may be experiencing heightened experience of pain (Pasero, 2004).

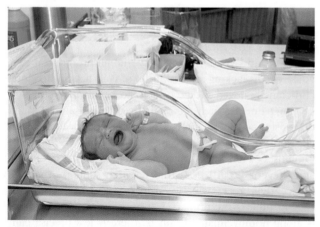

FIG 15-1 Neonates and infants have a total-body response to pain. Parents can frequently distinguish the infant's cry of pain from other cries because it is tense, high-pitched, and harsh sounding.

The nurse must be cognizant of this information to make a beginning assessment of pain through observation of an infant's facial expressions, motor response, and cry.

Physiologic changes may be more difficult to assess. Increases in blood pressure, heart rate, and respiratory rate and decreases in arterial oxygen saturation have been associated with pain in neonates, although these changes can be linked to other alterations in the infant's body, such as agitation. Crying may also affect the infant's physiologic response. Rawlings, Miller, and Engel (1980) reported that oxygenation will decrease in response to pain but may increase after vigorous crying; accordingly, such data can be confusing. Distinguishing between pain and agitation is sometimes difficult. If an infant is simply agitated, yet is treated for pain, the cause of the agitation will be untreated, the intervention is inappropriate, and the agitation will likely increase. The nurse should realize that physiologic changes are just one part of the assessment of pain in the neonate and infant and should suspect that an infant is in pain before physiologic changes occur. The behavioral and physiologic indicators discussed are components in several different assessment tools used for the preverbal or nonverbal child. Increasing research and anecdotal experiences have provided data to support the reliability and validity of such assessment tools. Accordingly, the nurse should implement use of these tools, as opposed to a personal, subjective assessment using only the behavioral and physiologic indicators.

CRITICAL THINKING EXERCISE 15-1

You are about to assume care for a 3500-gram term female neonate who is 24 hours postoperative for a fundoplication and placement of a gastrostomy device. You receive report from the nurse who has been taking care of the child for the previous shift. The nurse states that the infant has slept for short periods throughout the shift, sucks vigorously on her pacifier, and occasionally cries. She also states that she has not medicated the infant for pain because the infant does have periods when she sleeps for 15 to 30 minutes. Her blood pressure is 98/74 mm Hg, pulse 170 beats/min, and respirations 50/min.

1. What would be your priority nursing action?
2. What principles related to pediatric pain control would apply to this infant?

Toddlers

The toddler in pain tends to cry longer than the infant does. As verbal abilities become more advanced, the toddler can verbally express displeasure when a painful experience occurs. The toddler asks for parents, verbalizes words that indicate discomfort ("ouch," "hurt") and may verbalize negative emotions about the nurse. The toddler may also try to delay the nurse's implementation of a procedure judged as painful. The older toddler can often localize the pain and point to the body part that hurts.

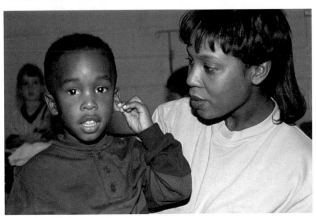

FIG 15-2 Toddlers and preschoolers may express pain by guarding or touching the painful area. Pulling on the ear is a characteristic expression of ear pain that accompanies otitis media. *(Courtesy University of Texas at Arlington School of Nursing.)*

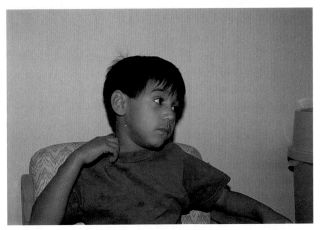

FIG 15-3 School-age children may withdraw and become very quiet when they are ill or in pain. Note how dull this boy appears. Although he has asthma, his mother knew something else was wrong because he was unusually quiet and withdrawn. *(Courtesy Parkland Health and Hospital System Community Oriented Primary Care Clinic, Dallas, TX.)*

Generalized restlessness, guarding the site, and touching the painful area are signs of pain in the toddler (Fig. 15-2). The toddler may associate discomfort with a particular procedure, such as a dressing change, and may run from the nurse when approached. The toddler's face may show anger and fear. The child may avoid eye contact or look sad. In response to discomfort and pain, the toddler may also demonstrate regression to earlier, more comfortable behaviors.

Preschoolers

Preschoolers are egocentric. Relating only to the present, they cannot associate discomfort with any positive outcome. For example, the preschooler will not understand that debriding a painful burn will ultimately have a positive effect. Not understanding the positive outcome of a painful procedure may cause a child in this age group to find pain more disorienting and be more profoundly affected than an older child (Schechter, 1988).

Preschoolers tend to think pain will magically go away and that they are being punished for some previous thought or deed. They also fear body mutilation, particularly the genitals. Preschoolers may deny pain to avoid an invasive, painful procedure. The preschooler may cry and struggle to avoid the procedure. Preschoolers may also regress to earlier, more comfortable behaviors as a response to pain or may withdraw and not participate in activities on the unit. However, the child can describe the location and intensity of pain.

School-Age Children

School-age children can describe pain and relate it to a body part as well as quantify the pain intensity. They are beginning to understand the need for painful procedures. They fear body harm and have an awareness of death. Therefore, they may appear to overreact to illness or injury. As in all age groups, the school-age child remembers previous pain experiences, which will affect the child's response. The child's culture, sex, and cognitive abilities will also affect the pain experience.

Nonverbal cues are very important in school-age children. The child may exhibit a stiff body posture, may withdraw, or may be found quietly sobbing (Fig. 15-3). If the school-age child resists a treatment, cries loudly, or otherwise acts in an aggressive manner, the child may later deny the behavior. School-age children may also attempt to procrastinate or bargain to delay a painful procedure. As with younger children, the school-age child may demonstrate regressive behaviors when experiencing pain.

Adolescents

Adolescents can think abstractly and understand cause and effect. They can describe and quantify pain intensity and their feelings about pain. They can also discuss the strategies that help manage their pain. They are able to perceive and understand pain at a physical, emotional, and mental level. Having these abilities does not mean the adolescent will exercise them. Adolescents are often confused by control issues and are uncertain of their role as they move from childhood to adulthood. Regression may also occur at this age in relation to pain.

Because adolescents are egocentric, they tend to think that others also focus on their behavior and so may suppress manifestations of pain. In addition, they may not report pain because they believe that the nurse is aware of when they hurt so they expect that they will receive the medication when they need it. Adolescents tend to exhibit fewer outward signs of pain than young children do. Signs observed in the adolescent include increased muscle tension, withdrawal, and decreased motor activity. Hospitalized adolescents use words such as "sore," "like an ache," "pounding," and "miserable" to describe pain. They complete the statement, "When I have pain, I most often feel . . . " with "sick to my stomach," "scared," "angry," "like crying, but I don't," "like hitting someone," and "like screaming" (Savedra, Tesler, & Wegner, 1988).

CRITICAL TO REMEMBER
Assessing Pain in Children

- The consistent use of an age and developmentally appropriate pain assessment tool is crucial for assessment of a child's pain. It is also necessary for the evaluation of pain management interventions. The tool is part of the child's chart.
- If the child is unable to express or quantify pain, use an appropriate tool designed for preverbal or nonverbal children. Also, include parents as a resource to assess the child's pain and response to interventions.
- Behavioral and physiologic changes may or may not be present for a child of any age. They are only one source of information and should not be relied on before intervention. Other states such as anxiety and fear may cause physiologic and behavioral changes.*
- Physiologic changes are only one source of information when pain is assessed in the neonate or infant and it should not be relied on before intervention. Other states, such as fear and anxiety, may also cause physiologic changes. Because physiologic changes tend to occur during the acute period and then return to normal, they may not be valid indicators of chronic pain.

*Children's Hospital, Boston. (2002). *Reference tool: Pain assessment tools.* Boston: Children's Hospital.

Assessment Tools

Consistent, appropriate use of a pain assessment tool is essential to pediatric pain management. A number of valid and reliable pain assessment tools are available to help the nurse make a more accurate pain assessment. Both self-report and behavioral instruments are available. Examples of these tools are detailed in Table 15-2. Children benefit when a pain assessment tool is used because they are given a simple and effective way to communicate the pain they are experiencing. Assessment tools provide more objective data, reducing the chance that more discreet signs of pain will be overlooked. Unfortunately, they are not always used consistently and appropriately in the clinical setting. Using a tool in a way other than the developer intended may invalidate the pain assessment.

An assessment tool should be selected according to the child's age and developmental abilities. The crucial factors concerning a pain assessment tool are that it is appropriate for the child's age and that an effective plan can be made using the information gathered from the assessment. Varieties of tools are available for infants and the preverbal or nonverbal child, such as those who are neurologically unresponsive, developmentally delayed, or unable to speak because of medical treatment such as intubation. Tools for infants and preverbal children usually are based on behavioral cues (e.g., facial expression, motor responses, intensity of cry). One such tool, the FLACC Scale, has been examined numerous times for reliability and validity. It has been shown to be an appropriate, effective tool for the preverbal and or nonverbal child (Manworren & Hynan, 2003; Merkel,

S., Voepel-Lewis, T., & Malviya, S., 2002; Voepel-Lewis, Merkel, Tait, Trzcinka, & Malviya, 2002; Willis, Merkel, Voepel-Lewis, Malviya, 2003). Accordingly, the tool is used with increasing frequency.

Children verbalize words for pain by approximately 18 months of age, and cognitive development is sufficient for reporting the extent of pain by 3 to 4 years of age. Self-report tools are effective in children older than 3 years. The Oucher, the Poker Chip Tool, and the FACES Scale are examples of tools for preschoolers and school-age children. For some children, the African American or Hispanic versions of the Oucher pain scale provide more culturally sensitive assessment (Fig. 15-4). The Wong-Baker FACES scale has been translated into 10 different languages. Matching the tool to the child's race and ethnicity can provide better information about pain experienced by children from nonwhite populations and so promote better pain control for these children (Beyer & Knott, 1998).

School-age children can understand concepts of order and number and can use numeric rating scales, horizontal word-graphic rating scales, and visual analog scales. Table 15-2 describes pain assessment tools and lists the appropriate age or developmental level for each tool (Figs. 15-5 and 15-6). The same tool should be used each time the child is assessed to obtain consistent data and to avoid confusing the child. Ideally, the child should be taught how to use the tool before pain is experienced (e.g., preoperatively). Obviously, in emergencies, such preparation will not be possible.

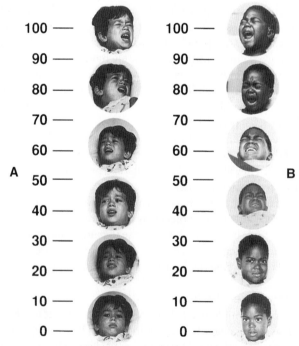

FIG 15-4   **A, The Hispanic (Latino) version of the Oucher pain scale. B, The African American version.** (*A, Developed and copyrighted by Antonia M. Villarruel, RN, PhD, & Mary J. Denyes, RN, PhD, 1991. B, Developed and copyrighted by Mary J. Denyes, PhD, RN, FAAN [Wayne State University], and Antonia Villarruel, PhD, RN, FAAN [University of Pennsylvania] at the Children's Hospital of Michigan in 1990. Cornelia P. Porter, PhD, RN, and Charlotta Marshall, MSN, RN, contributed to the development of this scale.*)

TABLE 15-2   Pain Assessment Tools

Tool	Description	Age
Adolescent and Pediatric Pain Tool: APPT[1,2]	Three-part tool composed of a body outline, an intensity scale, and a pain descriptor word list (see Fig. 15-6)	8-17 yr
CRIES Pain Scale[3]	Five behavioral categories—**C**rying, **R**equires O2 for SAO2 <95%, **I**ncreased vitals signs, **E**xpression, **S**leepless—each scored from 0-2, resulting in a total score of 0-10. A higher score indicates higher pain or distress.	Neonates (0-6 months)
COMFORT Scale[4]	Nine behavioral categories—Alertness, Calmness, Crying, Physical Movement, Muscle Tone, Facial Tension, Blood Pressure, Heart Rate—each category is scored from 1-5, resulting in a total score from 9-45. A higher score indicates higher pain or distress.	Infants and children in a critical care or operative setting who are unable to use the Numeric Rating Scale or the Wong-Baker Faces Pain Rating Scale
FLACC[5]	Five behavioral categories—**F**ace, **L**egs, **A**ctivity, **C**ry, **C**onsolability—each scored from 0 to 2, resulting in a total score of 0 to 10. A higher score indicates higher pain or distress.	Infants and preverbal or nonverbal children.
FACES Pain Rating Scale[6]	Six cartoon faces with a number under each, ranging from a happy face (0 or No Hurt) to a crying face (5 or Hurts Worst) (see Fig. 15-5)	3 yr and older. It may be more helpful if the child is able to understand number order or "greater than." This is usually seen in children of kindergarten or school age.
FACES Pain Scale—Revised[6]	Six faces with neutral to gradually increasing painful expressions, corresponding to an analog scale of 0 to 10	
Numeric Rating Scale (NRS)	Uses numbers (e.g., 0 to 10 or 0 to 100) to indicate increasing pain.	Child must know numbers
The Oucher[7-10]	A poster with two scales: one is numeric, for use by children who can count to 100; the other is a photographic scale to be used by children who cannot count to 100. The bottom picture (or 0) is no pain; the top picture (or 100) is the greatest pain (see Fig. 15-4).	3-12 yr
Poker Chip Tool[11]	Four poker chips are used; each chip represents a piece of hurt. One poker chip represents a little hurt, and four chips represent the most hurt the child could have.	4-12 yr
Visual Analog Scale (VAS)[12]	Usually a 10-cm line with one end representing "no pain" and the opposite end "the worst pain."	Older school-age children and adolescents. May be used by younger school-age children, but less abstract tools are more appropriate.

[1]Savedra, M. C., Tesler, M. D., Holzemer, W. L., & Ward, J. (1992). *Adolescent and pediatric pain tool: User's manual.* San Francisco: University of California, San Francisco, School of Nursing.

[2]Savedra, M. C., Tesler, M. D., Holzemer, W. L., Wilkie, D. J., & Ward, J. (1989). Pain location: Validity and reliability of body outline markings by hospitalized children and adolescents. *Research in Nursing and Health, 12,* 307-314.

[3]Ambuel, H., Marx, C. M., & Blumer, J. L. (1992). Assessing distress in pediatric intensive care environments: The COMFORT scale. *Journal of Pediatric Psychology, 17,* 95-109.

[4]Krechel, S. W., & Bildner, J. (1995). CRIES: A new neonatal postoperative pain measurement score—Initial testing of validity and reliability. *Paediatric Anaesthesia, 5,* 53-61.

[5]Merkel, S., Voepel-Lewis, T., & Malviya, S. (2002). Pain assessment in infants and young children: The FLACC scale: A behavioral tool to measure pain in young children. *American Journal of Nursing, 102,* 55-58.

[6]Wong, D. L., Hockenberry-Eaton, M., Wilson, D., & Winkelstein, M. L. (2005). *Essentials of pediatric nursing* (7th ed.). St. Louis: Mosby.

[7]Beyer, J. (1984). *The Oucher: A user's manual and technical report.* Evanston, IL: Judson Press.

[8]Beyer, J., & Aradine, C. (1986). Content validity of an instrument to measure young children's perceptions of the intensity of their pain. *Journal of Pediatric Nursing, 1,* 386-395.

[9]Beyer, J., Denyes, M., & Villarruel, A. (1992). The creation, validation, and continuing development of the Oucher: A measure of pain intensity in children. *Journal of Pediatric Nursing, 7,* 335-346.

[10]Beyer, J. E., & Knott, C. B. (1998). Construct validity estimation for the African-American and Hispanic versions of the Oucher Scale. *Journal of Pediatric Nursing, 13,* 20-31.

[11]Hester, N. O. (1979). The preoperational child's reaction to immunization. *Nursing Research, 4,* 250-254.

[12]Spagrud, L., Piira, T., & Von Baeyer, C. (2003). Children's self-report of pain intensity. *American Journal of Nursing, 103,* 62-64.

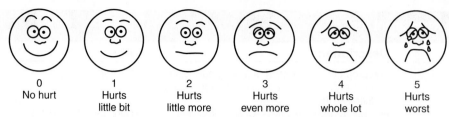

0	1	2	3	4	5
No hurt	Hurts little bit	Hurts little more	Hurts even more	Hurts whole lot	Hurts worst

FIG 15-5 **FACES Pain Rating Scale.** *Instructions:* **Explain to the child that each face is for a person who feels happy because he has no pain (hurt) or sad because he has some or a lot of pain. Face 0 is very happy because he doesn't hurt at all. Face 1 hurts just a little bit. Face 2 hurts a little more. Face 3 hurts even more. Face 4 hurts a whole lot. Face 5 hurts as much as you can imagine, although you don't have to be crying to feel this bad. Ask the child to choose the face that best describes how he is feeling. Recommended for persons age 3 years and older.** *(From Hockenberry, M. J., Wilson, D. [2007]. Wong's nursing care of infants and children [8th ed.]. St. Louis: Mosby.)*

CODE _____

DATE _____

Adolescent and Pediatric Pain Tool (APPT)

INSTRUCTIONS:

1. **Color in the areas on these drawings to show where you have pain. Make the marks as big or small as the place where the pain is.**

Right   Left   Left   Right

2. Place a straight, up and down mark on this line to show how much pain you have.

No pain	Little pain	Medium pain	Large pain	Worst possible pain

3. Point to or circle as many of these words that describe your pain.

1	5	10	15
annoying	blistering	awful	off and on
bad	burning	deadly	once in a while
horrible	hot	dying	sneaks up
miserable	**6**	killing	sometimes
terrible	cramping	**11**	steady
uncomfortable	crushing	crying	
2	like a pinch	frightening	If you like,
aching	pinching	screaming	you may add
hurting	pressure	terrifying	other words:
like an ache	**7**	**12**	
like a hurt	itching	dizzy	_____
sore	like a scratch	sickening	
3	like a sting	suffocating	_____
beating	scratching	**13**	
hitting	stinging	never goes away	_____
pounding	**8**	uncontrollable	
punching	shocking	**14**	For office use only.
throbbing	shooting	always	
4	splitting	comes and goes	
biting	**9**	comes on all of	
cutting	numb	a sudden	
like a pin	stiff	constant	
like a sharp knife	swollen	continuous	
pin like	tight	forever	
sharp			
stabbing			

For office use only.			
BSA: _____			
IS: _____			
#S (2-9) _____ /37= ____ %			
#A (10-12) _____ /11= ____ %			
#E (1,13) _____ /8= ____ %			
#T (14,15) _____ /11= ____ %			
Total _____ /67= ____ %			

FIG 15-6 **Adolescent and Pediatric Pain Tool, appropriate for use with 8- to 17-year-olds.** *(From Savedra, M. C., Tesler, M. D., Holzemer, W. L., & Ward, J. A. [1992]. Adolescent and pediatric pain tool: User's manual. San Francisco: University of California, San Francisco, School of Nursing. Copyright © 1989, 1992. For original tools, write or call 415-476-4040.)*

In assessing pain and obtaining the pain history, the nurse should first question the child to determine which word, or words, is used for pain. Such words must be used consistently in any future discussions with a child regarding pain. This chapter will refer to either pain or hurt, with the understanding that the nurse always uses the child's word of choice (e.g., "owie," "ouchie"). In questioning the parents, one of the first issues the nurse should address is the presence of family, cultural, or spiritual beliefs and practices regarding pain. Box 15-3 describes how to obtain a pain history from both child and parent. After pain terminology and special beliefs or practices have been addressed, the nurse should:

- Question the child (pain history).
- Question the parent (pain history, other factors affecting the child).
- Observe and note behavioral changes.
- Observe and note physiologic changes.

| BOX 15-3 | **Pain Experience History** |

Child Form*

Can you tell me what pain is?

Can you tell me about the hurt you've had before?

Do you tell others when you hurt? Who do you tell?

What do you do for yourself when you are hurting?

What do you want other people to do for you when you hurt?

What don't you want other people to do for you when you hurt?

What helps the most to take your hurt away?

Is there anything special that you want me to know about you when you hurt? (If yes, have child describe.)

Parent Form

What word or words does your child use to describe pain?

Describe the pain experiences your child has had in the past.

Does your child tell you or others when hurting?

How do you know when your child is in pain?

How does your child usually react to pain?

What do you do when your child is hurting?

What does your child do when she is hurting?

What works best to take away your child's pain?

Is there anything special that you would like me to know about your child and pain? (If yes, describe.)

*Use the word(s) to describe pain that are developmentally and personally appropriate for the child. In addition to "pain" or "hurt," this may include terms appropriate for younger children, such as "owie."
Modified from Hester, N. O., & Barcus, C. S. (1986). Assessment and management of pain in children. *Pediatrics: Nursing Update, 1,* 2-8.

NONPHARMACOLOGIC AND PHARMACOLOGIC PAIN INTERVENTIONS

At times, nonpharmacologic interventions may be the only action needed to relieve certain types and intensities of pain. At other times, the only way to break the cycle of pain is to use a pharmacologic agent. The nurse's assessment helps determine the suitable intervention. If pharmacologic interventions are determined to be the first and best option, nonpharmacologic interventions may always be presented as an adjuvant for the chosen analgesic. Doing so may offer the child a sense of accomplishment and control that can replace the sense of helplessness that often accompanies the presence of pain, illness, and hospitalization. Additionally, Rusy and Weisman (2000) note that children are highly responsive to pain management strategies that involve use of their imagination and their sense of play and that use of nonpharmacologic or complementary therapies may reduce the amount of medication required to treat pain.

Nonpharmacologic Interventions

The nurse caring for a child in pain can provide nonpharmacologic interventions in addition to pharmacologic interventions Furthermore, use of nonpharmacologic in preparing the child for procedures and treatments can help minimize or relieve pain by reducing anxiety and fear of the unknown (see Chapter 11). Nonpharmacologic interventions must be suitable for the child, considering stage of development, the child's personality, and the circumstances surrounding the child.

Parents play a very important role in assessing and providing pain management for children (Box 15-4). They are a resource for determining what methods of pain relief were effective in the past. They can help the nurse assess their child's current pain status and need for intervention. Repositioning, holding, touching, massage, warm or cold compresses, breathing techniques, distraction, guided imagery, and muscle relaxation are all techniques that can be used by the person the child usually trusts the most—a parent. Many techniques require preliminary instruction by the nurse or other qualified individuals but then are easily learned and put into practice by parents. This is also a mechanism to give parents "hands on" involvement and a sense of control when their child is hospitalized.

| BOX 15-4 | **PARENTS WANT TO KNOW** About Pain Management for Their Child |

- Parents are given a pain assessment tool with instructions on accurate use. They should verbalize understanding about the tool and give a return demonstration using the tool with their child.
- The dose, route, and schedule for all pain medications are explained to the parents verbally and in writing. **All instructions should be in the appropriate language, given in the simplest terms possible, at an educational level suitable for the parents.**
- Nonpharmacologic interventions that are appropriate and comforting for the child's pain (e.g., massage,

warm or cold compresses, repositioning) are explained and demonstrated. Written instructions are provided as necessary.

- Parents are instructed to notify the primary health care provider if interventions for pain management are ineffective or if the child shows behavior or physiologic changes not consistent with the expected pain management outcomes for the child.
- Parents are given a phone number where they can contact a nurse if they have any questions about their child's condition once the child in the home setting.

Breathing Techniques

Regulated breathing techniques can help provide a focal point for distraction, produce relaxation, be a simple mode of biofeedback, or be a component of imagery. The child is instructed about and assisted to achieve a rhythmic pattern of breathing. This pattern must also be easily sustainable. Parents can demonstrate and participate in the breathing technique themselves.

Distraction

Distraction can be one of the more effective adjuvants for pain management (Fig. 15-7). It is also one of the simplest to accomplish. Distraction works by refocusing the child from the pain to something else. It does not imply total pain relief, and children with severe pain may not be able to be distracted. The child's ability to use distraction does not mean that the child is not experiencing pain. Children may distract themselves with activities such as playing, reading, or watching television, to ignore or "forget" their pain. However, this does not mean the child is pain free. The form of distraction should be appropriate for the child's developmental level.

Distraction may be accomplished with blowing bubbles, looking through a kaleidoscope, music, stories, number games, video games, board games, watching a video, or even doing multiplication tables or spelling words. If a child has a favorite doll or stuffed animal, it may be used to create a story or a game. Children love to talk about their pets, and the nurse can ask the child to tell a favorite story about the pet. Another distraction technique is to allow the child to help by handing, opening, or holding objects. This technique should be used only when it is safe and there is no danger of contamination of materials or of a site.

For example, a child brought to the emergency department after an accident is invariably frightened. Even if the injury is minor by emergency department standards, the fear and pain are real to the child. By use of distraction, the nurse can decrease both anxiety and pain. Although each child is different, cues or verbal instruction from the child and the parent can indicate whether the nurse should hold the child's hand, touch the child's head, or provide some other interventions that are appropriate and comforting for the child.

> Once both the child and nurse can communicate personally, the nurse might say, "I see you have a baseball shirt on. Do you play baseball?" If the child expresses an interest in the game, the nurse can continue, "Which team is your favorite? What was the most exciting play you saw this year? Have you been to a game?" The nurse should be comfortable with the topic because the child will sense a lack of genuine interest. If it is appropriate on the basis of the child's developmental level and degree of egocentricity, the nurse might interject a personal note: "I love baseball also. When I was a child, it was my biggest treat to go with my father to see the St. Louis Cardinals." This conversation could go on for 10 to 15 minutes, certainly long enough for sutures to be put in or other minor procedures completed. The child will not be focusing as much on the procedure as on baseball. The topic should be of interest to the child because the important idea is to focus the child on something other than the injury and procedure.

Guided Imagery

Guided imagery is a process involving relaxation and focused concentration on mental images. The child can be encouraged to think of a favorite place and imagine the sounds, sights, and smells of that place. The nurse, in a quiet, soothing voice, can guide the child on a "make-believe" trip. Breathing techniques can also relax the child. The child is instructed to take several slow, deep breaths while thinking pleasant thoughts. Children often need guidance, and the nurse may suggest remembering a birthday or a special time with family, friends, or a pet.

Biofeedback

Biofeedback provides visual or auditory evidence that physiologic changes are taking place. Special instruments detect and magnify body states that a person cannot usually notice. It also helps the person bring them under control. Visual feedback involving changes in colors or numbers or involvement in computer games is an effective way to use this technique. Biofeedback gives the child an instant response, which can hold the child's interest. Biofeedback does require specialized equipment, trained instructors, and is more often useful for chronic pain as opposed to acute pain (Rusy & Weisman, 2000).

Progressive Muscle Relaxation

Children can achieve relaxation, decrease anxiety, and decrease pain by identifying and decreasing the body tension that can accompany pain. They are taught a progressive,

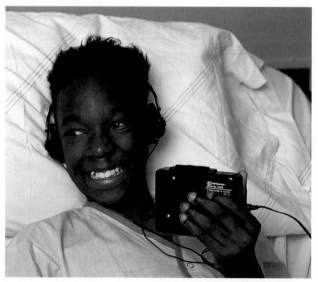

FIG 15-7   **Distraction effectively reduces pain by helping the child refocus attention. This boy listens to the radio through earphones, allowing him to be distracted without annoying others.** *(Courtesy Children's Medical Center, Dallas, TX.)*

systematic, purposeful relaxation of their body, part by part. This involves tensing and relaxing specific muscles, usually beginning with the arms and moving down the body. Learning this method can require ability to practice frequently and a degree of skill that may only be seen with older children.

Hypnosis

Hypnosis is a form of focused and narrowed attention, an altered state of consciousness, or a trance, often accompanied by relaxation. Hypnosis is effective in relieving pain and symptoms in children undergoing painful procedures associated with cancer, burns, and sickle-cell disease (Cravero, Manzi, & Rice, 1998). Hypnosis has also been shown to have positive effects on children undergoing surgery (Jones, 1997; Lambert, 1996). Hypnosis combined with acupuncture has also shown efficacy for chronic pediatric pain (Zeltzer et al., 2002). Typically, a licensed psychologist or health care personnel who have undergone special training perform hypnosis. Children can be taught self-hypnosis. Hypnosis and self-hypnosis are being used with increasing frequency and with positive results among children.

Transcutaneous Electrical Nerve Stimulation

In transcutaneous electrical nerve stimulation (TENS), a unit with electrodes delivers small amounts of electrical energy to the skin. The stimulation interferes with the transmission of pain signals and helps suppress the sensation of pain in that area. Rusy and Weisman (2000) note that TENS has proven effective in pain management, alone or with analgesics. Typically, a physical therapy department provides TENS therapy.

Pharmacologic Interventions

Many nurses are reluctant to administer analgesics. Some nurses and physicians believe, incorrectly, that children will become addicted to the analgesic. Others fear respiratory depression or do not believe the child has enough pain to justify analgesic administration. If a procedure, surgery, or trauma causes pain in an adult, it will cause pain in a child and analgesic medications are necessary. However, it is important to ensure that the correct medication and dose are ordered and administered. In some cases, the analgesic is underdosed and the child still experiences untreated, unwarranted pain. Increased pain management experience and research have taught that combination or multidrug therapy is often far more effective than a single analgesic. However, not one analgesic or combinations of analgesics will be ideal for all circumstances requiring pain management. The chosen analgesic therapy must have a prompt onset of action, a predictable duration of action, manageable side effects, and an appropriate reversal agent.

Administration of Analgesics

Analgesics can be administered by various routes—oral, rectal, intranasal, topical, transdermal, intravenous (IV), intramuscular (IM), subcutaneous, and epidural (see Chapter 14 for a discussion of the common routes). The least invasive route that provides optimum analgesia should always be chosen. In as many situations as possible, as soon as the child can tolerate oral nutrition, the medication should be given by the oral route. Rectal medication can be very frightening to children and is generally disliked. It should be avoided as much as is feasible.

CRITICAL TO REMEMBER
Disadvantages of Intramuscular Analgesics

- Altered tissue absorption leads to peaks and troughs in analgesia.
- Children quickly run out of suitable sites for injection.
- IM analgesics have a shorter duration of action than do orally administered analgesics.
- IM analgesics are contraindicated in children with low platelet counts.
- Children hate IM injections.
- Nurses dislike administering IM injections.

Modified from Eland, J. (1990). Pain in children. *Nursing Clinics of North America, 25,* 871-884.

Patient-Controlled Analgesia. One of the most effective ways of administering analgesic is by use of a patient-controlled analgesia (PCA) pump. The pump administers an IV bolus of pain medication either with or without a continuing infusion of the same medication. PCA can be used in a child as young as 5 years who is developmentally appropriate (McCaffery & Pasero, 1999). In some institutions, children younger than 5 years use PCA with parents or nurses activating the pump for them. Further research and anecdotal experience are needed on the use of PCA in children younger than 5 years.

When the child needs pain medication, a small dose of the medication is received after a button connected to the pump is pushed (Fig. 15-8). After each dose, there is "lockout" time during which the pump will not release the medication even if the button is pushed. The pump also has a maximum amount of medication that can be given over a designated period—usually 1 hour. If the maximum amount of medication for the time has been reached, the pump will not release medication even if the button is pushed.

After checking to ensure that all doses are within appropriate range, two registered nurses (RNs) must check the bag or syringe of medication before hanging it. After a PCA pump is programmed, it must then be double-checked by a second RN. Box 15-5 gives an example of orders for a PCA infusion. The opioid bag or syringe is locked into the PCA pump, and the pump itself is locked to the IV pole. Typically, the PCA tubing is special tubing that does not have IV port access.

The child is monitored frequently to ensure that pain control is effective and that the equipment is functioning correctly. The nurse should also carefully monitor the child for

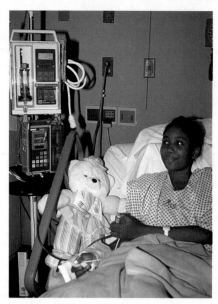

FIG 15-8   **PCA gives the older child greater control over pain management. The child presses the button when pain medication is needed, and the machine delivers a preprogrammed bolus through the IV line. The child cannot overdose because the controller has a lock-out feature to prevent excess analgesic administration.** (Courtesy Children's Medical Center, Dallas, TX.)

BOX 15-5	**Aspects of Patient-Controlled Analgesia Orders**

Medication/concentration: _____
Mode: PCA only _____ PCA and basal infusion _____
Continuous infusion only _____
Doses:
• Bolus _____ mg by RN every _____ minutes or _____ (recommended dose is 0.05 mg/kg/dose)
• PCA bolus _____ mg (recommended starting dose is 0.02 mg/kg/dose for morphine)
• Basal rate or continuous infusion _____ (recommended starting dose is 0.02 mg/kg/hr)
Lockout: _____ minutes (usual is 6-10 min as needed)
One-hour limit: _____ mg PCA and basal rate combined (usual is 0.075 mg/kg)

---

signs of overmedication (especially depressed respiratory rate or inability to rouse) and the side effects that may accompany opioid administration. Vital signs should be assessed every 15 to 30 minutes when PCA therapy is first initiated and then every 2 to 4 hours thereafter. Some institutions require hourly documentation of respiratory rate.

Additionally, many institutions' policies require that children receiving PCA therapy be placed on continuous pulse oximetry, cardiac and respiratory monitoring, or both. Oxygen, a bag and mask, and naloxone (Narcan) should be readily available. Naloxone will reverse the opioid-related analgesia and the respiratory depression. For this reason, it is administered slowly until it is first noted that the respiratory depression is reversed. It has a short half-life and so may need

to be repeated every 30 to 60 minutes. Many institutions will mandate that naloxone must be given in the presence of a physician because too-rapid infusion can result in cardiac arrest.

Frequent pain assessment is also necessary, usually every 4 hours and with any bolus dose, with subsequent reassessment as to the bolus's effectiveness. Charting will include hourly documentation as to the number of boluses received and possibly the number of bolus attempts made by the child. Total milligram dosages of the medication received will be noted anywhere from every hour to every 4 hours. This will be documented on the medication administration record.

Topical Anesthetic Cream. There are several non-injection-based transdermal topical numbing anesthetics agents available for use before painful invasive procedures. These can be used to reduce the pain associated with selected procedures, such as scheduled injections and immunizations, venipuncture, lumbar puncture, and bone marrow aspiration. Many pediatric institutions also mandate that a numbing agent be used for all IV starts, unless it is on an emergency basis. One such agent is lidocaine-prilocaine 5% cream (eutectic mixture of local anesthetics). This agent was the first of these newer agents to demonstrate efficacy for managing pain with certain invasive procedures. Newer, similar cream agents are 4% amethicaine (Ametop) and liposomal lidocaine 4% cream (ELA-MAX, Maxiline). The cream agents are applied to intact skin in a mound, not rubbed in, and covered with an occlusive dressing 30 to 60 minutes before the procedure. The numbing effect lasts from 2 to 4 hours. Parents may apply the analgesic cream at home before scheduled IV starts, injections, or venipuncture to help decrease or eliminate pain. Care should be taken with small children to avoid their removing the dressing and rubbing the cream in their eyes or eating the cream, which to some children may look like cake frosting.

There is also dichlorodifluoromethane and lidocaine hydrochloride 2% with 1:100,000 epinephrine topical solution (Numby Stuff) and trichlorodifluoromethane vapocoolant (Fluori-Methane or cold spray). Numby Stuff comes in an electrode patch. The medication is delivered by iontophoresis, a mild electrical current, to push the lidocaine and epinephrine to levels of 10 mm, producing a deeper numbing effect. This method can only be applied in the health care setting. Cold spray vapocoolant is used to directly spray the procedure site or saturate a sterile cotton ball, which is then applied to the site for 15 seconds. This has an immediate onset of action and lasts approximately 15 seconds. Accordingly, this anesthetic is used immediately before the procedure. The main side effect of all of these topical numbing agents is skin redness or blanching, with normal skin color returning in a few hours. There is research to support the effectiveness of many of these numbing agents (Koh et al., 2004; Lindh, Wiklund, Blomquist, & Hakansson, 2003; Mawhorter et al., 2004; O'Brien, Taddio, Ipp, Goldbach, & Koren, 2004; Taddio, Soin, Schuh, Koren, & Scolnik, 2005). Research related to the use these agents for the treatment of acute pain in neonates is in progress.

Even with the decreased or absence of pain from topical numbing agents, children may still fear needles; therefore, distraction or another nonpharmacologic method may also be necessary to help them through the painful procedure. Parents may need reassurance that the numbing effect does decrease or eliminate pain but that anxiety and fear also cause the behaviors typically associated with reaction to pain. Older children may have a noted preference for the agent used. Although the iontophoresis use to administer Numby Stuff may seem frightening to some children, others do prefer Numby Stuff to one of the numbing creams. To the degree possible, such choices should be honored.

Nonsteroidal Anti-Inflammatory Drugs

Nonsteroidal anti-inflammatory drugs (NSAIDs) are ibuprofen or aspirin-like drugs that reduce pain and inflammation. Ibuprofen, naproxen/naproxen sodium (Naprosyn, Anaprox) (see Chapter 26), ketorolac (Toradol), and choline magnesium trisalicylate (Trilisate) are some of the most commonly used drugs in this category. Because aspirin has been associated with Reye syndrome, it is not recommended for children.

It is questionable whether acetaminophen can be classified as an NSAID at all because it has a minimal

---

DRUG GUIDE

IBUPROFEN

Classification: NSAID, analgesic.
Action: Blocks prostaglandin synthesis.
Indications: Chronic, symptomatic rheumatoid arthritis and osteoarthritis; relief of mild to moderate pain.
Dosages and Route: By mouth: 5-10 mg/kg/dose every 6-8 hr. Do not exceed 40 mg/kg/24 hr. For juvenile arthritis: 30-50 mg/kg/24 hr. Medication comes in liquid form for young children.
Absorption: 80% absorbed from gastrointestinal (GI) tract; peak action in 1-2 hr.
Excretion: Excreted primarily in urine; some biliary excretion.
Contraindications: Contraindicated in children in whom urticaria, severe rhinitis, bronchospasm, angioedema, nasal polyps are precipitated by other NSAIDs; active peptic ulcer; bleeding abnormalities.
Precautions: Hypertension, history of GI ulceration, impaired hepatic or renal function, chronic renal failure.
Adverse Reactions: Heartburn, nausea, vomiting, epigastric or abdominal discomfort or pain, GI ulceration.
Nursing Considerations: Give on an empty stomach 1 hr before or 2 hr after meals. If GI intolerance occurs, it may be taken with meals or milk. If the child is unable to swallow a tablet, administer the medication in liquid form. Non–enteric-coated ibuprofen can be crushed and mixed with a very small amount (1 tablespoon) of food or liquid before swallowing.

GI, Gastrointestinal.

DRUG GUIDE

KETOROLAC

Classification: NSAID, analgesic.
Action: Blocks prostaglandin synthesis.
Indications: Short-term management of moderate pain.
Dosages and Route: Children older than 2 years IV: 0.4-1 mg/kg one time, followed by 0.2-0.5 mg/kg/dose every 6 hr, up to a maximum of 120 mg/24 hr.
Absorption: Absorbed rapidly; peak action in 1 to 2 hr.
Excretion: Excreted in the urine; effects last 4-6 hr.
Contraindications: Contraindicated in patients in whom urticaria, severe rhinitis, bronchospasm, angioedema, nasal polyps are precipitated by other NSAIDs.
Precautions: Cautious use with history of ulcers, impaired hepatic or renal function.
Adverse Reactions: Drowsiness, dizziness, nausea, GI pain, hemorrhage.
Nursing Considerations: Do not administer longer than 5 days; monitor liver function studies, signs and symptoms of GI upset or bleeding.

GI, Gastrointestinal.

DRUG GUIDE

ACETAMINOPHEN

Classification: Analgesic, antipyretic.
Action: Unknown, thought to produce analgesia by blocking generation of pain impulses.
Indications: Mild pain or fever.
Dosages and Routes: By mouth or rectal suppository: 10-15 mg/kg/dose every 4-6 hr up to a maximum of 5 doses/24 hr.
Absorption: Rapid and almost complete absorption from GI tract; less complete absorption from rectal suppository; peak effects in 1-1½ hr.
Excretion: 90%-100% of drug excreted as metabolites in urine; excreted in breast milk; effects last 4-6 hr.
Contraindications: Hypersensitivity to acetaminophen or phenacetin; administration to patients with anemia or hepatic disease; cautious use in arthritic or rheumatoid conditions affecting children younger than 12 yr; thrombocytopenia.
Adverse Reaction: Negligible with recommended dosage; rash.
Nursing Considerations: May be crushed. Chewable tablets need to be thoroughly chewed and wetted before swallowing. With high doses or long-term therapy, periodic tests of hepatic, renal, and hematopoietic function are advised. Caution the parent about giving other medications containing acetaminophen without medical advice. No more than 5 doses in 24 hr should be given to children unless prescribed by physician. Available in infant strength (drops). Be sure to advise parents to check the strength before administering liquid acetaminophen (Tylenol) to avoid overdosing.

GI, Gastrointestinal.

anti-inflammatory effect and does not inhibit prostaglandin. However, it is frequently listed with NSAIDs. The short-term use of acetaminophen is safe, even in neonates. It does not have the gastric side effects of aspirin, and although it can cause hepatic damage, this effect is usually related to overdosage. It is the drug of choice for treating fever in children in the United States and is the most commonly used analgesic for mild to moderate pain. However, ibuprofen may be the drug of choice for conditions where there is bone pain, such as may be seen with bone injuries, arthritis-like conditions, or certain types of cancer.

Opioids

Opioids are natural or synthetic opium derivative analgesics that bind to central nervous system (CNS) opioid receptors and control pain by depressing pain impulse transmission. Opioids are the cornerstone drugs in the management of most forms of moderate to severe acute and chronic pain, including postoperative pain, posttraumatic pain, the pain of sickle-cell vaso-occlusive crisis, and cancer pain. Some of the more commonly used opioids are codeine, fentanyl, hydrocodone, hydromorphone, meperidine, methadone, morphine, and oxycodone. Opioid is the term of choice in pain management, as opposed to the antiquated, but possibly more familiar term, "narcotic." Narcotic is an older term for medications that depress the CNS to relieve pain and produce sleep.

Opioids can be administered by most routes. However, the oral route should be used when it is appropriate and the child is able to take and tolerate oral opioids. Sustained-release forms of morphine and oxycodone, which last 12 hours, are available. These are supplemented with a short-acting liquid for "break-through" pain. The use of these two forms of morphine and oxycodone can help ensure longer pain-free periods for children, such as those with cancer pain. The short-acting liquids may also be used for children who cannot effectively swallow tablets. When the oral route is contraindicated, an IV route, a subcutaneous route, or both can be used. IV and subcutaneous opioids may be given by bolus or continuous infusion, either separately or in combination with another analgesic or sedative agent. Morphine, fentanyl, hydromorphone, methadone, and meperidine can be given IV or subcutaneously.

The nurse should remember that opioids could produce sedation and respiratory depression, in addition to analgesia. Other side effects can include constipation, pruritus, nausea, vomiting, cough suppression, urinary retention, and vasodilation. Although these side effects must be closely monitored, most children can tolerate these drugs if their dosages are adjusted. It has been noted that side effects such as pruritus, nausea, and sedation are inclined to be time limited and will resolve spontaneously within 3 to 4 days. Until that time, antiemetics and antipruritics can be used to control such side effects.

Codeine is the most commonly given oral opioid for moderate pain. It is usually given in combination with acetaminophen or aspirin. It can cause constipation, nausea,

---

DRUG GUIDE

CODEINE
Classification: Opioid analgesic.
Action: Binds with opiate receptors in the CNS; alters both perception of and emotional response to pain.
Indications: Mild to moderate pain.
Dosage and Routes: By mouth, IM, subcutaneous: 0.5-1 mg/kg/dose every 4-6 hr; maximum dose 60 mg/dose.
Absorption: Readily absorbed from GI tract, with peak action in 1-1½ hr.
Distribution: Crosses placenta; distributed into breast milk.
Excretion: Effects last approximately 4-6 hr; excreted in urine.
Contraindications: Hypersensitivity to codeine or other morphine derivatives; hepatic or renal dysfunction.
Precaution: Use cautiously in very young children.
Adverse Reactions: Primarily with CNS symptoms: dizziness, lightheadedness, drowsiness, sedation, lethargy, euphoria, agitation, restlessness, respiratory depression; GI: nausea, vomiting, constipation; genitourinary: urinary retention.
Nursing Considerations: To reduce possibility of GI upset, administer oral codeine with milk or other food. Because dizziness and lightheadedness may occur, supervision of ambulation and other safety precautions may be necessary. Nausea is a common side effect; report if this is accompanied by vomiting. Change to another analgesic may be necessary.

GI, Gastrointestinal.

---

vomiting, and pruritus. Oxycodone and hydrocodone have side effects similar to those of codeine. They are combined with acetaminophen as an oral medication. However, oxycodone also comes as a sustained-release tablet and immediate-release solution.

Morphine is the preferred opioid for children. It reaches its peak effect 10 to 20 minutes after IV administration and 1 hour after oral administration. It can produce sedation along with the analgesia. If it occurs, maximum respiratory depression will happen 7 minutes after IV administration. Naloxone (Narcan) should be available to reverse the sedation or respiratory depression if necessary.

Fentanyl and its analogs (sufentanil, alfentanil) have a shorter duration of action than morphine and are 50 to 100 times more potent. Because much less histamine is released, these agents may cause less vasodilation and pruritus. The short duration of effect makes IV use of these drugs appropriate when a brief, painful procedure is to be performed (e.g., bone marrow aspiration, inserting a chest tube, changing a burn dressing) and when children are critically ill. Fentanyl should be administered in a closely monitored setting. Experience with the use of the fentanyl patch (Duragesic) is limited in children. Most often, it is used in adolescents whose weight is closer to that of an adult. The fentanyl patch

DRUG GUIDE

MORPHINE

Classification: Opioid analgesic.

Action: Binds with CNS opiate receptors; alters physical and emotional response to pain.

Indications: Acute and chronic pain.

Dosages and Routes: Intermittent dose. By mouth or rectal: 0.2-0.5 mg/kg/dose every 4-6 hr. IM, IV, subcutaneous: 0.1-0.2 mg/kg/dose every 2-4 hr, up to a maximum of 15 mg/dose. Continuous IV infusion: 0.01-0.04 mg/kg/hr (average 0.06 mg/kg/hr). Begin with the lowest dose; increase up to 2 mg/kg/hr as required. Patient controlled: maintenance: 0.02 mg/kg/hr; increase if child requires more than 2 bolus doses per hour. Bolus at 0.02 mg/kg/dose at intervals of at least 10 min as needed.

Absorption: Variable absorption from the GI tract; peak action 60 min orally, 20 min IV.

Excretion: Excreted primarily in the urine; 7%-10% excreted in bile. Effects last up to 7 hr.

Contraindications: Hypersensitivity to opioids, increased intracranial pressure, seizure disorders, chronic pulmonary disease, respiratory depression.

Precautions: Cautious use with cardiac arrhythmias, reduced blood volume.

Adverse Reactions: Sedation, dizziness, euphoria, paradoxical CNS excitation, respiratory depression, hypotension, bradycardia, nausea, vomiting, constipation, urinary retention.

Nursing Considerations: Carefully and frequently assess respiratory status. Assess cough reflex; monitor intake and output carefully for urinary retention and constipation.

GI, Gastrointestinal.

DRUG GUIDE

FENTANYL

Classification: Opioid analgesic.

Action: Narcotic agonist with actions similar to morphine and meperidine but action is faster and less prolonged.

Indications: Moderate to severe pain, particularly for brief procedures and when children are critically ill or high risk. Transdermal fentanyl is for severe chronic pain only; experience with children is very limited.

Dosages and Routes: IM and IV intermittent doses: 1-2 μg/kg/dose every 30-60 min. IV patient-controlled: maintenance 1 μg/kg/hr continuous infusion, increased if the patient requires more than 2 bolus doses per hour. Bolus: 0.1-0.4 μg/kg/dose at intervals of at least 5 min. Transdermal patch used only in children older than 12 years.

Absorption: Absorbed rapidly after IV administration, 6-8 hr transdermally.

Excretion: Excreted in the urine. Lasts 30-60 min IV; 72 hr transdermally.

Contraindication: Patients who have received monoamine oxidase inhibitors within 14 days.

Precautions: Use cautiously in children with head injuries, increased intracranial pressure, respiratory problems, liver and kidney dysfunction.

Adverse Reactions: Sedation, dizziness, euphoria, seizures with high doses. Hypotension, bradycardia, circulatory depression, respiratory depression, bronchoconstriction.

Nursing Considerations: Watch carefully for signs and symptoms of respiratory distress, depression; have oxygen, resuscitative equipment, and naloxone available.

---

is indicated for chronic pain. Transdermal fentanyl, 25 μg/hr, is approximately equal to parenteral morphine at 15 mg/24 hr or oral morphine at 90 mg/24 hr.

Hydromorphone (Dilaudid) is very similar to morphine. It is approximately six times more potent than morphine. It may be used to control pain in patients with cancer.

Methadone is metabolized very slowly and therefore has a prolonged duration of action. It is absorbed well after both oral and IV administration. Because of its long duration, it must be carefully titrated according to pain level (moderate, minimal alert, minimal somnolent). It is equal in potency to morphine.

Meperidine (Demerol) should be used only for short-term pain control in children who have shown an allergy or intolerance to other opioids. It has no advantages to morphine. The duration of analgesia is shorter than with morphine. Normeperidine, a metabolite of meperidine, has been associated with convulsions and dysphoria after as few as two doses. In addition, it has been shown to cause hallucinations and agitation. Meperidine is used minimally; it is most often used postoperatively and in combination with other medications for procedural pain.

CRITICAL TO REMEMBER

Pain Management for Children

- The preferred route of administering analgesics to children is oral or IV.
- As soon as the child can tolerate oral intake, switch the medication to the oral route.
- After starting with the recommended starting dose for opioids, the dose is adjusted to achieve best pain management with the fewest side effects
- Opioids do not have a dose limit. The maximum dose is the dose that causes intolerable side effects.
- Infants and children receiving epidural opioids should be monitored by a cardiac apnea monitor and pulse oximetry.
- Certain infants and children receiving IV opioids may require a cardiac apnea monitor and pulse oximetry, typically neonates, those who are opioid naïve, or those with a history of apnea or other respiratory difficulties. The risk of respiratory depression is greatest during the first 24 hours of administration.
- If respiratory depression occurs with opioid use, naloxone hydrochloride should be used for reversal if oxygen and stimulation of the child are ineffective.

DRUG GUIDE

HYDROMORPHONE
Classification: Opioid analgesic.
Action: Inhibits ascending pain pathways in CNS, increases pain threshold, alters pain perception
Indications: Moderate to severe pain
Dosage and Routes: By mouth, IM, subcutaneous, or IV; 0.03-0.08 mg/kg every 4-6 hr by mouth, maximum 5 mg/dose; IV dose 0.015 mg/kg/dose
Absorption: Onset, 15-20 minutes, peak 0.5-1 hr, duration 4-5 hr
Excretion: Excreted in the urine, half-life 3.5-4.5 hr
Contraindications: Hypersensitivity, addiction
Precautions: Addictive personality, increased intracranial pressure, respiratory depression, hepatic disease, renal disease. Cautious use in head injuries, increased intracranial pressure, asthma, and other respiratory conditions. Impaired renal or hepatic function.
Adverse Reactions: Dizziness, lightheadedness, confusion, hallucinations, mood changes, sedation, respiratory depression, dependence, increase urine output, urinary retention, seizures, palpitations, bradycardia, tachycardia, hypotension, other changes in blood pressure.
Nursing Considerations: Assess respiratory status carefully; assess for CNS changes and implement appropriate safety measure, monitor intake and output carefully for oliguria or assess for urinary retention.

DRUG GUIDE

OXYCODONE
Classification: Opioid analgesic
Action: Inhibits ascending pain pathways in the CNS, increases pain threshold, alters pain perception
Indications: Moderate to severe pain
Dosage and Routes: By mouth 0.05-0.15 mg/kg/dose every 4-6 hr; maximum 5 mg/dose
Absorption: Onset, 10-20 min, duration 4-6 hr
Excretion: Excreted in the urine, half-life 3.5-4.5 hr
Contraindications: Hypersensitivity, addiction
Precautions: Addictive personality, increased intracranial pressure, respiratory depression, hepatic disease, renal disease. Cautious use in head injuries, increased intracranial pressure, asthma, and other respiratory conditions. Impaired renal or hepatic function.
Adverse Reactions: Dizziness, lightheadedness, confusion, hallucinations, mood changes, sedation, respiratory depression, dependence.
Nursing Considerations: Assess respiratory status carefully; assess for CNS changes, and implement appropriate safety measures.

DRUG GUIDE

HYDROCODONE
Classification: Opioid analgesic.
Action: Binds to opiate receptors in CNS to diminish pain
Indications: Mild pain
Dosage and Routes: By mouth, maximum doses of 1.25 mg (children <2 years old)-5 mg (children >2 years old) every 4-6 hours as needed or 0.2 mg/kg every 3-4 hr
Absorption: Onset, 10-20 min, duration 4-6 hr
Excretion: Excreted in the urine, half-life 3.5-4.5 hr
Contraindications: Hypersensitivity, addiction
Precautions: Addictive personality, increased intracranial pressure, respiratory depression, hepatic disease, renal disease. Cautious use in head injuries, increased intracranial pressure, asthma, and other respiratory conditions. Impaired renal or hepatic function.
Adverse Reactions: Dizziness, lightheadedness, confusion, hallucinations, mood changes, sedation, respiratory depression, dependence.
Nursing Considerations: Assess respiratory status carefully; assess for CNS changes and implement appropriate safety measures.

DRUG GUIDE

METHADONE
Classification: Opioid analgesic
Action: Depresses pain impulse transmission at the spinal cord level through interaction with opioid receptors, thus producing CNS depression
Indications: Severe acute and chronic pain, opioid withdrawal
Dosages and Routes: 0.05-0.1 mg/kg/dose every 6-12 hr
Absorption: Variable absorption from the GI tract; peak action 60 min orally, 20 min IV
Excretion: Excreted in the urine, crosses the placenta, excreted in breast milk, half-life 15-30 hr
Contraindications: Hypersensitivity to this drug, chlorobutanol injection, addiction.
Precautions: Cautious use with addictive personalities, increased intracranial pressure, respiratory depression, hepatic or renal disease
Adverse Reactions: Sedation, dizziness, confusion, euphoria, seizures, respiratory depression, hypotension, bradycardia, palpitations, nausea, vomiting, constipation, urinary retention.
Nursing Considerations: Carefully and frequently assess respiratory status. Assess cough reflex; monitor intake and output carefully for urinary retention and constipation.

GI, Gastrointestinal.

Conscious Sedation

Conscious sedation is a medically controlled state of depressed consciousness that allows appropriate responses to physical stimulation or verbal commands and maintenance of protective reflexes. This means that the child retains the ability to maintain a patent airway continuously and independently (AAP, 2002). It generally is achieved using an amnesic, sedative, or both, administered IV. With conscious sedation, children usually have little or no recollection of the procedure they have undergone.

Midazolam (Versed) is a short-acting drug that can be given by multiple routes—IV, intranasal, rectal, IM, oral, or sublingual. It can be used for conscious sedation and for preoperative sedation and as an induction agent for general anesthesia. Advantages to using midazolam include minimal side effects, short duration of sedation, and ability to administer without an IV access. It may be used alone or in combination with other medications used for conscious sedation, including ketamine, fentanyl, and propofol. During and after conscious sedation, the child's vital signs, oxygen saturation, and level of consciousness should be closely monitored.

Epidural Analgesia

Pain medication (usually an opioid, a local anesthetic, or both) can be administered through an epidural catheter inserted into the epidural space and secured to the child's back with an occlusive dressing. Because the medication is administered directly to the nerves that transmit pain, smaller doses are required for pain control, with fewer side effects than usually associated with systemic opioid administration. It is suggested for children undergoing abdominal, anal, or urogenital procedures; open-heart surgery; and thoracic surgery, or orthopedic surgeries of the lower limbs. Nursing

---

NURSING CARE PLAN

The Child in Pain

Focused Assessment

The nursing assessment for the verbal child begins with questioning to determine what word or words are used for pain. Then the parents are questioned as to cultural or spiritual beliefs or practices that might have an impact on pain issues. The nurse should remember that parents are the first resource to help assess the child's pain and the child's response to pain management interventions. Then a pain history is taken from child and parent, including physical, emotional, and psychosocial factors that might affect the child with regard to pain.

Assess the current pain as to onset, duration, location, intensity, and quality. An age-appropriate pain tool assesses the intensity of pain. The same tool is used consistently, and it becomes a part of the child's chart as a future reference. Behavioral and physiologic changes are noted also. If the child is preverbal or nonverbal, complete a behavioral assessment along with use of an assessment tool designed for preverbal or nonverbal children. Response to the interventions, pharmacologic and nonpharmacologic, is assessed with the pain tool, parents' input, and, as appropriate, observation of behavioral and physiologic data.

NURSING DIAGNOSIS   Acute Pain related to physical or biologic factors: edema, disease process, infection, invasive procedure, surgery, trauma.

EXPECTED OUTCOMES   The child will:
- Experience a decrease in pain to an acceptable level, as evidenced by reduced pain level based on assessment with a developmentally appropriate, verbal or nonverbal, pain assessment tool, and a relaxed body posture and decreased crying, fussiness, restlessness, and facial grimacing.
- Return to the activity level experienced before the onset of pain.
- Achieve uninterrupted sleep periods of at least 90 minutes to experience a complete REM (rapid eye movement) cycle.

Intervention	*Rationale*
1. Assess child by use of a developmentally appropriate pain assessment tool. The tool should be a part of the child's chart for easy reference.	1. Infants and children may have difficulty communicating about their pain. Pain assessment tools provide more consistent, objective, and quantitative information.
2. Observe and document behavioral and physiologic signs of pain in the child. Note both verbal and nonverbal responses. Assess vital signs.	2. Assessment of pain in children is based on the child's report of pain and on behavioral and physiologic changes. Children may have difficulty verbalizing pain. The nurse will have to depend on behavioral changes alone to assess infants and other children who are nonverbal or unable to communicate clearly. Physiologic changes vary in response to pain and should be evaluated together with a behavioral assessment.
3. Determine other factors that might be affecting the child: separation, fear, anxiety, loss of control, and spiritual or cultural beliefs regarding pain.	3. The child's perception of pain and ultimate reaction to pain may be influenced by other factors.

Continued

NURSING CARE PLAN—cont'd

4. Monitor pain on the basis of the child's developmental stage.
5. As possible, question the child to assess the onset, duration, location, and type of pain and what type of pain relief measures works best.
6. Note whether the child's pain level is different when at rest, ambulating, playing, or during procedures.
7. Administer the appropriate analgesic. Give by oral or IV route. Avoid injections.

8. Implement nonpharmacologic pain reduction strategies:

   a. Distraction
   b. Relaxation techniques
   c. Cutaneous stimulation, such as massage or warm or cold compresses
   d. Quiet, calm environment

   e. Repositioning

   f. Decreased environmental noise and light

   g. Comfort measures (touch, holding, rocking)

9. Involve parents in care.

10. Record the response to both pharmacologic and non-pharmacologic pain reduction measures by use of the appropriate pain assessment tool.
11. Observe for side effects of medication.

---

4. Infants and children at each developmental level have a unique way of reacting to and coping with pain.
5. These factors will influence the choice of analgesic.

6. Pain relief measures can be improved by a thorough understanding of cause and effect.
7. Nonopioids are appropriate for mild to moderate pain. Opioid analgesics should be given for moderate to severe pain. Children fear injections and may deny pain to avoid an injection.
8. Pharmacologic analgesia can be enhanced through the use of nonpharmacologic pain management strategies as adjuvant therapy.
   a. Distraction interrupts the transmission of pain.
   b. Relaxation is also thought to interrupt pain.
   c. Cutaneous stimulation blocks pain transmission.

   d. A quiet, calm environment is more conducive to rest and sleep, which enhance the effects of analgesia.
   e. A change in position may relieve pressure or provide for a more relaxed, comfortable body.
   f. A quiet, comfortable environment can have a soothing, relaxing effect on the child and parent.
   g. Comfort measures can be provided by parents that can help to decrease anxiety and the skeletal muscle tension that often accompanies pain.

9. The presence of the child's parents may reduce fear and anxiety, thus reducing the amount of pain felt. Parents also know their child best. They can assist in the assessment of pain and the child's response to interventions.

10. Documentation aids in determining the effectiveness of pain relief measures and continuity in the management of pain.
11. Respiratory depression is the most serious side effect of opioids but is rare. Other side effects include sedation, nausea and vomiting, and constipation.

Evaluation

- Does the child verbalize or demonstrate decreased?
- Has the child been able to return to the level of activity seen before the onset of pain?

- Has the child been able to achieve uninterrupted sleep for appropriate lengths of time?

---

care of the child with an epidural catheter is similar to that for a child receiving PCA therapy. The child is monitored with a cardiac monitor and pulse oximetry. The nurse assesses the child for adequate pain relief and the presence of undesired side effects (particularly decreased respirations) and for complications that might accompany the catheter placement. It is important to avoid any action that would pull or place tension on the catheter. The nurse assesses the dermatome level (the level of sensory blockade) every 4 hours and as needed. The nurse also monitors the catheter site frequently for slippage, bleeding, loss of cerebrospinal

fluid, or a hematoma at the insertion site—a rare but serious complication that needs to be reported immediately. Other side effects include constipation, nausea, vomiting, urinary retention, motor block, and sensory block.

┤ KEY CONCEPTS ├

- Pain is whatever the experiencing person says it is, existing whenever the person says it does (McCaffery & Pasero, 1999) and "an unpleasant sensory and emotional experience associated with actual or potential tissue damage or described in terms of such damage" (International Association for the Study of Pain, 1979).

- The gate-control theory of pain postulates that gating mechanisms at the level of the dorsal horn can facilitate or inhibit pain transmission. The theory further states that stimulation of the larger afferent nerves, which carry benign sensations, can dull pain. The theory lends support for the use of both physiological and psychological interventions in pain management.

- Two of the most prevalent myths that interfere with the provision of adequate pain medication to infants and children are the fear of addiction and the fear of respiratory depression. Neither belief is supported by research.

- Pain assessment in infants and children takes a multidimensional approach. The child and parent should be questioned, and behavioral and physiologic changes should be noted.

- A pain assessment tool should be used for each child to assess, implement, and document pain management effectively. The tool should be developmentally correct for the child and must be used consistently, according to instructions, for the results to be valid.

- Both pharmacologic and nonpharmacologic measures should be used in the treatment of pain in children. Acetaminophen is used for mild to moderate pain and morphine is the opioid of choice for severe pain. Nonpharmacologic interventions include biofeedback, breathing techniques, distraction, guided imagery, hypnosis, progressive muscle relaxation, and TENS.

ANSWERS TO CRITICAL THINKING EXERCISE 15-1

1. An assessment to determine objective and subjective data should be performed, starting with use of a pain assessment tool designed for preverbal children. You will also be looking at behavioral (crying, facial expression, motor responses) and physiologic cues. When the infant cries, describe the crying and duration. Note whether holding and cuddling can quiet her. If not, her behavior could be an indication of discomfort. Obtain current vital signs and compare them with earlier signs. One clue from the nurse giving report is that the infant is not able to experience periods of *uninterrupted* sleep. This information, together with information from the assessment tool, vital signs, type of surgery, and postoperative day, strongly indicates that the infant should be medicated for pain. After the assessment has been completed, a nursing decision can be made. Documentation should also be checked to confirm that pain medication was not given during the previous shift.

2. Research has shown that neonates do experience pain. Because they are preverbal, pain assessment is based on an appropriate assessment tool and physiologic and behavioral responses. This information, plus an understanding of the type of surgery and postoperative day, presents a picture of pain in an infant of this age.

REFERENCES AND READINGS

Agency for Health Care Policy and Research, Acute Pain Management Guideline Panel. (1992a). *Acute pain management in infants, children, and adolescents: Operative and medical procedures. Quick reference guide for clinicians* (AHCPR Publication No. 92-0020). Rockville, MD: Public Health Service, U.S. Department of Health and Human Services.

Agency for Health Care Policy and Research, Acute Pain Management Guideline Panel. (1992b). *Acute pain management: Operative or medical procedures and trauma. Clinical practice guideline* (AHCPR Publication No. 92-0032). Rockville, MD: Public Health Service, U.S. Department of Health and Human Services.

Ambuel, H., Marx, C. M., & Blumer, J. L. (1992). Assessing distress in pediatric intensive care environments: The COMFORT scale. *Journal of Pediatric Psychology, 17,* 95-109.

American Academy of Pediatrics, Committee on Drugs. (2002). Guidelines for monitoring and management of pediatric patients during and after sedation for diagnostic therapeutic procedures. *Pediatrics, 110,* 836-838.

American Academy of Pediatrics, Committee on Psychosocial Aspects of Child and Family Health, & American Pain Society. (2001). The assessment and management of acute pain in infants, children and adolescents. *Pediatrics, 108,* 793-797.

Anand, K., & Hickey, P. (1987). Pain and its effects in the human neonate and fetus. *New England Journal of Medicine, 317,* 1321-1347.

Beyer, J. (1989). *The Oucher: A user's manual and technical report.* Denver: University of Colorado Health Sciences Center.

Beyer, J., & Aradine, C. (1986). Content validity of an instrument to measure young children's perceptions of the intensity of their pain. *Journal of Pediatric Nursing, 1,* 386-395.

Beyer, J., Denyes, M., & Villarruel, A. (1992). The creation, validation, and continuing development of the Oucher: A measure of pain intensity in children. *Journal of Pediatric Nursing, 7,* 335-346.

Beyer, J. E., & Knott, C. B. (1998). Construct validity estimation for the African-American and Hispanic versions of the Oucher Scale. *Journal of Pediatric Nursing, 13,* 20-31.

Bishop-Kurylo, D. (2002). Pediatric pain management in the emergency department. *Topics in Emergency Medicine, 24,* 19-30.

Children's Hospital, Boston. (2002). *Reference tool: Pain assessment tools.* Boston: Children's Hospital.

Collins, J. J. (2005). Pain control options in palliative care: Special considerations for children. *American Journal of Cancer, 4,* 77-85.

Cravero, J. P., Manzi, D. J., & Rice, L. J. (1998). The management of procedure-related pain in the child. In M. A. Ashburn & L. J. Rice (Eds.), *The management of pain* (pp. 667-681). Philadelphia: WB Saunders.

Craig, K. D. (1998). The facial display of pain in infants and children. *Pain Research and Management.* 10, 103-121.

Eland, J. (1990). Pain in children. *Nursing Clinics of North America, 25,* 871-884.

Foster, R. L., Yucha, C. B., Zuk, J., & Vojir, C. P. (2003). Physiologic correlates of comfort in healthy children. *Pain Management Nursing, 4,* 23-30.

Franck, L. S., Greenberg, C. S., & Stevens, B. (2000). Pain assessment in infants and children. *Pediatric Clinics of North America, 47,* 487-512.

Gharaibeh, M., & Abu-Saad, H. (2002). Cultural validation of pediatric pain assessment tools: Jordanian perspective. *Journal of Transcultural Nursing 1,* 12-18.

Giger, J. N., & Davidhizar, R. E. (2004). *Transcultural nursing* (4th ed.). Philadelphia: Mosby.

Golianu, B., Krane, E. J., Galloway, K. S., & Yaster, M. (2000). Pediatric acute pain management. *Pediatric Clinics of North America, 47,* 559-587.

Grunau, R., Johnston, C., & Craig, K. (1990). Neonatal facial and cry responses to invasive and non-invasive procedures. *Pain, 42,* 295-305.

Halimaa, S. (2003). Pain management in nursing procedures on premature babies. *Journal of Advanced Nursing, 42,* 587-597.

Hockenberry, M., Wilson, D., & Winkelstein, M. L. (2005). *Wong's essentials of pediatric nursing* (7th ed.). St. Louis: Mosby.

Hockenberry, M., Wilson, D., Winkelstein, M. L., & Kline, N. E. (2003). *Wong's nursing care of infants and children* (7th ed.). St. Louis: Mosby.

Hooke C., Hellsten, M. B., Stutzer, C., and Forte, K. (2002). Pain management for the child with cancer in end-of-life care: APON position paper. *Journal of Pediatric Oncology Nursing, 19,* 43-47.

Howard, R. F. (2003). Current status of pain management in children. *JAMA: Journal of the American Medical Association, 290,* 2464-2469.

International Association for the Study of Pain. (1979). Pain terms: A list with definitions and notes on usage. *Pain, 6,* 249.

Jacob, E., & Puntillo, K. A. (1999). A survey of nursing practice in the assessment and management of pain in children. *Pediatric Nursing, 25,* 278-286.

Jansaithong, J. (2002). *Northern Thai school-aged children pain experience: Pain descriptions and pain management.* Unpublished doctoral dissertation, University of Washington, Seattle.

Johnson, L. (2005). Clinical knowledge: Managing acute and chronic pain in sickle cell disease. *Nursing Times, 101,* 40-43.

Joint Commission on Accreditation of Healthcare Organizations, National Pharmaceutical Council, Inc. (2001). *Pain: Current understanding of assessment, management and treatments.* Retrieved May 20, 2005, from *www.jcaho.org.*

Joint Commission on Accreditation of Healthcare Organizations (2001). *Pain standards for 2001.* Retrieved May 20, 2005, from *www.jcaho.org.*

Jones, C. (1997). Hypnosis and spinal fusion by Harrington rod instrumentation. *American Journal of Clinical Hypnosis, 19,* 155-157.

Jordan-Marsh, M., Hubbard, J., Watson, R., Hall, R. D., Miller, P., & Mohan, O. (2004). The social ecology of changing pain management: Do I have to cry? *Journal of Pediatric Nursing, 19,* 193-203.

Koh, J. L., Harrison, D., Myers, R., Dembinski, R., Tuner, H., & McGraw, T. (2004). A randomized, double-blind comparison study of EMLA and ELA-MAX for topical anesthesia in children undergoing intravenous insertion. *Pediatric Anesthesia, 14,* 977-982.

Krechel, S. W., & Bildner, J. (1995). CRIES: A new neonatal postoperative pain measurement score-initial testing of validity and reliability. *Paediatric Anaesthesia, 5,* 53-61.

Lambert, S. (1996). The effects of hypnosis/guided imagery on the post-operative course of children. *Developmental and Behavioral Pediatrics, 17,* 307-310.

Lindh, V., Wiklund, U., Blomquist, H. K., & Hakansson, S. (2003). EMLA cream and oral glucose for immunization pain in 3-month-old infants. *Pain, 104,* 381-388.

Long, C. O. (2005). Infobytes: From the internet to informatics. Seeking out pain management resources. *Nursing, 35,* 74-75.

Luffy, R., & Grove, S. K. (2003). Examining the validity. Reliability and preferences of three pediatric pain measurement tools in African-American children. *Pediatric Nursing, 29,* 54-59.

Lyon, V. B. (2005). Approaches to procedures in neonates. *Dermatologic Therapy, 18,* 117-123.

Manworren, R. C. B. (2001). Unacceptable pain levels. *American Journal of Nursing. 102,* 75-77.

Manworren, R. C. B., & Hynan, L. S. (2003). Clinical validation of FLACC: Preverbal patient pain scale. *Pediatric Nursing, 29,* 140-146.

Mawhorter, S., Daugherty, L., Ford, A., Hughes, R., Metzger, D., & Easley, K. (2004). Topical vapocoolant quickly and effectively reduces vaccine-associated pain: Results of a randomized, single-blinded, placebo-controlled study. *Journal of Travel Medicine, 11,* 267-272.

McCaffery, M., & Pasero, C. (1999). *Pain clinical manual* (2nd ed.). St. Louis: Mosby.

McCarthy, P., Chammas, G., Wilimas, J., Alaoui, F. M., & Harif, M. (2004). Managing children's cancer pain in Morocco. *Journal of Nursing Scholarship, 36,* 11-15.

McCleary, L., Ellis, J., & Rowley, B. (2004). Evaluation of the pain resource nurses' role: A resource for improving pediatric pain management. *Pain Management Nursing, 5,* 29-36.

Merkel, S., Voepel-Lewis, T., & Malviya, S. (2002). Pain assessment in infants and young children: The FLACC scale: A behavioral tool to measure pain in young children. *American Journal of Nursing, 102,* 55-58.

O'Brien, L., Taddio, A., Ipp, M., Goldbach, M., & Koren, G. (2004). Topical 4% amethocaine gel reduces the pain of subcutaneous measles-mumps-rubella vaccination. *Pediatrics, 114,* e720-e724.

Pasero, C. (2004). Pain relief for neonates. *American Journal of Nursing, 104,* 44-47.

Pasero, C., & McCaffery, M. (2005). No self-report means no pain-intensity rating. *American Journal of Nursing, 105,* 50-54.

Pietila, A., & Polkki, T. (2003). Hospitalized children's descriptions of their experiences with post-surgical pain relieving methods. *International Journal of Nursing Studies, 40,* 33-44.

Polkki, T. (2002). Nurses' perceptions of parental guidance in pediatric surgical pain relief. *International Journal of Nursing Studies, 39,* 319-327.

Rawlings, D., Miller, P., & Engel, R. (1980). The effect of circumcision on transcutaneous Po2 in term infants. *American Journal of Diseases of Children, 134,* 676-678.

Rusy, L. M., & Weisman, S. J. (2000). Complementary therapies for acute pediatric pain management. *Pediatric Clinics of North America, 47,* 589-599.

Savedra, M. C., Holzemer, W. L., Tesler, M. D., & Wilkie, D. J. (1993). Assessment of postoperative pain in children and adolescents using the Adolescent Pediatric Pain Tool. *Nursing Research, 42,* 5-9.

Savedra, M. C., Tesler, M. D., Holzemer, W. L., & Ward, J. (1992). *Adolescent and pediatric pain tool: User's manual.* San Francisco: University of California, San Francisco, School of Nursing.

Savedra, M. C., Tesler, M. D., Holzemer, W. L., Wilkie, D. J., & Ward, J. (1989). Pain location: Validity and reliability of body outline markings by hospitalized children and adolescents. *Research in Nursing and Health, 12,* 307-314.

Savedra, M. C., Tesler, M. D., & Wegner, C. (1988). How adolescents describe pain. *Journal of Adolescent Health Care, 9,* 315-320.

Schechter, N. L. (1988). An approach to the child with pain. *Patient Care, 3,* 116-131.

Schechter, N. L., Berde, C. B., & Vaster, M. V. (Eds.). (2003). *Pain in infants, children and adolescents* (2nd ed.). Philadelphia: Lippincott Williams & Wilkins.

Simons, J., & Roberson, E. (2002). Poor communication and knowledge deficits: Obstacles to effective management of children's post-operative pain. *Journal of Advanced Nursing, 40,* 78-86.

Skidmore-Roth, L. (2005). *Mosby's drug guide for nurses* (6th ed.). Philadelphia: Mosby.

Spagrud, L., Piira, T., & Von Baeyer, C. (2003). Children's self-report of pain intensity. *American Journal of Nursing, 103,* 62-64.

Stanford, E. A., Chambers, C., & Craig, K. D. (2005). A normative analysis of the development of pain-related vocabulary in children. *Pain, 114,* 278-283.

Stevens, B., Gibbins, S., & Franck, L. S. (2000). Treatment of pain in the neonatal intensive care unit. *Pediatric Clinics of North America, 47,* 633-650.

Stevens, B., Yamada, J., Beyene, J., Gibbins, S., Petryshen, P., Stinson, J., Narciso, J. (2005). Consistent management of repeated procedural pain with sucrose in preterm neonates: Is it effective and safe for repeated use over time? *Clinical Journal of Pain, 21,* 543-548.

Taddio, A., Soin, J. H. K., Schuh, S., Koren, G., & Scolnik, D. (2005). Liposomal lidocaine to improve procedural success rates and reduce procedural pain among children: A randomized controlled trial. *CMAJ: Canadian Medical Association Journal, 172,* 1691-1694.

Thompson, D. (2005). Utilizing an oral sucrose solution to minimize neonatal pain. *Journal for Specialists in Pediatric Nursing, 10,* 3-10.

Venes, D., Thomas, C. L., & Taber, C. W. (Eds.) (2005). *Tabers cyclopedic medical dictionary*. Philadelphia: FA Davis.

Voepel-Lewis, T., Merkel, S., Tait, A. R., Trzcinka, A., & Malviya, S. (2002). The reliability and validity of the Face, Legs, Activity, Cry, Consolability observational tool as a measure of pain in children with cognitive impairment. *Anesthesia & Analgesia, 95,* 1221-1229.

Von Baeyer, C. L., Marche, T. A., Rocha, E. M., & Salmon, K. (2004). Children's memory for pain: Overview and implications for practice. *Journal of Pain, 5,* 241-249.

Von Hulle, J., & Denyes, M. (2004). Relieving children's pain: Nurses' abilities and analgesic administration practices. *Journal of Pediatric Nursing, 19,* 40-50.

Wang, X., Tang, J., Zhao, M., Guo, H., Mendoza, T., & Cleeland, C. (2003). Pediatric cancer pain management practices and attitudes in China. *Journal of Pain Symptom Management, 26,* 748-759.

White, K., Coyne, P., & Patel, U. (2001). Are nurses adequately prepared for end-of-life care? *Journal of Nursing Scholarship, 33,* 147-151.

Willis, M., Merkel, S., Voepel-Lewis, T., & Malviya, S. (2003). FLACC behavioral assessment scale: A comparison with the child's self-report. *Pediatric Nursing, 29,* 195-199.

World Health Organization Expert Committee. (1998). *Cancer pain relief and palliative care in children*. Geneva, Switzerland: World Health Organization.

Zeltzer, L. G., Tsao, J. C., Stelling, C., Powers, M., Levy, S., & Waterhouse, M. (2002). A phase one study on the feasibility and acceptability of an acupuncture/hypnosis intervention for chronic pediatric pain. *Journal of Pain and Symptom Management, 24,* 437-446.

Zempsky, W. T., Cravero, J. P, Committee on Pediatric Emergency Medicine, & Section on Anesthesiology and Pain Medicine (2004). Relief of pain and anxiety in pediatric patients in emergency medical systems. *Pediatrics, 114,* 1348-1356.

Zisk, R. Y. (2003). Our youngest patient's pain—From disbelief to belief? *Pain Management Nursing, 4,* 40-51.

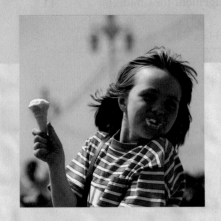

CHAPTER **16**

The Child With an Infectious Disease

Learning Objectives

After studying this chapter, you should be able to:
- Analyze the infectious process.
- Compare the modes of transmission of infectious diseases.
- Analyze the pathophysiology, clinical manifestations, complications, and nursing management of childhood infectious diseases.
- Analyze the pathophysiology, clinical manifestations, complications, and nursing management of sexually transmissible diseases.
- Use the nursing process to describe the nursing care of a child with an infectious disease.

Definitions

antitoxin A particular kind of antibody produced by the body in response to the presence of a toxin.
epidemiology The study of health, illness, and the factors that determine health and illness in a selected population.
exanthem An eruption or rash on the skin.
host The organism from which a parasite obtains its nourishment.
immune globulin Vaccine made from the pooled blood of a large number of people to ensure a broad spectrum of antibodies.
immunity Resistance of the body to the effects of a harmful organism or its toxin.
infection Condition resulting from invasion of the body by pathogenic or nonpathogenic organisms, such as bacteria, viruses, protozoa, helminths, or fungi.

inflammation A tissue response to injury or destruction of cells.
pathogen A disease-producing microorganism.
prodrome The initial stage of a disease; symptoms indicating an approaching disease.
toxin A poison produced by pathogenic microorganisms.
vector A carrier that transfers an infective agent from one host to another.
virulence Strength of effect produced by a pathogenic organism.

Electronic Resources

Additional information related to the content in Chapter 16 can be found on:

the interactive companion CD-ROM
- Audio Glossary
- NCLEX Review Questions

or the companion website at *evolve*
http://evolve.elsevier.com/james/ncoc
- NCLEX Review Questions
- WebLinks

CLINICAL REFERENCE

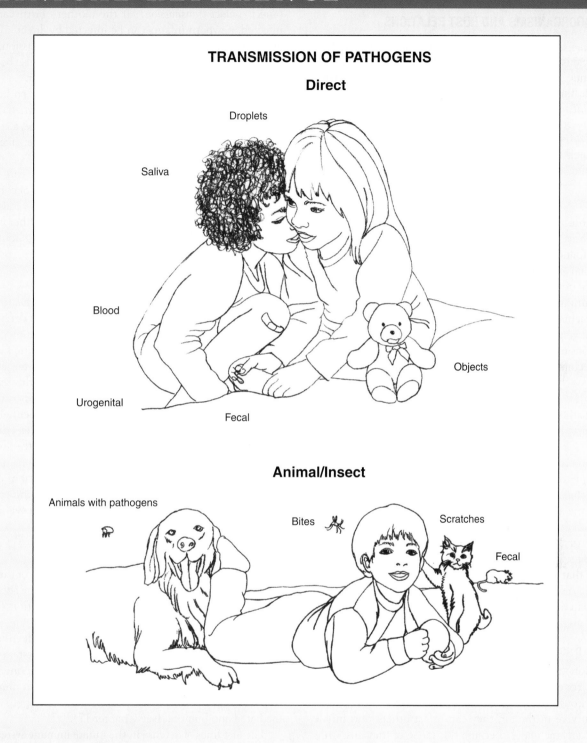

TRANSMISSION OF PATHOGENS

Direct

Droplets

Saliva

Blood

Urogenital

Fecal

Objects

Animal/Insect

Animals with pathogens

Bites

Scratches

Fecal

REVIEW OF DISEASE TRANSMISSION

Microorganisms exist throughout the environment. Most are harmless residents and a normal part of human flora. An organism that invades body tissue, causing tissue damage and disease, however, is a pathogen. For pathogens to invade a host, they must breach the normal host defenses, either by attaching to or penetrating the host. The power of these pathogens, known as their *virulence*, depends on their ability to overcome the host defense mechanisms. Thus a highly virulent organism can cause disease with relative ease.

Microorganisms can have one of several relations with the host: *commensalism, mutualism,* or *parasitism.* Those that cause infectious disease are classified into five types: bacteria, viruses and rickettsiae, fungi, protozoa, and helminths.

Exogenous pathogens are transmitted from outside the body to the host by various mechanisms. Exogenous organisms exist in contaminated air, food, water, and body fluids and on objects contaminated by these substances. *Endogenous pathogens* are found within the human body. Microorganisms (normal flora) exist on the skin and in the nose, mouth,

MICROORGANISMS AND HOST RELATIONS

Commensalism: host provides shelter and food for the organism; organism retains the ability to exist independently (e.g., nonpathogenic bacteria living in human intestines).

Mutualism: host provides shelter and food for the organism; both benefit.

Parasitism: host provides shelter and food; the parasite benefits, but the host may be harmed (e.g., a tapeworm living at the expense of its human host).

gastrointestinal tract, and urogenital tract. For example, *Staphylococcus epidermidis* inhabits the skin, and *Escherichia coli* is found in the intestines. These microorganisms are beneficial and play an important role in the body's defenses. They help prevent virulent pathogens from colonizing by maintaining an acidic pH environment to discourage pathogen attachment, taking up epithelial space to prevent growth of pathogens, and stimulating the immune system. However, situations may arise in which these normally benign organisms become virulent and harmful to the host.

Chain of Infection

For a pathogen to maintain its infectious state, it must be transmitted to another host. Certain factors and conditions must be present for a disease (infection) to begin. These components and their relations are often referred to as a *chain of infection*. The major variables in the chain of infection include the agent (organism), reservoir (environment in which the agent exists and multiplies), portal of exit (route by which the agent leaves the host), transmission mode, portal of entry (route by which the agent enters the new host), and host susceptibility (internal and external environmental factors that increase or decrease the likelihood the host will develop disease). Changes in any one variable result in a change in the presence, intensity, and frequency of the entire infectious disease process.

Transmission of Pathogens

Infection transmission occurs through several modes, or routes. For example, pathogens from the respiratory tract are shed through sneezing, coughing, and talking. If the pathogens survive in the air, they can infect others who inhale them (*airborne route*). Because this mode of transmission is relatively uncontrollable, infections can easily be spread in crowded conditions.

Pathogens may also be shed through fecal matter. When personal hygiene is poor and handwashing is not routinely practiced, pathogens have ample opportunities to enter through the mouth (*fecal-oral transmission*). Unclean hands can also contaminate food, which is then ingested.

In the urogenital tract, pathogenic transmission does not generally occur through infected urine. Rather, sexual activity involving direct mucosal contact is the most common means of transmission of sexually transmissible diseases (STDs)

(*direct contact transmission*). If the mother's birth canal is infected, newborn infants can be infected by direct contact during birth. Saliva is another avenue of transmission, as is direct contact with infected skin. Pathogens can also be present in breast milk and can infect a nursing infant.

A tick, mosquito, mite, or animal can inject pathogens into the skin and blood of the host. Organisms carried in this way are considered to be *vector borne*. For example, a certain species of mosquito carries the malaria parasite; likewise, certain bats carry the rabies microorganism.

Contamination by blood of an infected host can occur through transfusions, blood products, and the use of contaminated needles (*direct inoculation*). A pregnant woman can transmit such pathogens through the placenta. Other modes of transmission also exist, such as through spores found in soil (e.g., tetanus).

Epidemiologic Investigations

Epidemiology is the study of the distribution of health and illness within a population and the factors that determine the population's health status. Recently, epidemiologic efforts have focused on identifying health-promoting factors, not just disease prevention (Stanhope & Lancaster, 2003). Nurses may not realize they are contributing to this process when they gather patient history information as part of the nursing assessment process. The data nurses collect help the entire health care team identify, treat, and prevent disease processes as well as promote health. Moreover, the specific steps of the epidemiologic process mirror the steps in the nursing process and include defining the condition; determining the condition's natural history; identifying critical control points; and designing, implementing, and evaluating control strategies.

INFECTION AND HOST DEFENSES

The first stage of *infection* begins with *colonization* of the host by the pathogen. Microorganisms invade either by adhering to tissues or by invading cells. Initially, replication of the pathogen does not cause tissue damage and colonization can occur without development of a clinical infection. As the host "recognizes" the invasion, the defense system—the immune response—is activated. The two components of the immune response are the innate, nonspecific immune response and the adaptive, specific immune response: cell mediated and humoral (see Chapter 17).

The first lines of defense in the innate immune system are the skin and intact mucous membranes. The skin serves as a barrier, preventing colonization of most pathogens. The acid secreted in sweat and by sebaceous glands inhibits pathogenic invasion. Smooth muscle contraction and ciliary actions, such as those seen in bladder and bowel emptying and coughing and sneezing, remove pathogens mechanically. Physical and chemical barriers are provided by mucus production by goblet cells in mucous membranes. Nevertheless, the innate system may be unable to prevent the invasion. *Phagocytosis,* the process by which phagocytic cells digest and thereby destroy foreign microorganisms, can be overwhelmed. Large numbers of pathogens or their *toxins* can inhibit phagocytosis. When this process occurs, the *adaptive immune system* is activated. This system "recognizes" and responds to pathogens by destroying them. The adaptive immune system "imprints" on these pathogens so that if the body encounters them again, the response will be rapid and specific.

IMMUNITY

Immunity is the body's resistance to the effects of harmful agents. It occurs as an antigen-antibody reaction that takes place whenever a foreign agent or its toxins enter the bloodstream. Immunity can be either active or passive (see Chapter 17).

Some childhood diseases have been significantly reduced and some nearly eliminated through the administration of vaccines producing active or passive immunity. A variety of preparations of disease-specific vaccines can accomplish active or passive immunity (see Chapter 4). Vaccines also can produce artificially active or artificially passive immunity, including the following:

- *Live or attenuated vaccines:* vaccines that have had their virulence (potency) diminished so as not to produce a full-blown clinical illness. In response to vaccination, the body produces antibodies and causes immunity to be established (e.g., measles vaccine).
- *Killed or inactivated vaccines:* vaccines that contain pathogens made inactive by either chemicals or heat. These vaccines, which are noninfectious, cause the body to produce antibodies. Their disadvantage is that they elicit a limited immune response from the body; therefore several doses are required (e.g., Salk polio, rabies, and pertussis vaccines).
- *Toxoids:* bacterial toxins that have been made inactive by either chemicals or heat. The toxins cause the body to produce antibodies (e.g., diphtheria and tetanus vaccines).
- *Human immune globulin:* a vaccine made from the pooled blood of many people. Large numbers of donors are used to ensure a broad spectrum of antibodies. This type of vaccine provides antibodies for a variety of diseases, including measles, rubella, and infectious hepatitis. Disease-specific immune globulin vaccines are also available and are obtained from donors known to have high blood titers of the desired antibody. Examples include hepatitis B immune globulin (HBIG), rabies immune globulin (RIG), and varicella-zoster immune globulin (VZIG). A disadvantage of human immune globulin is that it offers only temporary passive immunity.
- *Animal serums (antitoxins):* vaccines derived from the serum of immunized animals. Antitoxin vaccines are used to stimulate production of antibodies. Examples include hepatitis, chickenpox, rabies, diphtheria, smallpox, cytomegalovirus (CMV) infection, botulism, snake bites, and spider bites. Animal serums have the disadvantage of being foreign substances, which may cause hypersensitivity reactions. Thus a history (including questions about asthma, allergic rhinitis, urticaria, and previous injections of animal serums) and skin sensitivity testing should always precede vaccine administration.

Infectious diseases are a major reason health care is sought for infants and children. Although most infections are not life threatening, fatal complications can develop. The infant or child with an immature or compromised immune system is at increased risk for developing life-threatening complications. Moreover, a child's illness directly affects the family and caregivers. Absence from work for the parent of a sick child can threaten job security, and the accompanying missed income can be devastating for both single- and two-income families.

Nurses play a major role in preventing pediatric infectious diseases and decreasing the incidence of disability and death in both community and hospital settings. Regardless of their clinical setting, nurses must be able to confidently recognize the sometimes subtle signs and symptoms of infectious diseases in children and initiate appropriate treatment and nursing care. Nurses must also provide education about accessing appropriate community resources and limiting exposure of other children and community members. For example, in the community-based setting, the consequences of an unrecognized case of meningococcemia can be devastating and deadly. In the hospital setting, relatively mild diseases, such as chickenpox, may pose potentially fatal problems for the immunosuppressed child.

In addition, because of the growing number of uninsured and underserved children in the United States, nurses may be the first and sometimes only health care professionals to evaluate and treat children in community-based settings. School nurses are frequently required to notify parents and caregivers when their children have been exposed to infectious diseases. Figure 16-1 illustrates an example of a notification letter from a school nurse written to inform parents and caregivers about an exposure to fifth disease. Regardless of the particular type of infection, underlying principles of nursing care are similar.

VIRAL INFECTIONS

Viruses are small parasitic organisms with unique characteristics that cause them to be quite different from other organisms. They contain only one type of nucleic acid—either deoxyribonucleic acid (DNA) or ribonucleic acid (RNA)—that prevents them from reproducing on their own. Instead, a host cell is needed to allow the virus to replicate.

The replication process begins with the virus first attaching itself to a host cell. After the initial attachment, a virus must invade the interior of the cell. Replication of the virus's nucleic material begins after the envelope and capsule (capsid) are shed and the nucleic material of the virus is released into the cell; the host cell then assists in the formation of the necessary nucleic material. New capsules are then formed and released into the host's cells. The infected host cell can respond to the viral invasion by cell death (lysis)

Text continued on p. 426

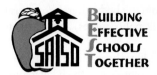

San Angelo Independent School District

HEALTH SERVICES

Ph: (915) 657-4049   Fax: (915) 657-4087

Susan Schultz, RN, BSN
Coordinator of Health Services

Dear Parent/Guardian:

Several students in our school district have been diagnosed as having Fifth Disease (Erythema Infectiosum). This is caused by a virus and can cause outbreaks, particularly among children, because the individual is infectious before symptoms appear. Symptoms are mild and it is usually recognized by a rash appearing on the cheeks resembling a "slapped cheek." There may also be a lacy rash on the trunk, arms and legs. Sometimes these characteristics are preceded by a low-grade fever, which lasts 5-7 days. No treatment is necessary. Children are no longer contagious and do not need to be excluded from school once the rash occurs.

Fifth Disease is generally a very mild disease. Please contact your primary care provider immediately if:

1. The rash becomes itchy

2. Your child develops a fever over 101°

3. You feel your child is getting worse

4. You have other concerns or questions

If you, a family member or a friend are pregnant and are exposed to a child with Fifth Disease, contact your obstetrician.

Please contact the nurse at your school if you have further questions or concerns.

Sincerely,

Susan Schultz, RN

Susan Schultz, RN, BSN
Coordinator, Health Services

Dr. Joe E. Gonzales, Superintendent • 1621 University • San Angelo, TX 76904

FIG 16-1   **Sample notification letter from school nurse informing parents and caregivers about an exposure to an infectious disease.** *(Courtesy Susan Schultz, RN, BSN, Coordinator, Health Services, San Angelo Independent School District, San Angelo, TX.)*

NURSING CARE PLAN

The Child With an Infection in the Community Setting

Focused Assessment

Most infectious diseases in children and adolescents are self-limiting and rarely produce devastating illness. Thorough assessment is always indicated. Many infectious diseases present with subtle and common symptoms that may be difficult to identify. Because rashes and fever can suggest many diseases, the nurse needs to begin assessment by obtaining a complete history, including the following:

- Child's usual state of health
- Any signs or symptoms of developing disease (prodrome)

- Vital signs, especially body temperature
- Description of any skin lesions or rashes, including color, pattern, or shape; size, location, and distribution on the body; presence of any drainage or erythema; and any changes since initial eruption
- Any other family members, classmates, or playmates (friends) showing signs or symptoms
- Any other associated signs or symptoms (arthralgia, malaise, pain, vomiting, headaches)
- Medications or treatments tried and their effects

NURSING DIAGNOSIS   Risk for Infection (cross contamination of self or others) related to insufficient knowledge of how to avoid the spread of infectious disease.

EXPECTED OUTCOMES   The child's contacts will:
- Remain free from symptoms of infection.

The child will:
- Demonstrate absence of infection, as evidenced by vital signs within normal parameters, resolving lesions with no evidence of complications, and age-appropriate behavior.

The family and child (if age-appropriate) will:
- State symptoms of infectious disease and symptoms of secondary bacterial infections and appropriate disease-containment procedures.
- Verbalize understanding of written health promotion information, including contact information for local community agencies and resources.

Intervention	*Rationale*
1. Teach the family and child (if old enough) the symptoms of secondary bacterial infections and complications of infectious diseases that should be promptly reported to their primary medical caregiver (e.g., redness, warmth, swelling, tenderness or pain, new onset of drainage or change in drainage from wound, increase in body temperature, malaise, abdominal pain, vomiting or diarrhea, enlarged glands, changes in skin lesions including sores or wounds that do not heal). Provide the phone number or numbers to call if complications occur.	1. Promptly recognizing and reporting signs and symptoms of secondary bacterial infections can decrease complications.
2. Teach the family and/or child about the underlying concepts of infection transmission, including how and to whom the infection should be reported (e.g., airborne, fecal-oral, direct contact).	2. Understanding promotes cooperation with infectious disease containment issues, policies, and procedures (e.g., child with chickenpox may not return to daycare or school until the sixth day after onset of rash or sooner if all lesions have dried and crusted).
3. Emphasize the importance and encourage the child and family to complete the full course of any prescribed medication unless experiencing adverse side effects.	3. Providing information and encouragement promotes understanding and compliance.
4. Role model and teach the child and family preventive behaviors, such as frequent and meticulous handwashing, disposal of used dressings to prevent spread of infectious disease to others, proper disposal of tissues, and coverage of the mouth when coughing or sneezing. (Follow Standard Precautions guidelines during any contact with blood, mucous membranes, nonintact skin, or any body substance except sweat; use goggles, gloves, and gowns when appropriate; help the family access these if needed.)	4. Demonstration and active participation are more effective teaching strategies (parents will retain better if they "use" the instruction) than verbal instruction alone. Nurses must assume all people are carrying blood-borne pathogens such as HIV or hepatitis B or C (HBV, HCV). Standard Precautions apply to everyone.

Continued

5. Review the infectious disease and the child's plan of care, including provision of rest, proper nutrition, fever control, and when the child can resume normal activities. Provide written information about any instructions for treatment, medication administration, and any scheduled follow-up visits with the child's primary health care provider.

5. Providing information and encouragement promotes understanding and adherence to the treatment plan.

6. Provide health promotion information and education (e.g., routine immunization schedule) for the family and child. Refer the family and child to local community agencies (health departments, clinics) as appropriate.

6. Maintenance of an ongoing relationship with a primary care provider provides continuity of care and methods for access to care for the well and sick child as needed.

Evaluation

- Have any of the child's contacts contracted the disease?
- Is the child free from infection, afebrile, and exhibiting age-appropriate behavior?
- Have the parents and/or child verbalized an understanding of the infectious process and disease-containment procedures?

- Is the family and/or child cooperative with written contact information and accessing follow-up and preventive health care and appropriate community resources?

NURSING DIAGNOSIS   Ineffective Health Maintenance related to insufficient knowledge about how to obtain needed information about infectious disease and its management.

EXPECTED OUTCOMES   The child and family will:
- Follow an agreed-on infection control plan.
- Meet goals for health maintenance.

Intervention

1. Teach the family or child skin and wound assessment and ways to monitor for signs and symptoms of infection, complications, and healing.

Rationale

1. Early assessment and intervention help prevent serious problems from developing (e.g., sexually transmissible diseases [STDs] in the adolescent girl can result in sterility). Providing information and encouragement promotes understanding and adherence to the treatment plan, thus preventing secondary infection or adverse consequences from infection.

2. Provide written instructions for comfort and prevention of secondary infections according to the child's specific condition.

2. Providing information and encouragement promotes understanding and cooperation with treatment plan.

3. Teach adolescents health-promoting and health-seeking behaviors to reduce the risk of contracting an STD; this includes a description of the direct contact transmission mode and recognition of complications.

3. Providing information and establishing a nonjudgmental environment encourage future health-seeking behaviors. Long-term complications (e.g., sterility, chronic abdominal pain from untreated STDs) can be avoided with early detection, treatment, and appropriate follow-up care.

4. Screen for STDs as appropriate (e.g., a prepubescent girl with signs and symptoms of an STD). For prevention, teach children that it is not all right for someone to look at or touch their private parts.

4. Signs and symptoms of problems with the genital area (itching, rash, vaginal or penile discharge) should always be explored by the nurse with a complete history of symptoms to rule out sexual abuse, especially in prepubescent children. Sexual abuse of a child is a reportable offense and must be ruled out.

5. Provide health promotion information and education (e.g., Papanicolaou [Pap] smears for sexually active adolescents). Refer the family or child to local community agencies (health departments, clinics) as appropriate.

5. Maintenance of an ongoing relationship with a primary care provider provides continuity of care and methods for access to care for health promotion and disease prevention.

NURSING CARE PLAN—cont'd

Evaluation

- Do the child and family follow the agreed-on infection control plan?

- Are they able to meet goals for health maintenance?

NURSING DIAGNOSIS Risk for Ineffective Thermoregulation related to infection.

EXPECTED OUTCOME The child will:
- Be afebrile and exhibit age-appropriate behavior.

Intervention	*Rationale*
1. Teach the family and/or child normal temperature parameters (e.g., what is a fever?) and temperature-monitoring techniques (see age-appropriate guidelines in Chapter 13).	1. Consistently monitoring and promptly recognizing and reporting signs and symptoms of hyperthermia complications promote prevention and early intervention and can decrease the potential for disability or death.
2. Teach the family the signs and symptoms of hyperthermia and the complications that should be promptly reported to their primary medical caregiver (e.g., visual disturbances, headache, nausea, vomiting, muscle flaccidity, absence of sweating, delirium, coma). Provide the phone number(s) to call if complications occur.	2. Understanding promotes cooperation and adherence to the child's treatment and care plan.
3. Teach the family about specific comfort measures (cool environment, light clothing, tepid baths) and medication administration (antipyretics) for hyperthermia. Teach parents the appropriate use of antipyretics (see Chapter 13). Use acetaminophen and/or ibuprofen as directed for fever control. Avoid aspirin products because of possibility of developing Reye syndrome (see Chapter 28). Check all over-the-counter medicines to be sure they do not contain aspirin or salicylate. Provide written information that explains the various preparations available (drops, suspension, chewable tablets, suppositories) and the appropriate dose and administration intervals for their child. For example: The dosage of acetaminophen for a 25-lb child is 160 mg. Any one of the following can be given every 4 to 6 hours as needed for fever or discomfort: • Concentrated drops (80 mg in 0.8 mL) = 0.8 mL + 0.8 mL = 1.6 mL • Suspension liquid (80 mg in ½ tsp) = 1 tsp • Children's chewable (80 mg each) = 2 tablets • Suppository (80 mg each) = 2 suppositories	3. Appropriate teaching promotes cooperation and adherence to the child's treatment and care plan and can also prevent innocent administration of readily available, potentially lethal over-the-counter medication to a child with a viral illness. Providing information and creating awareness of self-care steps the family or adolescent can take to maintain or regain health promotes positive health-seeking behaviors. Because of the many different formulations of both of these over-the-counter medications, parents are frequently confused and inadvertently give the wrong dose, sometimes resulting in overdosing or underdosing and inadequate fever control.
4. Teach the importance of and specific techniques for maintaining adequate hydration (monitoring the child's intake and output, frequently offering cool liquids, ice pops).	4. Maintaining adequate hydration will help maintain a normal body temperature. An elevated temperature is associated with increased metabolism and fluid use.
5. Provide written health promotion information and education about fever control and when to access the health care system.	5. Maintenance of an ongoing relationship with primary care provider provides continuity of care and methods for access to care for well and sick child care as needed.

Evaluation

- Has the child maintained a body temperature within normal parameters?

- Is the child's behavior within normal parameters for age?

Continued

NURSING CARE PLAN—cont'd

NURSING DIAGNOSIS   Fatigue related to discomfort associated with the infectious disease.

EXPECTED OUTCOME   The child will:
* Experience an increase in comfort level and energy, as evidenced by verbalization of decreased discomfort, a relaxed body posture, ability to rest appropriately, decreased crying and irritability, and an interest in age-appropriate activities.

Intervention	*Rationale*
1. Teach and provide written information for comfort measures (cool environment; tepid, not cold, baths; lightweight, cool clothing); treatments (monitoring the child's temperature); or medication administration (antipruritics, antipyretics).	1. Appropriate teaching promotes cooperation and adherence to the child's treatment and care plan. Maintaining adequate hydration will help maintain a normal body temperature. An elevated temperature is associated with increased metabolism and fluid use.
2. Encourage bed rest and energy conservation during healing process of an infectious disease. Provide age- and energy-appropriate activities depending on the child's level of wellness.	2. Bed rest and energy conservation promote the healing process and provide comfort to children with discomfort, pain, or fever. Nonpharmacologic techniques, such as distraction, provide diversion.
3. Teach the child's family personal hygiene principles to promote the healing process and maintain health after the infectious disease process. Keep the child's skin clean, and change linens and clothing frequently. Wash clothes and linen in mild detergent, and double rinse.	3. Clean clothing helps prevent the spread of secondary infections. Double rinsing reduces the potential irritants in the clothing, thereby minimizing irritation.

Evaluation

* Has the child experienced relief from discomfort by demonstrating a relaxed body posture, an interest in age-appropriate play, and verbalization of an increased comfort level?

NURSING DIAGNOSIS   Social Isolation related to the confinement for the duration of the communicable disease.

EXPECTED OUTCOMES   The child and family will:
* Describe the reasons for isolation and will incorporate the resulting restrictions into their home management.

The child will:
* Participate in age-appropriate activities within the restrictions imposed.

The family will:
* Contact community agencies for assistance if appropriate.

Intervention	*Rationale*
1. Encourage the family and child to maintain contact with friends and family by telephone, mail, or e-mail while the child is isolated.	1. Maintaining contact with family and friends helps the family adjust to activity limitations, reduces boredom, and provides emotional support.
2. Provide written information to family about age- and energy-appropriate activities.	2. Providing age-appropriate activities prevents boredom and promotes normal growth and development.
3. Provide information about community resources for respite and/or sick child care.	3. Providing resources for family provides caregiver relief and could result in the family's primary wage earner (especially in single-parent families) returning to work with less loss of income and decrease in the financial burden on the family.

Evaluation

* Can the child and family describe the reasons for the isolation, and have they incorporated the appropriate restrictions?
* Is the child engaging in age-appropriate activities?

* Is the family able to maintain contact with family and friends?
* Have support systems been mobilized, both within the family and in the community?

and destruction, or the infected cells can remain alive and continue to function while new viral particles are slowly released. This slow release occurs in an asymptomatic person who is a carrier of the virus. Some viruses are selective about the cells to which they attach. For example, the human immunodeficiency virus (HIV) prefers to attach to the T cell.

A virus can also invade a host and remain dormant until a trigger stimulates the virus to begin replicating. Many triggering factors are not fully understood. However, some triggers have been identified. An example of this triggering effect is the effect of stress in herpes simplex (a viral disease), resulting in the formation of cold sores.

Nursing Considerations for the Child With a Viral Exanthem Infection

An *exanthem* is an eruption or rash on the skin. Several childhood infectious diseases are characterized by rashes with distinctive characteristics. Nurses need to be aware that rashes have more than one characteristic and obtain a detailed history of the characteristics of the rash, including its onset, initial location, and progression as well as any associated physical signs or symptoms. Specific characteristics of the rash should be documented, including color, elevation, pattern or shape, size (in centimeters), location and distribution on the body, and any drainage. Vital signs, including temperature, should be taken and recorded. Also record the child's general state of health, any recent exposures to illnesses, and any prescribed or over-the-counter medications and treatments taken and their results. The child's eyes, ears, nose, and throat should be examined for signs of inflammation, swelling, and secretions. Auscultate the lungs for any abnormal sounds, and palpate the child's spleen, liver, and lymph nodes, documenting any enlargement or tenderness.

Children with typical uncomplicated viral exanthems are usually cared for at home. Hospitalization is indicated when complications occur. High-risk (immunosuppressed) children and children with an infectious disease should not be cared for by the same nurse to prevent any possible cross transmission by the nurse.

Whether the child is cared for in the hospital or at home, any specific isolation measures will be determined by the child's specific infectious disease process.

Rubeola (Measles)

Causative agent: RNA virus
Incubation period: 8 to 12 days from exposure to onset of symptoms
Infectious period: Ranges from 3 to 5 days before the appearance of the rash to 4 days after appearance of the rash
Transmission: Transmitted between individuals by direct contact with infectious droplets or less frequently by airborne spread
Immunity: Natural disease or live attenuated vaccine
Season: Late winter and spring

Manifestations

The measles virus enters the body and slowly spreads. Respiratory symptoms appear after an average of 10 days. Typically, children have a prodrome period with fever and "the three Cs" (coryza [profuse runny nose], cough, conjunctivitis) that lasts between 1 and 4 days. Children are usually quite ill during this time. *Koplik spots* appear approximately 2 days before the appearance of the rash (Fig. 16-2). Koplik spots are small, blue-white spots with a red base that cluster near the molars on the buccal mucosa. These spots last approximately 3 days, after which they slough off. As prodromal symptoms reach a peak, the exanthem appears and is characterized by a deep-red, macular rash that usually begins on the face and neck and spreads down the trunk and extremities to the feet. The rash blanches easily with pressure and will gradually turn a brownish color. The duration of the rash is approximately 6 to 7 days.

A partially immune child, such as an infant younger than 9 months who has passively acquired maternal antibodies or a child given immune gamma-globulin, may contract modified measles. The prodromal period is shorter and the symptoms are minimal, with few to no Koplik spots. The rash progression follows the pattern of regular measles.

Complications

Because of respiratory involvement, secondary bacterial infections such as otitis media, bronchopneumonia, and laryngotracheobronchitis (croup) can occur, especially in infants and younger children. Central nervous system (CNS) complications, including acute encephalitis, are rare but can occur.

Therapeutic Management

The treatment of measles is symptomatic, whether the child is hospitalized or remains at home. If hospitalized, the child will require airborne isolation precautions. During the febrile period, the child should be restricted to quiet activities and bed rest.

The World Health Organization and the United Nations International Children's Emergency Fund recommend administration of vitamin A to all children diagnosed with measles in communities where vitamin A deficiency is a recognized problem or where the measles case fatality rate is 1% or greater. In the United States, low blood levels of vitamin A have been found in children with more severe cases of measles. Although vitamin A deficiency is not recognized as a major problem in the United States, the American Academy of Pediatrics (AAP) (2003f) has recommended that vitamin A supplementation should be considered in the following circumstances:

- Children ages 6 months to 2 years who are hospitalized with complications (pneumonia, croup, diarrhea)
- Children older than 6 months with measles who are not already receiving vitamin A supplementation and who have the following risks: immunodeficiency, evidence of vitamin A deficiency, impaired intestinal absorption, moderate to severe malnutrition, or recent immigration from an area with high mortality from measles

Parenteral and oral formulations of vitamin A are available in the United States. The following are recommended dosages:

- Children 6 months to 1 year of age should receive a single dose of 100,000 IU orally.
- Children 1 year and older should receive a single dose of 200,000 IU orally.
- Additional doses are recommended at 24 hours and again 4 weeks later for children with ophthalmologic evidence of vitamin A deficiency. Vitamin A toxicity is rare and usually associated only with extremely large doses (>1 million IU) (AAP, 2003f).

Children can be protected against measles and other vaccine-preventable diseases by receiving *all* their routine

First day   Third day

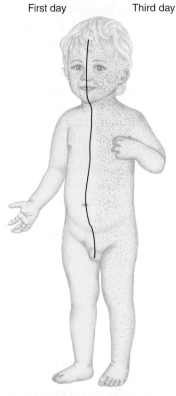

- Preceded by Koplik's spots on buccal mucosa
- Begins behind ears, at hairline, and on upper neck and spreads downward toward feet
- Red, maculopapular rash that gradually turns brownish
- Duration: 6-7 days

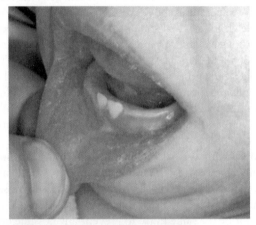

Measles Rash Distribution

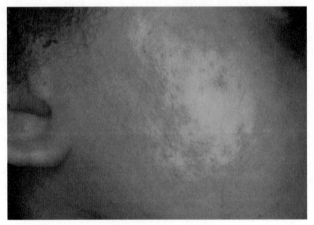

Measles Rash, Dark Skin

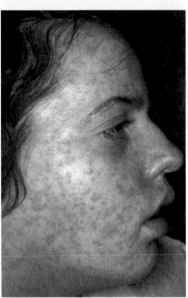

Measles Rash, Light Skin

FIG 16-2 **Rubeola (measles) lesions and rash distribution.** *(Reprinted from Feigin, R. D. & Cherry, J. D. [Eds.]. [1998]. Textbook of pediatric infectious diseases [4th ed.]. Philadelphia: Saunders; Hurwitz, S. [1993]. Clinical pediatric dermatology: a textbook of skin disorders of childhood and adolescence [2nd ed.]. Philadelphia: Saunders.)*

immunizations during their routine well-child check-ups. Two doses of measles, mumps, and rubella vaccine (MMR) are required to be fully protected. The first MMR is recommended routinely at 1 year of age. The second dose of MMR is recommended at 4 to 6 years but may be administered during any visit if at least 4 weeks has

elapsed since the first dose and both doses are administered beginning at or after 12 months of age. Children who have not previously received their second MMR dose should complete the schedule no later than their 11- to 12-year health maintenance visit (Centers for Disease Control and Prevention, 2006).

Rubella (3-Day Measles, German Measles)

Causative agent: RNA virus

Incubation period: 14 to 21 days

Infectious period: Ranges from 7 days before onset of symptoms to 14 days after appearance of the rash

Transmission: Airborne particles or direct contact with infectious droplets, transplacental transmission; small number of infants with congenital rubella continue to shed the virus for months after birth

Immunity: Natural disease or live attenuated vaccine

Season: Late winter and early spring

Manifestations

Rubella is usually a mild disease for children and adults. The virus enters the host, producing a rash after approximately 14 to 16 days. Young children are often asymptomatic until the appearance of the rash. Older children may report profuse nasal drainage, diarrhea, malaise, sore throat, headache, low-grade fever, polyarthritis, eye pain, aches, chills, anorexia, and nausea. Children of all ages usually have impressive posterior cervical, posterior auricular, and occipital lymphadenopathy.

The rash presents as a pinkish rose maculopapular exanthem that begins on the face, scalp, and neck (Fig. 16-3). It spreads downward to include the entire body within 1 to 3 days. As the rash spreads to the trunk, the rash on the face begins fading. Petechiae (spots), which are reddish and pinpoint, may occur on the soft palate. Their appearance is sometimes referred to as *Forschheimer's sign*.

Complications

Rubella has relatively few complications. The most common are arthritis and arthralgia, which occur more often in adult women than in children or adolescents. Mild thrombocytopenia may also occur but is usually self-limiting and of short duration. A rare complication is encephalitis, which is usually less severe than measles-related encephalitis.

The importance of recognizing and respecting this viral illness is not the morbidity of the disease itself but rather the consequences that can occur to a fetus during maternal infection. The most devastating form of rubella is congenital rubella that occurs after maternal infection. Congenital rubella can result in growth retardation, cataracts, retinopathy, and cardiac anomalies. The most common complication is sensorineural deafness. Some manifestations may not be present at birth but may develop at a later time, including mental retardation, diabetes mellitus, thyroid disorders, and encephalopathy. The risk for damage to the developing fetus is greatest in the early weeks of the pregnancy. Kenner and Lott (2003) report when infants born to mothers who were infected during the first 8 weeks of gestation were monitored for 4 years, 85% were affected. When infection occurred in

First day   Third day

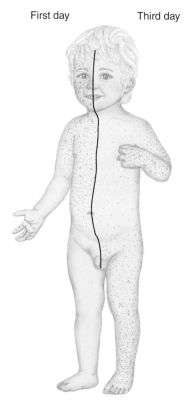

- Begins on face, neck, and scalp and spreads downward to entire body; fades on face as it spreads to trunk
- Pinkish, maculopapular
- Reddish, pinpoint petechiae may occur on soft palate (Forschheimer's sign)

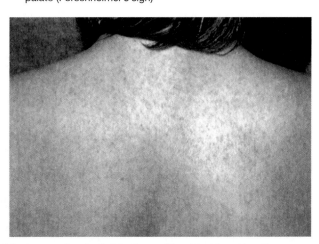

German Measles Rash Distribution

FIG 16-3 **Rubella (German measles) lesions and rash distribution.** *(Reprinted from Hurwitz, S. [1993]. Clinical pediatric dermatology: a textbook of skin disorders of childhood and adolescence [2nd ed.]. Philadelphia: Saunders.)*

the ninth through twelfth week of gestation, the risk of infant anomalies dropped to 52% and the risk of defects virtually disappeared after the twentieth week of gestation.

Therapeutic Management

Treatment is generally supportive and symptomatic, with the disease being self-limiting. Children with postnatal rubella should be excluded from school or childcare for 7 days after the onset of the rash. Infants with congenital rubella should be considered contagious until they are at least 1 year old unless nasopharyngeal and urine cultures are repeatedly negative for the rubella virus. Parents should be made aware of the potential risks their infants pose for pregnant women with whom they come into contact (AAP, 2003j). Primary prevention of rubella can be accomplished through administration of the rubella vaccine in combination with measles and mumps vaccine (MMR), as previously discussed.

CRITICAL TO REMEMBER
Congenital Rubella
The rubella virus can cross the placenta and infect the fetus, causing fetal death or abnormalities.

Erythema Infectiosum (Parvovirus B19, Fifth Disease)

Causative agent: Parvovirus B19
Incubation period: 4 to 14 days but can be up to 21 days
Infectious period: Unknown but thought to extend from the prodromal period until the rash appears
Transmission: Airborne particles, respiratory droplets, blood, blood products, transplacental transmission
Immunity: Natural disease is thought to provide antibodies for immunity
Season: Winter and spring

This disease is most common in children ages 5 to 14 years but may also occur in adults.

Manifestations

Fifth disease is a relatively mild systemic disease. Typically the child may appear well but presents with an intense, fiery red, edematous rash on the cheeks, which gives a "slapped cheek" appearance (Fig. 16-4) or the history of a rash that "comes and goes." Before the appearance of the rash, many children are asymptomatic or have nonspecific symptoms such as headache, runny nose, malaise, and mild fever. Approximately 1 to 4 days after the facial rash appears, an erythematous, maculopapular, lacy rash appears on the trunk and extremities. The rash fades with a central clearing area, resulting in a lacy appearance. The rash may last 2 to 39 days and reappear when aggravated by environmental factors, such as heat, exercise, warm baths, rubbing of the skin, and stress.

Complications

Because the disease is mild complications are not usually reported, especially in children. A careful history should be obtained, with an emphasis on identifying any pregnant family members, teachers, or friends to prevent intrauterine infection and death. Pregnant women are at risk for intrauterine infection. Many school districts notify pregnant staff if they have been exposed to a child with fifth disease and recommend that they contact their health care provider. Fifth disease has resulted in fetal death, but parvovirus-associated fetal anomaly has not been established. The risk of fetal death is estimated to be between 2% and 6%, with the greatest risk when infection occurs during the first half of the pregnancy (AAP, 2003d). Parvovirus 19 also can cause a transient aplastic crisis in children with sickle cell anemia and some other forms of hemoglobinopathy.

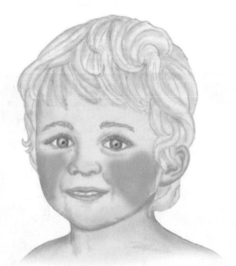

Erythema Infectiosum: "Slapped Cheek" Appearance

- Presents with fiery-red, edematous rash on cheeks—"slapped cheek" appearance
- Followed in 1-4 days by erythematous, maculopapular, lacy rash on trunk and extremities

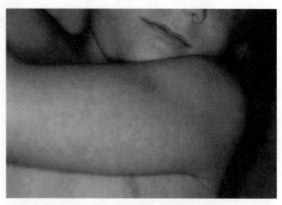

FIG 16-4   **Erythema infectiosum lesions and rash distribution.**   *(Reprinted from Hurwitz, S. [1993]. Clinical pediatric dermatology: a textbook of skin disorders of childhood and adolescence [2nd ed.]. Philadelphia: Saunders.)*

Therapeutic Management

The disease is generally benign and self-limiting. Treatment is symptomatic and supportive.

Roseola Infantum (Exanthem Subitum, Sixth Disease, 3-Day Fever)

Causative agent: Human herpesvirus 6 (HHV-6)

Incubation period: Unknown but estimated to be 9 to 10 days

Infectious period: Unknown but thought to extend from the febrile stage to the time the rash first appears

Transmission: Most likely by contact with secretions (saliva, cerebrospinal fluid [CSF]) of asymptomatic close contacts

Season: Throughout the year without a distinctive seasonal pattern

Manifestations

Roseola was the sixth childhood exanthem identified. Although HHV-6 appears to be the major causative agent, other viruses have been linked to the disease. Most clinical cases of roseola occur in children 6 to 18 months old. The child has a sudden high fever (39.4° to 41.1° C [103° to 106° F]), malaise, and irritability but may remain active and alert. An intermittent or constant fever may persist for 3 to 5 days. The child may also have a mild cough, runny nose, abdominal pain, headache, vomiting, and diarrhea. After 3 to 5 days the fever subsides, and within several hours to 2 days a rash appears. The rash consists of rose-pink maculopapules or macules that blanch with pressure (Fig. 16-5). The rash occurs predominantly on the neck and trunk and may be surrounded by a whitish ring. It normally persists for 24 to 48 hours before fading.

Complications

Complications associated with roseola are uncommon. Seizures related to the high fever may occur. Rare cases of encephalitis, hemiplegia, paresis, and mental retardation have been reported.

Therapeutic Management

Treatment is symptomatic. Family members should be taught about fever control management.

Generally, fever can be controlled with antipyretic medications, tepid sponge baths, decreased clothing, environmental temperatures, and increased fluid intake. Temperature monitoring, medication administration (prescription and over-the-counter), and other comfort measures should be discussed. The nurse should make sure the child's family has access to a thermometer and knows how to use it. In addition, parents should be given information regarding the absolute avoidance of any form of aspirin (including over-the-counter medications containing salicylates) because of

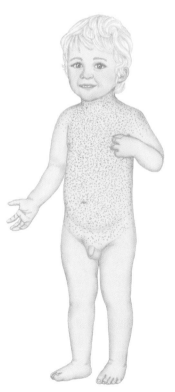

Roseola Infantum Rash Distribution

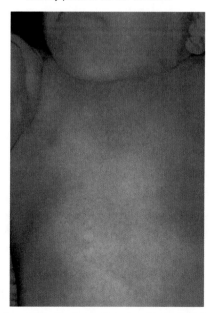

- Rash appears several hours to 2 days after fever subsides
- Erythematous maculopapular or macular, may be surrounded by whitish ring
- Blanches with pressure
- Predominantly on neck and trunk
- Usually persists for 24-48 hours

FIG 16-5 **Roseola infantum lesions and rash distribution.** *(Reprinted from Hurwitz, S. [1993]. Clinical pediatric dermatology: a textbook of skin disorders of childhood and adolescence [2nd ed.]. Philadelphia: Saunders.)*

- For elevated temperature, the child's activity should be restricted to age-appropriate, quiet activities and bed rest. As the fever decreases, the activity level can be gradually increased to a normal level.
- Generally, fever can be controlled with acetaminophen or ibuprofen (no aspirin products because of the possible risk of developing Reye syndrome), sponge baths, decreased clothing, decreased environmental temperature, and increased fluid intake. Bed linens may need to be changed frequently during periods of high fevers. Over-the-counter antipyretic acetaminophen comes in several different formulations. Read the label carefully and ask your primary care provider if you have any questions regarding medication administration. Seizure precautions should be taken if your child has had a seizure previously.
- The amount of skin irritation and discomfort will vary. Lukewarm baths with colloid preparations (Aveeno), oatmeal, or baking soda (½ cup in tub of water) may help relieve itching. Soothing lotions (Lubriderm, Curel, Moisturel) may also provide comfort. Avoid the use of topical corticosteroids unless ordered by your primary care provider. Use superfatted soaps for sensitive skin (Dove, Basis, Neutrogena, Aveeno). Fingernails should be short. If the child continues to scratch, cotton mittens

or socks can be applied to the child's hands. Integrity of the skin must be maintained to prevent any secondary infections. If secondary infections occur, antibiotic therapy may be necessary.
- Administer antihistamines or antipruritics as prescribed.
- Dress your child in lightweight clothing that is not irritating. Avoid wool and scratchy materials.
- Coughing can be managed with cool humidification of the room and antitussives.
- For arthralgia, antiinflammatory medications may be used. Involvement of weight-bearing joints may warrant bed rest.
- Some viral exanthems cause photophobia. In such cases, keeping the room dimly lit or providing sunglasses for the child may be helpful. If the child has conjunctivitis, secretions or crusts should be removed with tepid water and a clean cloth to prevent contamination.
- Fluid intake is important for successfully managing febrile stages of the disease. Encourage your child to drink cool liquids frequently. If the child's mucous membranes are involved, soft, bland foods may be beneficial.
- As your child progresses through the stages of illness, diversional activities will be necessary during the period of isolation. Choose activities that your child likes and can participate in without becoming unduly tired.

---

the potential risk of developing Reye syndrome (see Chapter 28). Anticipatory guidance should include alerting the parent to the possibility of febrile seizures (caused by the sudden high fevers) and teaching about seizure precautions (especially if the child has a history of previous febrile seizures) (Box 16-1).

Parents' understanding of the care necessary for their child is important. Parents need to be educated about immunizations and measures to prevent the spread of infectious diseases. They should also be taught to recognize the signs and symptoms of complications so they can seek medical treatment when warranted. Providing parents with written instructions that they can refer to at home may prove helpful.

Enterovirus (Nonpolio) Infections (Coxsackieviruses, Group A and Group B), Echoviruses, and Enteroviruses

Causative agent: RNA viruses including 23 group A coxsackieviruses (types A1 to A24, except type A23), six group B coxsackieviruses (types B1 to B6), 31 echoviruses (types 1 to 33, except types 10 and 28) and four enteroviruses (types 68 to 71).
Incubation period: Usually 3 to 6 days
Infectious period: Unknown but fecal viral excretion and transmission can continue for several weeks after the onset of infection.

Transmission: Spread by fecal-oral and possibly by oral-oral (respiratory) routes
Season: In temperate climates infections are most common in the summer and fall but no seasonal pattern is evident in the tropics.

Manifestations

Common presentations in both infants and children include nonspecific febrile illnesses with a wide variety of respiratory, gastrointestinal, cardiac, neurologic, skin, oral, and eye signs and symptoms.

A frequently seen pattern of illness in young children is hand-foot-and-mouth disease, caused by coxsackievirus A16 or other enteroviruses. Inflammation and lesions in the mouth (Fig. 16-6), on the palms of the hands, and the soles of the feet are the hallmarks of this syndrome, along with mild fever. Lesions become vesicular over the course of several days and usually resolve by 1 week. If lesions are particularly widespread in the oropharynx, the child may refuse to eat or drink; the potential for dehydration exists in very young children.

Complications

Although each of these groups of symptoms can be associated with different enteroviruses, complications can occur from specific strains. These complications include acute hemorrhagic conjunctivitis (coxsackievirus A24 and enterovirus

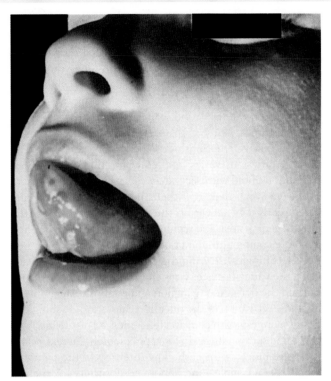

FIG 16-6 **Coxsackievirus mouth lesions.** *(Reprinted from Fegin, R., Cherry, J., Demmler, G., & Kaplan, S. [2004]. Textbook of pediatric infectious diseases. Philadelphia: Elsevier.)*

70), encephalitis (enterovirus 71), petechial exanthema and meningitis (echovirus 9), myopericarditis (coxsackieviruses B1 to B5), and neonatal complications (AAP, 2003c).

Therapeutic Management

No specific therapy exists for enteroviral infections. However, enteric precautions are indicated for any affected hospitalized infant or child. Parents and caregivers should be given educational information regarding the importance of handwashing and personal hygiene, especially after diaper changes and trips to the bathroom. Additionally, in immunocompromised children and for life-threatening infections in the neonate, intravenous immunoglobulin that contains antibodies specific to the causative virus has shown promise for limiting the course of severe infections (AAP, 2003c; Abzug, 2004).

Management of hand-foot-and-mouth disease is symptomatic. The parent can provide comfort and pain relief with acetaminophen and frequent administration of cool liquids. Milk-based ice cream is especially palatable. Extensive oropharyngeal lesions that prevent adequate oral intake can be treated with a salt and water mouth rinse or a topical solution of equal parts lidocaine gel, Benadryl liquid, and Maalox (mixed by prescription) either applied directly to lesions or used as a mouthwash.

Nursing Considerations

The nurse needs to obtain a detailed history of the onset of symptoms with a focused assessment on the particular body systems involved. The child's vital signs (including temperature) should be monitored and documented.

Community-based children with an enterovirus infection can be challenging because of the wide variety and degree of signs and symptoms. Parents and caregivers should be given educational information about disease transmission, supportive care, school or daycare attendance policies, any available community resources (sick child care), and specific guidelines to determine when they should seek additional medical care if their child's symptoms increase or their child's condition deteriorates (high fever, nonresponsiveness, decreased urinary output).

Mumps

Causative agent: Paramyxovirus
Incubation period: Usually 16 to 18 days but may extend to 25 days
Infectious period: From 7 days before swelling to 9 days after onset
Transmission: Airborne droplets, salivary secretions, possibly urine
Immunity: Natural disease or live attenuated vaccine
Season: Late winter and spring

Manifestations

Prodromal manifestations include fever, muscular pain, headache, and malaise. The classic clinical sign of parotid glandular swelling (parotitis) often follows these, although a substantial number of individuals have no such swelling. When parotid swelling does occurs, it may be accompanied by fever.

Complications

Mumps generally affects the salivary glands but can involve multiple organs. The most common complication is aseptic meningitis, with the virus identified in the CSF. Signs of CNS involvement include nuchal rigidity, lethargy, and vomiting. Children with these manifestations usually completely recover. A less common CNS complication is meningoencephalomyelitis manifested by fever, headache, nausea, vomiting, nuchal rigidity, and changes in sensorium. These complications are treated symptomatically and generally have an uneventful recovery period.

The potential complication of most concern to parents is orchitis (inflammation of a testis). Orchitis is a common complication in adolescents, with sterility occurring rarely. Although deafness does not occur frequently, mumps can cause hearing impairment. Other rare complications include pancreatitis, nephritis, thyroiditis, myocarditis, arthritis, and mastitis.

Therapeutic Management

Uncomplicated mumps may require only symptomatic care. Droplet Precautions are indicated until 9 days after the onset of the parotid swelling. Parents should be given educational information regarding the absolute avoidance of any form of aspirin (including over-the-counter medications containing salicylates) because of the potential risk of developing Reye syndrome.

Orchitis requires bed rest, intermittent application of ice packs, emotional support, and diversional activities. CNS complications require neurologic evaluations and vital sign measurement as indicated by the child's condition when the complications require hospitalization.

Nursing Considerations

The nurse needs to obtain a history of the onset of symptoms, examine the child's ears and throat, and perform a neurologic assessment. The child's vital signs (including temperature), usual state of health, and characteristics of the lymph nodes in the neck should be documented. In boys, an examination of the testes should be included in the initial assessment.

Typically, children with mumps are not hospitalized unless they have complications. Therefore good handwashing technique should be taught to the child, the family, and close contacts to prevent transmission. Hospitalized children are placed in isolation according to the facility's policies.

Primary prevention of mumps can be accomplished through administration of the mumps vaccine in combination with measles and rubella vaccine (MMR), as previously discussed.

Varicella-Zoster Infections (Chickenpox, Shingles)

Causative agent: Varicella-zoster virus
Incubation period: 10 to 21 days
Infectious period: 1 to 2 days before the onset of rash until all lesions are dried (crusted over), usually 5 to 7 days
Transmission: Direct contact, droplet, airborne particles
Immunity: Natural disease of varicella; same virus causes zoster, and child may contract zoster at a later time; varicella vaccine
Season: Late winter through early spring

Primary infection with the varicella-zoster virus causes chickenpox. Before a vaccine was available, this was one of the most common childhood diseases in children 5 to 9 years old. Zoster (shingles), which is the reactivation of the latent varicella-zoster virus, occurs most frequently in the elderly population but can occur also in children, especially adolescents and young adults. Generally, varicella and zoster in children are not life threatening. However, varicella is a major risk factor for severe invasive group A streptococcal disease (AAP, 2003m). Secondary bacterial infections, frequently group A streptococcal disease, can occur and are considered life-threatening complications. Severe, sometimes fatal cases of varicella have been reported in otherwise healthy children who have received short courses of steroids (for asthma and other chronic illnesses) before becoming infected with the disease. Children who are immunosuppressed and contract varicella are at risk for developing serious, potentially fatal complications.

Manifestations

Varicella. During the 24 to 48 hours before the appearance of lesions, symptoms may include a slightly elevated body temperature, malaise, and anorexia. The macular rash generally first appears on the trunk and scalp (Fig. 16-7). The lesions may be in various stages of development, beginning as macular and developing into a red papular rash. The lesions soon become teardrop vesicles with an erythematous base. The vesicles then become pustular, after which they begin to dry and develop a crust. The lesions appear in crops, beginning on the trunk and scalp and moving (sparsely) to the extremities. These crops of lesions generally appear in three successive eruptions over a period of 3 to 4 days. The number of lesions varies from child to child, but children in the household with secondary cases generally have more extensive rashes than does the child with the primary case. The lesions may appear on the mucous membranes in the mouth, genital area, and rectum. Second attacks are rare and are more common in immunocompromised children.

Zoster (Shingles). During the primary infection with varicella, the varicella-zoster virus enters the sensory nerve ending and the dorsal root ganglion and establishes a latent infection. Activation of the infection causes zoster (shingles). Zoster manifests with pain and tenderness along the involved nerve and surrounding skin for approximately 2 weeks before the appearance of the rash. The intensity of the pain can range from an unpleasant, abnormal sensitivity to touch to burning, tingling, itching, sharp knifelike prickling, or even deep pain. Unilateral crops of lesions appear along the nerve. These macules and papules progress through the same stages as varicella. There may be enlargement and tenderness of the lymph nodes in the same region.

Zoster is generally thought to be a disease of elderly people, but it can also occur in children, especially those who are immunocompromised, have HIV infection, were exposed in utero, or were infected before their second birthday (AAP, 2003m).

Complications

The most common complication of varicella-zoster virus infection is secondary bacterial infection of the skin lesions. Staphylococci and group A beta-hemolytic streptococci are the usual causative agents. CNS complications have been associated with mild to severe varicella infections. Encephalitis with ataxia, tremor, and nystagmus may occur in the first week. The prognosis is generally good unless CNS involvement is severe—usually manifested by convulsions and coma. Children with these complications may have future CNS difficulties, including seizures, mental retardation, or behavior disorders.

Varicella pneumonia, a common complication in adults, rarely occurs in children. Reye syndrome has been known to occur after varicella infection (see Chapter 28). Corneal involvement can occur if lesions involve the eye.

Complications of zoster are rare but may involve the same difficulties with secondary infections that occur with varicella.

Parents should be given educational information regarding the absolute avoidance of any form of aspirin (including over-the-counter medications containing salicylates) because of the potential risk for developing Reye syndrome.

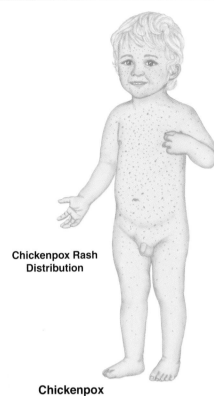

- Macular rash 24-48 hours after slight fever, malaise, anorexia
- Lesions appear in "crops," first on trunk and scalp, then moving sparsely to extremities; may appear in mucous membranes (mouth, genital area, rectum)
- Generally three successive eruptions over 3-4 days
- Lesions begin as a macular rash, develop into a red papular rash, then move quickly into teardrop vesicles with erythematous base; vesicle becomes pustular and begins drying, and a crust develops
- Rash varies from child to child

Chickenpox Rash Distribution

Chickenpox

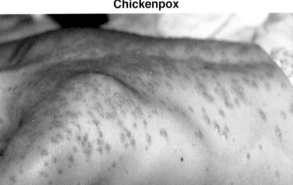

Shingles

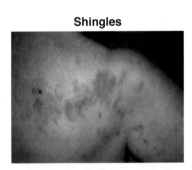

FIG 16-7 **Chickenpox and shingles lesions and rash distribution.** *(Reprinted from Moschella, S. L. & Hurley, H. J. [1992]. Dermatology [3rd ed.]. Philadelphia: Saunders [shingles photo].)*

Therapeutic Management

Treatment is symptomatic and supportive for the healthy child. Oral acyclovir is not recommended for routine use in otherwise healthy children with varicella. However, varicella and zoster can be treated with intravenous (IV) or oral antiviral drugs (acyclovir being the most common). The decision to use these medications, along with the duration and route, is individually determined by the primary health care provider. Antiviral drugs have a limited "window of opportunity" to affect the infection's outcome and, if administered, should be started as soon as symptoms are present. Oral acyclovir should be considered for those at high risk for moderate to severe varicella (those older than 12 years, persons with chronic illnesses, and persons receiving long-term aspirin therapy or short courses of steroids) (AAP, 2003m).

In the hospital setting, children with varicella or zoster infections should be placed in strict isolation. The nurse assigned should not simultaneously care for immunocompromised clients to decrease the risk of varicella transmission. Early initiation of IV acyclovir therapy (within 24 hours of onset of rash) is recommended for immunocompromised clients.

For children at high risk for developing severe varicella or zoster, varicella-zoster immune globulin (VZIG) should be given within 96 hours for maximal effectiveness. Immunocompromised children, newborns of mothers having active varicella infections at the time of birth or with siblings at home with active varicella infection, and HIV-positive children are considered to be at increased risk.

Primary prevention of varicella includes screening and administering the vaccine at routine well-child visits. Varicella vaccine (one dose) is recommended at any visit on or after the first birthday for all susceptible children without a reliable history of actual disease or immunization. Susceptible children 13 years or older should receive two doses of vaccine given at least 4 weeks apart (CDC, 2006).

Nursing Considerations

The nurse needs to obtain a detailed history of the onset of symptoms and examine the skin lesions. The appearance, distribution, and stages of the lesions should be documented. The child's vital signs (including temperature) and a general physical assessment should also be noted.

Community-based care of children with varicella can be challenging. Parents and caregivers should be given educational information regarding disease transmission, supportive care, school or daycare attendance policies, and any available community resources (sick child care). Missing work can be especially difficult for single, working parents and can affect their job security.

Hospitalized children with varicella infections are placed in strict isolation, which requires that the nurse wear a mask, gown, and gloves for all contacts with the child. All contaminated materials must be bagged and labeled before reprocessing. Hands should be washed after contact with the child and before contact with another client. Hospitalized children who have been exposed to varicella should be kept in strict isolation for 8 to 21 days after the onset of rash in the infected individual. At birth, neonates with mothers who have active varicella infections should be placed in strict isolation. In addition, Airborne Precautions and Contact Precautions should be in effect for children with zoster infections.

The nurse needs to educate parents of children with varicella about skin care to prevent secondary bacterial infections and emphasize the importance of absolute avoidance of any form of aspirin (including over-the-counter medications containing aspirin). Resource identification to provide a plan for access to acute or follow-up well-child visits should be discussed, along with any community childcare alternatives.

CRITICAL TO REMEMBER
Varicella and the Immunocompromised Child

Immunocompromised children who contract varicella may have large hemorrhagic lesions. Primary varicella pneumonia is a frequent complication. Some children may develop an acute form of varicella with disseminated intravascular coagulation (DIC) that is fatal, often before antiviral therapy can be started.

Smallpox (Variola)

Worldwide eradication of smallpox (variola) was declared in 1980. The last naturally occurring smallpox case was in Somalia in 1977, followed by two cases attributable to laboratory exposure in 1978. The United States discontinued routine childhood immunization against smallpox in 1971 and routine immunization of health care workers in 1976. The U.S. military continued to immunize military personnel until 1990. Since 1980, the vaccine has been recommended only for people working with nonvariola orthopoxviruses (AAP, 2003l). Increasing concern has been raised that the virus and the expertise to use it could be used as a bioterrorism weapon.

This concern is the reason that smallpox is included in this discussion of infectious diseases.

Causative agent:	Smallpox (variola virus)
Incubation period:	Averages 12 days, with a range of 7 to 17 days
Infectious period:	As the rash in the mouth breaks down, a skin rash becomes visible and the client is the most contagious during this time and remains contagious until all of the lesions have scabbed over and the scabs have dried and fallen off.
Transmission:	Transmitted through direct and prolonged face-to-face contact with an infected person; less commonly, smallpox can also be transmitted through contact with contaminated objects
Immunity:	Live vaccinia virus
Season:	Not confined to a particular season

Manifestations

Smallpox is an acute, contagious disease that can sometimes be fatal. The prodrome of the illness begins abruptly with fever, malaise, headache, muscle pain, prostration, and often nausea, vomiting, and backache. Fever is usually at least 101° F (38.3° C) but can be higher. The client usually appears quite ill. At approximately day 4 of the illness, the first signs of rash appear as red spots in the mouth and on the tongue, which develop into sores and break open. As the rash in the mouth breaks down, a skin rash becomes visible. The client is most contagious during this time. The skin rash typically appears first as a few macules, known as "herald spots," on the face, particularly on the forehead. Within a few days of rash onset, clients with smallpox develop a distinctive generalized vesicular rash (Fig. 16-8). By the third or fourth day of illness, the temperature usually falls and the client feels somewhat better. The rash progresses into pustules, which then form scabs. By the end of the second week, the pustules have all scabbed over. The person continues to be contagious until all the scabs have dried and fallen off.

Therapeutic Management

Variola virus can be detected in vesicular or pustular fluid by culture or polymerase chain reaction assay. Variola diagnostic testing is conducted only at the Centers for Disease

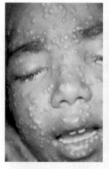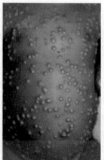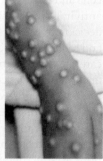

FIG 16-8   Lesions of variola are at the same stage of development on all body parts. *(Reprinted from Centers for Disease Control and Prevention. [2002]. Evaluating patients for smallpox. Atlanta, GA: Author.)*

Control and Prevention (CDC) but may be expanded in the future. If a client is suspected of having smallpox, Standard Precautions, Contact Precautions, and Airborne Precautions should be implemented immediately and the state and local health departments should be alerted at once. Postexposure immunization (within 3 to 4 days of exposure) provides some protection against disease and significant protection against a fatal outcome. A smallpox immunization plan has been implemented in the United States (*www.bt.cdc.gov*). The plan does not include immunizing children. However, children may be at risk of complications related to coming in contact with vaccinated individuals (Onieal, 2003). Additional information can be found at the CDC's website (*www.cdc.gov/smallpox*).

Cytomegalovirus

Causative agent: Human cytomegalovirus (CMV)
Incubation period: Unknown, except for 3 to 12 weeks after blood transfusions and 4 weeks to 4 months after organ (tissue) transplantation
Transmission: Saliva, urine, blood, semen, cervical secretions, breast milk, organ transplants
Immunity: None, although CMV immune globulin, used only in seronegative transplant clients, has had moderate effectiveness
Season: Can occur during any season

CMV infection is a common cause of congenital infection in infants. A child may become infected with the virus during the prenatal, perinatal, or postnatal period. Congenital infection has a wide variety of manifestations but those who are affected are usually asymptomatic. Some congenitally infected infants who are asymptomatic at birth are later found to have hearing loss or a learning disability. Approximately 10% of infants with congenital CMV infection have profound involvement evident at birth (AAP, 2003a).

Signs and symptoms in the infant can include jaundice, lethargy, seizures, enlarged spleen and liver, petechial rash, respiratory distress, microcephaly, and intracerebral calcifications. Complications include mental retardation, hearing loss, blindness, and learning disabilities. Some of these conditions may not be apparent until the child is older. The child can continue to shed the virus for up to 5 years.

During the postnatal period, the infant may acquire CMV from a maternal or nonmaternal source. The virus can be transmitted through the breast milk of an infected mother. Blood transfusions, which can be numerous in the premature infant, can also be a source of CMV infection. Children who are not infected congenitally or perinatally often acquire the virus during their toddler or preschool years. Because of sexual activity, the teen years may be another period of acquisition. Affected adolescents are generally asymptomatic but can present with a mononucleosis-like syndrome with fever, hepatosplenomegaly, mild hepatitis, and absence of heterophil antibody.

Therapeutic Management

Specific therapy for CMV is still in the experimental stage but includes immunoglobulin therapy, vaccines, and chemotherapy. Intravenous immunoglobulin therapy provides passive immunity to at-risk infants but not to those already infected. Limited research has been performed on two live attenuated vaccines that could, theoretically, prevent vertical transmission of CMV. Chemotherapy offers the most promise for treatment of neonatal CMV infection, but it has so far not been shown to be clinically effective or improve outcomes (Kenner & Lott, 2003). An antiviral drug (ganciclovir) has been beneficial in treating acquired or recurrent retinitis in the immunocompromised client. Experience with this drug in the pediatric population has been limited, and more research is needed (Kenner & Lott, 2003). Toxicity, associated immunosuppression, and neurologic sequelae are major concerns with use in the neonatal population (Stagno, 2004).

Nursing Considerations

The nurse needs to obtain a history of the child's symptoms and possible exposures. Children with congenitally acquired CMV may develop a wide range of manifestations, so nursing care will vary according to the child's specific needs. When developmental delays, mental retardation, neurologic deficits, or hearing losses occur, the nurse can help coordinate the health care team's efforts to meet the child's needs. Parents will need support and education in caring for a child with developmental deficits. The nurse will play a key role in identifying the need for referral and any resources available in the community, including parental support groups.

Epstein-Barr Virus (Infectious Mononucleosis)

Causative agent: Epstein-Barr virus (EBV, a herpeslike virus)
Incubation period: 4 to 7 weeks
Infectious period: Unknown; the virus is commonly shed before clinical onset of disease until 6 months or longer after recovery; asymptomatic carriers are common
Transmission: Saliva, intimate contact, blood
Immunity: Natural disease
Season: Can occur during any season

The primary sites of infection in mononucleosis are the epithelial cells and the B lymphocytes. EBV has been well recognized as the causative agent in infectious mononucleosis. It has also been associated with other diseases, especially outside North America. It has been identified as a co-factor in Burkitt lymphoma, often seen in Africa, and in cases of nasopharyngeal carcinoma seen in China and Southeast Asia. EBV alone cannot cause the lymphomas or the carcinoma, but it acts in association with other factors.

Manifestations

Infectious mononucleosis typically occurs in otherwise healthy individuals, most commonly in older children and young adults. Clinical signs include fever, exudative pharyngitis, lymphadenopathy, and hepatosplenomegaly. The severity of the clinical signs can range from asymptomatic and mild to severe and fatal. Some children develop a maculopapular rash. Children may report malaise, headache, fatigue, nausea, and abdominal pain. The acute illness usually lasts 2 to 4 weeks and is followed by a gradual recovery. The prognosis is generally excellent if no complications occur.

Complications

The risk of splenic rupture associated with EBV infection occurs most frequently during the second week of the illness. Swelling of the pharynx and tonsils can be severe enough to compromise respiration. The outcome of these complications depends on the severity of the infection and the course of the complications.

Therapeutic Management

The illness is generally self-limiting; therefore treatment is supportive. Complications are addressed with appropriate medical treatment. Steroids may be indicated for tonsillar swelling associated with complications. Strenuous physical activity and contact sports should be avoided during the acute illness and as long as the spleen is enlarged to minimize the risk of splenic rupture.

Nursing Considerations

The history should include presenting signs and symptoms. Physical examination of the pharynx should be performed, with documentation of any redness or swelling. Note any rashes, including a description of their distribution and appearance. The spleen and liver should be evaluated for enlargement. The child's body temperature should be recorded and nutrition and hydration status evaluated.

Because EBV infection is self-limiting, nursing care is mainly supportive. Most children are cared for at home. Hospitalization for hydration therapy may be necessary if the child is unable to swallow. Care in both settings involves bed rest, hydration, and relief of discomfort.

Education and reinforcement regarding the importance of avoiding contact sports, including roughhousing at home with family and friends, should be given to older children or adolescents to help them understand the risks involved (Box 16-2).

Poliomyelitis

Causative agent:	Poliovirus (an enterovirus)
Incubation period:	3 to 6 days for abortive poliomyelitis; 7 to 21 days for paralytic poliomyelitis
Infectious period:	Shortly before and after the onset of clinical illness when the virus is in the throat and in high concentration in feces; the virus is shed in the pharynx for 1 week after onset and in the feces for several weeks to months
Transmission:	Fecal-oral, oral-oral (respiratory)
Immunity:	Inactivated poliovirus (IPV) and oral poliovirus (OPV) vaccines
Season:	Summer and fall

The three forms of poliovirus are Brunhilde, Lansing, and Leon. The virus, which enters the body through either ingestion or inhalation, has a preference for the CNS, affecting only certain cells, such as the anterior horn cells of the spinal cord.

Manifestations

The initial signs and symptoms of poliomyelitis are fever, malaise, anorexia, nausea, headache, sore throat, and generalized abdominal pain. This stage, referred to as *abortive poliomyelitis*, is generally so mild and brief that it may go unrecognized. The second stage is *nonparalytic poliomyelitis*. The signs and symptoms are the same as in the abortive stage but are more intense, with soreness and stiffness of the trunk, neck, and limbs. Without further progression to paralysis, the temperature will fall and the meningeal symptoms will decrease. Recovery may begin within 3 to 10 days. In the third (*paralytic*) stage, flaccid paralysis is the most obvious sign. With paralysis, muscles deteriorate and atrophy. Distribution of signs and symptoms may be asymmetric. Generally, the lower extremities and the large muscle groups are affected. Cervical involvement, called *bulbar polio*, may also occur. This is the most life-threatening form of polio because it affects the respiratory and vasomotor centers. Damage to the respiratory center can result in inability to breathe.

BOX 16-2	**PARENTS WANT TO KNOW** How to Care for the Child With Infectious Mononucleosis

- Bed rest is indicated during the acute stage of the illness.
- Acetaminophen may be useful in controlling discomfort caused by fever and enlarged tonsils.
- Activity restrictions include no contact sports of any type, including no roughhousing at home with siblings or friends, to protect the child's enlarged spleen from rupture. With improvement in clinical signs, the child should be allowed to resume normal activities as tolerated.
- The parents and child need to be prepared for a slow and gradual recovery. Fatigue may continue, necessitating a gradual return to school activities.
- Hydration should be monitored and encouraged.

- In children with a sore throat, soothing liquids, bland foods, and milkshakes may be better tolerated than a regular diet.
- Anxiety related to missed schoolwork should be anticipated. Home-bound school programs should be arranged if the child will be absent from school for a prolonged period.
- The parents should have an understanding of the disease and the usual course of recovery. They may need support in exploring options for caring for their child during a lengthy recovery period, including referrals for alternative childcare arrangements, to decrease lost income and maintain job security.

Therapeutic Management

Poliomyelitis has no specific treatment. Rather, treatment is specific for each child's needs. For paralytic polio, hospitalization may be necessary. In children with respiratory paralysis, mechanical ventilation is necessary. Physical therapy helps maintain muscle integrity and prevent contractures.

The prognosis for polio depends on the severity of nerve damage. Months may pass before the full extent of damage and the probable degree of recovery can be determined.

Primary prevention of polio includes administering the vaccine at routine well-child visits. The two types of poliovirus vaccines are inactivated vaccines (IPV) given parenterally (subcutaneously [SC] or intramuscularly [IM]) and live-virus vaccine (OPV) given orally. Inactivated poliovirus vaccine is now the only poliovirus vaccine available in the United States. OPV can cause vaccine-associated paralytic poliomyelitis (VAPP). Before the expanded use of IPV vaccine in the United States, the overall risk of VAPP was approximately 1 case in 2.4 million doses of OPV vaccine distributed. The AAP (2003g) recommends a four-dose, all-IPV vaccine schedule for routine immunization of all infants and children in the United States (see Chapter 4 and Evolve website).

Nursing Considerations

The nurse should obtain a history of symptoms along with an immunization history. A family immunization history is also important to identify any unvaccinated adult family members.

In immunocompromised children, a history of contact with anyone who recently received the active polio vaccine is important to obtain. The child should be observed for neurologic symptoms and respiratory distress, and the body temperature should be recorded.

The primary focus of nursing should be preventive because the development and use of the polio vaccine have drastically reduced the incidence of polio. In addition, the AAP (2003g) recommends the use of inactivated poliomyelitis vaccine for the prevention of vaccine-acquired poliomyelitis cases.

For the child with paralytic polio, hospitalization may be necessary and nursing care should focus on preventing muscle and skeletal deformities. Active and passive range-of-motion exercises are indicated. Constipation is common, and fluid intake and nutrition should be monitored. If mechanical ventilation is indicated, the nursing care is the same as for any child on ventilatory support.

Nursing care of children with abortive polio focuses on reducing the parents' and child's fear and on minimizing muscular deformities. The child can be treated at home with analgesics, sedatives, and bed rest until the fever subsides. Nonparalytic polio can also be treated at home.

Rabies

Causative agent: Rhabdovirus
Incubation period: 5 days to more than 1 year; incubation can extend to 6 years, but the average is 2 months
Infectious period: 10 days (if the animal is still healthy, rabies is unlikely); however, bats may harbor the virus for a longer period
Transmission: Bites with contaminated saliva, scratches from claws of infected animals, airborne transmission in laboratory settings and in bat-infested caves, transplantation of corneas from undiagnosed donors
Immunity: Human diploid cell vaccine (HDCV)
Season: Can occur during any season

Rabies is caused by a virus that can infect any warm-blooded animal. In the United States, the reservoir consists of skunks, bats, raccoons, foxes, squirrels, and woodchucks. Dogs and cats may also be reservoirs, but the use of animal vaccines makes them a less common source of infection.

Manifestations

The rhabdovirus results in a slowly developing infection. The virus travels up the axons of the motor or sensory neurons to the brain. For this reason, bites that occur on the feet or lower extremities are associated with longer incubation periods than are bites on the face. Incubation periods are shortened in children.

When left untreated, the virus will cause vague signs and symptoms. The child may report not feeling well. The child may have a sore throat, headache, fever, discomfort at the site of the bite, hyperactivity, anxiety, muscle spasms, or convulsions. The decreased ability to swallow results in drooling or aspiration, which explains the use of the term *hydrophobia* in connection with rabies. Once the disease has established itself, it is fatal. Once symptoms appear, the disease generally lasts 5 to 6 days before progressing to death.

Therapeutic Management

The focus of rabies management is preventive and includes educating adults and children to avoid touching and petting strange animals, especially those in unusual settings exhibiting strange behaviors. When an animal bites a child, a determination must be made regarding whether to treat that child. Factors to be considered include the geographic area, type of animal, circumstances of the bite, and the animal's vaccination record. If the animal is available, it can be observed for 10 days or killed for microscopic examination of the brain.

The bite wound should be cleaned with copious amounts of soap and water. Human rabies immune globulin (HRIG) is given. One half of the dose is infiltrated locally around the wound, and the other half is administered intramuscularly. The vaccine (HDCV) should be administered as early as possible after exposure, preferably within 48 hours. The injection is given into the deltoid muscle on days 3, 7, 14, and 28. Rabies vaccine is the only vaccine that can be given after exposure and result in successful vaccination.

Nursing Considerations

A complete history of the event should be obtained, including the type of animal involved, identification of the animal as wild or domestic, immunization record of the animal, and the present location of the animal (if known). This information will determine the course of action. The wound should be examined and a description noted in the child's record.

For the child who will undergo a complete series of vaccinations, the nurse may use a variety of distraction techniques (e.g., counting, singing). Allowing the child to administer injections to a doll may help relieve some anxiety associated with multiple injections. For the older child, an explanation of the injection process and reasons for treatment may be adequate.

Primary prevention of rabies includes anticipatory guidance focusing on teaching children to avoid petting or touching unknown animals.

For the child who develops rabies, nursing actions are supportive, including support of the child and family through the dying process (see Chapter 12). The child is placed in strict isolation, and Standard Precautions are instituted. The family will need support in preparing for the child's inevitable death and in coping with feelings of guilt.

BACTERIAL INFECTIONS

Bacteria are abundant in the environment, yet relatively few cause diseases that have an impact on human beings. Bacteria are organisms that contain both DNA and RNA. They lack a nuclear membrane but have a complex cell wall. The properties of the cell wall determine the bacterium's classification as either gram positive or gram negative. Gram-positive bacteria have a thicker wall that helps resist bile activity, drying, and other environmental factors. Gram-positive bacteria can cause chronic inflammation of dermal tissue, fever, and shock. Gram-negative bacteria have a thinner cell wall.

Outside the cell wall, many bacteria have flagella, which help propel the bacteria through their environment. They may also have pili—rigid projections that assist in attachment to the host cell or other bacteria. The capsules help hide the bacteria's presence from the host and make phagocytosis by the host cell more difficult.

Bacteria excrete toxins. Exotoxins are highly poisonous substances that cause cell damage by cell lysis, inhibition of protein synthesis, or interference with passage of nerve impulses. Endotoxins, which are a portion of the gram-negative cell, cause fever, shock, and disseminated intravascular coagulation (DIC).

CRITICAL TO REMEMBER
Classification of Bacteria

Bacteria are classified by three characteristics:
- Shape (rods or cocci)
- Reaction on Gram stain (positive or negative)
- Ability to grow in the presence of oxygen (aerobic or anaerobic)

Neonatal Sepsis

Neonatal sepsis occurs when bacteria or their poisonous products, known as *endotoxins*, gain access to the bloodstream, causing systemic signs and symptoms. Evaluation of the newborn for the presence of bacterial sepsis is a common occurrence in the newborn nursery and presents challenges for the health care team in both the evaluation and treatment procedures. The challenges are the result, in part, of the varied and frequently nonspecific subtle signs and symptoms of the infant with neonatal sepsis. Available research demonstrates that the rapidity of deterioration in neonates with true sepsis and the success of treatment if instituted early warrant early and aggressive treatment. Early signs of infection must be recognized so that the infection can be diagnosed and appropriate therapy started. Treatment of asymptomatic infants at high risk may also be warranted if clinical judgment determines the benefits are greater than the risk of "watchful waiting." Outcome of neonatal sepsis is improved with early diagnosis and implementation of therapy (Kenner & Lott, 2003).

Etiology

The infant is at risk for sepsis because of a number of maternal, neonatal, and environmental factors (Box 16-3). The microorganisms that cause newborn infection have changed over the past 60 years, and major regional variations exist. Microorganisms commonly identified in early-onset infection include group B streptococcus, other streptococci, and *Escherichia coli*. Common causes of nosocomial infections include coagulase-negative staphylococci, gram negative bacilli, enterococci, *Staphylococcus aureus* and *Candida*. Community-acquired pathogens such as *Streptococcus pneumoniae* and *Escherichia coli* are common late onset pathogens (Stoll, 2004).

Incidence

Before antibiotic use, the mortality rate from bacterial sepsis was 95% to 100%, but early recognition of signs and symptoms, vigorous initiation of antibiotic therapies, and supportive care have reduced the mortality rate to less than

---

PATHOPHYSIOLOGY

NEONATAL SEPSIS

An infection occurs when a susceptible host comes in contact with a potentially pathogenic organism. When the encountered organism proliferates and overcomes the host defenses, infection results. A pathogenic organism (bacteria) can reach the fetus or infant and cause infection in one of three ways: (1) bacteria passing through the maternal bloodstream by way of the placenta (intrauterine infection); (2) perinatal acquisition during labor and delivery (intrapartum infection); and (3) hospital acquisition in the neonatal period (postnatal infection) from the mother, hospital environment, or personnel. Intrauterine infections may result in abortion, stillbirth, and disease present at birth or in the neonatal period. The main goal must be to prevent infections (Stoll, 2004).

BOX 16-3	**Risk Factors for Neonatal Sepsis**

Maternal

Premature or prolonged rupture of amniotic membranes
Chorioamnionitis
Endometritis
Peripartum infection or fever
Urinary tract infection
Leukocytosis
Uterine tenderness
Fetal tachycardia
Precipitous delivery
Prolonged or difficult labor
Abruptio placentae
Colonization of organisms in genital tract
Cardiovascular disease
Poor or no prenatal care
Poor nutrition

Low socioeconomic status
Recurrent abortion
Substance abuse
Premature labor
Foul-smelling amniotic fluid

Neonatal

Prematurity
Perinatal asphyxia
Congenital defects causing an opening in the skin or mucosa
Prolonged hyperalimentation
Concurrent neonatal diseases
Male sex
Low birth weight
Developmental or congenital immune defects
Congenital heart disease

Intracranial bleeding
Difficult or traumatic labor or delivery
Meconium staining
Prenatal or intrapartal stress
Multiple gestation
Immature immune system
Antimicrobial therapies
Galactosemia

Environmental

Exposure to bacteria from caregivers
Exposure to bacteria from contaminated equipment
Invasive procedures (e.g., use of venous or arterial catheters, endotracheal tubes)
Surgical procedures
Resuscitation

50%. However, the infant's survival remains highly variable and dependent upon the organism and underlying or associated conditions. Preterm and sick neonates are at greater risk and have a higher incidence of morbidity and mortality than term healthy neonates (Stoll, 2004).

Manifestations

The early signs and symptoms of sepsis may be vague and nonspecific. Often, the mother or nurse first recognizes that something is wrong or "just not right" but is unable to describe any one specific physical sign or symptom. The infant may have respiratory or gastrointestinal symptoms. Common clinical manifestations of sepsis include the following:

- Temperature instability: hypothermia, hyperthermia
- Lethargy, irritability, poor feeding, change in muscle tone or activity, an abnormal Moro reflex
- Respiratory distress: grunting, flaring, retractions, tachypnea, cyanosis, apnea
- Persistent pulmonary hypertension
- Tachycardia; bradycardia; cold, clammy skin; cyanosis; decreased perfusion; pallor; mottling; hypotension; shock
- Vomiting, increasing gastric residuals, diarrhea, ileus, abdominal distention, bloody stools
- Jaundice, hepatosplenomegaly
- Jitteriness, tremors, high-pitched cry, full or bulging fontanel, decreased response to stimuli (does not respond to parents), seizures
- Petechiae, purpura, rashes
- Hypoglycemia, hyperglycemia
- Metabolic acidosis

Therapeutic Management

The treatment approach used for evaluation of infants for neonatal sepsis is generally called a *sepsis* (or *septic*) *workup*.

The exact management plan or treatment approach varies with each infant, but all are based on assessment of clinical signs, careful history, and appropriate laboratory findings. Diagnostic tests, including cultures (blood, urine, nasopharyngeal, CSF [if indicated]) and additional blood tests (complete blood count [CBC] with white blood cell count [WBC] and complete differential count, C-reactive protein [CRP]) are obtained, and a lumbar puncture is always performed in the symptomatic neonate and may be done in asymptomatic infants if the infant's condition warrants. Neonates with suspected sepsis or meningitis are started on antibiotics as soon as the appropriate cultures and IV access are obtained. Once appropriate cultures have been obtained, antibiotic therapy should be initiated as soon as possible. Ampicillin and an aminoglycoside, usually gentamicin, are one of the combinations that have proved to be a highly effective combination against a majority of causative organisms. Once the pathogen or pathogens are identified and sensitivities identified, antimicrobial therapy is modified accordingly. Aminoglycoside levels should be monitored to avoid toxic levels and long-term side effects (hearing impairment). The duration of antimicrobial therapy depends on the culture results and the infant's response to treatment with most continued for 7 to 10 days (Stoll, 2004).

Specific risk-based guidelines were approved by the Centers for Disease Control and Prevention, the American College of Obstetricians and Gynecologists (ACOG) and the AAP in 1997 and updated in 2002 (CDC, 2002a) to screen for prevention of early-onset group B streptococcal disease in newborns. One of the major recommendations in these guidelines is universal screening of pregnant women for vaginal and rectal group B streptococcal colonization at 35 to 37 weeks. Some women for whom screening is positive for group B streptococci, or who have diagnosed group B streptococcal bacteriuria, will require intrapartum penicillin prophylaxis to reduce exposure for the newborn. These guidelines have resulted in a significant decline in the number of early-onset group B streptococcal cases (approximately 70%) and provide a foundation for the development of uniform approaches in individual institutions caring for mothers and infants in the perinatal period (Kanto & Baker, 2003). The complete CDC and AAP recommendations are available online at http://www.cdc.gov/mmwr/preview/mmwrhtml/rr5111a1.htm.

In all care scenarios supportive measures make up a large part of the treatment of septic infants. Once neonates are symptomatic, they should be treated in an intensive care nursery, with full cardiopulmonary monitoring and respiratory and cardiac support as needed. Monitoring the effectiveness of any therapy is an essential part of the supportive care for the neonate with sepsis. Constant environmental temperature control is essential because the neonate's thermal regulation system is immature. Respiratory support with supplemental oxygen, blood gas and oxygen saturation determinations with subsequent intubation, and mechanical ventilation may be necessary. In addition, vital signs (blood pressure, centrally if indicated), blood glucose levels, and hydration status (urine output, hourly if indicated) must also be assessed, documented, and reported to the primary care provider when normal parameters are exceeded so supportive treatment can be rapidly initiated. The infant's hematocrit level should be maintained at 40% or greater to help ensure adequate oxygen-carrying capacity. Serial platelet counts should be monitored to help identify the development of DIC. Anemia, thrombocytopenia, and DIC are treated with the appropriate transfusions, and aggressive nutritional support is given (Kenner & Lott, 2003).

NURSING CARE

The Infant With Neonatal Sepsis

Assessment

The nurse should carefully and thoroughly review the maternal history (including labor and delivery) to identify any risk factors for the development of sepsis. All infants considered at risk should be closely observed for the development of the often subtle signs and symptoms of sepsis. Thorough documentation of the infant's behavior during each shift allows nurses to determine whether the behavior they observe is different or abnormal for that infant. The nurse should immediately notify the physician if any changes are observed in the infant's respiratory status, muscle tone, activity level, or temperature or if the infant lacks interest in or does not tolerate feedings.

Nursing Diagnosis and Planning

Nursing diagnoses for the infant with neonatal sepsis are the following:

- Risk for Injury related to effect of sepsis on all body systems.
  Expected Outcome: Harmful effects of sepsis on the infant will be avoided or minimized, as evidenced by lack of complications.
- Ineffective Thermoregulation related to stress of infection and unstable central temperature control.
  Expected Outcome: The infant's temperature will remain within the normal range.
- Imbalanced Nutrition: Less Than Body Requirements related to lack of interest in nipple feedings or feeding intolerance.
  Expected Outcome: The infant's growth will progress appropriately along established growth curves for postconceptual age.

Interventions

Infants at risk for sepsis should be closely observed to ensure early recognition and treatment.

In most cases, early identification and treatment can prevent the complications of sepsis. Diagnostic tests should be completed before antibiotic therapy is initiated. Antimicrobial therapy cannot be specific for the invading organism until the cultures have grown and antimicrobial sensitivities have been determined.

Extra measures may be necessary to warm or cool the infant to minimize the harmful effects of temperature extremes.

Early in the clinical course of sepsis, the infant may be unable or unwilling to take oral feedings. Adequate fluid and caloric intake should be ensured by administering gavage feedings or IV fluids as ordered.

CRITICAL TO REMEMBER
The Infant With Neonatal Sepsis

The infant's condition can deteriorate rapidly from apparently normal to fulminant septic shock and death, especially if the causative agent is group B streptococcus. When diagnostic tests are ordered, the nurse should evaluate the results and bring any abnormal values to the immediate attention of the infant's physician. Monitoring culture results promptly and notifying the physician of any positive results and antibiotic sensitivities can help ensure prompt institution of specific therapy.

CRITICAL TO REMEMBER
Monitoring Temperature

The infant's temperature is monitored closely because both hypothermia and hyperthermia may be signs of sepsis. Hyperthermia is rare.

Evaluation

- Have severe complications of sepsis been avoided?
- Were changes in the infant's condition recognized and reported to the physician in a timely manner?

- Has the infant been able to maintain body temperature within normal limits without extraordinary nursing intervention?
- Has the infant shown the expected weight gains for age?

Diphtheria

Causative agent: *Corynebacterium diphtheriae* (a gram-positive, nonmotile bacillus)

Incubation period: 2 to 7 days

Infectious period: Ranges from 2 weeks or less to several months in an untreated individual

Transmission: Contact with carrier or disease, droplets

Immunity: Vaccine with boosters, passive immunity from maternal antibodies, natural disease

Season: Fall and winter

Manifestations

Nasal manifestations of diphtheria include discharge of foul-smelling mucopurulent material. Low-grade fever is common. Thin, gray membranes appear on tonsils and pharynx, causing "bull neck," or neck edema.

Therapeutic Management

Treatment includes the administration of IV diphtheria antitoxin and antibiotics.

Primary prevention of diphtheria can be accomplished through administration of the diphtheria vaccine in combination with DTaP. Immunization of children ages 2 months to 7 years should consist of five doses of the DTaP vaccine (see Chapter 4 and Evolve website). After the initial childhood immunization series is completed, a booster dose of diphtheria and tetanus toxoids and pertussis (given as Tdap) is recommended at 11 to 12 years of age and should be given no later than age 18 years (AAP, 2005). Subsequently, booster doses of diphtheria and tetanus toxoids (given as Td) should be administered every 10 years. For children older than 7 years receiving primary immunization, three doses plus a booster dose of Td are administered. Tdap may be substituted for one of these doses, although if used as a booster dose, it should be given no earlier than 5 years after the last Td (CDC, 2006).

Nursing Considerations

The nurse should obtain a history of symptoms and an immunization history. The nurse should teach parents and give them information about monitoring for any increased respiratory efforts, mode of transmission, and prevention of spread of the disease to family and close contacts. Nursing care of the hospitalized child with diphtheria involves Droplet Precautions, bed rest, and monitoring of the child's respiratory status (patency of the airway).

The primary focus of nursing should be preventive because the development and use of the diphtheria vaccine have drastically reduced the incidence of diphtheria in the United States. In addition, the AAP (2003b) recommends the use of DTaP for the prevention of any adverse reactions to the whole-cell pertussis vaccine available as DTP.

Pertussis (Whooping Cough)

Causative agent: *Bordetella pertussis* (a gram-negative bacillus)

Incubation period: 6 to 20 days

Infectious period: Catarrhal stage (1 to 2 weeks) until the fourth week

Transmission: Direct contact or respiratory droplets from coughing

Immunity: Bacteria or vaccine, both of which provide varying degrees and duration of immunity against pertussis

Season: Can occur during any season

Manifestations

The three stages of pertussis are catarrhal, paroxysmal, and convalescent (Box 16-4).

Complications

The most common complication of pertussis is pneumonia. Other respiratory complications may occur to varying degrees, ranging from atelectasis to interstitial or subcutaneous emphysema to pneumothorax. Approximately 90% of the deaths attributable to pertussis are related to respiratory complications. Anoxia can lead to CNS involvement. Malnutrition and dehydration may result from extensive vomiting and can be quite dangerous, especially for infants. Other complications include otitis media, ulcers of the frenulum of the tongue, epistaxis, hernia, and rectal prolapse.

Therapeutic Management

Primary prevention of pertussis can be accomplished through administration of the pertussis vaccine in combination with DTaP, as previously described. In 2005 the AAP issued a new policy on adolescent pertussis vaccine. Recognizing that pertussis infection has become a significant and costly illness in the adolescent population (because of waning immunity), the AAP recommends immunizing children at age 11 to

BOX 16-4	Stages of Manifestation of Pertussis

Catarrhal
Duration: 1-2 weeks
Symptoms: Symptoms of upper respiratory tract infection (rhinorrhea, lacrimation, mild cough, low-grade fever).

Paroxysmal
Duration: 2-4 weeks or longer
Symptoms: Increased severity of cough. Repetitive series of coughs during a single expiration, followed by massive inspiration with a whoop. Cyanosis, protrusion of tongue, salivation, distention of neck veins. Coughing spells may be triggered by yawning, sneezing, eating, or drinking. Coughing may induce vomiting.

Convalescent
Duration: 1-2 weeks
Symptoms: Episodes of coughing, whooping, and vomiting that decrease in frequency and severity. Cough may persist for several months.

12 years with a newly approved tetanus and diphtheria toxoids and pertussis vaccine (Tdap), as previously described. Tdap is primarily to be used as a booster dose, replacing the Td formerly given at that age (AAP, 2005).

Erythromycin, Azithromycin, or clarithromycin, if given early in the course of the disease, will eliminate the organism from the nasopharynx within a few days, thereby reducing communicability. Erythromycin, Azithromycin, or clarithromycin are also given to all nonimmune close contacts, which include most children older than 13 years, because the immunity conferred by the childhood immunization declines by that age. Corticosteroids and albuterol have been used to reduce paroxysmal coughing.

Hospitalization and supportive care for the infant may be necessary to monitor airway patency, whereas older children can usually be cared for at home. Respiratory status is monitored with a cardiopulmonary monitor and pulse oximeter. Droplet Precautions are observed.

CRITICAL TO REMEMBER
Immunity to Pertussis

Because infants do not receive maternal immunity to pertussis, they are quite susceptible to pertussis. Pertussis is a highly contagious illness that is associated with a high infant mortality rate.

Nursing Considerations

The nurse should obtain a complete immunization history and any recent known exposures to illnesses. Documentation should also include the parent's description of any respiratory events before admission and indicators such as coughing, secretions, cyanotic episodes, and the child's activity level. Assessment of the child's respiratory, fluid, nutrition, output, and neurologic status should be done.

The child's respiratory status needs monitoring with a cardiopulmonary monitor and pulse oximeter. If the child is hospitalized, the limits of the monitor should be frequently checked. Explain any monitoring devices to the child (if age appropriate) and parents to help alleviate anxiety. Suction and oxygen equipment should be readily available. Supplemental oxygen therapy could be ordered if the child's oxygen saturation falls below an acceptable range (especially during any coughing episodes). If the child needs oxygen therapy, parents should receive instructions about any oxygen equipment and the timing and possible length of treatment. Some children will need additional oxygen only during the paroxysmal spells.

Because the child's coughing paroxysms may be triggered by noises or frightening experiences, a quiet environment and a calm, reassuring approach should be used when caring for the child and supporting the parents. Paroxysmal episodes should be monitored for any drop in oxygen saturation levels. Parents and children will need additional support and reassurance that assistance is near and ready if needed during the child's coughing spells because these episodes can be extremely frightening.

The infant's nutritional status should be closely monitored. Small, frequent feedings may benefit infants if the feeding process becomes exhausting. If the child's intake becomes insufficient, nutritional support (gavage or parenteral nutrition) may be needed to prevent dehydration or weight loss. If the child has vomiting episodes when coughing, frequent oral care will be necessary.

Nursing care activities should be clustered, if possible, to allow the child and parent or parents to rest. Diversional activities should be age appropriate. Parents may need emotional support to deal with feelings of guilt, especially if they chose not to immunize their child.

Scarlet Fever (Scarlatina)

Causative agent:	Group A beta-hemolytic streptococci
Incubation period:	1 to 7 days (average of 3 days)
Infectious period:	Acute stage until 24 hours after antimicrobial therapy has begun
Transmission:	Airborne (inhalation or ingestion), direct contact
Immunity:	None
Season:	Late fall, winter, and spring

Manifestations

Abrupt fever, vomiting, headache, abdominal pain, pharyngitis, and chills may characterize the onset of scarlet fever. The fever reaches a peak by the second day and returns to normal within 5 to 6 days. Within 24 hours a fine red papular rash appears in the axillae, groin, and neck. The rash then spreads peripherally to cover the entire body (Fig. 16-9). The rash will blanch on pressure except in areas of deep creases (Pastia's sign). Desquamation begins on the face at the end of the first week, and flaking proceeds down the trunk. This process may continue for up to 6 weeks. The tongue is initially coated with a white, furry covering with red projecting papillae (so-called *white strawberry tongue*). By the fourth day the papillae slough off, leaving a red, swollen tongue (so-called *strawberry tongue*). The tonsils are edematous and may be covered with a gray-white exudate, which may spread to the pharynx. Petechial hemorrhages cover the soft palate.

Complications

Complications generally result from extension of the streptococcal infection. They may include sinusitis, otitis media, mastoiditis, peritonsillar abscess, bronchopneumonia, meningitis, osteomyelitis, rheumatic fever, and glomerulonephritis.

Therapeutic Management

The preferred treatment for any streptococcal infection is penicillin. Children allergic to penicillin can be given erythromycin. Supportive care for symptoms is indicated. Laboratory confirmation (generally by a throat culture) is recommended for children with sore throats because of the similarity of symptoms between viral and group A streptococcal throats. Children with streptococcal

First day   Third day

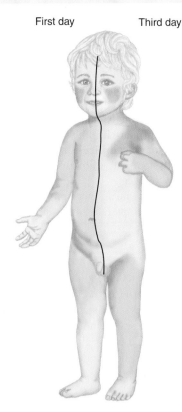

**Scarlet Fever Rash
Distribution**

- Red, fine, papular rash appears within 24 hours of fever and other symptoms; in dark skin, rash is often seen as punctate papular elevations
- Begins in axillae, groin, and neck and spreads to cover entire body
- Desquamation begins on face at end of first week, and flaking proceeds down trunk; may continue up to 6 weeks
- Tongue: initially presents with white, furry coat with red, projecting papillae (white strawberry tongue); by the fourth day, the white sloughs off, leaving a red, swollen tongue (strawberry tongue)

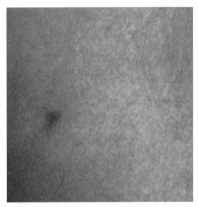

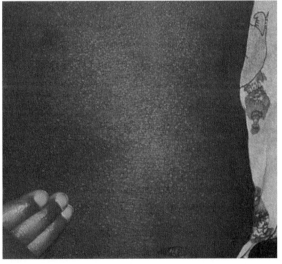

Rash, Light Skin

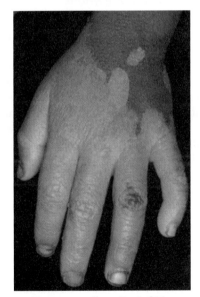

Desquamation, Dark Skin

Rash, Dark Skin

FIG 16-9 **Scarlet fever rash distribution and appearance. Note the characteristic skin peeling.** *(Reprinted from Hurwitz, S. [1993]. Clinical pediatric dermatology: a textbook of skin disorders of childhood and adolescence [2nd ed.]. Philadelphia: Saunders.)*

infections (throat, skin) may return to school or daycare 24 hours after beginning antibiotics when they are no longer considered contagious. Droplet Precautions should also be observed until the child has been on antibiotics for 24 hours.

Nursing Considerations

The nurse should obtain and document a complete history of symptoms. The nurse should also assess the child's throat, tongue, rash, nutritional and fluid intake, vital signs, and level of general wellness. Any history of sensitivity to

- The entire course of antibiotic therapy (usually 10 to 14 days) must be taken to destroy all the bacteria and decrease the risk of complications. If a partial course of antibiotics is given (antibiotic stopped by parent when child is feeling better), the bacteria can become resistant and fail to be eradicated with subsequent attempts.
- Cool drinks and liquid refreshments (ice pops, milkshakes) may be soothing and help maintain hydration.
- Acetaminophen, ibuprofen, throat lozenges, antiseptic throat spray (e.g., Chloraseptic), and cool mist may be used to relieve discomfort.

- Encouraging quiet activities will help prevent fatigue.
- In providing oral care, acidic preparations should be avoided. Saline rinses may provide comfort and promote hygiene.
- A soft, bland diet should be offered.
- Call your primary health provider if your child develops drooling or great difficulty swallowing or acts very sick. After 48 hours of antibiotic therapy, your child should not have a fever.
- Your child is no longer contagious after 24 hours of antibiotic therapy. The rash is not contagious.

penicillin should be thoroughly explored and prominently noted on the child's records.

Generally, children with scarlet fever are cared for at home. Comfort measures include encouraging fluids (especially cool, nonacidic liquids) and administering antipyretics for fever control.

Analgesics may be given for discomfort, and antipruritic comfort measures may be necessary. Parents should understand the typical course of disease and any treatment measures, including the importance of completing the full course of any antibiotics prescribed (to prevent growth of resistant bacteria). Bed rest and quiet activities may be beneficial during the acute stage (Box 16-5).

Children with severe symptoms and complications may, however, need hospitalization and supportive care. In such cases, vital signs, especially body temperature, should be monitored.

RICKETTSIAL INFECTIONS

Rickettsiae are small, parasitic bacteria that are transmitted to human beings by blood-sucking arthropods. A vertebrate is not necessary for the survival of the bacteria, and the host arthropod appears not to be affected adversely by the rickettsiae. Replication of the rickettsiae in the new host cell causes cell death, which may be accompanied by vasculitis with thrombosis, increased permeability, tissue edema, hemorrhage, circulatory failure, and meningoencephalitis. Rickettsial diseases cannot be transmitted from person to person.

Rocky Mountain Spotted Fever

Causative agent:	Rickettsia rickettsii
Reservoir:	Wild rodents, dogs
Vector:	Tick (wood, dog, Lone Star)
Incubation period:	2 to 14 days (average of 7 days)
Transmission:	Bite of infected tick
Season:	April through October

Manifestations

The onset of Rocky Mountain spotted fever is marked by nonspecific signs and symptoms such as headache, fever, anorexia, and restlessness. Generally, on the third day a characteristic maculopapular or petechial rash appears. This rash begins on the extremities (usually the wrists, palms, ankles, and soles) and spreads to the rest of the body. As the rash progresses, hemorrhagic and necrotic lesions can appear. Gangrene of the distal parts of the body can result from thrombosis. Edema develops, beginning in the periorbital area and progressing to a generalized edema of the body and extremities. Delayed treatment can lead to a mortality rate of 25%.

Therapeutic Management

With early detection in children (within 5 days of the beginning of the illness), the likelihood of positive resolution increases. Doxycycline is the drug of choice; chloramphenicol is an alternative. Chloramphenicol and tetracycline are both used less frequently because of the side effects (including staining of teeth) in children younger than 8 years. If vascular damage has already occurred, however, the drugs may not alter the course of the disease. Treatment before day 5 of illness in children with clinical signs and symptoms is more likely to achieve a good outcome. No licensed vaccine or role for antibiotics in the prevention of Rocky Mountain spotted fever is available in the United States.

Nursing Considerations

The assessment of children presenting with symptoms indicating Rocky Mountain spotted fever should include obtaining a complete history of skin eruptions, medications taken, exposure to infectious diseases, and recent hiking or other activities in wooded areas. Any rashes or skin lesions should then be examined, with documentation of distribution and morphology. The child's vital signs, especially body temperature, should also be assessed and noted.

Hospitalized children will require supportive care for their presenting symptoms. Straws should be used, and the mouth should be flushed if tetracycline is administered because it can stain the teeth. Parents should be cautioned to give the full course of any antibiotic to decrease the risk of complications and ensure that the disease is eradicated.

Education regarding the control measures for prevention of tick-borne infections is vital (Box 16-6).

BOX 16-6	Preventive Measures to Avoid Insect and Tick Bites

- Children should wear tightly woven clothing consisting of long pants, long-sleeved shirts, long socks, and a hat when in woods and grassy areas. Pants should be tucked into socks. Clothing should also be light-colored so ticks are easily visible.
- Paths should be followed and dense areas avoided if possible. Avoid known tick-infested areas.
- Insect repellents that contain diethyltoluamide (DEET) and permethrins should be used; apply before any possible exposure and every 1 to 2 hours sparingly according to manufacturer's directions. Care should be taken to avoid contact of repellent with the child's eyes or mouth. The repellent should not be applied to the hands to avoid contact with the eyes and mouth. Wash hands and skin after the child goes indoors.
- Repellents should be used with caution in infants because of the risk of encephalopathy.
- Insect repellent should not be applied to wounds or irritated skin.
- The body (especially exposed hairy regions) should be inspected periodically for ticks, which may resemble small moles or blood blisters. Early removal can prevent transmission of disease from an infected tick.
- Ticks should be removed with tweezers. The tick should be removed as close to the skin as possible.
- Care should be taken to avoid handling the tick with bare hands or crushing the tick's body.
- Ticks may be preserved in alcohol for later identification.
- Pets should be kept free of ticks by dipping and spraying during tick season. Yards should be kept free of brush and undergrowth.

BORRELIA INFECTIONS

Borrelia is a genus of spiral bacteria that are transmitted to human beings by arthropods. The diseases caused by *Borrelia* are relapsing fever and Lyme disease.

Relapsing Fever

Relapsing fever is spread from person to person by lice or ticks. The bacteria are introduced into a bite wound when the bite is rubbed. This infection is spread when people fail to wash thoroughly and do not change clothes.

Tick-borne relapsing fever (*Borrelia hermsii, B. turicatae*) results from tick exposures in rodent-infested cabins in western mountainous areas of the United States, including state and national parks. *B. turicatae* infections occur less frequently, with the majority of cases in Texas.

Manifestations

The sudden onset of high fever, shaking chills, sweats, headache, muscle and joint pains, and progressive weakness characterize relapsing fever. A macular rash on the trunk and petechiae of the skin and mucous membranes may occur.

Therapeutic Management

Several antibiotics provide effective treatment. These include penicillin, tetracycline, erythromycin, and chloramphenicol in children older than 8 years. For children younger than 8 years and for pregnant women, penicillin or erythromycin is the preferred drug.

Nursing Considerations

Assessment should include a complete history of rash onset and characteristics, medications taken, and living environment, including available bathing and washing facilities. Fever, headache, and arthralgia should be treated with antipyretics and analgesics. Antibiotics should be given as ordered. Education includes personal hygiene, the use of pediculicides, and eradication methods.

Lyme Disease

Lyme disease is spread by tick bites and is the most frequently reported vector-borne disease in the United States (Shapiro, 2004). Lyme disease is a multisystem illness that affects the skin and the musculoskeletal, cardiovascular, and nervous systems.

Causative agent: *Borrelia burgdorferi* (spirochete)
Vector: Tick (Fig. 16-10)
Incubation period: 3 to 32 days
Transmission: Bite of infected tick (person-to-person transmission not possible)
Season: April to October

Manifestations

The manifestations of Lyme disease can be divided into three stages (early localized, early disseminated, late disseminated). In the first stage (early localized), the skin lesions are most prominent; in the second stage (early disseminated), cardiac and neurologic findings are prominent; and in the third stage (late disseminated), arthritis is the main manifestation (Shapiro, 2004).

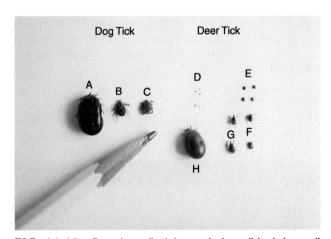

FIG 16-10 **Dog (wood) ticks and deer (black-legged) ticks compared with a pencil. Dog ticks: *A*, engorged female; *B*, female; *C*, male. Deer ticks: *D*, larvae; *E*, nymphs; *F*, males; *G*, females; *H*, engorged female.** *(Courtesy Lyme Disease Foundation,* www.lyme.org.)

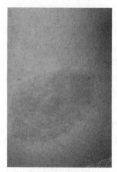

FIG 16-11   Characteristic lesion of Lyme disease. *(Reprinted from Larson, W. G., Adams, R. M., & Maibach, H. I. [1991]. Color text of contact dermatitis. Philadelphia: Saunders.)*

In the early localized stage of Lyme disease, local reactions to an infected tick bite occur, along with vague, flulike symptoms (headache, chills, fatigue, vague muscle aches and pains). An erythematous macula or papule forms at the site of the tick bite within 3 to 30 days (Fig. 16-11). This rash can enlarge to 16 to 68 cm in diameter, with a clearing in the center (erythema migrans, or "bull's eye" rash). It may itch, prickle, or burn. The rash generally lasts for 3 weeks, during which time it gradually fades.

In the early disseminated stage (generally 1 to 4 months after the bite), neurologic symptoms may be the first to occur. CNS symptoms may include severe headaches with myelitis, nausea, vomiting, facial nerve paralysis (Bell palsy), forgetfulness or decreased concentration, and cerebral ataxia. General lymphadenopathy and joint and muscle pain may also be present. Lyme arthritis generally affects the large joints, with the knee being the most often involved. Cardiac disease is usually brief and uncommon in children. The signs and symptoms generally resolve over a few days, but many individuals have recurrences. Skin lesions may recur but are smaller and more diffuse than the initial ones.

Symptoms of late disseminated Lyme disease (occurring months to years after the initial infected tick bite) occur intermittently and include chronic arthritis, profound fatigue, and chronic neurologic manifestations. The debilitating effects frequently affect a child's ability to participate in normal activities (e.g., sports) because of extreme fatigue or cardiac complications.

Therapeutic Management

Primary prevention of Lyme disease includes anticipatory guidance and information about routine preventive measures to avoid insect bites. A vaccine that had been approved for use in the United States in those between the ages of 15 and 70 years was withdrawn from the market by the manufacturer in 2002. Currently, no other vaccine for Lyme disease is available (Shapiro, 2004).

Early detection and antibiotic treatment in any of the disease's stages are highly effective and are usually highly successful in positively affecting the course of the disease (Shapiro, 2004). In addition, disease identified in early stages and treated with antibiotics does not progress to the more debilitating stages. The characteristic rash of Lyme disease linked to other symptoms leads to a diagnosis except in cases where the child has atypical manifestations of the disease (e.g., one septic joint, usually the knee).

Presently, treatment for early localized disease involves the use of doxycycline for children older than 9 years and amoxicillin for children younger than 9 years and pregnant or lactating women, with the course of treatment lasting 14 to 21 days. For those allergic to penicillin, cefuroxime axetil and erythromycin are alternate drugs. For early disseminated and late Lyme disease with additional systemic complications (persistent or recurrent arthritis, carditis, meningitis, encephalitis), IV or IM ceftriaxone or penicillin is indicated.

Nursing Considerations

Assessment should include a complete history of rash onset and characteristics; medications taken; recent exposures to infectious diseases; and recent hiking, working (forestry, farming, outdoor construction or maintenance), or vacationing (camping [e.g., Boy or Girl Scouts], hunting) in a known endemic area or heavily wooded area. Rashes should be examined for characteristics and distribution and documented (Shapiro, 2004). Fever, headache, and arthralgia should be treated with antipyretics and analgesics. Parents should have a complete understanding of the course of treatment, including the importance of administering medications and antibiotics as prescribed. The importance of completing the entire course of antibiotic treatment should be stressed. Generally, affected children will be treated at home. Parental and caregiver education is important to prevent further exposures and to facilitate early recognition of disease symptoms.

HELMINTHS

Helminths are worms that live as parasites. The three groups with the greatest impact on human beings are tapeworms, flukes, and roundworms (Table 16-1). Children are more commonly infected than adults, primarily as a result of frequent hand-to-mouth activity and the likelihood of fecal contamination. Transmission may occur by oral-fecal ingestion, ingestion of contaminated tissue from another host, skin penetration, or the bite of a blood-sucking insect.

Therapeutic Management

Treatment consists of the administration of oral medications effective against a specific helminth. Treatment is provided to the entire family. Anticipatory guidance to prevent reinfestation and education about the prevention of the spread of disease (basic enteric isolation procedures) for the family and primary caregivers, along with personal hygiene and sanitary practices, are also necessary (Box 16-7).

Nursing Considerations

A thorough history, including the child's general wellness, personal hygiene practices, availability of running water and bathing and laundry facilities, along with nutritional intake, should be obtained.

TABLE 16-1 Common Helminths				
Class and Typical Agent	**Transmission**	**Manifestations**	**Diagnosis**	**Treatment**
Roundworm (*Ascaris lumbricoides*)	Ingestion of eggs from contaminated soil or food, transfer to mouth from fingers, toys, or other vectors	Abdominal pain or distention, abdominal obstruction, vomiting with bile staining, pneumonitis	Fecal smear	Mebendazole, pyrantel pamoate
Pinworm (*Enterobius vermicularis*)	Ingestion or inhalation of eggs, transfer from hands to mouth	Nocturnal anal itching, sleeplessness	Adhesive tape test and microscopic examination	Pyrantel pamoate, mebendazole
Tapeworm (*Taenia saginata*)	Ingestion from handling or eating infected beef or pork	Asymptomatic, segments of worms seen in stool, abdominal pain, nausea, anorexia, weight loss, insomnia	Fecal smear or microscopic examination	Praziquantel (safety in children younger than 4 years not established; use is being investigated)
Hookworm (*Necator americanus*)	Skin penetration from direct contact with contaminated soil	Dermatitis, anemia, pneumonitis, blood loss, malnutrition	Fecal smear or microscopic examination	Pyrantel pamoate

---

BOX 16-7   **PARENTS WANT TO KNOW**   How to Prevent Parasitic Infections

- Handwashing (including under the fingernails) with soap and water should be done before eating or handling of food and after using the toilet.
- Placing hands in the mouth and nail biting should be discouraged.
- Toilets or other appropriate bathroom facilities should be used for elimination.
- Toilets or bathroom facilities should be cleaned with agents containing bleach.
- Scratching the anal area with bare hands should be discouraged.
- Dogs and cats should be kept at a distance from play areas and sandboxes, and the latter need to be covered when not in use.

- Shoes should be worn when outside.
- All fruits and vegetables should be washed before being eaten.
- Diapers should be changed frequently and disposed of properly (out of children's reach).
- Swimming facilities that allow diapered children should be avoided.
- Only bottled water should be used during camping outings.

Most parasites are identified in fecal smears obtained from stool specimens. If the family or caregiver is to bring a stool specimen in for laboratory testing, the nurse needs to provide specific, clear instructions and provide a container if needed. Sample size and number, as well as proper storage, should be clearly explained. Stool specimens that have not been contaminated with urine are ideal. Obtaining urine-free specimens may be difficult, especially in infants or very young children. Plastic wrap can be placed over the toilet bowl or a potty chair, or specimens can be collected from a diaper using a clean tongue blade and placing in a container. The container should be marked with the child's name and the date and time of collection. It should then be refrigerated until it is delivered to the laboratory.

Education for the parents and primary caregivers should focus on medication administration, primary prevention of future reinfestations, and resource identification with referral to available community and social services for any basic living needs (running water, bathing facilities). The rationale for evaluating and treating the entire family for infection and the usual mode of transmission must be discussed to prevent future reinfestation or cross contamination of family members. Anticipatory guidance regarding primary prevention and teaching about prevention (personal hygiene and health habits) should be covered with the child's family. The nurse should help the family identify any resources (access to care, social services) necessary and initiate referral if appropriate.

FUNGAL INFECTIONS

Fungi are free-living organisms that can be found throughout the environment. Some species of fungi are part of the normal human flora, especially those in the mouth, intestine, vagina, and skin. A fungus is transmitted through inhalation or penetration of tissue as a result of trauma. Fungi grow quite slowly, so clinical symptoms may appear only after a prolonged period. They are aerobic, can grow in a wide range of temperatures, and are resistant to most antibiotics. They exist in two forms: *molds* and *yeasts*.

Infections caused by fungi are classified into four groups:
- Opportunistic: caused by a defect in host immunity
- Systemic: involving deep tissues and organs
- Subcutaneous: limited to deep subcutaneous tissue
- Superficial: limited to skin, hair, and nails

Common fungal infections include tinea capitis, tinea pedis, and candidal infections (see Chapter 26).

SEXUALLY TRANSMISSIBLE DISEASES

The rates of infection of many STDs, or diseases transmitted through sexual activity, are highest among adolescents. Those adolescents at highest risk are male homosexuals, sexually active heterosexuals, younger sexually active adolescents, and IV drug users. Adolescents are at greater risk because they have frequent unprotected intercourse, are biologically more susceptible to infection, and face multiple obstacles regarding access to health care (Eissa & Cromwell, 2003). Often adolescents lack knowledge of methods for preventing STDs. Moreover, the use of drugs and alcohol makes unsafe, unprotected sex more likely to occur. In addition, adolescents' inherent developmental stage and sense of invulnerability lead to risky behavior and risk taking (Box 16-8).

Neonates are at risk for transplacental transmission of STDs from an infected mother or from direct contamination during the birthing process. Sexual abuse should be suspected in children who acquire STDs after the neonatal period. These children may present without the typical genital symptoms but with a variety of physical or behavioral complaints. Related changes in behavior may include insomnia, eating disorders, bed-wetting, or emotional withdrawal.

A careful, complete history and physical examination are required. The examination should include inspection of oral, anal, and genital mucosa for any signs of trauma or infection. Because obtaining a complete history may be difficult, children should undergo a complete laboratory evaluation and all potentially infected areas should be cultured if sexual abuse is suspected.

Gonorrhea

Causative agent: *Neisseria gonorrhoeae* (gram-negative diplococcus)
Incubation period: 2 to 7 days
Transmission: Intimate contact (perinatally, through sexual abuse, by sexual intercourse)

Gonorrhea may be transmitted three different ways:
- *Perinatally:* Transmission can occur during birth of a neonate whose mother is infected or with premature rupture of the membranes. The neonate can acquire the disease through aspiration of vaginal secretions, which leads to sepsis; through direct contact through the conjunctiva; or through direct contact through attachment of a fetal scalp electrode.
- *Sexual abuse:* Any child with a positive culture and without a prior history of voluntary sexual behavior should be considered a potential sexual abuse victim until proven otherwise. Transmission through sexual play with children has been documented but is rare. Almost all children diagnosed with gonorrhea at the age of 1 year or older have experienced sexual abuse.
- *Voluntary sexual activity:* This route of transmission remains the primary route of infection among adolescents. Sexual abuse should not, however, be excluded as a possibility.

BOX 16-8 | **TEENAGERS WANT TO KNOW**   About Sexually Transmissible Diseases

- STDs are diseases that can be transmitted through body fluids (semen, vaginal fluids, blood) and contact with infected mucous membranes (mouth, vagina, anus).
- Not all STDs have symptoms. Many people with chlamydia (an STD infection) do not have any symptoms. Transmission of an STD that you do not know you have to someone else is possible.
- STDs can be painful, ugly, and dangerous to those who have them. Some can even cause sterility, neurologic (brain) damage, cancer, or death.
- STDs can infect anyone, regardless of race, religion, sexual preference, social status, or gender.
- Because many STDs can be transmitted through sexual intercourse as well as skin-to-skin contact, even the most careful individuals can be susceptible to infections.
- Some STDs, such as gonorrhea, chlamydia, and syphilis, can be cured fairly easily by completing a course of medication. Others, such as herpes, genital warts, and human immunodeficiency virus (HIV), cannot be cured, although some treatments are available to reduce their symptoms.

- Abstinence is the *only* 100% effective way to prevent both pregnancy and STD transmission.
- Abstinence means never engaging in any form of sexual contact with a partner.
- Deciding if and when to have sex is an important issue to think about.
- No one should ever be pressured to have sex.
- If you choose to have sex, a male or female condom can reduce (*not eliminate*) your chances of acquiring or passing on an STD.
- Some symptoms that might mean you have an STD are unusual discharge, swelling, pain, sores, or a rash in your genital area; unusual nonmenstrual bleeding; pain when you urinate or have a bowel movement; or a sore throat for several weeks.
- If you are sexually active and note any of these symptoms, see your primary health care provider as soon as possible. Detecting and treating an STD early will decrease the chances of permanent damage.

Manifestations

Ophthalmia neonatorum is the most common type of gonorrheal infection in the infant, presenting 1 to 4 days after birth. A thick, purulent discharge from the eyes may be present and, if not treated promptly, will progress to corneal ulceration, rupture, and blindness. Ophthalmia neonatorum has been controlled through prophylactic treatment with an ophthalmic antibiotic given immediately after birth. In older children, ophthalmic infection can be the result of self-inoculation from the genital site.

Girls with gonorrheal infection may present with a purulent vulvovaginitis, whereas boys often have urethritis. A history of purulent discharge with burning during urination is often elicited. Adolescent girls may present with cervicitis, urethritis, perihepatitis, and salpingitis. Gonorrhea in adolescent and younger girls may progress to pelvic inflammatory disease (PID). PID is the most common cause of infertility in young women (Eissa & Cromwell, 2003).

Therapeutic Management

Because syphilis and chlamydial infection are also often present in individuals with gonorrhea, testing should take place for those diseases. Penicillin-resistant *N. gonorrhoeae* strains have influenced the choice of therapy. Currently, the drug of choice for gonorrhea is a third-generation cephalosporin, such as ceftriaxone. Ceftriaxone is effective in treating syphilis but not chlamydial infections. A course of tetracycline or doxycycline is recommended in conjunction with ceftriaxone for those with chlamydial infection. Sexual partners should be treated.

Syphilis

Causative agent: Treponema pallidum
Incubation period: Acquired primary infection—10 to 90 days
                                 (average 21 days)
Transmission: Intimate contact, transplacentally, or
                                 sexually

Congenital syphilis may be transmitted transplacentally by an infected mother at any time during pregnancy or birth. Acquired syphilis is contracted through sexual contact. In children, syphilis diagnosed after the neonatal period can almost always be linked to sexual abuse.

Manifestations

Infants with congenital syphilis may be asymptomatic or may exhibit signs and symptoms within the first 3 months of life. The classic signs are rhinitis, a maculopapular rash, and hepatosplenomegaly. Diagnostic radiographs may show osteochondritis, periosteitis, or metaphyseal changes, especially in the long bones of the femur and humerus. Late manifestations are a result of the scarring from the systemic disease process. The bones, teeth, eyes, and eighth cranial nerve are involved. The teeth are notched (Hutchinson's teeth), and hearing loss can occur suddenly near the age of 8 to 10 years. Acquired syphilis has the same clinical course in children as in adults.

Therapeutic Management

Syphilis responds well to a single dose of benzathine penicillin G intramuscularly (the preferred treatment for children and adults). Aqueous crystalline penicillin G or procaine penicillin is effective with congenital syphilis. Acquired syphilis can be treated with benzathine penicillin G. Tetracycline and doxycycline are options for the client older than 8 years but should not be used in younger children because of the greater risks of permanent tooth staining. In addition, the effectiveness of drugs other than penicillin and tetracycline remains unproven. When follow-up cannot be guaranteed, especially for children younger than 8 years, consideration should be given to hospitalizing the child and consulting a specialist (for potential desensitization followed by penicillin G administration) (AAP, 2003k).

Education regarding potential long-term effects of partially or untreated syphilis must be discussed. Resources should be available and care should be accessible to ensure completion of treatment and eradication of disease.

Chlamydial Infection

Causative agent: Chlamydia trachomatis, Chlamydia psittaci,
                                 Chlamydia pneumoniae
Incubation period: 7 to 21 days
Transmission: During birth if mother is infected, through
                                 sexual activity

Chlamydial infection has become one of the most prevalent STDs. Infants are infected during the birthing process. Chlamydial infection can cause morbidity in the infant and is responsible for neonatal eye infections and interstitial pneumonia.

Manifestations

Many people with a chlamydial infection have few or no symptoms. As a result, the disease may go undiagnosed until complications develop.

Neonatal conjunctivitis manifests with a watery discharge that becomes purulent. Eyelids are edematous, and the conjunctiva may become inflamed. Mucoid rhinorrhea may be associated with the infection. Many infants with conjunctivitis will develop infection of the nasopharynx, which can progress to pneumonia. These infants may have a history of a cough and congestion. Long-term abnormalities of pulmonary function may result in chronic respiratory problems.

Urethritis with dysuria, urinary frequency, or mucopurulent discharge may indicate chlamydial infection. Any identification of this organism in young children indicates possible child abuse.

Therapeutic Management

In infants with conjunctivitis or pneumonia, a 14-day course of oral erythromycin is recommended. For uncomplicated genital tract infection, azithromycin is effective for children younger than 8 years and doxycycline may also be used for older children and teenagers.

Trichomoniasis

Causative agent: *Trichomonas vaginalis* (flagellated protozoan)
Incubation period: 4 to 28 days (average of 1 week)
Transmission: Perinatal contact during delivery, sexual activity

Manifestations

Infections with *Trichomonas* are frequently asymptomatic. Only 25% to 50% of female clients with trichomoniasis will exhibit symptoms. Most male clients are asymptomatic. When symptoms occur, they may include dysuria, vaginal itching and burning (in female clients), and a frothy, yellowish green, foul-smelling discharge. Infected mothers can infect their newborn infants during birth. Children with a positive culture for *Trichomonas* should be investigated for possible sexual abuse.

Therapeutic Management

A single dose of metronidazole (Flagyl, Protostat) is the treatment of choice for adolescents and adults; it has an approximate cure rate of 95%. For prepubertal girls, the drug is given in two or three divided doses. Sexual partners should also be treated. Metronidazole should not be used during the first trimester of pregnancy.

Education regarding the potential presence of other STDs should be thoroughly discussed, especially with the adolescent client, in a respectful and confidential manner.

Human Papillomavirus

Causative agent: Human papillomavirus (HPV)
Incubation period: 4 weeks to many months
Transmission: Direct sexual contact, perinatal contact during delivery

Human papillomavirus is responsible for the common wart and for venereal warts (condylomata acuminata). These anogenital warts may be contracted through direct sexual contact or perinatally during the delivery process. Children with anogenital warts should be investigated for sexual abuse. A person can get warts through autoinoculation from other body sites. A break in skin integrity is necessary for infection to occur.

Manifestations

Anogenital warts begin as small papules that grow into soft, clustered lesions. They are found in moist areas, such as the labia minora, vagina, cervix, anus, rectum, and glans penis. Most warts in children resolve within several years.

Therapeutic Management

Treatment can include surgery, cryotherapy, electrocautery, and laser therapy or chemical ablation. For sexually active individuals, transmission can be decreased by the use of condoms.

Herpes Simplex Virus

Causative agent: Herpes simplex virus, type 2 (see Chapter 25)
Incubation period: 2 to 20 days
Transmission: Direct sexual contact with an infected person

Herpes simplex virus, type 2, is the cause of genital herpes. Genital herpes is one of the most frequently seen STDs in the United States. It is especially problematic because an infected mother can transmit it to her newborn during vaginal delivery, causing multisystem disease. Women with active HSV infection as labor and delivery approach may be advised to have a cesarean delivery.

Manifestations

At the initial infection, lesions occur in the genital area, usually on the vulva, perineum, or perianal area. However, lesions may also occur in the vagina and on the cervix, areas where they cannot be seen. Pain and tenderness in the affected area may coincide with lesion eruption. Vesicles erupt, rupture, and then ulcerate over the course of 1 to 7 days. The virus is shed for 2 to 3 weeks. Occasionally, flulike symptoms (fever, malaise, enlarged lymph nodes) can accompany vesicular eruption. After the acute phase has passed, the virus can remain dormant in the nerve ganglia, where it can reappear later in response to stressful triggers.

Therapeutic Management

Viral culture from vesicular fluid can confirm the diagnosis. There is no cure for HSV 2, but administration of acyclovir (Zovirax) can diminish symptoms and reduce shedding time. Infected neonates are treated with parenteral acyclovir; those with ocular involvement receive a topical ophthalmic drug as well. Infected individuals should refrain from all sexual contact until the lesions have healed completely. Because shedding time in an initial infection is prolonged, abstinence is recommended for several weeks.

CRITICAL THINKING EXERCISE 16-1

Adolescents with an STD may seek out school- or community-based health care. Their symptoms may be vague, with generalized feelings of malaise or fever; or specific, with reports of painful urination or vaginal or penile discharge. Often they hope that the nurse will ask about sexual activity because they feel they cannot trust other adults. What challenges does the nurse face when caring for these adolescents?

Bacterial Vaginosis

Causative agent: Specific cause is not clearly identified; however, the normal vaginal flora is replaced by an overgrowth of organisms such as *Gardnerella vaginalis, Mycoplasma hominis,* or anaerobic bacteria; a corresponding decrease in the concentration of lactobacilli occurs (AAP, 2003k)
Incubation period: Unknown
Transmission: Presumed to be transmitted through sexual contact because it is uncommon in sexually inexperienced females

Bacterial vaginosis is the most prevalent vaginal infection in sexually active adolescents and adults. It may occur with other conditions associated with vaginal discharge, such as trichomoniasis or cervicitis.

Manifestations

Bacterial vaginosis is characterized by a profuse, white, malodorous (having a fishy smell) vaginal discharge that sticks to the vaginal walls. Bacterial vaginosis may be asymptomatic and is not associated with abdominal pain, skin rashes, itching, or painful urination. Other STDs may occur simultaneously.

A diagnosis of bacterial vaginosis in a prepubertal girl raises concern and warrants further investigation but does not prove sexual abuse. Occasionally, vaginal foreign bodies (forgotten tampons at the end of a menstrual period) and other infections are found.

Bacterial vaginosis may be a risk factor for PID. Pregnant women with bacterial vaginosis are at increased risk for chorioamnionitis and premature delivery. Sexually active women with bacterial vaginosis should be evaluated for the presence of other STDs.

Therapeutic Management

Bacterial vaginosis responds well to metronidazole or clindamycin orally (2- and 7-day schedules) or with vaginal gels and creams (5- and 7-day administration schedules). Clindamycin cream is oil-based and may weaken latex condoms for at least 72 hours after the last application.

Nursing Considerations

Prevention, early identification, and treatment are the goals of nursing care associated with any STD. The nurse plays a key role in educating young people about STDs. Often, the school nurse is the health care professional whom adolescents feel they can trust, so school nurses may be the care providers in the best position to educate this population. Establishing rapport with the teenager by using a nonjudgmental approach and reassurance of confidentiality is key. The nurse must be aware of symptoms and assist in identifying those adolescents who are at risk for STDs. Encouraging abstinence in those who are not sexually active and condom use in sexually active adolescents is a way to prevent STDs. The nurse may be the one to assume responsibility for helping the adolescent obtain proper medical treatment and gain an understanding

---

USING RESEARCH TO IMPROVE PRACTICE

From an infectious disease perspective, the trend of adolescents increasingly engaging in oral sex has become an issue of concern for health care providers. It is a problem that is especially important to school nurses because they provide health care and health education within the school setting. Always a sensitive issue for nurses in public schools, discussions about sex with adolescents requires establishing a trusting relationship between nurse and teen and an awareness of "popular" activities that put adolescents at risk. Think about how nurses can obtain information about sexuality trends in adolescents. How might you as a nurse find information about this issue? What challenges might you encounter from parents or community members?

Research that provides an accurate assessment of oral sexual experience in adolescents is scarce in the literature for many reasons, not the least of which is that the Youth Risk Behavior Surveillance system, which is given to high school students to monitor health trends, and other types of surveys about sexual activity do not ask specifically about oral sex. Two research studies published recently have provided some insight about the prevalence of oral sex in adolescents and the health implications of this trend.

Boekeloo & Howard (2002) collected data from 335 adolescents who were interviewed about sexual activity in conjunction with a well visit to their physician. Before developing the questionnaire, the researchers conducted focus groups with adolescents and their caregivers to devise precise and understandable terminology for the questions. Their questionnaire demonstrated appropriate reliability and validity. Study results illustrated a significant trend of both passive and active oral sexual activity as the adolescent aged, with the highest prevalence in 14- and 15-year-olds.

Although overall the prevalence for engaging in oral sex among this sample of adolescent boys and girls was 17% (male) to 20% (female), only a small percentage (<10%) reported using any type of barrier protection to prevent STDs. Furthermore, nearly one third of the adolescents in this sample did not regard oral sex as a significant risk for contracting HIV or other communicable STDs.

Halpern-Felsher, Cornell, Kropp, and Tschann (2005) conducted a similar study with 580 ethnically diverse ninth graders from two California high schools who were participating in a longitudinal study that looked at perception of risks and benefits associated with engaging in sexual activity (e.g., risks of STDs, pregnancy, adverse social and emotional consequences; benefits of pleasure, popularity). Students completed questionnaires in the classroom setting that explored their intentions to have oral sex, actual oral sexual activity, and attitudes about oral sex. Similar to the Boekeloo and Howard study, prevalence of engagement in oral sex was 20%. Approximately 14% of adolescents in this sample believed that contracting HIV or chlamydia is not possible from having oral sex versus vaginal sex. In general, adolescents in this study viewed oral sex to be more acceptable socially and emotionally than engaging in vaginal sex; this study did not investigate use of barrier protection.

Both these studies confirm that adolescent sexual behavior is changing and suggest the need for health providers to be more comprehensive in their assessment of and intervention with sexually active adolescents to reduce the risks for STDs. Both studies also suggest that health care providers must be more specific when performing a health history to obtain needed information about noncoital forms of sexual activity.

of the importance of completing the entire course of medication as well as treatment of partners.

An issue that has become increasingly concerning is the number of young adolescents who practice oral sex (Halpern-Felsher, Cornell, Kropp, & Tschann, 2005). Research on this subject, although scarce, suggests that between 7% and 20% of young adolescents have been either active or passive participants in oral sex (Boekeloo & Howard, 2002; Halpern-Felsher, Cornell, Kropp, & Tschann, 2005), and many of these teens do not understand or believe that they are at risk for STDs from this behavior. Health providers need to assess adolescents for oral sex participation and provide appropriate information about the risks involved in the same way information is provided about vaginal sex.

KEY CONCEPTS

- Microorganisms that cause infectious disease are classified as bacteria, viruses, fungi, protozoa, and helminths.
- The skin is the first line of defense in the innate immune system.
- Infectious diseases can be transmitted by direct contact with another infected person, by contact with animal or insect carriers, by ingestion of contaminated food or water containing the pathogens, and by contact with a contaminated object.
- Exogenous pathogens are transmitted by direct contact, by animal or insect contact, through contaminated water or food, or by contact with a contaminated object.
- Vaccines can be live or attenuated, killed or inactivated toxoids, human immune globulin, or animal serums or antitoxins.
- Assessment of the child with an infectious disease includes a thorough history (recent exposure, other family members or friends exhibiting signs or symptoms) and documentation of the type, configuration, and distribution of lesions; the child's temperature; and any associated signs and symptoms.
- Children with infectious diseases usually can and should be cared for at home.
- Neonates with sepsis frequently display subtle signs and symptoms. Recognition and sensitivity on the part of the nurse can lead to early and life-saving interventions.
- Children who acquire an STD after the neonatal period should always be evaluated for possible sexual abuse.
- Gonorrhea can be transmitted during delivery of a neonate or with premature rupture of the membranes, through sexual abuse, and through voluntary sexual activity.
- Abstinence is the only 100% effective way to prevent both pregnancy and STD transmission. Sexually active individuals need to use barrier protection to prevent STDs.
- Not all STDs have symptoms. Many people with chlamydia (an STD infection) do not have any symptoms. It is possible to transmit an asymptomatic STD.

ANSWERS TO CRITICAL THINKING EXERCISE 16-1

Frequently, the community-based or school nurse is the only health care provider to have an ongoing relationship with an adolescent. The school nurse's vital role in risk assessment for STDs is challenging. The following two major challenges are involved:

- Establishing rapport and providing educational information in an easily understood, nonjudgmental manner. This includes maintaining confidentiality and providing guidance and referral to community resources. All 50 states in the United States allow minors to give their own consent for confidential STD diagnosis and treatment (AAP, 2003k).
- Striking a balance between school district policies and guidelines for distributing sex education materials to students in the school setting and the nurse's personal philosophy about what teens should know. Some school districts, under pressure from parents, do not allow school nurses to give any information to students about STD and pregnancy prevention. In this instance, the school nurse may need to advocate for adolescents' rights to have appropriate information.

REFERENCES AND READINGS

Abzug, M. (2004). Nonpolio enteroviruses. In R. Behrman, R. Kliegman, & H. Jenson (Eds.). *Nelson textbook of pediatrics* (17th ed., pp. 1042-1048). Philadelphia: Elsevier.

Ackley, B. J., & Ladwig, G. B. (Eds.). (2003). *Nursing diagnosis handbook: a guide to planning care* (6th ed.). St. Louis: Mosby.

American Academy of Pediatrics. (2003a). CMV. In L. K. Pickering (Ed.), *Red book: 2003 report of the Committee on Infectious Diseases* (26th ed., pp. 259-262). Elk Grove Village, IL: Author.

American Academy of Pediatrics. (2003b). Diphtheria. In L. K. Pickering (Ed.), *Red book: 2003 report of the Committee on Infectious Diseases* (26th ed., pp. 263-266). Elk Grove Village, IL: Author.

American Academy of Pediatrics. (2003c). Enterovirus (nonpolio) infections, group A & B coxsackieviruses and echoviruses. In L. K. Pickering (Ed.), *Red book: 2003 report of the Committee on Infectious Diseases* (26th ed., pp. 269-270). Elk Grove Village, IL: Author.

American Academy of Pediatrics. (2003d). Fifth disease—human parvo 19. In L. K. Pickering (Ed.), *Red book: 2003 report of the Committee on Infectious Diseases* (26th ed., pp. 459-461). Elk Grove Village, IL: Author.

American Academy of Pediatrics. (2003e). Group B streptococcal infections. In L. K. Pickering (Ed.), *Red book: 2003 Report of the Committee on Infectious Diseases* (26th ed., pp. 584-591). Elk Grove Village, IL: Author.

American Academy of Pediatrics. (2003f). Measles. In L. K. Pickering (Ed.), *Red book: 2003 report of the Committee on Infectious Diseases* (26th ed., pp. 419-429). Elk Grove Village, IL: Author.

American Academy of Pediatrics. (2003g). Poliomyelitis. In L. K. Pickering (Ed.), *Red book: 2003 report of the Committee on Infectious Diseases* (26th ed., pp. 505-509). Elk Grove Village, IL: Author.

American Academy of Pediatrics. (2003h). Preventing tickborne infection. In L. K. Pickering (Ed.), *Red book: 2003 report of the Committee on Infectious Diseases* (26th ed., pp. 186-187). Elk Grove Village, IL: Author.

American Academy of Pediatrics. (2003i). Rabies. In L. K. Pickering (Ed.), *Red book: 2003 report of the Committee on Infectious Diseases* (26th ed., pp. 514-521). Elk Grove Village, IL: Author.

American Academy of Pediatrics. (2003j). Rubella. In L. K. Pickering (Ed.), *Red book: 2003 report of the Committee on Infectious Diseases* (26th ed., pp. 536-541). Elk Grove Village, IL: Author.

American Academy of Pediatrics. (2003k). Sexually transmitted diseases in adolescents and children. In L. K. Pickering (Ed.), *Red book: 2003 report of the Committee on Infectious Diseases* (26th ed., pp. 157-167). Elk Grove Village, IL: Author.

American Academy of Pediatrics. (2003l). Smallpox. In L. K. Pickering (Ed.), *Red book: 2003 report of the Committee on Infectious Diseases* (26th ed., pp. 554-558). Elk Grove Village, IL: Author.

American Academy of Pediatrics. (2003m). Varicella. In L. K. Pickering (Ed.), *Red book: 2003 report of the Committee on Infectious Diseases* (26th ed., pp. 672-686). Elk Grove Village, IL: Author.

American Academy of Pediatrics. (2005). *Policy statement: prevention of pertussis among adolescents: recommendations for use of tetanus toxoid, reduced diphtheria toxoid, and acellular pertussis (Tdap) vaccine.* Retrieved December 27, 2005, from *www.aap.org/advocacy/releases/Tdap121205.pdf*

Boekeloo, B., & Howard, D. (2002). Oral sexual experience among young adolescents receiving general health examinations. *American Journal of Health Behavior, 26*(4), 306-314.

Carpenito-Moyet, L. J. (2003). *Nursing diagnosis: application to clinical practice.* (10th. ed.). Philadelphia: Lippincott Williams & Wilkins.

Centers for Disease Control and Prevention [CDC]. (2002a). *2002 guidelines for prevention of perinatal group B streptococcal disease.* Retrieved February 1, 2006, from *http://www.cdc.gov/mmwr/preview/mmwrhtml/rr5111a1.htm.*

Centers for Disease Control and Prevention. (2002b). *Early-onset group B streptococcal disease in newborns.* Retrieved June 5, 2005, from *www.cdc.gov/groupbstrep.com.*

Centers for Disease Control and Prevention. (2002c). *Smallpox fact sheet: disease overview.* Retrieved June 5, 2005, from *www.bt.cdc.gov/agent/smallpox/overview/disease-facts.asp.*

Centers for Disease Control and Prevention. (2002d). *Smallpox fact sheet: vaccine overview.* Retrieved June 5, 2005, from *www.bt.cdc.gov/agent/smallpox/vaccination/facts.asp.*

Centers for Disease Control and Prevention. (2006). *Recommended immunization schedule for children and adolescents who start late or who are more than 1 month behind.* Retrieved February 3, 2006, from *http://www.cdc.gov/mmwr/preview/mmwrhtml/mm5451-Immunizationa1.htm.*

Chamberlain, L. J. (2003a). Bacterial meningitis is less prevalent but still dangerous. *Infectious Diseases in Children, 16*(5), 55.

Chamberlain, L. J. (2003b). Varicella epidemiology may be changing. *Infectious Diseases in Children, 16*(5), 15-19.

Cherry, J. (2004). Enteroviruses and parechoviruses. In R. Fegin, J. Cherry, G. Demmler, & S. Kaplan (Eds.). *Textbook of pediatric infectious diseases* (5th ed., pp. 1984-2027). Philadelphia: Elsevier.

Choma, K. (2003). ASC—US HPV testing. *American Journal of Nursing, 103*(2), 42-50.

Colyar, M. (2003). Testing for sexually transmitted diseases. *Advance for Nurse Practitioner, 11*(5), 28-31.

Eftychiou, V. (2003). Sexually transmitted disease treatment update: a closer look at the CDC guidelines. *Advance for Nurse Practitioners, 11*(1), 43-45.

Eissa, M., & Cromwell, P. (2003). Diagnosis and management of pelvic inflammatory disease in adolescents. *Journal of Pediatric Health Care, 17*(3), 145-147.

Halpern-Felsher, B., Cornell, J., Kropp, R., & Tschann, J. (2005). Oral versus vaginal sex among adolescents: perceptions, attitudes, and behavior. *Pediatrics, 115*(4), 843-851.

Jarvis, C. (2003). *Physical examination and health assessment* (4th ed.). Philadelphia: W. B. Saunders.

Kanto, W., & Baker, C. (2003). Commentary: new recommendations for prevention of early-onset group B streptococcal disease in newborns. *Pediatrics in Review, 24*(7), 219-221.

Kenner, C., & Lott, J. W. (2003). *Comprehensive neonatal nursing: a physiologic perspective* (3rd ed.). Philadelphia: Elsevier.

Mack, T. (2003). A different view of smallpox and vaccination. *New England Journal of Medicine, 348*(5), 460-463.

Moorehead, S., Johnson, M., & Maas, M. (Eds.). (2003). *Nursing outcome classification (NIC)* (3rd ed.). St. Louis: Mosby.

Onieal, M. E. (2003). Smallpox update: educate yourself. *Advance for Nurse Practitioners, 11*(2), 70.

Pender, N. J., Murdaugh, C., & Parsons, M. (2005). *Health promotion in nursing practice* (5th ed.). Upper Saddle River, NJ: Prentice-Hall.

Shapiro, E. (2004). Lyme disease. In R. Behrman, R. Kliegman, & H. Jenson (Eds.), *Nelson textbook of pediatrics.* (17th ed., pp. 986-990). Philadelphia: Elsevier.

Stagno, S. (2004). Cytomegalovirus. In R. Behrman, R. Kliegman, & H. Jenson (Eds.), *Nelson textbook of pediatrics.* (17th ed., pp. 1066-1069). Philadelphia: Elsevier.

Stanhope, M., & Lancaster, J. (2003). *Community and public health nursing* (6th. ed.). St. Louis: Mosby.

Stoll, B. (2004). Infections of the neonatal infant. In R. Behrman, R. Kliegman, & H. Jenson (Eds.), *Nelson textbook of pediatrics* (17th ed., pp. 623-640). Philadelphia: Elsevier.

Trossman, S. (2003). The return of the smallpox vaccination: nurses report on plans, concerns. *The American Nurse, 35*(2), 1-3.

Weigand, J. (2003). Pushing the edge of viability: treatment dilemmas in neonatology. *Advance for Nurse Practitioners, 11*(5), 59-62.

Wexler, D. L. (2003). *Needle tips and the Hepatitis B Coalition News, 13*(1). Retrieved June 5, 2005, from *www.immunize.org/nslt.d/n27/n27.pdf.*

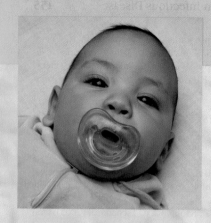

CHAPTER 17

The Child With an Immunologic Alteration

Learning Objectives

After studying this chapter, you should be able to:

- Describe how the immune system attempts to maintain homeostasis of the internal and external environment and what happens when it overfunctions or underfunctions.
- Explain how neonates acquire active and passive immunity.
- Delineate how to prevent the spread of organisms in children with an immune deficiency.

- Describe how to prevent, test for, care for, and support children with human immunodeficiency virus and their families throughout the entire spectrum of illness.
- Outline critical information needed by families with children receiving long-term corticosteroid therapy.
- Describe nursing interventions to help prevent the sudden death of a child having an anaphylactic reaction.

Definitions

active immunity   Protection that forms in response to exposure to natural antigens or vaccines; protection can last months, years, or a lifetime.

allergy   A hypersensitivity reaction in various body systems resulting from the immune system's response to exposure to an irritant (allergen).

antibody   A protein that the immune system produces to bind to specific antigens and eliminate them from the body.

antigen   A substance that possesses unique configurations enabling the immune system to recognize it as foreign.

autoimmune disease   Disease that occurs when the immune system produces antibodies—called autoantibodies—against cells of the body.

complement   An accessory system to a humoral response that is composed of serum proteins that facilitate enzyme action and antigen death.

immune (lymphoreticular) system   The body's internal defense against foreign substances, such as bacteria, viruses, parasites, and fungi.

immunodeficiency   A defect in the immune system leading to increased susceptibility to multiple and repeated infections.

leukocytes   White blood cells, whose chief function is to protect the body against foreign substances; includes five types: lymphocytes, monocytes, neutrophils, eosinophils, and basophils.

lymphocytes   The primary white blood cells of the immune system (e.g., B lymphocytes or B cells; and T lymphocytes or T cells).

nonspecific immune functions   Protective barriers, such as chemicals, interferon, inflammation, and phagocytosis, that are activated in the presence of an antigen but are not specific to that antigen.

passive immunity   Protection that occurs when serum containing an antibody is given or transmitted to a person who does not have that antibody.

specific immune functions   Humoral (B cell and antibody production) and cell-mediated (T cell) responses that are activated in a highly discriminatory way to antigens that survive in the body.

Electronic Resources

Additional information related to the content in Chapter 17 can be found on:

the interactive companion CD-ROM

- Audio Glossary
- NCLEX Review Questions

or the companion website at *evolve*
http://evolve.elsevier.com/james/ncoc

- Common Pediatric Laboratory Tests and Normal Values
- NCLEX Review Questions
- WebLinks

REVIEW OF THE IMMUNE SYSTEM

The body's network of first-line, or external, defenses—intact skin and mucous membranes and processes such as sneezing, coughing, and tearing—helps keep it free of disease. When a foreign substance penetrates first-line defenses, the immune, or internal defense system, provides secondary and tertiary protection through nonspecific and specific responses. The immune system is able to distinguish the body's own cells, or self, from foreign substances, or nonself; activate a response to detect and destroy foreign substances; suppress a response against the self; and memorize and store information.

Foreign substances, or antigens, possess unique configurations on their cell surfaces that mark them as foreign. The immune system first responds to the invader through nonspecific

immune functions. If the antigen survives the action of the nonspecific response, the immune system initiates specific immune functions. It begins producing proteins called *antibodies* or *immunoglobulins*. Each antibody is specific for a particular antigen, contains sites that are complementary, and can combine, or bind, with the antigen. This combination of antigen and antibody is called the *antigen-antibody complex* or *immune complex*. The immune complex prevents the antigen from binding with receptors on vulnerable cells.

The major organs and tissues of the immune system include the bone marrow, thymus, spleen, lymph nodes, and lymphoid tissue. Both the circulatory system and the lymphatic system connect these organs and tissues to one another. Specific types of cells are also important to the immune system.

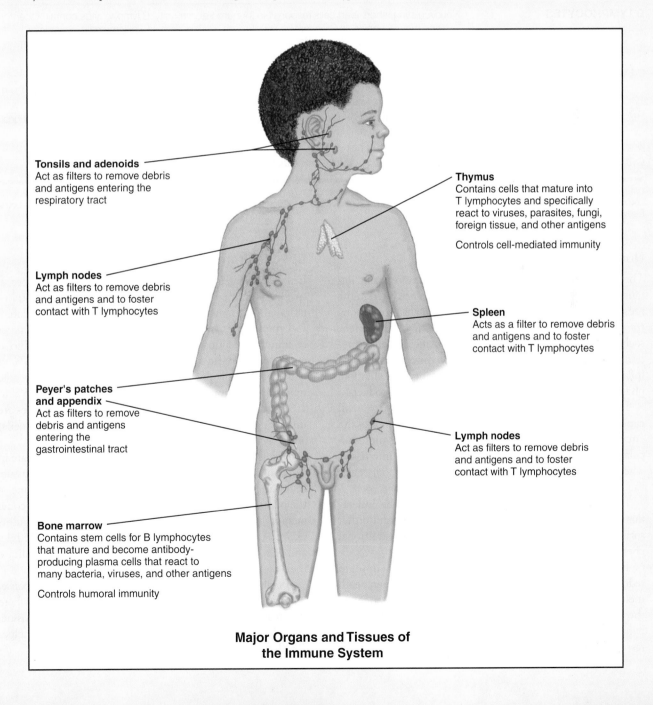

Tonsils and adenoids
Act as filters to remove debris and antigens entering the respiratory tract

Lymph nodes
Act as filters to remove debris and antigens and to foster contact with T lymphocytes

Peyer's patches and appendix
Act as filters to remove debris and antigens entering the gastrointestinal tract

Bone marrow
Contains stem cells for B lymphocytes that mature and become antibody-producing plasma cells that react to many bacteria, viruses, and other antigens

Controls humoral immunity

Thymus
Contains cells that mature into T lymphocytes and specifically react to viruses, parasites, fungi, foreign tissue, and other antigens

Controls cell-mediated immunity

Spleen
Acts as a filter to remove debris and antigens and to foster contact with T lymphocytes

Lymph nodes
Act as filters to remove debris and antigens and to foster contact with T lymphocytes

Major Organs and Tissues of the Immune System

Cells Involved in the Immune Response

Cell Type	Nonspecific Immune Response
GRANULOCYTES	
Neutrophils	First leukocytes to respond to tissue damage. Ingest and destroy antigens, especially bacteria, by phagocytosis. Increase in number during acute inflammation, bacterial infection, and necrosis. Immature neutrophils are called *bands*. Increased bands (shift to the left) indicate infection.
Eosinophils	Help control the inflammatory response. Neutralize histamine. Increase in number during hypersensitivity reactions and kill parasites directly.
Basophils	Secrete histamine, heparin, and serotonin in inflammation and immediate hypersensitivity reactions. Basophils located in tissue rather than in blood are called *mast cells*, which activate the inflammatory allergic response.
AGRANULOCYTES	
Monocytes/macrophages	Monocytes, immature macrophages, are large phagocytic agranulocytes. Monocytes ingest and introduce antigens into the circulation for recognition by B and T lymphocytes. Macrophages engulf bacteria and cellular debris to finish the cleanup process started by the neutrophils.

Cell Type	Specific Immune Response
B LYMPHOCYTES	Noncirculating, short-lived cells responsible for humoral immunity. B lymphocytes contain receptor sites that recognize specific foreign substances. Differentiate into plasma cells capable of secreting antibodies against bacteria. First responder to viral infection. Some become memory cells for long-term recognition of specific antigens.
T LYMPHOCYTES	Responsible for cellular immunity. Interact with specific antigens on cell surfaces and directly attack invading microorganisms. Respond to viruses, fungi, parasites, and foreign tissue. T-cell regulatory functions mobilize or deactivate the other cells in the immune system.
Helper (CD4$^+$) T cells	Recognize antigens that have been processed and presented to them by B cells or macrophages. CD4$^+$ cells secrete cytokines that stimulate B cells to manufacture antibodies.
Suppressor T cells	Inhibit the actions of helper T cells and B cells. Help keep the immune system cells in check.
Cytotoxic (CD8$^+$) T cells	Kill target cells directly. Particularly effective with viruses and malignant cells.

Data from Rote, N. (2002). In K. McCance & S. Huether (Eds.). *Pathophysiology: The biologic basis for disease in adults and children* (pp. 168-225). St. Louis: Mosby; Banasik, J. (2005). Inflammation and immunity. In L. Copstead & J. Banasik (Eds.). *Pathophysiology* (3rd ed.; pp. 203-243). St. Louis: Elsevier/Saunders.

Nonspecific Immune Functions

The body's innate immune system consists of nonspecific immune functions, which are protective barriers activated in the presence of an antigen but not specific to that antigen. Among these nonspecific immune functions are chemical barriers, such as bactericides and fungicides and enzymes in body secretions; interferon, a protein produced in response to viruses; and inflammation, increased capillary permeability, vasodilation, phagocytosis (cell eating), and elimination of cell products.

During an inflammatory response, vasodilation of small capillaries at the site of the organism invasion increases the circulation to the site. The resulting alteration in microvascular pressure facilitates movement of plasma cells into tissue, where they accumulate. Neutrophils are the first phagocytes that arrive at the site.

Phagocytosis can occur alone or as part of the inflammatory response. Phagocytes ingest the antigen and either survive or die. In dying, the phagocytes release additional chemicals that draw more phagocytes to the area.

Increased capillary permeability and vasodilation result in redness and edema. The products of phagocyte antigen death include toxins that give rise to fever, pain, and purulence. As the antigens are destroyed, the toxins are cleared from the lymph nodes, which often become enlarged. If the immune response is effective, the inflammation subsides.

Specific Immune Functions

If the antigen survives within the phagocyte, two types of specific immune functions can recognize and destroy it: humoral and cell mediated. Both responses are closely related.

Lymphocytes (white blood cells) function in both types of immune response. Lymphocytes circulate in the blood and the lymphatic system. They make up 53% to 57% of white blood cells during the first year of life, when specific immunity develops rapidly, but they make up only 25% to 30% after 12 months of age. Two classes of lymphocytes are involved in the immune response: B lymphocytes (B cells) and T lymphocytes (T cells).

B cells, which promote the humoral response, originate in the bone marrow or liver but mature in the lymphoid tissue, becoming plasma cells. When exposed to antigens, some of the plasma cells produce antibodies, whereas others become memory cells. Antibodies are classified as immunoglobulins G, M, A, D, and E, often abbreviated IgG, IgM, IgA, IgD, and IgE. Immunoglobulins bind to antigens and facilitate their destruction.

T cells, which are responsible for the cell-mediated response, originate in the bone marrow and mature in the thymus, where they react specifically to viruses, fungi, parasites, foreign tissue, and other antigens. The three major types of T cells are helper T cells, cytotoxic T cells, and suppressor T cells.

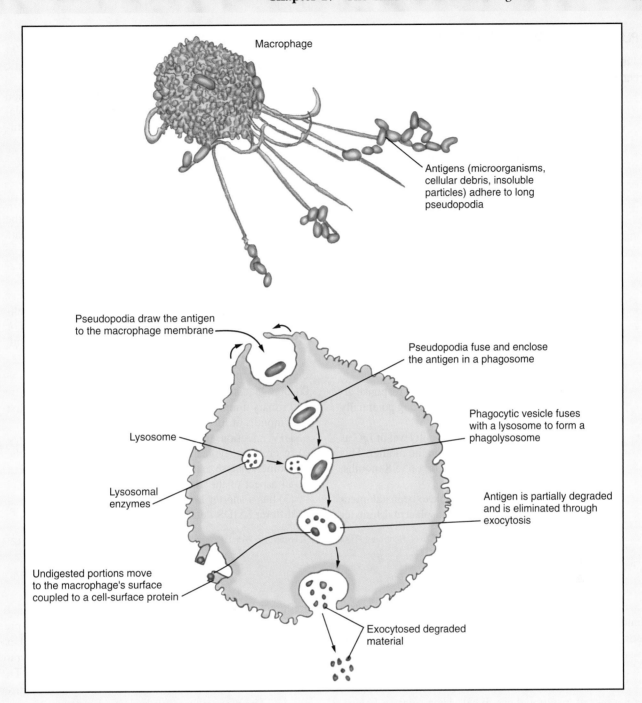

Macrophage

Antigens (microorganisms, cellular debris, insoluble particles) adhere to long pseudopodia

Pseudopodia draw the antigen to the macrophage membrane

Pseudopodia fuse and enclose the antigen in a phagosome

Lysosome

Phagocytic vesicle fuses with a lysosome to form a phagolysosome

Lysosomal enzymes

Antigen is partially degraded and is eliminated through exocytosis

Undigested portions move to the macrophage's surface coupled to a cell-surface protein

Exocytosed degraded material

Natural killer cells, or large granular lymphocytes that resemble T lymphocytes, can recognize and directly destroy infected or malignant cells. They are not antigen-specific (Buckley, 2004).

The Humoral Response

The humoral response involves chiefly B cells, although the cooperation of helper T cells is almost always necessary. Macrophages ingest antigens and introduce them into the circulation. In response, the B cells and helper T cells interact. The helper T cells secrete substances that cause B cells to multiply and differentiate into plasma cells, which produce vast quantities of antibodies specific to the antigen.

These antibodies combine with the antigens to form immune complexes. The antibodies promote phagocytosis, destroy the antigens, or activate an accessory system called *complement*, a series of serum proteins involved in enzyme action and antigen death. Destruction and elimination of antigen eventually result in a decrease in the chemical factors that enhance the humoral response, "turning off" the response when it is no longer needed (Banasik, 2005).

The Cell-Mediated Response

A cell-mediated response is also initiated by macrophages presenting antigens. Once activated, helper T cells secrete substances that spur additional T cells to grow. One set of

PEDIATRIC DIFFERENCES IN THE IMMUNE SYSTEM

The Organs of the Immune System Mature During Infancy and Childhood:

- Lymphoid tissue increases in mass during infancy and early childhood. It reaches adult size by 6 weeks of age, grows larger during the prepubertal years, and involutes at puberty.
- The thymus reaches its peak mass before puberty and then involutes.
- The spleen reaches its full size during adulthood.
- The number of Peyer's patches increases until the adult mean is exceeded during adolescence.

Immaturity of the Immunologic System Places the Infant and Young Child at Greater Risk for Infection:

- The infant has a limited capacity to mount an antibody response. The ability to respond to infections develops gradually as the infant acquires immunity actively and passively.
- Because of the immaturity of the inflammatory response in neonates, the more common signs and symptoms of infection (e.g., fever) are less pronounced, making diagnosis more difficult.
- Neonates' diminished nonspecific immune response allows a more rapid spread of infection, leading potentially to sepsis.
- The term newborn infant receives an adult level of IgG as a result of transplacental transfer from the mother. This level begins to disappear during the first 6 to 8 months, causing a physiologic drop in IgG.
- Premature infants are more susceptible to neonatal infections because of lower levels of transplacental transfer of IgG from the mother and a more severe physiologic drop in IgG.
- IgM, IgE, and IgD are normally in low concentration at birth. IgM, IgE, IgA, and IgD do not cross the placenta. The immunoglobulins reach adult levels at different ages*:
  —IgM: 1 year
  —IgA: 6 to 7 years
  —IgG: 7 to 8 years
  —IgE: 6 to 7 years
- Absolute lymphocyte counts reach a peak during the first year. Helper T cells reach adult levels by 6 years of age.
- Passive placental transfer of IgG may affect infants' response to active immunization (i.e., pertussis or diphtheria).
- Immature or inexperienced immune cells affect the reliability of delayed hypersensitivity skin reactions. For this reason, allergy skin tests are not routinely used with infants.

Disorders of the Immune System Present Differently in Children than in Adults:

- Primary immunodeficiencies typically present in the first 6 months of life.
- HIV infection, the major secondary immunodeficiency in children, typically (1) infects an infant through the mother, not sexually; (2) is diagnosed by measuring an aspect of the virus, not antibodies as in adults; and (3) has a shorter latency period in infants, with several different AIDS-defining illnesses.

*Buckley, R. (2004). The T-, B-, and NK-cell systems. In R. Behrman, R. Kliegman, & H. Jenson (Eds.), *Nelson textbook of pediatrics* (17th ed., pp. 683-689). Philadelphia: WB Saunders.

T cells, called *cytotoxic T cells*, tracks down and kills viruses, tumor cells, and other pathogens. Suppressor T cells, interacting with other immune components, draw the immune response to a close (Rote, 2002).

Development of Immunity

By 8 weeks of gestational age, B cell differentiation begins. The normal fetus can produce IgM by 20 to 24 weeks of gestation. The neonate's immune protection comes from prenatal transfer of maternal antibodies (IgG) and breast milk transfer of IgA. Gradually, the normal newborn infant's own humoral and cell-mediated responses to infections begin; immunity is acquired both actively and passively.

Active Acquired Immunity

When the body reacts to an antigen through either a humoral or a cell-mediated response, it is developing active immunity. Active immunity is long lived and measured in months, years, or even a lifetime; it follows exposure to environmental antigens or vaccines. Immediately after exposure, there is a latency period when antibody levels are low. When the body recognizes the antigen as foreign, it makes antibodies. The first antibodies produced are predominantly IgM and subsequently IgG. After a second exposure to the antigen, antibodies appear at a faster rate and the latency period is shortened or nonexistent. The antibody levels remain high and persist for much longer periods. The predominant antibody in a secondary response is IgG.

Infants receive specific live or attenuated vaccines on a recommended schedule to induce immunity against the antigens in the vaccine (see the recommended schedule on the Evolve website).

Passive Acquired Immunity

Passive immunity results from antibody transfer from one person to another. Transfer of antibodies from a woman to her fetus is an example of passive immunity. The fetus receives maternal IgG antibodies across the placenta and becomes protected against many infections. Most maternal antibodies dissipate in the infant by 6 to 9 months of age, but some persist for up to 18 months. The duration depends on the level of a particular antibody in the maternal plasma. Protection against measles, for example, may last through the second year of life, whereas protection against certain bacterial infections may last only 1 to 2 months. The reason neonates are so susceptible to infections by bacteria such as *Escherichia coli* is that the respective antibodies do not cross the placenta.

Other sources of passive acquired immunity include administration of immune globulin to produce temporary protection after an exposure and certain other disease-specific antibodies (e.g., rabies).

COMMON LABORATORY AND DIAGNOSTIC TESTS OF IMMUNE FUNCTION
Immunodeficiencies

A variety of laboratory tests evaluate immune system function. Laboratory evaluation determines intactness of its major functions: B-cell immunity, T-cell immunity, and phagocytosis. Many values vary significantly with age, especially during infancy. Among these are the differential in the complete blood cell count, the amount of various immunoglobulins, the lymphocyte surface antigen count (e.g., CD4+ count), and the total lymphocyte count.

Allergy

Measurement of eosinophilia and IgE levels, along with a radioallergosorbent test and skin testing, is helpful in diagnosing allergic reactions.

Laboratory and Clinical Screening Tests for Allergy

Test	Findings Suggestive of Allergy
CBC, differential	Excess eosinophils (>5% of WBCs)
Total eosinophil count	>450 μL eosinophils
Nasal smear	Excess eosinophils (>4% in young children, >10% in adolescents)
Serum IgE	Elevated for age
RAST, antigen-specific IgE	Increase in antigen-specific IgE in the serum
Skin testing	Urticarial wheal appears on skin within 20 to 30 min after administration of selected potential allergens; reaction can be immediate or delayed and can even include anaphylaxis

CBC, Complete blood cell count; *WBC,* white blood cell.

Immunoglobulin Function and Pediatric Implications

Immunoglobulin Type*	Percent (%) of Total Ig*	Function and Pediatric Significance	Location
IgG	70-80	Comprises approximately 80% of circulating immunoglobulin Contains most antibodies against bacteria, viruses, and fungi in blood and body spaces Crosses the placenta; provides maternal antibody protection to infants Responsible for Rh reactions IgG response is longer and stronger than that of the other immunoglobulins	Appears in all internal body fluids; present in majority of B cells
IgM	5-10	Earliest immunoglobulin produced in response to bacterial and viral infections Responsible for transfusion reactions in the ABO blood typing system Does not cross placenta, so values are low in neonates. However, IgM is produced early in life, and level increases after 9 mo of age. Presence in cord or infant blood may mean infection in utero or newborn period.	Appears mostly in the circulation Attached to B cells; released into plasma during immune response
IgA	10-15	Prevents infection across mucous membranes (local immunity) Especially important in antiviral protection Passes to neonate in breast milk	Appears in body secretions (nasal and respiratory secretions, saliva, tears, breast milk)
IgE	0.004	Leads to release of histamines, producing an allergic response Elevation may indicate allergy in children Plays a role in defense against parasites	Found on the surface membranes of basophils and mast cells Produced by plasma cells in mucous membranes and tonsils and in lymphoid tissue
IgD	0.2	Poorly understood Thought to influence B-cell differentiation	Appears in small amounts in serum Attached to B cells

Data from Tosi, M. (2004). Immunologic and phagocytic responses to infection. In R. Fegin, J. Cherry, G. Demmler, & S. Kaplan (Eds.). *Textbook of pediatric infectious diseases* (5th ed., pp. 25-27). Philadelphia: WB Saunders.
*Normal immunoglobulin values differ for age.

Common Laboratory and Diagnostic Tests of Immune Function

Test	Function	Nursing Considerations
Serum immunoglobulins (IgG, IgM, IgA, IgE)	Tests humoral immunity function Measures levels of immunoglobulins by separating them through immunoelectrophoresis	Immunization and toxoids received in the last 6 mo and blood transfusions, tetanus antitoxin, and gamma globulin received can affect results and should be noted on the laboratory requisition.
Lymphocyte surface antigen	Determines the types and subtypes of lymphocytes present in blood Names of lymphocyte surface antigens are based on "clusters of differentiation" (CDs). CD antigens on a lymphocyte allow its identification. The two most frequently found surface antigens and the cell types they identify: CD4: helper T cells CD8: suppressor T cells	To determine the number of a particular type of cell, a CBC must also be done.
Serum antibody titer to commonly received antigens in vaccines (e.g., tetanus, diphtheria)	Used to evaluate humoral immune function	Tests antibody level to specific antigens
Skin tests to *Candida,* tuberculosis	Used to evaluate cell-mediated immune function	Administered intradermally Size of induration is measured at daily intervals for 3 days
Differential WBC count	Part of the CBC, describes the relative amount of the five types of WBCs (leukocytes) in the blood: neutrophils, eosinophils, basophils, monocytes, and lymphocytes. The differential WBC count is expressed in number per cubic millimeter (mm^3) and as a percent of the total number of WBCs.	Helps identify infection, immune status, and allergy
Allergy skin tests	On administration of minute amounts of antigen into the skin, tests either immediate or delayed-type hypersensitivity	Because anaphylactic reactions can occur even in the presence of minimal allergen exposures, emergency equipment and medications should be immediately available
RAST	Measures the quantity and increase of antigen-specific IgE present in the serum. Exact quantities of antibodies to pollens, foods, etc., can be tested.	More expensive than traditional allergy skin testing but provides precise information without risk for hypersensitivity reaction

CBC, Complete blood cell count; *WBC,* white blood cell.
Data from Pagana, K., & Pagana, T. (2002). *Mosby's manual of diagnostic and laboratory tests* (2nd ed.). St. Louis: Mosby.
Refer to Evolve website for normal values.

Immunologic alterations typically are chronic, lasting from months to years and interfering with a child's life. Physical signs range from simple, such as impaired skin integrity, to complex, such as overwhelming infection. Intervals of wellness, relapses, and sometimes a decline in health should be expected. Repeated office visits and hospitalizations, disruptions in family routines, altered social interactions, and emotional and financial strain often are coupled with anxiety about the future.

Initially, the nurse helps the family adjust to a new, often devastating diagnosis. Care during the acute phase of the illness may be critical in nature, as underlying organisms are diagnosed and treated and fevers and pain are controlled. Once the acute crisis has resolved, the nurse prepares the family for discharge by teaching home management and identifying community resources and referrals for continuing support. The nurse also teaches the family how to prevent the spread of microorganisms through infection control practices at home and describes parameters for when to call the physician. The nurse discusses ways to maintain the child's skin integrity—the body's first line of protection against microorganisms—and

recommends a diet that supports immune cell growth. The nurse must keep abreast of current information because the field of immunology continues to evolve. Nurses also play a vital role in advocating for children with conditions such as human immunodeficiency virus (HIV) infection.

Despite all efforts, rehospitalization is often inevitable. The family is an integral part of the multidisciplinary team, keeping the physicians, nurses, and social workers informed of changes in the child's condition, administering medications, providing respiratory care, and often making difficult decisions about continued treatment and comfort.

HUMAN IMMUNODEFICIENCY VIRUS INFECTION

HIV infection is an acquired cell-mediated immunodeficiency disorder that causes a wide spectrum of illness in children, ranging from no signs or symptoms to mild and moderate to severe signs and symptoms. Acquired immunodeficiency syndrome (AIDS) is the most advanced manifestation of this illness.

Etiology

HIV, present in an infected individual's blood or body fluids, can enter an uninfected adult's or adolescent's body in several ways, including sharing of needles or syringes, engaging in unprotected sexual activity with an infected person where body fluids are shared, or receiving an infected blood product. Infected women can transmit the virus to a fetus across the placenta during pregnancy, to the infant at delivery, and to the young child through breastfeeding. Since 1994, when it became practice to administer zidovudine (ZDV) to mothers prenatally and intrapartally and to the newborn infant, the incidence of perinatal transmission has decreased by two thirds (Table 17-1) (Fowler, Garcia, Hanson, & Sansom, 2004). An antiretroviral regimen during pregnancy, combined with specific obstetric interventions designed to prevent transmission during labor, has reduced the transmission risk to less than 2% (Fowler et al., 2004). The risk for children acquiring HIV infection through sexual abuse exists.

Historically, children, especially those with hemophilia, acquired HIV/AIDS through infected blood products. Most of those children have died, having been infected before widespread and accurate screening of donor blood was routinely done. Of those approximately 10,000 children who acquired HIV infection perinatally and have survived through effective management, many are currently reaching the age of middle school and beyond, which brings new challenges for clients, families, and health professionals alike (Fowler et al., 2004; Menting, 2000).

Incidence

In the United States through 2004, approximately 9443 children younger than 13 years have been diagnosed with AIDS, and 58% of them have died. Of the reported cases, 8779 (93%) were acquired perinatally (Centers for Disease Control and Prevention [CDC], 2006). Heterosexual intimacy and infection through intravenous drug use are the most common transmission modes of HIV for women and adolescent girls. African American and Hispanic women are disproportionately represented among women living with AIDS in the United States, as are their infected children (Fowler et al., 2004). The prevalence of new perinatally acquired pediatric AIDS cases has declined steadily in the United States since 1994 (Fowler et al., 2004); the transmission rate is less than 2% (Working Group on Antiretroviral Therapy and Medical Management of HIV-Infected Children, 2005).

Manifestations

Box 17-1 lists general findings associated with immunodeficiency. Children with HIV manifest most or all of these signs. HIV infection in children and adults differs in several ways (Yogev & Chadwick, 2004; Working Group on Antiretroviral Therapy and Medical Management of HIV-Infected Children, 2005):

- The progression of HIV infection to AIDS is faster in infants and young children; most untreated infants have symptoms associated with HIV infection by 1 year of

---

BOX 17-1	**Clinical Findings Associated With Immunodeficiency**

Frequently Present, Highly Indicative Signs
- Repeated or persistent respiratory tract infection
- Repeated or persistent otitis media or sinusitis
- Severe bacterial infections
- Opportunistic infections, such as PCP or cryptosporidiosis
- Poor response to appropriate therapy

Frequently Present, Somewhat Suggestive Signs
- Skin lesions
- Failure to thrive or grow
- Chronic diarrhea
- Thrush
- Hepatosplenomegaly
- Anemia, thrombocytopenia, neutropenia
- Small or absent lymph nodes, tonsils, and adenoids

TABLE 17-1 Pediatric AIDS Clinical Trials Group 076 Zidovudine Regimen

Time of ZDV Administration	Regimen
Antepartum	Oral administration of 100 mg of ZDV five times daily,* initiated at 14-34 weeks' gestation and continued throughout the pregnancy
Intrapartum	During labor, intravenous administration of ZDV in a 1-hour initial dose of 2 mg/kg body weight, followed by a continuous infusion of 1 mg/kg body weight/hr until delivery
Postpartum	Oral administration of ZDV to the neonate (ZDV syrup at 2 mg/kg body weight/dose every 6 hr) for the first 6 weeks of life, beginning at 8-12 hours after birth†

Data from Perinatal HIV Guidelines Working Group. (2006). U.S. Public Health Service Task Force recommendations for use of antiretroviral drugs in pregnant HIV-1-infected women for maternal health and interventions to reduce perinatal HIV-1 transmission in the United States: (Table 1). Retrieved July 28, 2006, from *www.aidsinfo.nih.gov.*
*Oral ZDV administered as 200 mg three times daily or 300 mg twice daily is currently used in general clinical practice and is an acceptable alternative regimen to 100 mg orally five times daily.
†Intravenous dosage for term infants who cannot tolerate oral intake is 1.5 mg/kg weight IV every 6 hours. ZDV dosing for infants <35 weeks' gestation at birth is 1.5 mg/kg/dose IV or 2 mg/kg/dose orally every 12 hours, advancing to every 8 hours at 2 weeks of age if >30 weeks' gestation at birth or at 4 weeks of age if <30 weeks' gestation at birth.

HIV INFECTION

HIV is a retrovirus composed of RNA and an enzyme, reverse transcriptase, which plays a key role in viral replication. HIV gains entry into a CD4⁺ cell by direct fusion of the viral envelope to CD4⁺ receptors on the cell surface. Within the CD4⁺ cell, reverse transcriptase causes the synthesis of HIV DNA. This integrates with the CD4⁺ cell's DNA. The HIV virus then uses the CD4⁺ cell to make more copies of itself. The new viruses assemble at the host cell's surface. As they bud through the cell membrane, the viruses mature, are released, and can infect other CD4⁺ cells. The most critical result of HIV entry into the CD4⁺ cell is cell incapacitation and death.* Because CD4⁺ cells primarily enhance cell-mediated immunity, severely infected infants and children will exhibit symptoms of viral or fungal infection. In addition, CD4⁺ helper cells interact with the humoral immune response. Immunoglobulins become nonfunctional, making the child extremely vulnerable to bacterial infections.

*Rote, N. (2002). Immunity. In K. McCance & S. Huether (Eds.). *Pathophysiology: The biologic basis for disease in adults and children* (4th ed., pp. 168-196). St. Louis: Mosby.

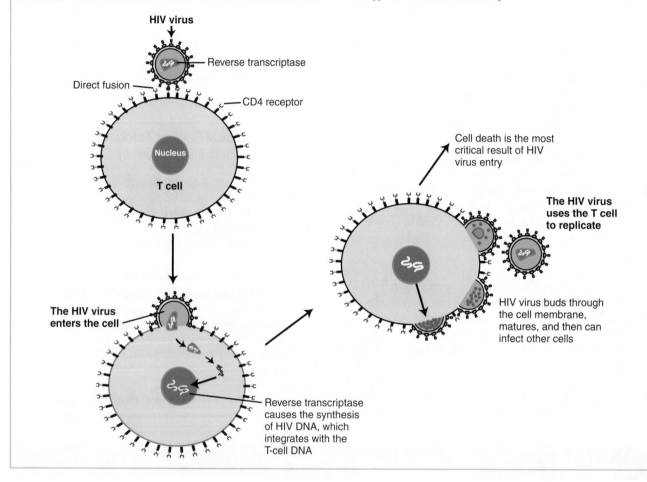

HIV virus

Reverse transcriptase

Direct fusion

CD4 receptor

Nucleus

T cell

The HIV virus enters the cell

Reverse transcriptase causes the synthesis of HIV DNA, which integrates with the T-cell DNA

Cell death is the most critical result of HIV virus entry

The HIV virus uses the T cell to replicate

HIV virus buds through the cell membrane, matures, and then can infect other cells

age and many young children with AIDS die before age 2 years. One factor contributing to the rapid progression in children is a higher viral load.

- Signs in children may include physical and developmental failure to thrive.
- Children have early opportunistic infections (e.g., chronic oral candidiasis), a greater number of bacterial infections from childhood illnesses, and lymphoid interstitial pneumonitis (LIP), a condition in which the child may be asymptomatic or may have parotid gland enlargement, hypoxia, and digital clubbing.
- *Pneumocystis carinii* pneumonia (PCP) in children with perinatally acquired HIV infection can occur early in

infancy, with the average age at onset being between 3 and 6 months.
- The CDC classifies the clinical manifestations of HIV infection as mild, moderate, or severe in children younger than 13 years. Mild signs of the illness may be nonspecific and include lymphadenopathy, hepatomegaly, splenomegaly, dermatitis, parotitis, and recurrent or persistent upper respiratory infection, sinusitis, or otitis media. In moderate disease, some signs are considered to be important if they persist or recur, particularly anemia, neutropenia, or thrombocytopenia; diarrhea; fever for longer than 1 month; herpes simplex; and oral candidiasis in children older than 6 months. Other signs of moderate infection

include bacterial meningitis, pneumonia, or sepsis (one episode); cardiomyopathy; complicated chickenpox; herpes zoster; hepatitis; nephropathy; LIP; and toxoplasmosis onset before age 1 month. In addition to LIP, the most common indicators of AIDS in children younger than 13 years are serious bacterial infections (multiple or recurrent), PCP, cytomegalovirus (CMV), encephalopathy, and wasting syndrome (seen most commonly in African children) (Yogev & Chadwick, 2004).

Diagnostic Evaluation

Because most HIV infections in infants and children occur as a result of perinatal transmission, HIV-positive pregnant women must be identified, educated, and treated. Early identification and treatment of women reduce the HIV transmission rate and enable early diagnosis and treatment for infected infants. If a woman does not receive HIV counseling during pregnancy, then counseling as soon as possible after delivery facilitates optimal management of the newborn (Working Group on Antiretroviral Therapy and Medical Management of HIV-Infected Children, 2005).

Diagnosing HIV through traditional HIV antibody measurement by enzyme-linked immunosorbent assay (ELISA) or Western blot assay is not accurate in infants younger than 18 months because of the presence of maternal antibodies. Viral diagnostic tests (culture, deoxyribonucleic acid [DNA] polymerase chain reaction [PCR], ribonucleic acid [RNA] assay) precisely diagnose most HIV-infected infants as early as 1 month of age and nearly all infected infants by 6 months of age. HIV DNA PCR is the preferred diagnostic method. Two positive virologic samples obtained on two separate occasions established a positive diagnosis. An infant who has had two or more negative tests, the first being at ≥ 1 month of age and others at ≥ 4 months of age in a non-breastfed infant usually suggests the child is not infected (Working Group on Antiretroviral Therapy and Medical Management of

HIV-Infected Children, 2005). Infants who have been exposed to HIV are tested before they are 48 hours old. If positive, the result is confirmed as soon as possible, and no later than 14 days of age, by viral assay on a second specimen. HIV-exposed infants should be retested at 1 to 2 months and again at 3 to 6 months (Table 17-2) (Working Group on Antiretroviral Therapy and Medical Management of HIV-Infected Children, 2005).

CD4$^+$ counts and HIV RNA assays assess an infected young child's immune status, response to therapy, risk for disease progression, and need for PCP prophylaxis after 1 year of age. CD4$^+$ counts are measured shortly after diagnosis and every 3 months thereafter. CD4$^+$ lymphocyte counts vary by age and the child's age is a basis for determining level of immune function or suppression. Although the absolute CD4$^+$ cell count varies with age, the CD4$^+$ cell percentage does not and the percentage is considered to be a more accurate assessment for childhood disease progression (Table 17-3) (Working Group on Antiretroviral Therapy and Medical Management of HIV-Infected Children, 2005).

The HIV viral burden in peripheral blood, measured by HIV RNA copy number, is determined by use of a quantitative HIV RNA assay. The HIV RNA copy numbers work in tandem with the CD4$^+$ percentage to provide independent information about prognosis and guide treatment decisions. HIV RNA copy number is assessed immediately after positive virologic diagnosis of HIV and every 3 to 4 months subsequently, or more often, depending on the child's clinical and treatment status (Working Group on Antiretroviral Therapy and Medical Management of HIV-Infected Children, 2005). Infants who are infected perinatally initially have a high viral burden; this burden decreases gradually over several years. A high viral burden in young infants may be related to more rapid disease progression seen in this age group (Working Group on Antiretroviral Therapy and Medical Management of HIV-Infected Children, 2005).

TABLE 17-2 Testing for the Presence of Human Immunodeficiency Virus	
Infants With Negative Viral Diagnostic Tests by 48 Hours of Age	**Infants With Positive Viral Diagnostic Tests by 48 Hours of Age**
Retest at 1-2 mo Retest at 3-6 mo HIV infection can be reasonably excluded in nonbreastfed infants with (1) two or more negative virologic tests at or after age 1 mo, with one of those tests performed at or after 4 mo, or (2) two or more negative HIV IgG antibody tests performed at age >6 mo with an interval of at least 1 mo between the tests also can be used to reasonably exclude HIV infection among children with no clinical evidence of HIV infection. HIV can be definitively excluded if HIV IgG antibody is negative in the absence of hypogammaglobulinemia at age 18 mo and if the child has both no clinical symptoms of HIV infection and negative HIV virologic assays.	Repeat the test as soon as possible after initial testing CD4$^+$ lymphocyte count and HIV viral load as soon as possible after first positive test Determine sequential CD4$^+$ lymphocyte counts every 2-3 mo HIV infection is diagnosed from two positive virologic tests performed on separate blood samples HIV DNA PCR is the preferred virologic method for diagnosing HIV infection during infancy

Data from Working Group on Antiretroviral Therapy and Medical Management of HIV-Infected Children. (2005, November 3). Guidelines for the use of antiretroviral agents in pediatric HIV infection. Retrieved July 18, 2006, from *www.aidsinfo.nih.gov.*

TABLE 17-3	**Revised Human Immunodeficiency Virus Pediatric Classification System: Immune Categories Based on Age-Specific CD4⁺ T-Cell Count and Percentage**					
	<12 Mo		**1-5 Yr**		**6-12 Yr**	
Immune Category	**No./mm³**	**%**	**No./mm³**	**%**	**No./mm³**	**%**
Category 1: No suppression	≥1500	≥25	≥1000	≥25	≥500	≥25
Category 2: Moderate suppression	750-1499	15-24	500-999	15-24	200-499	15-24
Category 3: Severe suppression	<750	<15	<500	<15	<200	<15

From Working Group on Antiretroviral Therapy and Medical Management of HIV-Infected Children. (2005). Guidelines for the use of antiretroviral agents in pediatric HIV infection: Table 1. Retrieved July 26, 2006, from *www.aidsinfo.nih.gov*.

Therapeutic Management

HIV-Exposed Infants

In addition to intravenous (IV) ZDV in the mother during labor, infants of known HIV-positive mothers should receive oral ZDV therapy within 6 to 12 hours after birth. This should continue for 6 weeks. Although some women may not be identified as being HIV infected until delivery, there are still prophylactic options for the neonate. The Perinatal HIV Guidelines Working Group (2006) describes clinical situations and therapeutic recommendations for women in the following categories. Updates of these recommendations are available from *http://AIDSinfo.nih.gov*:

- HIV-1–infected pregnant women who have not received prior antiretroviral therapy
- HIV-1–infected women receiving antiretroviral therapy during the current pregnancy
- HIV-1–infected women in labor who have had no prior therapy
- Infants born to mothers who have received no antiretroviral therapy during pregnancy or intrapartum (see Table 17-1).

Discussion about treatment options and recommendations should not be threatening. The mother makes the final decision about the use of antiretroviral medications. Women who decide not to accept treatment with ZDV or other drugs should not face punitive action or denial of care (Perinatal HIV Guidelines Working Group, 2006).

Because PCP can affect an infant as young as 2 months, PCP prophylaxis is initiated when an exposed infant is 4 to 6 weeks old, regardless of HIV status. Treatment with trimethoprim-sulfamethoxazole usually continues until the infant is 1 year old or is determined to be HIV-negative, usually by 6 months of age (CDC, 1995).

HIV-Infected Infants and Children

The Working Group on Antiretroviral Therapy and Medical Management of HIV-Infected Children updates treatment recommendations regularly. The underlying principles for the guidelines for antiretroviral treatment of infants and children infected with HIV include, but are not limited to the following (2005, p. 3):

Preventing Transmission and Ensuring Optimal Therapy

- Identification of HIV-positive women before or during pregnancy
- HIV testing with consent and counseling offered during pregnancy or as soon as possible after delivery, if not available prenatally.
- Accessibility of Clinical Trials and Appropriate Medication
- Accessible clinical trials specifically designed for HIV-infected women, HIV exposed neonates and infected infants, children and adolescents
- Availability of antiretroviral drug trials that identify the drug's impact on specific manifestations of HIV in children, including effects on growth and development and the child's neurologic system. Absence of Phase III efficacy trials for childhood manifestations of HIV does not preclude using approved antiretroviral drugs in children.
- Cooperation between the federal government and pharmaceutical companies to develop and evaluate effective and safe medication formulations specific for infants and children

CRITICAL THINKING EXERCISE 17-1

Some states in the United States have begun considering mandatory HIV antibody testing of newborn infants. This test is done at the same time as the other mandatory newborn screenings (e.g., phenylketonuria, sickle cell disease). Because recent HIV medication protocols have produced a marked decrease in the perinatal infection transmission rate and because very early treatment of HIV-infected infants has been shown to prolong intact immune status, universal HIV testing appears warranted.

What are the major issues, positive and negative, that legislators should consider before approving legislation for mandatory universal HIV testing for infants?

- Enrollment in clinical trials to be discussed by the health care provider and child's caregivers. Information about clinical trials for children and adults is available from *www.aidsinfo.nih.gov/clinical_trials/* or by telephone 1-800-448-0440.

Management Challenges

- Effective management of the complex and diverse care required by HIV-infected infants, children, adolescents and their families to be provided by a multidisciplinary team of health professionals (physicians, nurses, dentists, social workers, psychologists, nutritionists, outreach workers, and pharmacists)
- Regular monitoring of assays that measure HIV RNA and CD4$^+$ T-cell levels to effectively modify antiretroviral treatment in infected children and adolescents
- Consideration of issues related to adherence:
  - a. the availability and palatability of pediatric formulations;
  - b. the impact of the medication schedule on the child's quality of life, including number of medications, frequency of administration, their compatibility with other prescribed medications, and whether they need to be taken with food;
  - c. the ability of the caregiver or the adolescent to administer complex drug regimens and the availability of effective resources to facilitate adherence; and
  - d. potential for drug interactions.
- Consideration of potential limitations in future treatment options related to the potential for antiretroviral resistance

Growth and Development

- Frequent and meticulous monitoring of growth and development, especially physical failure to thrive and neurologic deterioration or developmental delay, for HIV-infected infants and children.
- Consideration of nutritional support, if needed, to enhance immune function, improve the child's quality of life, or assist the bioactivity of antiretroviral medications

More potent and improved antiretroviral medications have benefited HIV-infected children who have immunologic or clinical symptoms of HIV infection. These benefits include enhanced survival, improvements in growth and development and reduced opportunistic infections and other complications related to HIV infection (Working Group on Antiretroviral Therapy and Medical Management of HIV-Infected Children, 2005). HAART, highly active antiretroviral therapy, has dramatically impacted HIV-infected children's health, although its rigorous treatment schedules are challenging for children and families to maintain. There are also associated short- and long-term toxicities, which can have an impact on children (Working Group on Antiretroviral Therapy and Medical Management of HIV-Infected Children, 2005). Because of this, management of pediatric HIV should be directed by or in consultation with a specialist in pediatric and adolescent HIV infection.

Many factors need to be considered when making decisions about starting antiretroviral therapy in children, and these include (Working Group on Antiretroviral Therapy and Medical Management of HIV-Infected Children, 2005, p. 14):

- Disease severity and risk of progression as assessed by CD4$^+$ cell count and viral load or clinical/historical evidence of serious HIV-related or AIDS-defining illnesses.
- Available and accessible appropriate (palatable) medications, along with pharmacokinetic information about age-appropriate dosing.
- Complexity of the recommended antiretroviral regimen (e.g., dosing frequency, food and fluid requirements) and associated potential long- and short-term adverse effects from the regimen, including the possible effect of treatment choice on future therapeutic intervention.
- Presence of other illness that could affect drug choice (e.g., tuberculosis, acute or chronic renal or liver disease) or the child's use of other medications that could adversely interact with the antiretroviral medications.

Perhaps the most important factor to consider is the child's and the caregiver's ability to adhere to the prescribed regimen because failure to follow the regimen can result in the development of drug resistance and subsequent treatment failure. Adherence issues need to be addressed before a decision to start therapy is made, even if this may cause a delay in the initiation of therapy. The Working Group on Antiretroviral Therapy and Medical Management of HIV-Infected Children (2005) describes strategies for improving adherence, which include incorporating adherence assessment in every visit, choosing a medication regimen that fits as much as possible into the child and family's lifestyle, and providing ongoing support and encouragement. A multidisciplinary team including physicians, nurses, pharmacists, and sometimes peers are the most helpful to families. Strategies focus on both the child and the caregiver and must address any social issue that is affecting the family's adherence to the prescribed regimen.

Experts agree that infected infants with clinical symptoms of HIV or evidence of immune compromise should be treated; however, treating asymptomatic infants with normal immunologic status remains controversial (Working Group on Antiretroviral Therapy and Medical Management of HIV-Infected Children, 2005). Because of a more rapid disease progression in children than in adults and the fact that laboratory studies are less precise in predicting disease progression, children are treated more aggressively (Working Group on Antiretroviral Therapy and Medical Management of HIV-Infected Children, 2005).

Recommendations from the Working Group (2005) include initiating therapy for infants younger than 12 months of age who demonstrate clinical or immunologic symptoms of HIV disease, irrespective of the HIV RNA level. Experts recommend considering therapy for HIV-infected infants younger than 12 months who are asymptomatic and have normal immunologic status, although others would treat all HIV-infected infants younger than 12 months because of the risk of rapid disease progression (Working Group on Antiretroviral Therapy and Medical Management of HIV-Infected Children, 2005).

The risk of disease progression diminishes in children over 1 year of age, making it possible to consider deferring treatment for older children. The Working Group (2005) recommends that treatment should be started for all children older than 12 months who have AIDS or severe immune suppression and be considered for children who have mild to moderate clinical symptoms, moderate immunologic suppression, or confirmed HIV RNA levels greater than 100,000 copies/mL. If treatment is deferred, the child's virologic, immunologic, and clinical status needs to be closely monitored.

Currently, 21 antiretroviral agents are available to treat HIV infection. The Food and Drug Administration has approved 13 of these for pediatric use. These drugs fall into several major classes: nucleoside analog reverse transcriptase inhibitors (NRTIs), nucleotide reverse transcriptase inhibitors (NtRTIs), nonnucleoside reverse transcriptase inhibitors (NNRTIs), protease inhibitors, and fusion inhibitors. Doses for infants and children are individualized according to age and growth considerations. Doses for adolescents usually are based on determination of pubertal status by Tanner staging (see Chapter 8).

Additional Issues Related to the Child With Human Immunodeficiency Virus

Multigenerational Problems. One of the unique aspects of perinatal HIV infection is the multigenerational nature of the disease, in which both the mother and child may be infected. An important but difficult area to be addressed is future planning. This can include exploring the efficacy of standby guardianship, kinship care, or foster and adoptive placement. In addition, for children with advanced HIV disease, families have to make difficult decisions about an infected child's continuing care. Should aggressive treatment continue, or should the goal of treatment be to make the child comfortable? These decisions are best made in consultation with a multidisciplinary team that can identify areas of concern and develop strategic approaches that incorporate family culture, beliefs, available physical and emotional resources, and knowledge.

Disclosure. Initial reactions to an HIV diagnosis include confusion, anger, denial, and despair. Informing a child about a shared HIV status may be intimidating in light of the parent's physical, emotional, and social experiences. Disclosure to children often leads to difficult questions about transmission, parents' sexuality, or drug use history and questions about death—their own as well as their parent's (Lewis, 2005). Nehring, Lashley, and Malm (2000) found three themes related to disclosure: telling for support, determining who should know, and telling children. Various challenges, along with concern about the child's ability to cope with the

knowledge of life-threatening illness, often cause families to struggle to keep the diagnosis a secret. Fear that their child will lose hope at learning of the diagnosis is a major concern for parents and guardians (Lewis, 2005).

Now that children with HIV are surviving into adolescence, the issue of disclosure becomes a vital part of their health care management, particularly considering the prevalence of adolescents who engage in sexual activity (Boatner, 2002). In 1999, the American Academy of Pediatrics (AAP) issued a policy statement regarding disclosure of illness status to HIV infected children and adolescents. The policy statement was reaffirmed by the AAP in 2005 (AAP, 1999/2005). Basing their recommendations on research that suggests more positive emotional status in both children and parents who have disclosed, the AAP recommends that disclosure be considered in light of the child's cognitive and psychosocial development and clinical status as well as the multitude of factors affecting parents' decision to disclose. Although health care professionals respect the wishes of parents regarding disclosure, it is important to create a continuing supportive environment in which disclosure issues can be discussed and adequate preparation for eventual disclosure can occur (AAP, 1999/2005). The AAP recommendations for disclosure strongly emphasize encouraging disclosure to school-age children and state the ethical responsibility of pediatricians to fully disclose HIV status to affected adolescents (AAP, 1999/2005). Parents and other guardians of an HIV-infected child should be counseled by a knowledgeable health care professional about disclosure to the child. This counseling may need to be repeated throughout the course of the child's illness.

HIV and School Settings. As the population of children living with HIV/AIDS gets older, there are more HIV-infected children in school systems. Parents of these children strive to maintain normal in-school and out-of-school routines as much as possible. Both parents of children who are infected and parents of children who are not infected have concerns regarding the school setting. Parents of children who are not infected worry about the risk of illness transmission. Parents of children with HIV are apprehensive that their child may be socially isolated or may be at higher risk of more easily acquiring common childhood illnesses (Jessee, Nagy, & Gresham, 2001). Balancing these issues is challenging for children, parents, and the school district. Children who have HIV are protected by the federal Individuals with Disabilities Education Act and may not be discriminated against in the school setting. Most state and local school agencies have policies that protect the rights of all ill children, but particularly children with HIV (National Association of State Boards of Education, 2001). The National Association of State Boards of Education, (2001) has produced an excellent guide to education policy and HIV infection that asserts that HIV is not a significant risk to others in the school setting when school personnel follow appropriate guidelines and affirms the right of children and adults with HIV to fully participate in both the education and extracurricular programs at school. Privacy provisions are clearly stated and maintain that no

Text continued on p. 472

NURSING CARE PLAN

The Child With HIV Infection in the Community

Focused Assessment

Nurses play a critical role in the care of the child with HIV infection and the child's family, primarily in home, school, and day care settings. In each of these settings, the nurse has an opportunity to listen, educate, and support the child and the family. Many children with HIV infection experience normal health, and it is of primary importance that families be encouraged to keep well-child visits and obtain appropriate immunizations (Table 17-4). Assessment of the child's developmental status also is imperative at each well visit.

If the immune system becomes more compromised and symptoms develop, hospitalization may become necessary. In that event, assessment and therapeutic management focus on the recognition and prevention of potentially serious infections (primary prophylaxis), the treatment of serious bacterial and opportunistic infections that might affect multiple organs and systems when they occur, and the prevention of recurrence of serious infections (secondary prophylaxis).

When caring for children with HIV and their families, the nurse should engage the family in a helping relationship and put aside any biases so that they do not interfere with listening, supporting, and providing care. The nurse should use an interpreter, if needed, to provide culturally sensitive care.

When an HIV diagnosis has been made, assess what the family understands about the HIV-related spectrum of illness, including immunologic status and treatment options. Under certain circumstances, the use of monthly IVIG may be recommended. Specific circumstances in which IVIG should be considered include children with hypogammaglobulinemia, recurrent serious bacterial infections, treatment of parvovirus B19 infections and treatment of thrombocytopenia; and single-dose administration of IVIG for measles exposure.*

At each well or ill visit, ask the caregivers about any fever, nausea, vomiting, diarrhea, ear pulling, or changes in appetite, sleep pattern, or behavior that might suggest a secondary infection. Should signs of a secondary infection be a concern, focus the physical examination on indicators of an infection:

- *Hydration status:* Assess the skin for turgor and the mucous membranes for moistness, drying, or cracking; confirm the absence or presence of tears; in infants, determine whether the anterior fontanel is palpable and soft; ask about intake and urine and stool output and check specific gravity.
- *Respiratory status:* Listen and observe for nasal flaring, retractions, cough, difficulty breathing, tachypnea, grunting, wheezing, rhonchi, and decreased breath sounds. Check oxygen saturation levels with a monitor.
- *Mouth lesions:* Observe for white patches on the tongue or inside the cheeks, blisters on the lips, or lesions on the tonsils or soft palate.
- *Skin lesions (especially in the diaper area):* Observe for blotchy, red, flat areas, blistering, dryness, rashes, or vesicles.

Assess pain by obtaining a self-report from the child, using faces, numbers, or color scales when appropriate; by observing the child's speech, facial expressions, body movements, and responses; and by talking with the family.

NURSING DIAGNOSIS	Deficient Knowledge about the natural history of pediatric HIV disease, potential complications associated with HIV infection, and current treatment modalities related to emotional reaction to the diagnosis.
EXPECTED OUTCOME	The family will: • Demonstrate knowledge acquisition, as evidenced by explaining what has been taught about HIV infection and playing an active role in determining the plan of care for the child.

Intervention	*Rationale*
1. Determine the family's knowledge about HIV infection, treatment modalities, and home care (Box 17-2).	1. Teaching needs to begin at the family's level of understanding. It is important to note that because the majority of HIV-infected children are infected perinatally, the nurse may also be educating parents about their own disease process.
2. Teach the family about HIV infection, its signs and symptoms, progression, and treatment.	2. Knowledge and understanding of HIV may increase cooperation and adherence to the often-complicated treatment regimens that are necessary to achieve viral suppression and will also serve to reduce anxiety.
3. Identify the family's areas of concern (e.g., a new diagnosis, fear of transmission by casual contact within the family).	3. Addressing family concerns decreases misinterpretation. First, educate about the lack of transmission by household contact and correct any myths or misperceptions that may exist.

Continued

NURSING CARE PLAN—cont'd

4. Use teaching strategies that will maximize potential for success (e.g., medication sheet that details medication name, dosage, how often to give, why the child is on the medication, and hints for administering bad-tasting medication).
5. Educate the family about what signs or problems necessitate calling the health care provider for management advice.

4. Written information may assist the family to ensure that the correct medication regimen is being followed.

5. Early identification of potential problems may prevent serious complications from developing.

Evaluation

Can the family describe the natural history of HIV, systems affected by HIV, current treatment modalities, and care for the child at home?
- Can the family administer the correct dosages of medications at the appropriate times?

- Does the family readily participate in developing and carrying out a plan of care for the child?
- Does the family contact health care providers when the child is ill and in need of services?

NURSING DIAGNOSIS Anxiety (primary caregiver) related to fear of disclosure.

EXPECTED OUTCOMES The family will:
- Share the diagnosis with those family members, health care professionals, and school staff who need to know.
- Move through the stages of disclosure and will feel comfortable sharing their feelings about the diagnosis with appropriate people.
- Answer the child's questions honestly and share the diagnosis when the time is right.

Intervention

1. Listen quietly when the family talks about the diagnosis of HIV. Note their stage of disclosure (secrecy, exploratory, readiness, or full disclosure).

2. Maintain confidentiality concerning the HIV diagnoses. Ask the primary caregiver what individuals know about the diagnosis and what they know. Encourage the family to share the diagnosis with health care professionals.
3. Help family members decide who needs to know the child's diagnosis and offer them education and support in the process of disclosure. Encourage peer support groups when the family is ready. Do not assume that all family or friends accompanying child to the clinic or hospital know the child or parent's diagnosis.
4. Encourage the family to be honest with the child and to explain the reason for physicians' visits and procedures.

5. Encourage the family to listen to the questions the child is asking and to answer the questions briefly, using words the child can understand. Look for readiness cues that indicate the child wants to know more.

Rationale

1. Sharing the diagnosis occurs on a continuum, with secrecy at one end and full disclosure at the other. Families initially may want to keep their feelings about the diagnosis private. However, a time may come when they wish to talk; the nurse should develop rapport and gain trust.
2. Health care professionals who plan and coordinate care need to know the diagnosis.

3. Although many people would like to know the diagnosis, only a handful needs to know. Ask families to consider the following when choosing whom to tell: the child's age, clinical condition, and health care requirements; the likelihood that bloody injuries will occur; the use of standard precautions.
4. When to tell the child the diagnosis is a personal choice, but families need to understand that children will worry more if no one talks with them or if they sense dishonesty; ethical considerations make it important that adolescents be aware of their diagnosis (American Academy of Pediatrics, 1999/2005).
5. It is important for families to understand what their children are asking and to answer their questions, keeping responses short and simple.

NURSING CARE PLAN—cont'd

6. Encourage the family to speak with a health care professional when the child asks questions that are difficult to answer. Suggest that the parent seek counseling to help find the appropriate language for answering the child.
7. Promote normal routines at home.

6. Role playing is a useful technique that allows families to practice potential responses to difficult questions. The nurse can offer to accompany them if they decide to share the diagnosis.
7. Children with HIV infection can go to school, church, and parties; play sports and games; and develop or maintain friendships.

Evaluation

- Is the family able to share the diagnosis with all appropriate health care professionals and at least one significant person?
- Does the family appear to be moving through the stages of disclosure and seeking out support from peers?

- Is the family able to seek social and health services for which they qualify on the basis of their HIV/AIDS status?
- Can family members answer the child's questions in a developmentally appropriate way?

NURSING DIAGNOSIS   Ineffective Therapeutic Regimen Management: Nonadherence related to lack of support systems or denial of the illness.

EXPECTED OUTCOMES   The mother who is infected with HIV will:
- Keep her own health care appointments and those of her child.

The family will:
- Work toward accepting the diagnosis.
- View themselves as valued members of the health care team.

The child/family will:
- Adhere to the medication regimen.

Intervention

1. Use language that shows respect. Offer information in a language that can be understood by the child and family. Use a translator as needed.

2. Encourage the HIV-infected mother to keep her own health care appointments.
3. Accept the parents' use of denial during periods of emotional respite. Refer for counseling to assist with the grieving process.
4. Maintain realistic hope when possible.

5. Refer the family to social services for assistance with finances, transportation, food, housing, clothing, medical care, and respite care as needed.

Rationale

1. Families affected by HIV do not want their children called *innocent victims* or *AIDS babies,* nor do they want to be judged as promiscuous or substance abusers. Labels can create barriers, which can result in nonadherence with health care recommendations.
2. HIV-infected women often neglect their own health care needs as they attend to those of their children.
3. The diagnosis of HIV brings a series of losses, including the loss of the future and all that the future holds for a child. Denial is a coping mechanism.
4. With new prophylaxis agents for HIV-positive pregnant women and their infants, HIV infection develops in fewer than 5% of all perinatally HIV-exposed babies, and antiretroviral treatments have been successful in preserving immune function in infected infants.
5. Although some women with HIV infection are judged to be uncaring because of missed appointments or because their children fail to gain weight, many simply lack the basic resources for adherence. Problems that affect the caregiver's ability to manage the therapeutic plan include inadequate or inconsistent housing or transportation and personal HIV disease. In some instances, substance use or abuse or mental illness can affect adherence. Guilt about passing HIV on to a child can interfere with providing the structure and discipline necessary for establishing a successful regular medication regimen.

Continued

NURSING CARE PLAN—cont'd

6. Teach the family how to give antiretroviral agents at home, keep a log, and adjust the schedule to accommodate school schedules, if necessary. Give suggestions about helpful devices, such as daily or weekly pill boxes that can be prefilled, alarm watches, and pictorial medication reminders. In some instances use of a gastrostomy tube or button may be effective (Weglarz & Boland, 2005).

7. Monitor medication adherence every visit.

8. Suggest ways to make medications more palatable to children.
   * Encourage early pill taking
   * Mix medication with chocolate syrup or follow with chocolate candy
   * Give ice or ice pop before giving the medication
   * Use an oral syringe to place the medication back in the mouth away from taste buds
   * Avoid mixing medications in food or drink, fighting with the child, and skipping medication doses

6. The antiretroviral regimen may include a combination of medications in addition to other medications a child may be taking. A daily log or other medication reminder device helps families keep track.

7. A multifaceted approach works best in adherence issues. Palatability of the medication, ability to meld the medication schedule with existing routines, denial, guilt, and embarrassment about the diagnosis are all barriers to appropriate cooperation with the medication regimen.

8. Liquid formulations of HIV medications may be foul tasting or have a gritty texture. Unlike short-course medications, these medications must become part of the family's everyday routine for years.

Evaluation

* Is the mother able to take care of herself?
* Has the patient or caregiver been able to move from denial to anger to acceptance of the diagnosis?
* Are the primary caregivers active, participatory, and valued members of the health care team?

* Does the child/family adhere to the medication regimen?

IVIG, Intravenous immune globulin.
*American Academy of Pediatrics. (2003). *2003 Red book: Report of the Committee on Infectious Diseases* (26th ed.). Elk Grove Village, IL: American Academy of Pediatrics.

one is required to disclose HIV status, nor will HIV antibody testing be required for any reason (National Association of State Boards of Education, 2001). Strict confidentiality and health record keeping and storage procedures will be followed for all in the school setting according to the law, and a person's HIV status will not appear in educational records without consent.

Schools will operate according to the standards promulgated by the U.S. Occupational Health and Safety Administration for the prevention of blood-borne infections. (For a complete copy of this guide, "Someone at School has AIDS," go to *http://www.nasbe.org.*) Because most HIV medications are now given once or twice daily under most circumstances, it is no longer necessary for school nurses to be involved in the administration of a child's medications.

CORTICOSTEROID THERAPY

Corticosteroids, given as part of a treatment regimen, act as natural products of the adrenal glands, reducing local and systemic inflammatory symptoms.

Incidence

Topical steroids are applied to the skin or mucous membranes to reduce edema and redness and to counteract itching. They may be used to treat ophthalmic reactions and skin conditions such as eczema. Hydrocortisone cream is one example of a topical steroid. *Systemic steroids* reduce the inflammatory symptoms of generalized allergic reactions (e.g., asthma, hives, severe contact dermatitis). Systemic steroids are also given increasingly to treat malignant or autoimmune disorders. An example of a systemic steroid is prednisolone (Drug Guide, p. 476).

Inhaled corticosteroids produce a very strong local action and can control symptoms in children with asthma and allergic rhinitis. An example of an aerosol steroid is beclomethasone (see Chapters 21 and 25). Studies have varied as to whether long-term use of inhaled corticosteroids results in growth delay, with the general consensus being that there may be an initial period of growth delay but little effect on eventual height (Randell et al., 2003; Salvatoni et al., 2000).

TABLE 17-4 **Recommendations for Routine Immunization of Human Immunodeficiency Virus—Infected Children in the United States**

Vaccines	Known Asymptomatic HIV Infection	Symptomatic HIV Infection
Hepatitis B	Yes	Yes
DTaP	Yes	Yes
IPV*†	Yes	Yes
MMR	Yes	Yes‡
Hib	Yes	Yes
Pneumococcal§	Yes	Yes
Influenza*‖	Yes	Yes
Varicella¶	Consider	Consider
BCG	No	No
Hepatitis A#	See text	See text

NOTE: Always check the most current immunization schedule. Administer immune globulin after measles exposure and varicella-zoster immune globulin after chickenpox exposure, unless administered during the previous 2 wk. Administer tetanus immune globulin in the management of tetanus-prone wounds. *DTaP,* Diphtheria and tetanus toxoids and acellular pertussis; *IPV,* inactivated poliovirus; *MMR,* live-virus measles-mumps-rubella; *Hib, Haemophilus influenzae* type b conjugate; *BCG,* bacille Calmette-Guérin.
Data from American Academy of Pediatrics. (2003). *Red book 2003: Report of the Committee on Infectious Diseases* (25th ed.). Elk Grove Village, IL: American Academy of Pediatrics.
*Including siblings and other family members.
†Only inactivated poliovirus vaccine should be used for HIV-infected children, HIV-exposed infants whose status is indeterminate, and household contacts of HIV-infected people.
‡Severely immunocompromised HIV-infected children should not receive live-virus measles-mumps-rubella vaccine.
§Pneumococcal vaccine should be administered to all age-appropriate HIV-infected children. Children who are older than 2 months of age should receive pneumococcal vaccine at the time of diagnosis. Reimmunization after 3 to 5 years is recommended in either circumstance.
‖Influenza vaccines should be provided each autumn for HIV-exposed infants 6 months of age and older, HIV-infected children and adolescents, and household contacts of HIV-infected people.
¶Consider for HIV-infected children in CDC class N1 and A1.
#Two doses 6-12 months apart after 2 years of age.

Pathophysiology

Corticosteroids have many different effects but are usually prescribed for their anti-inflammatory or immunosuppressive properties. As anti-inflammatories, they inhibit chemical mediators and the occurrence of edema, capillary dilation, phagocytic activity, and the migration of leukocytes associated with the inflammatory response. As immunosuppressives, they decrease monocyte and macrophage differentiation and block lymphokine production, leading to T-cell inhibition.

The side effects of steroids vary widely with the child and the medication. Generally, the higher the dose and the longer the medication is taken, the more serious are the side effects. More knowledge about reactions and a broader selection of steroids and alternatives have significantly reduced untoward reactions in recent years.

Manifestations

Clinical manifestations of excess topically administered steroids include skin atrophy, delayed wound healing, telangiectasis or dilation of the cheek blood vessels, striae, and excess absorption leading to any of the clinical manifestations of systemic use.

Some clinical manifestations of excess steroid administered systemically include the following:
- Edema, particularly in the face
- Gastrointestinal irritation, even bleeding
- Bruising and delayed wound healing

- Susceptibility to infections
- Growth limitations
- Hypertension
- Loss of muscle mass
- Increased appetite and weight gain
- Amenorrhea
- Pancreatitis
- Joint pain and osteoporosis (may lead to bone fractures)
- Cataracts

Diagnostic Evaluation

The diagnosis of corticosteroid excess is suspected when clinical manifestations appear and it is confirmed by administering a bolus of adrenocorticotropic hormone (ACTH) to the child. ACTH challenges the adrenal gland to respond to pituitary stimulation. If serum cortisol levels do not rise after administration of ACTH, adrenal suppression (cortisone excess) is present.

Therapeutic Management

Every effort is made to prevent corticosteroid excess by observing the following:
- Short-term, high-dose therapy (for 1 week or less) is preferred over long-term therapy if there is a strong indication for the use of steroids.
- If long-term use is necessary, alternate-day administration may be prescribed.

Text continued on p. 476

NURSING CARE PLAN

The Adolescent With HIV Infection

Focused Assessment

Adolescents with HIV infection pose unique and important challenges for nurses. Although some teens who have had HIV since childhood continue to enjoy relatively good health, others may have advanced HIV disease, which can interfere with normal daily activities. Newly diagnosed adolescents, who may have entered the health care system because of the consequences of high-risk behavior (e.g., sexually transmitted diseases, pregnancy), usually are healthy with normal immune systems; some may not even have been aware that they are infected.

In addition to assessing needs related to their diagnosis and normal development, special attention must be directed to assessing the adolescent's knowledge of the disease process, risk-taking behaviors that could potentially transmit the virus to others, and how to prevent such occurrences. The adolescent's understanding of the importance of regular medical follow-up must also be assessed. It is critical that the adolescent be involved in all aspects of decision making, especially in discussions and plans for antiretroviral therapy options.

NURSING DIAGNOSIS   Deficient Knowledge about the effect of HIV on adolescents, current treatment options available, and preventing transmission of virus to others.

EXPECTED OUTCOME   The adolescent and family will:
- Explain in their own words what has been taught about HIV infection, including potential treatment regimens, goals of preserving or restoring immune function, and issues related to adolescent risk taking and adolescent sexuality.
- Adhere to a mutually agreed on treatment regimen.

Intervention

1. Determine the adolescent's and family's knowledge of HIV infection and associated concerns and emphasize the necessity for regular well care, developmental monitoring, nutritional support, and immunizations.
2. Identify the adolescent's specific concerns and address them first.

3. Educate the adolescent about potential symptoms and problems to report to the health care provider.
4. Establish readiness to adhere to medication regimen. Include the adolescent in decision making about a treatment routine that will maximize adherence (e.g., compatibility with daily routine, minimum number of required pills and capsules, fewest side effects).

5. Discuss high-risk behaviors that could result in transmission of HIV to others (e.g., sexual activity, IV drug use) and methods of prevention of transmission.

6. Offer participation in peer support groups.

7. Encourage school attendance and promote normal routines at home.

Rationale

1. Teaching needs to be geared toward the adolescent's cognitive and emotional readiness to learn about HIV, its treatment, and prevention of complications.

2. Acknowledging the adolescent's concerns may help allay fears and anxiety and help begin to develop a trusting relationship.
3. Early identification of problems may prevent development of serious complications.
4. Adherence to medication regimens is critical to prevent development of viral resistance. Medication dosages for adolescents are based on Tanner stage (see Chapter 8), not age. Doses for those in Tanner stage 1 or 2 are similar to pediatric dosages; for those in Tanner stage 5 dosages are based on adult dosages. For adolescents in other Tanner stages of development, dosages are monitored and adjusted for effectiveness (Working Group on Antiretroviral Therapy and Medical Management of HIV-Infected Children, 2005).
5. Frank discussions may empower the adolescent to assume responsibility for reducing the risk for transmission to others by encouraging safer behaviors in sexual practices and drug use.
6. The adolescent may benefit from sharing thoughts and feelings about living with HIV, difficulties in taking medications, and so on with others.
7. When possible, promoting normalcy assists in meeting developmental needs as well as preventing social isolation.

Evaluation

- Can the adolescent and family explain what HIV is and its treatment goals?
- Can the adolescent describe appropriate measures to reduce disease transmission to others?

- Does the adolescent state adherence with the prescribed therapeutic regimen?

| BOX 17-2 | PARENTS AND CAREGIVERS WANT TO KNOW | How to Care for the Child With an HIV Infection |

Review the following information and health practices at the time of initial testing and subsequent visits.

Transmission

HIV can be spread by:
- Unprotected sexual activity
- Sharing of needles
- An infected mother to her baby
- Breastfeeding
- Open wounds (if there is blood-to-blood contact)

HIV cannot be spread by:
- Sharing knives, forks, spoons, or cups
- Using the same toilet seats, bathtubs, or showers
- Coughing or sneezing
- Hugging, holding, or touching people

Prevention

The best way to prevent the spread of HIV is to:
- Abstain from sex and from sharing needles, or
- Use latex condoms with nonoxynol 9, and
- Wash needles in a 1:10 bleach solution

The best way to prevent pregnancies is to:
- Abstain from sex, or
- Use a latex condom
- Use contraception
- Undergo tubal ligation

If infected with HIV, follow these precautions:
- Do not breastfeed
- Do not donate blood, sperm, or organs

Testing
- The most common HIV tests used for older children and adults are the ELISA and the Western blot assay, which measure levels of antibodies to the virus.
- The most common HIV tests used for infants and children younger than 18 months are the HIV DNA qualitative PCR and HIV RNA quantitative assays, which detect the presence of the virus itself.
- $CD4^+$ counts indicate how well the immune system is working.

Illness (AIDS)

Children with HIV infection might initially be asymptomatic. Mild and moderate symptoms include the following:
- Persistent upper respiratory and ear infections
- Thrush
- Skin conditions
- Vomiting and diarrhea
- Enlarged liver, spleen, lymph nodes, and parotid gland
- Growth and development problems
- LIP—a rare lung disease

Some severe symptoms of the illness include the following:
- Opportunistic infections, such as PCP and CMV
- Recurrent bacterial infections, such as sepsis, meningitis, and pneumonia
- Severe developmental delay or neurologic symptoms
- Wasting syndrome/failure to thrive

Medications
- Adherence to schedule
- Proper administration
- Safe and proper storage
- Side effects

Home Care

Offer a high-calorie, high-protein diet if growth is a problem:
- Mix formula as directed.
- Do not add extra water or cereal to formula.
- Give supplemental vitamins and minerals as ordered.

Practice basic infection control measures and follow standard precautions, including the following practices:
- Avoid touching blood.
- Do not share toothbrushes, pierced earrings, razors, or nail clippers.
- Use a barrier when caring for a cut or a bloody nose.
- Cover open sores.
- Leave scabs alone.
- Wipe up blood spills with a paper towel, wash the area with soap and water, rinse with bleach and water, and air dry.
- Wrap disposable materials soiled with blood in newspaper, tie off in a plastic bag, and throw away in a plastic-lined trash can.
- Wash hands with soap and water if you touch blood.
- Rinse blood-soiled clothing with hydrogen peroxide or cold water and then wash as usual.
- Allow blood to air dry on dry-clean-only clothing.

Keep your child's immunizations up to date. Your child should also receive the following:
- Pneumococcal vaccine at 2 years of age, if not given during infancy
- Flu shot each fall
- Immune globulin after measles exposure
- Varicella-zoster immune globulin after chickenpox exposure
- Tetanus immune globulin for tetanus-prone wounds

Call the physician if any of the following symptoms occur:
- Fever higher than 101° F
- Vomiting and diarrhea
- Decreased appetite, difficulty swallowing, drooling
- Rashes, bumps, lumps, or sores on the skin
- Coughing or chest congestion
- Ear pain, pulling on the ears, or drainage from the ears
- Wounds that will not heal
- Exposure to measles or chickenpox

Give prophylaxis against PCP and antiretroviral drugs as ordered.

DRUG GUIDE

PREDNISOLONE (PEDIAPRED, PRELONE)

Classification: Corticosteroid.

Action: Decreases inflammation; suppresses the immune response; affects bone marrow and the metabolism of proteins, carbohydrates, and fats.

Indications: Given for severe allergic and inflammatory conditions (e.g., asthma, eczema, juvenile arthritis), immunosuppression, and some autoimmune disorders.

Dosage and Route: Pediatric, oral: 0.5-2 mg/kg daily in divided doses; comes in syrup (15 mg/5 mL) or tablets (1 mg, 5 mg, 25 mg).

Absorption: Rapid absorption from the gastrointestinal tract.

Excretion: Half eliminated in 2-4 hr; metabolized in the liver and excreted in the urine.

Contraindications: Do not give if the child has a systemic fungal infection or is sensitive to any of the ingredients.

Precautions: Children taking prednisolone are more prone to infection. Avoid exposure to measles or chickenpox while on prednisolone; immunize the child with live virus vaccines (measles, mumps, rubella; varicella) before beginning corticosteroid treatment. Avoid giving with nonsteroidal anti-inflammatory drugs or aspirin because it may increase the risk for gastrointestinal bleeding.

Adverse Reactions: Gastrointestinal distress, cushingoid state (moon face, buffalo hump), delayed wound healing, skin eruptions, carbohydrate intolerance, fluid retention, growth delay in children. *Acute adrenal insufficiency can occur when the child is under stress or if the medication is withdrawn abruptly. Do not discontinue this medication without tapering the dose.*

Nursing Considerations: Teach the parent to have the child take the medication with food or milk. Store the medication in a cool, dry location. Teach the parent to notify the physician if the child exhibits any of the following: fever, other signs of infection, fatigue, muscle weakness, sudden weight gain, severe gastric irritation, slow wound healing, or growth delay, or if the child is experiencing increased stress.

• At the time of an acute infection or surgery, supplementary steroids are indicated for children who have received them over a long period.

Because of immunosuppression, killed-virus vaccines are substituted for live-virus vaccines for children receiving high-dose or long-term steroids.

NURSING CARE

The Child Receiving Corticosteroids

Assessment

Assessment of a child receiving long-term steroid therapy includes measuring height, weight, and blood pressure at each visit. In addition, the nurse observes the child for facial puffiness, abdominal pain, increased appetite, blurred vision, and increased thirst or urination. Families may report recent illnesses, bruising, or delayed wound healing.

Nursing Diagnosis and Planning

The nursing diagnoses and expected outcomes that may be appropriate after assessment of a child receiving corticosteroid therapy are

• Ineffective Therapeutic Regimen Management: Nonadherence related to associated complications.

Expected Outcome: The child will take all medications as directed.

• Disturbed Body Image related to changes caused by treatment.

Expected Outcome: The child will share feelings about any changes in appearance.

• Risk for Infection related to immunosuppression.

Expected Outcome: The child will be afebrile and free of signs of secondary infections.

• Risk for Injury (adrenal insufficiency, delayed wound healing) related to insufficient knowledge.

Expected Outcomes: The child will not experience injury as a result of too-rapid withdrawal of medication or delayed wound healing. The parent can explain the reason for not withdrawing the medication abruptly.

• Risk for Delayed Growth and Development related to growth suppression and muscle wasting.

Expected Outcome: The child will continue to grow according to his or her own height and weight curve.

Interventions

The nurse should provide the family with written instructions that specifically state what to do if a dose is missed and when to decrease dosages. In general, if a dose is missed, the child should take it as soon as it is remembered; if it is almost time for the next dose, the child should skip the dose altogether. The nurse should emphasize not to discontinue corticosteroid therapy abruptly.

The child needs to take the medication with foods or milk to minimize the risk for gastrointestinal bleeding. Because the child's appetite may be increased, encouraging low-calorie snacks throughout the day is appropriate. (The nurse should remind the family that salt may increase fluid retention.) Liquid forms of systemic corticosteroids can seem unpalatable to children. In this instance, the child may prefer a crushed tablet that has been put in a very small amount of a sweet food, or the liquid can be mixed with a sweet drink. Be sure to tell parents to mix the medication in 1 teaspoon or less of food or only a small amount of liquid to ensure that the child receives all the medication.

Changes in appearance are temporary and reversible. The nurse can compare changes in appearance and weight gain at each visit and encourage expression of the child's feelings. Weight and height monitoring of the child receiving long-term corticosteroid therapy is important; fluid retention can mask muscle wasting and growth suppression.

Corticosteroids can also mask infections. The family should be instructed to call the physician in the event of temperature elevation, cough, runny nose, ear tenderness, decreased appetite, nausea, vomiting, diarrhea, or behavioral change, or even if the child just "does not seem right." The child's skin should be checked routinely for bruising and signs of wound infection, and lesions that do not resolve as expected should be reported. The family should not treat the child with over-the-counter products without consulting the physician. The child receiving long-term therapy should avoid others who are sick; parents should promptly report any exposure to a communicable disease, such as measles or chickenpox, to the health care provider.

Potential environmental hazards and accident prevention strategies based on the child's developmental age should be emphasized. If the child gets a cut, the parent may hold gentle pressure to the site for 3 to 5 minutes to stop the bleeding and prevent hematoma formation. The child should wear a Medi-Alert bracelet stating the key clinical manifestations of corticosteroid excess or adrenal insufficiency.

Evaluation

- Is the child taking corticosteroids as directed?
- Is the child able to express feelings about any changes in appearance?
- Does the child remain afebrile and free of any signs of secondary infection?
- Are any wounds healing at a normal rate?
- Is the child displaying any signs of adrenal insufficiency, and can the parent explain why the medication should not be withdrawn abruptly?
- Is the child growing at a rate appropriate for age as measured on a standard growth chart?

CRITICAL TO REMEMBER
The Child Taking Oral Corticosteroids

Long-term corticosteroid therapy causes adrenal insufficiency because exogenous (outside the body) use reduces the need for endogenous (within the body) production. Abrupt cessation of corticosteroid use without allowing for a gradual increase in adrenal production can cause insufficiency.

- Taper the dose to allow for a gradual return of adrenal function.
- Carefully monitor the child during the tapering process for the following: fatigue, muscle weakness, joint pain, dizziness, anorexia, nausea.
- Supplemental glucocorticoids might be necessary during times of increased stress to prevent adrenal insufficiency.

IMMUNE COMPLEX AND AUTOIMMUNE DISORDERS
Immune Complex Disorders

Immune complexes are clusters of interlocking antigens and antibodies. Under normal conditions, immune complexes are removed from the blood. In some circumstances, however, immune complexes continue to circulate. Eventually they become trapped in the tissues of the kidneys, lungs, skin, joints, or blood vessels. There they set off reactions that lead to tissue inflammation and damage.

Deposition of immune complexes is considered to be a precipitator for several different conditions in childhood. Both Kawasaki disease (see Chapter 22) and acute poststreptococcal glomerulonephritis (see Chapter 20) are thought to be caused by immune complex deposition in tissue.

Autoimmune Disorders

Sometimes the immune system's ability to differentiate self from nonself breaks down and the body begins to make antibodies against its own cells, tissues (particularly connective tissue), and organs. Such antibodies are known as *autoantibodies*. Autoantibodies are common in conditions such as rheumatic fever (see Chapter 22), juvenile arthritis (see Chapter 26), and systemic lupus erythematosus.

It is still unclear what initiates an autoimmune response. Several theories have been proposed:
- Activation of immature B cells that do not develop antigen-specific receptors
- Alteration of normal tissue cells by infection or another process, which causes them to become antigenic
- Similarity between the structures of some infectious organisms and self-antigens, causing a cross-reaction
- Genetic predisposition of defective immune regulation

The response is exacerbated by a malfunction of helper T and suppressor T cells when there are too many helper cells and not enough suppressor cells to turn off the immune response. Some autoimmune disorders also manifest with increased tissue deposits of immune complexes.

SYSTEMIC LUPUS ERYTHEMATOSUS

Systemic lupus erythematosus (SLE) is a chronic, multisystem autoimmune disease characterized by inflammation of the connective tissue. SLE varies in severity and is marked by remissions and exacerbations.

Etiology

Although the etiology of SLE is not known, genetic, environmental, hormonal, and immune response factors are likely to be responsible. Environmental factors can include exposure to the sun, ultraviolet light, stress, fatigue, viruses, bacteria, certain medications, and some food additives.

Incidence

The overall incidence of SLE in the United States is up to 250 cases per 100,000 population (Klein-Gitelman & Miller,

2004). The condition is relatively rare in young children. In young children, the female to male ratio is 4:1; after puberty, this ratio increases to 8:1 (Klein-Gitelman & Miller, 2004). Onset in girls is most common between the ages of 9 and 15 years. More African American, Hispanic, and Asian children are affected than white children.

Manifestations

Malaise, arthralgia, and recurrent fever of unknown etiology frequently are among the early manifestations of SLE. The symptoms, however, depend on what organs the immune

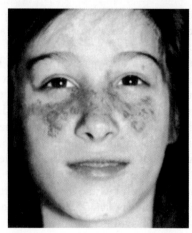

FIG 17-1 **The butterfly rash of systemic lupus erythematosus.** *(From Behrman, R. E., Kliegman, R. M., & Arvin, A. M. [1996]. Nelson textbook of pediatrics [15th ed.]. Philadelphia: WB Saunders. Color Plate Fig. 150-1.)*

PATHOPHYSIOLOGY

SYSTEMIC LUPUS ERYTHEMATOSUS

Many abnormalities in the immune system are associated with SLE. Autoantibodies, referred to as *antinuclear antibodies (ANA),* act against DNA and other cell nucleus components. Abnormal immune complex formation and nonspecific activation of B lymphocytes cause an increase in immune globulins, a process that triggers autoantibodies. This response is exacerbated by a reduction in the number of suppressor T cells. These autoantibodies produce inflammation and damage tissues and organs, including the skin, joints, heart, lungs, kidneys, brain, and circulatory vessels.

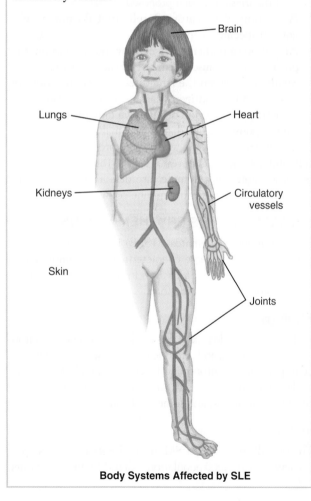

Body Systems Affected by SLE

complexes affect and can include (Klein-Gitelman & Miller, 2004; Rote, 2002):

- Malar butterfly rash—a fixed, red, flat or raised rash over the cheeks and bridge of nose (Fig. 17-1)
- Discoid rash—red, round, raised patches that spread
- Photosensitivity—skin rash from sun exposure
- Oral and nasal ulcers—usually painless lesions
- Arthritis—painful, swollen joints with edema
- Pleuritis, pericarditis, or peritonitis
- Renal disorder—protein, casts, or red blood cells in urine
- Neurologic disorders—headaches, personality changes, seizures, or psychosis
- Hematologic disorders—anemia, leukopenia, lymphoma, or thrombocytopenia
- Immunologic disorders
- Positive antinuclear antibody (ANA) assay

A child with SLE also might have weight loss, growth impairment, headache, and memory problems. Occasionally, children will have Raynaud's phenomenon, in which the digits of the hands and feet suddenly change color (mottled to white to blue) in response to cold. The most serious complications of SLE include renal disease and neurologic problems.

Diagnostic Evaluation

The presence of four or more of the clinical manifestations just listed, regardless of whether they occur simultaneously, is suggestive of SLE. In addition, a number of tests can be used to diagnose and monitor the progress of SLE. A positive ANA test and the presence of anti-DNA antibody are highly suggestive of SLE but can occur also in other autoimmune disorders. Blood urea nitrogen levels, gamma-globulin levels, and the erythrocyte sedimentation rate might be elevated. Complement levels (C3 and C4) can be decreased. Pathologic changes compatible with SLE may be confirmed by electrocardiography, computed tomography, and magnetic resonance imaging and by skin and renal tissue biopsy specimens demonstrating immune complexes.

Therapeutic Management

The treatment of SLE is tailored to the organ system or systems affected and is aimed at preventing exacerbations and complications. The goal of treatment is to use the least amount of pharmacologic intervention needed. Helping the child and family develop long-term coping strategies is important.

Systemic corticosteroids are most often given to control the inflammatory response. When steroid treatment is not effective or renal progression is rapid, cyclophosphamide (Cytoxan) might be considered. Nonsteroidal anti-inflammatory drugs, excluding ibuprofen, are sometimes used to treat arthritis, serositis, and febrile attacks. Because they can cause liver damage, they are used with caution and careful monitoring. Children with renal and neurologic disorders generally receive anticonvulsant and antihypertensive therapy, whereas those with skin lesions and joint problems take antimalarial drugs such as hydroxychloroquine (Plaquenil). Killed-virus vaccines rather than live-virus vaccines are used in affected children. A low-salt diet may reduce fluid retention and prevent elevated blood urea nitrogen levels; a low-protein diet helps preserve renal function.

The long-term prognosis for children with SLE is positive; the 10-year survival rate is 95% (Szer & Athreya, 2002). Close monitoring is essential for positive outcomes.

NURSING CARE

The Child With Systemic Lupus Erythematosus

Assessment

During a period of disease exacerbation, a child can become acutely ill. The nurse should monitor the child's vital signs, mobility, activity level, and pain and should complete a neurologic examination that assesses for decreased sensation, weakness in the extremities, and changes in behavior. Of equal importance is evaluation of the effect of living with a chronic illness on a young child's self-image and interaction with peers.

Nursing Diagnosis and Planning

The nursing diagnoses that apply to the child with SLE are
- Disturbed Body Image related to changes secondary to the disease process and treatments.
  Expected Outcome: The child will share feelings about altered appearance or function.
- Powerlessness related to memory and emotional alterations.
  Expected Outcome: The child and family will seek assistance in managing memory or emotional problems.
- Activity Intolerance related to the effects of the disease process.
  Expected Outcome: The child will participate in activities to the extent possible.
- Chronic Pain related to arthritis and numbness of the hands and feet.
  Expected Outcome: The child will be free of pain, demonstrating an acceptable level on an age-appropriate pain

assessment tool and the ability to gain appropriate rest and participate in age-appropriate activities.
- Ineffective Therapeutic Regimen Management: Nonadherence related to associated complications and developmental level.
  Expected Outcome: The child will take all medications as directed and describe the medication plan and any medication side effects.

Interventions

The nurse needs to help the child and family understand the importance of drug therapy and activity restriction during acute exacerbations. Avoiding triggers that cause exacerbations is essential (e.g., avoiding exposure to sun or avoidable sources of infection). Wearing an appropriate sunscreen is a necessity (sun protection factor above 15, waterproof, para-aminobenzoic acid free, ultraviolet A and ultraviolet B protective). Raynaud's phenomenon can be prevented by dressing warmly in cold weather, paying particular attention to hat, gloves, and warm socks.

An adolescent will have difficulty achieving a balance between the need to take risks and be accepted by peers and the realities of a chronic illness (see Chapter 12). The teenager with a chronic illness needs to participate as fully as possible in activities at home, at school, and in the community. Documenting episodes of fatigue along with associated activities allows young people to gain some control. They can then use this information to make sensible decisions about participation in extracurricular activities. The adolescent should be encouraged to plan an appropriate and convenient medication self-administration schedule and should be able to describe the side effects of the prescribed medications.

Anger about the diagnosis and alienation from peers are common. Wearing makeup can mask rashes and improve appearance. Keeping a diary also helps the young person vent anger. An affected peer who is in remission can offer support, as can national SLE organizations (see Evolve website). The Internet is also a source of support and information.

Evaluation

- Does the child share feelings about her (or his) appearance or function?
- Do the child and family seek assistance as needed for related memory or emotional problems?
- Does the child participate in sports and extracurricular activities without becoming overly fatigued?
- Is the child free of pain as documented on an age-appropriate pain assessment tool?
- Is the child taking all medications as directed, and can the child describe the medication plan and side effects from the medications?

ALLERGIC REACTIONS

Allergy is the immune response to an antigen called an *allergen* that causes a hypersensitivity reaction in various body systems. This hypersensitivity reaction, which occurs with

TABLE 17-5   Classification of Allergic Reactions

Type	Pathophysiology	Examples
I Immediate (anaphylactic) hypersensitivity	IgE attaches to mast cells and basophils, causing rupture and release of all contents (i.e., histamines).	Allergic rhinitis, acute anaphylaxis, hives, eczema, asthma
II Cytotoxic hypersensitivity	An allergen (e.g., red blood cell) stimulates IgE or IgM to react and mobilize complement to destroy the allergen.	Transfusion reaction after receiving incompatible blood
III Arthus hypersensitivity (immune complex)	Immune complex is formed and can destroy tissues.	Serum sickness, glomerulonephritis
IV Delayed cell-mediated hypersensitivity	An allergen reacts with T lymphocytes, and these lead other cells to produce damage.	Contact dermatitis (e.g., poison ivy)

TABLE 17-6   Common Allergic Conditions in Children

Allergens	Manifestations	Diagnosis
INHALANTS Pollen, dust, mold, dander	Sneezing; red, itchy nose, eyes, pharynx, and palate; edematous nasal passages; tongue clicking; runny or congested nose; mouth breathing; chronic cough; dark circles under eyes; nose wrinkling; pale, boggy nasal mucous membranes	Allergic rhinitis
APPLICANTS Heat, cold, wool, cosmetics, solutions for hair permanents, sunscreens, plants, grasses	Well-defined red, raised skin or mucosal lesions	Hives Contact dermatitis
FOODS Milk, wheat, eggs, strawberries, tomatoes, oranges, chocolate, nuts, shellfish	Intestinal cramping, nausea, vomiting, diarrhea Bronchospasm Red patches on cheeks, face, wrists, neck, hands, extremities; swelling; itching; weeping; scales and crust Well-defined red, raised skin or mucosal lesions Vascular headaches	Colic Asthma Eczema Hives Migraines Possible anaphylaxis
MEDICINES Penicillin, cephalexin, immunizations, allergy immunotherapy, chemotherapy	Redness, swelling, pain Weakness, restlessness, edema, laryngospasm, cardiovascular collapse	Local inflammation Anaphylaxis
INSECTS Stings of bees, wasps, hornets	Redness, swelling, pain Weakness, restlessness, edema, laryngospasm, cardiovascular collapse	Local inflammation Anaphylaxis

a second exposure to an antigen, can be immediate or delayed. The classification of allergic reactions often reflects the pathophysiologic features of each type (Table 17-5). In most children with allergies, there is a genetic link. Common allergic conditions include allergic rhinitis, hives, eczema, asthma, colic, and migraines (Table 17-6).

Allergic rhinitis is an immediate hypersensitivity reaction to allergens trapped by the hairs and mucus that line the inside of the nose (see Chapter 21). Anaphylaxis is a life-threatening allergic response. Allergic reactions are related to the antibody IgE.

ANAPHYLAXIS

Anaphylaxis, a severe, immediate hypersensitivity reaction to an excessive release of chemical mediators, affects the entire body.

Etiology

Food allergy has become the primary cause of anaphylaxis in children (Sampson & Leung, 2004). Other causes include penicillin or other antibiotics, insect stings, immunizations, allergy immunotherapy (desensitization), chemotherapeutic agents, blood products, and diagnostic contrast media.

Peanuts (including peanut butter) and tree nuts (e.g., cashew, almond, walnuts, pecans, pistachios) are particularly potent substances, causing anaphylaxis in increasing numbers. Other frequently seen food allergies include milk, eggs, wheat, shellfish, and other fish. Anaphylactic reactions to products containing latex have increased in incidence, especially among children with spina bifida (see Chapter 28) and children with abnormalities of the urinary tract.

Incidence

Approximately 6% to 8% of children younger than 3 years in the United States have severe allergic reactions to foods (Sampson & Leung, 2004). In many cases, previous exposure to the allergen is undocumented, so the child has anaphylaxis presumably on first documented exposure. For example, studies suggest that exposure to peanut allergens can occur in a breastfeeding child whose mother has a high intake of nuts (Zeiger, 2003), but the child only has anaphylaxis when peanut butter is introduced into the diet at about age 2 years. In the child who is allergic to peanuts or other nuts, anaphylactic reaction can occur with exposure to nut oils, surfaces contaminated with nuts, shell fragments, or cooking and serving utensils used previously for nut products.

The incidence of anaphylaxis in the United States from all causes is considered to be 30 per 100,000 (Sampson & Leung, 2004).

Manifestations

The onset of anaphylaxis is sudden, usually occurring within seconds to minutes after exposure to an allergen. Initial symptoms of impending anaphylaxis include the following:
- Sneezing
- Tightness or tingling of the mouth or face, with subsequent swelling of the lips and tongue
- Severe flushing, urticaria, and itching of the skin, especially on the head and upper trunk
- Rapid development of erythema
- A sense of impending doom

PATHOPHYSIOLOGY

ANAPHYLAXIS

Anaphylaxis occurs when an allergen binds with IgE on mast cells and basophils, causing degranulation and release of histamines and other chemical mediators. Histamine action precipitates respiratory signs of bronchoconstriction with bronchospasm and edema (especially laryngeal edema) from increased vascular permeability. Other systems most affected during an anaphylactic response include gastrointestinal (itchiness and tingling along the gastrointestinal tract, vomiting, diarrhea, pain) and integumentary (urticaria). Anaphylaxis can lead to circulatory collapse and death if not promptly managed. An allergen that has previously provoked a response, or one that has not, can cause anaphylaxis.

These symptoms might be followed by gastrointestinal and respiratory symptoms, which include nausea, vomiting, diarrhea, and cramping, as well as rhinorrhea, stridor, wheezing, and hoarseness.

The most serious features of anaphylaxis are laryngospasm, edema, cyanosis, hypotensive shock, vascular collapse, and cardiac arrest. Several hours after the initial phase of anaphylaxis resolves, a second, or biphasic, reaction can occur. This second reaction can be as severe as the initial reaction, affects similar body systems, and can occur hours up to several days after the initial episode.

Diagnostic Evaluation

Anaphylaxis occurs suddenly, allowing no time for diagnosis. The etiology is determined later by obtaining a history of the exposure. Serum studies may reveal an elevated IgE for the agent of exposure. In some cases the allergen can be confirmed by skin tests or radioallergosorbent test (RAST).

Therapeutic Management

Treatment of anaphylaxis must begin immediately because it may be only a matter of minutes before shock occurs. In the community setting, immediately activate the emergency response system. Injectable epinephrine is the first drug of choice in the acute treatment of anaphylaxis. In addition to epinephrine, oral diphenhydramine and a histamine inhibitor (e.g., cimetidine) may be indicated.

Epinephrine (0.01 mg/kg/dose of 1:1,000 concentration) is administered to children with suspected anaphylaxis. Children with known severe allergic reactions need to have an EpiPen or other preloaded, automatic delivery system available at all times. The EpiPen (0.3 mg) is appropriate for children who weigh more than 66 pounds, whereas the EpiPen Jr. (0.15 mg) can be administered to children who weigh at least 22 pounds (Sampson, 2003).

In a hospital or emergency setting, managing anaphylactic shock includes the following:
- Ensure an adequate airway, possibly by endotracheal intubation (see Chapter 10).
- Administer epinephrine. If reaction is caused by an insect sting, place a tourniquet proximal to the site of the sting and administer epinephrine in the uninvolved extremity and in the area of reaction, with repeat dosing within 5 to 10 minutes.
- Administer oxygen if available.
- Administer corticosteroids and antihistamines as ordered.
- Keep the child warm and lying flat or with feet slightly elevated.
- Start an IV line.

Children who have had life-threatening insect sting anaphylaxis and demonstrate venom-specific IgE antibodies on skin studies or RAST are candidates for venom immunotherapy. All children experiencing episodes of anaphylaxis in the community should be transported by ambulance to an emergency facility (see Chapter 10) and kept for observation at least 4 hours after the episode is resolved.

NURSING CARE

The Child With Anaphylaxis

Assessment

The child should be monitored closely for airway obstruction and vascular collapse during the acute phase of anaphylaxis. Assessment includes noting airway patency, respiratory rate and effort, heart rate, peripheral pulses, capillary refill time, oxygen saturation, urine output, and level of consciousness. After emergency efforts, the nurse can try to determine the cause of the attack by correlating when the symptoms first occurred with foods ingested, medications administered, and the possibility of an insect sting.

Nursing Diagnosis and Planning

The nursing diagnoses that apply to the child with anaphylaxis and to the family are

- Ineffective Breathing Pattern and Decreased Cardiac Output related to an excessive hypersensitive reaction to an allergen.

  Expected Outcome: The child will maintain a patent airway and adequate cardiac output (short term).
- Deficient Knowledge about allergens and prevention through risk reduction related to inexperience.

  Expected Outcome: The child and family will describe the child's allergic reaction and initiate a management plan for avoiding allergens and treating reactions (long term).

Interventions

Initially, the nurse maintains an adequate airway by administering oxygen and assisting with aerosol treatments and intubation as necessary. A laryngoscope, intubation tray, and tracheostomy kit should be available, and the code cart should be nearby. In the case of an insect sting or injected medication, a tourniquet applied to the affected extremity just proximal to the site might help confine the allergen. It is important to have IV access, with a large-bore needle, in at least one site, preferably two, for medication administration. The nurse administers IV fluids, epinephrine, corticosteroids, and antihistamines as ordered and informs the physician of the child's improvement or deterioration. Extra fluids (crystalloids or colloids) and plasma expanders should be administered if the child shows signs of vascular collapse (see Chapter 10).

Because epinephrine causes vasoconstriction and an increase in cardiac output, a child receiving the drug might have heart palpitations and tachycardia. This is frightening and aggravated by the emergency nature of the situation. The nurse should offer gentle reassurance to the child and provide the family with frequent reports about the child's condition.

After an initial anaphylactic episode, the nurse should assure the child and family that they were not at fault for the anaphylactic reaction and discuss how to prevent recurrences. Any child who has experienced anaphylaxis should have and learn to use an injectable epinephrine. The Epi-Pen Jr. for children delivers 0.15 mg of epinephrine through a spring-loaded injector, and the Epi-Pen provides 0.3 mg of epinephrine. The dose chosen by the provider is based on the child's weight. Teach the parent or child to hold the injector against the skin of the upper outer region of the child's thigh for 10 seconds after administering the injection to deliver the medication completely. The Epi-Pen can be injected through clothing. A Medi-Alert bracelet alerts others to the child's allergy.

Caring for the child at school presents an additional challenge (Box 17-3). The school nurse must be aware of and communicate to appropriate others information

---

BOX 17-3	**PARENTS WANT TO KNOW** About Communicating With the School About Peanut Allergies

- If your child has had a severe reaction to peanuts or other nuts, it is important for you to talk to your health care provider about whether the child should have medication available at home and school.
- Epinephrine, the medication that relieves a severe allergic reaction, is available in an easy-to-use automatic injector, which older children can self-administer and teachers or other school personnel can be taught to administer.
- Important things to remember when using automatically injected epinephrine are:
  1. If using an Epi-Pen, the injection can be given through the child's clothing.
  2. After starting the injection, you must continue to hold the Epi-Pen against the child for at least 10 seconds for all the medication to be delivered.

- Your child should have an allergy action plan readily available at school. You can obtain a sample action plan from *www.foodallergy.org*.
- Talk to the school nurse about the severity of your child's reaction and work with the nurse to create a way your child can avoid contact with peanuts while not singling the child out for special attention.

  Many school districts have policies that prohibit sharing of food or eating food on school buses. Other practices available at certain schools include peanut-free classrooms and a peanut-free area in the school cafeteria. Your school nurse can help you decide what modifications are appropriate for your child.

BOX 17-4	**CHILDREN WANT TO KNOW** How to Prevent Insect Stings

- Select clothes with white or khaki colors, not dark or brightly decorative ones.
- Wear fitted clothes with long sleeves, pants, and shoes.
- Use unscented soaps, lotions, and deodorants.
- Apply insect skin protection.
- Avoid orchards, flowers, blooming trees, and shrubs.

- Stay away from picnic areas.
- Keep out of the garden.
- Keep car windows closed while driving.
- Place screens on all windows.
- Cover all garbage cans.
- Move away slowly from approaching insects.

about any child who has had anaphylaxis. Policies about storage of and access to the Epi-Pen in the school setting differ in each school district. Some school districts train nonmedical personnel to administer the epinephrine if the child goes on a field trip; other school districts require a parent of a child who cannot self-administer epinephrine to accompany the child on a field trip. It is necessary for the school nurse to notify teachers and school nutrition personnel if a child or children in the school have allergies to peanuts or other foods. In some instances, the child may be so highly allergic that lunch needs to be eaten in the school health office, away from even the odor of peanut butter. Most commercial fast-food establishments post signs if pastries or other foods contain peanuts or other allergenic substances.

Evaluation

- Is the child awake and alert with adequate oxygenation and a patent airway?
- Are the child's vital signs within normal limits for age?
- Is the family taking appropriate steps to reduce the risks of another anaphylactic reaction (Box 17-4)?
- Do the child, family, and other appropriate adults demonstrate the proper use of the insect sting kit?

KEY CONCEPTS

- The immune system maintains homeostasis of the internal and external environment through nonspecific functions (inflammation, phagocytosis) and specific functions (humoral and cell-mediated immunity). Any derangement results in an immunologic imbalance whereby the immune system either underfunctions or overfunctions.
- When the immune system underfunctions, susceptibility to infections is increased (immunodeficiency). When the immune system overfunctions, it produces antibodies against cells of the body in autoimmune disease or against external sensitizing agents, forming the basis for allergies.
- The immune response is produced either actively or passively. Active immunity means the body has reacted to

antigens in nature or vaccines. The effect of active immunity lasts months to a lifetime. Passive immunity results from antibody transfer from a person with active immunity to a person who does not have that antibody. The effect of passive immunity is transitory.

- Children with acquired or congenital immunodeficiency are vulnerable to bacterial and viral infections. The best way to prevent the spread of organisms is to practice appropriate hand hygiene routinely and to follow basic infection control practices on the basis of three principles: (1) prevent contact with organisms, (2) create barriers if contact is unavoidable, and (3) kill organisms if contact is made.
- HIV infection is the best-known acquired immunodeficiency disease. It causes a wide spectrum of illness in children, ranging from no symptoms to mild and moderate symptoms to severe symptoms.
- Standard treatments for HIV infection include a modified immunization program, antiretroviral therapy, PCP prophylaxis, and aggressive use of antibiotics.
- For children with HIV, nurses have the challenging tasks of respiratory management, promoting normal growth and development, preventing infections, and providing comfort. In addition, nurses must support families in dealing with a stigmatizing illness that is ultimately terminal.
- Adolescents who acquired HIV when they were born are now reaching teen years. Nurses must discuss issues of infection transmission and medication adherence with these teens.
- Corticosteroids have immunosuppressive and anti-inflammatory properties. Tapering the dose during both long-term and short-term therapy regimens allows for the gradual return of adrenal function.
- Emergency treatment takes priority in an anaphylactic reaction because it is only a matter of minutes before the child will go into shock. In a community setting, epinephrine is administered to children with a known prior anaphylactic episode and the emergency service system is activated. Initially, the goal is to maintain an adequate airway, sometimes necessitating endotracheal intubation. This is followed by the administration of epinephrine.

ANSWERS TO
CRITICAL THINKING EXERCISE 17-1

Negative Considerations

HIV antibody testing in infants younger than 18 months is unreliable because antibodies (indicating infection) are passed from the mother to the child. HIV antibody testing in infants only indicates the HIV infection status of the mother. Several problems are associated with this:

- The mother might not know or suspect that she is HIV positive.
- Her denial on learning of her diagnosis might delay her and the baby's treatment.
- Early discharge of mother and infant from the hospital complicates follow-up.
- Some infants are not brought for well-child care, and the mother does not receive the information.
- HIV testing without consent might violate the mother's rights.

Positive Considerations

HIV testing allows for early identification and treatment of potentially infected infants and their mothers. This is especially important for PCP prophylaxis initiation and treatment with combination antiretroviral agents. The CDC has recommended education about voluntary HIV testing for pregnant women. If the nurse's first contact with an infant, particularly the infant of a high-risk mother, is after delivery and HIV testing was not done during pregnancy, HIV testing should be offered for both the mother and the newborn infant.

REFERENCES AND READINGS

Agertoft, L., & Pedersen, S. (2005). Short term lower-leg growth rate and urine cortisol excretion in children treated with ciclesonide. *Journal of Allergy and Clinical Immunology, 115,* 940-945.

American Academy of Pediatrics. (2003). *2003 Red Book: Report of the Committee on Infectious Diseases* (26th ed.). Elk Grove Village, IL: American Academy of Pediatrics.

American Academy of Pediatrics Committee on Pediatric AIDS. (1999, reaffirmed 2005). Disclosure of illness status to children and adolescents with HIV Infection. *Pediatrics, 103,* 164-165.

Bader-Meunier, B., Armengaud, J., Haddad, E., Salomon, R., Deschenes, G., Kone-Paut, I., Leblanc, T., Loirat, C., Niaudet, P., Piette, J. C., Prieur, A. M., Quartier, P., Bouissou, F., Foulard, M., Leverger, G., Lemelle, I., Pilet, P., Rodiere, M., Sirvent, N., & Cochat, P. (2005). Initial presentation of childhood-onset systemic lupus erythematosus: A French multicenter study. *Journal of Pediatrics, 146,* 648-653.

Banasik, J. (2005). Inflammation and immunity. In L. Copstead & J. Banasik (Eds.). *Pathophysiology* (3rd ed., pp. 203-243). St. Louis: Elsevier/Saunders.

Behrman, R., Kliegman, R., & Jenson, H. (Eds.). (2004). *Nelson textbook of pediatrics* (17th ed.). Philadelphia: WB Saunders.

Berrin, V., Salazar, J., Reynolds, E., & McKay, K. (2004). Adherence to antiretroviral therapy in HIV-infected pediatric patients improves with home-based intensive nursing intervention. *AIDS Patient Care and STDs, 18,* 355-363.

Boatner, L. (2002). To tell or not to tell: The ethics of disclosure in pediatric AIDS via vertical transmission. *Journal of the Association of Nurses in AIDS Care, 13,* 80-82.

Brady, M. (2005). Infectious disease in pediatric out-of-home child care. *American Journal of Infection Control, 33,* 276-285.

Buckley, R. (2004). The T-, B-, and NK-cell systems. In R. Behrman, R. Kliegman, & H. Jenson (Eds.), *Nelson textbook of pediatrics* (17th ed., pp. 683-689). Philadelphia: WB Saunders.

Centers for Disease Control and Prevention. (1995). 1995 Revised guidelines for prophylaxis against PCP for children infected with or perinatally exposed to HIV. *MMWR: Morbidity and Mortality Weekly Report, 44,* 1-11.

Centers for Disease Control and Prevention. (2006). *HIV/AIDS surveillance report HIV infections and AIDS in the United States, 2004.* Retrieved July 18, 2006 from *www.cdc.gov.*

Clarke, S. (2005). Anaphylaxis and severe allergy. *Practice Nurse, 29,* 18-23.

Ellis, A., & Day, J. (2004). Biphasic anaphylaxis: A prospective examination of 103 patients for the incidence and characteristics of biphasic reactivity. *Journal of Allergy and Clinical Immunology, 113(Supplement),* 259.

Fowler, M. G., Garcia, P., Hanson, C., & Sansom, S. (2004). Progress in preventing perinatal HIV transmission in the United States (Conference Summary). *Emerging Infectious Disease,* Retrieved January 21, 2006, from *www.cdc.gov/ncidod/EID/vol 10no11/04-062202.htm.*

Hammami, N., Nostlinger, C., Hoeree, T., Lefevre, P., Jonckheer, T., & Kolsteren, P. (2004). Integrating adherence to highly active antiretroviral therapy into children's daily lives: A qualitative study. *Pediatrics, 114,* e591-e597.

Jackson, P. (2002). Peanut allergy: An increasing health risk for children. *Pediatric Nursing, 28,* 496-500.

Jessee, P. O., Nagy, M. C., & Gresham C. (2001). Public opinion concerning group involvement for children with aids. *Early Child Development and Care, 166,* 29-38.

Jones, S. (2004). Mothers' voices: Culturally diverse mothers' experiences talking with their children about HIV. *Journal of Cultural Diversity, 11,* 58-64.

Kelly, W., Strunk, R., Donithan, M., Bloomberg, G., McWilliams, B., & Szefler, S. (2003). Growth and bone density in children with mild-moderate asthma: A cross-sectional study in children entering the Childhood Asthma Management Program. *Journal of Pediatrics, 142,* 286-291.

Klein-Gitelman, M., & Miller, M. (2004). Systemic lupus erythematosus. In R. Behrman, R. Kliegman, & H. Jenson (Eds.). *Nelson textbook of pediatrics* (17th ed., pp. 809-813). Philadelphia: WB Saunders.

Larson, E., Lin, S., & Gomez-Pichardo, C. (2004). Predictors of infectious disease symptoms in inner city households. *Nursing Research, 53,* 190-197.

Lewis, S. (2005). Commentary on the AAP disclosure of illness status to children with HIV. Retrieved May 6, 2005, from *www.apa.org.*

Lupus Foundation of America. (2005). Lupus facts and overview. Retrieved September 5, 2005, from *www.lupus.org.*

Menting, A. (2000). Children and AIDS. *Harvard AIDS Review.* Retrieved June 19, 2005, from *www.aids.harvard.edu/news _publications/har/spring_2000/spring00-2.html.*

Munoz-Furlong, A. (2003). Daily coping strategies for patients and their families. *Pediatrics, 111,* 1654-1662.

National Association of State Boards of Education. (2001). Someone at school has AIDS. Retrieved September 1, 2005, from *www.nasbe .org.*

Nehring, W. M., Lashley, F. R., & Malm K. (2000). Disclosing the diagnosis of pediatric HIV infection: mother's views. *JSPN, 5,* 5-13.

Pagana, K. D., & Pagana, T. (2002). *Mosby's manual of diagnostic and laboratory tests.* St. Louis: Mosby.

Perinatal HIV Guidelines Working Group. (2006). U.S. Public Health Service Task Force recommendations for use of antiretroviral drugs in pregnant HIV-1-infected women for maternal health and interventions to reduce perinatal HIV-1 transmission in the United States. Retrieved July 18, 2006, from *www.aidsinfo.nih.gov.*

Randell, T., Donaghue, K., Ambler, G., Cowell, C., Fitzgerald, D., & VanAsperen, P. (2003). Safety of the newer inhaled corticosteroids in childhood asthma. *Pediatric Drugs, 5,* 481-504.

Rote, N. (2002). In K. McCance & S. Huether (Eds.). *Pathophysiology: The biologic basis for disease in adults and children* (4th ed., pp. 168-225). St. Louis: Mosby.

Salvatoni, A., Piantanida, E., Nosetti, L., & Nespoli, L. (2000). Inhaled corticosteroids in childhood asthma. *Pediatric Drug, 5,* 351-361.

Sampson, H. (2002). Peanut allergy. *New England Journal of Medicine, 346,* 1294-1299.

Sampson, H. (2003). Anaphylaxis and emergency treatment. *Pediatrics, 111,* 1601-1609.

Sampson, H., & Leung, D. (2004). Adverse reactions to foods. In R. Behrman, R. Kliegman, & H. Jenson (Eds.). *Nelson textbook of pediatrics* (17th ed., pp. 789-792). Philadelphia: WB Saunders.

School guidelines for managing students with food allergies. (2003). Retrieved Sept. 21, 2003, from *www.foodallergy.org/school/guidelines.html.*

Sheets, A., Goldman, P., Millett, P., Franks, J., McIntyre, J., Carroll, C., et al. (2004). Guidelines for managing life-threatening food allergies in Massachusetts schools. *Journal of School Health, 74,* 155-161.

Sicherer, S., Munoz-Furlong, A., & Sampson, H. (2003). Prevalence of peanut and tree nut allergy in the United States determined by means of a random digit dial telephone survey: A 5-year follow-up study. *Journal of Allergy and Clinical Immunology, 112,* 1203-1207.

Storm, D., Boland, M., Gortmaker, Y., Skurnick, J., Howland, L., & Oleske, J. (2005). Protease inhibitor combination therapy, severity of illness, and quality of life among children with perinatally acquired HIV-1 infection. *Pediatrics, 115,* e173-e182.

Students with chronic illness: Guidance for families, schools, and students. (2003). *Journal of School Health, 73,* 131-132.

Szer, I. S., & Athreya, B. (2002). Systemic lupus erythematosus in children. In F. Burg, J. Ingelfinger, R. Polin, & A. Gershon (Eds.). *Gellis & Kagan's current pediatric therapy* (17th ed., pp. 754-757). Philadelphia: WB Saunders.

Tosi, M. (2004). Immunologic and phagocytic responses to infection. In R. Fegin, J. Cherry, G. Demmler, & S. Kaplan (Eds.). *Textbook of pediatric infectious diseases* (5th ed, pp. 25-27). Philadelphia: WB Saunders.

Weglarz, M., & Boland, M. (2005). Family-centered nursing care of the perinatally infected mother and child living with HIV infection. *JSPN, 10,* 161-170.

Working Group on Antiretroviral Therapy and Medical Management of HIV-Infected Children. (2005, November). Guidelines for the use of antiretroviral agents in pediatric HIV infection. Retrieved July 18, 2006, from *www.aidsinfo.nih.gov.*

Yogev, R., & Chadwick, E. (2004). Acquired immunodeficiency syndrome (human immunodeficiency virus). In R. Behrman, R. Kliegman, & H. Jenson (Eds.). *Nelson textbook of pediatrics* (17th ed, pp. 1111-1121). Philadelphia: WB Saunders.

Zeiger, R. (2003). Food allergen avoidance in the prevention of food allergy in infants and children. *Pediatrics, 111,* 1662-1671.

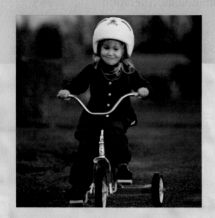

CHAPTER 18

The Child With a Fluid and Electrolyte Alteration

Learning Objectives

After studying this chapter, you should be able to:

- Identify the regulatory mechanisms that maintain fluid and electrolyte balance in the body.
- Compare those differences in body fluid and electrolyte composition and regulation between infants/children and adults that make infants and children more vulnerable to imbalances.
- Describe dehydration and acid-base imbalance.

- Differentiate among the various types of acid-base disturbances.
- Describe the processes and nursing care of a child with diarrhea or vomiting.
- Integrate assessment findings with nursing implementation to determine the success of therapy.
- Describe nursing interventions to prevent fluid and electrolyte imbalances.

Definitions

acidosis Abnormal accumulation of acid in, or loss of base from, the body, with serum pH less than 7.35.

alkalosis Abnormal accumulation of base in, or loss of acid from, the body, with serum pH more than 7.45.

anuria Absence of urine formation; usually indicative of kidney failure but may be the result of severe dehydration.

extracellular fluid Fluid found outside the cell, composing approximately one third of the body's fluid in older children and about one half of the body's fluid in infants.

hypernatremic (hypertonic) dehydration State in which the sodium concentration is above that of normal body fluids (i.e., 150 mEq/L).

hyponatremic (hypotonic) dehydration State in which the sodium concentration is below that of normal body fluids (i.e., 130 mEq/L).

interstitial fluid Extracellular fluid surrounding the cell, including lymph fluid.

intracellular fluid Fluid found within the cells, composing approximately two thirds of the body's fluid in older children and about one half of the body's fluid in infants.

intravascular fluid Extracellular fluid contained within a blood vessel (e.g., plasma).

isonatremic (isotonic) dehydration State in which the sodium concentration is practically identical to that of body fluids (i.e., between 135 and 145 mEq/L).

oliguria Diminished urine output.

Audio Glossary

Electronic Resources

Additional information related to the content in Chapter 18 can be found on:

the interactive companion CD-ROM

- Audio Glossary
- NCLEX Review Questions

or the companion website at *evolve*
http://evolve.elsevier.com/james/ncoc

- Common Pediatric Laboratory Tests and Normal Values
- NCLEX Review Questions
- Resources for Health Care Providers and Families
- WebLinks

CLINICAL REFERENCE

REVIEW OF FLUID AND ELECTROLYTE IMBALANCES IN CHILDREN

Characteristics unique to children affect fluid and electrolyte balance. Infants and young children are more vulnerable than adults to changes in fluid and electrolyte balance. Under normal conditions, the amount of fluid ingested during a day should equal the amount of fluid lost through sensible water loss (e.g., urine output) and insensible water loss (through the respiratory tract and skin). Insensible water loss per unit of body weight is significantly higher in infants and children. The faster respiratory rates of infants and young children also result in higher evaporative water losses. Any condition that prevents normal oral fluid intake (e.g., vomiting) or results in fluid losses (e.g., diarrhea, hyperventilation, burns, hemorrhage) is especially significant because it depletes the body's store of water and electrolytes much more rapidly in infants and young children than in adults.

Body water is located in two major compartments: within the cell, in the intracellular compartment; and outside the cell, in the extracellular compartment. These two compartments are separated by the cell membrane, across which body fluid is continually exchanged. Extracellular fluid (ECF) is located in several places: in interstitial spaces (surrounding the cells, e.g., lymph fluid), intravascularly (within the blood vessels or plasma), and transcellularly (e.g., cerebrospinal fluid, pericardial fluid, pleural fluid, synovial fluid, sweat, digestive secretions). A child is more likely to lose ECF than intracellular fluid (ICF). ECF is lost first when fluid loss occurs (e.g., through illness, trauma, fever). The intracellular compartment is more difficult to dehydrate.

In the neonate, approximately 40% of body water is located in the extracellular compartment compared with 20% in the adolescent and adult. In the infant, one half of the ECF may be exchanged compared with an adult exchange of one sixth of the ECF in a similar time. Because approximately 50% of this ECF is exchanged daily in an infant, dehydration can occur very suddenly and rapidly if fluid intake is inadequate or fluid losses are excessive. Because of the infant's higher metabolic rate, the rate of water turnover is rapid. Depletion of ECF, often caused by gastroenteritis, is one of the most common problems among infants and young children. In adults and older children, because a greater proportion of fluid is located in the intracellular compartment, severe fluid depletion does not occur as rapidly. Maturity in body space distribution is usually reached around age 3 years.

Body fluids are basically composed of two elements, water and solutes. *Water* is the primary constituent, with the infant's weight being approximately 75% water to the adult's 55% to 60%. In general, the volume of total body water to total body weight decreases with increasing age. An inverse relationship exists between total body water and total body fat. Compared with adults, neonates, particularly premature infants, have a lower proportion of fat.

Solutes are composed of both electrolytes and nonelectrolytes. Most of the body's solutes are electrolytes, primarily sodium (Na^+), potassium (K^+), chloride (Cl^-), calcium (Ca^{++}), and magnesium (Mg^{++}). The primary electrolyte of the ECF is sodium; potassium and magnesium are the primary electrolytes in the ICF. The extracellular compartment contains more sodium and chloride during infancy, which increases the vulnerability of infants to electrolyte imbalances. Changes in the concentration of these electrolytes may result in cellular dysfunction and illness. Problems of fluid and electrolyte balance involve both water and electrolytes; thus treatment includes replacement of both, calculated according to serum electrolyte laboratory values.

PEDIATRIC DIFFERENCES RELATED TO FLUID AND ELECTROLYTE BALANCE

Infants
- Because of the higher percentage of water in the ECF, infants can lose fluids equal to their ECF within 2 to 3 days.
- Infants are less able to concentrate urine because of immature renal function.
- Infants have a higher rate of peristalsis than do older children.
- Infants have an immature lower esophageal sphincter, making them more prone to gastroesophageal reflux, which can lead to dehydration and electrolyte disturbances.
- Infants have a harder time compensating for acidosis because of their decreased ability to acidify urine.

Infants and Young Children
- Infants and young children have a higher metabolic turnover of water relative to adults because of a higher metabolic rate. (If losses are not replaced rapidly, imbalance occurs.)
- Infants and young children are unable to verbalize or communicate thirst.

Infants and Children
- In comparison with adults, infants and children have a proportionately greater body surface area in relation to body mass, resulting in a greater potential for fluid loss through the skin and gastrointestinal tract.
- Infants and children have a higher proportionate water content (premature infants have 90%, term infants 75% to 80%, preschool children 60% to 65%, and adolescents and adults approximately 55% to 60%), with a larger proportion of fluid in the extracellular space.
- The immune system of infants and children is not as robust as an adult's immune system, rendering young children more susceptible to infectious diseases, fever, gastroenteritis, and respiratory infections, all of which can result in fluid and electrolyte disturbances and fluid-volume deficit.
- Infants and children are at higher risk because of increased exposure to infections in a day care or nursery setting.

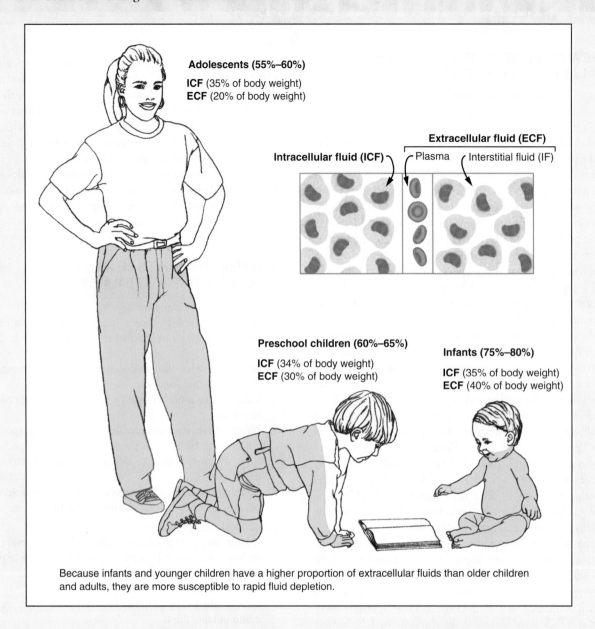

Adolescents (55%–60%)

ICF (35% of body weight)
ECF (20% of body weight)

Extracellular fluid (ECF)

Intracellular fluid (ICF)   Plasma   Interstitial fluid (IF)

Preschool children (60%–65%)

ICF (34% of body weight)
ECF (30% of body weight)

Infants (75%–80%)

ICF (35% of body weight)
ECF (40% of body weight)

Because infants and younger children have a higher proportion of extracellular fluids than older children and adults, they are more susceptible to rapid fluid depletion.

ALTERATIONS IN ACID-BASE BALANCE IN CHILDREN

Alterations in acid-base balance can affect cellular metabolism and enzymatic processes. The body's ability to regulate this status is crucial. Children can have acid-base imbalance as a result of many pathologic conditions. The pH, or measure of acidity or alkalinity of body fluids, is regulated within a narrow range (normal blood pH is 7.35 to 7.45). Maintenance of serum pH within normal limits is crucial to maintaining cellular function, enzyme activity, and neuromuscular membrane potentials. Chemical buffers, the respiratory system, and the kidneys work together to keep the blood pH within normal range. Acid is constantly produced as a byproduct of metabolism. The body attempts to maintain blood pH within normal limits by reducing the buildup of acid. Chemical and cellular buffer systems minimize the effect of alterations in blood pH by neutralizing excess acids

and bases that accumulate in body fluids. Two of the most significant buffers are bicarbonate and proteins. Bicarbonate, the most important buffer for plasma and interstitial fluids, is responsible for most ECF buffering and can exert its effects relatively quickly (within minutes).

When alterations in pH become too much for the buffer systems to handle, compensatory mechanisms in the respiratory and renal systems are activated. The lungs remove carbon dioxide from the blood, reducing the amount of carbonic acid and raising the blood pH. The respiratory system works rapidly to compensate for acid-base disturbances. If the blood pH drops below normal (causing *acidosis*), the respiratory rate and depth will increase, removing carbon dioxide and raising blood pH. Conversely, in the presence of alkalosis, the respiratory rate and depth decrease, thus lowering blood pH.

Kidneys regulate bicarbonate and remove hydrogen ions from the blood. If the blood is too alkaline, the kidneys

Overview of Fluid and Electrolyte Disorders

Disorder	Precipitating Events	Clinical Manifestations
Hyponatremia (sodium <135 mEq/L)	Fever Increased water intake without electrolytes Decreased sodium intake Diabetic ketoacidosis Burns and wounds SIADH Malnutrition Cystic fibrosis Renal disease Vomiting, diarrhea, nasogastric suction	Neurologic: • Usually do not show signs until sodium reaches 125 mEq/L • Behavioral changes: irritability, lethargy, headache, dizziness, apprehension Cardiovascular: • Increased heart rate • Decreased blood pressure • Cold, clammy skin Muscle cramps (especially abdominal) Nausea
Hypernatremia (sodium >150 mEq/L)	Water loss or deprivation High sodium intake Diabetes insipidus Diarrhea Fever Hyperglycemia Renal disease	Intense thirst Oliguria Agitation, restlessness Flushed skin Peripheral and pulmonary edema Dry, sticky mucous membranes Nausea and vomiting Serum sodium 150 mEq/L: disorientation, seizures, hyperirritability when at rest
Hypokalemia (potassium <3.5 mEq/L)	Stress Starvation Malabsorption Excessive loss of GI fluids through vomiting, diarrhea, sweat, nasogastric tube Administration of diuretics (especially furosemide, ethacrynic acid, thiazide diuretics) IV fluids without added potassium Administration of corticosteroids Diabetic ketoacidosis	Muscle weakness, paralysis Leg cramps Decreased bowel sounds Weak and irregular pulse, tachycardia or bradycardia, cardiac arrhythmias Hypotension Ileus Irritability, fatigue
Hyperkalemia (potassium >5 mEq/L)	Increased intake of potassium (e.g., salt substitutes) Decreased urine excretion Kidney failure Metabolic acidosis Hyperglycemia Potassium-sparing diuretics Dehydration (severe) Too-rapid IV administration of potassium Burns	Irritability, anxiety Twitching, hyperreflexia Weakness, flaccid paralysis Nausea, diarrhea Bradycardia Cardiac arrest (concern if potassium >8.5 mEq/L) Apnea, respiratory arrest
Hypocalcemia (calcium <8.5 mg/dL, ionized calcium <4.5 mg/dL)	Inadequate intake of calcium Vitamin D deficiency Renal insufficiency Calcium losses (e.g., infection, burns) Alkalosis Administration of diuretics Hypoparathyroidism	Numbness and tingling of fingers, toes, nose, ears, circumoral area Hyperactive reflexes, seizures Muscle cramps, tetany Laryngospasm Lethargy and poor feeding in the neonate Positive Trousseau's and Chvostek's signs Hypotension Cardiac arrest
Hypercalcemia (calcium >11.0 mg/dL, ionized calcium >5.5 mg/dL)	Milk-alkali syndrome (chronic ingestion of calcium carbonate antacids or milk) Excessive IV or oral calcium administration Acidosis Prolonged immobilization Hypoproteinemia Renal disease Hyperparathyroidism Hyperthyroidism	Lethargy, weakness, anorexia Thirst Itching Behavioral changes: confusion, personality change, stupor Nausea, vomiting, constipation Bradycardia, cardiac arrest

SIADH, Syndrome of inappropriate secretion of antidiuretic hormone; *GI,* gastrointestinal.

Assessment of Fluid and Electrolyte Disturbances

Parameter Evaluated	Clinical Manifestations	Possible Fluid or Electrolyte Disturbance
Heart rate	Rapid, weak, thready	Fluid volume deficit
	Rapid, bounding	Fluid volume excess
	Weak, irregular, slowing	Severe hyperkalemia
	Weak, irregular, rapid	Severe hypokalemia
Respirations	Rapid, deep	Metabolic acidosis
	Slow, shallow	Metabolic alkalosis
Blood pressure	Increased	Fluid volume excess
	Decreased	Late stages of shock, fluid volume deficit, hypokalemia or hyperkalemia, hyponatremia
Skin	Poor elasticity	Fluid volume deficit
	Pallor	Fluid volume deficit
	Cool to touch	Fluid volume deficit, increased or decreased sodium
	Poor capillary refill	Fluid volume deficit
	Edema	Fluid volume excess (usually)
Mucous membranes	Dry	Fluid volume deficit
Salivation or tearing	Decreased	Fluid volume deficit
Behavioral changes	Lethargy	Fluid volume deficit
	Irritability	Fluid volume deficit
	Increased restlessness	Hyperkalemia
	Coma	Markedly increased acidosis or alkalosis
Sensorium changes	Thirst	Fluid volume deficit, increased sodium or calcium
	Tingling in extremities	Hypocalcemia, alkalosis
	Abdominal cramps	Hyponatremia, hyperkalemia
	Muscular cramps	Hypocalcemia, hypokalemia
	Lightheadedness or dizziness	Respiratory alkalosis
	Nausea	Hypercalcemia, hypokalemia, or hyperkalemia
Neurologic changes	Hypotonia	Hypokalemia, hypercalcemia
	Weakness	Metabolic acidosis
	Hypertonia:	Hypocalcemia
	• Positive Chvostek's sign	Hypocalcemia, alkalosis
	• Tremors, cramps, tetany	

Data from Kee, J. L., & Paulanka, B. J. (2000). *Fluid and electrolytes: Clinical applications*. Albany, NY: Delmar; Greenbaum, L. (2004). Electrolyte and acid base disorders. In R. Behrman, R. Kliegman, & H. Jenson (Eds.). *Nelson textbook of pediatrics* (17th ed.). Philadelphia: Elsevier Saunders.

Common Pediatric Laboratory Tests and Normal Values

Common Laboratory and Diagnostic Tests for Fluid and Electrolyte Imbalance

Test	Description	Indications	Normal Findings	Nursing Considerations
Urine osmolality	24-hr urine collection or random test	Altered fluid status	300-900 mOsm/kg	No preparation Done by nurse
Urine sodium	24-hr urine collection or random urine specimen	Altered fluid status, hyponatremia	50-130 mEq/L	No preparation Done by nurse
Urine specific gravity	Random urine specimen	Altered fluid status	1.002-1.030	No preparation Done by nurse
Urea nitrogen	Random blood specimen	Altered fluid status, renal function	5-18 mg/dL	No preparation Draw blood needed for sample
Serum osmolality	Random blood specimen	Altered fluid status Measures solute concentration of blood	275-295 mOsm/kg	No preparation Draw blood needed for sample

Acid-Base Disturbances: Principal Causes, Clinical Manifestations, and Treatment

Condition	Principal Causes	Clinical Manifestations	Principal Treatment Methods
Metabolic acidosis	Ketoacidosis (DKA, alcohol-induced ketoacidosis) Increasing metabolic rates from fever, RDS, seizures Interference with normal metabolism: ketosis, tissue hypoxia Loss of bicarbonate from diarrhea, ileostomy, or fistula drainage Acute and chronic renal failure ECF expansion and decreasing HCO_3^- concentration	Increasing heart rate, arrhythmias (fibrillation) Hyperventilation Kussmaul respirations Cold, clammy skin (mild to moderate acidosis) Warm, dry skin (severe acidosis) Level of consciousness changes from fatigue and confusion to stupor and coma	Identify and treat the underlying disorder Provide $NaHCO_3$, K^+ replacement, and mechanical ventilation as indicated
Metabolic alkalosis	Volume depletion related to various conditions, such as vomiting, pyloric stenosis, gastric drainage, and diuretics Increased alkali intake Medical conditions, such as cystic fibrosis	Arrhythmias (atrioventricular with prolonged QT interval) Increasing heart rate Decreased respiratory rate and depth Change in level of consciousness from apathy and confusion to stupor Muscular weakness	Treatment depends on underlying cause; mild to moderate alkalosis usually does not require treatment Use of fluids with NaCl and KCl, along with isotonic saline solution, an H_2-receptor antagonist (e.g., cimetidine) to decrease gastric hydrochloric acid, acidifying agents, and potassium-sparing diuretics (e.g., spironolactone [Aldactone], mannitol)
Respiratory acidosis	Pulmonary disease (BPD, RDS, asthma, cystic fibrosis, croup) Airway obstruction Chest conditions, such as flail chest, pneumothorax Acute and chronic respiratory failure Neuromuscular abnormalities such as Guillain-Barré syndrome, toxins, drugs, paralysis CNS depression from sedative overdose, trauma, anesthesia	Increasing heart rate Arrhythmias with hypotension Increasing rate and depth of respirations, forceful use of accessory muscles with retraction and cyanosis Increasing intracranial pressure	Correction of ventilation problem: use of oxygen, intubation, mechanical ventilation, $NaHCO_3$
Respiratory alkalosis	Hyperventilation from CNS stimulation, such as emotions, fear, hysteria, pain, salicylate poisoning Decreased lung compliance and hypoxemia from conditions such as pulmonary edema, CHF, pneumonia, asthma, pulmonary emboli Pregnancy Compensation from metabolic acidosis Sepsis	Dizziness, paresthesias, lightheadedness, diaphoresis Arrhythmias (changes in ST-T wave)	Mild to moderate respiratory alkalosis usually does not require specific treatment For hyperventilation-induced conditions, provide oxygen, rebreathing oxygen masks, breathing into a paper bag, psychologic reassurance Institute mechanical ventilation if condition is severe Give sedatives or tranquilizers for anxiety-induced condition, acetazolamide to prevent motion sickness

DKA, Diabetic ketoacidosis; *RDS,* respiratory distress syndrome; *HCO_3^-,* bicarbonate; *$NaHCO_3$,* sodium bicarbonate; *NaCl,* sodium chloride; *KCl,* potassium chloride; *BPD,* bronchopulmonary dysplasia; *CNS,* central nervous system; *CHF,* congestive heart failure.

Selected Laboratory Values for Acid-Base Disturbances

Test	Metabolic Acidosis	Metabolic Alkalosis	Respiratory Acidosis	Respiratory Alkalosis
ABG: pH	<7.35	>7.45	<7.35	>7.45
$Paco_2$ (mm Hg)	<40	>45	>45	<35
Pao_2 (mm Hg)	WNL or slightly decreased	Decreased	Decreased	Decreased
HCO_3^- (mEq/L)	<22	>26	WNL or slightly increased	Decreased
K^+ (mEq/L)	>4.0	Decreased	WNL	Slightly decreased
Na^+ (mEq/L)	Varies according to condition	Decreased	WNL	Slightly decreased
Cl^- (mEq/L)	Usually increased	Decreased	WNL	Slightly decreased

ABG, Arterial blood gas; *Paco₂,* partial pressure of carbon dioxide in arterial blood; *Pao₂,* partial pressure of oxygen in arterial blood; *WNL,* within normal limits; *HCO₃⁻,* bicarbonate.

Mechanisms of Acid-Base Disturbances*

Principal	Primary Disturbance	Principal Compensatory Response
Metabolic acidosis	Decreasing HCO_3^-	Hyperventilation causes decreased $Paco_2$
Metabolic alkalosis	Increasing HCO_3^-	Hypoventilation causes increased $Paco_2$
Respiratory acidosis	Increasing $Paco_2$	Release of HCO_3^- and increased renal reabsorption of HCO_3^-
Respiratory alkalosis	Decreasing $Paco_2$	Decreased renal reabsorption of HCO_3^-

HCO₃⁻, Bicarbonate; *Paco₂,* partial pressure of carbon dioxide in arterial blood.
Modified from Kee, J. L., & Paulanka, B. J. (2000). *Fluid and electrolytes: Clinical applications.* Albany, NY: Delmar.
*Important items to remember when acid-base compensation occurs:
- Normal values from which to interpret blood gases: $Paco_2$ 35-45 mm Hg; pH 7.35-7.45; bicarbonate 22-26 mEq/L.
- When metabolic compensation occurs, assume origin in respiratory alteration.
- When respiratory compensation and release of tissue buffers occur, assume metabolic origin.

conserve hydrogen ions, thus lowering blood pH. In the presence of acidosis, the kidneys excrete hydrogen ions and conserve bicarbonate, raising blood pH. Renal compensatory processes work more slowly than respiratory mechanisms—usually within 1 to 2 days. If compensatory mechanisms are ineffective, acid-base imbalances occur. When a dysfunction results in decreased hydrogen ion concentration in the blood, the arterial pH increases (causing *alkalosis*). When a dysfunction results in an increase in hydrogen ions, the arterial pH decreases (causing *acidosis*).

CRITICAL TO REMEMBER
Treatment Goals in Acid-Base Imbalance

The treatment of metabolic acid-base disturbance is oriented toward correcting the underlying problem. The treatment of respiratory imbalance is directed toward reestablishing alveolar ventilation.

DEHYDRATION

Dehydration, or fluid loss in excess of fluid intake, is one of the most common causes of hospitalization in infants and children (Centers for Disease Control and Prevention [CDC], 2003). Decreased fluid intake or increased fluid loss may cause it. Dehydration produces both fluid and electrolyte deficiencies. Dehydration is classified as isonatremic, hyponatremic, or hypernatremic (Table 18-1), according to the status of the serum sodium concentration. In *isonatremic dehydration,* the most common type of dehydration in children, water and electrolytes are lost in approximately the same proportion as they exist in the body, and serum sodium levels remain within the normal range of 138 to 145 mEq/L. In *hyponatremic dehydration,* the electrolyte loss is greater than the water loss, resulting in a serum sodium concentration of

less than 135 mEq/L. In *hypernatremic dehydration,* the water loss is greater than the electrolyte loss and the serum sodium concentration is more than 150 mEq/L.

Etiology and Incidence

Dehydration has many varied causes. Common alterations that may lead to dehydration reflect disturbances in the following systems:
- Gastrointestinal tract: vomiting, diarrhea, pyloric stenosis, malabsorption
- Endocrine system: fever, diabetes mellitus, cystic fibrosis
- Skin: burns
- Lungs: tachypnea
- Kidneys: renal failure
- Heart: congestive heart failure

TABLE 18-1	Types of Dehydration: Etiology, Clinical Manifestations, and Laboratory Values	
Isonatremic Dehydration	**Hyponatremic Dehydration**	**Hypernatremic Dehydration**
Etiology		
Vomiting, diarrhea	***Renal Losses***	***Renal Losses***
Insensible fluid loss from respiratory and integumentary systems	Diuretics, hyperglycemia, nephritis, adrenal insufficiency	Diuretics, diabetes insipidus, adrenal insufficiency
Decreased oral intake with increased activity	***Extrarenal Losses***	***Extrarenal Losses***
	Vomiting, diarrhea, third spacing, burns, tube drainage	Vomiting, diarrhea
	Other	***Other***
	CHF, SIADH, nephrosis; administration of large amounts of electrolyte-free solutions (plain water) during illness or postoperatively	Fever, increased sodium in formula, diet, or tube feeding; administration of hypertonic sodium IV fluids
Clinical Manifestations		
Mild thirst	Increased thirst	Thirst very increased
Skin turgor poor	Skin turgor very poor	Skin turgor fair
Dry skin	Skin usually clammy	Skin texture thickened or "doughy"
Decreased urine output	Decreased urine output	Decreased urine output
Dry mucous membranes	Mucous membranes dry to slightly moist	Mucous membranes parched
Skin temperature cold	Skin temperature cold	Skin temperature cold or hot
Body temperature afebrile or febrile	Body temperature afebrile or febrile	Body temperature afebrile or febrile
Lethargy	Very lethargic, possible seizures	Lethargic, hyperirritable with stimulation
Laboratory Values		
Serum sodium: 138-145 mEq/L	***Renal Losses***	***Renal Losses***
	Serum sodium <135 mEq/L	Serum sodium >150 mEq/L
Urine		
Sodium usually within normal limits	Urine sodium increased	Urine sodium increased
Specific gravity slightly elevated	Urine specific gravity decreased	Urine specific gravity decreased
Osmolality usually within normal limits	Urine osmolality decreased	Urine osmolality decreased
Volume usually within normal limits or slightly decreased	Urine volume increased	Urine volume increased
	Extrarenal Losses	***Extrarenal Losses***
	Serum sodium <135 mEq/L	Serum sodium >150 mEq/L
	Urine sodium decreased	Urine sodium decreased
	Urine specific gravity increased	Urine specific gravity increased
	Urine osmolality increased	Urine osmolality increased
	Urine volume decreased	Urine volume decreased
	Other	***Other***
	Serum sodium <135 mEq/L	Serum sodium >150 mEq/L
	Urine sodium decreased	Urine sodium decreased
	Urine specific gravity increased	Urine specific gravity increased
	Urine osmolality increased	Urine osmolality increased
	Urine volume decreased	Urine volume decreased

CHF, Congestive heart failure; *SIADH,* syndrome of inappropriate secretion of antidiuretic hormone.
Data from Greenbaum, L. (2004). Electrolyte and acid base disorders. In R. Behrman, R. Kliegman, & H. Jenson (Eds.). *Nelson textbook of pediatrics* (17th ed.). Philadelphia: Elsevier Saunders.

Any age group can be affected, but neonates and infants, as discussed previously, are especially vulnerable to the effects of dehydration. In the United States, more than 200,000 children a year are hospitalized for gastroenteritis, most because of secondary dehydration (CDC, 2003).

Manifestations

For infants and young children with isonatremic dehydration, the fluid deficit is described as mild, moderate, or severe dehydration, depending on the percentage of body weight lost:
- *Minimal dehydration:* <3% loss of body weight
- *Mild dehydration:* 3% to 5% loss of body weight; fluid volume loss of less than 50 mL/kg

- *Moderate dehydration:* 6% to 10% loss of body weight; fluid volume loss of 50 to 100 mL/kg
- *Severe dehydration:* 10% or more loss of body weight; fluid volume loss of 100 mL/kg or more

One milliliter of body fluid is approximately equal to 1 g of body weight, so a weight loss or gain of 1 kg (2.2 lb) in 24 hours represents a 1-L fluid loss or gain.

Older children have a lower total body water content and ECF volume than do infants and younger children. Therefore an equivalent percentage of body weight lost from dehydration represents a more severe fluid depletion in the older child. Isonatremic dehydration in the older child is classified as *mild* if 3% of body weight is lost, *moderate* if

PATHOPHYSIOLOGY

DEHYDRATION

In the early phases of dehydration, fluids, with some electrolytes, are lost from the ECF. If the fluid loss continues, loss of ICF can occur. Dehydration can lead to shock (see Chapter 10).

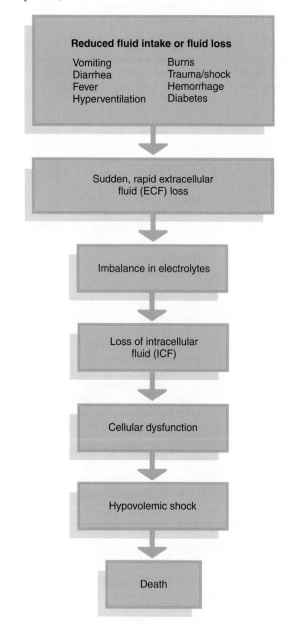

Reduced fluid intake or fluid loss

Vomiting   Burns
Diarrhea   Trauma/shock
Fever   Hemorrhage
Hyperventilation   Diabetes

↓

Sudden, rapid extracellular fluid (ECF) loss

↓

Imbalance in electrolytes

↓

Loss of intracellular fluid (ICF)

↓

Cellular dysfunction

↓

Hypovolemic shock

↓

Death

6% of body weight is lost, and *severe* if 9% of body weight is lost.

The signs and symptoms associated with degree of isonatremic dehydration are listed in Table 18-2. As with impending shock, the most essential manifestations are changes in heart rate; general appearance, behavior, or sensorium; urine output; skin and mucous membrane qualities, and, in infants, fontanels. Sunken eyes and decreased tears are definitive signs of dehydration (Friedman, Goldman, Srvastava, &

> **CRITICAL TO REMEMBER**
> **Signs of Impending Shock in the Dehydrated Child**
> Because of the child's ability to compensate and maintain an adequate cardiac output, changes in heart rate, sensorium, and skin color are earlier indicators of impending shock than is blood pressure.

Parkin, 2004), but lack of tears is not an accurate sign in very young infants, who do not produce tears.

Diagnostic Evaluation

Key factors to consider in determining the type and severity of dehydration in children include the following:
- A history of acute or chronic fluid loss
- Clinical manifestations
- Child's weight
- Serum electrolyte values for moderate to severe dehydration

Abnormal serum electrolyte values, which include decreased bicarbonate, decreased potassium, and decreased glucose, are not unusual in the dehydrated child, although in isonatremic dehydration the sodium level remains within normal limits (Wathen, MacKenzie, & Bothner, 2004). Serum pH levels provide information about acid-base balance in an infant or child suspected of being acidotic or alkalotic. An elevated urine specific gravity (>1.020) suggests dehydration.

Therapeutic Management

Management is directed toward correcting the fluid and electrolyte imbalance and then treating the causative factors. In 2003, the CDC published evidence-based guidelines for addressing dehydration; these guidelines were accepted as policy in 2004 by the American Academy of Pediatrics.

Minimal Dehydration

Treatment of minimal dehydration consists of continuing breastfeeding or age-appropriate diet, along with fluid replacement for each episode of fluid loss (stool, emesis) (Table 18-3). Regardless of the child's age, fluids are replaced with an oral rehydration solution (ORS), such as the World Health Organization's solution, Rehydralyte, Pedialyte, or Infalyte (CDC, 2003). The oral rehydration solutions have changed from the days of homemade recipes (mixtures of water, salt, sugar, and cereals) to today's commercially available, lower-osmolality fluids. Because of their osmotic effect, the high-carbohydrate content in fluids such as apple juice or colas may further aggravate diarrhea and cause additional fluid loss.

Electrolyte or sports drinks (e.g., Gatorade) have long been accepted oral rehydration formulations for older children. Recent studies, however, suggest that sports drinks are not the best solutions for rehydration and may in fact worsen diarrhea because of their high percentage of sugar and carbohydrates. These supplements greatly increase the osmotic load in the intestines and further aggravate diarrhea (Bender, Skae, & Ozuah, 2005).

TABLE 18-2	**Assessment of the Severity of Dehydration**		
Clinical Signs	**Mild**	**Moderate**	**Severe**
Weight loss	3%-5%	6%-10%	>10%
Vital signs:			
Pulse	Normal	Increased	Increased and weak
Blood pressure	Normal	Normal to low	Very low, orthostatic, shock
Respiratory rate	Normal	Normal to deep	Rapid and deep
General appearance:			
Infants	Fussy, thirsty, alert	Fussy, restless, thirsty, lethargic but arousable	Drowsy to comatose, not arousable, gray color, limp, cold, and sweaty
Older children	Thirsty, restless, alert	Thirsty, restless, postural hypotension	Apprehensive, comatose, cold, mottled skin, cyanotic
Mucous membranes	Normal to slightly dry	Dry	Parched
Anterior fontanel	Normal	Sunken	Markedly depressed
Eyes	Normal	Sunken	Markedly sunken
Capillary refill	<3 sec	3-5 sec	>5 sec
Skin turgor (see Fig. 18-1)	Normal	Decreased (may have a doughy feel in hypernatremic dehydration)	Tenting (may have a doughy feel in hypernatremic dehydration)
Urine output	Mildly decreased, diaper may be dry	Decreased, diaper is dry, concentrated urine with specific gravity of 1.020-1.030	Decreased, diaper is dry, decrease in the number of diapers changed during the day, concentrated urine with specific gravity >1.030

Modified from Dabbagh, S., Atiyeh, B., Fleischmann, L. E., & Gruskin, A. B. (1999). Fluid and electrolyte therapy. In F. D. Burg, J. R. Ingelfinger, E. R. Wald, & R. A. Polin (Eds.), *Gellis & Kagan's current pediatric therapy* (16th ed.). Philadelphia: WB Saunders.

Mild to Moderate Dehydration

Treatment of fluid and electrolyte imbalances in children with mild to moderate dehydration should include rapid oral rehydration therapy (ORT) with an ORS in addition to replacing fluid losses. Suggested rehydration for children with mild to moderate dehydration is 50 to 100 mL/kg of ORS over 3 to 4 hours with frequent evaluation of the child's hydration status (Berman, 2003; CDC, 2003). Breastfeeding infants should continue to breastfeed during oral rehydration; an age-appropriate diet should be offered to all other children once the hydration status has improved (CDC, 2005). The resumption of solid food promotes mucosal repair caused by acute gastroenteritis and helps maintain the child's nutritional status (Berman, 2003).

Severe Dehydration

If the child is severely dehydrated or unable to take fluids by mouth and continuing fluid replacement is needed, parenteral fluid and electrolyte therapy is initiated. Initial therapy is aimed at treating or preventing shock. Either lactated Ringer's solution or 0.9% sodium chloride solution is the fluid of choice for parenteral rehydration and restoration of circulation. Sodium chloride (0.9%) solution may be ordered initially in boluses (20 mL/kg; 10 mL/kg in frail or ill infants) until the child's hydration status has improved (as assessed by improved level of consciousness), at which time ORT (100 mL/kg) can be initiated (CDC, 2005). If the child cannot tolerate oral fluids, the remainder of the fluid losses is provided by 5% dextrose in 0.45% normal saline solution at twice the hourly maintenance rate (CDC, 2003). Once

rehydrated, the child's additional fluid losses are replaced intravenously (IV) with 5% dextrose and 0.225% normal saline solution, if the child cannot tolerate ORT (CDC, 2005). If necessary, potassium is added to the IV solution once urine output is adequate. See Box 18-1 for daily fluid requirements by body weight and age-appropriate urine output.

The type of dehydration determines the rate of administration of replacement fluids. For the child with hyponatremic dehydration, lost fluids are replaced over 24 hours (in addition to the child's maintenance fluid requirements). Half the amount of estimated fluid loss is replaced over the first 8 hours and the remaining half over the next 16 hours

BOX 18-1	**Maintenance Fluid Requirements and Minimum Urine Output**

Daily Fluid Requirements by Body Weight

≤10 kg: 100 mL/kg

10-20 kg: 1000 mL + 50 mL/kg for each additional kilogram between 10 and 20 kg

>20 kg: 1500 mL + 20 mL/kg for each additional kilogram over 20 kg

Minimum Urine Output by Age Group

Infants and toddlers: >2-3 mL/kg/hr

Preschoolers and young school-age children: >1-2 mL/kg/hr

School-age children and adolescents: 0.5-1 mL/kg/hr

TABLE 18-3   Oral Replacement and Rehydration Therapy in Children With Vomiting or Diarrhea

	Minimally Dehydrated	Mild to Moderate Dehydration	Severe Dehydration
ORT	Not necessary unless not taking other fluids well	50-100 mL/kg of ORS plus replace continuing losses rapidly over a 3- to 4-hr period	IV therapy: bolus of 20 mL/kg of normal saline or lactated Ringer's solution; begin ORT for the remaining deficit (100 mL/kg over 4 hr) when child is stable and alert and can take oral fluids; alternatively, infuse 5% dextrose in half-strength normal saline solution at twice maintenance fluid rate; keep IV line in place until child is drinking well
Continuing losses	60 to 120 mL ORS for child weighing <10 kg, 120 to 240 mL for child weighing >10 kg to replace fluid loss from each episode of diarrhea **or** vomiting, or lost volume is measured and replaced (1 mL/g fluid loss)	60 to 120 mL ORS for child weighing <10 kg, 120 to 240 mL for child weighing >10 kg to replace fluid loss from each episode of diarrhea or vomiting, **or** lost volume is accurately measured and replaced (1 mL/g fluid loss)	60 to 120 mL ORS for child weighing <10 kg, 120 to 240 mL for child weighing >10 kg to replace fluid loss from each episode of diarrhea or vomiting, **or** lost volume is accurately measured and replaced (1 mL/g fluid loss); if unable to drink, administer replacement through nasogastric tube **or** infuse 5% dextrose and quarter-strength normal saline solution; potassium 20 mEq/L may be needed after urination established
Feeding	Continue age-appropriate diet	Continue breastfeeding; resume age-appropriate diet as soon as dehydration is corrected	Continue breastfeeding; resume age-appropriate diet as soon as dehydration is corrected
Re-evaluate hydration and estimate continuing fluid losses	As necessary	Every 1 to 2 hr	Continuous evaluation; must evaluate after each bolus of IV solution

Modified from Centers for Disease Control and Prevention. (2003). Managing acute gastroenteritis among children: Oral rehydration, maintenance, and nutritional therapy [Electronic version]. *MMWR: Morbidity and Mortality Weekly Report 52,* 1-16.

CRITICAL TO REMEMBER
Guidelines When Administering Potassium

- Do not administer potassium chloride if urine output is not age appropriate. See Box 18-1 for adequate urine output.
- *Never* give potassium by IV push.
- Give no more than 40 mEq/L, at a rate no faster than 1 mEq/kg/hr.
- Always check the dose and dosage calculations of potassium chloride. (Incorrect placement of a decimal point can result in a dose lethal to a child.)
- To avoid the risk of inadequate mixing, add potassium chloride to IV fluids with the plastic IV bag in the upright (noninfusion) position rather than in the down (infusion) position. (Inadequate mixing could result in the child's receiving an excessive amount of potassium chloride in the first few minutes.)
- Because of irritation of the vessel walls and potential phlebitis, IV solutions containing more than 30 mEq/L of potassium chloride should not be given through a peripheral IV line.

(Greenbaum, 2004). With hypernatremic dehydration, lost fluids are replaced more slowly, over 48 hours, to prevent a sudden decrease in serum sodium level. Potassium losses must also be replaced; this process should proceed slowly to avoid hyperkalemia. Potassium replacement should begin only after urine output is adequate (see Box 18-1) and should be administered with extreme caution. If the child is anuric, potassium is retained, causing elevated potassium levels.

NURSING CARE

The Child With Dehydration

Assessment

Because dehydration can develop very quickly in infants and young children, the nurse must be alert for early signs of dehydration in children with conditions in which fluid losses are likely to occur, such as diarrhea, vomiting, burns, diabetes, trauma, and fever. The condition of infants and young children can change rapidly when fluid and electrolyte imbalances occur.

The general appearance of the child should be assessed, as well as specific parameters:

- *Intake and output:* Measure all fluid intake and losses accurately (including vomitus, urine, stools, nasogastric drainage, wound drainage). The practitioner must also consider insensible water loss.
- *Urine output and specific gravity:* Output of less than 2 to 3 mL/kg/hr in infants and toddlers, 1 to 2 mL/kg/hr in preschoolers and young school-age children, and 0.5 to 1 mL/kg/hr in school-age children or adolescents or a specific gravity greater than 1.020 may indicate dehydration. Glucose, large amounts of protein, and radiographic dyes, however, elevate the specific gravity and may interfere with its accuracy.
- *Weight:* Weight is a crucial indicator of fluid status. Accurate measurements of the weight of the unclothed child, using the same scale at the same time of day, are essential. Changes in weight related to changes in IV lines or dressings should be identified by recording "with IV." Weight gain during illness may indicate fluid retention or pulmonary or generalized edema. The weight should be rechecked, and the child should be assessed for pulmonary crackles and periorbital edema.
- *Stools, vomitus:* Frequency, type, amounts, and consistency should be assessed and recorded.
- *Sweating:* Estimate from dampness of clothing and linen.
- *Serum electrolytes:* See p. 492.
- *Skin:* Assess color, temperature, turgor (Fig. 18-1), moisture, and capillary refill.
- *Mucous membranes and presence of tears:* Dry or sticky mucous membranes and the absence of tears indicate dehydration. Absence of tears is not significant in an infant younger than 2 to 4 months because infants of this age often do not manufacture tears.
- *Anterior fontanel:* A sunken or depressed fontanel in infants indicates dehydration. Cranial suture lines may also become prominent with dehydration.
- *Vital signs:* Fever increases the metabolic rate and fluid requirements. With dehydration, the pulse is rapid, weak, and thready. An increase in the respiratory rate compensates for metabolic acidosis, which often accompanies dehydration.

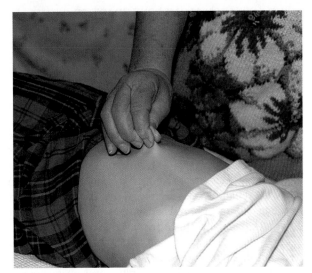

FIG 18-1   **Testing skin turgor. Turgor refers to the elasticity of the skin, which is affected by the extent of hydration. The nurse tests turgor by gently grasping the skin. When the skin is released, it should instantly spring back into place; if it does not, tissue turgor is considered poor.** *(Courtesy University of Texas at Arlington School of Nursing.)*

Blood pressure may be decreased in moderate and severe dehydration, but it is a late sign of hypovolemia.
- *Behavior:* Irritability, lethargy, confusion, or seizures may be present. The child's cry may be high pitched and weak.

Nursing Diagnosis and Planning

- Deficient Fluid Volume related to gastric or intestinal infection or inflammation, hemorrhage, burns, or failure of fluid regulatory mechanisms.

Expected Outcome: The infant or child will display adequate fluid volume, as evidenced by age-appropriate urine output, age-appropriate urine specific gravity, elastic skin turgor and moist mucous membranes, serum pH and electrolyte levels within normal limits, and weight gain.

Interventions

Teach parents how to prevent dehydration (Box 18-2). Parents should be taught to give infants and young children

---

BOX 18-2 | **PARENTS WANT TO KNOW**   About Dehydration

Signs and Symptoms of Dehydration
Watch for the following signs and symptoms of dehydration:
- Fewer wet diapers (especially no wet diaper for more than 6 to 8 hours)
- No tears when your child is crying if older than 2 to 4 months
- Inside of mouth dry or sticky
- Irritability; high-pitched cry
- Difficulty in awakening
- Increased respiratory rate or difficulty breathing
- Sunken fontanel, sunken eyes with dark circles
- Abnormal skin color, temperature, or dryness

Because a young child's condition may worsen faster than an older child's, seek professional assistance early if your child is younger than 6 months old.

Oral Rehydration Therapy
Giving plain water alone or in large amounts can be extremely dangerous because it does not contain needed electrolytes. Instead, commercially available oral rehydration solutions, such as Rehydralyte, Infalyte, or Pedialyte, should be given.

USING RESEARCH TO IMPROVE PRACTICE

It is an important part of contributing to evidence-based nursing practice for nurses not only to conduct research but also to participate in research carefully conducted by others. In the emergency department setting, finding a rapid, but accurate, way of assessing the severity of dehydration in young children (younger than 3 years old) would facilitate the initiation of an appropriate rehydration method. Researchers in a children's hospital in Toronto recruited experienced nurses to assist with developing a three-category dehydration assessment scoring method, which could improve the reliability of detecting the degree of dehydration in young children. For research purposes, each dehydration descriptor (similar to Table 18-2) was given a score of 0 to 2. For example, mucous membranes were scored a 0 if they were moist, a 1 if they were "sticky," and a 2 if they were dry. Each characteristic of dehydration was given a precise definition so that well-trained nurses could reliably assign a score.

The parents of 137 children diagnosed with gastroenteritis and isonatremic dehydration consented to participate. To prevent measurement error, research nurses weighed all children before the assessment of dehydration on a scale that was calibrated specifically for the study. One or more research nurses then scored the child with the new dehydration scoring method. To establish validity (e.g., that the scoring system accurately measured dehydration severity), the child was rescored independently by the emergency department nurse or physician with another scale that assessed the degree of dehydration. Then the child received either ORT or IV fluid replacement. The weight after rehydration was measured on most of the children and the percent of weight gained confirmed the degree of dehydration.

After statistically measuring the reliability and validity of all of the dehydration items on the scale, the researchers determined that scores on four characteristics of dehydration—general appearance (level of consciousness), eyes, mucous membranes, and presence of tears—most accurately predicted the response to rehydration. The researchers state that the scoring scale can be used to both precisely assess degree of dehydration and evaluate response to treatment (e.g., moving from a prehydration score of 8 to a posthydration score of 0).

A strength of this study is that dehydration characteristics were precisely defined so that research nurses and physicians could easily assign each a score. Only a limited number of research nurses and physicians participated, so the quality of the assessments was controlled and the chance for error reduced. In this study, the scoring method was not used to determine the method of rehydration but was used to assess the child's response to rehydration. Additional studies would be needed to use this scoring system to assess degree of dehydration for purposes of calculating rehydration.

Think about the ways in which nurses can participate in clinical research. What types of clinical problems might you identify that would be of interest to a nurse researcher? Think about how sources of error could be controlled in clinical research studies.

Friedman, J., Goldman, R., Srvastava, R., & Parkin, P. (2004). Development of a clinical dehydration scale for use in children between 1 and 36 months of age. *Journal of Pediatrics,* 145, 201-207.

extra fluids during hot weather, to avoid overdressing their children, and to encourage frequent rest periods during high-energy playtimes. During minor illness, providing additional fluids to a child with fever may prevent the development of more serious problems. Teach parents how to identify the early signs and symptoms of dehydration and instruct them to seek professional help if these signs and symptoms should occur.

Also, teach parents how to replace fluids when the child is mildly dehydrated. Oral rehydration formulations, such as Rehydralyte, Infalyte, or Pedialyte, contain the appropriate concentration of electrolytes and should be used. Parents need to understand that giving plain water alone or in large amounts can be extremely dangerous and why it is dangerous. The infant or child needs to continue to eat as tolerated.

When caring for the hospitalized child with fluid and electrolyte imbalance, the nurse assumes the responsibility of continuously monitoring the child's condition and administering oral and IV fluids safely (see Chapter 14 for a discussion of IV therapy). When caring for children with conditions such as fever, burns, diarrhea, vomiting, or trauma, the nurse must continuously assess for signs of dehydration.

Evaluation

- Is the child alert?
- Is urine output appropriate for age with a specific gravity within normal limits?
- Is the skin elastic and soft?
- Are the mucous membranes moist?
- Are serum pH and electrolyte levels within normal limits?

DIARRHEA

Diarrhea, one of the most common disorders in childhood, is defined as an increase in the frequency, fluidity, and volume of stools. In the United States and Canada, children have an average of 1.3 to 2.5 episodes of diarrhea per year, with 49.4 hospitalizations for every 10,000 children and 325 to 425 deaths annually (Berman, 2003). Diarrhea accompanies many childhood disorders. Diarrhea in children may be acute or chronic, inflammatory or noninflammatory. Diarrhea caused by infection is usually called *gastroenteritis.* Viral gastroenteritis is the cause of approximately 80% of all cases, making it the most common cause of diarrhea in children older than 1 year. Rotavirus infections account for approximately one third of hospitalizations of children in industrialized countries, due to the resulting fluid imbalances (Parashar, Gibson, Bresee, & Glass, 2006).

If not treated, acute diarrhea can lead to dehydration, electrolyte imbalance, and hypovolemic shock. Acute diarrhea can be life threatening in infants and small children if gastrointestinal fluid losses are not adequately replaced.

Etiology and Incidence

There are many causes of both acute and chronic diarrhea (Table 18-4). Diarrhea with ensuing dehydration is the leading killer of children worldwide and is a major cause of morbidity as well as a primary sign of many other conditions. In the United States, diarrhea accounts for approximately 1.5 million acute-care visits by children younger than 5 years, with 200,000 hospitalized annually (CDC, 2003). It can be either a short-term or a long-term condition. In infants and young children, diarrhea can be life threatening if the losses are not replaced.

Manifestations

Diarrhea may manifest either quickly or insidiously. Its manifestations include the following:

- *Integumentary:* dry, hot skin; changes in skin texture and turgor; dry mucous membranes

- *Small intestine:* cramps, nausea, vomiting; large-volume stools, light in color, loose to watery in texture; stools that tend to be soupy, greasy, or foul-smelling
- *Large intestine:* the urge to defecate with insignificant stool present; mushy, jellylike, or even bloody fecal matter; stool that is usually dark in color; stool that is rarely foul-smelling
- *Other:* increased heart and respiratory rates, decreased tearing, fever

Diagnostic Evaluation

Most infectious causes of diarrhea are self-limiting, making comprehensive testing of minor cases of diarrhea impractical. Because of the different possible causes, the diagnostic workup is frequently geared toward ruling out infectious agents and anatomic and physiologic reasons, such as allergies, food intolerance, and bowel problems. Tests to be performed after an initial history has assessed for food intolerance, stress, or school- or work-related problems include the following:

- *Stool:* cultures (for bacteria, ova, parasites, rotavirus), pH, red blood cells, leukocytes, glucose (Clinitest), blood (guaiac test or Hemoccult)
- *Blood tests:* especially blood cell counts, electrolytes, blood urea nitrogen, glucose, and blood cultures (if an infectious agent is suspected)
- *X-rays:* check for possible bowel abnormalities

TABLE 18-4 Causes and Manifestations of Diarrhea in Infants and Children

Causes of Diarrhea	Manifestations
Intestinal infection: Bacterial (*Campylobacter jejuni,** *Salmonella,** *Shigella,** *Escherichia coli*) Viral (rotavirus,* cause of more than 50% of cases of acute diarrhea in children; enteric adenovirus) Parasitic (*Giardia lamblia,** *Cryptosporidium**—high incidence of both in day care centers) Fungal overgrowth	Watery stools containing mucus and possibly blood Pain, cramps, nausea, vomiting, fever (>101.6 °F [38.7 °C] with bacterial infection); risk of dehydration, electrolyte imbalance, and shock
Food intolerance (lactose intolerance, overfeeding, introduction of new foods)	Diarrhea, increased mucus in stools, flatus, pain after ingestion of lactose or offending food
Malabsorption (cystic fibrosis, disaccharide deficiencies, celiac disease)	Diarrhea, cramps, distention, steatorrhea occurring after meals Anorexia, weight loss, fatigue
Medications (antibiotics, chemotherapy)	Diarrhea after administration of medications, which usually stops when medications are discontinued
Colon disease (ulcerative colitis, Crohn's disease, enterocolitis)	Inflammation and ulceration of intestinal walls, increased motility May have 10-20 stools per day Abdominal pain, fever, chills, anorexia, weight loss
Irritable bowel syndrome	Diarrhea alternating with constipation or normal bowel function Pain, distention, nausea may be present
Intestinal obstruction (including intussusception)	Partial obstruction may result in diarrhea caused by increased intestinal motility Pain, nausea, and sometimes bloody stool; may note mucus in stools
Emotional stress (anxiety, fatigue)	Increased motility
Infectious disease (otitis media, upper respiratory infection, urinary tract infection)	Diarrhea frequently accompanies other infections

*Most common causative organisms.

PATHOPHYSIOLOGY

DIARRHEA

Increased motility and rapid emptying of the intestines result in impaired absorption of nutrients and water and in electrolyte imbalance. Water, sodium, potassium, and bicarbonate are drawn from the extracellular space into the stool, resulting in dehydration, electrolyte depletion, and metabolic acidosis.

Diarrhea occurs when there is excess fluid in the small intestine. This condition can result from a number of processes:

- Bacterial toxins stimulating active transport of electrolytes into the small intestine: cells in the mucosal lining of the intestines are irritated and secrete increased amounts of water and electrolytes.
- Organisms invading and destroying intestinal mucosal cells, decreasing intestinal surface area, and impairing the intestine's capacity to absorb fluids and electrolytes.
- Inflammation, which decreases the intestine's ability to absorb fluid, electrolytes, and nutrients. This condition occurs in malabsorption syndromes.
- Increased intestinal motility, resulting in impaired intestinal absorption.

Therapeutic Management

The treatment of diarrhea is aimed at maintaining and restoring fluid and electrolyte balance and returning the bowel to normal function. Preventing the spread of infection to others is an important component of care, with meticulous handwashing being critical. Parents must be informed of specific fluid intake requirements and signs of dehydration, which would signal a worsening of the child's condition. Treatment of diarrhea and prevention of dehydration include replacing fluids, continuing feedings, and close monitoring and observation. Infants should continue to be given breast milk or regular-strength formula.

The continued feeding of a normal diet can prevent dehydration, reduce stool frequency and volume, and hasten recovery. It does not prolong diarrhea, and there is evidence that it may reduce the duration of diarrhea. Normal diets replace much-needed nutrients lost during diarrheal events; not continuing a normal diet could lead to altered growth or malnutrition, particularly in children from some underdeveloped countries (CDC, 2003). If adding milk to the diet increases diarrhea, transient lactose intolerance may be considered, although it is not as common as was once thought. If lactose intolerance is present, it may be necessary to give the infant a soy formula until the deficiency resolves, usually within several weeks (Berman, 2003). Common foods that are especially well tolerated during diarrhea are bland but nutritional foods, including complex carbohydrates (e.g., rice, wheat, potatoes, cereals), yogurt, cooked vegetables, and lean meats. Fatty foods and foods high in simple sugars (e.g., tea, juices, soft drinks) should be avoided (Bender et al.,

2005). This recommendation is a change from the formerly recommended BRAT diet, which consisted of bananas, rice, applesauce, and toast. The BRAT diet can be tolerated but is low in energy, density, fat, and protein.

Preventing dehydration is a primary issue in the management of the infant or child with diarrhea. ORS is given to replace each loose stool. In addition to continuing an age-appropriate diet, children weighing less than 10 kg should have losses replaced with 60 to 120 mL of ORS for each episode of diarrhea. Children weighing more than 10 kg should receive 120 to 240 mL of ORS (CDC, 2003). For infants with mild to moderate diarrhea who have not become dehydrated, fluid loss replacement is started at home.

If an infant or child has become mildly to moderately dehydrated and requires a visit to a clinic or emergency department, ORT is recommended as described previously and in Table 18-3. At the end of each hour of rehydration, hydration and replacement losses should be assessed. Initial rehydration may require limiting the intake to smaller volumes (sips) to reduce any incidence of associated vomiting (e.g., 5 mL every 2 to 5 minutes) with a gradual increase in volume as tolerated. Nasogastric administration of ORS may be necessary to provide slow, steady, continuous administration to rapidly hydrate child and prevent hospitalization.

Feeding of solids or formula is started as soon as the child is rehydrated. Children should be encouraged to eat frequently—every 3 to 4 hours. Parents should be instructed that, although stool output may increase, feeding will not prolong diarrhea and the child will be absorbing necessary nutrients and calories. For a child with severe dehydration and continuing losses, ORT is not recommended. Such children are usually admitted to a hospital for observation and IV therapy.

If bacteria, parasites, or fungi cause the diarrhea, other types of medication along with antibiotics may be ordered. The use of antidiarrheal medication is not recommended in children because of the binding nature of these products and the potential for toxicity. Antidiarrheal medications have not been found to shorten the course of the diarrhea, and in cases where the diarrhea is caused by pathogens, they may increase fluid and electrolyte loss by interfering with the body's attempt to rid itself of the organism and allowing the pathogen to remain in the body longer. *Lactobacillus* supplementation has demonstrated effectiveness in shortening the course of diarrhea from nonbacterial causes, and many pediatricians recommend this as an adjunct to ORS (Berman, 2003).

Prognosis

Most children with diarrhea and subsequent dehydration usually have a relatively quick recovery, provided that the cause of the diarrhea is determined and therapy is started as soon as possible. A vaccine to prevent rotavirus infection was removed from the market in late 1999 because of the risk of unacceptable side effects. The CDC recommends a newly approved vaccine for rotavirus to be given to infants at age 2, 4, and 6 months (CDC, 2006).

NURSING CARE

The Child With Diarrhea

Assessment

When a child is admitted to a hospital setting, the child's condition and hydration status should be the first area of assessment. The concern about dehydration is the potential for shock. The child and family should be questioned about possible food allergies, intolerance to foods, food eaten over the past 24 hours, and outbreaks of diarrhea in the nuclear or extended family or day care setting. If diarrhea is present, stools should be assessed for amount, color, consistency, and time—abbreviated as ACCT—and odor. When assessing and monitoring for ACCT, note the quantity and quality of the stool, its color (e.g., green, brown, clear, blood tinged), consistency (watery, loose), the presence of mucus, and the length of time since the stool's consistency has changed.

Other continuing assessments include monitoring intake and output; assessing the current weight and comparing it with the last known weight; assessing for thirst, along with skin turgor and texture and mucous membranes; and monitoring the child's level of activity. If diarrhea is severe, it may be necessary to apply a urine bag to measure urine output and to obtain urine to measure specific gravity. Skin integrity must be monitored if a urine bag is to be used. Observe the skin in the perineal area for color, texture, lesions, or drainage with each diaper change. Assess family members' knowledge of the transmission of infection by questions or testing. Observe family members as they use contact precautions. Ask family if any members have cramping or diarrhea.

Nursing Diagnosis and Planning

The following nursing diagnoses and expected outcomes may be appropriate in the treatment of diarrhea in a child:

- Deficient Fluid Volume related to increased stool output.

  Expected Outcomes: The child will maintain fluid balance within normal limits, as evidenced by age-appropriate urine output, capillary refill time less than 2 seconds, elastic skin turgor, moist mucous membranes, and weight gain.

- Impaired Skin Integrity related to exposure to stool

  Expected Outcomes: The child will have no sign of skin breakdown, as evidenced by intact perineal and perianal skin, or will exhibit signs of healing on affected or excoriated areas.

- Risk for Infection (in others) related to lack of knowledge about transmission prevention.

  Expected Outcomes: Family members will show no signs of infection and demonstrate correct precaution technique (contact precautions).

- Imbalanced Nutrition: Less than Body Requirements related to decreased intake and inability of body to absorb fluids.

Expected Outcomes: The child will tolerate the diet, as evidenced by weight gain and no recurrence of diarrhea.

Interventions

The child with diarrhea should be weighed unclothed on admission and daily on the same scale and at the same time each day to precisely determine changes in weight. To accurately determine fluid losses with each episode of diarrhea in untrained infants and children, weigh the diaper after each voiding and liquid stool (each gram of diaper weight is equal to 1 mL of fluid output). Measuring amounts of liquid stool may be required for the older child. Accurate accounting of losses is necessary to maximize the effectiveness of the ORT and to prevent deficits and imbalances in electrolytes. Document the child's intake as well as output.

Vital signs should be measured every 4 hours, or as needed. Changes in vital signs and signs of dry mucous membranes, decreased tearing, and sunken fontanel (if appropriate) or eyes are often the first of indicators of dehydration. Determining the causes of diarrhea may include obtaining stool cultures and other tests to determine specific management approaches.

Infants and young children may have skin excoriation resulting from continual contact with loose stools. Nursing intervention includes providing meticulous skin care. Gently wash the area with warm water and mild soap after each loose stool and pat dry. If ordered, apply a medicated cream or ointment to protect and heal the skin. Some children benefit from exposing damaged skin to the air for small periods of time to promote healing. Turning every 2 hours keeps pressure off the skin and facilitates circulation to the affected area.

Nursing interventions, along with the prescribed therapy, work together to achieve the expected outcomes of managing any dehydration, decreasing the number of stools, and returning the bowel to normal function. ORT may be initiated in a hospital setting after IV rehydration. Administer the ORS as ordered, increasing the volume as tolerated. If the child refuses or is unable to tolerate the ORS, nasogastric therapy may be considered.

Most cases of diarrhea in children can be managed at home. Parent teaching needs to be clear, concise, and specific (Box 18-3). Education about appropriate oral replacement fluids should include avoidance of sugary drinks, apple juice, sports beverages, and colas. Fluids should be offered in small amounts to prevent gastric distention and at room temperature to prevent increased peristalsis stimulation.

Additional education needs to occur regarding prevention of illness in the nuclear and extended family or day care setting. Instruction in careful handwashing technique before and after caring for the sick child will prevent spread of infection or reinfection. Proper disposal of and cleaning of contaminated articles decreases spread of infection.

BOX 18-3	**PARENTS WANT TO KNOW** About Caring for a Child With Diarrhea

Diet

Diet depends on the age of the child and the severity of the diarrhea.

Mild Diarrhea (Mushy Stools) in Children of Any Age

Continue with an age-appropriate diet. Continue breast-feeding, formula, or milk. Encourage increased intake of fluids. Avoid fruit juices, because they may worsen diarrhea. Provide a variety of nutritious foods, including foods containing complex carbohydrates, such as rice, potatoes, bread, and cereals. Avoid fatty or spicy foods.

Moderate Diarrhea (Watery or Frequent Stools) in Children Younger than 1 Year

Continue breastfeeding or formula and age-appropriate diet. Provide additional fluids by using Infalyte, Pedialyte, Rehydralyte, or other similar commercially prepared oral rehydration solutions if urine output begins to decrease. If the diarrhea is severe or it does not improve after 3 days on regular formula, give the infant soy formula (Isomil, Pro-Sobee) instead of cow's milk formula. Soy formula should be continued until the diarrhea is gone for 3 days. Foods include the ABCs (applesauce, bananas, strained carrots), mashed potatoes, rice cereal, yogurt, and other bland foods. Watch closely for signs of dehydration and report these immediately to your health care provider.

Moderate Diarrhea (Watery or Frequent Stools) in Children Older than 1 Year

Continue age-appropriate diet with foods that are nutritional, bland, and high in starch. Suggested foods include breads, crackers, rice, mashed potatoes, noodles, yogurt, cooked vegetables, and lean meats. Avoid beans, spices, and fatty foods. Avoid sports drinks, colas, and apple juice. Give additional fluids in the form of Infalyte, Pedialyte, or Rehydralyte. Watch closely for signs of dehydration and report these immediately to your health care provider.

Preventing the Spread of Infection

Infectious diarrhea is very contagious. Some of the infectious agents can live on toys, water fountains, and other inanimate objects for several days. Thorough handwashing after diaper changing or using the toilet is crucial to prevent others in the household from getting diarrhea. All family members should be taught the importance of thorough and frequent handwashing. Diapers should be changed on a surface designated for that purpose, *not* on the kitchen counter where food is prepared. Changing areas should be cleaned with disinfectant after each diaper change.

Skin Care

To prevent breakdown of the sensitive skin in the diaper area, diarrhea stools should be completely washed off with mild soap and water after each bowel movement. (Washing the child under running water in the bathtub makes the job easier. The tub should be cleaned with disinfectant before anyone else uses it.) The skin should be patted dry and a layer of A & D ointment or other protective or "barrier" ointment applied.

Changing diapers immediately after bowel movements is important to prevent skin breakdown. The use of commercial baby wipes should be avoided because they may further irritate and cause additional breakdown of the skin. To prevent overflow of diarrhea from the diaper, diapers should be applied snugly.

When to Call the Physician

Call the physician immediately if any of the following occurs:

- The child does not urinate for longer than 6 hours.
- Crying produces no tears, or the mouth becomes dry.
- The infant's fontanel appears sunken.
- The child's behavior or mental status changes.
- Blood appears in the diarrhea, or the diarrhea becomes severe (e.g., a bowel movement every hour for more than 8 hours, or more than 10 watery bowel movements in 1 day).
- Severe abdominal cramps occur.
- The child becomes dizzy when standing.
- The child starts acting very sick.
- A fever unexpectedly develops (>101° F).
- Mild diarrhea lasts more than 1 week.

Data from Centers for Disease Control and Prevention. (2003). Managing acute gastroenteritis among children: Oral rehydration, maintenance, and nutritional therapy [Electronic version]. *MMWR: Morbidity and Mortality Weekly Report, 52,* 1-16; Centers for Disease Control and Prevention. (2005). Guidelines for the management of acute diarrhea. Retrieved January 31, 2006, from *www.cdc.gov;* Berman, J. (2003). Heading off the dangers of acute gastroenteritis. *Contemporary Pediatrics, 20,* 57-68.

Evaluation

- Are weight, urine output, and specific gravity within normal limits for age?
- Is the capillary refill less than 2 seconds?
- Is skin turgor elastic, and are mucous membranes moist?
- Have signs of excoriation, redness, blisters, pruritus, and infection been reduced or eliminated?
- Are family members free of infection?
- Do family members correctly practice contact precaution technique on a consistent basis?
- Can the child retain food and fluids?
- Are normal bowel elimination patterns present?
- Has the child maintained or shown an increase in weight?

CRITICAL THINKING EXERCISE 18-1

Mrs. Peters calls the clinic about 8-month-old David. She states that David has had diarrhea for 2 days and that she does not know what to do. She also states that her neighbor said she should stop breastfeeding and give David clear liquids. Mrs. Peters tells you that she is afraid she may have done something to cause David to get sick.

1. What questions should you ask Mrs. Peters about her infant?
2. What teaching can you do to help Mrs. Peters?

VOMITING

Vomiting is the forcible ejection of stomach contents through the mouth. It involves a complex reflex associated with sweating, salivation, and often tachycardia (all symptoms of autonomic nervous stimulation). Other terms that may be used to differentiate vomiting episodes include *spitting up* (or *chalasia*, which is a normal process during infancy), *regurgitation* (associated with gastroesophageal reflux or overfeeding), and, if severe, *projectile vomiting* (usually indicative of obstruction, tumor, pyloric stenosis, or increasing intracranial pressure). Isolated incidents of vomiting are usually of little concern. The consequences of persistent or prolonged vomiting, however, can be serious.

Etiology

Vomiting, which occurs frequently in children, is usually a sign of some other underlying problem or disease. Vomiting has many possible causes. Some of them are infections, obstructions, motion sickness, metabolic alterations, and psychologic alterations. If vomiting occurs in association with diarrhea, it may be related to gastroenteritis. Vomiting can also result from allergic reactions or occur as a side effect of medications (e.g., chemotherapy), as a toxic effect of medications or ingested substances, and from certain eating disorders.

Manifestations

Sour milk curds without green or brown color and undigested food from the stomach are manifestations of vomiting. Green emesis usually indicates the presence of bile and possible intestinal obstruction below the ampulla of Vater. A fecal odor indicates lower intestinal obstruction or peritonitis. Emesis may be blood tinged, or the color may be bright red or look like coffee grounds. Bright red blood indicates that the blood has not been in contact with gastric juices.

The force of vomiting varies. Regurgitation, a backward flow of undigested food, could be caused by overfeeding. Forceful vomiting could indicate some obstruction. Projectile vomiting may indicate obstruction, tumor, or increased intracranial pressure. Continuous vomiting in a young child, in the absence of diarrhea, can contribute to metabolic alkalosis.

Diagnostic Evaluation

Vomiting in children is usually of brief duration and not severe. If vomiting continues and the child starts to look deficient in fluid or electrolytes, however, the following tests may be indicated:

- Complete blood cell counts and electrolyte studies, blood urea nitrogen, glucose levels, and urine tests
- Radiographic studies (if an obstructive or neurologic process is suspected)
- Blood cultures (if an infectious disease is suspected)
- Arterial blood gas determinations

Therapeutic Management

The primary focus of managing vomiting is detecting and treating the cause, with the secondary intent of preventing complications. ORT, as indicated for the treatment of diarrhea (see Table 18-3), is also appropriate for the vomiting child. Even with continued vomiting, most children can maintain hydration with small frequent feedings of an ORS and an age-appropriate diet as tolerated (Bender et al., 2005), and therefore the vomiting can be managed at home. Adequate fluid intake and replacement of continuing losses from emesis are necessary. The practitioner and parents must estimate the volume of emesis and replace it. Re-evaluation and continuing loss replacement should be done every 1 to 2 hours for a mild to moderately dehydrated child. As the vomiting decreases in frequency, the amount and interval between feedings can increase. If the vomiting is severe or prolonged in neonates and young infants, however, IV therapy may be initiated. Most children will respond well to treatment, but some will need antiemetics. To rid the mouth of the hydrochloric acid, and to freshen the mouth, the parent should rinse the child's mouth and brush the child's teeth after each time the child vomits.

PATHOPHYSIOLOGY

VOMITING

Vomiting is under the control of the emetic center, located in the reticular core of the medulla (in the brainstem). The emetic center receives stimuli from one of three sources:
- From the vagal and sympathetic afferent nerves, such as the stimulation of irritation, distention, obstruction, or inflammation
- Chemically, from drugs (e.g., ipecac, other opioids), cerebral hypoxia, inner ear disturbances, or increased intracranial pressure
- From the higher cortical centers, with stimuli such as sights, odors, and fright or fear
- The mechanism of vomiting occurs in the presence of several complex reflexes:
  - Autonomic nervous system discharge, which causes salivation, sweating, pallor, and an increased heart rate
  - Contraction of the stomach antrum and duodenum
  - Relaxation of the remainder of the stomach, esophagus, and sphincters
  - Closure of the glottis and soft palate
  - Contraction of the diaphragm and abdominal muscles, which increases intra-abdominal pressure and compresses abdominal contents, thus propelling them into the esophagus and out the mouth

---

NURSING CARE

The Vomiting Child

Assessment

Major concerns with vomiting are dehydration and fluid and electrolyte imbalance; therefore, it is essential that hydration status be carefully assessed, including accurate assessment of intake and output, weight, fontanels in infants, general behavior, dryness of mucous membranes, skin turgor, eyes, and urine output. Ask the parent to describe the type and force of vomiting (e.g., "spitting up" as opposed to regurgitation, forceful vomiting, or projectile vomiting) and the character (using the acronym ACCT: amount, color, consistency, time) of the vomitus. Because vomiting is often associated with gastric distention, the relationship, if any, with infant feeding should be assessed (e.g., poor feeding techniques, failure to bubble or burp, regurgitation with burp or "wet burp," improper positioning). Inquire about any other signs or symptoms the child may have.

Nursing Diagnosis and Planning

The following nursing diagnoses and expected outcomes may be appropriate in the treatment of the vomiting child:

- Deficient Fluid Volume related to increased loss of gastrointestinal contents.

Expected Outcomes: The child will maintain fluid balance within normal limits, as evidenced by age-appropriate fluid intake, and will have age-appropriate urine output, a capillary refill time of less than 2 seconds, elastic skin turgor, and moist mucous membranes.

- Imbalanced Nutrition: Less Than Body Requirements related to vomiting.

Expected Outcomes: The child will maintain electrolyte and acid-base balance within normal limits, as evidenced by adequate amount of calories absorbed, steady weight gain or lack of weight loss, and decreased vomiting episodes.

CRITICAL TO REMEMBER

Caring for the Child Who Is Vomiting

Nursing care of the child who is vomiting is directed toward the following:

- Observing and reporting vomiting
- Assessing for associated problems, such as dehydration
- Implementing measures to reduce the vomiting
- Recording accurate intake and output
- Evaluating the effectiveness of therapy
- Preventing aspiration

Interventions

The vomiting child should be placed in an upright or side-lying position to prevent aspiration. Nursing interventions are frequently determined by the cause of the vomiting and therefore may be very specific. For example, if the vomiting is found to be caused by incorrect feeding techniques, the nurse's role is to educate the family regarding appropriate feeding techniques (e.g., adequate bubbling and burping and positioning after the feeding) and preparation of formulas.

Once the cause of vomiting has been determined, nursing interventions are directed toward ensuring a continued reduction in the vomiting and preventing dehydration. Advise the parent to offer an ORS (see Table 18-3) in small, frequent feedings to avoid gastric distention and to continue age-appropriate diet as tolerated. The parent can gradually increase the amount of fluids and foods as vomiting episodes decrease. Another important consideration is education for the child and family about avoiding certain foods (e.g., fatty, acidified, or seasoned foods) and minimizing stimuli such as stress, anxiety, or unfavorable-smelling foods, which might lead to nausea and subsequent vomiting. Antiemetic medications, decreased stimuli, and avoidance of food or activities that might tend to upset the stomach, either directly or by association, may be helpful in decreasing nausea and vomiting. If the child repeatedly vomits or vomits large volumes, or if the child begins to exhibit signs of dehydration, the parent should notify the physician.

Evaluation

- Is the child taking age-appropriate amounts of fluid without vomiting?
- Is the child's urine output age appropriate?
- Is the child's skin turgor elastic, with a capillary refill time of 2 seconds or less?
- Does the child have moist mucous membranes?
- Is the child tolerating an age-appropriate diet?

KEY CONCEPTS

- Infants and children are at a much greater risk than adults for fluid and electrolyte disturbances.
- The three mechanisms by which acid-base balance is maintained are chemical buffering, respiratory control of carbon dioxide, and renal regulation of bicarbonate and secretion of hydrogen ions.
- The two major forms of acid-base disturbance are acidosis and alkalosis, either of which may be respiratory or metabolic.
- The treatment of metabolic disturbances is directed toward correcting the underlying problem. Interventions for respiratory alterations are implemented toward reestablishing alveolar ventilation.
- Dehydration may be classified as isonatremic (the most common form), hyponatremic, or hypernatremic.
- Monitoring of intake and output, vital signs, and level of activity (or sensorium) is crucial in appropriately assessing the child with a fluid or electrolyte disturbance.
- Diarrhea can lead to loss of bicarbonate (and subsequently to acidosis).
- Oral rehydration therapy is indicated for the child with diarrhea, dehydration of any degree, and vomiting.

ANSWERS TO
CRITICAL THINKING EXERCISE 18-1

1. When taking a history related to diarrhea, it is very important that you have accurate information. One person's definition of diarrhea may be very different from that of the next person. David may indeed have severe diarrhea, or he may have just an increase in stools. Ask Mrs. Peters the following questions:
   - How long has David had diarrhea?
   - How many stools has he had? What is the color, amount, and consistency of the stools?
   - How many wet diapers has David had in the last 24 hours?
   - Is David playing and acting normally?
   - What is David's temperature?
   - When David cries, does he have tears?
   - Has David been in a day care setting or a church nursery?
   - Does anyone else in the family have diarrhea?
   - What solids does David eat?
2. On the basis of Mrs. Peters' response, you can develop a teaching plan. Three areas need to be addressed: diet, infection control, and emotional support. Although you may think diet and infection control are priorities, until Mrs. Peters is less anxious she will not be able to give full attention to the information you are about to give her. For that reason, you should provide emotional support and assurance.

Emotional Support

Mrs. Peters seems to be blaming herself for David's illness. Provide an environment that encourages her to talk about her feelings. The use of therapeutic communication will build trust and allow her to share her concerns. You can commend her for breastfeeding and point out that breastfeeding provides extra help in fighting infections. Because David is now 8 months old, the antibodies that Mrs. Peters passed to him during her pregnancy are gone, and he is more susceptible to infections. As you talk with Mrs. Peters, you are constantly assessing her emotional needs and responding to her questions.

Diet

Mrs. Peters should continue to breastfeed David and provide an age-appropriate diet of solids. Fruit juices and raw fruits and vegetables should be discontinued because they may increase the diarrhea. Foods given should be nutritional and include complex carbohydrates. Suggested foods include cereal, mashed potatoes, strained bananas, strained carrots, and applesauce. Mrs. Peters should be given instructions regarding signs of dehydration and should be advised to call back if David's condition worsens. If he is mildly dehydrated and urine output is decreased, Mrs. Peters should be encouraged to breastfeed at more frequent intervals. She may be advised to add an ORS in amounts appropriate for David's weight to replace fluid lost from the diarrhea. Mrs. Peters should closely watch David for signs of increasing dehydration; if his condition worsens, he should be seen by the health care provider.

Infection Control

Instructions should also cover handwashing and infection control. Instruct Mrs. Peters in the disposal of contaminated linens and other soiled items. Instruct her in the cleaning of areas where diapers are changed and where children play with toys. Instruct her to clean the bathtub after use. Reinforce the importance of not sharing toys among children who have diarrhea.

REFERENCES AND READINGS

Atherly-John, Y. C., Cunningham, S. J., & Crain, E. F. (2002). A randomized trial of oral vs. intravenous rehydration in a pediatric emergency room. *Archives of Pediatric Adolescent Medicine, 156,* 1240-1243.

Banks, J. B., & Meadows, S. (2005). Intravenous fluids for children with gastroenteritis. Retrieved June 15, 2005, from *http://www.aafp.org/afp/20050101/fpin.html.*

Bender, B., Skae, C., & Ozuah, P. (2005). Oral rehydration therapy: The clear solution to fluid loss. *Contemporary Pediatrics, 22,* 72-77.

Berman, J. (2003). Heading off the dangers of acute gastroenteritis. *Contemporary Pediatrics, 20,* 57-68.

Brewster, D. R. (2002). Dehydration in acute gastroenteritis. *Journal of Pediatric Child Health, 38,* 219-222.

Centers for Disease Control and Prevention (2003). Managing acute gastroenteritis among children: Oral rehydration, maintenance, and nutritional therapy [Electronic version]. *MMWR: Morbidity and Mortality Weekly Report, 52,* 1-16.

Centers for Disease Control and Prevention (2005). *Guidelines for the management of acute diarrhea.* Retrieved January 31, 2006, from *www.cdc.gov.*

Centers for Disease Control and Prevention (2006). Prevention of rotavirus gastroenteritis among infants and children. *MMWR, 55*(RR-12), 1-13.

Dale, J. (2004). Oral rehydration solutions in the management of acute gastroenteritis among children. *Journal of Pediatric Health Care, 18,* 211-212.

Farthing, M. J. G. (2002). Oral rehydration: An evolving solution. *Journal of Pediatric Gastroenterology and Nutrition, 34,* 564-567.

Friedman, J., Goldman, R., Srvastava, R., & Parkin, P. (2004). Development of a clinical dehydration scale for use in children between 1 and 36 months of age. *Journal of Pediatrics, 145,* 201-207.

Fuchs, G. J. (2002). Reduced osmolarity oral rehydration solutions: New and improved ORS? *Journal of Pediatric Gastroenterology and Nutrition, 34,* 252-253.

Greenbaum, L. (2004). Electrolyte and acid base disorders. In R. Behrman, R. Kliegman, & H. Jenson (Eds.). *Nelson textbook of pediatrics* (17th ed.). Philadelphia: Elsevier Saunders.

Kee, J. L., & Paulanka, B. J. (2000). *Fluid and electrolytes: Clinical applications.* Albany, NY: Delmar.

Leung, A. K. C., & Sigalet, D. L. (2003). Acute abdominal pain in children. *American Family Physician, 67,* 2321-2326.

Miller, K. E. (2003). *Oral or IV rehydration in children with gastroenteritis.* Retrieved June 15, 2005, from *http://www.aafp.org/afp.*

Nager, A. L., & Wang, V. J. (2002). Comparison of nasogastric and intravenous methods of rehydration in pediatric patients with acute dehydration. *Pediatrics, 109,* 566-572.

Nalin, D. R., Hirshhorn, N., Greenough, W., Fuchs, G. J., & Cash, R. A. (2004). Clinical concerns about reduced-osmolality oral rehydration solution. *Journal of the American Medical Association, 291,* 2632-2636.

Ozuah, P. O., Avner, J. R., & Stein, R. K. (2002). Oral rehydration, emergency physicians, and practice parameters: A national survey. *Pediatrics, 109,* 259-261.

Parashar, U., Gibson, C., Bresee, J., & Glass, R. (2006). Rotavirus and severe childhood diarrhea. *Emerging Infectious Diseases [serial on the Internet].* Retrieved February 1, 2006, *from www.cdc.gov.*

Phavichitr, N., & Catto-Smith, A. G. (2003). Acute gastroenteritis in children: What role for antibacterials? *Pediatric Drugs, 5,* 279-290.

Robertson, J., & Shilkofski, N. (Eds.). (2005). *The Harriet Lane handbook.* St. Louis: Elsevier Mosby.

Santosham, M. (2002). Oral rehydration therapy. *Archives of Pediatric Adolescent Medicine, 156,* 1177-1179.

Spandorfer, P. R., Alessandrini, E. A., Joffe, M. D, Localio, R., & Shaw, K. N. (2005). Oral versus intravenous rehydration of moderately dehydrated children: A randomized, controlled trial. *Pediatrics, 115,* 295-301.

Taylor, J. A. (2004). *Oral rehydration: In pediatrics, less is often better.* Retrieved June 27, 2005, from *http://www.archpediatrics.com.*

Wathen, J., MacKenzie, T., & Bothner, J. (2004). Usefulness of the serum electrolyte panel in the management of pediatric dehydration treated with intravenously administered fluids. *Pediatrics, 114,* 1227-1234.

Wellbery, C. (2005). Diagnosing dehydration in children. *American Family Physician, 71,* 1010.

Willock, J., & Jewkes, F. (2000). Making sense of fluid balance in children. *Paediatric Nursing, 12,* 37-42.

CHAPTER 19

The Child With a Gastrointestinal Alteration

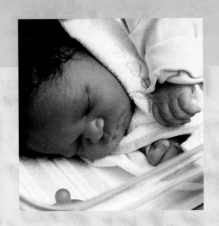

Learning Objectives

After studying this chapter, you should be able to:

- Describe the development of the gastrointestinal system and its relation to selected congenital defects.
- Describe the anatomy and physiology of the gastrointestinal system in the infant and child.
- Describe the common diagnostic and screening tests used to detect alterations in gastrointestinal function.
- Discuss and demonstrate an understanding of the structural and functional alterations in the gastrointestinal system.
- Discuss and demonstrate an understanding of the pathophysiology, etiology, clinical manifestations, diagnostic evaluation, and therapeutic management of malabsorption and infectious problems affecting the gastrointestinal system.
- State expected nursing diagnoses for gastrointestinal alterations.
- Use the nursing process to develop nursing care plans and teaching guidelines for the child with gastrointestinal alterations.
- Develop home care guidelines for the child with gastrointestinal alterations.
- Implement child and family teaching.
- Develop nursing implications for common medications used with the child with gastrointestinal alterations.
- Demonstrate critical thinking skills to manage a given patient care situation.

Definitions

achalasia Failure of smooth muscle fibers of the gastrointestinal tract to relax, resulting in a functional obstruction and difficulty in passage of food and chyme along the tract.

anastomosis Surgical connection of separate tubular hollow organs to form a continuous channel, as between two parts of the intestine or esophagus.

atresia Absence or abnormal closure of a normal body orifice or passage.

azotemia The presence of urea and other nitrogenous bodies in the blood; an elevated blood urea nitrogen or creatinine level.

dysphagia Inability to swallow or difficulty in swallowing.

encopresis Incontinence of feces.

fistula Abnormal passage or communication between two organs or tissues.

fundoplication A 270- to 360-degree wrap of the stomach fundus around the distal esophagus to tighten the lower esophageal sphincter and prevent gastric reflux.

hematemesis Vomiting of bright red blood or of denatured blood that looks like coffee grounds; usually represents a bleeding source proximal to the jejunum.

melena Rectal passage of black, tarry stools, indicating denatured blood from the upper gastrointestinal tract.

occult bleeding Bleeding in such minute quantity that it can be recognized only by microscopic or chemical means.

peristalsis Progressive, wavelike movements caused by contraction and relaxation of the longitudinal and circular muscles of the gastrointestinal tract; propels a bolus of food or fluid forward.

projectile vomiting Vomiting that is projected with force, perhaps 2 to 4 feet away from the mouth; may be preceded by deep gastric left-to-right peristaltic waves characteristic of pyloric stenosis.

pylorus The distal opening of the stomach where the stomach contents pass into the duodenum; the pylorus is surrounded by muscle bands.

tenesmus Ineffective, painful, or continuous urge to defecate.

REVIEW OF THE GASTROINTESTINAL SYSTEM
Upper Gastrointestinal System

The upper gastrointestinal (GI) system includes the mouth, esophagus, and stomach. Its primary functions are to take in food and fluids, begin the digestive process, and propel food into the intestines, where nutrients are absorbed. The *mouth*, or buccal cavity, is the entrance to the GI tract. Here food is broken up and mixed with saliva. This process starts the digestion of carbohydrates. The submandibular, parotid, and sublingual glands secrete saliva in response to the smell, taste, or thought of food. The tongue contains taste buds that distinguish salt, sweet, sour, and bitter sensations. The tongue is essential for swallowing.

At birth, the *esophagus* measures approximately 10 cm in length; it lengthens to 18 to 25 cm by adulthood. The upper third of the esophagus consists of striated voluntary muscle;

the lower two thirds consist of smooth muscle. The upper esophageal sphincter (UES) prevents the reflux of esophageal contents into the pharynx and lungs and prevents esophageal distention during respiration; the lower esophageal sphincter (LES, or cardiac sphincter) prevents the reflux of gastric contents into the lower esophagus.

Swallowing is under both voluntary and involuntary control. As food is chewed, it forms a small bolus, or mass; the tongue propels the bolus toward the oropharynx. The presence of this mass in the oropharynx stimulates the medulla, causing the soft palate to rise. The nasal passages close, the pharyngeal muscles contract, the larynx closes, and respiration is inhibited. As a result of these processes, food is propelled to the esophagus. Through peristalsis, the bolus moves on to the LES, the muscle relaxes, and the bolus enters the stomach.

The *stomach* lies in the epigastric, umbilical, and left hypochondrial regions of the abdomen. It is a muscular pouch,

Animation: Passage of Food Through the Digestive Tract

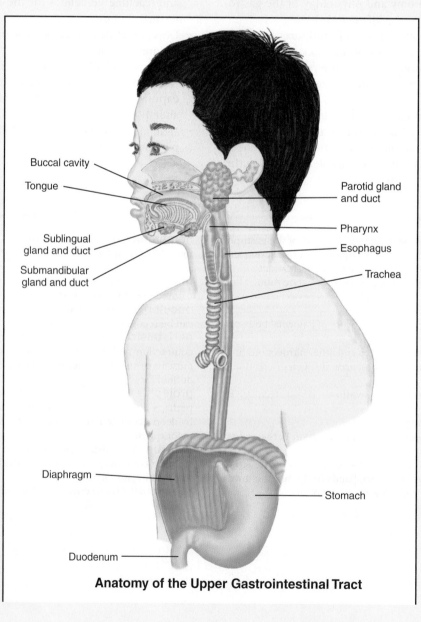

Buccal cavity
Tongue
Sublingual gland and duct
Submandibular gland and duct
Parotid gland and duct
Pharynx
Esophagus
Trachea
Diaphragm
Stomach
Duodenum

Anatomy of the Upper Gastrointestinal Tract

shaped somewhat like a gourd, where the bolus is received. As the LES and the pylorus contract, the stomach muscles churn the contents. The contents mix with the digestive juices to form chyme. The chyme moves on to the pylorus and into the duodenum.

A mucus-bicarbonate barrier in the stomach provides a thick layer of mucus and a buffer zone to neutralize acid. Stomach acids diffuse slowly through this layer toward the gastric wall. They are neutralized by bicarbonate ions from the surface epithelial cells. Thus a neutral pH is maintained at the gastric epithelial surface.

Lower Gastrointestinal System

The lower GI system includes the duodenum, liver, gallbladder, pancreas, jejunum, ileum, cecum, appendix, ascending colon, transverse colon, descending colon, sigmoid colon, rectum, and anus. The primary functions of the lower GI tract are to digest and absorb nutrients, detoxify and excrete unwanted waste, and aid in fluid and electrolyte balance.

The *duodenum*, the first part of the small intestine, extends from the pylorus to the jejunum. Partially digested chyme from the stomach enters the duodenum, where pancreatic enzymes and bile are excreted to further break down fats, carbohydrates, and proteins. The *pancreas* is an oblong gland lying behind the stomach that secretes enzymes to digest food and secretes glucagon and insulin to control motility and absorption.

The *liver*, the largest organ in the body, is located under the right diaphragm. The liver lies predominantly in the right upper quadrant, with the left lobe extending into the left upper quadrant. It is divided into two lobes separated by the falciform ligament. Within each lobe are numerous lobules, which form the functional units of the liver.

The liver is unique in that it is supplied with blood from two sources: (1) the hepatic artery, which supplies oxygenated blood; and (2) the hepatic portal vein, which supplies deoxygenated blood with absorbed nutrients from the GI tract. The liver has numerous functions, including phagocytosis, bile production, detoxification, glycogen storage and breakdown, and vitamin storage. The production of bile is essential for the absorption of fat and the excretion of the end products of blood cell breakdown. The primary function of the *gallbladder*, a saclike structure attached to the underside of the right lobe of the liver, is to store bile for secretion into the duodenum when stimulated by the presence of fat in its lumen.

The *jejunum* and *ileum* form the remainder of the small intestine. Absorption of all nutrients and vitamins occurs here through the villi and microvilli by the processes of diffusion and active transport. Absorption of vitamin B_{12} occurs only in the terminal ileum.

The large intestine starts with the *cecum*. This blind pouch, 2 to 3 inches long, begins at the ileocecal valve, which prevents reverse peristalsis into the small intestine. Attached to it is the *appendix*, a wormlike tube about 3 inches long. The open end of the cecum attaches to the remainder of the colon, which is divided into four sections: the *ascending, transverse, descending,* and *sigmoid colon*. One major function of the large intestine is water reabsorption, which occurs mostly in the cecum and ascending colon. Intestinal bacteria ferment the remaining carbohydrates and aid in the synthesis of vitamins B and K. Final breakdown of bile occurs here. Mucus secretion and peristalsis of wastes are also important functions.

The *rectum* is the last 7 to 8 inches of the intestine, and the *anal canal* refers to the last 1 to 2 inches. Stool is stored in the rectum until distention of the rectal walls initiates the defecation reflex—the final stage of the GI processes.

Prenatal Development

The primitive gut is formed from the endoderm in the first 4 weeks of embryonic development. The primitive gut then gives rise to the following three sections of the GI tract, each having an individual blood supply and rate of development:
- *Foregut*—from the pharynx to the duodenum, including the liver, pancreas, and biliary tract
- *Midgut*—from the duodenum to the transverse colon
- *Hindgut*—descending colon, rectum, and anal canal

Problems in the development of each of these three sections give rise to specific malformations and disease states. Anatomically, development is complete at birth, but physiologically, the neonate's GI tract is immature.

Fetal swallowing, intestinal motility, and defecation are detectable in the second trimester of gestation, but the most rapid and extensive development of the GI system occurs in the third trimester. The newborn must be able to adapt from total parenteral nutrition to total enteral nutrition because the placenta no longer performs nutrient exchange and waste removal.

Major Digestive Enzymes		
Location	**Enzyme**	**Function**
Mouth	Amylase	Converts complex carbohydrate to simple carbohydrate
Stomach	Pepsin	Converts proteins to proteases
Small intestine	Enterokinase	Activates trypsin
	Peptidases	Convert peptides to amino acids
	Sucrase, maltase, lactase	Convert disaccharides to monosaccharides
Pancreas	Trypsin	Converts peptides to amino acids
	Lipase	Converts fat to fatty acids and glycerol
	Amylase	Converts carbohydrates to disaccharides
Liver, gallbladder	Bile	Emulsifies fat, allowing the lipase to function. Increases fat and fat-soluble vitamin absorption

Common Laboratory and Diagnostic Tests for GI Disorders

Test	Description	Normal Findings	Indications	Preparation and Nursing Considerations
Stool				
Culture and sensitivity	Organisms from a small sample of stool are grown in culture media.	Normal GI flora	To identify infectious organisms and determine their antibiotic sensitivity.	No patient preparation is necessary. The sample is delivered to the laboratory immediately; it must be kept free from contamination.
Reducing substances (Clinitest)	Stool is diluted with water and then tested for undigested carbohydrates with Clinitest tablets.	Negative	Used to diagnose malabsorption syndromes.	No preparation is necessary. The test is done by the nurse, who checks for a color change in the solution.
Occult blood (guaiac, Hematest)	Stool is smeared on filter paper and prepared with solution.	Negative	Used in inflammatory conditions, bowel necrosis.	No preparation is necessary. The test is done by the nurse; a blue color is positive.
Ova and parasites (O&P)	Stool is examined microscopically for presence of parasites or their eggs.	Negative	To identify enteric parasites in child with diarrhea or abdominal pain.	No patient preparation is necessary. Sample must be free from water or urine contamination. The sample is delivered to the laboratory either fresh or in preservatives. Barium, antacids, mineral oil, and antibiotics may interfere with results. 1-3 samples collected.
Urine				
Urobilinogen	Dipstick or laboratory analysis is performed to determine bile byproducts in urine.	Negative	Levels determined in hepatic dysfunction and obstruction.	No preparation is necessary. The test is done by the nurse.
Blood				
Liver function tests	Serum levels are measured to give an indication of liver function.	AST: <9 yr, 15-55 U/L; >9 yr, 5-45 U/L ALT: 5-45 U/L Total bilirubin: 0.2-1.0 mg/dL Ammonia: 29-70 µg/dL children; 90-150 µg/dL newborns	Studies are performed when liver problems are suspected.	No preparation is necessary. Venipuncture is performed.
Endoscopy				
Fiberoptic upper GI endoscopy	Study allows direct viewing of the lining of the esophagus, stomach, and proximal duodenum. It also provides a means to obtain material for biopsies and cultures.	Normal mucosa	Used to rule out various upper GI tract disorders.	Preparation includes teaching, keeping the child on NPO status for at least 6 hr before the examination, providing conscious sedation, and monitoring child's respiratory function during sedation.
Colonoscopy	The colon is viewed directly by a fiberoptic scope and camera inserted rectally.	Normal mucosa, patent bowel	Performed to detect mucosal changes and abnormalities in the lumen of the colon.	Preparation includes teaching, keeping the child on NPO status, bowel cleansing, and providing conscious sedation.

Procedure	Description	Purpose	Normal Findings	Preparation/Nursing Considerations
Biopsy (gastric, jejunal, rectal, liver)	A small piece of tissue is removed for analysis.	Study determines the amount of mucosal inflammation and the absence of ganglion cells.	No abnormal tissue	Preparation includes teaching, bowel cleansing, and providing sedation or anesthesia if the procedure is done percutaneously (liver).
Radiologic Examinations				
Abdominal flat plate	Anterior and posterior radiographs are obtained.	Radiographs demonstrate stool and gas patterns, inflammation, and patency of the GI tract. It is commonly performed in cases of abdominal pain, imperforate anus, intussusception, and appendicitis.		Usually no preparation is necessary other than teaching.
Barium swallow examination	Radiopaque contrast medium or air (or both) is swallowed.	Study identifies esophageal abnormalities, swallowing difficulties, and sphincter function.	Normal swallowing, no anatomic defects	Preparation includes teaching and keeping the child on NPO status for 2-4 hr before the examination. Adequate fluids are essential after the examination to prevent barium impaction.
Upper GI examination	Radiopaque contrast material is swallowed or inserted by NG tube.	Study outlines the stomach and pyloric canal and can be used to determine gastric emptying time.	Normal gastric emptying, no abnormalities	Preparation includes teaching and keeping the child on NPO status for 4 hr before the examination. Adequate fluids are essential after the examination to prevent barium impaction.
Barium enema, air-contrast barium enema examination	Radiopaque contrast material or air (or both) is placed in the large intestine via the rectum.	Study used to identify abnormalities on the surface of the bowel lumen and to determine bowel patency. It also provides hydrostatic reduction of intussusception.		Preparation includes teaching, keeping the child on NPO status, and bowel cleansing. Adequate fluids are essential after the examination to prevent barium impaction.
CT scan	Oral radiopaque contrast material often used. May also use IV or rectal contrast.	Used to identify inflammatory conditions, appendicitis.	Normal anatomy without evidence of inflammation	No patient preparation other than teaching. Sedation may be used if child unable to remain still. Can be completed in less than 15 min.
Other				
Ultrasound	Study uses sound waves noninvasively to image anatomy and inflammation.	Performed to identify anatomic abnormalities and inflammatory conditions.		Preparation includes teaching. For pelvic ultrasound, a full bladder is needed to improve imaging of pelvic organs.
Breath hydrogen test	Carbohydrate solution is given by mouth and exhaled. Breath samples are collected over 3 hr.	Used to diagnose maldigestion or malabsorption syndromes. Inadequately digested carbohydrate produces hydrogen when acted on by GI flora.	Less than 20 ppm above baseline	Nursing preparation entails teaching about the procedure. The child prepares by fasting for 4½ hr. The study is noninvasive. A face mask may be worn to collect expired air.

PEDIATRIC DIFFERENCES IN THE GI SYSTEM

- Infants have minimal saliva.
- Swallowing is not under voluntary control until 6 weeks.
- Infants and children have less stomach capacity:

Age	Stomach Capacity (mL)
Newborn	10-20
1 wk	30-90
2-3 wk	75-100
1 mo	90-150
3 mo	150-200
1 yr	210-360
2 yr	500
10 yr	750-900
16 yr	1500
Adult	2000-3000

- The stomach lies transversely and is horizontal in infants' abdomens; the abdomen is round in infants and toddlers.
- Peristaltic waves may reverse in infancy, causing regurgitation and vomiting. Peristalsis is faster; food remains in the stomach for a shorter period.
- Hydrochloric acid concentration is low until school age.
- Fever increases the rate of propulsion.
- The immature neonatal liver is not yet efficient in its detoxifying ability, which results in less vitamin and mineral breakdown than in older children.
- The large intestine is relatively short, with less epithelial lining to absorb water from a fecal mass. As a result, stools have a soft consistency and peristalsis is more rapid.

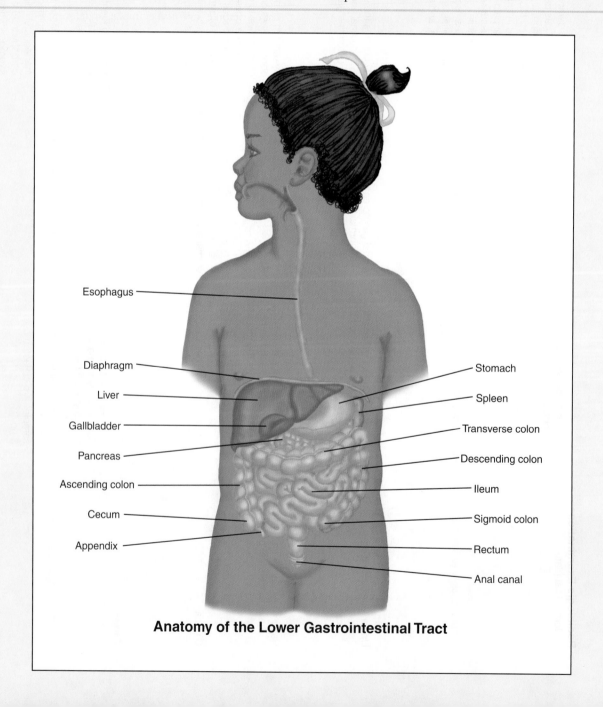

Anatomy of the Lower Gastrointestinal Tract

Children with GI alterations and their families have many special needs. Some GI problems begin at birth, with life-threatening consequences. Some require the parents to accept their child's altered appearance. Other problems develop after birth and provide long-term challenges in management and treatment. Sudden, unexpected surgery may be necessary. GI alterations cause anxiety and affect nutrition, elimination, respiratory status, skin integrity, body image, family processes, growth and development, and educational needs.

Upper and lower GI conditions can be categorized as follows:
- Developmental problems, such as cleft lip and palate, hernias, esophageal atresia, tracheoesophageal fistula, imperforate anus, and abdominal wall defects
- Problems affecting motility, such as gastroesophageal reflux, constipation, encopresis, and irritable bowel syndrome
- Inflammatory or infectious conditions, including ulcers, gastroenteritis, appendicitis, inflammatory bowel disease, and necrotizing enterocolitis
- Obstructive disorders, such as pyloric stenosis, intussusception, and Hirschsprung disease
- Malabsorption conditions, such as lactose intolerance and celiac disease
- Hepatic disorders, such as hepatitis, biliary atresia, and cirrhosis

Disorders that involve the liver and biliary tract may be the result of congenital malformations or acquired infection. Because the liver is important to metabolism, alterations in its function can affect many body systems, including the cardiovascular, integumentary, renal, neurologic, hematologic, and immunologic systems. These disorders can also have significant effects on growth and development. Nursing care may involve nutritional support, infection control, developmental stimulation, family support, and intensive physiologic care during a period of crisis or transplantation.

DISORDERS OF PRENATAL DEVELOPMENT
Cleft Lip and Palate

Cleft lip, cleft palate, and cleft lip and palate are separate anomalies that are closely related in etiology, pathophysiology, and nursing care. These distinct problems are all abnormal openings in the lip or palate. The defects may occur unilaterally (on either side) or bilaterally and are the most common congenital craniofacial deformity.

Incidence
The incidence ranges from 1 in 700 to 1000 births for cleft lip and palate and 1 in 2000 for cleft palate alone (Cleft Palate Foundation, 2005; March of Dimes, 2006). Cleft lip is seen predominantly in male infants and cleft palate in female infants. The prevalence of clefts is higher in Asians and Native Americans and has a lower frequency in African Americans. A genetic pattern or familial risk seems to exist (Tinaroff, 2004). Many infants who are affected with cleft lip and palate have other associated defects.

Manifestations and Diagnostic Evaluation
Cleft lip has the following manifestations: a notched vermilion border, variably sized clefts that involve the alveolar ridge, and dental anomalies (usually deformed, supernumerary, or absent teeth). Cleft palate includes nasal distortion, midline or bilateral cleft with variable extension from the uvula and soft and hard palates, and exposed nasal cavities.

The diagnosis of cleft lip and cleft palate is based on observation at birth and complete examination in the neonatal period. Diagnosis may also be made *in utero* with ultrasound. Cleft lip is readily diagnosed through inspection of the lip. The first sign of cleft palate may be formula coming from the nose. A gloved finger placed in the mouth to feel the defect or visual examination with a flashlight confirms the diagnosis.

Therapeutic Management
Management is based on the severity of the defect. A number of professionals are involved in this process, including surgeons; nurses; geneticists; psychologists or psychiatrists; ear, nose, and throat specialists; audiologists; and occupational and speech therapists. Orthodontists and plastic surgeons become involved in the lengthy management. Pediatricians provide ongoing child health care.

The first intervention involves modifying feeding techniques as needed to allow adequate growth. Use of special

PATHOPHYSIOLOGY

CLEFT LIP AND PALATE

Cleft lip and cleft palate occur from embryonic developmental failures related to multiple genetic and environmental factors. These developmental failures result in an abnormal opening in the lip, palate and, sometimes, nasal cavity. Cleft lip results when the medial nasal and maxillary processes fail to join at 6 to 8 weeks of gestation. Cleft palate results from failure of the primary palatal shelves, or processes, to fuse at 7 to 12 weeks of gestation.

Each of these abnormalities appears as a distinct malformation, but they may also appear together. Achieving suction during feedings may be impossible, and fluids may enter the nose, putting the child at risk for aspiration, feeding difficulties, and respiratory distress.

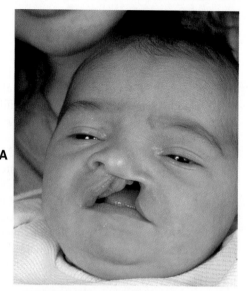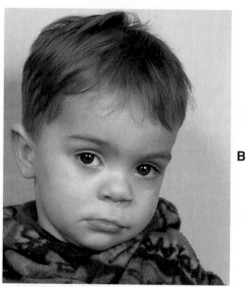

Child born with a cleft lip and palate, before **(A)** and after **(B)** repair. Repair of facial clefts usually requires multiple surgeries at different stages in the child's growth. Early repair of a cleft lip facilitates parent-infant bonding and improves feeding. Results are generally quite good with today's surgical, orthodontic, and speech therapy techniques. *(Courtesy Children's Medical Center, Dallas.)*

feeding techniques, obturators, and unique nipples and feeders can usually accomplish this goal and allow early discharge with parents (Fig. 19-1). These modified techniques can decrease the energy required for the infant to take in adequate nutrition. Before surgical repair, removable orthopedic devices such as a Latham device may be used to expand and realign parts of the palate or decrease the size of a wide lip cleft.

Cleft lip repair is usually performed by age 3 to 6 months. Early repair may improve bonding and makes feeding much easier. The surgical technique involves the use of a staggered suture line to minimize scarring. Some cosmetic modifications may be needed again at age 4 to 5 years.

Cleft palate repair is individualized and based on the degree of deformity and size of the child. Closure is completed between ages 6 and 24 months. Most teams recommend repair by 1 year. Earlier closure facilitates speech development.

Concurrent treatment of altered dentition, recurring otitis media, speech dysfunction, emotional issues, and cosmetic concerns completes the ongoing therapy. Children with cleft palate are at high risk for developing chronic otitis media, which can cause long-term hearing loss.

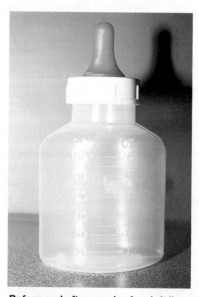

FIG 19-1   **Before and after repair of a cleft lip or palate, special feeding techniques are essential for adequate nutrition. A feeder with compressible plastic sides allows the person feeding the baby to gently squeeze the sides of the bottle to help eject the breast milk or formula. A slightly longer nipple allows the milk to be swallowed with less chance of entering the nasopharynx and yet is not so long that it stimulates the gag reflex.**

Text continued on p. 519

NURSING CARE PLAN

The Child With a Cleft Lip or Palate

Focused Assessment

Cleft lip and cleft palate are readily apparent at birth, and the degree of involvement should be documented during the newborn examination. After identifying this condition, assess the infant's ability to suck, swallow, and breathe without distress and handle normal secretions. Because the occurrence of cleft lip and palate is usually unexpected and its appearance can be frightening to parents and families, assess and record parents' reactions as well as their interactions with the neonate.

Parents of an infant with a cleft lip or palate may need help to resolve feelings about their infant's appearance. The parents might need to deal with many questions from family members, stares from strangers, and expressions of pity from other new parents. Providing information about the cause of the defect and showing them pictures of other children before and after surgical repair can give them some relief from these fears and concerns. In addition, modeling and encouraging bonding through touching, holding, and examining their newborn can be very reassuring. Pointing out the newborn's positive attributes can help decrease the focus on the defect. For example, emphasize how alert the baby is or the infant's responsiveness or beautiful eyes.

NURSING DIAGNOSES Imbalanced Nutrition: Less Than Body Requirements related to inability to suck and to the surgical repair.
Deficient Knowledge about feeding techniques and surgery related to unfamiliarity with the information.

EXPECTED OUTCOMES The child will:
- Drink the desired amount of fluid within 30 minutes.
- Be content during and after feeding.
- Gain weight and height according to the normal growth curve.

The parents will:
- Express satisfaction with progress of feedings.
- Understand expected preoperative and postoperative feeding techniques.

Intervention	*Rationale*
1. Describe the degree of cleft and impairment of sucking.	1. Infants with cleft lip alone or simple cleft dental arch may be successful with breastfeeding or bottle feeding without modifications.
2. Keep care and teaching simple and as closely related to normal infant feeding as possible.	2. Nutrition, parent-infant relationship, and adherence may be improved if normal techniques can be used.
3. Provide alternative assistive feeding devices as needed and ordered. Some infants may be able to breastfeed successfully.	3. Techniques and equipment vary among institutions. Use what is available and effective for each child. Encourage breastfeeding first.
4. Burp the infant frequently, and hold the infant in a more upright position.	4. Burping minimizes air swallowing and GI flatus and minimizes risk of aspiration.
5. Document the feeding program in written form for parents to use at home, and provide the plan to other health professionals.	5. Documentation provides consistency at home and at other times when the family is in contact with numerous medical professionals treating the child.
6. Provide emotional support and positive reinforcement to parents as they learn to feed their child.	6. Self-care and bonding are improved when parents can assume total care.
7. Keep an accurate record of the child's growth by using a growth chart.	7. A chart identifies growth changes early, when intervention can be most effective.
8. Explain preoperative and postoperative procedures: oral feedings withheld for 6 hours, placement of IV lines, use of arm restraints, appearance of repair in the immediate postoperative period (see Box 19-1).	8. Explanation decreases parental anxiety and encourages involvement.
9. Postoperatively:	9. For postoperative care:
a. Keep straws, pacifiers, spoons, or fingers away from the child's mouth for 7 to 10 days. Do not take temperatures orally.	a. Avoiding contact with the incision site reduces stress on surgical repair and prevents accidental tearing of very fine sutures.
b. Advance the child's diet as ordered and tolerated from clear liquids to a normal *soft* diet within 48 hours.	b. A normal diet minimizes nutritional deficits and stress on the child. No foods that can tear surfaces are offered.

Continued

NURSING CARE PLAN—cont'd

c. After repair of a cleft lip, resume preoperative feeding techniques.

d. After repair of a cleft palate, provide short nipples that do not rest on palatal sutures; give baby food or baby food mixed with water.

c. Little evidence shows that sucking causes excess suture stress.

d. Prevents direct contact with surgical site.

Evaluation

- Is the infant following the appropriate growth curve?
- Is the infant happy and content during and after feedings?
- Do the parents express satisfaction with the feeding technique used and the time required to complete a feeding?

- Can the parents explain and demonstrate expected preoperative and postoperative care?

NURSING DIAGNOSIS   Interrupted Family Processes related to the emotional reaction to an infant with a visible defect.

EXPECTED OUTCOMES   The parents will:
- Demonstrate positive behaviors toward the infant.
- Access appropriate support.

Intervention	Rationale
1. Encourage parents to discuss their fears, concerns, and negative emotions.	1. Grief, anxiety, confusion, guilt, denial, and anger are not uncommon and should be expressed.
2. Encourage touching and holding.	2. Contact encourages bonding and prevents a delayed attachment.
3. Make appropriate referral to a cleft lip and palate team of nurses, physicians, and other specialists as soon as possible.	3. A health care team can provide accurate information and begin to outline a plan of action.
4. Express acceptance of the baby by modeling feeding and close physical contact.	4. These interventions assist parents with the adaptation process.
5. Refer parents to community resources and parent groups (see Evolve website).	5. Sharing with others in similar situations facilitates acceptance and adaptation.
6. Encourage parents to share concerns about long-term care and emotional and financial stress.	6. Long-term concerns require extensive follow-up and can strain many families' resources. Identifying concerns early can increase problem-solving options.

Evaluation

- Can the parents identify their infant's positive characteristics?
- Do the parents hold, cuddle, and make eye contact with the infant?

- Have the parents sought personal, community, or organizational support?

NURSING DIAGNOSIS   Impaired Skin Integrity related to the surgical repair.
Risk for Infection related to the surgical repair and aspiration.

EXPECTED OUTCOMES   The repair site will:
- Heal without complications.
The infant will:
- Show no signs of infection as evidenced by a clean and intact suture line, absence of fever, and clear breath sounds.

Intervention	Rationale
1. Clean the lip repair site according to physician protocol. Many physicians recommend cleaning with sterile water by using a cotton swab or saline after feeding and as ordered. Use a rolling motion vertically down the suture line. Have parents demonstrate this cleaning technique.	1. The procedure decreases the medium for bacterial growth, decreases crusting, and minimizes scarring.
2. Apply anti-infective ointment as ordered.	2. Anti-infective ointment prevents infection, crusting, and scarring.

NURSING CARE PLAN—cont'd

3. Use elbow restraints (no-no's) to keep the child from touching the repair site. Continue for 6 to 8 days. Remove every 2 hours for 10 to 15 minutes. Remove restraint from only one elbow at a time, with a parent or nurse in constant attendance.
4. Do not brush the child's teeth for 1 to 2 weeks.

5. Keep the child in a supine position, on the side opposite to the repair, or in an infant seat.
6. Observe for redness, swelling, excessive bleeding, drainage, respiratory distress, or fever.
7. To clean the palate repair site, rinse the child's mouth with water after feedings.
8. Encourage the parents to hold and cuddle the child as the child desires.
9. Maintain lip protective devices if ordered.

3. Elbow restraints prevent accidental rupture or tear of sutures. Periodically removing restraints promotes contact with the child, decreases anxiety, and allows the nurse to assess skin integrity and circulation.

4. Avoiding brushing prevents accidental tear of palatal sutures.
5. Careful positioning prevents contact of suture lines with bed linens.
6. Signs of infection must be identified early because additional inflammation can increase scarring.
7. Rinsing after feeding removes food and residual sugars from suture lines, reducing the risk of infection.
8. Crying puts additional stress on the suture line.

9. Protective devices prevent separation of lip suture lines.

Evaluation

- Is the suture site clean, dry, and without redness, heat, or drainage?
- Is the suture site intact and healing without crusting or excessive scarring?

- Is the infant afebrile and demonstrating clear breath sounds?

NURSING DIAGNOSIS Acute Pain related to the surgical incision and elbow restraints.

EXPECTED OUTCOME The child will:
- Be free from pain as evidenced by ability to sleep, eat, and respond in a positive way.

Intervention

1. Describe and document pain with appropriate tools (see Chapter 15).

2. Provide comfort measures, especially holding, rocking, and parental voices.

3. Provide analgesics and sedatives on a regular basis as ordered. Pain should decrease significantly after 24 to 48 hours.
4. Report pain not managed by usual means.

Rationale

1. Infants and young children do not react to pain in typical adult ways, so alternative observations are needed to validate assessment findings. Parents are the best resource to validate the nurse's assessment of their infant.
2. Comforting increases parental involvement, relieves discomfort, and reduces stress on sutures caused by crying.
3. Medication can prevent peaks of pain that cannot be managed appropriately.

4. Pain may indicate hematoma formation or other complications of the repair.

Evaluation

- Does the child participate in age-appropriate activities?
- Is the child responding well to pain medication?

- Does the child appear relaxed and content at rest?
- Does the parent describe a child who is not in pain?

NURSING DIAGNOSIS Ineffective Health Maintenance related to the need for long-term care.

EXPECTED OUTCOMES The parents will:
- Seek continued follow-up care to evaluate and manage long-term complications.
The child will:
- Demonstrate normal speech and hearing.

Intervention

1. Make appropriate and early referrals for any problems with speech impairment or language-based learning disabilities.
2. Monitor for recurrent or chronic otitis media. Schedule frequent hearing tests.

Rationale

1. Speech and language-learning impairments are common complications of cleft lip and palate. Early intervention minimizes harm.
2. Because of craniofacial deformities, otitis media can occur frequently and must be treated to prevent language and learning problems.

Continued

NURSING CARE PLAN—cont'd

3. Encourage early speech attempts. Arrange speech therapy as needed.

3. Cleft palate can make speech difficult to understand, and the child may feel self-conscious about speech errors. Practice improves development.

4. Encourage good dental care.

4. With abnormalities of teeth and the alveolar ridge, malocclusion and dental caries are a major concern.

Evaluation

- Do the parents continue to seek follow-up care (ear, nose, and throat [ENT]; speech therapy; dental)?
- Does the child demonstrate age-appropriate speech?

- Does the child have normal hearing?
- Does the child have normal dentition?

NURSING DIAGNOSIS Anxiety (parental) related to special care needs and surgery.

EXPECTED OUTCOMES The parents will:
- Express concerns and fears.
- Express control over special care needs.

Intervention

1. Use a calm, reassuring, accepting approach with the infant and family.
2. Explain all procedures and their rationale, including sensations likely experienced by their child.
3. Listen actively to parents and their concerns. Encourage verbalization of feelings, perceptions, and fears.
4. Encourage parents to stay with their child in the immediate preoperative and postoperative periods.

Rationale

1. Being calm and accepting encourages communication and reinforces to parents that their child is worthwhile.
2. Uncertainty and loss of control contribute to increased levels of anxiety.
3. Talking and sharing may decrease anxiety.

4. Staying with the child encourages parent participation and control over as much as possible.

Evaluation

- Do the parents express concerns and fears?
- Do the parents seek information to decrease anxiety?

- Do the parents demonstrate ability to care for their child?

BOX 19-1 | **PARENTS WANT TO KNOW** About Home Care of the Child With Cleft Lip or Palate

Your infant may require a special feeding method to maximize growth while waiting for surgery, and you may need to practice the feeding method to be used after surgery until the incision heals. The feeding method you use will be based on what works for your child and what your physician recommends. In general, the following apply:

- Breastfeeding may be possible if your child has a small cleft lip or palate.
- A compressible bottle will prevent your child from having to suck because the breast milk or formula can be squeezed into the mouth.
- A longer nipple may allow the milk to be swallowed without entering the nose. It must not be so long that it causes gagging. Making a larger hole or "cross-cutting" a nipple may also be effective.
- A syringe with a rubber tip may also be used, especially after surgery.
- Try to keep your child in an upright position during feedings to allow gravity to assist in the feeding and decrease the chance that your child might choke.
- Burp your child frequently because excess air is often swallowed.

Before surgical repair, devices may be placed in your child's mouth to help line up the cleft in the palate for better surgical repair of decrease the size of the lip cleft. These devices may require special care and cleaning. Consult your cleft team and nurses for specific instructions about your child's device.

After surgery, elbow restraints ("no-no's") may be used so that your baby cannot touch the stitches. The following are recommendations:

- Do not apply the restraints too tightly. They should be loose but still prevent elbow bending.
- Remove no-no's every 2 hours for 10 to 15 minutes and play games with your child that encourage movement of the elbows. Look for any skin irritation every time you remove the no-no's.
- Remove only one no-no at a time.

Position your child for sleep with blankets to prevent rolling onto the abdomen so the child cannot rub the stitches on the linens. An infant seat may be used.

Do not brush your child's teeth for 1 to 2 weeks after surgery. Feeding a small amount of water after meals will help keep the teeth clean. Clean your child's lip as recommended by your physician. Use a cotton swab and a gentle rolling motion down the suture line. Apply anti-infective ointment with the same technique.

Make use of the many support professionals in following your child for speech, hearing, dental, or orthodontic problems.

Contact the American Cleft Palate-Craniofacial Association and the Cleft Palate Foundation at *www.cleft.com* for further information.

Esophageal Atresia with Tracheoesophageal Fistula

Esophageal atresia and tracheoesophageal fistula (TEF) are congenital malformations in which the esophagus terminates before it reaches the stomach and/or a fistula is present that forms an unnatural connection with the trachea. Figure 19-2 reviews types of TEF.

Etiology and Incidence

The cause of TEF and esophageal atresia is unknown. Esophageal atresia with or without TEF occurs in 1.2 to 4.67 in 10,000 births, with no difference by sex (National Birth Defects Prevention Network, 2005). Nearly half of infants born with esophageal atresia have other associated anomalies of the cardiac, GI, and central nervous systems. Prematurity and low birth weight are frequent concomitant problems that have a significant impact on long-term prognosis.

Manifestations

- Failure to pass suction catheter, nasogastric (NG) tube at birth
- Excessive oral secretions
- Vomiting
- Abdominal distention
- Airless, scaphoid abdomen (atresia without fistula)

Diagnostic Evaluation

A history of maternal polyhydramnios is a significant prenatal clue. If TEF is suspected prenatally, diagnosis can be made at the ideal time—in the delivery room. Atresia should be suspected if an NG tube cannot be passed 10 to 11 cm beyond the gum line. This suspicion is confirmed with an abdominal radiograph that will identify a proximal esophagus dilated with air (atresia) or abdominal distention (fistula). The radiologist can identify the specific type of defect after instilling less than 1 mL of a water-soluble contrast medium into the NG tube and documenting its movement into the tracheal tree and the proximal pouch.

PATHOPHYSIOLOGY

ESOPHAGEAL ATRESIA AND TRACHEOESOPHAGEAL FISTULA

Tracheoesophageal fistula is the result of an embryonal failure to differentiate the foregut into the trachea and esophagus and the incomplete fusion of them into distinct organs. The failure occurs between the fourth and fifth week of pregnancy and is manifested in several ways (see Fig. 19-2).

The presence of a fistula between the esophagus and trachea causes oral intake to enter the lungs or large amounts of air to enter the stomach. Coughing, choking, and severe abdominal distention can occur. Eventually, aspiration pneumonia and severe respiratory distress will develop in the untreated child, and death may occur without surgical intervention. Esophageal atresia occurring by itself causes respiratory distress attributable to aspiration of saliva and any oral fluids that may be given before diagnosis.

This is then withdrawn from the pouch to minimize the risk of aspiration. Bronchoscopy and endoscopy are also used to identify and assess fistulas.

Therapeutic Management

Keeping the infant supine with the head of the bed elevated decreases the chance of gastric secretions entering the lungs. An NG tube must be in place and aspirated every 5 to 10 minutes to keep the proximal pouch clear of secretions. Intravenous (IV) fluids are essential. Normal newborn care is appropriate, with special attention to keeping the infant warm and oxygenated.

Surgical repair is the mainstay of treatment. Initial repair includes the ligation of the fistula and end-to-side anastomosis of the atresia to decrease the severity of stricture formation. If the gap between the two parts of the esophagus is too large, primary anastomosis may not be possible. Newest advances use traction suture ends to stimulate rapid growth of the esophageal ends over a 7- to 10-day period and allow primary anastomosis. If a staged repair is necessary a gastrostomy tube (G-tube) and cervical esophagostomy are placed. Later anastomosis, colon interposition, and dilation can be expected. Evaluation and treatment of esophageal motility dysfunction, gastroesophageal reflux, strictures, bronchitis, and pneumonia may occur as the child grows.

NURSING CARE

The Infant With TEF

Assessment

The infant with TEF is at constant risk for aspiration. Assessment for respiratory distress in the immediate period after birth is essential. The nurse must examine the infant for excessive oral secretions, choking, and cyanosis. Difficulty swallowing, regurgitation, vomiting, and unexplained cyanosis after an initial feeding in the infant who is not diagnosed at birth are important assessment findings that must be reported to the physician immediately. Abdominal distention should be measured and the infant continually assessed for distress (vital signs, respiratory effort, nasal flaring, retractions, cyanosis). A newborn assessment should be completed, with special attention to identifying any concomitant congenital defects.

Family assessment of anxiety levels, fears, concerns, and knowledge level will provide important information for planning nursing care and teaching.

CRITICAL TO REMEMBER

Assessing and Managing the Child With Esophageal Atresia and Tracheoesophageal Fistula

Any child who exhibits the "3 Cs" of *c*oughing, *c*hoking with feedings, and *c*yanosis should be suspected of tracheoesophageal fistula (TEF). Esophageal atresia and TEF represent a critical neonatal surgical emergency. While the baby is awaiting transfer to a neonatal unit and surgery, management centers on prevention of aspiration.

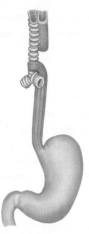

Esophageal Atresia With Distal TEF

Incidence: 85%–88%
Clinical Manifestations: Feeding causes regurgitation and coughing. Constant flow of saliva. Gastric distention.
Diagnostic Findings: Contrast reveals blind pouch. Air on abdominal x ray.
Surgical Treatment: One-stage surgical repair to ligate fistula and anastomose esophagus.

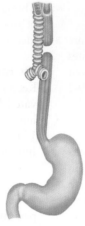

Esophageal Atresia Without Fistula

Incidence: 6%–8%
Clinical Manifestations: Excess oral secretions. Regurgitation of feedings.
Diagnostic Findings: Blind pouch. No air in abdomen.
Surgical Treatment: Two-stage repair: (1) Gastrostomy and cervical esophagostomy; (2) colon interposition to create patent esophagus.

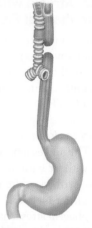

Proximal Esophageal Fistula With Trachea; Distal Segment Has No Communication

Incidence: 1%
Clinical Manifestations: Excessive oral secretions. Immediate respiratory distress with oral intake.
Diagnostic Findings: PO contrast outlines tracheal tree. No air in abdomen.
Surgical Treatment: One- or two-stage repair depending on length of separation.

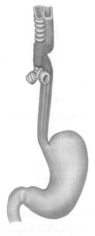

Proximal and Distal Esophageal Fistulas With Trachea

Incidence: 1%
Clinical Manifestations: Excessive secretions. Respiratory distress with feedings.
Diagnostic Findings: PO contrast outlines tracheal tree. Air in abdomen.
Surgical Treatment: Ligation of fistulas and anastomosis of esophagus.

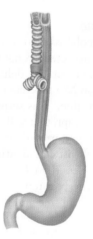

TEF Without Atresia (Also Called "H Type")

Incidence: 4%
Clinical Manifestations: Minimal symptoms unless regurgitation occurs. Choking, coughing. Abdominal distention.
Diagnostic Findings: Bronchoscopy demonstrates fistula.
Surgical Treatment: Ligation of fistula.

FIG 19-2   **Types of esophageal atresia and tracheoesophageal fistulas (TEFs).**

Nursing Diagnosis and Planning

The nursing diagnoses and expected outcomes appropriate after assessment of the infant with TEF include the following:

• Risk for Aspiration related to TEF.

Expected Outcome: The infant will not aspirate, as evidenced by control of oral secretions without coughing, cyanosis, or adventitious breath sounds.

• Imbalanced Nutrition: Less Than Body Requirements related to possible feeding difficulties.

Expected Outcome: The infant will gain weight and follow growth chart at appropriate level.

- Risk for Impaired Skin Integrity related to G-tube and esophagostomy.

  Expected Outcome: The infant will maintain skin integrity, as evidenced by intact skin around the G-tube and esophagostomy.

- Risk for Infection related to surgical repair.

  Expected Outcome: The infant will have surgical site, G-tube site, and esophagostomy free from infection, as evidenced by clean, intact skin without drainage, exudate, or redness.

- Acute Pain related to surgical repair.

  Expected Outcome: The infant will be free from pain, as evidenced by resumption of normal activities, ease of comforting, and relaxed facial features.

- Anxiety (parental) related to neonatal surgical emergency.

  Expected Outcome: The parents will express feelings and concerns.

- Deficient Knowledge related to home care needs and follow-up care.

  Expected Outcome: The parents will demonstrate safe G-tube feedings and esophagostomy care.

Interventions

Nursing interventions are different in the preoperative and postoperative periods. In the immediate period after birth, placing the newborn in a radiant warmer and administering humidified oxygen are essential to relieve respiratory distress. The child is prepared for surgery, remains on nothing-by-mouth (NPO) status, and is hydrated with IV fluids. Maintaining thermoregulation and fluid balance is essential, so monitoring temperature and other vital signs, using radiant warmers, and keeping accurate intake and output records are important.

The risk of aspiration must be minimized. A chalasia board that helps keep the child at a 30-degree angle while supine can be useful to decrease reflux. Placing a suction catheter in the proximal pouch and mouth will keep secretions to a minimum. Constant assessment of respiratory status is essential. Even after surgical repair, these children are prone to gastroesophageal reflux.

In the immediate postoperative period, monitoring respiratory status, supporting fluid balance and nutrition, maintaining thermoregulation, providing pain relief, monitoring for infection, and promoting bonding with parents take priority. The child will likely have a chest tube in place. Patency must be maintained, suction monitored, and output documented. Respiratory rate, effort, and the presence of abnormal breath sounds should be documented. Thermoregulation can significantly affect respiratory status in the newborn, so monitoring and maintaining temperature with a radiant warmer may be needed.

IV fluid, antibiotics, and parenteral nutrition may be ordered. The nurse must maintain patency of the IV line; monitor intake and output; and assess for signs of fluid and electrolyte alterations, including sunken fontanel and increased urine specific gravity measurements. Daily weights and measurement of head circumference can aid in assessing growth. Pain medications must be administered as needed on the basis of objective assessment measures used in each institution.

If a cervical esophagostomy has been performed as the first stage of a surgical repair, keep it covered with gauze to absorb saliva and provide skin care. Frequent cleaning with half-strength hydrogen peroxide and assessing for redness, breakdown, or exudate are essential because this wet area can easily become macerated and infected. Referral to an enterostomal therapist can be helpful in teaching parents esophagostomy care.

In the immediate postoperative period, the gastrostomy tube is elevated to allow gastric contents to pass to the small intestine and air to escape; this promotes comfort and decreases risk of leakage at the anastomosis. A pacifier satisfies sucking needs, provides early training in swallowing, makes later feeding easier, and provides comfort through distraction. Pacifiers should not be offered until the child can tolerate oral secretions.

Numerous types of G-tubes are available for placement, either percutaneously or during surgery. Among these are traditional gastrostomy tubes and Foley catheters, which are anchored in place by an air- or saline-inflated balloon, as well as more innovative tubes that use a variety of means for anchoring, depending on the manufacturer (Fig. 19-3). Tube selection is usually made by the physician, but long-term successful care and use of the tube are nursing and parental responsibilities.

Parents should be taught the techniques of G-tube feeding and care (Box 19-2). Skin care at the site may include cleaning with half-strength hydrogen peroxide, rotating the tube, and using a skin barrier product as well as other ostomy skin care products. Redness, exudate, pus, heat, or leakage of formula should be reported.

Parent education and support are critical components. Home care between stages of repair requires extra support from community health care givers and demonstration of parental proficiency in skin care, suctioning, gastrostomy feedings and

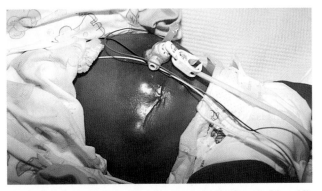

FIG **19-3** **The skin level gastrostomy button is good for children who require long-term gastrostomy feeding. It is relatively flat, reduces skin breakdown, increases comfort, and is fully immersible in water.** *(Courtesy Parkland Health and Hospital System, Dallas.)*

BOX 19-2 | **PARENTS WANT TO KNOW** About Home Care of the Child With Esophagostomy or Gastrostomy Tube

Your child's esophagostomy will require the following special but simple care:
- Cover the stoma with gauze.
- Change gauze frequently to prevent constant wetness.
- Clean with half-strength peroxide daily.
- Use skin barriers, such as Skin-Prep protective dressing, to prevent breakdown.
- Look at the stoma daily and observe for redness, drainage, swelling, and pain. Call your physician if these develop.
- Call your enterostomal therapist for support or help.

Remember to use a pacifier or small amounts of fluid in a bottle to allow your baby to practice swallowing. This should be done every day.

Your child's gastrostomy tube will also require special care depending on the type of tube that is used. Your nurse and physician will help you learn the following skills:
- For a new gastrostomy, clean the site daily with half-strength peroxide, rinse with water, and apply antimicrobial ointment. Rotate the tube every day.

- After 1 to 2 weeks, soap and water and tub baths may be used to clean the site. Stomahesive powder may be used to decrease moisture.
- Keep the tube open in the postoperative period.
- While the site is healing, make sure it is stabilized by using a Hollister tube drainage attachment, nipple with gauze at the base, or silicone retention disks as determined by the tube used.
- When the tube is well healed, it can be secured with tape or OpSite.
- Use skin barriers around the stoma to prevent breakdown.
- Report any drainage, leakage of formula, redness, or pain to your physician.
- Ask your enterostomal therapist for help in making the best choices for your child.

---

cardiopulmonary resuscitation (Aziz, Schiller, Gerstle, Ein, & Langer, 2003). These should include discussing feelings and anxieties, providing information about home care, practicing special techniques, providing stimulation, and using appropriate resources such as enterostomal therapists and dietitians.

Evaluation
- Can the child coordinate sucking and swallowing?
- Is the child tolerating oral feedings without choking, coughing, or becoming cyanotic?
- Is the child growing according to the growth chart?
- Is the surgical site clean, dry, intact, and free of redness, drainage, or exudate?
- Is the skin intact without breakdown around the gastrostomy tube and esophagostomy?
- Is the child resting contentedly without pain medication?
- Can the parents explain the need for the surgical procedure?
- Do parents demonstrate appropriate care of the gastrostomy tube or esophagostomy?
- Have parents assumed all care responsibilities?

Upper Gastrointestinal Hernias

A hernia is an abnormal protrusion of part of an organ or tissue through the structures that normally contain it. Hernias can be either congenital or acquired. Some hernias can be reduced, whereas others become incarcerated and cannot be returned by manipulation. A medical emergency occurs when a hernia becomes strangulated and blood supply is cut off. This condition can occur suddenly and requires immediate treatment. The most common hernias of the upper GI tract are discussed in Table 19-1.

Other Developmental Disorders

Table 19-2 discusses other developmental disorders of the upper and lower GI tracts.

MOTILITY DISORDERS
Gastroesophageal Reflux Disease

Gastroesophageal reflux (GER) is regurgitation of gastric contents back into the esophagus. GER is a normal physiologic phenomenon; all adults and infants periodically experience reflux, especially after meals. GER disease (GERD) is a more severe and chronic form. Reflux can be divided into two types: physiologic GER and pathologic GERD (Box 19-3).

BOX 19-3 | **Types of Gastroesophageal Reflux**

Physiologic (GER)
Painless emesis after meals
Parents may not be concerned or may think it is normal
Rarely occurs during sleep
No failure to thrive
40% asymptomatic by 3 months
70% asymptomatic by 18 months
Pharmacologic and medical management very effective

Pathologic (GERD)
Failure to thrive
Aspiration pneumonia, asthma
Apnea, coughing, and choking
Frequent emesis, amount varies
May require surgery and pharmacologic treatment

| TABLE **19-1**   **Upper GI Hernias** | | | |

Description	Clinical Manifestations	Therapeutic Management	Nursing Management
Hiatal Hernia Protrusion of a portion of the stomach through the esophageal hiatus of the diaphragm	Vomiting Coughing, wheezing, short periods of apnea Failure to thrive	Medical management similar to that for the child with reflux Surgical repair of defect	Monitor intake and output, document vomiting, observe for respiratory distress, provide routine postoperative care for GI surgery Teach parents about surgery and medical treatment of reflux
Congenital Diaphragmatic Hernia (CDH) Opening in the diaphragm through which abdominal contents herniate into the thoracic cavity during prenatal development *and* some degree of pulmonary hypoplasia, determined by the timing and size of the herniation Mortality rate: 50%-80%; 40% if ECMO used Degree of pulmonary hypoplasia determines outcome Incidence: 1 in 2200-5000 live births	Clinical findings depend on severity of defect: • Abdominal organs in chest (by fetal ultrasonography) • Diminished or absent breath sounds on affected side • Bowel sounds that may be heard over the chest • Cardiac sounds that may be heard on the right side of the chest • Respiratory distress developing soon after birth: dyspnea, cyanosis, nasal flaring, tachypnea, retractions • Scaphoid abdomen	If diagnosed prenatally, mother moved to tertiary care center before delivery In utero surgery may be performed *Neonatal emergency* NG intubation with suction Ventilate with high-frequency ventilation; manage acidosis with bicarbonate and ventilation ECMO Inhaled nitric oxide Liquid ventilation Manage pulmonary hypertension, inhaled nitric oxide may be used Surgical reduction of hernia after physiologically stable May wait 6-18 hr after birth Respiratory support, ECMO until lungs functioning after surgery	Identify clinical findings and report immediately Place child in semi-Fowler position on affected side with head of bed elevated Maintain patency of NG tube Monitor IV fluids Maintain mechanical ventilation, ECMO, chest tubes, assess oxygenation Do not use face mask/bag for ventilatory support because air can enter stomach and further impair respiratory function Provide minimal stimulation Provide routine postoperative care Monitor for signs of infection, respiratory distress, and feeding difficulties; report to physician Support family mourning loss of perfect child Provide clear, truthful information Encourage the parent to see and touch the infant Provide referral to support groups Provide discharge teaching Use prescribed feeding techniques

ECMO, Extracorporeal membrane oxygenation.

Etiology

Many factors contribute to the development of GERD. Neurologic impairment, such as cerebral palsy, Down syndrome, and head injury, may affect the transmission of neural signals to the LES. Delayed gastric emptying of a liquid meal because of distention may also contribute. Partial or incomplete swallowing dysfunctions or drugs such as theophylline or caffeine can also trigger LES relaxations. Increased intraabdominal pressure incurred while straining, crying, coughing, or slumping tends to promote increased episodes of GER. These postural effects are most likely primary contributing factors in infants. Obesity and hiatal hernias also promote

GERD. Finally, during the first 6 months of life, the LES pressure undergoes maturational development. Because infants have a short abdominal LES, they have GER more often. As the infant grows, the LES matures and the reflux improves. The prognosis is likely related to the severity of symptoms. Reflux from maturational causes will likely resolve by 1 to 2 years of age.

Incidence

Approximately 45% to 50% of healthy infants have signs of GER (Salvatore, Hauser, Vandemaele, Novario, & Vandenplas, 2005) with most experiencing regurgitation

Text continued on p. 526

TABLE 19-2   Developmental GI Defects

Imperforate Anus	Gastroschisis	Omphalocele	Umbilical Hernia
Pathophysiology, Etiology, and Clinical Manifestations			
Incomplete development or absence of the anus in its normal position in the perineum. Defect can be high (above the levator ani muscle) or low (below the levator ani muscle). Symptoms include failure to pass meconium stool, absence of anorectal canal, presence of an anal membrane, external fistula to the perineum. Condition is diagnosed during the newborn examination with radiography, ultrasound, or CT used to determine the level of the lesion and associated anomalies.	Embryonal weakness in abdominal wall causes herniation of gut on one side of umbilical cord during early development, most commonly on right side. Viscera are outside the abdominal cavity and are not covered with the sac.	Large herniation of gut into umbilical cord. Viscera are outside the abdominal cavity but inside translucent sac, covered with peritoneum and amniotic membrane.	Imperfect closure of umbilical ring allows gut to push outward at umbilicus during straining and crying. Viscera are inside the abdominal cavity and under the skin. The hernia is usually 1-3 cm and easily reduced.
Incidence			
1 in 4000-5000 live births. More common in male infants.	1 in 4000 live births.	1 in 5000 to 10,000 live births.	Most common in low-birth-weight and African-American infants.
Associated Anomalies			
Genitourinary, sacral, or additional GI anomalies.	Prematurity. Malrotation of intestines. Decreased abdominal capacity. Atresia, stenosis rare. Higher incidence of Meckel diverticulum. Other anomalies rare.	Malrotation of intestines. Decreased abdominal capacity. Atresia, stenosis common. Higher incidence of Meckel diverticulum. Cardiac, genitourinary, or chromosomal anomalies in one third to one half of cases. Associated with Beckwith syndrome (hypoglycemia, macrosomia, macroglossia).	Commonly occurs in children with Down syndrome, hypothyroidism, Hurler syndrome.
Morbidity and Mortality			
Prognosis depends on the level of the lesion. Complete continence may be impossible.	Mortality rate 10%-15%.	Mortality rate 20%-30%. Common complications include sepsis and intestinal obstruction.	Minimal.
Therapeutic Management			
Anal stenosis is treated with repeated dilatation. All other defects require surgical intervention. High defects may require a colostomy and bowel pull-through procedure.	IV and NG tubes are placed immediately. Total parenteral nutrition is provided. Synthetic material (Silastic) is used to cover the gut in a sac (if the sac has ruptured or the omphalocele is large). If defect is large, the sac is suspended over the child's abdomen and gravity is used to return the gut slowly to the abdominal cavity over 28 days or longer.	Same as for gastroschisis.	Most umbilical hernias disappear spontaneously by 1 yr. No surgical repair is necessary unless the hernia causes symptoms, persists past age 5 yr, becomes strangulated, or continues to grow.

CT, Computed tomography.

TABLE 19-2	Developmental GI Defects—cont'd		
Imperforate Anus	**Gastroschisis**	**Omphalocele**	**Umbilical Hernia**
Therapeutic Management—cont'd			
	The defect is closed surgically after all contents have been returned to the abdominal cavity. Even if the defect is small, immediate surgical repair may be done in several stages. If the condition is diagnosed prenatally, surgical delivery is recommended. Necrotic bowel may need to be removed surgically.		
Nursing Care			
Report any skin dimples or the presence of stool in the urine or vagina. Determine anal patency if meconium is not passed in the first 24 hr after birth. Assess for other GI or genitourinary anomalies. Facilitate bonding. Provide appropriate postoperative care, including care of the colostomy.	Thermoregulation is critical because significant heat loss can occur through the exposed intestines. Use warmers and monitor the child's temperature. Use sterile technique in dealing with the defect. Immediately cover with warm, moist, sterile gauze and wrap with plastic to keep moist. Minimize movement of the infant and handling of the intestines. Assess for circulatory compromise, obstruction, sepsis: monitor temperature, pulses, capillary refill time, skin color, changes in respiratory patterns, heart rate. Observe for respiratory distress from high intraabdominal pressure as the gut returns to the peritoneal cavity. Fluid-volume management is a crucial nursing responsibility: monitor intake and output and daily weights, assess fontanels, monitor electrolytes, maintain IV line. Postoperatively, monitor and manage ileus, which commonly lasts for 2-4 wk: maintain NG tube for decompression, monitor bowel sounds and stools, measure abdominal girth. Maintain parenteral nutrition to sustain growth. Offer pacifier to meet sucking needs. Provide emotional support for parents as they deal with the loss of the "perfect child."	Same as for gastroschisis.	Binding is not effective in reducing or minimizing the bulge. Monitor for changes in size of hernia. Assess for changing bowel sounds and an irreducible mass, which may indicate strangulation.

Continued

TABLE 19-2 Developmental GI Defects—cont'd			
Imperforate Anus	**Gastroschisis**	**Omphalocele**	**Umbilical Hernia**
Nursing Care—cont'd			
	Encourage parents to provide care as they are able, talk to and touch infant, and hold the infant when appropriate.		
Teaching and Home Care			
Teach parents colostomy care.	Encourage parents to hold, cuddle, and bond with infants as soon as possible.	Same as for gastroschisis.	Teach parents signs of strangulation: vomiting, pain, irreducible mass at umbilicus.
Demonstrate anal dilatation (use only prescribed dilator, insert no more than 1-2 cm, and use a water-soluble lubricant).	Provide developmental stimulation for long-term hospitalization.		Contact physician immediately if strangulation is suspected.
Refer parents for counseling and support: March of Dimes Birth Defects Foundation *www.modimes.org*.	Assist parents in dealing with feelings of guilt and disappointment.		
Provide guidance for toilet training.	Use pictures to help parents understand the defect.		
	Contact national support groups and community resources (e.g., March of Dimes).		
	Teach parents signs of bowel obstruction: vomiting, pain, irritability, anorexia, firm abdomen.		
	Provide follow-up from nutritional support personnel as needed.		

accompanied by crying. The peak incidence of GER occurs at approximately 4 months of age and decreases thereafter (Orenstein, Peters, Kahn, Youssif, & Hussain, 2004). Pathologic GERD occurs in approximately 5% to 8% of all newborns (Salvatore et al., 2005). GERD has been associated with episodes of apnea and apparent life-threatening events (ALTE) (GER Guideline Committee, 2001; Orenstein et al., 2004).

PATHOPHYSIOLOGY

GASTROESOPHAGEAL REFLUX

The LES, a zone of tonically contracted smooth muscle surrounding the distal esophagus, is innervated by vagal nerves and receives signals from multiple organs. A defect in this neural control may result in a dysfunctional LES with periods of transitory spontaneous relaxation. These periods of relaxation allow gastric contents to reflux back into the esophagus.

In addition, the esophagus traverses both the abdominal and thoracic cavities, with the LES positioned strategically between the two. Most of the LES is abdominal. The greater the length of intraabdominal esophagus, the more competent this valve becomes. Any condition that shortens the abdominal segment of the LES will increase the likelihood of reflux.

Manifestations and Diagnostic Evaluation

Vomiting or spitting up after a meal, hiccupping, and recurrent otitis media related to pooled secretions in the nasopharynx during sleep are the hallmarks of all types of GERD. In addition, the infant with pathologic GERD can experience weight loss, failure to thrive, irritability, discomfort, and abdominal pain. Severe GERD can result in hematemesis or melena and anemia. Frequently, respiratory illness or asthma is associated with GERD, and the child may experience coughing, choking, asthma, wheezing, pneumonia, apnea, or bradycardia.

A variety of chronic and acute illnesses have been associated with GERD. GERD should be confirmed only after other major conditions have been ruled out. Diagnostic tests include barium swallow examination, upper GI study, fiberoptic endoscopy, esophageal manometry, ambulatory pH studies, and gastroesophageal scintigraphy (radionuclide scan), ultrasound, and chest computed tomography (CT).

Therapeutic Management

Therapy for GERD is based on the severity of symptoms and includes dietary alterations, positional changes, medications, and surgery. Early treatment may prevent or lesson complications such as failure to thrive, esophagitis, and strictures. Many infants suspected of functional GER are treated conservatively with pharmacologic support, without time-consuming and costly diagnostic testing. The American

Academy of Pediatrics supports the North American Society for Pediatric Gastroenterology and Nutrition (2001) guidelines for managing the child with gastroesophageal reflux.

Diet. Small, frequent feedings of predigested formulas, such as Nutramigen or Pregestimil, will reduce the amount of formula in the stomach, decrease distention, and minimize reflux. These smaller, more frequent feedings with frequent burping are often tried as the first line of treatment. Feedings thickened with rice cereal may reduce episodes of emesis but do not affect reflux time. In fact, thickened feedings actually may increase the risk of GER by delaying gastric emptying time. However, thickened feedings do tend to decrease crying and the number of episodes of vomiting (Hassall, 2005; Henry, 2004). Concentrated formulas and NG tube feedings provide nutritional supplementation for the child with failure to thrive. Caffeine and fatty foods lower LES pressure and should be eliminated.

Positioning. Much attention has been given to the best positioning for GER. Although prone positioning more effectively reduces reflux, current recommendations from the American Academy of Pediatrics and the North American Society for Pediatric Gastroenterology and Nutrition are that infants younger than 12 months should be placed supine to sleep to reduce the risk of sudden infant death syndrome (SIDS), even if an infant is diagnosed with GERD. The only exception to this recommendation would be if the risk of death from aspiration or other complications of GERD greatly outweighed the increased risk from the prone positioning (Henry, 2004).

Medications. Although the Food and Drug Administration (FDA) has not approved most medications used in the treatment of GERD for children, their use in children is quite common and many are now available over the counter. Medications are often added to the treatment protocol. Antacids for symptom relief, H_2-receptor antagonists (e.g., cimetidine, ranitidine) to decrease acid secretion, mucosal protectants (e.g., sucralfate) for barrier protection, proton pump inhibitors (e.g., omeprazole) to suppress gastric acid secretion, and prokinetic agents (e.g., metoclopramide) to accelerate gastric emptying may be used. Higher doses may be necessary in children because of their greater hepatic metabolic efficiency (Gold, 2004).

Treatment of Acute Bleeding. Bleeding is a complication of long-standing GERD and esophagitis. Stomach lavage (washing) with an NG tube is commonly performed to evacuate blood and blood clots during an episode of upper GI bleeding. The use of iced saline lavage to stop bleeding is no longer advocated. Radiologic procedures or surgery to coagulate bleeding vessels may be needed.

Surgery. Up to 15% of infants with GERD will require fundoplication. A 270-degree to 360-degree wrap to the stomach fundus is made around the distal esophagus. This procedure tightens the LES and prevents gastric reflux. Gas bloat syndrome may develop because of the child's inability to burp, and a gastrostomy tube may be temporarily needed for gastric decompression. Continuance of the pharmacologic treatment regimen may be needed after surgery.

NURSING CARE PLAN

The Infant With Gastroesophageal Reflux in the Community Setting

Focused Assessment

Nursing assessment begins with a thorough history, including the amount and frequency of feedings, changes in formula, and position during feedings. The frequency and pattern of emesis should be recorded, including documentation of whether it is projectile, is painful, or contains blood. A medical history of frequent respiratory problems or pneumonia, apnea, choking, or cyanosis should be gathered. Observing the child during a feeding can provide critical information about choking, gagging, coughing, color change, and comfort during feeding.

Plot the child's length, weight, and head circumference on a growth chart. Assess the infant for *Sandifer movements,* or unusual postural habits that may be observed in infants with severe reflux-induced esophagitis. These typically irritable infants may demonstrate head cocking, arching, and arm thrashing. Drawing the head to one side may relieve pain by keeping gastric secretions from entering the esophagus or mouth. If a history of respiratory symptoms is present, assess the infant for abnormal breath sounds or retractions.

Assessment of the family should not be overlooked. Assessment should include observations of parent-child interactions and feeding styles and a discussion of feelings and concerns about the child who vomits frequently, is difficult to feed, and may have failure to thrive.

NURSING DIAGNOSES
Risk for Aspiration related to GER.
Impaired Swallowing related to esophagitis.
Acute Pain related to esophagitis.

EXPECTED OUTCOMES
The infant will:
- Maintain a patent airway without signs of aspiration or respiratory distress.
- Swallow effectively without choking, coughing, or cyanosis.
- Remain free from the discomfort of esophageal irritation, as evidenced by calm appearance, ability to sleep well, and participation in usual play activities.

The parents will:
- Demonstrate CPR.

Continued

NURSING CARE PLAN—cont'd

Intervention	*Rationale*
1. Provide continuous cardiac and/or apnea monitoring.	1. Monitoring reduces risk of silent apnea or respiratory distress.
2. Provide repeated instructions, written materials, home health visits, and emotional support in managing monitoring.	2. Parents of infants with GERD may feel overwhelmed by doubt and anxiety over their ability to care for their child. This support can significantly increase their competency.
3. Train all caretakers in infant CPR.	3. Apnea is a serious complication of GERD, and all caretakers must be able to provide support as needed.
4. Have parents keep a log of episodes of apnea, bradycardia, or color change.	4. Because this is a home care issue, accurate parental reporting is essential.
5. Position infant on right side after feeding and minimize handling of infant after feedings. Position supine for sleeping.	5. Proper positioning reduces the risk of aspiration.
6. Encourage parents to offer pacifiers so that infant can "practice" swallowing.	6. Pacifier use decreases crying and reflux episodes and may increase clearance of refluxed stomach contents.

Evaluation

- Is the child's airway patent, without choking, coughing, cyanosis, or retractions?
- Have the parents and all caregivers demonstrated infant CPR?
- Can the child swallow without incurring respiratory distress?

- Is the child content and comfortable during feedings, able to sleep appropriately, and able to participate in usual play activities?

NURSING DIAGNOSES Deficient Fluid Volume related to reflux of stomach contents.
Imbalanced Nutrition: Less Than Body Requirements related to anorexia, reflux, and dysphagia.

EXPECTED OUTCOMES The infant will:
- Retain feedings with regurgitation of less than 10 mL.
- Maintain and gain weight according to growth charts.

Intervention	*Rationale*
1. Explain to parents that several different formula and feeding routines may need to be tried before success is found.	1. Frustration will be avoided if parents know that this may be a trial-and-error process with their infant.
2. Feed infant small, frequent feedings with predigested formulas or breast milk.	2. This reduces amount of formula or breast milk in stomach, decreases distention, and minimizes reflux.
3. Try thickened formula or breast milk by adding 1 to 3 tsp of rice cereal per ounce.	3. Thickened formula is more difficult to reflux high into the esophagus.
4. Show parents how to cross-cut nipples to improve feeding of thickened formulas. Several tries may be necessary to determine what works best for their infant.	4. Nipple holes must be enlarged or infant will not be able to exert enough force to receive formula. Too large a hole can increase risk of aspiration.
5. Use thickened feedings only with infants who are not on solid foods. Give toddlers solids first, followed by liquids.	5. This decreases the chance of reflux or aspiration.
6. Eliminate chocolate and caffeine from the diets of older children. Offer alternative treats.	6. Caffeine relaxes the LES.
7. Help parents position infants properly after feedings. Side-lying is preferred. Older children should remain in an upright position, standing or sitting, while awake.	7. Proper positioning assists in preventing reflux.
8. Have parents keep a log of feeding successes and any reflux.	8. Success of interventions relies on accurate information from parents. A log eliminates the need to remember details.
9. Teach parents signs of dehydration: sunken fontanels, decreased number of wet diapers, no tears when crying. Have them call immediately if child becomes dehydrated.	9. Early detection is essential.

NURSING CARE PLAN—cont'd

Evaluation

- Can the child retain feedings with regurgitations of less than 10 mL?
- Is the child growing according to growth charts?

- Is the child well hydrated as evidenced by flat fontanels, good skin turgor, moist mucous membranes, and adequate urine output for age?

NURSING DIAGNOSES   Deficient Knowledge related to unfamiliarity with the disease process, home care, and medications.
Anxiety (parental) related to special needs of infant and possible need for surgery.
Impaired Home Maintenance Management related to complex, long-term care.

EXPECTED OUTCOMES   The parents will:
- Explain GERD and the reasons for diagnostic tests, medications, dietary changes, and surgery.
- Demonstrate effective coping mechanisms for dealing with the long-term consequences of GERD.
- Express confidence in their ability to deal with their infant's special needs.

Intervention

1. Teach parents about each medication their child is taking, including mechanism of action, dosage, times, relation to feedings, side effects.
2. Help parents rearrange mealtimes so that medications can be given correctly.
3. Encourage parents to continue medications for the full period and not to discontinue them if their child improves.
4. Help parents modify positioning at home with supplies that are readily available.

5. Encourage parents to practice medication administration, positioning, feeding techniques, and assessment with supervision until they are confident in their abilities to provide total care for the infant.
6. Allow and encourage parents to share their concerns and worries.
7. Provide community referral as needed.

Rationale

1. Parent education is essential for appropriate home care.

2. Some medications must be given in relation to meals to have maximum effect.
3. This is a long-term problem that may require several months to resolve. Esophagitis may be present after reflux has resolved.
4. What works in the hospital may be difficult to achieve at home without special equipment. Parents will need support and suggestions to make these modifications work in their own homes.
5. Return demonstration and positive reinforcement can significantly increase compliance at home and decrease parental anxiety.

6. This decreases anxiety.

7. Support and continued communication with other parents and children experiencing the same stresses can increase coping.

Evaluation

- Is the child receiving medications as prescribed at the correct times and in the correct dosage?
- Can the parents explain GERD and the reasons for positioning and dietary modifications?
- Have the parents assumed all care responsibilities?

- Do the parents demonstrate correct feeding techniques?
- Have the parents expressed their concerns and feelings related to caring for their child?
- Are the parents demonstrating confidence in their abilities to care for the many needs of their child?

Constipation and Encopresis

Constipation is the infrequent and difficult passage of dry, hard stools. A major concern with constipation is the development of encopresis, or fecal incontinence. Encopresis is repeated and involuntary defecation in a child older than 4 years who has normal colon and rectal anatomy. With encopresis, children often report that soiling occurs without warning. Parents find the situation frustrating, and soiling often becomes a major issue between parent and child. Often encopresis causes children to feel ashamed or embarrassed, and they may avoid situations in which embarrassment might

be heightened, such as spending the night with a friend or even going to school. If the condition persists over a long period, it usually affects the child's self-esteem and may impair social relations. Often, the parents experience guilt and shame or revulsion, disgust, or anger, and they may project these feelings onto the child.

Etiology and Incidence

Constipation can have many causes, such as changes in diet, dehydration, lack of exercise, emotional stress, certain drugs, pain from anal fissure, or excessive milk intake. If the child

CONSTIPATION AND ENCOPRESIS

When stool passes into the rectum, distention of the walls stimulates mass peristaltic movements in the bowel. This process is called the *defecation reflex*. If defecation is not desired, the external sphincter contracts and voluntary retention of stool occurs. As the stool remains in the rectum, the rectum relaxes and the defecation reflex wanes. Water reabsorption from the colon continues, resulting in hard, dry stool that is difficult to pass. The eventual passage of that stool may result in pain or anal fissures. If retention of stool continues, more fissures may develop or become worse, so that eventually even soft stool may produce pain. A cycle of pain develops in which the stool is retained to avoid pain but the retention leads to even more difficult defecation. Over time, the rectum becomes enlarged. An enlarged rectum can result in failure to control the external sphincter, which in turn results in encopresis.

has no neurologic or anatomic disorders, encopresis is usually the result of recurrent fecal impaction and an enlarged rectum caused by chronic constipation. Factors predisposing to encopresis include inadequate or inconsistent toilet training or some type of psychological stress, such as starting school or the birth of a sibling.

Constipation can affect any child at any time. Encopresis generally affects 3- to 7-year-olds with three to six times more boys than girls affected. The incidence of encopresis is higher in lower socioeconomic classes and among children with learning disabilities. Constipation accounts for up to 3% of visits to pediatric clinics and 30% of visits to pediatric gastroenterologists (Borowitz et al., 2005).

Manifestations

Constipation. The principal symptoms of constipation are absence of stool, abdominal pain and cramping without distention, and palpable, movable fecal masses with large amounts of stool in an enlarged rectum. The child may also experience diarrheal overflow; normal or decreased bowel sounds; malaise, anorexia, and headache; nausea and vomiting; or anal fissure.

Encopresis. Children with encopresis have evidence of soiled clothing and fecal odor without apparent awareness. Anal irritation leads to scratching or rubbing of the anal area. Social withdrawal and avoidance of extended contact with others (e.g., overnight stays, camp) are common. Urinary incontinence and urinary tract infections may also be present.

Diagnostic Evaluation

Abdominal radiographs may demonstrate an enlarged rectum with large amounts of stool and gas. The definitive diagnostic procedure is a rectal examination. This is rarely performed because of its emotional impact on the child and the possibility of pain from anal fissure. A thorough history is usually sufficient for the diagnosis.

Therapeutic Management

The best form of treatment is preventing development of the chronic problem through appropriate diet, exercise, and regular toileting habits. Education about "normal" bowel function can prevent a psychogenic component from compounding the problem. The focus of management is to remove the impaction, retrain the rectum to be aware of when it is full, and help the child overcome the pain-retention cycle.

Treatment usually involves the following three phases:
1. Disimpaction: critical for success of management
   a. Enemas until impaction is cleared; use Fleet, 1 oz/5 kg; if the child is larger than 20 kg, use an adult size
   b. Stool softener or laxative including magnesium hydroxide, senna syrup, lactulose, sorbitol, mineral oil
2. Maintenance:
   a. Mineral oil, 2 mL/kg twice daily, up to 180 to 240 mL/day for children older than 1 year; the dosage is adjusted depending on results achieved. Mineral oil may be contraindicated in children who resist taking it or who vomit frequently after it is taken; aspiration of mineral oil can lead to aspiration pneumonia in these children (Coughlin, 2003).
   b. Lactulose (10 g/15 mL), 1 or 2 mL/kg twice daily, or milk of magnesia (according to physician direction) for children older than 6 months and younger than 1 year.
   c. Dietary changes, including limiting milk intake, increasing water intake, and increasing residue.
3. Changing the retention habit:
   a. Sitting on the commode for 5 to 10 minutes approximately 20 to 30 minutes after meals
   b. Keeping a behavioral chart with positive rewards (daily stars may be helpful)
   c. Avoiding negative reinforcement
   d. Biofeedback may be a useful tool to reteach the feeling of rectal fullness

The goal is for the child to pass two or three soft stools per day without pain within the first month. Medications are withdrawn slowly over a 3- to 6-month period after the fear of pain has been lost.

For infant constipation, rectal stimulation is discouraged. For example, rectal thermometers and glycerin suppositories should not be used. Barley cereal can be substituted for rice cereal. Fructose, such as prune juice, or lactulose can help. High-fiber fruits and vegetables will also decrease constipation.

NURSING CARE

The Child With Constipation or Encopresis

Assessment

Obtain a thorough history of the soiling events, including frequency, intensity, and duration. Because parent-child relationships are often strained, interview the parents and child separately to reduce the child's embarrassment. The nurse can explain to parents that a medical history and examination will be performed to rule out organic causes of the chronic constipation, such as Hirschsprung disease.

Nursing Diagnosis and Planning

The following nursing diagnoses and expected outcomes may be appropriate after assessing for constipation or encopresis in the child:

- Constipation or Bowel Incontinence related to inconsistent patterns of elimination, anxiety, or pain during elimination.

  Expected Outcome: The child will have normal bowel function, as evidenced by the passage of soft stools without pain or incontinence, maintenance of a well-balanced diet high in fiber and sufficient fluid intake, and decreased reliance on laxatives.

- Compromised or Disabled Family Coping related to persistent stress, guilt, and embarrassment about the child's elimination difficulty.

  Expected Outcomes: The family will function effectively as a unit, openly discuss problems, and develop a plan to achieve control over incontinence.

- Social Isolation related to embarrassment, peer teasing, and odor from bowel incontinence.

  Expected Outcomes: The child will verbalize positive, realistic feelings about self and verbalize appropriate ways to achieve control over bowel incontinence.

- Impaired Skin Integrity related to poor hygiene in anal area, bowel incontinence, and lack of knowledge.

  Expected Outcome: The child will maintain skin integrity, as evidenced by clean, intact skin.

Interventions

Because constipation and encopresis represent a continuum of the same problem, a variety of approaches can be tried as needed to deal with the problem. Simple constipation may resolve with only dietary changes or changing a habit of retention. Severe encopresis may require that all interventions be continued for 3 to 6 months.

Overcoming Withholding

Before bowel retraining can begin, the child's bowel must be evacuated of all hard stool and impactions. This goal is best accomplished with the use of appropriate-size Fleet or isotonic enemas every 12 hours until the impaction is cleared, usually within 48 hours. Teach parents to administer enemas at home. During this time, the child should be monitored for hypernatremia or hyperphosphatemia, which could result from repeated use of Fleet enemas (see Chapter 13 for a discussion of enema administration).

After bowel cleansing has been achieved, the child older than 1 year may be started on mineral oil or another maintenance laxative. Lactulose or milk of magnesia may be used in infants at least 6 months old but younger than 12 months. Mineral oil is best tolerated when it is given chilled or mixed with cold drinks. Mixing the oil with ice cream or chocolate

milk, blending it with ice cubes and fruit juice, or chilling it helps disguise the taste. The child may leak oil when dosages are high, and parents and children need to be aware that leakage does not constitute encopresis. At the end of this intervention, the child should be passing soft stool without pain or incontinence. Parents should be advised to adjust doses of laxatives based on characteristics of stool.

Dietary Changes

Dietary modifications are used as a part of the treatment. Increasing water and fiber intake by offering granola bars, dried fruits, whole-grain cereals, and fresh vegetables with low-fat dip can increase the bulk in stool and make it easier to pass. Decreasing sugar and milk intake also helps keep stools soft. Advise supplementing with fat-soluble vitamins when mineral oil is being used because the oil can theoretically interfere with vitamin absorption in the small intestine.

Changing the Retention Habit

To help reestablish a normal bowel habit, the child should sit on the toilet for 5 to 10 minutes after breakfast and dinner. This routine will allow the normal gastrocolic reflex to assist with defecation and will eliminate the need to be involved with retraining during school hours. Star charts and small prizes may be helpful in rewarding success. These interventions are continued for at least 3 to 6 months, during which the rectum will resume its normal size and the child will relearn to attend to the defecation reflex. If fecal impaction occurs at any time, enemas are again administered and the dosage of mineral oil is adjusted.

Emotional Support

Allow the child and parents to express their feelings of success and failure with the ongoing program. To minimize the damage to the child's self-esteem, encourage self-care as much as possible. To decrease embarrassment, school-age children should have a complete change of pants and underwear at school if leakage or an accident occurs. Age-appropriate support groups may be available in a center with a large population or encopresis clinic.

Teaching is a major intervention. Encouraging the child and parents to share feelings of embarrassment is equally important. Allow the child to verbalize any concerns, and provide developmentally appropriate anatomic information to assist with understanding the cause of the problem. Drawings and books may be an effective way to begin this sharing of feelings and information. Relieving the child of shame and embarrassment may improve cooperation with the plan of care.

Home Care

Because this condition is managed at home, teaching parents is a critical intervention. The parents need to understand the correct way to administer enemas (see Chapter 13). They also need support in implementing and documenting the child's successes and setbacks. The child and parents need encouragement to continue, even when the successes seem few. This problem develops over time and takes time, patience, and perseverance to resolve.

Evaluation

- Is the child passing soft stools without pain?
- Does the food diary indicate a well-balanced, high-fiber diet?
- Is the child experiencing any incontinence?
- Are enemas, laxatives, or mineral oil still needed?
- Is the child experiencing success with bowel control as a result of implementation of a family-designed plan?
- Does the child more readily participate in age-appropriate activities and express increasing control over bowel incontinence?
- Is the skin in the anal area clean and intact?

Irritable Bowel Syndrome

Irritable bowel syndrome (IBS) is the result of increased intestinal motility, which can lead to spasm and pain.

Etiology and Incidence

Stress and emotional factors are thought to be the most common causes of this disorder. In infants, it may be related to a lactase deficiency. It is not associated with any psychopathology.

IBS occurs after infancy and is most common in toddlers (in whom it is sometimes called *chronic nonspecific diarrhea of childhood*) and adolescents. The condition tends to occur in families with a history of other bowel disturbances or infantile colic. The condition tends to resolve by late adolescence but is sometimes present in adults. IBS is the most common diagnosis in children with recurrent abdominal pain and occurs as either diarrhea predominant or constipation predominant (Kohli, 2004).

Manifestations and Diagnostic Evaluation

Manifestations of IBS include diffuse abdominal pain unrelated to meals or activity; alternating constipation and diarrhea, with undigested food and mucus present in the stool; and normal growth.

The diagnosis is made on the basis of elimination of major GI pathologic conditions, including Crohn disease, giardiasis, lactose intolerance, and genitourinary abnormalities. Abdominal ultrasound, stool for ova and parasites (O&P) and cultures, abdominal radiography, and a complete gynecologic assessment (if age appropriate) are often ordered.

Therapeutic Management and Nursing Considerations

No definitive treatment exists for this poorly understood functional bowel problem. Management is aimed at identifying and reducing triggers and reducing bowel spasms, which decreases symptoms. The primary nursing intervention should be reassurance that it is a self-limiting, intermittent problem.

Unless lactose intolerance is suspected, no dietary modifications are required other than the maintenance of a healthy, well-balanced, moderate-fiber, lower-fat diet. Encourage the child to eat slowly and not drink carbonated beverages.

PATHOPHYSIOLOGY

IRRITABLE BOWEL SYNDROME

The precipitating factors in irritable bowel syndrome are unknown but result in two distinct problems. The first is *disorganized contractility,* which causes spasmodic peristaltic rushes and lulls. This disorganization causes alternating diarrhea and constipation with intermittent abdominal pain. The second component is *excess mucus production in the lumen of the bowel.* This produces maldigestion and the passage of incompletely digested food and nutrients.

Because carbohydrate malabsorption from fruit juice may also trigger symptoms in some children, eliminating juice or changing from apple to white grape juice can help eliminate symptoms (Moukarzel, Lezicka, & Ament, 2002).

Medications are not typically used in the treatment, but pH-dependent, enteric-coated peppermint oil capsules have been used successfully in initial trials to reduce IBS pain (Kline, Kline, DiPalma, & Barbero, 2001). Antispasmodics, such as Levsin, Donnatol, and Pro-Banthine, and antidepressants may also be used in severe cases.

Family and psychosocial assessment may reveal a family that is worried about a serious life-threatening disease and is quite focused on the child's bowel habits. The family may not be reassured by the normal findings on a physical and developmental examination.

The primary nursing interventions are teaching and reassurance. Health promotion activities such as exercise, balanced nutrition, and school activities have the best influence on the disease. Because of the associated psychosocial component, referral to mental health and family counseling services can be effective in cases that are unresponsive to other measures. The child and family will express feelings and concerns that will assist in evaluating the interventions.

INFLAMMATORY AND INFECTIOUS DISORDERS
Ulcers

A peptic ulcer is an area of sharply circumscribed loss of the mucosa, submucosa, or muscular tissue occurring in areas of the digestive tract exposed to acid and pepsin. Peptic ulcers can be primary or secondary, gastric or duodenal. Primary, or idiopathic, ulcers occur in the absence of underlying systemic disease. Secondary, or stress, ulcers are acute and are found in conjunction with other illnesses, such as shock, respiratory failure, sepsis, hypoglycemia, severe burns, or intracranial lesions.

Gastric ulcers occur in the stomach, particularly the gastric antrum, and are uncommon in childhood. Duodenal ulcers occur in the pylorus or duodenum, are often chronic, frequently lead to complications, and are the most commonly encountered ulcers in children.

Etiology

Known factors that can alter the mucus-bicarbonate barrier in children include the following:

- *Excessive acid secretion:* Zollinger-Ellison syndrome or gastrinoma may cause excess acid secretion and multiple ulcers. Hyperparathyroidism may also contribute to increased acid secretion.
- *Bile salts:* Bile breaks down the adherent mucous structure of the gastric-duodenal lining and exposes the mucosa to acid.
- *Lack of prostaglandins:* Prostaglandins augment both the mucous gel lining and bicarbonate secretion. Deficiencies in mucosal prostaglandins may cause impairment of the mucus-bicarbonate barrier.
- *Genetic factors:* Duodenal ulcers show a familial tendency. This, together with environmental factors, may predispose children to ulcer formation. An association between ulcer activity and type O blood has also been noted.
- *Bacteria: Helicobacter pylori* is a gram-negative spiral bacterium that has been identified in the gastric antrum of children with duodenal ulcer. It infects most adults with ulcer disease and acts by weakening the gastric mucosal barrier and allowing acid and peptic digestion of the susceptible mucosa.
- *Psychological factors:* The importance of psychological factors is questionable. They likely influence exacerbations or complications but not initial ulcer activity.
- *Stress:* Stress accounts for at least 80% of secondary ulcers encountered during infancy and early childhood. They tend to be acute and occur in seriously ill children.
- *Diet:* Diet does not seem to influence the development of ulcer disease in children. Although certain foods may cause indigestion, no convincing data show that dietary factors cause, perpetuate, or reactivate ulcers, especially duodenal. Colas, teas, and chocolate do, however, increase acid secretions and may be contributing factors.
- *Medications:* Many medications, such as aspirin, nonsteroidal anti-inflammatory agents, and indomethacin, as well as tobacco and alcohol, are known to affect the gastroduodenal mucosa adversely in adults but appear to have little importance in pediatric ulcer disease.

PATHOPHYSIOLOGY

ULCERS

A thick mucus-bicarbonate barrier, a layer of mucus that provides a buffer zone for acid neutralization, lines the stomach and duodenum. Stomach acids diffuse slowly through this layer toward the gastric wall but are encountered and neutralized by slowly diffusing bicarbonate ions liberated from surface epithelial cells. The establishment of a neutral pH at the gastric epithelial surface provides protection from the combined effects of acid and pepsin. Ulcers result when any imbalance in the process occurs and erosions develop on the surface of the gastric or duodenal mucosa.

Incidence

The true incidence of peptic ulcer disease in children is unknown because ulcers often spontaneously heal before a diagnosis is made. The average age for onset of ulcer activity is 11 to 12 years, with boys affected two to three times more than are girls. Duodenal ulcers occur more frequently in children older than 6 years. *H. pylori* gastritis has been found in 90% to 100% of children with duodenal ulcers (Wyllie, 2004a). Stress ulcers account for 80% of ulcers occurring during infancy and early childhood, affect both sexes, and are equally distributed between the stomach and duodenum.

Manifestations and Diagnostic Evaluation

Manifestations of ulcer disease in children are burning, cramping pain when the stomach is empty, awakening during the night or early morning with abdominal discomfort, and vomiting in children younger than 6 years. Hematemesis and melena are common in infants and young children.

Fiberoptic upper endoscopy is the diagnostic tool of choice for all children, including neonates. Endoscopy provides direct visual observation of the lining of the esophagus, stomach, and proximal duodenum and also is a means for obtaining biopsy or culture material. Ultrasound may be performed to rule out gallstones, tumors, or mechanical obstruction. The fecal occult blood test may be performed to check for GI bleeding.

Therapeutic Management

Medical management is the most common treatment for ulcer disease in children. Factors considered in ulcer treatment include drug safety, symptom relief, patient and parent adherence, and the prevention of complications or ulcer recurrence. A bland diet with milk and small, frequent feedings was long thought to be the mainstay of ulcer therapy. However, the protein and calcium in milk actually stimulate more acid secretions than they buffer. A regular diet low in caffeine is now generally prescribed because caffeine is a potent stimulant of acid secretion and exacerbates GERD. A diet high in fiber and polyunsaturated oils may also play a role in ulcer prevention.

Medications are now considered the first line of treatment. They include antibiotics, antacids, H_2-receptor antagonists, and mucosa-protective agents. Vaccines to prevent *H. pylori* infections are currently under development.

Surgery is indicated for the management of ulcer complications, such as hemorrhage, perforation, or obstruction. Vagotomy, pyloroplasty, ligation of a bleeding vessel, or closure of a perforation may be performed.

If the child is actively bleeding, an NG tube is inserted to remove blood, decompress the stomach, and estimate blood loss. IV fluids, oxygen, blood replacement, and vasoactive drugs such as vasopressin (Pitressin) may be given. Balloon tamponade with a Sengstaken-Blakemore tube may be indicated. Blood or clots are removed with room-temperature gastric lavage. The use of iced saline lavage to stop GI bleeding is no longer advocated because it increases bleeding and clotting times and prolongs the prothrombin time. It also imposes a risk of hypothermia on an already compromised child.

The long-term prognosis for children diagnosed with peptic ulcer disease remains controversial. Marked improvement in symptoms, however, is noted with the use of H_2-receptor blockers and other medications. Without adequate treatment, peptic ulcer disease frequently persists into adult life.

Nursing Considerations

Nursing assessment of the child with peptic ulcer disease begins with a thorough history, including a family history of ulcer disease, past episodes of abdominal pain, or recent stressful events in the home, school, or community. A complete assessment of pain includes a description of the nature of the pain and its location; its relationship to meals, defecation, or voiding; episodes of nocturnal pain; and medications used to effectively relieve the pain. The child is examined for the presence of epigastric tenderness, nausea, vomiting, abdominal distention, hematemesis, melena, or recent changes in appetite or eating habits.

All stools and emesis fluid should be checked for the presence of blood. Bowel sounds are auscultated for 5 minutes. If vomiting is present, the child is assessed for signs of dehydration. If bleeding is observed, the child is monitored for changes in vital signs and the physician is notified immediately. Finally, the nurse assesses family members for their understanding of the disease, the presence of a viable support system, and their ability to participate in their child's care.

Providing Information. The major focus of nursing interventions is teaching. The nurse reviews pathophysiology, medication administration, and diet and assesses for complications.

Preparing the child for diagnostic tests also is an important nursing intervention. Because fiberoptic endoscopy is often performed, the child must be prepared for conscious sedation. Keeping the child on NPO status for at least 6 hours, maintaining an IV line, and monitoring vital signs and respiratory function during the procedure are nursing responsibilities. Upper GI examinations and ultrasonography may also be performed.

Home Care. Ulcers are managed almost exclusively in the home environment, so teaching, follow-up, and home health referral are essential. The correct use of medications and dietary modifications are parental responsibilities that may require educational materials, emotional support, help with time organization, and encouragement to continue even when symptoms are relieved (Box 19-4).

Infectious Gastroenteritis

Infectious gastroenteritis is caused by a group of viruses, bacteria, and parasites capable of causing serious communicable diarrhea, massive fluid and electrolyte loss, sepsis, and death (for further discussion of fluid and electrolyte alterations, see Chapter 18).

Etiology

Ingestion of contaminated food or water and person-to-person contamination are the most frequent causes of infectious gastroenteritis in the United States. High-risk groups include children in daycare centers, preschools, and long-term care facilities and those infected with the human immunodeficiency virus (HIV). *Giardia* is the most common pathogen seen in children in daycare settings, and rotavirus is the most common GI pathogen seen in infants and young children (Parasher, Gibson, Bresee, & Glass, 2006). In most cases the pathogen is not identified (Table 19-3).

BOX 19-4	**PARENTS WANT TO KNOW** About Care of the Child With an Ulcer

Parents need to understand the pathophysiology, causes, diagnosis, and therapeutic management of ulcers. When educating the parent and older child, follow these guidelines:

- Emphasize the relation of the ulcer to acute illness.
- Help the older child identify sources of excess stress that can be modified.
- Teach stress-reduction activities such as relaxation and exercise and refer parents to support groups.

Directions for administering medications include the following:

- Do not administer antacids within 1 hour of other anti-ulcer medications.
- Do not stop medications when symptoms improve; continue for the full prescribed course.
- Do not use aspirin or other nonsteroidal antiinflammatory drugs because they may cause bleeding.
- Do not use over-the-counter medications without your physician's knowledge.

- Do not add other drugs because your child's metabolism and absorption may be altered by ulcer medications.

Help parents make changes in diet as prescribed by teaching the following:

- If your child has a poor appetite, provide a well-balanced diet with many choices.
- Seek assistance from dietary services as needed.
- Provide meals and snacks every 2 to 3 hours.
- Make sure your child avoids coffee, chocolate, and caffeine and any other foods that might cause discomfort.

Instruct parents to call their physician if their child experiences any of the following problems:

- "Coffee grounds" vomitus
- Weight loss
- Tarry stools
- Increased pain
- Diarrhea
- Vomiting

TABLE 19-3 Characteristics of Infectious Gastroenteritis

Infectious Agent	Characteristics	Clinical Manifestations	Diagnostic Findings	Treatment
Shigella (enteroinvasive with cytotoxin)	Incubation period 1-7 days Most common in summer Fecal-oral spread Remains communicable for 1-3 wk	Symptoms last 5-10 days Diarrhea begins as watery, progresses to small, bloody, with mucus Severe abdominal pain High fever Neurologic symptoms (headache, nuchal rigidity, convulsions) Risk for sepsis, hemolytic uremic syndrome, rectal prolapse, DIC	Blood, mucus, WBCs in stool Positive culture in some cases	Bactrim, 8-10 mg/kg/day × 5 days OR Ampicillin, 50- 100 mg/kg/day × 5 days Contact Precautions Identify source if possible
Salmonella (enteroinvasive)	Incubation 6 hr to 3 days Most common in summer, fall Usually foodborne Infectious for duration of illness and variable period afterward	Symptoms last 2-5 days Rapid onset Secretory diarrhea Abdominal pain, nausea, vomiting common	Blood and PMNs in stool	For infants younger than 12 wk, same as for *Shigella* Contact Precautions Identify source if possible
Escherichia coli (enteroinvasive with enterotoxin)	Variable incubation Most common in summer Foodborne most common	Green, watery, secretory diarrhea May cause hemorrhagic colitis Fever	Blood and PMNs in stool	Same as for *Shigella* Contact Precautions
Campylobacter	Incubation 1-8 days Most common in infants and adolescents	History of consumption of contaminated shellfish Severe abdominal pain Foul-smelling, watery diarrhea	Blood and PMNs in stool	Possibly treated with erythromycin for 7 days Contact Precautions
Giardia lamblia	Most common cause of parasitic diarrhea Spread in water	Afebrile Abdominal distention, flatulence Variable diarrhea	Ova and parasites found in stool but no blood or PMNs Parasites found on duodenal biopsy	Metronidazole (Flagyl) for 7 days Contact Precautions Treat all unknown water sources with chlorine/iodine before drinking
Rotavirus	Incubation 1-3 days Common in winter months Accounts for 50% of cases of acute diarrhea in children	Symptoms usually last 2-6 days History of preceding or concurrent respiratory illness	Virus in stool detected by enzyme immunoassay	No pharmacologic treatment Contact Precautions
Clostridium difficile	Antibiotic-associated Most common nosocomial diarrhea	Fever for 24-48 hr Diarrhea develops after antibiotic treatment	Blood and PMNs in stool	Cholestyramine used to enhance mucosal recovery and decrease length of diarrhea Possibly treated with vancomycin or metronidazole (Flagyl) for 10 days
Norwalk	Incubation 1-2 days Common in winter in schools and other group settings Fecal-oral route of transmission	Symptoms last 1-2 days Nausea, vomiting, diarrhea Headache, low-grade fever, muscle aches, chills	Virus in stool	No pharmacologic treatment Contact precautions

WBCs, White blood cells; *DIC,* disseminated intravascular coagulation; *PMNs,* polymorphonuclear leukocytes.

PATHOPHYSIOLOGY

INFECTIOUS GASTROENTERITIS

As the pathogen adheres to the mucosa of the intestine, it is no longer affected by peristaltic waves and is not removed from the site. Epithelial invasion occurs, causing an inflammatory response and epithelial cell death. This leads to ulcerations, pseudomembranes, bleeding, and possibly sepsis. As the pathogens multiply, they may produce toxins. Enterotoxins (e.g., cholera, *Shigella*) cause fluid and electrolyte shifts that result in increased secretion into the intestine and simultaneous decrease in absorption caused by edema. The absorptive capacity of the colon is exceeded, and massive diarrhea and dehydration result. Cytotoxins (e.g., *Salmonella*) produce local edema, malabsorption, and dehydration. Some pathogens are also capable of producing neurotoxins (e.g., *Shigella*) that act outside the GI tract.

Incidence

Gastroenteritis is one of the most common outpatient infectious diseases in children. In children younger than 5 years in the United States, gastroenteritis accounts for in excess of 1.5 million outpatient visits a year and 300 deaths (CDC, 2003a). Infections peak in the summer and have an equal gender distribution. Worldwide, gastroenteritis is a significant cause of death for children younger than 5 years old (CDC, 2003a).

Manifestations

Gastroenteritis likely manifests with diarrhea of varying amount and consistency, vomiting, and abdominal pain. In addition, the child may experience tenesmus and fever. Dehydration is a severe consequence of gastroenteritis and occurs mainly in children younger than 2 years. A history of travel to other regions of the world can provide clues to the causative organism.

Diagnostic Evaluation

A definitive diagnosis can be made when a rectal or stool culture yields a pathogen, but these cultures are expensive and result in many false-negative findings. Ova and parasites are more reliably found. Usually only children who appear to be in a toxic condition or have bloody stools, abdominal pain, or tenesmus undergo a diagnostic work-up. The presence of white blood cells (WBCs) and blood in the stool can support the presumptive diagnosis on the basis of clinical findings. Blood cultures may also be needed in the acutely ill infant and young child. An unprepared sigmoidoscopy can be useful in determining the amount of mucosal involvement, obtaining more reliable samples for culture, and diagnosing the disease.

Therapeutic Management

The priority therapy is to replace water and correct acid-base or fluid and electrolyte disturbances with IV fluids or oral (PO) electrolyte replacement liquids. The rate of replacement may be as high as 50 to 100 mL/kg over a 4- to 6-hour period (1 to 2½ times maintenance requirements). Because diarrheal fluid is high in sodium, potassium, and bicarbonate, oral rehydration solutions should be used to match losses (see Chapter 18). Hospitalization for treatment is not uncommon, especially for the infant or small child, to allow for continued assessment and management of symptoms or sepsis. Antimicrobial therapy is useful in cases of infection with *Shigella* and *Giardia*, and in some cases of infection with *Salmonella*, *Clostridium difficile*, and *Escherichia coli* but not for rotavirus infection. The US Food and Drug Administration has licensed a rotavirus vaccine for use among infants in 2006. The Advisory Committee on Immunization Practices (ACIP) is recommending that all infants be immunized with 3 doses of the vaccine at 2, 4, and 6 months of age.

NURSING CARE

The Child With Infectious Gastroenteritis

Assessment

Obtain an adequate history of the event, including the length of symptoms, the frequency and consistency of stools, and the presence of blood or mucus in stools. Noting the amount, color, consistency, and time (ACCT) of each stool or episode of vomiting is a consistent way to document findings. The concurrent appearance of symptoms in other members of the family can be helpful in the diagnosis. Any travel to other countries or wilderness areas should be recorded. Evaluating formula and food preparation at home and in daycare facilities as well as examining sanitation and hygiene in these places can provide valuable information.

The child may appear moderately to severely dehydrated with hyperactive bowel sounds and severe diarrhea, which is often bloody. Blood in the stool usually appears after the maximal fluid loss has occurred and can be useful in determining the stage of illness. The presence of abdominal pain, vomiting, tenesmus, and fever should be assessed. Headache, nuchal rigidity, irritability, and seizures are important symptoms of the neurotoxic effects of *Shigella*.

Assessment of hydration status is critical. Poor urine output, high urine specific gravity, poor skin turgor, dry mucous membranes, crying without producing tears, a sunken or depressed fontanel in infants, and skin tenting can occur quickly with the large amount of fluid lost through diarrhea. Loss of bicarbonate from severe diarrhea and dehydration makes metabolic acidosis a major concern. The compensatory mechanisms of increased respiratory rate and effort are important to document.

Nursing Diagnosis and Planning

The following nursing diagnoses and expected outcomes may be appropriate for the infant or child with gastroenteritis:

- Deficient Fluid Volume related to severe diarrhea.

  Expected Outcomes: The child will be adequately hydrated without electrolyte disturbance, as evidenced by moist mucous membranes; good skin turgor; urine output appropriate for age; return to normal weight; and normal serum sodium, potassium, and bicarbonate levels; the child will have soft, formed stools without diarrhea, blood, or mucus.

- Risk for Infection related to exposure of family members and others to infectious agents.

  Expected Outcome: The child will not transmit pathogens to others.

- Acute Pain related to hyperactive motility.

  Expected Outcome: The child will be free from abdominal pain, as evidenced by a return to normal activity and no reports of pain.

- Deficient Knowledge related to inadequate information about the disease and its control.

  Expected Outcomes: The parents will describe how to prevent transmitting the condition to others and will use Standard and Contact Precautions when handling the child's excretions.

- Imbalanced Nutrition: Less Than Body Requirements related to malabsorption.

  Expected Outcomes: The child will resume a normal diet and will regain weight lost during the acute phase within 1 week after symptoms abate.

- Risk for Impaired Skin Integrity related to skin contact with feces and the necessity for frequent cleansing.

  Expected Outcome: The child will maintain skin integrity, as evidenced by clean, dry, intact skin without redness, drainage, or breakdown.

Interventions

Maintaining Fluid Balance

Critical nursing interventions are related to the fluid volume deficit. Oral or parenteral rehydration with correction of acid-base imbalances is essential to establish homeostasis. Accurate intake and output and weight measurements are important. Monitoring skin turgor, urine output, and serum electrolyte levels provides evaluation criteria in this area (see Chapter 18 for a further discussion of fluid and electrolyte alterations).

Decreasing Risk

Providing safety, assessing neurologic symptoms, and monitoring for seizures are also priorities for the child with *Shigella* infection. Preventing the spread of infection remains a critical nursing intervention. Thorough handwashing is a must. Contact Precautions must be strictly enforced for all staff and family members to minimize the risk of infection. These precautions must be maintained at home for up to 2 weeks or for less time if antibiotics are given. Pain and fever may be treated with acetaminophen, but symptomatic treatment with antidiarrheals is not recommended because it tends to increase the length of symptoms. Symptomatic care of the febrile child may include tepid sponging and light dressing.

Parents and children need to be taught these interventions and given information about the disease process during this period. Depending on the organism causing the gastroenteritis, follow-up by the public health department may be necessary. Organisms such as *Salmonella* and *E. coli* can be found in food and present a significant public health concern. A dietary recall for possibly contaminated foods can be important in establishing the cause and minimizing the risk of spread to the public.

Home Care

The most important intervention that can be implemented at home is proper rehydration to prevent the need for hospitalization and IV therapy (see Chapter 18 for a discussion of oral rehydration fluids and care for the child with dehydration).

Dietary changes for vomiting and diarrhea may not be necessary if the child does not demonstrate dehydration. Breast milk may be offered as needed, and formula should be given full strength. Oral rehydration therapy (ORT) may also be used in addition to usual diet to replace GI losses and prevent dehydration (see Chapter 18). Vomiting does not prevent oral rehydration because the child can be successfully rehydrated with 5 to 10 mL of rehydrating solution every 2 minutes. When diet is continued, fats and high sugar concentrations should be avoided. Complex carbohydrates, starches, lean meats, and vegetables should be encouraged.

Children who demonstrate mild or moderate dehydration may require ORT at a rate of 50 to 100 mL/kg rapidly over a 3- to 4-hour period in addition to replacing fluid losses from vomiting or diarrhea (CDC, 2003a). Regular diet may be resumed as just described once the fluid deficit has been corrected. Once a dehydrated child has been rehydrated, resuming an age-appropriate diet enhances recovery (CDC, 2003a). Severe dehydration may require parenteral therapy and hospitalization.

Preventing the spread of infection is also essential for home care (Box 19-5). Good handwashing; the disinfection of contaminated linens, clothes, and diapers; and the use of surface disinfectant sprays are important preventive measures.

Evaluation

- Has the child returned to preinfection weight within 1 week after symptoms subside?
- Does the child have good skin turgor, moist mucous membranes, and a urine specific gravity of less than 1.030?
- Does the child have a serum sodium level of 135 to 145 mmol/L and a serum potassium level of 3.5 to 5 mmol/L?
- Is the child passing soft, formed stools without diarrhea, blood, or mucus?
- Are other family members free from infectious diarrhea, and is the family following the appropriate precautions to prevent transmission?
- Is the child reporting abdominal pain?
- Does the child guard the abdomen during palpation?
- Are parents and staff at the daycare facility practicing infection control procedures, if appropriate?
- Can the child tolerate an age-appropriate regular diet?
- Is the child's skin intact and free from irritated areas?

BOX 19-5 | **PARENTS WANT TO KNOW** About Care of the Child With Infectious Gastroenteritis

If your child has infectious gastroenteritis, you must do the following:
- Wash your hands frequently and thoroughly and insist that your child do so as well. Always wash your hands after changing diapers.
- Allow your child to use a separate bathroom if available.
- Continue to follow these measures for several weeks because bacterial diarrhea may be communicable for several weeks after symptoms disappear.
- Administer oral fluids with appropriate rehydration solutions (e.g., Rehydralyte) in small, frequent amounts (every 30 min). If your child is vomiting, administer 1 tsp of fluid every 5 to 10 minutes. Give one-half cup for each watery stool.
- Do not give your child fruit juices, cola, sports drinks, tea, or sugary drinks.

- Continue to feed your child but avoid high-fat or high-sugar foods. Breast milk and formula may be continued.
- Do not give over-the-counter medications without notifying your physician.

Call your physician if the following pertain:
- Your child is younger than 6 months.
- Your child has a fever.
- Diarrhea worsens.
- Diarrhea has blood in it.
- Vomiting increases or your child cannot keep down any fluid.
- Your child reports severe abdominal pain.
- Your child shows signs of dehydration, such as no tears, sunken eyes, or decreased urination.

PATHOPHYSIOLOGY

APPENDICITIS

Obstruction of the appendix allows normal mucus secretions to accumulate in the appendix, producing distention. Distention eventually causes occlusion of the capillaries and engorgement of the walls of the appendix. Microabscesses form and can progress to abscesses and fistulas. Perforation occurs as a result of tissue breakdown and swelling. Bowel contents then contaminate the mesenteric bed and peritoneum, leading to peritonitis and sepsis.

Appendicitis

Appendicitis is the inflammation and infection of the vermiform appendix, a small lymphoid, tubular, blind sac at the end of the cecum. It is the most common cause of emergency surgery in children and adolescents.

Etiology and Incidence

Common causes of obstruction and subsequent appendicitis include lymphoid swelling related to viral infection, impacted fecal material, foreign bodies, and parasites. In most cases no definitive cause can be identified at the time of surgery.

Appendicitis occurs with equal frequency in both sexes, with most cases occurring during adolescence and early adulthood. Appendicitis is uncommon in children younger than 4 years, but in young children it is associated with a high frequency of perforation by the time of the first visit, most likely related to the difficulty in establishing the diagnosis.

Manifestations and Diagnostic Evaluation

The cardinal symptom of appendicitis is pain, progressing in intensity and localizing to the right lower quadrant at McBurney point (Fig. 19-4). Associated signs and symptoms include nausea and vomiting, anorexia, diarrhea or constipation, and fever and chills. If the appendix perforates, the

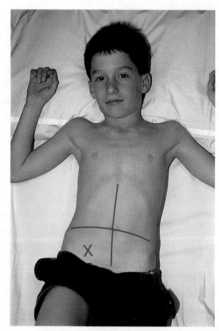

FIG 19-4 **McBurney point is midway between the right anterior superior iliac crest and the umbilicus. It is usually the location of greatest pain in the child with appendicitis.** *(Courtesy The University of Texas at Arlington School of Nursing.)*

child will initially experience relief of pain. Other signs and symptoms will worsen, so that the child will appear acutely ill with high fever and signs of dehydration.

The diagnosis is usually made on the basis of classic abdominal findings of pain localizing at McBurney point, guarding, rebound tenderness, nausea, vomiting, and fever. A WBC count of 15,000 to 20,000/mm^3 can support the clinical findings. A quick, safe, and accurate diagnosis can usually be made with ultrasound, which shows an enlarged, incompressible appendix that may be fluid filled and locally inflamed. This has also been shown to predict the severity of the disease (Kaneko & Tsuda, 2004).

CRITICAL TO REMEMBER
Assessing Appendicitis in the Young Child

Because symptoms of appendicitis can be vague and develop slowly over approximately a 12-hour period, the condition can be quite difficult to assess in young children. The complaint that "my tummy hurts" often is the only initial symptom. Appendicitis should be suspected if pain, anorexia, or nausea and vomiting and fever occur simultaneously. If pain occurs before vomiting, appendicitis should be suspected. However, if vomiting precedes abdominal pain, gastroenteritis is more likely. The young child will usually refuse to play, preferring instead to lie down. Often, the child will lie in a knee-chest position to be comfortable. One way of helping the child describe the pain focus is to ask the child to stand on tiptoes and then drop to flat feet. The pain location elicited from this maneuver usually will be in the right lower quadrant.

Therapeutic Management

The definitive treatment for appendicitis and suspected appendicitis is appendectomy. Preoperatively the child is managed with fluid therapy, immobilization to control pain, NPO status, and antibiotics. The procedure may be done laparoscopically or through an open abdominal approach if perforation is suspected.

NURSING CARE

The Child With Appendicitis

Assessment

The nursing assessment will reveal a history of pain, fever, vomiting, and diarrhea or constipation. The physical examination discloses abdominal tenderness and guarding. The child may assume a supine position with the right leg flexed to decrease tension on the abdominal wall. The nurse must be keenly aware of the symptoms of perforation, including a sudden relief from pain followed by an increase in pain, rigid abdomen, and early shock symptoms. Behavioral changes and refusal to eat are important indicators in infants.

Assess anxiety in the child and family members, who are most likely facing unexpected surgery. Because of the pain, the child may be uncooperative with abdominal assessment. The parents may have financial concerns related to the unplanned surgery.

Nursing Diagnosis and Planning

The following nursing diagnoses and expected outcomes may be appropriate after assessing the child with appendicitis:

- Acute Pain related to abdominal inflammation and surgical incision.

  Expected Outcome: The child will be free from pain, as evidenced by resumption of normal activity and movement with no reports of pain.

- Risk for Infection related to rupture and surgery.

  Expected Outcomes: The child will have a clean, dry surgical incision that is free from redness, heat, or exudate, and the child will be afebrile with a WBC count of 5,000 to 15,000/mm^3.

- Deficient Fluid Volume related to vomiting or diarrhea.

  Expected Outcome: The child will be well hydrated, as evidenced by moist mucous membranes, good skin turgor, and hourly urine output appropriate for age (see Chapter 18).

- Anxiety related to unplanned surgery.

  Expected Outcomes: The parent or child will express feelings about surgery and will verbalize the need for emergency hospitalization.

Interventions

Uncomplicated Appendicitis

On admission, vital signs should be taken to monitor for sepsis or shock. Institute comfort measures, including topical cold application, pain medications, and positions of comfort. Enemas or laxatives should not be administered. No heat should be applied to the abdomen because it may increase the chance of perforation as a result of vasodilation. IV fluid therapy is started to prepare the child for surgery and correct any existing acid-base disturbance related to vomiting and diarrhea.

If the procedure is performed by laparoscopy, the nurse can expect the child to be discharged within 24 hours. Open surgery may be followed by several days of recovery in the hospital. After either operation, the child will be on NPO status until bowel function has returned.

Ruptured Appendix

The child with a ruptured appendix needs special care (Fig. 19-5). If perforation is suspected, prepare the child for NG tube insertion. The NG tube provides decompression before surgery and allows gastric content drainage postoperatively. The child will need IV antibiotics, which may be started preoperatively. For the child with a perforation, IV antibiotics are continued and hospitalization may last 5 to 14 days. During this time and after the NG tube is removed, the diet should be advanced gradually as tolerated so that the child can tolerate a normal diet without vomiting or diarrhea.

Depending on the extent of the peritonitis, the child is likely to have postoperative incisional drains. These drains may be attached to suction, and aseptic technique and maintenance of patency are essential. Carefully document the drainage amount each shift. The wound is often left open and treated with sterile wet-to-dry (saline-soaked gauze) dressings and wound irrigation with antibacterial solutions.

Round-the-clock opioid analgesics provide relief from incisional pain and from pain caused by frequent dressing changes (see Chapters 14 and 15). Continued reassessment of abdominal pain is essential for evaluating the presence of abscess or fistula.

Monitor vital signs, including temperature, every 2 to 4 hours. NG suction will likely be continued postoperatively until normal bowel sounds return. Positioning the child to

APPENDECTOMY-PERFORATED
(Uncomplicated-without multi-system problems)
ICD-9 Codes 540.0 and 540.1

Expected LOS-5 Days
D#.#=Key interventions for this study.

Examples of appropriate Co-morbidities
Otitis Media
Acute Sinusitis
Pharyngitis
chronic illness not in active stage

Examples of Co-morbidities that are not appropriate:
HIV
Pneumonia
Sickle Cell
Hemophilia
Immuno-compromised patients
cardiac patients
reflux
oncology diagnoses

Refer to Variance Sheet for Recording

Aspect of Care	Admission Day Date___ Unit___ ED/OR_____	Day 2 Date___Unit___	Day 3 Date___Unit___	Day 4 Date___Unit___	Day 5 Date___Unit___
DAILY OUTCOME			Ambulating	NG tube out	Afebrile Discharge *(D 7.1 If not d/c by* *Day 7. record on* *tracking sheet)*
TESTS	CBC BUN, Cr Sonogram (if ind)	BUN,Cr		CBC (+/-)	CBC (+/-)
CONSULTS	Surgeon		Consider Home Health		
FLUID/ELECTROLY TE MANAGEMENT	Strict I&O	Strict I&O	Routine I&O	Routine I&O	Routine I&O
TREATMENTS/ PROCEDURES	Appendectomy NG Irrigation Wound Care	NG Irrigation Wound Care	NG Irrigation Wound Care	Wound Care	Wound Care
MEDICATIONS	IV (pump, site check) *D1.1 Gentamicin* *w/* *Clindamycin q 8* *hrs.* *+/-Ampicillin q 6* *hrs* *+/- Mefoxin q 6* *hrs.* *Methadone or* *morphine for pain.*	IV (pump, site check) *D2.1 Gentamicin* *w/* *Clindamycin q 8* *hrs.* *+/-Ampicillin q 6* *hrs* *+/- Mefoxin q 6* *hrs.* *Methadone or* *morphine for pain.*	IV (pump, site check) *D3.1 Gentamicin* *w/* *Clindamycin q 8* *hrs.* *+/-Ampicillin q 6* *hrs* *+/- Mefoxin q 6* *hrs.* *Methadone or* *morphine for pain.*	IV (pump, site check) *D4.1 Gentamicin* *w/* *Clindamycin q 8* *hrs.* *+/-Ampicillin q 6* *hrs* *+/- Mefoxin q 6* *hrs.* *Methadone or* *morphine for pain.*	Hep lock *D5.1 Gentamicin* *w/* *Clindamycin q 8* *hrs.* *+/-Ampicillin q 6* *hrs* *+/- Mefoxin q 6* *hrs.* *Methadone or* *morphine for pain* *Analgesics p.o. if* *tol.*
CLINICAL SUPPORT	NPO Parent Support Bed/Chair Extra Patient Checks Routine Safety	NPO Parent Support Chair Routine Safety	NPO Parent Support Ambulate Routine Safety	NPO/Cl liq (+/-) Parent Support Ambulate Routine Safety	Full liq/Regular Parent Support Ambulate Routine Safety Pain Control Wound Care Activity Follow-up Visit

Original 7/22/1994   Revised 11/2/1995 5/1/97

Disclaimer: This clinical pathway is provided as a general guideline for use by physicians and staff in planning the care and treatment of patients and their families. **It is not intended to be and does not establish a standard of care.** Each patient's care is individualized according to specific needs.

Cook Children's Medical Center
M:\WPFILES\PATHWAYS\APPYPERF.WPD

This pathway is not a permanent part of the patient's medical record.

FIG 19-5   **Clinical pathway for a child undergoing an appendectomy.** *(Courtesy Cook Children's Medical Center, Fort Worth, TX.)*

facilitate drainage and minimize the spread of infection into the upper abdomen should be done by elevating the head of the bed or having the child lie on the operative side.

Home Care

After surgery and discharge, parents must be prepared to assume responsibility for the child's care. The surgical incision and any drain sites must be assessed for redness, drainage, dehiscence, or suture infections. Report any problems to the physician. Parents should advance the child's diet slowly, beginning with liquids and soft foods and progressing to the child's normal diet if tolerated without nausea or vomiting. Teach parents to watch for vomiting, abdominal pain, or distention as possible signs of bowel obstruction or peritoneal infection.

Evaluation

- Does the child report pain?
- Does the child demonstrate guarding on abdominal palpation?
- Has the child returned to normal activity level?
- Is the surgical incision clean, dry, and free from redness, heat, purulent drainage, or dehiscence?

- Is the child afebrile, with a WBC count of 5,000 to 15,000/mm³?
- Is the child tolerating an age-appropriate regular diet without vomiting, diarrhea, or increased abdominal pain?
- Are the child and parents able to express relief from anxiety?

Inflammatory Bowel Disease

Inflammatory bowel disease is a chronic inflammatory condition of the small or large intestine. It includes two distinct conditions: ulcerative colitis and Crohn disease. Ulcerative colitis affects only the colon and involves both the mucosal and submucosal layers of the intestine. Crohn disease can occur anywhere in the GI tract, from the mouth to the anus, and is transmural, involving all layers of the intestine.

Etiology

The exact cause of inflammatory bowel disease is not known. Several triggers have been identified, including viral and other infectious agents, food allergies, vasculitis, increased

---

PATHOPHYSIOLOGY

INFLAMMATORY BOWEL DISEASE

The triggering factor, whether viral, allergic, or immunologic, causes the bowel to "respond" as if to an injury and results in capillary vasoconstriction and histamine release within the bowel. The histamine has two effects on the bowel. The first is *vasodilation,* which results in swelling that can cause malabsorption by distorting the surface area of the villi. Swelling then produces cell death and

ulceration, which can progress to the development of fissures, strictures, fistulas, adhesions, and bowel obstruction. The second effect of histamine release is *increased capillary permeability,* which results in increased fluid in the intestine and subsequent diarrhea. Crohn disease affects all layers of the bowel; ulcerative colitis affects the mucosa and submucosa only.

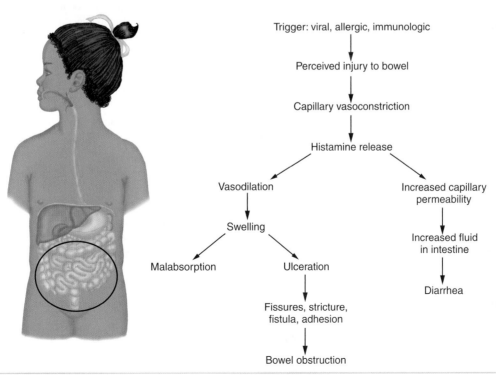

intestinal permeability, immunologic dysfunction, and genetic factors. Increasing evidence demonstrates a connection between inflammatory bowel disease and the effects of stress on the immune response.

Incidence, Manifestations, and Diagnostic Evaluation

The incidence, manifestations, and diagnostic evaluation for both ulcerative colitis and Crohn disease are summarized in Table 19-4.

Therapeutic Management

Management for inflammatory bowel disease is multidimensional and includes medication, dietary and nutritional support, and symptomatic treatment. Pharmacologic treatment includes anti-inflammatory, antibacterial, antibiotic, and immunosuppressive drugs. The principal medications used to treat inflammatory bowel disease include the following:

- 5-Aminosalicylic acid (5-ASA) medications such as sulfasalazine

- Corticosteroids such as prednisone
- Immune-modulating agents such as azathioprine, 6-mercaptopurine (6-MP), methotrexate, and cyclosporin A
- Tumor necrosis factor-α antibody (Infliximab)
- Antibiotics such as metronidazole (Flagyl) and ciprofloxacin

Infliximab (Remicade) has been approved for treatment of ulcerative colitis and Crohn disease in children. It binds to tumor necrosis factor-α to decrease inflammation and increase intestinal healing. It has been shown to be effective in moderate to severe acute disease (Eidelwein, Cuffari, Abadom, & Oliva-Hemker, 2005; Russell & Katz, 2004). It is safe with mild reactions that respond rapidly to intervention (Friesen et al., 2004).

5-ASA and 6-MP are first-line immunosuppressants that allow selected patients with Crohn disease to avoid steroids and their side effects.

For ulcerative colitis, avoidance of milk products and ingestion of a hypoallergenic, low-fiber, low-fat, low-residue, high-protein, elemental diet can be useful. Elemental diets

---

TABLE 19-4   Crohn Disease and Ulcerative Colitis

Crohn Disease	Ulcerative Colitis
Pathophysiology	**Pathophysiology**
Affects entire GI tract, most common in the terminal ileum	Involves only colon, starting at the rectum and moving upward
Transmural involvement	Mucosa and submucosa only
Cobblestone appearance of mucosa	Mucosa lacking in most cases
Fistulas common	Fistulas rare
Remissions and exacerbations	Remissions uncommon
Diagnostic Evaluation: Colonoscopy, Rectoscopy, Barium Enema, Biopsy	
"Skip" lesions with deep fissures and granulomas	Continuous spreading with superficial ulceration
Normal	No normal mucous membrane
Incidence	
5 per 100,000 and increasing	5 per 100,000
Equal gender distribution	Equal gender distribution
Not seen in infants; peaks in teens, early 20s	Peaks between ages 15 and 40 yr
Clusters in families	Clusters in families
Associated with higher standard of living	Affects whites more than others
Clinical Manifestations	
Abdominal pain	Abdominal pain unusual
Diarrhea, nonbloody	Diarrhea, occasionally with hemorrhage and anemia
Fever	
Palpable abdominal mass	No masses
Anorexia and severe weight loss	Moderate weight loss
Significant growth impairment	Mild growth impairment
Perianal and anal lesions	Perianal and anal lesions rare
Fistulas and obstructions	Fistulas and obstructions rare
Extraintestinal symptoms (arthralgia, arthritis)	Risk of toxic megacolon
Morbidity and Mortality	
Life expectancy not reduced	12%-15% mortality rate
50%-70% will eventually require surgery for obstruction or fistula	10% chance of cancer after 10 yr
Surgery does not cure disease	Removal of colon cures intestinal disease

may be as useful as corticosteroids in inducing remission in children (Rayhorn & Rayhorn, 2002). These diets may include Tolerex, Vivonex, Peptamen, or Modulen. Nutritional therapy is a useful component with no side effects. Total parenteral nutrition (TPN) may be needed during acute flareups or surgery to maintain nutritional support. Total colectomy is the only true cure.

Crohn disease is best managed before permanent structural changes have developed. Malnutrition is a common problem and can involve protein, fat, carbohydrate, and vitamin deficiencies. Nutritional support and teaching are essential. Surgery is not curative but may be necessary to treat abscesses, fistulas, or chronic recurrent obstruction. Bowel resection is the usual procedure.

NURSING CARE

The Child With Inflammatory Bowel Disease

Assessment

Recurrent or chronic diarrhea is the primary finding in the nursing history of a child with inflammatory bowel disease. The major assessment findings are related to this diarrhea and the associated malabsorption that occurs. Weight loss, dehydration, anorexia, growth failure, vitamin deficiencies, and anemia are common. The severity of the GI symptoms and the amount and length of steroid use will have a significant influence on a child's growth rate. Remissions and exacerbations of symptoms are common. Frank bleeding is possible in ulcerative colitis. Intermittent cramping discomfort exacerbated by eating is common in Crohn disease. The child with Crohn disease may have oral lesions and perianal skin breakdown.

Inflammatory changes also can occur outside the GI system. Arthralgia and arthritis, especially of the lower extremities, can cause discomfort and mobility problems.

Depression, anxiety, fears about social interactions, and low self-esteem occur and are most likely related to the need to have quick access to restrooms at all times and to be close to home if an accident occurs. The chronic nature of this condition and its unknown prognosis can lead to family stress and tax the family's financial resources and support systems. Assessment should include questions about family and peer support, resources, and knowledge about the disease.

Nursing Diagnosis and Planning

The following nursing diagnoses and expected outcomes may be appropriate for the child with inflammatory bowel disease as well as the child's family:

- Imbalanced Nutrition: Less Than Body Requirements related to chronic malabsorption.

  Expected Outcomes: The child will have acceptable bowel patterns, as evidenced by passing no more than four stools per day and being free from nocturnal diarrhea; the child will receive adequate nutrition, as evidenced by normal hemoglobin values and normal growth that follows the growth curve.

- Acute Pain related to cramping.

  Expected Outcome: The child will be free from abdominal pain, as evidenced by resumption of normal activity and no reports of pain.

- Chronic Low Self-Esteem related to chronic diarrhea and colostomy.

  Expected Outcome: The child will have a positive self-concept, as evidenced by leading an active lifestyle without depression.

- Delayed Growth and Development related to malnutrition, chronic illness, and steroid use.

  Expected Outcome: The child will meet normal developmental milestones, as evidenced by progress on standard developmental screenings.

- Disturbed Body Image related to weight loss, water retention from steroid therapy, and colostomy or ileostomy.

  Expected Outcome: The child will state reasons for changes in body appearance and will share concerns about changes with family and support personnel.

- Anxiety related to chronic diarrhea and risk for surgery.

  Expected Outcomes: The child will express concerns about the future and will contact support services as needed.

- Deficient Knowledge related to management of chronic disease.

  Expected Outcomes: The child will explain day-to-day management of disease and will demonstrate ability for self-care that is age appropriate.

Interventions

Nursing interventions focus on maintaining pharmacologic interventions, developing long-term nutritional management, educating, and providing emotional support.

Medications

Teaching appropriate administration of medications is an important nursing role. Enemas are used before critical diagnostic tests and as a method of medication administration. Any child who will be taking steroids (see Chapter 17) needs to understand the importance of regular administration. Steroids should be given with food or antacids if GI distress becomes a problem. The steroids, although beneficial in suppressing symptoms, may actually exacerbate the growth delays associated with inflammatory bowel disease.

Nutritional Management

Nutritional support varies with the disease and the child's tolerance of changes. In general, maintaining a low-fiber, low-residue, low-fat, milk-free elemental diet provides some relief, although strict restrictions do not alleviate symptoms. A balanced, nutritious diet is recommended, as are vitamin, iron, and folate supplements.

During acute flareups or surgery, TPN and lipids may be needed to restore a seriously malnourished child. These interventions do not change the course of the inflammation in the bowel but provide essential nutritional support. Elemental diets, which can be absorbed without significant digestion, may be used during acute episodes of Crohn disease to allow the bowel to rest. NG or gastrostomy tube feedings during the night may be necessary during puberty to prevent further growth impairment (see Chapter 13).

Continued assessments of nutritional status, growth patterns, and development are important elements of nursing care for children with this chronic problem. Assessing the number of stools, nutritional status, weight, developmental milestones, and pain will help evaluate the child's response to treatment.

Family Education and Support

Appropriate community resources can provide education and support. The Crohn's and Colitis Foundation of America supplies educational materials and family information on local resources and support groups (see Evolve website). Long-term nursing care can be improved by providing consistent caregivers and encouraging the child to form relationships. Self-care and management should be major goals in working with children with inflammatory bowel disease, as with other chronic diseases. A team approach that includes medical, educational, rehabilitative, and psychological support is essential for success.

The parents and child will assume responsibility for home care. Because Crohn disease is a long-term health problem with numerous medical, pharmacologic, and surgical interventions required, family support and financial resources can be strained to the limit. National and local support groups may be able to give essential support to the family in these areas. In addition, emotional support for caregivers becomes quite important.

Another important resource for children with inflammatory bowel disease is Camp MAGIC (Many Adventures at GI Camp), Children's Medical Center of Dallas, 1935 Motor Street, Dallas, TX 75235.

Home Care

Home care is a mainstay of treatment. Teaching parents to administer steroids, including providing information on their inherent side effects and the importance of not discontinuing their use abruptly, should be a high priority. Also teach techniques of enema administration and skin care for perianal lesions. Nutrition diaries can provide useful information. TPN may be administered at home, and parents need complete instructions.

In addition, helping children and parents know when to seek care is important. Sudden exacerbations of symptoms, weight loss, blood loss, and severe abdominal pain should be reported to health care professionals. Stress management and the avoidance of triggers can help minimize the symptoms of the disease and its impact on the child.

Evaluation

- Is the child free from nocturnal diarrhea?
- Is the child passing fewer than four stools per day?
- Is the child gaining weight appropriately and following the growth chart?
- Is the child's hemoglobin value between 11 g/dL and 16 g/dL?
- Does the child report abdominal pain?
- Does the child participate in age-appropriate activities without evidence of depression?
- Is the child's development normal for age?
- Is the child able to share body image concerns with appropriate family members?
- Has the child or family sought external support through appropriate referral groups?
- Do the child and parent demonstrate appropriate skills for day-to-day management and make appropriate future plans for long-term management of disease?
- Do the child and family seek help when exacerbations occur?
- Does the child manage self-care age appropriately?

OBSTRUCTIVE DISORDERS
Hypertrophic Pyloric Stenosis

Pyloric stenosis results when the circular area of muscle surrounding the pylorus hypertrophies and obstructs gastric emptying. This condition is one of the most common surgical disorders of early infancy.

Etiology and Incidence

The exact cause of pyloric stenosis remains unknown, but muscular hypertrophy is not present at birth. Pyloric stenosis may be associated with other GI anomalies such as malrotation, short-gut syndrome, esophageal and duodenal atresia, anorectal anomalies, hiatal hernia, and GER. Heredity and family predisposition seem to increase the risk of pyloric stenosis.

The incidence of pyloric stenosis is 3 in 1000 births (NBDPN, 2004). Children and offspring of an affected parent are at highest risk. Male infants are affected more often than female infants, and term infants are affected more often than premature infants. The incidence is also higher in white infants than in African-American or Asian infants.

Manifestations

Progressive projectile, nonbilious vomiting in a previously healthy infant is the major manifestation of pyloric stenosis. The vomitus may become blood tinged if esophageal irritation occurs. A movable, palpable, firm, olive-shaped mass is felt in the right upper quadrant. This mass is most easily palpated when the stomach is empty and the infant is relaxed. Deep gastric peristaltic waves from left upper quadrant to right upper quadrant may be visible immediately before vomiting. The infant will be irritable and hungry a short time after being fed. If the condition progresses, the infant may become dehydrated and experience metabolic alkalosis.

Diagnostic Evaluation

The diagnosis is made on the basis of a history of vomiting, visible peristaltic waves, and a palpable pyloric mass. When the mass cannot be palpated, radiography and

---

PATHOPHYSIOLOGY

HYPERTROPHIC PYLORIC STENOSIS

Pyloric spasms cause milk curds to be propelled against a narrowed pyloric channel and subsequently irritate its sensitive mucosal lining. Edema of the pyloric mucosa results. This edema further reduces the size of the pyloric canal and creates resistance to the flow of milk. To promote gastric emptying and compensate for this resistance, the pylorus contracts with more force and gradually enlarges. This enlarged pyloric muscle slowly begins to constrict the pyloric channel, and when the mucosal edema subsides the resistance to flow still remains. A vicious cycle develops and progresses to a high-level obstruction of the pyloric canal.

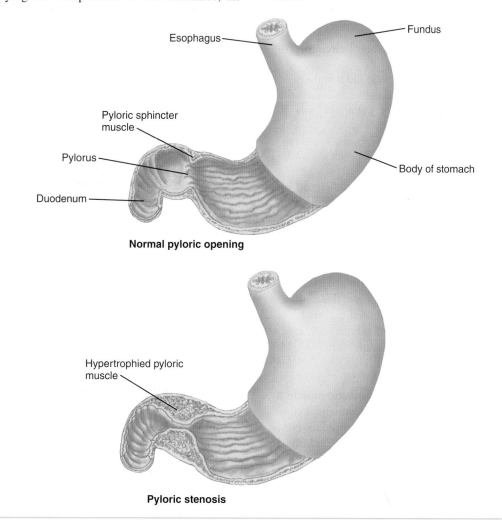

Esophagus — Fundus

Pyloric sphincter muscle

Pylorus —

Duodenum —

— Body of stomach

Normal pyloric opening

Hypertrophied pyloric muscle —

Pyloric stenosis

---

ultrasonography are helpful. A flat plate of the abdomen will show a narrow pylorus with a dilated stomach and the absence of gas distal to the pylorus. Ultrasonography can confirm the presence of a pyloric mass. A barium swallow examination will disclose the long, narrow pyloric canal and detect delayed gastric emptying. Laboratory findings may indicate metabolic alkalosis as a result of vomiting, including decreased serum potassium and sodium levels, increased pH and bicarbonate, and a decreased chloride level. Indirect bilirubin may be elevated.

Therapeutic Management

Because pyloric stenosis is usually diagnosed early, few infants are seen in advanced stages of dehydration, malnutrition, and alkalosis. If present, these conditions must be corrected before surgery. An infant who is slightly dehydrated with a total serum or plasma carbon dioxide (CO_2) of 25 mEq/L or less or an infant who is moderately dehydrated with a CO_2 of 26 to 35 mEq/L is managed with replacement parenteral fluids and electrolytes and an NG tube for stomach decompression. Once the stomach is empty, most

**Gathering Information from a
Parent about Infant Vomiting**

Eliciting a description of the amount and characteristics of vomiting can be difficult because descriptive terms are nonspecific and estimation of amounts is very inconsistent. Useful questions include the following:

- Could you wipe the vomitus off the child with a diaper or cloth?
- Did it require a change of clothes for the infant or caregiver?
- If it was on a bed or sheet, how big a circle did it make?
- If it was on the floor, how big a circle did it make?
- Did it happen after every feeding?
- Did it look like what was just eaten, or was it curdled?
- What color was it?
- Did it appear to be under force and projected away from the child?

Encouraging the parents to keep a written record of answers to these questions can provide essential assessment information.

infants will stop vomiting. Surgery is usually delayed 24 to 48 hours until fluid and electrolyte deficits and the acid-base balance are corrected. Severely dehydrated and malnourished infants with CO_2 levels above 35 mEq/L may need a 3- to 5-day course of IV fluids, electrolyte replacement, and infusions of plasma or packed red blood cells (RBCs) before surgical repair.

A *pyloromyotomy*, an incision of the pyloric muscle to release the obstruction, is the definitive treatment. Pyloromyotomy is not considered an emergency procedure but is usually performed without delay in well-hydrated infants. It is usually performed laparoscopically.

NURSING CARE

The Child With Hypertrophic Pyloric Stenosis

Assessment

Hypertrophic pyloric stenosis is suspected in infants with a history of projectile vomiting, especially after meals. A thorough nursing history includes the infant's feeding schedule with the type, amount, and frequency of fluid taken. Determine and document the relation of feedings to vomiting. Vomiting is assessed for frequency, amount, color, and consistency as well as projection.

Assess for signs of dehydration, such as the absence of tears, a weak cry, a depressed fontanel, poor skin turgor, and dry mucous membranes. Signs of potassium, sodium, and chloride depletion should be noted. The abdomen is checked for distention, tenderness, bowel sounds, the presence of a pyloric mass, or gastric peristaltic waves. Assess family members for their understanding of the disorder, a viable support system, and the ability to participate in their child's care.

Nursing Diagnosis and Planning

The following nursing diagnoses and expected outcomes are appropriate after assessment of the child with hypertrophic pyloric stenosis:

- Deficient Fluid Volume related to vomiting.

  Expected Outcomes: The infant will have a balanced intake and output, be free of signs of dehydration, and have a urine output greater than 2 to 3 mL/kg per hour.

- Imbalanced Nutrition: Less Than Body Requirements related to persistent vomiting.

  Expected Outcomes: The infant will tolerate regular feedings and will continue to show growth according to a growth chart.

- Impaired Skin Integrity and Risk for Infection related to a surgical incisions.

  Expected Outcome: The infant will have clean, dry, intact incisions without redness or exudate.

- Deficient Knowledge related to insufficient information about the need for surgery or about pyloric stenosis.

  Expected Outcomes: The parents will describe pyloric stenosis and the expected preoperative and postoperative care and will assume total care of the infant before discharge.

- Acute Pain related to surgery.

  Expected Outcomes: The child will not exhibit guarding to palpation and will be calm and content in parent's arms. The parent will be confident that the infant is pain free.

- Anxiety (parental) related to need for hospitalization and surgery.

  Expected Outcomes: The parent will express feelings about the surgery and will list the reasons the infant needs to be hospitalized.

Interventions

Preoperative Care

Preoperatively, the infant is on NPO status and is stabilized with IV fluids and electrolytes. Measuring the vital signs, weighing the infant daily, and monitoring laboratory values and intake and output are essential nursing interventions. Intake and output should include all IV and PO fluids, blood products, emesis, urine output, stools, and NG drainage. Keep the dehydrated infant warm and quiet. The nurse should provide oral care because membranes are more susceptible to breakdown in their dehydrated state.

Elevate the head of the bed to reduce the risk of aspiration. Use blankets or towel rolls to maintain desired position. The NG tube should be patent and properly positioned. Record the amount, color, and type of drainage. Assess for respiratory distress.

Explain procedures and plans to parents. Encourage their participation in holding and caring for their infant.

Postoperative Care

Postoperatively, the care varies with each surgeon. Most surgeons remove the NG tube immediately and order feedings within the first 4 to 6 hours after surgery if bowel sounds are normal. Because gastric peristalsis is normally depressed for 12 to 18 hours after the pyloromyotomy, others delay feedings for 24 hours and leave the NG tube in place.

Feeding is started with small amounts of an oral electrolyte solution, such as Pedialyte, and the amount is slowly increased. Formula is offered in half-strength concentrations and advanced to full strength within 48 hours after surgery. If the child is receiving breast milk, dilution is not necessary. Feedings are not advanced until the child can tolerate the previous amount without vomiting. IV fluids are continued until the infant is taking and retaining sufficient amounts of formula or breast milk. Many infants have some vomiting during the early postoperative periods, but it is usually temporary and without complications.

Ad lib feedings within 6 hours postoperatively are now being recommended to decrease time to full diet and discharge, but these protocols vary by institution (Morash, 2002).

Postoperative nursing care follows the same guidelines as preoperative care, with accurate monitoring of all vital signs, laboratory values, respiratory problems, and hydration. In addition, the nurse assesses the small surgical or laparoscopic incisions for redness, swelling, or drainage. Encourage parents to participate as much as possible in their infant's care, but they may need emotional support in the unfamiliar environment of the hospital.

Home Care

Because symptoms normally abate in the immediate postoperative period, parents may find taking care of their infant much easier than before repair. They need to be instructed, however, to report any excessive vomiting, abdominal tenderness, fever, incisional redness, or drainage. If the child is discharged before the diet has been advanced to full strength, written instructions for advancing the diet are essential.

Evaluation

- Does the child have a flat fontanel, good skin turgor, moist mucous membranes, a urine specific gravity of less than 1.030, and a sodium level within normal limits?
- Is the child tolerating oral feedings without vomiting?
- Has the child's weight returned to preillness level within 1 week?
- Is the surgical site clean, dry, intact, and without drainage or redness?
- Can the parents explain the need for surgery and routine preoperative and postoperative care?
- Is the child calm, content, and free from pain?
- Have the parents assumed all care responsibilities at home without assistance?

CRITICAL THINKING EXERCISE 19-1

Andrew, age 5 weeks, is seen in the outpatient clinic of a large hospital. This is his first visit to the clinic since birth. Andrew's mother states that Andrew is her first child and that she has been concerned that Andrew "spits up" so much. She states she called the clinic approximately 2 weeks ago, but the nurse told her that all babies spit up and that she could talk with someone when she came in for Andrew's 1-month checkup. She missed the appointment because she could not get a ride to the clinic. She further states that the "spitting up" has increased, and for the past 2 days she has not been sure whether Andrew was keeping any of his feedings in his stomach; he has also been very fussy. After several unsuccessful attempts to speak to someone at the clinic by phone, she decided to bring Andrew in to be seen.

1. What will be your priority nursing action?
2. Identify two issues that you should address with Andrew's mother related to seeking care when health care information is needed.

Intussusception

Intussusception is an invagination of a section of the intestine into the distal bowel that causes bowel obstruction. In children, this condition most often occurs as a section of terminal ileum telescopes into the ascending colon through the ileocecal valve. It is the most common cause of bowel obstruction in children younger than 2 years (Wyllie, 2004a). Although relatively rare, it does represent a pediatric emergency with classic assessment findings.

Etiology and Incidence

In young children, the cause of intussusception is unknown. Contributing factors include a preexisting upper respiratory tract infection or other viral infection. A pathologic condition within the colon, such as a mass or anatomic defect, is the most likely cause in children older than 6 years.

Intussusception generally affects infants and young children, with most cases occurring before age 2 years and rarely before 3 months. This incidence is 1 to 4 per 1,000 births, but the condition is more common in children with celiac disease and cystic fibrosis (Wyllie, 2004a). The male/female ratio is 4:1. Recurrence is a risk.

Manifestations and Diagnostic Evaluation

Intussusception occurs in children who are well nourished and without a history of GI problems. Paroxysms of pain occur, subside, and recur during the first several hours and then progress to a more constant severe pain. The child may vomit. The following are classic signs of intussusception:

- Passage of bloody mucus ("currant jelly") stool and diarrhea, which may not occur until the postoperative period
- A sausage-shaped abdominal mass

Symptoms of shock and sepsis are present if obstruction has been present for longer than 12 to 24 hours. The child

PATHOPHYSIOLOGY

INTUSSUSCEPTION

As the bowel telescopes inside itself, obstruction develops. In addition, the mesenteric vessels become trapped between the walls of the two layers, and ischemia occurs. This pressure on the bowel leads to bleeding and "currant jelly" stools. Mesenteric ischemia also causes edema and possible strangulation or infarction of the bowel, which can progress to perforation, peritonitis, sepsis, shock, and death.

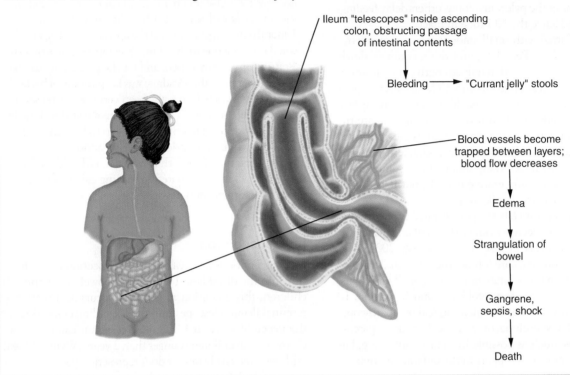

Ileum "telescopes" inside ascending colon, obstructing passage of intestinal contents

Bleeding ⟶ "Currant jelly" stools

Blood vessels become trapped between layers; blood flow decreases

Edema

Strangulation of bowel

Gangrene, sepsis, shock

Death

may be listless. Older children may have pain without other symptoms.

Abdominal radiographs may show abnormal gas patterns related to the bowel obstruction or a soft tissue mass. Ultrasonography is useful in identifying the location of the intussusception and the amount of edema in the area. A definitive diagnosis can be made and treatment provided simultaneously with a barium enema or air enema examination.

Therapeutic Management

The goal of treatment is to restore the bowel to its normal position and function as quickly as possible. In children who do not show symptoms of shock or sepsis, attempts at hydrostatic reduction are made with a barium or air enema until free flow of barium into the terminal ileum is evident. This procedure can be performed in approximately 80% of cases. Ultrasound-guided isotonic saline enema may also be used (Wyllie, 2004a). If reduction fails or findings indicate damage to the bowel, immediate surgery is performed. If the intussusception is detected and reduced within 24 hours, morbidity is minimal. Laparoscopy is now being used if the enema fails to reduce the intussusception except where bowel necrosis is present.

NURSING CARE

The Child With Intussusception

Assessment

The nursing history typically reveals a previously healthy infant who suddenly began crying and flexing the legs in severe pain. This problem may resolve, only to recur a short time later and become more constant. Assess any child with the following signs for indicators of bowel obstruction: vomiting, nausea, distention, and hypoactive or hyperactive bowel sounds. A palpable abdominal mass and passage of "currant jelly" stools will help confirm the diagnosis. Assess the child's hydration status on admission. Fever, an increased heart rate, changes in level of consciousness or blood pressure, and respiratory distress should be reported immediately as possible indicators of sepsis or peritonitis.

Nursing Diagnosis and Planning

The following nursing diagnoses and expected outcomes may be appropriate for the child with intussusception and the family:

• Ineffective Tissue Perfusion (GI) related to bowel compression.

Expected Outcome: The child will have a patent bowel, as evidenced by the passage of soft, formed, Hematest-negative stools.

- Acute Pain related to bowel obstruction and surgery.

Expected Outcomes: The child will be free from abdominal pain, as evidenced by age-appropriate play and activity, and will not exhibit guarding during palpation.

- Deficient Fluid Volume related to vomiting and diarrhea.

Expected Outcomes: The child will tolerate age-appropriate food and fluids without vomiting or recurrence of symptoms and will be free from fluid and electrolyte disturbances, as evidenced by return to normal weight, moist mucous membranes, good skin turgor, and normal serum sodium level and hematocrit.

- Deficient Knowledge related to possibility of surgery and the need for immediate intervention.

Expected Outcomes: The parents will verbalize an understanding of the need for immediate intervention and will explain the mechanisms of intussusception and hydrostatic reduction.

- Anxiety (parental) related to the child's hospitalization or possible surgery.

Expected Outcomes: The parents will express concerns and fears and will seek appropriate support as needed.

- Disturbed Sleep Pattern related to colicky abdominal pain.

Expected Outcome: The child will return to normal sleep patterns.

Interventions

Once the diagnosis is made, immediate plans are made to admit the child to the hospital for hydrostatic reduction. Prompt assessment for dehydration, shock, or sepsis is essential, including documenting mental status, capillary perfusion, and urine output. The child is given IV fluids, and an NG tube is inserted if distention is present. During reduction, pain medications or sedation may be needed to decrease spasm. After reduction, clear liquids are started and the diet is advanced gradually as tolerated.

Observe for the passage of barium, and note the characteristics of stool. Also note the recurrence of previous symptoms of bowel obstruction; the risk of recurrence after nonsurgical reduction is approximately 10%. Resumption of a normal diet and normal activity and the passage of stool without blood indicate a successful outcome. If hydrostatic reduction is unsuccessful, the child must be prepared for abdominal surgery or laparoscopy. If hydrostatic reduction is unsuccessful, continue to monitor for return of normal bowel function because spontaneous resolution could occur, eliminating the need for surgery.

Postoperatively, the child is kept on NPO status until bowel function returns. NG suction and IV therapy, pain medications, maintenance of respiratory function, frequent assessment, and meeting developmental needs remain nursing responsibilities.

During this difficult time for parents, relieving their anxiety by providing appropriate information is essential. This effort should include a description of the pathophysiology of intussusception, the usefulness of hydrostatic reduction, and the expected recovery care for their child, including the need for IV fluids, NG suction, and frequent vital sign checks and assessments. In addition, emotional support can be provided by encouraging them to participate in their child's care, listening to their concerns, and encouraging expression of their feelings during this stressful time.

To help parents understand intussusception, use a hospital glove. As you press one finger (representing the terminal ileum) into the inflated glove (the distal colon) and cause it to go inside itself, the parents can visualize the telescoping. The same mechanism can show how hydrostatic reduction works. As you press on the glove (the distal portion) with your hand, you can see and feel how the telescoped portion is pushed back to its normal position.

Evaluation

- In the preoperative period, does the child have moist mucous membranes, good skin turgor, and a urine specific gravity of less than 1.030?
- Is the child passing soft, formed, Hematest-negative stools?
- Does the infant guard the abdomen during palpation?
- Is the child demonstrating age-appropriate activity levels, sleep patterns, and play?
- Is the child tolerating age-appropriate food and fluids without vomiting or recurrence of symptoms?
- Can the parents explain the rationale for hydrostatic reduction?
- Are all the parents' questions answered to their satisfaction?
- Are the parents able to resume care of their infant without stress or anxiety?
- Has the child returned to normal sleep patterns?

Volvulus

Volvulus is a condition caused by a malrotation or twisting of the bowel that results in a bowel obstruction. It is the result of a defect in fetal development in which the midgut, which normally rotates 270 degrees around the superior mesenteric artery, fails to rotate and fixes itself to the abdominal wall.

Affected infants usually manifest pain, bilious vomiting, and other signs of bowel obstruction. Surgery is essential to prevent bowel ischemia. The nursing care is similar to that for the child with intussusception who has undergone surgery.

Hirschsprung Disease

Also known as *congenital aganglionosis* or *megacolon*, Hirschsprung disease is the result of an absence of ganglion cells in the rectum and, to varying degrees, upward in the colon. Hirschsprung disease is the major cause of lower bowel obstruction in newborns (Wyllie, 2004b).

PATHOPHYSIOLOGY

HIRSCHSPRUNG DISEASE

Ganglia provide parasympathetic innervation of the colon. In Hirschsprung disease, ganglia are absent from a variable length of colon extending proximally from the anus. Adequate peristalsis cannot occur in the affected colon, leading to a tonic contraction of the lumen. This produces a functional bowel obstruction, chronic constipation, and the passage of ribbon like stools. It can lead to a complete bowel obstruction. Because of the constriction of the lumen, huge amounts of feces and gas collect proximal to the aganglionic portion, resulting in a gross enlargement of this segment. The enlarged segment of colon is actually normal in its function.

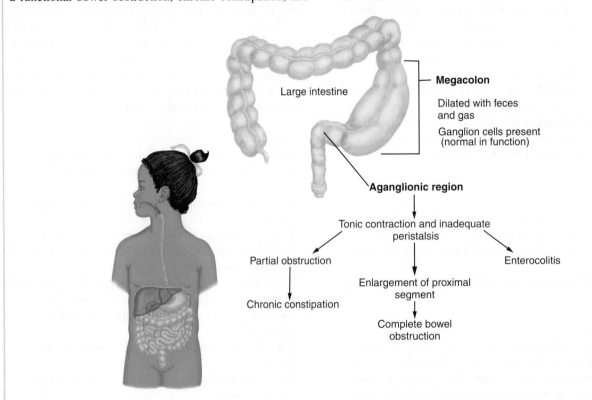

Large intestine

Megacolon

Dilated with feces and gas

Ganglion cells present (normal in function)

Aganglionic region

Tonic contraction and inadequate peristalsis

Partial obstruction

Chronic constipation

Enlargement of proximal segment

Complete bowel obstruction

Enterocolitis

Etiology and Incidence

The disease is a result of embryonic failure of migration of the hindgut ganglion cells to the most caudal portion of the GI tract, the rectum. The initiating factor in this failure is unknown.

Hirschsprung disease occurs in 1 in 5000 live births, with a 4:1 male/female ratio (Wyllie, 2004b). It has a strong hereditary component and a higher incidence in children with Down syndrome.

Manifestations and Diagnostic Evaluation

Delayed passage or absence of meconium stool in the neonatal period is the cardinal sign of Hirschsprung disease. Any child who does not pass meconium within the first 24 hours and who is prone to constipation or stool infrequency in the first month after birth is suspected of having Hirschsprung disease. The neonate, infant, or older child may exhibit signs of bowel obstruction, abdominal pain and distention, vomiting, and failure to thrive. Chronic constipation beginning in the first month of life results in pelletlike or ribbon stools that are foul smelling.

A rectal examination reveals a tight internal sphincter and the absence of stool, followed by an often explosive release of gas and feces related to the sudden but transient increase in rectal size. Barium enema examination demonstrates an abrupt change in the size of the colon from a distended ganglionic proximal portion to the contracted, saw-toothed appearance in the aganglionic distal portion, with a transitional zone of tapered bowel between them. Significantly, the child will not evacuate barium after the examination. The definitive diagnosis is made by rectal biopsy. During biopsy, a small core or punch sample that contains all layers of the bowel mucosa is removed. Absence of ganglionic cells in the sample confirms the diagnosis of Hirschsprung disease.

Therapeutic Management

Treatment for mild to moderate Hirschsprung disease is based on relieving the chronic constipation with stool softeners and rectal irrigations. Treatment for moderate to severe Hirschsprung disease involves removing the aganglionic portion of the intestine in a two-step surgical intervention.

In the neonatal period, performing a temporary colostomy with the most distal section of normal bowel relieves the obstruction. A complete surgical repair is delayed until the child weighs 8 to 10 kg (18 to 20 lb), at which time a pull-through procedure is performed to excise all aganglionic portions of the bowel and reanastomose the normal bowel to the anal canal. The colostomy is closed during this procedure, and normal bowel function returns shortly thereafter. If the child is older before diagnosis and surgery, the physician will most likely wait 3 or 4 months before the pull-through procedure.

If diagnosis is made early enough before the bowel becomes severely dilated, a one-stage pull-through procedure, which eliminates the necessity of a temporary colostomy, may be used. In addition, some medical centers are now performing this surgery by using minimally invasive or laparoscopic techniques that have less morbidity and shorter recovery times.

NURSING CARE

The Child With Hirschsprung Disease

Assessment

The child with Hirschsprung disease will have constipation that has been present since the neonatal period and frequent passage of foul-smelling ribbonlike or pelletlike stools. Nutritional status should be assessed because malnutrition can develop as a result of extreme distention or enterocolitis. Thin extremities, abdominal distention, and a history of poor feeding should be noted.

If the child is acutely ill on presentation, enterocolitis must be suspected. *This is a life-threatening complication and, if it is suspected, must be reported immediately.* Document the assessment of bowel sounds and abdominal distention, the frequency of vomiting and diarrhea, and changes in abdominal circumference. Assess temperature by a route other than rectal.

Assess family members' concerns and their methods of dealing with the problem. This disease can drain family and financial resources during the diagnosis and surgical treatment. Mild disease may not be diagnosed until the child is older. Assessing the older child's feelings about chronic constipation and its treatment is important.

Nursing Diagnoses and Planning

The following nursing diagnoses and expected outcomes may be appropriate for the child with Hirschsprung disease:

* Constipation related to aganglionic bowel and inadequate peristalsis.
  Expected Outcome: The child will pass soft, formed stools without retention.
* Risk for Deficient Fluid Volume or Excess Fluid Volume related to surgical preparation.
  Expected Outcome: The child will be free from fluid or electrolyte disturbances related to bowel cleansing.

* Impaired Skin Integrity related to colostomy and surgical repair.
  Expected Outcomes: The surgical and colostomy sites will be clean and free from exudate, redness, or drainage; the colostomy site will be intact without bleeding or skin irritation.
* Risk for Infection related to surgical repair.
  Expected Outcome: The child will be afebrile without signs of infection at the site.
* Imbalanced Nutrition: Less Than Body Requirements related to GI surgery.
  Expected Outcomes: The child will have normal bowel sounds, will pass stool, and will tolerate a regular diet.
* Acute Pain related to surgical incisions.
  Expected Outcomes: The child will be free from pain and will be able to participate in usual activities of daily living.
* Deficient Knowledge related to incomplete information about the need for surgery, irrigation, or care of the ostomy.
  Expected Outcomes: The parent will state the necessity for rectal irrigations or surgical intervention; the parent or child will assume responsibility for care of the ostomy.
* Disturbed Body Image related to colostomy and irrigations.
  Expected Outcome: The child and family will express feelings about irrigations, ostomy care, and the impact the condition has had on the child's body image.
* Anxiety (parental and child) related to the loss of the perfect child or need for surgery.
  Expected Outcomes: The parents will express fears and concerns and seek support as needed.

Interventions

Preparing the Child for Surgery

The nurse closely monitors and records the child's bowel elimination pattern. Isotonic saline enemas are administered preoperatively until the return is clear (see Chapter 13). An alternative bowel-cleansing regimen is to administer a polyethylene glycol-electrolyte lavage solution (GoLYTELY) orally or through the NG tube. This regimen is used only in children older than 5 years and is given at a dosage of 25 to 40 mL/kg per hour. Sodium phosphate (Fleets Phosphosoda) is another alternative requiring only approximately 200 mL at one time for children older than 5 years. After bowel cleansing, keep the child on NPO status until surgery. Provide IV fluids as needed and keep strict intake and output records.

Preventing Infection and Maintaining Skin Integrity

Neomycin 1.0% solution given by rectum or stoma is administered preoperatively to sterilize the bowel for surgery. Additional sterilization is provided by IV antibiotics, which also prevent infection at the surgical incision site. Monitor vital signs carefully, and measure the child's abdominal circumference with each vital sign measurement. Use tympanic or axillary methods for taking the temperature to avoid traumatizing the rectal mucosa. Monitor the surgical site for redness, swelling, and purulent drainage.

If the child has a colostomy, monitor the stoma site for bleeding and impaired skin integrity. After a pull-through procedure, which pulls the healthy bowel to the anal opening, monitor the anal site carefully for redness, discharge, and the presence of stool. To prevent skin breakdown, provide meticulous skin care of abdominal, perineal, and ostomy sites by changing dressings and appliances as needed. Use the appropriate-size hypoallergenic ostomy supplies. Encourage the parent and child to begin ostomy care as soon as possible.

Maintaining Nutritional and Hydration Status

Postoperatively, keep the child on NPO status until bowel sounds return or the child passes flatus; set the NG tube to intermittent suction until peristalsis returns. Monitor the child for signs of dehydration and acid-base disturbances. Begin advancing the diet from clear liquids to a regular diet as ordered. To prevent dehydration, keep the child on IV fluids until the child tolerates oral fluids well.

Relieving Pain

Provide pain medications on a regular basis as ordered. Most school-age children can use patient-controlled analgesia for effective pain control (see Chapter 15). The nurse should encourage the parents to institute nonpharmacologic pain control measures such as repositioning, back rubs, music, holding, rocking, massage, and quiet talking. If pain is not controlled by usual means, the child may have a bowel obstruction or infection.

Providing Education and Relieving Anxiety

Before the time of scheduled surgery, the parents may need to manage rectal irrigations at home. The parents must learn the procedure and observe for distention and signs of obstruction. Encourage the parents to express any concerns they may have about the need for irrigations or their ability to perform them. Teach the parents and child about the surgery and recovery process. If the child is to have a colostomy, the child and parents may find seeing and manipulating the equipment to be helpful.

Postoperatively, encourage preschoolers and young school-age children to draw pictures, use dolls, and play to express concerns about body appearance, irrigations, and the colostomy. Teach colostomy care in the immediate postoperative period, and encourage the parents to participate in the child's care as quickly as possible in the supervised setting. Promote self-care as soon as possible for the older child. Referral to an enterostomal therapist can be helpful. The nurse also can refer the family to support groups for children with ostomies.

Provide parents time to share their fears, concerns, and questions. Active listening is a critical nursing intervention. Referral to community resources may be useful (see Evolve website).

Evaluation

- Does the child pass soft, formed stools without retention after completion of the surgical correction?
- Has the child tolerated the bowel-cleansing regimen without signs of fluid and electrolyte imbalance, as evidenced by moist mucous membranes, good skin turgor, and an hourly urine output appropriate for age?
- Is the child afebrile, and are surgical sites free from redness, purulent drainage, excess heat, and dehiscence?
- Is the colostomy or anal pull-through area free from bleeding and skin breakdown?
- Are bowel sounds active and present in all four quadrants, and is the child tolerating a developmentally appropriate diet without vomiting or diarrhea?
- Does the child appear to be free of pain, as evidenced by the ability to sleep comfortably and participate in appropriate play activities when awake?
- Can the parents and child demonstrate all procedures needed for appropriate care?
- Is the child able to express feelings about body changes related to treatments or procedures?
- Are the parents calm and able to resume all care of their child without anxiety?

MALABSORPTION DISORDERS
Lactose Intolerance

An inability to tolerate lactose, the sugar found in dairy products, is the result of an absence or deficiency of lactase, an enzyme found in the secretions of the small intestine and needed for the digestion of lactose. The two types of lactose intolerance are congenital and developmental. Congenital lactose intolerance, which is quite rare, appears at birth, with a complete absence of lactase. Developmental lactose intolerance, which is more common, is a deficiency of lactase that appears in early to late childhood.

Etiology and Incidence

Most cases of lactose intolerance are the result of inadequate levels of lactase. The exact reason for this deficiency is unknown. The condition is likely to be more severe during and after other illnesses affecting the GI mucosa, such as viral gastroenteritis or food poisoning.

The condition appears to have an ethnic association, with a 50% to 90% incidence in Asians, American Indians, Arabs, Jews, African Americans, and southern Europeans (NDDIC, 2003).

PATHOPHYSIOLOGY

LACTOSE INTOLERANCE

An absence or deficiency of lactase leads to inability to digest lactose and the subsequent accumulation of lactose in the lumen of the small intestine. As a result, water is drawn into the colon, resulting in watery osmotic diarrhea containing undigested lactose. In addition, GI bacteria break down lactose and release hydrogen, which causes excess gas production, bloating, and abdominal pain.

| BOX 19-6 | **PARENTS WANT TO KNOW**   About Care of the Child With Lactose Intolerance |

- Your child must avoid all high-lactose foods (e.g., milk, ice cream). If you are unsure about whether a food contains lactose, examine labels for milk or milk products.
- You can use soy-based, lactose-free formulas as needed for your infant (Isomil, Nursoy, Nutramigen, Prosobee). If you are breastfeeding, limit your own intake of dairy products.
- Soy-based beverages (Silk) are available in most grocery stores.

- You or your older child can obtain calcium through other foods besides milk. They include egg yolks, green leafy vegetables, dried beans, cauliflower, and molasses. Calcium supplements are also available.
- Once your child's symptoms have disappeared, you can gradually add yogurt, hard cheeses, and small amounts of milk to assess tolerance.
- If you are having difficulty determining what foods are lactose free or need help finding recipes that use lactose-free foods, ask for a dietary consultation.

Manifestations and Diagnostic Evaluation

Manifestations of lactose intolerance include diarrhea that is frothy but not fatty, abdominal distention, cramping abdominal pain, and excessive flatus. The symptoms are not usually seen until lactase activity begins to decrease after age 3 years or during other GI insults. If the child has congenital lactose intolerance, symptoms will be immediate and may be severe.

A history of improvement after a lactose-free diet has been implemented provides a presumptive diagnosis. The finding of 1+ or greater sugar values on Clinitest examination of the stool can support the diagnosis. Breath hydrogen testing may indicate the amount of lactase available by indirectly measuring the amount of undigested carbohydrate.

Therapeutic Management

The treatment for lactose intolerance is removal of lactose from the diet. In most cases, total elimination is unnecessary. Removing milk as the beverage of choice can provide enough relief from symptoms. Additional dietary changes may be necessary to provide adequate sources of calcium and, in the infant, protein and calories. Formulas that do not contain lactose (Isomil, Nursoy, Nutramigen, Prosobee, and other soy-based formulas) may be given to the infant suspected of having lactose intolerance. Breastfeeding mothers are urged to eliminate lactose products from their diet.

These dietary changes can be supplemented with the use of commercial lactase preparations (Lactaid, Dairy Ease, Lac-Dose) that can be taken with lactose-containing food to provide adequate lactase levels and variable relief from symptoms.

NURSING CARE

The Child With Lactose Intolerance

Assessment

Assessment will reveal a healthy-looking child with episodic abdominal pain and occasional diarrhea without any nutritional deficiencies or other health problems. If the problem is congenital and thus likely to be more severe, diarrhea may be a major concern. The neonate or infant may appear extremely dehydrated, with severe diarrhea and weight loss. The child and family may or may not be able to correlate symptoms with food intake.

Nursing Diagnosis and Planning

The following nursing diagnoses and expected outcomes may be appropriate for the infant or child with lactose intolerance:
- Acute Pain related to bloating and flatus.
  Expected Outcomes: The child will be free from abdominal pain, as evidenced by developmentally appropriate play and activity; the child will have normal bowel sounds with a soft abdomen that is not painful during palpation.
- Diarrhea related to maldigestion.
  Expected Outcome: The child will have soft, formed stools.
- Deficient Knowledge related to incomplete understanding about needed dietary changes.
  Expected Outcome: The child will take in a minimum of 800 mg of calcium per day, as reported in the dietary history. The family will state foods to be avoided or provided in small amounts and will provide adequate calcium sources in diet and select appropriate lactase products.

Interventions

The principal nursing intervention is teaching. Symptoms are often relieved after a lactose-free diet is followed for a short period. Foods containing small amounts of lactose may be added gradually after this time to assess the child's reaction. If small amounts of milk are tolerated, offer food or lactase preparations simultaneously with milk. These simple changes can offer instant relief.

After diagnosis and initial management, this condition is often perceived to be only a minor nuisance. Emotional support for the family, however, may be needed. Referring the family to self-help and information groups and encouraging family members to share successes and concerns are important nursing interventions (Box 19-6).

Evaluation

- Is the child happy, content, and free of excess gas and bloating?
- Can the parent state what foods are essential to avoid?
- Are the child's stools normal and formed?
- Does the food diary indicate an intake of at least 800 mg of calcium daily for a child aged 1 to 10 years?
- Does the parent express satisfaction with control of the child's condition?

Celiac Disease

Celiac disease, also known as *gluten enteropathy* or *tropical sprue,* results from the inability to digest fully the gliadin or protein part of wheat, barley, rye, and oats. This is a lifelong deficiency requiring dietary modification to prevent chronic maldigestion and malabsorption.

Etiology and Incidence

Celiac disease is considered genetic. From 80% to 90% of children with celiac disease have the genetic marker HLA-B8, a human leukocyte antigen complex located on chromosome 6. This chromosomal variation results in the inability to digest gliadin, causing severe GI mucosal changes that continue on exposure to gluten. Delaying the introduction of gluten into the infant's diet and breastfeeding before and during that introduction can delay the appearance of symptoms in at-risk individuals (Norris et al., 2005).

The incidence of celiac disease varies in different regions. In the United States the incidence is approximately 1 in 1000 live births. The incidence is much higher in Europe. Siblings and children of affected individuals are at highest risk for the disease (Garcia-Careaga & Kerner, 2004).

Manifestations

The major manifestations in the child with celiac disease include diarrhea and growth failure. The child's growth usually is below the twenty-fifth percentile on growth charts.

The child may also have abdominal distention, vomiting, anemia, irritability, anorexia, muscle wasting, edema, and folate deficiency. Symptoms are not seen until 3 to 6 months

---

PATHOPHYSIOLOGY

CELIAC DISEASE

Gluten—the protein found in rye, oats, barley, and wheat—breaks down into gliadin and other byproducts. Celiac disease results from an inability to digest gliadin. This results in the accumulation of glutamine in the intestine, which has a toxic effect on the mucosal cells. This leads to atrophy of the villi and a marked decrease in the absorptive surface. Malabsorption of fats, carbohydrates, and vitamins develops. *Celiac crisis* is a result of sudden accumulation of glutamine and the subsequent destruction of the mucosal cells, causing severe diarrhea and dehydration.

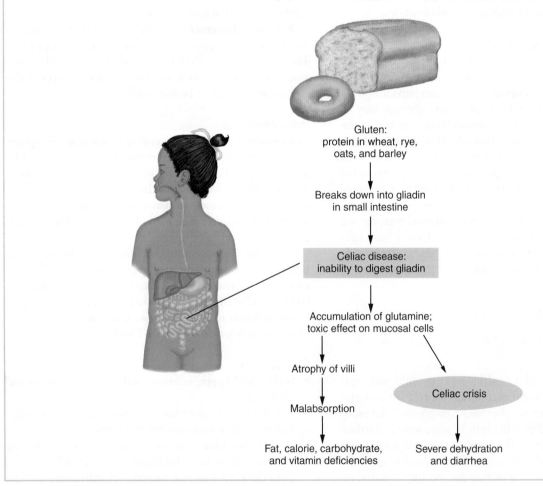

Gluten:
protein in wheat, rye,
oats, and barley

↓

Breaks down into gliadin
in small intestine

↓

Celiac disease:
inability to digest gliadin

↓

Accumulation of glutamine;
toxic effect on mucosal cells

↓   ↘

Atrophy of villi   Celiac crisis

↓   ↓

Malabsorption

↓

Fat, calorie, carbohydrate,   Severe dehydration
and vitamin deficiencies   and diarrhea

after the introduction of grains to the diet, usually at age 9 to 12 months. The child in celiac crisis exhibits profuse, watery diarrhea and vomiting.

Diagnostic Evaluation

The serum antigliadin antibody (AGA) assay is a diagnostic test that allows continued assessment and evaluation of dietary changes. In the past, this test required specialized laboratory equipment. Now, the strip AGA test requires only a single drop of blood, and results can be determined quickly and inexpensively. Its ease of use makes the diagnosis of celiac disease simpler and more cost effective. A newer, more accurate test measures tissue transglutaminase (tTG) through enzyme-linked immunosorbent assay (ELISA). The test is also effective in evaluating the adequacy of dietary changes. Jejunal biopsy will unequivocally identify ulcerations in the GI tract. Monitoring the reaction to a gluten-free diet supports the diagnosis. Symptoms are often relieved in 1 week by removal of gluten from the diet.

Further diagnostic testing may include the breath hydrogen excretion test to identify the amount of carbohydrate malabsorption occurring. This test is not specific for sprue. D-Xylose testing indicates the amount of mucosal damage; the remaining absorptive surface can be estimated.

Therapeutic Management

Dietary management is the mainstay of treatment. All wheat, rye, barley, and oats should be eliminated from the diet and replaced with corn and rice. To correct deficiencies, vitamin supplements, especially with fat-soluble vitamins and folate, may be needed in the early period of treatment.

Dietary restrictions are likely to be lifelong, although small amounts of grains may be tolerated after the ulcerations have healed. Adolescents have difficulty maintaining a gluten-free diet without having an unbalanced diet high in protein and fat. An adolescent on a strict gluten-free diet still has a risk for dietary imbalance, and supplements or support from dietary services is essential for maintenance.

Occasionally the nurse is the first to see a child in celiac crisis. Celiac crisis causes profuse, watery diarrhea and vomiting and can quickly lead to severe dehydration and metabolic acidosis. The cause of the crisis, usually an infection or a hidden source of gluten, must be identified. The child is given fluids IV to correct fluid and acid-base imbalance, albumin to treat shock, and corticosteroids to decrease severe mucosal inflammation.

NURSING CARE

The Child With Celiac Disease

Assessment

Assessment of the infant with celiac disease usually reveals an irritable, malnourished infant who exhibits failure to thrive by 9 to 12 months. Any child with diarrhea, especially one with foul-smelling, fatty stools and significant growth delays, should be suspected of having this disorder. A noticeable

decline in the child's rate of growth as charted on the growth curve, associated with the addition of grains to the diet, is essential supportive evidence.

Abdominal assessment reveals distention and ascites with an increasing girth; observation identifies other signs of malnutrition, such as thin, edematous extremities; pallor; and muscle wasting. Anemia is a common finding.

The child with severe diarrhea, foul-smelling stools, vomiting, poor perfusion, edema, or changes in vital signs (shock or metabolic acidosis) should be referred for emergency care of celiac crisis.

Nursing Diagnosis and Planning

The following nursing diagnoses and expected outcomes may be appropriate for the infant or child with celiac disease:
- Imbalanced Nutrition: Less Than Body Requirements related to malabsorption.

  Expected Outcome: The infant or child will have soft, formed stools without diarrhea.
- Acute Pain or Chronic Pain related to abdominal distention.

  Expected Outcome: The infant or child will be free from abdominal pain, as evidenced by age-appropriate play and activity.
- Delayed Growth and Development related to malnutrition.

  Expected Outcome: The infant or child will return to and follow a normal growth pattern according to a growth chart.
- Deficient Knowledge related to dietary changes.

  Expected Outcomes: The family will offer appropriate foods to the infant or child, as evidenced by a food diary; will state the need for lifelong dietary changes; and will seek emotional and educational support as needed.
- Deficient Fluid Volume related to celiac crisis.

  Expected Outcome: The infant or child will be adequately hydrated, as evidenced by moist mucous membranes and good skin turgor.

Interventions

The most important nursing intervention is teaching parents to modify their child's diet (Box 19-7). Pain will likely be quickly relieved by eliminating gluten in the diet. Involvement of nutritionists in teaching and follow-up is helpful. Careful and consistent follow-up will be necessary to ensure the infant resumes a normal growth and development pattern as soon as possible. When the child has normal stools without diarrhea and resumes a normal growth pattern, teaching will have been effective.

Because celiac disease is a lifelong condition, support groups can be useful in managing the problem. The American Celiac Society is an excellent source of information and support (see Evolve website). Referral to this group and other family support organizations is essential. Encourage the parents to share their fears and concerns about the chronic nature of the disease and its impact on family life.

Evaluation

- Does the child have soft, formed stools without diarrhea or signs of dehydration?
- Is the child participating in age-appropriate activities?
- Has the child resumed a normal growth pattern according to a growth chart?
- Is the family able to verbalize an understanding of the child's dietary and emotional needs?
- Does a food diary indicate an intake of approximately 100 kcal/kg for the infant and for the child up to age 3 years?
- Do the parents use available support and education groups?
- Do the parents express satisfaction with the way they are coping with dietary changes?
- Does the child have good skin turgor, moist mucous membranes, and a urine output appropriate for age (see Chapter 18)?

HEPATIC DISORDERS
Viral Hepatitis

Hepatitis is an acute or chronic inflammation of the liver caused by several different viruses and some toxins or disease states. Although each type of hepatitis is unique, assessment findings and treatment have many similarities.

Etiology

The most common causes and modes of transmission of viral hepatitis are discussed in Table 19-5. Rubella, cytomegalovirus (CMV), herpes simplex virus, and Epstein-Barr virus may also occasionally produce hepatitis in children.

In children, hepatitis A virus (HAV) is highly contagious and spreads readily in households and daycare centers. Infection with hepatitis B virus (HBV) can be transmitted perinatally. The incidence of HBV infection transmitted by blood transfusions has decreased in recent years as a result of improved blood product screening procedures. Contaminated body fluids splashed into the mouth or eyes can cause HBV infection. HBV can survive in the dried state for 1 week or longer, and percutaneous contact with contaminated objects can transmit infection.

Incidence

In the United States and other Western industrialized countries, HBV infection occurs most often in adolescents and adults. The incidence of hepatitis B infection in the United States has declined over the past 10 years to 2.8 in 100,000 in adults and 0.3 in 100,000 in children (Centers for Disease Control and Prevention [CDC], 2004). In developing countries where sanitation is poor, HBV occurs most often in infants and children younger than 5 years. In the United States, perinatal exposure to a hepatitis B–positive mother is the major cause of infection in young children (Snyder & Pickering, 2004). The incidence of hepatitis A is 4 in 100,000 (CDC, 2003b). Because the virus may be excreted for 2 to 3 weeks before the appearance of clinical signs and for 2 to 3 weeks afterward, outbreaks are common wherever good handwashing is not practiced.

Manifestations

In infants and preschool-age children, HAV infection usually causes no symptoms or mild, nonspecific symptoms such as anorexia, malaise, and easy fatigability. In adults, the disease causes the more severe symptoms of nausea, jaundice, and malaise. Because most children with HAV infection are asymptomatic or have mild, nonspecific symptoms, the disease may not be diagnosed until an outbreak of hepatitis occurs. Thus spread of HAV infection in a daycare center often occurs before the initial case is identified.

HBV infection may cause a wide range of clinical manifestations, from asymptomatic infection to fatal acute fulminant hepatitis. Symptomatic acute hepatitis occurs in two stages: the anicteric (without jaundice) phase and the icteric (jaundiced) phase.

During the anicteric phase, manifestations include anorexia, nausea and vomiting, right upper quadrant or epigastric pain, fever, malaise, fatigue, depression, and irritability. The anicteric phase lasts approximately 5 to 7 days. During the icteric phase, manifestations include jaundice, urticaria, dark urine, and light-colored stools. The child begins to feel better as jaundice becomes more apparent. Acute fulminating hepatitis is marked by bleeding problems, encephalopathy, ascites, and acute hepatic failure. Fulminant hepatitis is caused primarily by hepatitis B and hepatitis C.

PATHOPHYSIOLOGY

VIRAL HEPATITIS

Hepatitis viruses cause necrosis of the parenchymal cells of the liver. The inflammatory response causes swelling and blockage of the drainage system in the liver. Biliary stasis and further destruction of the hepatic cells occur. Because the liver cannot excrete bile into the intestine, bile appears in the blood (causing hyperbilirubinemia), urine (as urobilinogen), and skin (causing hepatocellular jaundice).

Hepatitis infection may result in asymptomatic or mild illness, in which complete regeneration of liver cells occurs within 2 to 3 months. More severe forms of hepatitis include (1) fulminant hepatitis, in which hepatic necrosis and death can occur within 1 to 2 weeks, and (2) subacute, or chronic, hepatitis, which can result in permanent scarring of the liver and impaired liver function. Chronically infected persons are carriers of the disease and are at increased risk for developing chronic liver disease (e.g., cirrhosis, chronic persistent hepatitis) or liver carcinoma later in life.

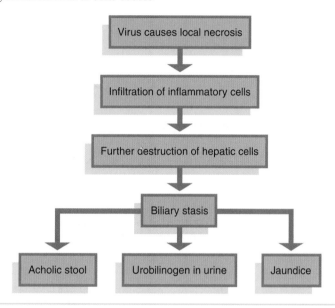

The symptoms and clinical changes should return to normal within 3 months of onset. If not, a chronic state should be suspected. Infection with hepatitis B, hepatitis D, and hepatitis C viruses (HBV, HDV, and HCV) can result in chronic hepatitis and cirrhosis. Chronic HBV infection can also cause hepatic carcinoma.

Diagnostic Evaluation

A history of exposure to jaundiced individuals, confirmed outbreaks in daycare centers, or percutaneous exposure to blood or body fluids should raise the suspicion of hepatitis. Although no liver function test is specific for hepatitis, tests of liver function, especially aspartate transaminase (AST), alanine transaminase (ALT), and bilirubin levels and sedimentation rate, can indicate liver damage caused by hepatitis. Serum bilirubin levels peak 5 to 10 days after jaundice appears. A history and the course of the disease are essential in making the appropriate diagnosis.

Hepatitis is diagnosed by identification of the antigens (e.g., HBsAg, HBeAg, HBcAg) responsible for the disease, antibodies (e.g., anti-HAV, anti-HBcAg, anti-HCV), or polymerase chain reaction (e.g., HCV RNA). In hepatitis A, immunoglobulin M (IgM) anti-HAV antibodies are present at the onset of illness and are diagnostic (Demmler, 2004).

They usually disappear within 6 months, but may persist for 12 months. Children with hepatitis B are diagnosed by the presence of antigen (HBsAg) and IgM antibodies to HBcAg. HCV serologic assays are used mainly to diagnose hepatitis C (Demmler, 2004).

Liver biopsy may be needed to evaluate the chronic active forms of the disease and to determine the extent of damage in advanced or fulminant cases. Liver fibrosis increases with the duration of HCV infection.

Therapeutic Management

Acute viral hepatitis has no specific treatment. In uncomplicated viral hepatitis, treatment is mainly supportive because the disease is self-limiting. Treatment is aimed at maintaining comfort and adequate nutritional balance. A low-fat, balanced diet can be helpful if the child is bothered by nausea and anorexia. Hospitalization is rarely needed. All nonessential medications should be discontinued and chemotherapy, corticosteroids, and alcohol should all be avoided during infection.

In fulminant hepatitis, intensive care may be needed to provide hemostasis, nutritional and fluid support, neurologic assessment, and management until the liver has had a chance to recover.

TABLE **19-5**	Differentiation of Viral Hepatitis				

Type/Etiology	Transmission	Incubation	Clinical Manifestations	Recovery Prognosis
Hepatitis A virus (HAV), previously called *infectious hepatitis*	Fecal-oral Food or water contaminated with HAV	15-50 days (average, 30 days) Most contagious 1-2 wk before symptoms Onset at 28-30 days	Mild, flulike symptoms Mostly asymptomatic in children No jaundice in children Adolescents: fever, malaise, anorexia, nausea, jaundice	Good prognosis Carriers do not occur Recovery provides lifelong immunity
Hepatitis B virus (HBV), previously called *serum hepatitis*	Blood and blood products Secretions Prenatally, perinatally Sexual contact Breast milk	45-180 days (average, 90 days)	Same as HAV Severity ranges from asymptomatic to fatal fulminant infection Anicteric or asymptomatic most common in children 90% of infected neonates will develop chronic carrier state	Generally a full recovery except in chronic carriers 30%-90% of infected children <10 yr old develop chronic hepatitis and are predisposed to cirrhosis and hepatocellular cancer
Hepatitis C virus (HCV), non-A, non-B hepatitis	Blood and blood products Perinatally IV drug use Unsterile tattoos and body piercings	14-115 days (average, 45 days)	Same as HAV	>50% progress to chronic hepatitis with risk of cirrhosis or cancer in adulthood Liver transplantation is an option for end-stage illness
Hepatitis delta virus (HDV), occurs only in patients with acute or chronic HBV infection	Blood and blood products More common in Mediterranean countries and among IV drug users and hemophiliacs	30-60 days; coincides with HBV infection	More than half of children have chronic hepatitis Occurs with HBV and causes it to be more severe Hepatitis B vaccination reduces risk	More likely to develop fulminating hepatitis than other strains
Hepatitis E virus (HEV), enterically transmitted non-A, non-B hepatitis	Fecal-oral More common in adults	Unknown	Epidemic with characteristics of HAV Uncommon in developed countries	High incidence of mortality in pregnant women Children usually asymptomatic
Hepatitis G virus (HGV)	Parenteral transmission Sexual contact	Unknown	Usually asymptomatic for liver involvement	Does not cause chronic hepatitis Little direct liver involvement

Data from Demmler, G. (2004). Hepatitis. In R. Feigin, J. Cherry, G. Demmler, & S. Kaplan (Eds.). *Textbook of pediatric infectious diseases* (5th ed., pp. 658-665). Philadelphia: Elsevier Saunders.

Hepatitis A. Control of further spread is essential. Because HAV can survive on contaminated objects for weeks, good handwashing and thorough disinfection of diaper-changing surfaces are imperative. Children and adults who have had direct contact with a person infected with HAV should receive immune globulin (IG) as soon as possible after exposure. A vaccine has been developed to prevent HAV infection, and immunization is currently recommended for all children at age 1 year as well other high risk groups (CDC, 2006). Cases of hepatitis should be promptly reported to local public health officials. Testing for IgM anti-HAV antibodies should be done in suspected cases of infected daycare center employees and household contacts of infected persons (American Academy of Pediatrics, Committee on Infectious Diseases, 2000).

Hepatitis B. Children with acute or chronic HBV infection should be cared for with scrupulous Standard Precautions. The most effective means of preventing HBV infection is immunization with HBV vaccine. HBV vaccination is recommended beginning in infancy as part of the routine childhood immunization schedule and for all unimmunized children before they reach adolescence. Other persons who should receive HBV immunization include IV drug users, health care and residential facility workers, household contacts and sexual partners of HBV carriers, inmates of correctional facilities, and international travelers. HBV immune globulin (HBIG) is effective in preventing HBV infection if given within 2 weeks after exposure. Hepatitis D can be prevented by preventing HBV (Table 19-6).

TABLE **19-6** Hepatitis Prophylaxis			
Infective Agent	**Prevention of Spread**	**Immunization**	**Postexposure Prophylaxis**

HAV	Handwashing
	Gloves
	Identifying infected food handlers
		Vaccine 97%-100% effective
		Given as two injections at age 1 yr
		  and at least 6 months later
		Recommended for all children at age
		  1 yr and specific populations in
		  high-risk areas
			Within 2 wk, give hepatitis A
			  immune globulin (HAIG), 0.02
			  mL/kg intramuscular (IM)

HBV	Sterilization of needles
	Blood Precautions
	Gloves
		Vaccine 80%-90% effective
		Three injections at 0, 1, and 6-18 mo
		Recommended for all infants,
		  children, and adolescents
			For neonates of infected mothers,
			  give hepatitis B immune
			  globulin (HBIG) within 12 hr of
			  birth followed by vaccines
			HBIG, 0.06 mL/kg, within 24 hr of
			  any percutaneous exposure

HCV	Standard Precautions	None	None
HDV	Same as for HBV	Protecting from HBV will protect because HDV cannot exist alone	None
HEV	Standard Precautions	Vaccine under animal trials	None

NURSING CARE

The Child With Viral Hepatitis

Assessment

The nursing history may identify a source of infection. In children, flulike symptoms of fever, malaise, anorexia, fatigue, and nausea may be the *only* symptoms of viral hepatitis. Abdominal assessment may disclose right upper quadrant tenderness and hepatomegaly. Stools will be pale and clay colored, and urine may be dark and frothy. Jaundice, if present, is best assessed in sclera, nail beds, and mucous membranes and usually follows a cephalocaudal progression. In HBV infection, arthralgias may be the presenting symptom.

Fulminant hepatitis will likely manifest as acute hepatic failure with associated encephalopathy, bleeding, fluid retention, ascites, and an icteric appearance.

Nursing Diagnosis and Planning

The following nursing diagnoses and expected outcomes may be appropriate after assessing the child with viral hepatitis and the child's family:

• Imbalanced Nutrition: Less Than Body Requirements related to anorexia.

Expected Outcomes: The child will tolerate an age-appropriate diet without weight loss, vomiting, or abdominal pain and will return to a normal activity level.

• Risk for Infection related to exposure of family members to infectious agents.

Expected Outcomes: The family will practice good handwashing and other necessary isolation procedures and will remain free from infection.

• Risk for Injury related to fulminant hepatitis.

Expected Outcome: The child will return to preillness weight and activity level.

• Deficient Knowledge related to incomplete information about home care and long-term prognosis.

Expected Outcome: The parents will verbalize a basic understanding of hepatitis and the importance of treatment and prevention.

Interventions

Unless fulminant hepatitis develops, children are usually treated at home, so parental education is crucial. Teaching parents the importance of a nutritious, low-fat diet as tolerated by the child, rest, and general supportive care is important. The child with hepatitis is often anorexic. Several small meals and snacks throughout the day are better tolerated than regular portions at mealtimes.

Fatigue and malaise can last for several weeks. Adequate rest and sleep are important for recovery. Because HAV is not infectious within 1 week after the onset of jaundice, the child may return to school at that time if well enough.

Child and Parent Teaching

Teach the parents the danger signals that could indicate a worsening of the child's condition—specifically, changes in neurologic status, bleeding, and fluid retention. Jaundice may worsen before it resolves, and parents should be prepared for this possibility. Also, teach parents not to give their child any over-the-counter medications because impaired liver function may result in inadequate metabolism and excretion of the medication. Caution adolescents not to drink alcohol during the illness or recovery period.

Preventing the spread of infection is an essential intervention for HAV. Prevention should include the use of Contact Precautions for at least 1 week after the onset of jaundice and excellent handwashing. Handwashing is the most important preventive measure. Teach family members to institute appropriate precautions and to clean exposed household surfaces with bleach. Diapers should not be changed on or near surfaces used for preparing or serving food. Explain to family members the ways in which HAV (fecal-oral route) and HBV (parenteral route) are spread to others. Provide education about the recommendations concerning hepatitis A and hepatitis B vaccination (see Evolve website).

If the child has HBV infection, especially neonatal HBV, prepare the parents for the possibility of a chronic carrier state and the development of cirrhosis and hepatocellular cancer in later years. If a child or adolescent with HBV infection has a history of illicit IV drug use, the nurse has the responsibility of teaching the dangers of such behaviors, including the risk of transmission of hepatitis and other infections. The youth should be assisted to obtain counseling through a drug program.

Home Care

Children with hepatitis are almost always managed at home. Nursing interventions include teaching parents handwashing skills, the use of gloves, and disinfection of contaminated surfaces and articles. Parents should be taught to monitor for complications, provide a well-balanced, low-fat diet, and monitor other family members for infection. All children in the family should be immunized against hepatitis.

Evaluation

- Has the child maintained a weight within 5% of the pre-illness weight?
- Is the child free of vomiting?
- Is the child participating in age-appropriate activities and play?
- Do family members practice good handwashing and adhere to procedures?
- Has the spread of hepatitis to other family members been avoided?
- Have all family members been immunized as appropriate?
- Can the parents describe the symptoms to watch for in other family members?

Biliary Atresia

Biliary atresia refers to the obstruction or absence of the extrahepatic bile ducts. At birth, the liver structure itself is normal without inflammation, but the structural problem

---

PATHOPHYSIOLOGY

BILIARY ATRESIA

Obstruction of the extrahepatic bile ducts causes obstruction of the normal flow of bile out of the liver and into the gallbladder and small intestine. As a result, bile plugs form, causing bile to back up in the liver. This process causes inflammation, edema, and hepatic degeneration. Eventually the liver becomes fibrotic, and cirrhosis and portal hypertension develop, leading to liver failure. The gradual degeneration of the liver causes jaundice, icterus, and hepatomegaly. Because bile is not present in the intestine, fat and fat-soluble vitamins cannot be absorbed. This condition leads to malnutrition, deficiencies in fat-soluble vitamins, and growth failure.

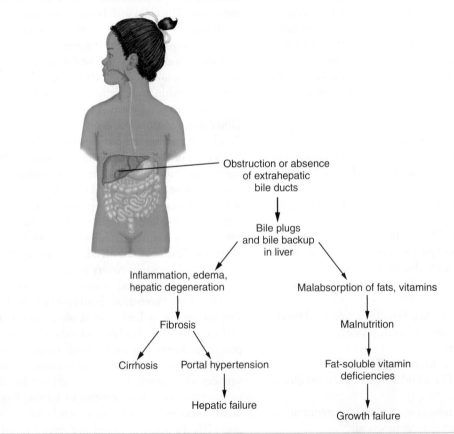

leads to significant cellular damage and eventual liver failure and death.

Etiology and Incidence

The cause of biliary atresia is unknown. Because the problem originates during the prenatal period, viruses, toxins, and chemicals cannot be ruled out. The condition is unlikely to recur within the same family.

Extrahepatic biliary atresia occurs in 1 in 10,000 to 15,000 births, with a slightly higher incidence in female infants than in male infants (A-Kader & Balistreri, 2004). It is the major indication for liver transplantation in children.

Manifestations

The child is apparently healthy at birth. Developing manifestations, however, include acholic stools (light in color because of the absence of bile pigment), bile-stained urine, and hepatomegaly.

Diagnostic Evaluation

Investigations of liver function (bilirubin, aminotransferases [ALT, AST]) and clotting studies (prothrombin time, partial thromboplastin time [PT, PTT]) are useful screening tools. Any newborn with conjugated hyperbilirubinemia should be evaluated completely. To rule out inborn errors of metabolism, such as galactosemia and α_1-antitrypsin deficiency, which can produce similar initial findings, metabolic screens are essential in these children. Hepatitis and other viral titers are also necessary so that neonatal hepatitis can be eliminated as the source of dysfunction. Urine and stool should be examined and urobilinogen levels determined as an indication of the degree of obstruction.

Percutaneous liver biopsy can provide a definitive diagnosis if bile plugs, edema, and fibrosis are found in the presence of normal hepatic lobular structure (A-Kader & Balistreri, 2004). Cholangiography may be used to determine the extent of atresia.

Therapeutic Management

During and after exploratory laparotomy, the size of the lesion can be identified and drainage can be attempted. If no correctable lesion is found, a hepatic portoenterostomy (Kasai procedure) will be performed to allow bile to drain from the liver. This procedure allows bile to flow directly into the intestine through an anastomosis of the jejunum to the porta hepatis, the point at which the hepatic ducts join to form the common bile duct. The Kasai procedure does provide some long-term benefits, but hepatic dysfunction will persist. The main goal of the procedure is to allow growth and development of the child until liver transplantation needs to be performed.

The medical management of the child involves managing the malnutrition and providing symptom relief. Medium-chain triglyceride (MCT) oil added to formula to increase calories or TPN provides essential nutrition. Vitamin malabsorption must be treated to prevent night blindness (vitamin A), neuromuscular degeneration (vitamin E), rickets (vitamin D), and hypoprothrombinemia (vitamin K). Assessment for and treatment of portal hypertension with its concomitant problems of ascites and variceal bleeding must be instituted. Controlling bleeding, restricting salt, and using diuretics are important in managing portal hypertension.

Nursing Considerations

During the early phase of disease, in the first months of life, the infant with biliary atresia will appear jaundiced, with mild hepatosplenomegaly and increased abdominal girth. As the disease progresses, the child may appear thin, with failure to thrive, marked jaundice, and evidence of rickets caused by chronic vitamin D deficiency. Pruritus becomes a major problem; the child may develop skin infections or xanthomas (lipid deposits in the skin) as a result of retention of cholesterol in the skin.

After the Kasai procedure, the child needs to be assessed for evidence of portal hypertension, which may include the development of ascites and GI bleeding. Even after repair, acholic stools and bile-stained urine are not uncommon.

Psychosocial and family assessment should have a high priority. Biliary atresia is a life-threatening, chronic problem that requires surgical intervention, contacts with numerous health care personnel, repeated hospitalizations, and eventually an extended wait for a transplant. The nurse gathers information about family and financial resources, emotional support available, and the feelings of the child and family about the progress and management of the disease.

Nursing interventions are directed toward six major areas: nutritional support, skin care, developmental stimulation, continued assessment, education, and emotional support.

Nutritional Support. Providing adequate calories, aiding in vitamin supply and absorption, and preventing hepatic encephalopathy are important goals. Calorie counts, daily weights, and abdominal girths are important assessments and will provide the data necessary to improve nutritional support. Concentrating calories with the use of Polycose and providing MCT supplements that do not require the presence of bile salts to digest will significantly change the child's nutritional status. NG tube feeding or TPN may become necessary at times. Supplements of vitamins A, D, E, and K as well as calcium, phosphate, and zinc are essential for adequate nutrition. Protein may need to be limited to avoid the development of hepatic encephalopathy. Growth charts and weighing on a monthly basis will provide evaluation criteria.

Skin Care. Bile acid binders, such as cholestyramine, aid in the excretion of bile salts and decrease pruritus and the development of xanthomas (A-Kader & Balistreri, 2004). Colloidal oatmeal baths (Aveeno) can relieve severe itching. Preventing skin breakdown from severe scratching is essential. Wearing gloves during sleep and applying soothing lotions and creams for dry skin may prevent infection.

Developmental Stimulation. Teaching parents activities to provide developmental stimulation and using resources available through physical and occupational therapy are essential nursing responsibilities. As the child awaits a transplant, efforts should be made to facilitate as much development as possible by providing stimulation for gross and fine motor skills and social and emotional growth. Routine screening tests can document developmental growth and help evaluate interventions.

Continued Assessment. Continued assessment for the development of portal hypertension is vital. The parents must be taught to watch for GI bleeding and the development of severe edema and ascites. If any of these occurs, sodium restriction, diuretics, IV albumin, and hospitalization may become necessary.

Family Education and Support. The family has many educational needs, and the nurse needs to help family members understand the disease process, deal with nutritional changes, manage skin care, assess for danger signs, and enhance the child's development. National resources are available to help these families. The Children's Liver Foundation can provide programs, educational materials, and referral to support groups as needed (see Evolve website).

The nurse plays a critical role by listening to parental concerns, providing resources and support, and encouraging participation and involvement. Provide information about daily care and focus the parents' attention on the future liver transplant and its long-term care and treatment. Because transplantation usually occurs within the first 2 years of life, age-appropriate explanations for the toddler are also indicated.

The child and family should be prepared for the eventual need for a liver transplant and the possible death of the child. The life-threatening condition requires numerous hospitalizations, and the many diagnostic tests place immense stress on families. Arranging the educational and emotional support needed by family members so that they can manage their child until liver transplantation becomes possible is a critical nursing intervention.

Home Care. The parents must be able to assume all home care responsibilities. They need to be able to monitor growth and nutritional intake, mix special formulas, manage NG feedings, provide skin care, and give medications. Their ability to assess for GI bleeding, ascites, edema, and skin infections is critical so that treatment can begin as soon as possible.

Cirrhosis

Cirrhosis is a chronic, degenerative condition of the liver that results in the development of bands of fibrous tissue, firm nodules, and connections between the central and portal areas of the liver. This scarring causes irreversible damage to the liver.

Etiology

Cirrhosis in children usually results from chronic liver disease, such as HBV infection or biliary atresia. Sickle cell disease, inborn errors in metabolism such as α_1-antitrypsin deficiency and disturbances in copper metabolism, cystic fibrosis, and Wilson disease are also possible causes in children.

> ## PATHOPHYSIOLOGY
>
> ### CIRRHOSIS
>
> Stasis of bile causes inflammation and hepatomegaly. If this continues, destruction of the liver begins. As the liver attempts to heal itself, fibrotic regeneration and nodules develop and function is impaired. This scarring can cause altered hepatic blood flow and decreased liver cell function. Changes in hepatic blood flow can cause scarring and collapse of the hepatic vasculature, increased vascular resistance, and eventually portal hypertension. As the liver cells decrease in function, more die and the liver cannot produce necessary proteins or bile, causing malabsorption and malnutrition. As liver cells continue to die, the cycle is repeated.

Incidence

Cirrhosis is uncommon in children, but as the life span of children with chronic disease continues to rise, it will become more common. Children with biliary atresia, chronic hepatitis, cystic fibrosis, or sickle cell disease are at risk.

Manifestations

The symptoms are often nonspecific, vague, and slow to develop. They result from either liver cell failure or portal hypertension. Liver cell failure results in jaundice, intense pruritus, steatorrhea, distention, edema, anemia, bleeding tendencies, anorexia, frequent infections, and poor growth. Portal hypertension may present as splenomegaly, varices, or GI bleeding. Both liver cell failure and portal hypertension contribute to the development of ascites.

Diagnostic Evaluation

Because the most likely cause of cirrhosis in children is chronic biliary obstruction, evaluation is based on the history of preexisting conditions, including biliary atresia and hepatitis. The presence of clinical manifestations of chronic liver disease and the history of one of these conditions are used for a presumptive diagnosis. Liver function tests, such as bilirubin, aminotransferases, ammonia, albumin, cholesterol, and prothrombin time, support the diagnosis. Definitive diagnosis is a liver biopsy, which will identify fibrous scarring and changes of hepatic vasculature.

Therapeutic Management

Because no effective treatment is available to halt the progression of cirrhosis, management is aimed at relieving the cause if possible. Any infectious agents should be treated and obstructive causes repaired. Supportive care includes rest, nutritional support, fluid management, and relief of symptoms. Management of life-threatening complications, especially bleeding varices, ascites, and hepatic encephalopathy, takes priority in medical management. Monitoring liver function is important to evaluate the child for eventual liver transplantation. Definitive therapy is a liver transplant.

Nursing Considerations

History and general appraisal will likely reveal a child with a history of failure to thrive and chronic biliary obstruction or HBV infection. The child may have varying degrees of distress and discomfort. Many children will have vague symptoms or be asymptomatic. The earliest findings are likely to be anorexia, nausea, indigestion, fatigue, and right upper quadrant (RUQ) pain or fullness. Monitoring height and weight with a growth chart, gathering information on a typical day's food intake, and assessing sleep habits and activity levels can help identify these more general problems and provide essential supportive evidence.

Abdominal palpation will likely reveal splenomegaly and RUQ tenderness or hepatomegaly. Distended superficial veins; tight, shiny skin; and edema may be present. Jaundice and pruritus may be detected, especially if the cirrhosis is the result of biliary obstruction. A complete skin assessment, including nail beds and sclera, will identify jaundice at its earliest stages. The skin should be examined for breakdown or infection caused by intense scratching. The amount and location of edema should also be noted. This skin assessment may also reveal bruises related to thrombocytopenia and pale color related to anemia. A stool specimen may be useful in identifying the degree of bile obstruction and malabsorption.

The most critical assessment needs to be centered on detecting signs of the three major complications of cirrhosis: ascites, varices, and encephalopathy. The child with significantly increased abdominal girth, edema, bloody emesis, or changes in level of consciousness should be referred for emergency medical care of these life-threatening complications.

The goal of nursing care is to sustain the child in optimal condition until liver transplantation can be achieved. The care can be divided into four areas: nutritional support, skin care, prevention of complications, and developmental and parental support.

Nutritional Support. Providing optimal nutrition for the child to grow and develop is a major nursing intervention. The diet needs to be high carbohydrate, high calorie, normal protein, and low fat. Protein may need to be limited in case encephalopathy develops. Because anorexia can be a problem, creative food options, NG tube feedings, and TPN may be needed. These changes put minimal stress on the liver while meeting the child's growth requirements. In addition, sodium restriction can help prevent edema. Multivitamins with vitamins A, D, E, and K supplements are essential. Vitamin K injections may be needed. Monitoring the child's weight on a daily and weekly basis and recording intake and output can provide critical information about edema and growth. Support from dietary personnel can be valuable when working with and teaching these families.

Skin Care. Pruritus can be intense in the child with cirrhosis. Continued assessment for open lesions, scratch marks, and bleeding is essential. Colloidal oatmeal baths and topical antipruritic lotions, such as calamine, may provide temporary relief. Drugs are not usually an option for itch relief because impaired liver function affects metabolism of drugs. Sedatives, opioids, acetaminophen (Tylenol), and alcohol are strictly avoided. Keeping the nails trimmed short or wearing cotton gloves during sleep can minimize damage to the skin from scratching. Ease of bruising should also be noted.

Prevention of Complications. The following are critical interventions:

- *Infection.* Prevent exposure to infection. Monitor for fever and report immediately.
- *Ascites.* Monitor for edema, give diuretics as ordered, maintain low-sodium diet, and give albumin as ordered. The child will likely have to be hospitalized for treatment; monitoring intake and output and weight, maintaining fluid balance, and monitoring abdominal girth and distention are nursing concerns.
- *Bleeding.* Administer stool guaiac tests, avoid injections, give vitamin K as ordered, and protect from injury. Identify bleeding as soon as possible. While the child is hospitalized, nursing care involves transfusing blood or blood products safely, maintaining fluid balance, monitoring pulse and blood pressure, administering oxygen therapy, and assisting with endoscopic sclerotherapy or the placement of a Sengstaken-Blakemore tube for compression of bleeding esophageal varices.
- *Encephalopathy.* This results from a buildup of ammonia in the blood from the incomplete breakdown of protein. Limiting protein in the diet, giving lactulose as ordered to decrease the GI bacteria that produce ammonia, administering antibiotics as ordered, and monitoring changes in behavior and level of consciousness are nursing responsibilities.

Developmental and Parental Support. Children with cirrhosis are chronically ill and require much time and effort to maintain optimal health. Providing developmental stimulation on a daily basis is essential, and parents need education and support services to achieve this. In addition, parents need to be educated about the disease, its prognosis, the feasibility of a liver transplant, and the risk of complications. As the parents cope with the potential loss of their child, community resources and national support groups, such as the Children's Liver Foundation, are helpful.

Home Care. The focus of home care is teaching. Because the child will be cared for at home unless a serious complication arises or the child is hospitalized for a liver transplant, parents need much information. Helping the parents develop meals and snacks that meet special nutritional needs on a day-to-day basis can be difficult, and dietary personnel can provide invaluable information. Preventing infection is something parents can control somewhat by sheltering the children from infected individuals as much as possible. The most critical intervention is helping parents identify when they should seek help, specifically if the child develops GI bleeding, changes in level of consciousness, or severe edema. The healthier the child can remain, the better the child and family can focus on developmental skills and preparation for liver transplant.

- The GI system is formed in the first 4 weeks of embryonic development. Congenital defects can be traced to this period.
- The GI system is anatomically fully developed at birth but physiologically immature, affecting enzymes, sphincter tone, permeability, secretion, and reabsorption.
- Assessment of GI distress is very difficult in small children and must include a thorough history, physical assessment, and general appraisal of the child's distress, as well as the parent's perception of the child's pain.
- Fluid balance is very quickly affected if the child is experiencing vomiting, diarrhea, or anorexia, so the nurse must assess changes quickly and completely.
- Gastroesophageal alterations often place the child at risk for respiratory distress from aspiration and compression of the abdomen into the pulmonary spaces. Assessment of respiratory function and airway maintenance are critical interventions.
- Medications play a crucial role in managing some upper GI alterations, so the nurse must be aware of dosages, indications, side effects, and teaching needs.

- The emotional needs of the parents need to be addressed quickly if the child has a congenital condition.
- Surgery to repair congenital defects and obstructive conditions requires nursing care similar to that for an adult but with special emphasis on nutrition, fluid status, pain control, parental involvement, and the developmental level of the child.
- Parental anxiety must be addressed with every GI alteration because it can have a significant effect on the child.
- The use of appropriate Standard Precautions is essential to prevent the spread of infection in children with GI disorders.
- Some malabsorption GI disorders are managed by simple dietary changes.
- Home care and teaching have a high priority because parents must have the necessary information to care for their child during the management of GI alterations.
- Community and home health resources are a critical part of nursing care for the child with GI alterations.

ANSWERS TO CRITICAL THINKING EXERCISE 19-1

1. An accurate history is essential to identify the cause of Andrew's problem and any pathophysiologic process that is occurring. Guide Andrew's mother in carefully describing the frequency, amount, and character of the emesis. Ask about the relation of feeding to vomiting, and determine whether the vomiting is projectile. A comparison of birth weight and current weight will determine whether Andrew is receiving normal nutrition to support weight gain and will assist in an assessment for dehydration. Assess the skin turgor, the fontanels, mucous membranes, and alertness appropriate for his age.

2. Parents, especially first-time parents, often are uncertain of when to seek health care advice. The nurse's responsibility is to set a tone that encourages questions and give guidelines regarding when to seek help. Andrew's mother had called the clinic, but either she did not give an accurate description of the problem or the nurse did not ask the questions that would have made that happen. Access to health care is often limited because clients do not have transportation and do not live near public transportation. Nurses can assist clients to identify resources that are more accessible or resources that assist them in other ways (e.g., financial aid, childcare). Stories of frustration told by parents seeking access to care should be a red flag for change within the system. Some clinics have hotlines that parents can use. Nurses can also manage caseloads of clients and track both preventive and acute care of those clients assigned to them. This process enables them to identify infants and children who are not receiving preventive care, monitor those receiving acute care, and respond to cues that additional intervention is needed.

REFERENCES AND READINGS

Ackley, B., & Ludwig, G. (2002). *Nursing diagnosis handbook* (5th ed.). St. Louis: Mosby.

A-Kader, H., & Balistreri, W. (2004). Cholestasis. In R. Behrman, R. M. Kliegman, & H. Jenson (Eds.), *Nelson textbook of pediatrics* (17th ed., pp. 1314-1319). Philadelphia: Saunders.

Allen, P. (2004). Guidelines for the diagnosis and treatment of celiac disease in children. *Pediatric Nursing, 30*(6), 473-477.

American Academy of Pediatrics, Committee on Infectious Diseases. (2003). *Report of the Committee on Infectious Diseases: 2003 Red Book* (26th ed.). Elk Grove Village, IL: Author.

American Academy of Pediatrics, Task Force on Infant Position and SIDS. (1992). Positioning and SIDS. *Pediatrics, 89,* 1120-1126.

Arguin, A., & Swartz, M. (2004). Gastroesophageal reflux in infants: a primary care perspective. *Pediatric Nursing, 30*(1), 45-71.

Aziz, D., Schiller, D., Gerstle, J., Ein, S., & Langer, J. (2003). Can long-gap esophageal atresia be safely managed at home while awaiting anastomosis? *Journal of Pediatric Surgery, 38*(5), 705-708.

Baron, M. (2002). Crohn disease in children. *American Journal of Nursing, 102*(10), 29-34.

Bercik, P., Verdu, E., & Collins S. (2005). Is irritable bowel syndrome a low-grade inflammatory bowel disease? *Gastroenterology Clinics of North America, 34*(2), 235-245.

Borowitz, S., Cox, D., Kovatchev, B., Ritterband, L., Sheen J., & Sutphen J. (2005). Treatment of childhood constipation by primary care physicians: efficacy and predictors of outcome. *Pediatrics, 115*(4), 873-877.

Bruzzese, E., Canani, R., DeMarco, G., & Guarino, A. (2004). Microflora in inflammatory bowel disease: a pediatric perspective. *Journal of Clinical Gastroenterology, 38*(6), 91-93.

Centers for Disease Control and Prevention (2003a). Managing acute gastroenteritis among children, oral rehydration, maintenance, and nutritional therapy. *MMWR, 52*(RR-16), 1-16.

Centers for Disease Control and Prevention (2003b). Summary of notifiable diseases United States, 2001. *Morbidity and Mortality Weekly Report, 50*(53), 1-108.

Centers for Disease Control and Prevention (2004). Incidence of hepatitis B—United States 1990-2002. *Morbidity and Mortality Weekly Report, 52*(51), 1252-1254.

Centers for Disease Control and Prevention (2006). Prevention of hepatitis A through active or passive immunization. *Morbidity and Mortality Weekly Report, 55*(RR07), 1-23.

Cleft Palate Foundation (2005). *About cleft lip and palate.* Retrieved February 12, 2006, from *www.cleftline.org.*

Coughlin, E. (2003). Assessment and management of pediatric constipation in primary care. *Pediatric Nursing, 29*(4), 296-302.

D'Agostino, J. (2002). Common abdominal emergencies in children. *Emergency Clinics of North America, 20*(1), 139-153.

Dale, J. (2004). Oral rehydration solutions in the management of acute gastroenteritis among children. *Journal of Pediatric Health Care, 18*(4), 211-212.

Davenport, M. (2005). Biliary atresia. *Seminars in Pediatric Surgery, 14*(1), 42-48.

Demmler, G. (2004). Hepatitis. In R. Feigin, J. Cherry, G. Demmler, & S. Kaplan (Eds.). *Textbook of pediatric infectious diseases* (5th ed., pp. 658-665). Philadelphia: Elsevier Saunders.

Eidelwein, A., Cuffari, C., Abadom, V., & Oliva-Hemker, M. (2005). Infliximab efficacy in pediatric ulcerative colitis. *Inflammatory Bowel Disease, 11*(3), 213-218.

Feldman, M., Friedman, L., Sleisenger, M., & Scharschmidt, B. (2002). *Sleisenger & Fordtran's gastrointestinal and liver disease: pathophysiology, diagnosis and management.* Philadelphia: Saunders.

Friesen, C., Calabro, C., Christenson, K., Carpenter, K., Welchert, E., Daniel, J., Haslag, S., & Roberts, C. (2004). Safety of infliximab treatment in pediatric patients with inflammatory bowel disease. *Journal of Pediatric Gastroenterology and Nutrition, 39*(3), 265-269.

Garcia-Careaga, M., & Kerner, J. (2004). Malabsorptive disorders. In R. Behrman, R. M. Kliegman, & H. Jenson (Eds.), *Nelson textbook of pediatrics* (17th ed., pp. 1257-1272). Philadelphia: Saunders.

Ghisham, F. (2004). Chronic diarrhea. In R. Behrman, R. M. Kliegman, & H. Jenson (Eds.), *Nelson textbook of pediatrics* (17th ed., pp. 1276-1281). Philadelphia: Saunders.

Gold, B. (2005). Asthma and gastroesophageal reflux disease in children: exploring the relationship. *Journal of Pediatrics, 146*(3), 13-20.

Gold, B. (2004). Gastroesophageal reflux disease: could intervention in childhood reduce risk of later complications. *American Journal of Medicine, 117*(5A), 23-29.

Gulanick, M., & Myers, J. (2002). *Nursing care plans: nursing diagnosis and intervention* (5th ed.). St. Louis, Mosby.

Hassall, E. (2005). Decisions in diagnosing and managing chronic gastroesophageal reflux disease in children. *Journal of Pediatrics, 146*(3), 3-12.

Henry, S. (2004). Discerning differences: gastroesophageal reflux and gastroesophageal reflux disease in infants. *Advances in Neonatal Care, 4*(4), 235-247.

Jones, M. (2002). Prenatal diagnosis of cleft lip and palate: detection rates, accuracy of ultrasonography, associated anomalies, and strategies for counseling. *Cleft Palate-Craniofacial Journal, 39*(2), 169-173.

Jones, S. (2003). A clinical pathway for pediatric gastroenteritis. *Gastroenterology Nursing, 26*(1), 7-20.

Josephson, K. (2004). Complications from gastroschisis: The untold story. *Pediatric Nursing, 30*(5), 424-425.

Jung, A. (2001). Gastroesophageal reflux in infants and children. *American Family Physician, 64*(11), 1853-1860.

Kaneko, K., & Tsuda, M. (2004). Ultrasound-based decision making in the treatment of acute appendicitis in children. *Journal of Pediatric Surgery, 39*(9), 1316-1320.

King, R. (2003). Pediatric inflammatory bowel disease. *Child and Adolescent Psychiatric Clinics of North America, 12*(3), 537-550.

Kinservik, M., & Friedhoff, M. (2004). The efficacy and safety of polyethylene glycol 3350 in the treatment of constipation in children. *Pediatric Nursing, 30*(3), 232-237.

Kline, R., Kline, J., DiPalma, J., & Barbero, G. (2001). Enteric-coated pH-dependent peppermint oil capsules for the treatment of irritable bowel syndrome in children. *Journal of Pediatrics, 138*(1), 125-128.

Kohli, R. (2004). Differential diagnosis or recurrent abdominal pain: new considerations. *Pediatric Annals, 33*(2), 113-122.

Lockridge, T., Caldwell, A., & Jason, P. (2002). Neonatal surgical emergencies: stabilization and management. *Journal of Obstetric, Gynecologic and Neonatal Nursing, 31*(3), 328-339.

March of Dimes. (2006). *Cleft lip and cleft palate.* Retrieved February 12, 2006, from *www.marchofdimes.com.*

Marx, G., Seidman, E., Martin, S., & Deslandres, C. (2002). Outcome of Crohn's disease diagnosed before two years of age. *Journal of Pediatrics, 140*(4), 470-473.

Mason D., Tobias, N., Lutkenhoff, M., Stoops, M., & Ferguson, D. (2004). The APN's guide to pediatric constipation management. *Nurse Practitioner, 29*(7), 13-21.

McCloskey, J., & Bulechek, G. (2000). *Nursing interventions classification* (3rd ed.). St. Louis: Mosby.

Moorhead, S., Johnson, M., & Maas, M. (2003). *Nursing outcomes classification* (3rd ed.). St. Louis: Mosby.

Morash, D. (2002). An interdisciplinary project that changed practice in feeding methods after pyloromyotomy. *Pediatric Nursing, 28*(2), 113-120.

Moukarzel, A., Lezicka, H., & Ament, M. (2002). Irritable bowel disease and nonspecific diarrhea in infancy and childhood: relationship with juice carbohydrate malabsorption. *Clinical Pediatrics, 41*(3), 145-150.

Nager, A. & Wang, V. (2002). Comparison of nasogastric and intravenous methods of rehydration in pediatric patients with acute dehydration. *Pediatrics, 109*(4), 566-572.

National Birth Defects Prevention Network. (2004). *Birth defects surveillance data from selected states 1997-2001.* Retrieved February 11, 2006, from *nbdpn.org.*

National Digestive Diseases Information Clearinghouse. (2003). *Lactose intolerance.* Retrieved February 12, 2006, from *www. digestive. niddk.nih.gov.*

Negai, B., & Feldstein, V. (2003). Ultrasound of the acute pediatric abdomen. *Applied Radiology, 32*(3), 13-19.

Norris, J., Barriga, K., Hoffenberg, E., Taki, I., Miao, D., Haas, J., Emery, L., Sokol, R., Erlich, H., Eisenbarth, G., & North American Society for Pediatric Gastroenterology and Nutrition. (2001). *Pediatric GE reflux clinical practice guidelines.* Retrieved February 12, 2006, from *www.naspgn.org.*

Orenstein, S., Peters, J., Kahn, S., Youssif, N., & Hussain, Z. (2004). Gastroesophageal reflux disease. In R. Behrman, R. M. Kliegman, & H. Jenson (Eds.), *Nelson textbook of pediatrics* (17th ed., pp. 1222-1224). Philadelphia: Saunders.

Parasher, U., Gibson, C., Bresee, J., & Glass, R. (2006). Rotavirus and severe childhood diarrhea. *Emerging Infectious Diseases.* Retrieved February 12, 2006, from *www.cdc.gov.*

Paton, E. (2003). Pediatric update: A 3-month-old with blood in the stool—a case scenario. *Journal of Emergency Nursing, 29*(1), 68-71.

Paton, E. (2005). Nontraumatic pediatric surgical emergencies: an overview of select presentations. *Advance for Nurse Practitioners, 13*(2), 22-27.

Raucci, J., Whitehall, J., & Sandritter, T. (2004). Childhood immunizations, part 1. *Journal of Pediatric Health Care, 18*(2), 95-101.

Rayhorn, N., & Rayhorn, D. (2002). Inflammatory bowel disease: symptoms in the bowel and beyond. *Nurse Practitioner, 27*(11), 13-29.

Redford-Badwal, D., Mabry, K., & Frassinelli, J., (2003). Impact of cleft lip and/or palate on nutritional health and oral-motor development. *Dental Clinics of North America, 47*(2), 305-317.

Rewers, M. (2005). Risk of celiac disease autoimmunity and timing of gluten introduction in the diet of infants at increased risk of disease. *JAMA, 293*(19), 2410-2412.

Russell, G., & Katz, A. (2004). Infliximab is effective in acute but not chronic childhood ulcerative colitis. *Journal of Pediatric Gastroenterology and Nutrition, 39*(2), 166-170.

Salvatore, S., Hauser, B., Vandemaele, K., Novario, R., & Vandenplas, Y. (2005). Gastroesophageal reflux disease in infants: how much is predictable with questionnaires, pH-metry, endoscopy and histology? *Journal of Pediatric Gastroenterology and Nutrition, 40,* 210-215.

Sandberg, D., Magee, W., & Denk, M. (2002). Neonatal cleft lip and palate repair. *AORN Journal, 75*(3), 490-501.

Snyder, J., & Pickering, L. (2004). Viral hepatitis. In R. Behrman, R. M. Kliegman, & H. Jenson (Eds.), *Nelson textbook of pediatrics* (17th ed., pp. 1324-1332). Philadelphia: Saunders.

Tinaroff, N. (2004). Cleft lip and palate. In R. Behrman, R. M. Kliegman, & H. Jenson (Eds.), *Nelson textbook of pediatrics* (17th ed., pp. 1207-1208). Philadelphia: Saunders.

Wald, E., & Marcy, M. (2002). Infections in day care environments. In F. Burg, J. Ingelfinger, R. Polin, & A. Gershon (Eds.), *Gellis and Kagan's current pediatric therapy* (17th ed., pp. 216-223). Philadelphia: Saunders.

Whitehill, J., Raucci, J., & Sandritter, T. (2004). Childhood immunizations: part 2. *Journal of Pediatric Health Care, 18*(4), 192-197.

Wyllie, R. (2004a). Ileus, adhesions, intussusception, and closed-loop obstructions. In R. Behrman, R. M. Kliegman, & H. Jenson (Eds.), *Nelson textbook of pediatrics* (17th ed., pp. 1241-1243). Philadelphia: Saunders.

Wyllie, R. (2004b). Motility disorders and Hirschsprung disease. In R. Behrman, R. M. Kliegman, & H. Jenson (Eds.), *Nelson textbook of pediatrics* (17th ed., pp. 1237-1241). Philadelphia: Saunders.

CHAPTER 20

The Child With a Genitourinary Alteration

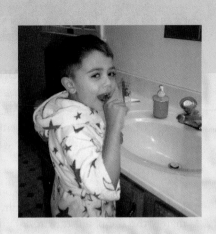

Learning Objectives

After studying this chapter, you should be able to:

- Describe the anatomy and physiology of the infant's and child's genitourinary system.
- Describe the most common diagnostic and screening tests used to assess alteration in genitourinary function.
- Discuss frequently seen alterations in the genitourinary system.
- Use the nursing process to assess, plan, and provide nursing care to children with common genitourinary alterations.
- Develop home care guidelines for the child with a genitourinary alteration.

Definitions

arteriovenous fistula A connection between an artery and vein, usually for the purpose of hemodialysis.

arteriovenous graft A U-shaped plastic tube inserted between an artery and vein, usually for the purpose of hemodialysis.

dysuria Pain on urination.

edema Presence of abnormally large amounts of fluid in the intercellular tissue spaces of the body.

frequency Urination at short time intervals.

hypercalciuria Excessive calcium in the urine.

hyperlipidemia High cholesterol and triglyceride levels in the blood.

hypoalbuminemia Low albumin levels in the blood.

proteinuria Protein in the urine.

urgency Sudden urge to urinate.

Audio Glossary

Electronic Resources

Additional information related to the content in Chapter 20 can be found on:

the interactive companion CD-ROM

- Audio Glossary:
- NCLEX Review Questions

or the companion website at *evolve*
http://evolve.elsevier.com/james/ncoc

- Common Pediatric Laboratory Tests and Normal Values
- NCLEX Review Questions
- Resources for Health Care Providers and Families
- WebLinks

REVIEW OF THE GENITOURINARY SYSTEM

The urinary system consists of the kidneys and ureters, or the upper urinary tract; and the bladder and urethra, or the lower urinary tract. The child's genitourinary system differs in structure and function from an adult's in several ways.

Structure

The bean-shaped kidneys lie one on each side of the spinal column. In an adolescent or adult, the kidney is approximately the size of a fist; in an infant, the size of the kidney is small but proportionally larger. The upper portion of the left kidney lies near the twelfth rib, with the right kidney slightly lower. The *hilum*, the indentation in the kidney, is the area where the blood vessels, lymphatics, nerves, and *ureter* enter the kidney.

A thin, fibrous capsule encases the kidney. The outer region of the kidney is the cortex, and the inner region is the medulla; both can be observed with the kidney dissected longitudinally. The cortex contains the glomeruli and tubules, whereas the medulla contains the renal pyramids. The renal pelvis, located in the area of the hilum, is an extension of the upper end of the ureter.

The ureters extend downward from the kidney and enter the bladder wall. As the bladder fills with urine, it compresses the distal ureters, preventing urine reflux. The bladder is a muscular vessel with a rich blood supply. The infant and child's bladder capacity is approximately equal to 10 mL/kg body weight. The urethra leads from the bladder and contains an internal sphincter and an external sphincter, which control urination. Boys have a longer urethra than do girls.

The *nephron* is the kidney's functional unit. It consists of Bowman's capsule, glomerulus, proximal tubule, loop of Henle, distal tubule, and collecting duct. Each kidney contains approximately 1 million nephrons.

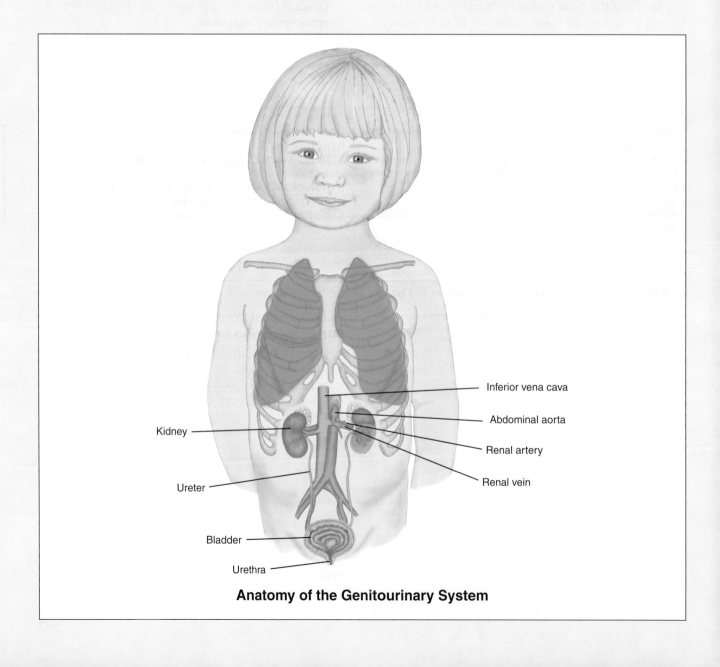

Kidney

Ureter

Bladder

Urethra

Inferior vena cava

Abdominal aorta

Renal artery

Renal vein

Anatomy of the Genitourinary System

PEDIATRIC DIFFERENCES IN THE GENITOURINARY SYSTEM

- In a healthy infant, the kidneys operate at a functional level appropriate for body size; however, function is reduced when the infant is under stress.
- By 6 to 12 months of age, kidney function is nearly like that of the adult.
- In premature infants, the reabsorption of glucose, sodium, bicarbonate, and phosphate is reduced.
- The young infant's kidneys cannot concentrate urine as efficiently as those of older children and adults because the loops of Henle are not yet long enough to reach the inner medulla, where concentration and reabsorption occur.* After the first few weeks of life, the kidneys' acidifying ability reaches the adult level. With acidosis, however, there is only a small increase in acid secretion, and susceptibility to acidemia rises.
- The neonate's bladder, which is in the lower abdominal cavity, gradually sinks into the pelvic cavity during early childhood.
- Young children have shorter urethras, which can predispose them to UTI.
- Children usually achieve complete bladder control by approximately 4 to 5 years of age.
- Unlike adults, most children with acute renal failure regain normal function.

*Banasik, J. (2005). Renal function. In L. Copstead & J. Banasik (Eds.). *Pathophysiology.* St. Louis, MO: Elsevier Saunders.

Blood enters the kidney through the renal arteries, which branch off the abdominal aorta. The renal artery divides and subdivides, eventually culminating in the afferent arterioles, which feed into the glomerular capillaries. The glomerular capillaries empty into the efferent arterioles.

Peritubular capillaries surround the proximal tubule, the loop of Henle, and the distal tubules. The capillaries drain into the venous system. Blood returns to the heart through the renal vein, which enters the inferior vena cava.

Function

The kidneys maintain fluid and chemical balance through glomerular filtration, tubular reabsorption, and secretion. The kidney also has important hormonal functions:

- Production of *renin*, which helps with the regulation of blood pressure. Release of renin is stimulated primarily by decreased pressure in the afferent arterioles of the glomerulus.
- Production of *erythropoietin*, which stimulates red blood cell (RBC) production by the bone marrow.
- Metabolism of vitamin D to its active form, which is important in calcium metabolism.

Adequate renal function is important to the function of other body systems. When assessing a child for a possible genitourinary dysfunction, the nurse should consider such nonspecific assessment data as altered growth, skeletal anomalies, hypertension, skin lesions, and immune dysfunctions.

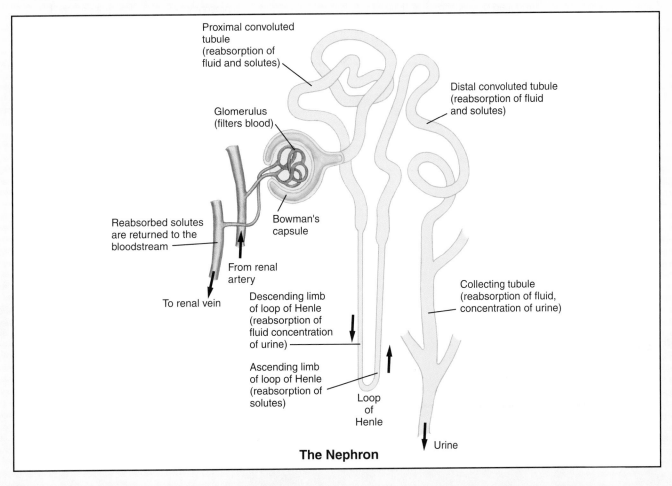

The Nephron

Common Laboratory and Diagnostic Tests for Genitourinary Disorders

Test	Description	Normal Findings	Indications	Nursing Considerations
Urinalysis				
Specific gravity	Measurement of concentration of urine	1.002-1.030	Provides information regarding hydration and renal concentration ability	Specific gravity is higher if protein or glucose is present
pH	Determines acidity and alkalinity	4.6-8.0	Increases in urinary infections	Affected by diet
Protein	Detection of protein in urine	Negative	May be first indication of renal disease	Early morning specimens preferable because they are more concentrated
Glucose	Detection of glucose in urine	Negative	Screens or confirms diabetes and monitors effectiveness of diabetes control; may be present in child with weight loss, dehydration, infection, renal disease	Nonspecific, needs further evaluation
Ketones	Formed in liver and completely metabolized; alteration in carbohydrate metabolism leads to excessive ketone production	Negative	Mainly associated with diabetes; may be present with fever, anorexia, diarrhea, fasting, starvation, prolonged vomiting	Children are more prone to development of ketonuria
Leukocyte esterase	Enzyme released during WBC breakdown	Negative	May be present when WBCs in urine	Indicates possible UTI
Nitrites	Produced by bacteria	Negative	May be present when bacteria in urine	In infant and child, bacteria may not be present in bladder long enough to produce sufficient nitrites to yield positive results
WBCs	Microscopic finding of WBCs in urine	0-2/high-power field	Seen with infection	Urine culture indicated
RBCs	Microscopic finding of RBCs in urine	0-2/high-power field	Trauma, stones, infection, glomerulonephritis	Normal in menstruating females
Bacteria	Microscopic presence of bacteria in urine	None	UTI	Urine culture indicated
Casts	WBC casts and RBC casts originate in kidney tubules	None	Pyelonephritis, glomerulonephritis, renal infarction, collagen disease, interstitial inflammation of kidney	Helps in diagnosis
Urine Culture and Sensitivity				
	Presence of bacteria or other pathogens	Negative or <100,000 colonies/mL urine from clean-catch or sterile bag specimen	Isolation and identification of pathogens in urinary tract; identification of antibiotic sensitivity	See Chapter 13 for specimen collection guidelines
Serum Studies				
BUN	End product of protein metabolism	0-6 mo: 4-15 mg/dL 6-24 mo: 5-15 mg/dL 2 yr to adult: 5-25 mg/dL	Gross indicator of renal function	Increases in renal insufficiency

Common Laboratory and Diagnostic Tests for Genitourinary Disorders—cont'd

Test	Description	Normal Findings	Indications	Nursing Considerations
Serum Studies—cont'd				
Serum creatinine	Byproduct of muscle metabolism; production is constant as long as muscle mass remains constant	0-2 wk: 0.2-0.8 mg/dL 2 wk to 2 yr: 0.2-0.4 mg/dL 2-4 yr: 0.3-0.6 mg/dL 4-6 yr: 0.4-0.8 mg/dL 6-10 yr: 0.4-0.8 mg/dL 10-12 yr: 0.5-1.0 mg/dL 12 yr to adult: *Female:* 0.5-1.1 mg/dL *Male:* 0.6-1.2 mg/dL	Increases in renal insufficiency	Should be assessed before giving nephrotoxic chemotherapeutic agents
Serum osmolality	Measurement of concentration of blood, determined by solute in blood	275-295 mOsm/kg	Indication of fluid and electrolyte balance	Helpful in evaluating hydration status, liver disease, antidiuretic hormone function
Radiography				
Kidney, ureter, bladder (KUB), flat plate scout film	Abdominal radiograph	Normal abdominal structures	Diagnoses renal stones; done before renal studies	No discomfort
Cystoscopy				
	Bladder and urethra examined with cystoscope—a tubular, lighted, telescopic lens	Normal appearance	Examination of bladder and lower tract; visualization of tumor and stones; removal of small stones; biopsy of bladder or tumors; fulguration of bladder tumors and posterior urethral valves	Usually performed with child under general anesthesia; little pain involved; encourage fluids; assess ability to void after procedure
Imaging Studies				
CT scan	Computerized calculations revealing a pattern of shades	Normal appearance	Renal tumors	Sedation may be required; child lies on back and should be still; oral contrast material may be administered; child is usually on NPO status because of sedation or oral contrast material
Voiding cystourethro-gram (VCUG)	Contrast dye instilled in bladder; child or infant voids after bladder is full; serial films taken	Negative for reflux and dilation of posterior urethra, complete bladder emptying	Detects reflux of urine into ureters and its severity; detects bladder emptying problems; detects urethral problems	Can be done in nuclear medicine department to decrease radiation exposure; procedure is invasive; provide support and diversionary activities for child
Dimercaptosuccinic acid (DMSA) renal scan	Injection of radioactive agent technetium-99m (^{99m}Tc)-DMSA to allow visualization of kidney structures and function; serial films taken	Prompt uptake and excretion of radioactive agent	Evaluates blood flow and renal function; assesses renal scarring; identifies pyelonephritis	Minimal radiation exposure; child must remain still for procedure

Continued

Common Laboratory and Diagnostic Tests for Genitourinary Disorders—cont'd

Test	Description	Normal Findings	Indications	Nursing Considerations
Imaging Studies—cont'd				
Renal ultrasonography	Noninvasive; high-frequency sound waves directed at kidneys, ureters, and bladder	Normal size, shape, position, function of kidneys	Assesses position, size, and contour of kidneys, ureters, bladder; detects obstruction and stones; localizes for renal biopsy	Child lies on abdomen; if for transplantation, child lies on back
Intravenous pyelogram (IVP)	IV injection of contrast material concentrates in urine and is seen in kidneys and urine; serial radiographic studies are done; a postvoid film is done after child has emptied the bladder	Normal appearance; activity in kidneys by 2-5 min; no residual urine on postvoid film	Determines bladder's ability to empty completely; provides information about kidneys, ureters, and bladder anatomy; identifies masses that compress urinary system	Child should be on NPO status for a period of time in preparation for receiving contrast material; assess child for hypersensitivity to contrast material; contraindications include decreased renal function
Urodynamic Studies	Invasive test involving urethral and rectal catheters and perineal surface electrodes; measures urine flow, bladder capacity, sensation, sphincter function, bladder pressures; measures voluntary and involuntary contractions	Normal bladder function	Voiding dysfunction, abnormal urinary tract	Inform child and family of procedure; provide support for child throughout procedure; provide diversionary activities

Genitourinary alterations in children encompass a wide range of conditions, from a single acute urinary tract infection (UTI) to end-stage renal disease (ESRD). The effects of illness on the child and family depend on the nature of the illness and on its severity and prognosis. Nursing care also varies. A child in an acute phase of nephrotic syndrome is hospitalized. Less-severe genitourinary disorders may be treated at home. There, the nurse can teach administration of an intravenous (IV) antibiotic or monitor adherence to a treatment plan.

ENURESIS

Children with difficulties in urinary control are defined as having enuresis. Nocturnal enuresis occurs at nighttime during sleep, whereas diurnal enuresis occurs during the day, or in waking hours. Primary enuresis is defined as a child never having experienced a period of dryness, whereas secondary enuresis occurs when a 6- to 12-month period of dryness has preceded the onset of wetting.

Etiology

Although there is no single cause for enuresis, several risk factors have been implicated. Physical factors include decreased bladder capacity, underlying urinary tract abnormalities, neurologic alterations, obstructive sleep apnea, constipation, UTI, pinworm infestation, diabetes mellitus, and voiding dysfunction. Emotional factors related to increased stress can contribute to secondary enuresis. These factors include family disruption, inappropriate pressure during toilet training, inadequate attention to voiding cues, and decreased self-esteem. Sexual abuse must be considered in a child with secondary enuresis.

PATHOPHYSIOLOGY

ENURESIS

Control of urination is related to the maturity of the central nervous system. By 5 years of age, most children are aware of bladder fullness and are able to voluntarily control voiding. Children usually achieve daytime urinary control first, with nighttime dryness occurring later. Girls seem to master this earlier than boys. Children who have primary nocturnal enuresis may have delayed maturation of this portion of the central nervous system.

A child with secondary nocturnal enuresis or with problems of daytime control and complaints of dysuria, urgency, or frequency should be evaluated for other conditions. Bladder infections can give rise to such symptoms. Excessive calcium loss in the urine can irritate the bladder and cause painful urination, urgency, frequency, or wetting. Secondary enuresis accompanied by excessive thirst and weight loss may indicate the onset of diabetes mellitus. Children whose bladders are very sensitive to urine volume may have uninhibited bladder contractions. Moderate to large amounts of urine in the bladder give rise to strong contractions of the bladder muscle. An anatomic abnormality in these cases is rare.

Incidence

Primary nocturnal enuresis is common, affecting approximately 3% to 7% of children at 5 years of age and decreasing to 2% to 3% of children older than 8 years (Boris & Dalton, 2004). It occurs more frequently in boys (Landgraf et al., 2004) and in children with a family history of bed-wetting. Most children eventually outgrow bed-wetting without therapeutic intervention. Some children have diurnal enuresis without nocturnal enuresis; this usually is related to waiting until the last minute to void and not being able to access a bathroom quickly (Boris & Dalton, 2004). Children with both nocturnal and diurnal enuresis are at increased risk for genitourinary abnormalities (Boris & Dalton, 2004). Primary enuresis often resolves spontaneously.

Manifestations

Nocturnal Enuresis

Children with a continuing history of bed-wetting are not able to sense bladder fullness and do not awaken to void. Because physical maturation varies, nocturnal enuresis is not a matter for excessive concern unless the child is older than 6 years or has markedly decreased self-esteem.

Diurnal Enuresis

Children with urgency, frequency, and inappropriate wetting during the day may be seen rushing to the bathroom or tightly crossing their legs. Often these children cannot sit still and they exhibit a constant odor of urine.

Diagnostic Evaluation

The diagnosis of enuresis is based on the history and presenting clinical symptoms. Urinalysis and urine culture can rule out possible UTI. Urine specific gravity and glucose measurement test for underlying diabetes. In addition, the child's urine should be checked for excessive calcium, and a pinworm preparation should be done to exclude infestation.

If the child has daytime enuresis, voiding dysfunction with urge incontinence is explored. Measures of urine flow and bladder capacity and bladder ultrasonography may be indicated. Children with UTIs should have a workup for underlying structural abnormalities.

Therapeutic Management

Treatment of primary nocturnal enuresis may begin with general interventions, such as explaining theories underlying the problem in terms the child can understand. The child is reassured that, with assistance, the problem can resolve. Common-sense approaches of limiting fluids after supper and voiding just before bedtime are encouraged. Also, the child can be trained to use imagery: thinking about what a full bladder feels like and picturing waking up and going to the bathroom. This imagery is done as the child lies in bed before drifting off to sleep. The child should keep a record of the number of dry and wet nights to measure progress.

Reward systems assume bed-wetting is a voluntary behavior and have had varying results for the child with primary nocturnal enuresis. The child may be given a roll of favorite stickers to mark the dry nights on the calendar. The family decides on a special reward or outing when the child has achieved a certain number of consecutive dry nights.

Behavioral conditioning with use of alarms has been successful in the older child with nocturnal enuresis A device worn on the child's pajamas contains a moisture-sensitive alarm. As the child starts to void, the alarm goes off, awakening the child. The alarm system may need to be used consistently over 15 weeks for resolution (Thiedke, 2003).

Imipramine hydrochloride, a tricyclic antidepressant, has been used effectively to treat nocturnal enuresis, although the mechanism of action is not completely understood. Because of the overdose potential with this medication, parents should be cautioned about safe storage. Desmopressin acetate (1-deamino-8-D-arginine vasopressin [DDAVP]) has also been helpful because of its antidiuretic effect. Desmopressin acetate is a nasal spray or tablet and is taken at bedtime. Pharmacologic treatment is not recommended for children under 6 years of age (Thiedke, 2003).

Voiding frequently to keep urine volume in the bladder low may benefit children who are affected by uninhibited bladder contractions during the day. The use of an anticholinergic such as oxybutynin chloride, which relaxes the smooth muscle of the bladder, can be helpful for children with diurnal enuresis related to underlying bladder instability or small bladder capacity. Biofeedback may also help children with diurnal enuresis, particularly those with dysfunctional voiding.

NURSING CARE

The Child With Enuresis

Assessment

The nurse should obtain a full set of vital signs and assess the child and parent for their understanding of enuresis, including the interventions they have already tried. The nurse asks the child and parent to describe voiding and bowel elimination patterns, establishing whether the enuresis is primary or secondary. The nurse should also ask whether the child participates in social activities with peers, such as sleepovers, and whether the child is concerned about the problem of wetting. Therapy is much more successful for the older child than for the younger child, who may not be bothered by bed-wetting. The nurse should assist the child in obtaining a urine specimen. The physical examination includes assessment for signs of sexual abuse or visible genital abnormalities. It also is important to observe the lower spine for the presence of a dimple or hair tuft that might suggest spina bifida occulta (see Chapter 28).

Nursing Diagnosis and Planning

The nursing diagnoses and expected outcomes that may be appropriate after assessment of the child with enuresis are as follows:

* Situational Low Self-Esteem related to bed-wetting or urinary incontinence.

Expected Outcome: The child will demonstrate positive self-esteem, as evidenced by a realistic description of the problem and positive self-statements.
* Impaired Social Interaction related to bed-wetting or urinary incontinence.

Expected Outcome: The child will participate in age-appropriate activities such as sleepovers and overnight camp.
* Compromised Family Coping related to negative social stigma and increased laundry load.

Expected Outcomes: The family will identify strengths and will describe positive problem-solving strategies.
* Risk for Impaired Skin Integrity related to prolonged contact with urine.

Expected Outcome: The child will have no rashes or redness in the perineal area.

Interventions

Enuresis can be a frustrating problem for both the child and family. The nurse can help by providing them with correct information about causes and therapeutic approaches. It is important that the family choose the treatment that will best meet its needs. Follow-up to determine the effectiveness of treatment is essential because becoming dry can be a long process and the nurse is instrumental in providing support to the child and family over the entire course of therapy.

Evaluation

* Is the child able to describe ways to manage the condition?
* Is the child verbalizing a decrease in stress related to the enuresis, and does the child make positive self-statements?
* Is the child showing an increased interest in peer activities?
* Is the family able to identify its strengths and demonstrate appropriate problem solving?
* Is the child having increased dry nights, and does the child's skin remain intact?

CRITICAL THINKING EXERCISE 20-1

Mr. Sampson brings his son Thomas in for his 5-year-old well-child visit. As the nurse is obtaining a history, Mr. Sampson expresses concern that Thomas wets the bed at night. He has been fully toilet trained for 1 year and does not have daytime urine accidents. Thomas refuses to wear a diaper at night because he "doesn't want to be a baby." As a result, he consistently sleeps in wet sheets and clothing.

1. What additional data would be helpful to obtain from Mr. Sampson?
2. What suggestions for an initial approach to the problem should the nurse give Mr. Sampson?

URINARY TRACT INFECTIONS

UTIs, which are characterized by the presence of bacteria in the urine along with systemic signs of infection, are commonly seen in children. In fact, they result in significant morbidity in infants and children (Ma & Shortliffe, 2004). These infections can have long-term complications that include renal scarring with decreased renal function, high blood pressure, and, rarely, ESRD.

Etiology

UTIs, except in newborn infants, are caused by bacteria ascending from outside the urethra into the bladder and from there into the upper urinary tract. Bacteria in the blood, which seed in the kidney, can cause UTIs in newborn infants.

Fecal bacteria cause most UTIs. *Escherichia coli* is implicated in approximately 80% of affected infants and children. Other bacteria known to cause UTIs are group B streptococci, *Klebsiella pneumoniae*, *Proteus* species, *Enterobacter* species, enterococci, and *Staphylococcus* species. Viruses and fungi, specifically *Candida* species, can rarely cause infections.

The following conditions predispose the infant or child to UTI:

- Urinary tract obstructions, which can be congenital or acquired. These include strictures, ureteropelvic narrowing, or other urinary tract anomalies. *Hydronephrosis* is dilation of the renal pelvis, usually caused by ureteropelvic junction obstruction. *Phimosis*, which is a narrowing of the prepuce opening, prevents the foreskin from being retracted.
- Voiding dysfunction resulting in urinary stasis. Conditions contributing to incomplete bladder emptying include neurogenic bladder and bladder instability. Constipation that causes pressure on the bladder can inhibit complete bladder emptying.
- Anatomic differences. Young girls have a short urethra, which expedites bacterial transit.
- Individual susceptibility to infection. Some infants and children have UTIs without any structural abnormality and may be more prone to bacterial adherence to epithelial cells in the urinary tract.
- Reflux. A primary contributing factor to upper UTI, or pyelonephritis, is vesicoureteral reflux (VUR).
- UTIs in toddler-age girls are more frequent during toilet training, most probably as a result of urinary retention or incomplete bladder emptying (Elder, 2004). It is generally accepted, however, that bacterial colonization of the prepuce of uncircumcised infants can increase the risk of UTI in infant boys younger than 1 year.
- Sexually active adolescent girls are at risk for UTIs.

Incidence

The overall prevalence of UTIs in the United States is 3% to 5% in girls and 1% in boys. During the first year of life, there is a higher incidence in males (Elder, 2004). Shaw et al. (1998) concluded that the incidence of UTI is greater than previously estimated because children younger than 2 years

with a febrile respiratory or gastrointestinal illness frequently have a coexisting undiagnosed UTI. Because scarring with reduced renal function can result from missed UTIs, the study authors suggest considering UTI in any young child with a febrile illness. VUR is a frequently seen underlying anatomical abnormality in children with UTIs. White girls are affected much more frequently than African American girls. Breastfeeding has been found to significantly reduce the risk of UTIs because of the protective factors observed in human milk that prevent microbial attachment to the mucosa (Hanson et al., 2002).

Manifestations

Clinical manifestations of UTI vary widely; factors include the child's age, sex, underlying anatomic or neurologic abnormalities, and frequency of recurrence. Signs in the young

---

PATHOPHYSIOLOGY

URINARY TRACT INFECTIONS

Fecal bacteria colonize the perineal area or under the prepuce of uncircumcised infant boys. Bacteria adhere to epithelial cells in the urinary tract and then ascend through the urethra into the bladder, causing a bladder infection, or *cystitis*. In most circumstances, the bladder is emptied on a regular basis, which decreases the opportunity for bacterial growth. In children with incomplete bladder emptying, bacteria grow in the residual urine.

Bacteria ascending from the bladder into the ureters and up into the renal parenchyma cause pyelonephritis. Pyelonephritis is more frequently seen in children with VUR but can occur in its absence.

Scarring, as an inflammatory consequence of pyelonephritis, is more frequently seen in infants younger than 1 year and is a significant cause of hypertension during childhood. Scarring causes decreased arterial perfusion to the kidney, mimicking volume depletion. This triggers the renin-angiotensin mechanism to increase aldosterone release and cause sodium and fluid retention. The subsequent increase in circulating blood volume results in hypertension.

PATHOPHYSIOLOGY

HYDRONEPHROSIS

Obstruction at the ureteropelvic junction or other parts of the ureter causes dilation of the kidney. As the renal dilation increases, the risk of renal parenchymal damage and decreased renal function increases as well. In some instances, the obstruction is only partial, causing an initial dilation but no progressive renal function loss. Hydronephrosis can be associated with VUR.

Ultrasonography has facilitated prenatal diagnosis of hydronephrosis. Many infants diagnosed prenatally have had spontaneous resolution of the condition.

┌───┐
│ **PATHOPHYSIOLOGY**   │

VESICOURETERAL REFLUX

A valvelike mechanism at the junction of the ureter and bladder prevents urine reflux into the ureters. As urine fills the bladder or as the bladder contracts during voiding, pressure in the bladder occludes the opening to the ureter. When a defect occurs at the vesicoureteral junction, VUR results. The defect at the vesicoureteral junction is considered a congenital abnormality, although transitory VUR associated with a lower UTI is also possible.

In VUR, two mechanisms contribute to UTI. Bacteria in the urine can be carried up to the kidney, causing pyelonephritis and renal damage with scarring. Also, when urine reflux into the lower ureter occurs, urine can return to the bladder, leaving a urine residual that becomes a medium for bacterial growth.

The severity of VUR determines the potential risk for pyelonephritis and kidney damage. The International Classification of Reflux grades reflux on a scale of I through V. Grade I describes reflux into the ureter only with no dilation. Grade V, the most severe, includes gross dilation and reflux involving the kidney.

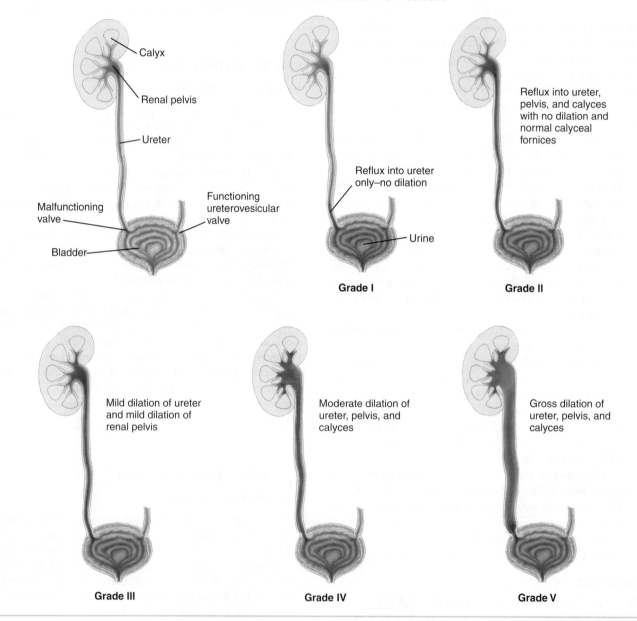

International Classification of Reflux

Calyx

Renal pelvis

Ureter

Malfunctioning valve

Functioning ureterovesicular valve

Bladder

Reflux into ureter only—no dilation

Urine

Grade I

Reflux into ureter, pelvis, and calyces with no dilation and normal calyceal fornices

Grade II

Mild dilation of ureter and mild dilation of renal pelvis

Grade III

Moderate dilation of ureter, pelvis, and calyces

Grade IV

Gross dilation of ureter, pelvis, and calyces

Grade V

child and infant are more vague and nonspecific. *Fever* (38° C [100.4° F]) without a focus for infection in infants and young children 2 to 24 months of age suggests a UTI.

An abdominal mass can suggest hydronephrosis in an infant. Other signs and symptoms of hydronephrosis are similar to those for an infant with a UTI (Box 20-1).

Diagnostic Evaluation

Bacteria in the urine establish a diagnosis of UTI. Symptoms of UTI in the absence of bacteriuria can be caused by perineal inflammation, vaginitis, pinworms, or chemical irritation from bubble baths.

Routine urinalysis that demonstrates hematuria, presence of white blood cells (WBCs), and positive nitrites can suggest a UTI. Urinalysis should be performed on a first morning urine specimen to be most accurate.

Urine culture is the single determining diagnostic study for a UTI. Any bacterial growth of a single-strain bacterium exceeding 10^5 colony-forming units/mL of a clean-catch urine specimen establishes a diagnosis of UTI. Obtaining a sterile urine sample is difficult in children, especially children who are not yet toilet trained. A child who can void on demand can provide a midstream clean-catch urine specimen. In infants and children who are not toilet trained, a sterile pediatric urine collection bag attached to the perineum can collect a urine specimen (see Chapter 13). Collecting urine by this method is less invasive but not as accurate as by other methods, and the urine specimen must be plated as quickly as possible. If the urine cannot be plated within 10 minutes of collection, it should be refrigerated.

When accurate determination of bacteria is the goal, more intrusive methods of bladder catheterization (see Chapter 13) or suprapubic aspiration are the collection methods of choice. If suprapubic aspiration is necessary, the area above the pubis is cleaned with an antiseptic solution, a needle attached to a syringe is inserted at a 90-degree angle into the bladder, and urine is aspirated. If catheterization or suprapubic aspiration is used to obtain a urine culture, the growth of any bacteria indicates infection.

More intensive evaluation for underlying structural abnormalities is necessary for certain infants and children with UTIs. Evaluative studies include ultrasonography (Giorgi, Bratslavsky, & Kogan, 2005) to detect kidney dilation resulting from obstruction and a voiding cystourethrography or radionuclide cystography to detect VUR.

Therapeutic Management

A 3- to 5-day course of oral antibiotics is the treatment of choice for an uncomplicated UTI without systemic symptoms (Chon, Lai, & Shortliffe, 2001; Elder, 2004). The antibiotic chosen should be sensitive to the specific bacterium (identified by culture), easily administered, and have minimal adverse effects. Oral trimethoprim-sulfamethoxazole and cephalosporins are frequently used. A follow-up urine culture evaluates treatment success.

Children with pyelonephritis require initial treatment with parenteral antibiotics followed by oral antibiotic treatment. The older child who does not need hospitalization can receive daily intramuscular ceftriaxone for 1 to 2 days, followed by 10 to 14 days of oral antibiotics. Infants and children admitted to the hospital for treatment usually receive an IV ampicillin or cephalosporin and an aminoglycoside (e.g., gentamicin). Oral antibiotics may follow this initial treatment.

When anatomic abnormalities are detected or UTIs recur, prophylactic antibiotic therapy might be initiated. Prophylactic antibiotics also are given to children after their initial course of treatment while they are waiting for imaging studies to confirm an underlying structural abnormality.

Because the majority of children with grades I through III VUR have a spontaneous resolution of the reflux, most physicians choose nonsurgical management of this condition (Elder, 2004). Children are given prophylactic antibiotics and screened for UTI every 2 to 4 months and when febrile. Cystography every 12 to 18 months monitors the progress of resolution.

First-line treatment for children with long-term VUR is the endoscopic injection of bulking material into the submucosa of the affected ureter. The material, Deflux injectable gel, builds a protective wall inside the ureter to prevent the backflow of urine (Lackgren, Whalin, Skoldenberg, & Stenberg, 2001). Children with grade III or greater after treatment receive up to two more implantations of Deflux, and those with persistent reflux are referred for open surgery.

Surgical intervention, or reimplantation of the ureters into the bladder, is indicated for persistent severe grades IV and V reflux. Other indications for surgical treatment include frequent UTIs, presence of renal scarring, or nonadherence with antibiotic therapy. Nonsurgical treatment of the child with hydronephrosis is similar to that for the child with VUR. Surgery is required for children with complete obstruction.

BOX 20-1	**Manifestations of Urinary Tract Infection in Infants and Children**

Infants

Nonspecific	Change in urine odor or color
Fever or hypothermia in neonate	Poor weight gain
Irritability	Feeding difficulties
Dysuria as evidenced by crying when voiding	

Children

Abdominal or suprapubic pain	Dysuria
Voiding frequency	New or increased incidence of enuresis
Voiding urgency	Fever

Children With Pyelonephritis

Same symptoms as for children with uncomplicated UTI plus	Back pain
	Costovertebral angle tenderness
	Nausea and vomiting
High fever, chills	Appears sick

CRITICAL TO REMEMBER
Evaluation After a Documented Urinary Tract Infection

Radiologic studies are indicated for infants and children who are likely to have renal damage associated with structural abnormalities. Studies can diagnose underlying abnormalities and monitor the extent of potential renal scarring. The following recommendations guide the necessity for follow-up:

* Radiographic imaging studies for at-risk infants and children (all boys with UTIs and all girls younger than 5 years) after the first UTI. Evaluation of older girls with recurrent UTIs.
* Renal ultrasonography before discharge in all infants and children hospitalized for treatment of a febrile UTI or suspected pyelonephritis.
* VCUG or isotope cystogram for at-risk children when symptoms have disappeared and the urine culture is negative. Some practitioners prefer to wait 4 to 6 weeks after the resolution of the UTI to allow transitory VUR to resolve.
* Renal scan for children diagnosed with VUR and children with suspected pyelonephritis.
* Evaluation of children after the first UTI who have hypertension, have a family history of urinary tract abnormalities, or exhibit delayed growth.

NURSING CARE

The Child With a Urinary Tract Infection

Assessment

The nurse obtains a history of signs and symptoms of UTI from the child and family, which will vary according to age. Determining bowel elimination patterns is important as well, because constipation can increase the risk for UTI in certain children.

Physical assessment includes temperature, blood pressure, abdominal examination for masses, examination for costovertebral angle tenderness, and examination for genital abnormalities. It is important to obtain a urinalysis and urine culture before initiating antibiotics.

Nursing Diagnosis and Planning

The nursing diagnoses and expected outcomes that apply to the child with UTI and family are as follows:

* Risk for Injury to the kidney related to complications from the infectious process.

Expected Outcome: The child will be free of recurrent UTIs, as evidenced by the absence of voiding frequency and urgency, dysuria, and fever and the presence of a negative urine culture.

* Deficient Fluid Volume related to decreased intake and increased fluid loss from fever.

Expected Outcome: The child will maintain adequate intake of fluids and electrolytes for age, as evidenced by an output normal for age (see Chapter 18).

* Deficient Knowledge related to incomplete understanding of the disease process, diagnostic tests, antibiotic administration, and preventive measures for UTI.

Expected Outcomes: The parent or child will explain the disease process, diagnostic tests, and preventive measures for UTIs. The family will follow through with appropriate follow-up care, including antibiotic administration and imaging studies, if recommended.

Interventions

Infants admitted to the hospital with fever of unknown origin often are evaluated to rule out a focal infection or septicemia, even though UTI is one of the most frequent causes of fever in infants. The evaluation includes blood studies and cultures, lumbar puncture, and urinary catheterization or suprapubic aspiration for urine culture. The parent already is anxious about the infant, so it is imperative that the nurse inform the parent about why procedures are being done. An IV line is established at the time of the septic workup because parenteral antibiotics are given while waiting for laboratory results and for several days thereafter if the child has a UTI.

Allow the parent to express concerns and provide reassurance about the infant's condition. Try to incorporate the infant's routine in care: the mother can continue to breastfeed, ensuring that the IV site is protected as she holds the infant. If the breastfeeding mother is unable to remain with the infant, she will need to pump her breasts. Allowing parents to participate in the infant's care provides them a measure of control in an uncertain situation. The infant with a documented UTI will require renal ultrasonography at the earliest convenient time.

Nursing care of the child who is not hospitalized includes ensuring administration of antibiotics, promoting comfort, maintaining good hydration, preparing the child and parent for diagnostic procedures, and monitoring for response to treatment and complications.

Give the child and family information on the prevention of UTIs (Box 20-2). Advise them to adhere to any treatment and recommended follow-up studies. Without causing anxiety, emphasize that repeated UTIs can contribute to renal damage, so prevention is especially important. For older children, once-daily antibiotics are best administered at bedtime because of urinary stasis during the night.

Good hydration is important, especially if the child has been febrile, nauseated, vomiting, or feeding poorly. Encourage oral fluids if possible. IV hydration may be required, especially for young infants. Observe the child for signs of dehydration: poor skin turgor, dry mucous membranes, a sunken fontanel, decreased output, and decreased peripheral perfusion. Daily weights, intake and output, and urine specific gravity are indicators of hydration. Acute renal infection with resulting renal impairment can alter the kidney's ability to concentrate urine, leading to falsely low specific gravity readings (American Academy of Pediatrics, 2000).

For children with VUR, explain the treatment plan, including medical or surgical management, to the parent

| BOX 20-2 | CHILD AND FAMILY WANT TO KNOW About How to Manage and Prevent Urinary Tract Infections |

If your child has been diagnosed with a urinary tract infection, it is most important for you to:

- Give your child the prescribed medication for the full number of days your physician or nurse practitioner recommends. Some children need to continue on a lower dose of the antibiotic after the initial treatment is finished.
- Take a follow-up urine culture to the laboratory if your physician or nurse practitioner has requested one. Use a sterile container to collect the urine. If the laboratory has not given you a sterile plastic container, you can use a glass container and a cover that have been sterilized. Make sure the urine stays refrigerated or in a cooler while you take it to the laboratory.
- Keep the appointment if the physician or nurse practitioner has ordered some follow-up studies of your child's urinary system. These studies can help diagnose a structural problem with your child's urinary system or monitor the kidney for any problems.
- Call your physician or nurse practitioner if your child has a fever or symptoms that make you think the infection has returned.

Preventing a urinary tract infection from recurring is important because repeated infections can cause kidney damage. Some suggestions that can help prevent a urinary tract infection are to:

- Wipe babies and teach young girls to wipe from front to back after going to the bathroom. This takes any germs away from the opening that leads into the urinary system. Be sure to keep the foreskin on uncircumcised baby boys as clean as possible without forcible retraction.
- Encourage your toilet-trained child to avoid "holding" urine and to urinate at least four times per day, emptying the bladder completely.
- Give your child lots of fluids throughout the day to help flush out the bladder.
- Avoid dressing your child in tight clothing or diapers. Use cotton underwear, rather than synthetic fabric.
- Avoid bubble baths, which can irritate your child's urinary system.
- Emphasize proper hygiene if your daughter is sexually active and encourage her to urinate immediately after having sexual intercourse.

and child in a simple, age-appropriate manner. If medical management is elected, both parent and child should understand that treatment may last for years and that adherence is important. Follow-up includes antibiotic therapy, urine cultures, renal function tests (blood urea nitrogen [BUN], serum creatinine), blood pressure monitoring, and imaging studies.

If surgical treatment is required, give the parent and child information regarding the procedure and preoperative and postoperative care. They need to understand that an inpatient hospitalization is required. Medications are given for pain and bladder spasms, which frequently occur after surgery. Follow-up care involves prophylactic antibiotics until a postsurgery cystogram indicates that the VUR has been corrected.

Evaluation

- Is the child free of frequency and dysuria?
- Is the urine culture negative?
- Is the child taking fluids on the basis of expected amounts for age, and is the child's urine output adequate (see Chapter 18)?
- Has the child received follow-up diagnostic testing and antibiotic therapy?
- Can the parent or child describe symptoms of recurrence and measures to take if infection occurs?

CRYPTORCHIDISM

Cryptorchidism (undescended or hidden testes) occurs when one or both testes fail to descend through the inguinal canal into the scrotal sac.

PATHOPHYSIOLOGY

CRYPTORCHIDISM

In normal fetal development, the testes begin their descent from the abdomen between 32 and 36 weeks' gestation. The exact reason for failure of the testes to descend is not known. It is generally agreed that endocrine, mechanical, and neural factors all play significant roles.* Sperm production is decreased in the undescended testis, and risk is increased for development of a malignancy when the child reaches adulthood. Inguinal hernias are commonly associated with cryptorchidism.

*Elder, J. (2004). Urologic disorders in infants and children. In R. Behrman, R. Kliegman, & H. Jenson (Eds.) *Nelson textbook of pediatrics* (17th ed., p. 1817). Philadelphia: WB Saunders.

Incidence

Cryptorchidism is a common urologic problem. Approximately 4% of normal healthy boys have undescended testes at birth (Elder, 2004). Premature infants (Nicholls, 2003) and low-birth-weight infants have a higher incidence of undescended testes (Leung & Robson, 2004). Most infants have spontaneous descent of their testes during the first year of life. Children with undescended testes are at increased risk for testicular malignancy and infertility (Leung & Robson, 2004).

Manifestations

Testes that are not palpable or not easily guided into the scrotum as well as a previously descended testis that ascends into an extrascrotal position are manifestations of cryptorchidism.

Diagnostic Evaluation

One or both testes may be undescended. If the testis is not palpable, in some instances ultrasonography, computed tomography scan, or magnetic resonance imaging can determine its location. The missing testis may be found at any point along the process vaginalis, may be located in the abdomen, or may follow an aberrant course and come to lie in the inguinal area, base of the penis, or perineum (Leung & Robson, 2004).

Location of an intra-abdominal testis may require surgical exploration by laparoscopy. When neither testis can be palpated, the child is evaluated for their presence by hormonal stimulation and measurement of testosterone response. Elevated follicle-stimulating hormone and luteinizing hormone levels accompanied by absent testosterone indicate testicular absence. True absence of both testes is rare.

Therapeutic Management

Initially, the infant with cryptorchidism is managed by observation because spontaneous descent of the testes during the first year of life is common. Medical or surgical treatment may be instituted after the child's first birthday. Human chorionic gonadotropin, the pituitary hormone that stimulates the production of testosterone, may be prescribed. It has shown limited success in stimulating the testis to descend.

The treatment of choice is surgical correction, or orchidopexy, which should be performed between 9 and 15 months of age (Elder, 2004). The testis is brought down and sutured in place. The most common complications from this surgery are bleeding and infection. The purpose of therapy is to preserve testicular function, provide a normal-appearing scrotum, and enable the child to perform testicular self-examinations as he matures, to screen for malignancy. A testicular prosthesis can be considered for the child with an absent testis on one side. The procedure is usually performed on an outpatient basis.

NURSING CARE

The Child With Cryptorchidism

Assessment

A physical examination should be performed, with careful attention given to the genitalia (Benjamin, 2002). Assess the parents' knowledge of undescended testes and the importance of treatment.

Nursing Diagnosis and Planning

The nursing diagnoses and expected outcomes that apply to the child with cryptorchidism and the family are as follows:

- Deficient Knowledge (parental) related to cause and management of cryptorchidism.

  Expected Outcome: The parents will be able to explain cryptorchidism, its management, and possible sequelae.
- Effective Therapeutic Regimen Management (individual) related to possible decreased fertility and increased risk of testicular malignancy.

CRITICAL TO REMEMBER
Assessing for Cryptorchidism

Testes can retract into the inguinal canal if the infant is upset or cold. The cremasteric reflex, or testicular retraction in response to tactile stimulation to the front inner thigh, can lead to a false diagnosis of cryptorchidism.

- Examine the infant in a warm environment. Be sure the infant is calm before the examination.
- Warm your hands before touching the infant.
- Milk the testis downward from the groin and document its distal point.
- Examine the older child in both a sitting and a frog-leg position.
- Most testes descend by the time the infant is 1 year old.

Expected Outcomes: The parents will help the child learn to perform regular testicular self-examination during adolescence and the individual will seek referral for fertility testing as warranted.

Interventions

Nursing care should be directed at educating parents and providing them with information and resources. If the child has bilateral undescended testes or absence of testes, referrals to a counselor, psychologist, or subspecialist may be appropriate. The nurse provides routine postoperative care after orchidopexy, paying particular attention to voiding patterns, pain and swelling, and signs of bleeding or infection.

Evaluation

- Are the parents able to explain cryptorchidism and its management?
- Do the parents state their responsibilities to guide their child when he is an adolescent to perform regular testicular self-examination and to seek fertility testing if appropriate?

HYPOSPADIAS AND EPISPADIAS

Hypospadias is a congenital anomaly in which the actual opening of the urethral meatus is below the normal placement on the glans of the penis (Fig. 20-1). The degree of misplacement of the urethral opening can vary. The urethra may open only slightly ventral to the glans or as far back as the penoscrotal junction. *Chordee,* or downward curvature of the penile shaft, can accompany hypospadias. Associated anomalies may include undescended testes and inguinal hernias. Dorsal placement of the urethral opening, or epispadias, also may occur but is less common.

Etiology and Incidence

Hypospadias is one of the most common congenital anomalies, occurring in 1 of every 250 male children (Manson & Carr, 2003). A greater frequency of hypospadias has uniformly been found in whites than in other races (Gallentine,

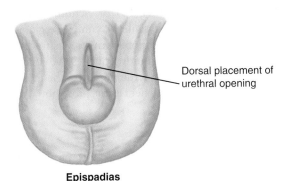

Epispadias

Dorsal placement of
urethral opening

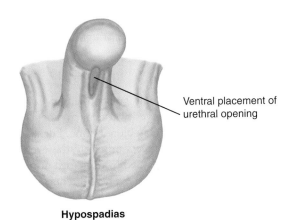

Hypospadias

Ventral placement of
urethral opening

FIG 20-1   **Epispadias and hypospadias are congenital anomalies in which the urethral opening is above or below its normal location on the glans of the penis. Stenosis of the opening could occur, leading to possible UTIs or hydronephrosis. Hypospadias might interfere with fertility if it is left uncorrected.**

Morey, & Thompson, 2001). Risk is increased if either the father or a sibling has the anomaly. Testes are undescended in 10% of affected children, and risk for inguinal hernias is increased. Epispadias is extremely rare and is often associated with bladder exstrophy.

Manifestations and Diagnostic Evaluation

Ventral or dorsal placement of the urethral opening, altered urinary stream, and chordee are physical manifestations of hypospadias. Diagnosis is based on physical examination (Stokowski, 2004).

Therapeutic Management

Correction of hypospadias is accomplished by surgical intervention, which is usually done in one stage and on an outpatient basis. The surgeon releases the chordee, lengthens the urethra, positions the meatus at the penile tip, and reconstructs the penis. The surgical procedure should be done before the age of toilet training because the location of the meatus may make it difficult for the child to urinate standing up. Surgery is ideally done when the child is between 8 and 12 months of age (Marrocco, Vallasciani, Fiocca, & Calisti, 2004). Infants with hypospadias should not be circumcised because the foreskin

PATHOPHYSIOLOGY

HYPOSPADIAS

Hypospadias occurs from incomplete development of the urethra in utero. The exact cause of the defect is not known, but it is thought to be related to genetic, environmental, and hormonal influences.*

The displacement of the urethral meatus does not usually interfere with urinary continence. Stenosis of the opening, however, would give rise to partial obstruction of out-flowing urine. Further, ventral placement of the urethral opening might interfere with fertility in the mature man if it is left uncorrected.

*Pierik, F., Burdorf, A., Deddens, J., Juttman, R., & Weber, R. (2004). Maternal and paternal risk factors for cryptorchidism and hypospadias: a case-control study in newborn boys. *Environmental Health Perspectives, 112,* 1570-1576.

may be used in the surgical reconstruction. After surgery, the child has some type of temporary urinary diversion to allow for healing of the meatus. Indwelling urinary catheters or urethral stents are commonly used. In addition, the child's activity must be restricted for several days. These treatments are tolerated better by the younger child. The goal of surgery is to make urinary and sexual function as normal as possible and to improve the cosmetic appearance of the penis.

Surgical correction of epispadias can include bladder neck reconstruction and lengthening of the penis and urethra.

NURSING CARE

The Child With Hypospadias

Hypospadias is usually discovered during the newborn examination. In the infant with hypospadias, palpate the abdomen for a distended bladder or enlarged kidneys. Assess urinary function by observing the urinary stream if possible. For the older infant with hypospadias, question the parents about UTIs, quality of urinary stream (whether it is steady or intermittent), dribbling, or family history of genitourinary problems. Assess the parents' understanding of hypospadias and the surgical procedure and follow-up care necessary for correction.

Nursing Diagnosis and Planning

The nursing diagnoses and expected outcomes that apply to the child with hypospadias and the family are as follows:

• Deficient Knowledge (parental) related to diagnosis of hypospadias, surgical procedure, and postoperative care.

Expected Outcomes: The parents will describe hypospadias and the reason for surgical correction. The parents will actively participate in the postoperative care.

• Risk for Infection related to indwelling catheter.

Expected Outcome: The child will remain free of UTI, as evidenced by normal urinalysis and culture and absence of fever.

- Acute Pain related to surgery.

  Expected Outcome: The child will exhibit infrequent episodes of crying and demonstrate normal sleep patterns.
- Impaired Physical Mobility related to surgical procedure on the penis.

  Expected Outcome: The child will tolerate activity restriction, as evidenced by participating in developmentally appropriate bedside play.

Interventions

The nurse should provide parents with detailed preoperative teaching and encourage them to participate in the postoperative care of their child. The child has a pressure dressing to decrease edema, which is removed by the physician after approximately 4 days. Some infants have a stent that drains directly into the diaper, whereas others require a closed drainage bag system. The parents should be able to demonstrate proper care of the catheter or stent before discharge.

The nurse advises parents to encourage the child to drink frequently. High fluid intake is necessary to maintain hydration and free flow of urine. Teach the parent to monitor the child's temperature and observe urine for cloudiness or foul smell. Any signs of a UTI should be reported immediately. Postoperative prophylactic antibiotics are usually prescribed.

The parent should provide the child with a variety of quiet diversional activities, being careful not to traumatize the site. The child can receive medication as ordered for pain. The parent can provide environmental stimulation and a feeling of mobility by transporting the child in a carriage, wagon, or cart. Encourage parents to bring favorite toys or music to help the child feel less anxious.

Evaluation

- Can the parents explain the surgical procedure and postoperative care of their child?
- Are the parents participating in the care of their child?
- Is the child afebrile, and are the child's urinalysis and culture within normal limits?
- Is the child happy, comfortable, and able to sleep?
- Is the child participating in age-appropriate play within restrictions?

MISCELLANEOUS DISORDERS AND ANOMALIES OF THE GENITOURINARY TRACT

Other disorders and anomalies associated with the genitourinary tract are described in Table 20-1. Most of them require surgical correction as noted. For both psychologic and mechanical reasons, these defects are usually corrected at a young age; some may require more than one surgery.

ACUTE POSTSTREPTOCOCCAL GLOMERULONEPHRITIS

The term *glomerulonephritis* refers to a group of kidney disorders characterized by inflammatory injury in the glomerulus. Infection or a systemic disease process, such as lupus erythematosus (see Chapter 17) or Schönlein-Henoch purpura (an autoimmune vasculitis), can cause glomerular inflammation. Acute glomerulonephritis refers to disorders that occur suddenly, are self-limiting, and resolve completely. Acute poststreptococcal glomerulonephritis, the most common type, is characterized by hematuria, proteinuria, edema, and renal insufficiency.

Etiology and Incidence

Acute poststreptococcal glomerulonephritis occurs as an immune reaction to a group A beta-hemolytic streptococcal infection of the throat or skin.

This disorder occurs most commonly in children aged 5 to 12 years and is uncommon before age 3 years. Clinical symptoms usually develop 1 to 2 weeks after a streptococcal pharyngitis or 3 to 6 weeks after a streptococcal pyoderma (Davis & Avner, 2004).

Manifestations

Hematuria, which is a cardinal sign of poststreptococcal glomerulonephritis, ranges in severity from microscopic to gross, as evidenced by smoky or tea-colored urine. Edema, which is worse in the morning, affects primarily the eyelids and ankles. This can be accompanied by decreased urinary output. Hypertension can be severe. The child may be febrile. Many children experience fatigue. Pulmonary edema can be a life-threatening complication.

Diagnostic Evaluation

History, presenting symptoms, and laboratory results can establish the diagnosis of acute poststreptococcal glomerulonephritis. A urinalysis reveals macroscopic or microscopic hematuria with red blood cell casts, which indicates glomerular injury. Proteinuria is also present but not severe. Blood chemistry values are usually within the normal range. If renal insufficiency is severe, however, BUN and creatinine levels are elevated. Electrolyte disturbances, such as high serum potassium and low serum bicarbonate levels, can result from inadequate glomerular filtration.

The complete blood cell count usually demonstrates normal WBCs and mild anemia. The lower hemoglobin and hematocrit values reflect the dilutional effect of extra fluid in the blood as a result of decreased glomerular filtration.

Immunologic studies are important in diagnosing acute poststreptococcal glomerulonephritis. Serum complement (C3) may be low because of the fixation of complement in immune complexes. An antistreptolysin (ASO) titer, which indicates the presence of antibodies to streptococcal bacteria, or a streptozyme test can be elevated. The ASO titer might not be elevated in a streptococcal skin infection. Culture of the throat or skin lesion (if present) may be helpful for isolating the bacterium. Again, this is useful only if the infection is recent and the child has not received antibiotics. A renal biopsy may be indicated for two reasons: (1) for those children whose signs and symptoms are not characteristic of acute poststreptococcal glomerulonephritis and (2) for those children whose symptoms do not improve as expected.

TABLE 20-1 Miscellaneous Disorders and Anomalies of the Genitourinary Tract	
Disorder or Anomaly	**Therapeutic Management**
Hydrocele: Painless swelling of the scrotum caused by a collection of fluid.	In the majority of infants, there is no indication for surgery within the first 12-24 months.[1] Some experts indicate repairing if, in the absence of a hernia, it is readily reducible by examination, progressively enlarging, or persisting as years pass.
Phimosis: Inability to retract the prepuce at an age when it should be retractable (usually 3 yr).	Accumulation of sebaceous gland secretions. Mild cases can be corrected through cleaning and gentle manual retraction. More severe cases require surgical enlargement of the phimotic ring or circumcision.
Testicular torsion: Rotation of the testicle that interrupts its blood supply, causing irreparable testicular damage if not corrected quickly. Manifests by sudden onset of severe, progressive scrotal pain, erythema, and edema. More common in adolescents and infants.	This is a surgical emergency. Surgery straightens and fixates the affected testicle and fixates the other testicle as well, to prevent torsion on the opposite side. If the affected testicle is necrotic, it is removed.
Bladder exstrophy: The extrusion of the urinary bladder to the outside of the body through a developmental defect in the lower abdominal wall. Associated with other genital anomalies, including a wide symphysis pubis.	Protect the exposed bladder tissue by covering it with nonadhering plastic wrap until surgical reconstruction. Surgical management is done in several stages, which include closing the abdominal defect and reconstructing the bladder and genitalia to allow the child to achieve urinary continence. It is important to address attachment issues with parents, who might be overwhelmed by their infant's appearance. Preventing UTI is essential.
Ambiguous genitalia: *Female pseudohermaphroditism:* Normal internal structures; is potentially fertile. Most common disorder of sexual differentiation, accounting for 60%-70% of all cases. May be associated with an inborn error in the biosynthesis pathway of cortisol.[2] *Male pseudohermaphroditism:* In some types of this disorder, fetal testes do not receive stimulation to produce testosterone. *True hermaphroditism:* Infant has both ovarian and testicular tissues, with abnormal internal and external genital structure. *Anatomic disruption of normal female or male structures:* The mechanism is neither hormonal nor chromosomal.	Cases require special attention, because life-threatening biochemical imbalances can be associated with this condition.[3] Traditionally, potential sexual function, fertility, and the cosmetic appearance of reconstructed genitalia have solely dictated gender assignment. However, new outcome data suggest that gender identity is influenced by androgens and sexual dimorphism of the brain and the external virilization is related to the degree of masculinization of the brain.[4] An external and internal masculinization scoring system provides a standardized format to summarize clinical features in newborn infants.[5] It is strongly implied that the prediction of the degree of masculinization of the brain will predict the likelihood of a child accepting his or her gender assignment. Decisions must be made cautiously with informed consent, emphasizing functionality over appearance.[6-10] A genetic workup is indicated because many of these conditions are inherited or autosomal recessive or X-linked traits. Psychologic support should also be provided regularly from birth onward.

[1]McCabe, A. J., Martin, D., & Glick, P. L. (2000). Insights: An "owl's eyes" view of hydroceles. *Journal of Pediatrics, 137,* 286.
[2]American Academy of Pediatrics, Committee on Genetics. (2000). Evaluation of the newborn with developmental anomalies of the external genitalia. *Pediatrics, 106,* 138-142.
[3]McCormack, K. (1999). A very special baby: Managing a baby with congenital adrenal hyperplasia. *Journal of Neonatal Nursing, 5,* 19-25.
[4]Reiner, W. G. (1999). Assignment of sex in neonates with ambiguous genitalia. *Current Opinion in Pediatrics, 11,* 363-365.
[5]Ahmed, S. F., Khwaja, O., & Hughes, I. A. (2000). The role of a clinical score in the assignment of ambiguous genitalia. *BJU International, 85,* 120-124.
[6]Beh, H. G., & Diamond, M. (2000). An emerging ethical and medical dilemma: Should physicians perform sex assignment surgery on infants with ambiguous genitalia? *Michigan Journal of Law, 7,* 1-63.
[7]Creighton, S. M., Minto, C. L., & Steele, S. J. (2001). Objective cosmetic and anatomical outcomes at adolescence of feminizing surgery for ambiguous genitalia done in childhood. *Lancet, 358,* 124-125.
[8]Hermer, L. (2002). Paradigms revised: Intersex children, bioethics & the law. *Annals of Health Law, 11,* 195-236.
[9]Martin, P. L. (2003). Moving toward an international standard in informed consent: The impact of intersexuality and the internet on the standard of care. *Duke Journal of Gender Law Policy, 10,* 135-169.
[10]Phornphutkul, C., Fausto-Sterling, A., & Gruppuso, P. A. (2000). Gender self-reassignment in an XY adolescent female born with ambiguous genitalia. *Pediatrics, 106,* 135-137.

Therapeutic Management

There is no specific therapy for acute poststreptococcal glomerulonephritis. Supportive care and medical management are directed to the associated signs and symptoms and guided by the degree of renal dysfunction. A 10-day course of antibiotic therapy may be required. Children with acute renal failure should be hospitalized to allow for fluid and electrolyte management until their renal function has stabilized.

Antihypertensive therapy may be necessary. This can be accomplished by limiting sodium and water intake or by administering diuretics or antihypertensive medication. The prognosis for children with acute poststreptococcal glomerulonephritis is excellent. The acute clinical episode is usually self-limiting, with diuresis signaling the beginning of resolution. Laboratory values usually return to baseline in 6 to 12 weeks. Most children have a complete recovery.

PATHOPHYSIOLOGY

ACUTE POSTSTREPTOCOCCAL GLOMERULONEPHRITIS

Acute glomerulonephritis after a streptococcal infection is thought to occur as a result of an immunologic response. The body responds to the *Streptococcus* bacteria by forming antibodies, which combine with the bacterial antigens to form immune complexes. As these antigen-antibody complexes travel through the circulation, they become trapped in the glomerulus and activate an inflammatory response in the glomerular basement membrane. Products of the in-

flammatory response damage the glomerular capillaries and reduce the size of the capillary lumen. This process causes a decrease in the glomerular filtration rate, leading to renal insufficiency. Sodium and fluid are retained, and the child exhibits edema and oliguria. In addition, injury to the capillary walls interferes with their permeability so that larger molecules and structures such as RBCs, casts, and proteins can pass through into the urine.

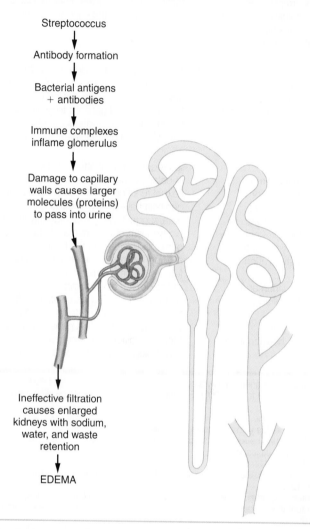

Streptococcus
↓
Antibody formation
↓
Bacterial antigens + antibodies
↓
Immune complexes inflame glomerulus
↓
Damage to capillary walls causes larger molecules (proteins) to pass into urine
↓
Ineffective filtration causes enlarged kidneys with sodium, water, and waste retention
↓
EDEMA

NURSING CARE

The Child With Acute Poststreptococcal Glomerulonephritis

Assessment

Assess the child for presence of periorbital or lower extremity edema. Obtaining vital signs and monitoring daily weight are important for assessing the degree of fluid retention and hypertension. Be sure to use the appropriate-size blood pressure cuff

for the most accurate blood pressure measurement (see Chapter 13). Monitor the child's level of fatigue and anxiety.

Assess the respiratory system for the presence of any respiratory difficulty, such as cough, increased respiratory rate, or increased work of breathing. Auscultate the breath sounds for crackles. Monitor laboratory values, especially urinalysis and serum electrolytes.

Determine what the child and family understand about the illness and the reason for hospitalization. The parents may be anxious about permanent damage to the child's kidneys as a result of this condition.

Nursing Diagnosis and Planning

The nursing diagnoses and expected outcomes that apply to the child with acute poststreptococcal glomerulonephritis and the family are as follows:

- Risk for Imbalanced Fluid Volume related to retention of sodium and fluid and dietary fluid restriction.

  Expected Outcome: The child will maintain normal fluid status, as evidenced by urine output normal for age group (see Chapter 18), moist mucous membranes, adequate skin turgor, normal blood pressure, no increase in weight, and no symptoms of respiratory distress.

- Risk for Activity Intolerance related to fatigue.

  Expected Outcome: The child will be rested, as evidenced by the ability to tolerate daily care and play activities.

- Risk for Impaired Skin Integrity related to edema and decreased activity.

  Expected Outcome: The child will exhibit no signs of skin breakdown, as evidenced by skin that is intact, normal color for race, and nontender to touch.

- Imbalanced Nutrition: Less Than Body Requirements related to diet restrictions.

  Expected Outcome: The child will have adequate nutrition, as evidenced by maintenance of weight at the preillness level.

- Anxiety related to insufficient knowledge about disease process or hospitalization.

  Expected Outcomes: The child and parents will demonstrate decreased anxiety, as evidenced by cooperation with daily care and interest in developmentally appropriate play. Parents or caregiver will describe the disease process and its usual resolution.

Interventions

Preventing the Consequences of Fluid Excess

Frequent, accurate assessment of intake and output is essential for evaluating fluid status. Children with severe renal impairment might require measurement of intake and output every 2 to 4 hours. Fluid intake includes oral intake and IV fluids. Report urine output of less than 1 mL/kg/hr, depending on the child's age (see Chapter 18) because oliguria suggests impending renal failure.

Accurate daily weights are important for determining fluctuation in fluid status. The nurse obtains daily weights, remembering to weigh the child on the same scale at approximately the same time every day for maximum consistency. Infants and young children should be weighed without diapers, and older children should wear only a gown.

Because hypertension from fluid overload and glomerular damage is a severe consequence of this condition, the nurse measures blood pressure with an appropriate-size cuff every shift and documents the results. Report increasing values immediately. More frequent readings might be required if the child has significant hypertension or receives antihypertensive medication.

Auscultate breath sounds every shift and document increased respiratory effort. Rapid respirations, retractions, nasal flaring, or crackles are signs of developing pulmonary edema, which can result from fluid overload.

Limit fluid intake if ordered. Limitation might be difficult if children are old enough to sneak drinks on their own or obtain them from people who are unaware of restrictions. The nurse should inform parents, visitors, and hospital staff of the need to limit fluids. Be sure to record the child's favorite fluids on the nursing care plan, so the child is able to enjoy the fluids given. Encourage the child to consume fluids gradually, rather than large amounts all at once. Provide the child with only the agreed-on amount for the period involved.

Excessive sodium can increase fluid retention. The nurse ensures that a low-sodium diet is followed if ordered. Inform parents and visitors of any dietary restrictions.

Providing Adequate Rest

If fatigue is a problem, it is important that the child has ample opportunity to rest. Children with glomerulonephritis may tire easily when first hospitalized, although most children participate in activities according to their level of fatigue. The nurse needs to arrange daily care so that the child has some uninterrupted time for sleep and naps. Encourage parents to bring a favorite sleep toy or blanket for the child and allow for nap time and bedtime to coincide with the child's home schedule as much as possible. Try to follow home rituals. If the child is unable to limit activity, the nurse can limit play time to short periods and extend that limit as the child's condition improves.

Maintaining Skin Integrity

Frequent position changes decrease pressure on bony prominences and help decrease edema in dependent areas. Encourage the child to change position at least every 2 hours during the day. If the child has edema of the lower extremities, elevate the extremities with pillows when the child is sitting or lying in bed. Promote activity as the child improves because activity increases the circulation and promotes reabsorption of fluid from edematous areas.

To prevent skin breakdown, the nurse maintains good hygiene for the child by giving baths and cleaning the skin well after bowel movements and diaper changes. Using a small amount of lotion to massage the skin prevents dryness and promotes active circulation.

Maintaining Nutritional Status

Low-sodium foods taste different, and children may refuse to eat them. Offering low-sodium foods or treats different from those available in the hospital may encourage the child to eat. Consult with the dietary department about palatable low-sodium food and drinks. Allow parents to bring favorite foods from home if these foods comply with dietary restrictions.

A small fluctuation in weight can indicate fluid loss or gain or weight loss from decreased food intake. After obtaining the child's preillness weight, the nurse weighs the child daily to monitor for any fluid shifts or underlying weight loss. In addition, the nurse monitors the child for signs of dehydration (dry mucous membranes, listlessness, poor skin turgor, tachycardia) that would coincide with fluid restriction, diuresis, or diuretic administration.

Relieving Anxiety

Allowing parents and the child to voice their concerns provides support and a basis for evaluating their understanding of the disease process and prognosis. Reassure the family that most children recover from this condition with no residual effects. Encourage them to participate in the child's care, helping to make the child comfortable and providing suitable play activities and emotional support.

Information enables the child and parents to understand the course of the condition and to anticipate procedures and events. Knowing what to expect helps decrease anxiety. It is especially important to provide information about the child's care at home because the child will be discharged quickly unless renal failure is a risk. If the child has been hypertensive or is to be discharged on antihypertensive medications, the nurse instructs parents on how to measure the child's blood pressure and emphasizes that blood pressure should be taken before medication administration. A blood pressure cuff of appropriate size and a stethoscope are ordered before discharge. The nurse explains the parameters for when to withhold medication or when to call the physician for high readings.

Evaluation

- Does the child demonstrate adequate urine output for weight and normal blood pressure for age?
- Are the child's mucous membranes moist, and does the child appear to be well-hydrated?
- Is the child's respiratory status stable?
- Has the child's weight changed from the preillness weight?
- Is the child able to tolerate usual activities for age?
- Is the child's skin intact, appropriate color for race, and nontender to touch?
- Is the child relaxed enough to cooperate with care activities and maintain interest in play?
- Do parents participate appropriately in the child's care, provide comfort to the child, and describe the disease process and care required?

NEPHROTIC SYNDROME

Nephrotic syndrome refers to a kidney disorder characterized by proteinuria, hypoalbuminemia, and edema. Nephrotic syndrome can be classified as primary or secondary. *Primary nephrotic syndrome*, or minimal change nephrotic syndrome (MCNS), results from a disorder within the glomerulus of the kidney and is the most common type seen in children. A child also can acquire nephrotic syndrome as the result of a systemic disease, such as hepatitis, systemic lupus erythematosus, heavy metal poisoning, or cancer.

Etiology

The cause of primary nephrotic syndrome is not fully understood, but it can arise from one of four types of renal lesions. Success in controlling the disease by the use of immunosuppressive drugs suggests the possibility of an immunologic component. In most children, minimal alterations of the glomerulus are seen on histologic examination. Accordingly, the most common disorder, MCNS, accounts for almost 85% of childhood nephrotic syndrome (Vogt & Avner, 2004a). Nephrosis develops in others as a result of focal segmental glomerulosclerosis or, more rarely, because of membranoproliferative glomerulonephritis or mesangial proliferation.

Incidence

Primary nephrotic syndrome occurs most frequently in children between ages 2 and 6 years. The incidence is slightly higher in boys. The prognosis for children with MCNS is very good. Manifestations of the disease usually decrease with age, so relapses are rare in adolescence. Focal segmental glomerulosclerosis carries a poorer prognosis; the disease is progressive and often results in ESRD.

Manifestations

Manifestations of primary nephrotic syndrome include edema, anorexia, fatigue, abdominal pain, respiratory infection, and increased weight. Unlike the child with glomerulonephritis, the child with nephrotic syndrome usually has normal blood pressure.

Edema is usually first noted in the periorbital spaces and dependent areas of the body; its onset is often insidious. Children often awaken with facial edema and, as the day progresses, become noticeably edematous in the abdomen, genital area, and lower extremities. The pitting edema is most noticeable over the bony prominences of the lower extremities. Abdominal pain can occur from the presence of extra fluid in the peritoneal area. Edema of the bowel may cause diarrhea and decreased absorption of nutrients. Many children are misdiagnosed with allergies because of periorbital edema and respiratory symptoms.

Diagnostic Evaluation

Nephrotic syndrome can be diagnosed on the basis of clinical presentation, age of the child, and laboratory results. Urinalysis demonstrates protein (3+ to 4+), and the urine appears dark and frothy. Microscopic hematuria may be present. Serum cholesterol, triglycerides, hematocrit, and hemoglobin values are elevated. Serum albumin is markedly decreased (<2.5 g/dL). The child has normal electrolyte levels and a negative ASO titer or streptozyme test. Serologic tests for hepatitis, human immunodeficiency virus, syphilis, and antinuclear antibody titers are done to rule out underlying systemic disease.

Because of an atypical presentation (a child older than 10 years or having gross hematuria or hypertension), a kidney biopsy might be done if a lesion other than MCNS is suspected. A biopsy is also indicated for the child who does not respond as expected to pharmacologic treatment.

Therapeutic Management

It is not unusual for the child with primary nephrotic syndrome to be hospitalized briefly during the initial onset of the disease to provide palliative treatment for the edema,

PATHOPHYSIOLOGY

NEPHROTIC SYNDROME

Primary nephrotic syndrome occurs from an insult to the glomerular basement membrane. Damage to the membrane causes increased permeability and loss of substances that would normally prevent negatively charged proteins from crossing the membrane. Negatively charged proteins, particularly albumin, are cleared at an increased rate, resulting in loss of plasma proteins and in proteinuria. Proteinuria is essential for the diagnosis of nephrotic syndrome.

Blood albumin values are low (hypoalbuminemia) because of the loss of albumin through the defective glomerulus and the liver's inability to synthesize proteins to balance the loss. Decreased levels of albumin reduce the plasma oncotic pressure so that the intravascular fluid moves into the interstitial spaces. This shifting of fluid reduces the intravascular volume, causing hypovolemia and subsequent decreased renal blood flow. In an effort to increase blood volume, the kidney stimulates renin production. Renin causes increased excretion of aldosterone, resulting in renal tubular reabsorption of sodium, which in turn causes water retention. The net effect of this phenomenon is edema.

In addition, the serum values of cholesterol and triglycerides are elevated. This change is thought to result from increased stimulation of lipoprotein production because of the decrease in oncotic pressure. Loss of immunoglobulins into the urine is common in nephrotic syndrome. Most notably, levels of immunoglobulin G are decreased, which makes these children more susceptible to infection. Before the use of antibiotics, infection was a frequent cause of death in these children.

Children with nephrotic syndrome are in a hypercoagulable state, predisposing them to venous thrombosis. This tendency occurs as a result of several factors, including decreased intravascular volume (hypovolemia), which causes increased concentration of RBCs and platelets and slowing of circulation. Urinary loss of proteins that inhibit coagulation also contributes to the risk of thrombus formation.

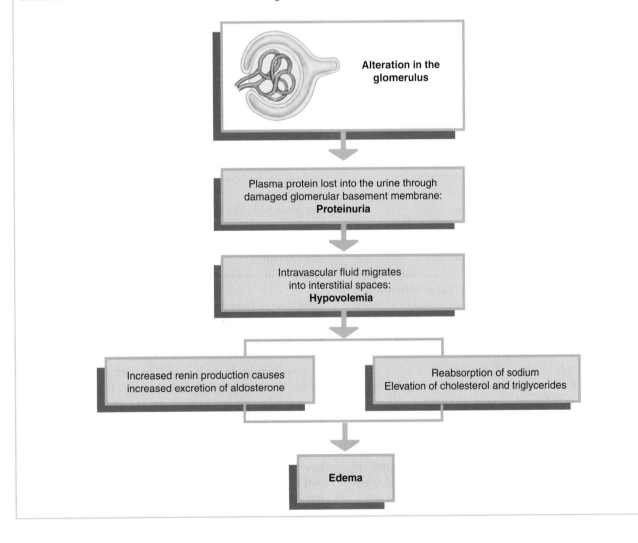

Alteration in the glomerulus

Plasma protein lost into the urine through damaged glomerular basement membrane: **Proteinuria**

Intravascular fluid migrates into interstitial spaces: **Hypovolemia**

Increased renin production causes increased excretion of aldosterone

Reabsorption of sodium Elevation of cholesterol and triglycerides

Edema

CRITICAL TO REMEMBER
Differences Between Children With Glomerulonephritis and Children With Nephrotic Syndrome

The signs and symptoms of glomerulonephritis and nephrotic syndrome in children can be confusing. It is important for nurses to be able to discriminate between the two. Remember the following:

The Child With Poststreptococcal Glomerulonephritis

Manifestations
- Hematuria—cola-colored urine
- Hypertensive
- Edema—abrupt onset, mild periorbital or lower extremity
- Usually young school-age child

Laboratory Findings
- RBCs, casts, small amount of protein in urine (0 to 2+)
- Normal serum albumin, cholesterol, and triglyceride levels; decreased or normal hemoglobin and hematocrit values
- Altered electrolytes, elevated blood urea nitrogen or creatinine levels
- Elevated ASO titer or Streptozyme, decreased complement

Management
- Supportive
- Administration of antihypertensives and diuretics; antibiotic treatment for active streptococcal infection
- Low-salt diet

The Child With Nephrotic Syndrome

Manifestations
- Proteinuria—frothy urine
- Edema—insidious onset, massive edema from shift of fluid into interstitial spaces, worsens during the day
- Hypovolemia
- Normotensive
- Pallor, fatigue
- Toddler or preschool-age child

Laboratory Findings
- Proteinuria (3+ to 4+), possible microscopic hematuria
- Hypoalbuminemia (<2.5 g/dL), elevated cholesterol and triglyceride, hemoglobin, hematocrit, and platelet levels
- Normal serum electrolytes, complement levels, ASO titer

Management
- Prednisone to initiate remission—0 to trace protein in urine for 5 to 7 days
- Diuretics, possible albumin administration
- Antibiotics to prevent infection
- No-added-salt diet

---

perform necessary diagnostic testing, and initiate therapy. Parents also may be educated about the disease process and necessary home care. Before treatment begins, the child is tested for exposure to tuberculosis and varicella because treatment suppresses the immune system.

Remission Induction

Therapy for remission includes prednisone at a dose of 2 mg/kg/day (maximum 60 mg) divided into two or three doses. This regimen is continued until the child is in remission (zero to trace urine protein for 5 to 7 consecutive days). Steroids usually are continued at the same daily dose for 4 to 6 weeks. After the initial treatment, the child's dose is decreased and changed to an alternate-day schedule and then slowly tapered.

In the event of a relapse, steroid therapy is less prolonged. Once remission is achieved, dosing decreases to alternate days and is tapered more quickly. This is done to minimize prednisone side effects (see Chapter 17).

Some children respond to steroids quickly and achieve remission in 5 to 7 days, whereas others may not respond for 4 weeks. If proteinuria continues beyond 8 weeks of daily steroid therapy, the child is said to be steroid resistant and a kidney biopsy is done to determine the exact nature of the disease.

Children who initially respond to steroid therapy but have relapses while on a tapering schedule or shortly after stopping steroids are said to be *steroid dependent* (Fig. 20-2). These children may benefit from a course of an alkylating agent such as cyclophosphamide or chlorambucil. The risks and benefits of this therapy must be carefully considered, and the parents should be informed of all possible side effects. A kidney biopsy is usually done before therapy is started. The use of cyclosporine in children who remain steroid dependent despite a course of an alkylating agent has proven to be effective in maintaining remission.

Additional Therapy

A no-added-salt diet is indicated. The caregiver should not use salt when cooking; the child should not be permitted to use the salt shaker; and the caregiver should avoid serving high-sodium foods, such as pickles, salted chips, and cured meats. If edema is severe or if the child is hypertensive, sodium intake may be further restricted and the child may be placed on fluid restriction.

Diuretic therapy is initiated until urinary protein loss is controlled. If the edema is marked and causes the child to have decreased mobility, poor oral intake, or decreased urine output, salt-poor albumin may be given intravenously. Albumin helps restore normal plasma osmotic pressure and promotes the movement of interstitial fluid back into the intravascular compartments. Furosemide is given intravenously after the albumin infusion to enhance diuresis and decrease the chance of fluid overload.

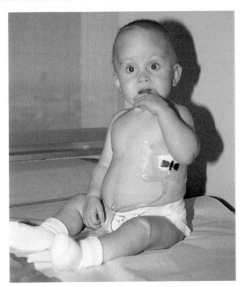

FIG 20-2 **This child has nephrotic syndrome that is in remission. She previously received steroid therapy and is now receiving cyclosporine chemotherapy to control the process. During the acute phase of the nephrotic syndrome, the child may have massive edema because blood proteins are lost in the urine. Skin pallor is also common.** *(Courtesy Children's Medical Center, Dallas, TX.)*

Oral penicillin is frequently given to reduce the likelihood of an infection developing. Severe edema in the lower extremities can give rise to cellulitis because of fluid stasis and poor circulation. Peritonitis, a severe complication, can develop from stasis of ascitic fluid, which is an excellent culture medium for organisms such as *Streptococcus pneumoniae*.

Live-virus vaccines are contraindicated in children receiving steroid therapy. In addition to routine killed-virus vaccines, the child should receive pneumococcal vaccine to prevent pneumococcal infection in the event of a relapse. It may also be beneficial for the child with nephrotic syndrome to receive an influenza vaccine each year because an exacerbation of the disease can occur after an infection.

ACUTE RENAL FAILURE

Acute renal failure is defined as the sudden, severe loss of kidney function. In acute renal failure, the kidneys can no longer filter waste products, regulate fluid volume, or maintain chemical balance. Most children with acute renal failure regain renal function.

Etiology and Incidence

Possible causes of prerenal failure are dehydration, perinatal asphyxia, hypotension, septic shock, hemorrhagic shock, and renal artery obstruction. Nephrotoxins (e.g., aminoglycosides,

Text continued on p. 592

NURSING CARE PLAN

The Child With Nephrotic Syndrome

Focused Assessment

The nurse should monitor the child's vital signs for early signs of infection or hypovolemia. Carefully document the child's fluid intake and urine output and obtain accurate daily weights. Nursing care should include assessing the amount of edema present in the child each shift, specifically in the periorbital areas, abdomen, genitalia, and lower extremities.

Monitor laboratory results to check urine daily for protein. The nursing history should include the child's immunization status and known recent exposures to communicable diseases. Assessment of the family's understanding of the disease process and treatment is important so that the nurse can make appropriate referrals and provide the parents with information.

NURSING DIAGNOSIS Risk for Impaired Skin Integrity related to edema and decreased circulation.

EXPECTED OUTCOME The child will:
* Remain free from skin breakdown, as evidenced by the absence of redness, tenderness to touch, and ulceration.

Intervention

1. Ensure that the child changes position every 2 hours.

2. Maintain good hygiene by giving daily baths and changing linen daily. Use non-alcohol-based lotion for dry skin.

3. Support or elevate edematous body parts with pillows while the child is in bed or sitting in a chair.

4. Promote physical activity as the child is able to tolerate by providing developmentally appropriate play activities.

Rationale

1. Frequent position change decreases pressure on body parts and helps relieve edema in dependent areas.

2. Body secretions and debris on linens can irritate the skin. Gentle massage when bathing and applying lotion helps increase circulation.

3. Edema is gravity dependent. Elevation helps move fluid away from dependent body parts.

4. Increased activity helps promote circulation.

Continued

NURSING CARE PLAN—cont'd

Evaluation

* Is the child's skin intact without redness or tenderness?

NURSING DIAGNOSIS Risk for Infection related to urinary loss of gamma globulins and immunosuppressive therapy.

EXPECTED OUTCOME The child will:
* Be free of signs of an infection, as evidenced by normal WBC count, normal body temperature, and absence of abdominal pain and cough.

Intervention	Rationale
1. Screen visitors for signs of infection, such as upper respiratory symptoms, sore throats, or exposure to communicable diseases.	1. Communicable diseases, especially varicella, pose a serious threat because the child receiving immunosuppressive therapy is not able to respond appropriately to infection.
2. Administer antibiotics as ordered.	2. Antibiotics are usually given for peritonitis prophylaxis during the edematous phase.
3. Use good hand hygiene techniques and instruct family members to do the same.	3. Handwashing helps decrease transmission of germs.
4. Monitor child for fever, cough, sore throat, or complaints of abdominal pain each shift. Monitor laboratory values.	4. Frequent monitoring ensures early detection of infectious processes. Abdominal pain can be an indication of peritonitis.

Evaluation

* Does the child maintain normal body temperature and exhibit normal laboratory values?
* Is the child free from cough, pain, or other signs of infection?

NURSING DIAGNOSIS Risk for Deficient Fluid Volume (intravascular) related to proteinuria, edema, and effects of diuretics.

EXPECTED OUTCOME The child will:
* Maintain adequate fluid volume, as evidenced by normal blood pressure measurement, urine output appropriate for age, and normal hematocrit and hemoglobin values.

Intervention	Rationale
1. Monitor vital signs, including blood pressure and pulse, every shift. Report variance from baseline.	1. Low blood pressure and increased heart rate are signs of hypovolemia. Blood pressure may be elevated because of renin release.
2. Monitor intake and output every shift. Report if child has output of less than 1 to 2 mL/kg/hr of urine (see Chapter 18).	2. Accurate intake and output measurement is essential for evaluating fluid status.
3. Monitor laboratory values, particularly hemoglobin and hematocrit.	3. Increasing values of hemoglobin, hematocrit, and platelets may indicate hemoconcentration or low intravascular volume.
4. Observe for signs of dehydration, such as appearance of mucous membranes, capillary refill, and level of activity. (Capillary refill may be altered because of edema; assess in nonedematous area.) Report positive findings.	4. The pathophysiologic mechanisms of nephrotic syndrome may predispose the child to decreased intravascular volume. This condition is compounded by the use of diuretics.

Evaluation

* Are the child's vital signs and hematocrit and hemoglobin within normal limits?
* Is the urine output normal for age group (see Chapter 18)?
* Does the child have moist mucous membranes and appropriate skin turgor?

NURSING DIAGNOSIS Excess Fluid Volume related to decreased excretion of sodium and fluid retention.

EXPECTED OUTCOME The child will:
* Not exhibit signs of fluid overload, as evidenced by stable daily weights and normal respiratory pattern.

NURSING CARE PLAN—cont'd

Intervention

1. Monitor intake and output each shift.

2. Obtain accurate daily weights. Weigh child on same scales, at same time each day, in a gown only.

3. Adhere to no-added-salt diet and fluid restriction if ordered.

4. Measure and record abdominal girth each day. Ensure accuracy by measuring in the same area each time.
5. Monitor blood pressure at least once each shift.

6. Administer diuretics as ordered. Ensure adequate potassium intake.
7. Monitor pulmonary status by listening to breath sounds for crackles and observing for signs of increased work of breathing and presence of cough.

Rationale

1. Accurate intake and output are essential for evaluating fluid status.
2. Daily weights are necessary to detect changes in fluid status. Clothing or presence of wet diaper can alter weight. Readings of weight can vary from scale to scale and time of day.
3. Excessive sodium intake can increase amount of water retention. If the child is hyponatremic, fluid restriction may be indicated (Vogt & Avner, 2004a).
4. Edema commonly occurs in the abdomen.

5. Increased total-body fluid volume and concurrent steroid therapy can result in increased blood pressure.
6. Diuretics may aid in the elimination of excessive fluid. Diuretics can increase excretion of potassium.
7. Fluid overload can result in pulmonary edema.

Evaluation

- Does the child maintain a stable weight?
- Is the child free from respiratory distress?

NURSING DIAGNOSIS   Anxiety (parental) related to hospitalization of child and caring for a child with a chronic disease.
Deficient Knowledge about home management related to anxiety or incomplete understanding.

EXPECTED OUTCOMES   The parents will:
- Demonstrate decreased anxiety, as evidenced by participating in the care of their child and explaining the normal course of the disease process.
- Be able to explain principles of home management.

Intervention

1. Allow parents to verbalize frustration and fears. Encourage them to ask questions and provide them with information about nephrotic syndrome and its treatment.
2. Incorporate the parents' help in the daily care of the child. Have them practice using Albustix, taking blood pressures, and assessing edema.
3. Arrange for a dietary consultation.

4. Teach parents how to maintain a daily calendar of protein readings, how to do a daily weight, what medications are appropriate for the child, and how to prevent infection. Encourage parents to report any exposure to communicable disease.

Rationale

1. Verbalization of fears is often therapeutic in itself. Information helps decrease anxiety because people often fear the unknown.
2. Nephrotic syndrome can be a chronic condition and it is usually managed at home. It is important for the parents to feel comfortable with caring for their child.
3. Steroid therapy stimulates appetite. Children should be informed about low-calorie snacks and portion size. Encourage the parent to cook without salt and remove the salt shaker from the child's access.
4. Providing appropriate information allows the family to manage the child's care. The child's urine protein results are monitored for signs of relapse. It is important to check with the nephrologist before giving the child any over-the-counter medications because some medications can aggravate hypertension. Children receiving steroids are unable to respond appropriately to viral or bacterial infections and may require additional treatment.

Evaluation

- Can the parents describe their child's condition and required treatment?
- Do the parents actively participate in the child's care?
- Do the parents accurately demonstrate procedures necessary to do at home?

contrast dye), ureterovesical obstruction, hemolytic uremic syndrome (HUS), glomerulonephritis, and pyelonephritis cause intrarenal acute renal failure. Postrenal acute renal failure is associated with structural abnormalities, such as ureteropelvic obstruction, ureterovesical obstruction, posterior urethral valves, neurogenic bladder, and outlet obstruction by stones, tumor, or edema.

HUS is the most frequent cause of acute renal failure in children. It is an acute disorder characterized by anemia, thrombocytopenia, and acute renal failure. Children with HUS become infected by *E. coli* in improperly cooked meat or contaminated dairy products. Acute renal failure in the child is uncommon.

Manifestations

Manifestations of acute renal failure include electrolyte imbalances, fluid imbalances, increased BUN and serum creatinine levels, acid-base imbalances, and nonspecific manifestations, such as poor feeding or decreased appetite, vomiting, lethargy, seizures, and pallor. In children with HUS, gastrointestinal illness characterized by abdominal pain, fever, vomiting, and bloody diarrhea may be present.

Diagnostic Evaluation

Determining the underlying cause of acute renal failure is very important. If the underlying cause can be reversed, renal function usually returns to normal.

PATHOPHYSIOLOGY

ACUTE RENAL FAILURE

Acute renal failure is categorized as prerenal, intrarenal, or postrenal. *Prerenal acute renal failure* is the result of decreased perfusion of the kidney. The kidney must have adequate blood flow for effective functioning. The decreased blood flow and subsequent ischemia cause cellular swelling and injury and possible cell death. *Intrarenal acute renal failure* is the result of actual ischemic damage to kidney tissue. *Postrenal acute renal failure* is the result of obstruction of urine outflow. The obstruction increases pressure within the kidney, which decreases renal function.

Impaired perfusion markedly decreases the glomerular filtration rate, triggering oliguria (markedly decreased urine output), azotemia (elevated blood levels of urea, creatinine, and uric acid), and associated electrolyte imbalances. Tissue injury further magnifies the damage and the decreased perfusion.

As the underlying problem is treated, recovery of the renal endothelial and tubular cells begins and renal function gradually returns.* Because the glomerular filtration rate returns to normal faster than the tubular transport mechanisms, the child begins to diurese, voiding large amounts of dilute urine. During this diuretic phase, the child is at increased risk for dehydration related to the fluid loss. Renal function gradually returns to normal.

*Choka, K. (2005). Renal failure. In L. Copstead & J. Banasik (Eds.). *Pathophysiology* (3rd ed.). St. Louis: Elsevier Saunders.

PATHOPHYSIOLOGY

HEMOLYTIC UREMIC SYNDROME

Most affected children have an associated prodrome of gastrointestinal symptoms, including bloody diarrhea, which suggests that an infectious agent may be the cause of HUS. Nearly all cases are the result of an antecedent infection by Shiga's toxin-producing strains of *E. coli*, especially the O157:H7 serotype.* Two important characteristics of *E. coli* O157:H7 contribute to the development of HUS. First, because this bacterium attaches itself to the intestinal mucosa, its clearance through normal intestinal peristalsis is decreased, allowing the bacteria to grow and multiply. Second, the bacteria produce a toxin that damages the endothelial cells of capillary walls, and the subsequent inflammatory response results in occlusion of capillaries. This is especially significant in the renal glomeruli. The occlusion of glomerular vessels decreases filtration and results in acute renal failure. However, it is important to understand that the vascular process seen in HUS can affect any organ. Anemia results from fragmentation of RBCs, which are damaged as they try to pass through the occluded vessels and are removed from circulation by the spleen. Thrombocytopenia occurs because the platelets get trapped within the small vessels.

*Thorpe, C. (2004). Shiga toxin-producing *Escherichia coli* infection. *Clinical Infectious Diseases, 38,* 1298-1303.

History

The history often gives an indication of the underlying cause of the acute renal failure. Vomiting, diarrhea, and fever may indicate dehydration and prerenal acute renal failure. It is necessary to ascertain any recent history of bloody diarrhea that might suggest HUS.

Fluid Status

Acute renal failure is usually associated with dehydration and oliguria (urine output <1 mL/kg/hr). Urine output might be normal or increased (see Chapter 18).

Laboratory Data

Serum creatinine and BUN levels are increased. BUN, an end product of protein catabolism, may reflect the child's nutritional status. Metabolic acidosis can occur, as indicated by low serum bicarbonate. Serum potassium may be increased. Serum sodium may be increased or decreased, depending on fluid status. The child with HUS exhibits hemolytic anemia, thrombocytopenia, hematuria, urine casts, proteinuria, and *E. coli* by stool culture.

Physical Examination

The child may be hypertensive. Edema resulting from decreased urine output and fluid overload may be present. The child may be in respiratory distress because of fluid overload.

Imaging Studies

Renal ultrasonography may help with the diagnosis of obstruction and postrenal acute renal failure. A renal scan can be helpful in determining the cause of renal failure. It can assess blood flow, function, and obstruction.

Therapeutic Management

Many children in acute renal failure are managed without dialysis. Management includes the following principles.

Fluid Imbalances

Fluid balance is an important component of the management of acute renal failure. If the child is dehydrated, careful fluid replacement is essential. Fluid restriction is necessary for a child who has decreased or absent urine output and is adequately hydrated or has fluid overload. Fluid intake is carefully calculated to replace insensible fluid loss and urinary output. Maintaining fluid restriction can be difficult for some children. It is helpful to give small amounts more frequently rather than a large amount occasionally. Older children can participate in decision making about the kind and frequency of fluids.

Electrolyte Imbalances

Potassium. Most children with acute renal failure have a high potassium level, requiring intervention when the serum potassium level reaches 6 mEq/L. Potassium is restricted from the diet and IV fluids. Interventions to remove potassium include instituting gastric suction; administration of an exchange resin, such as Kayexalate; or administration of sodium bicarbonate, glucose, and insulin.

Sodium. The sodium level may be elevated or decreased. It is more common for the level to be decreased because of water overload. Fluid restriction helps improve the serum sodium level. Any replacement sodium is adjusted to maintain a normal sodium level.

Acid-Base Imbalances. Children with acute renal failure are unable to excrete hydrogen ions and ammonia through the kidney, so metabolic acidosis (low serum bicarbonate) develops. Additional sodium bicarbonate can be administered orally or by IV.

Nutrition

Nutritional support of children with acute renal failure is critical. Foods should be low in sodium and potassium.

CRITICAL TO REMEMBER
Indications for Dialysis in Acute Renal Failure

- Severe fluid overload
- Pulmonary edema or congestive heart failure caused by fluid overload
- Severe hypertension
- Metabolic acidosis not responsive to medications
- Hyperkalemia not responsive to medications
- Blood urea nitrogen level greater than 120 mg/dL

The underlying principle of nutritional therapy for these children is to provide maximum calories and moderate restriction of protein. If the child is critically ill, parenteral hyperalimentation with essential amino acids may be administered (Vogt & Avner, 2004b).

Dialysis

Dialysis is a process of removing waste products and excess body fluid and regulating electrolytes and minerals. Two types of dialysis are hemodialysis and peritoneal dialysis.

Nursing Considerations

Most children with acute renal failure are cared for in special-care units. Principles of nursing care include (1) monitoring and maintaining fluid, electrolyte, and acid-base balance, (2) preventing infection, (3) providing adequate nutrition, (4) reducing parent and child anxiety, and (5) teaching about dialysis (Box 20-3).

CHRONIC RENAL FAILURE AND END-STAGE RENAL DISEASE

Chronic renal failure is an irreversible loss of kidney function that occurs over months to years. It can be managed conservatively with medications and diet restrictions. Chronic renal failure progresses to ESRD, which is the permanent, irreversible loss of kidney function that can no longer be managed conservatively to maintain life and health. Dialysis or transplantation is required to treat ESRD. Treatment usually occurs when only 5% to 10% of kidney function remains.

Etiology

The causes of chronic renal failure in children are different from those in adults. The most common causes, especially in younger children, are congenital anomalies, such as obstruction, VUR, and renal dysplasia. Chronic renal failure can develop in children from diseases such as glomerulonephritis, pyelonephritis, and HUS. In general, secondary causes of ESRD, such as diabetes and high blood pressure, are not seen in children.

Incidence

The incidence of chronic renal failure with ESRD among children younger than 19 years is approximately 18 in 1 million (Vogt & Avner, 2004b). The incidence is higher in adolescents, in boys, and in whites.

Pathophysiology

Regardless of the cause of kidney damage, chronic renal failure progresses to ESRD. The exact mechanisms are unclear. Negative contributing factors include continuing immunologic injury, hyperfiltration (the overwork of the remaining nephrons), high dietary protein and phosphorus intake, persistent proteinuria, and hypertension.

Manifestations

Manifestations of chronic renal failure and ESRD include electrolyte imbalance, fluid imbalance (dehydration or fluid

---

BOX 20-3 | **Dialysis**

Dialysis is a process of removing waste products and excess body fluids and regulating electrolytes and minerals. It is sometimes necessary in acute renal failure. When chronic renal failure progresses to ESRD, dialysis or kidney transplantation is required. The two types of dialysis are hemodialysis and peritoneal dialysis.

Hemodialysis

Hemodialysis cleanses the blood by circulating it through a special filter called an *artificial kidney.* Blood is pumped through the artificial kidney and returned to the body. Hemodialysis occurs through a vascular access, such as a double-lumen central line or an arteriovenous fistula or shunt. The access is surgically placed. Children who receive long-term dialysis usually receive treatments three times per week for 3 to 4 hours each time.

The major complications of hemodialysis include access infection and access obstruction. In addition, school, peer, and family life are disrupted because of the treatment schedule. However, children treated with hemodialysis in a specialized pediatric unit can thrive. In infants and small children, hemodialysis is technically more difficult and fluid and electrolyte shifts are more pronounced.

Hemodialysis is more efficient and requires less time than peritoneal dialysis. In addition, the family has less responsibility.

Peritoneal Dialysis

In peritoneal dialysis, fluid enters the peritoneal cavity through a catheter, which may be placed in the child at the bedside or in the operating room. The dialysis fluid remains in the cavity for a prescribed time, during which waste products, chemicals, and fluid pass through the peritoneal membrane into the fluid. The fluid is then drained, and the process is repeated.

In children receiving long-term dialysis, the exchanges can be performed overnight with an automated cycler or they can be done manually four or five times per day. The treatments usually are performed at home.

Peritoneal dialysis is technically easier than hemodialysis. Advantages over hemodialysis include more independence for the child and family and a more stable physiologic state because of frequent dialysis. The disadvantages include the risk of infections (peritonitis, catheter exit site) and family and child fatigue from treatment demands.

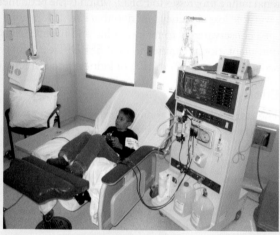

Child receiving hemodialysis.
Photo courtesy Cook Children's Medical Center, Fort Worth, TX.

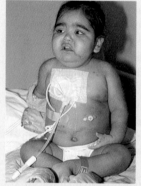

Peritoneal dialysis. Implanted lines allow instillation of the dialyzing fluid into this child's peritoneal cavity. This child has rejected a transplanted kidney and receives peritoneal dialysis until another transplant will be attempted, She previously received steroids in an attempt to control rejection, which accounts for the characteristics typical of Cushing syndrome.
Photo courtesy Children's Medical Center, Dallas, TX.

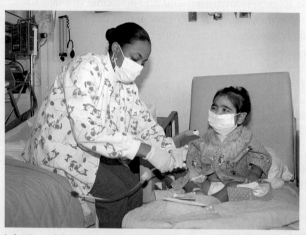

Infection of the peritoneal cavity is the chief hazard of peritoneal dialysis. When the lines are open to begin or end the dialyzing cycle, both adult and child wear masks.
Photo courtesy Children's Medical Center, Dallas, TX.

overload), acid-base imbalance, renal bone disease (osteo-dystrophy) and rickets, anemia, poor growth, hypertension, fatigue, decreased appetite or poor feeding, nausea and vomiting, and neurologic symptoms from accumulation of wastes.

Diagnostic Evaluation

Chronic renal failure may present nonspecifically. Physical examination may reveal short stature and failure to thrive. The child may be hypertensive. Blood work reveals electrolyte abnormalities (varying according to the underlying disease process), calcium and phosphorus abnormalities (decreased calcium and bone calcium resorption, elevated serum phosphorus), or anemia. Rising creatinine and BUN levels suggest ESRD. Creatinine clearance testing measures the ability of the renal system to excrete metabolic products. Bone radiographs diagnose renal osteodystrophy. The child may have normal fluid volume, be dehydrated, or have fluid overload.

The history may or may not include known renal disease. Diagnostic tests may be performed to determine etiology and prognosis. These may include a voiding cystourethrogram (VCUG), renal ultrasonography, renal scan, and renal biopsy.

Therapeutic Management

Chronic Renal Failure

The diet of a child with chronic renal failure is modified because of the decreased ability of the kidney to regulate fluids, electrolytes, minerals, and waste products. This might include the following restrictions: salt and fluid to prevent fluid overload and hypertension, protein because of the kidneys' inability to remove waste products, phosphorus to help prevent bone disease, and potassium because of the kidneys' inability to remove it.

Diuretics also are indicated to control fluid balance, and antihypertensives are given for hypertension. Sodium bicarbonate may be necessary to maintain acid-base balance. Vitamin D and phosphorus-binding medications may be helpful in preventing bone disease.

Children with chronic renal failure should receive all childhood immunizations and yearly influenza vaccine, unless immunosuppressive treatment precludes live-virus vaccines. Immunization with live-virus vaccines as soon as possible within the normal childhood schedule is desired because after kidney transplantation the child will be taking immunosuppressants (Vogt & Avner, 2004b).

Advances in the treatment of infants and children with chronic renal failure, such as recombinant erythropoietin and recombinant growth hormone, have improved the quality of life of these children (Vogt & Avner, 2004b). Recombinant erythropoietin is used to treat anemia, thus improving the energy level and avoiding repeated blood transfusions. The use of recombinant growth hormone has significantly improved the growth of children with chronic renal failure (Chan, Williams, & Roth, 2002).

End-Stage Renal Disease

Once a child reaches ESRD, dialysis or kidney transplantation is required for health and life. The diagnosis of ESRD is made by monitoring serum creatinine levels, glomerular filtration rate, and the quality of the child's life. ESRD usually is diagnosed when the glomerular filtration rate decreases to about 10%.

Kidney Transplantation

Transplantation is the goal for most children with ESRD; it offers the best opportunity to have a normal lifestyle. Unfortunately, transplantation is not a cure. Children who have received transplants must continue to take immunosuppressive medication, have blood tests, and keep clinic appointments.

Kidneys come from two types of donors: living donors and cadaveric donors. A living donor is someone in the child's family, such as a parent or grandparent. A person who donates must be in good health and have healthy kidneys. A cadaveric donor kidney is a healthy kidney obtained from someone who is brain dead and whose family has consented to the transplantation. The blood and tissue types of the donor and recipient need to be compatible. Transplantations with kidneys from a relative have been more successful in children than transplantations with cadaveric kidneys.

Rejection is the most common complication of kidney transplantation. Immunosuppressive medications, taken to help prevent rejection, include cyclosporine, azathioprine, and prednisone. Other examples of immunosuppressive drugs include tacrolimus (Prograf), mycophenolate mofetil, and a new form of cyclosporine (Neoral).

As with all medications, immunosuppressive medications have side effects. When the immune system is suppressed, risk of infection is increased, related to the body's decreased ability to fight infection. Children with renal transplants should be monitored for infection and may take anti-infective medications routinely.

High blood pressure is also a complication of transplantation. Underlying renal disease, the transplanted kidney, or immunosuppressive medication side effects can cause high blood pressure.

NURSING CARE

The Child With Chronic Renal Failure and End-Stage Renal Disease

Assessment

The assessment of the child with chronic renal failure or ESRD is directed toward clinical manifestations of the renal failure and its possible complications. Blood is monitored for abnormalities and response to interventions. Monitoring hemoglobin and hematocrit assesses for potential anemia and assesses response to therapy in the child receiving recombinant erythropoietin. Serum calcium and phosphorus, alkaline phosphatase, and parathyroid hormone levels and bone radiographs are obtained to monitor for renal osteodystrophy.

The nurse assesses fluid status for fluid overload and dehydration by obtaining weight, monitoring blood pressure and heart rate, and observing and recording edema, skin turgor, mucous membranes, and fontanels.

Obtain accurate weights and height measurements regularly to assess growth and development. Ask the parent about the child's dietary and caloric intake. Information regarding attainment of development tasks, school performance, and peer relationships is helpful.

Nursing Diagnosis and Planning

The nursing diagnoses and expected outcomes that apply to the child with chronic renal failure and the family are as follows:

- Imbalanced Nutrition: Less Than Body Requirements related to decreased appetite and dietary restrictions.

  Expected Outcome: The child will receive adequate nutrition for growth and health as measured by appropriate growth for age.
- Deficient Knowledge about disease process, treatment, or diet restrictions related to anxiety or incomplete understanding of principles.

  Expected Outcome: The child or parents will be able to explain the disease process, its treatment, and dietary restrictions.
- Risk for Imbalanced Fluid Volume related to fluid and electrolyte shifts secondary to renal dysfunction.

  Expected Outcome: The child will exhibit no signs of fluid overload or deficit, as measured by weight, blood pressure, and absence of edema or signs of dehydration.
- Delayed Growth and Development related to restricted diet, chronic illness, and anemia.

  Expected Outcome: The child will attain maximum development according to normal growth and development measuring instruments.
- Interrupted Family Processes related to having a child with a chronic and potentially life-threatening disease.

  Expected Outcome: The child and family will achieve successful coping strategies, as measured by their ability to care for the child, meet the needs of other family members, and access appropriate support.
- Risk for Impaired Skin Integrity related to edema and poor nutrition.

  Expected Outcome: The child's skin will not show signs of a break in integrity (redness, irritation, breaks).

Interventions

The care of the child with chronic renal failure or ESRD is complex and requires a multidisciplinary team. Maintaining adequate nutritional intake within the dietary restriction parameters is a challenge. The nurse individualizes the diet of the child with chronic renal failure and includes foods the child likes. Small, frequent meals may be helpful. Diet supplements may be necessary to meet caloric needs. Recombinant growth hormone may allow the child to have adequate growth.

Children with chronic renal failure and their families have multifaceted information requirements. The parents need information regarding diet, medications, potential effects of the renal failure, and its treatment. They need to be informed regarding treatment options, such as hemodialysis, peritoneal dialysis, and transplantation.

Provide appropriate fluid intake and continuing assessment of fluid status. Instruct the child and family about fluid restriction and hydration assessment, such as weight, blood pressure, and appearance of edema.

Encourage the child to participate in school and age-appropriate activities. Parents may find it difficult to allow the child autonomy and will need support to do so.

The child with chronic renal failure and the family need support. They need opportunities to ask questions, verbalize feelings, and express concerns. Involving children in their own care and decisions regarding treatment is beneficial. Determine the family's prior successful coping strategies and encourage family members to use those. A social worker, psychologist, or psychiatrist may provide additional support.

Evaluation

- Does the child maintain the age-appropriate growth percentile on a growth chart despite dietary restrictions?
- Can the parents and the child discuss the disease course and management and how well the child is adapting to diet restrictions?
- Is the child free of edema?
- Does the child have moist mucous membranes and adequate urine output (see Chapter 18)?
- Does the child continue to achieve age-appropriate developmental milestones?
- Is the family involved in the child's care?
- Has the family demonstrated appropriate problem-solving strategies to meet the needs of all family members and do they access appropriate support?
- Has the integrity of the child's skin been maintained?

⌐ KEY CONCEPTS ¬

- The kidney reaches near-adult function at 6 to 12 months of age.
- The kidneys of infants cannot concentrate urine as efficiently as those of older children and adults.
- Most children eventually outgrow enuresis with therapeutic intervention.
- The clinical manifestations of UTIs vary according to the child's age, underlying anatomic or neurologic abnormalities, and frequency of recurrence.
- UTI is the most common clinical manifestation of VUR. Medical management includes low-dose prophylactic antibiotic therapy to prevent renal scarring.
- Nursing care of the child with a UTI includes giving information to the parents and child about perineal hygiene, increased fluid intake, emptying the bladder, and wearing cotton underwear.

- Most infants with cryptorchidism have spontaneous descent of their testes during the first year of life.
- The goals of surgery to correct hypospadias are to make urinary and sexual function as normal as possible and to improve the cosmetic appearance of the penis.
- Children with glomerulonephritis should be assessed for hypertension and the presence of any respiratory difficulty, such as cough, increased respiratory rate, and difficulty breathing, which may indicate fluid overload.
- Children at risk for fluid volume excess should be weighed daily on the same scale, at the same time, wearing only a gown. Infants should have their diapers removed.
- Children with edema should have their position changed at least every 2 hours and their lower extremities elevated when they are sitting or lying in bed.
- Edema related to nephrotic syndrome is first noted in the periorbital spaces and dependent areas of the body. The child may awaken with facial edema; as the day progresses, edema becomes more noticeable. Prednisone usually induces a remission in the child with nephrotic syndrome.
- Most children with acute renal failure regain renal function.
- Children with chronic renal failure and ESRD and their families require multidisciplinary care and extensive nursing support.

ANSWERS TO CRITICAL THINKING EXERCISE 20-1

1. The nurse should first determine whether Thomas has ever been able to be dry at night. This information helps discriminate between primary and secondary nocturnal enuresis. Other information the nurse will need includes whether Thomas has experienced any excessive thirst or weight loss (signs of diabetes mellitus), whether he complains about anal itching (rule out pinworms), and whether he has a fever or other signs of a UTI. It would also be helpful to know what approach the parents used during toilet training and whether either parent had enuresis as a child.

2. After underlying problems have been ruled out, the nurse can reassure Mr. Sampson that nighttime wetting is not unusual in children of this age and that the initial approach should be one of benign neglect. Focusing too much on the problem can create anxiety in the child and decreased self-esteem if the problem persists later into childhood. The nurse can suggest that the parents encourage Thomas to wear a disposable diaper or waterproof pull-up at night. They can explain to Thomas that lots of children this age need to be in pull-ups for a while and that it does not mean that he is a baby. When he has stayed dry, he can decide to try going without the pull-up. Putting a plastic draw sheet covered by a regular draw sheet over the middle portion of the bed can reduce the amount of laundry required and preserve the mattress.

REFERENCES AND READINGS

American Academy of Pediatrics. (1999). Practice parameter: The diagnosis, treatment, and evaluation of the initial urinary tract infection in febrile infants and young children. *Pediatrics, 103,* 843-852.

American Academy of Pediatrics, Action Committee for Determining Timing of Elective Surgery on the Genitalia of Male Children. (1997). Timing of elective surgery on the genitalia of male children with particular reference to the risks, benefits, and psychological effects of surgery and anesthesia. *Pediatrics, 95,* 590-594.

American Academy of Pediatrics, Committee on Genetics. (2000). Evaluation of the newborn with developmental anomalies of the external genitalia. *Pediatrics, 106,* 138-142.

Beh, H. G., & Diamond, M. (2000). An emerging ethical and medical dilemma: Should physicians perform sex assignment surgery on infants with ambiguous genitalia? *Michigan Journal of Law, 7,* 1-63.

Benjamin, K. (2002). Scrotal and inguinal masses in the newborn period. *Advances in Neonatal Care 3,* 140-148.

Boris, N., & Dalton, R. (2004). Enuresis (bedwetting). In R. Behrman, R. Kliegman, & H. Jenson (Eds.). *Nelson textbook of pediatrics* (17th ed., pp. 74-75). Philadelphia: WB Saunders.

Chan, J. C. M., Williams, D. M., & Roth, K. S. (2002). Kidney failure in infants and children. *Pediatrics in Review, 23,* 47-60.

Chon, C. H., Lai, F. C., & Shortliffe, L. M. D. (2001). Pediatric urinary tract infections. *Pediatric Clinics of North America, 48,* 1441-1459.

Cohen, A. L., Rivara, F. P., Davis, R., & Christakis, D. A. (2005). Compliance with guidelines for the medical care of first urinary tract infections in infants: A population-based study. *Pediatrics, 115,* 1474-1478.

Davis, I. D., & Avner, E. D. (2004). Nephrology: Glomerular disease. In R. Behrman, R. Kliegman, & H. Jensen (Eds.). *Nelson textbook of pediatrics* (17th ed., pp. 1783-1826). Philadelphia: WB Saunders.

DiCenso, A., Guyatt, G., & Ciliska, D. (2005). *Evidence-based nursing: A guide to clinical practice.* St. Louis: Elsevier.

Elder, J. (2004). Urologic disorders in infants and children. In R. Behrman, R. Kliegman, & H. Jensen (Eds.). *Nelson textbook of pediatrics* (17th ed., pp. 1783-1826). Philadelphia: WB Saunders.

Elenberg, E. (2002). Enuresis and voiding dysfunction. In F. Burg, J. Ingelfinger, R. Polin, & A. Gershon (Eds.). *Gellis & Kagan's current pediatric therapy* (17th ed., pp. 768-772). Philadelphia: WB Saunders.

Elenberg, E., & Travis, B. (2002). Urinary tract infection and perinephric/intranephric abscess. In F. Burg, J. Ingelfinger, R. Polin, & A. Gershon (Eds.). *Gellis & Kagan's current pediatric therapy* (17th ed., pp. 772-777). Philadelphia: WB Saunders.

Gallentine, M. L., Morey, A. F., & Thompson, I. M. (2001). Hypospadias: A contemporary epidemiologic assessment. *Urology, 57,* 788-790.

Giorgi, L. J., Bratslavsky, G., & Kogan, B. A. (2005). Febrile urinary tract infections in infants: Renal ultrasound remains necessary. *Journal of Urology, 173,* 568-570.

Hanson, L. A., Korotkova, M., Haverson, L., Mattsby-Baltzer, I., Hahn-Zoric, M., Silfverdal, S., Strandvik, B., & Telemo, E. (2002). Breast-feeding, a complex support system for the offspring. *Pediatrics International, 44,* 347-352.

Hermer, L. (2002). Paradigms revised: Intersex children, bioethics & the law. *Annals of Health Law, 11,* 195-236.

Ingelfinger, J. (2002). Disorders of the bladder and urethra, ureter, and collecting system. In F. Burg, J. Ingelfinger, R. Polin, & A. Gershon (Eds.). *Gellis & Kagan's current pediatric therapy* (17th ed., pp. 762-767). Philadelphia: WB Saunders.

Lackgren, G., Whalin, N., Skoldenberg, E., & Stenberg, A. (2001). Long-term followup of children treated with dextranomer/hyaluronic acid copolymer for vesicoureteral reflux. *Journal of Urology, 166,* 1887-1892.

Landgraf, J. M., Abidari, J., Cilento, B. G., Cooper, C. S., Schulman, S. L., & Ortenburg, J. (2004). Coping, commitment, and attitude: Quantifying the everyday burden of enuresis on children and their families. *Pediatrics, 113,* 334-344.

Langer, J., & Coplen, D. (1998). Circumcision and pediatric disorders of the penis. *Pediatric Clinics of North America, 45,* 801-812.

Leung, A. K. C., & Robson, W. L. M. (2004). Current status of cryptorchidism. *Advances in Pediatrics, 51,* 351-377.

Lieberman, K. V. (2000). A practical guide to acute glomerulonephritis. *Office and Emergency Pediatrics, 13,* 151-154.

Ma, J. F., & Shortliffe, L. D. (2004). Urinary tract infection in children: Etiology and epidemiology. *Urologic Clinics of North America, 31,* 517-526.

Manson, J. M., & Carr, M. C. (2003). Molecular epidemiology of hypospadias: Review of genetic and environmental risk factors. *Birth Defects Research, 67,* 825-836.

Marrocco, G., Vallasciani, S., Fiocca, G., & Calisti, A. (2004). Hypospadias surgery: A 10-year review. *Pediatric Surgery International, 20,* 200-203. Published on-line April 9, 2004.

Martin, P. L. (2003). Moving toward an international standard in informed consent: The impact of intersexuality and the internet on the standard of care. *Duke Journal of Gender Law & Policy, 10,* 135-169.

McCormack, K. (1999). A very special baby: Managing a baby with congenital adrenal hyperplasia. *Journal of Neonatal Nursing, 5,* 19-25.

Nicholls, E. (2003). Inguino-scrotal problems in children. *The Practitioner, 246,* 226-230.

Pagana, K. D., & Pagana, T. J. (2005). *Mosby's diagnostic & laboratory test reference* (7th ed., pp. 952-976). St. Louis: Elsevier.

Phornphutkul, C., Fausto-Sterling, A., & Gruppuso, P. A. (2000). Gender self-reassignment in an XY adolescent female born with ambiguous genitalia. *Pediatrics, 106,* 135-137.

Pierik, F., Burdorf, A., Deddens, J., Juttman, R., & Weber, R. (2004). Maternal and paternal risk factors for cryptorchidism and hypospadias: a case-control study in newborn boys. *Environmental Health Perspectives, 112,* 1570-1576.

Pillai, S., & Besner, G. (1998). Pediatric testicular problems. *Pediatric Clinics of North America, 45,* 813-830.

Reiner, W. G. (1999). Assignment of sex in neonates with ambiguous genitalia. *Current Opinion in Pediatrics, 11,* 363-365.

Schnaper, W., Daouk, G., & Ingelfinger, J. (2002). In F. Burg, J. Ingelfinger, R. Polin, & A. Gershon (Eds.). *Gellis & Kagan's current pediatric therapy* (17th ed., pp. 798-804). Philadelphia: WB Saunders.

Shaw, K. N., Gorelick, M., McGowan, K. L., Yakscoe, N. M., & Schwartz, J. S. (1998). Prevalence of urinary tract infection in febrile young children in the emergency department. *Pediatrics, 102*(2), e16 (5 pages).

Slutsker, L., Ries, A. A., Maloney, K., Wells, J. G., Greene, K. D., & Griffin, P. M. (1998). A nationwide case-control study of *Escherichia coli* O157:H7 infection in the United States. *Journal of Infectious Disease, 177,* 962-966.

Somers, M. (2002). Acute renal failure. In F. Burg, J. Ingelfinger, R. Polin, & A. Gershon (Eds.). *Gellis & Kagan's current pediatric therapy* (17th ed., pp. 809-814). Philadelphia: WB Saunders.

Sparrow, M. (2002). Nephrology. In V. Gunn & C. Nechyba (Eds). *The Harriet Lane handbook* (16th ed., pp. 397-416). Philadelphia: Mosby.

Stokowski, L. (2004). Hypospadias in the neonate. *Advances in Neonatal Care, 4,* 206-215.

Thiedke, C. C. (2003). Nocturnal enuresis. *American Family Physician, 67,* 1499-1506.

Thorpe, C. (2004). Shiga toxin-producing *Escherichia coli* infection. *Clinical Infectious Diseases, 38,* 1298-1303.

Tobias, N. E. (2000). Management of nocturnal enuresis. *Nursing Clinics of North America, 35,* 37-60.

Vogt, B., & Avner, E. (2004a). Conditions particularly associated with proteinuria. In R. Behrman, R. Kliegman, & H. Jensen (Eds.), *Nelson textbook of pediatrics* (17th ed., pp. 1751-1762). Philadelphia: WB Saunders.

Vogt, B., & Avner, E. (2004b). Toxic nephropathies—Renal failure: Renal failure. In R. Behrman, R. Kliegman, & H. Jensen (Eds.), *Nelson textbook of pediatrics* (17th ed., pp. 1767-1775). Philadelphia: WB Saunders.

Wallace, M. (2003). What is new with renal transplantation. *AORN J, 77,* 945-958.

The Child With a Respiratory Alteration

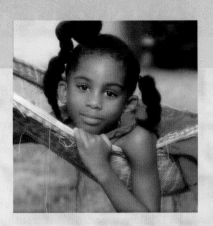

Learning Objectives

After studying this chapter, you should be able to:

- Describe the differences in the anatomy and physiology of the infant or child's respiratory system that increase the risk for respiratory disease.
- Outline nursing care for a child with allergies to inhalants.
- Discuss the pathophysiology, clinical manifestations, and therapeutic management of common acute and chronic respiratory alterations.
- Identify the nursing care needs of infants and children with acute and chronic respiratory alterations.
- Develop guidelines for the home care of a child with an acute respiratory alteration.
- Identify common triggers of asthma symptoms.

- Apply measures that can be taken to prevent and treat asthma episodes.
- Identify teaching needs for children with asthma and their families.
- Describe the nursing care of the child with cystic fibrosis.
- Discuss measures to maintain adequate oxygenation and provide appropriate developmental stimulation for the child with bronchopulmonary dysplasia.
- Describe the correct method of administering and evaluating tuberculosis skin tests.
- Identify ways to prevent the transmission of tuberculosis and explain the importance of administering antituberculosis medications as prescribed.

Definitions

atelectasis A collapsed or airless state of the lung that may involve all or part of the lung.

crackles Abnormal, discontinuous, nonmusical sounds heard on auscultation, primarily during inhalation; also called rales.

dysphagia Difficulty swallowing.

dyspnea Difficulty breathing.

grunting A sound similar to a grunting noise that can be heard with or without a stethoscope.

hypercapnia Increased levels of carbon dioxide in the blood, as indicated by an elevated $Paco_2$ as determined by blood gas analysis.

hypocapnia Decreased levels of carbon dioxide in the blood.

hypoxemia Decreased levels of oxygen in the blood.

hypoxia Decreased oxygenation of cells and tissues.

nasal flaring A serious sign of air hunger demonstrated by widening of the nares to enable an infant or young child to take in more oxygen.

nasal polyps Semitransparent herniations of respiratory epithelium.

orthopnea Difficulty breathing except in an upright position.

retractions An abnormal movement of the chest wall during inspiration that may occur intercostally and substernally.

rhonchi Adventitious breath sounds caused by the passage of air through an airway obstructed by thick secretions; sounds do not clear with coughing.

stridor A shrill, harsh sound that can be heard during inspiration, expiration, or both; produced by the flow of air through a narrowed segment of the respiratory tract.

tachypnea Increased respiratory rate.

wheezing High-pitched, musical whistles that can be heard with or without a stethoscope; may be inspiratory or expiratory; caused by bronchial constriction or obstruction of the airway and commonly occurs in asthma.

REVIEW OF THE RESPIRATORY SYSTEM

The respiratory system consists of the nose, pharynx, larynx, trachea, bronchi, and lungs. It is further divided into the *upper respiratory tract* (nose, pharynx, larynx) and the *lower respiratory tract* (trachea, bronchi, lungs).

The Upper Airway

Air enters the body through the *nares*, or nostrils, two nasal cavities lined with mucous membrane. In older infants and children, air can also enter through the mouth into the *pharynx*, or throat. The *nasopharynx* is located immediately behind nasal cavity; the *oropharynx* is located behind the mouth. The *laryngeal pharynx* lies below the oropharynx and opens into the larynx toward the front and into the esophagus toward the back.

The *larynx* is located between the pharynx and the trachea. The vocal cords are at the upper end of the larynx. The proximity of the upper esophagus to the upper respiratory system can put an individual at risk for inhaling food or liquids, but the *epiglottis* covers the larynx during swallowing and helps keep food out of the lower respiratory tract.

Cilia are hairlike processes that move mucus and fluid. Damage to cilia interferes with the removal of mucus from the respiratory tract. Ciliated mucous membranes line the larynx and filter dust and other particles from the air. The particles are then carried to the pharynx to be removed by sneezing, blowing, or coughing. After being filtered, the air that enters the respiratory system is humidified and warmed before proceeding into the lungs. The three types of tonsils are: the oval *palatine tonsils*, located on either side of the

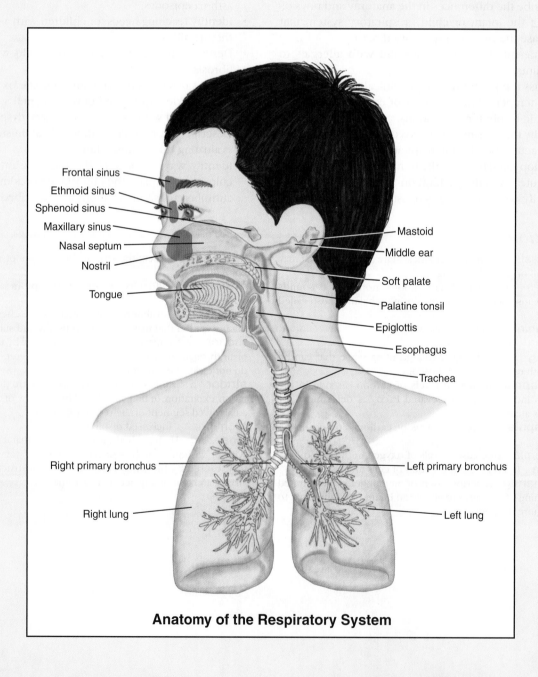

Frontal sinus

Ethmoid sinus

Sphenoid sinus

Maxillary sinus

Nasal septum

Nostril

Tongue

Mastoid

Middle ear

Soft palate

Palatine tonsil

Epiglottis

Esophagus

Trachea

Right primary bronchus

Left primary bronchus

Right lung

Left lung

Anatomy of the Respiratory System

pharynx; the *lingual tonsil,* located below the palatine tonsils at the base of the tongue; and the *pharyngeal tonsils,* or *adenoids,* located at the nasopharyngeal border. The tonsils are composed mainly of lymphoid tissue. They help filter the circulating lymph of bacteria and other foreign material that enter the body, especially through the mouth and nose.

The Lower Airway

The *trachea* conducts air between the larynx and the lungs. It divides into right and left main *bronchi* at its lower end, the *carina.* The right main bronchus is shorter and wider than the left. The main bronchi divide into *lobar bronchi, segmental bronchi,* and *bronchioles* and terminate in *alveoli.* Mucus-secreting goblet cells line the bronchi and protect the lungs from dust and bacteria.

The *lungs* are two conical structures within the thoracic cavity. The right lung has three *lobes* (upper, middle, lower); the left has two lobes (upper, lower). The *pleura* consists of two layers, the *parietal pleura* and the *visceral pleura.* The parietal pleura lines the entire thoracic cavity; the visceral pleura encases each lung. The pleura helps maintain lung stability. Negative pressure within the intrapleural space prevents the lungs from separating from the thorax. *Diffusion* of gases takes place in the lungs. Terminal bronchioles lack mucus-secreting goblet cells and cilia, and gas exchange does not take place here.

Distal to the terminal bronchioles are the alveoli, where most gas exchange occurs. Thinness of the alveolar walls aids in gas exchange. An almost solid sheet of capillaries is within the alveolar walls, so the alveolar gases are proximate to the capillary blood.

Prenatal Respiratory Development

The respiratory system must mature before birth for the neonate to survive. The placenta performs oxygenation *in utero,* but to adapt to extrauterine life the neonate must be able to inflate the lungs, establish continuous breathing, and transfer the gases needed to meet metabolic needs.

Postnatal Respiratory Changes

Postnatal changes in the respiratory system occur as follows:
1. Compression of the thorax during vaginal delivery forces out some fetal lung fluid.
2. Respirations are stimulated by hypoxemia; hypercarbia; cold, tactile stimulation; and a possible decrease in the concentration of prostaglandin E_2.
3. Inflation of the normal lung is complete within a few breaths, and most alveoli have expanded within the first hour of life.
4. Surfactant in the lung liquid lowers surface tension and facilitates lung expansion.
5. Pulmonary blood flow increases.
6. Closure of the foramen ovale and the ductus arteriosus (see Chapter 22) establishes the pulmonary and circulatory systems.

Gas Exchange and Transport

Two-way diffusion takes place between the walls of the alveoli. In *diffusion,* molecules move from an area of greater concentration to one of lesser concentration. Blood entering the lung capillaries is somewhat low in oxygen. Oxygen will diffuse from the alveoli, where its concentration is higher, into the blood. Similarly, carbon dioxide moves out of the blood and into the alveoli. Most oxygen that diffuses into the capillary blood in the lungs is bound to the hemoglobin of red blood cells. A small percentage is dissolved in plasma. For oxygen to enter the cells, it must separate from hemoglobin. Carbon dioxide diffuses into the blood from the tissues and is

---

PEDIATRIC DIFFERENCES IN THE RESPIRATORY SYSTEM

- Surfactant is lacking in premature infants. Infants born before 34 weeks' gestation have a higher risk for RDS.
- Smaller lower airways and undeveloped supporting cartilage predispose the child to an increased risk for obstruction by mucus, edema, and foreign bodies. The neonate's airway is 50% smaller than that of adults. A premature infant has a more compliant chest wall and weaker respiratory muscles than those of a term infant.
- Lung size is proportional to body height. Therefore, lung volumes and capacities do not vary from age to age.
- Infants are obligatory nose breathers; they have difficulty breathing through the mouth. If the infant has nasal congestion, breathing becomes more difficult.
- The diaphragm is the neonate's major respiratory muscle. Intercostal muscles are not well developed. Retractions are more common in the infant than in older children and adults.
- Brief periods of apnea (10-15 sec) are common in the neonate. The respiratory pattern may be irregular.
- Children's normal respiratory rate is higher than that of adults.
- An increased metabolic rate increases oxygen needs.
- Alveoli develop from approximately 20 million to 200 million by age 3 years. Alveolar development gradually decreases after age 3 years; few develop after age 8 years.
- The lung surface increases until 5 to 8 years. Actual lung growth continues into the adolescent years.
- Eustachian tubes are relatively horizontal, which increases the risk for bacteria entering the middle ear.
- Tracheal size approximately triples by adulthood.
- Tonsillar tissue is normally enlarged in early-school-age children.
- Infants and children use abdominal muscles to inhale until about age 5 to 6 years.
- The child's flexible larynx is more susceptible to spasm.

transported to the lungs by the blood. In this activity, hemoglobin is a buffer that enables blood to take up carbon dioxide without altering the blood pH significantly. The uptake and delivery of gases by the blood is a continuous process.

Ventilation occurs through *inspiration* and *expiration*. In inspiration, the diaphragm contracts and flattens, expanding the vertical dimension of the chest; the lung volume increases. In expiration, the diaphragm and chest wall relax, decreasing thoracic volume. Intrathoracic pressure increases, and gas flows out of the lungs, taking with it the carbon dioxide that was delivered to the lungs by the blood. Ventilation of the lungs is intermittent. Inspired air is 21% oxygen; end-expired air is 16% oxygen and 35% carbon dioxide.

DIAGNOSTIC TESTS

In most instances, respiratory tract disorders are diagnosed from the findings on physical examination and the clinical manifestations. Sometimes, however, specific diagnostic tests are needed.

Blood Gas Analysis

Arterial blood gas analysis plays an important role in the investigation of pulmonary function. Arterial blood gas values most frequently determined include the partial arterial oxygen tension (PaO_2), the partial pressure of carbon dioxide in arterial blood ($PaCO_2$), the acid-base balance (pH), and bicarbonate (HCO_3^-). Arterial blood is more reliable than capillary or venous blood for these tests, especially in children with poor peripheral perfusion. Arterial blood gas values are used primarily to determine acid-base balance, not oxygen saturation (see Chapter 18).

Pulmonary Function Tests

Probably the most useful measures of ventilatory function are the *vital capacity* and the *expiratory flow rate*, both measured by spirometry. Most children can perform these tests

by 6 years of age (Tee & Hui, 2005). Accurate measurements are difficult to obtain in younger children because they are unable to follow commands. Infant pulmonary function testing is now being performed at many institutions with use of conscious sedation (Castile, 2004). Pulmonary function tests assess the degree of pulmonary disease, the response to therapy, and the presence of restrictive or obstructive disease. They are also done to test the child's response to bronchodilators should pulmonary function be affected.

The child must be given instruction and practice in blowing, pushing, and holding respirations. The child should become familiar with the mouthpiece and the nose clip to feel comfortable with their use.

Pulse Oximetry

Pulse oximetry is a simple, noninvasive, intermittent or continuous method for measuring oxygen saturation for the purpose of determining the need for or response to oxygen therapy (see Chapter 13). The goal of treatment for most respiratory conditions is an oxygen saturation value greater than 95%. For children with chronic respiratory disease, however, a realistic goal may be slightly lower.

Transcutaneous Monitoring

Transcutaneous monitoring continuously checks oxygen and carbon dioxide concentrations in the body through an electrode placed on the child's skin. Electrode sites must be changed every 3 to 4 hours to prevent burning the skin, and the machine must be recalibrated each time electrodes are changed. The readings may not be accurate if tissue perfusion is poor. End-tidal carbon dioxide monitoring is a newer technology, often used in conjunction with pulse oximetry, that measures carbon dioxide in the exhaled breath noninvasively. It is useful in verifying endotracheal tube position, in evaluating asthma, and during procedural sedation (Yldzdas, Yapcoglu, & Ylmaz, 2004).

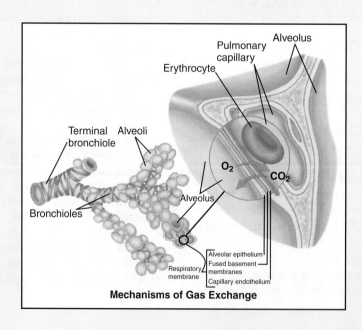

Mechanisms of Gas Exchange

Common Laboratory and Diagnostic Tests for Respiratory Disorders

Test	Description	Normal Findings	Indications	Nursing Considerations
Chest radiography, posteroanterior and lateral views	Shows airways, lungs, heart, great vessels.	Normal appearance of internal structures of chest.	To detect respiratory disease of lungs.	Assist in holding child.
Computed tomography	Shows lesions in chest wall, pleural space, mediastinum, and lung parenchyma.	Normal cross-section of lung tissue.	To image tumors or masses; to evaluate response to therapy aimed at defined lesions.	Assist with sedation and immobilization of child. Withhold feedings 3-4 hr before the test because of frequent use of contrast medium.
Bronchoscopy	Provides viewing of tracheobronchial tree through a scope.	Normal appearance of tracheobronchial tree or successful removal of foreign body or mucous plugs.	To view a lesion and obtain biopsy material for culture; to remove foreign body or mucous plugs.	Rigid bronchoscopy is usually performed with child under general anesthesia. Fiberoptic flexible bronchoscopy can be performed while child is awake or sedated. Observe child closely for signs of airway obstruction. Mist may be given to decrease swelling and edema.
Laryngoscopy	Provides direct viewing of larynx with a scope.	Normal appearance of larynx.	To identify cause of stridor and local abnormalities.	Mirror (indirect) laryngoscopy can be performed on children age 4 yr or older. In infants and younger children, direct laryngoscopy or transnasal laryngoscopy with flexible bronchoscope will give much better results. General anesthesia is usually required; topical anesthesia and mild sedation may be provided for fiberoptic examination. Fluids and foods are withheld until effects of local anesthetic have worn off and gag reflex has returned.
Cultures	Throat, blood, nasopharyngeal, sputum, induced sputum (hypertonic saline solution delivered by nebulizer).	No culture growth or normal flora only.	To isolate and identify pathogens.	See Chapter 13 for procedures.

Continued

Common Pediatric Laboratory Tests and Normal Values **EVOLVE**

Common Laboratory and Diagnostic Tests for Respiratory Disorders—cont'd

Test	Description	Normal Findings	Indications	Nursing Considerations
RAST for IgE	Measures quantity of IgE antibodies in serum after exposure to specific antigens.	If the child is not allergic to the antigen, IgE antibody is not detected. A test result is positive in relation to a specific antigen if the value is above 400% of control.	To identify specific allergens; systemic reactions to insect venom, drugs, and chemicals; to monitor response to desensitization procedures; also performed at the onset of asthma, hay fever, or dermatitis.	Prepare child for peripheral blood sample to be drawn. Determine whether child has undergone any radioisotope tests within past week because such tests may alter the results.
Pilocarpine iontophoresis (sweat test)	Measures sweat electrolyte concentration for diagnosis of CF. Sweating is stimulated on the child's forearm with a small electrical current and pilocarpine; a sweat sample is then collected on preweighed, dry, sterile gauze or filter paper and the amounts of sweat sodium and chloride are measured.	*Normal chloride:* <40 mEq/L. *Suggestive of CF:* 40 to 60 mEq/L. *Positive for CF:* ≥60 mEq/L.	To diagnose cystic fibrosis.	No physical preparation is needed. Offer parents and child support as they face the implications of a positive diagnosis. Inform child and parents that the test is painless and that it is usually performed twice to ensure accurate results. Because an adequate amount of sweat is difficult to obtain from infants, the sweat test is usually unreliable in infants younger than 4 weeks.
Mantoux test	Skin test for TB. PPD, 5 TB units (0.1 mL) is injected intradermally into volar surface of forearm with short, 26- to 27-gauge needle, beveled side up. A wheal 6-10 mm in diameter should appear during injection. The site is checked in 48-72 hr by a health care professional. Results are recorded in millimeters (not simply as positive or negative). The reading is based on induration (hardness), not redness.	*Positive result:* in area of induration ≥15 mm (in children 4 years of age and older); area of induration ≥10 mm in children younger than 4 yr or at high risk for exposure; area of induration ≥5 mm in highest risk group. *Negative result:* Mantoux test cannot rule out the presence of TB, particularly in young infants.	To screen and test individuals suspected of having TB or of having been exposed to TB.	Test is fairly difficult to administer. After PPD is injected, withdrawal of needle should be delayed 2-3 sec to minimize leakage of PPD at the puncture site. In most children, skin testing will elicit positive reaction 3-6 wk after initial infection. Steroids and immunosuppressants given within 4-6 wk can cause false-negative skin test results. Positive tuberculin reactivity usually continues for person's lifetime, even with treatment.

Electronic Resources

Additional information related to the content in Chapter 21 can be found on:

the interactive companion CD-ROM

- Animations: Asthma
            Intubation
            Intubation in Children
- Audio Glossary
- NCLEX Review Questions

or the companion website at *evolve*
http://evolve.elsevier.com/james/ncoc

- Common Pediatric Laboratory Tests and Normal Values
- NCLEX Review Questions
- Resources for Health Care Providers and Families
- WebLinks

Respiratory alterations are the most common causes of illness in the infant and child. Upper respiratory disorders affect the ears, nose, pharynx, and larynx; lower respiratory disorders include those disorders that involve the trachea, bronchi, and lungs.

Infants and children younger than 3 years are at greater risk than older children and adults for development of respiratory infections because of their immature immune systems, smaller upper and lower airways, and underdeveloped supporting cartilage. Although most respiratory infections are self-limiting, in infants and young children respiratory distress can occur quickly as mucus and edema obstruct their small airways.

Parents should be taught preventive measures, including adequate rest, good nutrition, and good hygiene, with an emphasis on handwashing. Even with the most careful hygiene and preventive practices, however, most children will have some type of respiratory infection each year. School nurses often see children with respiratory problems in the school health office and may be the primary health care providers for these children.

Most children can be cared for at home by their parents and do not need hospitalization. Those children who are hospitalized are being discharged from the hospital earlier in their recovery than in the past. The current health care environment underlies the need for nurses to teach parents good home care techniques, including careful observation and recognition of signs that indicate the need to contact health care providers. Parents, especially first-time parents, often are frightened by the sudden onset of respiratory symptoms, which may indicate a severe problem. Teaching them the signs and symptoms of serious illness will help them develop appropriate decision-making skills.

Children with chronic conditions have many special needs, and the child with a chronic respiratory disease is no different. Medications and treatments become a way of life for many of these children. Their activity level is often altered, and some may have a shortened life span.

The nurse plays an important role in the care of the child with a chronic respiratory disease. Beyond giving acute care to the hospitalized child, the nurse must coordinate and facilitate the child's long-term care. Because of advances being made in the treatment of chronic pediatric respiratory conditions, the treatment and care of children affected by these disorders are constantly changing and improving, requiring the nurse to stay current in these areas.

ALLERGIC RHINITIS

Allergic rhinitis is an inflammatory disorder of the nasal mucosa. It is usually seasonal, recurrent, and triggered by specific allergens (see Chapter 17). It is sometimes referred to as *seasonal allergic rhinitis*, *seasonal pollinosis*, or *hay fever*. Some children have symptoms year round (*perennial allergic rhinitis*).

Etiology and Incidence

Common causative agents of allergic rhinitis include dust mites, feathers, animal dander, mold spores, and pollens of trees, grasses, and weeds. There is usually a family history similar to that seen in individuals with atopic dermatitis and asthma. Unlike atopic dermatitis, however, allergic rhinitis does not predispose to the development of asthma.

The onset of allergic rhinitis usually occurs during childhood but rarely before age 2 years. It is estimated that 20% to 40% of children have this type of allergic response (Milgrom & Leung, 2004).

Manifestations

The classic symptoms of allergic rhinitis are watery rhinorrhea, associated with itching of nose, eyes, ears, and palate, and paroxysmal sneezing. Additional signs and symptoms include the "allergic salute"—an upward rubbing of the nose with the palm of the hand, which can leave a crease below the bridge (Fig. 21-1); allergic shiners—dark circles under the eyes from congestion and edema; dry lips from mouth breathing; pale, boggy nasal mucous membranes; and nasal obstruction. Children with allergic rhinitis have symptoms as long as they are exposed to the allergen.

It is important to distinguish allergic rhinitis from viral *nasopharyngitis* (the common cold), which is usually caused by a

---

PATHOPHYSIOLOGY

ALLERGIC RHINITIS

Allergens (pollens, molds, spores, dust mites, animal dander) are deposited on the nasal mucosa, causing local inflammation and increased capillary permeability. Local IgE is produced, and sensitization of the respiratory tissues occurs. Mast cell mediators are released, producing vasodilation, mucosal edema, mucus secretions, stimulation of itch receptors, and a reduced threshold for sneezing.

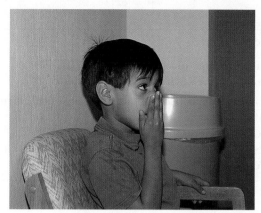

FIG 21-1 Children with allergic rhinitis often have dark circles under their eyes, called *allergic shiners,* and may be seen rubbing their noses upward with the palm—the "allergic salute." *(Courtesy Parkland Health and Hospital System Community Oriented Primary Care Clinic, Dallas, TX.)*

rhinovirus and is spread by droplet or by contact with contaminated items. Usually children with nasopharyngitis have the associated symptoms of sore throat, fever, cough, and fatigue. The condition is self-limiting and usually resolves within 2 weeks. The quality of the nasal discharge in children with nasopharyngitis often changes from clear to cloudy or yellow. Management is supportive. Because young infants are obligatory nose breathers, the infant's blocked nasal passages can be relieved with instillation of normal saline solution drops followed by gentle bulb suction.

Diagnostic Evaluation

A thorough personal and family history usually elicit a description that suggests an allergic rather than infectious pattern. The nasal smear may demonstrate eosinophils. Allergy skin testing is done if signs and symptoms continue after treatment with medication. The radioallergosorbent test (RAST) is used only when skin testing is difficult because of generalized dermatitis, the child is very young, or the child is too ill for skin testing. A complete blood cell count might reveal elevated eosinophils, a finding associated with allergic manifestations.

Therapeutic Management

The treatment of choice is to eliminate the allergen from the child's environment (Halken, 2004). When this is impossible, as in the case of pollen in the air, medication can control symptoms. Finally, immunotherapy (allergy shots) may be considered for children whose condition is not responsive to either environmental modification or medication. Immunotherapy involves injecting the child with progressively larger doses of the allergen in an effort to reduce the magnitude of the body's allergic response. Injections are given once or twice a week until a maintenance dose is reached; monthly maintenance injections can continue for several years.

Antihistamines or intranasal corticosteroids are the treatment of choice (Berger, 2004). Antihistamines are most effective when given before or very early in an allergic episode. Because they can cause drowsiness, they should be given at night. Some of the newer antihistamines (e.g., loratadine, cetirizine, fexofenadine, desloratadine) are long acting and require only one or two doses daily. A decongestant can be given in conjunction with an antihistamine if nasal congestion is a problem. Short-term topical intranasal corticosteroids (e.g., fluticasone, mometasone) are quite effective and seem to actually offer better relief than antihistamines and decongestants (Blaiss, 2004). It usually takes several days of treatment before the child feels the effects of topical corticosteroids. Children with severe symptoms that do not respond to treatment may be given systemic corticosteroids; relief is usually attained within 24 hours.

BOX 21-1	**PARENTS WANT TO KNOW** How to Implement Environmental Modifications

To reduce your child's exposure to allergens, take the following measures:

Pollen and Dust
- Wash your child's sheets and blankets weekly in hot water.
- Avoid using wool and down blankets.
- Encase pillows and mattresses in dust-proof covers.
- Replace carpet with wood, tile, slate, or vinyl.
- Replace drapes and blinds with curtains and shades.
- Replace upholstered furniture with wood or plastic.
- Keep closet doors shut.
- Cover hot air vents with filters.
- Install air cleaners.
- Use multilayer vacuum bags.
- Clean with a towel treated to attract dust.
- Run an air conditioner.
- Keep household humidity at 40% to 50%.

Mold
- Clean with a mold inhibitor.
- Dry everyone's shoes thoroughly.
- Use a moisture remover in closets.
- Encourage your child to stay out of the basement.
- Replace foam rubber mattresses with inner spring mattresses.
- Run an air conditioner.
- Keep the humidity below 35%.
- Run a dehumidifier.
- Ventilate the house.
- Store firewood outside.
- Limit the number of indoor plants.

Dander
- Keep pets outside if possible.
- Ventilate the house.
- Install air cleaners.
- Encase mattresses and pillows in dust-proof covers.

For further information, contact:
Allergy & Asthma Network/Mothers of Asthmatics, Inc. website: *www.aanma.org.* A family site that provides information on asthma, products, kits, and books.

Nursing Considerations

Nursing care focuses on early identification of clinical signs and symptoms of allergic rhinitis and support of the therapeutic management of the condition. The nurse assesses and records the applicable history and helps the family identify allergens to which the child is sensitive. Once the allergens are known, the nurse counsels parents regarding administration of medications, environmental control, and immunotherapy as appropriate. Allergic rhinitis can negatively affect quality of life and school performance—not only does allergic rhinitis impair cognitive function but allergies are also one of the most common reasons for lost school days (Schoenwetter, Dupclay, Appajosyula, Botteman, & Pashos, 2004).

Side effects of medications used to treat allergic rhinitis can further impair functioning. Drowsiness, the most common side effect of antihistamines, can usually be overcome if the child takes a combination antihistamine and decongestant or takes the medication at night. Some children have dry mucous membranes or excitability. Warm water or saline solution irrigations of the nasal passages can be used to moisten mucous membranes, soften crusted secretions, and wash out irritants. Saline solution can be mixed by adding ¼ teaspoon of salt to a cup of warm water. Saline solution nose drops are also available without prescription.

When specific allergens have been identified, they should be eliminated or controlled (Box 21-1). During the pollen season, the child should stay indoors as much as possible and the windows should be kept closed if the house is air conditioned. After being outdoors, the child should shower and wash the hair to remove pollens from the body. Animals that have been outside may also be a source of contamination.

Receiving immunotherapy can be a traumatic experience for the child. It is often difficult for children to understand how an injection will help them. Allergy injections must be given in a physician's office because some children can have an anaphylactic reaction to the allergy serum. Monitor the child closely (vital sign changes, difficulty breathing) for 20 to 30 minutes after the injection in case anaphylaxis develops. Keep emergency epinephrine ready.

SINUSITIS

Sinusitis, although not itself a serious disorder, can lead to life-threatening complications. Inflammation and infection of the sinuses can be acute or chronic.

Etiology and Incidence

Acute sinusitis often follows an upper respiratory tract viral infection. Children with chronic sinusitis often have allergic rhinitis or otitis media with effusion (OME). Hypertrophied adenoids, immune deficiencies, and foreign body obstruction in the nose also predispose to sinusitis. Children with cystic fibrosis have a high incidence of sinusitis because of highly viscous mucous secretions and nasal polyps. The most common causative organisms are *Streptococcus pneumoniae*, *Haemophilus influenzae*, and *Moraxella catarrhalis*, and less frequently, group A *Streptococcus* species (Huang & Fang, 2004).

Sinus infections can occur in infancy as well as in childhood but are most common during the school-age years.

Manifestations

Sinusitis is characterized by signs and symptoms of a cold that do not improve after 14 days, low-grade fever, nasal congestion with purulent nasal discharge, halitosis, cough (which usually increases when the child is lying down), and headache, tenderness, and a feeling of fullness over the affected sinuses; young children may become irritable. Occasionally, children have facial edema. Children with chronic sinusitis have many of the same symptoms except that the cough is chronic and the headache is recurrent. The child's sense of taste or smell may be impaired, and the child may be fatigued.

Diagnostic Evaluation

Sinus radiographs show mucosal thickening, opacification, and air-fluid levels in children older than 1 year. Sinus radiographs are of no value in younger children because of their small sinuses. Computed tomography has become the gold standard for diagnosis of sinus disease because it provides detailed anatomic information (Bhattacharyya, Jones, Hill, & Shapiro, 2004). Because of the thick bone of the maxilla in the anterior part of the face and the small size of the sinus, transillumination of the sinuses is not useful.

Therapeutic Management

Most cases of acute sinusitis are self-resolving and do not require antibiotics (Contopoulos-Ioannidis & Ioannidis, 2004). When a prescription is required, amoxicillin or amoxicillin–potassium clavulanate (Augmentin) is used most frequently. In addition to antibiotics, treatment includes analgesics, hydration, the application of moist heat, and decongestants. The use of antihistamines in the treatment of sinusitis is

---

PATHOPHYSIOLOGY

SINUSITIS

Acute sinusitis occurs when the sinus cavity is invaded by bacteria, causing mucosal inflammation and edema that block narrow sinus channels. The volume of secretions increases, and the affected sinuses fill with purulent material. Inflammation and infection interfere with the protective cleansing action of the cilia covering the sinus mucous membranes. Impaired mucociliary transport leads to stagnation of secretions within the sinuses; the stagnant secretions provide a medium for bacterial growth.

Chronic sinusitis is usually a complication of acute sinusitis. Prolonged or repeated infections result in irreversible changes in the mucosal lining of the sinus. Nasal polyps, a deviated septum, and enlarged adenoids inhibit sinus drainage, which can lead to infections. The frontal and sphenoid sinuses are most often involved in children.

Infection from sinusitis can spread to the middle ear, causing otitis media. Serious complications occur when infection spreads either directly through the bone or along the venous channels of the skull into adjacent structures, such as the orbit or the central nervous system.

controversial (Contopoulos-Ioannidis, Ioannidis, & Lau, 2003). Antihistamines may be used to treat allergy symptoms associated with chronic sinusitis, but they tend to impair sinus drainage by thickening secretions. Steroid nasal sprays may be used to reduce inflammation while avoiding the rebound effect of decongestant nose drops.

Obstructive deformities, such as enlarged adenoids or polyps, are sometimes surgically corrected (Sobel, Samadi, Kazahaya, & Tom, 2005). If orbital cellulitis develops, the child should be hospitalized immediately and parenteral antibiotic therapy begun.

Nursing Considerations

The nurse should assess the location of pain or fullness. Pain can occur in the forehead or over the cheek bones or upper teeth, or it may radiate to the top of the head. The nurse should inspect and palpate the face for edema, document any fever, and inspect the nose and throat for purulent discharge. The nasal mucous membranes are inspected for erythema and edema.

Nursing care focuses on teaching the parents antibiotic administration, comfort measures, how to monitor for response to treatment, and how to identify complications. Emphasize the importance of the child's taking the antibiotics as prescribed. Sinus drainage is facilitated by increasing the child's intake of clear fluids and by using a bedside humidifier.

Warm, moist compresses applied two or three times daily help decrease swelling and pain. Acetaminophen is given for fever and discomfort. Breathing warm mist in a hot shower or through hot, moist towels can help liquefy and mobilize nasal mucus, as can saline solution nose drops. The nurse teaches the parent to administer nose drops after the nasal passages have been gently cleaned. The amount, color, and consistency of nasal drainage should be noted and evaluated to determine whether the child is responding to treatment.

Carefully evaluate the child's response to treatment and the development of complications. Advise parents to contact the physician promptly if symptoms become worse, if the child has any periorbital redness or edema, or does not seem to be feeling better after 3 to 4 days.

OTITIS MEDIA

Otitis media is one of the most common illnesses of infancy and childhood. The term *otitis media* refers to effusion and infection or blockage of the middle ear. *Acute otitis media* is effusion in the middle ear that occurs suddenly and is associated with other signs of illness. *Otitis media with effusion* refers to the presence of fluid behind the tympanic membrane without signs of infection. Otitis media with effusion often follows an episode of AOM and usually resolves in 1 to 3 months.

Etiology

The bacterial pathogens that usually cause AOM are S. pneumoniae, H. influenzae, and M. catarrhalis. H. influenzae has become the predominant pathogen since 2000 when universal immunization with the pneumococcal conjugate vaccine was begun (Casey & Pichichero, 2004). Although viruses do not cause otitis media, they are thought to predispose the child to ear infection by altering host defenses and contributing to eustachian tube dysfunction. Allergies are also thought to precipitate otitis media. Exposure to a household member who smokes increases the risk.

Attendance at day care centers predisposes children to otitis media. Infants younger than 1 year who attend day care have a significant risk for acquiring AOM (Vernacchio et al., 2004). The risk for ear infections is up to three times higher in those who use a pacifier (Adair, 2003).

Bottle-feeding contributes to ear infection because of the position of the infant during feeding. Reflux of formula into the eustachian tube from the nasopharynx occurs when the infant swallows while supine. Breastfeeding offers some protection from ear infection by providing maternal antibodies and by decreasing the incidence of allergy; also, the more upright position of the infant while nursing is protective against ear infection (Bowd, 2005).

Incidence

The incidence of otitis media peaks between ages 6 months and 6 years, with most episodes occurring in children younger than 3 years. Most initial episodes occur at about age 6 months, when maternal antibody levels decline. Early onset of AOM (during infancy) increases the risk for recurrent episodes (Pettigrew et al., 2004).

By the end of the third year of life, 50% to 70% of all children have had at least one episode of AOM. Most children younger than 5 years have two or three episodes of otitis media each year. Boys have a slightly higher incidence of otitis media than girls. American Indian and Eskimo children, especially infants, have higher otitis media–associated outpatient and hospitalization rates than those for the general U.S. population of children (Bowd, 2005). The incidence of otitis media is highest in winter and spring and lowest in the summer months.

Manifestations

AOM is characterized by the following:

- Otalgia (earache); infants may pull their ears or roll their heads.
- A bulging, opaque tympanic membrane that usually looks red, with decreased mobility; diffuse light reflex; and obscured landmarks (Fig. 21-2).
- Drainage, usually yellowish green, purulent, and foul-smelling (indicates perforation of the tympanic membrane).

These signs and symptoms might also be accompanied by irritability, sleep disturbances, persistent crying in infants, fever, vomiting, anorexia, or diarrhea (especially in infants).

Otitis media with effusion (OME) differs from AOM in that there are no signs of acute infection. The tympanic membrane appears retracted and either dull gray or yellow, and an air-fluid level or air bubbles may be visible through the tympanic membrane. The mobility of the tympanic membrane is decreased, and landmarks are distorted. Associated signs and symptoms can be subtle and can include the following:

- Tinnitus, popping sounds.

PATHOPHYSIOLOGY

OTITIS MEDIA

The immature anatomy of the child's middle ear and eustachian tube predisposes infants and toddlers to otitis media. When the eustachian tube is obstructed, as frequently occurs with enlarged adenoids or mucosal edema from an upper respiratory tract infection, effective drainage and ventilation of the middle ear cannot occur. Air that is normally present in the middle ear is absorbed by the blood, causing a vacuum or negative pressure in the middle ear. Fluid (effusion) accumulates within the middle ear space, creating a medium for bacterial growth. After an upper respiratory tract infection, pathogens travel from the nasopharynx to the eustachian tube. In the presence of effusion, negative pressure in the middle ear draws mucus through the eustachian tube whenever the child cries, yawns, or sucks forcefully on a nipple. Purulent fluid accumulates in the middle ear space, causing the pressure and pain of acute otitis media.

If the eustachian tube remains nonfunctional for a prolonged period, the fluid within the middle ear becomes thick and dark (glue ear). Mild temporary conductive hearing loss (see Chapter 31) often occurs in otitis media with effusion because of the decreased mobility of the ossicles and the tympanic membrane. Permanent conductive hearing loss can result from repeated episodes of otitis media and may interfere with the development of language and cognitive skills. Chronic otitis media with effusion is the most common cause of hearing loss in children.

Complications of otitis media include conductive hearing loss and sensorineural hearing loss. The infection of acute otitis media can spread to surrounding tissues, causing mastoiditis or intracranial complications such as meningitis or brain abscess. Inflammation and pressure from otitis media may result in *tympanosclerosis* (scarring of the tympanic membrane), perforation of the tympanic membrane, and *cholesteatoma* (pus and debris in the middle ear).

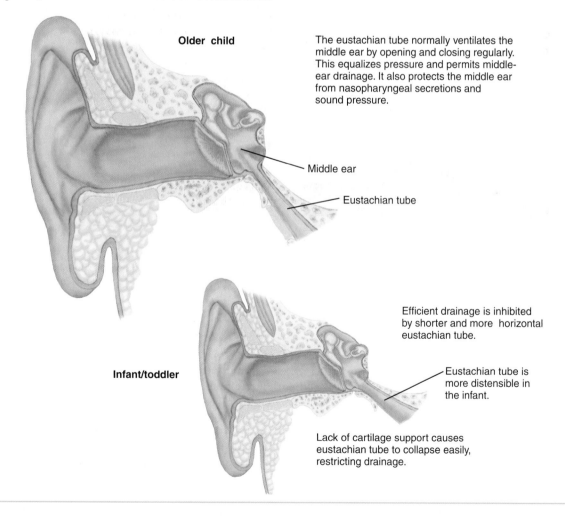

Older child

The eustachian tube normally ventilates the middle ear by opening and closing regularly. This equalizes pressure and permits middle-ear drainage. It also protects the middle ear from nasopharyngeal secretions and sound pressure.

Middle ear

Eustachian tube

Efficient drainage is inhibited by shorter and more horizontal eustachian tube.

Eustachian tube is more distensible in the infant.

Infant/toddler

Lack of cartilage support causes eustachian tube to collapse easily, restricting drainage.

- Hearing loss (usually conductive) below 35 decibels, with delays in speech development possible from prolonged hearing loss; in the older child, hearing loss may manifest as behavior problems, poor school performance, disturbed sleep, irritability, and decreased responsiveness.

- Mild balance disturbances that may result in delays in motor skills.
- A flattened tracing and negative pressure on the tympanogram (a graphic representation of tympanic mobility and middle ear pressure).

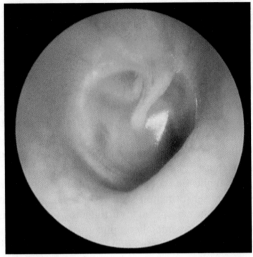

Normal right tympanic membrane and middle ear.

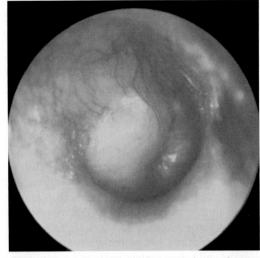

Acute otitis media: bulging right tympanic membrane.

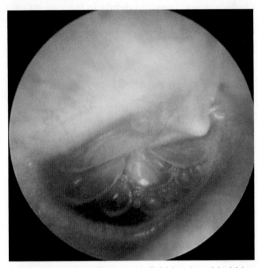

Otitis media with effusion: air-fluid level and bubbles visible through right retracted, translucent tympanic membrane.

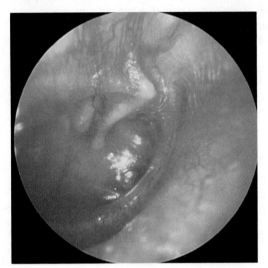

Otitis media with effusion: severely retracted, opaque right tympanic membrane.

FIG 21-2 **Appearance of tympanic membrane in otitis media compared with normal tympanic membrane.** *(From Bluestone, C. D., & Klein, J. O. [1995]. Otitis media in infants and children [2nd ed.]. Philadelphia: WB Saunders.)*

Diagnostic Evaluation

The diagnosis of otitis media is based on the history of signs and symptoms and pneumatic otoscopy. In pneumatic otoscopy, a small puff of air is blown into the ear canal through the otoscope; the examiner can discern the appearance and mobility of the tympanic membrane. In addition to pneumatic otoscopy, tympanometry can be used to confirm what was seen with the eye.

Therapeutic Management

The emergence of resistant organisms has created much discussion around the use of antibiotics to treat AOM because spontaneous resolution of the infection occurs in about 80% of children. In 2004, the American Academy of Pediatrics

(AAP) issued two policy recommendations regarding identification and management of AOM and OME in healthy children ages 2 months to 12 years (AAP, 2004; American Academy of Family Physicians, American Academy of Otolaryngology-Head and Neck Surgery, American Academy of Pediatrics Subcommittee on Otitis Media With Effusion, 2004). Recommendations include the following:

- Accurate discrimination between AOM and OME before treatment decisions are made
- Adequate pain relief for children with AOM
- Symptomatic treatment and observation for 48 to 72 hours after diagnosis as an alternative to initiating antibiotic therapy for selected children older than age 6 months with AOM

- Reassessment and treatment initiation for children with positive AOM after the 48- to 72-hour observation period
- Use of amoxicillin at a dose of 80 to 90 mg/kg/day for 5 to 10 days when treatment is indicated
- Encourage reduction of risk factors as a method for preventing AOM episodes
- Treat children with OME who are not at risk for hearing, language, or learning problems with 3 months of "watchful waiting"

Alternative antibiotics, such as erythromycin-sulfisoxazole (Pediazole), trimethoprim-sulfamethoxazole (e.g., Bactrim, Septra), cefaclor (Ceclor), cefixime (Suprax), or a macrolide (Zithromax), may be prescribed for penicillin-resistant organisms or in cases of penicillin allergy (Toltzis, Dul, O'Riordan, Toltzis, & Blumer, 2005). The pneumococcal conjugate vaccine was recently approved for use in children and should be administered to all children younger than 2 years according to the recommended schedule (see Evolve website).

The usefulness of decongestants and antihistamines in the prevention and treatment of otitis media is controversial. Although these medications are widely prescribed, new policy recommendations do not support their use (American Academy of Family Physicians, American Academy of Otolaryngology-Head and Neck Surgery, American Academy of Pediatrics Subcommittee on Otitis Media With Effusion, 2004). Acetaminophen is given to help relieve the pain and fever of AOM.

In children with persistent ear infection despite antibiotic therapy or with OME that persists for more than 3 months and is associated with hearing loss, *myringotomy* with insertion of *tympanostomy tubes* (pressure-equalizing tubes) may be performed (Rovers, Schilder, Zielhuis, & Rosenfeld, 2004). During this operation, mucoid material is removed from the middle ear and a tympanostomy tube is inserted through the tympanic membrane. A tympanostomy tube is a small polyethylene tube that is inserted into the middle ear to equalize the pressure on both sides of the tympanic membrane and to keep the ear aerated. Negative pressure in the middle ear is relieved, allowing the middle ear mucosa to return to normal and growth of the eustachian tube to occur. The tube usually falls out spontaneously in 6 to 12 months. This period may provide enough time for the effusion process to resolve, but some children need repeated insertions of tympanostomy tubes because of persistent eustachian tube dysfunction. Tympanostomy tubes are inserted with the child under general anesthesia, usually in an outpatient surgery setting.

NURSING CARE

The Child With Otitis Media

Assessment

Ask the parent whether the child has had a recent upper respiratory tract infection or previous ear infections. Assess the child for fever and pain. Because signs of ear infection may be subtle in infants, the nurse should assess not only for obvious signs of ear pain, such as head rolling and pulling at the ear, but also for nonspecific findings, such as irritability, diarrhea, or decreased appetite. Older children may complain of pain or a feeling of fullness in the affected ear. The nurse examines the ear with a pneumatic otoscope, noting the color, mobility, and translucency of the tympanic membrane and the appearance of the external canal. The tympanic membrane should be inspected carefully for signs of perforation. The nurse obtains a culture of any drainage and notes the color, consistency, and odor. Hearing and language development should be assessed.

Nursing Diagnosis and Planning

The nursing diagnoses and expected outcomes that may be appropriate for the family and infant or child with otitis media are as follow:

- Acute Pain related to inflammation and pressure in the middle ear.

  Expected Outcomes: The child will be free of pain, as evidenced by sleeping through the night, not pulling at the ears, and crying less. The child's tympanic membranes will appear shiny and pearl-gray, with normal landmarks, a visible light reflex, and normal mobility on tympanography.

- Deficient Knowledge related to incomplete understanding of the disease process and treatment regimen.

  Expected Outcomes: The parents will demonstrate (1) methods of feeding the infant that decrease the risk for otitis media, (2) how to keep the child's ears dry if tympanostomy tubes are in place, and (3) ways to follow the treatment regimen, including administering the entire course of antibiotics.

- Risk for Imbalanced Body Temperature related to inflammation.

  Expected Outcome: The child will display a normal body temperature.

- Risk for Deficient Fluid Volume related to elevated temperature and decreased intake.

  Expected Outcomes: The child will have moist mucous membranes, good skin turgor, and appropriate intake and output for age.

Interventions

Teach the parents the importance of giving prescribed antibiotics on time and for the prescribed number of days. Because the child usually feels much better after a few days of medication, parents may believe that the antibiotics are no longer necessary and stop giving them. Increase adherence by giving written and oral instructions for administering medications. Providing a medication record form on which to record doses taken and a calibrated measuring device for liquid medications is also helpful.

The nurse also advises the parents to discard any unused antibiotic rather than save it and not to give the child an antibiotic without consulting the physician first.

Acetaminophen can be given to relieve discomfort. The child's fluid intake should be increased if fever is present. Advise the parents to notify the physician if the child's condition has not improved after 48 hours of observation without antibiotics, after 48 hours of antibiotic treatment without improvement in symptoms, or if there is drainage from the affected ear. If a follow-up visit is recommended, emphasize the importance of keeping the appointment.

The nurse can enhance medication adherence through specific teaching about administration of antibiotics. For example, the nurse might say, "After a few days, your child may seem to be well and show no signs of the ear infection. If you stop giving the antibiotic at that time, some of the germs that caused the otitis media might still be alive and your child can have a relapse."

If the child is undergoing myringotomy with insertion of tympanostomy tubes, the nurse should prepare the child and parents as for any outpatient surgical procedure. Explain the procedure in clear terms and answer questions simply and honestly.

Postoperatively, the child is monitored for ear drainage. A small amount of reddish drainage is normal for the first few days after surgery, but the parents should report any heavier bleeding or bleeding that occurs after 3 days. The parents should also be instructed to report any fever or increased pain. The child should avoid blowing the nose for 7 to 10 days.

Most physicians prefer that the child's ears be kept dry if tubes are in place, but some feel that a small amount of water in the ears is not harmful. Bath and lake water are potential sources of bacterial contamination, however, and chlorinated swimming pool water can be irritating to tympanic membranes with tubes. The usual recommendation is to place ear plugs or cotton balls covered with petroleum jelly in the ears during baths and shampoos. Swimming is allowed only with ear plugs and the physician's approval. Diving and swimming deep under water are prohibited. The size and appearance of the tympanostomy tubes should be described to the parents, and they should be reassured that if the tubes fall out it is not an emergency but that the physician should be notified.

Otitis media is usually a chronic problem, with frequent recurrences of infection and effusion. The nurse should teach the parents the early signs of ear infection and the importance of seeking care if these signs should occur. Because hearing impairment from middle ear effusion can be very difficult for parents to detect, the child with chronic otitis media should undergo periodic hearing evaluations.

The nurse should teach parents methods to decrease the risk for recurrent otitis media, such as breastfeeding during infancy, discontinuing bottle-feeding as soon as possible, feeding the infant in an upright position, and refraining from giving a bottle to the infant in bed. Parents should be told not to smoke in the child's presence because passive smoking increases the incidence of otitis media.

Evaluation

- Is the child sleeping an appropriate amount of time for age with decreased episodes of crying or pulling at ears?
- Have otoscopic findings returned to normal?

- Did the parents complete the treatment regimen by giving the entire dose of the prescribed antibiotic, and are they able to demonstrate appropriate feeding methods?
- Were follow-up appointments kept to determine the resolution of the otitis media?
- Is the child afebrile?
- Does the child appear well hydrated with moist mucous membranes and good skin turgor?

PHARYNGITIS AND TONSILLITIS

Pharyngitis, inflammation of the pharynx and surrounding lymphoid tissue, can be viral or bacterial in origin. Although pharyngitis is a self-limiting and relatively minor disorder, streptococcal infections can have serious complications—among them, rheumatic fever and acute glomerular nephritis.

Tonsillitis is the term commonly used to describe inflammation and infection of the two palatine tonsils. *Adenoiditis* refers to infection and inflammation of the pharyngeal tonsils, or adenoids, which are located above the palatine tonsils on the posterior wall of the nasopharynx. The purpose of these lymphoid tissues is to filter and protect the respiratory and digestive tracts from invasion by pathogens, but often the tonsils become a site for infection.

Etiology

Pharyngitis can be caused by adenoviruses, parainfluenza virus, influenza virus, coxsackieviruses, respiratory syncytial virus, *Mycoplasma pneumoniae*, *Streptococcus pyogenes*, or *Chlamydia pneumoniae* (Esposito et al., 2004). Streptococcal pharyngitis is rare before age 3 years. Streptococcal infection is spread by close droplet transmission. Tonsillitis, like pharyngitis, may be bacterial or viral in origin. The most common bacterial agent is group A beta-hemolytic *Streptococcus*.

Incidence

The incidence of pharyngitis and tonsillitis peaks between ages 4 and 7 years, when most children begin preschool and elementary school and have increased exposure to microorganisms. Group A beta-hemolytic streptococcal infection

---

PATHOPHYSIOLOGY

PHARYNGITIS

Pharyngitis often accompanies the common cold. Tonsillitis is usually present with pharyngitis. Infection and inflammation of the tonsils cause them to enlarge. The palatine tonsils may meet in the midline (i.e., kissing tonsils) and cause difficulty swallowing and breathing. If adenoids enlarge, they can obstruct the eustachian tubes, resulting in otitis media and hearing impairment. Hypertrophy of the adenoids can also block the passageway between the nose and the throat, causing mouth breathing or obstructive sleep apnea.

occurs most frequently in the winter and is spread more readily in crowded living situations. The incidence of tonsillitis decreases during middle childhood as the lymphoid tissue undergoes normal shrinkage.

Manifestations

Signs and symptoms differ between viral and bacterial pharyngitis (Table 21-1). *The only reliable means of determining whether a case of pharyngitis is viral or bacterial in origin is with a throat culture.* Not all children with pharyngitis complain of a sore throat, particularly if they are of preschool age. Instead, the child may complain of a stomachache or simply refuse to eat. The child with tonsillitis demonstrates the following:

* Sore throat, which may be persistent or recurrent
* Tonsils enlarged and bright red; may be covered with white exudate or cryptic plugs
* Difficulty swallowing
* Mouth breathing and an unpleasant mouth odor
* Enlarged adenoids, which may cause a nasal quality of speech, mouth breathing, hearing difficulty, otitis media, snoring, or obstructive sleep apnea

Older children and adolescents can have a *peritonsillar abscess* associated with pharyngitis or tonsillitis. Peritonsillar abscess usually is unilateral, with the enlarged tonsil displacing the uvula to the opposite side. The child might refuse to talk or swallow because of severe pain that often radiates to the ear. There is a risk for airway obstruction and dehydration.

Diagnostic Evaluation

Rapid streptococcal antigen tests ("rapid strep test") can accurately screen for group A beta-hemolytic streptococcal infection, but because rapid strep tests have an approximately 20% incidence of false-negative results, if the child's symptoms suggest a streptococcal infection, culture of a throat specimen obtained by swab should be done simultaneously (Gerber & Shulman, 2004). Because approximately 10% of children carry group A beta-hemolytic streptococci in their throats, a positive throat culture is not proof of active infection.

Therapeutic Management

During the acute phase of pharyngitis or tonsillitis, treatment is symptomatic, focusing on pain relief and rest. Acetaminophen or ibuprofen is used for pain; older children may find gargling with warm saline solution comforting. Cool, bland liquids are tolerated best because of the discomfort caused by swallowing solids or irritating liquids.

Antibiotics should be restricted to those children who test positive on antigen detection tests or cultures. Streptococcal pharyngitis is most commonly treated orally with penicillin given two or three times daily for 10 days. Recent studies have shown that shorter courses of antibiotics (amoxicillin, cephalosporins, azithromycin) were as effective or more effective than the traditional 10-day penicillin therapy because of superior compliance and adherence, lower incidence of side effects, improved patient/parent satisfaction, and lower drug costs (Low, Pichichero, & Schaad, 2004; Cohen, 2004; Casey & Pichichero, 2004). Erythromycin may be used in children who are allergic to penicillin. A single intramuscular dose of procaine penicillin and benzathine penicillin G might be considered in children for whom adherence is expected to be a problem. Children given penicillin therapy are noninfectious to others 24 hours after therapy is initiated.

Surgical removal of the tonsils, or tonsillectomy, is controversial. Although some physicians think that a tonsillectomy is warranted in cases of recurrent tonsillitis, the prevailing attitude is more conservative, and the procedure is generally reserved for cases of upper airway obstruction, peritonsillar abscess, obstructive sleep apnea, or other serious problems. Electrosurgical tonsillectomy is a newer technique that uses electromagnetic radiation to generate heat within tissue for cutting and coagulation. This technique may reduce the risk for bleeding and produce less patient discomfort than traditional surgical procedures (Isaacson, 2004). Tonsillectomy is generally not performed in children younger than 3 years because of the tendency for remaining tonsillar tissues to hypertrophy. Contraindications to tonsillectomy include active infection and cleft palate (see Chapter 19). Surgical removal of the tonsils while they are infected can result in spread of the infecting organism and sepsis. In children with cleft palate, the tonsils help prevent air escape during

TABLE 21-1 Comparison of Viral and Bacterial Pharyngitis	
Viral Pharyngitis	**Bacterial Pharyngitis**
Gradual onset	Abrupt onset (may be gradual in children <2 yr old)
Sore throat (reaches a peak on the second or third day)	Sore throat (usually severe)
Erythema and inflammation of the pharynx and tonsils (may be slight), vesicles or ulcers on tonsils	Erythema and inflammation of the pharynx and tonsils
Fever (usually low grade but may be high)	Fever (usually high, 39.4° C to 40° C [103° F to 104° F], but may be moderate), begins early in illness and usually lasts 1-4 days
Hoarseness, cough, rhinitis, conjunctivitis, malaise, anorexia (early)	Abdominal pain, vomiting, headache
Cervical lymph nodes may be enlarged and tender	Cervical lymph nodes may be enlarged and tender
Usually lasts 3-4 days	Usually lasts 3-5 days

speech. Adenoidectomy alone may be performed in cases of recurrent otitis media caused by eustachian tube obstruction or for persistent nasal or airway obstruction.

Many parents believe that a tonsillectomy will solve their child's problems of frequent sore throats, mouth breathing, and poor weight gain. There is no evidence that a tonsillectomy reduces the incidence of recurrent pharyngitis. The nurse should be prepared to discuss the current treatment philosophy with parents and address their concerns. If tonsillectomy is chosen as the method of treatment, the procedure is often done in a day surgery setting.

Nursing Considerations

Assessment of the child with pharyngitis or tonsillitis includes inspecting the pharynx for erythema, exudate, or petechiae. The skin should be inspected for rash and color changes. Some children with streptococcal pharyngitis have a pink, sandpaper-like rash on the trunk (see Chapter 16). The child is questioned about the onset and location of throat, ear, or abdominal pain. The parent of a preverbal child may report that the child refuses to eat or begins to cry during feedings. The nurse also assesses the child's temperature and respiratory status and asks the older child or parent about the onset of symptoms and any known contact with streptococcal infection in the school or family. Also ask whether the child has been taking any antibiotics at home because antibiotics will interfere with the results of the throat culture.

Measures to relieve throat discomfort include administering acetaminophen, warm salt water gargles (¼ teaspoon of salt per 8-oz glass of water), and warm or cool compresses applied to the neck. Recent studies demonstrate pain relief with one dose of oral steroids (Olympia, Khine, & Avner, 2005). The child should not be forced to eat. Offer cool, bland liquids to prevent dehydration. Soft foods such as gelatin, soup, mashed potatoes, puddings, Cream of Wheat, and flavored ice pops appeal to children the best. Bed rest is advisable while the child has a fever. The nurse should advise the parent to call the health care provider if the child has difficulty breathing or increased difficulty swallowing or if the fever has lasted more than 3 days. If a fever, sore throat, or headache develops in any family members, they should have a throat culture. Instruct the parents that leftover antibiotics from siblings or friends should never be used.

Moist mucous membranes and adequate urine output are signs of proper fluid balance. At the end of treatment, the child should be free of signs of infection and show no signs of complications of the disease.

NURSING CARE

The Child Undergoing a Tonsillectomy

Assessment: Preoperative Period

A complete history is taken, with special attention given to allergy symptoms, difficulty swallowing, or airway obstruction. The child is assessed for signs of active infection (fever, elevated white blood cell [WBC] count) and redness and

---

CRITICAL TO REMEMBER
Caring for the Child Who Has Had a Tonsillectomy

Monitoring the child for postoperative bleeding is most important. Because the operative site is not as readily visible as other sites, the nurse needs to look for the following:
- Excessive swallowing
- Elevated pulse; decreasing blood pressure
- Signs of fresh bleeding in the back of the throat
- Vomiting bright-red blood
- Restlessness that does not seem to be associated with pain

---

exudate of the throat. The child should be questioned about the presence of pain in the throat or ears. Because the tonsillar area is so vascular, any bleeding history must be recorded and communicated to the primary physician.

Laboratory results (prothrombin time, partial thromboplastin time, platelet count, hemoglobin, hematocrit, urinalysis) are reviewed, and the child should be checked for loose teeth to decrease the risk for aspiration during surgery.

Nursing Diagnosis and Planning: Preoperative Period

The nursing diagnoses and expected outcomes that may be appropriate for the child undergoing a tonsillectomy and the child's family are as follow:
- Anxiety related to surgery.
  Expected Outcome: The child and parents will exhibit a decreased level of anxiety, as evidenced by relaxed body posture and involvement in play activities.
- Deficient Knowledge related to surgery and procedures.
  Expected Outcome: The child and parents will restate preoperative teaching.

Interventions: Preoperative Period

The nurse reassures the child that talking will not be a problem after surgery. Emphasize to the child that it is important to drink liquids after surgery, although the child's throat will be sore (see also Chapter 18). Teach the child's family about postoperative pain assessment and appropriate analgesia administration because many parents undermedicate their children. Undermedication can interfere with optimal postoperative recovery.

Evaluation: Preoperative Period

- Does the child demonstrate relaxed body posture and the ability to engage in play while waiting for surgery?
- Can the parents describe what to expect during the postoperative period?

Assessment: Postoperative Period

Immediately after surgery, the child should be assessed for bleeding and ability to swallow secretions. Postoperative hemorrhage is the most serious and life-threatening complication of tonsillectomy (Windfuhr, Chen, & Remmert,

2005). If bleeding occurs, the child is returned to surgery for recauterization. The rate and quality of respirations and breath sounds should be assessed. Vital signs, including blood pressure, should be monitored frequently until discharge. Suction equipment should be available, but do not suction unless there is airway obstruction. The child is assessed for bleeding (frequent swallowing; restlessness; a fast, thready pulse; or vomiting bright red blood). When visually assessing the site for clots or bleeding, use a flashlight for illumination and avoid using a tongue depressor if at all possible. If a tongue depressor is necessary, use a sterile tongue depressor and keep it as forward in the mouth as possible.

Nursing Diagnosis and Planning: Postoperative Period

The nursing diagnoses and expected outcomes that may be appropriate for the child who has undergone a tonsillectomy and the child's family are as follow:

- Risk for Injury (hemorrhage) related to surgery.

  Expected Outcome: The child will experience minimal postoperative bleeding, as evidenced by vital signs within normal limits and absence of excessive swallowing, bright red vomitus, or restlessness.

- Ineffective Airway Clearance related to throat discomfort.

  Expected Outcome: The child will maintain a clear airway without jeopardizing the operative site.

- Acute Pain related to surgical removal of tonsils.

  Expected Outcomes: The child will describe relief from pain and will be able to rest.

- Risk for Deficient Fluid Volume related to difficulty swallowing and nothing-by-mouth (NPO) status before surgery.

  Expected Outcomes: The child will have adequate fluid intake for age and minimal fluid loss.

- Deficient Knowledge related to home care.

  Expected Outcome: The parents will describe how to care for their child at home.

Interventions: Postoperative

The child should be placed in a prone or side-lying position to facilitate drainage. Although not all clinicians are in agreement, straws and forks may be withheld to prevent trauma to the surgical site. If bleeding occurs, the child is turned to the side and the physician notified.

Vomiting of old blood ("coffee grounds" emesis) is common. Antiemetics are given as ordered to decrease throat pain caused by retching. If vomiting occurs, keep the child on NPO status for 30 minutes and then resume clear liquids.

Nonaspirin analgesics (e.g., acetaminophen) are given as ordered. In some instances, the surgeon prescribes acetaminophen with codeine liquid to provide adequate analgesia (avoid administering oral medications in suspension that are colored red because they can be confused with blood in vomitus). Adequate analgesia increases fluid intake. It is common to prescribe the analgesic every 4 hours for the first 24 hours because throat discomfort is expected. An ice collar can be applied for comfort.

Provide clear, cool liquids when the child is fully awake. Avoid citrus drinks, carbonated drinks, and extremely hot or cold liquids because they may irritate the throat. Milk and milk products (puddings, ice cream) can coat the throat, causing a need to clear the throat and thus increasing the risk for bleeding. Adequate fluid intake promotes healing and maintains hydration. The nurse teaches the parents the principles of home management and ensures that the child is keeping fluids down before discharging the child from the surgical unit. Be sure to tell the parent to monitor the child for postoperative bleeding both within the first 24 hours and again 7 to 10 days after surgery (Box 21-2).

BOX 21-2 | **PARENTS WANT TO KNOW** About Caring for a Child After a Tonsillectomy

- Encourage your child to participate only in quiet activities for 1 week after surgery.
- Encourage abundant liquid intake. Avoid citrus juices, which irritate the throat, for 10 days.
- Avoid red liquids, which will give the appearance of blood if your child vomits.
- Add full liquids (cream soups, gelatin, puddings, other soups) on the second day and soft foods (mashed potatoes, soft cereals, eggs) as your child tolerates them. Avoid rough or scratchy foods (bacon, chips, popcorn), citrus foods, or spicy foods for 3 weeks.
- Encourage your child to chew and swallow because this exercises pharyngeal muscles and promotes healing.
- Do not give your child any straws, forks, or sharp pointed toys that could be put in the mouth.
- Use acetaminophen for pain relief; your child may have a prescription for acetaminophen with codeine for sore throat. Do not use aspirin or any medicine containing aspirin because it might affect the clotting time of the blood.

- Pain should not persist past the first week. Notify your physician if pain persists.
- Discourage your child from coughing, clearing the throat, or gargling.
- Bad mouth odor is normal and may be relieved by drinking more liquids.
- Earache and slight fever are common.
- Call your physician for any bleeding, persistent earache, or fever greater than 101° F (38.3° C).
- Bleeding caused by tissue sloughing during the healing process can occur 7 to 10 days after surgery. Such bleeding requires immediate medical attention.
- To protect your child from catching a cold, keep the child away from crowds for 2 weeks.
- Your child may return to school when directed by the physician, usually in about 10 days.
- Bring your child for a follow-up appointment in 1 to 2 weeks.

Evaluation: Postoperative

- Does the child have minimal bleeding, nausea, and vomiting, and are vital signs within normal limits?
- Is the child taking clear liquids and avoiding liquids that irritate the throat?
- Are the child's complaints of pain and irritability minimal?
- Can the parents describe home care measures?

CRITICAL THINKING EXERCISE 21-1

Discharge teaching following a tonsillectomy should include pain management. Inadequate pain relief at home is a major nursing concern.
1. What factors may contribute to this occurring?
2. What effects might inadequate pain relief have on the child?

LARYNGOMALACIA (CONGENITAL LARYNGEAL STRIDOR)

Flaccidity of the epiglottis and supraglottic aperture and weakness of the airway walls contribute to laryngomalacia, the most common cause of inspiratory stridor in the neonatal period (Midulla et al., 2004). Laryngomalacia may be caused by immature neuromuscular development in the airway.

Manifestations

Noisy, crowing inspiratory respiratory sounds (stridor) are present, with or without retractions. The infant usually does not become cyanotic despite the stridor. Stridor is usually present at birth but may begin as late as age 2 months. Symptoms increase when the infant is supine or when the infant is crying. The diagnosis is based on a thorough history and on findings on direct laryngoscopy.

Therapeutic Management

Symptoms usually resolve without treatment by age 18 to 24 months. In rare instances, endotracheal intubation or tracheostomy may be required.

Nursing Considerations

The nurse observes the neonate for stridor, retractions, and dyspnea, noting any signs of acute respiratory distress. Because some infants have feeding problems, the infant should be observed for feeding difficulties. The infant's respiratory status is assessed, and findings are recorded every 2 hours and as needed. Obstruction increases during crying when the child has a respiratory infection, and stridor increases when the child is supine with the neck flexed. Positioning with the neck hyperextended improves the child's breathing. A respiratory tract infection might place undue stress on the infant's system.

As part of discharge teaching, parents are taught the signs of respiratory distress so that they can monitor for changes that might indicate respiratory tract infection. If the bottle-fed infant has feeding difficulties, the parents can try using a smaller nipple. Smaller, more frequent feedings are sometimes better tolerated by infants with respiratory difficulties. Reassure the parents that the condition usually resolves by the time the child is 2 years old. The ability of parents to comfortably care for their child indicates the effectiveness of the discharge teaching.

CROUP

Croup refers to a group of conditions characterized by inspiratory stridor, a harsh (brassy or croupy) cough, hoarseness, and varying degrees of respiratory distress (Table 21-2). The major types of croup are acute spasmodic croup, laryngotracheobronchitis, bacterial tracheitis, and epiglottitis. Although epiglottitis is a type of croup, it is discussed separately because it is a bacterial infection with unique symptoms and treatment.

Etiology and Incidence

Parainfluenza viruses cause most cases of viral croup. The cause of acute spasmodic croup is unknown.

Laryngotracheobronchitis, the most common form of croup, usually affects infants and toddlers, and it is a common cause of airway obstruction in children ages 6 months to 6 years. The incidence of croup is higher in boys than in girls, and the disease occurs more often during the winter than in other seasons.

Acute spasmodic croup occurs most often in children ages 1 to 3 years. Spasmodic croup occurs more often in anxious and excitable children. There seems to be hereditary predisposition to spasmodic croup.

Bacterial tracheitis is less common than laryngotracheobronchitis and acute spasmodic croup. It progresses from an upper respiratory tract infection and may be confused with laryngotracheobronchitis because of similar manifestations. Treatment for laryngotracheobronchitis is not effective if the child has bacterial tracheitis.

The following discussion focuses on acute spasmodic croup and laryngotracheobronchitis, the most common types of croup leading to hospitalization.

Manifestations

Croup often begins at night and may be preceded by several days of symptoms of upper respiratory tract infection. The child with laryngotracheobronchitis may have a gradual onset and a fever along with other signs and symptoms; occasionally the fever is as high as 40° C (104° F). Children with spasmodic croup do not have a fever. Other manifestations include the following:

- The sudden onset of a harsh, metallic barky cough; sore throat; inspiratory stridor; and hoarseness
- The use of accessory muscles (substernal, intercostal, suprasternal retractions) to breathe
- Frightened appearance
- Agitation
- Cyanosis

TABLE 21-2	Comparison of Types of Croup			
	Acute Spasmodic Laryngitis (Spasmodic Croup)	**Acute Laryngo-tracheobronchitis (LTB)**	**Acute Epiglottitis**	**Acute Tracheitis**
Age usually affected	1-3 yr	3 mo–3 yr	3-7 yr	1 mo–6 yr
Location of swelling and inflammation	Subglottic (below vocal cords)	Vocal cords, subglottic, and tissue below vocal cords, including bronchi	Supraglottic (above vocal cords)	Mucosa of upper trachea
Cause	Viral, emotional, or genetic predisposition	Usually viral but may be bacterial	Bacterial (usually Hib)	*Staphylococcus* (most common)
Assessment	Sudden onset, usually at night Child awakens with harsh cough, inspiratory stridor, dyspnea, and hoarseness	Gradual onset, usually at night Child awakens with harsh cough and inspiratory stridor	Sudden onset, which may rapidly progress to complete airway obstruction and death Sore throat, dyspnea, high fever	Progresses from upper respiratory infection (1-2 d) High fever Stridor Croupy cough Purulent secretions
Treatment	Humidity Increased fluids May treat at home	Humidity Racemic epinephrine IV fluids during respiratory distress Hospitalization may be necessary	IV antibiotics Artificial airway IV fluids Emergency hospitalization	Humidified oxygen Antipyretics IV antibiotics May require intubation

Symptoms are usually worse at night and better in the day; they may recur for several nights. Croup usually lasts 3 to 4 days.

Diagnostic Evaluation

The diagnosis is made mainly from observation of clinical symptoms. Differentiation between viral croup and bacterial epiglottitis is very important because treatment differs (Hammer, 2004). However, the use of the *H. influenzae* type b (Hib) vaccine has reduced the incidence of epiglottitis. A croup score is often used to describe the severity of respiratory distress. Arterial blood gas values or pulse oximetry readings may be monitored to detect decreased PaO_2 levels.

Therapeutic Management

The goal of treatment is to maintain a patent airway. Children with acute spasmodic croup can usually be cared for at home. Treatment for acute spasmodic croup includes a calm approach and increased oral fluid intake if the child is not in respiratory distress. The benefits of providing mist, either from steam produced by hot running water in a closed bathroom or cool mist from a bedside humidifier, appear to provide more of a psychologic effect than a physiologic one. If mist is used, cool mist humidifiers are recommended rather than steam vaporizers, which pose a danger of scald burns. Taking the child out into the cool, humid night air may relieve mucosal swelling.

Crying aggravates the airway obstruction. Children who develop stridor at rest, cyanosis, severe agitation or fatigue, or moderate to severe retractions or who are unable to take oral fluids should be seen in the emergency department.

Children with laryngotracheobronchitis, usually a more severe type of croup, are more often hospitalized than are those with acute spasmodic croup. Racemic epinephrine nebulized with oxygen may be given to decrease the laryngeal edema and bronchospasm. The child must be observed closely for changes in respiratory status and should not be treated with epinephrine on an outpatient basis because the effects of epinephrine are temporary. Children who receive epinephrine should be observed in the emergency department for at least 3 hours after treatment and should not be discharged if stridor or retractions are present.

Oral or parenteral corticosteroid therapy may be used in children with croup to reduce inflammatory edema and to prevent destruction of ciliated epithelium (Leung, Kellner, & Johnson, 2004). Nebulized budesonide may also be used (Cetinkaya, Tufekci, & Kutluk, 2004). Antibiotics are not indicated unless a bacterial infection is present. Acetaminophen is given to reduce fever.

The benefits of mist tent or hood therapy remain controversial, particularly if placing the child in a tent increases agitation. Cool mist in the room may be more effective. Intravenous (IV) fluids are given until respiratory distress subsides and the child can take adequate fluids by mouth. Sedatives are contraindicated because they depress respirations and could mask restlessness, an early sign of hypoxia.

If signs of moderate or severe hypoxia develop, the child is intubated immediately and is transferred to an intensive care unit. Usually the tube remains in place from 3 to 5 days and is removed when the child can breathe around the tube.

PATHOPHYSIOLOGY

CROUP

Croup is a viral infection of the upper airway. Although the entire upper, or nonreactive, airway is involved to some extent in all forms of croup, each type is named according to the anatomic area most severely involved. For example, laryngotracheobronchitis affects the larynx, trachea, and bronchi. In acute spasmodic croup, the larynx is the area of most severe inflammation.

In all forms of croup, mucosal inflammation and edema cause narrowing of the airway. This narrowing is more dangerous in infants and young children than in adults because of their small airway diameter and flexible larynx, which is more susceptible to spasm.

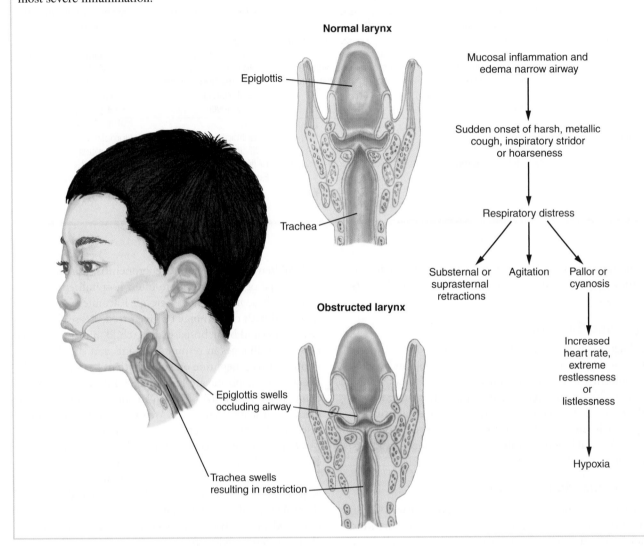

Normal larynx

Epiglottis

Trachea

Obstructed larynx

Epiglottis swells occluding airway

Trachea swells resulting in restriction

Mucosal inflammation and edema narrow airway

↓

Sudden onset of harsh, metallic cough, inspiratory stridor or hoarseness

↓

Respiratory distress

↓

Substernal or suprasternal retractions   Agitation   Pallor or cyanosis

↓

Increased heart rate, extreme restlessness or listlessness

↓

Hypoxia

NURSING CARE

The Child With Croup

Assessment

A nursing history typically reveals a recent upper respiratory tract infection. Assess the child for inspiratory stridor, barking cough, hoarseness, and increased heart rate and respiratory rate. Record any signs of respiratory distress, such as the use of accessory muscles; substernal, intercostal, and suprasternal retractions; nasal flaring; restlessness and irritability; and pallor or cyanosis. Cyanosis, increased heart rate and respiratory rate, extreme restlessness, or evidence

of fatigue or listlessness may be signs of hypoxia and should be reported to the physician immediately. The lungs should be auscultated for adventitious breath sounds or areas of decreased breath sounds. Temperature and hydration status should also be assessed.

Nursing Diagnosis and Planning

The diagnoses and expected outcomes that may be appropriate for the child with croup and the child's family are as follow:

- Ineffective Airway Clearance related to mucosal swelling and obstruction of the upper respiratory tract.

Expected Outcome: The child will breath without difficulty and have a heart rate and respiratory rate within normal limits for age.

- Risk for Deficient Fluid Volume related to inadequate oral intake and tachypnea.

Expected Outcome: The child will have adequate fluid intake for age and weight.

- Fear related to dyspnea and hospitalization.

Expected Outcome: The child will appear less fearful, as evidenced by resting quietly, crying less, and cooperating with nursing care as appropriate for age. The parents will demonstrate decreased fear, as evidenced by their ability to assist the child to deal with stressors of hospitalization and illness.

- Deficient Knowledge related to the course of croup and home care.

Expected Outcomes: The parents will have accurate knowledge of croup symptoms, state they are comfortable in home management of croup, and seek assistance appropriately if symptoms become severe.

Interventions

Facilitating Airway Clearance

The nurse monitors the child's breathing continuously for signs and symptoms of increased respiratory distress (increased respiratory rate, stridor at rest, nasal flaring, retractions, cyanosis, changes in level of consciousness or increased irritability, decreased or adventitious breath sounds, tachypnea). A child with respiratory distress should never be left alone and the physician should be notified immediately. If epiglottitis is suspected, the physician should be contacted and the throat should not be inspected because this may result in laryngospasm and airway obstruction. The nurse should administer humidified oxygen at the ordered flow rate and mist only if ordered. Monitor vital signs, pulse oximetry readings, or transcutaneous oxygen concentration hourly. There should be emergency intubation equipment (e.g., intubation tray, oxygen, suction, manual-resuscitation bag-valve-mask) closely available should the child's condition change rapidly. Aerosolized racemic epinephrine is often administered to decrease laryngeal edema and dexamethasone is given as an anti-inflammatory agent. The child should be observed for recurrence of obstruction, which may occur within a few hours after administration of racemic epinephrine.

The child should be kept as quiet as possible because crying aggravates laryngospasm and increases hypoxia. Encourage parents to stay nearby or even to climb inside the mist tent (if used) with the child if the child is frightened and refuses to stay inside the tent. If the use of a tent or hood is causing distress, treatment may be more effective if the child is held by a parent and cool mist is directed toward the child's face. Maintain a calm, quiet environment. Observe the child closely but disturb as little as possible. Support the child in an upright position with the head of the bed elevated to facilitate respiration.

Maintaining Fluid Balance

Tachypnea causes insensible water loss, and difficulty swallowing leads to decreased intake. Therefore, the nurse monitors

the child's hydration status with intake and output and urine specific gravity measurements. Check mucous membranes, skin turgor, and presence of tears. Weigh the child daily on the same scale and at same time of day. Offer the child clear, room temperature liquids as tolerated when the child no longer exhibits signs of respiratory distress. Observe the child's ability to swallow because tachypnea and laryngospasm often cause dysphagia. IV fluids are administered in the acute phase of croup because oral fluids are contraindicated in the setting of severe respiratory distress because of the risk for aspiration. The child's temperature is monitored every 4 hours and acetaminophen is administered as ordered.

Decreasing Fear

Maintain a calm, restful environment for the child and organize nursing care so as to disturb the child as little as possible and allow for periods of uninterrupted rest. Encourage parents to touch and cuddle the child because a parent's presence is important in reducing fear in infants and young children. Also, encourage parents' participation in care and explain ways that they can make their child more comfortable. Caring for a child in the hospital is exhausting to parents, and fatigue magnifies feelings of anxiety and helplessness. Therefore, provide parents with breaks as needed and assure them that their child will be cared for in their absence. Allow the child to keep a favorite toy or blanket and use developmentally appropriate communication techniques (e.g., play, puppets) when explaining treatments and procedures. Allow the child and parents to ask questions and to discuss fears and concerns because croup symptoms can be frightening and parents sometimes feel guilty for not having brought the child in for treatment sooner.

Providing Teaching

The nurse determines the parents' level of understanding of croup and previous experiences in coping with the illness. Teach the parents that once a child has had an attack, croup tends to recur. Teach the parents that maintaining a stable environmental temperature and humidity and keeping the child well hydrated may help decrease the severity of attacks. Teach that croup is a viral infection and that avoiding large groups of people and practicing good health habits to prevent infection may decrease the risk for recurrence of croup. Teach parents the signs and symptoms of respiratory distress and symptoms that should prompt a call to the physician:

- Increased difficulty breathing or seems to be getting worse
- Retractions (tugging in of the skin between, above, or below the ribs with inspiration)
- Lips turn bluish or dusky
- Breathing cool or warm mist does not improve symptoms in 20 minutes
- Inability to drink much over the past 24 hours
- Drooling or difficulty swallowing
- Fever (greater than 39.4° C [103° F])
- Seems exhausted, listless, or very agitated

The nurse reviews ways to provide a humidified environment in treating croup symptoms to help thin secretions and decrease swelling and explain the importance of

Animation: Intubation in Children

adequate hydration and nutrition. Parents are taught that acetaminophen is effective in reducing fever and will help the child feel more comfortable. Cough syrups and cold medicines are avoided because they can dry and thicken secretions.

Evaluation

- Are the child's respiratory rate and heart rate within normal limits for age and is the oxygen saturation greater than 95%?
- Does the infant have moist mucous membranes, good skin turgor, and urine output appropriate for age (see Chapter 18)?
- Does the child exhibit decreased signs of agitation or being upset (less crying) and is the parent able to comfort the child?
- Can the parents explain the appropriate treatment of croup and when medical help is needed?

EPIGLOTTITIS (SUPRAGLOTTITIS)

Epiglottitis, the acute inflammation and swelling of the epiglottis and surrounding tissue, is a life-threatening, rapidly progressive condition that may cause complete airway obstruction within a few hours of onset.

Etiology and Incidence

Epiglottitis is almost always caused by *H. influenzae*. Other organisms, such as *Staphylococcus aureus, Haemophilus parainfluenzae, S. pneumoniae,* and group A beta-hemolytic streptococci, cause the infection less frequently. Viral epiglottitis is rare.

Epiglottitis occurs most often in children ages 3 to 7 years. The incidence is about equal in boys and girls. The incidence has decreased markedly with use of the Hib vaccine (Shah, Roberson, & Jones, 2004).

Manifestations

Unlike croup, epiglottitis has an abrupt onset with rapid progression of symptoms. Often parents report that the child was put to bed well and awakened with a severe sore throat and difficulty swallowing. The child demonstrates a high

---

CRITICAL TO REMEMBER

Cardinal Signs and Symptoms of Epiglottitis

- **D**rooling
- **D**ysphagia (difficulty swallowing)
- **D**ysphonia (difficulty talking)
- **D**istressed inspiratory efforts

Do not examine or obtain material for culture from a child's throat if epiglottitis is suspected because any stimulation with a tongue depressor or culture swab could trigger complete airway obstruction.

Do not leave a child with epiglottitis unattended.

---

fever (39° C to 40° C [102.2° F to 104° F]) and appears to be in a toxic condition and very ill. The accompanying sore throat can progress to acute respiratory distress in a few hours. The child appears anxious and frightened and may be irritable or lethargic. One of the classic signs of epiglottitis is that the child insists on sitting upright, often in a tripod position (leaning forward supported on the arms), with the chin thrust out and the mouth open. Respiratory symptoms include nasal flaring; suprasternal, substernal, and intercostal retractions; pale skin color to cyanosis (depending on the degree of airway obstruction); and tachycardia. The epiglottis appears edematous and cherry red.

Diagnostic Evaluation

The most reliable diagnostic sign of epiglottitis is an edematous, cherry red epiglottis. However, examination and visual observation of the epiglottis *are contraindicated* until emergency intubation equipment and qualified personnel are available to support the child in case of sudden airway obstruction. The child's WBC count is usually elevated (20,000 to 30,000/mm^3).

Therapeutic Management

Treatment for epiglottitis should achieve a patent airway as quickly as possible. The child with epiglottitis has an edematous epiglottis, which can completely obstruct the airway at any time. Radiographs are best obtained at the bedside, where the child can be constantly monitored and emergency equipment is readily available. The danger of airway obstruction is so great that usually all invasive procedures, such as venipuncture, are postponed until the child is intubated. Once the airway is secured, the child is transferred to the intensive care unit. Oxygenation status is closely monitored with arterial blood gas values or pulse oximetry, and humidified oxygen is administered. Mechanical ventilation is sometimes instituted.

Throat and blood specimens are obtained for culture after the child is intubated. Antipyretics are given for fever. Antibiotics are administered IV until the child is extubated. Usually the child improves dramatically after 48 hours of antibiotic therapy and can be extubated at this time. The usual course of treatment is 7 to 10 days. Discharge occurs in about 3 to 7 days, and the child is sent home on a regimen of oral antibiotics.

Nursing Considerations

The nurse should continuously assess for signs of respiratory distress (stridor, nasal flaring, tachypnea, tachycardia, retractions, drooling, changes in level of consciousness, cyanosis). A sudden decrease in respiratory effort may be a sign of exhaustion and impending respiratory arrest. Arterial blood gas values and pulse oximetry findings are monitored. On pulse oximetry, the oxygen saturation should remain above 95%, with the PaO$_2$ between 80 and 100 mm Hg.

Maintenance of a patent airway is essential. The nurse should also keep the child as calm and quiet as possible. If

PATHOPHYSIOLOGY

EPIGLOTTITIS

Epiglottitis is a bacterial form of croup. The epiglottis and surrounding structures become inflamed as bacterial infection invades the soft tissue. The epiglottis becomes edematous and cherry red and may become so swollen that it completely covers the glottis and obstructs the airway. Secretions pool in the hypopharynx and larynx. As the disease rapidly progresses, swelling becomes so severe that the child is unable to swallow and begins to drool. The child's voice is muffled, and the throat is very sore. Inspiratory stridor, cough, and irritability are present. Complete airway obstruction can occur rapidly, resulting in hypoxia, acidosis, and death.

The onset of epiglottitis is usually sudden. The child may have had symptoms of a mild upper respiratory tract infection for a few days before symptoms began. Children with epiglottitis can progress from wellness to complete airway obstruction within 2 to 6 hours.

Clinical manifestations

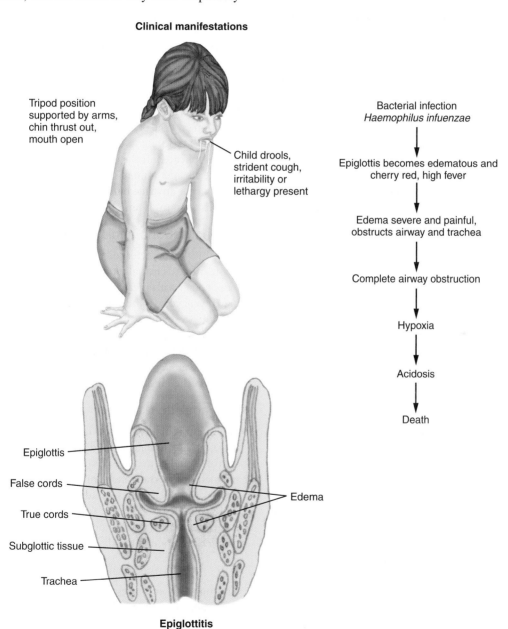

Tripod position supported by arms, chin thrust out, mouth open

Child drools, strident cough, irritability or lethargy present

Bacterial infection
Haemophilus infuenzae

↓

Epiglottis becomes edematous and cherry red, high fever

↓

Edema severe and painful, obstructs airway and trachea

↓

Complete airway obstruction

↓

Hypoxia

↓

Acidosis

↓

Death

Epiglottis
False cords
True cords
Subglottic tissue
Trachea
Edema

Epiglottitis

temperature is taken, it should be by the axillary or tympanic route rather than the oral route. The child should be supported in a position of comfort, usually sitting straight up (orthopneic); never force the child to lie down. Children who are anxious and in respiratory distress are often less fearful on their parents' laps. Parents should be encouraged to hug and comfort their child. The parents' anxiety level must be assessed and controlled because their anxiety is easily transferred to the child.

Humidified oxygen is delivered in high concentrations. Oxygen therapy is usually less upsetting if the parent holds the oxygen tubing in front of the child's face. All procedures should be explained to the parent and child clearly, calmly, and according to the child's level of understanding.

Emergency intubation equipment (oxygen, laryngoscope, endotracheal tube, suction equipment) should be immediately available in case of complete airway obstruction. Worsening of the child's condition should be reported to the physician immediately.

Antipyretics are given rectally for fever. Because of the risk for aspiration, the child is kept on NPO status and fluids are given IV. The nurse must closely monitor the ordered IV rate and the urine specific gravity and other indicators of hydration. IV antibiotics are administered as ordered.

If the child has an artificial airway, either with an endotracheal tube or a tracheostomy, the nurse must observe the child closely for respiratory distress and suction the airway as needed. The endotracheal tube must be securely taped to decrease movement of the tube and to minimize the chance of accidental extubation. Once intubated, the child needs to be restrained to prevent accidental extubation. It may be impossible to reintubate the child because of the severe swelling of the epiglottis. The endotracheal tube is usually kept in place for approximately 24 to 40 hours. After extubation, the child must be watched carefully and is usually placed in a mist tent for 24 hours before being transferred to a pediatric unit. Normal respiratory rate and rhythm and normal color serve as evaluation criteria.

Because epiglottitis progresses rapidly and acute respiratory distress is frightening, both parents and child have high anxiety levels. The nurse should care for the child calmly and efficiently and offer the family much-needed support during hospitalization. On discharge, the parents need to be taught how to administer the child's oral antibiotics. They should be reassured that epiglottitis rarely recurs. The child should be free of respiratory difficulty, resting well, and without other distress. The nurse should encourage parents of young children to have their children immunized against *H. influenzae* (see Chapter 4) to decrease the risk for contracting epiglottitis.

BRONCHITIS

Bronchitis is a disease that rarely exists by itself but occurs together with other conditions of the upper and lower respiratory tracts. It can be confused with asthma. A cough is the major sign; it usually resolves without therapy in approximately 2 weeks.

PATHOPHYSIOLOGY

BRONCHITIS

Inflammation of the trachea and major bronchi is present in bronchitis. Mucus production is increased, and the mucosa is congested. Because of nonspecific leukocytic migration, purulent secretions can occur even in the absence of a bacterial infection.

Acute bronchitis is a self-limiting disease. Chronic bronchitis in children may indicate an underlying chronic respiratory dysfunction.

Etiology and Incidence

Acute bronchitis is usually viral in origin. Rhinoviruses are the most common causative organisms. Other viruses thought to cause bronchitis include respiratory syncytial virus, influenza virus, parainfluenza virus, and adenovirus. Most bacterial infections occur secondary to a primary viral infection or some other airway problem. They may also occur as a result of foreign body aspiration. Air pollution has also been implicated in the disease.

The disorder is more common in young children and boys. It can occur anytime but is more common during the winter months than in other seasons.

Manifestations and Diagnostic Evaluation

Bronchitis is characterized by the gradual onset of rhinitis and a cough that is initially nonproductive but may change to a loose cough with increased mucus production. Auscultation may reveal coarse and fine, moist crackles and high-pitched rhonchi (resembling the wheezing of asthma). Associated symptoms include malaise, low-grade fever, and increased mucus, which may be purulent.

Chest radiographs are usually normal. The diagnosis is based on the clinical picture.

Therapeutic Management

Treatment is mainly symptomatic and includes rest, humidification, and increased fluid intake. Exposure to cigarette smoke should be avoided. Cough suppressants are not recommended unless the cough interferes with the child's ability to rest. Antihistamines should be avoided because of their drying effect on secretions. Antibiotics should be given only if a bacterial infection is confirmed by culture or if the clinical picture supports the diagnosis.

Nursing Considerations

The nurse should assess temperature, appearance of secretions, and respiratory effort every 2 to 4 hours. The child's intake should be monitored, and the nurse should observe for signs of sleep deprivation related to the persistent cough.

Advise the parents to encourage fluids by frequently offering small amounts of the child's favorite liquids and to humidify the child's room. The child should be monitored for signs of dehydration; monitoring includes taking daily weights if the child is hospitalized. Acetaminophen is administered for an elevated temperature (usually >38.3° C [101° F]). Quiet activities should be provided for diversion.

BRONCHIOLITIS

Bronchiolitis, or inflammation of the bronchioles, is a significant cause of hospitalization in infants younger than 1 year (Holman et al., 2004). Respiratory syncytial virus (RSV) is the causative agent in more than 50% of cases.

Etiology and Incidence

Infants usually acquire the disease from an older child or adult, particularly a family member or day care contact, who has a minor respiratory illness. RSV infection is easily communicable and is acquired mainly through contact with contaminated surfaces. Nosocomial outbreaks in pediatric hospitals are common. RSV can live on skin or paper for up to 1 hour and on cribs and other nonporous surfaces for up to 6 hours. Although it is not airborne, it is highly communicable. It is usually transferred by inadequately washed hands. Meticulous handwashing decreases the spread of organisms.

In addition to RSV, other causative organisms include *Mycoplasma,* parainfluenza virus, and some adenoviruses (Garofalo et al., 2005). RSV infection occurs in annual epidemics during the winter and early spring. The incidence peaks at age 6 months. By age 2 years, nearly 100% of children will have had RSV. Immunity does not occur, but the incidence and severity decrease with age.

Manifestations

A mild upper respiratory tract infection usually precedes the development of bronchiolitis. Serous nasal drainage, sneezing, low-grade fever, and anorexia are present for several days, followed by the onset of acute respiratory distress, manifested by the following signs and symptoms:

- Tachypnea—respiratory rates of 60 to 80 breaths/min
- Tachycardia—heart rate >140 beats/min
- Wheezing, crackles, or rhonchi
- Intercostal and subcostal retractions with or without nasal flaring
- Cyanosis

Feeding may be difficult because of increased respirations, which interfere with sucking and swallowing. The body temperature varies from hypothermic to as high as 41° C (105.8° F).

Diagnostic Evaluation

The clinical presentation and the age of the child suggest the diagnosis. Rapid virus identification can be performed on respiratory secretions obtained by nasal or nasopharyngeal washing (see Chapter 13). The diagnostic test is the enzyme-linked immunosorbent assay.

Chest radiographs show hyperinflation of the lungs and an increased anteroposterior chest diameter on lateral views. There are scattered areas of consolidation in some infants, a finding attributable to atelectasis caused by obstruction or inflammation of the alveoli. In some infants, the chest radiographs appear normal.

Therapeutic Management

Infants with mild bronchiolitis can be treated at home with fluids, humidification, and rest. Infants with respiratory distress are hospitalized for supportive treatment (Panitch, 2003). Cool, humidified oxygen is delivered to relieve dyspnea, hypoxemia, and insensible water loss from tachypnea.

Parenteral administration of fluids may be necessary for acutely ill infants who are dehydrated from tachypnea or poor intake. The infant should be positioned with the head and chest at a 30- to 40-degree angle and the neck slightly extended to maintain an open airway and decrease pressure on the diaphragm.

Antibiotics are not given unless there is a secondary bacterial infection. Although some health care providers routinely prescribe bronchodilators, epinephrine, or corticosteroids, randomized clinical trials have failed to demonstrate clinical efficacy in the use of these medications (Scarfone, 2005).

Ribavirin (Virazole) is an antiviral respiratory drug that appears to interfere with ribonucleic acid and deoxyribonucleic acid (DNA) synthesis, inhibiting viral replication. It is used primarily in hospitalized children with severe RSV and in high-risk children (those with congenital heart disease, chronic respiratory disease, prematurity, or immunodeficiency). Administration is by hood, face mask, or oxygen tent over 18 to 20 hours per day for a minimum of 3 days and a maximum of 7 days. The drug is most effective if it is administered within the first 3 days of the beginning of the disease. It is very expensive and has proved to be teratogenic in some animal studies, so pregnant health care workers or visitors should not be in the room where ribavirin is being delivered. Some caregivers have reported headaches, burning nasal passages and eyes, and crystallized soft contact lenses. The use of ribavirin is controversial because a majority of studies have demonstrated neither dramatic nor cost-effective results (Fitzgerald & Kilham, 2004).

RSV prevention is of the utmost importance to reduce hospitalizations for young, at-risk infants and children. IV RSV immune globulin (RSV-IG, RespiGam) or intramuscular RSV monoclonal antibody (Synagis) administered monthly throughout the RSV season has significantly reduced the hospitalization risk for premature infants (<35 weeks' gestation) younger than 6 months and children younger than 24 months with chronic lung disease (Domachowske & Rosenberg, 2005). Prophylaxis is done on an outpatient basis. The measles, mumps, rubella and varicella vaccines must be postponed for 9 to 10 months after the last dose of RSV-IG.

NURSING CARE

The Child With Bronchiolitis

Assessment

The nurse should assess the infant for signs and symptoms of respiratory distress (tachypnea, dyspnea, retractions, cyanosis, nasal flaring) every 1 to 2 hours during the

PATHOPHYSIOLOGY

BRONCHIOLITIS

In bronchiolitis, edema and the accumulation of mucus and cellular debris cause obstruction of the bronchioles. Infants' bronchioles are very small and can become obstructed quickly. Airway resistance is increased during the inspiratory and expiratory phases of respiration because of the small air passages. Hyperinflation of the lungs results from air trapping because the bronchioles constrict during expiration. Atelectasis can occur if obstruction becomes complete and trapped air is absorbed. Normal gas exchange is impaired, and the infant becomes hypoxic. Some infants have mild respiratory alkalosis; more frequently, metabolic acidosis is observed.

The child with bronchiolitis is most acutely ill during the first 48 to 72 hours after the onset of the disease. Improvement usually occurs in a few days. Mortality is less than 1%, and hospitalization is rare.* Some infants' lung function studies remain abnormal for months.

*Panitch, H. B. (2003). Respiratory syncytial virus bronchiolitis: Supportive care and therapies designed to overcome airway obstruction. *Pediatric Infectious Disease Journal, 22(Suppl. 2),* S83-S87.

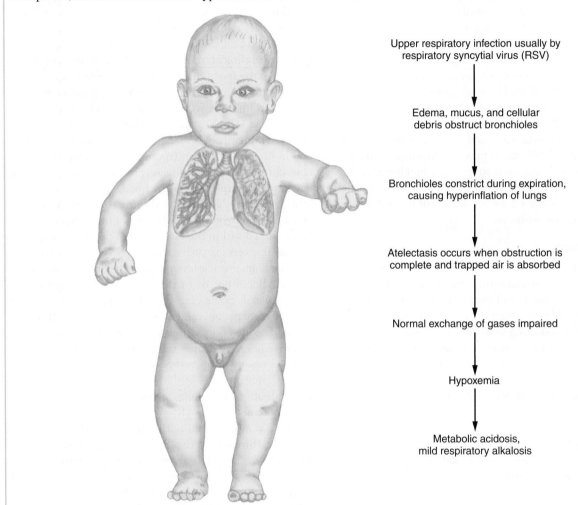

Upper respiratory infection usually by respiratory syncytial virus (RSV)

↓

Edema, mucus, and cellular debris obstruct bronchioles

↓

Bronchioles constrict during expiration, causing hyperinflation of lungs

↓

Atelectasis occurs when obstruction is complete and trapped air is absorbed

↓

Normal exchange of gases impaired

↓

Hypoxemia

↓

Metabolic acidosis, mild respiratory alkalosis

acute phase and as needed if changes occur. Auscultate the lungs for breath sounds. Apnea monitoring and cardiorespiratory monitoring are indicated for the infant with acute disease. Make sure that the alarms on the cardiorespiratory monitor are appropriately set and document any periods of apnea.

Assess the infant for signs of dehydration (dry mucous membranes, decreased urine output, sunken fontanel, weight loss) and monitor body temperature. The temperature in oxygen tents should be monitored, as well as the moisture in the tent, in the tubing, and on the bedding and infant. The infant should be placed in a room near the nurses' station for easy observation.

Assess the family's understanding of the disease and family members' level of anxiety. Observe the infant for signs of anxiety, restlessness, or irritability.

Isolate the infant with RSV infection in a single room or place the infant in a room with other RSV-infected infants.

Meticulous handwashing is imperative. Nurses caring for these infants should not care for other high-risk children. Maintaining contact precautions (i.e., wearing a gown and gloves) reduces nosocomial transmission of RSV.

Nursing Diagnosis and Planning

The diagnoses and expected outcomes that may be appropriate for the infant with bronchiolitis and the infant's family are as follow:

- Impaired Gas Exchange related to airway edema and increased mucus.

  Expected Outcome: The infant will have increased gas exchange, as evidenced by oxygen saturation above 95% on room air.

- Ineffective Airway Clearance related to increased secretions.

  Expected Outcome: The infant will exhibit clear breath sounds and normal respiratory rate, depth, and rhythm.

- Deficient Fluid Volume related to decreased intake and insensible loss.

  Expected Outcome: The infant will maintain adequate hydration, as evidenced by moist mucous membranes, a flat fontanel, urine output normal for age, and stable weight.

- Ineffective Thermoregulation related to illness.

  Expected Outcome: The infant will demonstrate a body temperature within normal limits.

- Anxiety related to hospitalization and the child's dyspnea.

  Expected Outcomes: The infant will demonstrate decreased anxiety, as evidenced by adequate sleep and stable vital signs. The parents will verbalize understanding of the infant's condition and be able to participate appropriately in the infant's care.

Interventions

Many hospitals are now using clinical pathways for children with respiratory disease. Figure 21-3 shows a clinical pathway for an infant with bronchiolitis. Even when using a clinical pathway, the nurse needs to focus on appropriate nursing interventions.

Facilitating Gas Exchange

The nurse monitors and documents the infant's vital signs and respiratory status every 1 to 2 hours or more often as needed. Particularly note the rate, quality, and depth of respirations along with any adventitious breath sounds and the presence of retractions. Close monitoring with a cardiorespiratory monitor or continuous pulse oximeter will ensure early identification of impending respiratory distress.

Monitor oxygen saturation and administer humidified oxygen (at 35%-40% concentration) in the manner most comfortable for the infant (by tent, hood, mask, or nasal prongs) to decrease hypoxia and bronchial edema. Positioning the infant's head at a 30- to 40-degree upright angle with the neck slightly extended will maintain an open airway and ease respirations by decreasing pressure on the diaphragm. If the infant is in an oxygen tent, change the bedding and infant's clothes regularly to keep the infant dry. Toys that might cause static electricity are kept outside the tent; provide the infant with appropriate safe toys.

Scheduling periods of uninterrupted rest between care episodes decreases oxygen demand. Chest physiotherapy should be performed (it may require coordination with the respiratory therapy department) before or at least 1 hour after meals. The use of chest physiotherapy in infants is controversial because it might increase their stress and oxygen demand.

Maintaining Fluid Balance

Most infants with bronchiolitis can take fluids orally; IV fluids are administered if respiratory distress is severe enough to risk aspiration. If the infant's nasal passages are blocked with mucus, instill saline solution nose drops (1 or 2 drops in each nostril, followed by gentle suctioning with a bulb syringe) before feeding. Offer the infant frequent, varied clear liquids (juices, Pedialyte, Ricelyte). Older infants may enjoy frozen electrolyte pops. The infant's hydration status (skin turgor, fontanel, mucous membranes) and electrolyte values are monitored, and daily weights and intake and output are documented.

Reducing Fever

The nurse monitors the infant's temperature every 2 to 4 hours and as needed. Control environmental temperature by maintaining the room temperature between 72° F and 75° F and dress the infant in light clothing. Fluid intake is encouraged, and liquid acetaminophen or ibuprofen is administered as ordered to reduce fever.

Decreasing Anxiety

Encourage the parent to stay with the infant when possible and to participate as much as possible in the infant's care. Hospital routines and all procedures and treatments should be explained to reduce fear of the unknown. Because adult anxiety can be transferred to the infant, maintain a calm environment and encourage parents to do the same. If the infant becomes anxious about being in an oxygen tent, the parent can hold the infant and direct the humidified oxygen toward the infant's face. If the infant remains in a tent, encourage the parent to play with the infant; the parent can get in the tent to maintain tactile contact with the infant. Parents need to be allowed to express concerns.

Evaluation

- Does the infant demonstrate adequate oxygenation (oxygen saturation >95%), clear breath sounds, and stable respiratory status?
- Does the infant have moist mucous membranes, good skin turgor, stable weight, a flat fontanel, and urine output of at least 2 to 3 mL/kg/hr? (For appropriate urine output in older children, see Chapter 18.)
- Is the infant's body temperature within normal limits?
- Does the infant demonstrate less crying or irritability and increased rest?
- Do the parents verbalize understanding of the disease, have a relaxed appearance, and demonstrate comforting behaviors toward the infant?

BRONCHIOLITIS & BRONCHIOLITIS (+) RSV
(Uncomplicated-without multi-system problems)
ICD-9 Codes 466.11 and 466.19

Expected LOS-3 Days
D#.#=Key interventions for this study.

Examples of appropriate Co-morbidities
Acute Pharyngitis
Acute Sinusitis NOS
Cellulitis
Other Specific Viral Infections
Otitis Media NOS

Examples of Co-morbidities that are not appropriate:
Asthma
Bronchopulmonary Dysplasia
Cardiac Conditions that extend the LOS
Cerebral Palsy
Cystic Fibrosis

Esophageal Reflux
HIV
Pneumonia
Respiratory Failure
Sickle Cell Anemia

Refer to Tracking Sheet for Recording

Clinical Pathway	Admission Day	Day 2	Day 3
Aspect of Care	Date ___ Unit___ ED	Date ___ Unit___	Date ___ Unit___
DAILY OUTCOME		↓ nebs if tolerated ↓ O2 if tolerated	*Discharge*

TESTS	CBC <2 mo.
	CXR
	CBG if resp distress or
	  ↑O2 requirements
	Possible:
	  Pertussis preps
	  Chlamydia preps
	  Viral culture
	  Blood Culture if fever (<2 mos)
		CBG if distress (↓oxygenation)
		Serum electrolytes if indicated	

CONSULTS	Case Manager:
	  Discharge needs and
	  possible home nebulizer
	Specialist:
	  Pulmonary or Infectious
	  Disease consult if hi-risk*
			Specialist if not improved

FLUID/LYTES MANAGEMENT	Possible IV fluids I/O	Hep lock if tolerating p.o.	
TREATMENTS/ PROCEDURES	*D1.0 Albuterol Nebs* Spot checks or Continuous oximeter if requiring 02 02 to keep Sat >92% Possible epi nebs CA monitor<2 mos or premature or severe respiratory distress Possible CPT	*D2.0 Albuterol or Epi Nebs* Wean 02 if tolerated Spot Check Oximetry w/vs	Albuterol or epi nebs *D3.0 Wean 02*
MEDICATIONS	*D1.2 Possible steroids* *(if hx recurrent wheezing)*	Review all IV meds and antibiotics	

CLINICAL SUPPORT	Diet p.o. if RR<60
	Contact Isolation during
	  season, even if viral studies
	  are (−) or not ordered, gown and
	  gloves when touching patient.
	R.T. to wear mask
	Education:
	  Exposure (smoke)
	  Follow-up
	  Neb treatments
		D2.1 Diet p.o. if RR <60	

Original 10/10/95   Rev. Date 11/9/95 5/1/97 8/18/97

*AAP guideline-CHD, parenchymal lung disease, infants less than 6 weeks old, prematurity, immunodeficiency, severely ill (impaired gas exchange)

Disclaimer: This clinical pathway document is provided as a general guideline for use by physicians and staff in planning the care and treatment of patients and their families. It is not intended to be and does not establish a standard of care. Each patient's care is individualized according to their specific needs.

Cook Children's Medical Center
M:\WPFILES\PATHWAYS\AUGBRONC.WPD

Privileged and Confidential Committee Document
TEX.REV.CIV.STAT.ANN. art. 4995b × 5.0

This pathway is not a permanent part of the patient's medical record.

FIG 21-3   **Clinical pathway for an infant with bronchiolitis.**   *(Courtesy Cook Children's Medical Center, Fort Worth, TX.)*

PNEUMONIA

Pneumonia is an inflammation of the lung parenchyma. It can occur as a primary or a secondary disease. Pneumonias can be classified by anatomic distribution or by the agents that cause them. Environment, immune system status, and the child's age are factors in the pathogenesis of the disease.

The two most common types of infectious pneumonia are *viral* and *bacterial* (Table 21-3). It is very difficult to differentiate clinically between viral and bacterial pneumonia. Viruses are the most common causative agents, but children with bacterial pneumonia tend to be more ill than are those with viral disease (Bradley, 2002). Community-acquired pneumonia is a significant problem worldwide. Difficulties related to treatment in children have increased greatly because of the emergence of resistant bacteria (Esposito & Principi, 2002). Children with chronic and acute conditions, such as acquired immunodeficiency syndrome, cystic fibrosis (CF), congenital defects, and foreign body aspiration, are at increased risk for development of pneumonia.

Opportunistic infections (*Pneumocystis carinii* pneumonia) may be associated with acquired immunodeficiency syndrome (see Chapter 17). Secondary pneumonia can result from aspiration of hydrocarbons contained in household products or lipids (e.g., mineral oil given to treat severe constipation).

NURSING CARE

The Child With Pneumonia

Assessment

Every 2 hours, assess the child's breath sounds, respiratory rate and rhythm, color, vital signs, and degree of restlessness. Immediately report any signs of respiratory distress, including dyspnea, tachypnea, cyanosis, use of accessory muscles of breathing, diminished breath sounds, and crackles. Also note any fever, tachycardia, malaise, anorexia, discomfort, and changes in condition.

TABLE 21-3   **Comparison of Types of Pneumonia**

Type	Etiology and Incidence	Pathophysiology	Manifestations	Therapeutic Management
Viral	Most often caused by adenoviruses, influenza viruses, cytomegalovirus (mainly in neonates), and RSV. Viruses cause 80% to 85% of all pneumonias. Most common in children younger than 3 yr.	Cell destruction with sloughing of cellular debris into lumen of terminal airways and alveoli causes patchy infiltrate that affects multiple lobes.	Low to high fever, cough, crackles, wheezing (more common with RSV), headache, malaise, myalgia, abdominal pain. Infiltrates seen on chest radiography. WBC count <20,000/mm³. Usually lasts 5-7 d.	Supportive. No antibiotics are prescribed. Severely ill infants and children may be hospitalized for oxygen and fluid therapy.
Bacterial and bacterial-like	Caused primarily by *S. pneumoniae* and *S. aureus* in infants and children younger than 5 yr. Pneumococcal infection is major type in children older than 5 yr. Also may be caused by *H. influenzae* and group A streptococci. Other bacteria-like organisms include *M. pneumoniae, C. pneumoniae,* and *Chlamydia trachomatis* (seen mainly in infants).	Alveoli fill with fluid and cells in small segment or entire lung. Bacteria enter bloodstream through pulmonary lymphatics. Vital capacity and lung compliance decrease as consolidation increases.	Preceded by upper respiratory infection. Abrupt onset of fever, chills, cough, decreased breath sounds, signs of respiratory distress (retractions, nasal flaring, tachypnea), restlessness, and apprehension. Symptoms may be vague in infants; older children can have gastrointestinal symptoms, chest pain, and abnormal breath sounds. Onset of the bacterial-like pneumonias may be more insidious. Radiography reveals consolidation; WBC count is elevated.	IV or oral antibiotic therapy, usually with penicillins, erythromycin (for penicillin-allergic children), or cephalosporins. Hospitalization for severely ill infants and children with oxygen and fluid therapy. Chest tube drainage of fluid or purulence from pleural cavity may be necessary (particularly for children with staphylococcal pneumonia).

Nursing Diagnosis and Planning

The nursing diagnoses and expected outcomes that may be appropriate for the child with pneumonia and the child's family are as follow:

- Ineffective Airway Clearance related to bronchial obstruction.

  Expected Outcome: The child will have clear airways, as evidenced by the absence of abnormal breath sounds and dyspnea.

- Ineffective Breathing Pattern related to increased mucus production.

  Expected Outcome: The child will demonstrate effective breathing, as evidenced by respiratory rate and rhythm within normal limits for age and absence of retractions.

- Impaired Gas Exchange related to increased mucus and accumulation of exudate.

  Expected Outcome: The child will maintain adequate gas exchange, as evidenced by decreased restlessness, appropriate oxygen saturation, and improved mucous membrane and nail bed color.

- Deficient Fluid Volume related to fever, decreased intake, and tachypnea.

  Expected Outcomes: The child will maintain fluid balance, as evidenced by moist mucous membranes, good skin turgor, urine output appropriate for age, and maintenance of age-appropriate weight.

- Deficient Knowledge related to the disease process and home care.

  Expected Outcome: The parents will explain the disease process and describe the child's care.

- Anxiety (parental) related to infant's dyspnea and hospitalization.

  Expected Outcomes: The parents will show a decrease in anxiety, as evidenced by decreased irritability and increased periods of rest. The parents will verbalize and demonstrate comfort and ease when caring for the child.

- Acute Pain related to coughing and difficulty breathing secondary to disease process.

  Expected Outcome: The child will have decreased pain, as evidenced by less irritability, verbalization of increased comfort (if age appropriate), and a relaxed body posture.

Interventions

The severity of the illness and the cause of the disease direct the nursing care of the child with pneumonia. Many children will be cared for at home, whereas others will be hospitalized on a general pediatric unit or special care area.

For the hospitalized child, chest physiotherapy, if needed, should be scheduled before meals and at bedtime. Elevating the head of the bed and changing the child's position every 2 hours assist respiratory effort and promote pulmonary drainage. Older children may assume a position of comfort but still must change their position every 2 hours. The use of infant seats should be avoided because pressure may be placed on the diaphragm, thus actually decreasing lung expansion.

The older child should be assisted with coughing and deep breathing and splinting as necessary to ease discomfort. Oxygen should be humidified and monitored. Pulse oximetry aids in monitoring oxygen saturation and the adequacy of air exchange. A cardiorespiratory monitor is used when available.

Oral or IV fluids are given as ordered. IV fluids may be indicated when oral intake increases the stress put on an already compromised body. The nurse monitors intake and output and observes for signs of dehydration (oliguria, poor skin turgor, dry mucous membranes, sunken fontanels, weight loss). Weight should be measured daily. The specific gravity of urine also is checked to monitor hydration status.

Because conserving energy aids oxygenation, nursing care is planned to provide for periods of rest. Quiet diversional activities, such as reading, puzzles, videos, and board games, are suggested. The nurse maintains a quiet and cool environment and limits visitors to allow the child maximum rest. Visits by anyone with an infection should be restricted.

Administer antipyretics (acetaminophen), antibiotics, and analgesics as ordered. Normal breathing may cause discomfort. If an analgesic is not ordered, the physician should be notified of any discomfort the child has. Splinting of the affected side by lying on that side may decrease discomfort. Diversional activities and manipulation of the environment are often effective for pain relief.

The family and child (if of appropriate age) need to receive information about the disease and its treatment. The nurse explains all procedures and treatments and encourages the parents to stay with their child and participate in the child's care. The nurse conveys empathy for the family's feelings and concerns. The nurse also teaches the family about home management of the infant or child (Box 21-3).

BOX 21-3	**PARENTS WANT TO KNOW** About Home Management of the Child With Pneumonia

- Provide rest.
- Increase your child's fluid intake. Offer favorite fluids more frequently than usual and be sure your child is urinating appropriate amounts. Warm liquids (lemonade, apple juice, Pedialyte, Ricelyte) help loosen secretions. Call your health care provider if the child's mucous membranes appear dry or if urination decreases.

- Administer acetaminophen for fever and discomfort.
- Use a cool mist humidifier and follow the manufacturer's instructions for cleaning.
- Administer antibiotics as ordered; give the correct dose and the entire prescribed amount.
- Avoid exposing your child to cigarette smoke.

Evaluation

- Are the child's vital signs and respiratory status within normal limits?
- Is the child's oxygen saturation greater than 95%?
- Does the child appear hydrated, with moist mucous membranes, good skin turgor, and adequate urinary output for age?
- Can the parents describe home care techniques?
- Do the parents appear relaxed, and are they able to fully participate in the child's care?
- Can the child comfortably participate in quiet activities and rest quietly when appropriate?

FOREIGN BODY ASPIRATION

Foreign body aspiration is seen most frequently in children ages 6 months to 5 years. Children who have objects in their mouths while they are playing, running, or laughing are at risk. Certain items have an increased incidence of aspiration by infants and children (Box 21-4).

Etiology and Incidence

Children's curiosity, oral needs, and occasionally lack of supervision contribute to the occurrence of foreign body aspiration. Infants and children love to explore and investigate objects. Exploration often includes putting objects into their mouths. Children also have the uncanny ability to remove small parts from toys and to find other objects that parents thought were out of their reach (e.g., pins, screws, nuts, coins, earrings). Adults may give infants and small children foods they are not developmentally prepared to ingest (hard candy, popcorn, uncooked carrots, hot dogs, peanuts). Latex balloons account for a significant number of deaths from aspiration per year. One hospital review of 1,160 children referred for foreign body aspiration found watermelon seeds, at 39%, to be the most common object (Eren et al., 2003). Childhood aspiration can occur at any age, but it occurs most frequently in children 1 to 3 years of age (Tokar, Ozkan, & Ilhan, 2004). Forty percent of accidental deaths in the home are caused by foreign body aspiration.

Manifestations

Immediate signs and symptoms include sudden, violent coughing; gagging; wheezing; vomiting; brief episode of apnea; and possibly cyanosis.

BOX 21-4	Common Items of Aspiration
<ul><li>Nuts</li><li>Pins</li><li>Screws</li><li>Coins</li><li>Seeds</li><li>Grapes</li><li>Bones</li><li>Earrings</li></ul>	<ul><li>Small toys</li><li>Chunks of food</li><li>Parts of toys</li><li>Hard candy</li><li>Latex balloons</li><li>Popcorn</li><li>Hot dogs</li><li>Carrots</li></ul>

> **PATHOPHYSIOLOGY**
>
> **FOREIGN BODY ASPIRATION**
>
> Most foreign bodies become lodged in the bronchi. The right main bronchus is a more common site than the left main bronchus because of its anatomic development. Objects lodged in the larynx cause edema and inflammation. Bronchial obstruction manifests as obstructive emphysema, pneumonia, or atelectasis. Failure to remove obstructing foreign objects is almost always fatal. Most can be removed mechanically without complications; a delay in treatment can lead to aspiration pneumonia and airway trauma.

After aspirating a foreign object, the child may remain asymptomatic for hours or weeks. If the object is not found and removed, signs and symptoms related to edema and increased irritation and obstruction may develop. Signs and symptoms of laryngeal and tracheal obstruction include choking, dysphagia, hoarseness, croupy cough, stridor, and possibly dyspnea with cyanosis. Coughing, wheezing, unilaterally decreased breath sounds, pneumonitis, and possibly respiratory arrest can indicate bronchial inflammation and obstruction.

Diagnostic Evaluation

The diagnosis is based on an accurate history and the clinical manifestations. Fluoroscopy and chest radiography are used to reveal the presence of a foreign object in the respiratory tract. Radiographs will reveal an opaque foreign body, and laryngoscopy or rigid bronchoscopy confirms the diagnosis and provides an avenue for removing the object.

Therapeutic Management

Foreign bodies are removed from the respiratory tract by direct laryngoscopy or bronchoscopy. After the procedure, the child should remain hospitalized for observation for laryngeal edema and respiratory distress. Antibiotics are unnecessary unless respiratory signs and symptoms suggest an infection. Cool mist and administration of bronchodilators or corticosteroids 24 to 48 hours after the removal of the foreign body may be indicated.

Nursing Considerations

The degree of obstruction should be assessed to determine the appropriate action to take. If the child is aphonic (not speaking) and not breathing, the nurse should follow the guidelines for managing an obstructed airway (see Chapter 10). Children with a partially obstructed airway are observed for signs of increasing obstruction.

After the object has been removed, the child is observed for signs of obstruction caused by laryngeal edema and soft tissue swelling (restlessness, dyspnea). The child should be placed on a cardiorespiratory monitor.

Liquids are withheld until the child's gag reflex returns after anesthesia. Oral fluids should be started slowly and increased as the child tolerates the intake. Intake and output should be recorded. If the child refuses to drink because of a sore throat or is unable to take fluids orally, the physician should be notified so that IV fluids may be started. The parents' knowledge of respiratory distress is also evaluated before discharge.

Parental anxiety and guilt are common after an episode of aspiration. In addition to supporting the parents, the nurse assesses their knowledge of safety. Prevention is the key to reducing the incidence of aspiration. Safety is discussed at every well-child visit (see Chapters 5 through 8).

PULMONARY NONINFECTIOUS IRRITATION

Although we think of foreign body aspiration as the most common type of pulmonary noninfectious irritation in children, other forms of irritation may cause respiratory difficulties. These include acute (adult) respiratory distress syndrome (ARDS), passive smoking, and smoke inhalation.

Acute (Adult) Respiratory Distress Syndrome

Although there is not uniform agreement as to what constitutes ARDS, it is generally agreed that ARDS represents severe diffuse lung injury precipitated by a variety of illnesses. The mechanism of lung injury in children is similar to that of adults and usually occurs from 8 to 48 hours after the initial illness, which may be but is not limited to aspiration, trauma, drug ingestion, shock, and massive transfusions.

Pathophysiology

The mechanism that initiates and perpetuates the lung injury is not understood. There is a breakdown in the alveolar-capillary barrier with fluid accumulation in the interstitium and alveoli. ARDS has acute and chronic stages. Initially there is capillary congestion and pulmonary edema. Fibrosis of the lungs develops in children who do not recover from the acute stage.

Table 21-4 discusses clinical manifestations, therapeutic management, nursing care, and prognosis.

Passive Smoking

Increased attention has been paid to the role of passive smoking in the development of respiratory disease in children. Children with a history of exposure to cigarette smoke have more episodes of airway obstruction, more frequent hospitalizations for respiratory complaints, onset of asthma at an earlier age, and more frequent upper respiratory complications than do nonexposed children (Cantani & Micera, 2005). There is increasing evidence that passive smoking increases the incidence of respiratory infections and bronchial hyperresponsiveness (Arshad, Kurukulaaratchy, Fenn, & Matthews, 2005). In utero exposure is associated with impaired lung growth and wheezing illnesses (Kukla, Hruba, & Tyrlik, 2004).

Pathophysiology

Smoke is an irritant that can cause increased airway reactivity and inflammation.

See Table 21-4 for a discussion of clinical manifestations, therapeutic management, nursing care, and prognosis.

Smoke Inhalation

As many as 50% of all fire-related deaths are caused by smoke injuries. The severity of lung injury is related to the nature of the material inhaled, the products of incomplete combustion that are generated, and the child's confinement in a closed space. Besides the noxious gases, fine particles of soot may also be inhaled, which may have toxic gases adsorbed on them or which may cause thermal burns.

Pathophysiology

Because the upper airway has a built-in cooling system, most thermal airway injury is limited to the areas above the larynx. Steam inhalation injury is an exception. Combustion of the materials involved causes a wide variety of noxious gases. These include but are not limited to oxides of sulfur and nitrogen, acetaldehydes, hydrocyanic acid, and carbon monoxide. Exposure to these gases can cause mucosal edema, activation of irritant receptors, necrosis, sloughing of airway mucosa, inspissation (thickening or drying) of sooty debris, and airway obstruction leading to further asphyxia, upper airway obstruction, and lung damage (Lynch & Thomas, 2004).

Carbon monoxide poisoning is a complication of smoke inhalation caused when carbon monoxide combines with hemoglobin to form carboxyhemoglobin, causing severe hypoxia.

See Table 21-4 for a discussion of clinical manifestations, therapeutic management, nursing care, and prognosis.

RESPIRATORY DISTRESS SYNDROME

Respiratory distress syndrome (RDS), also known as *hyaline membrane disease*, occurs when there is immature development of the respiratory system or an inadequate amount of surfactant in the lungs. Infants with RDS are unable to keep their lungs expanded and the alveoli open. RDS is the leading cause of respiratory failure in the preterm infant.

RDS occurs in infants with immature lung development or insufficient amounts of surfactant. Predisposing factors include prematurity, asphyxia at birth, cesarean delivery, a diabetic mother (especially <38 weeks' gestation), acute antepartum hemorrhage, multiple gestation, and a sibling who had RDS. Affected boys outnumber affected girls 2 to 1.

Incidence

The incidence of RDS increases as gestational age decreases. In premature infants less than 28 to 30 weeks' gestation, the incidence is approximately 50% to 70%. At greater than 34 weeks' gestation, the incidence is decreased markedly. Maternal diabetes is another risk factor, as is perinatal asphyxia and birth by cesarean delivery (Zanardo et al., 2004). On the other hand, factors that tend to cause chronic fetal stress, such as maternal hypertension, drug abuse, and prolonged rupture of membranes, decrease the incidence of RDS.

TABLE 21-4 **Pulmonary Noninfectious Irritants**

	Acute Respiratory Distress Syndrome (ARDS)	Passive Smoking	Smoke Inhalation
Clinical manifestations	Acute, subacute, and chronic phases Pulmonary manifestations may be minimal during acute phase but will move toward respiratory distress (dyspnea, tachypnea, retractions, grunting, cyanosis) Severe hypoxemia and, occasionally, hypercapnia may develop Note that there is a primary disease and manifestations of that disease process will also be present	Increased respiratory infections An effect on respiratory function and growth in infants and small but significant reduction in airway function in older children Possible negative effect on linear growth of children with CF	Singed nasal hair Cough Hoarseness Hemoptysis Soot in sputum Cyanosis Wheezing Carbon monoxide: Mild—headaches, mild dyspnea, visual changes, confusion Moderate—irritability, diminished judgment, dim vision, nausea Severe—hallucinations, confusion, ataxia, collapse, coma
Therapeutic management	Need to be treated in ICU Treat underlying cause Oxygen/mechanical ventilation Pulse oximetry Maintain cardiac function Stabilize hematocrit Prevent infection	Awareness of problem and preventive teaching Effective programs to prevent smoking in parents and minors	100% oxygen by mask Arterial blood gases Intubation and tracheostomy equipment available Aerosolized bronchodilators Balance fluid therapy between need for large volume of fluid and need to limit fluid to decrease pulmonary edema Prophylactic antimicrobial therapy is controversial
Nursing care	Monitor respiratory status Monitor blood gas analysis Psychologic support of child and parents Monitor urine output, capillary filling, perfusion	Involvement in community projects to designate "no smoking" ordinances in public places School-based prevention programs Education of parents as part of anticipatory guidance of dangers of smoking, both active and passive Role modeling no smoking	Respiratory assessment Support of pulmonary therapy Psychologic support of child and family as a result of the fear of the trauma of the fire or insult that caused the injury Children who have lost a family member will need long-term psychologic support
Prognosis	High mortality, usually more than 50% Those who survive have a good chance of full recovery	Increased numbers of studies have shown correlation between smoking and respiratory disease; more studies needed to show long-term effects	Most will return to near-normal pulmonary function, and few will have long-term problems associated with the injury

ICU, Intensive care unit.

Manifestations

Symptoms of RDS usually appear at or shortly after birth, worsen over the first 24 to 48 hours, and gradually improve over the next 3 to 5 days. Signs and symptoms include tachypnea, inspiratory retractions (e.g., suprasternal, substernal, intercostal), paradoxic seesaw respirations, inspiratory nasal flaring, and an audible expiratory grunt. Chest x-ray findings show overall hypoventilation and a reticular granular pattern (i.e., ground-glass appearance). Apnea occurs as lung function worsens. Central cyanosis (a late, ominous sign) indicates increased hypoxemia and an advanced stage of deterioration. Blood gases initially show a decrease in the concentration of oxygen in the blood. Carbon dioxide levels in the blood rise as respiratory failure occurs from repeated apnea or poor air exchange. As respiratory failure progresses, metabolic acidosis slowly develops, and, as the concentration of carbon dioxide in the blood increases, a mixed metabolic and respiratory acidosis develops. Respiratory failure may result in death if supportive management is not timely and appropriate.

PATHOPHYSIOLOGY

RESPIRATORY DISTRESS SYNDROME

In the preterm infant, anatomic immaturity of the chest wall, lung parenchyma, and capillary endothelium contributes to the development of RDS.* The immature chest wall anatomy increases the chances of lung collapse at the end of expiration. Immaturity of the lung parenchyma and capillary endothelium results in less surface area for gas exchange. In the preterm as well as the term infant, RDS may be caused by a decreased total amount of pulmonary surfactant or a qualitative alteration of the surfactant present. The resulting inability to keep the lungs expanded causes the lung to be relatively noncompliant with changes in intrathoracic and extrathoracic pressure, decreasing air exchange. Lung repair begins after 24 to 48 hours, even as further cell damage takes place. Hyaline membranes, consisting of debris from necrotic cells enmeshed in a proteinaceous filtrate of serum, are phagocytosed by macrophages. Cuboidal cells replace the damaged alveolar and airway epithelium and eventually flatten. New capillaries develop and make contact with the regenerating cells of the alveoli. Surfactant synthesis begins and helps the repaired alveoli remain expanded. Diuresis is usually a sign that the acute phase of RDS has ended and recovery is taking place. The differential diagnosis of RDS should include transient tachypnea of the newborn, pulmonary insufficiency of prematurity, group B streptococci pneumonia, and anatomic malformations.

Contributing Factors in the Pathophysiology of RDS

Immature Chest Wall

- The ribs and costal cartilages are relatively soft and pliable.
- The intercostal muscles have a low total muscle mass and are prone to fatigue, providing inadequate stabilization of the rib cage.
- The highly compliant rib cage allows the lower chest wall to collapse when the diaphragm contracts, inadequately expanding the lungs.
- The diaphragm is easily fatigued because it has a decreased number of fatigue-resistant muscle fibers.

Immature Lung Tissue

- Alveoli are few in number and poorly developed, providing less surface area for gas exchange.
- Type 1 epithelial cells lining the alveoli are relatively thick, impeding their ability to exchange gases.
- The walls of the capillaries surrounding the alveoli are relatively thick, impeding gas exchange.
- Few of the capillaries surrounding the alveoli actually touch the alveoli, making them unavailable for gas exchange.
- The lung lymphatic system is poorly developed, resulting in decreased clearance of fetal lung fluid and pulmonary edema.

Decreased Surfactant

- In the preterm infant, an insufficient amount of surfactant is produced.
- Numerous factors can adversely affect the production and metabolism of surfactant, including acidosis, hypercapnia, hypoxia, shock, pulmonary edema, mechanical ventilation, overinflation or underinflation of the lungs, and infection.

Complications of RDS

Pulmonary	*Acute:* pneumothorax, pneumomediastinum, pulmonary interstitial emphysema
	Chronic: BPD
Cardiovascular	Patent ductus arteriosus, hypotension
Renal	Decreased urine output
Metabolic	Acidosis, hyponatremia, hypernatremia, hypocalcemia, hypoglycemia
Hematologic	Anemia, disseminated intravascular coagulation
Neurologic	Seizures, intraventricular hemorrhage
Other	Secondary infection, retinopathy of prematurity, complications of umbilical vessel catheterization

*Boyd, S. (2004). Causes and treatment of neonatal respiratory distress syndrome. *Nursing Times, 100,* 40-44.

Therapeutic Management

Supportive Care

The goals of supportive care are to keep oxygen consumption as low as possible and to maintain adequate nutrition and hydration. Every effort should be made to maintain the infant in a neutral thermal environment. Oxygen consumption increases rapidly above or below the neutral thermal environment. Evaporation is a significant contributor to fluid loss in premature infants. Measures should be taken to minimize fluid loss by evaporation and loss of heat. Because handling stimulates movement and oxygen consumption, the infant should be handled as little as possible. For ventilated infants with evidence of asynchronous respiratory efforts, initiating neuromuscular paralysis with pancuronium, a neuromuscular blocking agent, may have favorable effect on complications such as intraventricular hemorrhage or air leak (Ozkan, Duman, Kumral, & Gulcan, 2004). A minimum of 60 kcal/kg/day should be provided with sufficient amino acids to prevent catabolism of endogenous proteins and ketoacidosis.

Respiratory Care

Oxygen should be given to maintain partial pressure of oxygen (PO_2) within the normal range. Interrupting oxygen administration, even briefly, may cause hypoxemia, pulmonary vasoconstriction, and reduced cardiac output. Mechanical ventilation should be started when the infant's respiratory system requires additional assistance. Apnea with brady-cardia that is unresponsive to stimulation, regardless of the blood gas values, is also an indication that mechanical ven-tilation is needed. With intubation and continuous positive airway pressure or positive-pressure ventilation, radiographic changes usually appear less severe.

Surfactant replacement is now standard therapy for both treating and preventing RDS (Lam, Ng, & Wong, 2005). In most infants with RDS, surfactant replacement therapy improves oxygenation and lung mechanics, thereby decreas-ing the need for supplemental oxygen and high ventila-tor pressures. The infant should be monitored closely for complications.

NURSING CARE

The Newborn With Respiratory Distress Syndrome

Assessment

The nurse should identify infants at risk for RDS by reviewing the perinatal history for risk factors. The respiratory system is assessed for signs of respiratory distress, including tachypnea, apnea, retractions, nasal flaring, and grunting. During aus-cultation of the chest, the nurse assesses the infant's breath sounds, comparing and contrasting the left and right sides and noting the equality of breath sounds, the quality of air entry, and the presence of rhonchi, crackles, and wheezes.

Assessment of the cardiovascular system includes deter-mining the heart rate and noting any murmurs that may indicate a cardiac malformation or patent ductus arteriosus. A shift in the location of the point of maximal impulse may indicate a shift in heart position from a pulmonary air leak.

Peripheral cyanosis may progress to central cyanosis, which in the neonate usually indicates severe hypoxia. Pe-ripheral cyanosis may become obscured as the infant's color further deteriorates to pale gray. Initially, extremely ill in-fants may have a blood pressure that is slightly higher than normal, progressing to hypotension as the infant's condition deteriorates.

The nurse discusses the results of laboratory tests for ab-normal findings. Blood gas abnormalities, acid-base imbal-ances, disturbances in electrolyte and glucose homeostasis, and early signs of complications, such as sepsis, require im-mediate intervention.

Nursing Diagnosis and Planning

The nursing diagnoses and expected outcomes that may be appropriate for the neonate with RDS and the family are as follow:

*   Impaired Gas Exchange related to immaturity of the lungs and chest wall or insufficient amounts of surfactant.
    Expected Outcome: The infant will be able to maintain adequate gas exchange, as evidenced by blood gas values and oxygen saturations within normal ranges.
*   Ineffective Airway Clearance related to obstruction or inappropriate positioning of an endotracheal tube.

Expected Outcome: The infant's artificial airway will be correctly positioned and patent, as evidenced by equal and adequate breath sounds and chest wall movement.
*   Ineffective Breathing Pattern related to asynchronous breathing between the infant and the ventilator, ventila-tor malfunction, or inappropriate ventilatory support.
    Expected Outcome: Ventilatory support will appropriately complement the infant's respiratory efforts, as evidenced by blood gas parameters within normal ranges.
*   Risk for Injury related to extremes in acid-base balance, oxygen levels, carbon dioxide levels, or barotrauma from mechanical ventilation.
    Expected Outcome: The respiratory assistance provided will prevent or promptly treat extremes in blood gas param-eters and will minimize potential barotrauma.
*   Risk for Impaired Parenting secondary to situational crisis (sick newborn infant).
    Expected Outcomes: The parent will exhibit signs of parent-child attachment and develop role identity as a parent.

Interventions

Infants with RDS are cared for in the special care nursery. The nurse monitors the infant's vital signs and respiratory status for evidence of respiratory distress. Continuous cardiorespiratory monitoring will provide for early recognition of respiratory dis-tress. Blood gas monitoring and pulse oximetry are also done, and results are reported to the physician. Proper positioning of the infant to maximize lung expansion is achieved in the supine position with the neck slightly extended and the nose pointed toward the ceiling to prevent narrowing of the airway. Suctioning of the endotracheal tube as needed optimizes ven-tilation. The nurse works closely with the respiratory therapist to administer and monitor respiratory support. If ventilatory support is indicated, settings are checked hourly and the nurse observes the infant to ensure synchronous breathing between the ventilator and infant. Ventilatory changes are made as ordered if blood gas results fall outside established parameters. The nurse encourages the parents to verbalize fears and con-cerns and to participate in caring for the infant as appropriate. The nurse may also consider directing the parents to contact outside resources for further support.

Evaluation

*   Does the infant maintain normal oxygen saturations on pulse oximetry?
*   Does the infant maintain a normal respiratory rate?
*   Are the infant's breath sounds and chest wall movements adequate and equal bilaterally?
*   Are the infant's blood gases within normal limits?
*   Are ventilatory settings adjusted in a timely manner when-ever blood gas results fall outside established parameters?
*   Does the family assume appropriate caretaking responsibilities?
*   Are the parents able to hold, feed, and interact with the infant?

APNEA
Manifestations

Apnea is the cessation of breathing for a period of 20 seconds or longer, or for a shorter period but accompanied by bradycardia or cyanosis. True apnea differs from periodic breathing, which might be seen in premature infants. In periodic breathing, there is a shift from regular rhythmic breathing to brief episodes of apnea. This type of breathing pattern consists of three or more respiratory pauses of longer than 3 seconds, with less than 20 seconds of respiration between pauses. Rarely, periodic breathing is associated with changes in heart rate or color. Periodic breathing is very common in premature infants and decreases as the infant's gestational age increases. The cause is unknown; periodic breathing may be a normal event.

Apparent life-threatening events are sudden episodes characterized by apnea, a color change, a change in muscle tone, choking, or gagging in an infant who otherwise appears healthy. The observer of the event relates the belief that the infant would have died if not for intervention. Apparent life-threatening events most often occur in infants of 37 weeks' gestational age or older while they are sleeping, feeding, or awake. Infants who have had such an event are usually hospitalized for observation and testing and are at increased risk for mortality (AAP Committee on Fetus and Newborn, 2003).

Two categories of true apnea events are apnea of prematurity and infant apnea (Table 21-5).

Diagnostic Evaluation

Tests are selected for the clinical indications and to rule out any underlying condition. Cardiorespiratory and neurophysiologic studies are commonly ordered. These studies include chest radiography, blood chemistry studies, electrocardiography, and electroencephalography. Pneumocardiography specifically tests for apnea by recording the heart rate and chest wall movements; however, the reliability of the test in predicting apnea has not been well established.

NURSING CARE
The Infant With Apnea

Assessment

The infant's heart rate and respirations are monitored continuously. The nurse should ascertain that the alarms on the cardiorespiratory monitor are set. Resuscitative equipment should be available.

If an apneic episode is observed, the nurse should record the time and duration of the episode, the skin color change, heart rate, and oxygen saturation. The nurse should also describe what the infant was doing before the episode and any actions the nurse took to stimulate breathing.

TABLE 21-5	Apnea of Prematurity Compared With Infant Apnea	
Etiology and Incidence	**Pathophysiology**	**Therapeutic Management**
Apnea of Prematurity		
Most common type of apnea; occurs in neonates of 24-32 weeks' gestational age, with onset usually within first week of life. It usually resolves by 38 wk. Although neonate's age may be related to higher incidence of SIDS, apnea of prematurity is not considered to predict risk.*	Varies among neonates but may be caused by upper airway obstruction, immaturity of central control mechanisms, compliant chest wall, or abnormal response during REM sleep. Apnea often occurs during feeding because of immaturity of breathing, sucking, and swallowing coordination.	Gentle cutaneous stimulation is used to stimulate breathing in neonates with mild apnea (<10 episodes/d with little desaturation). For persistent apnea, use oxygen administration, cardiorespiratory monitor; consider CPAP for neonates with severe apnea. Drug therapy may include caffeine, oral theophylline, or IV aminophylline to increase central respiratory drive and improve carbon dioxide sensitivity.
Infant Apnea		
Most infant apnea has no known cause. Underlying conditions such as gastroesophageal reflux, seizures, or hypoglycemia should be ruled out.	Three types: • *Central*—absence of respiratory effort and air movement. • *Obstructive*—apparent respiratory efforts without air movement or sound. • *Mixed*—absence of respiratory effort and nasal air movement followed by resumption of respiratory effort without air movement. Short episodes of apnea are usually central apnea; apnea episodes that last 15 sec or more are usually mixed.	If no underlying disorder is identified, home monitoring with a respiratory stimulant (caffeine, theophylline).

REM, Rapid eye movement; *CPAP,* continuous positive airway pressure.
*Bhatt-Mehta, V., & Schumacher, R. E. (2003). Treatment of apnea of prematurity. *Paediatric Drugs, 5,* 195-210.

Nursing Diagnosis and Planning

The nursing diagnoses and expected outcomes that may be appropriate for the infant with apnea and the family are as follow:

- Ineffective Breathing Pattern related to apnea secondary to prematurity of respiratory control mechanisms (premature infant) and related to apnea of known or unknown etiology (term infant).

  Expected Outcome: The infant will have regular breathing patterns, as evidenced by respiratory rate and rhythm within normal limits for age.

- Anxiety (parental) related to the possibility of the infant's death.

  Expected Outcome: The parents will verbalize feelings concerning the infant's periods of apnea.

- Deficient Knowledge (parental) related to unfamiliarity with apnea monitoring equipment and cardiopulmonary resuscitation (CPR).

  Expected Outcome: The parents will learn how to perform infant CPR and how to operate the apnea monitor.

Interventions

The nurse sets the heart rate parameters of the cardiorespiratory monitor according to the infant's age and the respiratory pause at greater than 15 seconds. Resuscitative equipment should be available, and the nurse should be proficient in using it.

The apneic infant can be stimulated by gently tapping the foot or trunk or turning the infant over. The infant should not be shaken vigorously. If breathing does not resume, institute bag-and-mask ventilation.

Maintain a neutral thermal environment while the infant is hospitalized and avoid suctioning if possible. Several studies have shown that feeding affects ventilation. Therefore infants should be monitored closely when being fed.

If home apnea monitoring is ordered, the family should be instructed in the use of the monitor and in CPR (Fig. 21-4) (Silvestri et al., 2005). Emphasize to the parents that

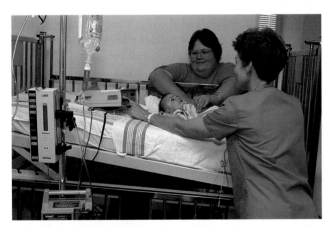

FIG 21-4   **Teaching the family about using an apnea monitor and how to respond to alarms is an important element in caring for the child with infant apnea. The nurse must assess the parents' ability to tolerate the stressors of living with a child who is prone to apnea and support them as they deal with these stressors.**

| BOX 21-5 | **Home Apnea Monitoring** |

Indications

- The infant is a survivor of an apparent life-threatening event (an event that required administration of CPR).
- The infant is a newborn sibling of an infant who died of SIDS.
- The infant is premature and has symptoms of idiopathic apnea of prematurity but is otherwise ready for hospital discharge.
- The infant has a tracheostomy
- The infant is dependent on a technologic resource for support
- The infant has sleep apnea syndrome caused by a neurologic disorder, periodic breathing, upper airway abnormality, or idiopathic syndrome.

Conditions

- The parents must be trained to do CPR and understand conditions for calling the health care provider.
- Twenty-four-hour medical and technical (equipment troubleshooting) coverage is mandatory.
- Parents should maintain a diary specifically describing each episode.

Modified from Silvestri, J. M., Lister, G., Corwin, M. J., Smok-Pearsall, S. M., Baird, T. M., Crowell, D. H., Cantey-Kiser, J. C., Hunt, C. E., Tinsley, L., Palmer, P. H., Mendenhall, R. S., Hoppenbrouwers, T. T., Neuman, M. R., Weese-Mayer, D. E., & Willinger, M. (2005). Factors that influence use of a home cardiorespiratory monitor for infants. *Archives of Pediatric and Adolescent Medicine, 159,* 18-24.; Brooks, J. (1998). SIDS and ALTE. In V. Chernick, T. Boat, & E. Kendig (Eds.), *Kendig's disorders of the respiratory tract in children* (6th ed., pp. 1166-1172). Philadelphia: WB Saunders.

when the monitor alarm is triggered, they should immediately assess the infant rather than focus on the machine (Box 21-5).

Evaluation

- Does the infant demonstrate normal respiratory rate and rhythm?
- Have the parents verbalized their fears associated with the infant's apnea?
- Have the parents demonstrated the ability to operate monitoring equipment and to perform CPR?

SUDDEN INFANT DEATH SYNDROME

Sudden infant death syndrome (SIDS) is defined as the sudden and unexplained death of an infant younger than 1 year. The exact cause is unknown despite a thorough investigation that includes a complete autopsy, examination of the death scene, and review of the clinical history. It is sometimes referred to by the public as *crib death*. SIDS usually occurs during sleep.

Etiology and Incidence

Although numerous theories have been proposed, the cause of SIDS is unknown. Proposed contributing factors include prematurity, brainstem defects, severe infant botulism, infections, reactions to immunizations, and hypersensitivity to cow's milk. Some studies have suggested a connection with lower socioeconomic status, cultural influences, lack of prenatal care, smoking, a sibling with SIDS, and season (winter).

Numerous reports from countries outside the United States have found a significant association between a prone sleeping position and the incidence of SIDS. On the basis of this information, the AAP (2005) updated its recommendations that healthy infants be placed on their backs to sleep, rather than prone. Since the AAP issued its initial recommendations in 1992, SIDS has declined 44% in the United States (Malloy & Freeman, 2004).

Risk factors are also associated with the use of soft bedding. Infants may suffocate by rebreathing carbon dioxide–laden expired air when sleeping face down on soft bedding (Pastore, Guala, & Zaffaroni, 2003). To reduce the risk of SIDS, the AAP (2005) recommends using mattresses with a firm sleeping surface, avoiding exposing the infant to second-hand smoke, and offering a pacifier for sleep. The AAP does not recommend bed sharing and advises parents to put the infant in a safe bassinet or crib in the parent's room for sleeping (AAP, 2005)

SIDS occurs most frequently between the second and fourth months of life, with 95% of cases occurring before age 6 months. It is more common in boys, low-birth-weight infants, and infants from lower socioeconomic groups. It occurs more often during the winter months. American Indians have the highest incidence, followed by African Americans.

Manifestations

The principal manifestation of SIDS is silent death. The child may be found in any position and may be clutching bedding.

Diagnostic Evaluation

Diagnosis is confirmed through autopsy. A medical history of the infant and family should be taken. The infant is examined for signs of illness or trauma. The death scene is also investigated.

PATHOPHYSIOLOGY

SUDDEN INFANT DEATH SYNDROME

Autopsy findings in infants who have died of SIDS have varied widely. Nonspecific findings such as mild pulmonary edema, vascular congestion, or pulmonary inflammation are common. Other consistent findings include retarded postnatal growth, increased pulmonary arterial smooth muscle, retention of brown fat, brainstem gliosis, and intrathoracic petechiae. Partial upper airway obstruction in association with rebreathing may be an explanation for many deaths from SIDS.* No single cause has been identified.

*Brooks, J. (1998). SIDS and ALTE. In V. Chernick, T. Boat, & E. Kendig (Eds.). *Kendig's disorders of the respiratory tract in children* (pp. 1166-1172). Philadelphia: WB Saunders.

NURSING CARE

The Family of the Infant With Sudden Infant Death Syndrome

Assessment

When an infant is brought into the emergency department with suspected SIDS, the family is often confused. If resuscitation was begun at home, they may assume that it was effective and that their infant is alive. Assessment of the family's understanding of the situation is necessary to plan for teaching and support. The nurse should assess the family's emotional status and coping strategies.

The nurse interviews the family in a calm, slow, and nonthreatening manner. Questions should not imply negligence or any involvement in the death. Parents need to be given time to think before they answer questions. Because the parents will be overwhelmed, questions may need to be repeated for clarity.

Nursing Diagnosis and Planning

The nursing diagnoses and expected outcomes that may be appropriate for the family of the infant victim of SIDS are as follow:

- Interrupted Family Processes related to death of a child.
  Expected Outcome: The parents and family will verbalize feelings related to the death of the infant.
- Compromised Family Coping related to death of a child.
  Expected Outcomes: The parents and family will identify strengths and accept support of other family members, friends, professionals, and support groups.
- Deficient Knowledge related to not understanding the cause of death.
  Expected Outcome: The parents will verbalize an understanding of the cause of their child's death.

Interventions

The nurse working with a family whose child has died of SIDS should provide calm and compassionate support. The parents are confused about the death and are trying to cope with many emotions. Most parents will experience a combination of guilt, anger, and emotional pain.

A quiet room with dim lighting and a rocking chair should be provided for the family, and someone should remain with them. Assist the family to call family, friends, or clergy. The nurse should accompany the physician when the parents are told their infant is dead. At this time the parents should also be told that the apparent cause of death is SIDS and that nothing could have been done to prevent the death. This information will help minimize feelings of guilt.

Parents should be given the opportunity to say good-bye to their child. Because the parents may not think to ask to see their infant, the nurse should provide this opportunity.

The nurse might say, "Would you like to have some time alone with your baby? We will bring him to you, and you can take as long as you would like to hold him."

The infant should be cleaned and wrapped in a blanket and brought to the parents. Parents who are not given the opportunity to hold their child and say good-bye often regret it later, but parents who do not want time alone with their baby should have their decision respected. The nurse should accept the parents' decision in this matter. Each parent will cope in an individualized way.

The need for an autopsy should be explained. The autopsy will verify the cause of death and confirm for the parents that they did not cause the death.

Before the parents leave the hospital, arrangements for follow-up care should be made. Many hospitals have a team consisting of a social worker, chaplain, and nurse that is called when a suspected SIDS death occurs.

Refer the family to a local SIDS program for information, support, and counseling (American SIDS Institute, 509 Augusta Dr., Marietta, GA 30067, website: *www.sids.org*). Nurses who are involved in home visiting can encourage the family to communicate their feelings. Siblings should not be overlooked; parents may be so overwhelmed with their own grief that they forget their other children. Another reaction might be to overprotect their other children. The nurse should guide the family in identifying the members' various responses and in treating them at the appropriate developmental level. Children in the family who perhaps resented the new baby may have tremendous guilt feelings. The loss of a sibling may be especially traumatic to a toddler, who does not understand the changes that are taking place in the family. Routines and rituals that are important to the toddler may be disrupted.

Evaluation

- Is the family able to verbalize feelings associated with the death of the child?
- Has the family joined a support group or identified a support system?
- Has the extended family mobilized to support the family?
- Is the family using effective coping skills to work toward an understanding of the child's death?

ASTHMA

Asthma is a leading cause of acute and chronic illness in children and the most frequent admitting diagnosis in children's hospitals. Despite advances in medical treatment, the incidence and death rate from asthma have increased markedly in recent years.

Etiology

It is unclear why some children's airways are more reactive than others. It is known, however, that heredity plays a role because asthma tends to appear in families. Other risk factors include male sex, African American or Hispanic ethnic background, crowded living conditions, poverty, prematurity, and exposure to environmental smoke (Federierico & Liu, 2003; Guilbert & Drawiec, 2003).

An asthma episode can be triggered by a variety of stimuli, among them cold air, smoke, fumes, viral infection, stress, exercise, odors, and medications (particularly aspirin and nonsteroidal anti-inflammatory drugs (Navaie-Waliser, Misener, Mersman, & Lincoln, 2004). Foods are occasionally the trigger in infants but less commonly in older children.

The immature anatomy of infants and small children predisposes them to increased distress from asthma. Children's smaller, narrower airways and decreased elastic lung recoil make them more prone to airway obstruction. The child's flexible rib cage and underdeveloped chest muscles and diaphragm lead to exhaustion when respiratory effort increases. Although asthma is not actually outgrown, the severity of asthma attacks often decreases as the child gets older because of increased airway size, improved diaphragmatic support, and better clearing of mucus. Asthma is considered a lifelong condition and may become increasingly severe after a period of remission.

Incidence

Since the early 1980s, the incidence of asthma has risen in the United States and other parts of the world. Asthma affects an estimated 9 million American children under the age of 18 years (NCHS, 2006b), with a 10% prevalence in all children in the United States (NCHS, 2006a). Asthma is more common among boys than girls until puberty, when the sex difference in incidence equalizes. Asthma is 26% more prevalent in African American children than in white children (American Lung Association, 2002).

Manifestations

The manifestations of asthma may vary. A child with an asthma episode may have only a dry cough. Wheezing is a classic sign of asthma, but other signs may be present, including shortness of breath, cough, or dyspnea on exertion. Other manifestations may have a sudden or an insidious onset:

- Retractions, nasal flaring, or stridor
- Nonproductive cough (with or without wheezing) that later becomes productive
- Tachypnea, orthopnea
- Restlessness, apprehension, diaphoresis
- Abdominal pain resulting from the strain placed on the abdominal muscles during labored breathing
- A hunched-over sitting position with arms braced (tripod position)
- Fatigue and difficulty performing simple tasks, such as eating, walking, or even talking, because of shortness of breath
- A feeling of chest tightness followed by a dry cough, wheezing, and dyspnea
- Worsening of symptoms after the child goes to bed at night because of increased narrowing of the airways at night and pooling of secretions

At the beginning of the asthma episode, wheezing may be heard only with a stethoscope. As the severity of the episode increases, wheezing may be audible to the unaided ear. Children in severe respiratory distress may not

PATHOPHYSIOLOGY

ASTHMA

Asthma is a reversible obstructive airway disease characterized by the following:

- Increased airway responsiveness to a variety of stimuli
- Bronchospasm resulting from constriction of bronchial smooth muscle
- Inflammation and edema of the mucous membranes that line the small airways and the subsequent accumulation of thick secretions in the airways

Immediate Reaction (Early-Phase Response)

Allergens or other trigger substances activate IgE receptors on sensitized airway mast cells, causing mast cell degranulation and release of chemical mediators (histamine, leukotrienes, prostaglandins). These mediators cause bronchoconstriction shortly after exposure to the trigger; the bronchoconstriction resolves within 1 to 2 hours.

Delayed Reaction (Late-Phase Response)

Chemical mediators attract immune system cells (eosinophils, neutrophils, basophils) to the respiratory tract. Infiltration by these cells and their release of additional inflammatory substances damage the epithelial and smooth muscle cells, causing airway edema, mucus plugging of small airways, and additional inflammation. Bronchoconstriction recurs and can persist for several hours. The airway hyperresponsiveness resulting from this inflammatory process can last several weeks or months.

Late asthmatic responses can occur without a previous early (immediate) response. When asthma is precipitated by nonallergenic stimuli (exercise, cold air), bronchospasm usually lasts less than 1 hour and is not followed by a late response.

During an asthma episode, the mucous membranes lining the bronchioles become edematous and secrete large amounts of thick mucus. As a result, the airways narrow, leading to increased airway resistance and respiratory distress. Because small airways are normally wider on inspiration than expiration, the child is able to inhale but has difficulty exhaling through the narrowed bronchioles. Wheezing can be heard as air is forced through the narrow passages during expiration. Air becomes trapped, causing hyperinflation of the alveoli.

Airway obstruction is more severe in some parts of the lungs than in others, and air flows more easily into areas with the least resistance. The blood that flows to the less-ventilated portions of the lungs is inadequately saturated with oxygen. Thus a mismatch between ventilation and perfusion in poorly ventilated areas of the lung occurs, resulting in incompletely saturated blood entering the systemic circulation and in decreased Po_2 levels (hypoxia).

As the child struggles to get enough air, the respiratory rate increases (tachypnea). Tachypnea lowers carbon dioxide levels in the blood (hypocapnia). As the child tires from the increased work of breathing, hypoventilation occurs and carbon dioxide levels increase. Increased levels of carbon dioxide in the blood (hypercapnia) during an asthma episode may be a sign of severe airway obstruction and impending respiratory failure.

---

demonstrate wheezing because of decreased air movement; decreased wheezing in a child who is not improving clinically may signal an inability to move air. This is referred to as a *silent chest* and is an ominous sign during an asthma episode. With treatment, increased wheezing may actually signal that the child's condition is improving.

Diagnostic Evaluation

Chest radiographs are usually normal except in cases of severe asthma, in which hyperinflation of the airways can be seen. Pulmonary function tests reveal a decreased forced expiratory volume in 1 second, increased residual volume from air trapping, and decreased vital capacity (the maximum amount of air exhaled after a maximum inhalation). Other pulmonary function test results might be altered as well. The peak expiratory flow rate (PEFR) is used to monitor children with chronic asthma. Because asthma can be triggered by gastroesophageal reflux, some children will be evaluated for its presence (see Chapter 19).

Rhinitis, sinusitis, and nasal polyps are often present in children with asthma. Eosinophilia is present in both the blood and the sputum. Skin tests are often performed to identify specific allergens. The RAST may be used to identify specific antigens. Arterial blood gas measurements may be ordered in children having a severe asthma episode because of initial respiratory alkalosis and subsequent metabolic acidosis. Pulse oximetry values provide information about oxygenation.

Therapeutic Management

Acute Asthma Episode

A child who is having an episode of wheezing along with other symptoms of asthma is usually seen at a physician's office or emergency department. First, a bronchodilator, usually a short-acting beta$_2$-adrenergic agonist such as albuterol, is administered by a powered nebulizer or metered-dose inhaler (MDI) as often as every 20 minutes for 1 hour or continuously. Close monitoring of the child's respiratory status after each course of medication assesses resolution of the episode. Beta$_2$-agonists, ipratropium bromide, and corticosteroids remain the most useful therapeutic agents for acute asthma episodes in children (Kallstrom, 2004).

If the child improves, the child can return home with an albuterol prescription and instructions for assessing respiratory status or with instructions for administering albuterol more frequently along with routine asthma medications. If symptoms do not improve or if the asthmatic child's PEFR is less than 70% of baseline, the child should receive a dose of an oral corticosteroid (liquid preparations are available for infants). If symptoms continue to worsen, administration of the bronchodilator every 20 minutes for an additional hour is warranted. Indicators for hospital admission include the following (Gorelick, Stevens, Schultz, & Scribano, 2004):

- PEFR less than 50% of baseline
- Inspiratory and expiratory wheezing
- Tachycardia and tachypnea
- Dyspnea, retractions, use of accessory muscles
- Oxygen saturation 91% or lower after aggressive treatment
- Child's mental status depressed
- Prolongation of expiration

Once the child is hospitalized, humidified oxygen is administered at 30%, either by nasal prongs or by face mask, to keep the oxygen saturation at 95% or greater. An IV line delivers fluids and provides venous access for parenteral medications (e.g., methylprednisolone) as ordered. Chest radiography, arterial blood gas determinations, or pulse oximetry may be performed to further evaluate the child's oxygenation status. The child receives a bronchodilator (albuterol) by nebulizer every ½ to 2 hours initially, with the interval between doses increased as the child's condition improves. Ipratropium bromide (Atrovent), an anticholinergic agent, has been found to be an effective bronchodilator when administered along with albuterol in children with severe exacerbations.

Increasingly severe asthma that is unresponsive to vigorous treatment measures is termed *status asthmaticus*. Status asthmaticus is a medical emergency that can cause respiratory failure and death. Hospitalization, usually in an intensive care unit, is indicated. The child is placed on a continuous cardiorespiratory monitor and continuous pulse oximeter. Blood gas and serum electrolyte values are monitored. In addition to the previously discussed measures, the child may receive continuous nebulized albuterol and ipratropium bromide every 6 hours. If the child's condition does not respond to these medications, oral or intravenous steroids are then administered. Levalbuterol is a relatively new treatment for acute asthma; it is delivered by a nebulizer.

Endotracheal intubation with mechanical ventilation may be necessary. Acidosis is corrected with IV administration of sodium bicarbonate. Antibiotics may also be administered to treat concurrent infection (e.g., pneumonia).

Long-Term Management

A partnership between the health care provider, parent, child, and school nurse is necessary for asthma to be managed effectively. Long-term asthma treatment should minimize symptoms, prevent acute asthma episodes, avoid the side effects of therapy, and help the child maintain a normal lifestyle. Children with asthma and their parents need to be taught methods of managing asthma, including

environmental control and monitoring symptoms and medication. A resource for parents is the Asthma and Allergy Foundation of America, 1233 20th St. NW, Washington, DC 20036, website: *www.aafa.org*.

Environmental Control

Irritants and Allergens. Children with asthma and their parents can decrease the frequency and severity of asthma episodes by recognizing and controlling the triggers that precipitate symptoms. Common environmental irritants include cigarette smoke, smoke from wood-burning stoves and fireplaces, fumes, deodorants, overhumidified air, and perfume. Allergenic triggers, such as animal dander, seasonal pollens, and molds, often cause problems. House dust can be both an irritant and an allergen (Arshad, Bateman, & Matthews, 2003).

The extent of environmental control needed depends on the severity of the asthma. If the asthma is mild, prohibiting smoking in the house and controlling dust with frequent house cleaning may be adequate. If the child continues to have problems after these interventions, additional steps should be taken to minimize environmental triggers.

Immunotherapy (allergy shots) can be helpful in decreasing asthma symptoms caused by specific allergens the child cannot avoid. Immunotherapy is used in conjunction with, not in place of, other asthma therapies.

Exercise. Exercise is a trigger of asthma in most asthmatic children. Exercise-induced asthma may be triggered by rapid breathing of large volumes of cool, dry air (e.g., with mouth breathing during exercise). The symptoms of exercise-induced asthma usually begin after 5 to 10 minutes of exercise and often last from 30 to 60 minutes.

Measures to prevent exercise-induced asthma include the following:

- Warming the air by breathing through the nose or covering the mouth and nose with a scarf when exercising in cold weather
- Using an inhaled beta$_2$-agonist or cromolyn before exercise
- Practicing techniques to decrease hyperventilation (e.g., progressive muscle relaxation, diaphragmatic breathing)

Because athletics and active play are important parts of a child's life, children with asthma should not be restricted from physical activity. Exercise not only increases physical fitness but also enhances self-esteem and offers valuable opportunities for socialization. Swimming is frequently recommended as an ideal sport for children with asthma because the air is humidified and exhaling underwater prolongs exhalation and increases end-expiratory pressure. Other sports that do not require sustained exertion, such as gymnastics, baseball, and weight lifting, are also well tolerated, and if asthma is well controlled, the child can usually participate in any type of sport.

Infection. Viral respiratory infections are the most frequent triggers of pediatric asthma. It is advisable for children with frequent or severe asthma to avoid exposure to individuals with a viral respiratory infection. Children with asthma also benefit from influenza vaccine.

Emotions. Asthma is not caused by psychosocial problems. Emotional upset, however, can exacerbate asthma symptoms. Laughing, crying, or shouting can act as mechanical triggers of bronchoconstriction. Also, a child with asthma may become angry or frustrated and refuse to take medication or adhere to a treatment regimen. Moreover, anxiety during an episode may cause the child to hyperventilate, aggravating asthma symptoms.

Monitoring Symptoms. Asthma symptoms can best be treated if they are detected early. Children and their parents should be taught the subtle early symptoms of an asthma episode (itchy chest or chin, cough, irritability or tired feeling, increased breathing rate, dry mouth, unusually dark circles under the eyes).

A useful device for monitoring breathing capacity is the peak flowmeter, which measures the flow of air in a forced exhalation in liters per minute. Peak flow monitoring can help identify the start of an asthma episode, often before the child is aware of symptoms. It can also help determine the need for treatment modification. Home monitoring of PEFR may be performed several times a day. The results can be compared with the child's normal predicted level and with results obtained over the preceding several days, providing an objective assessment of respiratory status (Box 21-6). Children with moderate to severe persistent asthma should do daily PEFR monitoring. Ideally, PEFR results should be compared with the child's "personal best" value. This value is the number on the meter reached most often over a 2-week period, when the child is feeling well.

Recent studies suggest that parents and children sometimes have difficulty recognizing asthma trouble signs, and even if signs are recognized they do not make appropriate treatment accommodations (Hogan & Wilson, 2003). This

---

CRITICAL TO REMEMBER
Emergency Asthma Management

The following symptoms indicate the need for emergency treatment of asthma:

- Worsening wheeze, cough, or shortness of breath
- NO improvement after bronchodilator use
- A peak flow rate that decreases or does not change (even after use of an inhaled beta$_2$-adrenergic agonist) or that is less than 60% of the child's predicted baseline level or personal best
- Difficulty breathing (the child's chest and neck are pulled in with each breath, or the child hunches over or struggles to breathe)
- Trouble with walking or talking
- Discontinuation of play without the ability to resume activity
- Listlessness and weak cry in an infant; refusal to suck bottle or breast
- Gray or blue lips or fingernails (in which case the child needs emergency treatment *immediately*!)

Modified from Gorelick, M. H., Stevens, M. W., Schultz, T. R., & Scribano, P. V. (2004). Performance of a novel clinical score, the Pediatric Asthma Severity Score (PASS), in the evaluation of acute asthma. *Academic Emergency Medicine, 11,* 10-18.

BOX 21-6 | Monitoring Breathing Capacity With a Peak Flow Meter

The peak flow meter is a device used to monitor breathing capacity in the child with asthma. It measures the flow of air in a forced exhalation in liters per minute. Peak flow monitoring can help identify the start of an asthma episode, often before symptoms are evident. To help children monitor their asthma, a zone system can be explained as a traffic light, making it easier for them to identify and understand differences in peak flow values.

Peak Flow Zones
Personal best: _____

(The personal best is the value reached most often over a 2-week period when the child is feeling well.)

Green: All clear—no asthma symptoms are present (80%-100% of personal best).

Yellow: Caution—acute episode may be present (50%-80% of personal best). A temporary increase in medication may be indicated. Asthma may not be under control. Medication may need to be increased.

Red: Medical alert (below 50% of personal best). An immediate bronchodilator should be taken. Practitioner should be notified if measurements do not return immediately to and stay in yellow or green zones.

How To Use a Peak Flow Meter
1. Remove gum or food from the mouth and stand up.
2. Move the pointer on the meter to 0.
3. Hold the meter horizontally, being sure to keep your fingers away from vent holes and the marker.
4. Relax and take a few moderately slow, deep breaths. Slowly take the deepest breath possible with your mouth wide open.
5. Hold your breath while placing the mouthpiece on your tongue. Seal your lips tightly around the mouthpiece.
6. Blow out as hard and fast as possible. Give a short, sharp blast—not a slow blow. (The meter records the fastest huff, not the longest.) Note the number by the marker on the numbered scale.
7. Repeat three times. Wait at least 10 seconds between attempts. (Be sure to move the pointer to 0 after each try.)
8. Record the highest of the three readings.
9. Ideally, peak flow values are obtained a minimum of once a day, preferably in the morning. Peak flow measurements should be done before and after administration of an inhaled bronchodilator. The number of measurements should be increased during a flare-up.

Modified from National Heart, Lung, and Blood Institute. (2002). *Guidelines for the diagnosis and management of asthma—Update on selected topics,* 2002. Bethesda, MD: National Heart, Lung, and Blood Institute.

observation underscores the need for thorough teaching guidelines for home asthma management, including the following (Burkhart, Rayens, & Bowman, 2005):

- A written asthma plan that includes details of home management and lists indications for seeking physician or emergency department care
- Daily use of a peak flowmeter (in children older than 5 years) to monitor pulmonary status and response to treatment
- Home initiation of inhaled beta$_2$-adrenergic agonists, and oral steroids when beta$_2$-adrenergic agonists and daily control medications are ineffective for resolving symptoms
- Prompt communication with the health care provider for deteriorating respiratory status or reduced response to medication

Medications. Generally, asthma is treated with a combination of medications from two categories: bronchodilators and anti-inflammatory agents. The medication regimen is based on the classification of the child's asthma and can be changed at home according to symptoms and peak flowmeter readings (Box 21-7). It is important to differentiate rescue medications (those used for immediate relief of an exacerbation) and routine medications.

Rescue Medications. Some medications used to relieve an asthma episode are described here:

- *Short-acting bronchodilators:* Beta$_2$-adrenergic agonists, such as albuterol (Ventolin, Proventil), metaproterenol (Alupent), terbutaline (Brethaire), bitolterol (Tornalate), and pirbuterol (Maxair inhaler), relax bronchial smooth muscle and inhibit the release of mediators from mast cells. They are delivered by MDIs or by nebulizer three or four times daily if the child is symptomatic or before exercise.
- *Anticholinergic:* Ipratropium bromide is used in combination with beta$_2$-adrenergic agonists.
- *Mast cell inhibitors:* Cromolyn sodium (Intal), an inhaled nonsteroidal anti-inflammatory drug, prevents asthma symptoms by blocking the release of mast cell mediators. It can be given 30 minutes before exposure to triggers. Another anti-inflammatory asthma medication, nedrocromil sodium (Tilade), is available for use in children age 12 years or older.
- *Systemic corticosteroids:* Prednisone or prednisolone decreases airway inflammation. They are preferably given in short-burst courses of 5 to 7 days.

Routine Medications. The medications used for long-term, routine control of asthma are the same as those used for relief but are administered in different dosages, depending on the classification of the child's asthma. Several additional medications have become available or are being tested for asthma control:

- *Long-acting bronchodilators:* Sustained-release albuterol, salmeterol (Serevent).
- *Inhaled corticosteroids:* Beclomethasone, triamcinolone, budesonide, and flunisolide deliver topical anti-inflammatory action directly to the airway.

BOX 21-7 | Classification of Asthma

Mild Intermittent
- Symptoms less than or equal to twice a week or only with exercise
- Asymptomatic with normal PEFR between episodes; PEFR 80% of predicted rate during exacerbation
- Brief episodes
- Infrequent use of bronchodilator
- Few missed school days
- Rare activity limitation
- Symptoms rarely disturb sleep (less often than twice monthly)

Mild Persistent
- Symptoms more often than twice a week but less than once a day
- Exacerbations may begin to affect activity
- Nighttime symptoms more than twice a month
- PEFR ≥80% predicted

Moderate Persistent
- Daily symptoms occur and bronchodilator used daily; exacerbations two or more times weekly
- More than 9 school days missed per year
- Frequent activity limitation (most days)
- Sleep disturbed by symptoms more than once a week
- PEFR 60% to 80% of predicted

Severe Persistent
- Daily symptoms
- Daily (or almost daily) use of bronchodilator for more than 6 months per year
- Limited physical activity
- Frequent sleep disturbance and exacerbations
- PEFR less than or equal to 60% of predicted

Modified from Kercsmar, C. (1998). Asthma. In V. Chernick, T. Boat, & E. Kendig (Eds.), *Kendig's disorders of the respiratory tract in children* (6th ed., p. 699). Philadelphia: WB Saunders; National Heart, Lung, and Blood Institute. (2002). *Guidelines for the diagnosis and management of asthma—Update on selected topics,* 2002. Bethesda, MD: National Heart, Lung, and Blood Institute.

- *Leukotriene blockers:* Montelukast, and zafirlukast diminish the mediator action of leukotrienes. Zileuton, another leukotriene blocker is given only to children older than 12 years and must be given four times a day to be effective, unlike other leukotriene blockers, which can be given once or twice daily. Montelukast is available in sprinkles and chewable tablets, and can be given to children as young as 1 year old. Zafirlukast is approved for children over the age of 7 years.
- *Anti-immunoglobulin (Ig) E antibody:* omalizumab (Xolair) for allergic-type moderate to persistent asthma is approved for use in children older than 12 years (Buhl, 2003).

Children with mild asthma use bronchodilators as needed for symptom relief. Children and families need to be cautioned not to overuse these medications and to notify the health care provider if the medications are needed more than twice a week or more frequently than every 3 to 4 hours during a 12-hour period.

Children with mild to moderate persistent asthma should take daily anti-inflammatory medications. The inhaled corticosteroid budesonide allows flexible once-daily dosing and is available for administration in ages 6 months and older (Szefler & Pedersen, 2003). It can take up to 3 weeks of daily dosing to realize a therapeutic effect. In addition, beta$_2$-adrenergic agonists are used to relieve symptoms. Long-acting bronchodilators or inhaled corticosteroids are also considered. Theophylline may be given to children who do not respond to mast cell inhibitors. PEFR monitoring helps the child with mild to moderate asthma monitor symptoms and pulmonary function. The family is given a written management plan.

Children with persistent severe asthma take daily mast cell inhibitors, inhaled corticosteroids, and long-acting bronchodilators or leukotriene blockers. Ipratropium bromide and oral corticosteroids are considered for management.

Medication Delivery. Inhaled medications are delivered either by nebulizer (Box 21-8) or by MDI (Box 21-9). Both can be used for older and younger children. A spacer attached to an MDI (see Chapter 14) prolongs the medication transit, effectively delivers the medication to the airway instead of the mouth, improves deposition of the medication by 50%, and makes it easier for younger children to use an MDI (Minai, Martin, & Cohn, 2004). If using a spacer, the child attaches the spacer to the outlet of the MDI, closes the lips around the spacer mouthpiece, activates the canister, and then inhales. Dry-powder inhalers (DPIs) require that patients have an inspiratory flow rate of at least 30 L/min, but they are easier to use and do not contain the ozone-damaging chlorofluorocarbons that some MDIs still use. In addition to the single-dose DPI, a multidose tubular inhaler (for budesonide) and a multidose disk-shaped inhaler (for fluticasone and salmeterol) are now available (O'Connell, 2005).

Text continued on p. 649

| BOX **21-8** | **PARENTS WANT TO KNOW**   Tips on Using a Nebulizer |

1. Use clean hands and a clean area.
2. Take slow, deep breaths through pursed lips to maximize deposition of aerosolized medication in the lungs.
3. Use all the medication in the nebulizer during one treatment. Do not store medication in the nebulizer for later use.
4. The length of the treatment is usually 10 to 15 minutes if the equipment is working properly and the correct amount of medication and diluent are used. If the length of treatments is prolonged, check the nebulizer or the compressor for defects.
5. Rinse the nebulizer in clean water after each treatment. Allow it to air dry after loosely covering it with a clean paper towel. Once daily wash the nebulizer in warm, soapy water and then rinse. Disinfect by boiling for 5 minutes in water or place in a dishwasher (temperature must be >158° F). Air dry the equipment. Never store the nebulizer in a closed plastic bag until it is completely dry. Storing wet equipment promotes the growth of mold and bacteria.

The powered nebulizer delivers a bronchodilator to the child who is having an acute asthma episode. This boy has a viral respiratory infection, which is a common trigger of acute asthma episodes in the pediatric population.

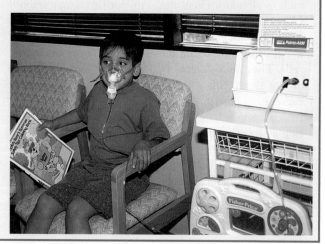

Modified from Brim, S. (1989). A quick guide for home use of inhalant medications. *Pediatric Nursing, 15,* 87-94, by permission of Janetti Publications, Inc. Photo courtesy Parkland Health and Hospital System Community Oriented Primary Care Clinic, Dallas, TX.

| BOX **21-9** | **THE CHILD WANTS TO KNOW**   How to Use a Metered-Dose Inhaler |

1. Stand up. Shake the inhaler well. Remove the cap.
2. Hold the inhaler upright and attach to a spacer device.
3. Tilt your head back slightly and breathe out fully.
4. Place your lips tightly around the mouthpiece of the spacer, press down on the inhaler, and start to breathe in slowly.
5. Breathe in slowly (3-5 seconds) because this allows the medicine to be inhaled more deeply.
6. Hold your breath for as long as possible—up to 10 seconds.
7. Remove the inhaler and breathe out slowly through your nose.
8. Wait at least 2 minutes and shake the inhaler again before repeating the dose.
9. Visible mist escaping from your open mouth indicates improper technique. Do not count that try. Relax and repeat.
10. Rinse your mouth with water if desired.

NURSING CARE PLAN

The Child Hospitalized With Asthma

Focused Assessment

Begin assessment with a thorough history that includes any family history of asthma or allergy and past episodes of asthma, allergy, or other respiratory problems. Ask the parents what treatment has been effective in previous asthma episodes. A new case of asthma may begin as a cough without wheezing. The child may have had recurrent bouts of pneumonia or sinusitis.

Assessment during an acute asthma episode should include vital signs and a careful evaluation of respiratory and oxygenation status. Note respiratory rate and effort, the presence or absence of retractions, the use of accessory muscles, nasal flaring, and pulse oximetry values. Level of consciousness is an important indicator of oxygenation and should be assessed carefully. The chest should be carefully auscultated for breath sounds, noting any adventitious sounds or areas of diminished breath sounds. The child should be assessed for neurologic signs of impending respiratory failure (changes in consciousness, increased fatigue, somnolence). As infants and children become more hypoxic, they may not recognize or interact appropriately with their parents. Inability to resist or struggle or lack of crying during painful interventions is an ominous sign.*

Because tachypnea and a decreased intake of oral fluids may cause dehydration, hydration status should also be assessed (urine output, status of mucous membranes, presence of tears, skin turgor, weight).

A record of the child's routines and habits should be included in the psychosocial history. Previous hospitalizations should be documented because a past experience may affect the child's perception of the current illness. An assessment of the family's knowledge of the disease, degree of adherence to treatment, and growth and development provides the basis for future teaching.

NURSING DIAGNOSES Ineffective Airway Clearance related to bronchospasm and mucosal edema.
Impaired Gas Exchange related to air trapping in the bronchioles.

EXPECTED OUTCOMES The child will:
- Be able to clear the airway, as evidenced by a respiratory rate and rhythm appropriate for the child's age, the ability to expectorate mucus, and normal vital signs for age.
- Have improved gas exchange, as evidenced by clear breath sounds, a pulse oximetry value of greater than 95% on room air, no use of accessory muscles, pink mucous membranes and nail beds, and a capillary refill time of less than 2 seconds.

Intervention

1. Monitor respiratory rate and effort, color, heart rate, and blood pressure every 15 to 30 minutes, with the interval lengthened as the child improves. Auscultate the chest for breath sounds. Monitor arterial blood gas values, pulse oximetry values, and pulmonary function test results. Notify the physician of any significant change (increased respiratory rate and effort, changes in wheezing, retractions, nasal flaring, severe cough, decreased alertness, cyanosis, increased dyspnea, apprehension).
2. Administer humidified oxygen at the ordered flow rate. If the child has chronic carbon dioxide retention, do not exceed 2 L/min.

3. Help the child assume an upright position or position of comfort. The older child may be most comfortable leaning forward on a pillow or overbed table.
4. Administer medications as ordered and monitor for effectiveness. Assess whether medications are effectively relieving the child's symptoms. Monitor the child for side effects.
5. Keep the child on NPO status during periods of respiratory distress, as ordered by the physician.

Rationale

1. Subtle changes in the child's condition may serve as an early warning of increased airway obstruction.

2. Supplemental oxygen decreases hypoxia caused by airway edema, mucus, and bronchospasm. Administration of oxygen to a child with chronic carbon dioxide retention may lead to respiratory depression by decreasing the stimulus to breathe.
3. An upright position aids in expansion of the lungs and decreases pressure on the diaphragm.

4. Short-acting bronchodilators provide relief fairly quickly. IV methylprednisolone begins to reduce airway inflammation.

5. Oral intake is contraindicated for the child in respiratory distress because of the risk for aspiration.

Continued

NURSING CARE PLAN—cont'd

6. Maintain an IV line.	6. IV access is necessary for administering medications and fluids.
7. Ensure that respiratory treatments are given as ordered. Listen to and document the child's breath sounds before and after treatments. Encourage the child to cough and deep breathe, especially after treatments. Suction as needed.	7. Breathing treatments help loosen or eliminate secretions and re-expand lung tissue. Mucous plugs can cause atelectasis and alveolar collapse.
8. Ensure that emergency equipment is available (e.g., appropriate-size ventilation bag, endotracheal tubes, laryngoscope, emergency medication).	8. The child's condition can deteriorate rapidly. Immediate resuscitation may be necessary in the event of severe respiratory distress.
9. Keep the child as calm as possible. Offer support during periods of respiratory distress.	9. Anxiety increases bronchospasms.

* Gorelick, M. H., Stevens, M. W., Schultz, T. R., & Scribano, P. V. (2004). Performance of a novel clinical score, the Pediatric Asthma Severity Score (PASS), in the evaluation of acute asthma. *Academic Emergency Medicine, 11,* 10-18.

Evaluation

- Does the child have clear breath sounds with free movement of air?
- Does the child expend minimal respiratory effort?
- Does the child maintain a patent airway?
- Is the respiratory rate within normal limits for age and is the oxygen saturation greater than 95%?

NURSING DIAGNOSIS Fatigue related to hypoxia and increased work of breathing.

EXPECTED OUTCOME The child will:
- Exhibit decreased fatigue, as evidenced by less irritability and restlessness, uninterrupted sleep periods, and ability to perform usual activities.

Intervention	Rationale
1. Observe the child for signs and symptoms of hypoxia, including restlessness, fatigue, irritability, increased heart rate, and increased respiratory rate.	1. Irritability and agitation may be early signs of hypoxia. Prompt treatment of hypoxia decreases fatigue.
2. Organize nursing care to provide periods of uninterrupted rest and sleep.	2. Periods of quiet decrease stress and promote rest.
3. Encourage the parents' presence, particularly if the child is young.	3. The parents' presence decreases fear and anxiety.
4. Provide for the child's physical comfort. Encourage quiet, age-appropriate play activities as the child's condition improves.	4. Physical and emotional comfort confers a sense of well-being and promotes rest.
5. Implement measures to relieve respiratory distress. Monitor the frequency of nebulized medications.	5. Restlessness, agitation, and inability to sleep are side effects of some asthma medications.

Evaluation

- Is the child able to play or perform usual activities without undue fatigue?

NURSING DIAGNOSIS Risk for Deficient Fluid Volume related to increased respiratory rate, diaphoresis, and decreased oral intake.

EXPECTED OUTCOMES The child will:
- Drink adequate fluid for age and weight.
- Not become dehydrated.

Intervention	Rationale
1. Monitor intake and output, status of mucous membranes, body weight, tearing, and urine specific gravity. Maintain urine specific gravity at 1.002 to 1.030. Monitor electrolyte levels. Observe the child's sputum for color, tenacity, and amount.	1. Rapid respiratory rate, diaphoresis, and increased pulmonary secretions may cause dehydration and increased viscosity of excretions.
2. Maintain IV infusion at the ordered flow rate. Avoid excessive amounts of fluid.	2. Adequate hydration enhances liquefaction of secretions, and thinner secretions are more easily expectorated. Excessive fluids may lead to pulmonary edema.

NURSING CARE PLAN—cont'd

3. Encourage oral fluids when the respiratory distress has decreased, with the amount consumed being determined by the child's calculated needs. Offer favorite fluids. Provide liquids at the bedside.
4. Offer liquids at room temperature. Avoid milk and milk products.

5. Provide a humidified atmosphere.

3. Oral fluids are contraindicated during acute respiratory distress to minimize the risk for aspiration. Children are most likely to drink fluids if they are offered fluids they like.
4. Cold liquids may aggravate bronchospasm. Milk sometimes causes increased coughing and production of mucus.
5. Humidification helps liquefy secretions and helps maintain hydration.

Evaluation

- Does the child ingest adequate fluid for age and weight?
- Does the child maintain a urine specific gravity of 1.002 to 1.030?
- Does the child maintain preillness weight?

- Are moist mucous membranes and good skin turgor present?
- Does the child have urinary output appropriate for age (see Chapter 18)?

NURSING DIAGNOSIS Anxiety related to hospitalization and respiratory distress.

EXPECTED OUTCOMES The child will:
- Exhibit reduced anxiety, as evidenced by a relaxed body position and a decrease in negative behaviors.

The parents will:
- Demonstrate reduced anxiety by verbalizing an accurate knowledge of asthma and participating in the child's care in a calm manner.

Intervention

1. Teach the child techniques to control panic and anxiety and to slow the breathing rate (e.g., visually imagining staying calm, breathing exercises, pursed-lip breathing, belly breathing).
2. Maintain a calm, quiet environment and a reassuring manner. Stay with the child. Provide care efficiently and calmly.
3. Reassure the child that there is someone nearby to assist if breathing difficulties develop. To allay any fears about going to sleep, tell the child that someone will be watching at night. Make the call light available for older children.
4. Use play therapy.

5. Encourage the parents to stay with the child. Praise the parents for rooming-in and supporting the child.
6. Keep parents informed of treatments, routines, and the child's condition.

7. Encourage expression of feelings by child and parents.
8. Avoid the use of sedatives.
9. Explain all procedures in an age-appropriate manner.

10. Facilitate trust by being truthful and acknowledging the discomfort of procedures.

Rationale

1. Concentration on such activities during an asthma episode calms the child and decreases the fear of suffocation.

2. The ability to remain calm decreases the child's oxygen demand and work of breathing.

3. Calm reassurance by the nurse can decrease the child's fear of suffocation and facilitate rest.

4. Therapeutic play allows the child to work through fears in a nonthreatening manner.
5. The presence of a familiar person can decrease fear and anxiety.
6. Reassuring the parents can help calm the child because parental anxiety is quickly transferred to the child. Frequent and accurate updating of the child's condition reassures parents and decreases fear of the unknown.
7. Expressing feelings can help relieve stress and guilt.

8. Sedatives may depress respirations.
9. Procedures and an unfamiliar hospital setting may produce anxiety. Explanations decrease fear of the unknown.
10. Honesty fosters trust.

Continued

NURSING CARE PLAN—cont'd

Evaluation

- Does the child cooperate with and participate in treatment and appear relaxed?
- Does the child obtain adequate rest and sleep?

- Do the parents verbalize decreased anxiety about the hospitalization and the child's condition?

NURSING DIAGNOSIS Interrupted Family Processes related to the possibility of a chronic illness.

EXPECTED OUTCOME The family will:
- Cope with the child's illness and comply with management in a way that promotes the child's normal growth and development.

Intervention

1. Provide opportunities for the family to express feelings. Recognize and accept negative feelings about the child and the illness.
2. Explore previous coping mechanisms used in times of stress.

3. Explain all procedures and treatments.

4. Keep parents informed of the child's condition.
5. Arrange for the family to meet with others affected by asthma. Identify available community resources (see Evolve website).

Rationale

1. This nonjudgmental approach helps the family work through fear, guilt, anxiety, and economic problems.

2. Identification and review of previously successful coping skills can assist the family in dealing with the current crisis.
3. A thorough explanation decreases fear of the unknown and anxiety.
4. Knowledge gives parents a sense of control.
5. Meeting others with asthma can assist with problem solving and provide support.

Evaluation

- Is the family able to provide necessary care?

- Can the family describe how to access helpful resources?

NURSING DIAGNOSIS Deficient Knowledge about the disease process and home management related to inexperience with asthma.

EXPECTED OUTCOMES The family will:
- Identify asthma triggers.
- Describe home management principles.

Intervention

1. Determine the child's and parents' understanding of asthma. Explain unfamiliar procedures and equipment at the child's level of understanding. Teach the family about the disease, its triggers, and prescribed medications and treatments.
2. Help the family identify precipitating factors (e.g., exercise, infections, allergens, weather changes).
3. Explain the role of emotions and stress in the development of asthma symptoms.
4. Teach the child and family about the importance of taking medications as prescribed. Assess ability to afford medications. Provide written information and instructions about medications (names, side effects, dosages, times of administration). Teach the family to recognize signs and symptoms that warrant notification of the physician. Reinforce the need to keep follow-up appointments.
5. Assist in developing an exercise program for the child. Medication may be needed before exercise. Teach the importance of a healthy lifestyle (regular exercise, adequate fluids and nutrition, rest, prevention of infection).

Rationale

1. Understanding increases adherence to treatment.

2. An awareness of triggers may decrease future asthma episodes.
3. Stress and emotional upset can trigger bronchospasm.
4. Knowledge of medications increases adherence to the therapeutic regimen; adherence helps maintain serum drug levels within a therapeutic range.

5. Exercise promotes pulmonary and cardiovascular health and assists the child in leading a normal life.

NURSING CARE PLAN—cont'd

6. Refer the family to a support group.

7. Teach self-management of asthma. Teach the necessary skills for home care. Encourage the child to take charge of asthma. The child should know what triggers to avoid, early warning signs of an episode, the correct use of treatment aids (MDI, DPI, nebulizer, peak flow meter), and proper administration of medications and techniques for stress reduction and relaxation. Encourage the child and family to participate in programs designed to develop effective self-management and decision-making skills.

8. Teach the importance of follow-up care and routine health maintenance, such as keeping immunizations up to date.

6. Meeting with other children and families affected by asthma provides an avenue for expressing feelings and sharing information.

7. Knowledge of asthma decreases anxiety during acute episodes. The frequency and severity of episodes will be minimized if the child knows the appropriate actions for controlling symptoms. Learning about the condition can help decrease anxiety during episodes and increase the child's ability to take appropriate action to control symptoms. The frequency and severity of asthma episodes will be minimized if the child knows what triggers to avoid, the early warning signs of an episode, and the correct treatment of symptoms.

8. Preventing infection and practicing healthy living habits help decrease asthma triggers.

Evaluation

- Do the child and family verbalize an accurate knowledge of asthma and its treatment?

- Do the child and family keep follow-up appointments?
- Does the child resume normal daily activities?

NURSING CARE PLAN

The Child With Asthma in the Community Setting

Focused Assessment

Parents and children usually are successful at managing asthma at home with the proper guidance from health care providers in the community. Whether in an outpatient facility or in a school health office, the nurse needs to know how to assess whether a child is having an asthma exacerbation. It is important to obtain information about the following:

- The child's baseline peak flow reading and the current reading (calculate the percentage of baseline to determine whether the child may need immediate intervention)

- Whether the child's respiratory effort has increased and whether the child complains of "feeling tight" or wheezing
- How often the child has taken an inhaled medication over the past 24 hours
- If the child has recently been exposed to an environmental trigger either at home or at school or whether the child has had a recent upper respiratory infection
- Whether the child is able to engage in usual activities and whether sleep has been interrupted because of respiratory signs

NURSING DIAGNOSIS Risk for Suffocation related to the child's response to environmental triggers and allergens.

EXPECTED OUTCOMES The child will:
- Avoid possible allergens.
The child and family will be able to:
- Detect signs of an impending asthma episode and implement appropriate interventions.

Intervention

1. Teach the child and family how to avoid situations that trigger an asthmatic episode.
2. Review potentially allergenic foods.

3. Remove or limit interaction with pets.

4. Assist the family in obtaining dehumidifier or air conditioner as needed.

Rationale

1. Knowledge about the disease process will decrease possible asthma exacerbations.
2. The child and family need to be knowledgeable about specific food items that trigger an asthmatic response to avoid the offending food items.
3. Removing pets will decrease potential asthma exacerbations because animal dander is a known allergen.
4. The proper electronic device for controlling the environment at home for molds and mildew will help minimize exacerbations.

Continued

NURSING CARE PLAN—cont'd

5. Eliminate the child's exposure to second-hand smoke.

6. Teach the child and family to recognize early signs and symptoms of an asthmatic episode.

5. Second-hand smoke is an irritant and thus minimizing exposure will minimize exacerbation of asthma symptoms.

6. Knowledge of asthma signals will enable the child or parent to control an impending episode before it becomes distressful.

Evaluation

* Is the family able to identify potential allergens that trigger episodes in the child?
* Is the family able to avoid or eliminate environmental triggers?

* Can the family and child describe what action they will take in the event of an asthma episode?

NURSING DIAGNOSIS   Ineffective Airway Clearance related to bronchospasm and mucosal edema.

EXPECTED OUTCOMES   The child will:
* Breathe easily without dyspnea.

The child and family will:
* Be able to use prescribed medications appropriately.

Intervention

1. Review correct use of prescribed medications; write down orders and directions for the family and the school nurse.

2. Teach proper use of peak flowmeter, nebulizer, MDI, DPI as indicated. Be sure the equipment is available for the child to use in school. Teach proper cleaning and maintenance of equipment.
3. Educate the family about prophylactic treatments when appropriate.
4. Review with the child and family the emergency plan if rescue medications are not effective.
5. Explain immunotherapy to the child and family if prescribed.

Rationale

1. It is important for the child and family to understand correct use of short-acting bronchodilators versus long-acting bronchodilators versus corticosteroids. Giving the school written directions improves management.
2. Teaching optimizes the therapeutic benefit of medications as well as adherence.

3. Education will minimize the need for rescue medications.
4. Having a plan of action will decrease the family's and child's anxiety.
5. Allergy shots are often prescribed in allergic asthma. It is important for the child and family to understand the benefits and reasons for frequent visits.

Evaluation

* Are the child and family able to demonstrate proper use of prescribed devices?
* Are the child and family able to discuss when and how to use prescribed medications?
* Does the family keep appointments for immunotherapy?

* Does the family contact the pediatrician or access the local emergency department when prescribed rescue medications are not effective?
* Does the child know when to visit the school health office if having problems at school?

NURSING DIAGNOSIS   Activity Intolerance related to fatigue and shortness of breath.

EXPECTED OUTCOME   The child will:
* Be able to participate in normal daily activities, obtain adequate rest and sleep, and participate in physical activity without shortness of breath.

Intervention

1. Encourage appropriate activities for the child's capabilities, including sports and other school or recreational activities.
2. Review with the child and family symptoms of difficulty breathing, times to take medication, and a plan for rest periods during the day as needed.
3. Discuss with the child and family a plan for adequate sleep and rest.

Rationale

1. Participating in activities will promote a sense of well-being and foster the child's independence.

2. Knowing when to administer rescue medications as prescribed or to limit activity will assist with managing an acute episode.
3. Scheduled rest and adequate nighttime sleep will promote health and minimize fatigue.

NURSING CARE PLAN—cont'd

Evaluation

- Is the child able to participate in normal daily activities?
- Does the child obtain adequate sleep and rest?

- Is the child able to engage in physical activity without excess fatigue?

NURSING DIAGNOSIS Deficient Knowledge related to unfamiliarity with the pathophysiological features of the disease and the treatment regimen.

EXPECTED OUTCOMES The family and child (if age appropriate) will:
- Describe the disease process.
- Demonstrate any associated treatment.

Intervention	*Rationale*
1. Reinforce proper use of medications and prescribed devices; give family members written instructions and advise them to keep a peak flow diary.	1. Having accurate knowledge will decrease anxiety and improve adherence.
2. Encourage verbalization of concerns and fears about diagnosis.	2. Expressing feelings will alleviate anxiety.
3. Reinforce the need to respond to early signs of an asthma episode with prescribed medications.	3. When the child and family have accurate knowledge, they will respond with preventive or emergency interventions in a timely fashion.
4. Encourage contact with day care or school personnel about the diagnosis and the treatment plan.	4. It is important to communicate the plan of care to all individuals caring for the child.
5. Refer the family to appropriate support groups.	5. It is helpful to meet with other children and families affected by asthma because they can offer support, suggestions, and information about the practical aspects of caring for a child with asthma.

Evaluation

- Can the family and child, if appropriate, demonstrate use of devices?
- Can the family describe the correct use of medications and their side effects?

- Have the family and child responded to early signs of an impending asthma episode in a timely and appropriate manner?

BRONCHOPULMONARY DYSPLASIA

Bronchopulmonary dysplasia (BPD) is a chronic obstructive pulmonary disease that occurs as a result of acute lung injury in some infants who have received supplemental oxygen and mechanical ventilation. BPD is now commonly referred to as *chronic lung disease of infancy.*

Etiology

Lung immaturity seems to be a key factor in the development of BPD, but many other factors affect its development as well. Four major risk factors for BPD include premature birth, respiratory failure, oxygen supplementation, and mechanical ventilation (D'Angio & Maniscalco, 2004). Infants with BPD often also have patent ductus arteriosus (see Chapter 22). Because lung development varies among infants, gestational age alone does not always predict the development of BPD.

Incidence

BPD is a significant cause of morbidity and mortality among very-low-birth-weight infants (<1000 g) and infants who have survived RDS. It is the most frequently seen chronic lung condition in infants. Because of treatment advances, the rates of severe BPD in infants with gestational age less than 33 weeks have declined from 9.7% in 1994 to 3.7% in 2002 (Smith et al., 2005).

PATHOPHYSIOLOGY

BRONCHOPULMONARY DYSPLASIA

The pressures of mechanical ventilation damage bronchial epithelium. Macrophages and polymorphonuclear inflammatory cells invade the airways, causing airway edema. Alveolar walls become thickened, and fibrotic changes occur in the airways and alveoli. The continued use of oxygen affects the growth and development of lung structures, significantly reducing the number of developing alveoli.

Cystic and atelectatic areas develop in the lungs, predisposing the infant to pulmonary hypertension. Loss of ciliated cells also may occur, which decreases the lungs' ability to remove mucus and leads to mucous plugs, atelectasis, and pneumonia.

Manifestations

Manifestations of BPD include tachycardia and tachypnea related to decreased oxygenation; an increased work of breathing, retractions, and prolonged exhalation with the increased use of abdominal and accessory muscles; pallor associated with chronic hypoxia; and cyanosis and activity intolerance (feeding, handling). Affected infants also exhibit weight loss or poor weight gain related to the increased metabolic workload, hypoxia, and poor feeding; restlessness and irritability related to hypoxia; wheezing (intermittent or chronic) associated with a hyperresponsive airway; and puckering or pursing of the mouth with flaring of the nares (early signs of impending respiratory distress).

Diagnostic Evaluation

The diagnosis is based on clinical manifestations and radiographic abnormalities. Infants with respiratory symptoms that persist beyond 28 days of life, who need supplemental oxygen by 1 to 2 weeks of age and are still oxygen dependent after 28 days, or who need mechanical ventilation during the first week of life are suspected of having BPD. Chest radiographs may show infiltrates.

Therapeutic Management

Treatment goals for the infant with BPD include maintaining adequate oxygenation to promote growth and development, preventing further lung disease, and promoting healing of the damaged lungs. Treatment consists of oxygen therapy, drug therapy, and nutritional support.

Positive-pressure ventilation should be discontinued as soon as possible. If mechanical ventilation is necessary to maintain life, the lowest possible inflation pressures should be used, together with expiratory times that allow the lung to empty completely. Weaning from the ventilator may be a slow process, requiring constant attention to subtle changes in the infant (Aly, Milner, Patel, & El-Mohandes, 2004).

Oxygen Therapy

Oxygen can be administered through a hood, tent, face mask, or nasal cannula. Oxygen saturation rates should be monitored closely and are usually maintained between 92% and 94%, although there is no consensus on an acceptable saturation for infants with BPD (Walsh et al., 2004). Many infants are discharged from the hospital while still oxygen dependent.

Medications

Diuretics and fluid restriction are initiated to treat pulmonary interstitial edema. Furosemide is the most common diuretic used, with some physicians attempting to change the medication to chlorothiazide and spironolactone once enteral feeding is tolerated. Because infants with BPD often have fluid overload and edema, fluid and electrolyte status should be monitored closely. Supplemental calcium, potassium, and chloride may be indicated for the infant receiving diuretics.

Inhaled bronchodilators, especially albuterol, when given in the early stages of BPD, can lessen airway resistance and decrease the possibility of lung damage. The corticosteroid dexamethasone is often administered during weaning from mechanical ventilation. Corticosteroids should not be given in the first 4 days of life because of the serious side effects of hyperglycemia, hypertension, and gastrointestinal complications (Grier & Halliday, 2005). Careful monitoring during steroid administration is needed because dexamethasone increases lung compliance, putting the infant at risk for pulmonary barotrauma. Administration of inhaled glucocorticoids early on has been shown to decrease the use of systemic glucocorticoid therapy and mechanical ventilation (Grier & Halliday, 2005).

Infants with BPD have frequent infections related to increased susceptibility and exposure to invasive treatments and procedures. After the initial stages of BPD, the risk for infection is probably the greatest risk to survival for these infants. Antibiotics are often needed. Palivizumab is highly recommended for the prevention of RSV in infants with BPD (Grimaldi, Gouyon, Michaut, Huet, & Gouyon, 2004).

Nutrition

The infant needs increased nutritional intake for lung growth and repair beyond that required for normal infant growth. Other factors, such as frequent respiratory exacerbations and feeding problems, also increase caloric needs. A calorie intake of about 150 kcal/kg/day to produce a weight gain of 20 to 30 g/day is an appropriate goal. High-calorie formulas (24 or 27 cal/oz) assist with meeting this requirement, especially in infants in whom fluids are restricted. Medium-chain triglyceride oil or glucose polymers, if added to the formula, increase the calories per ounce.

Prognosis

Most infants with BPD do improve. The mortality ranges from 10% to 25%; death usually is a result of pulmonary complications. Most infants with BPD will require continuing therapy at home, and in some chronic airway hyperreactivity will develop, which may progress to bronchial asthma. Many infants with BPD are rehospitalized during the first year of life because of acute respiratory tract infections. Infants have growth retardation and developmental delay for the first 24 to 36 months of life (D'Angio & Maniscalco, 2004).

Nursing Considerations

Because of their low birth weight and possible RDS, most neonates with BPD are initially cared for in a special care nursery. Nursing intervention before discharge includes meticulous planning for home care, coordinating referrals, and teaching home management.

Home care of the infant with BPD decreases the risk for hospital-acquired infection and reduces health care costs. Care at home also improves social development by encouraging interaction between the child and family.

Preparation for discharge and home care requires a great deal of education and reassurance. Educating the family with a chronically ill or technology-dependent child must begin early with basic care—feeding, bathing, holding, and playing. This care progresses to medical, nursing, and respiratory procedures. The infant may continue to receive supplemental oxygen at home or may have a tracheostomy. Some infants are discharged while they are still ventilator dependent. Families must be taught the necessary precautions for safe use of oxygen in the home (Box 21-10). Before hospital discharge, the nurse contacts emergency services, utility companies, and the telephone company to notify them that a technology-dependent child will be living in their area (Fig. 21-5). Required actions for contacting these services in case of emergency should be reviewed with the family.

ELECTRIC COMPANY
REQUEST FOR SPECIAL CONSIDERATION

Date: _____

Name: _____

Address: _____

_____

Phone: _____

Account Number: _____

Attention: Customer Service

Our infant/child, _____, is under the care of Dr. _____ at _____ for _____.
This condition(s) requires the use of a cardiorespiratory monitor and/or other life support equipment, specifically:

_____

The necessary equipment selected for home care is equipped with a battery back-up system that will power the equipment in the event of a power failure for a **limited period of time.** If a power failure occurs, it is imperative to restore service to this home as soon as possible. Please place this home on a priority list for restoration of electric service. If you have advance warning of a temporary interruption in electric service, please notify the parents so alternative arrangements can be made. If you have questions regarding the specifications of the equipment provided, please contact our equipment provider, Pediatric Home Care Associates.

Thank you for your cooperation.

Sincerely yours,

OUR EQUIPMENT PROVIDER IS: _____

FIG 21-5 **Example of a letter that can be used to notify the local public service company that a technology-dependent child is living in the service area.** *(Courtesy Pediatric Home Care Associates, Garfield, NJ. From Barnhart, S. L., & Czervinske, M. P. [1995]. Perinatal and pediatric respiratory care [p. 662]. Philadelphia: WB Saunders.)*

BOX 21-10	**PARENTS WANT TO KNOW** About Safe Use of Oxygen at Home

Safety Guidelines	Rationale
Secure the oxygen tank in an upright position.	Oxygen tanks are highly explosive. If a horizontally positioned tank explodes, the rapid release of oxygen can catapult it through both animate (human bodies) and inanimate (walls) objects.
Keep oxygen tanks at least 5 feet from heat sources and electrical devices (e.g., space heaters, heating vents, fireplaces, radios, vaporizers).	
Ensure that no one smokes in the room or in the area of the oxygen tank.	Smoking increases the risk for fire, which could cause the tank to explode; escaped oxygen would feed the fire.
Avoid using alcohol-based substances or oil to relieve dryness around your child's mouth (e.g., petroleum jelly, vitamin A & D ointment, baby oil).	Both alcohol and oil are flammable and increase the risk for fire.
Keep a fire extinguisher readily available.	A fire extinguisher may be needed to put out a fire immediately.
Turn off both the volume regulator and the flow regulator when oxygen is not in use.	If the volume regulator is on when the oxygen is turned on, the child might receive a rapid, forceful flow of oxygen in the face that could be frightening and uncomfortable. Oxygen leakage, which might not be detected because oxygen is odorless, can cause a fire.

Evaluating the family's response to the infant's illness and their coping strategies is critical for optimal home management of the infant with a chronic condition. The nurse should help the family identify physical and psychological strengths and weaknesses. Because the care of an infant with BPD can be extraordinarily expensive, the nurse should consider referring the family to social services for access to potential financial assistance.

CYSTIC FIBROSIS

Cystic fibrosis (CF), the most common lethal genetic disease in whites, is a chronic multisystem disorder affecting the exocrine glands. The mucus produced by the exocrine glands (particularly those of the bronchioles, small intestine, and pancreatic and bile ducts) is abnormally thick, causing obstruction of the small passageways of these organs. Although CF is incurable, the life expectancy of affected children has increased dramatically. The median survival age is 33 years, making CF a disease not only of children but also of young adults. The discovery of the mutated gene encoding a defective chloride channel in epithelial cells (named *cystic fibrosis transmembrane conductance regulator*) has improved clinicians' understanding of the disorder's pathophysiologic features and has significantly aided diagnosis.

Etiology

CF is transmitted as an autosomal recessive trait, which means that both parents must carry the gene for the child to be affected. If both parents carry the CF gene, each pregnancy has a 25% chance of producing an affected child. The CF gene has been localized to the long arm of chromosome 7.

Incidence

The incidence of CF in white children is approximately 1 in 4000 live births (Ratjen & Doring, 2003). The prevalence in African Americans is considerably lower, and CF rarely affects Hispanics or Asians. It is estimated that 1 in 28 white Americans carries the gene for CF. Of all patients with CF in the United States, 50% are diagnosed by 6 months of age and 90% by 8 years (Ratjen & Doring, 2003).

Manifestations

Signs and symptoms of CF, the extent of specific organ system involvement, and age at which symptoms begin vary widely among affected children. Symptoms gradually worsen as the disease progresses, and the outcome is eventually fatal.

Respiratory System

Signs and symptoms of respiratory involvement include wheezing and a dry, nonproductive cough (earliest pulmonary manifestations), repeated bouts of pneumonia and bronchitis, and purulent and copious sputum accompanying chronic bacterial infections. The cough at this stage is wet and paroxysmal and may be followed by vomiting. Crackles, wheezes, and diminished breath sounds; accessory muscle use, retractions, hypoxia, and cyanosis; and increased cough, dyspnea,

tachypnea, and cyanosis occur as the disease progresses. Emphysema and atelectasis may develop as the airways become increasingly obstructed with secretions; cor pulmonale and congestive heart failure resulting from fibrotic lung changes can be seen in later stages of the disease. Spontaneous pneumothorax or hemoptysis (blood-stained sputum) is seen in later stages as well. Nasal polyps (10%-25% of patients), sinusitis (evident on radiography in nearly 90% of patients), digital clubbing (Fig. 21-6), and a barrel chest (increased anteroposterior chest diameter) are also noted.

Digestive System

Digestive system involvement is marked by steatorrhea (frothy, foul-smelling stools two to three times bulkier than normal) and flatus. Malnutrition and growth failure are evident despite normal caloric intake; deficiencies in the fat-soluble vitamins A, D, E, and K are caused by an inability to absorb fats. Vitamin A deficiency may lead to xerophthalmia (abnormal thickening of eye tissue), and vitamin K deficiency may result in bleeding, especially in infants. Children with CF are usually thin and underweight, but with adequate treatment most attain normal height. Sixteen percent of children with CF are assigned to less than the 5th percentile for height or weight (Cystic Fibrosis Foundation, 2004). A protuberant abdomen, barrel chest, wasted buttocks, and thin extremities are common.

Meconium ileus in the neonate is the earliest clinical manifestation of CF. Intestinal obstruction later in life, called *meconium ileus equivalent*, may occur and is the result of impacted feces at the ileocecal junction. Rectal prolapse and intussusception may also occur. Liver disease, as manifested by biliary cirrhosis, portal hypertension, and esophageal varices, resulting from obstruction of the bile ducts, is commonly see in the first decade of life, with a prevalence of 41% of patients by age 12 years (Lamireau et al., 2004). Diabetes mellitus has evolved as a complication because of increased longevity. The prevalence of diabetes has been reported upward of 15%, but it is unusual in patients below the age of 10 years (Cystic Fibrosis Foundation, 2004).

Exocrine Glands

Abnormally high concentrations of sodium and chloride in sweat are an early sign of CF (mothers often report that their infants taste salty when kissed). The risk for electrolyte imbalance during hot weather is high; infants are especially prone to development of hyponatremia and hypochloremia as well as dehydration. Many children complain of dry mouth and have an increased susceptibility to infection.

Reproductive System

Reproductive system involvement is marked by an average of 2 years' delay in the development of secondary sex characteristics. Females with CF may have difficulty becoming pregnant because of the thick cervical mucus, which acts as a barrier to sperm. This impairment of fertility should not be relied on as a birth control method. An increased incidence of fetal loss and preterm birth and an increased neonatal mortality are also seen, although a woman with mild CF can carry a pregnancy to term with conscientious prenatal care (Virgilis et al., 2003). Sterility caused by lack of sperm is noted in approximately 98% of male patients with CF; otherwise sexual function is normal.

Diagnostic Evaluation

CF has been called the great imitator because signs of failure to thrive and chronic respiratory infection are signs of many other childhood conditions. In some infants, CF is evident at birth because of symptoms of severe bowel obstruction (meconium ileus) caused by intestinal plugging by thick, tenacious secretions. Many U.S. states now test for CF with the routine newborn screening. Thus the diagnosis is often made in the first 2 to 3 weeks of life (Ratjen & Doring, 2003). The current test uses the immunoreactive trypsinogen assay and has a high number of false-positive results. In those states that do not perform newborn screening for CF, the diagnosis is made as a result of poor growth; bulky, greasy stools; and frequent colds or bouts of pneumonia. The early diagnosis and treatment of CF make a difference in the quality and length of life for these children.

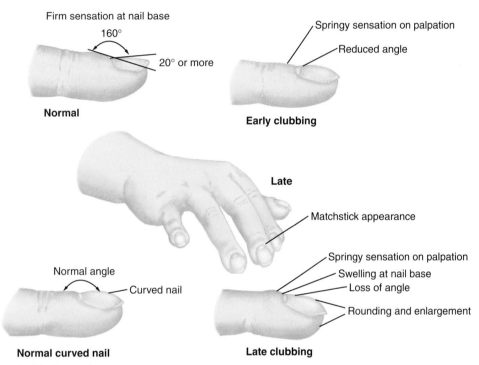

FIG 21-6   **Digital clubbing may be an indication of hypoxia, which often occurs in cystic fibrosis and other respiratory disorders.**

PATHOPHYSIOLOGY

CYSTIC FIBROSIS

CF affects the exocrine glands throughout the body and causes respiratory, digestive, integumentary, and reproductive dysfunction and damage.

Respiratory System

Abnormally thick, sticky secretions cause obstruction of both the small and large airways. Stasis of secretions from bronchial obstruction provides a medium for bacterial growth. Chronic infection causes the release of toxic chemicals that damage lung tissues and alter host defenses within the airways, thus exacerbating the infection and inflammation. Inflammation may also cause bronchospasm, worsening airway blockage. Because airways dilate on inspiration and constrict on exhalation, air trapping occurs in the peripheral airways narrowed by mucous secretions. Hyperinflation is one of the first findings on chest radiographs of a child with CF. Chronic infection leads to atelectasis and eventual fibrosis and destruction of pulmonary tissue.

As the disease progresses, the lungs of almost all children with CF eventually become colonized with *P. aeruginosa,* an organism that most clinicians believe can never be completely eradicated from the respiratory tract but can be controlled with vigorous antibiotic therapy. Chronic respiratory tract infection, impaired oxygen and carbon dioxide exchange causes varying degrees of hypoxia, hypercapnia, and acidosis. Fibrotic lung changes occur as the disease worsens and hypoxia increases. Alveolar hypoxia leads to pulmonary vasoconstriction, increasing pulmonary vascular resistance. Increased pulmonary vascular resistance causes the right side of the heart to work harder to pump blood into the lungs. Enlargement of the

Continued

PATHOPHYSIOLOGY

CYSTIC FIBROSIS—cont'd

Respiratory System—cont'd

right ventricle in response to increased pulmonary resistance (cor pulmonale) results. Congestive heart failure may develop. Pulmonary complications include sinusitis, spontaneous pneumothorax, and hemoptysis. Death in individuals with CF is almost always the result of respiratory failure.

Digestive System

The pancreatic ducts, blocked by thick mucus, are unable to secrete trypsin, amylase, and lipase into the small intestine. Without these digestive enzymes, proteins, carbohydrates, and fats are poorly absorbed. Bowel obstruction from thickened intestinal mucus and pancreatic insufficiency may be present at birth (meconium ileus). The islets of Langerhans in the pancreas are normal in patients with CF, but they

may decrease in number as the disease progresses and the pancreas undergoes fibrotic changes. Type 1 diabetes sometimes develops in older children with CF. Abnormalities of the gallbladder are common.

Integumentary System

The sweat glands of children with CF secrete normal amounts of sweat. The levels of sodium and chloride in the sweat, however, are two to five times the normal range.

Reproductive System

Ninety-eight percent of males with CF are sterile because of obstruction of the deferent ducts and seminal vesicles. Females have reduced fertility because of abnormally thick cervical mucus, which impedes sperm penetration of the cervical canal.

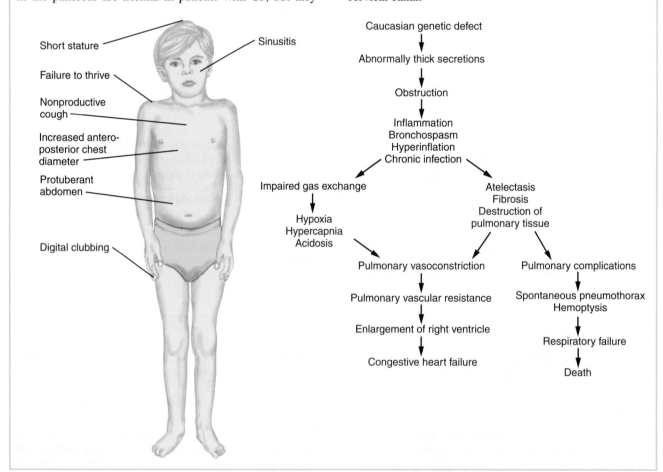

The diagnosis of CF requires a positive sweat test result and either a family history of CF or clinical signs consistent with CF. The sweat test, *pilocarpine iontophoresis*, measures the amount of sodium and chloride in sweat and is simple, painless, and reliable. It is usually performed twice to ensure accuracy. A chloride level greater than 60 mEq/L is considered to be diagnostic for CF; a level of 40 to 60 mEq/L is suggestive of CF and requires repeating the test. A sample of at least 50 mg of sweat is required for accurate results. Because this amount is difficult to obtain from small infants, the sweat test is usually not reliable in infants younger than 3 weeks.

In addition to the sweat test, the following studies may also be performed: 72-hour fecal fat determination; liver function tests (alanine transaminase, aspartate transaminase); fasting blood glucose test; chest radiography; sputum culture (for identification of infective organisms); and pulmonary function tests.

DNA analysis of chorionic villi samples or amniotic fluid testing can establish a diagnosis prenatally. DNA analysis (by buccal smear or blood sample) can also determine whether siblings of the affected child are carriers.

Therapeutic Management

Therapy is individualized for each child and is aimed at preventing and treating pulmonary infections, maintaining optimal nutritional status, and promoting psychologic adjustment. Children with CF are cared for at home most of the time. They are hospitalized during acute pulmonary infections, periodically for IV antibiotic treatment and vigorous chest physical therapy (CPT), and for end-stage disease.

Respiratory Problems

Because chronic respiratory infection is a major cause of lung damage in patients with CF, treatment goals are to relieve airway obstruction by mobilizing secretions, to decrease the number of bacteria by removing secretions, and to treat infections by administering antibiotics.

Segmental percussion and postural drainage (see Chapter 13) with inhalation therapy are performed several times a day to loosen secretions and move them from the peripheral airways into the central airways where they can be expectorated. Newer airway management techniques, such as forced exhalation and positive expiratory pressure devices (PEP valve, Flutter device, acapella device), have been successful in mobilizing mucus. Mucolytic agents (inhaled recombinant DNase or Pulmozyme), inhaled bronchodilators, and anti-inflammatory agents (ibuprofen, steroids, macrolides) are often used with postural drainage to decrease the viscosity of secretions or increase the size of the airways (Bush, Accurso, Macneem, Lazarus, & Abrahamm, 2005).

Exercise is an important part of pulmonary treatment. Some researchers suggest that aerobic exercise, such as jogging or swimming, may be as effective as traditional CPT in relieving pulmonary obstruction and that adherence is more likely (Wagener & Headley, 2003). Children with CF who exercise regularly have fewer pulmonary exacerbations and generally feel better than those who do not.

Antibiotics have played a major role in increasing the life expectancy of children with CF. Some physicians prescribe antibiotics prophylactically, whereas others use them only during periods of active infection (Smyth & Walters, 2003). IV antibiotics are the usual treatment of choice during acute pulmonary exacerbations. Children with CF frequently need higher-than-usual doses of antibiotics because of their rapid metabolism of these drugs. IV antibiotics are usually administered during hospitalization, but home IV therapy is becoming more widely accepted, offering substantial savings and minimizing disruption of daily activities. Oral or aerosolized antibiotics (tobramycin solution for inhalation) may be used instead of IV therapy.

Because they decrease inflammation in the lung, steroids are sometimes prescribed when pulmonary symptoms are unresponsive to antibiotics and increased CPT. Because of the side effects of steroid therapy, including growth retardation and altered glucose tolerance, oral steroids are most often prescribed in short courses of 5 to 7 days (Boat, 2004). High-dose ibuprofen has also been used for its anti-inflammatory properties (Ratjen & Doring, 2003). Azithromycin (administered orally, three times per week) has been shown to improve lung function and decrease the need for IV antibiotics in adults and children older than 6 years. Nebulized hypertonic saline solution (3%-7%) has been well studied in Europe and research suggests that it improves pulmonary function over the short term (Suri, Metcalfe, Wallis, & Bush, 2004). Oxygen therapy is used with caution because many children with CF have chronic carbon dioxide retention and are at risk for oxygen-induced carbon dioxide narcosis.

Digestive Problems

Early in the course of CF, the child may exhibit a huge appetite but not gain weight. Chronic pulmonary infections, increased work of breathing, and malabsorption place an increased caloric and protein demand on the child with CF. The child's calorie requirements are approximately 150% of the normal recommended daily allowance. Children with CF are managed with a high-calorie, high-protein diet, pancreatic enzyme replacement therapy, fat-soluble vitamin supplements, and, if nutritional problems are severe, nighttime gastrostomy feedings or total parenteral nutrition. Fats are not restricted unless steatorrhea cannot be controlled by increased pancreatic enzymes.

Infants are sometimes given a predigested formula (Pregestimil, Nutramigen), which is more easily absorbed than regular formula. Formulas may also be concentrated to provide increased calories. For the older child, caloric intake may be increased with food supplements or enteral tube feedings. The administration of growth hormone has had significant improvement in both height velocity and weight gain in children with CF (Hardin et al., 2005).

Enteric-coated microencapsulated pancreatic enzyme preparations (Ultrase, Creon, Pancrease) are administered with every meal and snack. Enzyme dosage is adjusted according to stool formation: less enzyme with constipation; more enzyme with loose, fatty stools. Still, the enzyme dosage should be individualized for each child and kept as low as possible while still maintaining the child's nutritional status. Only brand-name enzymes should be used because generic enzymes are not bioequivalent. Often, histamine-2 receptor blockers (ranitidine) or proton-pump inhibitors are prescribed to decrease the overly acidic intestines because enzymes will only work in an alkaline environment. Extra salt is added to the diet in extremely hot weather or when the child exercises vigorously.

The Child With Cystic Fibrosis

Assessment

The child with CF should be assessed for signs and symptoms in each of the systems usually affected by the disease and for psychosocial adaptation to this chronic condition.

Respiratory Assessment

The child may have had frequent episodes of pneumonia or bronchitis. Auscultate the chest to detect any crackles, wheezes, areas of diminished breath sounds, or a prolonged expiratory phase of respiration. Note signs of long-standing respiratory difficulty, such as barrel chest or digital clubbing. The respiratory status is assessed by noting the rate, depth, and ease of respirations; the color of the nail beds and mucous membranes; and pulse oximetry. The characteristics of the child's cough and the color, amount, and quality of sputum should be documented, along with any fever. Exercise tolerance and the child's ability to sleep lying down at night should also be assessed.

Digestive Assessment

The nurse weighs and measures the child, plotting the results on a standardized growth chart. Signs of malabsorption (e.g., steatorrhea; loose, bulky stools; protuberant abdomen with thin extremities) should be noted. A diet history is useful in assessing the child's caloric intake. The use of vitamins and dietary supplements should be recorded. Determining the number and consistency of stools assesses the adequacy of intestinal enzyme replacement. Because ulcers and intestinal obstruction often accompany CF, complaints of abdominal pain, blood in the stools, and constipation should be noted. Use of antacids, H_2-receptor blockers, or antireflux medications should also be assessed.

Reproductive Assessment

Girls should be assessed for vaginal itching or drainage, which may indicate a vaginal infection. Contraception should be discussed with adolescents.

Nursing Diagnosis and Planning

The nursing diagnoses and expected outcomes that often apply to children with CF are as follow:

* Ineffective Airway Clearance related to increased pulmonary secretions.

  Expected Outcome: The child will be able to remove secretions from the airway.

* Impaired Gas Exchange related to air trapping within the alveoli secondary to obstruction of the airways by thick mucus.

  Expected Outcome: The child will maintain an oxygen saturation level of greater than 95%.

* Risk for Infection related to tenacious secretions and altered body defenses.

  Expected Outcome: The child will remain free of infection.

* Imbalanced Nutrition: Less Than Body Requirements related to poor intestinal absorption of nutrients.

  Expected Outcomes: The child's nutritional status will improve, and the child will exhibit normal growth; the child's stools will be of normal consistency, frequency, and color.

* Activity Intolerance related to pulmonary congestion and poor absorption of nutrients.

  Expected Outcomes: The child will rest comfortably and will engage in age-appropriate activities.

* Situational Low Self-Esteem related to physical changes from chronic illness.

  Expected Outcome: The child will demonstrate a positive self-concept and feelings of independence, as demonstrated by participating in self-care and in age-appropriate activities.

* Ineffective Coping (individual) and Compromised Family Coping related to chronic illness.

  Expected Outcomes: The child and family will adhere to the treatment regimen, will verbalize feelings about the impact of the illness on their lives, and will use available support systems and community resources.

* Anticipatory Grieving related to a potentially fatal diagnosis.

  Expected Outcomes: The child and family will make realistic plans for the future and will be able to discuss feelings about the child's prognosis.

Interventions

Facilitating Airway Clearance and Gas Exchange

Perform CPT two or three times a day and as needed; perform treatments at least 1 hour before or 2 hours after meals to reduce gastrointestinal upset. The child's respiratory status should be determined before and after CPT. Note the child's tolerance of the procedure. Teach "huffing" (forced expiration) to mobilize secretions. The child should take a deep breath and then exhale rapidly while whispering the word "huff." Administer ordered bronchodilators or mucolytics in conjunction with CPT or as ordered. There are now many techniques from which to choose to facilitate airway clearance (Phillips, Pike, Jaffe, & Bush, 2004). These include PEP valve, autogenic drainage, active cycle of breathing, Flutter valve, Acapella, and the ThAIRapy® vest.

To facilitate gas exchange, administer humidified, low-flow (2 L/min or less) oxygen as ordered. The recommended amount of oxygen should not be exceeded because too much oxygen administered to children who are chronically hypoxic can depress respirations. Elevate the head of the bed, or support the child in an upright position, if the child is dyspneic. Be sure to stay with the child during coughing episodes.

Preventing Infection

Children with CF are prone to respiratory infection, especially airway colonization with *Pseudomonas aeruginosa*, and oral or inhaled antibiotic therapy may be routine. IV antibiotics may be required during acute exacerbations. Pay meticulous attention to hygiene measures, especially handwashing, and teach the child and family to do the same. Monitor the child for signs of respiratory infection (fever, chills, increased respirations, dyspnea, cough, purulent secretions, increased WBC count). Advise the family to avoid exposing the child to others who are ill. Children with CF should receive all routine childhood immunizations at ages recommended by the AAP (see Evolve website). An annual influenza vaccine also is appropriate, on the basis of the recommendations by the Centers for Disease Control and Prevention.

Providing Optimal Nutrition for Growth

Provide a well-balanced diet that is high in calories, protein, and carbohydrates and that includes the child's favorite foods. Oral or enteral high-calorie supplements can increase the child's calorie intake.

The child needs to take pancreatic enzymes (which come as enteric-coated capsules containing the enzyme beads) as ordered within 30 minutes of eating all meals and snacks. The child should not mix the enzymes with hot or starchy foods because enzymes are inactivated by heat. Most older children can swallow the enteric-coated pancreatic enzyme capsules. For children who cannot swallow capsules, the capsules may be opened to display the beads, which can then be mixed with a small amount of a nonprotein food. Because prolonged contact with enzyme beads may cause excoriation of oral mucosa, wipe off any beads that remain on the child's lips. Advise the family to note the color, consistency, and frequency of the child's stools because enzyme replacement is correlated with the child's bowel elimination pattern (e.g., an acceptable pattern is one or two stools daily in older children and more often in infancy). The enzyme dosage should be increased when high-fat foods are eaten. Administer multivitamins, water-miscible, fat-soluble vitamins, and iron supplements as ordered. Monitor the child's appetite and food intake. Extra salt and fluid are required when the weather is hot.

Promoting Increased Exercise Tolerance

For the child in acute exacerbation, provide rest periods between treatments and organize nursing care to ensure periods of uninterrupted rest. The child's activity level is increased as tolerated. Arrange age-appropriate activities geared to the child's energy level. When the child is feeling well, encourage active play and activities, such as swimming and gymnastics.

Meeting the Child's and Family's Emotional Needs

Encourage the child to express feelings about the chronic illness and its effect on feelings of self-worth. Identifying a support system is especially important for adolescents as they begin to take responsibility for their health. Helping the child identify personal strengths and areas of accomplishment will increase the child's self-esteem. Teach parents the importance of fostering their child's independence. As the child grows, encourage discussion about areas of concern, such as dating, sexuality, and peer acceptance. Assist families with the child's transition from pediatric to adult health care providers.

Introducing the family to other families affected by CF can increase problem-solving strategies and facilitate support. Provide information about available community resources, such as the Cystic Fibrosis Foundation and the American Lung Association (see Evolve website). The family also should be encouraged to communicate with personnel at the child's school to ensure coordination of care between home and school.

Although tremendous progress has been made in treating CF, it remains a chronic disease with no cure. Provide the family with honest information about the disease and its prognosis. Refer the family for counseling and listen if they wish to discuss feelings about the disease, the future, and possible death.

Home Care

Preparation for home care involves teaching family members how to carry out CPT, how to provide breathing treatments, and how to give medications at home. Written instructions should describe the specifics of all aspects of the child's care. Families may need assistance in obtaining home care equipment.

Evaluation

- Does the child exhibit improved breath sounds, oxygen saturation greater than 95% on room air, and stable respiratory status?
- Are the child's body temperature and WBC count within normal limits? Has the sputum amount decreased?
- Is the child growing in height and weight along the normal growth curve?
- Are the child's stools of normal consistency, frequency, and color?
- Is the child able to engage in appropriate physical activity?
- Does the child appear to be developing age-appropriate cognitive, emotional, and social skills and an appropriate level of self-care?
- Does the child demonstrate an attitude of acceptance of self and of the illness?
- Does the family demonstrate appropriate coping strategies, adherence to the child's treatment plan, and the ability to access needed resources?
- Can the parents demonstrate CPT, inhalation therapy, and other treatments to be performed at home?
- Are the child and family able to appropriately express feelings of anger, sadness, and fear without guilt?

TUBERCULOSIS

Tuberculosis (TB) is a reportable contagious disease with a high morbidity and mortality throughout the world. Between 1985 and 1992, cases of TB in the United States increased by 20%. From 1992 through 2001, the incidence of TB decreased by 40% as a result of prompt identification of persons with TB and prompt initiation of appropriate therapy (National Center for HIV, STD, and TB Prevention, 2005). The World Health Organization estimates that there are approximately 8 million new cases of TB each year, with 3 million people dying from this disease (Munoz & Starke, 2004). Left untreated, each person with active TB will infect between 10 and 15 people each year.

Etiology

Mycobacterium tuberculosis, an acid-fast bacillus, causes TB. Contamination occurs chiefly through inhalation of droplets from a person with active TB. Droplets produced by coughing and sneezing remain suspended in the air. When they are inhaled, they can reach the bronchioles and alveoli.

The risk for infection by the organism is thought to depend on several physiologic and socioeconomic factors. Most children are infected by a family member, babysitter, or other person with whom they have frequent contact (Box 21-11).

Incidence

Almost 1.3 million cases and 450,000 deaths from TB occur among children each year. Although TB diagnosis and treatment in the United States has improved significantly, it is tempered by TB in foreign-born persons residing in this country. TB in this population is eight times higher than in U.S.-born persons (National Center for HIV, STD, and TB Prevention, 2005). In the pediatric population, TB occurs most commonly in infants and adolescents and in children with immunosuppressive conditions. Of particular concern is the increase in multidrug-resistant TB. Because this is most often caused by poor adherence to drug therapy, directly observed therapy is indicated for anyone being treated for tuberculosis disease (Gupta, Berg, de Lott, Kellner, & Driver, 2004).

Manifestations

Children ages 3 to 15 years are usually asymptomatic, have normal chest radiographs, and can be identified only through a positive skin test. Some children have malaise, fever, night sweats, a slight cough, weight loss, anorexia, lymphadenopathy, or more specific symptoms related to the site of extrapulmonary infection (e.g., kidneys, brain, bone).

Diagnostic Evaluation

Skin testing is the initial method of screening and testing for TB. In most children, skin testing will become positive

---

BOX 21-11	**Risk Factors for the Development of Tuberculosis**

- Contact with adults with infectious TB
- Chronic illness, immunosuppression, HIV infection
- Malnutrition
- Age (infancy, adolescence)
- Nonwhite racial and ethnic groups; immigration from areas with a high incidence of TB
- Urban, low-income living conditions
- Incarcerated adolescents
- Children in close contact with any of the following groups of adults: HIV-infected persons, users of IV or other street drugs, poor or medically indigent city dwellers, residents of nursing homes, migrant farm workers

---

PATHOPHYSIOLOGY

TUBERCULOSIS

The bacillus multiplies in lung tissue, alveoli, and regional lymph nodes. After an incubation period of 2 to 12 weeks, hypersensitivity develops; at that time, skin tests of the infected child will test positive. Most infected children are asymptomatic at the time of the initial positive skin test result.

The *disease* of TB is differentiated from TB *infection* by the presence of clinical manifestations. The risk for development of TB disease is highest in the first 2 years after infection, but many infected children never progress to clinical disease.

The immunologic response of most people is usually strong enough to keep the bacteria from multiplying and spreading. If the host response is adequate, the organism is walled off and the tubercle becomes a healed calcified mass. TB bacilli can remain dormant and cause active disease at a later time if the child's resistance is lowered. If the lesion does not heal and is not walled off, it may continue to enlarge and spread into nearby tissues or it may enter the blood and spread to other sites (middle ear, brain, kidney, bones, joints, skin).

TB disease destroys host tissue. When tubercle bacilli multiply, they may damage tissue so badly that the center of the infected area turns to liquid pus. When this liquid escapes through an airway, it is coughed up as sputum, leaving a tiny hole (cavitation) in the lung. The bacteria-laden sputum is infectious. Children rarely have active TB with cavitation, in which case they can be infectious to others. Because children with primary pulmonary TB have small lesions and minimal cough, they are not contagious.* The duration of infectivity of treated adults and adolescents depends on the drug susceptibility of the infecting organism and cough frequency. Although infectivity usually lasts only a few weeks after treatment is begun, it may last longer if the person fails to take the prescribed medication or is infected with a resistant strain.

*American Academy of Pediatrics, Committee on Infectious Diseases. (2003). *Report of the Committee on Infectious Diseases, 2003 Red Book* (26th ed.). Elk Grove Village, IL: American Academy of Pediatrics.

---

2 to 12 weeks after the initial infection, and once positive, tuberculin reactivity usually continues throughout life, even with treatment.

Skin testing with 5 tuberculin units of purified protein derivative (Mantoux test) is the preferred method of screening. The PPD is administered by intradermal injection on the forearm. The skin reaction is read by an experienced professional 48 to 72 hours after placement. A 15-mm induration in any child older than 4 years is considered a positive sign of TB. Induration of more than 5 mm suggests TB in children younger than 4 years and in certain populations of children. A negative tuberculin skin test does not rule out TB, particularly in infants (Box 21-12).

BOX 21-12	Definition of a Positive Mantoux Skin Test in Children

Area of Induration ≥5 mm
- Children in close contact with persons who have known or suspected infectious cases of TB
- Children suspected of having TB disease (based on positive chest x-ray findings or clinical manifestations of TB)
- Children receiving immunosuppressive therapy or with immunosuppressive conditions, including HIV infection

Area of Induration ≥10 mm
- Children younger than 4 years
- Children with chronic illness (malignant disease, diabetes mellitus, chronic renal failure, malnutrition)
- Children known to have environmental exposure (those born [or with parents born] in regions of the world where TB is highly prevalent; those in close contact with adults who are HIV infected, homeless, users of illicit drugs, migrant farm workers, nursing home residents, or incarcerated or institutionalized persons)

Induration ≥15 mm
- Children 4 years old or older without any risk factors

Modified from American Academy of Pediatrics, Committee on Infectious Diseases. (2003). *Report of the Committee on Infectious Diseases, 2003 Red Book* (26th ed., p. 643.). Elk Grove Village, IL: American Academy of Pediatrics. Used with permission of the American Academy of Pediatrics.

Children with positive skin test results undergo follow-up examinations, which include periodic chest radiography and sputum cultures and smears. Because children often swallow sputum rather than expectorate it, gastric washings to obtain swallowed sputum are sometimes done. A thorough history should be obtained, and all contacts of the affected child should be tested for the disease.

Therapeutic Management and Nursing Considerations

It is important to understand the differences between TB exposure, infection, and disease. *Exposure* is recent and significant contact with an individual diagnosed with contagious TB. The skin test is often negative at this point, and the child is asymptomatic. TB *infection* is defined by a positive skin test. The child continues to lack signs and symptoms of TB, and there may be no chest radiograph changes at this time. Prophylactic treatment is instituted to prevent the progression to disease. TB *disease* is defined by chest radiograph changes along with signs and symptoms of disease and a positive skin test.

Tuberculosis Infection

After a chest radiograph is obtained, asymptomatic children with positive tuberculin tests and no previous history of TB

receive isoniazid (INH) for 9 months. For children with human immunodeficiency virus (HIV) infection, a minimum of 12 months of treatment is recommended. Children with drug-resistant TB need an individualized treatment regimen. Household contacts (especially children younger than 4 years), immunosuppressed contacts, and contacts who were exposed during the previous 3 months should undergo skin testing and chest radiography. Even if the skin test is negative, asymptomatic contacts should receive INH for at least 12 weeks after contact has been broken until a negative skin test can be confirmed (AAP, Committee on Infectious Diseases, 2003). Reporting cases of TB is required by law in all states in the United States. Nurses should assist in searching for the source case and others infected by the source case.

Bacillus Calmette-Guérin vaccine is the only anti-TB vaccine available. Unfortunately, the vaccine varies in the immunity it provides and has resulted in serious reactions. In the United States, it is used mainly for (1) children with negative chest x-ray readings and skin test results who have had repeated exposures to untreated or ineffectively treated contagious TB who cannot be removed from the exposure or treated with INH and (2) children who are exposed continually to a person with contagious pulmonary tuberculosis resistant to INH and rifampin and the child cannot be removed from this exposure (AAP, Committee on Infectious Diseases, 2003).

Tuberculosis Disease

A 6-month course of antituberculous medications (INH, rifampin, and pyrazinamide for the first 2 months; INH and rifampin for the next 4 months), optimal nutrition, and preventing exposure to infection, which could further compromise the child's already challenged immune system, are the mainstays of treatment (AAP, Committee on Infectious Diseases, 2003). Most children are treated at home. The nurse needs to emphasize to the family the importance of following the prescribed medication regimen meticulously and for the appropriate length of time because inappropriate medication dosing contributes to the growth of drug-resistant organisms.

Children with TB may be hospitalized, depending on the severity of the disease, the age of the child, the need for more extensive testing, or the child's family and social environment. Unless the child is acutely ill, bed rest is not required. Isolation usually is not required because children with TB are rarely contagious.

Prevention and Screening

Promptly identifying cases and treating appropriately are the focus of disease prevention (Hoskyns, 2003). Because most children are infected by a family member, the best way to stop transmission of the disease is to identify those who are infected and to provide TB therapy.

Early detection of the disease is accomplished by screening. Children at high risk for TB should be tested annually with the Mantoux test. Annual skin testing of children in low-prevalence areas who have no risk factors is not indicated.

KEY CONCEPTS

- Infants and children younger than 3 years are at increased risk for development of respiratory tract infections because of their immature immune system, smaller airways, and underdeveloped supporting cartilage.
- At birth, the neonate must inflate the lungs, establish continuous breathing, and transfer the gases needed to meet metabolic needs.
- The severity of allergic rhinitis can be decreased through the early identification and treatment of manifestations.
- Respiratory obstruction increases during crying, and stridor increases when the child is supine with the neck flexed.
- The only reliable way to determine whether pharyngitis is viral or bacterial in origin is with a throat culture.
- Manifestations of bleeding after a tonsillectomy include frequent swallowing; restlessness; a fast, thready pulse; and the vomiting of bright-red blood.
- The mucosal edema associated with croup can sometimes be decreased by steam from hot running water in a closed bathroom or by a cool humidifier or by taking the child out into the cool, humid night air.
- Children with croup who have stridor at rest, cyanosis, severe agitation or fatigue, or moderate to severe retractions or who are unable to take oral fluids should be seen in the emergency department.
- The four Ds of epiglottitis are drooling, dysphagia, dysphoria, and distressed inspiratory efforts.
- Visual examination of the epiglottis is contraindicated if epiglottitis is suspected because the examination tools can provoke laryngospasm and airway obstruction.
- Because RSV infection is highly communicable, during RSV season hospitalized infected children should be placed in contact isolation. Good handwashing should be emphasized and gowns worn when there is a chance that clothing might be soiled.
- Oxygen needs can be decreased in the child in respiratory distress by scheduling nursing care to allow the child periods of rest.
- If a child is aphonic and not breathing, the guidelines for management of an obstructed airway should be followed.
- During an apneic episode, the time and duration of the episode, color change, bradycardia, oxygen saturation, what the infant was doing before the apneic period, and any actions that stimulated breathing should be recorded.
- Healthy infants should be placed on their sides or backs for sleeping to reduce the risk for SIDS.
- When interviewing parents of an infant suspected of dying of SIDS, the nurse should avoid any implication of fault on the part of the parents.
- Asthma is the most common chronic disease of childhood. Asthma is characterized by bronchospasm, edema of the bronchiolar mucous membranes, and increased secretion of mucus in the airways.
- Asthmatic symptoms signaling spasm of the smooth muscle of the bronchi and bronchioles may be triggered by a variety of stimuli, including allergens, cold air, weather changes, infection, exercise, fatigue, and emotional distress.
- Status asthmaticus, or continued severe respiratory distress despite medical treatment, places the child in imminent danger of respiratory arrest and requires immediate hospitalization.
- Nursing care of the child with a severe asthma episode includes administration of inhaled or IV bronchodilators or corticosteroids, as ordered; providing oxygen therapy; providing IV fluids; and assisting with intubation and mechanical ventilation.
- Nursing care of the child with chronic asthma includes administration of prescribed medications and treatments and education of the child and family about medications, how to avoid triggers of asthma symptoms, how to recognize early warning signs of an asthma episode, and measures that can be taken to prevent severe asthma episodes.
- BPD is a chronic obstructive pulmonary disease characterized by thickening of the alveolar walls and bronchiolar epithelium. BPD occurs primarily in premature and low-birth-weight infants who have been mechanically ventilated with high concentrations of oxygen for prolonged periods.
- Nursing care of the infant with BPD includes supportive interventions to maintain adequate oxygenation and the provision of appropriate stimulation to promote normal growth and development.
- CF is an inherited (autosomal recessive), multisystem disorder characterized by widespread dysfunction of the exocrine glands. Abnormal secretion of thick, tenacious mucus causes obstruction and dysfunction of the pancreas, lungs, salivary glands, sweat glands, and reproductive organs.
- Nursing care of the child with CF includes maintaining a patent airway by administering bronchodilators and performing or supervising respiratory treatments, administering antibiotics and pancreatic enzymes, and teaching the child and family about CF and its treatment.
- Nursing care of the child with TB includes administering and evaluating TB skin tests and administering anti-TB medications as ordered. The nurse also instructs the child and family about the importance of adequate rest, a nutritionally adequate diet, adherence to the medication regimen, and ways to prevent the transmission of TB infection.

ANSWERS TO
CRITICAL THINKING EXERCISE 21-1

1. Children often leave the hospital with pain medication (usually liquid acetaminophen with codeine) ordered to be given as needed. Ordering the medication this way relies on the parent or caregiver to assess the child's pain before administering the analgesic. Further research is needed to determine how well parents understand and accurately assess their child's pain during the initial postoperative period. In addition, undermedication can be related to the following*:

   - Inadequate doses ordered
   - Parents' fear of overmedication
   - Parents' fear that the child will become addicted to the medication
   - Inadequate instructions for medicating
   - Expectations regarding the amount of pain associated with the procedure
   - Difficulty getting the child to swallow the medication

2. Inadequate pain relief can adversely affect the child's behavior and ability to rest. In the child who has had a tonsillectomy, more serious effects are related to the refusal of fluids. Children who have had tonsils removed can have moderate to severe postoperative pain. For most effective postoperative progress, pain medication should be administered regularly around the clock and not as needed. Nurses should emphasize this to parents before discharge. If the facility allows, a postoperative phone call to the child's home to inquire about the child and remind the parent about continuous pain relief may be helpful.

*Helgadottir, H. L., & Wilson, M. E. (2004). Temperament and pain in 3 to 7-year-old children undergoing tonsillectomy. *Journal of Pediatric Nursing, 19*, 204-213.

REFERENCES AND READINGS

Adair, S. M. (2003). Pacifier use in children: A review of recent literature. *Pediatric Dentistry, 25*, 449-458.

Aly, H., Milner, J. D., Patel, K., & El-Mohandes, A. A. (2004). Does the experience with the use of nasal continuous positive airway pressure improve over time in extremely low birth weight infants? *Pediatrics, 114*, 697-702.

American Academy of Family Physicians, American Academy of Otolaryngology–Head and Neck Surgery, American Academy of Pediatrics Subcommittee on Otitis Media With Effusion. (2004). Otitis media with effusion. *Pediatrics, 113*, 1412-1429.

American Academy of Pediatrics. (1992). *AAP Task Force on Infant Positioning and SIDS*. Elk Grove Village, IL: American Academy of Pediatrics.

American Academy of Pediatrics. (2004). Clinical practice guideline: Diagnosis and management of acute otitis media. *Pediatrics, 113*, 1451-1465.

American Academy of Pediatrics. (2005). The changing concept of sudden infant death syndrome: Diagnostic coding shifts, controversies regarding the sleeping environment, and new variables to consider in reducing risk. *Pediatrics, 116*, 1245-1255.

American Academy of Pediatrics, Committee on Fetus and Newborn. (2003). Apnea, sudden infant death syndrome, and home monitoring. *Pediatrics, 111*, 914-917.

American Academy of Pediatrics, Committee on Infectious Diseases. (2003). *Report of the Committee on Infectious Diseases, 2003 Red Book* (26th ed.). Elk Grove Village, IL: American Academy of Pediatrics.

American Lung Association. Epidemiology and Statistics Unit, Best Practice and Program Services. (2002). *Trends in asthma morbidity and mortality*. New York: American Lung Association.

Arshad, S., Bateman, B., & Matthews, S. (2003). Primary prevention of asthma and atopy during childhood by allergen avoidance in infancy: A randomised controlled study. *Thorax, 58*, 489-493.

Arshad, S. H., Kurukulaaratchy, R. J., Fenn, M., & Matthews, S. (2005). Early life risk factors for current wheeze, asthma, and bronchial hyperresponsiveness at 10 years of age. *Chest, 127*, 502-508.

Baroody, F. M. (2003). Allergic rhinitis: broader disease effects and implications for management. *Otolaryngology and Head and Neck Surgery, 128*, 616-631.

Berger, W. E. (2004). Allergic rhinitis in children: Diagnosis and management strategies. *Paediatric Drugs, 6*, 233-250.

Bhattacharyya, N., Jones, D. T., Hill, M., & Shapiro, N. L. (2004). The diagnostic accuracy of computed tomography in pediatric chronic rhinosinusitis. *Archives of Otolaryngology, Head and Neck Surgery, 130*, 1029-1032.

Bhatt-Mehta, V., & Schumacher, R. E. (2003). Treatment of apnea of prematurity. *Paediatric Drugs, 5*, 195-210.

Blaiss, M. (2004). Current concepts in therapeutic strategies for allergic rhinitis in school-age children. *Clinical Therapeutics, 26*, 1876-1889.

Boat, T. (2004). Cystic fibrosis. In R. Behrman, R. Kliegman, & H. Jenson (Eds.). *Nelson textbook of pediatrics* (17th ed., pp. 1437-1450). Philadelphia: WB Saunders.

Bowd, A. D. (2005). Otitis media: health and social consequences for aboriginal youth in Canada's north. *International Journal of Circumpolar Health, 64*, 5-15.

Bradley, J. S. (2002). Old and new antibiotics for pediatric pneumonia. *Seminars in Respiratory Infections, 17*, 57-64.

Buhl, R. (2003). Omalizumab (Xolair) improves quality of life in adult patients with allergic asthma: A review. *Respiratory Medicine, 97*, 123-129.

Burkhart, P.V., Rayens, M. K., & Bowman, R. K. (2005). An evaluation of children's metered-dose inhaler technique for asthma medications. *Nursing Clinics of North America, 40*, 167-182.

Bush, A., Accurso, F., Macneem W., Lazarus, S. C., & Abrahamm E. (2005). Cystic fibrosis, pediatrics, control of breathing, pulmonary physiology and anatomy, and surfactant biology in AJRCCM in 2004. *American Journal of Respiratory and Critical Care Medicine, 171*, 545-553.

Cantani, A., & Micera, M. (2005). Epidemiology of passive smoke: A prospective study in 589 children. *European Review for Medical and Pharmacologic Sciences, 9*, 23-30.

Casey, J. R., & Pichichero, M. E. (2004). Meta-analysis of cephalosporin versus penicillin treatment of group A streptococcal tonsillopharyngitis in children. *Pediatrics, 113*, 1816-1819.

Castile, R. (2004). Novel techniques for assessing infant and pediatric lung function and structure. *Pediatric Infectious Disease Journal, 23*(11 Suppl), S246-S253.

Centers for Disease Control and Prevention. (1997a). Case definitions for infectious conditions under public health surveillance. *MMWR: Morbidity and Mortality Weekly Report, 46*, 1-55.

Centers for Disease Control and Prevention. (1997b). Screening for tuberculosis and tuberculosis infection in high-risk populations: Recommendations of the Advisory Council for the Elimination of Tuberculosis. *MMWR: Morbidity and Mortality Weekly Report, 46*, 18-34.

Cetinkaya, F., Tufekci, B. S., & Kutluk, G. (2004). A comparison of nebulized budesonide, and intramuscular, and oral dexamethasone for treatment of croup. *International Journal of Pediatric Otorhinolaryngology, 68*, 453-456.

Chernick, V., Boat, T., & Kendig, E. (Eds.). (1998). *Kendig's disorders of the respiratory tract in children* (6th ed.). Philadelphia: WB Saunders.

Cohen, R. (2004). Defining the optimum treatment regimen for azithromycin in acute tonsillopharyngitis. *The Pediatric Infectious Disease Journal, 23(2 Suppl.),* S129-S134.

Contopoulos-Ioannidis, D. G., & Ioannidis, J. P. (2004). Treatment options for acute sinusitis in children. *Current Allergy and Asthma Report, 4,* 471-477.

Contopoulos-Ioannidis, D. G., Ioannidis, J. P., & Lau, J. (2003). Acute sinusitis in children: Current treatment strategies. *Paediatric Drugs.* 5 (2), 71-80.

Cystic Fibrosis Foundation. (2004). *Patient registry 2003 annual data report.* Bethesda, MD: Cystic Fibrosis Foundation.

D'Angio, C. T., & Maniscalco, W. M. (2004). Bronchopulmonary dysplasia in preterm infants: Pathophysiology and management strategies. *Paediatric Drugs, 6,* 303-330.

Domachowske, J. B., & Rosenberg, H. F. (2005). Advances in the treatment and prevention of severe viral bronchiolitis. *Pediatric Annals, 34,* 35-41.

Eren, S., Balci, A. E., Dikici, B., Doblan, M., & Eren, M. N. (2003). Foreign body aspiration in children: Experience of 1160 cases. *Annals of Tropical Paediatrics, 23,* 31-37.

Esposito, S., Blasi, F., Bosis, S., Droghetti, R., Faelli, N., Lastrico, A., & Principi, N. (2004). Aetiology of acute pharyngitis: The role of atypical bacteria. *Journal of Medical Microbiology, 53,* 645-651.

Esposito, S., & Principi, N. (2002). Emerging resistance to antibiotics against respiratory bacteria: Impact on therapy of community-acquired pneumonia in children. *Drug Resistance Updates, 5,* 73-87.

Federierico, M., & Liu, A. (2003). Overcoming childhood asthma disparities of the inner-city poor. *Pediatric Clinics of North America, 50,* 655-675.

Fitzgerald, D. A., & Kilham, H. A. (2004). Bronchiolitis: Assessment and evidence-based management. *The Medical Journal of Australia, 180,* 399-404.

Garofalo, R. P., Hintz, K. H, Hill, V., Patti, J., Ogra, P. L., & Welliver, R. C., Sr. (2005). A comparison of epidemiologic and immunologic features of bronchiolitis caused by influenza virus and respiratory syncytial virus. *Journal of Medical Virology, 75,* 282-289.

Gerber, M. A., & Shulman, S. T. (2004). Rapid diagnosis of pharyngitis caused by group A streptococci. *Clinical Microbiology Reviews, 17,* 571-580.

Gorelick, M. H., Stevens, M. W., Schultz, T. R., & Scribano, P. V. (2004). Performance of a novel clinical score, the Pediatric Asthma Severity Score (PASS), in the evaluation of acute asthma. *Academic Emergency Medicine, 11,* 10-18.

Grier, D. G., & Halliday, H. L. (2005). Management of bronchopulmonary dysplasia in infants: Guidelines for corticosteroid use. *Drugs, 65,* 15-29.

Grimaldi, M., Gouyon, B., Michaut, F., Huet, F., & Gouyon, J. B. (2004). Severe respiratory syncytial virus bronchiolitis: Epidemiologic variations associated with the initiation of palivizumab in severely premature infants with bronchopulmonary dysplasia. *The Pediatric Infectious Disease Journal, 23,* 1081-1085.

Guilbert, T., & Drawiec, M. (2003). Natural history of asthma. *Pediatric Clinics of North America, 50,* 523-538.

Gupta, S., Berg, D., de Lott, F., Kellner, P., & Driver C. (2004). Directly observed therapy for tuberculosis in New York City: Factors associated with refusal. *International Journal of Tuberculosis and Lung Disease, 8,* 480-485.

Halken, S. (2004). Prevention of allergic diseases in childhood: Clinical and epidemiological aspects of primary and secondary allergy prevention. *Pediatric Allergy and Immunology, 15(Suppl. 16),* 4-5, 9-32.

Hammer, J. (2004). Acquired upper airway obstruction. *Paediatric Respiratory Reviews, 5,* 25-33.

Hardin, D. S., Rice, J., Ahn, C., Ferkol, T., Howenstine, M., Spears, S., Prestidge, C., Seilheimer, D. K., & Shepherd, R. (2005). Growth hormone treatment enhances nutrition and growth in children with cystic fibrosis receiving enteral nutrition. *The Journal of Pediatrics, 146,* 324-328.

Helgadottir, H. L., & Wilson, M. E. (2004). Temperament and pain in 3 to 7-year-old children undergoing tonsillectomy. *Journal of Pediatric Nursing, 19,* 204-213.

Hogan, M. B., & Wilson, N. W. (2003). Asthma in the school-aged child. *Pediatric Annals, 32,* 20-25.

Holman, R. C., Curns, A. T., Cheek, J. E., Bresee, J. S., Singleton, R. J., Carver, K., & Anderson, L. J. (2004). Respiratory syncytial virus hospitalizations among American Indian and Alaska Native infants and the general United States infant population. *Pediatrics, 114,* e437-e444.

Hoskyns, W. (2003). Paediatric tuberculosis. *Postgraduate Medical Journal, 79,* 272-278.

Huang, W. H., & Fang, S. Y. (2004). High prevalence of antibiotic resistance in isolates from the middle meatus of children and adults with acute rhinosinusitis. *American Journal of Rhinology, 18,* 387-391.

Isaacson, G. (2004). Pediatric intracapsular tonsillectomy with bipolar electrosurgical scissors. *Ear, Nose and Throat Journal, 83,* 702, 704-706.

Kallstrom, T. J. (2004). Evidence-based asthma management. *Respiratory Care, 49,* 783-792.

Kercsmar, C. (1998). Asthma. In V. Chernick, T. Boat, & E. Kendig (Eds.), *Kendig's disorders of the respiratory tract in children* (6th ed., p. 699). Philadelphia: WB Saunders.

Kukla, L., Hruba, D., & Tyrlik, M. (2004). Influence of prenatal and postnatal exposure to passive smoking on infants' health during the first six months of their life. *Central European Journal of Public Health, 12,* 157-160.

Lam, B. C., Ng, Y. K., & Wong, K. Y. (2005). Randomized trial comparing two natural surfactants (Survanta vs. bLES) for treatment of neonatal respiratory distress syndrome. *Pediatric Pulmonology, 39,* 64-69.

Lamireau, T., Monnereau, S., Martin, S., Marcotte, J. E., Winnock, M., & Alvarez, F. (2004). Epidemiology of liver disease in cystic fibrosis: A longitudinal study. *Journal of Hepatology, 41,* 920-925.

Lee, T., Brugge, D., Francis, C., & Fisher, O. (2003). Asthma prevalence among inner-city Asian-American schoolchildren. *Public Health Report, 118,* 215-220.

Leung, A. K., Kellner, J. D., & Johnson, D. W. (2004). Viral croup: A current perspective. *Journal of Pediatric Healthcare, 18,* 297-301.

Low, D. E., Pichichero, M. E., Schaad, U. B. (2004). Optimizing antibacterial therapy for community-acquired respiratory tract infections in children in an era of bacterial resistance. *Clinical Pediatrics, 43,* 135-151.

Lynch, E. L., & Thomas, T. L. (2004). Pediatric considerations in chemical exposures. *Pediatric Emergency Medicine, 20,* 198-208.

Malloy, M. H., & Freeman, D. H. (2004). Age at death, season, and day of death as indicators of the effect of the back to sleep program on sudden infant death syndrome in the United States, 1992-1999. *Archives of Pediatric and Adolescent Medicine, 158,* 359-365.

Midulla, F., Guidi, R., Tancredi, G., Quattrucci, S., Ratjen, F., Bottero, S., Vestiti, K., Francalanci, P., & Cutrera, R. (2004). Microaspiration in infants with laryngomalacia. *Laryngoscope, 114,* 1592-1596.

Milgrom, H., & Leung, D. (2004). Allergic rhinitis. In R. Behrman, R. Kliegman, & H. Jenson (Eds.). *Nelson textbook of pediatrics* (17th ed., pp. 759-760). Philadelphia: WB Saunders.

Minai, B. A., Martin, J. E., & Cohn, R. C. (2004). Results of a physician and respiratory therapist collaborative effort to improve long-term metered-dose inhaler technique in a pediatric asthma clinic. *Respiratory Care, 49,* 600-605.

Munoz, F., & Starke, J. (2004). Tuberculosis *(Mycobacterium tuberculosis).* In R. Behrman, R. Kliegman, & H. Jenson (Eds.). *Nelson textbook of pediatrics* (17th ed., pp. 956-972). Philadelphia: WB Saunders.

National Center for Health Statistics [NCHS] (2006a). *Early release of selected estimates based on data from the January-March, 2006 National Health Interview Survey.* Accessed October 29, 2006 at *www.cdc.gov/nchs/.*

National Center for Health Statistics [NCHS] (2006b). *Summary health statistics for U.S. children: National Health Interview Survey, 2004.* Accessed October 29, 2006 at *www.cdc.gov/nchs/.*

National Center for HIV, STD, and TB Prevention. (June 13, 2005). *The changing epidemiology of TB.* Retrieved June 20, 2005, from *www.cdcnp.org/scripts/tb/tb.asp.*

National Heart, Lung, and Blood Institute. (2002). *Guidelines for the diagnosis and management of asthma—Update on selected topics, 2002.* Bethesda, MD: National Heart, Lung, and Blood Institute.

Navaie-Waliser, M., Misener, M., Mersman, C., & Lincoln, P. (2004). Evaluating the needs of children with asthma in home care: The vital role of nurses as caregivers and educators. *Public Health Nursing, 21,* 306-315.

O'Connell, E. J. (2005). Optimizing inhaled corticosteroid therapy in children with chronic asthma. *Pediatric Pulmonology, 39,* 74-83.

Olympia, R. P., Khine, H., & Avner, J. R. (2005). Effectiveness of oral dexamethasone in the treatment of moderate to severe pharyngitis in children. *Archives of Pediatric and Adolescent Medicine, 159,* 278-282.

Ovetchkine, P., & Cohen, R. (2003). Shortened course of antibacterial therapy for acute otitis media. *Paediatric Drugs, 5,* 133-140.

Ozkan, H., Duman, N., Kumral, A., & Gulcan, H. (2004). Synchronized ventilation of very-low-birth-weight infants; report of 6 years' experience. *Journal of Fetal and Neonatal Medicine, 15,* 261-265.

Panitch, H. B. (2003). Respiratory syncytial virus bronchiolitis: Supportive care and therapies designed to overcome airway obstruction. *Pediatric Infectious Disease Journal, 22(Suppl. 2),* S83-S87.

Pastore, G., Guala, A., & Zaffaroni, M. (2003). Back to sleep: risk factors for SIDS as target for public health campaigns. *Journal of Pediatrics, 142,* 453-454.

Pettigrew, M. M., Gent, J. F., Triche, E. W., Belanger, K. D., Bracken, M. B., & Leaderer, B. P. (2004). Association of early-onset otitis media in infants and exposure to household mold. *Paediatric Perinatal Epidemiology, 18,* 441-447.

Phillips, G. E., Pike, S. E., Jaffe, A., & Bush, A. (2004). Comparison of active cycle of breathing and high-frequency oscillation jacket in children with cystic fibrosis. *Pediatric Pulmonology, 37,* 71-75.

Ratjen, F., & Doring, G. (2003). Cystic fibrosis. *Lancet, 361,* 681-689.

Rovers, M. M., Schilder, A. G., Zielhuis, G. A., & Rosenfeld, R. M. (2004). Otitis media. *Lancet, 363,* 465-473.

Scarfone, R. J. (2005). Controversies in the treatment of bronchiolitis. *Current Opinions in Pediatrics, 17,* 62-66.

Schoenwetter, W. F., Dupclay, L., Appajosyula, S., Botteman, M. F., & Pashos, C. L. (2004). Economic impact and quality-of-life burden of allergic rhinitis. *Current Medical Research Opinions, 20,* 305-317.

Shah, R. K., Roberson, D. W., & Jones, D. T. (2004). Epiglottitis in the *Hemophilus influenzae* type B vaccine era: Changing trends. *Laryngoscope, 114,* 557-560.

Silvestri, J. M., Lister, G., Corwin, M. J., Smok-Pearsall, S. M., Baird, T. M., Crowell, D. H., Cantey-Kiser, J., Hunt, C. E., Tinsley, L., Palmer, P. H., Mendenhall, R. S., Hoppenbrouwers, T. T., Neuman, M. R., Weese-Mayer, D. E., & Willinger, M. (2005). Factors that influence use of a home cardiorespiratory monitor for infants: The collaborative home infant monitoring evaluation. *Archives of Pediatric and Adolescent Medicine, 159,* 18-24.

Smith, V. C., Zupancic, J. A., McCormick, M. C., Croen, L. A., Greene, J., Escobar, G. J., & Richardson, D. K. (2005). Trends in severe bronchopulmonary dysplasia rates between 1994 and 2002. *Journal of Pediatrics, 146,* 469-473.

Smyth, A., & Walters, S. (2003). Prophylactic antibiotics for cystic fibrosis. *Cochrane Database of Systematic Reviews,* CD001912.

Sobel, S. E., Samadi, D. S., Kazahaya, K., & Tom, L. W. (2005). Trends in the management of pediatric chronic sinusitis: Survey of the American Society of Pediatric Otolaryngology. *Laryngoscope, 115,* 78-80.

Sockrider, M. (2003). Asthma prevalence among inner-city Asian American school children. *Public Health Reports, 118,* 215-220.

Suri, R., Metcalfe, C., Wallis, C., & Bush, A. (2004). Predicting response to rhDNase and hypertonic saline in children with cystic fibrosis. *Pediatric Pulmonology, 37,* 305-310.

Szefler, S. J., & Pedersen, S. (2003). Role of budesonide as maintenance therapy for children with asthma. *Pediatric Pulmonology, 36,* 13-21.

Tee, A. K., & Hui, K. P. (2005). Effect of spirometric maneuver, nasal clip, and submaximal inspiratory effort on measurement of exhaled nitric oxide levels in asthmatic patients. *Chest, 127,* 131-134.

Tokar, B., Ozkan, R., & Ilhan, H. (2004). Tracheobronchial foreign bodies in children: Importance of accurate history and plain chest radiography in delayed presentation. *Clinical Radiology, 59,* 609-615.

Toltzis, P., Dul, M., O'Riordan, M. A., Toltzis, H., & Blumer, J. L. (2005). Impact of amoxicillin on pneumococcal colonization compared with other therapies for acute otitis media. *Pediatric Infectious Disease Journal, 24,* 24-28.

Vernacchio, L., Lesko, S. M., Vezina, R. M., Corwin, M. J., Hunt, C. E., Hoffman, H. J., & Mitchell, A. A. (2004). Racial/ethnic disparities in the diagnosis of otitis media in infancy. *International. Journal of Pediatric Otorhinolaryngology, 68,* 795-804.

Virgilis, D., Rivkin, L., Samueloff, A., Picard, E., Golberg, S., Faber, J., Kerem, E., & Wilschanski, M. (2003). Cystic fibrosis, pregnancy, and recurrent, acute pancreatitis. *Journal of Pediatric Gastroenterology Nutrition, 36,* 486-488.

Wagener, J. S., & Headley, A. A. (2003). Cystic fibrosis: current trends in respiratory care. *Respiratory Care, 48,* 234-245.

Walsh, M. C., Yao, Q., Gettner, P., Hale, E., Collins, M., Hensman, A., Everette, R., Peters, N., Miller, N., Muran, G., Auten, K., Newman, N., Rowan, G., Grisby, C., Arnell, K., Miller, L., Ball, B., & McDavid G. (2004). Impact of a physiologic definition on bronchopulmonary dysplasia rates. *Pediatrics, 114,* 1305-1311.

Windfuhr, J. P., Chen, Y. S., & Remmert, S. (2005). Hemorrhage following tonsillectomy and adenoidectomy in 15,218 patients. *Otolaryngology–Head and Neck Surgery, 132,* 281-286.

WHO annual report on global TB control—Summary. *Weekly Epidemiology Record, 78,* 122-128.

Yldzdas, D., Yapcoglu, H., & Ylmaz, H. L. (2004). The value of capnography during sedation/analgesia in pediatric minor procedures. *Pediatric Emergency Medicine, 20,* 162-165.

Zanardo, V., Simbi, A. K., Franzoi, M., Solda, G., Salvadori, A., & Trevisanuto, D. (2004). Neonatal respiratory morbidity risk and mode of delivery at term: Influence of timing of elective caesarean delivery. *Acta Paediatricia, 93,* 643-647.

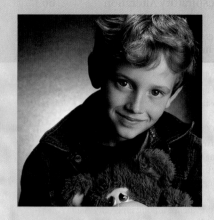

CHAPTER 22

The Child With a Cardiovascular Alteration

Learning Objectives

After studying this chapter, you should be able to:

- Describe the anatomy and physiology of the normally functioning heart.
- Describe the major circulatory changes that occur in the fetus during the transition from intrauterine to extrauterine life.
- Discuss specific techniques used in a comprehensive cardiac assessment.
- Explain the various classifications of congenital heart disease, describe their underlying mechanisms, and list the associated congenital cardiac defects.
- Discuss the nursing process used for an infant or child with congestive heart failure.
- Discuss the major physiologic features and the therapeutic management of a child with a heart defect,
- including left-to-right shunting lesions and obstructive or stenotic lesions.
- Discuss the major physiologic features, therapeutic management, and nursing care of a child with a cyanotic heart defect.
- Discuss the importance of early recognition and treatment of infective endocarditis.
- Describe nursing care of a child with rheumatic fever, Kawasaki disease, or hypertension.
- Explain why high cholesterol is an important health issue for children and adolescents and describe the assessment and nursing management of this problem in children in the community.
- Explain the effects of childhood obesity on future cardiovascular health.

Definitions

ablation Destruction of diseased tissue.

afterload The amount of force against which the ventricles contract.

angioplasty Procedure that dilates vessels.

arrhythmia Disturbance of rhythm.

cardiomegaly An enlarged heart.

central venous pressure Pressure measured in the right atrium; helpful in determining the amount of circulating blood volume.

chronotropic Affecting the time or rate.

compensation Maintenance of an adequate blood flow without distressing symptoms; accomplished by cardiac and circulatory adjustments, such as tachycardia, cardiac hypertrophy, and increased blood volume from sodium and water retention.

decompensation Inability of the heart to maintain adequate circulation; may be marked by dyspnea, venous engorgement, cyanosis, and edema.

gradient Difference.

inotropic Affects the force of muscular contractions; can cause a positive or negative effect.

myocardial contractility Ability of myocardial cells and tissues to shorten in response to an appropriate stimulus; force of contraction of the myocardium.

palpitations Sensation of rapid or irregular heartbeat.

preload Amount of stretch of the myocardial fibers before contraction; most easily measured by determining central venous pressure.

pulmonary edema Collection of excessive fluid in the alveoli of the lungs.

pulmonary hypertension Increased pressure in the pulmonary arteries and arterioles.

pulmonary vascular resistance Amount of resistance in the pulmonary vascular bed against which the right ventricle must pump to achieve blood flow to the lungs.

pulmonary venous congestion Increased pulmonary pressure leading to the accumulation of excessive fluid and blood in the pulmonary veins.

regurgitation Abnormal backward flow of blood through a heart valve.

shunt Abnormal blood flow from one part of the circulation to another.

systemic vascular resistance Amount of resistance in the systemic vascular bed against which the left ventricle must pump to achieve cardiac output.

systemic venous congestion Increased systemic venous pressure leading to the accumulation of excessive fluid in the systemic veins.

valvotomy An opening surgically created in a valve.

valvuloplasty Mechanical procedure to open a valve.

REVIEW OF THE HEART AND CIRCULATION
Normal Cardiac Anatomy and Physiology

The heart is a muscular pump divided into four chambers. The two upper chambers are the atria, and the two lower chambers are the ventricles. There are two atrioventricular (AV) valves, the tricuspid valve and the mitral valve. There are two semilunar valves—the pulmonary valve and the aortic valve. In normal blood flow, desaturated venous blood returning from the body flows from the superior vena cava and inferior vena cava into the right atrium. It then moves through the tricuspid valve into the right ventricle and is pumped into the main pulmonary artery and branch pulmonary arteries to the pulmonary circulation (the lungs). In the lungs, carbon dioxide is removed and oxygen added to the blood. This richly oxygen-saturated blood returns from the pulmonary circulation to the left side of the heart through the pulmonary veins and into the left atrium. From the left atrium, it flows through the mitral valve into the left ventricle and is pumped into the aorta and systemic circulation.

Electrical stimulation is required before mechanical contraction of the heart muscle can occur. This electrical stimulation is normally initiated by a group of cells called the *sinus node,* located at the superior vena cava and right atrial junction. The electrical impulse spreads through the atrium to the relay station, the AV node, and is then transmitted to the ventricles through the bundle of His, the bundle-branch system, and finally the Purkinje fibers. The result is rhythmic atrial electrical stimulation and then contraction, followed by ventricular stimulation and contraction. The P wave reflects atrial depolarization, the QRS wave reflects ventricular depolarization, and the T wave reflects ventricular repolarization.

Each cardiac cycle consists of this electrical activity, which produces depolarization and subsequent repolarization of the cardiac muscle—more simply, a heartbeat.

The venous (or right) side of the heart is normally a lower pressure system compared with the higher arterial (or left) side of the heart. The right ventricle has a range of normal pressure of 18-30/0-5 mm Hg and pulmonary artery pressure of 20-30/8-12 mm Hg. The left ventricle has a range of normal pressure of 90-140/5 mm Hg (age dependent), and the aorta has a normal pressure of about 100/60 mm Hg (age dependent). On average, the left-sided pressures are four to five times higher than those on the right side.

In addition, the venous circulation normally has lower oxygen saturations, in the range of 65% to 80%. This compares with the arterial circulation, which has a normal range of 95% to 100%. Congenital or acquired malformations or anomalies in any of the cardiac structures can affect blood flow, pressures, and oxygen saturations, thereby altering hemodynamic stability.

Fetal Circulation

Fetal circulation differs from neonatal circulation in three areas: the process of gas exchange, the pressures within the systemic and pulmonary circulations, and the existence of anatomic structures that assist in the delivery of oxygen-rich blood to vital organ systems. In the fetus, oxygenation (gas exchange) takes place at the placenta. Oxygen and nutrients are carried by blood in the umbilical vein, which travels through the fetal liver to the inferior vena cava.

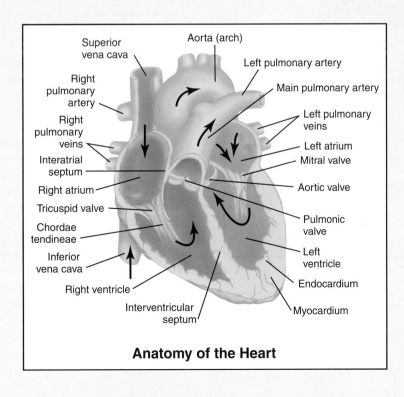

Anatomy of the Heart

Superior vena cava · Aorta (arch) · Left pulmonary artery · Right pulmonary artery · Main pulmonary artery · Right pulmonary veins · Left pulmonary veins · Interatrial septum · Left atrium · Mitral valve · Right atrium · Aortic valve · Tricuspid valve · Chordae tendineae · Pulmonic valve · Inferior vena cava · Left ventricle · Right ventricle · Endocardium · Interventricular septum · Myocardium

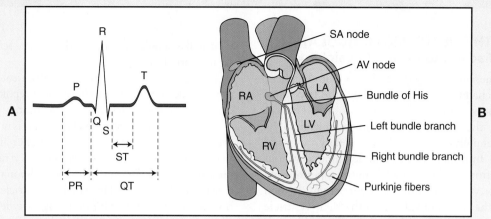

A, Normal heart cycle, represented as an electrocardiographic configuration. **B,** Cardiac electrical conduction system. *(Modified from Park, M. K., & Guntheroth, W. G. [1992]. How to read pediatric ECGs [3rd ed., p. 1], St. Louis: Mosby.)*

A small amount of blood travels into the hepatic circulation to provide oxygen and nutrients to the hepatic tissue. Liver function is minimal in the fetus, so very little blood supply is required. The remainder of the blood flows into the inferior vena cava through a fetal structure, the *ductus venosus*.

The inferior vena cava empties blood into the right atrium. The trajectory (direction) of the blood flow, as well as the pressure in the right atrium, propels most of this blood through a second fetal structure, the *foramen ovale*, into the left atrium. This richly oxygenated blood travels through the left ventricle into the aorta, feeding the coronary arteries and the brain—the two most oxygen-needy organ systems.

Blood returning from the upper body enters the right atrium through the superior vena cava. This blood is directed primarily through the tricuspid valve and the right ventricle into the pulmonary artery. Resistance in the pulmonary circulation is very high because the lungs are collapsed and filled with fluid. A very small amount of blood flows through the branch pulmonary arteries to provide oxygen and nutrients to the pulmonary tissue. Most of the blood flows through a third fetal structure, the *ductus arteriosus*, to the descending aorta. This blood is then distributed to the organ systems and tissues in the lower portion of the body and returns to the placenta for gas exchange through two umbilical arteries.

Transitional and Neonatal Circulation

Major changes in the circulatory system occur at birth. With the neonate's first breath, gas exchange is transferred from the placenta to the lungs.

In the normal neonate, the fetal shunts (ductus venosus, ductus arteriosus, foramen ovale) functionally close in response to pressure changes in the systemic and pulmonary circulations and to increased blood oxygen content. Pulmonary vascular resistance begins to decrease, and pulmonary blood flow markedly increases. Closure of the ductus arteriosus, along with the increased pulmonary blood flow, enhances left ventricular filling. The increase in systemic arterial pressure as a result of clamping the umbilical cord at delivery and placental separation from the fetus increases the workload of the left ventricle, and the neonatal heart now functions on its own. The neonatal circulation is now normal. In some neonates, it may take several days for the fetal shunts to close.

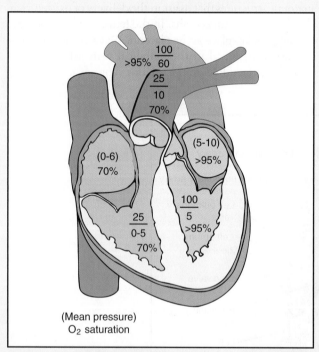

(Mean pressure)
O₂ saturation

Normal pressures (in millimeters of mercury) and saturations (percents). *(Modified from Ko Chiang, L., & Ensor Dunn, A. [2000]. Cardiology. In G. K. Siberry & R. Iannone [Eds.], The Johns Hopkins Hospital Harriet Lane Handbook [15th ed., p. 154]. St. Louis: Mosby.)*

Common Diagnostic Tests for Cardiac Disorders

Test	Description	Preparation and Nursing Considerations	Comments
ECG	Provides recording of heart's electrical activity from outside surface of body. Electrodes are placed over precordium and on the four extremities; electrodes are attached to lead wires. Lead wires are attached to an electrocardiogram that records and prints electrical activity.	Best done when the child is quiet and cooperative. Skin should be free of lotions and oils.	Detects chamber enlargement and deviations in axis that may be caused by congenital or acquired heart defects or disease. Displays heart rate and rhythm.
Holter monitor	Continuously records heart rate and rhythm for 24 hours. Electrodes and leads are attached to the child, who wears a compact recorder.	Same as for ECG.	Child or parent records times of activities, symptoms, or other events in a diary to be returned with the monitor. Important that diary be accurately completed.
Chest radiography	Provides x-ray picture of heart and associated organs and structures in the chest cavity.	Remove electrodes and lead wires if attached. Encourage the parent or family member to accompany the child to x-ray department.	Provides information about heart size, blood flow to lungs, sidedness of the stomach, liver, and heart.
Echocardiography	Uses high-frequency sound waves (ultrasound) to generate an image of the heart and associated structures. The study assesses location and relationship of intracardiac and extracardiac structures, cardiac function; measures size of cardiac chambers, valve function, size of septal or other defects; estimates gradients across structures and blood flow direction.	Must be done when the child is quiet and cooperative. If not cooperative, sedation may become necessary.	Methods of echocardiograms: • M-mode • Two-dimensional • Doppler Types of echocardiograms: • Transthoracic • Transesophageal • Directly on cardiac muscle • Fetal
Magnetic resonance imaging	A strong magnetic field surrounds the child; the field promotes rotation of nuclei (that normally spin) at predictable speed, allowing visualization of soft tissue, tumors, shunts, myocardial thickness, structure, valve function.	Teaching about the procedure. Nothing-by-mouth status for at least 4 hr before procedure if requiring sedation. Assessment for allergy if contrast medium is to be used. All metallic items must be removed.	The child must be able to lie still for up to 1 hr or will require sedation.
Ventilation-perfusion scan	IV injection of isotope, which reveals distribution of pulmonary blood flow and ventilation; assists in quantifying percentage and pattern of pulmonary blood flow.	Requires an IV line for radioisotope injection.	The child must be able to lie still for a short time for the scan.
Pulse oximetry	A bandage probe is attached to a digit; measures oxygen saturation of blood noninvasively.	No specific preparation. The extremity needs to be relatively motion free for accurate reading. All nail polish must be removed.	If low or high saturation level alarms, validate that the child's heart rate corresponds to the monitor and the expected saturation range for the child's cardiac defect.

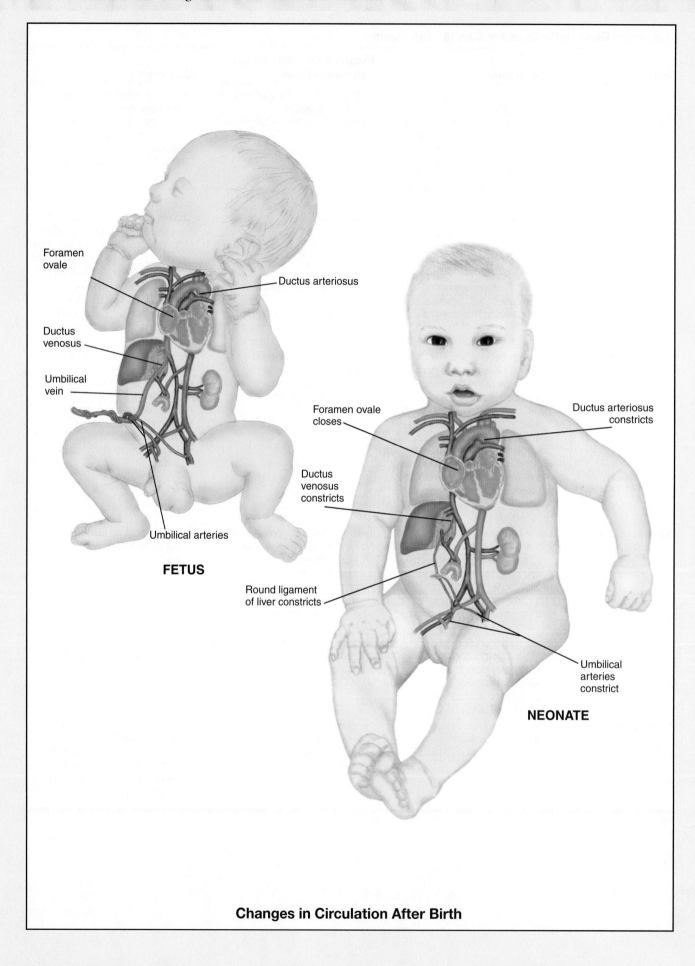

Foramen ovale

Ductus arteriosus

Ductus venosus

Umbilical vein

Umbilical arteries

FETUS

Foramen ovale closes

Ductus arteriosus constricts

Ductus venosus constricts

Round ligament of liver constricts

Umbilical arteries constrict

NEONATE

Changes in Circulation After Birth

DIFFERENCES IN THE HEART AND CIRCULATION OF NEONATES AND INFANTS

- The heart and the great vessels develop during the first 3 to 8 weeks of gestation. The fetus is most vulnerable to cardiac malformations during this period.
- Heart sounds in the neonate are higher pitched and of greater intensity than in the adult, and the pulse rate is higher. Many variations in these parameters are both possible and normal. The intensity of the murmur does not necessarily correlate with the degree and severity of the congenital or acquired heart disease.
- The chest wall of infants and young children is thin because of the relative lack of subcutaneous fat and muscle tissue. Innocuous murmurs can be auscultated in structurally normal hearts because of the wall thinness.
- The neonate's and infant's myocardial muscle is less efficient. The myocardial cells are smaller and contain fewer contractile elements; therefore, neonatal and infant hearts have decreased myocardial contractility. This makes neonates and infants particularly dependent on adequate heart rate and rhythm to maintain their cardiac output because they cannot increase their stroke volume

as effectively as the older child or adult (Cardiac output = Stroke volume × Heart rate).
- The neonatal heart is very dependent on calcium, glucose, and volume for optimal cardiac function.
- In a very sick child, the cardiac output should be evaluated as either adequate or inadequate to meet metabolic demands. Shock may be present even when the cardiac output is normal or high.
- Blood pressure not a reliable indicator of clinical decompensation. Hypotension may indicate decompensated shock.
- Increased pulmonary vascular resistance in the neonate increases pressure on the right side of the heart. This may delay detection of left-to-right shunts in the newborn period because increased right-sided pressure decreases the left-to-right shunting and the intensity of cardiac murmurs. Normally, pulmonary vascular resistance decreases to the adult range over the first 4 to 6 weeks of life. Obvious signs and symptoms of left-to-right shunting may not be present until that time.

Electronic Resources

Additional information related to the content in Chapter 22 can be found on:

the interactive companion CD-ROM

- Animations: Structure of the Heart
        Subaortic Stenosis
- Audio Glossary
- NCLEX Review Questions

or the companion website at *evolve*
http://evolve.elsevier.com/james/ncoc

- Common Pediatric Laboratory Tests and Normal Values
- NCLEX Review Questions
- Pediatric Assessment Video Clips
- Resources for Health Care Providers and Families
- WebLinks

Heart disease in children is either congenital or acquired. Congenital heart disease denotes one or more structural abnormalities that develop before birth, although the clinical symptoms may not be present in the newborn period. Acquired heart disease, such as the cardiomyopathies, Kawasaki disease, or acute rheumatic fever (RF), develops after birth and may be seen both in children with normal hearts and in those with congenital heart disease; however, the risk for development of a cardiomyopathy is increased in the child with a history of congenital heart disease.

The nurse's role includes the astute and vigilant assessment, monitoring, and collaborative treatment of a child with known or potential cardiovascular alterations. Rapid changes in acuity and decompensation can occur in certain congenital and acquired heart diseases. Thus, the skills required of the pediatric nurse must be focused and refined to identify clinically significant changes that may have an impact on this often-complex population.

ASSESSMENT OF THE CHILD WITH A CARDIOVASCULAR ALTERATION

Serious congenital cardiac lesions usually become symptomatic early in infancy. Remarkable technologic advances in the understanding of the cardiovascular system's function and needs have led to refinements in the tools and techniques for detecting, diagnosing, and treating congenital heart defects. Invasive procedures are now required less for initial diagnosis but rather to obtain more detailed hemodynamic information and for interventional procedures. Nevertheless, no tool or technique replaces obtaining a comprehensive history from both the child and the parents and performing a thorough physical examination (Table 22-1).

The cardiac assessment should take place in a quiet and nonthreatening environment with a parent present if possible. Parents know their children best, and they can offer a timeline of events and subtle clinical information that may

Text continued on p. 672

TABLE **22-1** **Cardiac Assessment***		
Parameter	**Assessment Guidelines**	**Findings and Comments**
Health history	Inquire about a family history of CHD, sudden death, or fetal/infant death.	There may be an increased incidence of CHD, cardiomyopathies, arrhythmias, or hypercholesterolemia in some families.
	Ask about prenatal care, maternal illnesses, infections, medications taken during pregnancy.	Chronic maternal illness such as diabetes, perinatal infections such as rubella, and certain medications such as lithium have been linked to CHD.
	Discuss pregnancy, birth history, associated birth defects or genetic anomalies.	There is an increased incidence of CHD with certain genetic anomalies or birth defects. Cyanosis, murmur, or other cardiac event present at birth may indicate cardiac disease.
	Discuss feeding difficulties (including decreased intake or increased rest periods during feeding), tachypnea or increased work of breathing, frequency of respiratory infections, poor weight gain, fatigue, exercise intolerance, color changes with crying or Valsalva maneuvers, diaphoresis.	Poor weight gain and failure to thrive are often associated with cardiac disease. Cyanosis may be more prominent with crying or Valsalva maneuvers.
Inspection	**Color:** Assess skin color in natural light if possible. Pay special attention to oral mucous membranes, nail beds, and conjunctiva, which can reflect central cyanosis. Assess hands, feet, and face. Assess body for differential or demarcated cyanosis or color differences.	Central cyanosis can reflect cardiac or pulmonary alterations. Differential cyanosis may indicate complex heart disease that is dependent on PDA blood flow for systemic or pulmonary blood flow. Pallor, mottling, or ruddiness may indicate cardiac disease. Acrocyanosis (a painless disorder caused by constriction or narrowing of small blood vessels in the skin) may be seen in the healthy newborn. Clubbing of nail beds may indicate chronic hypoxia. Usually present after 6 months of arterial desaturation (see Fig. 21-6).
	Activity level: Assess child while sitting and lying down. Observe level of activity and position of comfort. Observe for color changes with activity, feeding, or crying. Observe for exercise tolerance, including any respiratory distress or frequent rest.	Lethargy, irritability, or restlessness may indicate poor cardiac function. Squatting may indicate cyanotic heart disease and attempts to improve hypoxia.
	Chest: Assess precordial activity, chest movement (including symmetry), and chest shape (including convex or concave). Assess for sternotomy or thoracotomy incisions.	PMI (apical pulse) may be seen in thin children. It is found at fourth left ICS in young children and fifth ICS in children older than 7 years. In neonate, PMI does not correspond with apical pulse. It is found at fourth ICS and can be more midline toward xiphoid because of right ventricular dominance in the fetal and neonatal heart. An active precordium may indicate cardiac disease. A convex chest cavity shape may indicate cardiac disease.
	Respiratory pattern: Observe work of breathing at rest and with activity, including feeding. Look for signs of respiratory alteration or distress. (Tachypnea, retractions, nasal flaring, crackles, grunting, and head bobbing are late signs of distress and may indicate impending respiratory failure.)	Increased work of breathing and respiratory difficulty may indicate CHF.
Auscultation	**Heart sounds:** Auscultate with both bell (for low-pitched sounds) and diaphragm (for high-pitched sounds) of stethoscope.	Heart sounds should be synchronous with palpable central or peripheral pulse. Rhythm normally is regular. A normal variation is sinus arrhythmia when the rhythm can alter and rate can increase with inspiration and decrease with expiration.

PMI, Point of maximal impulse; *ICS,* intercostal space; *LLSB,* left lower sternal border.
*A thorough cardiac workup will often include chest radiography, ECG, and echocardiogram.

TABLE 22-1   Cardiac Assessment*—cont'd

Parameter	Assessment Guidelines	Findings and Comments
Auscultation—cont'd	**Heart sounds—cont'd**	Ask the older child to briefly hold a breath to allow the nurse to hear more clearly.
	Identify first and second heart sounds.	S_1 is heard best at apex of heart (fourth or fifth ICS at left midclavicular line) and reflects closure of mitral and tricuspid valves. Correlates with palpable pulse. S_2 is heard best at base (right and left of sternum at second ICS) and reflects closure of aortic and pulmonic valves.
	Identify additional heart sounds (S_3, S_4). These can be assessed with the child lying supine or on the left side.	S_3 can be heard at the LLSB or apex and can be a normal finding or reflect CHF. S_4 can be heard at the LLSB or apex and reflects cardiac disease. A gallop is an extra heart sound (S_3 or S_4), common in CHF.
	Identify presence of murmurs, clicks, precordial friction rubs.	Murmurs are caused by turbulent blood flow. Murmurs are described according to location, timing within cardiac cycle, intensity, pitch, quality, and duration. Clicks reflect abnormal valve motion. Precordial friction rubs can reflect pericardial inflammation.
Palpation	**Temperature:** Compare temperature of trunk with temperature of extremities.	Cooler extremities may indicate poor perfusion because of decreased cardiac output. If room is cold, cool extremities may indicate vasoconstriction to conserve heat.
	Pulses: Compare central and distal pulses. Assess pulses in all four extremities.	Peripheral pulses may be diminished if cardiac output is impaired. Causes include CHF or dehydration. Weak or absent pulses in the lower extremities may indicate coarctation of the aorta.
	Blood pressure: Assess in all four extremities during initial assessment.	Discrepancies between upper and lower extremity blood pressure may indicate cardiac disease, including coarctation of the aorta.
	Capillary refill: Assess capillary filling in extremities; use fingertips to compress skin.	Normal is less than 2 seconds.
	Chest: With fingertips, locate the PMI. Assess for presence of vibratory thrills, heaves or lifts, or friction rubs.	PMI located farther down than normal may indicate cardiac enlargement. Thrills, described as a palpable murmur, are vibratory in nature. Heaves or lifts are palpable chest wall movement, separate from the PMI, and reflect hyperactive precordium. Friction rubs, caused by the presence of fluid in the cardiac or pleural space, produce a grating sound.
	Abdomen: Locate the liver border. It should be at or slightly below the right costal margin in infants and young children. In the neonate the liver can be 2 to 3 cm below the right costal margin and still be normal.	**Abdomen:** Normally the border should be firm and smooth. Liver may be boggy with a poorly defined edge and palpable more than 1-2 cm below the right costal margin when CHF is present.
Percussion	Percussion of the chest provides little useful data in a cardiac assessment.	PMI is a better indicator of heart size.

not be evident on examination. The nurse needs to establish an atmosphere of trust and cooperation—cardiac assessment is best and most easily performed on a cooperative infant or child.

The room should be warm and well lit. Natural light from windows will allow the nurse to accurately assess skin color.

The assessment should begin with the least threatening steps—the history and inspection. During the parent interview, the child has the opportunity to observe the interaction between nurse and parent and has time to become comfortable with the nurse's presence. The child should be allowed to participate in the assessment and encouraged to touch and inspect each piece of equipment to be used during the examination.

Assessment progression includes inspection, auscultation, and palpation; each step requires more touching. The nurse must remember to warm the stethoscope used for auscultation, as well as the hands before touching the child's skin. This is particularly important when assessing a resting infant, who may become startled by the cold touch of the hands and stethoscope.

CRITICAL TO REMEMBER
Assessing Murmurs

Develop a systematic approach to assessing heart sounds with every examination. Abnormal heart sounds will be easier to detect once you can recognize a normal heart sound. Consider other clinical findings, including fatigue associated with anemia and fever, which can intensify a murmur by altering cardiac output.

Organic murmurs reflect an abnormality in the heart structures. Innocent (functional) murmurs do not reflect heart abnormalities but are the sounds made as the blood flows through the structurally normal heart. They can be loud or soft and are often vibratory in quality. Innocent murmurs do not affect growth or well-being and are quite common in children.

CARDIOVASCULAR DIAGNOSIS

Tests used to diagnose cardiac problems in children have been described previously (see p. 667). Cardiac catheterization is still considered the gold standard by which all other therapeutic modalities are measured. It usually constitutes the final definitive diagnostic test for many patients.

Cardiac Catheterization

Cardiac catheterization is an invasive diagnostic procedure. It also is both an interventional and therapeutic procedure. Catheters are advanced, generally through the femoral vein or artery, into the venous or arterial system and directed into the heart. Data obtained and interventions performed during the procedure include the following:

- Measurement of oxygen saturations in cardiac chambers and great arteries
- Measurement of pressures in cardiac chambers and great arteries and determination of gradients

- Evaluation of cardiac output
- Angiography to identify detailed images of structures and blood flow patterns
- Electrophysiologic studies to map the cardiac conduction system and identify the locus of arrhythmia-producing cells; radiofrequency catheter ablation is used for destruction of these cells
- Corrective or palliative interventional procedures include pulmonary artery or valve and aortic valve balloon angioplasty, stent placement to maintain patency of vessels, balloon/blade septostomy for creation of an atrial septal defect (ASD) (indicated for certain complex congenital heart defects), percutaneous pulmonary valve replacements, and device closure of septal defects or coil embolization of a patent ductus arteriosus (PDA) or collateral vessels

Complications

Complications may result both during and after the procedure. Potential complications of which the nurse should be aware include arrhythmias, hemorrhage, vascular damage, vasospasm of the catheterized vessel, thrombus or embolus formation, infection, reaction to the dye, and catheter perforation. Arrhythmias may be hemodynamically compromising. Vasospasm of the vessel results in poor perfusion to the affected leg. Thrombus (stationary blood clot) formation at the catheter insertion site may impair perfusion to the affected limb and may shed emboli (mobile blood clots) that may travel anywhere in the vascular system depending on the cardiac anatomy, including the lung or brain. A thrombus in the venous system can be associated with swelling or inflammation of the affected limb. A thrombus in the arterial system may be associated with coolness or discoloration of the extremity and loss of pulses distal to the thrombus. Thrombus formation may occur in the systemic–to–pulmonary artery shunts that provide pulmonary blood flow. Reactions to the dye may be rash, pruritus, mild (vomiting) or, very rarely, severe (anaphylaxis). Perforation by the catheter of the heart or vessels during the procedure can result in cardiac tamponade and cardiac arrest. Additional minor reactions to the procedure include nausea and vomiting related to anesthetics or sedatives or pressure ulceration of pressure points related to prolonged immobility and decreased subcutaneous tissue.

Nursing Care

Because impaired peripheral perfusion is a possible consequence of a cardiac catheterization, it is important for the nurse to locate and mark distal pulses before the procedure. Marking the location of pulses will assist the nurse with rapid postprocedure assessment.

After the procedure, the child is positioned with the affected leg straight for 4 to 6 hours; infants may be held prone on a parent's lap. Older children remain in bed with the head of the bed raised at only a 20-degree incline. Intravenous (IV) fluid administration continues until the infant or child is taking and retaining adequate amounts of oral fluids.

Vital signs should be obtained frequently (every 5-15 min) for the first hour, with continuous initial monitoring of heart rate, blood pressure, respiratory rate and oxygen saturation, and temperature.

The insertion site dressing should be observed frequently, at least every 5 to 15 minutes, during the early postprocedure hours. Assess for bleeding not only on the dressing but also on sheets. Look under the child to check for pooled blood. Pull back bed linens and remove the infant's diaper (if applicable) to check the perineal area for bleeding under the skin. If bleeding occurs, place a gloved heel of the hand firmly on the insertion site. Apply pressure for at least 10 to 15 minutes and assess distal perfusion of the extremity. Immediately notify the cardiologist. Assess blood loss and the child's hemodynamic status.

Peripheral perfusion is also monitored. The affected extremity will frequently be mottled in appearance and cooler to touch than the other extremities. Distal pulses should, however, be palpable, although they may be weaker than in the contralateral extremity. Nonpalpable distal pulses should be checked with Doppler technology. Notify the cardiologist if distal pulses are absent on the affected extremity or the temperature or degree of mottling has changed or the child complains of increasing pain.

Heparin drip infusions are initiated under certain circumstances that may be related to the catheter route or to placement of stents, coils, or closure devices.

Children who have undergone a diagnostic cardiac catheterization are often discharged the same day. Children undergoing interventional procedures or electrophysiologic studies may remain hospitalized overnight. The following day, the pressure bandage is removed and is replaced with an adhesive bandage (Band-Aid). Discharge instructions vary according to the institution but may include the following:

- Inspecting the catheter insertion site to assess healing or the presence of local infection
- Bathing limited to a shower, sponge bath, or brief tub bath (no soaking) for the first 1 to 3 days after the procedure
- Avoiding strenuous exercise (climbing trees, swimming, contact sports) for up to 1 week after the procedure
- Returning to school on the third day after the procedure
- Notifying the cardiologist if the child has a fever above 38.3° C (101° F); bleeding or drainage (pus) from catheter insertion site; or pallor, coolness, or numbness of the affected extremity
- Resuming normal feeding patterns and medication therapy, if applicable
- Reviewing the need to continue antibiotic prophylaxis for dental or other specific medical procedures
- Follow-up with a cardiologist at a scheduled visit

CONGENITAL HEART DISEASE

Congenital heart defects are some of the most frequently seen congenital defects in infants and children, with the incidence reported in approximately 1% of pregnancies and approximately 8 to 10 per 1000 live births (Green, 2004). Of the cardiac problems in children, the majority result from congenital heart disease—structural defects within the heart that are present at birth. The precise etiology of congenital heart disease is not known. The majority of cases ($\approx$90%) are thought to be multifactorial.

Investigations into environmental and genetic causes of congenital heart disease are in progress. The genetic component of congenital heart disease has been investigated more thoroughly than the environmental aspect. Children with certain genetic defects have an extremely high incidence of cardiac disorders, including children with chromosome aberrations, most specifically trisomy 21 (Down syndrome), in which the incidence of congenital heart disease is approximately 50% (Bernstein, 2004). Other children who have an increased risk of having congenital heart disease include girls with *Turner's syndrome* (genetically having only a single X chromosome) and boys with *Klinefelter's variant* (genetically having additional X chromosomes), children with velocardiofacial syndrome *(DiGeorge syndrome)*, and children with Marfan syndrome. Some children with nonhereditary conditions, such as fetal alcohol syndrome (25% to 30% incidence) are at increased risk for congenital heart disease (CHD), as are infants of diabetic mothers (3% to 5%) (Park, 2002).

A family history of CHD increases the risk for giving birth to a child with CHD. Having a parent or sibling with CHD increases the risk (2% to 6%) (Bernstein, 2004).

The current approach to CHD is to return the child to normal or near-normal anatomy and physiology as soon as possible. Corrective and palliative procedures are now performed earlier in life because of a number of advances in surgical techniques and medical management. In addition, the impact on the natural history of uncorrected, palliated, and corrected defects and the effect on the child's morbidity and mortality are now better understood given the past four to five decades of surgical intervention. Also, there is an increased awareness and understanding of the impact of chronic illness on the child and family.

Classification of Congenital Heart Disease

Congenital cardiac defects can be classified according to structural abnormalities, functional alterations, or both (Table 22-2). Historically, defects were classified according to whether they were acyanotic or cyanotic. This classification is generally imprecise because children who may be acyanotic initially can become cyanotic as an uncorrected lesion worsens cardiac status. Clinical signs of congenital cardiac defects are not always apparent at birth; they can manifest any time during infancy or early childhood. The degree of symptoms, indications for medical and surgical interventions, and chronicity of condition depend on the diagnosis.

Shunting: Saturation Considerations

Shunting, or blood flow through an abnormal opening in the heart or great vessels, occurs when (1) there is an abnormal opening or connection between the cardiac chambers or great arteries, (2) the pressure is higher on one side of the heart compared with the other, and (3) the oxygen saturation is

TABLE 22-2	Classification of Congenital Heart Disease	
Defect	**Underlying Mechanism**	**Examples**
Left-to-right shunting lesions (lesions that increase pulmonary blood flow)	Left-sided heart pressures, which normally exceed right-sided pressures, cause saturated blood to shunt through any abnormal opening in the heart, aorta, or pulmonary artery. This left-to-right shunting of blood results in a volume overload in the right side of the heart and in the pulmonary artery; cardiac workload (including ventricular strain, dilation, hypertrophy) increases to manage the additional volume (pressure overload). A "step-up" oxygen saturation (abnormal increase because of the addition of more highly saturated blood), combined with the increased fluid volume in the lungs, results in altered gas exchange. One of the major consequences of left-to-right shunting lesions is CHF. Other consequences include pulmonary vascular disease, pulmonary hypertension, Eisenmenger's syndrome, and frequent upper and lower respiratory infections that can progress to respiratory failure.	ASD VSD PDA AVSD, endocardial cushion defect
Obstructive or stenotic lesions, or lesions that decrease cardiac outflow	*Stenosis,* the narrowing or constriction of an opening, can occur in a valve or vessel constricting or obstructing blood flow through the area. Pressure rises in the area behind the obstruction; blood flow distal to the obstruction may be decreased or absent. Stenotic lesions can occur in the right or left side of the heart; obstruction on the left side of the heart decreases the amount of available blood for systemic perfusion. Physiologic effects of stenotic lesions include increased cardiac workload and ventricular strain, with clinical consequences of CHF, decreased cardiac output, and pump failure.	Pulmonary stenosis Aortic stenosis Coarctation of the aorta
Cyanotic lesions with decreased pulmonary blood flow	These lesions arise from an error in fetal development that results in *hypoplasia* (incomplete development), malalignment, or obstruction on the right side of the heart, and decreased amount of blood volume to the lungs. Pulmonary blood flow may rely on having a PDA. There is a "step-down" (abnormally decreased) oxygen saturation in the left side of the heart. Physiologically, the child manifests hypoxemia, increased cardiac workload, and ventricular strain. The hypoxemia results in cyanosis (baseline saturations often as low as 75%-85%), and, even with oxygen administration, saturations do not approximate normal. Other clinical findings may include upper respiratory infection, severely limited pulmonary blood flow, and marked exercise intolerance.	Tetralogy of Fallot Tricuspid valve abnormalities Pulmonary atresia with intact ventricular septum
Cyanotic lesions with increased pulmonary blood flow	When the fetal heart fails to develop into separate pulmonary and systemic circulations (so that there is a mixing of saturated and desaturated blood) or when there is a reversal of circulation so that desaturated blood goes to the systemic circulation and saturated blood to the pulmonary circulation, cyanosis occurs. Sometimes classified as mixing lesions, these defects cause increased cardiac workload, ventricular strain, and decreased cardiac output. Usually discovered early in the neonatal period, the infant might appear ruddy or cyanotic, with increased respiratory effort, or, if systemic circulation is compromised, may be dusky or gray and in cardiogenic shock (see Chapter 10). To support life, these complex cardiac defects may require intervention that allows for mixing of arterial and venous blood.	Truncus arteriosus Hypoplastic left heart syndrome* Transposition of the great arteries

*Also classified as a lesion that decreases cardiac outflow.

increased or decreased in the normally desaturated or fully saturated blood. It is important to remember that the venous side (normally the right side) is usually a low-pressure, desaturated (average 70%) system and the arterial side (normally the left side) is usually a high-pressure, fully saturated (95% to 100%) system. The combination of pressure differences and the size of the abnormal opening determine the extent of shunting. Understanding the principles of shunting and normal saturations helps clarify the blood flow direction in CHD.

Blood Flow Considerations

Generally, the amount of blood flow to the lungs through the pulmonary artery is the same as to the systemic circulation through the aorta. This ratio of pulmonary to systemic blood flow is described as the *pulmonary-to-systemic ratio* (QP/QS ratio), which is usually 1:1. Congenital heart defects have normal, increased, or decreased pulmonary-to-systemic blood flow ratios. Left-to-right shunts or obstructive lesions have normal or increased pulmonary-to-systemic blood flow ratios. Right-to-left, or complex, cyanotic lesions may have normal, decreased, or increased pulmonary-to-systemic blood flow ratios.

PHYSIOLOGIC CONSEQUENCES OF CONGENITAL HEART DISEASE IN CHILDREN
Congestive Heart Failure

Congestive heart failure (CHF) is a clinical syndrome that reflects the heart's inability to maintain cardiac output sufficiently to meet the metabolic demands of the body. The incidence of heart failure as a result of congenital heart disease is 0.1% to 0.2% of all live births (Kay, Colan, & Graham, 2001). The defects that are most likely to cause CHF in infants include left-to-right shunts (e.g., ventricular septal defects [VSD], AV defect, and PDA) and left heart obstructive lesions (e.g., critical aortic stenosis, severe aortic coarctation, congenital mitral stenosis) (Park, 2002). CHF is often what is diagnosed first in an older infant with a previously undiagnosed congenital cardiac defect. CHF results when hemodynamic and neurohumoral responses attempt to compensate for inadequate cardiac output. Symptoms are related to these responses. In infants and children decreased cardiac output is most often caused by effects of volume overload or pressure overload caused by underlying defects (e.g., large left-to-right shunts or palliated complex defects).

Pediatric CHF can develop from many other etiologies, including congenital and acquired anatomic anomalies (including cardiomyopathies), arrhythmias, infections (e.g., endocarditis, myocarditis), inborn metabolic disorders, tumors, drugs, and toxins (Park, 2002).

Manifestations

The clinical manifestations of CHF are related to the degree of hemodynamic and neurohormonal responses. Manifestations include tachycardia and gallop rhythm; tachypnea, increased work of breathing demonstrated by intercostal and subcostal retractions, grunting, nasal flaring, rales, and rarely wheezing or cough; periorbital and facial edema, neck vein

PATHOPHYSIOLOGY

CONGESTIVE HEART FAILURE

In CHF, hemodynamic and neurohormonal changes occur in response to decreased cardiac output; these changes determine the clinical manifestations. The hemodynamics affected include preload, afterload, contractility, and cardiac output. Cardiac output is the amount of blood ejected with each heartbeat. The neurohormonal responses include the stimulation of both the sympathetic nervous system and the renin-angiotensin system.*

Maintaining blood pressure, blood flow, and oxygen delivery to vital organs is the goal of the compensatory systems. With decreased cardiac output, there is stimulation of the sympathetic nervous system. This initially leads to increased heart rate, contractility, and stroke volume; increased systemic vascular resistance (afterload); and selective peripheral vasoconstriction. Tachycardia, although beneficial to compensate for early CHF, increases myocardial oxygen consumption, decreases the diastolic filling time and resting phase of the heart, and decreases coronary artery perfusion.†

Decreased cardiac output also causes the renal system to have a diminished glomerular filtration rate and a decreased renal blood flow. This leads to increased stimulation of the renin-angiotensin-aldosterone system. Sodium and water are reabsorbed, leading to fluid retention and thereby increasing intravascular volume. Initially, this volume retention increases preload and cardiac output. Later, the myocardium becomes more edematous, and ventricular function decreases from volume and pressure overload.

The pulmonary system is also affected by this increased volume, and interstitial edema develops. In addition, myocardial oxygen consumption increases and may exceed the oxygen availability. Finally, myocardial muscle can undergo cellular and muscular mass changes, or hypertrophy. Without intervention, heart failure progresses until the compensatory mechanisms are no longer effective.

*Balaguru D., Artman, M., & Auslender M. (2000). Management of heart failure in children. *Current Problems in Pediatrics, 30,* 5-30.
†Bernstein, D. (2004). The cardiovascular system. In R. E. Behrman, R. M. Kliegman, & H. Jenson (Eds.), *Nelson textbook of pediatrics* (17th ed., pp. 1475-1591). Philadelphia: WB Saunders.

distention (in children), hepatomegaly, and splenomegaly; and decreased peripheral perfusion, decreased urine output, diaphoresis, mottling, and cyanosis or pallor. The infant or child may be lethargic, be irritable, or fatigue more easily.

The earliest clinical manifestations of CHF are often subtle. The infant may have mild resting tachypnea and increasing difficulty feeding. Feedings take longer, requiring frequent rest periods, and less is consumed while more energy is expended, resulting in fewer calories being consumed although metabolic demands are increased. Feedings therefore provide little satisfaction. The infant may appear hungry and irritable soon after a feeding. Over time, the infant fails to gain weight and eventually has failure to thrive.

Diagnostic Evaluation

The diagnosis of CHF is established on the basis of clinical history, physical examination, chest radiographic appearance, electrocardiography (ECG), and echocardiography. Chest x-ray films may reveal cardiomegaly and increased pulmonary vascular markings reflecting increased interstitial pulmonary fluid, but it is not as sensitive in diagnosing ventricular hypertrophy as ECG. Laboratory studies that may be indicated to determine the presence of heart failure in children include determinations of arterial blood gas values, serum electrolyte levels, complete blood cell count, sedimentation rate, serum glucose and calcium levels, and urinalysis.

Therapeutic Management

Management of a child with CHF involves correcting the underlying problem as soon as it is feasible to do so. The medical management of CHF is directed toward decreasing cardiac workload and improving cardiac output through the manipulation of the hemodynamics and neurohormonal responses. Supplemental oxygen can be helpful for increasing oxygen saturation, but it should be used with caution in children with left-to-right shunting lesions because oxygen is a vasodilator and may increase pulmonary blood flow. Pharmacologic agents used include positive inotropes, diuretics, and angiotensin-converting enzyme (ACE) inhibitors. In addition, optimizing nutritional intake to meet the metabolic demands and improve growth is of paramount importance. Inability to decrease symptoms and achieve weight gain is an indication for surgical intervention.

Initial medication therapy depends on the presenting symptoms. Diuretics and a positive inotropic agent (e.g., digoxin) are used most commonly.

Diuretics are administered to eliminate excess water and sodium through increased urine production, thereby reducing systemic and pulmonary congestion. Furosemide is a potent loop diuretic and is frequently the initial diuretic therapy. Another classification of diuretics, the thiazides, acts at the distal renal tubules. These can be less potent than loop diuretics. These drugs cause the kidneys to waste potassium, placing the child at risk for hypokalemia. Potassium-sparing diuretics, such as spironolactone, are weak diuretics. This class of diuretics is often given with loop diuretics or thiazides to decrease the potential for hypokalemia. Potassium supplements can also be given in tandem with diuretics to replace these losses.

Digoxin is a cardiac glycoside that increases cardiac output and improves cardiac effectiveness by several mechanisms. It has a positive inotropic effect that strengthens the force of ventricular contractions. It has a negative chronotropic effect that slows the heart rate and, at higher doses, conduction of cardiac impulses through the AV node, allowing the ventricles more time to fill with blood. It also improves blood flow to the kidneys and enhances diuresis.

Obtain a baseline ECG before initiating digoxin. Digoxin may be administered IV or orally. The effectiveness of digoxin depends on achieving and maintaining a therapeutic serum drug level. A loading or digitalizing dose is administered in divided doses over 12 to 18 hours, and maintenance doses are given daily, usually in two divided doses. The range between therapeutic and toxic levels is narrow, with the therapeutic range 0.8 to 2.0 ng/mL (Robertson & Shilkofski, 2005). To avoid a falsely elevated serum digoxin level, serum levels should be measured at a minimum of 6 hours from the previous dose of digoxin; measurement in the first 3 to 5 days after digitalizing could also result in elevated results (Park, 2002). Levels are generally obtained when assessing for toxicity or medication adherence. Digoxin levels may be difficult to measure and monitor in preterm infants (Park, 2002). If a child is receiving digoxin and is having arrhythmias, a digoxin level should be obtained. Hypokalemia and hypomagnesemia can potentiate digoxin toxicity. In addition, the dose needs to be decreased in children with altered renal function.

Vasodilators, such as captopril or enalapril, may be used to relax vascular smooth muscles and reduce afterload (Bernstein, 2004). This class of vasodilators is called ACE inhibitors because they block the conversion of angiotensin I to angiotensin II and reduce vasoconstriction and sodium retention. In addition, ACE inhibitors also decrease norepinephrine release from the sympathetic nervous system.

CRITICAL TO REMEMBER
Feeding the Infant or Child With Congestive Heart Failure

Feed the infant or child in a relaxed environment. Time the feedings before multiple other activities to preserve the infant's energy. The infant with CHF tends to tire easily during feedings. Frequent, small feedings may be less tiring. Holding the infant in an upright position may provide less stomach compression and improve respiratory effort during the feeding. If the child is unable to consume an appropriate amount during a 30-minute feeding period every 3 hours, nasogastric feeding should be considered. Monitor for increased tachypnea, diaphoresis, or feeding intolerance (vomiting). Concentrating formula from the basic level of 20 kcal/oz to 27 kcal/oz can increase caloric intake without increasing the infant's work.

CRITICAL THINKING EXERCISE 22-1

Lin, a 2-month-old infant, is seen in the pediatrician's office. She has gained 1 pound since birth and has a murmur. She is admitted to the pediatric unit with a diagnosis of CHF. You will obtain a health history and perform an admission assessment.

1. What specific questions should you ask Lin's parents about her feeding patterns and behavior?
2. What physical assessment findings would you expect in an infant with CHF?
3. List nursing interventions that would address Lin's nutritional and comfort needs.

Text continued on p. 681

NURSING CARE PLAN

The Child With Congestive Heart Failure

Focused Assessment

Assessment of the child with CHF includes close monitoring of vital signs and a thorough cardiovascular, pulmonary, nutritional, and fluid status evaluation. Children being medically treated for CHF are often admitted because of worsening symptoms, including failure to thrive. In the newborn period, recognizing the early signs of CHF will expedite timely treatment. The early symptoms of tachycardia, tachypnea, poor feeding, and diaphoresis during feeding and increased irritability or fatigue should be noted and the physician or nurse practitioner alerted. Strict monitoring of intake and output and daily weights is also important in assessment and management.

NURSING DIAGNOSIS Decreased Cardiac Output related to CHF or decreased myocardial function.

EXPECTED OUTCOME The child will:
- Have adequate cardiac output, as evidenced by pink or baseline cyanotic (in cyanotic heart disease) mucous membranes and nail beds, a capillary refill time of less than 2 seconds, warm extremities, easily palpable peripheral pulses, adequate urinary output, no edema, appropriate heart rate, and an activity level within the normal limits of the defect.

Intervention

1. Monitor peripheral perfusion by palpating peripheral pulses, noting temperature, color changes, and capillary refill time.

2. Assess whether heart rate is appropriate for level of activity.
3. Monitor and document hourly urine output.

4. Maintain a neutral thermal environment; use a warmer bed or incubator for the neonate; treat fever promptly.
5. Time nursing interventions to allow the infant or child rest periods. Anticipate and respond quickly to stressful events, crying, or restlessness.
6. Administer digoxin (Lanoxin) as prescribed. Ascertain that the dosage is within safe limits. Count the apical rate for 1 full minute. Check the dosage with a second nurse. Withhold the dose and notify physician if the heart rate is less than 100 beats/min in infants; the heart rate at which the medication should be withheld varies in older children and adolescents. In general, if the withholding pulse rate is not ordered, withhold the medication and call the physician if the pulse rate is progressively decreasing or markedly lower than previous rates. Observe for signs of toxicity, and monitor for hyperkalemia in the child taking potassium-sparing diuretics.

Rationale

1. Poor peripheral perfusion is usually evidenced by decreased or absent pulses in the extremities. Color and temperature changes (e.g., cyanosis, coolness, mottling) may be present in all extremities. Prolonged capillary refill time is an additional sign of poor perfusion.
2. Tachycardia occurs in an attempt to maintain adequate cardiac output.
3. Altered renal perfusion caused by decreased cardiac output results in decreased urinary output.
4. Episodes of hypothermia or hyperthermia increase oxygen demands and increase the cardiac workload.
5. Rest periods reduce cardiac workload. Organizing nursing activities to promote rest results in decreased stress and fatigue for the child.
6. Digoxin is effective within a narrow therapeutic range (0.8-2 ng/mL*), although the pediatric range is not well defined. Safety in dosing is achieved by double checking the dose and counting the apical heart rate for a full minute. Digoxin toxicity can manifest with slow pulse, vomiting, and arrhythmias.

Evaluation

- Are mucous membranes and nail beds pink or baseline cyanotic?
- Is the capillary refill time less than 2 seconds?

- Are peripheral pulses easily palpated, and is the child alert and active?
- Is the heart rate in the expected range for activity?

*Park, M. K. (2002). *Pediatric cardiology for practitioners* (4th ed.). St. Louis: Mosby.

Continued

NURSING CARE PLAN—cont'd

NURSING DIAGNOSIS   Excess Fluid Volume related to volume overload and CHF.

EXPECTED OUTCOME   The infant or child will:
* Remain free of evidence of fluid overload (e.g., infrequent urination, inappropriate water weight gain, inadequate balance between intake and output, edema [periorbital, hepatomegaly], respiratory distress, poor feeding).

Intervention	*Rationale*
1. Administer diuretics as prescribed, ensuring correct dosage, route, and effectiveness.	1. Diuretics help the body eliminate excess fluid. Their effectiveness is evaluated from the urine output (either by measuring the amount of urine or by weighing diapers), weight, decreasing edema, decreasing respiratory distress, and improved feeding.
2. Maintain accurate intake and output records.	2. The fluid intake and output should be about the same. If intake grossly exceeds output, the diuretics may need to be altered, the child may need fluid restriction, or both.
3. Maintain fluid restriction, if ordered.	3. Fluid restriction will decrease pulmonary and liver edema.
4. Using the same scales, weigh the child daily at approximately the same time. Notify the physician of excessive weight gain (>50 g/day in infants, >200 g/day in children).	4. Excess fluid volume is not always overtly visible. Weight changes may indicate fluid retention. Weighing the infant or child on the same scales at the same time each day ensures consistency.
5. Provide skin care and change position frequently.	5. Edematous areas are extremely prone to skin breakdown because of stretching and opacity. Frequent position changes will prevent undesirable pooling of fluid in certain areas.
6. Monitor for increased or decreased edema (In infants and young children, edema is usually periorbital) and hepatomegaly; generalized edema in the preoperative patient is extremely rare.	6. Changes in the amount of edema can indicate the effectiveness or ineffectiveness of therapies and interventions.
7. Monitor serum electrolyte levels, especially potassium.	7. Diuretics may stimulate potassium loss.

Evaluation

* Is the child urinating frequently in comparison with age-related norms (see Chapter 18)?
* Is the child edematous?

* Has the child lost or gained weight?
* Are intake and output balanced?

NURSING DIAGNOSIS   Ineffective Breathing Pattern related to pulmonary congestion.

EXPECTED OUTCOMES   The child will:
* Demonstrate a respiratory rate within normal limits for age and a normal respiratory effort.
* Have satisfactory rest periods.
* Have color that remains pink or baseline cyanotic.

Intervention	*Rationale*
1. Monitor respiratory rate and rhythm, the presence or absence of retractions or nasal flaring, the use of accessory muscles, and the presence or absence of crackles or rhonchi.	1. Infants and children with CHF have changes in their breathing pattern because of increased fluid retention in the lungs, liver, and other areas of the body.
2. Position the infant or child with the head of the bed elevated 30 to 45 degrees. Avoid clothing that constricts the chest.	2. An elevated position lowers the diaphragm and maximizes chest expansion.
3. Administer oxygen as needed.	3. Supplemental oxygen administration improves oxygen saturation and delivery to tissues. Cautious use of oxygen is indicated in left-to-right shunting lesions because of the effect of oxygen on lowering pulmonary vascular resistance, which can increase pulmonary blood flow and increase the degree of pulmonary congestion and symptoms of CHF.

NURSING CARE PLAN—cont'd

4. Plan nursing interventions to allow maximum rest for the child. Feed the child when the child is rested. Avoid performing multiple interventions at any one time.
5. Prevent exposure to individuals with respiratory illnesses. Prevent nosocomial exposures and infections.

4. Clustering nursing activities decreases the child's fatigue, promotes feeding effort, and conserves metabolic demands.
5. Respiratory infections with associated CHD can have a severe adverse impact on respiratory stability. Children with CHD are at a higher risk for nosocomial infections.

Evaluation

- Is the child's respiratory rate within normal limits for age?
- Are the child's mucous membranes and nail beds pink or at baseline cyanosis?

- Is the child breathing easily?
- Is the child able to obtain an appropriate amount of rest?

NURSING DIAGNOSIS   Imbalanced Nutrition: Less Than Body Requirements related to increased energy expenditure and increased feeding effort.

EXPECTED OUTCOME   The infant or child will:
- Demonstrate appropriate weight gain and no significant loss of weight over a short period.

Intervention

1. Weigh the infant or child daily or before and after each feeding for breastfed infants. Use the same scale.
2. Breastfeed or feed smaller volumes of concentrated formula (24-27 cal/oz) every 3 hours.

3. Use a nipple that the infant can comfortably adjust for flow rate and energy to express milk. May need a soft, large-hole nipple.

4. Implement gavage feedings if the infant tires before the recommended amount of feedings is consumed, takes longer than 30 minutes to feed, displays increased fatigue during or after feeding, or demonstrates poor weight gain on adequate caloric intake.
5. Time the feedings to allow for adequate rest. Every 3 hours is a frequently used interval.

6. Monitor for feeding intolerance.

Rationale

1. Using the same scale ensures consistency.

2. Increased caloric content of formula increases caloric consumption and enhances weight gain. May require 120 to 150 kcal/kg/day for adequate weight gain. Additives are available that increase the caloric content of breast milk.
3. Infants with CHF tire easily. An appropriate nipple for the infant minimizes the level of energy required to express milk at a rate of flow the baby can swallow comfortably. A soft nipple with a large hole may facilitate easy sucking and decrease energy expenditure during feeding.
4. Gavage feedings decrease energy expenditure and allow calories consumed to be used for growth. Can be used in conjunction with timed nipple periods to maintain feeding skills.

5. Frequent disturbances increase oxygen consumption. Too frequent feedings disturb rest, whereas less frequent feedings require increased intake, which tires the infant.
6. May not tolerate concentrated formulas. Also, gastroesophageal reflux may be present.

Evaluation

- Has the infant or child maintained a steady weight gain?
- Is the feeding pattern stable or changing?

- Is the infant or child tolerating feedings without vomiting or other signs of intolerance?

NURSING DIAGNOSIS   Deficient Knowledge related to anxiety and unfamiliarity with the disease process, treatment, interventions, and home care.

EXPECTED OUTCOMES   Parents will:
- Describe the cardiac defect and current and future interventions.
- Demonstrate an ability to perform treatments, including medication administration.

Continued

NURSING CARE PLAN—cont'd

Intervention	*Rationale*
1. Determine the parents' readiness to learn, anxiety level, knowledge needed to care for their child, and specific concerns.	1. A baseline assessment of prior knowledge should be considered before developing a teaching plan. Addressing special concerns initially can facilitate parents' comfort level and receptiveness to new knowledge. Decreasing anxiety assists with information processing.
2. Provide brief, factual explanations of the child's defect or any treatments and interventions. Do so frequently.	2. Parents are most likely to retain consistent, repetitive explanations.
3. Allow the parents and child to verbalize feelings and concerns related to hospitalization and caring for the child at home.	3. Hospitalization is a frightening experience. By allowing verbalization of feelings and concerns related to the experience, nurses can assist in allaying fears and addressing concerns. Discussing care at home can also assist in allaying fears and addressing concerns.
4. Teach the parents to administer all necessary cardiac medications and explain their associated actions and potential adverse effects. Provide demonstrations and obtain return demonstrations by parents. Explain the use of oral syringes for accurate measurement of drugs. Provide a daily medication chart (which can be color-coded for specific medications) for children receiving multiple medications. Provide parents with written information (Box 22-1).	4. Family members should be taught how to administer all cardiac medications before discharge. This allows for teaching appropriate medication dosage, questions, answers, and evaluation of their home care techniques. Written information provides an adjunct to individual teaching and a reference for the caregiver at home. Written information can be referred to during less stressful times, when it may be more likely to be retained or used as a reference.
5. Assess parents' understanding of instructions through return demonstrations and repeated information. This includes signs and symptoms requiring medical or nursing assessment.	5. Return demonstrations and repeated information validate that learning has occurred and that the parents are competent to provide care.

Evaluation

- Have the parents verbalized adequate and correct knowledge of the diagnosis and interventions?
- Have the parents demonstrated confidence and competence in caregiving activities, including medicine administration?

- Are the parents able to describe conditions that necessitate a call for medical or nursing advice?

BOX 22-1 | PARENTS WANT TO KNOW   About Giving Your Child Digoxin Elixir

Medication: Digoxin (Lanoxin)
Your child's dosage: _____ mL twice a day. Your child will be taking this medicine twice a day for several months to years.
What it does: Digoxin (Lanoxin) helps the heart pump blood more efficiently.
What you need to know:
- Digoxin (Lanoxin) is usually given every morning and evening. You may adjust the times to fit your and your child's schedule.
- Give the digoxin 20 to 30 minutes before a feeding. Give it at the same time every day so that it becomes part of your routine.
- The amount of digoxin you give your child must be measured carefully with a syringe, not the dropper provided with the medicine.
- Put a few drops of digoxin in your child's mouth and let the child swallow it before giving more.

- If you forget to give your child a single dose of digoxin, give the dose when you remember it; then resume your original schedule.
- If your child vomits after taking the digoxin, do not repeat the dose. Resume the digoxin at the next dosage time.
- *If you miss or your child vomits two doses in a row, call the cardiology department.*
- Rarely, children have too much digoxin in their body and can have vomiting. If your child vomits, call your pediatrician or cardiologist. You will be instructed what to do about your child's dosage.
- Keep the digoxin in a place where children living or playing in your home will not be able to reach it.
- If someone accidentally takes the digoxin, call poison control or take the person and the digoxin bottle to the emergency department.
- Obtain refills at least 1 week before you are out of medicine. Ask for new prescriptions as needed.

Modified and used with permission from Children's Hospital Oakland, Department of Cardiology, Oakland, CA. Developed and revised by Lili Cook, RN, MS, and Sally Higgins, PhD, RN, FAAN.

Pulmonary Hypertension

Pulmonary hypertension is defined as an elevated mean pulmonary artery pressure of greater than 25 mm Hg at rest or ≥30 with exercise (Rosenzweig, Widlitz, & Barst, 2004). Initially, in children with significant left-to-right shunting, there is reversible pulmonary vasoconstriction and increased pulmonary blood flow that causes elevated pulmonary artery pressure. Pulmonary vascular disease occurs when vascular changes lead eventually to vessel wall thickening, severe irreversible vasoconstriction, and vascular obstruction. This severe condition leads to a reversal of the cardiac shunting, becoming right to left (called *Eisenmenger syndrome*), with less blood being pumped to the lungs, so that the child becomes cyanotic although the defect was previously acyanotic. It is critical to time any surgical intervention before the development of irreversible vascular changes. This information is assessed clinically and in the cardiac catheterization laboratory. Repair of lesions with large left-to-right shunts is generally recommended in the first 3 to 6 months of life.

Pulmonary hypertension has multiple etiologies. In children with congenital heart disease, the causes include pulmonary overcirculation, pulmonary vasoconstriction, and pulmonary vascular disease. Other conditions leading to pulmonary hypertension include alveolar hypoxia, such as pulmonary parenchymal disease or airway obstruction that leads to vasoconstriction. Pulmonary venous hypertension is seen in left heart outflow obstructive lesions and connective tissue disorders. Some children have pulmonary arterial hypertension. When no underlying disease can be found, it is referred to as idiopathic. Additionally, newborns may have idiopathic pulmonary arterial hypertension.

Children with large left-to-right shunting lesions, particularly at the ventricular level, have high pulmonary artery pressures but low pulmonary vascular resistance; initially CHF develops. Management is directed toward treating the CHF. Additionally, the families are advised to have the child avoid strenuous exercise and high altitudes. Treatment with vasodilators or oxygen may, or may not, be helpful (Park, 2002). Inhaled nitric oxide has been shown to be an effective pulmonary vasodilator and is used in the treatment of persistent pulmonary hypertension of the newborn. With early surgical intervention, children with reversible pulmonary hypertension can have a return of normal pulmonary pressures postoperatively. As increasing pulmonary vascular resistance caused by pulmonary vascular changes develops, children have a higher risk for surgical morbidity and mortality and for development of irreversible pulmonary hypertension.

Cyanosis

Significant CHD manifests with central cyanosis (hypoxemia). Cyanosis, a bluish discoloration of the skin, nail beds, and mucous membranes, appears when tissues are deprived of adequate amounts of oxygen. Cyanosis becomes visible when hemoglobin, approximately 5 g/dL blood, circulates unbound to oxygen and the measured oxygen saturation drops below

85%. The degree of cyanosis varies; some children will appear pale and mildly cyanotic, whereas others will be quite dusky. In anemic infants or children, desaturation will be higher before cyanosis is apparent (lower hemoglobin level in anemia, so a higher percentage needs to be desaturated before cyanosis is visible). Concurrently, with significant polycythemia, children will appear cyanotic when less desaturated (higher hemoglobin in polycythemia, so a lower percentage needs to be desaturated before cyanosis is visible).

Cardiac lesions produce cyanosis when desaturated blood from the venous system enters the saturated arterial system without passing through the lungs. Cyanosis can occur when blood flow to the lungs is decreased (e.g., in severe pulmonary artery stenosis, pulmonary atresia, tetralogy of Fallot, or tricuspid atresia) or desaturated blood is pumped to the body (e.g., in total anomalous pulmonary venous return, truncus arteriosus, and hypoplastic left heart syndrome). Cyanosis intensifies with crying in children with these defects and is not alleviated by the administration of 100% oxygen.

The clinical consequences of cyanosis include polycythemia, anemia, clotting abnormalities, hypercyanotic episodes, central nervous system (CNS) injury caused by abscess or embolic events, pulmonary hypertension, and endocarditis. Developmental delay can be related to CNS injury, severe hypoxic events, or chronic illness.

Polycythemia is a compensatory response of the body to chronic hypoxia. The body attempts to improve tissue oxygenation by increasing the oxygen-carrying capacity of the blood—in other words, by producing additional red blood cells. Accelerated red blood cell production increases the viscosity of the blood and crowds the vascular space so there is less room for plasma and clotting factors. Children who are polycythemic are at greater risk for bruising and prolonged bleeding because of decreased specific clotting factors.

Increased blood viscosity makes the peripheral circulation sluggish and places the child at risk for CNS injury from a brain abscess or cerebrovascular accident. Depletion of iron stores may also result, and anemia may develop if iron is not available to participate in hemoglobin formation.

Dehydration can occur rapidly in cyanotic heart disease. Hyperthermia (fever or environmental), poor oral intake, vomiting, and diarrhea can cause acute dehydration. Dehydration can be life threatening for the child with cyanotic heart disease who is shunt dependent for pulmonary blood flow. Once the shunt closes off, there is no pulmonary blood flow and metabolic acidosis and severe hypoxemia will develop and degenerate to cardiopulmonary arrest.

Hypercyanotic Episode

A serious, clinically significant, and dramatic event seen in children with cyanotic heart disease is the hypercyanotic episode. These events are often called *tet spells* because they frequently occur in children with unrepaired tetralogy of Fallot. The exact cause is unknown, but it is thought that the child has acute spasm of the right ventricular outflow tract as a result of agitation or another adverse event that dramatically decreases pulmonary blood flow, causing hypoxia and metabolic acidosis (Bernstein, 2004). These episodes include rapid and deep respirations (tachypnea, hyperpnea), irritability and crying, peripheral vasodilation, increased systemic venous return, increasing cyanosis that can be very severe, and a decrease in the systolic murmur, reflecting decreased pulmonary blood flow (Bernstein, 2004). As the child becomes more cyanotic, the child has increased tachypnea and hyperpnea, which increase the degree of right-to-left shunting. The incidence of hypercyanotic spells is not directly related to the degree of baseline desaturation and cyanosis.

Hypercyanotic episodes are seen most frequently in the first 2 years of life and seem to occur mainly in the morning. Often the episode is preceded by crying, feeding, or defecation. The infant becomes agitated and may eventually lose consciousness. Although usually self-limiting, the spells can progress to a vicious cycle that can be fatal if not recognized and treated. Frequent or prolonged episodes may lead to diminished cerebral oxygenation and ischemic brain injury.

Treatment of the episode includes calming the infant, placing the infant in the knee-chest position, and administering oxygen. Morphine sulfate is administered to suppress the respiratory center and decrease the degree of hyperpnea (which contributes to vasodilation) (Park, 2002). Potent medications that cause vasoconstriction (e.g., phenylephrine) may be needed to increase systemic vascular resistance, decrease the degree of right-to-left shunting, and force blood into the pulmonary system. Preventing or treating hypovolemia is also an important factor. Ultimately, however, hypercyanotic episodes indicate the need to surgically repair or palliate the defect.

NURSING CARE

The Child With Cyanosis

Assessment

The nurse must know the source of pulmonary blood flow when caring for a child with cyanotic heart disease. Infants and children who are shunt dependent for pulmonary blood flow are at risk for shunt thrombosis (as just detailed). Infants with right-to-left shunts are at risk for air embolus in IV lines.

Evaluation of the child with cyanotic heart disease includes an assessment of baseline cyanosis and general appearance. Assess the level of activity, including irritability. Visible cyanosis is most easily seen in natural light and is evaluated by observing the skin of the central mucous membranes of the mouth and conjunctiva and the nail beds. General skin color is also assessed. Cyanotic children may be smaller than their peers and may demonstrate clubbing, thickening, and flattening of the fingertips and toes as a result of polycythemia (see Fig. 21-6). Oxygen saturations should be obtained and compared with the children's baselines. Some children with cardiac defects require life-long daily antibiotic prophylaxis, for example, children with infective endocarditis or patients with asplenia; therefore, the nurse needs to document this.

The child may become dyspneic during feeding, crying, and other exertional activities and may have difficulty keeping up with peers. Children with cyanosis may have frequent respiratory infections, may miss more school days, and may, as a result, academically lag behind their classmates although they are often developmentally normal. They are also at greater risk for development of infective endocarditis and may need continuing antibiotic prophylaxis. If the child requires an IV line for hydration or another indication, it is imperative the nurse assess IV line patency and inspect IV tubing for the presence of air in the line because the risk of systemic air emboli causing a stroke or heart attack is always present. The use of an air filter is recommended.

Nursing Diagnosis and Planning

Nursing diagnoses and expected outcomes typical for the child with cyanosis and the child's family include the following:

- Deficient Knowledge related to inexperience with the management of a child with a life-threatening illness.

  Expected Outcomes: The parents, and child if age appropriate, will explain the disease process, treatment, and interventions and will demonstrate the ability to perform home care treatments, including medication administration.

- Interrupted Family Processes related to impact of an acute, chronic, or life-threatening disease.

  Expected Outcomes: The parents will express positive feelings for their child and for each other and will demonstrate the ability to meet the needs of the child, each other, and other family members.

- Delayed Growth and Development related to altered oxygenation or inadequate cardiac output to meet metabolic needs.

  Expected Outcomes: The child will demonstrate adequate growth according to an optimal growth curve for age and condition and will perform motor, social, and expressive skills typical of age group within the scope of the child's present capabilities. The parents will describe any developmental delay or deviation and make plans for intervention.

- Ineffective Tissue Perfusion related to hypercyanotic episodes.

  Expected Outcomes: The child will remain free of decreased tissue perfusion, as evidenced by the absence of profound cyanosis and by the child's activity level, affect, respiratory status, and oxygenation all being normal. The parents will list signs and symptoms that would signal the onset of hypercyanotic episodes.

- Risk for Infection related to the presence of infection-promoting conditions created by the underlying defect.

  Expected Outcomes: The child will remain free of endocardial infection. The parents will understand and carry out the ordered antibiotic prophylaxis; and the parents will list when to seek medical attention for fevers.

- Deficient Knowledge related to unfamiliarity with the systemic complications from increased risk of clotting.

Expected Outcome: The parents will describe the signs and symptoms to report immediately, including increasing cyanosis, vomiting, and fever (signs of clotting of the pulmonary shunt), and new-onset facial or extremity weakness, slurred speech, clumsiness, or breathing difficulty (signs of a CNS clot).

Interventions

Cyanotic heart disease is usually diagnosed in the newborn period. The initial nursing interventions are directed toward stabilizing the child hemodynamically and preparing the child for medical or surgical intervention. Pulmonary blood flow in cyanotic heart disease may depend on the persistence of the ductus arteriosus. Prostaglandin (PG) E_1, a vasodilator, is often administered IV to maintain ductal patency. The nurse is responsible for monitoring PGE_1 infusion flow and evaluating peripheral perfusion and respiratory status.

Parental teaching and support at the time of diagnosis are paramount. Parents receive complicated information and are often asked to make important decisions that may affect their child's current therapy and, perhaps, future interventions. Parents need simple yet thorough explanations to help them make informed choices. The nurse may need to repeat the information several times. Help parents identify sources of emotional support and encourage communication within the family.

Parents of children with cardiovascular disease respond with a variety of reactions. Knowing this, the nurse has a responsibility to educate parents about their child's disease and to stress the importance of the child interacting with the environment as normally as possible. For effective planning and provision of care, the child's condition must be placed in the context of the family's life.

In the child with cyanosis, careful monitoring of fluid status is necessary to prevent hemoconcentration. Intake and output are closely monitored, and daily weights may be recorded during hospitalization. Teach parents to recognize illnesses that place their child at risk for dehydration and to seek medical attention when their child has fluid losses.

Parents have concerns about worsening cyanosis and fear hypercyanotic episodes. Teach parents to recognize events that may trigger an episode and to respond calmly and place the infant in a knee-chest position. Review indications to seek medical care. Because most children with cyanosis limit their own physical activities, parents do not need to strictly limit the child's activities.

Prevention of infective endocarditis is accomplished through antibiotic prophylaxis. Parents may be given copies of the American Heart Association's guidelines for infective endocarditis prophylaxis.

Children with cyanosis are prone to frequent respiratory infections. Respiratory infections may increase cardiac workload and lead to increased cyanosis and desaturation. Careful handwashing is necessary to reduce the risk of infection. Teach parents to avoid crowded areas and contact between their child and other people with respiratory infections.

Evaluation

- Can the parents, or child if appropriate, describe the cardiac defect and its implications?
- Are the parents able to monitor their child's condition, provide home treatments, administer medications, and support the child's fluid and nutritional needs?
- Are family members appropriately expressing feelings and supporting each other and the child, and can the parents meet the needs of siblings and each other?
- Is the child showing a steady increase in physical growth and attaining age-appropriate developmental milestones?
- Is the child undergoing any change in the level of cyanosis, activity, or respiratory status and oxygenation?
- Can the parents describe signs, symptoms, and management of hypercyanotic episodes?
- Is the child afebrile and free of other signs and symptoms of infection, and can the parents explain the necessity for seeking medical attention for any fevers?
- Are the parents able to list complications related to possible pulmonary shunt or CNS clotting?

LEFT-TO-RIGHT SHUNTING LESIONS
Patent Ductus Arteriosus (PDA)

Incidence and Pathophysiology

As an isolated lesion, PDA (Fig. 22-1) accounts for 5% to 10% of all congenital heart disease (Park, 2002). In the preterm infant, however, the incidence is inversely related to gestational age; PDA affects up to 60% of neonates less than 28 weeks' gestation (Overmeire & Chemtob, 2005). PDA can also be present with all other types of congenital heart defects. In certain CDHs (e.g., tetralogy of Fallot, hypoplastic left heart syndrome), keeping the ductus arteriosus patent is critical to ensure viability through maintaining pulmonary or systemic blood flow.

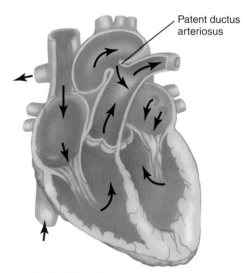

Patent ductus arteriosus

FIG 22-1 **Patent ductus arteriosus.**

PDA is caused by failure of the fetal ductus arteriosus to close completely after birth. The stimuli for this closure are the increased oxygen levels in the blood when the infant begins to breathe normally, a decrease in PG levels after birth, and a decrease in blood pressure within the ductus lumen. Normally, closure of the ductus arteriosus occurs in 50% of term neonates by 24 hours of life, in 90% by 48 hours of life, and in 100% by 72 hours of life and the ductus arteriosus degenerates to a ligament (anatomic closure) within the first few weeks of life (Clyman, 2005).

Altered Hemodynamics

In utero, the pulmonary vascular resistance is high and the lungs receive only about 5% to 8% of blood flow from the aorta. The blood flows from the pulmonary artery through the PDA to the aorta (right-to-left shunting). After birth, the pulmonary vascular resistance drops and the systemic pressure is higher than the pulmonary pressure. Then oxygenated blood from the aorta returns through the PDA to the pulmonary arteries (left-to-right shunting) to the lungs and on to the left atrium and left ventricle. The effects of this altered circulation include increased cardiac workload on the left side of the heart and increased pulmonary blood flow. There can also be decreased systemic blood flow if the PDA is large. The degree of left-to-right shunting depends on the pulmonary vascular resistance, the size and shape of the ductus, and the systemic blood pressure.

Manifestations

The degree of CHF symptoms depends on the amount of left-to-right shunting. Many children can be clinically asymptomatic. The classic murmur is a machinery-like one that can be heard throughout both systole and diastole, called a *continuous murmur*. This murmur may be accompanied by a suprasternal thrill. Continuous "runoff" of the aortic blood flow to the pulmonary arteries produces a widened pulse pressure (increased difference between systolic and low diastolic blood pressures) and bounding pulses. With significant left-to-right shunting, the heart will be enlarged and there will be increased pulmonary vascular markings on chest radiographs. Also, the infant may have tachypnea, poor feeding and weight gain, frequent respiratory tract infections, fatigue, and diaphoresis.

Preterm infants frequently are seen with CHF and increased respiratory distress. They may require ventilatory support and intensified medical and surgical interventions.

Therapeutic Management

The symptomatic term newborn infant is treated with diuretics and digoxin to control CHF. Caloric density may be increased in the formula to improve weight gain. The infant should be given rest periods to conserve energy, placed in a position of comfort to optimize respiratory effort, and monitored for signs and symptoms of increasing CHF. It is important to prevent exposure to others who have respiratory illnesses.

Medical Management. In premature, symptomatic infants, ductal closure may be achieved by the use of indomethacin (Indocin), a PG inhibitor that promotes ductal constriction. Renal function can be adversely affected and needs to be monitored. Contraindications to therapy may include abnormal renal function, thrombocytopenia, bleeding disorders, necrotizing enterocolitis, and sepsis. Intracranial hemorrhage is not a contraindication to the use of indomethacin in an infant with a symptomatic ductus arteriosus (Clyman, 2005).

Interventional Cardiac Catheterization. Nonsurgical closure of ductus arteriosus can be performed during cardiac catheterization; this type of closure has become the corrective measure of choice because it is less invasive than surgical closure and it has positive results. A coil is placed that promotes embolization (occlusion) of the ductus arteriosus. Occasionally, closure is incomplete and either additional coil placement or surgical intervention is required. Antibiotics for endocarditis prophylaxis (see p. 703) continue for 6 months until the coil endothelializes.

Surgical Management. For PDAs that cannot be closed with coils or indomethacin, surgical closure is necessary. Surgical closure is performed through a left thoracotomy. The ductus is ligated (circumferential sutures) or divided (surgically cut and the ends oversewn). Surgery is usually performed within the first year of life in symptomatic term infants who were either not candidates for or not responsive to medical management of CHF. The ductus is also ligated in preterm infants for whom indomethacin therapy is unsuccessful.

The major complication of uncorrected PDA is CHF. In addition, there is the risk for endocarditis or aneurysm if the PDA persists.

Atrial Septal Defect (ASD)

Incidence and Pathophysiology

ASD (Fig. 22-2) accounts for approximately 5% to 10% of all congenital heart disease. It is seen approximately twice as often in females than in males (Moake, 2005). This lesion consists of an abnormal opening between the atria. The

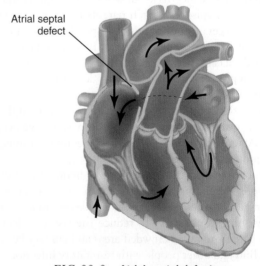

FIG 22-2 **Atrial septal defect.**

three types are (1) ostium secundum, which is located in the middle of the atrial septum (fossa ovalis) and is the most common type seen; (2) ostium primum, which is located low in the atrial septum, results from a defect in endocardial tissue formation, and is often associated with a cleft mitral valve malformation; and (3) sinus venosus, which is located high in the septum close to the superior vena cava. More commonly, the right pulmonary vein may enter normally into the left atria at the point near the ASD and give the appearance of an anomalous entry of this vein into the right atria. Mitral regurgitation is associated with some ASDs.

Altered Hemodynamics

Lower right ventricular *compliance*, which is the ease of ventricular diastolic (relaxation) filling, compared with left ventricular compliance leads to left-to-right shunting at the atrial level through the ASD. This increased blood flow through the ASD leads to an enlarged right atrium and ventricle and increased pulmonary blood flow.

Manifestations

Most infants and children are asymptomatic but, over years to decades, may have fatigue and dyspnea on exertion. Other symptoms can include palpitations or atrial arrhythmias. Recurrent respiratory infections can occur when there is a large amount of pulmonary blood flow. A murmur may not be present in infants. The characteristic systolic murmur is produced by increased blood flow across the pulmonary valve. A diastolic murmur is present with large shunts. The second heart sound usually displays fixed splitting. The chest wall may be mildly hyperactive. CHF is a rare finding in childhood (Park, 2002). It can develop in young adults because of pulmonary vascular disease and decreased right ventricular function after the second decade of life if the lesion is unrepaired. Atrial arrhythmias have been reported, usually as the result of atrial enlargement. Rarely, stroke or major organ damage can occur because of embolization of a thrombus, air, or other material that is shunted right to left at the atrial level. This is called a *paradoxical embolism*.

Therapeutic Management

The asymptomatic child is followed by the cardiologist. Spontaneous closure can occur in the first years of life for smaller-size secundum ASDs. Elective surgical repair may be performed around 2 to 5 years of age. Surgical repair is recommended for all sinus venosus and ostium primum defects. Infective endocarditis prophylaxis should be provided when indicated for 6 months after surgical repair.

Medical Management. Asymptomatic infants with moderate-size secundum ASDs are monitored for spontaneous closure in the first years of life without medication. Symptomatic infants and children are treated with diuretics and digoxin as indicated for CHF. Atrial arrhythmias are treated with appropriate antiarrhythmics.

Interventional Cardiac Catheterization. Devices to achieve transcatheter closure of ASDs are showing promising results in children with ASD, particularly of the osteum secundum type (Andrews & Tulloh, 2004; Moake, 2005). The U.S. Food and Drug Administration has approved such devices. Other devices have been used in human research trials; research is continuing on a variety of device models.

Surgical Management. Surgical closure with either sutures or a pericardial or prosthetic patch is performed on an elective basis early in childhood. This is an open heart procedure, through a sternal incision, in which cardiopulmonary bypass is used. The mortality rate is less than 2%; at most centers it is near 0%. For the young adult with ventricular dysfunction or pulmonary hypertension, the risk can be significantly higher.

Surgical complications include sinus node and atrial arrhythmias (early and late development) and postpericardiotomy syndrome (an inflammatory process with the development of pericardial effusion).

Ventricular Septal Defect (VSD)

Incidence and Pathophysiology

VSDs (Fig. 22-3) account for approximately 15% to 20% of all CHD (Park, 2002). The type of VSD is based on the location. These types include conoventricular, AV canal type, and muscular. VSD is the most common congenital cardiac lesion and it is often accompanied by other cardiac defects. The lesion consists of an abnormal opening between the right and left ventricles, which may vary in size from a minuscule hole to complete absence of the septum, resulting in a common ventricle. VSDs that are part of complex lesions are discussed in those sections.

Altered Hemodynamics

The degree of left-to-right shunting through the VSD depends on the size of the defect and the pulmonary vascular resistance compared with the systemic vascular resistance. Pulmonary vascular resistance is high in the neonate, but over the first few weeks of life the resistance decreases. As this occurs, an increased amount of blood shunts left to right at the VSD level. The pulmonary vascular circulation

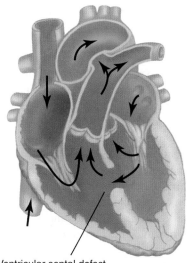

Ventricular septal defect

FIG 22-3   **Ventricular septal defect.**

receives increased pulmonary blood flow. With large defects the pulmonary arteries are exposed to systemic pressures, causing pulmonary hypertension and, over time, progressive pulmonary vascular disease (see "Pulmonary Hypertension," p. 681).

Manifestations

Signs and symptoms vary with the size of the defect and the presence of associated cardiac lesions. Clinical symptoms are usually not seen at birth because of continued high pulmonary vascular resistance in the neonate. Infants with moderate to large defects will become symptomatic within the first few weeks of life. Children with small defects will remain asymptomatic.

A murmur may not be heard in the newborn infant. The characteristic murmur is loud and harsh and can be heard over the entire systole, but the murmur can vary in duration and intensity on the basis of the degree of shunting and the size of the defect. The murmur can have an associated palpable thrill. In children with large defects, a diastolic murmur and a gallop rhythm may be present.

Infants with moderate to large defects may develop CHF that is accompanied by poor feeding and failure to thrive. An associated ASD or PDA may increase the symptoms.

Therapeutic Management

From 20% to 80% of all VSDs close spontaneously (Park, 2002). Most small lesions do not require surgical intervention. Occasionally, there is aortic valve regurgitation related to VSD position near the valve, and even if the defect is small, surgery is indicated (Bernstein, 2004). Surgical timing is based on the location of the VSD, the symptoms, and the incidence of spontaneous closure of certain types of VSDs. Generally, surgery is performed in the first year of life. Antibiotic prophylaxis is indicated for all VSDs.

Medical Management. Infants in whom CHF develops are managed with digoxin, diuretics, and, increasingly, afterload reduction (e.g., ACE inhibitors). Nutritional status is a concern, and supplements are often added to the infant's formula to increase caloric intake. Some infants have such poor energy reserves that they are unable to obtain adequate calories orally. These infants may require nasogastric tube or gastrostomy tube feedings. In addition, decreasing the infant's exposure to respiratory infections is very important.

Interventional Cardiac Catheterization. There are some interventional devices that may be used to close VSDs, similar to those used for ASDs, that have received approval from the Food and Drug Administration and others are currently under investigation.

Surgical Management. Young infants with severe CHF and failure to thrive undergo total repair, with patch closure of the defect, on cardiopulmonary bypass. Children with multiple muscular VSDs, which make complete repair more complicated, may be candidates for pulmonary artery banding. In this palliative procedure, a band is placed around the main pulmonary artery, decreasing pulmonary blood flow, reducing the severity of CHF, and decreasing the risk for pulmonary

vascular disease. The current trend is to perform corrective surgery earlier in life, and consequently, pulmonary artery banding is performed less frequently than in the past.

Total correction is accomplished by placing sutures to close small defects or by placing a pericardial or prosthetic patch over moderate and large defects. Both procedures require cardiopulmonary bypass. The surgical approach is usually through the right atrium to avoid a right ventricular incision, which could impair the contractility of the ventricle. VSDs just below the pulmonary valve are closed through an incision in the main pulmonary artery. The mortality rate is 2% to 5% after the age of 6 months. The mortality rate is higher for small infants younger than 2 months of age, in infants with associated defects, or in infants with multiple VSDs (Park, 2002).

Surgical complications include residual VSDs, pulmonary hypertension in the postoperative period, heart block that may require a pacemaker (temporary or permanent), and an abnormal rhythm called *junctional ectopic tachycardia*. In both these arrhythmias, the atria and ventricles do not conduct in the normal sequence. Cardiac output can be significantly decreased if arrhythmias are persistent. Postpericardiotomy syndrome can also occur.

Atrioventricular Septal Defect (AVSD) (Endocardial Cushion Defect)

Incidence and Pathophysiology

AV septal defects (Fig. 22-4) account for 2% of all CHD in live births (Park, 2002). These defects are often associated with genetic syndromes, with a high incidence in children with Down syndrome. Inappropriate development of the endocardial cushion tissue produces abnormalities in the atrial and ventricular septum and the AV valves (the tricuspid and the mitral valves). The three major classifications of AVSDs are (1) partial/incomplete, which is marked by an ostium primum ASD, two AV valves with a cleft in the

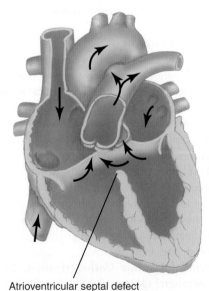

Atrioventricular septal defect
FIG 22-4   **Atrioventricular septal defect.**

mitral; (2) intermediate or transitional, in which the AV valve configuration is between two AV valves and a common AV valve, an ASD, and no significant VSD; and (3) complete, marked by a single common AV valve orifice as well as an ASD and VSD. The term *canal* has been used to describe this lesion because the defect creates a large opening in the center of the heart. *Endocardial cushion defect* is another term used to describe this defect.

Altered Hemodynamics

The direction and magnitude of the intracardiac shunting are determined by the combination of defects and the difference between aortic and pulmonary pressures. Partial defects produce left-to-right shunting with increased pulmonary blood flow and the risk of CHF; complete defects produce CHF as a result of greatly increased pulmonary blood flow and have a risk for developing into early pulmonary vascular disease in association with pulmonary hypertension. Also, there can be significant AV valve regurgitation that increases the risk of pulmonary vascular disease. Mixing of oxygenated and unoxygenated blood also occurs in very large defects, along with right-to-left shunting, so mild cyanosis may be seen. The risk of systemic air or thrombus embolization to the systemic circulation is present with right-to-left shunting.

Manifestations

The child with a partial defect may be asymptomatic. A systolic pulmonary flow murmur, however, may be heard. Children with complete AV canal can have no significant murmur as a neonate, with a murmur developing over the first few weeks of life. The symptoms seen in a child with a complete defect depend on the pulmonary artery pressure (presence or absence of pulmonary hypertension) and the size of the septal defects and degree of shunting. CHF will develop when pulmonary pressures are low and there is a large amount of left-to-right shunting. If pulmonary hypertension is present, the child may have borderline normal saturations and be intermittently cyanotic. If there is associated Down syndrome, concurrent airway compromise may be present (e.g., upper airway obstruction, hypoventilation, tracheomalacia), leading to an increased risk for pulmonary hypertension and pulmonary vascular disease.

Therapeutic Management

Medical Management. CHF is treated symptomatically with digoxin, diuretics, and afterload reduction. As in large VSDs, poor feeding and failure to thrive may occur. Nutritional recommendations include increasing caloric density, with the need for nasogastric feedings based on feeding capabilities and weight gain.

Surgical Management. If the child with a partial defect is asymptomatic, an elective surgical repair is planned in later infancy or early childhood. The ostium primum defect is closed with sutures or a prosthetic patch, and the mitral valve cleft is sutured. The infant with a complete defect undergoes surgery preferably around 3 to 4 months of age, depending on the presence of severe CHF or increased pulmonary vascular

resistance. Total correction involves closing the atrial and ventricular septal defects and constructing two AV valves from the common valve. If the mitral valve remains severely deficient (mostly regurgitation), a replacement valve may be used (although rarely performed, this is associated with higher morbidity and mortality). Correction for less-symptomatic children is generally at an age older than 3 months but before pulmonary vascular disease develops.

Children with small left or right ventricles may not be candidates for complete repair and may require palliation, such as a Fontan procedure (a surgical procedure that directs venous return directly to the pulmonary artery). Children with Down syndrome have a higher incidence of pulmonary vascular disease, and surgery is performed ideally by 3 to 6 months of age, regardless of the clinical course.

The surgical mortality may be as high as 10% in complete AV canal. For partial AV canal, the risk of death is less than 5%. Postoperative complications include those listed for VSDs. In addition, postoperative pulmonary hypertension or significant low cardiac output related to mitral valve regurgitation may develop.

OBSTRUCTIVE OR STENOTIC LESIONS
Pulmonary Stenosis

Incidence and Pathophysiology

Isolated pulmonary stenosis occurs in about 10% of congenital heart defects; however, pulmonary stenosis occurs frequently in conjunction with other congenital cardiac lesions (Daller, 2004) (Fig. 22-5). Obstructive lesions are marked by narrowing at the entrance to the pulmonary artery, which may be valvular, subvalvular, or supravalvular. The valve may be a normal tricuspid or bicuspid or dysplastic.

Altered Hemodynamics

Resistance to blood flow at the right ventricular outflow tract or valve leads to right ventricular hypertrophy. In severe pulmonary stenosis, right ventricular pressures may be

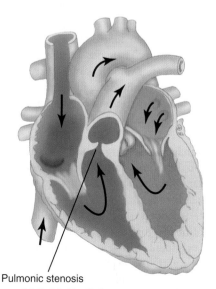

Pulmonic stenosis

FIG 22-5 **Pulmonary stenosis.**

severely elevated and may cause blood to regurgitate through the tricuspid valve into the right atrium, increasing right atrial pressure and forcing the foramen ovale open to allow blood to flow from the right to left atrium. This will lead to systemic desaturation and cyanosis. "Critical" pulmonary stenosis denotes very severe pulmonary stenosis that leads to low cardiac output. Also, in severe forms the right ventricle may be underdeveloped, which will influence the choice of medical and surgical interventions.

Manifestations

Many children are clinically asymptomatic. They have a systolic ejection murmur that may be accompanied by a palpable thrill. The heart is enlarged on chest radiographs.

Children with moderate to severe pulmonic stenosis may have exercise intolerance. Severe pulmonary stenosis may manifest with right ventricular failure, CHF, and, if there is right-to-left shunting through the foramen ovale, mild to severe cyanosis.

Therapeutic Management

Medical Management. In the clinically asymptomatic child, cardiac follow-up and appropriate antibiotic prophylaxis are the usual treatment. Over time, an increasing pressure gradient across the pulmonary valve may develop in children with pulmonic stenosis. The timing of intervention is based on the gradient across the valve, even if the child is asymptomatic. Severe pulmonary stenosis in the neonate requires emergency intervention, through either balloon dilation or surgical valvotomy. These neonates often require PGE_1 infusion to maintain ductus arteriosus patency so that there is a way for a sufficient amount of blood to return to the lungs for oxygenation (see p. 683 for a discussion of PGE_1). This infusion is often maintained for a certain stabilization period after interventional cardiac catheterization.

Interventional Cardiac Catheterization. Balloon valvuloplasty is often cited as the treatment of choice for isolated valvular pulmonary stenosis (Andrews & Tulloh, 2004). Pressure gradients are obtained during the cardiac catheterization. The valve is then dilated, with a goal of significantly decreasing the pressure. There may be some degree of pulmonary regurgitation afterward. It is often very successful and carries a low risk. Mortality rates are higher in the neonate with critical pulmonary stenosis. Reintervention because of continued significant stenosis or recurrent stenosis is sometimes necessary.

Surgical Management. Surgical valvotomy is performed when balloon dilation is unsuccessful or there is associated supravalvular stenosis. The mortality rate is very low for surgical repair. For neonates with critical pulmonary stenosis who remain dependent on PGE_1 after balloon dilation because of continued significant cyanosis related to subvalvular obstruction or a small right ventricle, surgical placement of a shunt from the aorta to the pulmonary artery may be necessary (called a *systemic-to-pulmonary artery shunt*).

Aortic Stenosis

Incidence and Pathophysiology

Aortic stenosis (Fig. 22-6) accounts for 3% to 6% of all cases of CHD. It is much more common in males than in females (Children's Hospital Boston, 2005). The level of obstruction to blood flow leaving the left ventricle can be at the valve level, supravalvular, or subvalvular. The majority of children with aortic stenosis have valvular stenosis. Severe aortic stenosis is often diagnosed in the neonatal period or first year of life. These children can be critically ill with CHF and decreased cardiac output. Children diagnosed after 1 to 2 years of age can be mostly asymptomatic with some exercise fatigue. In this lesion, the aortic valve is thickened and rigid, with some fusion of the commissures (leaflets); the valve frequently is bicuspid.

Altered Hemodynamics

Stenosis creates a pressure gradient across the aortic valve. Left ventricular hypertrophy develops. In children with severe aortic stenosis, cardiac output and myocardial blood supply through the coronary arteries may be diminished. In neonates with critical aortic stenosis, the left ventricle may not be large enough to eject a normal or adequate cardiac output.

Manifestations

Aortic stenosis may be classified as mild, moderate, or severe, depending on the degree of stenosis and the pressure gradient across the aortic valve. The diagnosis may be made with echocardiography or cardiac catheterization.

Very severe aortic stenosis manifests in early infancy and is called *critical aortic stenosis*. The infant exhibits profoundly decreased cardiac output with faint peripheral pulses, poor peripheral perfusion, severe CHF, and feeding difficulties. Older children with severe, uncorrected, aortic stenosis may have chest pain, dizziness, and syncope on exertion. Sudden death has been reported (Bernstein, 2004).

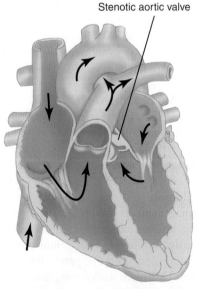

Stenotic aortic valve

FIG 22-6 **Aortic stenosis.**

Children with mild to moderate aortic stenosis are frequently clinically asymptomatic with normal growth and development, although they may manifest ECG abnormalities with strenuous exercise. A systolic ejection murmur, sometimes accompanied by a thrill or an ejection click, is heard on examination. Cardiomegaly is seen on chest radiographs.

Therapeutic Management

Medical Management. Aortic stenosis can increase over time, so continuing follow-up with the cardiologist is recommended. Treatment with antibiotics for endocarditis prophylaxis is indicated. The timing for intervention is based on the pressure gradient at the valve level, the ventricular function, and symptoms. Because approximately 3% of sudden cardiac deaths in competitive athletes are related to aortic stenosis, competitive physical activity is often limited in children with aortic stenosis on the basis of their degree of stenosis and symptoms (Maron & Zipes, 2005). Guidelines include the following: if severe stenosis, no competitive sports; if moderate stenosis, the child may compete in certain competitive sports with permission of the cardiologist subsequent to echocardiography, ECG, and exercise tolerance testing; and if mild aortic stenosis without symptoms or ECG changes, competitive sports may be allowed, although not encouraged (Graham et al., 2005).

Interventional Cardiac Catheterization. Aortic balloon valvuloplasty is performed to treat moderate to severe aortic stenosis. Decreasing the stenosis can improve cardiac output, decrease the degree of left ventricular dysfunction and hypertrophy, and reduce the risk of sudden death.

Interventional cardiac catheterization can be performed in neonates as well as older children. It is often performed in an attempt to delay surgical intervention. Complications can include the development of aortic insufficiency, artery damage or thrombosis, and infection.

Surgical Management. Surgical valvotomy may be performed in infants and children with severe aortic stenosis. Many children have aortic valvular insufficiency and restenosis after either surgical or balloon procedures and may need additional intervention.

For recurrent stenosis or progressive insufficiency, aortic valve replacement may be indicated. This becomes a very complex situation in neonates and younger children. Mechanical aortic valves require warfarin (Coumadin) for anticoagulation to decrease the risk of systemic thrombosis or valve failure because of thrombus. In addition, mechanical valves do not grow with the child and often need to be replaced. There is also an increased risk of endocarditis.

Another approach is the resection of the native aortic valve and reimplantation of the child's own pulmonary valve into the native aortic position. A pulmonary valve from a donor, called a *homograft*, is implanted from the right ventricle to the main pulmonary artery. This is called the *Ross procedure*. It does not require anticoagulation. The newly positioned "aortic" valve will grow with the child. The homograft will require replacement over time, and sometimes the new "aortic" valve will develop insufficiency. Data from a recent long-term study of a small cohort of infants who underwent a Ross procedure suggest that this procedure is an effective approach for infants with aortic stenosis (Williams et al., 2005). However, aortic root dilatation can be a significant long-term problem.

Coarctation of the Aorta

Incidence and Pathophysiology

Coarctation of the aorta (Fig. 22-7) accounts for 8% to 10% of cases of CHD (Park, 2002). Many children with coarctation of the aorta have a bicuspid aortic valve that may later become stenotic. This lesion consists of localized constriction of the aorta at or near the insertion site of the ductus arteriosus, termed the *juxtaductal region*. This improper development of the aorta creating narrowing of the aortic wall causes obstruction to left ventricular output. This narrowing can be localized to the area opposite the ductus arteriosus or there may be a more extensive area of narrowing. Narrowing increases the afterload and work on the left ventricle. Blood supply is decreased to the abdominal organs.

Altered Hemodynamics

Aortic narrowing impedes systemic blood flow and in severe cases can lead to CHF with low cardiac output as a result of left ventricular failure. Pulmonary congestion or edema can also occur as the left-sided heart pressures increase. Aortic pressure is high proximal to the constriction and low distal to the constriction. In severe cases, the neonate depends on the ductus arteriosus being patent to provide adequate systemic blood flow (circulation) to the descending aorta and abdominal organs (especially the mesenteric and renal systems). In less-severe coarctations, collateral blood vessels develop over time to provide channels for blood flow past the constricted area.

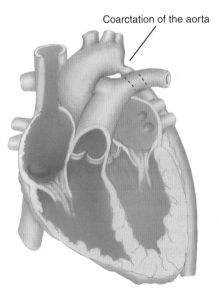

FIG 22-7 **Coarctation of the aorta.**

Manifestations

The clinical symptoms seen are directly related to the severity of the constriction and the presence of associated cardiac lesions. In the neonate with severe coarctation of the aorta, the PDA helps maintain systemic blood flow. When the ductus closes, signs of poor lower body perfusion, metabolic acidosis, CHF, and shock may develop. The infant may require PGE_1 infusion to maintain ductal patency. If a PDA is present, there may be right-to-left shunting and differential cyanosis (significant differences in color and oxygen saturation between upper and lower body parts) may result. The upper extremity saturations will be higher and reflective of left ventricular outflow and cerebral blood oxygenation. The lower extremity saturations will be lower and reflective of right ventricular outflow and descending aorta oxygenation.

Children who are diagnosed after infancy are frequently asymptomatic. They may be referred to the cardiologist after systolic hypertension (in the upper extremities) is detected on routine screening. The right upper extremity is the preferred location for blood pressure checks because the left subclavian artery can be involved in coarctation and may not accurately reflect hypertension. The classic finding in these children is a disparity in pulses and blood pressures between the upper and lower extremities. Frequently, femoral pulses are weak or absent. The child may describe weakness, tingling in the lower extremities, and muscle cramps on exertion. A systolic murmur may be heard on auscultation and may be accompanied by an ejection click (if there is a bicuspid aortic valve) or thrill.

Therapeutic Management

Treatment of the symptomatic neonate depends on the severity of the coarctation, symptoms, degree of CHF, and systemic circulation. Treatment of the older child includes hypertension management and corrective interventions.

Medical Management. Medical management of the neonate or infant with CHF includes the use of diuretics, digoxin, or other inotropic medications to improve cardiac output. In addition, the newborn infant may require PGE_1 infusions to maintain ductal patency and improve perfusion to the lower body.

Interventional Cardiac Catheterization. The use of balloon dilation of the coarctation as a primary intervention remains controversial. Balloon dilation, with possible stent placement, for children who have had a recurrence of coarctation is a well-accepted treatment option. It is a safe procedure, with low morbidity and mortality. Risks include artery thrombosis or damage, tear in the aorta, or inadequate relief of coarctation. In some instances the risk of subsequent aortic aneurysm increases in children who have had balloon angioplasty (Cowley, Orsmond, Feola, McQuillan, & Shaddy, 2005).

Surgical Management. Surgical intervention for the neonate may require cardiopulmonary bypass through a midline sternotomy incision if an extensive region of the aorta requires reconstruction or if associated intracardiac defects need repair. Elective surgical repair occurs near the time of diagnosis for significant coarctation of the aorta. The repair is performed through a left thoracotomy. Several surgical techniques are available: end-to-end anastomosis if the constricted area is short, use of a prosthetic patch to widen the constriction, or a subclavian flap in which the left subclavian artery provides the patch. Children undergoing the subclavian flap procedure will no longer have a palpable pulse in their left arm. Blood pressures should not be taken in the left arm.

Mortality rates after surgical repair in children are low but are slightly higher in infants or children with other associated congenital defects (Park, 2002). Renal failure, among other postoperative complications, can increase the mortality rate (Park, 2002). The rate of recurrence of the coarctation is elevated in children whose repairs were performed in infancy (Bernstein, 2004). These children may benefit from balloon dilation performed in the cardiac catheterization laboratory.

CYANOTIC LESIONS WITH DECREASED PULMONARY BLOOD FLOW

Cyanotic lesions permit unoxygenated, or desaturated, blood to enter the systemic circulation. Infants with complex or mixing cyanotic heart lesions who are dependent on having a PDA for all or the majority of their pulmonary or systemic blood flow can become severely symptomatic within the first few days of life as the ductus arteriosus begins to close. They often need emergency management with medical or surgical intervention to survive the neonatal period.

PGE_1 is a potent vasodilating drug that is administered to prevent closure of the ductus or to reopen the ductus arteriosus and restore pulmonary or systemic blood flow. Continuous infusion of the drug may improve arterial oxygen saturation and tissue perfusion, allowing the infant to be stabilized in anticipation of further diagnostic and treatment interventions. It is rapidly metabolized through the pulmonary circulation and excreted through the renal system. It must be infused by continuous IV administration. The major side effect is apnea, and infants frequently require intubation.

Tetralogy of Fallot

Incidence and Pathophysiology

Tetralogy of Fallot (Fig. 22-8) accounts for 10% of all cases of CHD; it is the most frequently seen cyanotic lesion in older infants and children (Park, 2002). Malalignment of the ventricular septum during fetal development results in the constellation of three of the four characteristics of this lesion: (1) a VSD, (2) pulmonary stenosis, and (3) overriding of the aorta (into the right ventricular side instead of over the left ventricle). The fourth characteristic, *right ventricular hypertrophy*, develops as a result of the pulmonary stenosis (also termed *right ventricular outflow tract obstruction*).

Altered Hemodynamics

The degree of pulmonary stenosis determines the resistance to blood flow out to the lungs through the pulmonary artery. The VSD is usually large, and the pressures in both ventricles

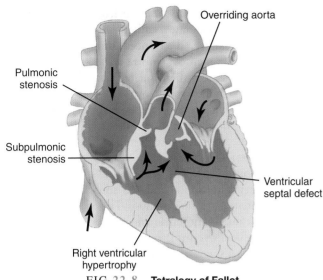

FIG 22-8 **Tetralogy of Fallot.**

Labels on figure: Overriding aorta, Pulmonic stenosis, Subpulmonic stenosis, Ventricular septal defect, Right ventricular hypertrophy

are equal. As desaturated blood enters the right ventricle (from the right atrium), it can flow into the pulmonary artery or shunt right to left across the VSD into the left ventricle (causing desaturated blood to enter the systemic circulation), depending on the relative resistance of the right heart versus the left heart.

Manifestations

The degree of pulmonary stenosis governs the onset and severity of the symptoms. The more severe the pulmonary stenosis, the less pulmonary blood flow, the greater the right-to-left shunting, the more desaturated is the blood and the more cyanotic is the child. If pulmonary stenosis is mild, there is little or no right-to-left shunting. The saturations can be normal or low normal. This is known as *pink tet.*

Some infants are cyanotic as neonates. When antegrade (forward) pulmonary blood flow is severely impeded because of pulmonary stenosis, blood flow to the lungs depends on a PDA. As the mixed saturated blood enters the aorta, a certain amount will shunt through the ductus arteriosus into the pulmonary arteries, allowing it to be oxygenated. As this structure closes, the infant becomes profoundly cyanotic.

Other infants become cyanotic over the first few months of life. Initially, they may tire easily, especially with exertion, and may have difficulty feeding and gaining weight before cyanosis develops. In time, these infants may have hypercyanotic episodes and other clinical signs of chronic hypoxemia. Auscultation reveals a harsh systolic murmur, often accompanied by a palpable thrill. The heart is boot shaped on chest radiographs because of the poor development of the pulmonary artery.

Therapeutic Management

The symptomatic neonate (severe desaturation related to decreased pulmonary blood flow or frequent tet spells) frequently needs continuous PGE_1 infusion to maintain ductal patency. Palliative or definitive surgical intervention is necessary in the first days of life.

Medical Management. Older infants need very close monitoring for signs and symptoms of worsening hypoxemia. Illnesses that put them at risk for dehydration must be treated promptly because secondary polycythemia can contribute to stroke. Hemoglobin levels and hematocrit values may be evaluated to assess for anemia. Close monitoring for hypercyanotic episodes may detect some very subtle and often self-limiting episodes lasting 10 to 15 minutes.

Surgical Management. Choices in surgical management include palliative procedures to increase pulmonary blood flow or a definitive intracardiac repair. Decisions and considerations regarding palliative or definitive repairs include institutional approach, associated anatomic issues such as abnormal coronary arteries, branch pulmonary artery size or stenosis, infant size, and whether pulmonary atresia is also present. Earlier surgical intervention is indicated for increasing or severe cyanosis, significant polycythemia, or hypercyanotic episodes. In recent years, primary surgical repair during early infancy has become the treatment of choice at many centers. Certain symptomatic infants undergo surgery during the newborn period (Bernstein, 2004). The rationale for early definitive repair is to normalize the cardiac anatomy and physiology sooner and promote normal growth of the pulmonary arteries. Definitive repair requires cardiopulmonary bypass. Postoperative complications include rhythm disturbances (e.g., a narrow complex tachycardia, varying degrees of heart block), residual VSD, low cardiac output related to right ventricular dysfunction, residual right ventricular outflow obstruction, and some degree of right-sided heart failure (Bernstein, 2004). The mortality rate for uncomplicated tetralogy of Fallot repair is reported at 2% to 3% (Park, 2002).

Some symptomatic neonates are poor candidates for primary repair. These infants may benefit from the lower-risk surgical creation of a systemic-pulmonary artery shunt to increase pulmonary blood flow. The most commonly performed is the modified Blalock-Taussig procedure. This usually is not done with the child on cardiopulmonary bypass. The complications are the same as for other thoracotomy incisions. In addition, shunt failure because of thrombosis or clot remains a potential major problem.

Tricuspid Atresia

Incidence and Pathophysiology

Tricuspid atresia (Fig. 22-9) represents approximately 1% to 3% of all (Park, 2002) and it is the third most common cyanotic cardiac condition. It is a complex lesion with many variations. In this lesion, the tricuspid valve does not develop. An ASD or patent foramen ovale must be present for the fetus or infant to survive. The right ventricle is hypoplastic (underdeveloped). The VSD can be of varying size. The pulmonary artery may be in the normal position or transposed with the aorta. There may be pulmonary stenosis of varying degrees. The newborn infant may rely on the ductus arteriosus for pulmonary blood flow. The degree of cyanosis and symptoms is related to these multiple factors.

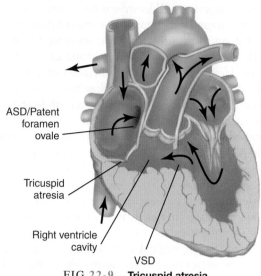

ASD/Patent foramen ovale

Tricuspid atresia

Right ventricle cavity

VSD

FIG 22-9 **Tricuspid atresia.**

Altered Hemodynamics

In a common form of tricuspid atresia, the desaturated blood enters the right atrium and is shunted right to left through the patent foramen ovale/ASD into the left atrium. It cannot flow into the right ventricle because the tricuspid valve is atretic or absent. In the left atrium, the desaturated blood mixes with the saturated blood (returning from the lungs). From the left atrium, it flows through the mitral valve into the left ventricle. Some of the mixed saturated blood flows out the aorta and to the systemic circulation. Some will flow through the VSD and into the right ventricular chamber, into the pulmonary artery, and to the lungs to become oxygenated.

For children with severe pulmonary stenosis and no VSD or other complex anatomy, the PDA is critical to ensure pulmonary blood flow.

Manifestations

Profound cyanosis may be present in the neonate and is usually visible within the first few hours of life in neonates with decreased pulmonary blood flow. Infants with increased pulmonary blood flow have milder cyanosis and increasing signs of CHF. A single first heart sound is present because there is no closure of the tricuspid valve. A systolic murmur of the VSD or a PDA murmur may be heard (if patent).

Therapeutic Management

Medical Management. For infants who depend on the PDA for pulmonary blood flow, continuous PGE$_1$ infusion is initiated. The infant is stabilized and readied for surgery. The foramen ovale can become restrictive over weeks to months, and the infant may require urgent intervention in the form of a balloon atrial septostomy during cardiac catheterization to allow blood to flow from the right atrium to the left atrium. This is a rare occurrence.

Interventional Cardiac Catheterization. To perform a balloon atrial septostomy, a catheter is inserted into the femoral vein (usually) and advanced into the right atrium and across the foramen ovale/intra-atrial septum. A balloon in this catheter is then inflated, and this balloon is pulled back through the foramen ovale, tearing the septum. If the balloon procedure is not effective, as can happen in infants beyond the newborn stage, a catheter blade septostomy can be performed to cut the septum (see "Transposition of the Great Arteries," p. 697).

Surgical Management. The goal of this staged palliative repair is to separate the desaturated and saturated blood, thereby eliminating systemic cyanosis. The equally important goal is to optimize ventricular function by decreasing the workload (volume overload) on the heart. The child will ultimately have a single ventricle.

The newborn may require a systemic–to–pulmonary artery shunt to provide adequate pulmonary blood flow if significant pulmonary stenosis is present (see discussion under "Tetralogy of Fallot," p. 691). This is the first procedure in a three-stage effort to palliate this defect.

A connection between the superior vena cava and the pulmonary arteries (bidirectional Glenn procedure) is performed at 4 to 6 months of age, once the pulmonary vascular resistance has decreased to normal pressures. This procedure reduces the volume in the left ventricle because, instead of crossing from the right atrium to the left side of the heart, the desaturated blood flows from the superior vena cava directly into the pulmonary artery and to the lungs. Pulmonary hypertension must be prevented and managed aggressively postoperatively to ensure adequate pulmonary blood flow. In addition, positioning the child with the head of the bed up to encourage passive blood flow to the lungs will help decrease the degree of venous congestion in the upper body. Pleural effusions can develop as the body adjusts to the flow and pressure changes. Occasionally, atrial arrhythmias are seen.

A third procedure, the Fontan operation, is usually performed between ages 18 months and 6 years. In this procedure, desaturated blood is directly channeled from the inferior vena cava to the pulmonary arteries. The goals with the Fontan procedure are (1) separation of the desaturated venous and saturated arterial blood and (2) volume unloading of the single ventricle. Sometimes, a small connection between the venous and arterial circulations is maintained, called a *fenestration*. This is placed in case the pressures are slightly higher than normal in the pulmonary arteries so that some desaturated blood can shunt right to left to the systemic circulation until the pulmonary arteries adjust to the new flow and pressures. At a later time, the fenestration may be closed.

Approximately 90% of children survive this procedure (Park, 2002), although postoperative and long-term complications (e.g., systemic venous pressures, pericardial and pleural effusions, supraventricular arrhythmias) are not unusual.

Pulmonary Atresia With Intact Ventricular Septum

Incidence and Pathophysiology

The incidence of pulmonary atresia with intact ventricular septum (Fig. 22-10) is less than 1% of cardiac defects seen in infants and children (Park, 2002). The causes of this lesion are the failure of the pulmonary valve to develop, accompanied by hypoplastic development of the pulmonary artery and right ventricle. The tricuspid valve may also be underdeveloped. The right ventricle pressures may be extremely high, and the coronary arteries may also be abnormal.

Altered Hemodynamics

As the blood enters the right ventricle, it cannot flow directly to the pulmonary arteries because of atresia of the pulmonary valve. The blood entering the right ventricle is propelled back through the tricuspid valve into the right atrium and shunted right to left through the foramen ovale to the left atrium. The desaturated and saturated blood mix in the left atrium and flow through the mitral valve and into the left ventricle, where the mixed blood is pumped to the aorta. From the aorta, this mixed saturated blood flows to the body and brain. Oxygenation of the blood occurs through the left-to-right shunting of blood in the aorta through the persistent PDA into the pulmonary arteries and to the lungs.

Manifestations

Profound cyanosis is seen during the early neonatal period. Survival depends on the presence of a PDA. On auscultation, the second heart sound (S_2) is single. The patent ductus murmur may be present as a soft systolic murmur or a continuous murmur.

Therapeutic Management

Medical Management. The neonate requires continuous PGE_1 infusion to maintain ductal patency. The primary treatment of this lesion is surgical.

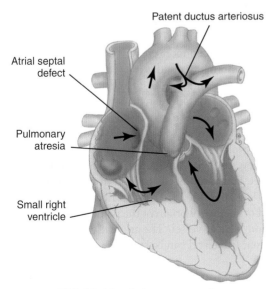

Patent ductus arteriosus

Atrial septal defect

Pulmonary atresia

Small right ventricle

FIG 22-10 **Pulmonary atresia.**

Interventional Cardiac Catheterization. As an alternative to surgical intervention, interventional cardiac catheterization with wire and radiofrequency-assisted valvulotomy achieves the same objective as surgical valvotomy but with a decreased risk for death (approximately 5%). Balloon dilatation of the valve follows the valvotomy (Bernstein, 2004; Park, 2002).

Surgical Management. Early surgical intervention involves pulmonary valvotomy or the creation of a systemic–to–pulmonary artery shunt (often a Blalock-Taussig shunt) (Bernstein, 2004). Valvotomy may encourage growth of the right ventricular chamber. Over time, right-to-left shunting at the atrial level may decrease as the right ventricle increases the amount of blood it pumps to the pulmonary system. If valvotomy is successful, future surgical interventions can include closing the ASD and the systemic-to-pulmonary shunt. The child will no longer be cyanotic. The surgical mortality rate is approximately 20% after the first procedure and 15% after the second (Park, 2002). If the right ventricle remains very small and cannot pump an adequate amount of blood to the lungs, a bidirectional Glenn procedure (as discussed earlier) or staging to the modified Fontan procedure is performed.

In children with a very small right ventricle and coronary sinusoids as the major source of coronary perfusion and in whom coronary anomalies are identified, the sinusoids are left alone and a systemic–pulmonary artery shunt is performed; a Fontan-type surgery may be performed in the future. If a child has a very small right ventricle and there is no evidence of anomalies of the coronary system, sinusoidal ligation or closure of the tricuspid valve may be performed. Sometimes, cardiac transplantation may be indicated for this subgroup of children with pulmonary atresia and intact ventricular septum.

Total Anomalous Pulmonary Venous Return (TAPVR)

Incidence and Pathophysiology

- Total anomalous pulmonary venous return is a congenital heart defect that is the result of abnormal development of the fetal heart during the first 8 weeks of pregnancy (Fig. 22-11). Total anomalous pulmonary venous return makes up about 1% of all children with congenital heart defects (Park, 2002). The pulmonary veins that bring blood back to the heart from the lungs are improperly connected, resulting in no direct communication between the pulmonary veins and the left atria. In TAPVR, the four pulmonary veins are connected somewhere besides the left atrium. There are several possible places where the pulmonary veins can connect. The most common connection is to the superior vena cava. The infracardiac type occurs predominantly in boys. TAPVR is classified according to Darling's classification of the location of the pulmonary veins.
- Type I = supracardiac (50%)—"Snowman heart"
- Type II = cardiac (20%)
- Type III = infracardiac (20%)
- Type IV = mixed (10%)

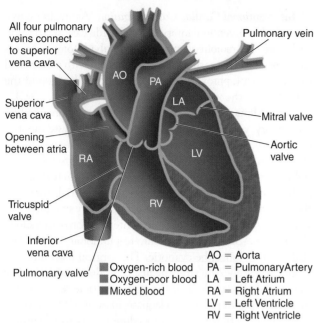

Labels on figure:
All four pulmonary veins connect to superior vena cava

Pulmonary vein

AO
PA
LA

Superior vena cava

Mitral valve

Opening between atria

Aortic valve

RA

LV

Tricuspid valve

RV

Inferior vena cava

Pulmonary valve

■ Oxygen-rich blood
■ Oxygen-poor blood
■ Mixed blood

AO = Aorta
PA = PulmonaryArtery
LA = Left Atrium
RA = Right Atrium
LV = Left Ventricle
RV = Right Ventricle

FIG 22-11   **Total anomalous pulmonary venous return.**

Altered Hemodynamics

In TAPVR, oxygen-rich blood that should return to the left side of the heart and then the body instead mixes with the oxygen-poor blood flowing into the right side of the heart. This situation by itself will not support life because there is no way for oxygenated blood to be delivered to the body. However, other heart defects that are often associated with TAPVR actually help the infant with TAPVR live until surgical intervention is possible:

- An ASD or a VSD will allow mixing of the blood from the right and left side of the heart, thereby allowing some oxygen to reach the body.
- A PDA will also allow mixing of blood. The oxygenated blood that results from this mixing is beneficial, providing at least a little oxygen to the body.

Manifestations

Presentation is determined by the classification. Infants can have severe respiratory distress, including tachypnea and cyanosis, usually at age 24 to 36 hours. Tachycardia may be present as well. Signs of pulmonary hypertension progress with worsening cyanosis. There is progressive clinical deterioration and early death in the first week or month of life, depending on the degree of pulmonary venous obstruction. Or they may have symptoms more similar to a very large AVSD. Mild failure to thrive with greater respiratory effort than normal with activity or recurrent respiratory infections may be present.

Physical symptoms may include severe cyanosis with significant respiratory distress. A murmur usually is not present, yet a systolic murmur over the pulmonary area or a tricuspid insufficiency murmur at the mid and lower left sternal border may be observed, and a gallop may be present. Peripheral pulses usually are normal after birth but may decrease as heart failure progresses. Liver enlargement commonly occurs, especially in TAPVR type III, with subdiaphragmatic drainage.

Therapeutic Management

Medical Management. CHF occurs in obstructive and unobstructive types of TAPVR. Neonates or young infants with obstructed TAPVR frequently have pulmonary edema with varying degrees of increases in pulmonary arterial and venous resistance. Pulmonary edema is treated with digitalis, diuretics, and oxygen. Some infants may require mechanical ventilation with oxygen and positive end-expiratory pressure. It is also important to correct any metabolic acidosis that may be present. No catheter-corrective treatment exists for TAPVR, although a balloon or blade atrial septostomy may be used in some patients when the foramen ovale is restricted to enlarge communication.

Surgical Management. Surgical repair of TAPVR with venous obstruction is necessary for all infants with this condition soon after birth. Infants who do not have obstructive TAPVR but who do have CHF usually undergo surgery between 4 and 6 months of age.

Procedures vary with the site of the anomalous drainage. However, all procedures attempt to redirect the pulmonary venous return to the left atrium. Surgery is performed with use of cardiopulmonary bypass, hypothermia, and total circulatory arrest.

In patients with a supracardiac or infracardiac connection, the common pulmonary vein is opened wide and a side-to-side anastomosis is made to the left atrium. The ASD is closed, and the ascending or descending vein is ligated. In a cardiac connection (to right atrium or coronary sinus), a coronary sinus may be separately tunneled to the right or left atrium to drain with the pulmonary veins, directing low-oxygen-saturated coronary sinus blood to the left atrium. The ASD is closed, directing pulmonary veins to the left atrium

CYANOTIC LESIONS WITH INCREASED PULMONARY BLOOD FLOW
Truncus Arteriosus

Incidence and Pathophysiology

Truncus arteriosus (Fig. 22-12) accounts for approximately 1% of all CHD (Park, 2002). It is marked by incomplete division of the common great vessel, the truncus arteriosus, which normally divides into the pulmonary artery and pulmonary valve and the aorta and aortic valve during fetal development. This failure in division results in a single large vessel and single valve, which gives rise to the pulmonary, systemic, and coronary circulations. The ventricular septum fails to develop at the same time, and therefore an associated VSD is present. The common truncal arteriosus vessel overrides the VSD and receives blood from both right and left ventricles. There are four classifications of truncus arteriosus related to the site of origin of the pulmonary artery from the common truncal vessel. The truncal valve is not a normal semilunar valve and can be stenotic or regurgitant.

Altered Hemodynamics

Desaturated blood enters the right atrium and flows through the tricuspid valve into the right ventricle. Saturated blood

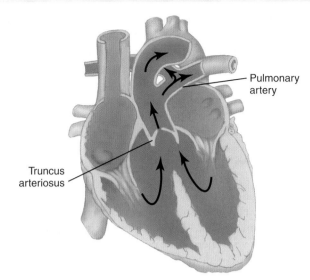

FIG 22-12 **Truncus arteriosus.**

from the left atrium flows through the mitral valve and into the left ventricle. The desaturated and saturated blood mix in the ventricles at the level of the VSD and common ventricular outflow tract. The common great vessel sends this mixed blood to the systemic, pulmonary, and coronary circulations. Oxygen saturation depends on the volume of pulmonary blood flow, related to the pulmonary vascular resistance; the greater this flow, the more symptoms of CHF, decreased cardiac output, and potential for coronary artery ischemia. The ventricles are under pressure and volume overload.

Manifestations

The infant presents, often in the neonatal period, with CHF and some degree of cyanosis. The volume of pulmonary blood flow determines the severity of symptoms. Unrestricted flow to the pulmonary artery results in pulmonary congestion and severe CHF. If undetected, pulmonary vascular disease can develop in early infancy. If pulmonic stenosis is present, pulmonary blood flow is limited and cyanosis increases.

A harsh systolic murmur is heard that may be accompanied by a thrill. A diastolic murmur of truncal valve insufficiency may be heard. The opening of the single truncal valve may produce a click. The infant may also have bounding pulses and a widened pulse pressure because of truncal valve insufficiency.

Therapeutic Management

Medical Management. Medical management is aimed at reducing the effects of CHF and preventing polycythemia. CHF is treated with digoxin and diuretics. Surgical repair is recommended in the neonatal period.

Surgical Management. Neonates who do not respond to early medical management may benefit from pulmonary artery banding; however, known risks and complications are associated with this procedure, and total corrective surgery is preferred (Park, 2002).

The corrective repair includes closing the VSD and placement of a conduit from the right ventricle to the pulmonary artery. A valvuloplasty of the truncal valve, which is the neoaortic valve, may be performed to improve valvular competence. Blood flow postoperatively is normal.

Surgical mortality depends on the type of truncus and the extent of the required repair. The risk for death is higher with truncal valve stenosis or insufficiency or other associated problems. Conduit replacement is necessary as the child grows, and a future truncal valve repair or replacement may be needed. Infective endocarditis prophylaxis is indicated.

Hypoplastic Left Heart Syndrome

Incidence and Pathophysiology

Hypoplastic left heart syndrome (Fig. 22-13) accounts for 1% of all CHD (Park, 2002). It is seen more frequently in males than in females. Most infants with untreated hypoplastic left heart syndrome die within the first few months of life (Bernstein, 2004).

Inadequate development of the left side of the heart results in only one effective ventricle. The syndrome may include aortic valve atresia, hypoplasia of the left ventricle, atresia or hypoplasia of the ascending aorta, and mitral valve stenosis or atresia. Most infants have an intact ventricular septum (Park, 2002).

Altered Hemodynamics

Saturated pulmonary venous blood return is unable to flow from the left atrium through the rest of the left side of the heart. It is shunted left to right through a patent foramen ovale into the right atrium, where it mixes with desaturated blood. Mixed saturated blood travels through the right ventricle to the main pulmonary artery. A portion of blood flows to the branch pulmonary arteries and to the lungs. A portion flows from the pulmonary artery through the PDA to the descending aorta. From the aorta this mixed saturated blood provides systemic and coronary blood supply. The coronary blood supply is from retrograde flow in the ascending aorta to the coronary arteries.

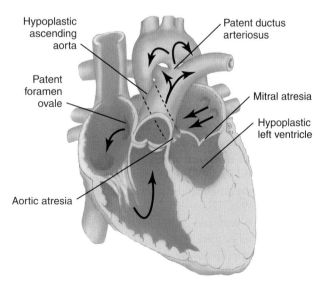

FIG 22-13 **Hypoplastic left heart syndrome.**

Manifestations

Most infants have, within the first few days of life, tachypnea and early CHF from increased pulmonary blood flow and, as the ductus arteriosus begins to close, systemic hypoperfusion and shock. The infant appears grayish blue in color, with dyspnea and hypotension.

Therapeutic Management

Management recommendations include options of supportive care only, surgical staged repair, or cardiac transplantation. The management options depend on the facility, team, and country. Over the past 20 years, progress in the stabilization, surgical interventions, and medical management has improved considerably and surgical intervention has become the preferred approach in many centers. Because parents often need to make the choice between the three options very rapidly, they may not be totally prepared to make such an important decision. Parents are likely to be highly anxious, responding to the severity of the child's condition, the prospect that their infant may die, and their own feelings of loss. Because these overwhelming feelings can interfere with effective decision making, health professionals need to be certain to fully inform the parents about the risks and benefits (both short-term and long-term) of each course of action, allow them the time to evaluate, and respect the parents' decision (Zeigler, 2003).

Medical Management. Emergency management addresses correction of the acid-base and electrolyte imbalances and re-establishment of ductal patency with use of PGE_1. If the family chooses not to have surgical or transplant intervention, PGE_1 is discontinued and supportive care is provided.

Surgical Management. Two surgical courses are available. Cardiac transplantation, as a single, definitive correction, has been successful, particularly when performed very early. The scarcity of neonatal donor hearts, however, greatly limits the number of infants who may receive transplants, and the prospect of life-long immunosuppression must be considered (Bernstein, 2004). The need for retransplant should be a consideration as well.

A three-stage palliative repair is known as the *Norwood procedure*. The child will have a single ventricle at the completion of the procedure. The stage I Norwood procedure provides unobstructed blood flow from the right ventricle to the main pulmonary artery, which is surgically connected to the ascending aorta, making a "neoaorta." This effectively allows the right ventricle to act as the systemic ventricle and the pulmonary artery to act as the aorta. Pulmonary blood flow is supplied through a systemic–to–pulmonary artery surgical shunt. This procedure is performed during the neonatal period.

The second stage, a bidirectional Glenn procedure, is performed at approximately 6 months of age (see "Tricuspid Atresia," p. 692). The palliation is completed, usually before the child is 6 years old, with a modified Fontan procedure (see "Tricuspid Atresia," p. 692). The surgical mortality rate for the staged procedure varies widely among institutions. The 4-year survival rate after staged repair is greater than 50% (Park, 2002).

Death remains a major factor after the stage I Norwood procedure and subsequent stages for single ventricle physiology. Postoperative and long-term complications include hypoxemia, CHF, right ventricular (systemic) dysfunction, pulmonary artery anomalies, systemic venous hypertension, pleural effusion, protein-losing enteropathy, arrhythmias, endocarditis, and developmental delays (Rosenthal, 2000). There is a risk of ventricle failure later in life.

Transposition of the Great Arteries (TGA)

Incidence and Pathophysiology

Transposition of the great arteries (Fig. 22-14) accounts for 5% of all CHD (Bernstein, 2004). It is more common in males than in females. Nearly half of affected children have a coexisting VSD (Bernstein, 2004). Improper septation and rotation of the common truncal vessel in fetal life cause this defect. In TGA the right ventricle gives rise to the aorta, and the left ventricle gives rise to the pulmonary artery.

Altered Hemodynamics

In this defect, the pulmonary and systemic circulations exist in parallel. Desaturated systemic venous blood returns to the right atrium, flows into the right ventricle, and pumps the desaturated blood into the aorta and back to the body. Saturated pulmonary venous blood returns to the left atrium (from the lungs), flows into the left ventricle, and is pumped through the pulmonary artery and back through the lungs. Survival depends on mixing of these two circulations through the fetal structures—the foramen ovale and ductus arteriosus. This allows oxygenated blood to be delivered to the body and deoxygenated blood to return to the lungs for oxygenation.

Manifestations

Most neonates with this defect have cyanosis during the first few hours or days of life. They demonstrate hypoxemia with a minimal response to oxygen administration. If intracardiac

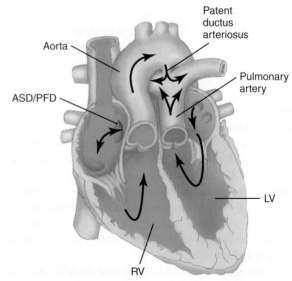

FIG 22-14   **Transposition of the great arteries.**

mixing is inadequate, they have progressive desaturation and acidosis. They can develop CHF. Prompt diagnosis and treatment are paramount for survival.

Therapeutic Management

Medical Management. A continuous infusion of PGE_1 is begun to maintain ductal patency and support mixing of oxygenated and unoxygenated blood at the level of the ductus. A Rashkind balloon atrial septostomy by interventional cardiac catheterization may be performed on some infants to enhance mixing of blood if there is not adequate intra-atrial mixing. Neonates with a VSD may have improved intracardiac mixing and improved oxygen saturation.

Surgical Management. The current surgical treatment of choice is the arterial switch procedure. This procedure anatomically corrects the defect by placing the pulmonary artery and aorta in their proper anatomic positions over the right ventricle and left ventricle, respectively. The critical component of this surgery is the reimplantation of the coronary arteries in the newly positioned aorta. The arterial switch survival rate is 90% to 95% for uncomplicated lesions (Bernstein, 2004). Coronary artery anomalies, associated coarctation, and multiple VSDs can increase mortality. Postoperative complications include low cardiac output related to poor left ventricular function and arrhythmias related to decreased coronary artery perfusion and myocardial ischemia.

THE CHILD UNDERGOING CARDIAC SURGERY

Most cardiac lesions are amenable to palliative or corrective repair, and the child with significant CHD will undergo a surgical or interventional catheterization procedure at some point during infancy or childhood. The timing of surgery is dictated by the child's clinical condition, but the trend in recent years is to intervene at an early age. The ultimate goal of intervention is for a two-ventricle repair, with physiologic and anatomic correction to normal or near-normal circulation. Complex lesions may require multiple, palliated stages with the goal of separating the saturated and desaturated blood, correcting cyanosis, and optimizing pulmonary and cardiac function.

Families anticipate surgery as a means of achieving a more normal lifestyle, but they also feel anxiety about the child's postoperative course and ultimate outcome. The nurse can help both the child and the parents cope with this stressful and traumatic event through support and education.

Preoperative Preparation

Preoperative teaching and preparation expose the child and family to the hospital environment and expected perioperative and postoperative care. The family should receive verbal, written, and visual information that describes the course of events throughout the hospitalization. Interpreter services should be used when indicated. It is important to evaluate the family's understanding of the surgical procedure and its expected outcomes. A multidisciplinary team, including physicians, nurses, child life specialist, and social services, provides a comprehensive approach in the assessment of and interventions for the child and family. Barriers to actual hospitalization (e.g., financial, social, transportation) and discharge can be identified and interventions begun before the actual hospitalization. In addition, identifying positive coping mechanisms and providing anticipatory guidance can help the child and parent be empowered in their understanding and participation in care while the child is hospitalized. In family-centered care the health care team works with the family in caring for the child.

The parents and child should tour the intensive care unit (Fig. 22-15) and other units in which the child will be during the hospitalization. This preparation allows them to become familiar with the physical environment and the noise and activity level. The visit should allow time for the family to meet members of the nursing staff and see equipment that will be used in the child's postoperative care. In addition, seeing other families and children who have undergone similar procedures as they progress and recover from the surgical process can be an encouraging experience.

Monitors, ventilators, and tubes should be described and shown to the family. Parents and children should be reminded that invasive monitoring lines, chest tubes, and an endotracheal tube are inserted during surgery while the child is anesthetized, and they should be reassured that these tubes and lines will be removed as soon as the child's condition permits.

The sequence of events surrounding the day of surgery—when and where to arrive and where to wait during the procedure—should be reviewed. Parents should be assured that they will receive updates about their child's condition throughout the procedure and will be permitted to visit soon after the surgery is completed.

Postoperative Management

Postoperative nursing management includes promoting hemodynamic and respiratory stability, preventing and identifying potential complications, providing comfort, ensuring pain assessment and interventions, and providing continuing educational and emotional support. Early postoperative care in the intensive care unit involves continuous monitoring of vital signs and cardiac output and frequent multisystem assessments. These assessments continue, with decreasing intensity, until discharge.

Cardiac surgical repair is either a closed heart procedure or an open heart procedure. The underlying cardiac defect and anticipated surgical intervention are the determining factors in the type of procedure performed.

In a closed heart surgery, the heart continues to pump and maintain cardiac function during the repair. Some closed heart procedures are repair of a PDA, coarctation of the aorta, and certain aorta-to-pulmonary shunts.

Potential complications include recurrent laryngeal nerve injury with associated vocal cord paralysis, pneumothorax, chylothorax, atelectasis, phrenic nerve injury and associated diaphragm paralysis, bleeding, infection, and rarely death.

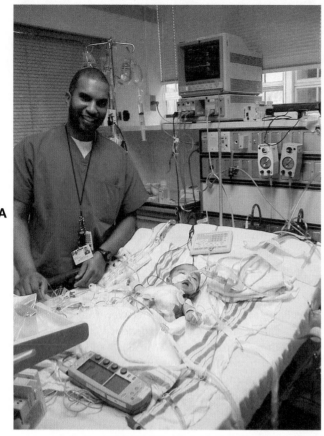

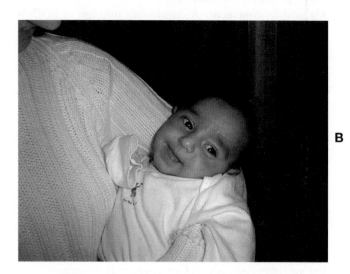

FIG 22-15 **A, A preoperative visit to the intensive care unit and other units should be directed at an age-appropriate level for the child and the family before the child undergoes cardiac surgery. The experience prepares the family for the sights and sounds of the unit. B, Going home.** *(Courtesy Children's Hospital Oakland, Oakland, CA.)*

Open heart surgery is done with the child on a cardiopulmonary bypass machine. The machine takes over the roles of the lungs and heart—oxygenation and the delivery of blood to the body. Special cannulas are placed in the venous side of the heart, and venous blood is diverted into the bypass circuit. In the circuit, the blood is oxygenated and filtered and returned to the aorta, where it is pumped to the brain and systemic circulation. The principles of hemodilution, hypothermia, and anticoagulation are critical to use of cardiopulmonary bypass. In addition, myocardial preservation is critical. The heart is generally not pumping during cardiopulmonary bypass, and all systems are supported. Potential complications from cardiopulmonary bypass include bleeding, stroke, myocardial infarction, arrhythmias, fluid and electrolyte imbalance, postpericardiotomy syndrome (an inflammatory process with the development of pericardial effusion), and death. Additional complications include those detailed for closed heart surgery (see previous paragraph). The majority of repairs are done with the child on cardiopulmonary bypass, including ASD, VSD, tetralogy of Fallot, and AVSD.

Monitoring Cardiac Output

The child's cardiac output is monitored through the assessment of vital signs and peripheral perfusion. Signs of low cardiac output include tachycardia, coolness and mottling of extremities, diminished peripheral pulses, delayed capillary refill time, hypotension, decreased urine output, metabolic acidosis, and changes in level of consciousness (difficult to assess in a sedated and intubated child). Intracardiac pressure monitoring is also used and assessed.

The components of cardiac output (heart rate times stroke volume) are heart rate, preload, contractility, and afterload. Problems with one or more of these components may develop during the early postoperative period. Changes in heart rate or rhythm affect cardiac function, and antiarrhythmic drugs or temporary cardiac pacing may be instituted to correct transient postoperative rhythm disturbances. Blood loss and leakage of fluid into the interstitial space influence preload. Transfusions of blood products, colloids, and crystalloids are frequently needed to maintain adequate circulating blood volume. Acid-base and electrolyte imbalances, as well as hypoxia, adversely affect contractility. Correction of these abnormalities may improve cardiac function, but most children will need some degree of continuous infusion of inotropic medications to support cardiac output. Changes in systemic and pulmonary vascular resistance influence afterload, and the use of inodilators (medications with inotropic and vasodilator effects), such as milrinone, sometimes proves necessary.

Supporting Respiratory Function

During cardiopulmonary bypass, the lungs are not ventilated and expanded, placing the child at risk for postoperative atelectasis. Also, fluid may accumulate in the pleural and interstitial spaces during and after cardiopulmonary bypass. For surgery, the child will be intubated and mechanically ventilated. The child often returns to the intensive care unit intubated.

Airway patency is maintained, in part, through prudent suctioning of the endotracheal tube. The nurse must pay strict attention to oxygen saturation readings (and know the anticipated saturations for the specific cardiac defect and surgical intervention), including during suctioning, to avoid episodes of transient hypoxia. Frequently, the child receives bolus or continuous infusions of analgesia (sedative medications) to help maintain comfort during this time.

Once extubated, the child is encouraged to deep breathe and cough. Incentive spirometry or therapy is often used to enhance lung expansion. Supplemental oxygen is administered initially and then tapered off as the child's condition permits. Pain medication is given before treatments and pulmonary exercises to allow the child to participate with minimal discomfort. The child can be encouraged to splint the chest during coughing by hugging a favorite stuffed animal.

Chest tubes are placed during surgery to evacuate drainage and air and assist with lung re-expansion. These tubes are inserted in either the mediastinal or pleural space, depending on the surgical approach, and are removed when lung re-expansion is confirmed and drainage has ceased.

Initial chest tube drainage is bloody and changes to serosanguineous and then serous over time. Drainage is heaviest during the first 12 to 24 hours postoperatively, and it is measured and the color evaluated hourly. Increased chest tube drainage may indicate surgical bleeding or clotting abnormalities and must be strictly monitored and rapidly resolved.

Chest tubes are uncomfortable while in place; they restrict movement and cause discomfort when the child's position is changed. Chest tube removal is a painful experience, and the child should be premedicated with an opiate analgesic before the procedure.

Pulmonary hypertension presents a complicated and potentially life-threatening problem postoperatively. Intensive monitoring of pulmonary status (while intubated and extubated), saturations, and pulmonary artery pressures is indicated. In addition, special precautions before suctioning or other noxious stimuli are indicated while caring for these children.

Maintaining Fluid and Electrolyte Balance

Cardiac surgery and cardiopulmonary bypass affect fluid and electrolyte status. Blood loss and fluid shifts reduce circulating blood volume. Cardiopulmonary bypass stimulates secretion of aldosterone and antidiuretic hormone, resulting in water and sodium retention and potassium loss. Stress can increase calcium deposition in bone, placing the child at risk for hypocalcemia. In addition, administration of blood products can bind circulating calcium and lead to hypocalcemia.

Accurate recording of intake and output monitors fluid balance. Urine output is measured hourly, and weight is often measured daily. Fluid requirements are calculated on the basis of the 24-hour intake and output and child's weight. The child with fluid-volume deficit may require fluid boluses of crystalloid, colloid, or blood, whereas the child with fluid-volume excess may require fluid restriction and diuretic therapy.

Electrolyte imbalances adversely affect cardiac contractility. Serum electrolyte values are determined at regular intervals in the early postoperative period, and IV boluses of calcium or potassium are administered to correct abnormalities. Calcium chloride continuous infusions are often instituted in neonates who have undergone open heart surgery. These medications are delivered through a centrally placed venous line and given according to precise guidelines.

In addition, glucose is a critical factor in maintaining cardiac contractility, especially in the neonate and infant. Monitoring for and treating hypoglycemia are critical.

Promoting Comfort

Postoperative pain management is an important nursing function in the care of the child undergoing cardiac surgery. The experience is frightening to both the child and parents. Parents worry that their child will be in constant, severe pain after the procedure.

Optimal pain management in the initial postoperative period may require the use of a continuous IV infusion of an opiate analgesic, such as morphine sulfate or fentanyl. This infusion is often accompanied by the administration of sedatives and antianxiety agents. In addition, nonsteroidal anti-inflammatory agents can be used. This combination of drugs controls pain, relieves anxiety, and allows the child to rest. Scheduled pain medication, along with as-needed doses, often provides better pain control than as-needed pain medication alone.

Once invasive monitoring lines and tubes have been removed, pain control can usually be achieved through the use of oral analgesics. Acetaminophen with or without an opiate additive or nonsteroidal anti-inflammatory agents are frequently the drugs of choice. The incision site sometimes determines the amount of pain medication the child will need to remain comfortable. A thoracotomy incision usually divides muscle and necessitates spreading of the ribs for exposure; children who have undergone this surgical approach frequently have more postoperative discomfort than those who have had a midsternotomy incision.

Pain should be assessed frequently throughout the hospitalization. Preverbal children are unable to express their discomfort, and older children may not be able to accurately describe their pain. Pain assessment tools should be used to accurately assess the child's pain. The nurse also must be alert to nonverbal pain behavior, which includes restlessness and irritability, difficulty resting and sleeping, guarding, rigidity, resistance to movement, an increase in heart rate and blood pressure, and disinterest in eating and other activities. Consulting the parents can help the nurse validate the assessment. Parents know their child best and are familiar with their child's response to stressful situations.

| BOX 22-2 | **PARENTS WANT TO KNOW** | About Care After Heart Surgery |

Activity
- Resume regular nap and sleep schedules and play activities (infants).
- Omit contact play for several weeks; allow quiet inside and outside play as tolerated. Avoid wrestling, jumping, tugging on arms. Also, avoid sandbox play or swimming until the incision is healed.
- Avoid activities where the child could fall (e.g., riding tricycles or bicycles, swinging, playing on monkey bars or jungle gyms, sliding) for 4 to 6 weeks after hospital discharge.
- Avoid ill contacts.
- Resume regular bedtime (children).
- Avoid large crowds of people for up to 4 to 6 weeks after discharge (including day care and places of public worship), especially during winter months.

Diet
- Resume regular or fortified formula (as instructed) and baby foods (infant).
- Do not give any new foods until after the first checkup (infant).
- Encourage adequate liquid intake.
- Appetite should improve at home.

Incision
- Do not bathe the infant or child until instructed to do so.
- When instructed, bathe the infant or child with soap and water in the usual way. Pat the incision, do not rub it while it is healing.

Incision—cont'd
- If the infant drools saliva or formula, cover incision with gauze to prevent excessive moisture.
- Do not use creams, lotions, or powders on incision until it is completely healed and without scabs.
- Report any redness, drainage, or signs of infection at the incision or suture sites.

School
- The child may return to school the second to third week after hospital discharge.
- The child may return to school for half days for the first few days.
- The child should not participate in physical education until 2 months after the operation.

When to Call the Physician
- Faster, harder breathing than normal when child is at rest.
- Temperature above 100° F (37.7° C).
- New, frequent coughing.
- Turning blue or bluer than normal.
- Any swelling, redness, or drainage of the incision.
- Frequent vomiting or diarrhea.
- Pain worse instead of better.
- Appetite worse than at time of discharge.

Checkup
- An appointment should be made for a 1- to 2-week follow-up at the time of discharge.
- No immunizations should be given for 4 to 6 weeks postoperatively.

Promoting Healing and Recovery

A balance between rest and activity is necessary to promote healing. Children often feel fatigue during their postoperative recovery and may benefit from a planned schedule of progressive activity. Parents should be encouraged to allow their child to gradually resume the preoperative activity level. Regularly scheduled administration of pain medication provides comfort during activity, allows the child to rest, and reduces fatigue and anxiety.

Nutritional intake is monitored, and the child is encouraged to resume normal eating patterns. Infants and children who were in significant CHF preoperatively from large left-to-right shunting lesions may demonstrate improved oral intake even before discharge home. Rarely, diet restrictions are implemented for the older child. These restrictions may be related to long-term anticoagulation with warfarin (Coumadin) or salt restrictions. Discharge teaching (Box 22-2) is important to ensure that parents feel comfortable managing their child at home.

ACQUIRED HEART DISEASE

Acquired heart disease encompasses all cardiac conditions that are not present at birth. Children with CHD may develop acquired cardiac problems, such as infective endocarditis and arrhythmias. Children with structurally normal hearts may be affected by these conditions and by other cardiac conditions such as rheumatic heart disease, Kawasaki disease, hypertension, and cardiomyopathies. Some factors that play a role in triggering these problems include genetic tendencies, autoimmune responses, and infection.

Infective Endocarditis (IE)

Infective endocarditis is an inflammation resulting from infection of the cardiac valves and endocardium by a bacterial or occasionally a fungal or viral agent. The infection can occur as the result of procedures such as dental work or surgery to the gastrointestinal tract; however, most cases are not attributable to an invasive procedure. Previously, distinction was made between acute bacterial endocarditis, with a rapid fulminant course of days to weeks, and infective endocarditis, with a slow, indolent course of several months' duration. The general term *infective endocarditis* is now more accepted, with further classification based on the organism responsible for the infection.

Etiology

IE in children occurs most commonly in the presence of CHD. Those with prosthetic heart valves, complex cyanotic heart

USING RESEARCH TO IMPROVE PRACTICE

In 2005, the AAP updated its policy on breastfeeding for infants. Asserting that the beneficial effects of breastfeeding include protection from infection and enhanced maternal infant bonding, among others, the AAP recommends exclusive breastfeeding, or provision of breast milk by bottle, for the first 4 to 6 months of life, preferably until the child reaches 1 year of age or beyond (AAP, 2005). In its report, the AAP (2005) recommends that health professionals provide support and education for breastfeeding mothers, promote policies that facilitate breastfeeding, and change policies that discourage breastfeeding (e.g., formula packages, discount coupons for formula, separating mother and infant in acute care settings).

As an important part of its policy on breastfeeding, the AAP states that breastfeeding should not be precluded for most high-risk neonates and infants. This includes infants with CHD who can derive the full benefits of breastfeeding from direct feeding or expressed milk (fortified or unfortified) from a bottle (AAP, 2005).

Little nursing research exists that specifically addresses the benefits or problems associated with breastfeeding infants who have CHD. In the review of literature section of a recent study looking at breastfeeding in this infant population, Barbas and Kelleher (2004) cite data suggesting benefits of breastfeeding that include higher and more stable oxygen saturation measurements, improved weight gain, and shorter hospital stays. The major impediment to breastfeeding infants with CHD appears to be health professionals' attitudes and in-hospital practices that are discouraging to mothers who wish to breastfeed their infants (Barbas & Kelleher, 2004).

The purpose of the Barbas and Kelleher study was to explore and describe breastfeeding outcomes, which included (1) length of time infants continued to breastfeed or receive expressed breast milk, (2) mothers' satisfaction with breastfeeding, and (3) perception of the level of breastfeeding support (Barbas & Kelleher, 2004, p. 285). Mothers of 68 infants with various types of CHD were surveyed by mail 6 months after their children's discharge from a large children's medical center that had initiated a lactation support program for mothers of high-risk infants. The study occurred over a 2-year time period. Included in the study were infants who had had cardiac surgery before 1 month of age, who breastfed during their hospitalization, and whose mothers received breastfeeding education and support. The objective questionnaire requested information about preoperative breastfeeding patterns, postoperative breastfeeding patterns, maternal breastfeeding goals, and breastfeeding satisfaction; qualitative comments also were collected (Barbas & Kelleher, 2004).

Results from this study demonstrated some important aspects about breastfeeding in the infant with CHD. Most mothers reported a prebirth breastfeeding goal compatible with the AAP policy recommendation of exclusive breastfeeding for 6 months followed by continued breastfeeding for as long as possible; approximately half revised and met their goal to include combined breastfeeding and bottle-feeding, fortifying with additional sources of calories, or expressing milk for bottle-feeding (Barbas & Kelleher, 2004). Significant factors that contributed to satisfaction included the ability to exclusively breastfeed and the ability to increase breastfeeding after the infant's discharge from the hospital. As the study progressed, qualitative comments indicated a more positive perception of the support provided by nurses and other professionals and a marked increase in the number of mothers who initiated and persisted with breastfeeding. The authors conclude that, despite a relatively small sample size, some self-selection and recall bias, and a sample drawn from a center committed to lactation support, breastfeeding rates in infants with congenital cardiac disease are positively related to accepting attitudes by nurses and other health professionals, improved knowledge and education about the benefits of breastfeeding in this population, and hospital facilities and policies that enhance and facilitate maternal breastfeeding goals (Barbas & Kelleher, 2004).

Think about the implication of this research on clinical practice. When a nurse cares for infants who have CHD in a hospital setting, what kinds of policies, procedures, and resources might need to be readily available to facilitate breastfeeding initiation or the provision of breast milk? What suggestions might a student nurse think about for continued research in this area?

AAP, American Academy of Pediatrics.

---

disease, or surgically constructed systemic–to–pulmonary artery shunts, and those with a previous history of endocarditis are at greatest risk (Park, 2002). At moderate risk are patients with PDA, VSDs, coarctation of the aorta, and bicuspid aortic valves. Acquired valvular disease (e.g., from RF) also presents a risk for IE, but the incidence of this is decreasing as the incidence of RF has decreased. The bacterial organisms most commonly responsible are gram-positive organisms, including *Streptococcus viridans, Streptococcus pneumoniae, Staphylococcus aureus,* and *Staphylococcus epidermidis.* Occasionally, fungi may be identified on culture (Baddour et al., 2005).

Incidence

The incidence of IE is variable depending on the population. The incidence is as high as 10% to 13% in children with unrepaired tetralogy of Fallot and VSD; however, the incidence in children who have undergone complete repair is much lower. The mean age of children with endocarditis has risen over the past several decades as survival has increased because of surgical intervention and the availability of corrective, as opposed to palliative, surgical options. The incidence of IE in neonates has increased over the past decade, probably attributable to the increased survival of at-risk neonates, such as those with CHD. The long-term use of central venous catheters in immunocompromised children is an additional risk. Bernstein (2004) enumerates reasons why endocarditis is still a significant cause of morbidity and mortality, despite the availability of antibiotic prophylaxis:

- Changes in the infecting organisms
- Lack of health provider knowledge or awareness of the threat of the disease and recommendations for prevention
- Delay in recognizing that subtle signs and symptoms may suggest the diagnosis
- Emergence of additional at-risk groups that include IV drug users, survivors of cardiac surgery, children and infants with lowered resistance to infection, and those who require long-term intravascular catheters

Manifestations

The clinical manifestations of IE are highly variable depending on the organism and the host immune response; manifestations include fever; nonspecific complaints of anorexia, nausea, fatigue, and malaise; arthralgias; chest pain; heart failure; petechiae; neurologic impairment as a result of embolic events; and presence of, or change in, a heart murmur (Bernstein, 2004). Because murmurs are present in many children with underlying CHD, it is important to detect a change in the quality of the murmur.

Diagnostic Evaluation

The diagnosis of bacterial endocarditis is established primarily on the basis of several blood cultures that yield the causative organism. In 90% of cases, the first two blood cultures will be positive if the patient has not received antibiotics (Park, 2002). The visualization of a *vegetation* (an abnormal growth of infected tissue) on echocardiographic studies helps considerably in establishing the diagnosis, but a study that is negative for vegetations does not rule out IE.

PATHOPHYSIOLOGY

INFECTIVE ENDOCARDITIS

Children with congenital heart defects often have pressure gradients between the structures of their hearts. A pressure gradient causes turbulence, which may erode underlying tissue and result in damage to the endocardium or endothelium. A clot composed of fibrin and entrapped platelets may form at the site of the disruption. If bacteria are present (most commonly *S. aureus* or *Streptococcus*), they also may become entrapped in the clot and encircled by the fibrin and platelets. This is known as a vegetation. The vegetation increases in size as the microorganisms, fibrin, and platelets proliferate within a protective sheath of fibrin. The contained and protected bacteria can quickly destroy the surrounding tissue and valve structures. Because the vegetation is constantly exposed to pressure from blood flow, the vegetation may break off and migrate to other tissues. Particularly dangerous is a cerebral infarct.

Echocardiography may help identify the subgroup of children who may require early surgical intervention to prevent further hemodynamic compromise or neurologic complications, such as those with large, mobile, left-sided vegetations. Other laboratory tests that may help confirm the diagnosis are an elevated erythrocyte sedimentation rate and C-reactive protein level (Baddour et al., 2005), but the development of AV block suggests extension of disease into the myocardium, which can be helpful in identifying another subgroup of children who may benefit from early surgery.

Therapeutic Management

Prevention is the most important therapeutic intervention for IE. Children at risk should establish and maintain an optimal oral hygiene routine to reduce the incidence of periodontal infections. Before any procedure that may increase the risk of introduction of organisms into the blood, endocarditis prophylaxis is recommended. Examples include dental procedures that may induce gingival or mucosal bleeding and certain respiratory, genitourinary, and gastrointestinal procedures. The standard general prophylactic agent is amoxicillin given orally 1 hour before the procedure. Clindamycin is the antibiotic of choice in children allergic to penicillin or amoxicillin (American Heart Association, 2005a) (Box 22-3).

Treatment for IE caused by bacteria invariably includes parenteral administration of antibiotics for 2 to 8 weeks, depending on the pathogen and the clinical circumstances. The prolonged course of antibiotics is necessary because total elimination of the bacteria is essential. Because the bacteria in vegetations are protected from host defense mechanisms by the deposition of platelets and fibrin, aggressive and prolonged treatment is necessary for bacterial eradication (Bernstein, 2004).

Surgical interventions such as excision of the vegetation or removal of an infected valve may be indicated, particularly in the acute forms of endocarditis such as those caused by *S. aureus* and *S. pneumoniae*. Indications for surgery include severe, unresponsive CHF and evidence of valve involvement (Baddour et al., 2005).

NURSING CARE

The Child With Infective Endocarditis

Assessment

Assessment of the child with IE requires close monitoring of temperature elevations and vital signs. Vital signs should be monitored every 2 to 4 hours, along with a thorough cardiovascular and neurologic assessment. If a heart murmur is present, any change in it should be reported to the physician.

Nursing Diagnosis and Planning

Nursing diagnoses and expected outcomes for the child with infective endocarditis include the following:

- Ineffective Tissue Perfusion (peripheral and cerebral) related to hemodynamic instability as a result of impaired

---

BOX 22-3 | **Recommendations for Infective Endocarditis Prophylaxis**

Defects Requiring Prophylaxis
- Prosthetic cardiac valves
- Previous bacterial endocarditis, even without heart disease
- Most congenital heart malformations
- Acquired valve abnormalities as a result of surgery, heart disease, RF
- Hypertrophic cardiomyopathy
- Persistent VSD despite surgery
- First 6 months after CHD repair

Defects Not Requiring Prophylaxis
- Isolated ostium secundum ASD
- Beyond first 6 months after ASD, VSD, or PDA repair
- Mitral valve prolapse *without* regurgitation
- Physiologic or functional heart murmurs
- Previous Kawasaki disease *without* valvular dysfunction
- Previous RF *without* valvular dysfunction
- Cardiac pacemakers and implanted defibrillators

Procedures Requiring Prophylaxis
- All dental procedures likely to induce gingival or mucosal bleeding, including professional teeth cleaning (not simple adjustment of orthodontic appliances or shedding of deciduous teeth)
- Tonsillectomy or adenoidectomy
- Surgical procedures or biopsy involving respiratory or intestinal mucosa
- Incision and drainage of infected tissue
- Genitourinary and gastrointestinal procedures, including most diagnostic and therapeutic procedures that are invasive (sclerotherapy for esophageal varices, esophageal dilation, cystoscopy, urethral dilation, urethral catheterization or surgery if urinary tract infection is present, prostatic surgery)

Modified from Dajani, A. S., Taubert, K. A., & Wilson, W. (1997). Prevention of bacterial endocarditis: Recommendations by the American Heart Association. *JAMA: The Journal of the American Medical Association, 227,* 1794-1801. Copyright 1997, American Medical Association.

---

valvular or myocardial function and effects of a cerebral infarction.

Expected Outcome: The child will have adequate peripheral tissue perfusion, as evidenced by pink mucous membranes and nail beds, a capillary refill time of less than 2 seconds, strong peripheral pulses, vital signs within normal limits, and adequate cerebral perfusion, as evidenced by mental status and a level of consciousness within normal limits and no evidence of focal neurologic deficits.

- Hyperthermia related to bacterial infection.

Expected Outcome: The child will maintain a body temperature that is within normal limits.

- Acute Pain or Chronic Pain (headaches, arthralgias, myalgias) related to the body's immunologic response.

Expected Outcome: The pain associated with headaches, arthralgias, and myalgias will be reduced or eliminated.

- Deficient Knowledge about home care of the child with IE related to unfamiliarity of the information.

Expected Outcomes: The parents will be able to administer medications and monitor the child's condition. They will explain the need for antibiotic prophylaxis and when it is indicated.

Interventions

The child will need vigilant monitoring of vital signs, peripheral perfusion, and hemodynamic stability. Any change in the vital signs, neurologic status, heart murmur, or tissue perfusion should be immediately reported to the physician. The child's activity level may be diminished, necessitating assistance with activities of daily living. Opportunities for quiet activities, such as reading, watching videos, drawing, and doing puzzles, should be provided.

The child's temperature should be monitored every 2 to 4 hours and plotted on a graph. If the child is receiving an aminoglycoside antibiotic, serum peak and trough levels may be monitored. The nurse must administer the antibiotics at the appropriate time, with trough levels determined before and peak levels determined 1 hour after the dose is administered. Acetaminophen is administered as needed for fever, as ordered by the physician, once the initial blood samples have been drawn for culture. Acetaminophen may also be administered for persistent headaches, arthralgias, and myalgias. Reassure the child and parents that the aches and malaise will resolve.

The child may be discharged home receiving parenteral antibiotic therapy. It is imperative that the parents have access to adequate community resources. The nurse must confirm that they have undergone formal instruction in the use of the IV mode selected (e.g., heparin lock, implanted venous access device, Hickman catheter, percutaneous line) and the proper administration of antibiotics. Provide reassurance and support to the family and child regarding the extensive and lengthy therapy that will be needed.

CRITICAL TO REMEMBER

Antibiotic Prophylaxis for Children at Risk for Infective Endocarditis

Children at risk for IE who are undergoing surgical intervention, dental procedures, or procedures involving the respiratory tract, genitourinary tract, or gastrointestinal tract will require prophylactic antibiotics before the procedure.

Evaluation

- Have the child's vital signs improved?
- Does the child have a capillary refill of less than 2 seconds?
- Does the child have a negative neurologic examination?
- Is the child's body temperature within normal limits?
- Have symptoms of anorexia, malaise, arthralgia, and fever subsided?
- Can the parents demonstrate administration of medications and verbalize an understanding of the need and indications for antibiotic prophylaxis?
- Are the parents demonstrating the ability to manage their child's condition at home?

ARRHYTHMIAS

The identification of an arrhythmia, a cardiac rhythm disturbance, in childhood is an important finding. The most important aspect is to recognize that an arrhythmia is present and classify it quickly as life threatening or non-life threatening. Assessing the child hemodynamically is a critical factor in determining the interventions. Often, the nurse will note an abnormal rhythm during a child's or adolescent's well examination. After the assessment of an abnormal or irregular radial pulse measurement, the nurse should obtain an apical pulse, counting for a full minute (if a pulse is present).

Etiology

Cardiac rhythm disturbances have numerous causes. Arrhythmias may be associated with underlying CHD or may occur in structurally normal hearts. Either an abnormal impulse formation or abnormal conduction or a combination of these two factors causes an arrhythmia. Rhythm disturbances can be classified as tachyarrhythmic (rapid) or bradyarrhythmic (slow) (Dubin, 2004).

Arrhythmias may be seen in the postoperative period after repair or palliation of a cardiac lesion. Postsurgical arrhythmias result from injury to the conduction system, edema, ischemia, incision or suture placement, and acid-base or electrolyte imbalances.

Underlying acquired heart disease, such as myocarditis or cardiomyopathy, sometimes produces arrhythmias. Abnormal electrical pathways in the heart can cause certain arrhythmias. *Wolff-Parkinson-White syndrome* is the most common example. Abnormal electrical repolarization of the heart can cause disturbances such as prolonged QT syndrome, which can result in a life-threatening ventricular tachycardia. This can have a genetic cause. Noncardiac causes of rhythm disturbances include fever, temperature instability, hypoxia, electrolyte and metabolic disturbances, increased intracranial pressure, hypovolemia, cardiac tamponade, and drug therapy or reactions.

Incidence

Arrhythmias in children are not uncommon, most are not life threatening, and most appear in children whose hearts are structurally normal. Supraventricular tachycardia (SVT) is the most common primary symptomatic rhythm disturbance seen in infants and children (Park, 2002).

Manifestations

In tachyarrhythmias and bradyarrhythmias, cardiac output is diminished. The clinical presentation is of low cardiac output syndrome with poor end-organ perfusion. The earliest signs and symptoms may be subtle; later they can be quite dramatic. Clinical manifestations for the infant and toddler may include poor feeding, irritability, lethargy, pale or mottled color, poor peripheral perfusion (diminished pulses, mottling, cool extremities, delayed capillary refill time), decreased urine output, and CHF.

In older children, palpitations, dizziness, syncope, and exercise intolerance may be demonstrated. Tolerance of rhythm disturbances is based on the type of rhythm, underlying cardiac condition, and duration of rhythm and the effect on cardiac output.

In absent rhythms there is no cardiac output. This is a medical emergency. Cardiopulmonary resuscitation (CPR) and medical intervention must be initiated if the child is to survive.

Diagnostic Evaluation

The primary tool for diagnosing pediatric arrhythmias is the 12-lead ECG. Twenty-four-hour Holter monitoring and transtelephonic monitoring may be useful for documenting intermittent episodes of cardiac rhythm disturbances.

Therapeutic Management

Pediatric rhythm disturbances should be treated as emergencies if they compromise cardiac output or have the potential to degenerate into lethal (collapse) rhythms (e.g., ventricular fibrillation) (Dubin, 2004). Management strategies include drug therapy, radiofrequency ablation, cardioversion, and pacemakers; the choice of treatment is guided by the origin of the arrhythmia and the clinical consequences.

Fast Pulse Rate

Supraventricular Tachycardia. SVT is a narrow QRS tachycardia. This narrow QRS configuration indicates that the impulse begins above the ventricles. Rates can be in the 220 to 300 beats/min range. Children who are asymptomatic and hemodynamically stable can be treated conservatively. Vagal maneuvers may be used to terminate an episode of SVT by eliciting the diving reflex. Immersing the older child's face in ice water stimulates a vagal response that may stop the tachycardia; briefly placing an ice bag or bag of frozen vegetables over the infant's face accomplishes the same result. This should be done only while constantly monitoring the child and with emergency equipment available in case the child has a prolonged slow heart rate while converting to a normal rhythm.

If vagal maneuvers do not convert the child's heart to a normal rhythm, antiarrhythmics need to be considered. Antiarrhythmic drug therapy may also be successful in

PATHOPHYSIOLOGY

ARRHYTHMIAS

Tachyarrhythmias

Primary tachyarrhythmias can originate in either the atria or the ventricles. The most common atrial tachyarrhythmia is SVT. SVT is triggered by an atrial ectopic focus (a group of irritable cells somewhere in the atrium) or a re-entry circuit (accessory pathway permitting abnormal conduction within the heart). Ventricular tachycardia is uncommon; it is seen in prolonged QT syndrome or in the preoperative or postoperative period in children with underlying structural heart disease.

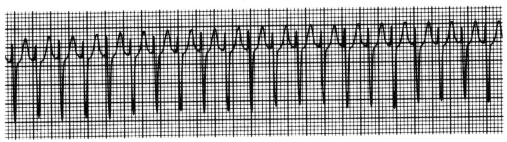

Supraventricular tachycardia.   *(From Park, M. K., & Guntheroth, W. G. [1992].* How to read pediatric ECGs *[3rd ed., p. 202]. St. Louis: Mosby.)*

Bradyarrhythmias

In children, bradyarrhythmias are most commonly the result of hypoxia resulting from respiratory failure or arrest. Primary cardiac bradyarrhythmias usually result from damage to the sinus node or the conduction pathway between the atria and the ventricles (AV block).

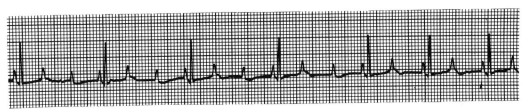

Heart block—two or three P waves for every QRS. Cardiac output is based on the rate of the QRS complexes—ventricular contraction.   *(From Park, M. K., & Guntheroth, W. G. [1992].* How to read pediatric ECGs *[3rd ed., p. 210]. St. Louis: Mosby.)*

Data from Zeigler, V. L. (1994b). Supraventricular tachycardia in children: A challenge for pediatric nurses. *Journal of Pediatric Nursing, 9,* 288-298; Chameides, L., & Hazinski, M. F. (1997). *American Heart Association pediatric advanced life support* (3rd ed., pp. 7.1-7.15). Dallas: American Heart Association.

suppressing further episodes. Older children who continue to have episodes of SVT may benefit from radiofrequency ablation of the ectopic focus or accessory pathway.

Infants and children who are hemodynamically unstable require emergency intervention. If vascular access is present, the drug adenosine may be given. Adenosine is an effective antiarrhythmic because of its ability to slow conduction through the AV node and, in many cases, successfully terminate episodes of SVT rapidly and safely (Park, 2002). Synchronized cardioversion, however, remains the treatment of choice for the child with profound cardiovascular compromise.

Ventricular Tachycardia. Ventricular tachycardia is a wide complex tachycardia. This indicates that the impulse originates in the ventricle. The emergency management of ventricular tachycardia in unconscious children is synchronized cardioversion. Children with a wide complex tachycardia and no pulse (absent pulse) require CPR until defibrillation is available. Lidocaine, 1 mg/kg, may be administered before cardioversion, followed by a continuous infusion of the drug to prevent further episodes (Park, 2002). Once the tachycardia has been terminated, underlying causes should be explored.

Slow Pulse Rate

Bradyarrhythmias. Most episodes of bradyarrhythmia during childhood are the result of noncardiac secondary causes. Hypoxia is a major cause of bradycardia in children, and the airway and breathing effort must be assessed in every situation. Airway management, oxygenation, ventilation, and cardiac compressions, if indicated, may successfully resolve the event. The use of epinephrine or atropine (or both) may be indicated if the rhythm has not improved once oxygenation and ventilation have been re-established.

Primary cardiac bradyarrhythmias include the varying degrees of heart block and junctional or ventricular "escape" rhythms caused by sinus node dysfunction. These arrhythmias are marked by dissociation between the P wave and the QRS complex, with the asynchrony between the atrial and ventricular contractions. They may be congenital, but are often seen in children who have undergone cardiac surgery. Temporary or permanent cardiac pacing may be necessary to maintain adequate cardiac output.

Absent Rhythms. The classification of absent or collapse rhythms includes asystole, ventricular fibrillation, and pulseless electrical activity. In asystole, electrical cardiac activity is absent. Epinephrine is administered to stimulate cardiac activity. The heart is in electrical standstill, and there is no myocardial activity or cardiac output. The ECG rhythm strip is a "flat line." The emergency management of asystole is CPR and medical management. Epinephrine is administered to stimulate cardiac activity. The drug may be given IV, intraosseously, or through an endotracheal tube.

Ventricular fibrillation, rare in children, is frequently the result of underlying cardiac disease. The emergency management of episodes of ventricular fibrillation is defibrillation and CPR. Drugs administered during resuscitation efforts include epinephrine, lidocaine, and other antiarrhythmic agents.

Pulseless electrical activity indicates a hemodynamically compromised state in which cardiac electrical activity is unable to generate effective myocardial contraction and cardiac output. The ECG rhythm strip shows what looks like a normal rhythm. When the nurse palpates for a pulse or listens for a heart beat, there will be none. CPR must be initiated. The underlying cause is usually noncardiac (e.g., respiratory arrest) and it must be identified and corrected for the child to survive the episode.

CRITICAL TO REMEMBER

Arrhythmias

If a child is having an arrhythmia, assess responsiveness and remember the ABCs:
- **AIRWAY** assessment.
- **BREATHING** assessment.
- If no breathing, begin ventilation.
- **CIRCULATION** assessment.
  —Palpate and auscultate pulses.
  —If no pulse, begin chest compressions.
  —If slow pulse, assess the child's tolerance of slow pulse (including perfusion and pulses).
  —Obtain an ECG rhythm strip for assessment.

NURSING CARE

The Child With an Arrhythmia

Assessment

Children with arrhythmias require a thorough cardiovascular assessment because they are at risk for development of cardiogenic shock. In a stable or compensated child with an arrhythmia, it is important to obtain a comprehensive and accurate history of activity tolerance. Older children may have unexplained episodes of dizziness, palpitations, or syncope. Irregular pulse may be noted. Nurses who have been trained to read pediatric ECG rhythm strips may observe signs of a particular arrhythmia.

Nursing Diagnosis and Planning

Nursing diagnoses and expected outcomes for the child with an arrhythmia include the following:
- Decreased Cardiac Output related to decreased ventricular filling or decreased rate of heart contractions.

  Expected Outcome: The child will have pink or baseline cyanotic mucous membranes and nail beds, brisk capillary refill, good-quality pulses, and a normal level of consciousness.
- Risk for Injury related to episodes of syncope.

  Expected Outcome: The child will remain free of injury during any episodes of syncope.
- Deficient Knowledge about care of a child with a potentially fatal condition related to unfamiliarity with the information.

  Expected Outcomes: The family will describe medication administration and an demonstrate an ability to identify signs and symptoms indicative of arrhythmias and will be able to perform CPR.

Interventions

Nursing interventions involve immediate care of the child who has the arrhythmia and education of the child and family. The child and family will need information regarding monitoring for future signs and symptoms of arrhythmias, administering medications as ordered, and appropriate emergency measures to initiate, including CPR, once the child has been discharged from the hospital.

Educating the child and family is imperative for those children with life-threatening arrhythmias. Teach the child and family how to take a pulse or listen to the heart rate with a stethoscope. Teach the child and family to identify the signs and symptoms of arrhythmia, including poor feeding, color changes, palpitations, syncope/dizziness, respiratory distress, and fatigue. These signs and symptoms should be reported to the parent or teacher as soon as possible, and medical attention should be sought. Children who take antiarrhythmics at home need to adhere to the prescribed medication schedule closely and must be careful not to skip any doses. Medical alert bracelets should be worn by children who are in preschool or school. Parents and teachers also need to be aware of signs and symptoms that may indicate the early appearance of arrhythmias. All caretakers should complete a formal course in CPR and know how to activate the emergency medical service system.

Evaluation

- Are the child's pulses of good quality and mucous membranes pink or baseline cyanosis and does the child have a normal level of consciousness?

- Has the child remained free of injury related to falling as a result of syncope?
- Have the child, parents, and other caregivers demonstrated an understanding of medications, activity limitations, and the possibility of a life-threatening episode and how to activate the emergency medical services system?
- Have the child and parents demonstrated how to listen to the heart rate with a stethoscope or palpate a pulse?

Rheumatic Fever (RF)

RF is a diffuse inflammatory condition, most probably of autoimmune origin (see Chapter 17), of the connective tissue, primarily of the heart, joints, subcutaneous tissues, brain, and blood vessels. The most serious complication is rheumatic heart disease, which can result in permanent damage to the cardiac valves, most commonly the mitral and aortic valves.

Etiology

RF characteristically manifests 2 to 6 weeks after an untreated or partially treated group A beta-hemolytic streptococcal infection of the upper respiratory tract. The initial infection may or may not produce symptoms of pharyngitis. Until recently, crowding in inadequate housing and decreased access to health care seemed to be the main risk factors for acquiring streptococcal infections and the resulting RF; however, recent outbreaks of RF in the United States have occurred in children from more affluent families who have access to appropriate health care (Guzman-Cottrill, Jaggi, & Shulman, 2004). These RF clusters appear to be the result of a change in the strains of group A beta-hemolytic streptococci (Guzman-Cottrill, Jaggi, & Shulman, 2004).

Incidence

RF is a disease in transition. Its incidence decreased dramatically in the late 1960s and 1970s but unexpectedly rose in the middle to late 1980s (Guzman-Cottrill, Jaggi, & Shulman, 2004). It is most often seen in susceptible children between

the ages of 5 and 15 years, and the annual incidence in the United States is less than 1 per 10,000 (Gerber, 2004). However, it is still the most common cause of heart disease in children in many developing countries (Tani, Veasy, Minich, & Shaddy, 2004). No differences in incidence have been found on the basis of sex or ethnic group. RF is seasonal in occurrence, with most new cases seen in late winter and spring.

Manifestations

Major manifestations of RF include the following (Fig. 22-16):

- Arthritis—tender, warm, erythematous joints, especially in the large joints, including the elbows, knees, ankles, and wrists; occurs in 75% of RF cases during the acute febrile period (first 1 to 2 weeks of illness). The typical presentation is a migratory polyarthritis, with inflammation moving rapidly from one joint to another and usually lasting less than 1 week for an individual joint before resolving.
- Carditis—inflammation of the endocardium, including the valves, myocardium, and pericardium; may be subclinical and is usually diagnosed by the development of a cardiac murmur, cardiac enlargement or failure, or a

---

PATHOPHYSIOLOGY

RHEUMATIC FEVER

Infection by group A beta-hemolytic streptococci located in the pharyngeal area triggers an abnormal humoral and cell-mediated immunologic response in children who have RF. Immune complexes cross-react with normal tissue in the heart, brain, skin, and joints, causing inflammation in these sites. The inflammatory response appears particularly intense in connective tissue. Eventually, although the disease is self-limiting, permanent damage to cardiac valve tissue can occur.

Data from Brashers, V. (2002). Alterations of cardiovascular function. In K. McCance & S. Huether (Eds.). *Pathophysiology the biologic basis for disease in adults & children* (4th ed., pp. 1025-1026). St. Louis: Mosby.

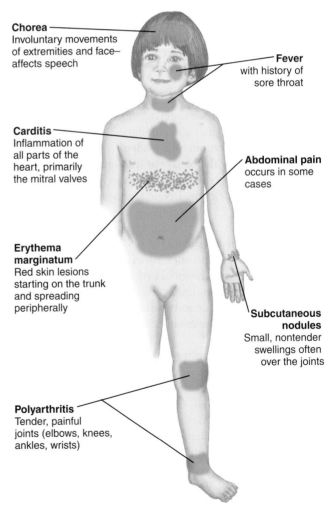

Chorea
Involuntary movements of extremities and face—affects speech

Fever
with history of sore throat

Carditis
Inflammation of all parts of the heart, primarily the mitral valves

Abdominal pain
occurs in some cases

Erythema marginatum
Red skin lesions starting on the trunk and spreading peripherally

Subcutaneous nodules
Small, nontender swellings often over the joints

Polyarthritis
Tender, painful joints (elbows, knees, ankles, wrists)

FIG 22-16   **Clinical manifestations of rheumatic fever.**

pericardial friction rub. Mitral valve involvement is the most frequent manifestation of carditis.

- Chorea—involuntary, purposeless, jerky movements of the legs, arms, and face, with speech impairment and emotional lability, caused by CNS involvement in RF. Also referred to as *Sydenham's chorea,* it is more common in girls and usually occurs in the absence of carditis or polyarthritis. Chorea has a longer latency period of up to 6 months after the initial streptococcal pharyngitis.
- Erythema marginatum—red, painless skin lesions that start as flat or slightly raised macules, usually over the trunk. The erythema spreads at the margins of the lesion with central clearing.
- Subcutaneous nodules—small, nontender lumps, attached to the tendon sheaths of joints and on bony prominences. They occur only rarely in RF and usually are associated with severe carditis.

Although arthritis is the most common manifestation, carditis is by far the most serious and the major cause of morbidity and mortality during both acute and chronic phases of the disease. Cardiac valvular disease is the major long-term consequence of RF (Tani et al., 2004). Children younger than 5 years of age are more likely than older children to have carditis, arthritis, or erythema marginatum (Tani et al., 2004).

Minor criteria that assist in making a diagnosis of RF include a history of previous RF; arthralgias (joint pain) without arthritis; fever; elevated acute-phase reactants, including C-reactive protein and erythrocyte sedimentation rate; and first-degree AV block on the ECG.

Diagnostic Evaluation

A diagnosis of RF is made using the Jones criteria in the presence of at least two major manifestations or one major and two minor manifestations, plus evidence of a recent streptococcal infection on the basis of at least one of the following diagnostic studies: positive throat culture; antistreptolysin O titer, Streptozyme, or anti-DNase B assay; or by a history of scarlet fever (Box 22-4). In children with suspected carditis, a chest radiograph may show enlargement of the heart. An ECG may show rhythm abnormalities or the decreased voltages and ST-T abnormalities associated with myocarditis. An echocardiogram is essential in determining the extent of valvular, myocardial, and pericardial involvement, including the severity of mitral or aortic insufficiency, decreased ventricular function, or pericardial effusions.

Therapeutic Management

The management of RF includes eradication of the streptococcal bacteria and treatment of other symptoms, such as joint inflammation, CHF, and chorea. Penicillin is the drug of choice for eradication of streptococcus. Erythromycin may be used in penicillin-allergic children. Once the diagnosis is firmly established, anti-inflammatory agents, including aspirin, or corticosteroids in the presence of significant carditis, are administered to speed resolution of the inflammatory process, although neither therapy has been proved to have an effect on the incidence or course of carditis. The duration

---

| BOX 22-4 | **Diagnosis of Acute Rheumatic Fever by the Jones Criteria—1992 Update** |

Major Manifestations
- Carditis
- Polyarthritis
- Chorea
- Erythema marginatum
- Subcutaneous nodules

Minor Manifestations
- Fever
- Arthralgia
- Elevated erythrocyte sedimentation rate or positive C-reactive protein
- Prolonged P-R interval

Plus supporting evidence of preceding streptococcal infection: history of recent scarlet fever, positive throat culture for group A streptococci, increased antistreptolysin O titer, or other streptococcal antibodies

From American Heart Association, Council on Cardiovascular Disease in the Young Special Writing Group of the Committee on Rheumatic Fever, Endocarditis, and Kawasaki Disease. (1992). Guidelines for the diagnosis of rheumatic fever: Jones criteria, 1992 update. *JAMA: The Journal of the American Medical Association, 268,* 2069-2073.

---

of therapy is tailored according to the clinical course of the child.

Children who have had RF are susceptible to recurrent attacks, risk further cardiac valve damage, and require secondary prophylaxis to prevent recurrence. The child without cardiac complications should receive antibiotic prophylaxis for 5 years or through age 21 to 25 years, whichever is longer. Those with rheumatic heart disease should continue prophylaxis for at least 10 years and at least until age 40 years. The American Heart Association recommends prophylaxis for life for those who have contact with children who may have group A streptococcal infection, such as teachers, health care workers, and parents of school-age children. Penicillin is the drug of choice, either by monthly intramuscular injection, which is more reliable in terms of adherence, or an oral dose of 250 mg twice daily.

NURSING CARE

The Child With Rheumatic Fever

Assessment

Initially, the nurse determines whether the child or any family members have had a sore throat or unexplained fever within the past 2 months. The child should be monitored for cardiac symptoms throughout the course of hospitalization. Temperature, pulse, respiration, and blood pressure are assessed, and the child is observed for signs of carditis, including tachycardia; heart murmur; friction rub; shortness of breath; or edema of the face, abdomen, or ankles. Examination of the joints may reveal very tender elbows, knees, ankles, and wrists, with subcutaneous nodules over extensor surfaces of the joints. Children with RF may have red skin lesions on the trunk or rapid, purposeless, involuntary movements (chorea), either on observation or by history.

Nursing Diagnosis and Planning

Nursing diagnoses and expected outcomes for the child with rheumatic fever include the following:

- Deficient Knowledge related to unfamiliarity with medications and activity restrictions.

  Expected Outcome: The child will adhere to the medication regimen and activity restrictions.

- Ineffective Coping related to confinement.

  Expected Outcomes: The child will participate in quiet activities and will maintain social contact.

- Acute Pain related to polyarthritis.

  Expected Outcomes: The child will verbalize an increase in comfort and will indicate a decrease in pain on an age-appropriate pain tool.

- Risk for Injury related to subsequent streptococcal infection.

  Expected Outcomes: The child will inform parents at the first sign of a sore throat, and the family will adhere to antibiotic prophylaxis.

Interventions

The nurse administers antibiotics, analgesics, and antipyretics as ordered and reports to the physician any fever or pain. In addition, children with RF require bed rest during the acute febrile stage of the illness and should not return to school while there is clear evidence of rheumatic activity. While the child's activities are restricted, the nurse and family should talk about limiting visitors and arranging for quiet yet enjoyable activities. Family members and friends may provide board and computer games, movies, puzzles, and crafts for the school-age child. Such activities will help minimize activity and cardiac demand. The child may benefit from a daily schedule that includes rest periods interspersed with these diverse activities and some limited exercise (e.g., passive range-of-motion exercises). An art or play therapist can work with the child who is extremely anxious because of confinement.

Nursing comfort measures include alternating application of heat and cold to affected joints, repositioning, massage, and providing distraction by use of guided imagery and relaxation. Seizure precautions are warranted if the child has chorea. At home, parents must practice safety measures. For example, the child who cannot control movements may need to sleep on a mattress on the floor and may need assistance going up and down stairs. The child may be embarrassed by uncontrolled movements, especially in front of peers, and will need reassurance that these symptoms are temporary.

Emphasize to parents the importance of adherence to antibiotic prophylaxis. The family may be allowed to offer an adolescent the choice of monthly injections versus daily oral administration. If the child chooses the oral route, instruct the family about the required dose, frequency of administration, duration, effects, side effects, and potential cardiac complications if the regimen is not followed precisely.

Evaluation

- Is the child taking antibiotics as ordered?
- Is the child following modified bed rest guidelines?
- Is the child playing board games, reading, and visiting with friends as tolerated?
- Has the child verbalized a decrease in pain and indicated decreased pain on an appropriate assessment tool?
- Does the child take antibiotic prophylaxis as ordered and notify the parent if experiencing a sore throat?

CRITICAL TO REMEMBER
Streptococcal Prophylaxis for the Child With Rheumatic Fever

Streptococcal prophylaxis is the most important aspect of therapeutic management in RF because damaged valves can become further damaged with repeated infections. This prophylaxis is life long if there is actual valve involvement. Intramuscular penicillin, administered monthly, is the drug of choice. Alternatives include oral penicillin taken twice daily or sulfadiazine taken orally once per day; either daily sulfadiazine or erythromycin taken twice a day is appropriate for children who are sensitive to penicillin.

Kawasaki Disease

Kawasaki disease, also called *mucocutaneous lymph node syndrome*, is an acute, febrile, exanthematous illness of children with a generalized vasculitis of unknown etiology. Kawasaki disease is a major cause of acquired heart disease in children in the United States. Coronary artery aneurysms are seen in 20% of children with untreated Kawasaki disease (Rowley & Shulman, 2004).

Etiology

The cause of Kawasaki disease remains unknown. However, recent evidence suggests that it is an immune-mediated vasculitis triggered by an acute infection or by a bacterial toxin. (See Chapter 17 for a discussion of immune complex disease.) Kawasaki disease also has a seasonal component; it is diagnosed most often in late winter and early spring.

Incidence

Kawasaki disease is seen most frequently in children younger than 5 years, with a peak incidence in the United States at 18 to 24 months (American Heart Association, 2005b). Kawasaki disease is diagnosed less frequently in children older than 8 years. Affected boys outnumber affected girls by at least 1.5 to 1, with an increased incidence in children of Asian ancestry (Rowley & Shulman, 2004).

Manifestations

Kawasaki disease manifests in three phases. The acute stage lasts approximately 10 to 14 days and is characterized by a high fever that persists longer than 5 days. The fever is unresponsive to antibiotic treatment. Clinical signs include

PATHOPHYSIOLOGY

KAWASAKI DISEASE

An infectious or possibly toxic trigger initiates an immune system response that affects medium-size arteries, especially the coronary arteries. A generalized immune response becomes more specific, with increasing numbers of T lymphocytes and B lymphocytes infiltrating the smooth muscle cells of the vascular walls. The infiltration causes edema and inflammation, which progressively weaken the vascular walls, leading to aneurysms. As the disease progresses, fibrous connective tissue forms at the inflammatory sites, eventually thickening and scarring the vascular walls. These vascular changes, along with the increased platelets that occur as part of the disease process, can cause thrombus formation, myocardial infarction, and death in some children.

bilateral, nonpurulent conjunctivitis; changes in the mucous membranes (i.e., erythema, fissures, and cracking of the lips; strawberry tongue); changes in the peripheral extremities, such as swelling of the hands and feet and erythema of the palms and soles; a generalized erythematous rash (Fig. 22-17); and enlarged cervical lymph nodes. Tachycardia and extreme irritability are also common.

The second or subacute phase lasts from approximately day 15 to day 25. The fever disappears, and most symptoms resolve. The phase is characterized by continued irritability, anorexia, desquamation of the fingers and toes, arthritis and arthralgia, and cardiovascular manifestations, including CHF, arrhythmias, and the typical coronary aneurysms (Rowley & Shulman, 2004).

Coronary aneurysm formation begins early in the second phase. A baseline echocardiogram at diagnosis with repeat studies at 2 weeks, 6 to 8 weeks, and 6 to 12 months (optional) will help identify those with coronary artery involvement (American Academy of Pediatrics & American Heart Association, 2004). Severe thrombocytosis occurs during this period and marks the period of highest risk for coronary artery thrombosis in the areas of aneurysm, resulting in myocardial infarction.

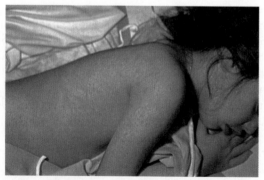

FIG 22-17   **Erythematous rash of Kawasaki disease.** *(From Lookingbill, D. P., & Marks, J. G., Jr. [1992]. Principles of dermatology [2nd ed., p. 223]. Philadelphia: WB Saunders.)*

The final or convalescent stage begins on day 26 and lasts until the erythrocyte sedimentation rate returns to normal and all signs of illness have disappeared. Deep transverse grooves, called *Beau's lines*, may appear on the child's nails.

Diagnostic Evaluation

Fever of 5 days' duration in conjunction with at least four of the five following primary clinical findings for the acute phase establishes the diagnosis of Kawasaki disease (Rowley & Shulman, 2004):

- Bilateral nonpurulent conjunctivitis
- Oral mucosal alterations (e.g., strawberry tongue; pharyngeal erythema; dry, fissured lips)
- Redness of the hands and feet followed by desquamation
- Rash on the trunk
- Cervical lymphadenopathy with large nodes
      AND
- No other known disease process to explain the signs and symptoms

Laboratory data are nonspecific. The white blood cell count is elevated during the acute phase, as is the erythrocyte sedimentation rate and C-reactive protein level. There is sterile pyuria. The ECG in the acute phase may demonstrate first-degree heart block. Platelet levels dramatically rise during the subacute phase. Aneurysms are detected with echocardiography.

Therapeutic Management

Therapeutic management is directed toward preventing or reducing the coronary artery damage from Kawasaki disease. High-dose intravenous immune globulin (IVIG) in combination with aspirin has been shown to lower the prevalence of coronary artery abnormalities when given within 10 days of fever onset. At diagnosis, IVIG is given in a dosage of 2 g/kg over a 10- to 12-hour infusion (Rowley & Shulman, 2004). High-dose aspirin therapy is begun at the same time. Initially, the dosage is in the anti-inflammatory range of 80 to 100 mg/kg/day in four evenly divided doses until fever resolves. The dosage is then reduced to an antiplatelet aggregation dose of 3 to 5 mg/kg/day once daily and continued through weeks 6 to 8 of the illness. If coronary artery abnormalities are identified, this dosage is continued indefinitely (Rowley & Shulman, 2004). Corticosteroids may be considered if the child is unresponsive to standard therapy.

NURSING CARE

The Child With Kawasaki Disease

Assessment

During the acute phase, the nurse must monitor the child's cardiac status closely, looking for clinical signs and symptoms of heart failure. Changes in pulse, respiration, blood pressure, and color, along with shortness of breath, chest pain, and decreased activity, may suggest cardiac complications. It is important to examine the child's eyes, mouth, and skin for signs of infection and the joints for redness, swelling, and tenderness.

The nurse should determine the parents' anxiety level. Parents are often frightened by how sick the child is and the threat of a possibly devastating outcome. Families appreciate talking about their fears; learning about the cause of the illness, the treatment plan, and the prognosis; and participating in the child's care.

Nursing Diagnosis and Planning

Nursing diagnoses and expected outcomes for the child with Kawasaki disease and the family include the following:
• Risk for Deficient Fluid Volume related to fever.
  Expected Outcome: The child will maintain fluid and electrolyte balance, as evidenced by normal laboratory values and intake and output appropriate for age.
• Acute Pain related to fever, skin manifestations, and joint inflammation.
  Expected Outcomes: The child will rest comfortably, as evidenced by periods of uninterrupted sleep, and will express decreased pain on an age-appropriate pain assessment tool.
• Fear related to changes in the child's behavior and uncertainty about the long-term prognosis.
  Expected Outcome: The parents and child will discuss their fears related to having a serious disease with a long recuperative period.

Interventions

The nurse should administer aspirin with milk or food and infuse IVIG as ordered. During the infusion, it is important to monitor the child's vital signs and any adverse reactions to IVIG, including facial flushing, tightness in the chest, chills, dizziness, nausea, vomiting, diaphoresis, and hypotension. Blood pressure is checked every 15 minutes for the first hour and every 30 minutes thereafter until the infusion is complete. A precipitous fall in blood pressure may occur 30 to 60 minutes after the infusion has begun; this is often related to the rate of infusion. The physician will usually lower the prescribed rate of infusion if such a reaction occurs and may order diphenhydramine (Benadryl) and acetaminophen to control side effects. Epinephrine is given for anaphylactic reactions. IVIG may interfere with achieving immunity from live-virus vaccines, so some immunizations (e.g., measles, mumps, rubella, varicella) should be delayed for 11 months after IVIG therapy (American Academy of Pediatrics, 2003).

Nursing care focuses on comfort measures and adequate hydration. The nurse and parents must encourage fluid intake by offering ice pops or ice to numb affected mucous membranes; giving liquids that are high in calories and low in acid through a straw (avoiding citrus drinks and sodas); and offering favorite foods that are soft and bland. The nurse or family can apply salve to soothe cracked, dry lips.

Sponge baths with tepid water often decrease fever and relieve discomfort from skin manifestations. The child should be handled gently and only when necessary. If itching is severe, the physician should be notified.

Toddlers and preschool children fear hospitalization and body changes, often exhibiting regressive behavior and sleeping poorly. In addition, children with Kawasaki disease also manifest increased irritability during the acute phase. If possible, keep the environment calm by talking in gentle tones, playing soft music, and avoiding bright overhead lights. It may help to line the bed with soft blankets from home. Assure the family that the fever, pain, and irritability will eventually resolve and praise their hard work in keeping the child comfortable. Because the child's extreme irritability is an area of concern for parents, the nurse should provide support so the parent can take periodic breaks. Discharge instructions (Box 22-5) should include provisions for a cardiac follow-up examination. Parents' fears can be decreased through an understanding of the disease and treatment.

BOX 22-5	**PARENTS WANT TO KNOW** About Kawasaki Disease

Review the following at the time of hospital discharge of a child diagnosed as having Kawasaki disease:
• Skin:
—Rinse with water only.
—Avoid soaps and lotions.
—Use salve on the lips.
—Call the physician for severe itching.
• Temperature:
—Record the child's temperature in the morning and evening before giving aspirin.
—Bring the temperature chart to all physician appointments.
• Arthritis:
—Look for hot, reddened joints.
—Observe for pain with touch or movement.
—Elevate affected joints.
—Call the physician if the child refuses to walk.

• Heart:
—Offer a low-cholesterol diet.
—Give aspirin as ordered.
—Call the physician for bleeding or bruising, color changes, shortness of breath, chest pain, or decreased activity level.
• Personality:
—Discuss personality changes with household members.
—Provide support and reassurance.
—Encourage quiet activities and rest periods.
—Eliminate stimulation at naptime and bedtime.
—Play soft music and use dim lights.
• Anorexia:
—Offer liquids high in calories but low in acid.
—Avoid citrus juices and sodas.
—Give bland foods initially.
—Prepare favorite dishes.

Modified from Lux, K. M. (1991). New hope for children with Kawasaki disease. *Journal of Pediatric Nursing, 6,* 159-165.

Evaluation

- Is the child taking adequate amounts of fluid and maintaining electrolyte balance?
- Is the child's urine output appropriate for age (see Chapter 18)?
- Is the child experiencing periods of uninterrupted rest?
- Does the child demonstrate decreased pain on an age-appropriate assessment tool?
- Are the parents able to verbalize their fears and discuss the course of the illness and their commitment to follow-up care?

Hypertension

Hypertension is defined as an average systolic or average diastolic blood pressure that exceeds or is equal to the 95th percentile for age, height, and sex on the basis of measurements obtained on at least three occasions. Children with systolic blood pressure or diastolic blood pressure between the 90th and 95th percentiles are considered to be prehypertensive; prehypertension in adolescents is defined as BP ≥120/80 mm Hg (National High Blood Pressure Education Program Working Group on High Blood Pressure in Children and Adolescents [NHBPEP], 2004). Normal blood pressure is defined as a systolic or diastolic pressure that is less than the 90th percentile for age and sex (see Appendix C).

The two primary categories of hypertension are *primary* (idiopathic) and *secondary* (symptom of underlying disease). Primary hypertension predominates in the older adolescent, whereas secondary causes are overwhelmingly more common in the younger age groups.

Etiology

Pediatric hypertension that is not the result of an underlying disease is referred to as essential hypertension, similar to that seen in adults. Essential hypertension is more prevalent among adolescents, teenagers, and those with moderately elevated blood pressure. The early development of essential hypertension is linked to childhood obesity, children with diabetes mellitus, and a strong family history of hypertension. Affected adults and children may exhibit exaggerated blood pressure responses to physical and emotional stresses compared with normotensive individuals. Some individuals (particularly the African American population) with essential hypertension are negatively affected by increased levels of dietary sodium (Bernstein, 2004).

Height and weight are additional determinations of blood pressure in children. Children with elevated blood pressure are usually taller and heavier than their age-matched peers. Obesity is a common concurrent condition in children with hypertension.

The causes of secondary hypertension in children include various renal and renovascular diseases, coarctation of the aorta, endocrine and metabolic disorders, neurologic disease, and drug-related causes.

Of children with significant blood pressure elevations, 80% to 90% have renal or renovascular disease as the underlying cause. Renal arterial disease is a common etiology in the sick neonate and is usually caused by renal artery thrombosis resulting from the use of umbilical artery catheters or from polycythemia. Renal parenchymal diseases, such as glomerulonephritis, obstructive uropathy, and hemolytic uremic syndrome (see Chapter 20), are the most common causes of hypertension in children before adolescence.

Coarctation of the aorta is the primary cardiovascular cause of hypertension. Coarctation should be ruled out early in the course of the evaluation because this is a treatable cause of hypertension but one that may result in fixed vascular changes if not detected before adolescence. The heart itself is primarily an *end-organ,* in which hypertension can have long-term detrimental effects, as opposed to having any important etiologic role in hypertension. Endocrine causes include pheochromocytoma and congenital adrenal hyperplasia. Diabetes mellitus is frequently complicated by renal involvement and associated hypertension. Increased intracranial pressure from a tumor, trauma, or meningitis will produce acute, severe hypertension and is a medical emergency. Common causes of elevated blood pressure include use of corticosteroids, oral contraceptives, and sympathomimetic drugs (e.g., those found in over-the-counter cold preparations) and cocaine or amphetamine abuse.

Incidence

Hypertension is increasingly seen in children, with an overall prevalence of between 1% and 3% (Cromwell, Munn, & Zolkowski-Wynne, 2005). The majority of these children have only mild elevations of blood pressure, and those with significant blood pressure elevations often have secondary hypertension. Because adult hypertension is more prevalent in the African American and Asian populations, adolescents from these racial groups should be monitored carefully. Children in families who have members with hypertension tend to have higher-than-normal blood pressures. Hypertension in children is closely associated with sleep pattern disturbances

---

PATHOPHYSIOLOGY

HYPERTENSION

Systolic pressure reflects the stroke volume of the heart, the rate of blood ejected, and the elasticity of the aorta. Diastolic pressure reflects the resting pressure of the arterial system; it is affected by the peripheral vascular resistance or the diameter of the arteries and the heart rate. An increase in the heart rate decreases the diastolic or ventricular filling time. Together, these measurements form the arterial blood pressure and provide information about arterial function.

Hypertension, or increased arterial blood pressure over time, may produce cardiac enlargement and subsequent cardiac failure, cerebrovascular disease, renal disease and failure, retinal disease, and accelerated atherosclerosis and coronary heart disease. These effects are seen predominantly with primary or essential hypertension.

(e.g., snoring, sleep apnea, daytime fatigue) (Hellekson, 2005). Because of increasing prevalence of hypertension in young children, the NHBPEP (2004) recommends blood pressure measurement for all children beginning at 3 years of age, and earlier in children with underlying cardiac or renal disease or certain other underlying medical conditions.

Manifestations

Children with primary hypertension rarely have clinical evidence of disease; the elevated blood pressure is usually detected on a routine physical examination. High elevations of blood pressure, however, can lead to the following manifestations:

- Essential or primary hypertension—dizziness, headaches, epistaxis, and visual disturbances. Late signs of severe or acute hypertension include neurologic deficits, extremity weakness, and cerebrovascular accidents.
- Secondary hypertension—*Renal:* weight loss or failure to gain weight, facial or pretibial edema, pale mucous membranes, and unilateral or bilateral abdominal mass. *Cardiovascular:* absent or decreased femoral pulses, decreased blood pressure in the lower extremities compared with the upper extremities, cardiomegaly, murmur, and signs and symptoms of CHF.

Diagnostic Evaluation

Differentiating primary from secondary hypertension requires a comprehensive medical history and physical examination. Blood pressure measurements are done on all four extremities and repeated twice if elevated. Blood tests (complete blood cell count; blood urea nitrogen, creatinine, uric acid, and electrolyte levels), urinalysis, echocardiography, ultrasonography of the kidneys, and arteriography can rule out causes of secondary hypertension. Urinary catecholamines may be considered to rule out pheochromocytoma.

The diagnosis of primary, or essential, hypertension is established primarily by excluding an underlying disease. A hypertensive preadolescent or adolescent with a family history of hypertension is more likely to have primary hypertension as opposed to secondary hypertension. For younger age groups, secondary causes of hypertension are much more prevalent.

Therapeutic Management

Primary Hypertension. Treatment of primary, or essential, hypertension in the adolescent emphasizes risk factor modification. Lifestyle counseling focuses on nonpharmacologic therapy that includes weight reduction, physical conditioning, dietary modifications, and stress modification. If the nonpharmacologic treatments are maximized, the need for pharmacologic therapy in children with hypertension should be reduced.

Weight Reduction. A direct relationship exists between obesity and hypertension. This relationship may be caused in part by increased sympathetic nervous system activity. Weight reduction plays an important role in lowering blood pressure. Weight loss requires a program of diet, exercise, and lifestyle changes, and it is often very difficult to achieve significant results in asymptomatic young people. Even so, a modest 5- to 10-pound weight loss can have a positive effect on blood pressure reduction. Because of the long-term nature of primary hypertension, efforts should focus on education regarding a healthy lifestyle and the gradual incorporation of good dietary habits and activity into the patient's everyday life. Success frequently depends on support from health care professionals, nutritionists, and family members.

Physical Conditioning. An exercise program should be initiated in conjunction with a dietary weight reduction plan. Not only does exercise facilitate weight loss but it also it lowers blood pressure independent of weight loss. Twenty to thirty minutes of aerobic exercise two or three times per week may result in a consistently lower resting blood pressure. Recently, studies have also suggested that any increase in total physical activity during the day, such as climbing a flight of stairs several times per day instead of using an elevator, can show measurable benefit over months and years. The most successful approach in children and adolescents is to focus on activities that they enjoy and that provide a social outlet, such as organized sports or bike riding. Exercise in which the whole family can participate, such as walking or hiking, is also more likely to be successful in terms of maintaining a consistent lifestyle change. Although research has not linked hypertension with sudden death in athletes, current recommendations limit participation in competitive sports for children and adolescents with severe hypertension (>99th percentile) until blood pressure is under control (Kaplan, Gidding, Pickering, & Wright, 2005).

Dietary Modification. Avoidance of a high-sodium intake is recommended in hypertensive and normotensive children and adolescents. The degree of sodium restriction necessary to decrease blood pressure has not been established, but it is recommended that the dietary intake should be not greater than 1.2 g/day for young children and 1.5 g/day in older children or adolescents, or a no-added-salt diet (NHBPEP, 2004).

Evidence suggests an association between alcohol and hypertension, believed to be related to alterations in the renin-angiotensin system and neurotransmitters. Smoking produces an aldosterone-like hypertension in young people. Therefore, avoidance of alcohol and tobacco is recommended.

Relaxation Techniques. Relaxation techniques have resulted in modest reductions in blood pressure in the adult population. Information on efficacy in children is not yet available.

Pharmacologic Treatment. Pharmacologic treatment of primary hypertension may be indicated if there is coexisting secondary hypertension, or if lifestyle modifications are ineffective (NHBPEP, 2004). The first-line drugs for children and adolescents are beta-adrenergic receptor blockers; angiotensin-receptor blockers; calcium channel blockers; diuretics; and vasodilators, primarily ACE inhibitors. To begin pharmacologic therapy, use of a single drug at the lowest effective dosage is preferred (Hellekson, 2005; NHBPEP, 2004).

CRITICAL TO REMEMBER
Infusing Intravenous Antihypertensive Medications
IV antihypertensive medications must be infused very slowly, and an arterial line must be in place for monitoring. Sudden hypotension may result after initiation of antihypertensive drugs.

Secondary Hypertension. Treatment of the underlying process is the focus of therapy in secondary hypertension. If the secondary disease is coarctation of the aorta or renal artery disease, surgery may be indicated. Therapy in patients with renal parenchymal or endocrine pathologic conditions focuses on the disease process. Effective treatment will often result in secondary control of blood pressure.

NURSING CARE

The Child With Hypertension

Assessment
Blood Pressure Screening
Blood pressure screening should be initiated when a child is 3 years old and should continue through adolescence. Blood pressure should be checked at least yearly. The environment should be as quiet as possible, and the child's arm should be supported at the heart level. If an elevated blood pressure is found, measurement should be repeated two more times, allowing a 2- to 3-minute interval between blood pressure checks.

Cuff size is of critical importance. A too-small blood pressure cuff will result in an inappropriately high blood pressure reading. (See Chapter 13 for cuff measurement and selection.)

Physical Assessment
Assessment of a child with hypertension includes inspection of the skin to detect evidence of underlying disease, including edema (renal disease) and the presence of café-au-lait spots (neurofibromatosis) or moon facies (Cushing's syndrome, steroid administration). The pulses should be palpated for symmetry and strength. A child with coarctation of the aorta is likely to have bounding upper extremity pulses and diminished or absent femoral and pedal pulses. The heart and chest are auscultated to determine the heart rate and to detect any heart murmur, gallop, or aortic bruit. The abdomen is auscultated for renal bruits. A neurologic examination is urgently indicated in children with acute, severe hypertension to rule out increased intracranial pressure.

Nursing Diagnosis and Planning
Nursing diagnoses and expected outcomes for the child with hypertension include the following:
- Ineffective Tissue Perfusion (peripheral and cardiovascular) related to elevation in systolic or diastolic arterial blood pressure.

Expected Outcome: The child will maintain normal tissue perfusion with blood pressure at a controlled level (below the 95th percentile for age).
- Ineffective Therapeutic Regimen Management related to excessive demands of dietary restrictions, physical conditioning, and a possible medication regimen.

Expected Outcomes: The child will describe and will engage in diet, physical conditioning, and medication therapy to lower blood pressure.

Interventions
Nursing interventions focus on education and family support and adherence to the treatment regimen. The nurse may consult a dietitian and collaboratively develop a teaching plan regarding a modified-sodium and weight-reduction diet if ordered. When the nurse counsels the family and child about dietary modifications, it is important to include the whole family in making dietary changes to increase motivation and adherence.

If a physical conditioning program is prescribed, physical activities the child enjoys are identified so that they can be incorporated into the plan. Family members and friends are encouraged to join the child in the exercise program. Praise the child for progress in weight loss and increased endurance. Encourage the child to express feelings about any possible problems related to home or school situations. Discuss methods for facilitating relaxation that may be helpful during periods of stress.

The child who is hospitalized with acute, severe hypertension may require medications. Once the child has been stabilized after an acute hypertensive crisis, oral antihypertensive medications will likely be prescribed. During discharge planning, reinforce the importance of adherence to the medication regimen and of periodic follow-up evaluations.

Evaluation
- Does the child maintain blood pressure below the 95th percentile for age?
- Has the child achieved weight loss?
- Is the child adhering to a modified-sodium diet?
- Is the child engaging in regular physical exercise according to the prescribed regimen?
- Is the child complying with the medication regimen?

CARDIOMYOPATHIES
The cardiomyopathies are diseases of the heart muscle in which the cardiac pathologic condition is not the result of CHD, coronary artery disease, or other systemic disease. Cardiomyopathy is classified into three types on the basis of the size and function of the ventricles:
- *Dilated:* Decreased contractility and dilation of the ventricles without an increase in wall thickness (hypertrophy). There are congenital or genetic forms and acquired forms caused by infection or toxin exposure.
- *Hypertrophic:* Hypertrophy of the ventricles, generally with improved contractility but impaired ventricular

filling because of increased "stiffness" of the ventricular walls. The interior chamber size of the ventricle may be decreased. Left ventricular outflow tract obstruction may occur and can be suddenly fatal. Hypertrophic cardiomyopathy is considered a genetic disorder.

- *Restrictive:* Impaired ventricular filling usually caused by infiltration of the muscle with abnormal material. The ventricular size and contractility are usually fairly normal. May be congenital or acquired.

Hypertrophic cardiomyopathy (HCM), with a prevalence in children of less than 1%, is nevertheless one of the major causes of sudden cardiac death in adolescents (Maron, 2004). Approximately 36% of cases of sudden death in athletes is related to hypertrophic cardiomyopathy (American Heart Association, 2005b). Predicting sudden cardiac death from this cause is difficult because children with this disorder may have completely normal physical examination findings.

The assessment data that best predict whether a child or adolescent may be at risk are a family history of early or sudden cardiac death or a family history of HCM (Maron, 2004). If the adolescent is symptomatic, the most frequently seen signs and symptoms include dyspnea or chest pain with exertion, palpitations, presyncope, and syncope. Infants and children may fatigue easily. The thickened left ventricle is poorly compliant (stiff) and has impaired filling, causing pulmonary venous congestion and associated exertional dyspnea and orthopnea (dyspnea when supine). On auscultation, the heart sounds are normal and there is often a systolic murmur at the left sternal border or apex. The murmur will characteristically vary in intensity depending on position or recent exertion.

The ECG may demonstrate left ventricular hypertrophy, deep Q waves, and ST-T abnormalities. Affected individuals should have a Holter monitor test to screen for asymptomatic ventricular arrhythmias. The chest radiograph may show mild cardiomegaly. The diagnosis is usually established by echocardiogram, often with concentric or localized ventricular hypertrophy, of the left and often the right ventricle.

All children with diagnosed HCM should be restricted from strenuous exertion and competitive sports. Beta blockade or calcium channel blockade (verapamil) is frequently used, especially in children with obstructive HCM, to decrease ventricular hypercontractility and outflow tract obstruction. Beta blockade is also used as prophylaxis against ventricular arrhythmias. Prophylactic therapy may be started in asymptomatic children with HCM, especially in the case of a family history of sudden death. Infective endocarditis prophylaxis is also indicated.

Surgery is indicated in children who are symptomatic or who have severe outflow tract obstruction despite medical management. The most common procedure is a septal myomectomy, which is resection of a portion of the left ventricular septum to relieve obstruction. This often results in an improvement in symptoms with low surgical mortality but does not decrease the mortality rate of the disease itself.

A newer intervention is insertion of a pacemaker, which, by depolarizing the ventricle, causes dyssynchronous ventricular contraction and decreased outflow tract obstruction. In addition, children with life-threatening arrhythmias may be offered an implantable defibrillator pacemaker. The surgical risk of pacemaker or defibrillator insertion is much lower than that of myomectomy, and these options are likely to be used increasingly as long-term outcome data become available.

HIGH CHOLESTEROL LEVELS IN CHILDREN AND ADOLESCENTS

Preventive cardiology has become increasingly important during childhood and adolescence. Developing heart-healthy habits during these years reduces the risk for coronary artery disease and other cardiovascular problems during adulthood. Several major risk factors during childhood and adolescence appear routinely in the literature. They include the following (Tershakovec & Rader, 2004):

- Tobacco use
- Total cholesterol levels >170% between the ages of 2 to 19 years old, dyslipidemia (elevated low-density lipoproteins [LDLs] and decreased high-density lipoproteins)
- Hypertension
- Decreased physical activity
- Obesity
- Type 2 diabetes mellitus

More than half the children in the United States are considered to be obese, and many of the recently updated national health objectives address the issue of obesity and dietary management in children (U.S. Department of Health and Human Services, 2000).

Assessment of Children at Risk

High cholesterol levels can be the result of genetic or dietary factors or a combination. Children at risk for high cholesterol levels should be screened during their developing years. According to guidelines from the National Cholesterol Education Program, the following children older than 2 years should be screened:

- Children whose parents or grandparents had vascular or cerebrovascular disease or who have been diagnosed with coronary atherosclerosis before the age of 55 years
- Children who have at least one parent with a total cholesterol level greater than or equal to 240 mg/dL
- Children who demonstrate other risk factors and whose parental history is unavailable
- Children or adolescents who have risk factors independent of family history (excessive smoking, decreased exercise, excessive fat intake) (American Academy of Pediatrics, Committee on Nutrition, 1998; Tershakovec & Rader, 2004)

Children with any of these risk factors should be followed with periodic cholesterol level measurements. Children whose total cholesterol measurement is 200 mg/dL or more, or 170 mg/dL or more on two successive measurements, need to have a follow-up fasting lipid profile.

Therapeutic Management

All children older than 2 years can follow a sensible low-fat dietary program. This includes using nonfat or low-fat dairy products, limiting red meat intake, and decreasing the amount of dietary saturated fat (see Chapter 4). The total daily fat intake should be no more than 30% of total calories, with saturated fat being no more than 10% of daily caloric intake. Children with borderline LDL measurements (110 to 129 mg/dL) need to have their food and fat intake carefully monitored by a health professional until cholesterol levels have improved. Children with high LDL measurements (>130 mg/dL) will need a more restrictive diet and comprehensive instruction and monitoring by a registered dietitian (American Academy of Pediatrics, Committee on Nutrition, 1998). Adequate intake of dietary fiber and avoidance of processed foods also can contribute to lowering LDL levels (Tershakovec & Rader, 2004).

Other factors that contribute to a healthy lifestyle in children and adolescents include increased physical activity and avoidance of sedentary lifestyle (e.g., excessive television watching) and monitoring for coronary heart disease risk factors (Tershakovec & Rader, 2004).

Cholesterol-lowering medications generally are not used in the pediatric population. Medications that bind bile acids in the intestine (cholestyramine, colestipol) are reserved for older children (>10 years old) who have very high LDL levels with or without associated risk factors (Tershakovec & Rader, 2004). A recent study of children with familial hypercholesterolemia, however, demonstrated that statin drugs in this population of high-risk children between 8 and 18 years were safe and effective (Wiegman et al., 2004)

Nursing Considerations

The most effective approach to decreasing risk factors during childhood and adolescence appears to be a population-based approach, with continuing education about risk factors occurring in communities, schools, physicians' offices, and the media. Nurses play an important part in educating parents and children about healthy diets, the importance of regular exercise, and reduction of other risk factors.

KEY CONCEPTS

- With the neonate's first breath, gas exchange is transferred from the placenta to the lungs. The fetal shunts (ductus venosus, ductus arteriosus, foramen ovale) close, and resistance to flow in the pulmonary system decreases as systemic resistance increases. Pulmonary vascular resistance decreases, and a marked increase in pulmonary blood flow follows.

- Stenosis can occur in a valve or a vessel and can result in obstruction of blood flow through the area.

- In left-to-right shunts, blood is shunted to the right side of the heart because the pressure is lower on the right side and higher on the left. Oxygenated and unoxygenated blood mix. Systemic saturations are normal.

- Poor weight gain with failure to thrive is a common sign of CHF.

- Hypercyanotic episodes, or "tet spells," are characterized by increased respiratory rate, depth of respiration, and severe hypoxemia.

- Assessment of the family of a child with a congenital cardiac defect should begin at diagnosis and continue throughout the care of the child.

- Common nursing diagnoses associated with infants with congenital heart defects and their parents include Decreased Cardiac Output, Imbalanced Nutrition: Less than Body Requirements, Activity Intolerance, Deficient Knowledge, Anxiety, Interrupted Family Processes, Risk for Infection, and Risk for Ineffective Health Maintenance.

- Signs of CHF include tachycardia, cardiomegaly, gallop rhythm, decreased peripheral perfusion, excessive diaphoresis, weight gain, ascites, liver and spleen enlargement, edema, neck vein distention, dyspnea, rales, tachypnea, intercostal muscular and sternal retractions, and wheezing.

- Measures to decrease the workload on the heart include limiting the time the child is allowed to breastfeed or bottle-feed, elevating the head of the bed, allowing for uninterrupted rest periods, allowing self-limiting activity, and providing oxygen (cautious use with left-to-right shunting lesions) during stressful periods.

- It is imperative to educate parents regarding medications, monitoring for signs and symptoms of CHF, increasing cyanosis, dehydration, infection, arrhythmias (when indicated), infective endocarditis prophylaxis, decreased nutritional intake, and decreasing ill contacts in the environment as the family is prepared for home discharge with infants or children with CHF and CHD.

- Prophylaxis with penicillin is the most important aspect of therapeutic management for RF. Intramuscular injection is the route of choice. Oral medication is an alternative, if given precisely and faithfully.

- In Kawasaki disease, coronary aneurysms may occur about 11 days after the onset of fever.

- Nursing management of a child with Kawasaki disease includes administering IVIG and aspirin to reduce the formation of the aneurysms and fever.

- The initial management of children with primary hypertension includes diet modification, reduction of weight (when needed), physical conditioning, and relaxation techniques.

- An appropriate-size blood pressure cuff, two repeat blood pressure readings on all four extremities, and a careful medical history are important in assessment for a diagnosis of hypertension.

- The heart rate is usually faster in infants and children than in adults and decreases with age.

- Population-based education of children and parents is the most effective way to prevent the cardiac consequences of high cholesterol levels.

ANSWERS TO
CRITICAL THINKING EXERCISE 22-1

1. Appropriate questions to ask concerning infant feeding patterns include the following:
   - How often does she eat?
   - How much does she eat at each feeding?
   - Does she tire easily?
   - Does she require frequent rest periods?
   - Do you notice beads of perspiration on her forehead during feedings?
   - Do you notice any change in her color or respiratory pattern during feedings?
   - Does she raise her eyebrows or wrinkle her forehead during feedings?

2. Some frequently seen physical assessment findings associated with CHF include tachycardia; tachypnea; increased work of breathing—nasal flaring, grunting, use of accessory muscles; pulmonary congestion, crackles; dry cough; hepatomegaly; distended neck veins; and periorbital, facial, or generalized edema.

3. Nutritional nursing care would include the following:
   - Finding an appropriate nipple for feeding; may need to enlarge the nipple hole to reduce the energy needed to suck
   - Feeding every 3 hours and allowing rest periods between feedings
   - Increasing the caloric content of the formula
   - May need to provide supplemental feedings through a nasogastric tube

Comfort measures include allowing rest periods between feedings. Do not overtire infants with multiple interventions at any one time. Place infants and children in a position of comfort, usually with the head of the bed elevated to decrease the work of breathing

REFERENCES AND READINGS

American Academy of Pediatrics. (2003). *2003 Red book: Report of the Committee on Infectious Diseases* (26th ed.). Elk Grove Village, IL: American Academy of Pediatrics.

American Academy of Pediatrics. (2005). Policy statement: Breastfeeding and the use of human milk. *Pediatrics, 115,* 496-506.

American Academy of Pediatrics, Committee on Nutrition. (1998). Cholesterol in childhood. *Pediatrics, 101,* 141-147.

American Academy of Pediatrics & American Heart Association. (2004). Diagnosis, treatment and long-term management of Kawasaki diseases: A statement for health professionals from the Committee on Rheumatic Fever, Endocarditis, and Kawasaki Disease, Council on Cardiovascular Disease in the Young, American Heart Association. *Pediatrics, 114,* 1708-1733.

American Heart Association. (2005a). *Endocarditis prophylaxis information.* A Report of the American College of Cardiology/American Heart Association Task Force on Practice Guidelines (Committee on Management of Patients With Valvular Heart Disease). Retrieved October 5, 2005, from *www.americanheart.org.*

American Heart Association. (2005b). *Youth and cardiovascular diseases—Statistics.* Retrieved October 5, 2005, from *http://www.americanheart.org/downloadable/heart/1110821457608FS11YTH5.REVDOC.DOC.*

Andrews, R., & Tulloh, R. (2004). Interventional cardiac catheterisation in congenital heart disease [Electronic version]. *Archives of Disease in Childhood, 89,* 1168-1173.

Baddour, L., Wilson, W., Bayer, A., Fowler, V., Bolger, A., Levison, M., et al. (2005). American Heart Association scientific statement: infective endocarditis. *Circulation, 111,* e394-e433. Retrieved October 5, 2005, from *www.circulationaha.org.*

Barbas, K., & Kelleher, D. (2004). Breastfeeding success among infants with congenital heart disease. *Pediatric Nursing, 30,* 285-297.

Bernstein, D. (2004). The cardiovascular system. In R. E. Behrman, R. M. Kliegman, & H. Jenson (Eds.), *Nelson textbook of pediatrics* (17th ed., pp. 1475-1591). Philadelphia: WB Saunders.

Carey, L., Nicholson, B., & Fox, R. (2002). Maternal factors related to parenting young children with congenital heart disease. *Journal of Pediatric Nursing, 17,* 174-183.

Chen, C., Li, C., & Wang, J. (2004). Growth and development of children with congenital heart disease. *Journal of Advanced Nursing, 47,* 260-269.

Chen, C., Li, C., & Wang, J. (2005). Self-concept: comparison between school-aged children with congenital heart disease and normal school-aged children. *Journal of Clinical Nursing, 14,* 394-402.

Children's Hospital Boston. (2005). Aortic stenosis. Retrieved September 20, 2005, from *www.childrenshospital.org.*

Clyman, R. I. (2005). Patent ductus arteriosus in the premature infant. In H. W. Taeusch, R. A. Ballard, & C. A. Gleason (Eds), *Avery's diseases of the newborn* (8th ed., pp. 816-820). Philadelphia: Elsevier.

Cowley, C., Orsmond, G., Feola, P., McQuillan, L., & Shaddy, R. (2005). Long-term, randomized comparison of balloon angioplasty and surgery for native coarctation of the aorta in childhood. *Circulation, 111,* 3453-3456.

Cromwell, P. F., Munn, N., Zolkowski-Wynne, J. (2005). Evaluation and management of hypertension in children and adolescents (part one): Evaluation and management. *Journal of Pediatric Health Care, 19,* 172-175.

Daller, J. (2004). Pulmonary valve stenosis. Retrieved September 19, 2005, from *www.nlm.nih.gov/medlineplus.*

Dooley, K., & Bishop, L. (2002). Medical management of the cardiac infant and child after surgical discharge. *Critical Care Nursing Quarterly, 25,* 98-104.

Dubin, A. (2004). Cardiac arrhythmias. In R. E. Behrman, R. M. Kliegman, & H. Jenson (Eds.), *Nelson textbook of pediatrics* (17th ed., pp. 1554-1565). Philadelphia: WB Saunders.

Fyfe, D., & Parks, W. J. (2002). Noninvasive diagnostics in congenital heart disease: Echocardiography and magnetic resonance imaging. *Critical Care Nursing Quarterly, 25,* 26-36.

Gerber, M. (2004). Group A *Streptococcus.* In R. E. Behrman, R. M. Kliegman, & H. Jenson (Eds.), *Nelson textbook of pediatrics* (17th ed., pp. 870-878). Philadelphia: WB Saunders.

Graham, T., Driscoll, D., Gersony, W., Newburger, J., Rocchini, A., & Towbin, J. (2005). 36th Bethesda conference eligibility recommendations for competitive athletes with cardiovascular abnormalities, Task force 2: Congenital heart disease. *Journal of the American College of Cardiology, 45,* 1326-1331.

Green, A. (2004). Outcomes of congenital heart disease: A review. *Pediatric Nursing, 30,* 280-284.

Griffin, K., Elkin, D., & Smith, C. (2003). Academic outcomes in children with congenital heart disease. *Clinical Pediatrics, 42,* 401-409.

Guzman-Cottrill, J., Jaggi, P., & Shulman, S. (2004). Acute rheumatic fever: Clinical aspects and insights into pathogenesis and prevention. *Clinical and Applied Immunology Reviews, 4,* 263-276.

Hellekson, K. (2005). Report on the diagnosis, evaluation, and treatment of high blood pressure in children and adolescents. *American Family Physician, 71,* 1016-1019.

Ikemba, C., Kozinetz, C., Feltes, T., Fraser, C., McKenzie, E., Shah, N., & Mott, A. (2002). Internet use in families with children requiring cardiac surgery for congenital heart disease. *Pediatrics, 109*, 419-423.

Kaplan, N., Gidding, S., Pickering, T., & Wright, J. (2005). Task force 5: Systemic hypertension. *Journal of the American College of Cardiology, 45*, 1346-1348.

Kay, J., Colan, S., & Graham, T. (2001). Congestive heart failure in pediatric patients. *American Heart Jounal, 142*, 923-928.

Maron, B. (2004). Hypertrophic cardiomyopathy in childhood. *Pediatric Clinics of North America, 51*, 1305-1346.

Maron, B., & Zipes, D. (2005). 36th Bethesda conference, Introduction: Eligibility recommendations for competitive athletes with cardiovascular abnormalities—General considerations. *Journal of the American College of Cardiology, 45*, 1318-1321.

Moake, L. (2005). Atrial septal defect treatment options [Electronic version]. *AACN Clinical Issues, 16*, 252-266.

National High Blood Pressure Education Program Working Group on High Blood Pressure in Children and Adolescents. (1987). Report of the Second Task Force on Blood Pressure Control in Children. *Pediatrics, 79*, 1-25.

National High Blood Pressure Education Program Working Group on High Blood Pressure in Children and Adolescents. (2004). The fourth report on the diagnosis, evaluation, and treatment of high blood pressure in children and adolescence. *Pediatrics, 114*, 1-24.

National Institutes of Health. (1996). *Update on the task force report (1987) on high blood pressure in children and adolescents: A working group report from the national high blood pressure education program.* Bethesda, MD: National Institutes of Health.

Neilson, D., & Robin, N. (2002). Advances in the genetics of pediatric heart disease. *Contemporary Pediatrics, 19*, 85-94.

Overmeire, B. V., & Chemtob, S. (2005). The pharmacologic closure of the patent ductus arteriosus. *Seminars in Fetal & Neonatal Medicine, 10*, 177-184.

Park, M. K. (2002). *Pediatric cardiology for practitioners* (4th ed.). St. Louis: Mosby.

Raja, S., & Basu, D. (2005). Pulmonary hypertension in congenital heart disease. *Nursing Standard, 19*, 41-49.

Robertson, J., & Shilkofski, N. (Eds.). (2005). *The Harriet Lane handbook* (17th ed.). St. Louis: Elsevier/Mosby.

Rosenthal, A. (2000). Hypoplastic left heart syndrome. In J. H. Moller & J. I. Hoffman (Eds.), *Pediatric cardiovascular medicine* (pp. 567-593). Philadelphia: Churchill Livingstone.

Rosenzweig, E., Widlitz, A., Barst, R. (2004). Pulmonary arterial hypertension in children. *Pediatric Pulmonology, 38*, 2-22.

Rowley, A., & Shulman, S. (1999). Kawasaki syndrome. *Pediatric Clinics of North America, 46*, 313-330.

Rowley, A., & Shulman, S. (2004). Kawasaki disease. In R. E. Behrman, R. M. Kliegman, & H. Jenson (Eds.), *Nelson textbook of pediatrics* (17th ed., pp. 823-826). Philadelphia: WB Saunders.

Second Task Force on Blood Pressure Control in Children. (1987). Report of the Second Task Force on Blood Pressure Control in Children: National Heart, Lung, and Blood Institute—1987. *Pediatrics, 79*, 1-25.

Sundel, R., Baker, A., Fulton, D., & Newburger, J. (2003). Corticosteroids in the initial treatment of Kawasaki disease: report of a randomized trial. *The Journal of Pediatrics, 142*, 611-616.

Tani, L., Veasy, G., Minich, L., & Shaddy, R. (2004). Rheumatic fever in children younger than 5 years: Is the presentation different? *Pediatrics, 112*, 1063-1068.

Tershakovec, A., & Rader, D. (2004). Disorders of lipoprotein metabolism and transport. In R. E. Behrman, R. M. Kliegman, & H. Jenson (Eds.), *Nelson textbook of pediatrics* (17th ed., pp. 445-453). Philadelphia: WB Saunders.

U.S. Department of Health and Human Services. (2000). *Healthy people 2010* (Conference edition in two volumes). Washington, DC: Department of Health and Human Services.

Wiegman, A., Hutten, B., de Groot, E., Rodenburg, J., Bakker, H., Büller, H., et al. (2004). Efficacy and safety of statin therapy in children with familial hypercholesterolemia: A randomized trial. *Journal of the American Medical Association, 292*, 331-337.

Williams, I., Quaegebeur, J., Hsu, D., Gersony, W., Bourlon, F., Mosca, R., et al. (2005). Ross procedure in infants and toddlers followed into childhood. *Circulation, 112*(I suppl), I390-I395.

Zeigler, V. L. (2003). Ethical principles and parental choice: Treatment options for neonates with hypoplastic left heart syndrome. *Pediatric Nursing, 29*, 65-69.

CHAPTER *23*

The Child With a Hematologic Alteration

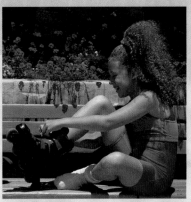

Learning *Objectives*

After studying this chapter, you should be able to:
- Describe the anatomy and physiology of the hematopoietic system.
- Discuss the pediatric differences related to blood and blood formation.
- Discuss the role of the nurse in the prevention of iron-deficiency anemia.
- Describe common factors in the care of a child with anemia.
- Discuss the pathophysiology and therapeutic management of common hematologic alterations.
- List possible nursing diagnoses for children with hematologic alterations.
- Describe possible nursing care for children with hematologic alterations.

Definitions

autoimmune disorder A disorder in which the body launches an immunologic response against itself.
chelation Binding of a metallic ion with a structure so that the ion is inactivated.
erythropoiesis Production of erythrocytes (red blood cells, RBCs).
extramedullary Outside the bone marrow.
granulocytes Polymorphonuclear leukocytes (neutrophils, eosinophils, basophils).
hematopoiesis Production of blood cells; normally occurs in the bone marrow but may occur in extramedullary sites.

hemolysis Breakdown of red blood cells.
hemostasis Process of vasoconstriction and coagulation to stop bleeding.
hemosiderosis Focal or general increase in tissue iron stores without associated tissue damage.
pancytopenia A reduction in all types of blood cells.
reticulocyte Immature red blood cell.
reticuloendothelial system The collection of cells, throughout the body, that are capable of phagocytosis.

Electronic Resources

Additional information related to the content in Chapter 23 can be found on:

the interactive companion CD-ROM
- Animations: Band Formation
           Hemophilia A
           Sickle Cell Anemia
- Audio Glossary
- NCLEX Review Questions

or the companion website at *evolve*
http://evolve.elsevier.com/james/ncoc
- NCLEX Review Questions
- Resources for Health Care Providers and Families
- WebLinks

REVIEW OF THE HEMATOLOGIC SYSTEM

Hematology is the study of the blood and blood-forming tissues. In fetal life, various tissues produce red blood cells (RBCs), but after birth, their production is controlled exclusively by the bone marrow, primarily in the long bones. With age, the more membranous bones of the vertebrae, sternum, and ribs assume RBC production. Age, sex, and the altitude at which a person lives affect the number of RBCs.

Normally, RBCs are biconcave disks that are capable of changing shape as they flow through the microvasculature of the body. They have a fairly uniform size that is determined mainly by the amount of cellular content of substances, primarily hemoglobin. Their function is to transport oxygen to tissues. Essential to this ability to carry oxygen is an appropriate amount of hemoglobin, whose production depends on sufficient amounts of circulating iron. Iron is absorbed from dietary intake by the intestines and stored by the liver in both soluble and insoluble forms, to be used when necessary.

The stimulus for production of RBCs is a decrease in circulating oxygen, which in turn stimulates the kidneys to produce a hormone called *erythropoietin*. Erythropoietin stimulates the production of RBC precursors and causes them to mature rapidly. Disorders of the kidney can affect the individual's ability to produce this hormone and thus can affect RBC production by the bone marrow.

Anemia is a decrease in the number of RBCs, reduction in their hemoglobin content, or reduced volume of packed RBCs. Anemia results from one of two problems: either too rapid a loss of RBCs (by covert or overt bleeding or destruction) or too slow a production of RBCs. Anemias are categorized according to the size of the RBC (macrocytic, microcytic, normocytic) and the content of hemoglobin in the RBC (hypochromic, normochromic).

Polycythemia, which is an increase in the number of RBCs, is less frequently seen than anemia. *Polycythemia* can occur as a result of hypoxia, such as that experienced at high altitude or when oxygen is not sufficiently directed to the tissues, as in cyanotic heart disease.

White blood cells (WBCs), or leukocytes, are formed in the bone marrow and in lymphatic tissue. They assist in the body's ability to distinguish "self" from "nonself." WBCs destroy foreign cells through the processes of phagocytosis and antibody production. Both phagocytes and antibodies destroy foreign cells and tissues perceived by the body as nonself (including, e.g., bacteria, fungi, viruses, parasites, transplanted tissue) (see Chapter 17). WBC disorders result from an altered rate of production of WBCs (lymphocytosis or lymphopenia) or an alteration in function of the cells.

Platelets are the cells that promote hemostasis—the prevention of blood loss. They are formed in the bone marrow from megakaryocytes. Megakaryocytes later fragment into smaller cells known as *platelets,* either in the bone marrow or shortly after release into the systemic circulation. Platelets can circulate in the blood for about 10 days before they die; however, disease, fever, and infection can shorten a platelet's lifetime. Platelet disorders occur when the bone marrow cannot meet the production demands of the body.

PEDIATRIC HEMATOLOGIC SYSTEM

- The life span of erythrocytes in neonates is shorter than in older infants and children because of increased destruction during rapid growth.
- By 2 months of age, erythropoiesis increases, leading to increased reticulocytes in the blood and a rise in hemoglobin.
- Erythrocytes are produced initially in the marrow of all bones. After 5 years of age, RBC production in the shafts of the long bones (tibia, femur) is reduced, and production ceases in these locations entirely at age 20 years. Hematopoiesis takes place primarily in the marrow of the ribs, sternum, vertebrae, pelvis, skull, clavicle, and scapulas.
- The number of erythrocytes varies according to age. The fetus has a higher oxygen-carrying capacity than an infant because of a considerably higher number of erythrocytes with proportionately elevated hemoglobin and hematocrit values.

TYPES AND FUNCTIONS OF WHITE BLOOD CELLS

- **Granulocytes:** Phagocytic cells produced in the bone marrow and found in the circulation.
  - *Neutrophils:* primary defense in bacterial infection; capable of phagocytizing and killing bacteria.
  - *Eosinophils:* influence the inflammatory process, fight parasites, and influence allergic hypersensitivity reactions.
  - *Basophils:* activate the inflammatory response; contain histamine; other roles are unclear.
- **Agranulocytes:** participate in inflammatory and immune reactions.
  - *Monocytes/macrophages:* phagocytize large cells, including necrotic tissue; they are therefore important in fighting chronic infection.
  - *Lymphocytes:* found in bone marrow, spleen, thymus, lymph glands, tissues, and circulation.
    - *T cells:* made in the thymus and responsible for cell-mediated immunity.
    - *B cells:* responsible for humoral immunity (antibody production).
    - *Natural killer cells*: lymphocyte-like cells that can kill certain type of tumor cells and viruses directly

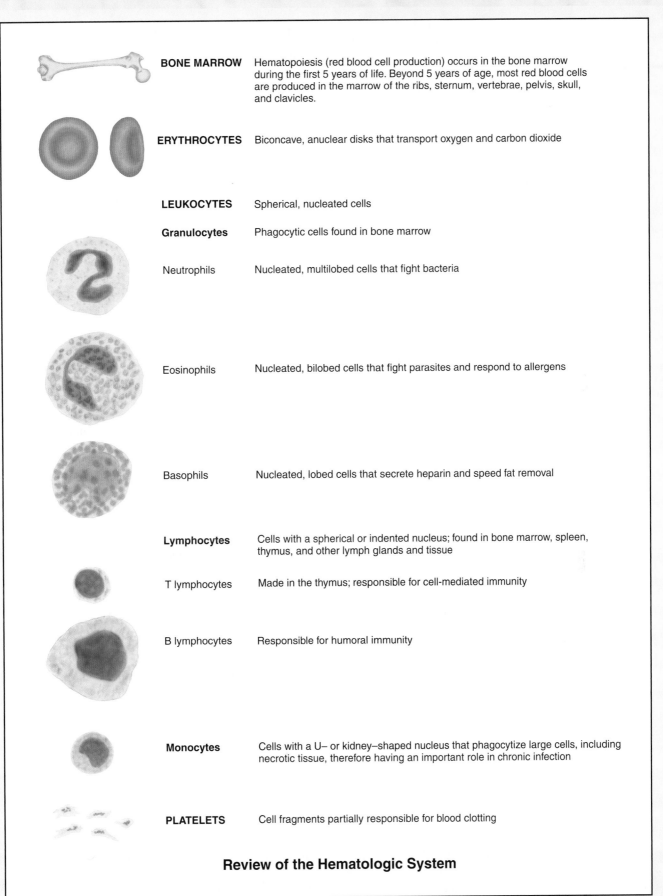

BONE MARROW — Hematopoiesis (red blood cell production) occurs in the bone marrow during the first 5 years of life. Beyond 5 years of age, most red blood cells are produced in the marrow of the ribs, sternum, vertebrae, pelvis, skull, and clavicles.

ERYTHROCYTES — Biconcave, anuclear disks that transport oxygen and carbon dioxide

LEUKOCYTES — Spherical, nucleated cells

Granulocytes — Phagocytic cells found in bone marrow

Neutrophils — Nucleated, multilobed cells that fight bacteria

Eosinophils — Nucleated, bilobed cells that fight parasites and respond to allergens

Basophils — Nucleated, lobed cells that secrete heparin and speed fat removal

Lymphocytes — Cells with a spherical or indented nucleus; found in bone marrow, spleen, thymus, and other lymph glands and tissue

T lymphocytes — Made in the thymus; responsible for cell-mediated immunity

B lymphocytes — Responsible for humoral immunity

Monocytes — Cells with a U– or kidney–shaped nucleus that phagocytize large cells, including necrotic tissue, therefore having an important role in chronic infection

PLATELETS — Cell fragments partially responsible for blood clotting

Review of the Hematologic System

(Photo from Behrman, R. E., Kliegman, R. M., & Arvin, A. M. [Eds.]. [1996]. Nelson textbook of pediatrics [15th ed., p. 1402]. Philadelphia: WB Saunders.)

When caring for infants and children with blood disorders, the nurse is challenged in the areas of preventive, acute, and chronic care. Depending on the disorder and the child's condition, care may be provided in the home, an outpatient setting, or the hospital. It is not unusual for a child to be seen in an outpatient setting (clinic, school), referred to a hospital for diagnosis and stabilization, and returned to the home for maintenance. Genetic counseling may be indicated for children or families with certain types of blood disorders.

Many medications for hematologic disorders can be given at home, including deferoxamine mesylate (Desferal), intravenous (IV) immune globulin (IVIG), IV antibiotics, coagulation factor products, and, in some instances, even blood transfusions. Parents are learning to manage infusion therapy in regard to initiating, monitoring, and discontinuing infusions when appropriate, with guidance from the collaborative efforts of the multidisciplinary health care team.

IRON-DEFICIENCY ANEMIA

Iron deficiency is the most common cause of anemia during infancy, childhood, and adolescence. Iron-deficiency anemia (IDA) may be characterized by mild or marked anemia.

Etiology and Incidence

Several factors can contribute to IDA, including decreased iron intake, increased iron or blood loss, and periods of increased growth rate.

IDA related to inadequate dietary iron intake is rare before age 4 to 6 months because of the presence of maternal iron stores; it occurs most often in children age 9 to 24 months as iron stores are depleted. Premature infants may develop iron deficiency early in life because they are born with insufficient maternal iron stores (Glader, 2004). Decreased iron intake is often related to the intake of large amounts of cow's milk instead of breast milk or fortified formula and inadequate intake of iron-fortified foods (Glader, 2004). The incidence has dropped in recent years because of increased education about and availability of iron-fortified formula and cereals. Early transition from breast milk or infant formula to cow's milk can precipitate chronic diarrhea with occult intestinal bleeding in children younger than 2 years. This results from exposure to a protein found in cow's milk (Glader, 2004). The rapid growth of infants and children younger than 2 years, combined with decreased iron intake, further contributes to the increased incidence in this age group.

Adolescents are also at risk for IDA because they too are undergoing increased growth and often have poor dietary habits. The situation is further complicated by the blood loss during menstruation in young women.

Manifestations

The clinical manifestations of IDA vary with the degree of anemia but may include extreme pallor with porcelain-like skin, pale mucous membranes and conjunctiva, tachycardia, tachypnea, lethargy, fatigue, and irritability. Children with lead poisoning often have associated IDA.

PATHOPHYSIOLOGY

IRON-DEFICIENCY ANEMIA

Iron is one of the components necessary for the synthesis of hemoglobin. Without an adequate amount of iron, the bone marrow continues to manufacture RBCs, but their content of hemoglobin is decreased, rendering these RBCs inefficient at carrying oxygen to the tissues. The constellation of clinical signs evident with IDA results from compromised tissue oxygenation.

The term neonate is born with enough stored maternal iron to produce adequate amounts of hemoglobin for 4 to 6 months. The average life of an RBC is about 120 days. Thus IDA is usually not seen in children before age 9 months.

As RBCs undergo *hemolysis*, intracellular iron is released into the circulation for use by the body. Adults are able to use this breakdown of RBCs as a primary source of iron. Children, however, grow very rapidly and expand their circulating blood volume at the same time. Because the breakdown of RBCs in children exceeds their ability to produce new RBCs and their need for iron to synthesize new hemoglobin for RBC production is increased, children must increase their dietary consumption of iron. The AAP recommends routine iron supplementation with iron-fortified formula in nonbreastfeeding term and preterm infants, as well as iron salt supplementation for all preterm infants (born before 32 weeks' gestation), who are at greater risk for anemia as a result of having less stored iron. Iron-fortified cereals are recommended when solids are introduced.

Various factors can contribute to a lack of absorption of iron by the gastrointestinal tract. When cow's milk is introduced into the diet before age 1 year in place of breast milk or formula, infants do not ingest sufficient iron because cow's milk is a poor dietary source of iron. Often, the potentially large amount of cow's milk replaces iron-fortified cereals and iron-rich baby food. Although iron from breast milk is well absorbed, it is not a complete source of iron, and dietary iron supplements must be introduced to augment its nutrients when the infant is approximately 4 to 6 months old.

Blood loss from an infant's intestine occurs very slowly and has several causes. The immature intestine may be unable to tolerate the protein in cow's milk or milk-based infant formula. Irritation of the bowel results in hemorrhages of the microvasculature, resulting in blood loss in the stool. Although unusual, parasitic infections can also irritate the intestinal lining.

Diagnostic Evaluation

Any child with anemia should first have a complete history taken, with particular emphasis on assessment of nutritional intake. The results of a complete blood cell count (CBC) in individuals with IDA will show low hemoglobin levels (6 to 11 g/dL) and microcytic, hypochromic RBCs, reflected in a decreased mean cell volume and decreased mean cell hemoglobin (see Evolve website). The reticulocyte count is usually normal or slightly elevated. With these findings, serum ferritin levels and serum iron or iron-binding capacity should be assessed. Iron-binding capacity is usually increased as a result of decreased serum iron levels. Hemoglobin electrophoresis may be done to rule out causes other than IDA.

Therapeutic Management

Therapy is directed toward increasing the dietary intake of iron and iron supplementation. The absorption of dietary iron-rich foods can be unreliable and will not rapidly provide the body with enough iron to correct the iron deficiency. Therefore, affected children are given a daily oral iron preparation (often three times per day) of one of the available ferrous salts (ferrous sulfate, ferrous gluconate, ferrous fumarate) on the basis of the content of elemental iron (dose should be 3 to 6 mg/kg/day [2 to 4 mg/kg/day for premature infants] in three divided doses). Iron therapy is continued for 3 months after the hemoglobin and hematocrit levels return to normal, after which a daily multivitamin with iron can be recommended.

Follow-up monitoring includes a CBC and reticulocyte count. The reticulocyte count should increase within days of the initiation of iron therapy. An increased hemoglobin level can be expected in 4 to 30 days. The response to iron therapy can often be positively predicted, so blood transfusions are rarely indicated to correct IDA. RBC transfusions are reserved for severe anemia and cardiovascular compromise.

CRITICAL TO REMEMBER
Obtaining a Dietary Intake History

Parents may not readily or accurately report their child's dietary questions. Ask the parent to begin the dietary history at the time the child awoke yesterday, describing the child's activities and exactly what the child ate. Correlating activities with diet may enable the nurse to obtain a better history and may alert the nurse to feeding patterns for which counseling may be indicated.

BOX 23-1 | **PARENTS WANT TO KNOW** About Home Care of the Child With Iron-Deficiency Anemia

Dietary Changes
- Provide iron-fortified formula or breast milk with iron-fortified food supplements if the child is younger than 12 months.
- If the child is older than 12 months, limit intake of cow's milk to 24 oz/day or less.
- Increase the child's intake of age-appropriate iron-rich foods, with selections based on the age of the child: liver, dried beans, Cream of Wheat, iron-fortified cereal, apricots and prunes (and other dried fruits), egg yolks, dark-green, leafy vegetables.

Administration of Iron
- Administer iron in three divided doses between meals.
- Give with vitamin C–rich fluids.
- Administer iron through a straw or medicine dropper placed at the back of the mouth, away from the teeth. Brush or wipe off teeth.
- Recognize that iron supplementation causes black, tarry stools.
- Avoid administration of iron with milk or formula and cereal because iron binds with calcium, thus impeding absorption.

Follow-Up Care
- Keep appointments for follow-up evaluations.
- Expect blood work to be done at follow-up visits.

NURSING CARE PLAN

The Child With Iron-Deficiency Anemia in the Community Setting

Focused Assessment

Parents may state that their child is more quiet than usual, with an increased desire to be held. In cases of extreme anemia, the parents may report that the child's heart races when the child is held. More often than not, there is a history of introduction to cow's milk before age 12 months and a history of increased milk consumption to the exclusion of solid foods.

On physical examination, the child is pale and appears tired, with mild to severe tachycardia. If the anemia is severe, a heart murmur may be heard; this will disappear as the anemic state is reversed.

NURSING DIAGNOSIS Imbalanced Nutrition: Less Than Body Requirements related to parents' lack of knowledge of age-appropriate nutritional needs.

EXPECTED OUTCOME The parents will:
- Have an understanding of the child's nutritional needs, as evidenced by verbal description of the child's dietary plan, including foods containing appropriate dietary iron.

Continued

NURSING CARE PLAN—cont'd

Intervention	*Rationale*
1. Obtain the child's past and current nutritional history. Instruct the caregiver to continue to give infant iron-fortified formula or breastfeed and give supplementary iron-fortified foods until age 12 months. In a child older than 12 months, milk intake should be decreased to 24 oz/day or less. Per the child's age, suggest intake of liver, dried beans, Cream of Wheat, iron-fortified cereal, apricots, prunes, egg yolks, and leafy, dark-green vegetables (Box 23-1). Advise the parent to keep a dietary diary.	1. Therapy is based on the child's history. Cow's milk is poorly digested and is not rich in iron. The AAP recommends continuing breast milk or iron-fortified formula until age 12 months. Decreasing milk intake will encourage the consumption of other iron-rich foods. Iron-fortified formula and food will establish healthier eating habits. Keeping a record of food and fluid intake assists with a dietary evaluation and identifies areas that need additional teaching.
2. Explain the need for iron in the manufacture of RBCs, the effect of iron therapy on laboratory test results, the potential outcome with no intervention, the lack of iron in cow's milk, and iron's effect on the body.	2. Providing explanations of the rationale for therapy can often help improve adherence to therapy.
3. Instruct the caregiver to administer oral iron supplements as ordered by the physician and allow opportunity to practice technique with assistance. Iron is usually given in three divided doses between meals (see Box 23-1).	3. The immediate need is to increase iron intake beyond that absorbed from formula or food. Do not assume the parents are able to administer iron effectively. Evaluate their technique of medication administration to build their skill and confidence.
• Encourage administration on an empty stomach, with fruit juice, and avoid administration with milk, formula, and cereals.	• An acid stomach environment facilitates absorption. Calcium in milk products binds with iron to decrease iron absorption.
• Instruct the caregiver to administer iron through a straw or medicine dropper placed at the back of the mouth. Brush or wipe teeth after administration.	• Iron temporarily stains teeth.
• Instruct the caregiver to administer vitamin C as ordered and encourage intake of foods rich in vitamin C.	• Vitamin C increases the absorption of iron by the body.
4. Instruct the caregiver to keep iron supplements (and all medications) out of reach of children.	4. Iron poisoning is possible with overdose. This can be serious and possibly fatal.
5. Instruct the caregiver to obtain follow-up laboratory examinations, including reticulocyte count and hemoglobin level.	5. The reticulocyte count should peak in 5 to 7 days. It serves as an objective test for determining the parents' degree of adherence to therapy. The hemoglobin level should increase in 4 to 30 days.*
6. Instruct the caregiver to expect black stools; inquire about their presence.	6. The absence of tarry stools may indicate lack of adherence to therapy.
7. Obtain a social services consultation for enrollment in a federal or state social services program if warranted.	7. Poor nutritional habits may be attributable to a lack of resources.

Evaluation

• Does the dietary diary reflect an increase in iron-rich foods in the child's daily meal plan?	• Do the parents demonstrate adherence to the prescribed therapy and verbalize appropriate questions?
• Does the child have normal iron, hemoglobin, and hematocrit levels?	• Has the child had a recurrence of IDA?

*Glader, B. (2004). Iron deficiency anemia. In R. Behrman, R. Kliegman, & H. Jenson (Eds.), *Nelson textbook of pediatrics* (17th ed., pp. 1614-1616). Philadelphia: WB Saunders.

CRITICAL THINKING EXERCISE 23-1

Mrs. Anders has brought 18-month-old Jacob to the clinic because he is irritable, running a low-grade fever, and has a cough. In the process of assessing Jacob, you note that he seems lethargic and his skin is very pale. A CBC count confirms a diagnosis of IDA.

1. What do you think Mrs. Anders is most concerned about?
2. What is the nurse's role when a child enters the health care system with an acute illness?
3. What opportunities present when a child is brought to an outpatient setting because of an acute illness?

SICKLE CELL DISEASE

Sickle cell disease (SCD) is the generic term that refers to a group of genetic disorders characterized by the production of sickle hemoglobin (HbS), chronic hemolytic anemia, and ischemic tissue injury. The more common forms of SCD include homozygous HbSS disease (sickle cell anemia), HbC disease (sickle C disease), and the sickle beta-thalassemia syndromes. SCD is an inherited, life-long disease that affects primarily African Americans but it can occur also in individuals of Mediterranean, Indian, and Middle Eastern descent. The morbidity and mortality rates from the severe forms of the disease have decreased as a result of newborn screening for the disease, routine prophylactic penicillin administration, and pneumococcal and *Haemophilus influenzae* vaccines.

Etiology

SCD is a group of hemoglobinopathies in which normal hemoglobin is partially or totally replaced by an abnormal hemoglobin, HbS. They are inherited, autosomal recessive conditions (see Chapter 4). If one parent has the HbS trait and the other parent does not, each pregnancy has a 50% risk of having the child inherit the trait. If each parent carries the trait, there is a 25% chance that the child will be unaffected, a 50% chance that the child will carry the trait, and a 25% chance that the child will have the disease. Although not a disease in and of itself, the carrier state of SCD—sickle cell trait—may produce clinical symptoms (e.g., hematuria, bacteriuria) in times of extreme stress, during extremely vigorous exercise, and at high altitudes.

Incidence

SCD affects approximately 1 in 600 African Americans. Sickle cell trait is found in 8% of African Americans and is prevalent also in persons of Mediterranean, Middle Eastern, Indian, Caribbean, and Central and South American descent (Lanzkowsky, 2005).

Manifestations

All the clinical manifestations of SCD are a result of the obstructions caused by the sickled RBCs and the increased destruction of sickled and normal RBCs caught in microcirculation obstructions. Large amounts of fetal hemoglobin (HbF) present in the first few months of life obscure the presence of HbS, so symptoms of the disease usually do not appear until age 4 to 6 months, when the infant begins to manufacture hemoglobin.

The disease affects most organ systems. Delayed growth and puberty are common. The child usually has small stature throughout adolescence but attains normal growth in the early 20s.

The general manifestations of SCD are chronic hemolytic anemia, pallor, jaundice, fatigue, cholelithiasis, delayed growth and puberty, avascular necrosis of the hips and shoulders, renal dysfunction, and retinopathy. However, sickling events may also progress to acute episodic exacerbations known as *sickle cell crisis*. Infection, dehydration, hypoxia, trauma, or general stress may precipitate a crisis episode. The crisis may take one of three forms: vaso-occlusive, acute sequestration, or aplastic. Repeated vaso-occlusive crises and a virtually continual state of anemia produce long-term problems later in the life of the individual with SCD. Table 23-1 presents the clinical manifestations of SCD.

Diagnostic Evaluation

In the past, many infants died from complications of SCD before being diagnosed with the disorder. However, newborn screening for SCD has significantly decreased the mortality rate. A laboratory diagnosis of SCD is established on the basis of a CBC, isoelectric focusing, hemoglobin electrophoresis, and high-performance liquid chromatography. Children with SCD have elevated reticulocyte counts because of the chronicity of loss and destruction as a result of the shortened life span of the sickled RBCs. Prenatal diagnosis is an option and is made by chorionic villus sampling at 8 to 10 weeks of gestation or amniocentesis at 15 weeks of gestation.

Therapeutic Management

In SCD, the spleen often does not function properly or has been surgically removed because of complications. Functional or actual asplenia places children and adults with SCD in an immunocompromised state at high risk for infection. Splenic dysfunction can begin at 6 months of age, and those with HbSS may have total dysfunction by age 5 years. Bacterial septicemia is associated with a 30% mortality rate in children younger than 5 years with SCD (Dover & Platt, 2003). The bacteria *Streptococcus pneumoniae* and *H. influenzae* are normally destroyed by the reticuloendothelial system of the spleen, but because children with SCD do not have a properly functioning spleen, they are considered to be more susceptible to infection with these bacteria.

The natural history of splenic dysfunction in children with HbSS places them at higher risk for fulminate septicemia and death during the first 3 years of life than children with HbC. Prophylactic daily penicillin therapy is recommended in all children with suspected or actual diagnosis by age 2 months and is continued until at least age 5 years (American Academy of Pediatrics [AAP], 2003b). Although views regarding the use of penicillin differ, some experts will continue penicillin prophylaxis throughout childhood in high-risk patients with asplenia. The pneumococcal polyvalent vaccine is recommended at age 2 years for children who did not receive it during infancy, with a booster after 3 to 5 years for children age 10 years or younger and for older children who were immunized at least 5 years earlier (AAP, 2003a). *H. influenzae* vaccine is recommended beginning at 2 months of age, as in healthy children, and for all previously unimmunized children with asplenia (AAP, 2003a). Routine immunization against hepatitis B is recommended, particularly in light of possible blood transfusions. Moreover, children with SCD should receive the influenza vaccine annually and immunization against meningococcal disease after age 2 years (AAP, 2003a) because of their increased risk for related complications.

PATHOPHYSIOLOGY

SICKLE CELL DISEASE

The normal RBC is a smooth, biconcave disk that is capable of changing shape to enable it to flow easily through the microvasculature of the circulation. Under conditions of low oxygen concentration, acidosis, and dehydration, the RBCs in a child with SCD assume a sickle shape, which prevents them from flowing easily through the smallest blood vessels. Sickled RBCs are stiff and nonpliable. These sickled cells clump together, causing occlusions in the small vessels. With reoxygenation, most of the sickled RBCs resume their normal shape. After repeated sickling and unsickling, however, the cells become irreversibly sickled and their life span is reduced from 120 days to 12 days.

Sickled cells cause microvascular occlusion, leading to tissue ischemia, infarcts, and organ damage. The lungs, spleen, and brain are the organs most seriously affected by the complications of SCD. The normal spleen functions to filter bacteria in the blood. The spleen of a child with SCD does not function properly much beyond age 5 years. The large vessels are also affected, leading to strokes and other vaso-occlusive events.

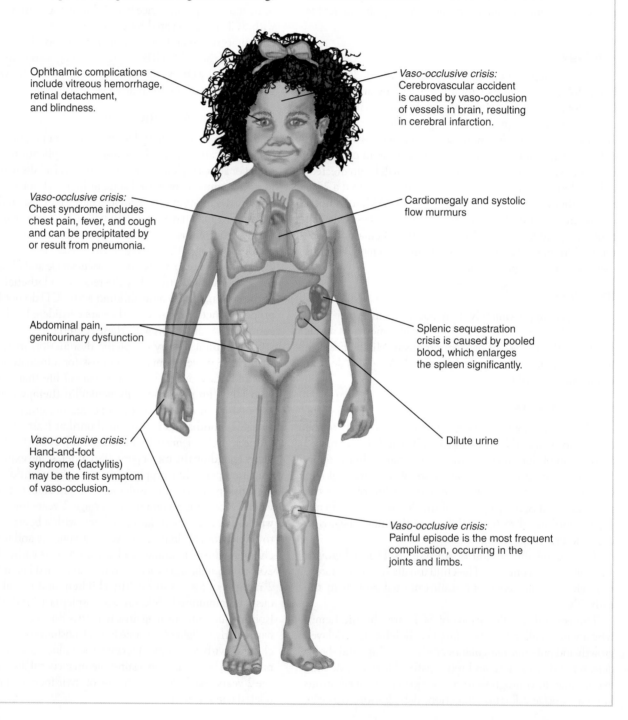

Ophthalmic complications include vitreous hemorrhage, retinal detachment, and blindness.

Vaso-occlusive crisis: Chest syndrome includes chest pain, fever, and cough and can be precipitated by or result from pneumonia.

Abdominal pain, genitourinary dysfunction

Vaso-occlusive crisis: Hand-and-foot syndrome (dactylitis) may be the first symptom of vaso-occlusion.

Vaso-occlusive crisis: Cerebrovascular accident is caused by vaso-occlusion of vessels in brain, resulting in cerebral infarction.

Cardiomegaly and systolic flow murmurs

Splenic sequestration crisis is caused by pooled blood, which enlarges the spleen significantly.

Dilute urine

Vaso-occlusive crisis: Painful episode is the most frequent complication, occurring in the joints and limbs.

TABLE 23-1   Clinical Manifestations and Therapeutic Management of Sickle Cell Disease Complications

Complication	Characteristics	Manifestations	Treatment
Vaso-Occlusive Crisis			
Painful episode	Most common type of crisis and reason for hospitalization Typically produces bone or joint pain, but pain can occur anywhere Pain may come and go Frequency of pain is individualized Pain is precipitated by infection, cold, stress, acidosis, local or generalized hypoxia	*Mild:* joint or bone pain lasting a few hours *Severe:* joint or bone pain lasting days	Oral analgesics initially and if ineffective, IV opioids (usually morphine), which may be given by either intermittent or continuous infusion Oral or IV NSAIDs Oral and IV hydration Oxygen in hypoxic patients Aggressive incentive spirometry use (10 breaths every 2 hr when awake) Consistent manner to assess subjective experience of pain is essential Use of nonpharmacologic pain management strategies in addition to medications
Acute chest syndrome	Common cause of hospitalization Sometimes confused with pneumonia Can recur	Chest pain, fever, cough, abdominal pain	IV hydration (1-1½ times maintenance), antibiotics, oxygen, RBC transfusion, analgesics
Dactylitis (hand-and-foot syndrome)	Occurs in children ages 6 mo to 4 yr Self-limiting complication	Swelling of hands or feet, pain, warmth in affected area	Oral analgesics, hydration (oral or IV), rest
Priapism (persistent erection of the penis)	Occurs if penile blood flow becomes obstructed	Persistent, painful erection	Analgesics; hydration Avoid hot and cold packs If prolonged, transfusion therapy
Cerebrovascular accident	Without treatment, mortality rate of 20%; 70% of patients have a recurrence	Hemiparesis or monoparesis, aphasia/dysphasia, seizures, alteration in level of consciousness, vomiting, vision changes, ataxia, headache	Long-term RBC transfusion therapy for indefinite period and possibly chelation therapy May require extensive rehabilitation
Acute Sequestration Crisis			
	Blood volume pooling in the spleen, causing splenic enlargement Life-threatening condition of hypovolemic shock Usually occurs in children ages 6 mo to 4 yr One episode increases the risk of future occurrences	Decreased hemoglobin level, acutely ill-looking child, pallor, irritability, tachycardia, impressively enlarged spleen, hypovolemic shock	Emergency treatment to restore circulating blood volume with crystalloid and colloid (blood) infusion Long-term transfusion therapy if recurrent Eventual splenectomy in cases of persistent recurrence
Aplastic Crisis			
	Profound anemia caused by diminished erythropoiesis Has been observed after parvovirus-like agent exposure	Pallor, lethargy, headache, fainting	RBC transfusions and treatment of symptoms

A child with SCD and a temperature of 38.5° C (101.3° F) or higher should receive prompt medical evaluation and treatment because of the overwhelming risk for infectious complications. Fever can be the first sign of bacteremia. Parenteral antibiotics, blood cultures, IV hydration, and general monitoring are the standard of care for children with SCD who have fever. Outpatient therapy with long-acting parenteral antibiotics may be provided in combination with rigorous evaluation and follow-up in those centers with the capabilities to do so. Children who are not eligible for outpatient therapy are those with the following signs and symptoms (and thus they are considered at high risk for sequelae):

- Ill appearance
- Cardiovascular instability
- Age younger than 1 year
- Pulmonary infiltrate
- Prior splenectomy or history of pneumococcal sepsis
- Hemoglobin less than 5 g/dL

- Family's or child's lack of ability to adhere to outpatient therapy
- WBC count less than 500/mm^3 or more than 30,000/mm^3
- Dehydration

Opioids and nonsteroidal anti-inflammatory drugs (NSAIDs) (i.e., ibuprofen, ketorolac) are the mainstay of analgesic treatment, particularly in combination for painful crises. Morphine is the current opioid of choice because meperidine (Demerol) is no longer recommended for long-term pain management due to its side effect profile. Opioids provide systemic relief, and the NSAIDS act locally to decrease inflammation at the site of vaso-occlusion and provide analgesia without the potential side effect of respiratory depression. Morphine has been very effective when administered IV, particularly when given in a patient-controlled analgesia fashion (see Chapter 15).

The treatment of SCD focuses on prompt diagnosis, education about the disease, prevention of exacerbations, prompt identification of exacerbation, and supportive care during crises (hydration, oxygenation, analgesia, RBC transfusion). Additional therapies currently under investigation include erythrocytapheresis (removal of sickled erythrocytes by an exchange transfusion technique), phenotyping RBCs for transfusion ("tissue typing" blood products that can potentially reduce alloimmunization), and hydroxyurea administration (augments HbF, which interferes with the RBC sickling process).

Research toward a cure continues; especially promising may be gene therapy. Another promising area of research is hematopoietic stem cell transplantation. It has been a successful treatment modality for a limited number of children. Logistic issues are related to candidate selection regarding this potentially curative strategy and ethical issues promoted by some.

Table 23-1 presents the therapeutic management of SCD.

Text continued on p. 731

NURSING CARE PLAN

The Child With Sickle Cell Disease

Focused Assessment

On initial diagnosis, the subjective data usually include parental concern that the child is in pain. The parents may have noticed swelling of the joints, the child's refusal to move an extremity, or the child's crying out when a joint is moved or touched. Fever and irritability may accompany the pain. Parents of a child already diagnosed with SCD who have been educated about the signs of complications will give a much more detailed history of the current illness that will likely include pain. A nurse familiar with the child can become adept at assessing the severity of that child's condition. The presence of SCD does not eliminate other serious causes of pain.

Despite teenagers' ability to verbalize symptoms, assessment of adolescents who are feeling pain is a unique challenge. During the developmental time in their lives when they most want to fit in with their peer groups, teenagers with SCD are different. After the initial pain of an episode has subsided, teens may seek attention from health care providers in an attempt to avoid their peer groups, verbalizing continued symptoms that would make them unable to return to their normal activities. Objective data will vary according to the type of painful episodes.

Parents should be taught to assess and report the size of the child's spleen for close monitoring of the child's condition.

NURSING DIAGNOSIS Ineffective Tissue Perfusion related to red blood cell sickling.

EXPECTED OUTCOMES The child will:
- Demonstrate adequate tissue perfusion, as evidenced by palpable peripheral pulses; warm, dry skin; adequate urinary output for age; and the absence of respiratory distress (oxygen saturation >95%).

The child and family will:
- Describe the treatment regimen, including medications and their actions and possible side effects.

Intervention	Rationale
1. Monitor the child's vital signs and respiratory status every 4 hours and as needed.	1. Vital signs and respiratory status are assessed frequently to detect changes in tissue perfusion and respiratory status. Signs of altered perfusion include increased respiratory rate, increased work of breathing, decreased oxygen saturation, poor color, mottled appearance, prolonged capillary refill time, decreased peripheral pulses, and altered level of consciousness. A change in the level of consciousness often indicates poor perfusion or oxygenation of the brain.

NURSING CARE PLAN—cont'd

2. Monitor pulse oximetry and administer oxygen to keep saturation >95%.

3. Ensure adequate hydration by measuring intake and output and administering crystalloids and colloids (RBCs) as ordered.

4. Determine the child's and family's understanding of SCD and the treatment regimen and provide information or clarification as necessary.

2. Oxygen saturation levels are monitored with pulse oximetry. Ensuring adequate oxygen can ease the child's work of breathing and facilitate tissue oxygenation. Oxygen does not reverse the sickling process but may prevent more sickling.

3. Measuring intake and output monitors renal function and level of hydration. Transfusions of crystalloids and (nonsickled) RBCs will increase the oxygen-carrying capacity of the blood and decrease the relative number of sickled cells.

4. Adequate understanding of SCD can increase adherence to preventive measures and prompt interventions during exacerbations and hospitalizations.

Evaluation

* Are the child's vital signs and oxygen saturation within normal limits?
* Does the child demonstrate palpable peripheral pulses, capillary refill less than 2 seconds, and warmth of extremities?

* Can the child and family demonstrate their ability to administer medication and describe possible side effects?
* Have the child and family requested additional information or clarification related to treatment?

NURSING DIAGNOSIS   Acute Pain related to vaso-occlusion.

EXPECTED OUTCOME   The child will:
  * Have decreased pain, as evidenced by a lowered score on the selected pain assessment tool.

Intervention

1. Monitor and record pain every 1 to 2 hours and more frequently if needed, using a pain assessment tool appropriate for the child's age.

2. Administer analgesics as ordered.

3. Increase oral fluids, if able to tolerate, or administer fluids IV at a rate that is 1 to 1½ times the maintenance rate.
4. Administer RBCs as ordered.

5. Incorporate the use of age-appropriate nonpharmacologic pain relief measures.
6. Perform passive range-of-motion exercises and avoid exertion.

Rationale

1. Pain can be severe in vaso-occlusive crisis and is relieved for only short periods. An assessment tool that measures the subjective experience of pain is helpful in determining the child's level of discomfort (see Chapter 15).
2. Analgesics may be administered intermittently, by a patient- or parent-controlled analgesic pump, or by continuous infusion through an IV line.
3. Increased fluid volume reduces the viscosity of the blood, thus alleviating sites of vascular occlusion and preventing further sickling caused by dehydration.
4. Maintaining an adequate hemoglobin level increases oxygen-carrying capacity to aid in further preventing sickling and microvascular ischemia.
5. Comfort measures often help distract the patient from discomfort (see Chapter 15).
6. Passive range-of-motion exercises promote circulation without exacerbating fatigue.

Evaluation

* Does the child verbalize or demonstrate decreased pain?

* Does review of the child's pain assessment tool rating show a decrease in discomfort?

NURSING DIAGNOSIS   Risk for Infection related to chronic immunocompromised state.

EXPECTED OUTCOMES   The child will:
  * Remain free from infection, as evidenced by normal vital signs and activity for age.
  The child and family will:
  * Verbalize signs and symptoms of infection and when to notify the medical team.

Continued

NURSING CARE PLAN—cont'd

Intervention	Rationale
1. Monitor vital signs every 4 hours and more frequently as needed. Report any temperature elevations to the physician.	1. Elevated temperature and increased respiratory rate may be signs of infection.
2. Administer antipyretics and antibiotics as ordered.	2. Antibiotics may be given prophylactically because of the high risk for infection. Prompt intervention is critical in children with HbSS and sickle beta-thalassemia during febrile illness.
3. Administer penicillin daily as ordered. Administer preventive immunizations to decrease the risk of infection (Pneumovax, meningococcal vaccine, *H. influenzae* type b, influenza vaccines).	3. Children are at a high risk for pneumococcal infections and should receive long-term penicillin therapy. The Pneumovax, meningococcal, and *H. influenzae* type b vaccines can prevent sepsis, and the influenza vaccine can prevent complications from influenza.
4. Teach the parents signs of infection to watch for and the proper way to obtain the child's temperature. Confirm that the parent has a thermometer.	4. Develop a teaching plan to address signs and symptoms of infection, including when to notify the physician. Do not assume that the parent has a thermometer or knows how to accurately obtain a temperature reading.

Evaluation

- Is the child's body temperature within normal limits?
- Can the child and family describe their plan to identify and respond to signs of infection?

NURSING DIAGNOSIS Ineffective Coping related to chronic illness.

EXPECTED OUTCOMES The child and family will:
- Adhere to the treatment plan and follow-up visits.
- Verbalize feelings about the impact of the illness on their lives.
- Use available support systems and community resources.

Intervention	Rationale
1. Teach the family the necessity of and rationale for following the treatment as outlined by the health care team (Box 23-2).	1. Conscientious adherence to the treatment regimen decreases the frequency of hospitalizations and improves the child's health and longevity.
2. Provide written instructions on all aspects of care and complications. Provide the address and phone number of the local chapter of the Sickle Cell Foundation (see Evolve website).	2. Education helps the family gain a sense of control by allowing them to make informed decisions regarding their child's health. Written instructions can be referred to later when the parent is less stressed and is able to comprehend.
3. Listen and encourage the child and family to verbalize their feelings and express their concerns regarding SCD. Answer questions honestly and openly. Encourage consultation with the social work team to provide additional support and referrals as necessary.	3. Identifying concerns and clarifying misconceptions will help the family cope with the stress of chronic illness.
4. Introduce the family to other families of children with SCD.	4. Families of other children with SCD can offer support, suggestions, and strategies for dealing with problems.
5. Provide parents with phone numbers of persons to contact if they have questions or problems. The Sickle Cell Foundation has information on the disease and on support groups in the area.	5. Knowing about resources decreases parents' feelings of frustration and helplessness.

Evaluation

- Are the child and family demonstrating adherence to the treatment plan?
- Do the child and family demonstrate positive coping mechanisms?
- Do the child and family use available resources?

- Is the family able to discuss problems related to caring for a child with a chronic disease?
- Does the child share fears and frustrations related to having SCD?

BOX 23-2 | **PARENTS WANT TO KNOW** About Home Care of the Child With Sickle Cell Disease

- Encourage fluid intake; increase fluid intake in hot weather or when there are other risks for dehydration.
- Expect frequent urination.
- Provide for adequate rest periods.
- Avoid cold, which can increase sickling, and extreme heat, which can cause dehydration.
- Avoid known sources of infection.
- Avoid prolonged exposure to the sun.
- Monitor the child's body temperature (know the proper use of a thermometer) and promptly notify the medical

- team in the event of a fever (avoid antipyretics until discussed with the medical team).
- Administer penicillin daily as ordered.
- Avoid use of aspirin; use acetaminophen or ibuprofen as an alternative.
- Be cautious when traveling with the child to avoid conditions or locations with decreased atmospheric oxygen.
- Call the primary caregiver if symptoms of infection are evident.
- Know the physician's telephone number.

USING RESEARCH TO IMPROVE PRACTICE

Children with SCD have exacerbations and remissions and are at risk for complications resulting from the disease. Frequently seen complications include severe pain, pneumonia and pulmonary infarction, dactylitis, and stroke (all related to vaso-occlusive crisis); infection and severe anemia (aplastic crisis); and hypovolemic shock (acute sequestration). Day (2004) constructed a numeric scoring system that would assist nurses who work with affected children to accurately and reliably assess the presence of factors that would both predict the level of risk for severe complications and classify the severity of disease manifestations. The focus and goal of this research was to construct and test for reliability, validity, and stability of the new scoring system. Justifying the necessity for such an instrument was an in-depth review of literature presenting evidence that early screening and recognition of risk factors could reduce morbidity and mortality from sickle cell disease. Although most states in the United States include SCD screening in their newborn screening panel, certain indicators can predict which children will need more complex and invasive treatments for the condition later in life.

Day's scoring system includes two domains: (1) identification of those at high risk, using carefully described

and defined critical attribute criteria for mean hemoglobin, mean leukocyte count, early dactylitis episodes, acute chest syndrome, and severe pain and (2) classification of disease severity criteria by using numbers of episodes of acute chest syndrome or severe pain. Each factor was given a numeric score between 1 and 2, with the total score for the high risk category being ≥ 1 (1 = high risk, 2 to 3 = very high risk), and the total score for the disease severity domain being ≥ 2 (severe disease). Through a carefully designed procedure, the scoring system was reviewed by experts for content validity, tested for interrater reliability, and pretested and posttested for stability. Experienced nurses and physicians participated in chart assessments and scoring. Although the sample of scores was small, the scoring system demonstrated acceptable content validity, reliability, and stability (Day, 2004).

Developing and testing a measuring instrument is a complex and challenging procedure for a researcher. Consider what might be the next steps to further establish reliability and the usefulness of this scoring system to help children at high risk for complications from SCD.

Day, S. (2004). Development and evaluation of a sickle cell assessment instrument. *Pediatric Nursing, 30,* 451-458.

BETA-THALASSEMIA

The thalassemias are a group of inherited disorders characterized by an abnormality in hemoglobin synthesis that results from a reduction in or absence of one of the chains found in normal hemoglobin. These disorders are categorized by the site of the aberrant globin synthesis (e.g., alpha-thalassemia, beta-thalassemia). The thalassemias are found primarily in people of Mediterranean descent, although the disease also has been reported in Asian and African populations. Beta-thalassemia, also known as *thalassemia major* or *Cooley's anemia,* is the most common and severe form of thalassemia.

Etiology and Incidence

Inheritance is through an autosomal recessive pattern. The child who inherits only one gene for beta-thalassemia may have only a mild anemia, hence the term *thalassemia minor.*

From 3% to 8% of Americans of Italian or Greek ancestry and 0.5% of African Americans carry a gene for beta-thalassemia (Quirolo & Vichinsky, 2004).

Manifestations

The clinical manifestations of beta-thalassemia include pallor, growth and maturation retardation, severe anemia, characteristic facies (enlarged head, frontal and parietal bossing, severe maxillary hyperplasia, malocclusion), hepatosplenomegaly, and a bronze skin tone (Box 23-3).

Diagnostic Evaluation

In addition to a CBC count, laboratory testing should include quantification of reticulocyte count, serum iron level, total iron-binding capacity, hemoglobin electrophoresis, and hemoglobin A and HbF levels to confirm the diagnosis. The

PATHOPHYSIOLOGY

BETA-THALASSEMIA

The abnormality of the beta-polypeptide chain in hemoglobin synthesis impairs the erythrocytes' ability to carry oxygen. Thalassemia is classified by the degree of imbalance in the globin chain and can be minor, intermediate, or severe.

Typically, during the second 6 months of life, a severe anemia develops. Erythrocytes are *hemolyzed* as they are produced. Because the body's natural response to a reduction in circulating hemoglobin is to try to produce more erythrocytes, the bone marrow begins massive production. Progressive disease constantly stimulates the bone marrow. The body perceives this as an inability to keep up with the need for erythrocytes. As a result, *extramedullary* (outside the bone marrow) sites of production of erythrocytes begin *erythropoiesis*. The result is a chronic state of production and destruction of erythrocytes, with a resulting inadequate amount of normal circulating hemoglobin.

Iron is necessary for the production of hemoglobin and it is a byproduct of the hemolysis of RBCs. Normally the intestines absorb small amounts of iron. In this disorder, however, the body increases the absorption of iron for some reason. When increased iron absorption is combined with increased iron from the breakdown of RBCs and the increased iron introduced into the circulation by the transfusions necessary to treat thalassemia, *hemosiderosis* occurs, usually during the second decade of life. Hemosiderosis is the deposition of excess amounts of iron in tissue.

The results of excessive erythropoiesis and hemolysis are considerable. The bones become thin and fragile from excessive erythropoiesis. Hepatosplenomegaly occurs as a result of extramedullary erythropoiesis and hemosiderosis. Growth is impaired and puberty delayed. Without proper management, multisystem organ dysfunction ensues.

BOX 23-3	Characteristic Features of a Child With Beta-Thalassemia

Features develop as a consequence of inadequate treatment:
- Frontal bossing (prominent and protruding forehead)
- Maxillary prominence
- Wide-set eyes with a flattened nose
- Hepatosplenomegaly
- Greenish yellow skin tone

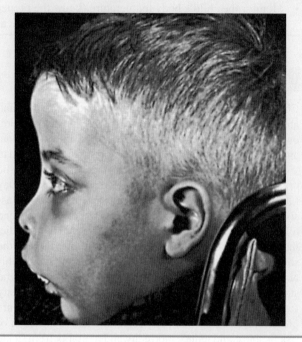

CBC count will often reflect microcytic hypochromic erythrocytes. A detailed family history may also reveal a history of anemia and delayed growth and maturation.

Therapeutic Management

The management of beta-thalassemia centers on three techniques: (1) erythrocyte transfusions, (2) chelation therapy, and (3) splenectomy. The use of neocyte transfusions is also being investigated. In neocyte transfusions, units of blood that contain young erythrocytes—neocytes—are preferentially separated and transfused. Theoretically, administration of neocytes provides erythrocytes with a longer life and increases the time between transfusions while decreasing the overall amount of transfusion. To prevent the severe side effects and bony changes associated with the disease, the hemoglobin is maintained at approximately 11 g/dL, although this parameter is often individualized.

The major complication of long-term transfusion therapy is hemosiderosis. To prevent organ damage from excessive iron overload, chelation therapy with deferoxamine (Desferal) is instituted. It is most effective when given subcutaneously or IV. To avoid hospitalizing children who require deferoxamine therapy, the drug is often administered in the home by continuous subcutaneous infusion (by pump) over an 8- to 12-hour period at night. This approach can preserve some degree of normalcy in lifestyle for the family. Therapy is continued until the iron returns to an acceptable level. This goal can be accomplished within months of initiating chelation therapy. Research continues in developing and improving the efficacy of oral iron chelation agents as well (Kwiatkowski & Cohen, 2004).

Splenectomy may be required as a result of sporadic or moderate transfusion therapy, whereas aggressive transfusion therapy may delay the need for splenectomy. Splenectomy is a therapy that should not be considered casually because susceptibility to infection with *S. pneumoniae, H. influenzae,* and *Neisseria meningitidis* increases after splenectomy in children, particularly in those younger than 5 years. Standard therapy for asplenic individuals includes immunizations, prophylactic penicillin, and a high index of suspicion and aggressive antibiotic therapy for febrile illnesses (AAP, 2003a). These children should also receive the influenza vaccine annually (AAP, 2003a). When splenectomy is performed, the transfusion requirements often drop moderately to significantly.

Bone marrow transplantation is the only available cure for thalassemia at this time. More than 1,000 successful transplants have been performed. Only a small percentage of patients (estimated at 30%) who have a matched donor and low risk factors, however, can undergo this procedure (Lanzkowsky, 2005).

NURSING CARE
The Child With Beta-Thalassemia

Assessment
Subjective data may include the parents' observation that their child is not as active as other children of the same age. The child may sleep more than other children or want to be held often. The child appears pale, with laboratory values reflecting a microcytic, hypochromic anemia. Clinical symptoms are related to the degree of anemia, ranging from mild to severe.

An older child with the disease or a child who has not received adequate treatment will likely have characteristic facial deformities, including maxillary hyperplasia and malocclusion. These characteristics develop from extramedullary marrow expansion, a consequence of the marrow's effort to keep up with the demand for RBCs as a result of anemia. Hepatosplenomegaly is usually seen at this time but is not a symptom in infancy.

Nursing Diagnosis and Planning
The nursing diagnoses and expected outcomes that may be appropriate after assessment of the child with beta-thalassemia are as follows:
- Ineffective Tissue Perfusion related to anemia.

  Expected Outcome: The child demonstrates adequate tissue perfusion, as evidenced by palpable peripheral pulses; warm, dry skin; urinary output appropriate for age; and the absence of cardiorespiratory distress (oxygen saturation >95%).
- Disturbed Body Image related to altered appearance and the perception of having a chronic disease.

  Expected Outcome: The child and family will verbalize feelings related to changes in appearance and the limitations imposed by the disease process.
- Anxiety related to the diagnosis.

  Expected Outcome: The child and family will express feelings about the disorder, lifestyle disruptions as a result of treatment, and possible genetic transmission of the disease.
- Deficient Knowledge related to inadequate information about the disorder.

  Expected Outcome: The child and family will describe the disorder and its treatment regimen, including medications and their actions and possible side effects.

Interventions
Expect transfusions to begin immediately for an affected child while cardiovascular compromise from the anemia is being assessed. Preparing the child and family for diagnostic procedures will help alleviate fears. Once the diagnosis is made, education should begin. Parents need to understand the importance of proper and continuing follow-up. The family needs much support as they begin chelation therapy (Box 23-4), which is very time consuming and interferes with family routines. Routinely monitor the family's adherence to therapy. If hematopoietic stem cell transplantation becomes an option, the parents will need referral to a specialty center and will need support from the entire health care team as they contemplate the course of therapy.

If parents are considering having another child, they should be offered genetic counseling. When both parents carry the defective gene, each pregnancy carries a 1 in 4 chance of producing another child with the disease. Genetic counseling should also be made available to the affected child on reaching maturity. If the affected individual conceives a child with someone who is a carrier of the thalassemia gene,

---

BOX 23-4	**PARENTS WANT TO KNOW** About Home Chelation Therapy

Subcutaneous Route By Infusion Pump
- Know the technique for placing the subcutaneous needle, medication preparation, and infusion pump operation.
- Check needle security and placement.
- Check pump for proper infusion rate.
- Call the home care, clinic, or physician resource if the site becomes inflamed, red, or painful.
- Know indications for medication and side effects that require health care team notification: hearing loss or ringing in the ears, fever, fever with diarrhea, visual disturbances, allergic reactions, respiratory compromise.

Intravenous Route: Totally Implantable or Tunneled Access Device
- Know the technique for placing access needle or catheter connection, medication preparation, and infusion pump operation.
- Call the home care, clinic, or physician resource if the site becomes inflamed, red, or painful or the specific access device is obstructed.
- Have a list of home care resources for technique assistance, supplies, and problematic pump functioning.
- Know indications for medication and side effects that require health care team notification: hearing loss or ringing in the ears, fever, fever with diarrhea, visual disturbances, allergic reactions, respiratory compromise.

with each pregnancy there is a 2 in 4 chance of producing a child with beta-thalassemia. Techniques for prenatal diagnosis are available and effective (Bain, 2001). Referral should be made to the Cooley's Anemia Foundation (see Evolve website).

Evaluation

- Are the child's peripheral pulses palpable and oxygen saturation increased to 95%?
- Is the child's hemoglobin level improving?
- Is the child able to verbalize feelings associated with the treatment or the psychosocial implications of the disease?
- Is the child sharing feelings related to changes in appearance, limitations imposed by the disease, and having a chronic disease?
- Has the family sought genetic counseling?
- Does the family readily verbalize feelings about having a child with beta-thalassemia?
- Has the family sought information and support from the Cooley's Anemia Foundation?

HEMOPHILIA

Hemophilia is a life-long hereditary blood disorder with no cure. Until 1952, hemophilia was associated solely with the deficiency of coagulation factor VIII. Since that time, the absence of two additional coagulation factors, factors IX and XI, has been associated with a constellation of symptoms similar to factor VIII deficiency. Congenital deficiencies in these three factors account for approximately 90% to 95% of the bleeding disorders referred to as *hemophilia*.

Etiology and Incidence

Hemophilia is an X-linked autosomal recessive disorder; carrier females pass on the defect to affected males. Women who never produce an affected male child may silently carry the gene for generations, but typically there is a history of hemophilia in the family. Rarely, female offspring are born with the disorder but only if they inherit an affected gene from the mother and are the offspring of a father with hemophilia. The prevalence of factor VIII deficiency is 1 in 5,000 males; factor IX deficiency prevalence is 1 in 35,000 males (National Hemophilia Foundation, 2006).

Manifestations

The disease severity is individual but tends to be familial. Bleeding occurs after surgery or serious trauma in all children with this disease. Bleeding occurs after tissue trauma in children with moderate and severe disease. Bleeding occurs for no apparent reason in children with severe disease. Affected children bruise easily, have episodes of epistaxis, and may have hematuria. They may also have bleeding with loss of deciduous teeth, from even minor lacerations, and from injections. Most commonly, bleeding develops in the muscles and joints, especially the knees, for moderate and severe disease (Fig. 23-1). Recurrent bleeding commonly occurs in the same joint in severely affected children. Swelling, pain, bleeding, and stiffness (hemarthrosis) occur.

Diagnostic Evaluation

Hemophilia is sometimes but not always diagnosed after circumcision, at which time prolonged bleeding may be observed. Because the most common sites of bleeding are in the muscles and joints, the diagnosis may be delayed until the toddler years, when the child becomes more active and the disease has an opportunity to manifest itself. By the preschool years, most affected children have had an episode of persistent bleeding from a minor traumatic laceration.

A diagnostic workup for the child with suspected hemophilia includes determining the prothrombin time (PT), partial thromboplastin time, bleeding time, fibrinogen level, and platelet count; quantitative immunoelectrophoretic assay; and factor VIII and factor IX assays.

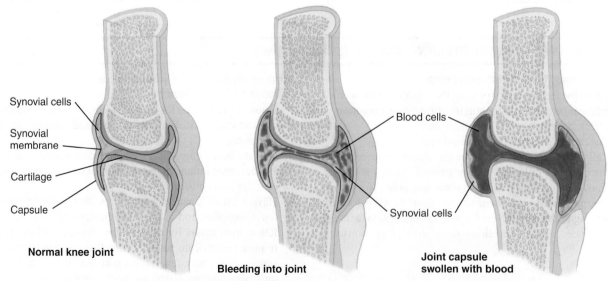

FIG 23-1   Hemarthrosis and joint destruction are characteristic of hemophilia.

PATHOPHYSIOLOGY

HEMOPHILIA

More than 10 factors in the blood work in sequence to produce blood clotting. Factor VIII, or antihemophilic factor, and factor IX, or plasma thromboplastin component, are the two missing or defective constituents in the blood that cause hemophilia A, or classic hemophilia, and hemophilia B, or Christmas disease. When these factors are missing or defective, blood does not clot as it should. The two disorders are inherited in the same way and have similar manifestations. Normal factor activity is described as a percentage. The percentage of factor activity is closely related to the level of factor in the blood (e.g., 100 units/dL factor equals 100% factor activity). Normal levels of factor VIII and IX are 50% to 150%. The severity of the disease is classified as follows:

- *Severe:* less than 1% factor activity
- *Moderate:* 1% to 5% factor activity
- *Mild:* 6% to 50% factor activity

Therapeutic Management

The management of hemophilia is very individual and depends on the severity of the illness. Therapy aims to prevent excessive bleeding and tissue damage by supplying the body with the missing or ineffective factors (VIII or IX).

Previously, treatment involved transfusions of blood products or administration of freeze-dried products manufactured from blood products. One of the major risks associated with this factor replacement therapy was contracting hepatitis or human immunodeficiency virus infection. Because of this risk, manufacturers began to heat-treat the blood factor to reduce the risk of viral transmission. Monoclonal products were then developed that were found to be even safer than the heat-treated products. The most recent development in the treatment of hemophilia is the availability of recombinant antihemophilic factor, which is not derived from human plasma but is produced synthetically from isolation of the gene. Recombinant factor eliminates the risk of virus transmission. The freeze-dried product is supplied with sterile water and must be reconstituted before being given IV.

Prophylactic therapy is now being started in infants and young children with severe hemophilia to prevent joint problems. Children age 1 to 2 years receive factor replacement on a regular schedule if clinical symptoms develop. Children with mild hemophilia A may be able to use desmopressin acetate (1-deamino-8-D-arginine vasopressin [DDAVP]) intranasal spray, because of its vasoconstrictor action, to stop bleeding. Children with hemophilias A and B can be given aminocaproic acid (Amicar) or tranexamic acid (Cyclokapron)—oral medications that stabilize oral clots and can also sometimes stop nosebleeds.

Aside from administration of factor, children with hemophilia must try to avoid activities that induce bleeding. For mild hemophilia, special precautions can be taken to protect joints, thereby allowing the child to lead a more normal life. Prophylactic replacement therapy should also be given before surgery and some dental procedures. Bleeding is treated with rest, ice, elevation of the affected part, and compression (also referred to as *RICE*: *r*est, *i*ce, *c*ompression, *e*levation).

CRITICAL TO REMEMBER
Acetylsalicylic Acid: Contraindication

Acetylsalicylic acid (e.g., aspirin, aspirin-containing products) should not be given to children with factor disorders because it inhibits platelet function. Because some over-the-counter medications may contain acetylsalicylic acid, it is important to read all labels carefully before giving the child the medication.

CRITICAL TO REMEMBER
Interviewing a Child With Hemophilia

Subjective data gathered for a child known to have hemophilia should include information about recent trauma and initial measures to stop bleeding. An important question is the length of time that pressure had to be applied before the bleeding subsided. Other questions to ask include whether the swelling increased after the surface bleeding stopped and whether swelling and stiffness occurred without apparent trauma.

Text continued on p. 738

NURSING CARE PLAN

The Child With Hemophilia

Focused Assessment

In a male neonate, observe the circumcision site or injection sites for prolonged bleeding. Notify the physician if prolonged bleeding is observed.

Be alert to the possibility of hemophilia when the parents of a child just learning to crawl or walk express concern that their child bruises easily on tumbling or falling down. Questions should be asked about previous cuts and scrapes to determine whether the child seemed to need more than the usual amount of pressure application or time for the bleeding to subside. The family should also be asked whether there is a family history of bleeding disorders.

Continued

NURSING CARE PLAN—cont'd

NURSING DIAGNOSIS Risk for Injury related to prolonged bleeding.

EXPECTED OUTCOME The child and family will:
- Recognize bleeding resulting from injury and promptly control it to prevent permanent tissue damage.

Intervention	*Rationale*
1. Monitor the area of injury frequently for bleeding over a 24-hour period.	1. Bleeding may be prolonged and, especially in the case of head trauma, may not manifest immediately.
2. Measure the injured joint.	2. Joint measurement provides objective rather than subjective data for future comparisons.
3. In the case of head trauma, assess the child's level of consciousness and note any behavioral changes.	3. Decreased level of consciousness and unusual behaviors are early indicators of increased intracranial pressure resulting from hemorrhage.
4. Apply gentle pressure for 10 to 15 minutes to small superficial wounds and assess the area for subcutaneous bleeding.	4. Small wounds may ooze blood into the subcutaneous tissue. Pressure facilitates clot formation.
5. Administer factor replacement as ordered.	5. Factor must be reconstituted just before infusion. It may be given as a prophylactic measure even if no bleeding is apparent.
6. Monitor factor levels as ordered.	6. With serious injuries warranting hospitalization, factor levels aid in prescribing dosages and in establishing thresholds for an individual child.
7. If a muscle or joint injury occurs, immobilize, elevate, and apply ice to the affected part, as ordered by the physician.	7. Initial immobilization will help prevent further injury until the bleeding resolves.
8. Offer suggestions for establishing a safe home environment for the child (Box 23-5).	8. A safe home environment will help prevent injuries.
9. Avoid rectal temperature measurement.	9. Rectal temperatures may cause bleeding from tissue trauma.
10. Provide for and expect behaviors consistent with normal growth and development for the child's age.	10. Parents may tend to overprotect or provide special treatment for their child. This unnecessarily limits the child's opportunities for normal psychosocial development and decreases self-esteem.

Evaluation

- Has the child had serious bleeding from injury?
- Has the child adhered to the treatment regimen to control injuries?

- Are there long-term complications from injury?

NURSING DIAGNOSIS Deficient Knowledge related to the need for information about disease diagnosis and treatment.

EXPECTED OUTCOMES The child and family will:
- Explain the diagnosis.
- Demonstrate adherence to the home care regimen.

Intervention	*Rationale*
1. Determine the child's and family's readiness for learning. Create an environment conducive to learning.	1. The family may need time to adjust to the initial diagnosis before they are ready to be educated. The appropriate setting for an educational session may be away from the child so that parents will be able to focus on the information.
2. On initial diagnosis and with subsequent follow-up visits, spend time with the family explaining the diagnosis, sequelae, and treatment. Offer written literature and educational tapes.	2. Education is continuing and will need to be reinforced with stressed parents. Explaining the rationale for treatment and the disease's sequelae will help ensure adherence to therapy.

NURSING CARE PLAN—cont'd

3. Offer encouragement and praise for prompt parental recognition and response to bleeding.
4. Teach techniques for reconstitution and infusion of factor at home. The instruction technique may be for peripheral infusion or infusion through a central venous access line, depending on the child's individual situation (see Box 23-5).
5. Consider using a topical anesthetic, such as eutectic mixture of local anesthetics, when accessing infusion ports or peripheral sites.

3. Written or taped information can be reviewed later, when comprehension is likely to be improved.
4. Praise will reinforce behavior. Parents want to know they are doing the right things for their child.

5. Parents are taught techniques for accessing the port, infusing the factor, and heparinizing the port. The use of topical anesthetics decreases pain, thus causing less trauma and anxiety.

Evaluation

- Are the child and family able to safely administer factor replacement at home?

- Do the child and family promptly recognize and react to bleeding?

NURSING DIAGNOSIS   Ineffective Coping related to chronic illness and guilt.

EXPECTED OUTCOMES   The child and family will:
- Adhere to the treatment plan, as evidenced by safety alterations being made in the home and community.
- Use available support systems and community resources.

Family members will:
- Verbalize concerns about the impact of the illness on the family.

Intervention

1. Teach the family the need for safety precautions, reacting cautiously to injury, administering medications properly, and following the treatment plan as outlined by health care providers (see Box 23-5).
2. Listen to and encourage the child and family to verbalize their feelings and express their concerns regarding hemophilia. Answer questions honestly and openly. Be particularly aware of feelings of guilt expressed by the mother.
3. Introduce the family to other families of children with hemophilia.
4. Provide referral to the National Hemophilia Foundation (see Evolve website).

5. Explore with the child feelings related to participation in some sports and other restrictions related to having hemophilia.

Rationale

1. Conscientious adherence to the treatment regimen decreases the potential for long-term complications.

2. Identifying concerns and clarifying misconceptions help families cope with the stress of chronic illness.

3. Other families of children with hemophilia can offer support, suggestions, and strategies for coping.
4. Access to information and assistance can help the family deal with the sometimes overwhelming financial and emotional burdens of caring for a child with hemophilia, especially if complications occur.
5. Discussing feelings related to a chronic disease provides an opportunity for the child to explore options and for the nurse to assess the child's needs and coping strategies.

Evaluation

- Does the older child avoid contact sports and participate in other activities, such as swimming?
- Has the family contacted the National Hemophilia Foundation?

- Is the child able to balance increased limitations and normal childhood?

| BOX 23-5 | **PARENTS WANT TO KNOW**   About Home Care of the Child With Hemophilia |

- Apply gentle, prolonged pressure to superficial wounds until the bleeding has stopped.
- Call the physician in the event of blunt trauma, especially trauma involving the joints.
- Establish an age-appropriate, safe environment:
  — Pad table corners.
  — Pad crib rails.
  — Provide extra joint padding on clothes.
  — Remove items that can tip over or be pulled down on the child.
  — Do not leave a crawling or toddling child unattended.
  — Use a toothbrush with soft bristles and a WaterPik for dental care.
- Instruct older children to avoid contact sports and to take precautions with other sports:
  — Pad the knees and elbows for physical education class.
  — Use protective helmets for any sport in which head injury could occur (e.g., bicycling, skating).
  — Use an electric razor for shaving.
- Call the physician if any head injury occurs.
- Reconstitute and administer factor through an IV line or the child's central venous access device.
- If a child has an implantable infusion device, caregivers should understand the following:
  — Site preparation.
  — Sterile technique for insertion of access needle.
  — Technique for verification of needle placement.

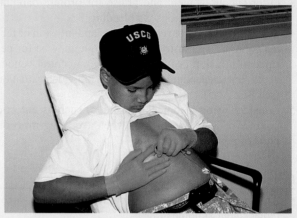

Control of deficient blood clotting in hemophilia requires injection of the missing clotting factors. This young man is injecting his factor into an implanted central venous access port. Sterile technique is essential.   *(Courtesy family of Jason Lee Davis.)*

  — Administration of factor by IV push.
  — Saline solution and heparin flush.
  — Removal and proper disposal of needle.
- Keep current with the schedule of immunizations, dental hygiene, and routine well-child care.
- Allow your child to set personal safety limits when possible.
- Provide for normal growth and development opportunities (safe activities, time with other children, limit setting, independence).

VON WILLEBRAND'S DISEASE

Von Willebrand's disease (VWD) is the most commonly inherited bleeding disorder (Cox, 2004). At least 20 subtypes of VWD have been identified (e.g., type 1, type IIA, type IIB). The most frequent subtype is type I; the other subtypes are rare.

Etiology

VWD is an autosomal dominant inherited disorder. It occurs in approximately 1% to 2% of the population and affects both males and females (National Hemophilia Foundation, 2006).

Pathophysiology

Children with VWD have either underproduction or dysfunction of von Willebrand's protein. The VWD protein occurs together with factor VIII in the circulation, making it a carrier protein for factor VIII. One of its most important functions is to bind and attract platelets to the site of endothelial tissue injury, thus facilitating the formation of a clot. Deficiency of von Willebrand's protein may result in a corresponding deficiency of factor VIII.

Manifestations

Clinical features and the need for treatment depend on the severity of the disorder. The clinical manifestations of VWD include a history of epistaxis, bleeding from the gums, prolonged bleeding from cuts, excessive bleeding after surgery or trauma, and menorrhagia (excessive menstrual bleeding) in females.

Diagnostic Evaluation

A thorough history will ascertain whether the episode of bruising is proportional to the degree of trauma. A family history of bleeding disorders is important.

Laboratory tests may include a bleeding time and a partial thromboplastin time, the results of which may be normal. The most clinically useful laboratory test for diagnosing this disorder is the quantitative immunoelectrophoretic assay, which, in the presence of the disease, will reveal a discrepancy in the quantity and function of von Willebrand's factor in the plasma.

Therapeutic Management

Therapy is aimed at replacing the missing or dysfunctional factor in the blood. In the past, cryoprecipitate or fresh-frozen plasma was given before surgery or after trauma with excessive bleeding. Currently, this treatment is recommended only if the cryoprecipitate is donated from a well-screened, unaffected family member or a repeat individual donor and the child is not responding to DDAVP.

The treatment of choice is DDAVP, which is administered IV or intranasally. The DDAVP products are given for type I and type IIA VWD only (Cox, 2004). High-purity (not monoclonal or recombinant) factor VIII products that are specifically known to contain von Willebrand's factor can be used to treat type IIB disease. (Only a minority of currently available factor VIII concentrates actually contain von Willebrand's factor.)

NURSING CARE

The Child With von Willebrand's Disease

Assessment

A careful history detailing episodes of bruising and bleeding is essential. Possible causes of any previous episodes of bleeding, if any can be identified, should also be discussed. Ask how many times the child has had a nosebleed, how long the child bleeds from "normal" trauma, and whether there is a history of prolonged bleeding associated with surgery or trauma.

Physical examination usually reveals a healthy child except for evidence of bruising greater than expected for the degree of trauma. If the child is being seen after a major bleeding episode, signs of hemorrhage or a decreased hemoglobin level (or both) will be seen.

Nursing Diagnosis and Planning

The nursing diagnoses and expected outcomes that may be appropriate after assessment of the child with von Willebrand's disease include:

- Ineffective Protection related to abnormal clotting.
  Expected Outcome: The child will remain free of life-threatening episodes of hemorrhage.
- Deficient Knowledge related to the disorder.
  Expected Outcome: The child and family will explain the disorder, its management, and its chronic nature.

Interventions

Education of the family is aimed at producing an understanding of the precautions to take with the child and knowledge of when prophylactic therapy should be given before elective procedures. The child should wear a medical alert tag at all times. The family should be referred to the Hemophilia Foundation for support services (see Evolve website). Avoidance of prescription and over-the-counter medications that affect platelet function, such as aspirin or NSAIDs, is also recommended. The nurse should advise the parent to check the labels of all over-the-counter medications for presence of aspirin or NSAIDs.

The degree of activity limitation will depend on the severity of the disorder. Limitations may include avoidance of contact sports, especially football.

Evaluation

- Are episodes of bleeding minimal and controlled?
- Does the family communicate an understanding of the importance of avoiding medications that affect platelet function and avoiding activities that increase the risk of bleeding?
- Does the family seek appropriate resources for information about the condition and its management?

IMMUNE THROMBOCYTOPENIC PURPURA

Immune thrombocytopenic purpura (ITP) is an acquired hemorrhagic disorder characterized by thrombocytopenia (platelet count <150,000/mm³), a purpuric rash, normal bone marrow, and the absence of signs of other identifiable causes of thrombocytopenia. It is classified as acute or chronic, with chronic being defined as the persistence of thrombocytopenia for more than 6 months.

Etiology and Incidence

ITP is estimated to be one of the most common acquired bleeding disorders in children. The incidence of symptomatic disease is approximately 3 to 8 per 100,000 children per year. Acute ITP is more prevalent among children younger than 10 years, affects males and females equally, and is more prevalent during the late winter and spring. Chronic ITP affects adolescents more than younger children, with females being affected more frequently than males (Bussel, & Cines, 2005). The etiology of ITP is unknown, although in the majority of children it follows a viral illness and is considered to be an autoimmune process.

Pathophysiology

In general, ITP is thought to occur as a result of the destruction of platelets by autoantibodies to glycoproteins normally expressed on platelet membranes. The spleen and other organs of the reticuloendothelial system subsequently destroy these antibody-coated platelets (Bussel & Cines, 2005).

Manifestations

Clinical manifestations of ITP include the sudden onset of bruising and petechiae, with bleeding involving the mucous membranes and gums, in a child who is in otherwise good health (Fig. 23-2).

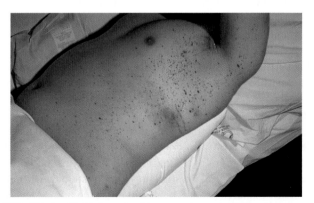

FIG 23-2 **Multiple petechiae are characteristic of immune thrombocytopenic purpura. This disorder results in the destruction of circulating platelets and decreased bone marrow production of new platelets.** *(Courtesy Cook Children's Medical Center, Fort Worth, TX.)*

Diagnostic Evaluation

The initial diagnostic evaluation should include a thorough history and a CBC count, including evaluation of a peripheral blood smear. The history should include information about any medications the child has taken that could cause thrombocytopenia, history of recent live virus vaccination, and any instances of illness, especially febrile illness, in the past month. In an affected child, the initial CBC count will reveal a low platelet count, often below 50,000/mm^3, but the results will otherwise be normal. The physical examination findings will be normal, aside from the signs of bleeding.

If any data in the history or CBC count are suggestive of a diagnosis other than ITP, the physician may obtain a bone marrow aspirate to rule out an oncologic disorder and to determine whether megakaryocytes, the precursors of platelets, are present. Routine bone marrow examination is not warranted in a child with findings consistent with acute ITP.

Physical examination of the affected child reveals bruising and petechiae, the severity of which depends on how low the platelet count is and the child's tolerance of the low platelet count. The spleen and liver are generally normal in size. The greatest risk of a low platelet count is intracranial hemorrhage, so a neurologic assessment is important.

Therapeutic Management

The goal of treatment is to prevent rare, life-threatening bleeding events, such as intracranial bleeding. Additional goals include restoration of the platelet count to above 20,000/mm^3 in children with mucocutaneous bleeding and a reduction in the duration of thrombocytopenia. Treatment is based on the child's presenting condition.

Treatment options have been an intense topic of discussion for years and have divided pediatric hematologists between what have been called *interventionists* and *noninterventionist* (Bussel & Cines, 2005). Because most cases of ITP are self-limiting, with a normal platelet count returning within 6 months, the noninterventionists recommend no therapy but frequent monitoring of platelet counts and bleeding status (Bussel & Cines, 2005).

Depending on whether the child is an inpatient or outpatient, IV or oral steroids may be administered over a 2- to 4-week period. For unknown reasons, the steroids block the autoimmune destruction of platelets. The other drug that may be used to treat ITP is IVIG, administered once daily for 1 to 2 days. Often, the platelet count is dramatically increased after one dose of IVIG. In children with Rh-positive blood types (A+, B+, and O+), IV anti-D immunoglobulin may be used.

ITP is considered to be acute if recovery of a normal platelet count is seen within 6 months. The condition becomes chronic if recovery takes longer than 6 months. Children with chronic ITP may initially respond to steroids with an increase in platelet count, but it will not reach normal levels. These children may go for long periods without problems with excessive bleeding or a low platelet count; the count will then begin to decline again, at which time steroid therapy should be resumed.

When steroids and IVIG do not control the thrombocytopenia in a child with chronic ITP, a splenectomy may be indicated. Splenectomy will cure most children with chronic ITP because the spleen synthesizes the antiplatelet antibody that results in the destruction of circulating platelets. The risk associated with removal of the spleen is sepsis from those organisms that the spleen's reticuloendothelial system fights as described previously, so ITP is managed without splenectomy, if possible, until age 5 years. Platelet transfusions are given in children only when active, uncontrolled bleeding occurs.

NURSING CARE

The Child With Immune Thrombocytopenic Purpura

Assessment

Parents usually bring their child to the physician because they have noticed excessive bruising or a "red rash" in the child's mouth or on the child's body. Although this "rash" may look remarkable to a nurse, it often evolves so gradually that it escapes the immediate notice of a parent who sees the child every day. As a result, health care may not be sought until very significant bruising and petechiae, even hematomas, are present.

Affected children usually demonstrate normal activity levels for their age because they do not "feel bad." Assessment should include observation for signs of any further bruising or bleeding, including epistaxis, hematuria, or blood in the stools, as well as for signs of a decreasing level of consciousness, which could indicate intracranial hemorrhage.

Nursing Diagnosis and Planning

The nursing diagnoses and expected outcomes that may be appropriate after assessment of the child with ITP are as follows:

- Ineffective Protection related to low platelet count.

  Expected Outcome: The child will exhibit no signs of active bleeding or intracranial hemorrhage, as evidenced by pulse and blood pressure within normal limits and an alert and responsive child.

- Risk for Infection related to chronic use of steroids or splenectomy.

  Expected Outcomes: The family will identify signs of infection and notify the health care team, and the child will respond rapidly to treatment for infection.

- Deficient Knowledge related to insufficient information about the disorder and its therapeutic management.

  Expected Outcome: The child and family will describe ITP and the treatment plan.

Interventions

The family is referred to a health care center to carry out medical treatments, and the family is educated about ITP and home care (Box 23-6).

BOX 23-6 | **PARENTS WANT TO KNOW** About Home Care of the Child With Immune Thrombocytopenic Purpura

- Eliminate participation in high-risk activities, such as contact sports, bicycle riding, roller-skating, and diving, if the child's platelet count is low.
- Avoid medications that can affect platelet function (ibuprofen, aspirin). Be sure to read over-the-counter medication labels to check for these medications, which can be included in combination products, such as cold, flu, and upset stomach remedies.
- Use an extra-soft toothbrush if the platelet count is less than 20,000/mm^3.

- Establish an age-appropriate, safe home environment.
- Pad table corners.
- Pad crib rails.
- Offer extra joint padding on clothes.
- For additional resources and information, contact national organizations (e.g., the ITP Society; see Appendix I on Evolve website).

An IV access line may be established for the purpose of administering IV steroids or IVIG. It can be quite challenging to establish IV access in children with ITP because merely puncturing the skin may result in a hematoma, which may be confused with "blowing" the vein. Careful evaluation of blood return and flushing of the IV catheter with normal saline solution will confirm proper placement of the catheter.

Restricting the activity of toddlers and young children can be a challenge. Extra-soft-bristle toothbrushes or toothettes should be used for mouth care on all children whose platelet count is less than 20,000/mm^3. Until the platelet count returns to normal, activities such as bicycle riding, contact sports, and roller skating should be curtailed.

Education includes teaching the family about the disease process of ITP; the side effects of steroids and IVIG, if used; the need to restrict the child's activity; and the importance of proper follow-up evaluations. Parents should be instructed regarding the signs and symptoms of infection and actions in the event of signs of fever because steroids may mask an infection.

Ensure that parents and the child's primary care physician are informed if the child receives IVIG. The AAP recommends delaying the administration of routine measles immunization for a minimum of 10 months to children who have received immune globulin preparations because these preparations may block the replication of live-virus vaccine immune response (AAP, 2003a).

If the child has had a splenectomy, pneumococcal vaccine or daily penicillin (or both) should be administered. Any signs and symptoms of infection should be reported immediately to the physician so that proper therapy can be initiated before the infection becomes life threatening.

Evaluation

- Are the child's vital signs within normal limits?
- Is the child responding in an age-appropriate manner?
- Have areas of ecchymosis and petechiae decreased?
- Does the family verbalize and implement a plan of care that decreases the risk of the child incurring an injury that is likely to cause hemorrhage?
- Does the family respond quickly to early signs of infection by notifying the primary health care provider?

CRITICAL TO REMEMBER

Actions to Avoid in Children With Low Platelet Counts

- Avoid administering intramuscular injections, aspirin, aspirin-containing products, and nonsteroidal anti-inflammatory medications (e.g., ibuprofen) to children with low platelet counts.
- Avoid taking temperatures rectally, and perform invasive procedures with extreme caution.

DISSEMINATED INTRAVASCULAR COAGULATION

Disseminated intravascular coagulation (DIC) is an acquired hemorrhagic syndrome characterized by uncontrolled formation and deposition of fibrin thrombi and by the resulting consumption of clotting factors leading to uncontrolled bleeding. In children, DIC does not have the overwhelming mortality rate that occurs in adults. The keys to recovery are identification and treatment of the underlying cause of the DIC.

Etiology

DIC is triggered by any factor that causes endothelial damage, liberation of tissue thromboplastin, circulating endotoxins, or immune complexes. In children, the most common causes are trauma, hypoxia, necrotizing enterocolitis, shock, liver disease, overwhelming viral or bacterial infections, and acute promyelocytic leukemia.

Manifestations

Manifestations of DIC involve an insidious onset, corresponding to platelet count and fibrinogen levels. Early indicators include excessive bruising and petechiae, oozing from puncture sites, oozing from sites of mild tissue trauma (e.g., site of insertion of a nasogastric tube), and mild gastrointestinal bleeding. As the disease progresses, manifestations of DIC include purpuric rash, worsening of bleeding, hemoptysis, hypoxemia, oliguria progressing to renal failure, progressive organ failure, and intracranial hemorrhage.

PATHOPHYSIOLOGY

DISSEMINATED INTRAVASCULAR COAGULATION

DIC is a consumptive disorder caused by abnormal activation of the clotting mechanism, which causes rapid depletion of platelets, prothrombin, and fibrinogen. It is a pathologic syndrome resulting from the formation of thrombin, subsequent activation and consumption of certain coagulant proteins, and the production of fibrin thrombi. DIC manifests with diffuse microvascular coagulation caused by depletion of clotting factors, resulting in impaired hemostasis.

The pathophysiology of DIC is complicated and often not easily understood because both excessive bleeding and excessive clotting are occurring at the same time. The syndrome of DIC leads to deposition of platelet and fibrin plugs in the vasculature and the simultaneous depletion of platelets and clotting factor proteins.

The process of blood coagulation follows either an intrinsic or an extrinsic pathway.* Both pathways ultimately lead to the common pathway of prothrombin forming thrombin, which, in the presence of fibrinogen, forms fibrin. Alternately, fibrinolysis (clot destruction) requires the presence of thrombin. During this process, the enzyme *plasmin* lyses fibrin into fragments called *fibrin degradation products,* which interfere with the ability of platelets to adhere to one another. In DIC, initiation of the clotting process is stimulated by endothelial damage or some form of tissue injury. Platelets and clotting factors are subsequently depleted. As clotting is stimulated, the body perceives the need to produce substances to dissolve those clots and there is an increase in the end result of clot lysis, fibrin degradation products. The overstimulation of both these normal processes has four major effects on the body:

- Increased, uncontrolled bleeding resulting from the depletion of platelets and clotting factors and overstimulation of the fibrinolytic process
- Anemia caused by the excessive bleeding and the mechanical fragmentation of RBCs
- Organ damage resulting from the formation of emboli
- Tissue hypoxia leading to tissue necrosis

*Guyton, A. C., & Hall, J. E. (2000). *Textbook of medical physiology* (10th ed.). Philadelphia: WB Saunders.

Diagnostic Evaluation

The diagnosis of DIC is confirmed by laboratory testing (Box 23-7).

Therapeutic Management

To control DIC, the clinician must identify and then treat the underlying cause of the condition. Treatment then becomes symptomatic and directed at replenishing consumed coagulation factors. Depleted fibrinogen and other coagulation factors are replaced (e.g., cryoprecipitate, fresh frozen plasma) to normalize the PT. RBCs and platelet transfusions can aid in replacing cells lost in hemorrhage. Exchange transfusions may

---

BOX 23-7	Confirmatory Laboratory Findings in Disseminated Intravascular Coagulation

- Decreased RBC count
- Low platelet count noted on CBC count
- RBC fragments on the smear
- Prolonged PT
- Decreased fibrinogen level
- Elevated levels of fibrin degradation products (e.g., D-dimer)

---

be used in neonates to minimize the excessive fluid volume required by replacing platelets, clotting factors, and RBCs. Vitamin K may also be administered to normalize the PT. The most familiar drug used to dissolve clots is heparin. However, heparin has a controversial role in the treatment of childhood DIC because it may increase the risk for bleeding.

Nursing Considerations

DIC typically develops in a child who is already hospitalized. The subjective and objective data assessed will depend entirely on the initial illness. The nurse must be cognizant of the patient who is at risk for DIC. Evidence of bleeding at any site of integumentary interruption and at every orifice should be assessed. The nurse also notes any changes in the pattern of vital signs. Adequate tissue perfusion should be confirmed because normal function of an organ is the end result of sufficient oxygenation of that organ. Children with full clinical manifestations of DIC are typically cared for in an intensive care setting owing to the complex multisystem sequelae and management of DIC.

Any areas of active bleeding should be located promptly and pressure applied, if possible. Continue to monitor the child for overt and covert signs of bleeding. Care should be taken to avoid any unnecessary tissue trauma or injury. IV lines and indwelling tubes should be secured and protected to eliminate the additional trauma caused by reinsertion. Frequent monitoring of vital signs is necessary to identify changing patterns and ensure adequate cardiac output and end-organ perfusion. Laboratory results are also monitored carefully, with particular attention to the trending of values. Medical orders are followed with regard to the administration of medicines, blood products, and treatments, including monitoring the child's tolerance and outcomes. Because hypoxemia and acidosis may actually cause DIC, adequate ventilation must be ensured to prevent or reduce compromised respiratory function.

Because DIC can be life threatening, the nurse helps parents deal with their anxiety about their child's condition. Being available to answer questions and updating the parents on the child's progress are essential.

The morbidity and mortality rates in children with DIC depend on the underlying causative condition. With prompt recognition of both the underlying cause and the diagnosis of DIC and with proper management of both, these children can have favorable outcomes.

APLASTIC ANEMIA

Aplastic anemia is a condition in which the bone marrow ceases production of the cells it normally manufactures. The result is peripheral *pancytopenia,* a condition in which all formed elements of the blood are simultaneously depressed.

Etiology and Incidence

Aplastic anemia can be congenital or acquired. Several rare, inheritable disorders are characterized by aplastic anemia. The most common of these is Fanconi's anemia. Aplastic anemia can also be acquired, with a number of agents and conditions implicated as the probable cause. These most often include drugs or chemicals and less often radiation exposure, viruses, and immune diseases. Most cases (approximately 70%) of aplastic anemia in children are idiopathic—without an identifiable cause. Aplastic anemia results in a physiologic and anatomic failure of the bone marrow preventing the development of granulocytes, erythrocytes, and megakaryocytes. Annually, in the United States and Europe the incidence of aplastic anemia is 2 cases per million per year. Leukemia, by comparison, has an incidence of 50 cases per million per year (Nathan, Orkin, Look, & Ginsburg, 2003).

Manifestations

The clinical manifestations of aplastic anemia include petechiae, ecchymosis, pallor, epistaxis, fatigue, tachycardia, anorexia, and infection.

Diagnostic Evaluation

Although the diagnosis of aplastic anemia may be suspected from the child's history and the results of a CBC count, bone marrow aspiration and biopsy must be performed to confirm the diagnosis. Biopsy results should reveal the presence or absence of precursors of the mature cells found in a peripheral blood sample. In aplastic anemia, these precursors are notably absent from the marrow sample. This type of marrow is described as *hypocellular* and often contains a predominance of lymphocytes and yellowish fatty tissue.

PATHOPHYSIOLOGY

APLASTIC ANEMIA

Aplastic anemia is characterized by cessation of hematopoiesis of granulocytes, erythrocytes, and megakaryocytes, by the bone marrow. The disease may be classified as mild, moderate, or severe, depending on how low the values are for absolute neutrophil count, platelet count, and absolute reticulocyte count. The diagnosis of severe aplastic anemia requires two of the following anomalies: granulocyte count less than 500/mm^3, platelet count less than 20,000/mm^3, and reticulocyte count below 1% (after correction for hematocrit). In addition, the bone marrow biopsy specimen must contain less than 25% of the normal cellularity.

Adapted from Hord, J. (2004). The acquired pancytopenias. In R. Behrman, R. Kligman, & H. Jenson (Eds.), *Nelson textbook of pediatrics* (17th ed., pp. 1644-1646). Philadelphia: WB Saunders.

Therapeutic Management

If the aplastic anemia is determined by history to be acquired, exposure to the causative agent is discontinued immediately. Treatment then is based on symptoms. Platelet and erythrocyte transfusions may be ordered. Granulocyte transfusions are not used routinely because of their short life span in the circulation. When signs and symptoms of infection are suspected or present, antibiotics are administered after appropriate cultures are obtained.

Bone marrow or allogeneic hematopoietic stem cell transplantation remains the treatment of choice for children with severe aplastic anemia for whom a suitable donor has been identified (Young, 2002). (See Chapter 24 for a discussion of hematopoietic stem cell transplantation.) A medication regimen of cyclosporine, antithymocyte globulin/antilymphocyte globulin, and colony-stimulating factors effectively treats acquired aplastic anemia for many children for whom a suitable bone marrow or stem cell donor is not available (Hord, 2004).

NURSING CARE

The Child With Aplastic Anemia

Assessment

The subjective assessment usually elicits parents' observations of bruising immediately after an event that would not normally result in a bruise. For example, an observant parent may have noted petechiae in the child's mouth while assisting the child in brushing the teeth. Information should be elicited about medications recently taken or recent exposures to environmental substances outside the child's usual realm in an effort to determine possible drug- or chemical-related causes for the pancytopenia.

Petechiae, bruising, pallor, lethargy, and tachycardia are the usual abnormal findings and are directly related to the degree of pancytopenia. Otherwise, the results of the physical assessment are usually normal.

Nursing Diagnosis and Planning

The nursing diagnoses and expected outcomes that may be appropriate for the child with aplastic anemia include the following:
- Risk for Infection related to inadequate secondary defenses or immunosuppression.

  Expected Outcome: The child remains free from infection, as evidenced by being in the expected range for body temperature, neurologic assessment, cardiorespiratory assessment, gastrointestinal status, and genitourinary status.
- Ineffective Protection related to thrombocytopenia.

  Expected Outcomes: The child will remain free of bleeding episodes and will demonstrate appropriate precautions to prevent or decrease bleeding.
- Ineffective Tissue Perfusion related to anemia.

  Expected Outcome: The child's tissues will be perfused, as evidenced by palpable peripheral pulses, capillary refill

<2 seconds, urine output appropriate for age, and absent respiratory distress.

- Deficient Knowledge related to incomplete information about the disease process.

  Expected Outcome: The child and family will describe the disease process and its potential complications.

Interventions

Nursing care initially focuses on providing supportive care and preventing any serious physiologic sequelae of pancytopenia. Because of the increased risk of bacterial infection, affected children should be assigned to a private room and instructed in meticulous handwashing. Precautionary measures should be taken as for any individual with a low platelet count, including no injections; no rectal temperatures, examinations, or medications; use of an extra-soft-bristle toothbrush or toothette; abstinence from any contact sports or activity; and periodic assessment for increased bleeding.

Physicians' orders should be followed with regard to blood transfusions, acquisition of blood cultures, and antibiotic administration. Usually, the platelet count will be maintained at a level greater than 20,000/mm^3 to prevent intracranial hemorrhage or signs of active bleeding. The hemoglobin level is typically maintained above 7 g/dL. However, if a child is to receive a hematopoietic stem cell transplant, efforts are made to use blood transfusions only as necessary to avoid possible alloimmunization. If any symptoms of infection are present, blood should be drawn for culture. The need for other cultures will depend on the child's clinical examination.

Antibiotics should be administered immediately to a febrile child with neutropenia, owing to the risk of rapid, overwhelming sepsis. Children who are hospitalized, febrile, and neutropenic should be assessed frequently for signs of septic shock. Assessment includes the quality of peripheral pulses compared with central pulses, extremity temperature, capillary refill time, level of consciousness, vital signs, condition of cannulation sites, and presence of skin breakdown.

Education of the family and child should include information about the disease process and the complications that should be reported promptly to the health care provider. Often, referral is made to a transplant center. If so, intense pretransplant education is indicated. The Aplastic Anemia & MDS International Foundation, Inc. is a good source of information for children, parents, and health care providers (see Evolve website). Follow-up studies should include frequent CBC counts and physical examinations.

Evaluation

- Is the child afebrile and do cannulation or other skin sites remain free of redness or swelling?
- Are assessment data related to other body systems within normal ranges?
- Has the child had any major bleeding?
- Is the child able to participate in age-appropriate activities without injury?
- Does the child demonstrate palpable peripheral pulses, capillary refill less than 2 seconds, urine output appropriate

for age (see Chapter 18), and oxygen saturation more than 95%?

- Has the family received instruction regarding the disease and home care and verbalized an understanding of the information?

ABO INCOMPATIBILITY AND HEMOLYTIC DISEASE OF THE NEWBORN

The possibility of blood incompatibility exists whenever the fetal blood type is different from the maternal blood type. The most common difference is among the major blood groups of A, B, and O. Differences in Rh factor, although less common, are the most common cause of severe hemolytic disease of the fetus and newborn infant. Both types of incompatibility involve a maternal antibody response to antigens in fetal circulation. This maternal antibody then crosses the placenta into fetal circulation and destroys fetal erythrocytes, resulting in fetal anemia, referred to as *hemolytic disease of the newborn* (HDN).

Three conditions must exist for HDN to develop: (1) maternal and fetal erythrocytes are antigenically incompatible, (2) maternal circulation contains or produces antibodies against fetal erythrocytes, and (3) immunoglobulin G (IgG) binds in sufficient amount to cause a widespread antigen-antibody–mediated hemolysis or splenic sequestration of erythrocytes.

Incidence

The risk for ABO incompatibility occurs in approximately 15% of pregnancies, with HDN developing in approximately 1% of neonates (Stoll & Kliegman, 2004). Rh incompatibility, the more serious cause of HDN, occurs in fewer than 5 per 10,000 pregnancies, although approximately 15% of women are Rh negative (Harrod, Hanson, VandeVusse, & Heywood, 2003). The prevalence of Rh hemolytic disease has decreased since the introduction of Rh$_o$(D) immune globulin.

Manifestations

Signs and symptoms of neonatal ABO and Rh incompatibility are the same and are listed in order of increasing severity of the hemolytic process:

- *Jaundice:* resulting from an excess of unconjugated bilirubin formerly excreted by the maternal circulation
- *Anemia:* resulting from an increased rate of destruction caused by incompatibility
- *Hepatosplenomegaly:* resulting from anemia and possibly sequestration of erythrocytes
- *Hydrops fetalis:* constellation of symptoms resulting from the above processes that results in overwhelming fetal edema and cardiovascular collapse

Diagnostic Evaluation

All women should have their blood typed before or during their initial pregnancies. The fetus affected by Rh incompatibility may be diagnosed with hydrops fetalis (a progressive condition related to hemolysis resulting in fetal hypoxia,

PATHOPHYSIOLOGY

ABO AND Rh INCOMPATIBILITY

The hemolytic process that occurs with hemolytic disease of the newborn begins in utero. In ABO incompatibility, the maternal blood type is usually O and the blood type of the fetus is either A or B, although it can also occur when the maternal type is either A or B and the fetal type is then B or A. The serum maternal type O contains antibodies against erythrocyte types A and B. These antibodies can cross the placenta and destroy the erythrocytes of the fetus. Most adults with type O erythrocytes also possess antibodies to types A and B, with ABO sensitization thereby occurring without fetal blood crossing into maternal circulation. Anti-ABO antibodies may in rare instances cross the placenta, but the potential for fetal harm is much less than what occurs with Rh factor incompatibility.

With Rh incompatibility, the maternal type is Rh negative and the fetal type is Rh positive. During placenta detachment (delivery or abortion), fetal and maternal circulation may mix. Unlike anti-ABO antibodies, Rh antibodies form only as the result of an actual exposure. When fetal blood cells enter the maternal circulation, the woman forms antibodies (IgG in nature) against the Rh factor that is perceived as foreign by the immune system. Once established, this anti-Rh antibody remains and recirculates through the reticuloendothelial system, crossing the placenta and causing an immune reaction during future pregnancies if the same Rh incompatibility exists between the maternal and fetal types. With this Rh incompatibility, serious consequences for the fetus may occur, such as hemolytic anemia, extramedullary erythropoiesis, hepatosplenomegaly, and the release of immature nucleated erythrocytes. Collectively, this is referred to as *erythroblastosis fetalis*. Without appropriate treatment, hydrops fetalis may occur, which can lead to fetal death as early as 17 weeks' gestation.

generalized edema, and eventual circulatory collapse) during prenatal ultrasonographic testing. This condition may cause death in utero during the pregnancy. Routine screening of the neonate's blood type and direct Coombs' test during the first hour after birth help to identify neonates with blood group incompatibilities (the direct Coombs' test evaluates for the presence of maternal antibody already bound to fetal erythrocytes). Assessment of the neonate's hematologic indices, such as reticulocyte count, hematocrit level, and RBC morphologic features, helps to determine the extent of hemolysis. Neonatal bilirubin levels can also help to determine the severity of disease. The greater the increases in the bilirubin level from one measurement to the next, the more severe the hemolysis.

Therapeutic Management

Some neonates with mild ABO incompatibility may not require treatment. Most neonates requiring treatment respond well to aggressive hydration and phototherapy. Rarely does

a neonate with ABO incompatibility have hemolysis severe enough to necessitate an exchange transfusion.

The best treatment for Rh incompatibility is prevention. $Rh_o(D)$ immune globulin (RhoGAM) suppresses the maternal immune response and antibody formation of Rh-negative individuals to Rh-positive erythrocytes. The specifics of dosing depend on the timing (prepartum, intrapartum, postpartum); however, the customary dose for postpartum prophylaxis is 300 μg intramuscularly to the mother (never the neonate) within 72 hours of delivery of *each* pregnancy. The widespread use of RhoGAM in women who are Rh negative and who give birth to Rh-positive neonates has decreased the incidence of Rh incompatibility. Miscarriages or missed abortions of Rh-positive fetuses can sensitize an Rh-negative woman and account for Rh incompatibility in future pregnancies if RhoGAM is not appropriately administered.

When preventive measures for Rh incompatibility are not taken, the hemolytic process is almost always severe. Most neonates require a minimum of one exchange transfusion, and possibly more, to remove antibody-coated erythrocytes. The neonates may also require phototherapy to treat elevated levels of bilirubin, which may approach toxic levels shortly after birth. Additional erythrocyte transfusions for recurrent anemia may be necessary during the slow resolution phase of Rh incompatibility.

Nursing Considerations

Determination of the maternal blood type should be made prenatally or as soon after admission as possible to identify women at risk for giving birth to neonates with ABO or Rh incompatibilities. Blood typing and the direct Coombs' test should be performed on cord blood soon after delivery whenever a neonate is identified as being at risk. Obtaining and assessing laboratory values in symptomatic neonates can help in the timely institution of appropriate treatment. Noting the rate of change in laboratory test results as well as the actual value can also help to determine the neonate's response to therapy.

If the neonate requires an exchange transfusion, the donor blood must be checked carefully to ensure that it is type O; Rh negative; low-titer anti-A, anti-B; and cross-matched with the maternal plasma and erythrocytes before transfusion. During the transfusion, the neonate should be monitored for changes in heart rate, blood pressure, oxygen saturation, body temperature, respiratory status, and integrity of indwelling catheters used for the exchange. Both during and after the exchange transfusion, the neonate must be monitored for evidence of complications, such as infection, thrombosis, air embolism, arteriospasms affecting the lower extremities, hypoglycemia, acid-base imbalance, hypernatremia, hypokalemia, hypocalcemia, coagulopathy, necrotizing enterocolitis, cardiac arrhythmias, volume overload, and hypothermia.

Ensure adequate hydration of the neonate by administering appropriate fluids in the necessary amounts. Administer phototherapy according to established guidelines (see p. 747). Monitor blood indices and bilirubin levels, and promptly report deviations from normal or expected values.

During an exchange transfusion, assess vital signs according to the established routine and monitor for evidence of complications (see Chapter 14).

HYPERBILIRUBINEMIA

Neonatal hyperbilirubinemia (also referred to as physiologic jaundice) is often a transient benign disorder occurring during the first week of life. It is often clinically significant, however, and does require follow-up to ensure that it is self-limiting. As bilirubin levels rise, the excess bilirubin is deposited in body tissues, resulting in a temporary yellow discoloration of the neonate's skin and sclerae. High bilirubin levels can penetrate and damage brain cells, a condition referred to as kernicterus.

Etiology

The most common causes of hyperbilirubinemia, including physiologic jaundice, are listed in Table 23-2. The discussion presented here will be limited to physiologic jaundice.

Incidence

Hyperbilirubinemia develops during the first few days of life in 45% to 60% of term neonates (Bhutani, Johnson, & Keren, 2004) and in as many as 80% of preterm neonates.

Manifestations

The yellow discoloration of the skin that is known as jaundice usually appears when the serum bilirubin level reaches 5 to 7 mg/dL. In the term neonate, peak levels are generally reached by the third to fifth day of life, followed by a gradual decrease in bilirubin levels until normal values are reached at about the tenth day of life. In the preterm neonate, peak levels are generally reached by the fifth day of life, followed by a slow decline in bilirubin levels until normal values are reached around the end of the first month of life.

PATHOPHYSIOLOGY

HYPERBILIRUBINEMIA

Physiologic jaundice in the neonate is caused by impaired bilirubin uptake and conjugation. The majority of the bilirubin produced in the neonate is derived from the normal breakdown of erythrocytes by enzymes in the liver and spleen. The hemoglobin in the erythrocytes is broken down into iron, protein, and bilirubin. The bilirubin then binds to albumin and is transported to the liver, where it undergoes conjugation, making it water soluble and able to be excreted from the body through the urinary and intestinal tracts. Conjugated bilirubin cannot be reabsorbed by the intestines; however, an enzyme present in the intestines of the neonate can convert the bilirubin back to the unconjugated form, which can be reabsorbed into the bloodstream. The process can contribute significantly to the amount of bilirubin the neonate must process. Unconjugated bilirubin is lipid soluble, not water soluble, and thus it is not as easily excreted from the body.

TABLE 23-2	**Common Causes of Hyperbilirubinemia**	
Mechanism	**Related To**	**Caused By**
Increased bilirubin availability	Overproduction of bilirubin	Polycythemia
		Decreased RBC life span
		Hemolysis (anemias, medication, infection)
		Extravascular blood (bruises, enclosed hemorrhages)
	Increased reabsorption of bilirubin from intestines	Delayed passage of meconium
		Increased enzyme activity
		Delayed enteral feedings
		Swallowed blood
Decreased bilirubin secretion	Altered liver metabolism of bilirubin	Prematurity indicates immature liver
		Decreased uptake by liver
		Inadequate perfusion of liver
		Decreased enzyme activity (deficiency or inhibition)
	Liver obstruction	Biliary atresia
		Cystic fibrosis
		Hyperalimentation
		Tumor
Combined overproduction and undersecretion of bilirubin	Congenital infection: toxoplasmosis, rubella, herpes, syphilis, hepatitis	
	Asphyxia	
	Neonate of diabetic mother	
Uncertain mechanism	Breast milk jaundice	
	Neonates of Chinese, Japanese, Korean, Greek, or American Indian descent	

Diagnostic Evaluation

Serum bilirubin levels should be obtained whenever clinical jaundice is present or in neonates with conditions known to cause hyperbilirubinemia. The direct bilirubin is a measurement of conjugated bilirubin, and the indirect bilirubin is a measurement of unconjugated bilirubin. The total bilirubin level is the direct level plus the indirect level. A total bilirubin level of 13 mg/dL or higher in premature neonates with clinical jaundice or in term neonates should be evaluated to determine the etiology of the jaundice. Total bilirubin levels are generally higher in breastfed neonates than in bottle-fed neonates and higher in neonates of Asian, African, or American Indian descent. Other diagnostic tests that may help to determine the etiology include a direct Coombs' test, peripheral blood smear, reticulocyte count, blood type, and Rh type of both mother and neonate.

Therapeutic Management

The therapeutic management of physiologic jaundice is often specific to the situation and is determined by the neonate's bilirubin level, gestational age, feeding pattern and the care-giving capabilities of the mother or family. In situations other than physiologic jaundice, the underlying cause of hyperbilirubinemia, the neonate's gestational age, chronologic age, clinical status, weight, history, and risk factors and the rate of rise in the bilirubin level must all be considered.

Prevention of hyperbilirubinemia includes preventing the neonate from becoming dehydrated. Breastfeeding mothers should be encouraged to nurse at least eight to twelve times a day (AAP, 2004) and bottle-fed babies should be fed the appropriate amount of formula. Newborn infants should be assessed routinely for the presence of jaundice, and follow-up laboratory studies should be conducted, if needed (AAP, 2004).

Treatment of hyperbilirubinemia usually begins with phototherapy, which consists of exposing the neonate to light from the blue part of the spectrum, ideally 420 to 470 nm. The light source can be a single quartz-halogen spotlight; a bank of fluorescent bulbs, either blue, cool white, or day bright; or a blanket of white light filaments with a fiberoptic light source. The phototherapy causes a chemical reaction in the skin that converts unconjugated bilirubin to a form that can be excreted by the body. Phototherapy also causes an oxidative reaction that allows unconjugated bilirubin removal by the liver and spleen. The therapeutic effect of phototherapy relies on the following factors: extent of hemolysis, amount of light energy used, distance from the neonate to the light source, amount of skin exposed, and the neonate's ability to excrete the bilirubin. Phototherapy is provided continuously with short breaks as dictated by other care needs, such as feeding, bathing, diapering, and visual stimulation.

If phototherapy does not reduce the bilirubin level or if the bilirubin level is dangerously high, the neonate may require an exchange transfusion. A double-volume exchange, in which the neonate's blood volume is replaced twice, can lower the bilirubin level to approximately one half the original value. Exchange transfusions should always be performed in a setting familiar with the procedure and one capable of providing intensive care nursing support. Small amounts of the neonate's blood are removed, alternating with administration of small amounts of donor blood, of the appropriate type, through a venous access device, often an umbilical venous catheter. After exchange transfusion, phototherapy is often administered as an additional measure to lower the bilirubin level.

Breastfed neonates may have elevated bilirubin levels that do not seem to decrease with the usual management. Stopping breast-milk feedings for 24 to 48 hours and instituting formula feedings instead can contribute to a decrease in the bilirubin level.

NURSING CARE
The Neonate With Hyperbilirubinemia

Assessment

The nurse can assess the neonate for the presence of jaundice by pressing lightly on the skin with a fingertip, observing for a slight to moderate yellowish discoloration of the skin with blanching. The yellow color of jaundice will be easier to see over the fingerprint area than over the surrounding skin. Common assessment sites are the nose and upper chest. Assessment for jaundice should take place in natural light whenever possible. In neonates with dark skin, the first evidence of jaundice may be yellowing of the sclera. The neonate should also be assessed for evidence of bruising, petechiae, cephalhematoma, pallor, plethora, and enlarged liver or spleen, as well as prematurity and perinatal risk factors, which may help to identify neonates at risk for hyperbilirubinemia.

Nursing Diagnosis and Planning

The following nursing diagnoses and expected outcomes may be appropriate for the neonate with hyperbilirubinemia:

- Risk for Imbalanced Fluid Volume: Deficit related to increased insensible losses from phototherapy

  Expected Outcome: The neonate will have moist mucous membranes, flat fontanel, and urine output of 2 to 3 mL/kg/hr.

- Ineffective Thermoregulation related to heat from phototherapy lights or lack of clothing to expose skin to phototherapy

  Expected Outcome: The neonate will maintain body temperature within a normal range.

- Risk for Injury to neurologic system related to deposition of bilirubin in brain tissue

Expected Outcome: The neonate will demonstrate resolving jaundice and decreasing bilirubin levels.

- Deficient Knowledge related to unfamiliarity with phototherapy equipment

Expected Outcomes: The parent will demonstrate proper use of home phototherapy equipment and describe when to contact appropriate support personnel.

Interventions

During hospitalization, to maximize the effectiveness of phototherapy, the neonate should be completely undressed or wearing only a diaper. While phototherapy is in use, the neonate's eyes are covered with an opaque mask that is usually secured in place with a headband or cloth adhesive. Several types of eye shields are commercially available. Care must be taken to ensure that the eye shield does not slip down and cover the neonate's nares, compromising nasal breathing efforts. Eye patches can be removed when the light source is off to assess the eyes and allow the neonate visual stimulation. The neonate's position is changed frequently to ensure maximal skin exposure to the light source. Monitoring the neonate's bilirubin level is performed one to four times daily to assess the effectiveness of phototherapy.

The nurse monitors the neonate's temperature every 2 to 4 hours to ensure maintenance within normal limits. The additional heat generated by the phototherapy unit places the neonate at risk for hyperthermia. The lack of clothing on the neonate increases the possibility of heat loss through convection, conduction, radiation, and evaporation and may lead to hypothermia. Any signs of feeding intolerance, such as diarrhea or lactose intolerance, are recorded and reported so that appropriate feeding changes can be made. Because neonates receiving phototherapy have increased insensible water losses, their intake and output should be closely monitored to ensure adequate hydration.

Term neonates who are otherwise healthy may be treated with phototherapy at home with the support of home health care. This practice not only saves health care costs and resources but also allows the family to interact with the neonate in a more natural environment. The equipment and care are the same as for the hospitalized neonate. The nurse ensures that the parent knows the precautions to take during home phototherapy treatments (Box 23-8). Technicians should be available to service equipment. Home health nurses make visits once or twice each day during treatment to assess the neonate, obtain bilirubin levels, and provide additional support to the parent as necessary.

CRITICAL TO REMEMBER
Care During Phototherapy

- During phototherapy, special care should be taken to ensure that the neonate is well hydrated to offset the effects of increased insensible water loss brought on by the phototherapy.
- The neonate's eyes must be protected at all times during phototherapy to prevent retinal damage from the light source.
- To maximize the effect of phototherapy, expose as much skin surface as possible; leave the neonate clothed only in a diaper.

BOX 23-8 | **PARENTS WANT TO KNOW**   About Home Care for the Infant Receiving Phototherapy

Position the phototherapy or "bili" light at the proper distance from your baby according to the manufacturer's directions. Placing it too close to the infant could result in fever or burns. Placing it too far away will make the treatment ineffective.

Close the baby's eyes and place patches over the eyes before placing the infant under the lights. Check at least every hour to see that the patches remain in place. They must cover the eyes but not press on the nose because they can interfere with breathing.

The infant may be removed from the lights for feedings, diaper changes, and other general care but should receive phototherapy for 18 hours every day (or the number of hours ordered by the physician). Hold and cuddle your infant during the time that the baby is out of the lights. When the infant is under the lights, you can talk to your baby. The sound of your voice will be comforting.

If you are using a fiberoptic blanket, keep it next to the baby's skin at all times. Be sure the baby does not roll off the blanket. You may wrap the baby with a receiving blanket over the "bili" blanket and hold the baby for feedings and other care. It is not necessary to cover the infant's eyes if the blanket alone is used.

Check your baby's temperature under the arm before every feeding. The temperature should remain between 97.7° F and 99.5° F. If it is abnormal, see whether the heat in the room is too low or high or if the "bili" light is out of position. Use warm blankets when you remove the baby from the warmth of the light. Call your physician if the baby has a temperature less than 97.7° F or more than 100° F.

Change your baby's position about every 2 hours so that the light reaches all areas of the body. Dress the baby in only a diaper to expose as much skin as possible to the lights.

Feed your baby every 2 to 3 hours because the lights cause the baby to lose fluid from the skin and have loose stools. This process could cause dehydration. The infant needs protein, which helps eliminate the bilirubin that causes the jaundice.

Keep a list of your baby's wet diapers and stools. Increase the feedings if the baby has fewer than six wet diapers per day or if the urine appears dark.

Call the physician or home care nurse if you have questions about care, if the baby has a fever or appears sick to you, if the mouth seems dry, or if the urine is dark or less than normal.

Evaluation

- Does the neonate have moist mucous membranes, a flat fontanel, and urine output of 2 to 3 mL/kg/hr?
- Has the neonate's body temperature remained within normal limits for age during phototherapy?
- Is the serum bilirubin level decreasing appropriately?
- Can the parent demonstrate proper home adaptations for phototherapy and describe situations that require notifying health care personnel?

KEY CONCEPTS

- For erythrocytes to carry oxygen there must be an adequate amount of hemoglobin, the level of which depends on sufficient circulating iron.
- Anemia results from blood loss, decreased production of erythrocytes or hemoglobin, or increased destruction of erythrocytes.
- Caring for children with blood disorders requires an understanding of the anatomy and physiology of blood and blood-forming tissues, genetics, and the care of children with a chronic disease.
- The number of erythrocytes varies according to age, sex, and the altitude at which a person lives.
- Iron-deficiency anemia can largely be prevented by teaching parents the importance of providing iron-fortified formula or breast milk with iron supplementary foods, such as iron-fortified cereal, to children until age 12 months.
- Morphine is the drug of choice for children with a painful episode associated with SCD.
- Complications associated with sickle cell anemia can be reduced through early screening; parent/child education; routine immunizations; pneumococcal, meningococcal, and influenza immunizations; penicillin prophylaxis; and early diagnosis and management of complications.
- Children with decreased platelet counts and factor disorders should not receive aspirin or aspirin-containing products or have their temperature taken rectally. Invasive procedures should be done only when necessary and then only with extreme caution to avoid hemorrhage.
- Factor prophylaxis is warranted in infants and young children with hemophilia who are at risk for development of joint problems as a result of bleeding.
- Bleeding associated with hemophilia is treated with rest, ice, elevation, compression, and factor replacement, as necessary.
- Education of the family about home care for the child with hemophilia should include information on the management of bleeding episodes, environmental safety, administration of medications, health promotion, and normal growth and development.
- Educating the family of a child with ITP about the need to restrict activity and to provide protection is a major nursing challenge.
- Treatment of DIC is directed toward treating the cause of the condition.
- Nursing care of the child with aplastic anemia focuses on the prevention of infection resulting from pancytopenia.
- Nursing care of the infant with ABO or Rh incompatibility or any other cause of hyperbilirubinemia is directed toward interventions that reduce serum bilirubin levels.

ANSWERS TO CRITICAL THINKING EXERCISE 23-1

1. Mrs. Anders is probably most concerned about Jacob's cough and fever. For that reason, the nurse will want to address the acute illness and then approach Mrs. Anders about concerns related to the anemia. Nurses must be sensitive to what parents perceive as priorities and should address those needs so that the parents will be able to give their attention to other concerns. In this case, even if Jacob has a minor common cold, the nurse can provide Mrs. Anders with information that will make Jacob more comfortable and then approach the treatment of anemia.

2. Although the priority is to take action related to the acute disease, it is also a time to assess the child and to provide preventive care. Some families see health care providers only when a family member is ill. Knowing the severity of the acute illness, the nurse can determine what can be achieved during the visit and what warrants a follow-up.

3. It is an opportunity to start or update a child's health records through assessment of the child and communicating with the parent and the child, if age appropriate. Such a visit also provides an opportunity to administer immunizations, if the child is not too ill, and to provide anticipatory guidance related to nutrition, safety, growth and development, and preventive care. For Jacob, the nurse will want to do a thorough nutrition assessment to determine whether diet is the causative factor in the anemia. To increase the chance of adherence, a system of tracking children with diseases that need long-term treatment should also be in place.

REFERENCES AND READINGS

Alter, B. P. (2003). Inherited bone marrow failure syndromes. In D. G. Nathan & S. H. Orkin (Eds.), *Nathan and Oski's hematology of infancy and childhood* (6th ed.). Philadelphia: WB Saunders.

American Academy of Pediatrics. (2004). Clinical practice guidelines: Management of hyperbilirubinemia in the newborn infant 35 or more weeks of gestation. *Pediatrics, 114,* 297-316.

American Academy of Pediatrics, Committee on Infectious Diseases. (2003a). Active and passive immunization. In *2003 Red Book* (26th ed., pp. 1-93). Elk Grove Village, IL: American Academy of Pediatrics.

American Academy of Pediatrics, Committee on Infectious Diseases. (2003b). Section III: Summaries of infectious diseases. In *2003 Red Book* (26th ed., pp. 189-771). Elk Grove Village, IL: American Academy of Pediatrics.

American Academy of Pediatrics, Committee on Nutrition. (2003). *Pediatrics nutrition handbook* (5th ed.). Elk Grove Village, IL: American Academy of Pediatrics.

Bain, B. (2001). *Haemoglobinopathy diagnosis.* Oxford: Blackwell.

Bhutani, V., Johnson, L., & Keren, R. (2004). Diagnosis and management of hyperbilirubinemia in the term neonate: for a safer first week. *Pediatric Clinics of North America, 51,* 843-862.

Brodsky, R. (2005) Acquired severe aplastic anemia in children: Is there a standard of care? *Pediatric Blood and Cancer, 45,* 361-362.

Bussel, J., & Cines, D. (2005). Immune thrombocytopenic purpura, neonatal alloimmune thrombocytopenia, and post-transfusion purpura. In R. Hoffman, E. Benz, S. Shattil, B. Furie, & H. Cohen (Eds.). *Hematology: Basic principles and practice* (4th ed.). Philadelphia: Elsevier.

Carley, A. (2003). Anemia: when is it iron deficiency? *Pediatric Nursing, 29,* 127-133.

Cox, G. (2004). Diagnosis and treatment of von Willebrand disease. *Hematology/Oncology Clinics of North America, 18,* 1277-1299.

Day, S. (2004). Development and evaluation of a sickle cell assessment instrument. *Pediatric Nursing, 30,* 451-458.

Dover, G., & Platt, O. (2003). Sickle cell disease. In D. G. Nathan, S. H. Orkin, A. T. Look, & D. Ginsburg (Eds.), *Nathan and Oski's hematology of infancy and childhood* (6th ed.). Philadelphia: WB Saunders.

Glader, B. (2004). Iron deficiency anemia. In R. Behrman, R. Kliegman, & H. Jenson (Eds.), *Nelson textbook of pediatrics* (17th ed., pp. 1614-1616). Philadelphia: WB Saunders.

Harrod, K., Hanson, L., VandeVusse, L., & Heywood, P. (2003). Rh negative status and isoimmunization update: A case-based approach to care. *Journal of Perinatal and Neonatal Nursing, 17,* 166-181.

Hord, J. (2004). The acquired pancytopenias. In R. Behrman, R. Kliegman, & H. Jenson (Eds.), *Nelson textbook of pediatrics* (17th ed., pp. 1644-1646). Philadelphia: WB Saunders.

Johnson, L. (2005). Managing acute and chronic pain in sickle cell disease. *Nursing Times, 101,* 40-43.

Kladny, B., Getting, E., & Krishnamurti, L. (2005). Systematic follow-up and case management of the abnormal newborn screen can improve acceptance of genetic counseling for sickle cell or other hemoglobinopathy trait. *Genetic Medicine, 7,* 139-142.

Kwiatkowski, J., & Cohen, A. R. (2004). Iron chelation therapy in sickle-cell disease and other transfusion-dependent anemias. *Hematology/Oncology Clinics of North America, 18,* 1355-1379.

Lanzkowsky, P. (2005). *Manual of pediatric hematology and oncology* (4th ed.). Amsterdam: Elsevier.

Lee, C., Berntorp, E., & Hoots, W. K. (2005). *Textbook of hemophilia.* Malden: Blackwell.

Nathan, D. G., Orkin, S. H., Look, A. T., & Ginsburg, D. (2003). *Nathan & Oski's hematology of infancy and childhood* (6th ed.). Philadelphia: WB Saunders.

National Hemophilia Foundation. (2006). *What is a bleeding disorder?* Retrieved February 15, 2006, from *www.hemophilia.org.*

National Institutes of Health, Division of Blood Diseases and Resource. (2002). *The management of sickle cell disease* (NIH Publication No. 02-2117). Bethesda, MD: National Institutes of Health.

Nursing 2005 Drug Handbook (25th ed.). Philadelphia: Lippincott Williams & Wilkins.

Quirolo, K., & Vichinsky, E. (2004). Hemoglobin disorders. In R. E. Behrman, R. M. Kliegman, & H. Jenson (Eds.), *Nelson textbook of pediatrics* (17th ed., pp. 1623-1634). Philadelphia: WB Saunders.

Stanley, I., et al. (2004). An evidence-based review of important issues concerning neonatal hyperbilirubinemia. *Pediatrics, 114,* e130-e153.

Stoll, B., & Kliegman, R. (2004). Blood disorders. In R. E. Behrman, R. M. Kliegman, & H. Jenson (Eds.), *Nelson textbook of pediatrics* (17th ed., pp. 599-606). Philadelphia: WB Saunders.

White, K. (2005). Anemia is a poor predictor of iron deficiency among toddlers in the United States; for heme the bell tolls. *Pediatrics, 115,* 315-320.

Young, N. (2002). Acquired aplastic anemia. *Annals of Internal Medicine, 136,* 534-546.

CHAPTER 24

The Child With Cancer

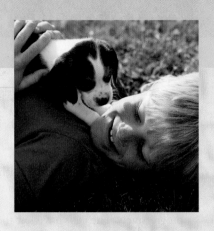

Learning Objectives

After studying this chapter, you should be able to:

- List common clinical manifestations of childhood cancer.
- Discuss the treatment modalities used in the treatment of children with cancer.
- Demonstrate an understanding of the nursing care associated with caring for a child with cancer.
- Discuss symptom management of the child with cancer.

Definitions

benign Slow-growing cells, often almost normal in appearance, forming a tumor with distinct borders.

blast cells Immature white blood cells, such as lymphoblasts, myeloblasts, or monoblasts.

clean margins Evidence of normal, disease-free tissue in the outermost layer of cells of a surgical sample.

extramedullary Outside the bone marrow.

hematopoiesis The normal formation and development of blood cells in the bone marrow.

hepatosplenomegaly Enlargement of the liver and spleen detected by palpation of the abdomen.

immunosuppression A weakening or cessation of the body's normal immune response.

intrathecal Within the spinal column.

leukocoria Appearance of a whitish reflex or mass in the pupillary area behind the lens of the eye.

lymphadenopathy Swelling of the lymph nodes detected by palpation.

malignant Abnormal cells that have invasive and unregulated growth and the potential to spread to distant locations in the body; life-threatening.

neutropenia Decrease in the number of circulating neutrophils that results in a decreased ability of the body to fight infection.

protocol A systematic plan of care outlining drug therapy and follow-up care based on research in cancer treatment.

thrombocytopenia A reduction in platelet count; places the individual at risk for increased bruising and bleeding.

Electronic Resources

Additional information related to the content in Chapter 24 can be found on:

the interactive companion CD-ROM

- Audio Glossary
- NCLEX Review Questions

or the companion website at *evolve*
http://evolve.elsevier.com/james/ncoc

- NCLEX Review Questions
- Resources for Health Care Providers and Families
- WebLinks

REVIEW OF CANCER

A *neoplasm* is any tumor that arises from new, abnormal growth. A tumor may be either benign or malignant. The distinguishing feature of cancer is its ability to invade surrounding tissue and spread to distant sites. Cancer cells spread in one of two ways: (1) by *invasion,* in which cells grow in unrestricted, disorderly fashion at the site of origin; and (2) by *metastasis,* in which the cells grow in sites other than the site of the primary cancer. The cancerous cells grow progressively. The cells have lost the ability to perform their intended functions because changes in the cell's deoxyribonucleic acid (DNA) cause "wrong" information to be transmitted. As the cancerous cells continue to proliferate, they crowd out normal cells and compress vascular structures and vital organs, which results in symptoms.

Tumor staging is based on the results of diagnostic studies and, in some cases, surgical examination. Staging describes the extent of disease locally, regionally, and systemically and guides the therapy for most solid tumors. Each tumor has its own specific system of staging, which assists in determining treatment and prognosis.

The cause of most childhood cancers is unknown. One underlying cause of cancer is genetic. Alterations in normal DNA occur that predispose the child to the development of cancer. A small percentage of cancers are associated with an inherited predisposition related to chromosomal

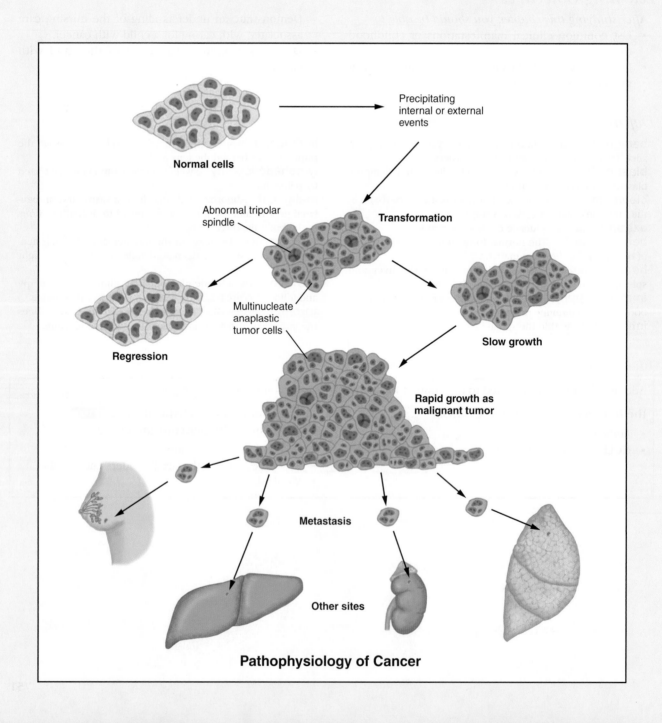

Pathophysiology of Cancer

abnormalities (Gurney & Bondy, 2004). A second, more controversial hypothesis contends that cancer develops as a result of failure of the immune system to distinguish between normal and abnormal cells. Inactivation of tumor suppressor genes is also thought to be implicated. Known carcinogens, such as radiation, physical irritation, and chemical irritants, contribute to the development of cancer. Certain environmental exposures known to cause cancer in adults have little correlation with the development of cancer in children.

The cardinal signs of cancer in children differ from those seen in adults. Most adult cancers are carcinomas, and more screening tools are available to assist with their early detection. The difficulty in diagnosing cancer in children is that symptoms resemble those of common childhood illnesses. Children are often not brought for medical care until obvious signs and symptoms are present. Primary care providers are understandably reluctant to think about cancer as the cause of the child's illness.

CARDINAL SIGNS AND SYMPTOMS OF CANCER IN CHILDREN

Overt Signs
A mass
Purpura
Pallor
Weight loss
Whitish reflex in the eye
Vomiting in early morning
Recurrent or persistent fever

Signs and Symptoms That May be Covert
Bone pain
Headache
Persistent lymphadenopathy
Change in balance, gait, or personality
Fatigue, malaise

Diagnostic Tests and Procedures for Cancer

Test	Description	Purpose	Nursing Considerations
Bone marrow aspiration	Bone marrow is aspirated from the anterior or posterior iliac crests (the tibia is sometimes used in infants).	Pathologic examination of the aspirated material shows the presence, absence, and ratio of cells that are specific to and diagnostic of certain diseases. Some conditions that can be diagnosed are leukemia, specific vitamin deficiencies, neoplastic diseases in which the marrow is invaded by tumor cells, and aplastic anemia.	1. Describe the procedure to the child and parents. Check the signed consent. Allow parents to stay with the child if they wish. 2. Depending on the protocol of the facility, the child may receive a wide range of sedative or anesthetic agents. Some centers use local anesthesia with no systemic sedation; others use a combination of a sedative and an analgesic. 3. The child should be positioned prone with a small pillow under the hips to facilitate access to the posterior iliac crest, the usual site. Tell the child that the physician will clean the site and that it will feel cold. Just before the needle insertion, the child should be told that some discomfort will be felt when the needle is inserted and the marrow aspirated but that the discomfort will last only a few seconds; it will help for the child to sing, count, or take slow, deep breaths. 4. Apply a dressing to the area. If the child's platelet count is less than 50,000/mm^3, use a pressure dressing. Monitor vital signs until stable, and monitor the puncture site for bleeding and later for signs of infection.
Bone scintigraphy	A radiolabeled nucleotide is injected into the bloodstream. This tracer migrates to areas of the body in a predictable pattern.	Pattern of uptake in the axial skeleton is evaluated for variation from normal. Areas of increased uptake indicate increased cellular turnover related to growth, infection, trauma, or tumor activity.	Preparation similar to steps 1 and 2 for bone marrow aspiration. The child will be asked to lie still for 45-60 min to complete testing.

Continued

Diagnostic Tests and Procedures for Cancer—cont'd

Test	Description	Purpose	Nursing Considerations
Gallium scan	Similar to bone scintigraphy.	Radiotracer uptake occurs in areas of active Hodgkin disease; 60%-70% of those with Hodgkin disease have uptake of this isotope at diagnosis, which can be used as a marker for disease during and after therapy.	Preparation similar to steps 1 and 2 for bone marrow aspiration. The child will be asked to lie still for 45-60 min to complete testing.
Positron emission tomography (PET)	This study combines conventional nuclear medicine techniques with tomography and adds double-photon imaging, which images metabolic activity.	PET scans reveal differences in metabolic processes. Tumor cells have accelerated glycolysis compared with the tissues of origin. PET can be useful for diagnosis, staging, and follow-up monitoring.	Be sure the patient is not pregnant. Younger children may need sedation. Older children should be told about the scan and allowed to see the equipment.
Single-photon emission computed tomography (SPECT)	This study combines the techniques of conventional nuclear medicine imaging with that of computed tomography (CT) using gamma-emitting radioactive isotopes.	SPECT displays a normal organ in axial, parasagittal, and coronal sections.	Same as for PET.

See Chapter 28 (CT, lumbar puncture, MRI) and refer to the Evolve website for other common tests (CBC, serum chemistry, urinalysis) used in the care of the child with cancer.

THE CHILD WITH CANCER

Cancer in children is often difficult to diagnose, and health care providers must be aware of the clinical manifestations that should raise the suspicion of cancer. The signs and symptoms depend on the type of tumor, the extent of the disease, and the child's age. Testing, diagnosis, and initiation of therapy may occur within a very short period. The diagnosis of cancer can be devastating to both the child and the family. The nurse becomes the informational lifeline for the child and the family as they go through the treatment process.

Incidence

Cancer is uncommon in children; nevertheless, pediatric cancer is the second leading cause of death in childhood, after unintentional injuries, and is the leading cause of death from disease. Childhood cancer represents only approximately 1% of all new cancers diagnosed annually (Fig. 24-1) (Gurney & Bondy, 2004). Treatment challenges include minimizing treatment-related side effects while maintaining the child's normal growth and development.

Childhood Cancer and Its Treatment

Children with cancer are treated in a multidisciplinary setting. Pediatric oncology nurses play a prominent role in the care of children with cancer and their families. They support and educate the children and their families as they move through a stressful process. Pediatric oncology nurses are challenged to maintain a high level of technical competence and an ability to provide the psychological support required by the child and family. Working with children with cancer can be an emotional experience. The nurse in this setting must have a support system and be aware of personal limitations and therapeutic relationship boundaries (Hawes, 2005).

A great deal of research has been done over the past 30 years to improve the outcomes for children with cancer. Current survival rates are attributed to cooperative, systematic research through the Children's Oncology Group (COG) and the International Society for Pediatric Oncology. Each group meets twice a year to develop new protocols and monitor the progress of current protocols; subgroups meet as needed throughout the year. Protocols direct when drugs are to be given, how frequently, and in what dosages, and which diagnostic and follow-up studies are to be performed. Research has shown that children have better outcomes if they are treated by a scientifically derived protocol.

Because of the efforts of cooperative pediatric clinical trials, approximately 74% of children diagnosed with cancer will survive 5 years or longer after their diagnosis (Gurney & Bondy, 2004). More than 270,000 survivors of childhood cancer are estimated to be living in the United States today (American Cancer Society, 2003). The marked improvement in childhood cancer survival rates has placed renewed emphasis on the importance of identifying the long-term sequelae of cancer treatment in children and initiating timely intervention (Friedman & Meadows, 2002).

Even after apparently successful treatment of cancer in children, the disease may recur. A recurrence may occur shortly after therapy has been completed or years later. A second tumor may represent a new (or second) malignancy. Recurrence represents the failure to cure the initial disease, whereas a second cancer is a likely result of the initial

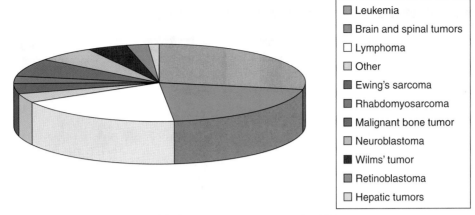

Leukemia
Brain and spinal tumors
Lymphoma
Other
Ewing's sarcoma
Rhabdomyosarcoma
Malignant bone tumor
Neuroblastoma
Wilms' tumor
Retinoblastoma
Hepatic tumors

FIG 24-1   **Incidence of cancers in children.**

treatment. For example, some children with acute lympho-cytic leukemia (ALL) develop acute myelocytic leukemia (AML) after therapy is complete. Brain tumors may develop in a small number of children with ALL who were treated with radiation to their central nervous system (CNS).

Therapeutic Management

Chemotherapy, surgery, and radiation therapy are the pri-mary treatment modalities for children with cancer. Hema-topoietic stem cell transplantation (HSCT) and biologic response modifiers are reserved for a specific subpopulation of children with cancer.

Chemotherapy

Chemotherapy is the use of drugs (antineoplastic agents) to kill cancer cells. Different drugs have different side effect profiles and modes of action. Combinations of drugs known individually to be active against the specific disease are used. Tumors possess the ability to develop resistance to chemo-therapy agents, so a variety of active drugs are frequently used. Chemotherapy may be given orally, intravenously, in-tramuscularly, subcutaneously, or intrathecally (through the spinal column). Depending on the protocol, a child may be hospitalized for chemotherapy, receive it on an outpatient basis, or be treated at home.

The side effects of chemotherapeutic agents represent challenges to caregivers. Chemotherapy nonselectively kills rapidly dividing cells. The cells most often affected include cells of the hematopoietic system, gastrointestinal (GI) tract, and integumentary system (Box 24-1).

The bone marrow cells are one of the rapidly proliferat-ing tissues adversely affected by many chemotherapy agents. Bone marrow production may become suppressed, resulting in neutropenia, anemia, and thrombocytopenia. The na-dir—the time of the greatest bone marrow suppression—gen-erally occurs 7 to 10 days after chemotherapy administration, depending on the specific agent used. The greatest concern during the period of bone marrow suppression is infection.

Neutropenia places the child with cancer at risk for the development of opportunistic infections. Opportunistic in-fections are caused by nonpathogenic bacteria and fungi that, because of compromised immunity, may invade and cause infection. Bacteria, generally present on the skin and within the gut, may invade the bloodstream through a break in the skin, leading to a life-threatening infection. In the presence of markedly decreased white blood cells (WBCs), the usual inflammatory response (erythema, edema, swelling) indica-tive of an infection is not present. Fever is frequently the only indication of infection. Health care providers and families must remain acutely aware of elevated body temperature and breaks in the skin during periods of neutropenia.

The GI tract is affected in a number of ways. Chemo-therapy represents a noxious stimulus that triggers nausea and vomiting. The treatment of nausea and vomiting was revo-lutionized in 1992 with the release of a class of nonsedating antiemetic drugs called *5-HT3 serotonin antagonists*. These drugs include ondansetron (Zofran), granisetron (Kytril), and dolasetron (Anzemet). They have been more effective in combating chemotherapy-induced nausea and vomiting than earlier antiemetics.

Anorexia is associated with nausea and a change in taste experienced by some people in response to certain chemo-therapeutic agents. Some children use anorexia as a way to exert what little control they have left after the diagnosis.

Certain chemotherapeutic agents cause sloughing of the mucosal tissue of the GI tract, leading to the development of mucositis and esophagitis. These conditions can be painful and can contribute to poor nutrition. Bacteria and yeasts, present as part of the normal digestive process in the mouth and gut, may cross the open skin and be absorbed into the bloodstream. The presence of breaks in the integument may lead to bacterial infections of the blood.

Decreased activity, pain medication, and poor oral intake may contribute to the development of constipation. Certain chemotherapeutic agents may also contribute to constipa-tion. Passage of hard stool may cause abrasion of the delicate mucous membrane of the rectum. The stool is loaded with microorganisms as part of the digestive process. Again, the presence of breaks in the integument may lead to bacterial infections of the blood.

BOX 24-1	**Common Side Effects of Chemotherapy and Radiation Therapy**

Chemotherapeutic drugs and radiation therapy affect normal and abnormal cells, primarily cells that divide rapidly, such as cells of the GI tract, hair follicles, and bone marrow. As a result, children undergoing these therapies frequently have the following:

Chemotherapy Side Effects

Bone marrow suppression
Alopecia
Malaise and fatigue
Nausea
Vomiting
Anorexia
Stomatitis

Radiation Side Effects

Skin reactions
Fatigue
Bone marrow suppression
Nausea
Vomiting
Anorexia
Mucositis

Side Effects of Radiation to the Brain

Acute (During and Shortly After Irradiation)

Brain edema
Transient increase in neurologic symptoms
General radiation side effects listed previously

Subacute (1 to 6 Months After Irradiation)

Somnolence syndrome—pronounced drowsiness, nausea, and malaise (typically 4 to 8 weeks after completing radiation therapy)
Fever
Irritability
Ataxia
Anorexia
Dysphasia

Late Effects (More than 6 Months after Irradiation)

Morphologic changes—cerebral atrophy, white matter degeneration, necrosis, calcification
Functional changes—encephalopathy, neuropsychological deterioration, focal neurologic deficits
Alopecia within the radiation field
Mucositis (inflammation of the mucous membranes) and mouth ulcers; any mucous membrane can be affected

(Photo courtesy Cook Children's Medical Center, Fort Worth, TX.)

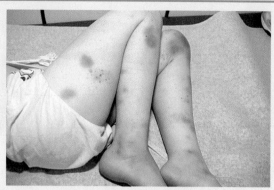

Suppression of the bone marrow because of chemotherapy or radiation therapy reduces the blood counts. Low platelet levels lead to spontaneous bruising, as shown. Nosebleeds and bleeding of the gums are other consequences. The nurse must make a special effort to observe for bruising in dark-skinned children because it will be more difficult to see.

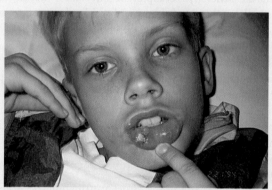

Mucositis (inflammation of the mucous membranes) and mouth ulcers are common side effects of chemotherapeutic drugs. Any mucous membrane can be affected.

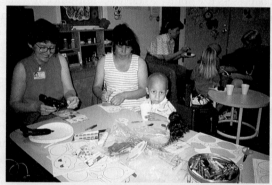

Hair loss is a distressing side effect of cancer treatment. School-age children and adolescents are most likely to feel this distress. Activities such as crafts or play groups help children feel more normal and provide interaction with others in an accepting environment.

Hair loss has a tremendous psychological effect, especially on the school-age and adolescent population. Some chemotherapeutic agents do not produce hair loss, but most do. Treatment-related fatigue, common in adult cancer patients, is poorly reported in the child and adolescent populations, although an increasing body of research has identified and described fatigue in adolescents with cancer (Erickson, 2004). Other side effects are specific to the agent being used as well as the dose.

Nurses administering chemotherapeutic agents should have evidence of special chemotherapy training by the institution in which they work. No nationally recognized chemotherapy administration certification is currently available. Nursing responsibilities and precautions related to chemotherapy administration are detailed in Box 24-2.

Surgery

Surgery is frequently part of cancer therapy for children. The surgery may be limited to a biopsy or be used to remove a solid tumor mass. The purpose of a biopsy is to obtain a small piece of the tumor for microscopic examination. Examination of the tissue by a pathologist confirms the tumor type and influences therapy decisions. Surgery may also be used to debulk or resect a solid tumor mass. In some diseases, the tumor cannot be resected at the beginning of therapy. After the child has received some chemotherapy, the mass may decrease in size and a less-extensive surgical procedure may be performed (see Chapter 13 for a discussion of preoperative care).

A central venous catheter is frequently placed during the initial surgical procedure to facilitate chemotherapy administration. A central venous catheter is a central line placed to provide easy access to the venous system; the proximal part of the catheter ends in the large vein just above the heart, the superior vena cava. Three types of central venous catheters are available. In an external catheter, the distal portion exits the skin and a tiny polyester cuff is located under the exit site where the skin will adhere and hold the catheter in place. In an implanted catheter, the distal portion ends in a well, which is placed in the subcutaneous tissue, frequently in the anterior chest wall. A percutaneously (peripherally) inserted central catheter (PICC) is not surgically placed. The proximal tip ends in the same large vein as other catheters, but the distal portion is not tunneled. The catheter is frequently inserted in the antecubital fossa by a technique similar to placement of a peripheral intravenous (IV) catheter.

Radiation Therapy

Radiation may be given curatively to eradicate disease or palliatively in low doses to prevent further growth of a tumor. To eradicate microscopic disease and promote bone marrow suppression, total body irradiation is given before some stem cell transplant attempts. Radiation may be given in hyperfractionated doses, in which the daily dose is split into smaller doses given more frequently to minimize side effects and increase tumor kill by decreasing time for cell repair between doses.

Preparing the child and family for radiation involves education about the process in addition to the side effects. Some institutions provide a preradiation tour so the child may experience the room and surroundings before therapy. During the tour, children should be shown the window or monitor through which they will be observed while undergoing radiation alone in the room. Some children need to be sedated for radiation treatments; others can be coached to lie still with the help of child life specialists and parents. The child must lie still for what may seem like long periods because the radiation oncologist must carefully control the depth and peripheral margins of the radiation site.

The side effects of radiation are dose and treatment site specific. As with chemotherapy, side effects are a result of radiation's effect on healthy, rapidly dividing cells. The side effects usually appear 7 to 10 days after the initiation of therapy. Acute side effects usually dissipate within days or a few weeks of cessation of the radiation therapy. The decision regarding radiation dose, frequency, and location depends on the purpose of the radiation and the disease process being treated. In general, radiotherapy is used more sparingly in children than in adults because developing tissues and organs are more vulnerable to its late adverse effects (Bleyer, 2004).

BOX 24-2	Nursing Responsibilities and Precautions for Chemotherapy

- Know Occupational Safety and Health Administration (OSHA) guidelines for administration of antineoplastic agents.
- Measure child's height and weight accurately.
- Confirm body surface area (BSA)—calculated in square meters and used to determine dosages.
- Always double check the ordered dosage against the BSA.
- Always double check the ordered dosage against protocol recommendations.
- Always double check the medication against the original physician's order.
- A CBC should be obtained within 48 hours preceding administration of chemotherapy.
- The WBC and platelet counts need to be at a predetermined level before chemotherapy is given.
- Know the potential side effects of the drugs being administered and appropriate actions to ameliorate those effects.
- Before giving any drugs, ensure the patency of IV tubing by checking for blood return.
- If using an implantable infusion device, ensure that needle placement is secure and blood returns.
- Vesicants (agents that produce blisters) should be given through a fresh IV site.
- Have emergency drugs available.

USING RESEARCH TO IMPROVE PRACTICE

Sometimes a clinical problem can be identified by anecdotal evidence, which provides the basis for beginning research into the specific clinical issue. For many years nurses have assessed and provided interventions for fatigue, one of the most distressing symptoms in adult cancer victims. Descriptions of fatigue and its effects on adolescents or children with cancer, however, have been only rarely documented until recently. Erickson (2004) suggests that fatigue in adolescents with cancer is an important and timely research area for exploration; learning more about how fatigue affects adolescents and their developmental trajectory enables nurses to appropriately tailor interventions to this population.

In an exploratory piece of research, Erickson (2004) conducts an integrative literature review of research related to the experience of fatigue in adolescents with cancer. Unlike a general literature review, an integrative review is focused on an issue of interest, usually includes only published research in the area, and has specific inclusion (or exclusion) criteria. The purpose of an integrative review is to identify what is known about the issue by analyzing and synthesizing information acquired in the published literature, thus building evidence for practice.* Erickson's review included 15 research studies that met the inclusion criteria of being published between 1980 and 2003, published in English, included the age range of 12 to 19 years (the generally defined age span for adolescence), and that examined or described physical symptoms related to cancer or its treatment.

Excluded from the review were studies focused on long-term survival, psychological experiences or symptoms, outcomes of treatment, and single case studies (Erickson).

Her results suggest that adolescents with cancer, like adults, frequently have fatigue and consider fatigue to be a distressing symptom during their adjustment to and management of cancer. In addition, some of the studies suggest a link between the experience of fatigue and anemia as well as the adolescent's altered nutritional status. Descriptions of fatigue in the reviewed research included "feeling tired," "lack of energy," "not wanting to be bothered" (Erickson, 2004, pp. 142-143). Fatigue was seen as a combination of physical symptoms and mental exhaustion.

Erickson's integrative review expands the base upon which additional research about fatigue in adolescents with cancer can occur. She offers some suggestions about helping the adolescent manage fatigue, such as being flexible with adolescent sleep routine, organizing activities to minimize energy expenditure, facilitating appropriate recreational activities that are interesting and healthy but conserve energy, improving nutritional status by providing nutritious adolescent-friendly foods, and assistance with relaxing and sleep promotion activities. Consider what the experience of fatigue would mean to an adolescent who continues to attend school. What types of modifications to the adolescent's schedule could facilitate learning while conserving energy? How might a school nurse work with the school administrators to advocate for the adolescent?

Erickson, J. (2004). Fatigue in adolescents with cancer: A review of the literature. *Clinical Journal of Oncology Nursing, 8*(2), 139-145.
*Burns, N., & Grove, S. (2005). *The practice of nursing research* (5th ed.). Philadelphia: Elsevier Saunders.

Erythema within the radiated area is the most common side effect. Fatigue associated with therapy may necessitate more frequent rest periods than parents are used to their child taking. Anorexia, nausea, and vomiting commonly occur. Radiation therapy will also cause bone marrow suppression depending on the dose and site of therapy.

Radiation therapy slows the growth of tumors and kills rapidly dividing cells nonselectively. Unfortunately, in a developing child normal cell development may not be complete when radiation exposure occurs. Radiation therapy to developing brain tissue may alter cognitive potential. In children younger than 3 years, the effect of radiation therapy can be cognitively devastating. Bone growth is altered if radiation therapy is delivered to areas of growth potential, such as facial bones, spine, or growth plates in long bones. The result many years later may be skeletal malformations.

The use of radiation as a treatment modality is not without risk. Radiation exposure has been linked to the development of certain types of cancer, and radiation exposure to treat cancer may lead to the development of a second malignancy. Approximately 8% of children treated for cancer will have a second malignancy develop. A subset of this 8% will be linked to the exposure to radiation as a primary treatment (Mettler & Stazzone, 2004).

Hematopoietic Stem Cell Transplantation

In recent years, the use of hematopoietic stem cell transplantation (HSCT) has become accepted therapy for the treatment of several hematologic and oncologic disorders. Transplantation allows extremely high doses of chemotherapy (with or without radiation) to be given without regard for bone marrow recovery because hematopoiesis will be restored through transplantation. Stem cells are harvested from bone marrow, peripheral blood, and umbilical cord blood. HSCT is often used interchangeably with bone marrow transplant (BMT) in the clinical setting even when the reference is toward stem cells from cord or peripheral blood.

BMT uses bone marrow to reconstitute the immunologic function of the patient after high-dose chemotherapy. Stem cell transplantation uses a unique immature cell present in the peripheral circulation to restore immunologic function in a similar manner. Stem cells are able to differentiate into any type of hematologic cell.

The healthy bone marrow cells or stem cells are infused into the bloodstream and migrate to the marrow space to replenish the patient's immunologic function. The decision regarding the source of marrow or stem cells depends on the disease process being treated and the availability of an appropriate donor source.

Recent advances in the understanding of histocompatibility and advances in supportive care have improved outcomes in allogeneic (matched related or unrelated donor) transplants. The patient's own harvested stem cells (an autologous transplant) using peripheral blood can be the source of stem cells in certain instances. This allows aggressive chemotherapy than could be safely given without fear of total bone marrow ablation. Peripheral blood stem cells (PBSCs) are then given back to "rescue" and restore hematopoietic function.

Umbilical cord blood is another source of transplanted stem cells. Because of the ability to "bank" or store umbilical cord blood, this source is becoming more significant. Cord blood from infants is easily harvested and banked. The donor undergoes no risk during harvesting of the cord blood, and the graft is thought to be more immunologically "tolerant" than stem cells from older donors. A national or international search for a matched, unrelated donor can be done through the National Marrow Donor Program (NMDP).

In preparation for a transplant, the child begins a regimen of chemotherapy with or without radiation (called *conditioning*). The goal of conditioning is to eradicate any disease from the body with high-dose chemotherapy and radiation therapy. WBC, red blood cell (RBC), and platelet counts begin to drop as the chemotherapy and radiation exert their effects on the bone marrow. When the conditioning phase is over, the child receives the donor marrow or stem cells by IV infusion.

Once the marrow is infused, nursing care focuses on preventing profoundly immunosuppressed children from developing life-threatening infections. The "waiting game" begins for parents and children until the daily complete blood cell count (CBC) begins to show signs of marrow engraftment. The production of WBCs, RBCs, and platelets from the transplantation of normal cells is evidence that the marrow has "engrafted," or been accepted by the body.

Common complications in the days and weeks after a HSCT include mucositis, diarrhea, fevers, and nosebleeds. Children receive aggressive nutritional support because most will not be able to take food and fluids as a result of severe mucositis and GI discomfort and diarrhea.

The major problem associated with allogeneic transplants is graft-versus-host disease (GVHD). GVHD is caused when the infused immunocompetent bone marrow recognizes the recipient's tissue as foreign. GVHD may affect numerous organ systems. Children can exhibit a wide variety of symptoms associated with GVHD, such as mild to severely elevated liver enzyme levels, mild to copious diarrhea, and maculopapular skin reactions ranging from rashes to full skin desquamation. Antirejection drugs such as prednisone, cyclosporine, and tacrolimus are given to prevent GVHD from occurring or lessen its severity.

Transplantation is currently standard therapy for children in first remission with Philadelphia chromosome–positive ALL (a genetically specific type of ALL with a 90% relapse rate), AML, stage IV neuroblastoma, severe aplastic anemia, severe combined immunodeficiency syndrome, and certain other hematologic disorders. Transplantation is also used for children with certain solid tumors, Hodgkin disease, and non-Hodgkin lymphoma resistant to conventional chemotherapy and radiation, as evidenced by relapse while the child is receiving therapy (Robertson, 2004).

Biologic Agents

Recent additions to cancer therapy are the biologic response modifiers. Biologic response modifiers are naturally occurring substances found in small quantities in the body that influence immune system functions (e.g., colony-stimulating factors [CSFs]).

Used to enhance cell recovery, different CSFs work on different types of blood cells to reduce the time and severity of bone marrow suppression. The granulocyte colony-stimulating factors (GCSFs) stimulate WBC recovery. GCSFs may reduce the length of time a child has neutropenia by stimulating production of neutrophils, a type of granulocyte. Other CSFs may promote recovery of platelets or RBCs to reduce the need for blood products.

Over the past few years, a number of immune-modulating agents have been examined in the laboratory with few translating into clinically beneficial treatment modalities. Some "targeted" monoclonal antibodies are being used for non-Hodgkin lymphomas. Interleukin, a protein that mobilizes the immune response, interferon, and activated T-cell antigens are all in ongoing clinical trials to evaluate their roles in the treatment of cancer (Bleyer, 2004).

CRITICAL THINKING EXERCISE 24-1

When caring for children with cancer, nurses often encounter families who want to try a method of complementary or alternative therapy to treat the child's cancer. If the family brings up the subject in conversation with the nurse, the family should be referred to the child's oncologist to explore motivation and acceptable use of therapies for the specific child. However, nurses must be aware of issues involved with complementary and alternative therapies. Think about the issues involved with the use of complementary and alternative therapies.
1. What is the difference between the two?
2. How does one learn about what particular therapies can be incorporated into the child's plan of care?
3. How can health professionals help families evaluate complementary and alternative therapies?

LEUKEMIA

Childhood leukemia was the first disseminated cancer demonstrated to be curable, and the approach to childhood leukemia set the standard for principles of cancer diagnosis, prognosis, and treatment (Tubergen & Bleyer, 2004). Leukemia is the most common form of cancer in children younger than 15 years. The cause of disease is an abnormal proliferation of immature WBCs (blasts), which compete with normal cells for space and nutrients. Bone marrow production is suppressed so very low numbers of WBCs (leukopenia), RBCs (anemia), and platelets (thrombocytopenia) may be seen at diagnosis. Considerable progress in treatment has been achieved through years of research. Leukemia was uniformly fatal in the 1960s. Today children diagnosed with the most common form of leukemia, ALL, can almost always achieve remission with a 5-year disease-free survival rate approaching 85% (Campana & Pui, 2004).

Etiology

The cause of childhood leukemia is unknown. Geographic distribution varies around the world, with leukemia being uncommon in developing countries but more common in industrialized countries. This variation may be correlated with underdiagnosis in developing countries or exposure to agents that may be implicated in the development of leukemia in industrialized countries.

Genetic factors appear to play a significant role in the development of leukemia. When karyotyped, the leukemic cells in most affected children with the disease reveal chromosomal abnormalities (Tubergen & Bleyer, 2004). The fraternal twin of a child who has had ALL has a two to four ~~times higher likelihood of~~ _____ _____ disease than other children. For identical twins, the unaffected twin has a 20% risk of developing the disease. Children with Down syndrome have a 10% to 20% greater risk of developing leukemia than the general population (Campana & Pui, 2004). Other less-common preexisting chromosomal abnormalities, such as Fanconi anemia and neurofibromatosis, have been correlated with the development of leukemia.

Exposure to ionizing radiation and certain chemical toxins has been shown to increase the risk of leukemia development. Leukemia was well documented in both the child and adult survivors of the atomic bomb detonations in Japan during World War II. Chemical exposure to alkylating agents, a drug class used to treat cancer, has been shown to increase the risk of developing AML.

Large epidemiologic studies are ongoing to examine links to pesticide exposure, electromagnetic fields, parental smoking, parental alcohol use, and parental exposures to occupational chemicals. Thus far relations to leukemia have not been demonstrated.

Incidence

Leukemia represents approximately 40% of all childhood cancers. Approximately 3,600 new cases of childhood leukemia are diagnosed each year in the United States (Tubergen & Bleyer, 2004). Overall incidence of ALL has been constant for the past 30 years and accounts for approximately 80% of all cases of leukemia; AML accounts for 15%, and chronic myelocytic leukemia (CML) and other subtypes are relatively rare. The peak incidence occurs between ages 2 and 6 years for ALL. Leukemia is more common in boys than in girls.

Manifestations

Clinical manifestations of leukemia include fever, pallor, excessive bruising, bone or joint pain (usually leg/knee pain), lymphadenopathy, malaise, hepatosplenomegaly, abnormal

WBC counts (either lower or higher than normal for age), and mild to profound anemia and thrombocytopenia. The severity of the clinical manifestations varies with the cell type of leukemia and the length of time before diagnosis.

Diagnostic Evaluation

The diagnosis can be strongly suspected from a history of the clinical manifestations and an initial CBC. The confirmatory test for leukemia is microscopic examination of bone marrow obtained by bone marrow aspiration and biopsy. A bone marrow aspirate alone usually provides sufficient material to establish the diagnosis of ALL. A lumbar puncture is also performed to look for blast cells in the spinal fluid that are indicative of CNS involvement.

Therapeutic Management

Combination chemotherapy is the preferred treatment for leukemia. The particular drugs used and their dose, route, and scheduling depend on the _protocol_ that will be used for that specific type of leukemia. Children are placed into prognostic categories with specifically designed therapies. Treatment of ALL is divided into phases: induction, consolidation, and maintenance. The aim of the first month of chemotherapy treatment, or induction, is to induce remission. Remission is the reduction of immature blast cells in the bone marrow to less than 5%. Approximately 98% of children achieve remission within 1 month (Tubergen & Bleyer, 2004).

Before induction, the child is treated for presenting signs, which may include sepsis, anemia, hemorrhage, and metabolic abnormalities. Serum electrolyte levels are determined to ensure metabolic stability before chemotherapy is initiated. An elevated uric acid level, indicating rapid cell turnover, can be expected if the WBC count is very high. As WBCs break down in reaction to chemotherapy, they release uric acid, which is poorly water soluble, into the serum, which can compromise kidney function (see discussion of tumor lysis syndrome, p. 773). Before receiving chemotherapy, allopurinol and IV fluids with sodium bicarbonate are given to decrease the serum uric acid level and alkalinize the urine. Parenteral urate oxidase may be given in situations when lysing of the tumor by chemotherapy is expected to be significant. This recombinant enzyme oxidizes uric acid into a water-soluble product that can be excreted (Taketomo, Hodding, & Kraus, 2005). This is especially important when the WBC count is extremely high. During induction, the hospitalized child receives the first doses of chemotherapy while the response to the drugs is assessed. Remission can be verified within the first 28 days after the initiation of chemotherapy by sequential bone marrow aspirates and lumbar punctures. If a significant number of blast cells are still present, a new and stronger drug regimen is given. The presence of more than 5% blasts in the marrow at day 28 is an ominous sign indicative of a poorer prognosis.

Once the child is medically stable, most chemotherapy treatment for ALL is given on an outpatient basis. Children are usually healthy and able to return to school and lead relatively normal lives.

PATHOPHYSIOLOGY

LEUKEMIA

Leukemia most likely arises from a fundamental alteration in the genetic makeup of the WBC. Cells produced from the altered cell have a defect that prevents maturation. These cells tend to replicate quickly, forming immature cells, or blast cells, in the bone marrow, which crowd out other normal cells produced. The blast cells do not respond properly to the body's feedback mechanism and continue to replicate in great numbers. Blast cells are then released into the peripheral circulation and appear in a CBC test.

In leukemia, normal bone marrow is replaced by malignant blast cells. As the blast cells take over the bone marrow, eventually RBC and platelet production is affected and the child becomes anemic and thrombocytopenic. The symptoms of the disease reflect bone marrow failure and organ infiltration.

In addition to being present in the blood and bone marrow, leukemia cells infiltrate extramedullary sites, most commonly the CNS and the testicles. Although extramedullary leukemia is not common at diagnosis, these are common sites of relapse.

Leukemias are classified by the type of WBC affected. Broadly, acute leukemias are classified as ALL and acute nonlymphocytic leukemia (ANLL). ALL is an abnormality of the lymphocytes. ANLL is a broad term for leukemias not originating from abnormal lymphocytes. AML is an example of an ANLL. AML can be further classified as acute promyelocytic leukemia (APL), acute myelomonocytic leukemia (AMMoL), and acute monocytic leukemia (AMoL). ANLL tends to be less common in children, less responsive to therapy, difficult to treat, and more likely to result in relapse than ALL.

Chronic leukemias are rare in children. The term *chronic* refers to the indolent nature of the disease. Whereas acute leukemias have a rapid onset to detectable disease, chronic leukemias have a slower onset of symptoms.

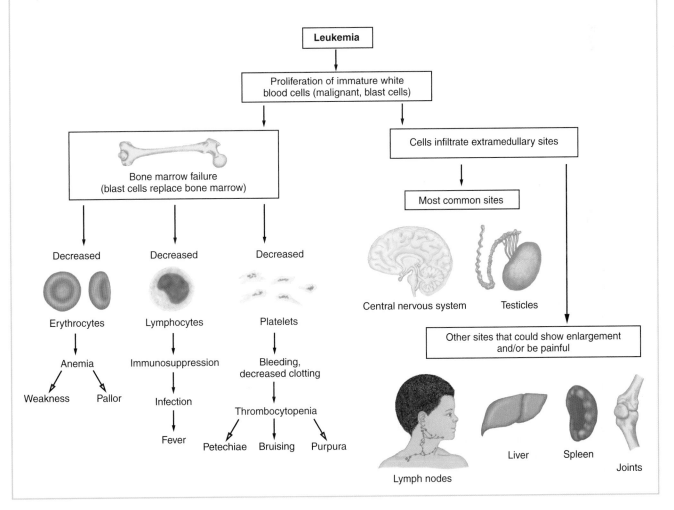

The goal of therapy after remission is to maintain remission and prevent disease in "sanctuary sites," including the testes and CNS. They are referred to as "sanctuary" because systemic therapy is poorly delivered to these areas. Intrathecal chemotherapy is given prophylactically to prevent relapse in the CNS. If the testes are involved, radiation therapy is delivered.

Generally, after the initial induction and consolidation phases, a maintenance phase of treatment is begun. Total treatment time for ALL is approximately 2½ years.

Text continued on p. 769

NURSING CARE PLAN

The Child With Leukemia

Focused Assessment

Subjective data almost always reveal an insidious onset of symptoms. The parents may have recognized the following: their child was less active than normal, had a persistent or recurrent fever of unknown cause, had more bruises than usual, reported an intermittent stomachache that the parents attributed to school avoidance, or had leg pain attributed to growing pains or laziness. Parents commonly express guilt because they did not recognize anything was wrong with their child sooner or, if they did notice, the manifestations were so vague they delayed seeking treatment. Psychosocial assessment of the family is ongoing.

Children often have fever, fatigue, pallor, bruising on the extremities, petechiae in the mouth and sclerae, and hepatosplenomegaly. Children with very high WBC counts or AML may have more pronounced manifestations, such as bleeding. The mental and neurologic status of the child is assessed because of the risk of infiltration into the CNS.

Observe both the child's and the parents' reactions to the disease. The emotional maturity of the child and the family affect how each person copes with the illness and treatment. The child's chronologic age and stage of development as well as previous experience with the health care system are critical factors in the assessment.

Parents who are unable to cope with the disease and who display a high level of anxiety will transfer this anxiety to their child. Children who have had previous negative experiences associated with hospitals, nurses, and physicians may exhibit increased anxiety. Families who have had prior experience with cancer may exhibit increased anxiety and need for support.

NURSING DIAGNOSIS   Risk for Infection related to the immunosuppressed state.

EXPECTED OUTCOMES   The child will:
- Be free of signs of infection, as evidenced by an afebrile state, no redness of the integument, no redness or swelling at the site of insertion of a central venous catheter, and negative culture results.

The parents and the child will:
- Recognize and verbalize early signs of infection.

Intervention	*Rationale*
1. Monitor vital signs every 4 hours and as necessary if the child is hospitalized. Instruct parents to measure the child's temperature as needed at home (by the oral, axillary, or tympanic routes only).	1. In the presence of markedly decreased WBCs, an elevated temperature may be the only sign of infection. The risk of injury to the fragile mucous membranes is so great that only oral, tympanic, or axillary routes should be used to measure temperatures. Rectal abscesses can easily occur to friable rectal tissue. Temperatures should not be measured rectally. Report a single temperature 38.5° C (101.3° F) or a temperature of 38.0° C (100.4° F) that continues for more than 1 hour.
2. Monitor CBC with differential as ordered. Report moderate to severe neutropenia. **Absolute Neutrophil Count (ANC) (cells/mm³)** **Risk** 1500-2000 Not significant 1000-1500 Minimal 500-1000 Moderate <500 Severe	2. The risk of infection increases significantly with moderate and severe neutropenia.
3. Practice proper handwashing and teach this to the family.	3. Proper handwashing is the best way to prevent the spread of infection.

4. Inspect the child's skin daily for breaks and redness.

5. Inspect the child's mouth daily for oral ulcers, and inspect the perineum for fissures. Teach older children to do self-examination. No suppositories should be given.

6. Encourage and monitor regular bowel habits.

7. Teach the parents and child meticulous oral hygiene at diagnosis:
   a. Use a soft-bristled toothbrush or toothettes.
   b. Perform oral hygiene four times a day.
   c. If the platelet count is low, use a cotton-tipped applicator, finger cot, or washcloth wrapped around a finger instead of a toothbrush.
8. At the first signs of mouth ulcers, begin a mouth care regimen three or four times daily, including an antifungal drug as ordered by the physician. Avoid alcohol-containing mouthwashes.

9. For the hospitalized neutropenic child, fresh flowers or plants are usually not permitted. Do not use humidifiers.
10. Use sterile techniques to change any dressings and IV lines.
11. In general, the child should not receive live-virus or live bacterial vaccines. Special circumstances exist when risks of the disease outweigh risks of the vaccine. Siblings should receive inactivated polio vaccine but may receive live measles-mumps-rubella (MMR) vaccine or varicella vaccine. Flu shots are recommended for family members and close contacts.

12. Keep any child with chickenpox or any child who has been exposed to the virus away from the child with cancer. Inform the teacher of the importance of notifying parents immediately if a case of chickenpox occurs in another child at school. Encourage vaccination of siblings who have not had varicella to create "herd" immunity.
13. Obtain specimens for culture as ordered and monitor the results.

14. Administer acetaminophen for fever.

15. Administer antibiotics as ordered after culture results are available.

4. Some neutropenic children will not produce erythema or purulent drainage. Because pus is made of WBCs, drainage cannot be used as a sign of infection. Skin provides a barrier against infection.
5. The mucous membranes are fragile and easily affected by chemotherapy and irradiation. Mouth ulcers and rectal fissures are common side effects of chemotherapy and radiation therapy and potential sites for bacteria entry because of the impaired mucosa.
6. Decreased activity, altered nutrition, and certain medications may predispose to constipation. The passage of hard stool may traumatize delicate rectal mucous membranes and create a potential site for entry of bacteria.
7. Preventing dental caries and ulcerations on fragile oral mucosa will help prevent infections.

8. Fungal infections originating from the mouth or GI tract can quickly become disseminated in immunosuppressed children. Over-the-counter mouthwashes may have a high alcohol content and may be drying to oral mucosa, thus increasing the risk of breaking down the protective barrier of the skin.
9. Standing water and damp soil harbor *Aspergillus* and *Pseudomonas,* to which these children are extremely susceptible.
10. Because the child with neutropenia is not able to fight infection normally, extra precautions must be taken.
11. Live virus is shed in the stool after administration of the oral polio vaccine. The live MMR vaccine could produce infection in the severely immunocompromised child, but no virus shedding occurs to create a threat if given to the sibling. Exposure to a rash produced by the varicella vaccine does have the potential of causing varicella disease in an immunocompromised child. If rash should occur in a vaccinated sibling, the immunocompromised child should be separated from the sibling until the rash resolves.
12. Immunocompromised patients are unable to fight varicella adequately. Chickenpox can be deadly to the immunocompromised child (see Fig. 24-2). If a child who has not had chickenpox is exposed to someone with varicella, the child should receive varicella zoster immune globulin within 96 hours of exposure.
13. Physicians will order blood, urine, stool, and wound cultures as signs appear when the neutropenic child has fever.
14. Aspirin and ibuprofen given to a child who is thrombocytopenic can cause platelet dysfunction.
15. Cultures identify the specific organism so that the most effective antibiotic can be given. Appropriate antibiotic treatment should begin promptly.

Continued

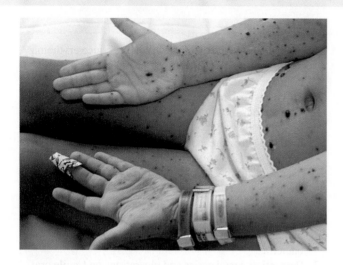

FIG 24-2 **Varicella (chickenpox) can be deadly in the immunocompromised child. Thrombocytopenia (low platelet count) associated with chemotherapy can cause the varicella lesions to be hemorrhagic, as those shown here. Secondary infections of the lesions are also common because of low WBC counts.** *(Courtesy Cook Children's Medical Center, Hematology-Oncology Clinic, Fort Worth, TX.)*

NURSING CARE PLAN—cont'd

Evaluation

- Is the child afebrile and free of redness or swelling at insertion sites or other integumentary sites?
- Have the child and parents promptly recognized and responded to warning signs of infection?

NURSING DIAGNOSIS   Risk for Injury related to thrombocytopenia.

EXPECTED OUTCOMES   The child will:
- Have no excessive, uncontrolled bleeding.

The parents and child will:
- Understand risk for hemorrhage, as evidenced by making the home environment safe and by their ability to respond appropriately to bleeding.

Intervention

1. Apply gentle, firm pressure to any puncture sites. Apply a pressure dressing to sites of bone marrow aspiration.
2. If the child is severely thrombocytopenic (platelet count <20,000/mm³), take the following steps:
   a. Limit any activity that could result in head injury; encourage the child to participate in quiet activities (e.g., reading books, watching videos, coloring). No contact sports are allowed.
   b. Provide a soft-bristled toothbrush only or toothettes.
   c. Give stool softeners to prevent straining with constipation.
   d. Do not use suppositories.
   e. Check urine and stools for blood.
   f. Avoid sharp foods such as chips.
3. Teach the child how to control nosebleeds and blow the nose gently.

4. Evaluate menstrual flow in adolescent girls.

Rationale

1. Additional pressure may be needed to stop bleeding if the platelet count is low.
2. A decreased platelet count increases the risk for bleeding. Intracranial hemorrhage is a potential risk.

3. One of the most common sites of bleeding is the nose. Blood loss can be reduced through avoidance of nosebleeds.
4. Menstrual bleeding can be severe when girls have low platelet counts. Occasionally hormone therapy is required to inhibit menses.

Evaluation

- Has the child had bleeding that could not be controlled?
- Have the parents demonstrated what to do for a nosebleed?

- Have the child or parents promptly recognized and responded to bleeding?

NURSING CARE PLAN—cont'd

NURSING DIAGNOSIS Imbalanced Nutrition: Less Than Body Requirements related to nausea and vomiting, mucositis, or taste changes.

EXPECTED OUTCOMES The child will:
- Experience no more than 5% weight loss.
- Eat palatable foods that provide appropriate nutrients for growth.

Intervention	*Rationale*
1. Administer antiemetics prophylactically and as needed or as ordered.	1. Antiemetics will decrease or prevent vomiting.
2. When the child is nauseated, offer cool, clear liquids. Offer bland, soft foods at room temperature, served in small portions. Be creative with the liquids and foods offered to make them more interesting and inviting.	2. Cool liquids and foods are soothing and better tolerated than hot ones, and the risk of burning fragile mucosa is eliminated.
3. Offer small, frequent meals of high-protein and high-calorie content. Fortify foods with nutritional supplements. Allow the family to bring favorite foods to the hospital.	3. Small, frequent meals are better tolerated than large ones. Protein promotes tissue healing. A large number of calories are needed for growth. Children are more likely to eat their favorite foods.
4. Avoid offering favorite foods when the child is nauseated.	4. Foods eaten within hours of nausea will be associated with being sick.
5. Administer ordered mouth analgesics before oral intake.	5. If mouth sores are present, analgesics will increase comfort and provide interest in eating.
6. Monitor daily weight. Keep strict intake and output records. Weigh the infant's diapers.	6. Strict measurement ensures adequate intake and provides an objective assessment to alert the nurse that further interventions may be needed.
7. Involve the child in food selection.	7. Food selection allows the child control over as much as possible and may increase interest and participation in eating.
8. Include a dietitian in the nutritional assessment and evaluation.	8. A dietitian provides specialized input into developing and evaluating nutritional status.

Evaluation

- Did the child have no more than 5% weight loss, as documented on a growth chart?
- Does the child eat foods that provide appropriate nutrients for growth?

NURSING DIAGNOSIS Deficient Knowledge related to unfamiliarity with the disease process and treatment plan.

EXPECTED OUTCOMES The child and parents will:
- Explain the diagnosis.
- Demonstrate adherence to treatment.

Intervention	*Rationale*
1. Assess the child's and parents' readiness for learning. Create an environment of learning.	1. On initial diagnosis, family members may need time to adjust before they are ready for education. Offer written supporting information.
2. On initial diagnosis and during subsequent follow-up visits, spend time with the family, repeating and explaining the diagnosis, its sequelae, and its treatment. Offer written literature or offer to tape educational sessions (Box 24-3).	2. Education is ongoing and will need reinforcing with stressed parents. Education should specifically include demonstrating procedures required for care, ways to approach nausea, managing fatigue and other side effects, and facilitating normal development (Moore & Beckwitt, 2004). Explaining the treatment rationale and sequelae helps ensure adherence to therapy. Written or taped information can be reviewed later for better absorption.
3. Keep explanations at the family's level of understanding.	3. Vary explanations to meet the family's educational level.
4. Offer encouragement for parents' recognition of danger signs and parents' appropriate use of medical care.	4. Praise reinforces behavior. Parents want to know they are doing the right thing for their child.

Continued

| BOX 24-3 | **PARENTS WANT TO KNOW**   About Caring for the Child With Cancer |

- Reinforce teaching concerning diagnosis, treatment, and side effects of chemotherapy.
- Encourage parents to participate actively in the child's care.
- Provide written and verbal instructions concerning home care, and provide ample opportunity for parents to give return demonstrations of the following:
  Central venous access dressing changes
  Oral medication administration
  Assessment of oral mucous membranes
  Temperature measurement by axillary, oral, and tympanic routes

- Teach the signs and symptoms of infection and bleeding that require immediate treatment and how to access after-hours emergency treatment.
- Provide telephone numbers needed for questions concerning the diagnosis, treatment, and side effects of chemotherapy.
- Make appropriate referrals to social services, a chaplain or other religious figure, and a home health nursing agency.
- Encourage parents to use community resources.
- Stress the importance of preventing infection (see Fig. 24-2) and bleeding and the need for follow-up visits.

NURSING CARE PLAN—cont'd

Evaluation

- Have the parents and child demonstrated an understanding of the treatment protocols by adhering to therapy and seeking appropriate medical care for danger signs?

NURSING DIAGNOSIS   Disturbed Body Image related to hair loss.

EXPECTED OUTCOMES   The child will:
- Adapt to alopecia, as evidenced by a return to socialization.
- Discuss concerns related to hair loss.

Intervention	*Rationale*
1. Instruct the child and parents on the progression of hair loss and potential changes in color and texture when the hair regrows. Suggest obtaining a wig before hair is lost or bringing a clipping of hair with a recent photograph.	1. Reassure that hair loss is temporary for most cancers, but some cranial irradiation can result in patches of permanent hair loss. Matching a wig to original hair color, texture, and style is easier before hair is lost.
2. Encourage verbalization of feelings about hair loss. Enlist the help of a child life specialist to engage the child in play therapy.	2. Allowing the child to verbalize concerns about returning to a social environment or school is important. Play therapy is a safe way for the child to express feelings and fears.
3. Discuss ways to minimize the reaction to alopecia by promoting creative solutions, such as hats, wigs, or scarves.	3. Allowing children to create their own headpieces may minimize the negative impact of hair loss.
4. Make visits to the child's classroom.	4. Preparation of classmates for the child's school reentry will lessen classmates' negative reactions, fears, anxiety, and lack of understanding. It will also increase the support they can give the ill child.
5. Encourage a return to school as soon as possible.	5. The sooner the child returns to school, the less likely the child will begin a pattern of absenteeism. If the child returns to school before major body changes take place, the changes may not be so noticeable to the other children, thus decreasing undesirable reactions.

Evaluation

- Is the child involved in prediagnosis social life?
- Has the child discussed hair loss and feelings connected with body image?

NURSING DIAGNOSIS   Ineffective Coping (individual) or Compromised Family Coping related to chronic illness.

EXPECTED OUTCOMES   The child will:
- Adhere to the treatment plan.
  The parents will:
- Verbalize concerns about the impact of the illness on their family.
  The child and parents will:
- Use available support systems and community resources.

NURSING CARE PLAN—cont'd

Intervention

1. Teach the family the necessity of adhering to the protocol. Teach the warning signs of problems and how to access after-hours emergency care.
2. Listen and encourage the child and family to verbalize their feelings and express their concerns. Answer questions honestly and openly.
3. Introduce the family to other families of children with cancer.
4. Consult social services and a chaplain or appropriate religious figure.
5. Offer a list of local support groups appropriate to the child's age and the family's individual needs.

Rationale

1. Conscientious application of the treatment plan increases the chance of a positive outcome.

2. Identifying concerns and clarifying misconceptions will help families cope with the stress of chronic illness.

3. Other families of children with cancer can offer suggestions and support.
4. The financial and emotional burden of caring for a child with cancer can be overwhelming.
5. Support groups of individuals in similar situations can provide much comfort and support to the child and the family.

Evaluation

- Is the family adhering to the treatment plan?
- Do the family and child verbalize appropriate concerns and questions?

- Has the family contacted a local support group?

NURSING DIAGNOSIS Acute Pain and Chronic Pain related to the disease process and procedures.

EXPECTED OUTCOME The child will:
- Experience decreased discomfort, as evidenced by periods of uninterrupted rest, verbalization of increased comfort, indication of increased comfort on an age-appropriate pain assessment tool, and participation in play activities.

Intervention

1. Explain procedures to the child in an age-appropriate manner before performing them.
2. Monitor for signs and symptoms of pain, such as inactivity for age, increased heart rate or blood pressure, grimacing, verbalization of discomfort, irritability, and crying. Use a developmentally appropriate assessment tool and nonverbal cues to evaluate pain.
3. Administer comfort measures as needed, such as positioning, adjusting room temperature, and offering distractions appropriate for age.
4. Administer analgesics promptly as ordered. Use topical anesthetics for procedural pain. Ensure analgesia or nonpharmacologic strategies before painful procedures.

5. Explain the pain-control regimen to the parents and child, as age appropriate.
6. Notify the physician if pain relief is not obtained with the ordered dose of analgesic.

7. Enlist a child life specialist's help before and during procedures.

8. Administer antianxiety drugs as ordered (see Chapter 15).

Rationale

1. Honest explanations build rapport and reduce fear.

2. Younger children will not be able to verbalize pain. Stoic children may not express discomfort. Nurses must watch for physiologic signs of pain.

3. Comfort measures can decrease the perception of pain and even decrease the amount of analgesic needed.

4. Analgesics reduce the pain of procedures and of the disease. Delays in analgesic administration can increase anxiety and thus increase pain. Nonpharmacologic interventions can decrease anxiety and pain.

5. Parents know their child and can help the nurse assess pain and report it promptly.
6. Pain tolerance varies greatly among children. Dosage increases may be needed, especially in the child with chronic pain or the dying child.

7. Child life specialists are trained to use distraction techniques with children and represent a "safe" person for the child to be with during repeated painful procedures.
8. Especially in the adolescent, anticipation of a painful procedure may worsen the pain. Giving an antianxiety drug may help calm the child so the procedure is better tolerated.

Evaluation

- Does the child express decreased levels of discomfort, and is this evident on an appropriate pain assessment tool?

- Is the child joining other children in play?

Continued

NURSING CARE PLAN—cont'd

NURSING DIAGNOSIS Impaired Skin Integrity related to radiation therapy, chemotherapy, and immobility.
EXPECTED OUTCOME The child and family will:
* Appropriately manage any problems with skin integrity.

Intervention	Rationale
1. Document the child's skin condition each shift.	1. Skin erythema is common with radiation therapy but should not progress to skin breakdown.
2. Use only approved lotions and creams on the skin and instruct parents in the same.	2. Some commercial lotions can increase skin irritation and redness.
3. Avoid excessive scrubbing of skin, hot water, and abrasive soaps.	3. Friction may increase skin breakdown. Hot water is uncomfortable to irritated tissue.
4. Offer loose clothing of soft materials.	4. Tight clothing or abrasive fabrics may further irritate the skin.
5. Notify the physician if skin breakdown occurs.	5. Additional orders for therapeutic creams may be needed.
6. If the child is immobile, gently turn and vary the position at least every 2 hours and teach parents to do the same.	6. Immobility may increase pressure on skin and promote breakdown.

Evaluation

* Has the child's skin remained intact, and can parents describe skin care techniques?

NURSING DIAGNOSIS Impaired Oral Mucous Membranes related to chemotherapy and radiation therapy.
EXPECTED OUTCOME The child will:
* Show no signs of side effects of treatment, as evidenced by intact oral and rectal mucous membrane.

Intervention	Rationale
1. Monitor the child's mouth and anus each shift for ulcers, erythema, or breakdown. Teach the parent or child, if age appropriate, the same. Report ulcerations to the physician.	1. A breakdown in mucous membranes usually begins with erythema and progresses to ulcerations. Home care should include this assessment for the duration of therapy. Additional medications, mouth rinses, or ointments are ordered if ulcerations occur.
2. Do not take a rectal temperature in a child undergoing chemotherapy or radiation therapy. Do not take oral temperatures if mouth ulcers are present. Teach parents how to take accurate axillary or tympanic temperatures.	2. The introduction of a thermometer into the rectum or mouth of a child with fragile mucous membranes, no matter how carefully done, can tear tissue.
3. Begin meticulous mouth care, avoiding alcohol-based mouthwashes, several times a day with a soft-bristled toothbrush or toothettes.	3. Frequent mouth care will help remove bacteria from the oral mucosa, decreasing the risk of infection of irritated tissue.
4. If the rectum becomes irritated, begin sitz baths several times a day and after bowel movements.	4. Lukewarm sitz baths keep the perineum clean and soothe irritated tissue.
5. In diaper-wearing children, use only diaper wipes that do not contain alcohol or perfumes. If the perineum is very irritated, use only warm water wipes of the area.	5. Alcohol and perfumes will further irritate the skin and can cause great discomfort. Very few commercial diaper wipes are safe for these children.
6. Offer bland, nonirritating foods and cool liquids.	6. Citrus products may be quite painful to an ulcerated mouth, as well as may spicy foods. Cool liquids are soothing. Ice pops and slushes are usually well tolerated.

Evaluation

* Has the child exhibited signs of oral mucositis or rectal ulceration?

BRAIN TUMORS

Brain tumors are the most common solid tumor and the second most common childhood malignancy after leukemia. Brain tumors are a diverse group of tumors described by their tissue of origin, location within the brain, and rate of growth. Unlike other neoplasms, primary brain tumors are confined to the brain and spine and rarely metastasize to bone marrow or other organs. The mortality rate is significant (approaching 45%), as is morbidity (primarily neurologic) associated with brain tumors and their treatment (Kuttesch & Ater, 2004).

Etiology

The cause of brain tumors remains unknown. Heredity and environment have both been associated with their development. Several inherited syndromes are associated with the development of brain tumors in children, such as neurofibromatosis and tuberous sclerosis. Additional risk factors include immune system suppression and cranial irradiation. Although exposure to electromagnetic fields has been suggested to increase a child's risk of a brain tumor, no confirming evidence supports this theory (Maity, Pruitt, Judy, & Phillips, 2004).

Incidence

In the United States, approximately 2,200 children younger than 20 years are diagnosed with brain tumors annually (Kuttesch & Ater, 2004). CNS tumors represent 35% of solid tumor malignancies diagnosed in children (Dome, Rodriguez-Galindo, Spunt, & Santana, 2004) and 24% of all pediatric cancers (Maity et al., 2004). More than 50% of pediatric CNS tumors develop in the posterior fossa—the lower part of the brain that contains both the cerebellum and the brainstem.

PATHOPHYSIOLOGY

BRAIN TUMORS

Brain tumors are classified according to cell histology and rate of tumor proliferation. Approximately 40% of pediatric brain tumors are astrocytomas, 20% to 25% are medulloblastomas, 10% to 15% are brainstem gliomas, 7% to 10% are craniopharyngiomas, and 10% are ependymomas (Kuttesch & Ater, 2004).

The histology of brain tumors ranges from benign to highly malignant. The impact these tumors have on the brain and the clinical symptoms they produce often have more to do with the tumor size and location than with the aggressiveness of the tumor. The majority of astrocytomas are low grade or slow growing; however, if they persist in spite of treatment, they can produce significant neurologic deficits.

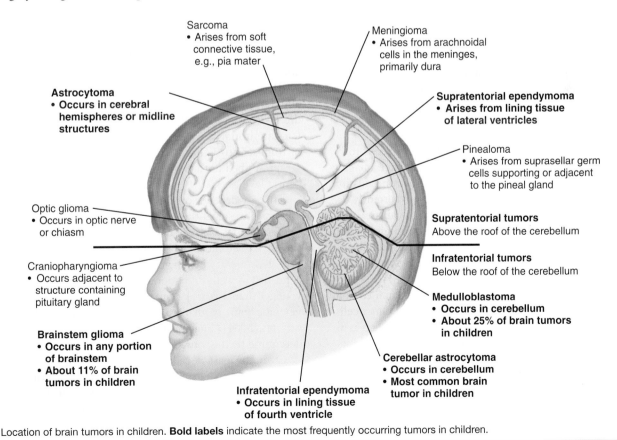

Location of brain tumors in children. **Bold labels** indicate the most frequently occurring tumors in children.

Manifestations

Manifestations of brain tumors vary with tumor location and the child's age and development. Symptoms produced by tumors in the posterior fossa include ataxia (unsteady gait), poor coordination of the upper extremities, visual changes (nystagmus, diplopia, strabismus), and occasionally head tilt. Tumors in this location are frequently associated with increased intracranial pressure (ICP) caused by the tumor mass itself or, more commonly, by the tumor obstructing the normal flow of cerebrospinal fluid (CSF). Increased ICP often causes headaches, vomiting, and lethargy. These symptoms are usually most intense on arising in the morning. Symptoms of increased ICP are frequently subacute and nonspecific.

Infants may be irritable, be lethargic, and feed poorly and have increased head circumference and bulging fontanel. Many younger children demonstrate loss of developmental milestones. School-age children may exhibit declining academic performance, fatigue, personality changes, and symptoms of vague, intermittent headache. Cranial nerve deficits and hemiparesis are usually associated with brainstem involvement. Supratentorial tumors characteristically present with headaches, seizures, or focal neurologic deficits. Especially with slow-growing tumors, symptoms may be subtle and initially attributed to more common childhood illnesses.

CRITICAL TO REMEMBER
Signs of Brain Tumor in Children

The hallmark symptoms of children with brain tumors are headache and morning vomiting related to the child getting out of bed. The sudden increase in intracranial pressure with the change in position causes the vomiting.

Diagnostic Evaluation

Once a tumor is suspected, evaluation is considered to be an emergency. Imaging with magnetic resonance imaging (MRI), computed tomography (CT), or positron emission tomography (PET) may be performed. MRI is currently the imaging modality most commonly used to evaluate brain tumors. During MRI, the child must lie motionless inside a dark tunnel for approximately 1 hour. This is especially difficult for young children. In general, children younger than 6 years need sedation. A spinal MRI is performed to look for metastatic disease in the spine. A CSF sample obtained from lumbar puncture is examined for the presence of tumor cells. In some cases, the tumor produces tumor markers such as alpha fetoprotein that can be identified in the CSF or blood.

Usually the diagnosis is suspected from the child's signs and symptoms and the location of the tumor (Fig. 24-3). Pathologic examination confirms the tissue type and tumor diagnosis. On the rare occasion when the tumor is not surgically accessible, the diagnosis must be made on the basis of location and radiologic evaluation alone.

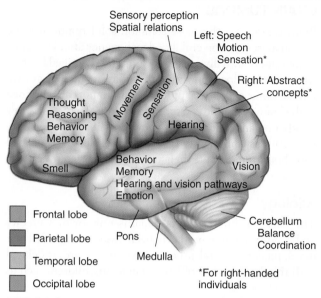

FIG 24-3 **Lobes of the brain (for right-handed individuals).**

Therapeutic Management

Initial intervention for a child with a brain tumor is surgery. The goal is to remove as much of the tumor as possible while minimally disturbing the surrounding brain tissue so that the child's neurologic functioning is preserved to the highest degree possible. Complete removal of the tumor is associated with the best prognosis. In the case of a brainstem tumor or optic pathway glioma, the risk to neurologic function outweighs the benefit of resection, so surgery is not performed. Depending on the location of the tumor and the extent of surgical resection, a ventriculoperitoneal (VP) shunt may be inserted to relieve the hydrocephalus and the symptoms associated with it (see Chapter 28). Children with tumors located above the roof of the cerebellum (supratentorial) are at risk for seizures from the tumor itself or from scar tissue formation after surgery. These children are prescribed anticonvulsants with monitoring of therapeutic levels.

Therapy depends on the type of tumor, its location, the amount of residual tumor after surgery, and the child's age. Benign tumors, such as low-grade astrocytomas, require only surgery if the tumor can be completely resected. Often, however, treatment with chemotherapy and radiation therapy is needed as well. Radiation therapy is avoided in children younger than 3 years because of the toxic effects on the developing brain, particularly in very young children (Kuttesch & Ater, 2004). Imaging is performed at intervals to help determine the response to therapy.

Over the past decade, chemotherapy has emerged as treatment for pediatric brain tumors, either in conjunction with radiation therapy or alone. Prognostic percentages vary with the type of tumor, the amount resected, metastatic spread, age and physical status of the child, and individual response.

NURSING CARE

The Child With a Brain Tumor

Assessment

A thorough neurologic examination is paramount for any child diagnosed with a brain tumor. Knowing the location of the tumor heightens the nurse's understanding of neurologic deficits the child may have (see Fig. 24-3). A good psychosocial and developmental history is important to obtain, including information regarding the child's neurologic symptoms, achievement of developmental milestones in younger children, and school performance in older children. Children who have insidious loss of vision may have learned to compensate well; excellent nursing skills will be needed to identify vision loss. Consider impaired balance and coordination, brainstem dysfunction, and any loss of vision when assessing the child's safety. The nurse should be especially vigilant for symptoms of increased ICP in children newly diagnosed with a brain tumor, in children in the immediate postoperative period, and in children who have a VP shunt in place. Many children with brain tumors have seizures at some time during their illness, so seizure precautions should be considered even in the child with no previous history of seizures (see Chapter 28). Depending on the length of time the child has been feeling ill, weight loss and poor nutrition may be present. Assess nutritional status throughout treatment.

Nursing Diagnosis and Planning

The following nursing diagnoses and expected outcomes may be appropriate for the child with a brain tumor and the child's family:

- Acute Pain and Chronic Pain related to increased ICP.
  Expected Outcome: The child will verbalize a decrease in the severity of headaches.
- Risk for Infection related to surgery or immunosuppression after chemotherapy.
  Expected Outcome: The child will remain free from signs of infection, as evidenced by body temperature within normal limits and demonstration of infection prevention measures.
- Anxiety (child and parent) related to the surgery and diagnosis.
  Expected Outcome: The child and parents will exhibit decreased anxiety about the outcomes of surgery and therapy, as evidenced by verbalization of less stress and an ability to problem solve.
- Deficient Knowledge about the disease process related to unfamiliarity with the information.
  Expected Outcome: The parents will describe the disease process and its management.
- Disturbed Body Image related to a shaved head, hair loss, and/or neurologic deficits.
  Expected Outcome: The child will demonstrate appropriate coping techniques for hair loss and changes in coordination or other abilities, as evidenced by maintaining social relationships and statements indicating adaptation to the changed appearance.

Interventions

Nursing care focuses on controlling acute symptoms, preparation for surgery, and postoperative management. The family will also need education and support to cope with the significant anxiety caused by the potential neurologic impact of surgery and the fear of treatment failure and death. Preoperative teaching at the child's developmental level prepares the child and family for the potential outcomes of surgery. The child should be educated about anesthesia and should be prepared to spend some time in the intensive care unit after surgery. (See Chapter 13 for a discussion of preoperative care.)

The child's head will be shaved before surgery. Although every effort is made to shave only as much hair as necessary, shaving may still be traumatic for the child. The nurse should be aware of this and assist the child in verbalizing fears. Some children enjoy wearing a favorite cap or hat or making an outing of going to buy a hat. Prepare the child to wake up with a large dressing covering the head.

In addition to postoperative concerns of pain, hemorrhage, and infection, the nurse must also monitor for signs and symptoms of increased ICP. Increased ICP (see Chapter 28) is a risk in the postoperative period related to cerebral edema, hydrocephalus, or hemorrhage. It can also occur at diagnosis or with recurrent tumor because of pressure from the tumor mass and associated edema or CSF obstruction. A shunt malfunction in any child with a VP shunt may result in hydrocephalus and increased ICP. Check and record vital signs, mental status, and neurologic status frequently when the child returns from surgery. Never place the child in Trendelenburg position because it increases ICP and the risk of bleeding. Symptoms that suggest increased ICP in any child diagnosed with a brain tumor should always be brought to the attention of the physician and generally require evaluation, including an MRI or CT scan.

Many children return from the surgical suite with external ventricular shunts in place that temporarily remove CSF as a means to reduce ICP. The external drains must be maintained at appropriate levels and CSF measured accurately. Normal CSF is colorless; bloody or discolored drainage can be a sign of contamination or bleeding. This should be reported to the physician immediately (Bowden & Greenberg, 2003). Many children require placement of a permanent shunt because of secondary hydrocephalus (see Chapter 28.)

After the child's condition has been stabilized, assess for functional deficits resulting from surgery or damage to normal brain tissue by the tumor. These deficits are somewhat predictable if the involved area of the brain and the function of that area are known (Box 24-4). If the deficits are significant, rehabilitative therapy may be necessary to help the child regain function. Studies have shown that radiation to the brain can affect cognitive abilities, with more significant deficits in children treated at a younger age (Kuttesch & Ater, 2004). Adequate academic support should always be considered for these children when they return to school.

If radiation therapy is delivered, the side effects of radiation merit special attention, as previously discussed. Families

After surgery, the child should be assessed for functional deficits in the following areas:
- Gait—look for ataxia, including head control and truncal stability
- Bilateral extremity strength and purposeful movement
- Speech
- Ability to swallow
- Vision and hearing
- Presurgical developmental task mastery
- Receptive and expressive language

If the deficits are significant, the child may need rehabilitative therapy to regain function.

should be aware of its potential side effects and understand that acute side effects will resolve. Chemotherapy may be delivered on an inpatient or outpatient basis, depending on the intensity, and the nursing care is similar for any child receiving chemotherapy.

Evaluation

- Are both verbal and nonverbal indications of a positive comfort level present?
- Does the child's rating on a pain assessment tool indicate decreased pain?
- Has the child remained afebrile, and do the child and family demonstrate infection prevention measures?
- Have the child and family expressed decreased levels of stress and the ability to rely on coping strategies?
- Is the family able to discuss the treatment plan and concerns related to the disease and treatment plan?
- Is the child relating with peers in the same manner as before the diagnosis and hospitalization, and is the child expressing adaptation to the changed appearance?

MALIGNANT LYMPHOMAS

Malignant lymphomas are neoplasms of lymphoid cells, a component of the immune system. Lymphomas represent 20% of childhood cancers in children younger than 20 years, making lymphomas the third most common childhood malignancy (Sandlund & Behm, 2004). Lymphomas are divided into two main types: non-Hodgkin lymphoma (NHL) and Hodgkin lymphoma.

The average occurrence of NHL in children younger than 20 years in the United States is approximately 500 new cases per year, with incidence higher in the white population than in the African-American population (Gilchrist, 2004). NHL originates from a proliferation of either B or T lymphocytes. The three subtypes of pediatric NHL are small, noncleaved cell (Burkitt, Burkitt-like) lymphomas; large-cell lymphomas; and lymphoblastic lymphomas.

Hodgkin lymphoma in 15- to 19-year-olds comprises approximately 15% of all cancers seen in this age group; it

accounts for 5% of all cancers seen in children younger than 15 years (Gilchrist, 2004). It represents approximately 40% of lymphomas. The presence of giant multinucleated cells (Reed-Sternberg cells) is the hallmark of Hodgkin disease.

The incidence of NHL increases gradually throughout life. Unlike Hodgkin disease, which has a bimodal incidence curve, the incidence of NHL increases with age (Sandlund & Behm, 2004). Because the incidence of Hodgkin disease peaks in children 15 years old and older, it accounts for a greater proportion of the lymphomas seen in older children. The incidence of either disease in children younger than 5 years is rare.

Non-Hodgkin Lymphoma

NHL differs greatly from Hodgkin disease in its clinical behavior, pathology, mode of metastasis, and responsiveness to therapy. This disease has a rapid onset with widespread involvement at diagnosis.

Etiology

Viral, immunologic, genetic, and environmental factors may contribute to the development of NHL. Although the exact cause is unknown, a link to the immune system is thought to exist. B-cell lymphoma has been associated with the Epstein-Barr virus, which suggests that delayed exposure to infectious agents may play a part (Gilchrist, 2004). Children with congenital immunodeficiency syndromes or acquired immunodeficiency syndrome (AIDS), as well as those who have undergone organ transplantation and have chronically suppressed immune systems, are at higher risk for developing NHL or other lymphoproliferative disorders (Sandlund & Behm, 2004).

Manifestations

Symptoms of abdominal disease include abdominal cramping, constipation, pain, anorexia, weight loss, ascites, and obstruction, with vomiting as a late sign. Painless, enlarged lymph nodes are found in the cervical or axillary region and less commonly in the inguinal area. If mediastinal disease is present, cough, respiratory distress, symptoms of bronchitis, and possibly significant tracheal deviation are seen. Bone marrow disease leads to a general decline in health and bone marrow suppression.

Diagnostic Evaluation

In addition to a physical examination looking for enlarged lymph nodes and hepatosplenomegaly, extensive laboratory work is necessary. Especially with Burkitt lymphoma, the uric acid level is often high, indicating a rapid turnover of cells.

A chest radiograph is obtained to look for mediastinal disease and tracheal deviation. The extent of disease is further evaluated with a CT scan of the chest, abdomen, and pelvis. Bone marrow aspirations and biopsies are performed to assess involvement of disease in the marrow. A lumbar puncture is performed to assess the CSF for disease. Pathologic findings are confirmed with a lymph node biopsy.

Therapeutic Management

Children with NHL, especially Burkitt lymphoma, often present in metabolic disarray because of the rapidity with which the disease progresses. These children are prone to tumor lysis syndrome from the large tumor burden and rapid tumor cell turnover and death. Before chemotherapy can be started, the metabolic state must be stabilized.

CRITICAL TO REMEMBER

Tumor Lysis Syndrome

In tumor lysis syndrome, the intracellular contents are dumped into the extracellular fluid as the tumor cells are lysed, or killed. Because the intracellular contents are a different electrolyte concentration from extracellular blood volume, electrolytes overload the kidneys and, if the condition is not monitored and treated carefully, cause kidney failure. Tumor lysis syndrome is most common in children with leukemias who have very high WBC counts and in children with non-Hodgkin lymphomas, especially when extensive disease is present.

In children susceptible to tumor lysis syndrome, intensive hydration with an IV fluid containing bicarbonate alkalinizes the urine to help prevent the formation of uric acid crystals, which damage the kidney. Oral allopurinol is started to decrease the uric acid level. Parenteral urate oxidase (Rasburicase) may be indicated to further degrade uric acid (Taketomo et al., 2005). With the initiation of chemotherapy, serum electrolyte levels may be checked several times a day to keep close surveillance on the child's metabolic state because these tumors respond rapidly to treatment. The urine may turn milky white as the tumor cells are filtered through the kidneys. Children who cannot be hemodynamically monitored on the general unit may be moved to the intensive care unit until metabolically stabilized.

The primary treatment modality for all histologic classifications and stages of NHL involves multiagent chemotherapy. Surgery is used to obtain a diagnostic biopsy. In general, these lymphomas present as generalized disease, making them less amenable to treatment with radiation therapy; irradiation is reserved for emergent situations resulting from CNS disease or airway compromise. Chemotherapy is given over a 6- to 24-month period, depending on the type of lymphoma. Typically, a central venous catheter is placed to assist in delivering chemotherapy drugs. Frequent follow-up visits are made after the completion of treatment because the risk of recurrent disease is greatest immediately after therapy is stopped.

Survival rates of children treated for Burkitt and Burkitt-like lymphomas are 70% to 90%. Those treated for lymphoblastic lymphoma have disease-free survival rates of 50% to 70% when disease is extensive at diagnosis and 90% when disease is limited. Large-cell lymphoma is the most difficult to cure, with 50% to 70% of patients achieving disease-free survival (Gilchrist, 2004).

NURSING CARE

The Child With Non-Hodgkin Lymphoma

Assessment

The parents of children with NHL will report an acute onset of symptoms that vary with the type of organ involved. Most parents will state that their child has become irritable and "just not himself." Children with metastatic disease often appear quite sick. Assess lymph nodes and closely check the respiratory system in a child with mediastinal disease, especially if the trachea is deviated. Signs of tumor lysis syndrome include subtle changes in behavior, such as restlessness and irritability, and changes in the sensorium, which are ominous signs of electrolyte imbalances that can include hyperuricemia, hyperkalemia, hyperphosphatemia, and hypocalcemia.

Nursing Diagnosis and Planning

The following nursing diagnoses and expected outcomes that to the child with NHL and the child's family:

- Ineffective Breathing Pattern related to mediastinal disease.
  Expected Outcome: The child's respiratory status will remain stable, as evidenced by normal breath sounds for age and stable respiratory rate and rhythm.
- Risk for Injury related to electrolyte imbalances secondary to tumor lysis syndrome.
  Expected Outcome: The child will maintain electrolyte balance, as evidenced by a stable metabolic state and urine output appropriate for age.
- Risk for Infection related to the state of immunosuppression.
  Expected Outcome: The child will exhibit no signs and symptoms of infection, as evidenced by normal body temperature.
- Deficient Knowledge related to unfamiliarity with the disease process.
  Expected Outcome: The parents will describe the disease process and its management.

Interventions

Initial nursing care focuses on following the physician's orders for maintaining a stable metabolic state before and during the induction phase of chemotherapy. All children undergoing induction chemotherapy should have intake and output and serum chemistry values strictly monitored. Occasionally, children with Burkitt lymphoma will need a urinary catheter inserted for measurement of output. If a fever develops, urine and blood should be cultured to rule out an infection. These children may be so sick that their nutritional status needs attention after induction, and many will receive enteral nutritional support. If necessary, total parenteral nutrition may be given.

Parents will need support because the chemotherapy may initially make the child more ill. Questions should be answered directly and honestly. Time to provide the child with extensive education about therapy may not exist until after the child has begun to recover from the initial chemotherapy.

Consultations with chaplains or other religious figures and social workers may enhance the psychosocial care of these families. Realistic expectations of therapy and of the child's response to therapy help parents deal rationally with their fears (see pp. 762-768 for other related nursing care).

Evaluation

- Has the child's respiratory status remained stable, with normal rate and rhythm and clear breath sounds?
- Is the child's urine output appropriate for age, and are electrolytes within normal range?
- Are the child's vital signs within normal limits?
- Are the parents asking questions about the disease process and the care of their child?

CRITICAL TO REMEMBER
Prevention of Urinary Tract Infections in the Immunocompromised Child

Urinary catheters are used very infrequently in immunocompromised children because of the risk of introducing organisms into the urinary system.

Hodgkin Disease

Hodgkin disease has a more indolent course than NHL. It frequently presents as localized disease. Systemic symptoms include unexplained fevers, weight loss, and night sweats. These systemic signs are used in diagnostic staging.

Etiology

The cause of Hodgkin disease is unknown. However, the possibility of an infectious agent is being investigated. Herpesvirus 6, cytomegalovirus, and Epstein-Barr virus (EBV) have been associated with Hodgkin disease, but the exact relation remains unknown. EBV readily infects Reed-Sternberg cells, and this infection can precede initiation of the malignant clone; however, this relation cannot be demonstrated in all cases (Connors, 2004). As with other cancers, no single environmental agent can be said to precipitate the disease process.

Manifestations

Painless, firm, movable adenopathy in the cervical and supraclavicular regions is the most common presentation. Mediastinal involvement, with or without airway obstruction, occurs in two thirds of children. Twenty to thirty percent of children have constitutional symptoms that include fever, drenching night sweats, and weight loss. Other manifestations are hepatosplenomegaly and fatigue.

Diagnostic Evaluation

Biopsy of an involved lymph node and histologic classification of the tissue confirm the diagnosis. Laboratory tests

include a CBC, renal and liver function tests, erythrocyte sedimentation rate (ESR), and serum copper and serum ferritin levels. Elevation of ESR or serum copper or ferritin level may be useful for follow-up evaluation if it correlates with disease activity at diagnosis. A gallium scan is performed to look for extent of disease. Gallium is a staging study as well as an excellent disease response marker when the tumor takes up gallium at diagnosis. PET scanning may be more sensitive and specific than CT or gallium scanning. Its use in diagnosis, staging, and follow-up surveillance imaging is being actively assessed (Connors, 2004). Chest radiography and CT of the chest, abdomen, and pelvis are performed to determine the extent of disease. Bilateral bone marrow aspirations and biopsies are done only if constitutional symptoms are present.

PATHOPHYSIOLOGY

HODGKIN DISEASE

Hodgkin disease originates in a single lymph node or a group of lymph nodes in the same anatomic region. Hodgkin disease is characterized by giant multinucleated cells called *Reed-Sternberg cells* that are thought to represent activated B and T lymphocytes. Hodgkin disease spreads predictably from lymph nodes to nonnodal sites such as the spleen, liver, bone, bone marrow, lungs, and mediastinum.

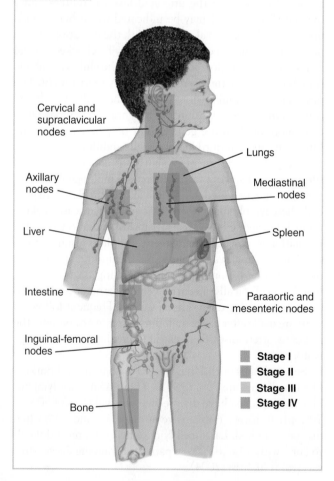

Cervical and supraclavicular nodes
Lungs
Axillary nodes
Mediastinal nodes
Liver
Spleen
Intestine
Paraaortic and mesenteric nodes
Inguinal-femoral nodes
Bone

Stage I
Stage II
Stage III
Stage IV

In the past, a surgical staging laparotomy was often performed. It is an invasive surgical procedure that involves splenectomy, liver biopsy, and sampling of the retroperitoneal and pelvic nodes; it was thought to define the extent of disease more precisely than radiographic studies alone. However, precise staging is less important now that most children receive systemic chemotherapy as part of their treatment. Universal staging laparotomy with splenectomy is no longer performed because of better diagnostic methods and better delivery of radiation therapy (Connors, 2004).

Some manifestations are of prognostic significance, and staging takes them into account. Children with unexplained weight loss of more than 10% body weight in the preceding 6 months, unexplained fevers greater than 38° C (100.4° F), and night sweats are considered to have B disease as opposed to A (local) disease. The presence of B symptoms is thought to impact prognosis negatively (Gilchrist, 2004). Four stages of the disease have been delineated, with stage I having limited disease and the most favorable prognosis.

Therapeutic Management

Therapy depends on the child's age at diagnosis, disease stage, and histologic type. If the mediastinal disease is expansive, it may compromise respiration. Radiation therapy may be used to shrink the tissue before any necessary procedure requiring general anesthesia.

Most children are treated with chemotherapy alone or chemotherapy and low-dose, involved-field radiation therapy. High-dose, extended-field radiation therapy alone may be used if the disease is detected in a single site or in fully grown children in whom growth and development are not a concern. Long-term survival rates in excess of 90% can be expected with stages I and II disease. For more advanced stages of disease, the long-term survival rate is approximately 70% (Gilchrist, 2004).

Nursing Considerations

The onset of Hodgkin disease is insidious. Frequently, when asked about activity level, children report not noticing any change until it was brought to their attention. Typically the child noticed lumps around the neck while bathing. Initial assessment of these children includes a thorough lymph node examination. Depending on the presence of the mediastinal disease, the respiratory system should be assessed for a change in status with the child both sitting and lying down.

Initially the nurse should prepare the child for the diagnostic procedures and a surgical biopsy. A central venous catheter may be inserted at the time of diagnosis. In older children, a peripheral IV line may be placed at the time of each chemotherapy treatment to avoid a central venous catheter placement.

At least two thirds of children have some degree of mediastinal involvement. As with NHL, management of the airway is a concern if the child has any mediastinal disease.

A staging laparotomy with splenectomy is generally avoided. If it is required, however, these children need special care. The spleen removes organisms such as *Streptococcus pneumoniae* and *Haemophilus influenzae*. Without the spleen, these organisms can produce fulminant infections. Ideally, children who undergo splenectomy receive a pneumococcal, meningococcal, and *H. influenzae* type B immunization before the procedure. Postoperative care includes assessing for bleeding at dressing sites and administering prophylactic antibiotics.

Induction chemotherapy is begun as soon as the child is stable and staging of disease has been completed. If the airway is compromised, radiation therapy will be given locally to provide immediate relief.

Education includes an explanation of the therapeutic protocol. Questions should be answered honestly. Realistic expectations of response to therapy help parents deal rationally with their fears. Hodgkin disease in first remission is treated in the outpatient setting at most centers. The nursing care is similar to that for a child with NHL.

NEUROBLASTOMA

Neuroblastoma is the second most common solid tumor of childhood. It is found exclusively in infants and children. Children who present at younger than 12 months may have spontaneous remission of the disease.

Etiology

The cause of neuroblastoma is unknown. Its prevalence is similar in various countries around the world, suggesting that environmental factors do not cause the disease. Evidence exists that a familial form of neuroblastoma may occur; children in families with one or more affected members may be at increased risk for the development of neuroblastoma.

Incidence

Neuroblastoma represents approximately 8% of all childhood cancers (Ater, 2004). Neuroblastoma occurs at a rate of 8.7 per 1 million children, or 500 to 600 new cases diagnosed each year in the United States. It is more common in boys than in girls and more common in white children than in African-American children. The peak age of presentation is 2 years, with the majority of cases being younger than 5 years.

Pathophysiology

Neuroblastoma arises from neural crest cells, which normally develop into the sympathetic nervous system and the adrenal medulla. Cells proliferate and begin to form a solid mass or tumor. These cells are immature and nonfunctional. Typically the tumor infringes and infiltrates into adjacent normal tissue and organs. Metastatic disease may be present in the bone marrow, bone, liver and skin, and rarely in the lung or brain (Ater, 2004). Greater understanding of the cellular genetic makeup of this tumor has given researchers insight into prognostic indicators, which help with treatment planning.

Manifestations

The manifestations of neuroblastoma depend on the extent of disease and the location of the tumor. In most cases, a primary abdominal mass and a protuberant, firm abdomen are present. Other manifestations include impaired range of motion and mobility with pain and limping. Chest tumors may produce cough and decreased chest expansion, with respiratory compromise. Compression of the superior vena cava results in facial and periorbital edema. Spinal cord compression may cause inability to walk and impaired bowel and bladder function. Tumor infiltration may cause dark circles under the eyes, giving an appearance of "raccoon eyes." Bruising, drooping eyelids, or small pupils may be evident, and possibly opsomyoclonus, or "dancing" eye movements and myoclonic jerks. These children act restless and uncomfortable.

Diagnostic Evaluation

The diagnostic workup includes chest radiography; CT of the chest, abdomen, and pelvis; and skeletal scintigraphy to determine the extent of disease. Bone marrow aspiration and biopsy, usually of both posterior iliac crests, are performed to evaluate marrow involvement. Urine catecholamine levels (homovanillic acid [HVA] and vanillymandelic acid [VMA]) are elevated in 95% of patients with neuroblastoma (Ater, 2004). In these patients, serial monitoring of HMA and VMA are helpful as markers during treatment and for follow-up when treatment is complete.

Definitive diagnosis is made when tissue is obtained by biopsy. Tumor samples are sent to special reference laboratories to look at the genetic makeup of the tumor. The genetic information may reveal the aggressiveness of the tumor and help determine the prognosis and treatment plan.

Therapeutic Management

The treatment of neuroblastoma depends on the presence and extent of metastasis. The International Staging System for Neuroblastoma is used to compare patients. Staging is graded I through IV, with stage I representing localized disease and stage IV distant spread. Staging criteria include the extent and location of metastases, lymph node involvement, and whether the tumor is unilateral or crosses the midline. Early-stage disease (stage I or II) without metastasis may require only surgical excision of the tumor and follow-up evaluations. Children with later-stage (stage IV) disease may undergo surgery to obtain tissue samples or for tumor debulking for pain control.

Age at diagnosis is an important prognostic indicator. Children diagnosed before they are 1 year old have a better prognosis than children diagnosed at a later age. Approximately half of the infants diagnosed with neuroblastoma at younger than 1 year have a genetically less-aggressive tumor type and may be watched carefully or treated with low-dose chemotherapy.

Treatment plans for children with advanced disease (stage III or IV) may include radiation therapy to tumor sites and systemic chemotherapy for several months. Another attempt may be made to resect the tumor after combination chemotherapy has been administered to reduce the tumor size. Peripheral blood stem cell transplant after myeloablative chemotherapy is part of the risk-based treatment for advanced-stage disease (Ater, 2004). This high-risk group may also receive 13-*cis*-retinoic acid orally after transplantation for possible minimal residual disease. This biologic modifier decreases proliferation and induces differentiation in neuroblastoma cell lines (Perry, Anderson, & Donehower, 2004).

Children with stage I or II disease and who are without poor prognostic factors have a long-term survival rate of 95%. Intermediate-risk children's long-term survival rate is approximately 80%. The long-term survival of high-risk children is approximately 25% even with aggressive treatment (American Cancer Society, 2003).

The Child With Neuroblastoma

Assessment

Parents may state their child has wanted to be held more often than usual. Activity level and appetite are usually decreased. Children with neuroblastoma typically appear pale, quite irritable, and uncomfortable. Because of large abdominal tumors, many present with protuberant abdomens in which hard masses crossing the midline can be palpated. Range of motion and mobility are often impaired, so much so that the child cannot bear weight. If the tumor is compressing a nerve, neurologic changes may be noted. If the tumor is causing compression within the abdomen, vascular drainage may be compromised and GI obstruction may be present. Periorbital infiltration can cause characteristic ecchymosis or "raccoon eyes" (Ater, 2004).

Nursing Diagnosis and Planning

The following nursing diagnoses and expected outcomes may be appropriate for the child with a neuroblastoma and the child's family:

- Acute Pain related to tumor pressure.
  Expected Outcome: The infant will exhibit pain relief, as evidenced by decreased crying and a relaxed body position.
- Anxiety (parents) related to a diagnosis of cancer, surgery, and treatment plan.
  Expected Outcome: The parents will express decreased anxiety about the outcomes of therapy.
- Deficient Knowledge related to unfamiliarity with the disease process and its management.
  Expected Outcome: The parents will describe the disease process and its implications.

Interventions

Nursing care initially focuses on support of family members as they react and adjust to the diagnosis of cancer. The nurse facilitates the educational process to allay fears of the unknown. The child's initial care includes pain management, both preoperatively and postoperatively. Expect the child with an abdominal tumor to return from surgery with a nasogastric (NG) tube in place. Assess the wound carefully for bleeding and signs of infection (see Chapter 13). With responsive tumors, the child's disposition will improve quickly.

Bowel habits may be altered because of pain, immobility, medication, surgery, and alteration in nutritional patterns. Children with large abdominal tumors may become obstructed because of tumor compression. The nurse should obtain a history of bowel habits and notify the physician if bowel habits are dramatically altered.

Management of the airway is of concern if the child has any mediastinal disease. Monitor respiratory effort, color, and pulses. Position for comfort.

Evaluation

- Has the child exhibited decreased crying and irritability?
- Does the child rest quietly and comfortably in the parent's arms and have uninterrupted periods of rest?
- Are the parents verbalizing their fears and expressing decreased anxiety?
- Are the parents asking questions related to the child's disease and treatment and seeking the support of family and friends?

OSTEOSARCOMA

Osteosarcoma (also called *osteogenic sarcoma*) is the most common primary bone malignancy in children. The symptoms of this disease in its earliest stage are almost always attributed to extremity injury or normal growing pains. Typically, unresolved pain related to trauma brings the tumor to the attention of medical personnel.

Etiology

The cause of osteosarcoma is unknown, although associations have been made between radiation therapy for other diseases and osteosarcoma. Familial tendencies have been seen, suggesting that genetic factors are involved (Arndt, 2004a).

Incidence

Osteosarcoma represents approximately 4 to 5 new cases per 1 million children per year (Arndt, 2004a), with a lower incidence in African-American children than other races. The incidence of osteosarcoma peaks in the teenage years. The rapid bone growth of the adolescent growth spurt is associated with the development of this tumor. Osteosarcoma occurs at an earlier age in girls than in boys, which corresponds to the earlier maturation of girls. Before adolescence, osteosarcoma is rare. If metastases are present, the lungs are the primary organ involved with bone metastases, with "skip lesions" (tumor nodules growing outside the reactive rim but within the same bone or across a neighboring joint) being the second. Approximately 20% of affected individuals have metastatic disease at diagnosis.

Pathophysiology

Osteosarcoma originates from bone-producing cells that invade the medullary canal of the bone and form a solid tumor. Incidence is higher in the most rapidly growing bones in adolescents—that is, the distal femur, proximal tibia, and proximal humerus. A possible association of rapid bone growth to malignant transformation can be suggested (Arndt, 2004a).

Manifestations

Manifestations of osteosarcoma include progressive, insidious, or intermittent pain at the tumor site; a palpable mass; limping, if a weight-bearing limb is affected; progressive, limited range of motion; and eventually pathologic fractures at the tumor site.

Diagnostic Evaluation

Initially radiographs of the primary site and chest are taken, and then CT or MRI and skeletal scintigraphy are performed. The CT scan includes the chest to search for pulmonary metastases, which helps stage the disease. A biopsy of the tumor must be performed with great care so that no local contamination of tissue by tumor occurs. Laboratory tests include a CBC, chemistry levels, and serum alkaline phosphatase (ALP) and lactate dehydrogenase (LDH) determinations. Surveillance ALP levels seem to correlate with osteoblastic activity and are therefore useful in monitoring response to therapy (Dome et al., 2004).

Therapeutic Management

The goals of therapy are to remove the tumor and prevent the spread of disease. Osteogenic sarcoma is treated with a combination of surgery and chemotherapy. Chemotherapy is administered before and after surgery. Radiation therapy is used only for palliative pain control in advanced-stage disease because osteosarcoma is generally unresponsive to irradiation.

Amputation was once the standard surgical intervention and is still necessary in some cases. Favorable tumor location allows specially trained orthopedic surgeons to perform a complex limb-salvage operation. The affected tissue is removed with the certainty of clean margins, and limb function is preserved. The diseased bone is removed, and either bone grafts or surgically placed orthopedic devices are implanted.

Early research on this disease found that 90% of patients developed recurrent disease after surgery alone. This finding alerted physicians to the presence of microscopic disease. Therefore chemotherapy is continued after surgery even if the procedure appears to have been successful. Chemotherapy is aimed at preventing the spread of disease by killing any microscopic tumor cells present anywhere in the body.

The extent of disease at diagnosis, elevated LDH and ALP levels, and tumor necrosis found on surgical resection are the three most significant prognostic indicators. The cure rate is approximately 50% to 75% for children who respond well to chemotherapy treatment. The 20% of children with metastatic disease at diagnosis have a substantially poorer outcome (Dome et al., 2004).

NURSING CARE

The Child With Osteosarcoma

Assessment

Subjective data to be gathered include a history of any injury to the affected limb and a history of discomfort. By the time children with osteosarcomas come to medical attention, they may be in considerable pain from the tumor. Warmth, erythema, and tenderness at the site of tumor are not uncommon. If the swelling is great, the skin may appear shiny and taut, with dilated blood vessels. Lung involvement is usually asymptomatic.

To prepare the child for outcomes of surgery, an assessment of physical activity and sports involvement is essential, as is the psychosocial history. As for any child with cancer, body image changes, especially if the affected limb must be amputated, are of paramount importance. Preoperatively, the nurse should assess the child's values and fears and begin the process of preparing the child for postoperative lifestyle modifications.

Nursing Diagnosis and Planning

The following nursing diagnoses and expected outcomes may be appropriate for the child with an osteosarcoma and the child's family:

- Acute Pain related to disease process and procedures.
  Expected Outcome: The child will have decreased pain, as evidenced by verbalization of adequate pain control and decreased pain rating on an age-appropriate pain assessment tool.
- Fear and Anxiety related to the potential loss or impairment of a limb and a diagnosis of cancer.
  Expected Outcome: The child and parents will express decreased fears and anxiety related to the surgery and diagnosis.
- Risk for Infection related to chemotherapy or surgery.
  Expected Outcome: The child will remain free from signs and symptoms of infection, as evidenced by normal body temperature and no redness or purulent drainage from the surgical site.
- Disturbed Body Image related to loss or impairment of a limb.
  Expected Outcome: The child will have a positive body image, as evidenced by a return to appropriate social situations and statements that indicate adaptation to the altered appearance and function.
- Impaired Physical Mobility related to loss or impairment of limb function.
  Expected Outcome: The child will regain maximal mobility, as evidenced by ability to perform activities of daily living.

- Deficient Knowledge related to unfamiliarity with the disease process and anxiety.
  Expected Outcome: The child and parents will describe the disease process and potential postoperative adaptations.

Interventions

Initial care is focused on making the child comfortable. Preoperative teaching is extensive and procedure specific. If limb salvage is the procedure of choice, the surgeon and nurse will spend considerable time with the family explaining what is to be done. The nurse reinforces the preoperative and postoperative teaching.

In addition to the usual postoperative care, pain, infection, and potential hemorrhage are nursing concerns. The potential for postoperative pneumonia may be greater in the child with pulmonary metastases than in the child without such metastases.

If amputation occurs, phantom limb pain is a temporary condition some children may experience. This sensation of burning, aching, or cramping in the missing limb is most distressing to the child. The child needs to be reassured that the condition is normal. Numerous pharmacologic agents are available to address postoperative neurogenic pain.

The child who undergoes amputation will be fitted with a permanent prosthesis once the surgical site has thoroughly healed. To begin to mold the stump for that, a temporary prosthesis may be used. A temporary prosthesis enables the child to maintain use and strength of surrounding muscles in preparation for the permanent device. A prosthesis will address the issue of body image disturbance and enable the child to become more quickly independent in activities of daily living. Prepare the child for extensive work with physical therapists to achieve mobility with the prosthesis. Teenagers especially may become discouraged if they expect the prosthesis to enable them to move normally. Prepare them for a limp or for awkward movements with the prosthesis.

Help the child verbalize feelings about changes in body image and function. Involve the child in age-appropriate decision making concerning care. Encourage interaction with other children of the same age who have the same disease (support groups). Provide opportunities for the family to participate in the child's care and provide support and encouragement.

Follow-up outpatient visits need to include a careful assessment of psychosocial adjustment. Questions should include the topics of social interactions, school attendance and performance, and behavioral changes.

Evaluation

- Does the child have discomfort related to the surgical procedures?
- Does the child's pain rating on the pain assessment tool show decreased pain?
- Are the family and child discussing fears related to the disease and treatment?
- Is the child afebrile, and is the surgical site free of redness and purulence?

- Is the child relating with peers?
- Has the child made positive statements indicating beginning adaptation to the physical impairment?
- Is the child readily participating in physical therapy and returning to performing activities of daily living?
- Are the child and family asking questions related to the disease process?
- Do the family and child accurately describe the treatment regimen?

EWING SARCOMA

Ewing sarcoma is the second most common bone tumor seen in children. The diagnosis is often challenging to make because this disease mimics infection and may be difficult to differentiate from other malignancies. Ewing sarcoma may also manifest as a soft tissue mass. This tumor may also be referred to as a peripheral primitive neuroectodermal tumor (PPNET).

Etiology

The cause of Ewing sarcoma is unknown. Interestingly, Ewing sarcoma has not been commonly associated with other preexisting congenital chromosomal abnormalities, suggesting chance rather than biology in the development of this tumor.

Incidence

The incidence of Ewing sarcoma is 2.1 per 1 million white children per year (Arndt, 2004a). The disease is extremely uncommon in African-American and Asian children. Ewing sarcoma is rare in children younger than 5 years and adults older than 30 years. The incidence peaks between ages 10 and 20 years, with typical presentation in the second decade of life.

Pathophysiology

The diagnosis of Ewing sarcoma is made after all other solid tumors have been excluded. Ewing sarcoma has no defining characteristics. As with osteosarcoma, this tumor invades the bone and is found most often in the midshaft of long bones, especially the femur, vertebrae, ribs, and pelvic bones. Gross metastasis is uncommon at diagnosis but does occur, most often to the lungs, bones, or bone marrow. As with osteosarcoma, microscopic disease is thought to be present early in the disease process.

Manifestations

Manifestations of Ewing sarcoma include pain, soft tissue swelling around the affected bone, and fever. If metastatic disease occurs, anorexia, fever, malaise, fatigue, and weight loss are seen. If a vertebral tumor is present, neurologic symptoms will be seen. If a rib tumor is present, respiratory symptoms may be seen.

Diagnostic Evaluation

The diagnostic workup is the same as for osteosarcoma, and biopsy is necessary to differentiate Ewing sarcoma from other neoplastic processes.

Therapeutic Management

A multidisciplinary approach with chemotherapy, surgery, and radiation is the basis of management. Treatment begins with chemotherapy to decrease the tumor bulk, followed by surgical resection of the primary tumor. Local control of the primary tumor site can be achieved with surgery or radiation therapy because this tumor is sensitive to radiation. Consideration is given to the expendability of the bone involved when surgery is a treatment option versus the potential late effects of radiation. Ribs and the proximal fibula are considered expendable and may be removed to excise the tumor without affecting function. Cure rates exceed 75% to 80% in children with small extremity tumors and no metastases (Dome et al., 2004). With gross metastasis, the cure rate is dramatically decreased.

Nursing Considerations

Nursing care is similar to that for children with osteosarcomas, with the addition of care for the child receiving radiation therapy.

RHABDOMYOSARCOMA

Rhabdomyosarcoma is a malignancy of muscle, or striated tissue, that most often occurs periorbitally, in the head and neck in younger children, or in the trunk and extremities in older children. Long-term survival rates vary with the child's age, the histologic subtype, and the location of the tumor.

Etiology

Although the exact cause is unknown, rhabdomyosarcoma has been associated with familial cancer syndromes.

Incidence

Rhabdomyosarcoma is the most common soft tissue malignancy in children and accounts for 5% to 8% of all pediatric cancers (Arndt, 2004b). The annual incidence in the United States is estimated at 4.3 cases per 1 million white children and 3.3 cases per 1 million African-American children. Two age groups predominate: children younger than 10 years and adolescents (American Cancer Society, 2003).

Pathophysiology

Four histologic subtypes of rhabdomyosarcoma exist. The embryonal type accounts for 50% to 60% of the tumors and has the best prognosis. Approximately 20% of cases are of the alveolar type, which is found most often in the perineal area, trunk, and extremities and has a less favorable prognosis. Alveolar-type disease is most often found in the adolescent age group.

The prognosis depends on several factors other than histologic type. If the tumor is in a location where manifestations appear early, rather than deeply buried in a body cavity, the prognosis is better because the tumor is usually found before it has metastasized. Abnormalities in the DNA content of the tumor cells have prognostic significance. Staging of the tumor is based on whether the tumor was resected completely, was resected with residual microscopic disease, was incompletely resected, or had metastasized to distant sites. Local failure is more common if the tumor cannot be completely resected.

Manifestations

The manifestations of rhabdomyosarcoma depend on the tumor location. Soft to hard, nontender, relatively immobile masses may be mistaken for a traumatic hematoma. If the lesion is periorbital, visual changes are present; the child may have ptosis, exophthalmos, or proptosis (bulging). Cranial nerve involvement may occur. If the lesion affects an extremity, range of motion will be limited. In the case of pelvic tumors, the function of organs around the tumor is disrupted.

Diagnostic Evaluation

CT, skeletal scintigraphy, and bone marrow aspiration and biopsy are performed to determine the extent of disease. The diagnosis is made after biopsy or attempted surgical resection of the tumor. A decision about treatment is made depending on the location of the tumor, histologic subtype, and the presence of distant metastases. Laboratory studies include a CBC, urinalysis, and renal and liver function tests.

Therapeutic Management

Rhabdomyosarcoma is treated with chemotherapy, surgery, and radiation therapy. Chemotherapy is used to decrease the tumor bulk and reduce the extent and morbidity of surgery. After surgical removal of the tumor, additional chemotherapy is provided. Like Ewing sarcoma, microscopic rhabdomyosarcoma is often present at the time of diagnosis. Discontinuation of chemotherapy after removal of the tumor generally results in recurrent disease. Tumor cells not removed by surgery are referred to as *residual disease*. Radiation therapy is used for children who have residual disease or whose tumor was not resectable. Approximately 50% of children with metastatic disease at the time of diagnosis do not achieve lasting remission (Arndt, 2004b).

Follow-up care involves periodic CT or MRI studies to assess tumor response to therapy and monitor any development of disease progression. Most relapses occur within 2 years of diagnosis and during therapy, although late relapse (more than 5 years from therapy) is occasionally reported.

Nursing Considerations

Parents may relate that their first indication that something was wrong was a decreased activity level in a young child unable to verbalize pain. If the tumor is more superficially located, parents may have discovered a lump or swelling.

The physical examination findings will depend on the location of the tumor, but typically a soft to hard, nontender mass will be palpated. The surrounding lymph nodes should be palpated for enlargement, which may indicate tumor involvement. The CBC is usually normal unless the tumor has extended into bone marrow, causing a decrease in hemoglobin and platelet values.

Nursing care initially focuses on support of family members as they react and adjust to the diagnosis of cancer. Second, the nurse facilitates the educational process to allay fears of the unknown.

Postoperative care of the biopsy or surgical site involves careful observation for signs of infection, hemorrhage, and edema. If surgery entailed excision of an abdominal or pelvic tumor, the child will return from the surgical suite with an NG tube and possibly drains in place.

WILMS TUMOR (NEPHROBLASTOMA)

Wilms tumor, or nephroblastoma, is the most common renal tumor in children. Much research has been done on this disease, and the subsequent changes in therapy have resulted in favorable outcomes. Prognosis is related to stage of disease at diagnosis, histopathologic features of the tumor, and patient age.

Etiology

The cause of Wilms tumor is unknown. Most Wilms tumors occur in children with no unusual physical features and no family history of the disease. These are considered sporadic cases. In some cases, however, a genetic predisposition exists. Approximately 1% to 2% of children in whom this disease develops have a family history (Jaffe & Huff, 2004). Bilateral disease is more common in familial cases than in sporadic cases. Wilms tumor has been associated with other congenital anomalies, including aniridia (absence of the irises), hemihypertrophy, cryptorchidism, and hypospadias. Wilms tumor is associated with a variety of other syndromes seen in childhood.

Incidence

Incidence is higher in African Americans and lower in East Asians. Approximately 8 new cases per 1 million are diagnosed annually, representing 5% to 6% of childhood cancers (Jaffe & Huff, 2004). The mean age at diagnosis is 2 to 5 years. Most children present before 7 years of age. Seven percent of children with Wilms tumor have bilateral tumors (Jaffe & Huff, 2004).

Pathophysiology

Wilms tumor arises from the renal parenchyma of the kidney. Categories of Wilms tumor are based on favorable and unfavorable histologic findings; children with favorable histologic findings (the majority of children with Wilms tumor) have a more positive prognosis (Jaffe & Huff, 2004). Wilms tumor may occur in one or both kidneys, although the latter is much less common. At the initial diagnosis, the disease is usually local, but metastasis to other organs occasionally occurs. The lungs are the most common site of metastasis. As with other tumors, a staging system directs treatment.

Manifestations

The most common clinical presentation of Wilms tumor is an asymptomatic, mobile, abdominal mass discovered by the parent or primary care provider during a routine physical examination. Additional manifestations include microscopic or gross hematuria, hypertension, abdominal pain, fatigue, anemia, and fever. The lungs are the primary site for distant metastasis.

Diagnostic Evaluation

The diagnosis can be suspected from a good history. Abdominal ultrasonography is the initial study done to detect a solid intrarenal mass. Abdominal CT or MRI, chest radiography, and chest CT are performed to evaluate extent of disease further. Laboratory tests include a CBC, electrolyte levels, liver and kidney function tests, and urinalysis. A definitive diagnosis is made at the time of surgery on the basis of pathologic findings. Palpation or any pressure on the tumor before surgery must be avoided to prevent possible rupture and spillage of tumor cells into the peritoneum.

Therapeutic Management

Treatment for Wilms tumor consists of surgery and chemotherapy alone or in combination with radiation therapy. In most cases the tumor can be completely removed by surgical resection at the time of diagnosis. During surgery, the surgeon is careful to prevent spillage of the tumor, which would necessitate more aggressive treatment (Jaffe & Huff, 2004). In a few cases, complete surgical resection is considered too great a risk at the time of diagnosis and only a biopsy is performed to determine pathology. The goal of the initial chemotherapy treatments in these children is to reduce the tumor size before definitive surgery. All children receive chemotherapy after the tumor is surgically removed. Radiation therapy is added to the treatment of larger, more extensive tumors or those with an unfavorable histologic classification.

Survival rates for Wilms tumor are much better than for many other forms of cancer. Histologic features remain the most important determinant of prognosis. Five-year survival rates approach 90% for children with favorable histology tumors (Dome et al., 2004).

NURSING CARE

The Child With Wilms Tumor

Assessment

Parents often report that when bathing or dressing their child they noticed the child's stomach seemed swollen. Some parents state the diapers no longer fit easily around the child's

---

CRITICAL TO REMEMBER

Assessing the Child With a Wilms Tumor

The tumor mass should not be palpated during the assessment because of the risk of rupturing the protective capsule. Excessive manipulation can cause seeding of the tumor and spread of cancerous cells.

---

abdomen. More often than not, the child's activity level and appetite have not changed. Except for a palpable abdominal mass that usually does not cross the midline, the child's physical examination is normal.

Nursing Diagnosis and Planning

The following nursing diagnoses and expected outcomes apply to the child with Wilms tumor and the child's family:
- Anxiety related to surgery with nephrectomy.
  Expected Outcome: The child and parents will express decreased anxiety about the outcome of surgery.
- Risk for Infection related to surgical interventions.
  Expected Outcome: The child will exhibit no signs and symptoms of infection, as evidenced by normal body temperature, intact incision site, and absence of purulent drainage.
- Deficient Knowledge related to unfamiliarity with the disease process and treatment plan.
  Expected Outcome: The child and parents will describe the disease process and treatment plan.
- Risk for Deficient Fluid Volume related to having only one kidney postoperatively.
  Expected Outcome: The child will demonstrate fluid balance, as evidenced by moist mucous membranes, normal electrolyte and urine values, and hourly urine output appropriate for age.

Interventions

Because the child usually feels well, nursing care initially focuses on preoperative teaching for the parents and child. Place a sign on the bed warning against palpating the abdomen. A nephrectomy is a serious surgical procedure, and family members will have anxiety about the child losing a kidney. Nurses must offer support and reassurance.

Postoperatively, monitor the child for GI activity, bowel sounds, stool production, abdominal distention, signs and symptoms of infection, hemorrhage, and changes in blood pressure. Careful assessment of output by the remaining kidney is important. Intake and output are precisely measured and totaled at least every 4 hours. These children will probably return from surgery with an NG tube in place and with an order for replacement IV fluid for the NG drainage. Typically NG tube output is totaled every 4 hours; that total is divided by 4, and either the resulting number is added to the current IV fluid rate or another IV solution is hung so that the amount lost by NG drainage is replaced over the next 4 hours. The process is repeated until the NG drainage has slowed enough that it does not affect overall fluid and electrolyte balance. The replacement fluid usually contains potassium because gastric contents are potassium rich. Serum electrolyte levels are checked every 8 to 12 hours during this process.

Once the tumor has been staged, the child is assigned to the appropriate therapeutic protocol. Teaching should center on the sequencing of tests and drugs on that protocol. Support for family members and assessment of their coping skills continue throughout therapy. Therapy for Wilms tumor is usually accomplished on an outpatient basis.

Evaluation

- Are the parents and child using coping skills and mobilizing support systems?
- Has the child remained afebrile?
- Is the incision site dry and intact and free from redness, swelling, and purulence?
- Is blood pressure within normal limits for age?
- Does the child have moist mucous membranes, electrolytes and urinalysis within normal limits, and hourly urine output appropriate for age?
- Is the family asking questions and sharing concerns and fears?

RETINOBLASTOMA

Retinoblastoma is a rare, malignant tumor of the embryonic neural retina. This tumor of the eye is found only in children. Observant parents may bring this disease to the attention of the physician when they look at a photograph and see a white reflection (leukocoria) in one of the child's eyes instead of the normal red color when the camera flash is reflected off the retina.

Etiology

Retinoblastoma is thought to result from a sequence of genetic mutations. The majority of these genetic mutations are sporadic, occurring within a single retinal cell that then multiplies to form the tumor. Hereditary, or familial, retinoblastoma occurs in individuals who have a germline mutation present. The mutation places the child at high risk of developing retinoblastoma as well as other associated malignancies. A second mutation occurs in one or more of the retinal cells, which then multiply to form a tumor. Advances in genetic studies of this disease have led to genetic research on other forms of childhood cancer.

Incidence

Retinoblastoma represents 3% of all pediatric cancers. Forty percent of retinoblastomas are the hereditary form, and sixty percent are the nonhereditary form (Dome et al., 2004). Bilateral involvement is found in 42% of those presenting when younger than 1 year but in 21% of those from 1 to 2 years of age and becomes even less common in older children (Herzog, 2004).

Pathophysiology

The human retina does not reach maturation until approximately age 3 years. During this early, differentiating process cells are at risk for abnormal division and neoplasia. The tumor develops on the retina, growing inward toward the vitreous humor or out toward the subretinal space. Retinoblastoma can develop at a single site or as multiple independent tumors that originate within the globe of the eye. The process of cells breaking off from the main mass and forming additional independent tumors is called *seeding*. Extension of the tumor down the optic nerve and into the CNS does not often occur in children living in the United States (Herzog,

2004). As with other cancers, a staging system has been developed to standardize descriptions of extent of disease confined to the eye and those tumors that have spread outside the eye and to other parts of the body. This system directs treatment and indicates prognosis.

Manifestations

The most common findings of retinoblastoma are leukocoria and strabismus resulting from vision loss. In general, young children will not report vision loss limited to one eye. Manifestations may also include pain, redness, and inflammation of the eye.

Diagnostic Evaluation

Leukocoria or strabismus discovered by the parent or on a routine physical examination results in a referral to an ophthalmologist. A funduscopic examination performed by the ophthalmologist with the child under general anesthesia is the best means of diagnosing and monitoring retinoblastoma. Ultrasound imaging confirms that the retinoblastoma tumors are present and determines their thickness and height. CT or MRI of the eyes, orbits, and brain is performed to evaluate the tumors within the eyes and search for extraocular spread. Skeletal scintigraphy, bone marrow aspiration and biopsy, and lumbar puncture generally are not necessary unless clinical evidence of metastasis is present (Dome et al., 2004).

Therapeutic Management

The goal of current treatment of retinoblastoma is to save the child's life and preserve the eye and useful vision when possible (Herzog, 2004). Enucleation, or removal of the eye, was standard therapy but is becoming less frequent as nonsurgical therapies improve. Enucleation may be indicated if the child has no chance for useful vision even if the tumor is destroyed. Another indication is failure of nonsurgical treatment. A disadvantage of enucleation in children younger than 3 years is that the orbit ceases to develop normally after the eye is removed and will look increasingly sunken as the child's face continues to grow. When enucleation is performed, the child does not require any further therapy and is monitored closely with serial examinations to confirm no tumor recurrence.

External beam radiation therapy is another treatment modality that can be used for multifocal disease. The disadvantages of radiation therapy are cosmetic deformities resulting from abnormal growth of the areas of skull exposed to radiation and a higher risk of secondary malignancies in children with familial retinoblastoma. Cryotherapy or photocoagulation may also be used for very small lesions.

The role of chemotherapy in treating intraocular disease has not been as useful in retinoblastoma because intraocular penetration of systemic drugs is poor and the tumors often develop multidrug resistance. Multiagent chemotherapy is used in certain circumstances. Chemotherapy is used to treat metastatic disease; however, these children are rarely cured. The long-term survival rate among children with retinoblastoma limited to the eyes is excellent, with a 5-year survival rate of 95% (Herzog, 2004). Retinoblastoma that extends to extraocular sites is associated with a poor prognosis.

NURSING CARE

The Child With Retinoblastoma

Assessment

Except for leukocoria (a whitish reflex in the pupillary area), the findings on physical examination may be normal. Assess for strabismus, esotropia, exotropia, or decreased vision. The child may have compensated for loss of vision in one eye; therefore the nurse must be very astute when assessing vision in these children.

Nursing Diagnoses and Planning

The following nursing diagnoses and expected outcomes apply to the child with retinoblastoma and the child's family:

* Anxiety (child and family) related to cancer and enucleation or fear of blindness.

   Expected Outcome: The child and family will express decreased anxiety about outcomes of therapy.

* Disturbed Sensory Perception (visual) related to visual changes caused by the tumor or enucleation.

   Expected Outcome: The child will develop compensatory mechanisms for vision, as evidenced by ability to perform activities of daily living.

* Deficient Knowledge related to unfamiliarity with the disease process and treatment.

   Expected Outcomes: The child and parents will describe the disease process and the treatment plan and will demonstrate use of any prosthetic device, if required.

Interventions

Nursing care initially focuses on support of family members as they react and adjust to the diagnosis of cancer. Second, the nurse facilitates the educational process to allay fears based on unknown factors.

Postoperative care of the enucleated orbit entails careful observations for signs of infection, hemorrhage, and edema. The child will wear a patch over the socket for approximately 1 week postoperatively. To preserve the shape of the orbit for prosthesis, which will be fitted 5 to 6 weeks after surgery, a conformer is placed in the orbit. Nursing interventions include teaching the parents (and child if old enough) how to remove, clean, and reinsert first the conformer and then the prosthesis.

The nurse can reassure parents that children can generally accommodate for vision in only one eye. These children must wear protective eyewear during sports or other hazardous activities to protect their remaining eye.

Whatever the extent of involvement by tumor or the treatment modality used, careful follow-up monitoring by retinal examination with the child under anesthesia and by CT is indicated. Genetic counseling is recommended. If the retinoblastoma is found to be genetically inherited, siblings should be periodically examined as well as any children the affected child should have.

Children with familial retinoblastoma have a high incidence of developing second malignancies (primarily osteosarcoma) later in life because of the genetic origin of the disease. Although no specific screening is recommended, signs and symptoms should be carefully evaluated with a high index of suspicion.

Evaluation

* Are the child and family verbalizing fears and a decrease in anxiety?
* Is the child able to compensate for loss of vision and continue daily activities?
* Is the child able to relate to peers and family?
* Are the child and family able to describe the disease and the treatment plan and demonstrate proper care of any prosthetic device?

RARE TUMORS OF CHILDHOOD

Several tumors not mentioned in this chapter occur infrequently in the pediatric population. These include soft tissue sarcomas other than rhabdomyosarcoma, primary tumors of the liver (e.g., hepatoblastoma and hepatocellular carcinoma), and gonadal and extragonadal germ cell tumors. Carcinomas, melanomas, and primary cancer of the lungs are a few of the cancers seen in adults that are exceptionally rare in children. Many of the key principles of nursing care—pain management, nutrition, comfort, infection control, and emotional support—remain constant for almost all pediatric cancer diagnoses.

KEY CONCEPTS

* The signs and symptoms of childhood cancer vary according to the child's age, the type of tumor, and the extent of the disease.
* Childhood cancer is difficult to diagnose because most symptoms can be attributed to common childhood illnesses.
* The decision to use allogeneic bone marrow, autologous peripheral blood stem cells, or umbilical cord blood stem cells is made with regard to the disease process being treated and available sources of hematopoietic cells. Increased screening for possible bone marrow donors through the NMDP has greatly increased the donor pool for stem cell and bone marrow transplantation.
* Nursing care of children with bone marrow transplants is complex and focuses on preventing infection until the marrow engrafts and the children produce their own WBCs with which to fight infection. All other organ systems must be monitored for GVHD and toxicities associated with preconditioning chemotherapy and radiation.

- Biologic response modifiers are naturally occurring substances found in the body that influence the immune system.
- Chemotherapy is nonselective in its cytotoxic effect.
- Fatigue is a common side effect of radiation therapy, and the child may need longer or more frequent periods of rest.
- Common nursing diagnoses associated with the child with cancer include Risk for Infection; Imbalanced Nutrition: Less Than Body Requirements; Deficient Knowledge; Ineffective Coping (individual); Compromised Family Coping; Acute and Chronic Pain; Impaired Skin Integrity; Disturbed Body Image; and Impaired Oral Mucous Membranes.

- The mouth and anus are at increased risk for breakdown in the child receiving chemotherapy or radiation therapy. Temperatures should be measured by means other than rectally, and meticulous mouth and anal care should be given.
- Postoperatively, the child with a brain tumor is at risk for increased intracranial pressure related to edema, hydrocephalus, or hemorrhage. Vital signs and mental and neurologic status are checked frequently.
- The abdomen of a child with a Wilms tumor should not be palpated because excessive manipulation can cause seeding of the tumor if the protective capsule is ruptured.

ANSWERS TO
CRITICAL THINKING EXERCISE 24-1

1. Complementary and alternative therapies are not the same. Complementary therapies are used in addition to conventional treatment and focus mainly on symptom relief. They are proven therapies (based on adequate research) or therapies that are not yet scientifically proven but are deemed to not be harmful as adjunctive treatment. Alternative therapies are those designed to replace conventional therapy in the treatment of individuals with cancer.

2. More people are using the Internet for information about various therapies for their specific health condition. The Internet is quite accessible; however, little control over information published on various websites exists. In the area of complementary and alternative therapies, any individual or group can publish information on a website; this information can be inaccurate, scientifically unfounded and, in some cases, dangerous. Become familiar with reputable websites that can provide necessary information. The following are respected websites that have information about complementary and alternative therapies along with conventional therapies:
   American Brain Tumor Association: *www.abta.org*
   American Cancer Society: *www.cancer.org*
   National Cancer Institute: *www.nci.nih.gov*
   National Institutes of Health: *www.nih.gov*
   National Center for Complementary and Alternative Medicine: *www.nccam.nih.gov*
   National Institute of Nursing Research: *www.nih.gov/ninr*

   Leukemia and Lymphoma Society: *www. leukemia.org*
   Children's Oncology Group: *www.childrensoncologygroup.org*

3. When assisting families in their thinking about complementary and alternative therapies, health professionals should help them consider the following questions*:
- What are the benefits and risks associated with the therapy?
- Do the benefits outweigh the risks?
- What side effects can be expected?
- What are the costs and will the therapy be covered by insurance?
- What training and other qualifications does the practitioner have?
- Are there scientific articles or references about using the treatment?
- Could the therapy interfere with or delay conventional treatments?
- How long will the treatment last and how often will it be assessed?
- Will it be necessary to buy equipment or supplies?
- Are there any conditions for which this treatment should not be used?

*National Center for Complementary and Alternative Medicine. (2006). *Key points in selecting a complementary and alternative medical (CAM) practitioner.* Retrieved September 9, 2006, from http://nccam.nih.gov/health/practitioner/index.htm.

REFERENCES AND READINGS

Abeloff, M., Armitage, J., Niederhuber, J., Kastan, M., & McKenna, W. (2004). *Clinical oncology* (3rd ed). Philadelphia: Elsevier.

American Academy of Pediatrics. (2003). Pickering, L. K. (Ed.), *Red Book: 2003 report of the Committee on Infectious Diseases* (26th ed., p. 73). Elk Grove Village, IL: Author.

American Cancer Society. (2003). How is osteosarcoma treated? Retrieved September, 9, 2006, from *http://www.cancer.org/docroot/CRI/content/CRI_2_4_4X_How_is_osteosarcoma_treated_52.asp.*

American Cancer Society. (2005). What are brain and spinal cord tumors in children? Retrieved February 19, 2006, from *http://www.cancer.org/docroot/CRI/content/CRI_2_4_1X_What_are_childrens_brain_and_spinal_cord_tumors_4.asp?sitearea=.*

Arndt, C. (2004a). Malignant tumors of bone. In R. Behrman, R. Kliegman, & H. Jenson (Eds.), *Nelson textbook of pediatrics* (17th ed., pp. 1717-1722). Philadelphia: Saunders.

Arndt, C. (2004b). Soft tissue sarcomas. In R. Behrman, R. Kliegman, & H. Jenson (Eds.), *Nelson textbook of pediatrics* (17th ed., pp. 1714-1717). Philadelphia: Saunders.

Ater, J. (2004). Neuroblastoma. In R. Behrman, R. Kliegman, & H. Jenson (Eds.), *Nelson textbook of pediatrics* (17th ed., pp. 1709-1711). Philadelphia: Saunders.

Bleyer, A. (2004). Principles of treatment. In R. Behrman, R. Kliegman, & H. Jenson (Eds.), *Nelson textbook of pediatrics* (17th ed., pp. 1688-1694). Philadelphia: Saunders.

Bowden, V., & Greenberg, C. (2003). *Pediatric nursing procedures.* Philadelphia: Lippincott Williams & Wilkins.

Boyer, H., & Whiles, L. (2004). Nurse-led assessment of children receiving chemotherapy. *Paediatric Nursing, 16*(5), 26-27.

Campana, D., & Pui, C. (2004). Childhood leukemia. In M. Abeloff, J. Armitage, J. Niederhuber, M. Kastan, & W. McKenna (Eds.), *Clinical oncology* (3rd ed., pp. 2731-2764). Philadelphia: Elsevier.

Connors, J. (2004). Hodgkin's lymphoma. In M. Abeloff, J. Armitage, J. Niederhuber, M. Kastan, & W. McKenna (Eds.), *Clinical oncology* (3rd ed., pp. 2985-3041). Philadelphia: Elsevier.

Dome, J., Rodriguez-Galindo, C., Spunt, S., & Santana, V. (2004). Pediatric solid tumors. In M. Abeloff, J. Armitage, J. Niederhuber, M. Kastan, & W. McKenna (Eds.), *Clinical oncology* (3rd ed., pp. 2661-2722). Philadelphia: Elsevier.

Eilersten, M., Reinfjell, T., & Vik, T. (2004). Value of professional collaboration in the care of children with cancer and their families. *European Journal of Cancer Care, 13,* 349-355.

Erickson, J. (2004). Fatigue in adolescents with cancer: A review of the literature. *Clinical Journal of Oncology Nursing, 8*(2), 139-145.

Friedman, D., & Meadows, A. (2002). Late effects of childhood cancer therapy. *Pediatric Clinics of North America, 49,* 1083-1106.

Gilchrist, G. (2004). Lymphoma. In R. Behrman, R. Kliegman, & H. Jenson (Eds.), *Nelson textbook of pediatrics* (17th ed., pp. 1698-1702). Philadelphia: Saunders.

Gurney, J., & Bondy, M. (2004). Epidemiology of childhood and adolescent cancer. In R. Behrman, R. Kliegman, & H. Jenson (Eds.), *Nelson textbook of pediatrics* (17th ed., pp. 1679-1684). Philadelphia: Saunders.

Hawes, R. (2005). Therapeutic relationships with children and families. *Paediatric Nursing, 17*(6), 15-18.

Herzog, C. (2004). Retinoblastoma. In R. Behrman, R. Kliegman, & H. Jenson (Eds.), *Nelson textbook of pediatrics* (17th ed., pp. 1722-1723). Philadelphia: Saunders.

Jaffe, N., & Huff, V. (2004). Neoplasms of the kidney. In R. Behrman, R. Kliegman, & H. Jenson (Eds.), *Nelson textbook of pediatrics* (17th ed., pp. 1711-1714). Philadelphia: Saunders.

Jennings, P. (2005). Providing pediatric palliative care through a pediatric supportive care team. *Pediatric Nursing, 31*(3), 195-200.

Kuttesch, J., & Ater, J. (2004). Brain tumors in childhood. In R. Behrman, R. Kliegman, & H. Jenson (Eds.), *Nelson textbook of pediatrics* (17th ed., pp. 1702-1709). Philadelphia: Saunders.

Maity, A., Pruitt, A., Judy, K., & Phillips, P. (2004). Cancer of the central nervous system. In M. Abeloff, J. Armitage, J. Niederhuber, M. Kastan, & W. McKenna (Eds.), *Clinical oncology* (3rd ed., pp. 1347-1387). Philadelphia: Elsevier.

Mettler, F., & Stazzone, M. (2004). Pediatric radiation injuries. In R. Behrman, R. Kliegman, & H. Jenson (Eds.), *Nelson textbook of pediatrics* (17th ed., pp. 2349-2353). Philadelphia: Saunders.

Moore, J., & Beckwitt, A. (2004). Children with cancer and their parents: self-care and dependent-care practices. *Issues in Comprehensive Pediatric Nursing, 27,* 1-17.

National Center for Complementary and Alternative Medicine. (2003). *Key points in selecting a complementary and alternative medical (CAM) provider.* Retrieved September 9, 2006, from *http://nccam. nih.gov/health/practitioner/index.htm.*

Perry, M., Anderson, C., Donehower, R. (2004). Chemotherapy. In M. Abeloff, J. Armitage, J. Niederhuber, M. Kastan, & W. McKenna (Eds.), *Clinical oncology* (3rd ed., pp. 483-535). Philadelphia: Elsevier.

Pizzo, P., & Poplack, D. (2002). *Principles and practice of pediatric oncology* (4th ed.). Philadelphia: Lippincott Williams & Wilkins.

Robertson, K. (2004). Hematopoietic stem cell transplantation. In R. Behrman, R. Kliegman, & H. Jenson (Eds.), *Nelson textbook of pediatrics* (17th ed., pp. 732-737). Philadelphia: Saunders.

Sandlund, J., & Behm, F. (2004). Childhood lymphoma. In M. Abeloff, J. Armitage, J. Niederhuber, M. Kastan, & W. McKenna (Eds.), *Clinical oncology* (3rd ed., pp. 2765-2792). Philadelphia: Elsevier.

Taketomo, C., Hodding, J., & Kraus, D. (2005). *Pediatric dosage handbook* (11th ed., pp. 1027-1028). Canada: Lexi-Comp, Inc.

Tubergen, D., & Bleyer, A. (2004). The leukemias. In R. Behrman, R. Kliegman, & H. Jenson (Eds.), *Nelson textbook of pediatrics* (17th ed. pp. 1694-1698). Philadelphia: Saunders.

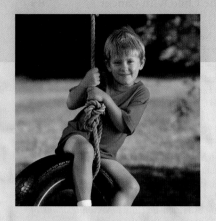

CHAPTER 25

The Child With an Integumentary Alteration

Learning Objectives

After studying this chapter, you should be able to:

- Describe the anatomy and physiology of normal skin.
- Contrast characteristics of the neonate's, child's, and adult's skin.
- Identify the manifestations of common skin disorders seen in infants and children.
- Discuss the management of skin disorders seen frequently in children, such as bacterial, fungal, and viral infections; infestations; inflammatory disorders; acne vulgaris; and insect bites and stings.

- Discuss common causes of burns in children and the prevention of burn injuries.
- Analyze the implications of burn injuries in children.
- Discuss the classifications of depth, extent, and severity of a burn injury.
- Describe the therapeutic management and nursing care of children with minor burns.
- Apply the nursing process to the care of infants and children with skin disorders.

Definitions

alopecia   Hair loss.
débridement   Removal of foreign material and devitalized or contaminated tissue from a traumatic or infected lesion to expose healthy tissue.
desquamation   Sloughing of the skin in scales or sheets; can lead to loss of the deeper skin layers.
ecchymosis   Discoloration of the skin or mucous membranes caused by leakage of blood into the subcutaneous tissue.
erythema   Redness of the skin.
eschar   Dark plaque associated with tissue necrosis, which can form an inelastic shell over wounds.
excoriation   Scratch or abrasion of the skin.
hydrotherapy   Therapy entailing water soaks to clean wounds, which removes old dressings and softens dead tissue for easier removal.

intertrigo   Maceration of two closely apposed skin surfaces.
keratosis   Overgrowth and thickening of the cornified epithelium.
lichenification   Thickening and hardening of the skin with accentuation of skin markings; often the result of chronic scratching.
pediculocide   An agent used to destroy lice.
petechiae   Tiny, flat, purplish red spots on the skin surface resulting from minute hemorrhages within the dermis.
pruritus   Itching.
urticaria (hives)   Vascular reaction of the skin characterized by pruritic wheals, often caused by allergy or emotional stress.
Wood light   Ultraviolet light used to help diagnose fluorescent skin lesions, including some superficial fungal infections.

Electronic Resources

Additional information related to the content in Chapter 25 can be found on:

the interactive companion CD-ROM

- Audio Glossary
- NCLEX Review Questions

or the companion website at *evolve*
http://evolve.elsevier.com/james/ncoc

- NCLEX Review Questions
- Resources for Health Care Providers and Families
- WebLinks

REVIEW OF THE INTEGUMENTARY SYSTEM

A knowledge of integumentary structure and function is necessary to understand the changes that occur with disease. There are a number of important differences between the skin of infants and young children and that of adults.

The skin has five major functions: (1) to protect the deeper tissues from injury, drying, and invasion by foreign matter; (2) to regulate temperature; (3) to aid in excretion of water; (4) to aid in production of vitamin D; and (5) to initiate the sensations of touch, pain, heat, and cold.

The skin is composed of two principal layers: the outer *epidermis* and the inner supportive *dermis*. Beneath these layers is the *subcutaneous layer*, which is composed largely of adipose tissue.

The *epidermis* is nonvascular stratified epithelium. It is divided into two major layers. The outermost layer, the *stratum corneum*, is a tough, horny collection of dead keratinized cells that have migrated up from the underlying layers. *Keratin*, a fibrous protein, is also the principal component of nails and hair. Skin cells are constantly being shed and replaced with new cells from the layers below.

The *stratum basale*, or basal cell layer, anchors the epidermis to the dermis. It contains dividing, undifferentiated cells that migrate upward toward the stratum corneum differentiating into keratinocytes on their way. Epidermal replacement is relatively rapid; the epidermis is completely replaced about every 4 weeks. The stratum basale also contains melanocytes—the source of melanin, the pigment that gives skin its color.

The *dermis*, composed of tough connective tissue, contains lymphatics and nerves. The highly vascular dermis nourishes the epidermis.

Appendages from the epidermis—sebaceous glands, sweat glands, and hair follicles—are embedded in the

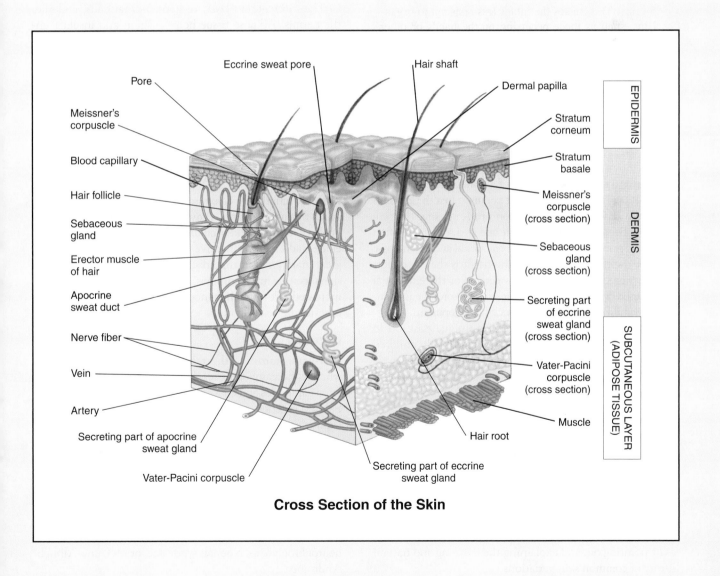

Cross Section of the Skin

PEDIATRIC DIFFERENCES IN THE SKIN

- The newborn's epidermis is thinner than that of adults. This results in increased permeability to topical agents and increased water loss through the skin.
- The ratio of skin surface area to body volume is greater in infants and small children than in adults, contributing to the risk of greater absorption through the skin. Topical medications should not be used without a physician's order.
- Premature infants have a proportionately greater body surface area than older infants and children, which increases evaporative fluid losses. Premature infants also have fewer cell attachments, which increases the tendency to blister.
- Eccrine glands do not reach mature function until age 2 or 3 years, making infants and young toddlers less able to regulate body temperature.
- Infants have fewer melanocytes than adults, which increases photosensitivity.
- IgA, secreted by the epithelial cells of the mucous membranes, does not reach adult levels until age 2 to 5 years. This makes the infant less resistant to organisms, such as those occurring on the hands or other objects the infant might mouth.
- Hormonal changes during adolescence increase sebum production, which contributes to acne vulgaris.

Modified from Cohen, B. (2005). *Pediatric dermatology* (3rd ed., p.15). Baltimore: Elsevier Mosby.

dermis. The sebaceous glands arise from the hair follicles and produce sebum, which lubricates the epidermis and is slightly bacteriostatic. Sebaceous glands are particularly abundant on the face and scalp. Hormones influence their activity, with testosterone increasing secretion and estrogen suppressing it.

There are two types of sweat glands. The *eccrine sweat glands* open directly onto the skin surface and produce sweat, which evaporates to reduce body temperature. Eccrine sweat glands are widely distributed over the body and are functionally mature by 2 months of age. The *apocrine sweat glands* produce a thick, milky secretion and open onto hair follicles. They are located mainly in the axillary and genital areas and become active during puberty.

Each hair is composed of a shaft and a root, which lie in a deep cavity of dermal cells called the *hair follicle*. There are several types of hair. *Lanugo* is the fine first hair that covers the body during fetal life and generally disappears before or shortly after birth. It is replaced by fine, nonpigmented *vellus* hair. *Terminal* hair covers all the ordinarily hairy parts of the body; it is coarse, long, and pigmented.

The *subcutaneous layer,* composed of fat cells, underlies the dermis. Adipose tissue helps cushion and insulate underlying structures.

The skin is a sensitive indicator of a child's general health. Skin disorders are among the most common health problems in children. They may cause pain, pruritus, or changes in local sensation. Because the skin is visible and its disorders are often disfiguring, skin disorders can cause emotional and psychologic stress for the child and family. Whether it is the discomfort and stress produced by an infant's eczema or the emotional upset caused by an adolescent's acne, these disorders can influence the child's psychologic and social development.

Nurses caring for children are in a unique position to assess the condition of children's skin and to help children and families cope with skin disorders. Nurses can play an important role by teaching parents and children strategies to maintain healthy skin and prevent future skin problems.

COMMON VARIATIONS IN THE SKIN OF NEWBORN INFANTS

Parents typically inspect every inch of their newborn infant's skin and continue to attend closely to variations in the skin of older infants. Regardless of whether the parent mentions it, the nurse may be sure the family is aware of spots, bumps, or rashes on the baby. Families frequently worry needlessly about skin lesions on infants, and the nurse can ease anxieties by pointing out and explaining the meaning and natural history of common skin variations.

COMMON BIRTHMARKS

Most birthmarks are composed of cells of one or more of the skin's normal elements. Any of the skin's components can produce a birthmark, including melanocytes, blood vessels, epidermal cells, connective tissue, and hair follicles. The great majority of birthmarks are benign, although some can signal congenital syndromes, some can be associated with an increased risk for malignancy, and others can interfere with function or be disfiguring.

Etiology

Port-wine stains are the result of capillary malformation, whereas hemangiomas result from the proliferation of dilated capillaries and endothelial cells of the capillary linings. Salmon patches (*nevus simplex*) represent distended dermal capillaries and are believed to result from persistent fetal circulation. Mongolian spots are not vascular but the result of collections of pigment deep in the dermis. They occur as a result of arrested migration of melanocytes from the neural crest to the skin during embryonic development. Café-au-lait spots, light-brown pigmented areas, can appear anywhere on an infant's body. Six or more of these lesions, if larger than 5 mm in diameter, suggest an underlying disorder, such as neurofibromatosis, Noonan syndrome, or McCune-Albright syndrome.

Incidence

Vascular birthmarks are extremely common, with most references estimating an incidence of occurrence in at least 20% to 40% of neonates. Port-wine stains occur in 3 in 1000 live births (Vascular Birthmarks Foundation, 2006), and about 1% to 2% of all newborn infants have hemangiomas (Darmstadt & Sidbury, 2004). The most common vascular lesion is the salmon patch, which some references estimate to occur in as many as 40% of neonates. The incidence of mongolian spots is proportional to the depth of the baby's pigmentation. As many as 80% of African American and American Indian infants are born with mongolian spots, and 70% to 80% of Asian and Latino infants have them. Fewer than 10% of white infants have mongolian spots (Darmstadt & Sidbury, 2004).

Manifestations

The port-wine stain is present at birth. At first it is only faintly colored and flat, but it becomes darker as the child grows. In some cases, underlying bone and tissue may enlarge as well. The port-wine stain is permanent, and by middle age, the mark may be dark purple and rough or nodular. Hemangiomas, on the other hand, are not usually visible at birth but appear during the first few weeks of life and then grow during the first year. Generally, they begin to disappear spontaneously after 1 year of age and are gone by age 5 or 6 years. The salmon patch is a flat, pink, irregular-shaped spot on the nape of the neck, on the forehead, between the eyes, on the eyelids, or around the nasolabial folds. Commonly called "stork bites" or "angel kisses," these lesions are benign and usually fade during the first year of life. Salmon patches typically appear darker when the child is crying. Mongolian spots are present at birth and appear as flat, gray-green or blue lesions similar to bruises. They are most commonly distributed on the lumbosacral regions or buttocks, although they can appear on any part of the body. Mongolian spots generally fade completely by the time the child is 4 to 5 years old.

Diagnostic Evaluation

The appearance of most birthmarks is sufficient to make a diagnosis, although biopsy and histologic evaluation are definitive. Although rare, some hemangiomas are signs of more serious underlying disorders. Worrisome hemangiomas include those with large, segmented facial distributions, those with a beard distribution, and those that involve the gluteal cleft. Magnetic resonance imaging is typically performed to rule out underlying anomalies (Guttman, 2005).

Therapeutic Management

Other than education, treatment for salmon patches and mongolian spots is not indicated. Treatment for port-wine stains is not indicated in the neonatal period, but their identification should prompt evaluation for associated congenital syndromes, such as Sturge-Weber, Beckwith-Wiedemann, and Klippel-Trenaunay syndromes. Conservative management of port-wine stains in older children includes instructions in concealing the lesions with makeup and psychotherapy if needed. Surgical excision and grafting of these lesions have been abandoned for the most part because of disfiguring scarring. Pulsed dye laser therapy has been used on port-wine stains since the 1980s with increasing success. It is generally most effective for port wine stains on the face and on lighter skin (Sommer, Seukeran, & Sheehan-Dare, 2003).

The treatment for hemangiomas includes simple observation as the lesion involutes on its own, pharmacotherapy, surgical excision, radiation, and laser therapy. Active intervention is reserved for hemangiomas that interfere with function, such as those that obstruct the nose, mouth, or eyes or lesions that tend to ulcerate and bleed frequently. Pharmacologic approaches include injection of steroids into the lesion, oral steroids, and topical imiquimod. The argon laser tends to relieve the symptoms of ulcerated hemangiomas in a matter of days, and involution typically follows. A rapidly growing, deep hemangioma may be a sign of Kasabach-Merritt syndrome, a consumptive coagulopathy that results in thrombocytopenia and collecting of platelets within the hemangioma. This may be life threatening. Treatment may include hospitalization and multimodal therapies to prevent bleeding and induce resolution of the lesion (Wananukul, Nuchprayoon, & Seksarn, 2003).

Nursing Considerations

Assess the child's entire body for distribution, size, and shape of lesions. Assess hemangiomas for symptoms such as ulceration or bleeding and for potential to obstruct function. Assess the extent of the parents' knowledge regarding the infant's birthmarks.

Parents are frequently anxious about newborn infants' skin lesions, and it is not unusual to discover that parents already have acquired misinformation from friends and family members about the meaning and prognosis of birthmarks. Common anxiety-provoking beliefs include the ideas that prominent lesions are malignant or that the mother caused the lesions by careless behaviors during her pregnancy.

The parents should receive a simple, scientific explanation for the skin lesions and instructions regarding the usual skin care for neonates (Box 25-1). Parents should be made aware of the expected course of their child's lesion, and their expectations should be explored. Parents should be reassured when the lesions are benign and educated thoroughly about what to expect when treatment is indicated.

INFECTIONS OF THE SKIN

Skin infections are common in childhood. Bacteria are normally present on healthy skin. The skin's susceptibility to bacterial infection depends on several factors, including the intactness of the skin, the virulence of the organisms, and the child's immune status. Children are susceptible to fungal and viral infections, as well. Unlike bacterial infections, which generally respond fairly quickly to treatment, fungal and viral infections can be more persistent and challenging to treat.

BOX 25-1 | PARENTS WANT TO KNOW About Care of Newborn and Infant Skin

Encourage parents to protect the infant's skin by teaching the following:

- Infants may be bathed and shampooed daily after the umbilical cord has fallen off. Use mild soap and warm water.
- Avoid overbathing, which dries the skin. Do not allow the infant to bathe longer than 10 minutes. Avoid bubble bath products; they dry and irritate the skin.
- Lotions, creams, and powders are not needed after the bath.
- Change diapers frequently and clean the diaper area with water at each change.

- Remove diapers for short periods during the day while the baby lies on a washable pad, to expose diaper area to air.
- Avoid hot environments and overbundling the baby. Infants do not sweat effectively, and heat results in rashes and problems with temperature regulation.
- Avoid direct exposure to the sun during the first 2 weeks of life and avoid sun exposure for more than 10 to 15 minutes daily thereafter during early infancy. Babies should wear hats or bonnets and shirts in the sun. Do not use sunscreen on infants younger than 6 months.

Although bacterial skin infections can be caused by a variety of microbes, *Staphylococcus* is a major pathogen, accounting for most of the skin infections of childhood. Skin infections predominantly caused by *Staphylococcus aureus* can range from minor, superficial lesions to severe generalized lesions with systemic effects. These skin infections include folliculitis, furuncles (boils), cellulitis, bullous impetigo, nonbullous impetigo, and staphylococcal scalded skin syndrome. Impetigo, a superficial, usually minor, staphylococcal infection, is the most common bacterial skin infection of childhood. Folliculitis is inflammation of hair follicles. Furuncles, or boils, develop when the infection of an existing folliculitis progresses deeper. Cellulitis is infection of the subcutaneous tissues.

IMPETIGO

Impetigo often occurs as a secondary infection from another skin lesion, such as an insect bite. Close contact contributes to the spread of impetigo, which is very contagious. Children in day care facilities, schools, or camps and adolescent athletes are at increased risk. The incubation period for impetigo is 7 to 10 days, and it may spread to other parts of the child's skin or to others who touch the child, use the same towel, or drink from the same glass. Spread of the infection is fostered by poor hygiene, crowded living conditions, and a hot, humid environment. Lesions resolve in 12 to 14 days with treatment.

Etiology

Impetigo can be caused by *S. aureus*, group A beta-hemolytic streptococci, or a combination of these bacteria. *S. aureus* is the primary pathogen in most cases. Nonbullous impetigo, sometimes referred to as crusted impetigo, was formerly thought to be a result of streptococcal infection. Studies have shown that *S. aureus* is the primary cause of both bullous and nonbullous impetigo (Ladhani & Garbash, 2005). Bullous impetigo is at the minor end of a spectrum of blistering disorders caused by the exfoliative toxins produced by some strains of *Staphylococcus*. Staphylococcal scalded skin syndrome is at the more severe end of that spectrum.

PATHOPHYSIOLOGY

IMPETIGO

Impetigo begins in an area of broken skin, such as an insect bite, scabies, or atopic dermatitis. The break in the skin allows for organism entry. The inflammatory process results in the formation of a pustular lesion. Honey-colored fluid from this lesion becomes crusted. In some children, nasal discharge containing the organism erodes healthy skin above the upper lip, allowing for organism entry.

Incidence

Impetigo occurs most often during hot, humid summer months. Toddlers and preschoolers are most commonly affected, often when recovering from an upper respiratory tract infection.

Manifestations

The primary lesions of impetigo occur in two forms. Bullous impetigo characteristically presents as small vesicles that can progress to bullae. The lesions are initially filled with serous fluid and later become pustular. The bullae rapidly rupture, leaving a shiny, lacquered-appearing lesion surrounded by a scaly rim. Crusted impetigo appears initially as a vesicle or pustule that ruptures to become an erosion with an overlay of honey-colored crust. The erosions bleed easily when crusts are removed (Fig. 25-1). Lesions are mildly pruritic. Scarring is uncommon but may occur if the child picks or scratches the lesions. Postinflammatory hyperpigmentation is a frequent sequela in dark-skinned children. The lesions are often located around the mouth and nose but can appear on any part of the body.

Diagnostic Evaluation

The characteristic appearance of the lesions usually confirms the diagnosis. A culture is not often done unless the child fails to respond to treatment. Failure to respond to treatment may indicate infection with community-acquired

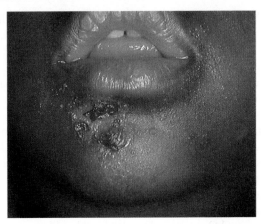

FIG 25-1   **Impetigo lesions are usually located around the mouth and nose but may be located on the extremities.**   *(From Hurwitz, S. [1993]. Clinical pediatric dermatology: A textbook of skin disorders of childhood and adolescence [2nd ed., p. 280]. Philadelphia: WB Saunders.)*

methicillin-resistant *S. aureus,* an increasingly common problem among children (Fridkin et al., 2005). If a culture is ordered, the specimen should be obtained from beneath the crust or from the fluid inside the lesions.

Therapeutic Management

Impetigo is treated with topical and oral antibiotics. The lesions should be gently washed three times a day with a warm, soapy washcloth and the crusts soaked and carefully removed. A topical ointment, such as mupirocin (Bactroban) or bacitracin (Baciguent), is then applied to the lesions. Topical therapy lasts 7 to 10 days. Severe cases of impetigo or cases of impetigo around the mouth are treated with oral antibiotics that are effective against both staphylococcal and streptococcal organisms. Impetigo that is extensive is treated with intravenous (IV) antibiotics. Antibiotic treatment of streptococcal impetigo does not prevent glomerulonephritis, but it does hasten healing of the lesions.

Good handwashing and careful hygiene are imperative to prevent spread of the infection and should be emphasized to the child and parents. The child should not attend school or day care for 24 hours after beginning treatment (American Academy of Pediatrics [AAP], 2003). The school should be notified of the diagnosis.

NURSING CARE

The Child With Impetigo

Assessment

Assess the child's skin for the size, distribution, and spread of impetigo lesions. If the child is taking systemic antibiotics, monitor for signs of adverse effects, such as rashes or diarrhea. Observe for periorbital edema or blood in the urine, which may signal the development of acute glomerulonephritis if the impetigo is caused by beta-hemolytic streptococci.

Nursing Diagnosis and Planning

The nursing diagnoses and expected outcomes that may be appropriate for the child with impetigo and the child's family are as follow:

- Impaired Skin Integrity related to destruction of skin layers secondary to bacterial infection.

  Expected Outcomes: The child will maintain skin integrity, as evidenced by confinement of the infection to the primary site. The area will heal without scarring or further infection.

- Deficient Knowledge related to unfamiliarity with measures to prevent spread of infection, care of impetigo lesions, and antibiotic administration.

  Expected Outcomes: The child and family will adhere to measures to prevent the spread of infection. The parent will demonstrate care of the lesions and administration of medications.

Interventions

Teach parents to soak the crusts and then wash them off with a warm, soapy washcloth three times a day. Advise them to gently remove the crusts after soaking, taking care not to spread the infection to other parts of the body with the contaminated washcloth. Antibiotic ointment should then be applied to the lesions and the affected areas left open to air. A small amount of bleeding after crust removal is common.

The child should sleep alone and should be bathed daily, alone, with antibacterial soap. The caregiver should wear gloves when caring for the child. Emphasize the importance of administering the full course of topical or systemic antibiotics as prescribed.

Evaluation

- Are the lesions healing, and have they remained confined to the primary site?
- Do the child and family members practice handwashing and other techniques to prevent the spread of infection?
- Do the parents appropriately explain the necessity for administering the full course of treatment?

CRITICAL TO REMEMBER
Caring for a Child With Impetigo

- The child can spread impetigo lesions merely by touching another part of the skin after scratching the infected area.
- Keep the child's fingernails short and wash the child's hands frequently with antibacterial soap.
- Emphasize good handwashing and careful hygiene for the child's entire household.
- Discourage family members from sharing towels, combs, or eating utensils with the infected child.

CELLULITIS

Cellulitis is bacterial infection of the subcutaneous tissue and the dermis. It is usually associated with a break in the skin, although cellulitis of the head and neck can follow an upper respiratory tract infection, sinusitis, otitis media, or tooth abscess. Cellulitis occurs most commonly in the lower extremities, the buccal (inside the cheek,) and periorbital (around the eye) regions. Complications of cellulitis include septic arthritis, meningitis, and brain abscess. Periorbital cellulitis can lead to blindness.

Etiology and Incidence

Since the introduction of the *Haemophilus influenzae* type B vaccine, group A streptococci and *S. aureus* are the most common causes of cellulitis. Cellulitis is most common in children age 2 years and younger.

Pathophysiology

Bacteria overwhelm the defensive cells that normally contain inflammation to local areas. The result is more extensive invasion of the causative organism as the infection moves from superficial tissue to deeper subcutaneous tissue.

Manifestations

The affected area is red, hot, tender, and indurated. If *H. influenzae* is the suspected organism, the affected area might have a purplish tinge. Edema and purple discoloration of the eyelids and decreased eye movement are present in periorbital cellulitis. Lymphangitis may be seen, with red "streaking" of the surrounding area and enlarged regional lymph nodes (lymphadenitis). The child usually exhibits fever, malaise, and headache.

Diagnostic Evaluation

Usually a complete blood cell count, blood cultures, and culture of the affected area are done. If no drainage is present, the affected area can be aspirated. Orbital cellulitis can be diagnosed by computed tomography of the orbit.

Therapeutic Management

After an initial intramuscular or IV dose of an antibiotic, such as ceftriaxone, the child with cellulitis of an extremity is usually treated at home with a 10-day course of oral antibiotics (cephalosporin, cloxacillin, or dicloxacillin) and warm compresses. If the cellulitis involves a joint or the face or if the child shows other signs of acute febrile illness, hospitalization and IV antibiotics are required. Incision and drainage of the affected area may be necessary.

NURSING CARE

The Child With Cellulitis

Assessment

Record the history and question the parent regarding recent ear infections, dental caries, or trauma to the skin surrounding the affected area. Other pertinent data include when the inflammation started and how rapidly it has progressed. Examine the skin, noting any temperature increase, swelling, redness, and drainage. Assess for fever, pain, guarding, and irritability.

Nursing Diagnosis and Planning

The nursing diagnoses and expected outcomes that may be appropriate for the child with cellulitis and the child's family are as follow:

- Impaired Skin Integrity related to bacterial invasion.
  Expected Outcome: The child will exhibit signs of healing, such as decreased redness, decreased swelling, and decreased fever.
- Acute Pain related to soft tissue swelling and inflammation.
  Expected Outcomes: The child will be able to sleep and will demonstrate decreased irritability.
- Deficient Knowledge related to unfamiliarity with the illness and treatment.
  Expected Outcomes: The family will describe measures to prevent the spread of infection, will describe how to administer antibiotics as prescribed, and will demonstrate the ability to carry out treatment measures.

Interventions

The child should rest in bed with the affected extremity elevated and immobilized. Warm, moist soaks applied every 4 hours increase circulation to the infected area, relieve pain, and promote healing. Acetaminophen can be given to control fever and pain. Frequent handwashing is essential to prevent the spread of infection. If the child is hospitalized, IV antibiotics should be administered accurately and on time to maintain a therapeutic blood level. If the child is being treated at home, the parents must understand the importance of administering the entire course of antibiotics as ordered. The child should be carefully monitored for signs of sepsis (increased fever, chills, confusion) and spread of infection.

Evaluation

- Does the child's skin exhibit signs of healing?
- Is the child free from signs of infection and pain?
- Does the parent administer prescribed medications and carry out appropriate home care?

CANDIDIASIS

Thrush (oral candidiasis) (Fig. 25-2) is a superficial fungal infection of the oral mucous membranes that is common in infants. Thrush occurs as a result of overgrowth of *Candida albicans*. In addition to oral lesions, the child may exhibit lesions in the diaper area, which are caused by *C. albicans* passing through the intestine. Moisture and heat in the diaper area create an environment favorable to the development of *Candida* dermatitis. Persistent candidiasis suggests that the child might be immunocompromised.

Etiology

A neonate can acquire candidiasis during delivery while passing through an infected vagina. An older infant may have a

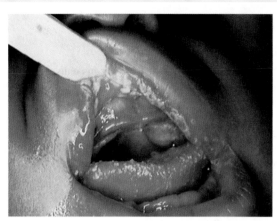

FIG 25-2   **White, curdlike plaques of thrush (oral candidiasis, oral moniliasis), a common fungal infection in infants.** *(From Hurwitz, S. [1993]. Clinical pediatric dermatology: A textbook of skin disorders of childhood and adolescence [2nd ed., p. 36]. Philadelphia: WB Saunders.)*

fungal overgrowth as a result of immunosuppression, during antibiotic therapy, from exposure to the mother's infected breasts, or from unclean bottles and pacifiers.

Incidence

Candidiasis occurs most often in infants. Predisposing factors in all age groups include antibiotic therapy, diabetes, and altered immune status.

Manifestations

White, curdlike plaques are noted on the tongue, gums, and buccal mucosa in children with thrush. They can be distinguished from milk curds by the difficulty encountered in removing them and the bleeding of an erythematous base when plaques are removed. A child with severe infection may have difficulty eating. The lesions of diaper dermatitis are usually bright red and coalesced, with some satellite lesions spreading out to the child's abdomen and thighs (Fig. 25-3).

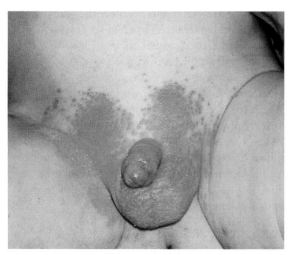

FIG 25-3   **Diaper candidiasis.** *(From Feigin, R. D., & Cherry, J. D. [Eds.]. [1999]. Textbook of pediatric infectious diseases [4th ed., p. 728]. Philadelphia: WB Saunders.)*

Diagnostic Evaluation

The diagnosis of thrush and candidal diaper dermatitis is made from the clinical appearance of the lesions.

Therapeutic Management

Nystatin oral suspension (100,000 U/mL), swabbed onto the mucous membranes of the mouth, is effective in treating thrush. Because *Candida* is present in the gastrointestinal tract, oral nystatin also may be ordered to decrease the likelihood of recurrence. Oral fluconazole is an alternative therapy. Candidal diaper dermatitis is treated with a topical antifungal agent, such as nystatin or clotrimazole (Lotrimin).

NURSING CARE
The Child With Candidiasis

Assessment

Nursing assessment includes obtaining a history of maternal and infant *Candida* infections. Question the mother regarding vaginal itching or discharge or any nipple tenderness or redness. Also discuss methods used to clean bottles and pacifiers. Examine the infant's mouth and diaper area and assess nutrition and hydration status.

Nursing Diagnosis and Planning

The nursing diagnoses and expected outcomes that may be appropriate for the child with candidiasis and the child's family are as follow:
* Impaired Skin Integrity related to the effects of fungal infection.
   Expected Outcome: The infant will exhibit signs of healing lesions, as evidenced by pink, intact mucous membranes or resolution of diaper rash.
* Acute Pain related to oral lesions or skin irritation.
   Expected Outcome: The infant will have reduced discomfort, as evidenced by ability to take feedings without difficulty, decreased fussiness, and improved ability to sleep.
* Deficient Knowledge related to incomplete understanding of the cause of the infection and administration of medication.
   Expected Outcomes: The family will demonstrate methods to prevent spread of infection and will administer the entire course of medication as prescribed.
* Imbalanced Nutrition: Less Than Body Requirements related to mouth irritation and altered taste.
   Expected Outcomes: The infant will accept feedings and will consume appropriate amounts of nutrients.

Interventions

Teach the parent to swab 1 mL of oral nystatin suspension onto the infant's gums, tongue, and buccal mucosa every 6 hours until 3 to 4 days after symptoms have disappeared. Because cotton-tipped applicators tend to absorb the medication, a more effective method of administration is to rub the suspension onto the mucous membranes with a gloved finger. To increase the amount of time the medication is in contact with the mucous membranes, nystatin should be applied after feedings. Alternatively, oral fluconazole administered once a day may be used for treatment of thrush in infants.

Pacifiers, nipples, and bottles should be thoroughly cleaned to decrease the chance of reinfection. Teach the parents the technique and importance of good handwashing. If the infant is breastfed, the mother's breasts should also be treated with nystatin.

Suggest small, frequent feedings for the infant or child with thrush who is uncomfortable. Cool liquids are soothing to the older child.

For the infant with candidal diaper dermatitis, suggest that the parent apply nystatin or clotrimazole cream. Leaving the diaper area exposed to air reduces the moisture that facilitates fungal growth.

Advise the parent to contact the health care provider if the infant refuses to eat or fever develops or if the candidiasis does not clear with treatment.

Evaluation

- Have the lesions disappeared, leaving intact skin and oral mucous membranes?
- Does the child appear to be comfortable, sleeping well, and less irritable?
- Can the parents demonstrate proper medication administration?
- Is the child increasing the amount of oral intake?

TINEA INFECTION

Tinea is a superficial skin infection caused by a group of fungi known as *dermatophytes*. Tinea infections are designated by the word *tinea* followed by the Latin word for the affected part of the body. Figure 25-4 illustrates various types of tinea infections.

Etiology

Two types of dermatophytes, *Trichophyton* spp. and *Microsporum* spp., cause the majority of tinea infections. *Trichophyton* affects all keratinized tissue, including skin, nails, and hair. *Microsporum* invades the hair.

Tinea infections are transmitted from person to person, by animal contact, or by contact with contaminated fomites (e.g., combs, hats, headrests, pillows). Tinea cruris (fungal infection affecting the groin and scrotal area) is not highly contagious. Poor hygiene, friction from tight clothing, and obesity are predisposing factors. Tinea pedis (athlete's foot) is a fungal infection of toes and feet. It is contagious but rarely develops on healthy, dry skin.

Incidence

Tinea capitis usually occurs in children ages 1 to 10 years, whereas tinea pedis and tinea cruris are most common in adolescent boys. Because a moist environment supports the growth of fungal infections, most tinea infections appear when the weather is hot and humid.

PATHOPHYSIOLOGY

TINEA INFECTION

Tinea infection occurs when the fungus causing tinea invades the hair, the stratum corneum of the skin, or the nails.

In *tinea capitis,* the fungus invades the hair shafts, causing the hairs to become brittle and to break off at the level of the scalp, leaving an area of stubby, black-dotted alopecia. An immune reaction to the fungus may develop in the form of a *kerion,* a boggy, red, tender scalp mass that may contain *S. aureus* and is often accompanied by fever and lymphadenopathy. Children with allergies seem to be more susceptible to tinea capitis.

Tinea corporis (ringworm) is a fungal infection of the face, trunk, or extremities. It can be transmitted by humans or by dogs and cats. Most lesions of tinea corporis clear without treatment in several months, but some may become chronic.

Tinea cruris (jock itch) is characterized by an intense inflammatory reaction with severe pruritus.

Tinea pedis (athlete's foot) may become chronic, particularly in adolescents who wear unventilated athletic shoes. Tinea lesions may become secondarily infected with bacteria or *Candida.*

Manifestations

Common manifestations of tinea capitis include erythema and scaling of the scalp and one or more round patches of alopecia that slowly increase in size. Small papules at the base of hair follicles become crusting pustules and red scales. In some cases, thick, broken hairs close to the scalp surface result in patches of "black dot" alopecia. Kerion formation may occur as a result of an inflammatory response to fungal antigens. A kerion is a boggy, fluctuant nodule, typically crusted and studded with pustules. Surrounding lymph nodes may be enlarged.

Tinea corporis, commonly seen on the trunk, face, and extremities, is characterized by ringlike plaques with clear centers and scaly, red margins. Lesions are usually ½ to 1 inch in diameter and mildly pruritic.

Manifestations of tinea cruris include pink papules and scales on the inner thighs, groin, scrotum, and buttocks (but not the penis). Pruritus is also present.

Tinea pedis, commonly referred to as "athlete's foot," produces fine vesiculopustular or scaly lesions on the soles of the feet, between the toes, and under the nails. The webs between the fourth and fifth toes are most commonly involved. Peeling, fissures, and maceration appear in severe cases, and pruritus and burning are typically present.

Diagnostic Evaluation

Most tinea infections can be diagnosed from the clinical appearance of the lesions. Fungal cultures or microscopic

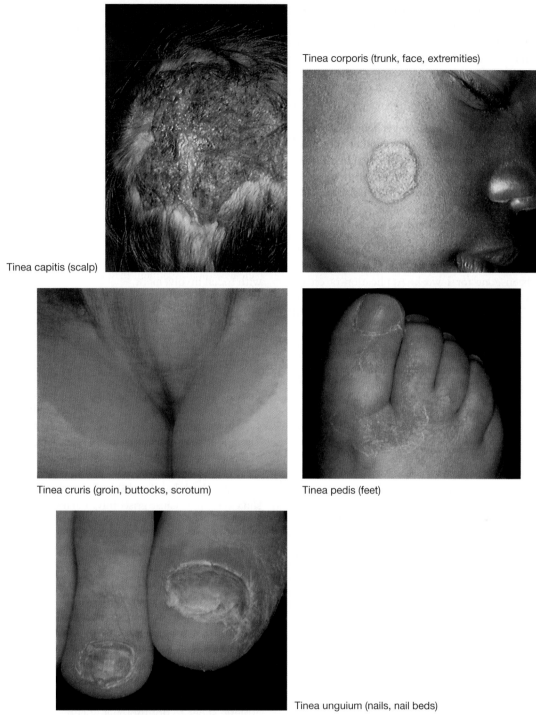

Tinea capitis (scalp)

Tinea corporis (trunk, face, extremities)

Tinea cruris (groin, buttocks, scrotum)

Tinea pedis (feet)

Tinea unguium (nails, nail beds)

FIG 25-4 **Tinea (ringworm) is an infection caused by dermatophytes, a group of fungi. Tinea is classified according to the part of the body affected. Five common types of tinea are shown here.** *(From Hurwitz, S. [1993]. Clinical pediatric dermatology: A textbook of skin disorders of childhood and adolescence [2nd ed., pp. 376, 380, 383, 385]. Philadelphia: WB Saunders.)*

examination of skin scrapings prepared with potassium hydroxide confirms the diagnosis. *Microsporum* lesions fluoresce as a bright blue-green under a Wood light. However, the most common organism causing tinea today, *Tinea tonsurans*, does not fluoresce.

Therapeutic Management

Tinea Capitis

For treatment to be effective, medication must penetrate the hair follicles. Topical therapy alone is not effective for tinea capitis. Oral griseofulvin administered daily for at least

6 weeks is the treatment of choice; it is the only drug approved by the U.S. Food and Drug Administration (FDA) for treating tinea capitis. Because griseofulvin is insoluble in water, its absorption is increased if it is taken with a high-fat meal or with milk. Other antifungals, such as ketoconazole (Nizoral), terbinafine (Lamisil), or fluconazole (Diflucan) may be prescribed for children who cannot tolerate griseofulvin or who fail to respond to it (Gupta et al., 2004). Ketoconazole and other azole antifungals are used with caution in children because of the risk of hepatotoxicity during long-term therapy. Selenium sulfide shampoo should be used twice per week for 2 weeks to eliminate spores and to decrease transmission.

Tinea Corporis

Local treatment is usually effective for tinea corporis. Antifungal preparations, such as clotrimazole (Lotrimin) or miconazole (Monistat), can be used three times a day until the lesions have been gone for 1 week. Application of cream should extend 1 inch beyond the lesion borders to prevent spread. Infected pets should be treated as well, and the child should avoid close contact with infected pets.

Tinea Cruris

Management for tinea cruris is similar to that for tinea corporis. Topical antifungal preparations should be applied twice a day to the lesions and at least 1 inch beyond the borders. Care should be taken to apply the medication to all creases, and the adolescent should be advised to wear loose clothing.

Tinea Pedis

A prescribed topical antifungal agent, such as clotrimazole (Lotrimin), miconazole (Monistat), or oxiconazole (Oxistat), is applied twice a day until the lesions have been cleared for 1 week. If the lesions do not respond to topical therapy, oral griseofulvin may be given for 1 month or longer, to promote healing. Newer systemic antifungals, such as itraconazole (Sporanox), have demonstrated improved success over a shorter time than griseofulvin. If the affected area is inflamed and oozing, soaking the feet in Burow's solution can promote healing.

NURSING CARE

The Child With a Tinea Infection

Assessment

Obtain a history that includes a description of the skin lesions and possible contacts. Animals with which the child has played should be carefully inspected for ringworm. The child's siblings and playmates should also be examined.

Nursing Diagnosis and Planning

The nursing diagnoses and expected outcomes that may be appropriate for the child with a tinea infection and the child's family are as follow:

- Impaired Skin Integrity related to inflammation and excoriation.

Expected Outcomes: The child will exhibit intact skin over impaired areas. The skin lesions will exhibit progressive healing.
- Impaired Comfort related to pruritic lesions.

Expected Outcomes: The child will remain calm and will exhibit no evidence of discomfort or pruritus; scratching will decrease.
- Deficient Knowledge of the cause, treatment, and spread of the infection related to lack of information.

Expected Outcomes: The child and family will verbalize accurate information about the child's skin condition. The child and family will demonstrate behaviors that prevent spread of the fungus. Treatments will be performed correctly.
- Disturbed Body Image related to alopecia or unattractive lesions.

Expected Outcome: The child will return to or continue with social involvement.

Interventions

Adequate teaching is essential for successful treatment of tinea infection (Box 25-2). In addition to teaching therapeutic management techniques specific for the child's particular type of tinea, emphasize to the parent that any prescribed oral medication regimen must be followed meticulously. Tinea infections are sometimes difficult to eradicate; discontinuing medication too soon risks recurrence. Treatment commonly continues for as long as 6 to 8 weeks and may continue for months for difficult infections of fingernails or toenails. It is important to advise the parent and the older child that the child taking griseofulvin must avoid sun exposure because griseofulvin makes the skin more susceptible to a photosensitivity reaction. If the child is taking itraconazole or longer courses of griseofulvin, the parent must ensure that the child undergoes the recommended liver function studies.

Fungus thrives in a warm, moist environment, so it is important to keep infected areas as dry as possible. Teaching proper hygiene is essential for preventing and treating fungal infections. Teach children to avoid sharing personal items, such as combs, hats, and hair ornaments. Children with tinea infections should sleep alone and should not share towels and washcloths with others. Feet should be washed daily and kept dry. Advise children to allow their nonventilated athletic shoes to dry thoroughly between wearings. Heavy cotton socks absorb sweat and keep the feet dry. If tinea pedis is present, the child should change socks at least twice a day and go barefoot or wear sandals as much as possible. Talcum powder or antifungal powder applied twice a day might help keep feet dry. If the child showers at school or at a gym, shower shoes should be worn.

Tinea cruris heals much faster if the groin area is kept dry. Loose-fitting cotton underwear should be worn, and athletic supporters and underwear should be washed frequently. The rash should be washed each day with plain water and carefully dried. Soap should be avoided. Scratching delays healing, so instruct the child to avoid scratching the area.

BOX 25-2	**THE CHILD & PARENTS WANT TO KNOW** About Home Care for a Child or Adolescent With a Tinea Infection

When providing information to the parent or older child with tinea, emphasize the following:
- Keep the infected areas as dry as possible.
- Do not share personal items, such as towels, washcloths, combs, hats, or hair ornaments.
- Athlete's foot: Wash the feet daily, and keep them dry. Nonventilated athletic shoes should dry thoroughly between wearing. Wear heavy cotton socks and change socks at least twice a day. Talcum powder or antifungal powder applied twice a day might help keep feet dry.

- Jock itch: Keep the groin area dry. Wear loose-fitting cotton underwear. Wash athletic supporters and underwear frequently. Wash the rash each day with plain water and dry carefully. Do not use soap on the affected area. Avoid scratching.
- Take oral medication as directed, even if the condition has improved. Discontinuing medication too soon can allow the infection to reappear.
- Call your physician if the infection has not improved in 4 weeks or if it continues to spread after 1 week of treatment.

Reassure the young man and his parents that tinea cruris is not associated with sexually transmissible disease.

Instruct parents to call the physician if the infection has not improved in 4 weeks or if it continues to spread after 1 week of treatment. Reassure parents that fungal infection is not an indication of poor hygiene or neglect. Avoid expressions of distaste or surprise when caring for children with severe alopecia or inflammation. Encourage parents to return the school-age child to school as soon as possible. Children with severe inflammatory tinea capitis may wish to wear a cap or scarf for a time until healing has progressed.

Evaluation
- Does the child have clean, intact skin?
- Is the child comfortable and without pruritus?
- Do the child and parents perform treatments correctly and verbalize ways to prevent the spread of infection?
- Does the child participate in usual social activities?

HERPES SIMPLEX VIRUS INFECTION

Herpes simplex types 1 and 2 (HSV-1, HSV-2) are responsible for a common, contagious, and often recurrent infection of the skin and mucous membranes. This infection can be asymptomatic or symptomatic and extremely painful. A wide spectrum of disease is caused by HSV: the common fever blister or cold sore (herpes labialis); corneal lesions; genital lesions (rare in children); and central nervous system infection.

Etiology

HSV is transmitted by infected body fluids and secretions coming in contact with breaks in the skin or mucous membranes. Delivery through an infected birth canal can cause infection in neonates. HSV can be transmitted by nurses who fail to practice careful handwashing. Children with burns, eczema, or diaper rash or those who are immunosuppressed are particularly susceptible to HSV infection.

Incidence

HSV is widespread. Infections in children are usually caused by HSV-1. Herpes labialis, commonly referred to as a "fever blister" is one of the most common manifestations of HSV-1. According to the Third National Health and Nutrition Study the annual prevalence of new herpes labialis manifesting is approximately 17% for children through the age of 17 years (Shulman, 2004). Infection with HSV-2, which affects primarily the anal-genital area, is rare before age 14 years. Child sexual abuse should be considered in any child with a genital herpes infection.

PATHOPHYSIOLOGY

HERPES SIMPLEX TYPE 1 INFECTION

The four types of human herpes viruses are HSV types 1 and 2; cytomegalovirus; Epstein-Barr virus, which causes infectious mononucleosis; and varicella-zoster virus. HSV-1 causes the "oral" type of herpes and usually affects areas above the waist, producing cold sores, fever blisters, and corneal lesions. HSV-2 affects areas below the waist (anal-genital area). However, either type can affect any region of the body. After an initial HSV-1 infection, the virus remains dormant but alive within nerve cells innervating that portion of the skin originally infected. Fever, stress, trauma, sun exposure, menstruation, or immunosuppression can reactivate the virus. When reactivated, the virus migrates to the skin area innervated by the ganglia that harbor it, near the site of the initial infection. The recurrent infection can be symptomatic or asymptomatic, but it is just as contagious as the initial infection. Recurrent infections tend to be less severe than the initial infection.

The immune status of the host determines the severity of HSV infection. HSV-1 infection in the neonate or immunocompromised child can be fatal. HSV-1 is a common cause of viral encephalitis in children.

Herpetic whitlow, a painful HSV-1 infection of the fingers, can be transmitted to a nurse during oral or tracheal care of a child with herpes infection. Thumb-sucking children with oral HSV-1 infection can also develop this condition. Health care personnel with herpetic whitlow should not have patient contact until the infection has healed because the infection is highly contagious.

Manifestations

Herpes Labialis ("Cold Sore," "Fever Blister")

Prodromal symptoms of herpes labialis are burning, itching, or tingling; these symptoms occur up to several days before lesions appear. Symptoms appear 2 days to 2 weeks after exposure. Lesions appear in clusters of fluid-filled vesicles that ulcerate, dry, and crust within 7 to 14 days (Fig. 25-5). Usually one or two lesions are present on the lips, tongue, gingiva, or buccal mucosa. Pruritus and pain are present. Approximately 85% of active HSV-1 infections are asymptomatic.

Herpetic Gingivostomatitis

Herpes gingivostomatitis is a severe oral infection that affects children younger than 5 years. Vesicles and ulcerations, an edematous throat, and enlarged, painful cervical lymph nodes are seen. Associated signs and symptoms include chills, fever, malaise, bad breath, and drooling.

Herpetic Ocular Infection

Herpetic ocular infection (keratitis) is typically the result of rubbing the eyes with contaminated fingers. Herpetic keratitis causes irritation and inflammation of the conjunctiva or cornea with associated tearing and photophobia. Vesicles appear on the eyelid and mucous membranes of the eye. Children with HSV keratitis are at risk for recurrent episodes and vision loss (Chong et al., 2004).

Herpetic Whitlow

Symptoms of herpetic whitlow appear 3 to 7 days after exposure and include vesicles, swelling, pruritus, and severe pain of the affected fingers. Discomfort may continue for weeks after the vesicles have healed.

Diagnostic Evaluation

Clinical manifestations and the child's history suggest the diagnosis. A Tzanck smear can confirm a herpes infection, but a positive smear cannot differentiate between varicella-zoster virus and HSV-1, and a negative smear does not rule out

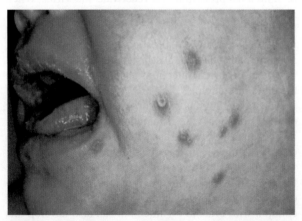

FIG 25-5   **Herpes simplex infection in an infant.**   *(From Feigin, R. D., & Cherry, J. D. [Eds.]. [1992]. Textbook of pediatric infectious diseases [3rd ed., p. 773]. Philadelphia: WB Saunders.)*

HSV infection. Immunofluorescence assay to detect HSV-1 antigen and polymerase chain reaction to detect HSV-1 deoxyribonucleic acid can be performed on blood samples, but tissue culture is still considered the gold standard for diagnosis (Subhan et al., 2004).

Therapeutic Management

Treatment is symptomatic. The child with oral HSV-1 infection is usually cared for at home if able to take adequate fluids. If the child becomes dehydrated, IV fluids are needed.

Topical or oral acyclovir (Zovirax), if given early enough in the course of the infection, can reduce the time to recovery. Although there is no cure for HSV-1 infection, acyclovir (Zovirax) given IV may be used in immunocompromised children, neonates, and children with encephalitis or ocular HSV to decrease the severity of the infection.

Antibiotic ointment may be used to treat secondary bacterial infection of lesions. Corticosteroids are contraindicated because they can worsen HSV-1 infection. Oral or rectal acetaminophen, with or without codeine, may be prescribed, and topical anesthetics may be dabbed on lesions to help relieve pain. A prescribed anesthetic mouth rinse of equal parts of diphenhydramine (Benadryl) elixir, Kaopectate, and 2% viscous lidocaine may decrease pain and help the child eat. Topical anesthetics, such as viscous lidocaine, must be used with caution. Overuse of topical anesthetics in small children can depress the gag reflex and increase the risk of aspiration

NURSING CARE

The Child With a Herpes Simplex Infection

Assessment

Obtain a history, and ask the parent or child about previous HSV infections or contact with an infected person. Examine the skin carefully for lesions. Inspect the eyes for corneal ulcerations and edema and assess the child's vision for blurring and photophobia. Referral to an ophthalmologist is necessary for suspected ocular HSV infection. For the child with herpes gingivostomatitis, pay particular attention to assessing hydration status.

Nursing Diagnoses and Planning

The nursing diagnoses and expected outcomes that may be appropriate for the child with a herpes simplex infection and the child's family are as follow:

- Impaired Skin Integrity related to inadequate secondary defenses.

  Expected Outcomes: The child will demonstrate healing of lesions. The child will have no other signs of infection.

- Acute Pain related to inflammation and infection.

  Expected Outcome: The child will have minimal pain, as evidenced by adequate fluid intake, decreased verbalization of pain, and decreased restlessness and irritability.

- Risk for Infection related to changes in skin integrity.

Expected Outcome: The child will have no signs of secondary bacterial infection, as evidenced by healing lesions and normal body temperature.

- Risk for Deficient Fluid Volume related to painful oral lesions.

Expected Outcomes: The child will maintain urine output appropriate for age and will exhibit moist mucous membranes and good skin turgor.

Interventions

Children with oral HSV infection may be extremely uncomfortable. Swallowing can cause severe pain, and dehydration is a real danger. Advise parents to contact the physician if the child has signs of dehydration. Fluid intake is very important, and the child must be encouraged to drink. Most children will accept Popsicles, noncitrus juices, milk, and noncarbonated or "flattened" soft drinks. Frequent small feedings of bland, soft foods can be offered. Reassure parents that a few days without solid food will not harm the child as long as fluid intake is adequate.

To prevent secondary infection, the child's mouth should be rinsed often with normal saline solution, especially after eating. Hospitalized children infected with HSV should be placed on contact precautions. The child is considered contagious until the scabs from visible lesions have fallen off. Because scabs do not form on mucous membranes, these lesions are considered contagious until they are completely healed. All personnel who have contact with the child should follow standard precautions and be particularly careful when touching the child near the lesions, during oral care or suctioning, and when handling bed linens or objects that might be contaminated with saliva or secretions from the lesions. Careful handwashing is essential.

Parents should take similar precautions when caring for the child at home to prevent spread of infection. Advise the parents to wash bottles, nipples, toys, eating utensils, and towels in hot, soapy water or in a dishwasher, if available. Family members should not share any of these items with the infected child.

Because the infection can be spread to other parts of the body, the child should not put his or her fingers near the mouth or infected area. Elbow restraints may be necessary for children too young to understand this. The child with HSV-1 infection is usually miserable and needs generous cuddling and comforting.

Evaluation

- Are lesions healed, with no sign of the infection spreading?
- Does the child demonstrate increased comfort?
- Does the skin remain free of signs of secondary infection (redness, swelling, drainage)?
- Is the child properly hydrated with adequate fluid intake and hourly urine output (see Chapter 18)?
- Can the parent or caregiver describe infection control measures?

LICE INFESTATION

Lice are small, blood-sucking insects about 2 to 4 mm in length. *Pediculosis* refers to infestation of lice on the scalp or body. Although pediculosis is not a serious health problem, it can cause embarrassment and often elicits an emotional reaction among parents and school personnel who may mistakenly associate it with poor hygiene. Head lice are not responsible for the spread of any disease, although body lice are known to serve as vectors of several pathogenic bacteria (La Scola & Raoult, 2004).

Etiology

Lice live only on humans and are transmitted by direct contact with infected persons and indirect contact with infested objects (e.g., brushes, hats). Lice cannot jump like fleas, and clean hair is no deterrent to head lice.

Incidence

The AAP (2002) reports approximately 6 to 12 million cases of head lice each year among children 3 to 12 years of age in the United States. Pediculosis rarely occurs in African Americans. Girls are affected twice as often as boys. All socioeconomic groups are affected. The peak incidence is in preschool and young school-age children. Pubic lice are usually seen in adolescents or young adults and are generally transmitted by sexual contact.

Manifestations

Pediculosis Capitis (Head Lice)

Nits are visible and are attached firmly to the hair shafts near the scalp. They are tiny, silvery or grayish white specks resembling dandruff but they are more difficult to remove. They are commonly found behind the ears and at the nape of the neck. In active infestation, nits are found approximately ¼ to ½ inch away from the scalp surface (Fig. 25-6). Adult

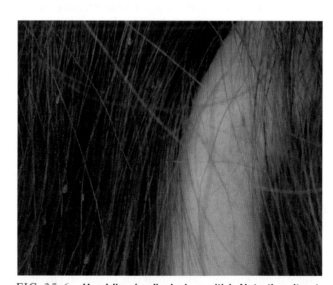

FIG 25-6 **Head lice (pediculosis capitis). Note the nits attached to the hair shafts.** *(From Calen, J., Greer, K. E., Hood, A. F., Paller, A. S., & Swinyer, L. J. [1993]. Color atlas of dermatology [p. 373]. Philadelphia: WB Saunders.)*

PATHOPHYSIOLOGY

PEDICULOSIS

Pediculosis may involve the scalp (pediculosis capitis), the body (pediculosis corporis), or the pubic area and eyelashes (pediculosis pubis). A specific type of louse, each of which has a similar life cycle, causes each of these infestations. All lice pierce the skin and suck blood. Severe itching caused by bites can predispose the child to secondary infection.

Head and pubic lice spend their life cycles on the skin of the human host; body lice live in clothing, coming to the skin only to feed. The female head louse lays eggs (nits) at the base of the hair shaft. The egg is covered with a gelatinous material, which hardens to semiopaque, tiny, pearly whitish masses that are stuck tight to the hair shaft (see Fig. 25-6). Eggs incubate for about 1 week, and lice reach sexual maturity in about 2 weeks.

Pediculosis pubis is spread through sexual contact. Half of all patients with pediculosis pubis have another sexually transmissible disease, usually gonorrhea.

Lice can spread as long as the lice and nits remain alive on the infested person or belongings. Lice can live only 48 hours off the human host. Nits shed into the environment are capable of hatching for 10 days.

lice are difficult to see because of their small size and the fact that they crawl very fast to avoid light. Scattered lesions on the scalp, behind the ears, or on the back of the neck cause intense pruritus. These lesions are often associated with posterior cervical lymph adenopathy. Secondary scalp infection may develop from scratching.

Pediculosis Corporis (Body Lice)

Papular, rose-colored dermatitis, causing intense pruritus, appears on the skin in areas under tight clothing. Nits attach firmly to seams of the child's clothing or bedding.

Pediculosis Pubis (Pubic Lice, Crab Lice)

Pediculosis pubis are lice that can be found in pubic hair and facial hair, in axillae, and on the body surface. The presence of pubic lice in the eyebrows or eyelashes of a prepubescent child suggests sexual abuse. Pubic lice also cause intense pruritus. *Maculae ceruleae* (blue spots) may be seen on the thighs and trunk in cases of heavy infestation. Dark-brown spots on underwear and sheets are insect waste materials.

Diagnostic Evaluation

The diagnosis of head lice is made by identification of nits or lice on the scalp. The examiner parts the hair with two tongue depressors and moves from side to side and front to back, paying particular attention to the crown, behind the ears, and the nape of the neck. The exposed scalp should be carefully examined under bright light or in a sunny area.

A magnifying glass can assist in identification. Unlike dandruff, nits are not easily removed from hair shafts. Pubic lice are diagnosed from a history of symptoms and visual inspection.

Therapeutic Management

Management of the child with pediculosis involves a three-tiered approach: (1) killing the active lice, (2) removing nits, and (3) preventing spread or recurrence by managing the environment.

Killing Active Lice

Approaches to treating pediculosis are changing as a result of the development of pediculicide-resistant strains of lice and because prescription lindane (Kwell) persists as a poison in the environment and can be neurotoxic if absorbed through the skin. Lindane, a hexachlorocyclohexane, has been nominated for elimination as a persistent organic pollutant under the provision of the Stockholm Convention on Persistent Organic Pollutants (United Nations Environmental Programme, 2005).

Over-the-counter products containing pyrethrins (RID, Triple X, R&C, Pronto) are safe and effective. Because they lack residual activity (i.e., they do not stay in the hair after treatment), treatment with these products must be repeated 1 to 2 weeks after the initial treatment. An over-the-counter pediculicide, permethrin 1% (Nix), kills head lice and pubic lice and eggs with one application and has residual activity for 10 days. Nix crème rinse is applied to the hair after it is washed with a conditioner-free shampoo. It is applied as a lotion to pubic hair. Crème rinse or lotion should be rinsed out after 10 minutes. The hair should not be shampooed for 24 hours after the treatment. Treatment and testing for other sexually transmissible diseases are required for sexual contacts of a person with pubic lice.

Body lice are treated with a prescription drug or an over-the-counter medication (RID, Pyrinate200, Triple X) according to the manufacturer's instructions. Clothing and bedding should be washed in hot water and dried for 20 minutes at a hot dryer setting.

The pesticide malathion (Ovide) is approved for the treatment of lice as well, but it requires prolonged contact (i.e., 8-10 hr) to be effective. It is also flammable, and families should be cautioned not to use hairdryers or allow the child near fires or heaters while hair is being treated. The AAP recommendations for the treatment of head lice are revised every 3 years, and the interested reader is referred to that source for current guidelines (*www.aap.org*).

Addressing the Environment

Environmental objects, clothing, and bedding should be treated or washed. It is important to examine and treat family members and others who might be in close contact with the infested child. Meticulous vacuuming of carpets in classrooms with affected children will help prevent continuation of an epidemic.

The Child With Pediculosis

Assessment

Examine children for lice in an unobtrusive and private manner. In a school setting, classmates should be brought to the school nurse's office and admitted one at a time, rather than being seen together in a general check in a classroom setting. Use disposable tongue depressors or Popsicle sticks to part the hair and discard these implements between children. Check all family members for the presence of nits or lice.

Assess adolescents with pubic lice for signs of other sexually transmissible diseases and ask about sexual contacts because they will need treatment as well.

Nursing Diagnosis and Planning

The nursing diagnoses and expected outcomes that may be appropriate for the child with pediculosis and the child's family are as follow:

- Acute Pain related to inflammatory response and pruritus.
  Expected Outcomes: The child will rest comfortably and be free of scratching.
- Risk for Infection related to scratching of scalp.
  Expected Outcome: The child will have no signs of secondary bacterial infection, as evidenced by intact skin and normal-size cervical lymph nodes.
- Deficient Knowledge about treatment of lice infestation and the prevention of recurrence related to anxiety or incomplete information.
  Expected Outcomes: The child or family will carry out the prescribed treatment. The parent will demonstrate measures taken to prevent reinfestation.
- Risk for Situational Low Self-Esteem related to social stigma associated with lice.
  Expected Outcomes: The child or family will verbalize self-acceptance and will engage in usual social activities.

Interventions

Advise parents to carefully follow directions that come with over-the-counter pediculicides or to follow the physician's instructions for using prescription products. Caution parents against applying the medication more frequently than recommended.

Reassure parents that lice infestation does not reflect poor hygiene or low socioeconomic status. Advise them that it is necessary to notify the school nurse if the child is infested.

Teach parents to remove nits by back-combing with a fine-tooth comb. One hour before combing, nits can be loosened with a mixture of half vinegar and half water or a commercial product, such as Clear or Step 2. It is easier to comb the child's hair for nit removal when the hair is damp rather than wet or dry. Lice and nits can be removed from eyelashes by applying petrolatum to the eyelashes twice a day for 8 days. Many schools have a "no nit" policy, which requires that a child be free of all nits before re-entry, although such policies are strongly discouraged by the AAP (2003).

Advise parents to wash clothing (especially hats and jackets), bedding, and linens in hot water and dry at a hot dryer setting. Dress-up clothes, bicycle helmets, batting helmets, headphones, and similar objects should be treated as well. Items that cannot be washed should be dry cleaned or sealed in plastic bags for 2 to 3 weeks.

Antilice sprays used for furniture and other environmental objects should *never* be used on a child. Thorough home cleaning is necessary to remove any remaining lice or nits. Parents should vacuum floors, play areas, and furniture to remove any hairs that might carry live nits. Combs and brushes should be boiled or soaked in antilice shampoo or hot water (>140° F) for at least 10 minutes. Routinely teach children not to share hats, combs, or hair ornaments with other children. At school, individually assigned lockers or separate hooks for coats can help inhibit spread of lice.

The child should be rechecked for infestation in 7 to 10 days. Advise parents to call the physician if itching interferes with the child's sleep, if the condition does not clear up after 1 week, or if scalp lesions look infected. The National Pediculosis Association provides information about this disorder (see *www.headlice.org*).

Evaluation

- Is the child free of infestation, pain, and pruritus?
- Is the skin intact, and does the child exhibit normal-sized cervical lymph nodes?
- Do parents carry out the prescribed treatments?
- Can parents describe measures to prevent the spread of lice to others?
- Do the parents and child realistically describe the cause of pediculosis and continue to engage in usual social activities?

CRITICAL THINKING EXERCISE 25-1

The pediatric clinic receives a phone call from an obviously upset mother about her 4-year-old daughter, who is in preschool. This is the third time in 1 month that the parent has been called at work to take her child out of school because the child was found to have lice. The mother states that she has properly treated her daughter and other family members, and she insists that the child is catching the condition from someone at school. The school maintains that no other child has this problem.
1. What should be the nurse's approach to this mother?
2. What kind of information will the nurse need to obtain to help this mother with her problem?

USING RESEARCH TO IMPROVE PRACTICE

Pediculosis is a worldwide problem and its treatment is challenging for families. The cost associated with treating a family for a lice infestation can be high. In addition, resistance to pediculocides is increasing, potentially reducing the effectiveness of existing treatments. Treatment is effective only when 100% of adult lice are killed and eggs are prevented from hatching. The frustration felt by families whose members are repeatedly infested with lice has resulted in an upsurge in use of traditional home remedies or remedies obtained by searching the Internet.

In a recent literature review of research on home treatment of pediculosis, Takano-Lee, Edman, Mullens, and Clark (2004) found only three research studies that addressed this topic; each of these studies contained methodologic or statistical flaws. To more accurately identify a home remedy that might kill lice within a reasonable contact time and with minimal danger (from flammability or chemical toxicity), these researchers tested the effectiveness of six commonly used home remedies: vinegar, isopropyl alcohol, olive oil, mayonnaise, melted butter, and petroleum jelly. Their experimental study was conducted in a laboratory setting, using cultivated human head lice colonies, which were allowed to infest hair tufts created from human hair.

Two different experiments that compared each home remedy with a control (deionized water) focused on different outcomes—impact of the remedies on live female lice and impact of the home remedies on eggs; the final study described the impact of prolonged water submersion on survivability of lice (Takano-Lee et al., 2004). Using a carefully controlled procedure of infesting the hair tufts, treating them with each home remedy, keeping them warm, and recording results after several different time periods, the researchers were able to statistically analyze differences between each of the home remedies and plain water.

Results from these experiments were interesting and have implications for teaching by nurses. None of the home remedies had a 100% kill of adult lice within the first 24 hours of treatment. Treatment with petroleum jelly significantly reduced the survival of lice compared with other remedies but not compared with water. Some of the home remedies delayed egg hatching but did not prevent it, and the remedies needed to remain on the hair for extended periods of time (9 to 10 days). Submersion of lice in water was not effective in killing adults either.

The researchers conclude that these common home remedies are ineffective in treating pediculosis, and, in some instances, are noxious or flammable. Nurses should discourage parents from using them on children. The only truly effective remedies that presently exist are treatment with an approved pediculocide, thorough combing and removal of nits, and meticulous environmental control (Takano-Lee et al., 2004).

Takano-Lee, M., Edman, J., Mullens, B., & Clark, J. (2004). Home remedies to control head lice: Assessment of home remedies to control the human head louse, *Pediculus humanus capitis* (Anoplura: Pediculidae). *Journal of Pediatric Nursing, 19,* 393-398.

MITE INFESTATION (SCABIES)

Scabies is a contagious condition that has been recognized for many centuries. It results from infestation with *Sarcoptes scabiei,* the "itch mite."

Etiology

Scabies is transmitted by close personal contact with infected persons. Persons who share a bed or live in crowded conditions are likely to transmit scabies to each other. The scabies mite cannot survive for more than 3 days away from human skin. For that reason, transmission of scabies by bedding or clothing is infrequent.

Incidence

Scabies is widespread throughout the United States and it is prevalent in many schools. All socioeconomic groups are affected.

Pathophysiology

The female mite burrows into the epidermis, lays her eggs, and dies in the burrow after 4 to 5 weeks. The eggs hatch in 3 to 5 days, and larvae migrate to the skin surface to mature and complete the life cycle. The mites, eggs, and their excrement cause intense pruritus. One of the major complications of scabies is impetigo resulting from scratching.

Manifestations

Intense pruritus occurs, especially at night. Infants may be cranky, sleep fitfully, and rub their hands and feet together. Burrows (fine, grayish, threadlike lines) can be difficult to see because they are usually obscured by secondary changes of excoriation and inflammation. Papules, vesicles, and nodules are common (Fig. 25-7) and are located mainly on the wrists, in the finger webs, on the elbows, in the umbilicus, in the axillae, in the groin, and on the buttocks. In infants, the head, palms, and soles may be affected.

Diagnostic Evaluation

The characteristic skin eruption and a history of intense pruritus, especially at night, are suggestive of scabies. The diagnosis is made by microscopic examination of scrapings of the lesions.

Therapeutic Management

Scabies can be treated with topical application of either permethrin 5% (Elimite) or lindane cream (Kwell, Scabene). Because of the risk of neurotoxicity, lindane should not be used in children younger than 2 years or in pregnant women. The medication is applied to the body and head, avoiding the eyes and mouth. The medication must remain on the child for 8 to 14 hours (depending on the medication

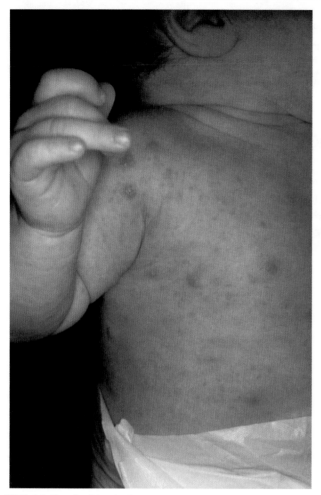

FIG 25-7 **Scabies lesions on an infant.** *(From Calen, J. P., Greer, K. E., Hood, A. F., Paller, A. S., & Swinyer, L. J. [1993]. Color atlas of dermatology [p. 301]. Philadelphia: WB Saunders.)*

prescribed) to be effective, so applying it at bedtime is most effective. It is washed off in the morning. Retreatment in 1 week is usually recommended. Pruritus may last for several days to weeks after treatment and can be relieved with corticosteroid cream (e.g., hydrocortisone cream) and oral antihistamines.

Family members, even if asymptomatic, and day care contacts (except for pregnant women) should also be treated. The child's bedding and clothing should be washed in hot water in a fashion similar to the environmental treatment for pediculosis.

Nursing Considerations

Nursing care of the child and family with scabies is similar to that for pediculosis. Inspect the child's hands, elbows, umbilicus, groin, and buttocks for burrows. Burrows may be difficult to see, however, and complaints of persistent itching may be the only symptom. Evaluate an adolescent with scabies for sexually transmissible disease.

Instruct parents to use the scabicide according to the manufacturer's instructions. The lotion is applied all over the child's body, including the soles of the feet, the scalp, behind the ears, in intertriginous areas, and under the toenails and fingernails. The lotion should be kept on for the recommended time (4-8 hr for lindane, 8-14 hr for Elimite), and then the child should be bathed. Infants should be clothed during treatment so they will not lick their skin. To minimize absorption and the risk of toxic effects from lindane, the lotion should not be applied for at least ½ hour after bathing and should be applied only to cool, dry skin. Advise the parent that persistent itching after treatment is expected for about 2 weeks and it is not a sign of reinfestation or an indication for repeated application.

Scabies is usually cured with one treatment; however, a repeat application in 1 week is recommended. Clothing and bed linen should be dry cleaned or washed in hot water and dried at a hot dryer setting.

ATOPIC DERMATITIS

Atopic dermatitis, or eczema, is a common chronic inflammatory disease of the skin characterized by severe pruritus. Atopic dermatitis can have distressing psychosocial effects on the child and family.

Etiology

The cause of atopic dermatitis is unknown, but the disease is thought to be genetically determined. Contributing factors include an inherited tendency for dry, sensitive skin; allergy; and emotional stress. Most children with atopic dermatitis have a family history of asthma, hay fever, or atopic dermatitis, and up to 80% of children with atopic dermatitis have asthma or allergic rhinitis (Eichenfield et al., 2003). Although the role of allergy in the etiology of atopic dermatitis is controversial, immunoglobulin E (IgE)–mediated food allergy has been shown to be an exacerbating factor in some children.

Incidence

The prevalence of atopic diseases, including asthma, allergic rhinitis, and atopic dermatitis has increased substantially in the last 30 years. Atopic dermatitis usually begins in infancy and clears by age 2 or 3 years, although it can persist through adolescence and adulthood. Data from the Prevention and Incidence of Asthma and Mite Allergy study show that high birth weight and day care attendance increase the risk for atopic dermatitis in infancy, whereas exclusive breastfeeding decreases the risk (Kerkhof et al., 2003). Atopic dermatitis affects all races. Symptoms tend to be worse during winter months.

Manifestations

During infancy, erythematous areas of oozing and crusting appear first on the cheeks and then on the forehead, scalp, and extensor surfaces of the arms and legs (Fig. 25-8). Papulovesicular rash and scaly, red plaques become excoriated and lichenified. The affected scalp area resembles seborrheic dermatitis, but unlike seborrheic dermatitis, atopic dermatitis is intensely pruritic. Infants begin manifesting symptoms at approximately age 1 to 4 months.

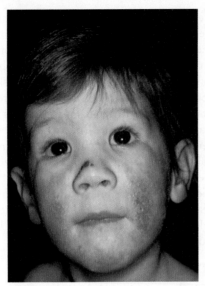

Lesions on cheeks often spread to the forehead, scalp, and extensor surfaces of arms and legs.

Flexor surfaces of wrists, ankles, knees, and elbows may be affected in the childhood form of the disease.

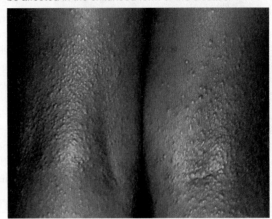

FIG 25-8   **Atopic dermatitis, an allergic skin condition, usually begins in infancy and clears by age 2 to 3 years. However, it can continue into childhood.** *(From Hurwitz, S. [1993].* Clinical pediatric dermatology: A textbook of skin disorders of childhood and adolescence *[2nd ed., pp. 49, 51]. Philadelphia: WB Saunders.)*

PATHOPHYSIOLOGY

ATOPIC DERMATITIS

Atopic dermatitis is an allergic skin condition. It has been suggested that infants who have atopic dermatitis have unusually slow maturation of T-cell function (Kerkhof et al., 2003). The skin of affected children releases more histamine than that of normal children. The high levels of histamine trigger an inflammatory response, resulting in erythema, edema, and intense pruritus. Scratching increases itching, leading to an itch-scratch-itch cycle. Continual scratching and rubbing excoriate and damage the skin. Oozing, weeping, crusting, and cracking lesions develop. The skin of children with atopic dermatitis carries a higher-than-normal colonization of *S. aureus,* and secondary infection is common. Impetigo and viral infections (herpes, molluscum contagiosum) occur frequently in these children.

Children who have atopic dermatitis after infancy have a rash pattern that differs from the rash seen during infancy. The flexor surfaces of the wrists, ankles, knees, and elbows are affected, as are the neck creases, the eyelids, and the dorsal surfaces of the hands and feet. There may be acute weeping areas, with or without secondary infection. Chronic lichenification results from persistent scratching.

Children and adolescents with atopic dermatitis readily experience intense itching, especially in response to sweating or contact with irritating fabrics, such as wool. Emotional upset increases sweating and precipitates itching and scratching. Dry skin is a hallmark of this condition.

Diagnostic Evaluation

The diagnosis is based on the clinical features of intense pruritus, the appearance of the lesions, the pattern of remissions and exacerbations, and a family history of allergy. IgE levels and eosinophils are often elevated. Skin testing for food allergies—usually milk, eggs, wheat, soy, peanuts, and fish—can help identify potential food triggers.

Therapeutic Management

The main goals of treatment are to control itching and scratching, moisturize the skin, prevent secondary infection, and remove irritants and allergens. Control of pruritus includes avoiding environmental triggers, such as overheating, soaps, wool clothing, and other skin irritants. Oral antihistamines, such as hydroxyzine (Atarax), diphenhydramine (Benadryl), and loratadine (Claritin), can be used to help break the "itch-scratch-itch" cycle. Nonsedating antihistamines, such as loratadine, may be preferred for school-age children. Itching is typically more severe at night; thus antihistamines should be given before bedtime. Secondary infection is treated with antibiotic therapy.

Proper skin hydration is essential. Either a "dry" or "wet" approach may be used. The dry approach depends on avoiding bathing and the liberal use of emollients on dry skin. The wet approach is currently more popular. It permits bathing for limited periods of time, and the use of wet compresses and occlusive creams and ointments are the mainstays of treatment. In humid climates bathing should be infrequent, and only lukewarm water and mild, nonperfumed soap (e.g., Purpose, white Dove, Basis) should be used. Emollients such as Eucerin cream or petroleum jelly applied immediately after bathing to damp skin help the skin retain moisture. Applying the moisturizer while the skin is still damp hydrates the skin. The child who lives in a dry climate should bathe frequently

DRUG GUIDE

TOPICAL CORTICOSTEROIDS

Classification: Topical anti-inflammatory.

Action: Reduce inflammation by causing vasoconstriction and inhibiting the movement of inflammatory cells from the bloodstream into local tissue.

Indications: Inflammatory skin diseases, such as atopic dermatitis.

Dosage and Route: Topical route; number of applications depends on the child's condition and the potency of the medication. Topical steroids are commonly divided into seven classes, with those of lowest potency assigned to the lowest (seventh) class.

- Class I: Optimized betamethasone dipropionate 0.05% (Diprolene cream or ointment)
- Class II: Triamcinolone acetonide ointment 0.5% (Kenalog); mometasone furoate ointment 0.1% (Elocon)
- Class III: Triamcinolone acetonide ointment 0.1% (Aristocort A); triamcinolone acetonide cream (Aristocort-HP); fluticasone propionate ointment 0.005% (Cutivate)
- Class IV: Hydrocortisone valerate ointment 0.2% (Westcort); mometasone furoate cream 0.1% (Elocon); desoximetasone cream 0.05% (Topicort-LP)
- Class V: Fluticasone propionate cream 0.05% (Cutivate); hydrocortisone valerate cream 0.2% (Westcort); triamcinolone acetonide cream 0.025% (Aristocort)

- Class VI: Desonide cream 0.05% (DesOwen); alclometasone dipropionate cream 0.05% (Aclovate)
- Class VII: Hydrocortisone cream 0.5%, 1% (Cortizone, Hytone, generic)

Absorption: Better absorbed through the skin immediately after bathing.

Contraindications: Never apply to diaper rashes or chickenpox lesions. Superpotent topical steroids (class I) are rarely used for children. Only low-potency agents should be used on the face.

Precautions: Unless directed by the physician, do not bandage, wrap, or otherwise cover areas being treated with topical steroids. In general, the more potent the medication, the shorter the treatment time will be.

Adverse Reactions: Systemic side effects can occur with short-term use of high-potency topical steroids or with long-term use of lower-potency topicals. Systemic effects include suppression of the hypothalamic-pituitary-adrenal axis, resulting in growth suppression; suppression of immune response; osteoporosis; moon face; and obesity. Locally, thinning of the skin, striae, telangiectasia, atrophy, and purpura can occur.

Nursing Considerations: Advise the parent to apply to the child's skin within 5 minutes of bathing, to meticulously follow the physician's directions for use, and to immediately report any side effects.

(several times a day), using a hydrophilic agent such as Cetaphil instead of soap, and should moisturize with a moisturizing ointment or cream immediately after bathing. The child should avoid lotions that contain alcohol because these can contribute to skin dryness. Regardless of the approach used, moisturizing the skin is maintenance therapy for atopic dermatitis and should become a daily routine for the child.

Anti-inflammatory corticosteroid creams and ointments are prescribed for inflamed or lichenified areas. These creams are more effective when applied to damp skin. The lowest potency that controls signs should be used, and topical steroids are usually reserved for treatment of episodic flares.

Topical calcineurin inhibitors, such as tacrolimus and pimecrolimus, suppress the release of inflammatory chemicals from lymphocytes without altering the function of other cells (Cohen, 2005). These drugs are approved by the FDA for children older than 2 years. They may be applied to 100% of the body surface if needed, and they may be used for longer periods of time than topical steroids may. Topical immunomodulators do not cause skin atrophy. Although they can penetrate the skin enough to suppress local inflammation, they are only minimally absorbed into the circulation.

Routine blood studies (to monitor for immunosuppression) in children using tacrolimus and pimecrolimus are not indicated. However, caution should be used in children whose skin integrity had widespread damage because immunosuppressives can be absorbed systemically in such cases

(Leung & Bieber, 2003). Topical calcineurin inhibitors have become popular for use in children with atopic dermatitis; however, postmarketing surveillance reveals risks. An FDA advisory panel recommended adding a black box warning to labels informing consumers that calcineurin inhibitors are associated with increased risk for certain cancers, especially in children (Nursing 2005, 2005).

Identifying and eliminating allergens can be helpful. Allergy proofing the home might be recommended (see Chapter 17). Because allergy to certain foods is an exacerbating factor in some children, those foods should be eliminated from the diets of sensitive infants. Breastfeeding for the first year is recommended for infants at risk for allergy. Solid foods should not be introduced until the infant is at least 6 months old.

NURSING CARE

The Child With Atopic Dermatitis

Assessment

Obtain a thorough history that includes information about allergies in the family. Question parents about any environmental or dietary factors that seem to worsen the child's condition. Determine what treatments have been tried and their effectiveness. Examine skin lesions for type, distribution, and evidence of any secondary infection. Assess the child's comfort level and the family's feelings and coping methods.

Nursing Diagnosis and Planning

The nursing diagnoses and expected outcomes that may be appropriate for the child with atopic dermatitis and the child's family are as follow:

- Impaired Skin Integrity related to environmental and immunologic factors.

  Expected Outcome: The child's skin will exhibit decreased evidence of dryness, irritation, and excoriation.

- Acute Pain related to dry skin, secondary infection, and external irritations.

  Expected Outcomes: The child will have minimal pain and pruritus, as evidenced by decreased irritability, absence of scratching, and uninterrupted periods of sleep.

- Risk for Infection related to skin excoriation.

  Expected Outcome: The child will have no signs of secondary bacterial infection, as evidenced by a normal body temperature and absence of purulent drainage.

- Deficient Knowledge about controlling itching, preventing secondary infection, and identifying aggravating factors related to anxiety or incomplete understanding of information.

  Expected Outcomes: The child and family will identify and eliminate allergens and aggravating factors. The family will carry out prescribed treatments correctly. Family members will express any anxiety related to the child's condition.

- Interrupted Family Processes related to the child's pruritus and involved treatment.

  Expected Outcome: The child and family will discuss their feelings and concerns.

- Disturbed Body Image related to perception of appearance.

  Expected Outcome: The child will engage in activities with other children. The child will verbalize positive ideas about self.

Interventions

Care of the child with atopic dermatitis is demanding, and the entire family routine may revolve around the affected child. Parents need support and reassurance as they care for an uncomfortable, often irritable child.

Keeping the child's skin hydrated will help relieve itching. Instruct parents to apply a moisturizing cream, such as Eucerin, several times a day and immediately after the child is bathed. Reassure parents that moisturizing creams contain no harmful drugs and should be applied whenever the child's skin looks dry. Soaks and cool, wet compresses are soothing and can be applied to remove crusts, reduce inflammation, and dry weeping areas. Provide parents with explicit instructions on the use of soaks and topical medications. Strips of old cotton sheets moistened in lukewarm or cool tap water work well for wet dressings. Wet compresses should not be used for more than 3 days.

Rough clothing can aggravate eczema, particularly wool or other fabrics that cause sweating. Soft cotton or cotton-polyester blends are tolerated best. Undergarments with irritating seams can be turned inside out so that the soft seam is against the skin. Heat and sweating increase pruritus, so instruct parents to be careful not to "bundle up" the child in heavy blankets or clothing. Because detergents and fabric softeners can also aggravate atopic dermatitis, clothes should be washed in mild detergent and rinsed twice.

Advise the parents to keep the child's fingernails clean and short. Cotton gloves or mittens might be needed to prevent excoriation from scratching but should be used with caution, preferably only at night, because overuse could interfere with fine motor development. Lightweight, long-sleeved tops and one-piece outfits discourage scratching.

The child's skin must be kept clean to minimize secondary infection. Avoid using soap. Bath oil or emulsifying ointment can be used as a soap substitute but must be used with caution because these cause both the child and the tub to become slippery. Tepid bath water helps prevent the child from becoming overheated and itchy. Instruct parents to contact the physician at the earliest signs of skin infection (weeping skin, pustules) and to administer topical and oral antibiotics as prescribed.

Children with atopic dermatitis who swim should apply moisturizer before swimming and immediately on exiting the pool. Prolonged immersion in water (more than 20 minutes) can have a drying effect. A humidifier in the child's room during winter months may decrease skin dryness. The child should avoid the drying effects of sun exposure.

Children and families of children with atopic dermatitis exhibit frustration when the condition does not resolve quickly. The parent or child might be concerned about the child's appearance as well as the child's discomfort.

> Help parents take control of the child's condition by empowering them with knowledge about therapeutic management. Allowing parents to verbalize frustrations and helping them learn management techniques that do not disrupt family routine are important interventions.

Although studies do not consistently support emotional upset as a direct cause of atopic dermatitis flares, it is helpful to teach an older child stress reduction techniques to help cope with the frustration and discomfort of the condition. A resource for families of a child with atopic dermatitis is the National Eczema Association for Science and Education.

Evaluation

- Is the child's skin intact and smooth?
- Have itching and pain been reduced?
- Is the child's skin free from redness or purulence that would indicate secondary infection?
- Do parents carry out prescribed treatments correctly?
- Are parents able to demonstrate appropriate coping techniques?
- Can the child demonstrate stress relief measures to decrease itching?

SEBORRHEIC DERMATITIS

Seborrheic dermatitis is a chronic inflammatory skin condition seen frequently in infants. It is referred to as "cradle cap" when located on the scalp. It often begins in the first 2 to 3 weeks of life and usually disappears by age 12 months. Seborrhea in older children might appear on the face, behind the ears, around the umbilicus, or in any other area with a large number of sebaceous glands. Although the precise cause is unknown, seborrhea appears to be related to sebaceous gland dysfunction and overgrowth of the fungus *Malassezia ovalis* (Abdulla & Brodell, 2005).

Seborrheic dermatitis is characterized by nonpruritic, oily, yellow scales that block sweat and sebaceous glands, causing retained secretions and inflammation in affected areas (Fig. 25-9). Confluent erythema might be present in the diaper and intertriginous areas and around the umbilicus (Fig. 25-10). Often, there is overgrowth of normal skin bacteria and yeast, which increases inflammation and leads to secondary infection.

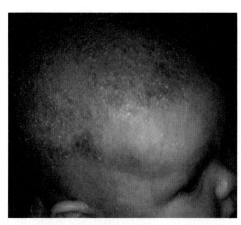

FIG 25-9   **"Cradle cap," the most frequent form of seborrheic dermatitis in infants. The condition often begins in the first 2 to 3 weeks of life and usually disappears by age 12 months.** *(From Hurwitz, S. [1993]. Clinical pediatric dermatology: A textbook of skin disorders of childhood and adolescence [2nd ed., p. 17]. Philadelphia: WB Saunders.)*

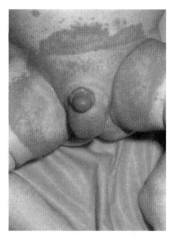

FIG 25-10   **Seborrheic diaper dermatitis.** *(From Moschella, S. L., & Hurley, H. J. [1992]. Dermatology [3rd ed., p. 239]. Philadelphia: WB Saunders.)*

The nurse inspects the infant's scalp or other affected areas for lesions and inflammation and questions parents about the frequency and technique of washing the infant's scalp. Instruct the parents to remove the scales daily by shampooing with a mild baby shampoo or an over-the-counter antiseborrheic shampoo containing sulfur and salicylic acid (Fostex Medicated Cleansing, P&S, Sebulex), selenium, or tar (Neutrogena T/Gel, Polytar). Massaging the scalp with warm mineral oil before shampooing helps loosen scales. Using a fine-tooth comb or a clean, soft-bristle toothbrush during the shampoo also helps loosen scales. Eyelid dermatitis (blepharitis) is treated with warm tap water compresses and cleansing with "no tears" baby shampoo. Care must be taken to keep topical medications out of the infant's eyes.

Teach the parents the importance of good hygiene of the infant's scalp and skin to prevent recurrence. Reassure them that the fontanel is not fragile and will not be damaged by gentle pressure and washing. Advise the parents to contact the physician if the sites become infected. Skin lesions that do not clear with frequent washing can be treated with hydrocortisone cream applied twice a day.

Seborrheic dermatitis of the diaper area is often secondarily infected with C. *albicans* and requires appropriate treatment. Lotions and creams tend to aggravate the condition and should not be used.

CONTACT DERMATITIS

Contact dermatitis is a skin inflammation that results from direct skin-to-irritant contact.

Etiology

Contact dermatitis can be caused by hundreds of substances. Among the most common causes of contact dermatitis are rubber products, clothing dyes, nickel (in jewelry, bra strap hooks, jeans fasteners), and plant oils. Scented or strongly alkaline soaps, skin lotions, cosmetics, and wool clothing also are irritating to many children.

Diaper dermatitis (diaper rash) is a contact dermatitis from irritants such as moisture, friction, and chemical substances. Urine ammonia, formed from the breakdown of urea by fecal bacteria, is extremely irritating to sensitive infant skin. Ammonia alone does not cause skin breakdown. Only skin damaged by infrequent diaper changes and constant urine and feces contact is prone to damage from ammonia in urine. Inadequate fluid intake, heat, and detergents in diapers aggravate the condition.

Incidence

Irritant contact dermatitis is more common in children than allergic contact dermatitis is. Diaper rash occurs in about 10% of infants, usually between the ages of 3 and 18 months, although it is most common between ages 6 and 9 months.

Manifestations

Manifestations of irritant contact dermatitis include dry, inflamed, and pruritic skin. The distribution of lesions correlates with the skin surface in contact with the offending

---

PATHOPHYSIOLOGY

CONTACT DERMATITIS

Contact dermatitis is an inflammatory reaction of the skin either caused by direct exposure to an irritant *(irritant contact dermatitis)* or as a result of a delayed hypersensitivity response to an allergen *(allergic contact dermatitis).*

Irritant contact dermatitis can occur in any person who has repeated or prolonged contact with a primary irritant. Examples of primary irritants include citrus juices, detergents, bubble bath formulations, and urine. Diaper dermatitis is an example of irritant dermatitis that results from prolonged exposure to urine. Teething infants can have dermatitis on the face and neck folds from drooling.

Allergic contact dermatitis, a delayed hypersensitivity reaction, occurs in susceptible individuals who are sensitized to a substance by a previous exposure to the contact allergen. *Rhus dermatitis* (caused by poison ivy, oak, and sumac), the most common type of allergic contact dermatitis in children, is caused by oleoresins contained in all parts of the plant. Lesions appear several hours to several days after contact.

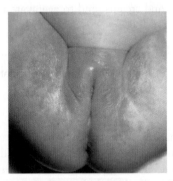

FIG 25-11   **Contact diaper dermatitis.**   *(From Moschella, S. L., & Hurley, H. J. [1992]. Dermatology [3rd ed., p. 239]. Philadelphia: WB Saunders.)*

agent (e.g., watchband, clothing). Diaper dermatitis begins with erythema in the perianal region and can progress to macules and papules, which form erosions and crusts (Fig. 25-11). Manifestations of allergic contact dermatitis include blistering, weeping lesions over an area of inflamed skin, intense pruritus, and crusted, scaly lesions that heal in 10 to 14 days without treatment. Rhus dermatitis may cause severe systemic reactions.

Diagnostic Evaluation

The characteristic appearance of the lesions and a history of exposure to an irritating substance establish the diagnosis. Skin testing might be performed in children with persistent or recurrent dermatitis.

Therapeutic Management

Discontinuing exposure to the offending agent treats contact dermatitis. The skin should be washed thoroughly if any irritant remains on the skin. Cool compresses of tap water or Burow's solution can soothe weeping, crusting lesions. Steroid cream (e.g., triamcinolone 0.1% or fluocinolone 0.025%) may be applied several times a day after application of compresses. Severe contact dermatitis might require treatment with oral steroids, which should be tapered gradually. Desensitization therapy is usually not effective in managing contact dermatitis.

NURSING CARE

The Child With Contact Dermatitis

Assessment

Investigate new or continuing exposure to any potentially irritating substances. Assessment of skin lesions includes noting their distribution and configuration and looking for evidence of pruritus.

For a child with diaper dermatitis, carefully inspect the diaper area, noting the type and extent of lesions. It is important to assess the infant's hygiene and the parents' knowledge of care related to the infant's skin integrity. Question parents about the type of diapers used, laundering practices, and frequency and method of cleaning the diaper area. Any recent changes in the infant's care, such as new foods, soaps, detergents, or lotions, should be investigated.

Nursing Diagnosis and Planning

The nursing diagnoses and expected outcomes that may be appropriate for the child with contact dermatitis and the child's family are as follow:

*   Acute Pain related to skin inflammation.

    Expected Outcomes: The child will have reduced skin irritation, as evidenced by decreased excoriation and increased healing. The child will exhibit decreased irritability, absence of scratching, and uninterrupted periods of sleep.

*   Risk for Infection related to scratching of pruritic lesions.

    Expected Outcome: The child will have no signs of secondary bacterial infection, as evidenced by clear intact skin.

*   Deficient Knowledge of management and prevention of future skin inflammation related to incomplete understanding of therapeutic principles.

    Expected Outcomes: The child and family will identify and avoid irritating substances and will carry out prescribed treatments correctly.

Interventions

Nursing care of the child with contact dermatitis is directed toward relieving itching, preventing infection, and identifying and removing offending substances. Cool compresses and tepid oatmeal (Aveeno) baths provide some relief from itching. Prescribed topical steroid creams should be applied in a thin layer after moisturizing with wet compresses to relieve inflammation. Antihistamines, such as diphenhydramine (Benadryl) or hydroxyzine (Atarax), also help the child rest. Because overheating increases itching, advise the parents to occupy the child with quiet activities and to keep the room temperature at a comfortable level.

Reassure the parents and child that the lesions are not contagious and cannot be spread to others or to other parts of the body by scratching. Oils from rhus plants (poison ivy, oak, sumac) that adhere to the skin, under the fingernails, and on clothing can cause new lesions if they are not removed with soap and water. Keep the skin clean and help the child avoid scratching to prevent secondary infection. Instruct the parents to contact the physician if the child has a fever or if the lesions produce purulent drainage.

Contact dermatitis is prevented by avoiding offending substances. Children should be taught to recognize plants of the rhus group. If the child is exposed to these plants, rinse the skin with cool water immediately (within 15 minutes) and wash clothing in hot, soapy water. Oleoresins in the plants can be spread not only by direct contact with the plant but also in the smoke of burning leaves or by touching pets that have contacted the plants.

Avoiding known irritants, such as cosmetics, jewelry, and canvas athletic shoes, can prevent other types of contact dermatitis. Nickel-sensitive children can usually tolerate 14-karat gold or sterling silver jewelry. Pierced earrings should have hypoallergenic or surgical stainless steel posts.

Diaper dermatitis is much easier to prevent than to treat. Successful treatment and prevention of diaper rash, regardless of the cause, depend on cleaning the diaper area thoroughly and keeping the skin dry. Prompt, gentle cleaning with water and mild soap (Dove, Neutrogena Baby Soap) after each voiding or defecation rids the skin of ammonia and other irritants and decreases the chance of skin breakdown and infection. Careful attention should be given to skin folds and creases. The parent should pat the skin dry with a soft cloth towel after washing. Air drying the skin and frequently exposing the skin to air and light promote healing of diaper rash. During bouts of diaper rash, the diaper may be left off during nap times.

A bland, protective ointment (A and D, Desitin, zinc oxide) can be applied to clean, dry, intact skin to help prevent diaper rash. Ointments should not be applied to inflamed areas because they retain moisture. Occlusion increases the risk of systemic absorption of steroid; thus steroid creams are rarely used for diaper dermatitis because the diaper functions as an occlusive dressing. Frequent diaper changes decrease irritation from urine and feces. Encourage the parents to check the newborn infant's diaper every hour and the older infant's diaper every 2 hours. Using disposable diapers does not eliminate the need for frequent diaper changes. Although the "wicking" action of disposable diapers pulls moisture away from the skin toward the liner, ammonia and other byproducts are left behind on the infant's skin, causing irritation. Rubber or plastic pants increase skin breakdown by holding in moisture and should be used infrequently.

If cloth diapers are laundered at home, the parents should wash them in hot water, using a mild soap and double rinsing. Soaking diapers before washing in a quaternary ammonium compound (Diaperene) decreases ammonia in the diapers. Using ¼ cup of vinegar in the rinse is also helpful.

Advise parents to contact the physician if the rash becomes solid and bright red, if it becomes raw or bleeds, if blisters or boils develop, if the rash does not improve in 3 days with treatment, or if the infant has a fever.

Evaluation
- Is the child's skin intact, with healed lesions and no evidence of pain or pruritus?
- Is the child's skin free from signs of secondary infection?
- Do the parents demonstrate understanding of proper skin and diaper area care?

ACNE VULGARIS

Acne is a disorder of the sebaceous hair follicles. Although acne is generally perceived as a minor disorder, it can cause significant anxiety and emotional pain for affected adolescents. The disfiguring lesions of acne can lead to physical and emotional scarring.

Etiology

Multiple factors play a role in the development of acne lesions, including abnormal sloughing of skin cells lining the sebaceous hair follicles, overgrowth of normal bacteria, and host factors, such as heredity, hormonal influences, and emotional stress. Acne of neonates may be triggered by infection with fungi, such as *Pityrosporum* species in some infants. Foods do not appear to cause or increase the severity of acne. Acne is unrelated to the general cleanliness of the skin.

PATHOPHYSIOLOGY

ACNE VULGARIS

Acne begins when sebaceous glands, stimulated by androgens at the onset of puberty, enlarge and secrete increased amounts of sebum. The sebaceous glands become plugged and dilated with sebum. When the enlarged gland is open to the skin surface, an open comedo, or blackhead, is formed. The characteristic black color is not a result of poor hygiene but is produced as fatty acids are oxidized on the skin. If the gland does not have an opening, a closed comedo, or whitehead, is formed. Closed comedones are small, nonerythematous papules just beneath the skin surface. Because a closed comedo has only a microscopic opening on the skin surface, pressure from excess sebum and keratin causes the comedo walls to rupture. Fatty acids produced by bacterial action on sebum are released into the surrounding tissues, causing inflammation. If the rupture occurs close to the surface, a pustule is formed. Ruptures deep in the dermis result in cysts and abscesses, which can lead to significant scarring.

Bacteria, particularly *P. acnes,* play a role in the development of acne lesions by increasing inflammation and disrupting the integrity of the follicle walls.

Incidence

Acne affects approximately 85% of adolescents and up to 20% of neonates. Although acne may begin at any age, it usually develops during puberty and lasts into early adulthood. Acne is more common in boys than in girls. It tends to improve in summer and flare up in winter. Acne of newborn infants typically resolves spontaneously by 3 months of age and does not seem to increase the risk for adolescent acne (Cohen, 2005).

Manifestations and Diagnostic Evaluation

Acne consists of closed whiteheads, blackheads, papules, pustules, nodules, and cysts (Fig. 25-12). Not all adolescents have all types of acne, and treatment is based on the type of acne. The areas most often affected are the face, neck, back, shoulders, and upper chest. The diagnosis is based on examination of the lesions and the child's history.

Therapeutic Management

The goal of treatment is to prevent scarring and to promote a positive self-image in the adolescent. Treatment must be individualized according to the severity of the condition, the types of lesion present, and the adolescent's gender. Improvement usually begins in 4 to 6 weeks, so the adolescent needs support to keep from feeling discouraged after treatment begins. Three to 5 months are needed for optimal results.

Topical therapy with a variety of agents is the primary treatment for acne. Commonly used agents include benzoyl peroxide, which reduces fatty acid production and is bactericidal for *Propionibacterium acnes*, and tretinoin (Retin-A),

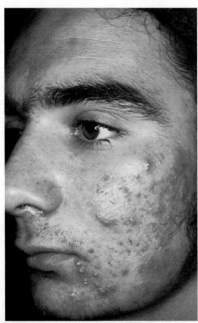

FIG 25-12   **An adolescent with acne vulgaris.**   *(From Hurwitz, S. [1993]. Clinical pediatric dermatology: A textbook of skin disorders of childhood and adolescence [2nd ed., p. 137]. Philadelphia: WB Saunders.)*

a vitamin A derivative. Tretinoin reduces comedo formation and eliminates the lesions already present. Benzoyl peroxide comes in a gel, cream, lotion, or soap in various strengths. Lower-potency formulas are available over the counter. Tretinoin is available in cream, gel, or liquid form by prescription. Sunscreen should be used with tretinoin to reduce photosensitivity. When applied together to the skin, benzoyl peroxide and tretinoin have a potentially offsetting effect and can reduce the overall effectiveness of each individual agent. For this reason, the physician may order that the two medications be applied on alternate days or that benzoyl peroxide be applied in the morning and tretinoin at bedtime.

Topical antibiotics, such as clindamycin and erythromycin, decrease the number of *P. acnes* organisms in hair follicles and are often used for inflammatory acne. Topical antibiotics are preferred over systemic antibiotics.

Oral antibiotics (tetracycline, minocycline, erythromycin, clindamycin) might be prescribed for adolescents with severe inflammatory acne or those who are unresponsive to topical treatment. Exposure to sunlight should be avoided if tetracycline is used. Oral isotretinoin (Accutane) has dramatically improved the condition of adolescents with severe nodular/cystic acne. This drug suppresses sebum production and sebaceous gland activity. Because of the severity of side effects, isotretinoin is not indicated for all adolescents. Side effects include cataracts, cheilitis, dry skin, pruritus, conjunctivitis, nosebleeds, and depression. In some instances, depression associated with isotretinoin has possibly resulted in suicide (Darmstadt & Sidbury, 2004). Young women who anticipate becoming pregnant should not take isotretinoin because of its teratogenic effects. Sexually active female adolescents should use an effective form of contraception, or combination of contraceptive methods, from 1 month before treatment until 1 month after discontinuing treatment. A negative pregnancy test must be obtained before initiating therapy. Informed consent is recommended for treatment with isotretinoin.

Estrogen may be prescribed for young women who are unresponsive to antibiotic therapy or who cannot take isotretinoin. Some combination (progestin and estrogen) oral contraceptives may also be indicated for acne treatment. Although the dermatologist may mechanically express comedones, the adolescent should be cautioned not to pick or squeeze lesions. Although scars cannot be completely removed, techniques such as dermabrasion, plastic repair, and collagen implants may improve appearance.

NURSING CARE

The Adolescent With Acne Vulgaris

Assessment

Obtain a history that includes how long acne lesions have been present and the effect of menses, stress, and other aggravating factors on the severity and frequency of the lesions.

Investigate acne treatments that have been tried and their effectiveness. Establish how often the adolescent washes the skin and hair and the type of cleansing agents used. Inquire about whether the adolescent uses cosmetics on a regular basis and what types of cosmetics are used. Try to assess the adolescent's understanding of the development and treatment of acne.

Examine the adolescent's face, chest, back, and neck for lesions. The depth of tissue involvement and the presence of pustules, papules, cysts, and scars should be noted. The adolescent's feelings about appearance and self-image and the effects acne may have had on social functioning should be explored.

Nursing Diagnosis and Planning

The nursing diagnoses and expected outcomes that may be appropriate for the adolescent with acne vulgaris are as follow:

- Impaired Skin Integrity related to increased sebaceous gland secretions, hormonal changes, and the action of bacteria on the contents of clogged follicles.
  Expected Outcome: Affected areas will exhibit signs of healing.
- Risk for Infection related to inflammation of skin lesions.
  Expected Outcome: The adolescent will have no signs of secondary bacterial infection, as evidenced by clear, intact skin.
- Disturbed Body Image related to appearance of skin lesions.
  Expected Outcomes: The adolescent will verbalize feelings and concerns and will participate in desired social activities.
- Deficient Knowledge about skin care and treatment regimen related to being too embarrassed to ask questions.
  Expected Outcome: The adolescent will carry out the prescribed treatment regimen to control excessive sebaceous gland activity.

Interventions

Because acne is a long-term condition, the affected adolescent needs support and encouragement if the treatment regimen is to be effective. Improvement may take as long as 12 weeks, and exacerbations are common. Although there is no cure for acne, much can be done to control inflammation and reduce scarring.

Explain the cause of acne and the rationale for treatment at the outset, so the adolescent can help plan the treatment regimen. Providing written instructions and involving the adolescent in care can help improve adherence. The treatment must be individualized, but all treatment regimens include measures to reduce oil on the skin. Gently cleaning the face twice a day with mild antibacterial soap and shampooing the hair daily are important facets of care. Warn the adolescent to avoid vigorous scrubbing and picking or squeezing of lesions, which can rupture pilosebaceous ducts

and cause secondary infection. Teach the adolescent how to apply topical medications and caution against overusing these products to speed results. Because oily cosmetics and creams add to the plugging of follicles, only water-based cosmetics should be used.

A healthy lifestyle, including adequate rest, exercise, and a balanced diet, promotes healing of lesions. Explore the adolescent's feelings about appearance and coping mechanisms. Reinforce positive self-image and self-esteem. Concerns and fears should be openly discussed and myths about acne dispelled. Provide parents with needed information about acne to clear up misconceptions and to prevent needless nagging of the adolescent.

Evaluation

- Do the acne lesions exhibit signs of healing without signs of infection?
- Is the adolescent able to express feelings and concerns about possible change in body image?
- Does the adolescent appear confident and assured as the process of healing is occurring?
- Does the adolescent carry out the treatment regimen to control acne and prevent scarring?

MISCELLANEOUS SKIN DISORDERS

There are a large number of less common skin disorders of varied causes and manifestations. Several of these disorders, along with their manifestations, management, and special considerations, are listed in Table 25-1.

INSECT BITES OR STINGS

Insects are found almost everywhere, and children often come in contact with them during play. The bites of most insects are not serious, usually causing only itching and mild pain; however, severe systemic reactions can occur in sensitized children. Systemic reactions to the venom of stinging insects, including wasps, honeybees, yellow jackets, hornets, and fire ants, is estimated to occur in about 1% of American children (David & Golden, 2003). Anaphylaxis from insect stings results in an estimated 40 to 100 deaths annually in the United States (National Institute of Allergy and Infectious Diseases, 2004).

Children who are allergic to insect stings should wear a medical alert bracelet and be provided with an epinephrine autoinjector (Epi-Pen) and information on avoidance. Parents should make sure the autoinjector is actually with the child or a responsible adult when the child is outdoors. The expiration date on the autoinjector must be checked regularly, and families must know how to obtain replacements when the autoinjector is outdated. Patients with a clear history of anaphylaxis after hymenoptera stings should be referred to an allergist for immunotherapy, which can reduce the risk of anaphylaxis to about 2% (Freeman, 2004) (see Chapter 17 for additional information about anaphylaxis).

TABLE 25-1 Skin Disorders			
Disorder/Etiology	**Manifestations**	**Management**	**Comments**
Stevens-Johnson Syndrome Acute, sometimes recurrent autoimmune disease. May be triggered by infections or medications, such as sulfonamides or anticonvulsants. New lesions continue to erupt for 2-3 wk, followed by healing during the next 6 wk.	After a prodromal respiratory illness, bullae appear on the lips, mouth, eyes, and genitalia. Fever, chills, malaise, neutropenia, anemia, weakness. Purulent conjunctivitis is common. Skin lesions rupture and may lead to significant fluid loss.	Withdraw the triggering medication. Treatment of skin lesions similar to treatment of extensive burns: aseptic technique, IV fluids, air/fluid bedding, nutritional support, pain management. Give antibiotics for secondary infections. Obtain ophthalmology consultation for eye lesions.	Reassure the child that the skin lesions will disappear. Inform parents about the possibility of recurrence and encourage them to avoid any implicated medications.
Psoriasis Chronic, inflammatory rash caused by rapid proliferation of keratinocytes. Hereditary predisposition; onset in first 2 decades of life. Remissions and exacerbations; lasts throughout life. Exacerbations associated with stress. Arthritis is sometimes a complication.	Pruritus; erythematous, elevated plaques and silvery scales on the scalp, face, knees, elbows, and gluteal folds. Scales are attached at the center rather than edges and may bleed when removed.	Topical corticosteroids and tar preparations; keratolytic agents. Exposure to ultraviolet light and sunlight. Skin care to prevent secondary infection. Keratolytic agents enhance penetration of topical steroids. Sunlight may cause phototoxic reactions with tar preparations. To prevent tar folliculitis, tar should be applied down an extremity rather than up.	There is no cure for psoriasis. Cutaneous trauma and streptococcal infections (e.g., tonsillitis) are common aggravating factors. A resource for families of children with psoriasis is the National Psoriasis Foundation: *http://www.psoriasis.org/home/*
Pityriasis Rosea Acute, inflammatory, self-limited skin disorder. Etiology unknown; may be viral.	Sudden eruption of salmon-pink, irregular patches on trunk and proximal portions of extremities. Symmetric distribution of lesions, "Christmas tree" appearance on back. "Herald patch" precedes rash by 7-10 days.	No treatment required for asymptomatic children. Pruritus can be treated with antipruritic lotions, ultraviolet light, or sunlight.	Child generally feels well. Rash may last 6-12 wk.
Warts Skin infection caused by human papillomavirus. Incubation period is 1-6 mo. Can persist from a few months to 5 or more years.	Painless, hyperkeratotic papule. Begins as a round, flesh-colored papule; later becomes brown or tan with a rough surface. Most common sites: dorsum of hands, fingers, feet, face, genitalia.	Various methods of treatment: daily application of lactic acid and salicylic acid (e.g., Compound W); freezing with liquid nitrogen; topical application of cantharidin for plantar or periungual warts.	Most warts disappear without treatment in 2-3 yr. With treatment, they usually resolve in 2-3 mo. Picking at warts may cause them to spread to other areas of the body. Warts are not highly contagious to other people. Immunocompromised children are more susceptible to warts.

Arachnids (scorpions, spiders, ticks, mites) are found in areas where children play. Most arachnids are not dangerous or aggressive. In the United States, only one type of scorpion and two types of spiders (black widow, brown recluse) cause life-threatening reactions.

Topical insect repellents are an important measure in preventing insect bites. The Centers for Disease Control and Prevention recommends the use of products that contain active ingredients registered with the Environmental Protection Agency. Repellents containing high concentrations of diethyl toluamide (DEET) should not be used on small children because of the risk of toxic encephalopathy. Likewise, products containing oil of eucalyptus are not indicated for children younger than 3 years (Centers for Disease Control and Prevention, 2005). Such repellents should not be applied near the face, and children should be cautioned not to put their fingers in their mouths when wearing diethyl toluamide.

The bites and stings of common insects and arachnids are discussed in Table 25-2. The table includes information on manifestations, treatment, and prevention.

TABLE 25-1   Skin Disorders—cont'd

Disorder/Etiology	Manifestations	Management	Comments
Molluscum Contagiosum Viral infection of the skin and mucous membranes. Transmitted by skin-to-skin and fomite-to-skin contact. May be transmitted by sexual contact.	Begin as pinpoint papules that increase in size to 2-3 mm or larger. Firm, solid, pink papules changing into soft, waxy, umbilicated papules. Curdlike core of the lesion can be expressed. Most common sites: face, trunk, extremities, oral mucous membranes, conjunctiva, genitalia.	Lesions may be treated with cantharidin, cryotherapy, tretinoin, or imiquimod. Condition usually responds well to treatment. Spontaneous disappearance is common.	Lesions may be spread to other parts of the body and may be transmitted to others. Lesions disappear spontaneously over time. Children with eczema or impaired immunity are at risk for generalized spread of lesions.
Frostbite Freezing of tissue resulting from exposure to extreme cold. Exposed areas (fingers, toes, nose, cheeks, ears) are most often affected. Cold causes arteriolar vasoconstriction, resulting in tissue anoxia and destruction.	*Early signs:* blanching of skin; stinging sensation followed by numbness and white, mottled appearance. Area feels cold, hard; may be without sensation. *First-degree:* redness and discomfort with return to normal in a few hours. *Second-degree:* redness; blisters and bullae 24-48 hr after rewarming. Pain during rewarming. *Third-degree:* cyanosis and mottling, followed by redness and swelling. Necrosis of epidermis, dermis, and subcutaneous tissue. Sensation is absent. Pain during rewarming. *Fourth-degree:* Complete necrosis with gangrene, possible loss of body part.	Immediately cover affected areas with warm hands and warm clothing. Massaging areas causes further damage and should be avoided. Rapidly rewarm areas by immersion in a warm water bath (90° F-106° F) until all frozen tissues are thawed and the skin appears flushed. Pain during thawing can be severe and should be treated with analgesics and sedatives. Severely damaged areas are treated as burns.	Children in cold climates should be taught to prevent frostbite by wearing adequate warm, layered clothing, hat, gloves, and two pairs of socks (one cotton, one wool). Children should be taught to warm themselves when hands or feet begin to sting. Young children should not be allowed to play outside in extremely cold temperatures.
Foreign Bodies Skin injury caused by penetration of splinters, gravel, cactus spines, bee stingers, glass, or other foreign objects.	Pain, erythema, possible secondary infection. Foreign body may or may not be visible.	Area surrounding foreign body should be washed with soap and water before removal. Superficial splinters can be removed with a needle and tweezers disinfected with alcohol or flame.	Deeply embedded foreign bodies, fishhooks, and other difficult-to-remove objects may require medical attention. Tetanus prophylaxis may be indicated.

BURN INJURIES

Burn injury may involve a small, painful area that hurts until healing occurs, or it may involve most of a child's body, with resulting severe trauma or death. Infants and toddlers are at greatest risk for sustaining burns because they depend totally on others for safety.

Recovery from a major burn injury requires many months, and the child's appearance might be altered for life. Caring for a burned child entails a multidisciplinary approach with a focus on the child and the family. Nursing care involves treating the physical injury and its psychologic effects on the child and family members. The challenges of burn nursing begin with acute burn care but continue through the rehabilitation phase until the child is restored to optimal function (Box 25-3).

Etiology

Burn injuries in children can be unintentional or intentional. In children younger than 5 years, unintentional burns are likely to occur as a result of environmental situations that are

TABLE 25-2   Skin Lesions Caused by Insects and Arachnids

Agent and Characteristics	Manifestations	Treatment and Prevention
Insects		
Mosquitoes, Fleas, Flies, Gnats Foreign protein in insect's saliva is injected as insect pierces skin to suck blood.	Itching, erythema, small wheal. Local reaction may occur that is difficult to distinguish from cellulitis.	Apply antipruritic lotions and cool compresses to relieve itching. Give antihistamines if needed for sleep. *Prevention:* Wear insect repellent when contact is anticipated. Treat potential breeding places (standing water for mosquitoes; pets, furniture, yard for fleas).
Hymenoptera (Bees, Wasps, Hornets, Yellow Jackets, Fire Ants) Venom is injected through a stinger.	Histamine and foreign proteins in venom cause local reaction of pain, swelling, redness, and itching. Systemic allergic reactions may be manifested by nausea, generalized edema, respiratory distress, and shock.	Carefully remove stinger by scraping it out horizontally. Avoid squeezing stinger, because more venom will be released. Wash with soap and water. Paste made of powdered meat tenderizer and water is soothing. Apply ice and analgesics for discomfort, antihistamines for itching. For a systemic allergic reaction, give epinephrine and corticosteroids immediately; transport to emergency facility. Children allergic to hymenoptera should wear medical identification. *Prevention:* Treat known hives or nests. Avoid wearing colorful clothing and perfumes when outside.
Arachnids		
Brown Recluse ("Fiddle Back") Spider Yellowish to reddish brown with a violin-shaped mark on its back. Venom injected by fangs. Bites only when threatened. Lives in dark, protected areas (woodpiles, basements, closets, trash heaps).	Mild stinging at time of bite. Within 2-8 hr, area around bite becomes painful and erythema develops, followed by a blister. Venom is necrotoxic. Edema, redness, and purpura may involve entire limb. Central portion of lesion develops an indurated wheal that progresses to deep, sloughing ulcer in 7-14 days. Ulcer often does not heal for several months. Usually results in a scar.	Immobilize and elevate affected extremity. Cool compresses, analgesics, tetanus prophylaxis. Observe for secondary infection. Skin graft may be necessary for large ulcers. No antivenin available. *Prevention:* Avoid areas inhabited by spiders.
Black Widow Spider Shiny black with a red hourglass-shaped mark on abdomen. Female's venom is very poisonous to humans. Males do not bite. Female builds irregular web in dark, sheltered spots and aggressively defends eggs.	Bite may be painless initially. Within 1 hr pain develops at site. Severe muscle pains and numbness spread from bite, and puncture site becomes red, swollen, and pruritic. Neurotoxic venom enters the bloodstream within 1 hr, causing dizziness, headache, nausea, vomiting, cramps, tremors, and rapid, shallow respirations. Shock and renal failure may develop in young children.	Hospitalization for children. Antivenin if no allergy to horse serum. Supportive care, including IV calcium gluconate, morphine, muscle relaxants. Tetanus prophylaxis. *Prevention:* Avoid areas infested by spiders (woodpiles, outhouses).
Ticks Brown or gray; live in fields, pastures, woods. Feed on blood of humans, dogs, livestock, or deer. Larvae feed on rodents. Tick buries head and mouth parts in the skin to suck blood.	Bites may cause local reactions or, rarely, systemic reactions (tick fever, tick paralysis). Ticks can transmit Lyme disease, Rocky Mountain spotted fever, Q fever, tularemia.	*Methods to remove ticks:* Remove with tweezers as close to the skin as possible, taking care to remove head. If mouth parts remain, remove with sterile needle. Wash site with soap and water. There is some evidence that prompt removal of ticks decreases chance of transmission of disease. *Prevention:* Wear long sleeves and pants and use insect repellent when walking in tick-infested areas. Inspect clothing and hair for ticks after walking through fields or woods.

TABLE 25-2   Skin Lesions Caused by Insects and Arachnids—cont'd

Agent and Characteristics	Manifestations	Treatment and Prevention
Arachnids—cont'd ***Scorpions*** Most scorpions are not dangerous. They rarely attack humans unless accidentally disturbed or stepped on. If disturbed, they inflict a painful sting. One type (found in Arizona), *Centruroides sculpturatus,* is extremely poisonous, and its sting can be fatal. Scorpions are found mainly in the southwestern United States. Scorpions hide by day in basements, garages, closets, crevices. Some varieties burrow and hide in gravel or children's sandboxes.	Sting is extremely painful. Local reaction of swelling at puncture site. Some species cause systemic reactions: tachycardia, hypertension, arrhythmias, irritability, seizures, pulmonary edema, coma. Fatal reactions most often occur in children younger than 3 yr.	Ice packs and tourniquet applied proximal to the site slow the spread of venom. Wound should not be excised. Topical steroids and antihistamines are used to relieve symptoms. For severe reactions, provide supportive care for pain, shock, seizures. Narcotic analgesics act synergistically with scorpion venom and are contraindicated. Antivenin is given for systemic reactions (available from the Antivenom Production Laboratory, Arizona State University). *Prevention:* Wear shoes to prevent stepping on scorpions. Inspect shoes and clothing before dressing. Apply creosote to garages, basements.
Chiggers (Harvest Mites) Live in tall grass and underbrush; burrow into hair follicles and skin pores to feed.	Tend to concentrate in warm areas where clothing is snug (underwear elastic). Cause erythematous papules and intense itching.	Antipruritic agents. Prevention of secondary infection. *Prevention:* Insect repellent on clothing, ankles, legs.

BOX 25-3 | Pediatric Differences in the Effects of Burn Injury

- Very young children who have been severely burned have a higher mortality rate than older children and adults with comparable burns.
- Because a child's skin is thinner than that of an adult, lower burn temperatures and shorter exposure to heat or chemicals can cause a more severe burn.
- A larger body surface area compared with that of adults places severely burned children at increased risk for fluid and heat loss. Children are also at increased risk for dehydration and metabolic acidosis from diarrhea, evaporative water loss, and increased fluid requirements.
- The higher proportion of body fluid to mass in children increases the risk of cardiovascular problems because of their less-effective cardiovascular response to changing intravascular volume.
- Burns involving more than 10% TBSA require fluid resuscitation.
- Infants and children are at increased risk for protein and calorie deficiency because they have smaller muscle mass and lower body fat than adults. If they are not eating and their metabolism is increased, their protein and calorie needs will not be met.
- Hypertrophic scarring is more severe, and scar maturation is prolonged.
- An immature immune system means an increased risk of infection for infants and young children.
- A delay in growth may follow extensive burns.
- In children, Curling (gastroduodenal) ulcer occurs in the third or fourth week after a burn, which is later than in adults.

---

not controlled by caretakers. The young child's curiosity and increasing mobility contribute to the risk (Table 25-3). A child can start a fire by playing with matches (Fig. 25-13) or flammable materials near open fires, or a child might be the victim of a house fire while sleeping or might be unintentionally scalded or electrocuted (Fig. 25-14). (See Chapters 5 through 8 for a discussion of safety.) Either inattentive supervision or purposeful abuse can cause intentional burns (Box 25-4).

The extent of the injury determines whether burn-related problems are local or systemic. Other factors, such as the location of the burned area, whether it is an electrical injury, whether there is a concurrent inhalation injury or trauma, and whether there is a pre-existing medical disease, contribute to morbidity and mortality rates. Morbidity and mortality rates are higher in children who have been burned than in adults.

Incidence

Fire and burn injuries are the fifth leading cause of unintentional deaths in children ages 1 to 14 years in the United States (National SAFEKIDS Campaign, 2004). Scald burns are the most common burn injuries seen in pediatrics (Allasio

TABLE 25-3	Age-Related Risks for Burn Injury	
Age	**Injury Type**	**Risk Factors**
<5 yr	Flame	Playing with matches and cigarette lighters
		Playing with fires in fireplaces, barbecue pits, trash fires
	Scald	Kitchen injury from tipping scalding liquids
		Bathtub scaldings associated with lack of supervision or child abuse
		Most pediatric burn patients are infants and toddlers younger than 3 yr burned by scalding liquids
5-10 yr	Flame	Boys at increased risk
		Often associated with fire play and risk-taking behaviors
	Scald	Girls at increased risk
		Likely to occur at home in kitchen or bathroom
Adolescent	Flame	Injury associated with male peer-group activities involving gasoline or other flammable products
		Gasoline sniffing possibly involved
		Rarely occurs in female adolescents except in house fires or automobile accidents
	Electrical	Occurs most often in male adolescents involved in dare-type behaviors, such as climbing utility poles or antennas
		In rural areas, may be associated with moving irrigation pipes that touch an electrical source

---

BOX 25-4 | THE CHILD & PARENTS WANT TO KNOW About Measures to Prevent and Initially Manage a Burn

Prevention
- Have periodic fire drills to teach your children how to evacuate the house in the event of a fire.
- Place child identification stickers, which can be obtained from most fire departments, on the outside of the bedroom door and in one window of each child's bedroom.
- Identify two or more exits from each room and a location to meet outside the house. Emphasize to your children that they should not return to the house under any circumstances, even if another family member or pet remains in the house.
- Be sure your child understands "stop, drop, and roll" as a measure to stop the burning process.
- Be sure to keep all matches and lighters out of reach. Check electrical cords regularly. Use outlet covers if children younger than 5 years are in the house.
- Check smoke detectors regularly and keep them clean. Replace the batteries regularly if they are battery operated.

- To reduce the number of scald burns, turn the hot water heater thermostat down to 120° F.
- Turn pot handles in and use back burners on the stove whenever possible.
- Do not sit a child on your lap while you are drinking a hot liquid.
- Keep your children away from outdoor grills and indoor wood- or coal-burning stoves. Keep older infants from crawling near floor heating grates.

Initial Emergency Burn Management
- Apply cool compresses or submerge minor burns in cool water, not ice.
- To prevent scalding, remove clothing soaked with hot water as quickly as possible.
- Contact the physician for any child with a burn that has blistered.
- Cover a child who has a major burn with a clean sheet while waiting for emergency personnel.
- Do not try to remove clothing that is adhering to burned skin.

& Fischer, 2005). Other burn injuries include those induced by flame, electrical, and chemical causes. Approximately 6% of burn injuries are related to child abuse (National Institute of Disability and Rehabilitation Research, 2003).

Most children with severe burns are treated in burn centers. The American Burn Association has outlined criteria for referral to a burn center (Box 25-5).

Pathophysiology

In burn injury the injuring agent, whether flame, chemical, ultraviolet light, or electrical energy, denatures cellular protein, which destroys collagen linkages in connective tissue. As a result, osmotic and hydrostatic pressure gradients are disrupted, and intravascular fluid moves into interstitial spaces. Inflammatory chemicals are released from injured cells, resulting in increased capillary permeability and adding to fluid shifts. Burn injuries are classified by depth and extent of tissue damage and by severity of injury (Johnson & Richard, 2003). The combination of these factors determines referral and therapeutic management decisions.

Depth of Burn Injury

Depth of burn injury describes local tissue damage and is largely a factor of the duration of exposure and the temperature or destructive potential of the agent causing the damage. Depth of injury is classified as superficial, superficial

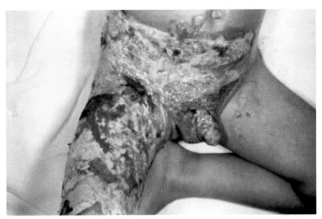

FIG 25-13 **These burns were sustained when the child's pajamas caught fire while he was playing with matches.** *(From Cosman, B. [1973]. Management of the burned patient. New York: MEDCOM.)*

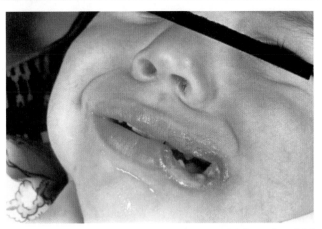

FIG 25-14 **These burns were sustained when the child sucked on an electrical socket.** *(From Cosman, B. [1973]. Management of the burned patient. New York: MEDCOM.)*

BOX 25-5	**Burn Center Referral Criteria**

The American Burn Association recommends that children with the following injuries be referred to a burn center after emergency assessment and stabilization:

- Second degree burns greater than 10% body surface area
- Burns that involve major joints, face, hands, feet, genitalia, or perineum
- Third-degree burns
- Electrical burns, including lightning injury
- Chemical burns
- Inhalation injury with burns
- Pre-existing medical disorders that might complicate recovery
- Coexisting trauma in which the burn injury poses the greatest risk to life or function
- Burned children in hospitals without qualified personnel to care for pediatric burn patients
- Children who will require specialized psychosocial or long-term rehabilitation

Modified from Committee on Trauma, American College of Surgeons (2006). Guidelines for the operations of burn centers. *Resources for optimal care of the injured patient:* 2006, p. 79.

partial thickness, deep partial thickness, or full thickness (Table 25-4).

Superficial burns, usually sunburns, affect only the epidermis. No blisters form in a true superficial burn, and the surface of the injury is dry. The pain of sunburns is usually delayed for several hours after sun exposure. Partial-thickness thermal, chemical, or electrical injury to the skin interferes with the skin's ability to carry out its normal physiologic functions of protection from infection or injury and preservation of fluid balance and temperature regulation. In addition, deep tissue injury damages sensory nerve endings and local circulatory patterns and adversely affects the skin's ability to regenerate or synthesize vitamin D.

Extent of Burn Injury

The extent of injury refers to the percent of total body surface area (TBSA) burned. The standard "rule of nines" used in adults gives an inaccurate estimate for children because of the differences in body proportion between children and adults. Many burn facilities use the Lund and Browder chart, which is a body surface chart corrected for age (Fig. 25-15). Another method estimates burn percentage by calculating the complete palmar surface of the child's hand and assumes the area of the palmar surface equals 1% of the TBSA. In fact, the palm is somewhat smaller, about 0.70% to 0.87% of the TBSA in children, so this method overestimates the extent of injury but is convenient for children or small or irregular burns (Johnson & Richard, 2003).

Severity of Burn Injury

Severity of burn injury is determined by the degree to which the skin's physiologic functions are disrupted beyond the body's normal ability to respond with compensatory mechanisms. Burn injuries are classified as minor, moderate uncomplicated, and major. The severity of burn injury is related to a combination of factors. These include age, medical history, extent and depth of burn, special care of the body area involved (e.g., face, hands), and the presence of concomitant trauma, such as fractures or head injury, sustained at the time of the burn. Burn severity relates to the child's eventual morbidity or mortality status.

Manifestations

Table 25-5 lists the clinical manifestations associated with burns of different severity. Assessment of the distribution of scald burns is of particular importance in infants and toddlers because of the possibility of child maltreatment. The classic forced immersion burn occurs when a child's extremity or buttocks are held under hot water. These burns have a "stocking" or "glove" appearance with a relatively sharp line dividing the burned from unburned skin. There are usually no smaller, scattered burns ("splash marks") that indicate attempts to remove the extremity.

TABLE 25-4 **Depth of Burn Injury**

	Superficial	Superficial Partial Thickness	Deep Partial Thickness	Full Thickness
Morphologic features	Destruction of epidermis; physiologic functions remain intact	Destruction of epidermis and some dermis	Destruction of epidermis and dermis	Destruction of epidermis, dermis, underlying tissue; may include fascia, muscle, tendon, bone
Blister formation	After 24 hr (e.g., from sunburn)	Within minutes; thin walled, fluid filled	May or may not appear as fluid-filled blisters; often they are flat, dehydrated, and like tissue paper; body fluids lost through burn tissue must be replaced	Rare; may appear as a tissue paper-like layer that is flat and dehydrated
Appearance	Peels after 24-48 hr	Red to pale ivory, moist surface	Mottled, waxy white, dry surface	White, cherry red, or black
Healing time	3-7 days	7-21 days if no infection develops	30 days to several months if no infection; if infected, this type of burn may convert to full-thickness	Will not heal; skin grafting required; very small areas may heal from edges after a period of weeks
Patient reaction	Moderate discomfort, pain; chills; nausea; vomiting	May cause considerable pain	Severe pain on exposure to air or water because nerve endings are intact	No pain in area of full-thickness burn because nerve endings are destroyed; surrounding areas of lesser depth are painful
Scarring	None	Minimal; influenced by genetic predisposition	Greatest because the slow healing of these burns increases scar tissue; scar formation influenced by genetic predisposition	Autograft scarring is minimized by early excision and grafting; scar formation influenced by genetic predisposition

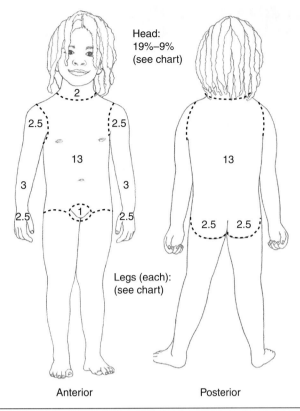

Head: 19%–9% (see chart)

Legs (each): (see chart)

Anterior   Posterior

Child Burn Size Estimation Table
(percent total body surface area)

Age in Years

	< 1yr	1	5	10	15	Adult
Head	19	17	13	11	9	7
Neck	2	2	2	2	2	2
Ant Trunk	13	13	13	13	13	13
Post Trunk	13	13	13	13	13	13
Buttock	2.5	2.5	2.5	2.5	2.5	2.5
Genitalia	1	1	1	1	1	1
Upper arm	2.5	2.5	2.5	2.5	2.5	2.5
Lower arm	3	3	3	3	3	3
Hand	2.5	2.5	2.5	2.5	2.5	2.5
Thigh	5.5	6.5	8	8.5	9	9.5
Leg	5	5	5.5	6	6.5	7
Foot	3.5	3.5	3.5	3.5	3.5	3.5

FIG 25-15 **Calculating TBSA burned in children. The standard "rule of nines" and standard body surface charts must be adapted because of the difference in body proportions between adults and children.** *(From Deitch, E., & Rutan, R. [2001]. The challenges of children: The first 48 hours. Chicago: American Burn Association.)*

Therapeutic Management

Superficial Burn Injuries

The most common cause of a superficial (epidermal layer only) burn is sunburn. Although uncomfortable, sunburn rarely requires intensive burn treatment. Cool compresses and application of soothing topical lotions (especially those containing aloe) or mild topical corticosteroids provide symptomatic treatment. If the discomfort is disturbing the child's sleep, acetaminophen or ibuprofen can provide relief.

Preventing sunburn is especially important in children because frequent sunburn causes long-term damage to the skin. Children who are susceptible to sunburn are also susceptible to the later development of melanoma and nonmelanoma skin cancers (Kennedy, Bajdik, Willemze, De Gruijl, & Bouwes Bavinek, 2003). Children should avoid sun exposure, especially between the hours of 10 AM and 3 PM during the summer. During sun exposure, parents should apply to the child's skin an appropriate ultraviolet A and ultraviolet B protective sunscreen with a sun protection factor greater

TABLE 25-5 Classification of Severity of Burn Injury in Children	
Type of Injury	**Clinical Manifestations**
Minor Partial-thickness burn of <10% of TBSA Full-thickness burn of <2% of TBSA that does not involve special care areas (eyes, ears, face, hands, feet, perineum, joints) Excludes electrical injury, inhalation injury, concurrent trauma, all poor-risk children (e.g., those of extremely young age or with concurrent disease)	**Minor** Localized pain and blister formation in the area of injury; white or black full-thickness injury No systemic effects Little or no scarring, except in areas of full-thickness injury
Moderate, Uncomplicated Partial-thickness burns of 10%-20% of TBSA Full-thickness burns of <10% of TBSA that do not involve special care areas Excludes electrical injury, inhalation injury, concurrent trauma, all poor-risk children (e.g., those of extremely young age or with concurrent disease)	**Moderate, Uncomplicated** Open wound that is a potential source of infection and a site for loss of fluids and electrolytes Pain that may interfere with routines of daily living Wound healing rate influenced by nutritional status Possible scarring in areas of partial- and full-thickness injuries
Major Partial-thickness burns of >20% of TBSA All full-thickness burns of ≥10% of TBSA All burns involving eyes, ears, face, hands, feet, perineum, or joints All inhalation injury, electrical injury, concurrent trauma, all poor-risk patients	**Major** Life-threatening injuries with risk for severe complications and death Volatile hospital course characterized by periods of relative physiologic stability followed, within hours, by life-threatening emergencies, such as shock Repeated operative procedures for skin grafting that are accompanied by major blood loss requiring multiple transfusions Potential risk for infection, either of the burn wound or related to pulmonary complications or systemic sepsis, until wound closure is achieved over 80% of the TBSA Much higher mortality rate associated with burn injury accompanied by inhalation injury than with burn injury alone

than 15. Hats and shirts are also desirable. Waterproof sunscreens are available for children who like to run in and out of the water, but frequent applications of sunscreen are still desirable. Sunscreen is contraindicated for infants younger than 6 months. Parents should keep infants in the shade, away from reflecting sun rays.

Minor Partial-Thickness Burn Injuries

In general, children with a minor burn injury are treated as outpatients in a physician's office, clinic, or hospital physical therapy department unless the extent of injury warrants hospital admission. Therapy is aimed at promoting wound healing, preventing infection, and providing pain relief. Burn wound care requires aseptic technique. Because anaerobic and aerobic bacteria can grow at the interface between burned and healthy tissue, tetanus toxoid is given to children who have not received tetanus immunization during the 5 years preceding the burn injury.

Wound Cleaning. Burn wounds receive care at least daily until closure is achieved. After old dressings are removed, the burned skin is cleaned with sterile saline solution or mild soap and water. If the child is hospitalized, hydrotherapy (Fig. 25-16) can be used to remove old dressings and clean the wound and the child. During this cleaning process, the child can perform active range-of-motion exercises. Hydrotherapy can be done in a tank, tub, or shower. Some facilities use disposable plastic liners to prevent contamination between

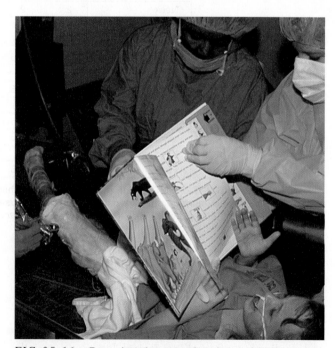

FIG 25-16   **Burn dressings can be changed in the hydrotherapy room. The room is kept warm because children who have been burned have poor body temperature control. The child life therapist reads a book to the child to distract her from the discomfort associated with the procedure.** *(Courtesy Parkland Health and Hospital System, Dallas, TX.)*

uses. Hydrotherapy should last no longer than 20 minutes to prevent electrolyte loss (through skin into water, as a result of osmosis). The room temperature is kept warm, and the child is covered and dried immediately after the procedure.

Debridement. *Debridement* is the removal of dead material within a wound to promote healing. In a burn injury, there is necrosis of skin and subcutaneous tissue. The burned tissue is called *eschar*. Eschar releases chemical mediators that stimulate leukocytes to digest debris, but this also damages capillaries and skin elements. Necrotic tissue within a wound prolongs inflammation and slows healing and epidermal coverage.

The initial debridement might be performed in the office, emergency department, or hydrotherapy treatment room. The burned area is debrided of loose debris and necrotic tissue. Blisters on palmar skin are usually left intact. Otherwise, it is currently recommended that blisters be removed to allow adequate examination and treatment of partial thickness wounds (Richard & Johnson, 2002). Old creams and ointments must be removed as part of the debridement, and loose tissue is trimmed around the burned area.

Application of Antimicrobial Agents and Dressings. Topical antibacterial agents (Table 25-6) are placed on burn wounds to penetrate the eschar and to control bacterial growth in and around the burn wound. Silver sulfadiazine (Silvadene) is the most commonly used topical agent, but it is not typically used on the face or on electrical burns. Facial burns are covered with a light layer of antimicrobial ointment. Mafenide (Sulfamylon) is the topical agent of choice for burns to the ear or electrical burns because of its deep penetration into the eschar. Mafenide should not be applied to the face.

After application of the topical antibacterial agent, a dressing usually is applied. Depending on the burn care protocol, dressings are changed one to three times a day. Because exposed nerve endings can cause significant pain, wound assessment and care should be done as quickly as possible. Narcotic or nonnarcotic pain medications are administered 20 to 30 minutes before dressing changes to ensure maximum pain control at the time of the procedure. The child life specialist can assist with teaching the child how to use nonpharmacologic pain relief techniques.

Besides pain control, measures to maintain the child's core body temperature, minimize shivering, and conserve energy also must be implemented as part of wound care activities. To the degree possible, the child's capacity for self-care should be optimized. Allowing the child to remove dressings provides a measure of control.

Aseptic technique is used during dressing changes. After dressings are applied to burn wounds, isolation is not necessary and the child does not need to be restricted to a room or to an area of the hospital.

Depending on the depth and extent of the burn, the physician might choose to cover the area with a biologic or synthetic dressing to reduce the chance of infection, provide pain relief, reduce evaporative fluid and heat loss, and promote healing. Such dressings are best used for partial-thickness burns. Commonly used biologic dressings include human skin, pig skin, and fresh human amniotic membrane (from the placenta). Synthetic dressings include plastic films, hydrocolloids, hydrogels, and collagen-impregnated dressings. The major risk associated with these dressings is infection; thus, the wound must be clean and dry before dressing application.

TABLE 25-6   Topical Antimicrobial Agents Commonly Used for Burns

Agent	Advantages	Side Effects and Disadvantages	Nursing Considerations
Silver nitrate solution	Effective against most gram-positive and some gram-negative organisms	Hyponatremia, hypokalemia, hypochloremia Decreased penetration of eschar Not effective against established infection Requires large, bulky dressings that limit mobility	0.5% solution in distilled water applied to wet dressing every 2 hr Dressing changes twice daily Can cause staining of linens and clothing and interferes with accurate wound assessment
Mafenide acetate cream (Sulfamylon)	Effective against a wide range of gram-positive and gram-negative organisms Rapid penetration through eschar (improved effectiveness in established infections) Permits open treatment of wound, thus increasing mobility	Painful on application May cause hypersensitivity reaction in 5%-7% of patients Associated with acid-base alteration (metabolic acidosis)	Applied to cleansed wound 1 or 2 times per day Treated area usually left open; a light dressing may be used Must be completely removed before reapplication Check sensitivity to sulfonamides
Silver sulfadiazine cream (Silvadene)	Effective against a wide range of gram-positive and gram-negative organisms Soothing on application Moderate eschar penetration Absorbed slowly, reducing the possibility of nephrotoxicity	May cause hypersensitivity reaction in 5%-7% of patients Associated with initial decrease in leukocyte count (transient)	Applied to cleansed wound 1 or 2 times per day Wound may be left open or covered with light dressing Check sensitivity to sulfonamides Must remove all medication before reapplication

NURSING CARE PLAN

The Child With a Minor Partial-Thickness Burn

Focused Assessment

In the first few seconds after the arrival of a child who has been burned, the severity of the burn is determined. If the burn is of minor severity, care focuses on pain management and wound care. Children with burns of moderate uncomplicated severity may need fluid resuscitation. Take vital signs, paying special attention to the child's body temperature. Without skin, the burned child, especially if very young, rapidly loses heat to the atmosphere and is at risk for hypothermia. The child should be awake, alert, and oriented unless some condition other than an uncomplicated burn injury exists.

Assessment for pain intensity takes place on a scheduled basis, and interventions to control pain are implemented as needed. Assess the wound with each dressing change and document any signs of decreased circulation or infection. Assessment also includes range-of-motion abilities and the frequency and effectiveness of any physical therapy treatments. It is important to assess the child's ability to assume independent activities, particularly when the burn affects the child's extremities. Young children tend to protect injuries, so the child might need encouragement to move appropriately. Children with minor partial-thickness burns may be managed completely on an outpatient basis, with parents bringing the child daily to the physician's office for burn assessment, debridement, and dressing changes.

NURSING DIAGNOSIS   Impaired Skin Integrity related to thermal injury.

EXPECTED OUTCOME   The burn will:
- Heal without infection, as evidenced by normal temperature, normal granulating tissue, and restoration of the epithelial layer.

Intervention	*Rationale*
1. Clean and debride the wound daily and apply antimicrobial ointments and dressings as ordered. Observe and assess the site and record findings.	1. Infection can be prevented by removing bacterial contamination, exudate, and previously applied medication.
2. Maintain aseptic technique for wound care by wearing protective gear and practicing meticulous handwashing techniques.	2. An open skin surface allows for organism entry.
3. Promote adequate fluid and nutritional intake. Offer, or encourage the parent to offer, high-calorie, high-protein meals and snacks. Provide foods that the child likes. Arrange the timing of meals so that they do not immediately precede or follow painful or distressing events.	3. Healing occurs only in the presence of a positive nitrogen balance. The child's protein and calorie needs are elevated because of increased metabolism and catabolism.
4. Perform active and passive range-of-motion exercises of the affected parts of the child's body; this can be done at the time of dressing change and between dressing changes.	4. Use of the burned area promotes edema reabsorption and prevents contracture deformity.
5. Make sure that the child's tetanus toxoid immunizations are current.	5. Anaerobic bacteria can cause infection at the interface between the burn wound and healthy tissue.
6. Monitor the child for signs and symptoms of infection: changes in sensorium, hypothermia, fever, or a change in wound appearance (drainage, odor). Obtain specimens for culture if ordered.	6. Early detection of infection will ensure prompt treatment.
7. Administer vitamins and minerals (vitamins A, B, and C and iron and zinc) as ordered, or encourage the parent to do so.	7. Vitamin and mineral supplements facilitate wound healing and epithelialization.
8. Instruct the child and parents to keep the healed burn wound out of the sun for at least 1 year.	8. Burned skin is more sensitive to sunlight, which increases the risk of sunburn.

Evaluation

- Does the burn wound show signs of progressive healing?
- Is the tissue pink and free from exudate?
- Is the child free of fever and other signs of infection?

NURSING CARE PLAN—cont'd

NURSING DIAGNOSIS Acute Pain related to thermal injury and related procedures.

EXPECTED OUTCOMES The child will:
- Describe decreased pain on an age-appropriate pain assessment tool, except during procedures and physical therapy.
- Exhibit age-appropriate behaviors, adequate nutritional intake, and appropriate sleep patterns.

Intervention	*Rationale*
1. Determine the child's pain level with an age-appropriate assessment tool.	1. The child's developmental stage affects response to pain, and the child's response to various pain assessment tools is related to developmental level.
2. Administer pain relief measures and medication on a scheduled basis rather than on demand. Premedicate the child at least 20 to 30 minutes before painful procedures and advise the parent to do the same before the physician visit.	2. The fact that burns hurt is irrefutable, so there is no need to wait until pain is behaviorally indicated before administering medication.
3. Minimize the time spent on wound manipulation and exposure.	3. Exposure of the burned area to air or water causes pain because the nerve endings are exposed. Dressing changes should be done as quickly as possible to minimize pain.
4. Use nonpharmacologic pain reduction measures.	4. Distraction, relaxation techniques, therapeutic touch, and other measures may help alleviate pain.
5. Perform passive and active range-of-motion exercises. Be careful that dressings are applied so as to preserve function of body parts.	5. Exercise, although painful in the acute stage, reduces the likelihood of contracture formation and increases functional ability.

Evaluation

- Except during times of direct wound care and physical therapy, is the child pain free, as evidenced by decreased pain assessment score and normal sleep, play, and eating patterns?
- Is the child able to cooperate with dressing changes and range-of-motion exercises?

NURSING DIAGNOSIS Risk for Deficient Fluid Volume related to fluid shifts into burned tissue.

EXPECTED OUTCOME The child will:
- Maintain normal fluid and electrolyte balance, as evidenced by intake and output measurements and serum electrolyte values within normal ranges, moist mucous membranes, and good skin turgor on unaffected area.

Intervention	*Rationale*
1. Administer fluids orally or IV as ordered.	1. Fluids help maintain capillary circulation to the viable skin appendages and general circulation to the vital organs. Fluid replacement continues until wound coverage is achieved.
2. Instruct the parents to monitor the child's intake and output frequently.	2. Close monitoring is necessary to determine whether fluid resuscitation is necessary or adequate. Fluid intake sufficient to produce age-appropriate hourly urine output (see Chapter 18) ensures adequate tissue perfusion.
3. Weigh the hospitalized child daily.	3. Weight is an accurate measurement of hydration status. Increasing weight indicates fluid overload.
4. Monitor laboratory values for elevated electrolyte or hemoglobin levels.	4. Early identification of abnormal laboratory values permits early treatment of fluid-volume imbalances.

Evaluation

- Is the child's urine output adequate for age (see Chapter 18)?
- Are serum electrolyte values within normal ranges?
- Does the child appear well hydrated with moist mucous membranes and good skin turgor?
- Does the child take fluids well?

Continued

NURSING CARE PLAN—cont'd

NURSING DIAGNOSIS   Risk for Infection related to scratching of healing tissue.

EXPECTED OUTCOMES   The child will:
- Not complain of itching.
- List the dangers associated with scratching healing tissue.

Intervention	*Rationale*
1. Administer antihistamines as ordered.	1. Itching persists for several months after burns heal as new nerve endings and dermal elements re-establish themselves. Antihistamines such as diphenhydramine hydrochloride (Benadryl) reduce itching.
2. Apply soothing lotions, such as Nivea or Eucerin, to healing skin.	2. These lotions reduce dryness, which is a factor contributing to itching.
3. Keep the child's hands clean at all times and the fingernails cut short. Encourage the child not to scratch or rub healing skin.	3. These actions reduce the risk of impairing skin integrity.

Evaluation

- Is the child's skin intact and healing as expected?
- Is itching reduced?

NURSING DIAGNOSIS   Disturbed Body Image related to altered appearance of the healing burn.

EXPECTED OUTCOMES   The child will:
- Re-enter previous social settings and will express a feeling of comfort in these areas.
- Discuss feelings about others' reactions to the change in appearance.

The family will:
- Provide emotional support for the child.

Intervention	*Rationale*
1. Encourage the child to verbalize feelings about appearance and about returning to school.	1. Identifying the child's concerns and anxieties is the first step in developing effective coping strategies.
2. Provide honest answers to the child's questions regarding appearance.	2. Honesty builds trust and helps the child develop realistic expectations.
3. Encourage the family's involvement in the child's care (Box 25-6).	3. Family involvement provides support for the child and decreases the child's feelings of separation from significant others.
4. Encourage the child to provide age-appropriate self-care.	4. Participating in self-care helps increase self-esteem.
5. Identify support systems and coping mechanisms used in previous times of stress or crisis.	5. Strategies that were previously effective can be mobilized to aid the child and family through a stressful period.
6. Engage the assistance of a child life specialist to work with the child to identify feelings.	6. Children can often best express feelings through play and art.
7. Discuss ways in which the child can "cover up" any disfigurement through clothing and makeup.	7. Cosmetics can decrease or minimize the disfigurement.
8. Visit the child's school before the child's return or remain in contact with the school nurse.	8. Visiting the school will prepare the child's classmates for the changes in the child's appearance and engage them in making the re-entry a positive experience through acceptance. If visiting is not possible, the school nurse can assist the child with the transition to school.

Evaluation

- Does the child express a desire to reengage social contacts?
- Is the child able to express fears related to the reactions of others?
- Does the family support the child emotionally and encourage the child to express feelings?

| BOX 25-6 | **PARENTS WANT TO KNOW** | About Home Care for a Child With Burns |

Often it is the parents' responsibility to care for the burn wound at home, supported by daily visits to the office or clinic for debridement and wound assessment.

Parents will need to know the following to adequately care for the child:
- Type of cleaning method used to remove old antimicrobial ointment
- Where to obtain the topical ointment and dressing supplies
- How often to visit the office or clinic (the nurse provides the telephone number and a list of scheduled appointments)

Teach the parents the following:
- Use principles of aseptic technique. Use sterile gloves and applicators and know where to obtain these supplies. Know how to put on the gloves; give a return demonstration.

- Give the child medication for pain (if needed) 20 to 30 minutes before changing the dressing. Enlist other family members to provide distraction or to help hold the child.
- Wash the area with mild soap and tepid water or sterile saline solution. The old dressing can be soaked in tepid water to loosen it and decrease the discomfort of its removal.
- Apply the prescribed ointment and a light gauze dressing. Cover the area with a tubular net bandage, if possible, rather than wrapping with flexible gauze.
- Recognize signs and symptoms of infection, provide adequate fluids, and be sure the child's nutritional needs are met.
- Encourage the child in activities appropriate for age and development.
- Keep follow-up appointments.

CONDITIONS ASSOCIATED WITH MAJOR BURN INJURIES

For a child with a major burn injury, initial assessment and care focus on the ABCs—establishing and maintaining the child's airway, breathing, and circulation. After an airway and IV access have been established, a catheter is inserted into the bladder to begin hourly urine output measurements and a nasogastric tube is inserted into the stomach to prevent aspiration.

Burn shock is a hypovolemic condition that develops after a burn injury that affects more than 15% to 20% of TBSA in children. Mechanisms of burn shock are not well understood, but the sequence of major burn injury followed by massive capillary leakage of circulating fluid into the surrounding tissues is well recognized.

Within minutes of a major burn injury, all the capillaries in the circulatory system, not just those in the area of the burn, lose their capillary seal, resulting in leakage of intravascular body fluid into the interstitial spaces. Erythrocytes and leukocytes remain in the circulation and produce an elevated hematocrit and leukocyte count. The process of burn shock continues for approximately 24 to 48 hours, at which time the capillary seal is restored.

Treatment for burn shock is aimed at supporting the child through the period of hypovolemic shock until capillary integrity is restored. To maintain adequate circulating volume, IV fluids are administered at a rate greater than the rate of fluid loss. Fluid resuscitation depends primarily on crystalloid solutions, particularly during the first 24 hours after injury, although recent studies show that colloid resuscitation (plasma) has the potential to decrease the amount of fluids needed to maintain adequate urine output and prevent complications, such as increased intra-abdominal pressure (O'Mara, Slater, Goldfarb, & Caushaj, 2005). Various formulas are used to calculate the rate of fluid administration. The specific protocol for fluid resuscitation remains controversial. In the absence of clinical trials to identify best burn resuscitation practices, protocols are determined by the burn unit or health care facility. In general, the amount of fluid replacement in children is calculated according to body surface area. Typically, half the calculated fluid amount is given over the first 8 hours after the burn, and the remaining half is given over the next 16 hours.

Because urine output reflects end-organ tissue perfusion, IV fluids are administered at a rate sufficient to maintain the child's urine output at a value appropriate for age (see Chapter 18). Inadequate urine output during burn shock is usually the result of insufficient administration of resuscitative fluids. Renal failure is not an expected component of burn shock if an adequate volume of IV fluids is being administered for burn shock resuscitation. It should be recognized that burn shock fluid resuscitation formulas are guidelines; individual children may need more fluids during the first 24 hours after the burn.

Table 25-7 lists additional physiologic effects caused by moderate to major burns. Once a child with a moderate or major burn has been stabilized, the child usually is transferred to a burn center for specialized care.

CONDITIONS ASSOCIATED WITH ELECTRICAL INJURY

Electrical injury is a major injury that often results in instant death because the electrical current disrupts the electrical rhythm of the heart. The child who does not die instantly is at risk for four major complications during the acute phase:
- Cardiac arrest or arrhythmia
- Tissue damage
- Myoglobinuria (globulin from muscle serum appearing in the urine)
- Metabolic acidosis

TABLE 25-7   Body System Alterations After Moderate to Severe Burns

System/Alteration	Cause	Management
Respiratory		
Upper airway tissue injury with respiratory distress, possible obstruction	Edema from inhalation of superheated air	Establish adequate airway, provide moist mist with oxygen as needed
Lower airway tissue injury	Inhalation of smoke	Give oxygen as needed, place child in a head-elevated position, intubate with ventilatory support if necessary
Carbon monoxide inhalation, hypoxia	End products of combustion	Give 100% oxygen by mask; intubate and provide ventilatory support if necessary
Limited chest expansion	Circumferential burns	Escharotomy
Cardiovascular		
Fluid volume deficit with decreased cardiac output; tachycardia	Fluid shifts from vascular to interstitial compartment; massive leaking of fluid through the burn wound	Provide fluid and electrolyte replacement with or without colloids; goal is to achieve urinary output appropriate for age and good capillary refill
Initial vasodilation, then vasoconstriction	Compensatory mechanism to preserve fluid volume and prevent shock	
Edema, compartment syndrome	Increased fluid in interstitial spaces	
Elevated hemoglobin, hematocrit levels	Hemoconcentration caused by fluid loss	
Increase followed by decrease in serum potassium levels	Release of destroyed tissue cells into extracellular space	
Decreased serum sodium levels	Trapped in edema fluids	
Gastrointestinal		
Gastric dilation, paralytic ileus	Decreased perfusion to gastrointestinal tract as a result of hypovolemia	Restore fluid and electrolyte balance
Thirst	Hypovolemia	
Renal		
Oliguria, elevated blood urea nitrogen and creatinine values	Reduced circulation to kidneys	Adequate fluid resuscitation
Risk for acute tubular necrosis	Obstruction of renal tubules	
Metabolic		
Increased metabolic rate with elevated body temperature and massive evaporative heat loss	Insult of open wound	Provide caloric requirements two or three times basal requirements; provide high-protein diet or protein supplements; tube feed or use parenteral nutrition as necessary; provide vitamin C and vitamin A supplements
Catecholamine release	Burn stress; increased temperature and metabolic rate	
Hyperglycemia	Mobilization of glucagon and decreased insulin production	
Hematologic		
Decreased hematocrit level follows initial hematocrit increase (from hemoconcentration)	Increased red blood cell (RBC) hemolysis, decreased RBC production, blood loss from wound care	Packed RBC transfusion for low hematocrit
Coagulation disorders	Decreased platelet count and serum clotting factors	
Increased immature neutrophils to digest products of injury	Depletion of mature neutrophils	
High risk for infection, wound sepsis, septic shock (disorientation, fever, diminished bowel sounds are first signs, temperature falls below normal as body's resistance to infection decreases)	Open wound; altered protective mechanisms; decreased circulation to the skin	Burn excision and debridement followed by application of topical antimicrobial agents; may need biologic or synthetic skin coverings, graft
Pain		
	Tissue injury exposing nerve endings; edema; burn treatments	Meticulous pain management both round-the-clock and before treatments

Cardiac Arrest or Arrhythmia

The immediate risk is cardiac arrest or arrhythmia resulting from damage to the heart's electrical conduction system. If cardiac arrest occurs, standard cardiac life support measures are initiated (see Chapter 10).

Tissue Damage

The electrical current follows the path of least resistance through the body. Entering through the skin, electricity causes heat damage to the skin layers, bone, nerves, tendons, and blood vessels. The heat of the electrical current coagulates blood vessels and leaves the affected area without a blood supply. Gangrene develops in necrotic tissue unless it is removed. Amputation is necessary in more than 90% of children sustaining electrical injuries. The location of the damage depends on the child's position and exposure. Electricity may enter one hand and exit from the other, for example, or it may travel through the body and exit from one or both legs. The greatest damage occurs at the entrance and exit sites.

Myoglobinuria

Myoglobinuria develops from release into the blood of products found in normal muscle; the release can be occasioned by electrical injury. Myoglobin is a large molecule that can mechanically obstruct the renal tubules and lead to acute tubular necrosis unless large amounts of IV fluid are administered to flush the myoglobin out of the kidney. Osmotic diuretics may be administered to promote increased urine volume. IV fluid is administered at a rate that maintains urine output at 2 mL/kg/hr until the myoglobinuria resolves.

Metabolic Acidosis

Metabolic acidosis follows electrical injury because of the associated cellular destruction and hypovolemic shock. Ringer's lactate solution, the fluid used for fluid resuscitation, contains sufficient bicarbonate to manage the acidosis that accompanies burn shock but not enough to correct that associated with shock after electrical injury (i.e., pathophysiologic hypovolemic shock, not a "shock" from the electrical current).

Other Complications

The four complications just described usually resolve within 24 hours after injury. Other complications that follow electrical injury include loss of short-term memory and altered emotional states. Children can usually remember events up to the time of injury, including the names of family members and their own address, telephone number, and personal information, but they are unable to recall more recent events. This loss of memory can be distressing to the child and frustrating to the family. For example, the child may be unable to remember visits by the family and so may feel abandoned by them. It is difficult for the child to follow instructions because of the inability to retain instructions, and this may lead to difficulty in planning care. Altered emotional states may include an absence of affect and blank stares or the opposite type of emotional response—manic behavior, hyperactivity, swearing, physical violence, and feelings of paranoia. Emotional responses usually become normal after about 1 week but may persist longer in some children. The electrical injury need not be to the head for these altered states to occur.

The long-term sequelae of electrical injury may include neurologic deficits, amputations, and ocular cataracts. Ocular cataracts may occur in one or both eyes at varying times from 3 months to 18 months after injury. In the very young child, changes in visual acuity may not be noticed; therefore, regular eye examinations should be scheduled every 3 months for the first year after injury.

KEY CONCEPTS

- The functions of the skin include protection, thermoregulation, excretion, production of vitamin D, and sensation.
- The skin comprises two major layers—the outer epidermis and the inner supportive dermis. The dermis contains blood vessels, nerves, and sweat glands. Beneath these layers is subcutaneous tissue, which attaches the dermis to the underlying structures.
- Developmental differences cause the skin of infants and children to be more susceptible to external irritants and infection than adults' skin.
- Impetigo, the most common skin infection of childhood, is highly contagious. Nursing care includes administration of topical or oral antibiotics and education regarding good handwashing and careful hygiene to prevent spread of infection.
- Because the fungus that causes tinea thrives where it is moist and warm, infected areas should be kept as dry as possible. Proper hygiene should be taught and maintained to minimize the spread of infection.
- Herpes simplex virus is transmitted by infected body fluids coming in contact with breaks in the skin or mucous membranes. Careful handwashing and attention to hygiene decrease the risk of spreading infection.
- Preventing reinfestation is a primary goal in the treatment of pediculosis and scabies.
- Nursing care for the child with eczema includes frequent skin moisturizing and cautioning against the use of clothing, fabrics, or soaps that might irritate the skin. Identifying and eliminating allergens may be helpful.
- Diaper dermatitis is much easier to prevent than to treat. Successful treatment and prevention of diaper rash entail thorough cleansing of the diaper area and keeping the skin dry.
- Nursing care of the adolescent with acne includes teaching about regular, gentle cleansing of the skin, applying topical medications, and encouraging a healthy lifestyle with adequate rest, exercise, and a balanced diet. The nurse must be sensitive to the effect of acne on the adolescent's self-image.
- Insect bites and stings can cause severe systemic reactions in a sensitized child.
- Young children are at increased risk for burn injuries because they are curious, mobile, and totally dependent on their caretakers for safety.

- The extent of a burn injury (depth, severity) determines whether the child will have a local or a systemic reaction.
- The depth of a burn injury is classified as superficial, superficial partial thickness, deep partial thickness, or full thickness.
- In comparison with adults, children who sustain burn injuries are at increased risk for fluid and heat loss, hypertrophic scarring, cardiovascular problems, infection, and protein and calorie deficiency.
- In calculating the TBSA burned, a body surface chart that is corrected for age should be used.
- A minor burn wound should be cleaned with mild soap and water, debrided of loose debris and tissue, and covered with an antimicrobial ointment and a sterile dressing.
- After stabilization, a child with a major burn is cared for in a burn treatment center because of multiple body system complications.

ANSWERS TO
CRITICAL THINKING EXERCISE 25-1

1. The nurse should first ask the mother what symptoms, if any, the child has. If the child is symptomatic with pruritus and visible nits or lice, treatment failure is a possibility. The nurse needs to ask what pediculicide was used, whether nits were fully combed out, whether family members were treated, and what environmental measures were taken to prevent reinfestation in the home. If the parent has followed the instructions meticulously, the nurse needs to explore other areas. Because of the child's age, the nurse needs to question whether the mother has treated her daughter's dress-up clothes and hair ornaments as well as the usual bedding, clothing, combs, brushes, and furniture. The parent should review her child's other contacts as well, such as neighborhood playmates or church play groups. If it appears the management has been thorough, the child may have developed pediculicide-resistant lice and will need a different treatment.

2. If the child is not symptomatic, the school official may be seeing dead nits in the child's hair. The nurse needs to ask the mother about the treatment used and whether all the nits were removed. Removing nits is especially difficult in preschool children because it is time consuming and these young children find sitting still that long difficult. Also, many preschool girls have long hair, which can prolong the process. The nurse should advise the mother to remove all the nits and check her child regularly to be sure that all the nits are gone. The nurse can give the mother suggestions about the most effective method of nit removal and encourage the mother to be persistent. Positive reassurance and encouragement are most important. The nurse may also contact the school official to discuss the concept of nonviable nits and explore the possibility of abandoning a "no-nit" policy.

REFERENCES AND READINGS

Abdulla, F. R., & Brodell, R. T. (2005). Seborrheic dermatitis. *Postgraduate Medicine, 117*, 43-45.

Allasio, D., & Fischer, H. (2005). Immersion scald burns and the ability of young children to climb into a bathtub. *Pediatrics, 115*, 1419-1421.

American Academy of Pediatrics. (2002). Head lice: Clinical report. *Pediatrics, 110*, 638-643.

American Academy of Pediatrics. (2003). *Red Book 2003: Report of the Committee on Infectious Diseases.* Elk Grove Village, IL: American Academy of Pediatrics.

Centers for Disease Control and Prevention. (2005). *Updated information regarding insect repellants.* Retrieved July 1, 2005, from http://www.cdc.gov/ncidod/dvbid/westnile/RepellentUpdates.htm.

Chong, E., Wilhelmus, K. R., Matoba, A. Y., Jones, D. B., Coats, D. K., & Paysse, E. A. (2004). Herpes simplex virus keratitis in children. *American Journal of Ophthalmology, 138*, 474-476.

Cohen, B. A. (2005). *Pediatric dermatology* (3rd ed.). Baltimore: Elsevier Mosby.

Darmstadt, G., & Sidbury, R. (2004). The skin. In R. Behrman, R. Kliegman, & H. Jenson (Eds.). *Nelson textbook of pediatrics* (17th ed., pp. 2243-2246). Philadelphia: WB Saunders.

David, B. K., & Golden, M. D. (2003). Stinging insect allergy. *American Family Physician, 67*, 2541-2546.

Edlich, R. F., Farinholt, H. A., Winters, K. L., Britt, L. D., Long, W. B., Werner, C. L., & Gubler, K. D. (2005). Modern concepts of treatment and prevention of chemical injuries. *Journal of Long-term Effects of Medical Implants, 15*, 303-318.

Eichenfield, L. F., Hanifin, J. M., Beck, L. A., Lemanske, R. F., Jr., Sampson, H. A., Weiss, S. T., & Leung, D. Y. (2003). Atopic dermatitis and asthma: Parallels in the evolution of treatment. *Pediatrics, 111*, 608-616.

Fore-Pfliger, J. (2004). The epidermal skin barrier: Implications for the wound care practitioner, part 1. *Advances in Skin and Wound Care, 17*, 417-425.

Freeman, T. M. (2004). Hypersensitivity to *hymenoptera* stings. *New England Journal of Medicine, 35*, 1978-1984.

Fridkin, S. K., Hageman, J. C., Morrison, M., Sanza, L. T., Como-Sabetti, K., Jernigan, J. A., Harriman, K., Harrison, L. H., Lynfield, R., Farley, M. M., & Active Bacterial Core Surveillance Program of the Emerging Infections Program Network. (2005). Methicillin resistant *Staphylococcus aureus* disease in three communities. *New England Journal of Medicine, 352*, 1436-1444.

Gupta, A. K., Cooper, E. A., Ryder, J. E., Nicol, K. A., Chow, M., & Chaudhry, M. M. (2004). Optimal management of fungal infections of the skin, hair, and nails. *American Journal of Clinical Dermatology, 5*, 225-237.

Guttman, C. (2005). Clinical, molecular features aid worrisome birthmark recognition. *Dermatology Times, 26*, 66-68.

Hainer, B. L. (2003). Dermatophyte infections. *American Family Physician, 67*, 101-108.

Johnson, R. M., & Richard, R. (2003). Partial thickness burns: Identification and management. *Advances in Skin and Wound Care, 16*, 178-186.

Karthikeyan, K. (2005). Treatment of scabies: newer perspectives. *Postgraduate Medical Journal, 81*, 7-11.

Kennedy, C., Bajdik, C. D., Willemze, R., De Gruijl, F. R., & Bouwes Bavinek, J. N. (2003). The influence of painful sunburns and lifetime sun exposure in the risk of actinic keratoses, seborrheic warts, melanocytic nevi, atypical nevi, and skin cancer. *Journal of Investigative Dermatology, 120*, 1087-1093.

Kerkhof, M., Koopman, L. P., van Strien, R. T., Wijga, A., Smit, H. A., Aaberse, R. C., Neijens, H. J., Brunekreef, B., Postma, D. S., Gerritsen, J., & PIAMA Study Group. (2003). Risk factors for atopic dermatitis in infants at high risk of allergy: The PIAMA study. *Clinical and Experimental Allergy, 33*, 1336-1341.

Ladhani, S., & Garbash, M. (2005). Staphylococcal skin infections in children. *Pediatric Drugs, 7*, 77-102.

La Scola, B., & Raoult, D. (2004). *Acinetobacter baumanii* in human body louse. *Emerging Infectious Diseases, 10,* 1671-1673.

Leung, D. Y. M., & Bieber, T. (2003). Atopic dermatitis. *The Lancet, 361,* 151-160.

National Institute of Allergy and Infectious Diseases. (2004). *Allergy statistics.* Retrieved June 28, 2005, from *http://www.niaid.nih.gov/factsheets/allergystat.htm.*

National Institute of Disability and Rehabilitation Research. (2003). *NIDRR model systems for burn injury rehabilitation, child facts and figures.* Retrieved February 25, 2006, from *http://bms-dcc.uchsc.edu.*

National SAFE KIDS Campaign. (2004). *Residential fire injury fact sheet.* Washington, DC: National SAFE KIDS Campaign.

Nursing 2005. (2005). Drug news. *Nursing 2005, 35,* 30.

O'Mara, M. S., Slater, H., Goldfarb, I. W., & Caushaj, P. F. (2005). A prospective, randomised evaluation of intra-abdominal pressures with crystalloid and colloid resuscitation inburn patients. *The Journal of Trauma, 58,* 1011-1018.

Richard, R., & Johnson, R. M. (2002). Managing superficial burn wounds. *Advances in Skin and Wound Care, 15,* 246-247.

Shulman, J. D. (2004). Recurrent herpes labialis in US children and youth. *Community Dentistry and Oral Epidemiology, 32,* 402-410.

Sommer, S., Seukeran, D. C., & Sheehan-Dare, R. A. (2003). Efficacy of pulsed dye laser treatment of port wine stain malformations of the lower limb. *British Journal of Dermatology, 149,* 770-775.

Stulberg, D. L., & Hutchinson, A. G. (2003). Molluscum contagiosum and warts. *American Family Physician, 67,* 1233-1240.

Subhan, S., Jose, R. J., Duggirala, A., Hari, R., Krishna, P., Reddy, S., Sharma, S. (2004). Diagnosis of herpes simplex virus-1 keratitis: Comparison of Giemsa stain, immunofluorescence assay and polymerase chain reaction. *Current Eye Research, 29,* 209-214.

Takano-Lee, M., Edman, J., Mullens, B., & Clark, J. (2004). Home remedies to control head lice: Assessment of home remedies to control the human head louse, *Pediculus humanus capitis* (Anoplura: Pediculidae). *Journal of Pediatric Nursing, 19,* 393-398.

United Nations Environmental Programme. (2005). *Governments take decisive action to rid the world of persistent organic pollutants (POPs) through the Stockholm Convention.* Retrieved June 16, 2005, from *http://www.pops.int/documents/press/pr5%2D05%20pops%20cop%201%20conclusion.doc.*

Vascular Birthmarks Foundation. (2006). *Port Wine Stain Information.* Retrieved September 9, 2006, from *http://www.birthmark.org/port_wine_stains.php.*

Wananukul, S., Nuchprayoon, I., & Seksarn, P. (2003). Treatment of Kasabach-Merritt syndrome: A stepwise regimen of prednisolone, dipyridamole, and interferon. *International Journal of Dermatology, 42,* 741-748.

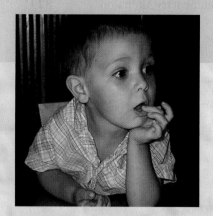

CHAPTER **26**

The Child With a Musculoskeletal Alteration

Learning Objectives

After studying this chapter, you should be able to:

- Describe the anatomy and physiology of an infant's and young child's musculoskeletal system.
- Describe the pathology, etiology, manifestations, diagnostic evaluation, and therapeutic management of musculoskeletal alterations frequently seen in infants and children.
- Select relevant criteria to determine the etiology and diagnosis of common musculoskeletal alterations.

- State appropriate nursing diagnoses for the child with alterations in musculoskeletal function.
- Identify characteristic behaviors that indicate alterations in musculoskeletal function.
- Summarize the treatment modalities used to manage the child with musculoskeletal alterations.
- Design, implement, and evaluate appropriate nursing interventions for the child with altered musculoskeletal function.

Definitions

abduction Movement of a limb away from the midline of the body.

adduction Movement of a limb toward the midline of the body.

ankylosis Condition in which a joint is stiff or difficult to move.

arthroscopic surgery (arthroscopy) Surgical procedure in which a lighted tubular scope is inserted into a joint to diagnose or treat traumatic soft tissue injury.

autologous blood transfusion Transfusion of one's own, previously harvested blood.

avascular necrosis Tissue damage caused by inadequate blood supply.

callus Tissue that joins fractured bone ends or repairs damaged bone; begins as cartilaginous tissue and becomes hardened through osteoblastic activity.

crepitus A grating sensation at a fracture site that occurs when the ends of a broken bone move against each other.

dislocation Displacement of a bone from its normal articulation within a joint.

dysplasia Abnormal development of tissue.

eversion Turned away from the midline.

external fixation Placement of pins, screws, or bars through bone and soft tissue to immobilize or correct a deformity.

external rotation Turning outward, or laterally, within a joint.

internal fixation Placement of instruments (wires, pins, rods, screws) inside the body to immobilize parts.

internal rotation Turning inward, or medially, within a joint.

inversion Turning toward the midline.

orthoses Braces, external supports, or artificial limbs made by a specialist to meet individual needs.

ossification The process of forming bone from osseous tissue or cartilage.

osteoblasts Mesodermal cells whose activity produces bone.

osteoclasts Cells found in bones that absorb and remove old bony tissue.

osteotomy Surgical cutting of bone.

paresthesia Sensation of numbness and tingling.

plantar flexion Bending toward the sole of the foot.

polydactyly Extra fingers or toes.

pseudarthrosis Failure of the bones to fuse.

reduction Repositioning of bone fragments into normal alignment followed by application of a device or mechanism that maintains alignment of bone until healing occurs.

subluxation Partial dislocation of a joint.

superior mesenteric artery syndrome A condition resembling intestinal obstruction caused by reduced blood supply to a segment of the mesentery.

syndactyly Fusion or webbing of two or more fingers or toes.

valgum Abnormal position of a limb in which it is bent away from the midline of the body.

varum Abnormal position of the limb in which it is bent toward the midline of the body.

REVIEW OF THE MUSCULOSKELETAL SYSTEM

Bones, joints, muscles, and cartilaginous tissues make up the musculoskeletal system. To understand alterations in musculoskeletal function, an understanding of normal musculoskeletal structure and function as well as patterns of growth and development is necessary.

Skeletal System

The bony skeleton provides a surface for the attachment of muscles, tendons, and ligaments. The pulling action on individual bones makes movement possible. The human skeletal system consists of 206 bones, which are classified as long bones (e.g., humerus, radius), short bones (e.g., carpals, tarsals), flat bones (e.g., ribs), irregular bones (e.g., vertebrae), and sesamoid bones (e.g., kneecaps).

Each long bone consists of a diaphysis (shaft) with an epiphysis (secondary ossification center) at each end. The muscles attach here and are responsible for joint stability. The metaphysis, or wide portion of the bone, is responsible for growth. The metaphysis consists of cartilage and actively produces bone through osteoblastic activity. Periosteum, a vascular connective tissue, covers the bone. The medullary cavity is located in the center of the diaphysis.

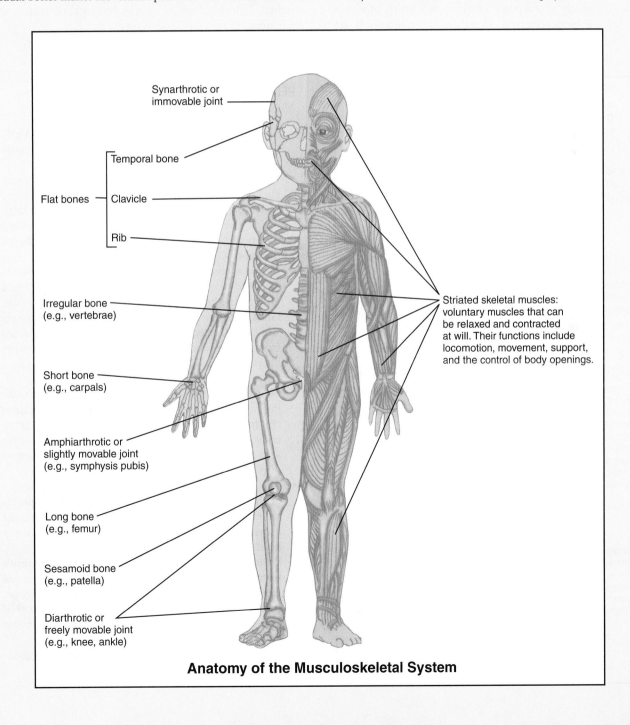

Anatomy of the Musculoskeletal System

Articular System

The joints, which are composed of connective tissue and cartilage, connect bones to one another and enable great freedom of movement. Joints are classified by their degree of movement: *synarthrotic*, or immovable (e.g., the skull); *amphiarthrotic*, or slightly movable (e.g., the symphysis); and *diarthrotic*, or freely movable (e.g., the knee). Muscles help stabilize joints and maintain contact between articular surfaces. The shape of the two ends of each muscle and of the joint determines the extent of movement or articulation. Ligaments bind one bone firmly to another, and the joints are further stabilized by the overlying tendons and muscles.

Muscular System

Muscle, which is composed of elongated fibers, produces movement by contraction. The three types of muscle are smooth muscle, found primarily in the internal organs; cardiac, or heart, muscle; and skeletal muscle. Smooth muscle and cardiac muscle are *involuntary* muscles because they are not willfully controlled. Skeletal muscle, which is controlled voluntarily, and cardiac muscle are striated muscles because of their striped appearance under the microscope.

Cartilage

Cartilage is dense connective tissue that develops at the epiphysis and is capable of withstanding considerable tension. The skeleton of an embryo is mostly cartilage. In time it will largely convert to bone by ossification. Bone is necessary for longitudinal growth. Growth in the length of the long bones continues at the epiphysis until adult height is reached. The epiphyseal plate absorbs shock, protecting the joint surfaces from serious fractures.

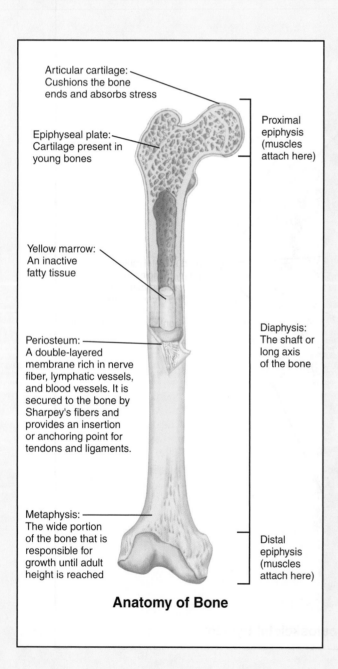

Articular cartilage:
Cushions the bone
ends and absorbs stress

Epiphyseal plate:
Cartilage present in
young bones

Yellow marrow:
An inactive
fatty tissue

Periosteum:
A double-layered
membrane rich in nerve
fiber, lymphatic vessels,
and blood vessels. It is
secured to the bone by
Sharpey's fibers and
provides an insertion
or anchoring point for
tendons and ligaments.

Metaphysis:
The wide portion
of the bone that is
responsible for
growth until adult
height is reached

Proximal
epiphysis
(muscles
attach here)

Diaphysis:
The shaft or
long axis
of the bone

Distal
epiphysis
(muscles
attach here)

Anatomy of Bone

PEDIATRIC DIFFERENCES IN THE MUSCULOSKELETAL SYSTEM

- Muscle tissue is almost completely developed at birth. Growth occurs because of an increase in size rather than number of the muscle fibers.
- In the fetus, bony tissue begins to develop as closely packed connective tissue. Connective tissue is replaced by cartilage, and cartilage is replaced by mineral salts, which give rise to solid bone. The infant's bones are only 65% ossified at 8 months of age and are neither as firm nor as brittle as those of the older child.
- New bony tissue is produced during periods of growth. The rate of growth varies at different ages. Skeletal growth is stimulated by pituitary growth hormone. Growth of the long bones occurs at the epiphyses, which are located at the ends of the bones and separated from the main portion of the bone by cartilage during the period of growth. Injury to the epiphyses can cause growth disturbances.
- Growing bones produce callus and heal quickly, making internal fixation of fractures unnecessary in most children. Fractures in children younger than 1 year are unusual because a large amount of force is necessary; abuse or underlying pathophysiology is often the cause of fractures in infants.
- The skull is not rigid during infancy, and the sutures of the cranium do not fuse completely until approximately 16 to 18 months of age. Increased intracranial pressure can separate the sutures, causing the infant's head to enlarge.
- Postural changes during infancy and childhood result from the development of neurologic control, bone and muscle growth, and the laying down of adipose tissue. Postural changes are a good indication of the level of development of the musculoskeletal and neurologic systems.
- Because soft tissues are resilient in children, dislocations and sprains are less common than in adults.

Common Diagnostic and Laboratory Tests and Procedures for Musculoskeletal Disorders in Children

Test	Purpose and Description	Nursing Implications
Radiography (x ray)	For detection of abnormalities or to determine bone age. X rays (gamma radiation) pass through the body, reach the film on the other side of the body, and turn the film black. Areas filled with air appear dark on the film. Different densities of tissue absorb various amounts of radiation. The four densities of x-ray: Air: blackish Fat: dark gray Water: lighter gray Bone: whitish	Food and fluids are not usually restricted. Clothing and jewelry should be removed; a paper or cloth gown is worn. Young children may require immobilization. Adequate preparation is essential to ensure cooperation.
Arthrography	To evaluate suspected joint damage, such as tears of cartilage. Dye is injected into the joint, usually the knee; sometimes the shoulder or other joint.	Performed with the child under local anesthesia. Check for allergies to iodine. May have mild to moderate discomfort after the procedure. Joint should rest for approximately 12 hr; compression dressing may be applied after procedure to reduce swelling.
Radionuclide scintigraphy (bone scan)	To detect tumors, infection, inflammation. Radioactive material given IV. In 2-4 hr, the entire body is scanned, both front and back.	Young children need sedation. Encourage fluids 2-4 hr before the test to ensure the child is well hydrated and quickly eliminate radioactive material not absorbed by the bones. Child must void before the scan so that the pelvic bones can be seen.
Computed tomography (CT)	To visualize anatomic details. Narrow-beam x rays are used to scan an area in successive layers. A computer processes readings and converts them to a picture shown on a screen, which is stored on disks. A three-dimensional cross section of body parts is shown.	Although the procedure is painless, it may be frightening. The child must remain still during procedure, so young children need sedation. Contrast medium may or may not be used. Tell the child the machine looks and sounds like a clothes dryer or washing machine. Remove clothing and jewelry.
Magnetic resonance imaging	Clearly defines organ structures; shows changes in tissue, such as edema, blood flow patterns, infarcts. Demonstrates marrow, bone and soft tissue tumors, structure of muscles, ligaments, bones. Huge magnet and radio waves create an energy field that can be translated into a visual image. Child is placed on a moving stretcher, which is pushed into the large cylinder that contains the magnet. A variety of noises are heard during the procedure.	Food and fluids are not restricted. Study is not done in children with metal implants, pacemakers, or prostheses. Procedure may take 1 hr or more, so young children need sedation. The child should void before procedure. Adequate preparation, relaxation techniques, and parental presence decrease fear and feelings of claustrophobia. Use of a music headset may promote relaxation.
Arthroscopy	To image the inside of a joint for diagnosis of injury or minor surgical repairs. Normally arthrography is performed before arthroscopy. Fiberoptic endoscope is inserted to examine interior of joint.	Requires local or general anesthesia. The child must be on nothing-by-mouth (NPO) status for 8 hr before the test if general anesthesia is used; NPO status recommendations for local anesthesia vary with the practitioner. Prepare the child for postoperative dressings, altered mobility, and pain. Assess for infection. Prophylactic antibiotics may be ordered. Use ice bags postoperatively to reduce swelling.
Joint aspiration	Fluid is withdrawn for analysis, usually to detect infection or relieve pain.	Requires local anesthesia. Prepare the child for some discomfort during and after procedure.
Ultrasound	To demonstrate body tissue structure or for waveform analysis of Doppler studies. Doppler probe is held over the skin surface or in a body cavity to produce an ultrasound beam in the tissues. Echoes reflected from the tissues are transformed by computer into a visual image or audible sounds (Doppler).	Noninvasive; food and fluid are not restricted except in small infants, who may be on NPO status for 2-3 hr before the procedure so they can eat during the test.
Alkaline phosphatase (ALP)	ALP is an enzyme found mainly in bone, liver, placenta, kidney; levels may be elevated in bone disease, fractures, trauma, or liver disease and during periods of rapid growth. Determinations may be ordered to differentiate between bone and liver problems.	Nonfasting

Continued

Test	Purpose and Description	Nursing Implications
Creatine kinase (CK)	CK is an enzyme found in heart and skeletal muscle; the CK assay is a specific test for cardiac and muscle damage. Levels are elevated in trauma, myocardial infarction, and muscular dystrophy. Determinations may be ordered to differentiate between cardiac (MB) and skeletal (MM) CK.	Nonfasting
Rheumatoid factor (RF)	RFs are antibodies that may be responsible for the destructive changes associated with rheumatoid arthritis. A positive RF supports the possible diagnosis of JA.	Nonfasting
C-reactive protein (CRP)	CRP is a protein that appears in blood because of an inflammatory process. It is not seen in healthy people. The measurement is nonspecific, merely indicating the presence of inflammation.	Nonfasting
Erythrocyte sedimentation rate (ESR)	ESR is the rate at which erythrocytes settle out of unclotted blood, measured in millimeters per hour. Inflammation and necrotic problems cause an elevation in ESR levels.	Nonfasting

Common Diagnostic and Laboratory Tests and Procedures for Musculoskeletal Disorders in Children—cont'd

Electronic Resources

Additional information related to the content in Chapter 26 can be found on:

the interactive companion CD-ROM
- Animation: Spine Structure
- Audio Glossary
- NCLEX Review Questions
- Pediatric Assessment Video Clips
- Skill: Monitoring Neurovascular Status

or the companion website at *evolve*
http://evolve.elsevier.com/james/ncoc
- Common Pediatric Laboratory Tests and Normal Values
- NCLEX Review Questions
- Pediatric Assessment Video Clips
- Resources for Health Care Providers and Families
- WebLinks

Musculoskeletal problems affect muscles, bones, joints, and tendons, all of which are necessary for movement and therefore are critical to a child's development. Many musculoskeletal problems occur because of vigorous motor activities that are part of a child's daily life, but the rapid growth of the skeletal system plays a significant role as well. Most musculoskeletal problems are short term, but a number of chronic musculoskeletal conditions require long-term treatment and nursing assistance.

CASTS, TRACTION, AND OTHER IMMOBILIZING DEVICES

Immobilizing a bone or joint helps achieve and maintain a more functional position or rests an affected area during bone healing. Because many musculoskeletal problems require the application of an immobilizing device, the nurse needs to understand general principles of care.

Casts

A cast provides support and maintains anatomic position for bone healing or correction of a deformity. Casts may also be used to ensure adherence to treatment protocols. Most casts are made of synthetic materials, such as fiberglass. They dry quickly and are lighter weight than materials formerly used for casting, such as plaster of Paris, and are water resistant (Fig. 26-1). They also come in varied colors and patterns that appeal to young children. If a synthetic cast becomes wet, inadequate airflow under the cast will prevent thorough drying of the skin, and damp skin is more susceptible to skin breakdown. The standard cast usually involves cast padding over a cotton stockinette. Waterproof casts are now also available, and when used for stable fractures provide acceptable immobilization with no increased associated risk (Shannon, Difazio, Kasser, Karlin, & Gerbino, 2005).

Most casts are applied on an outpatient basis. The type of the fracture or injury and the amount of weight bearing the extremity can tolerate dictate the size of the cast. Short or long leg or arm casts are generally used for fractures of the upper and lower limbs. Fractures of the hip and knee may require a body, or *spica*, cast.

The following equipment needed for cast application includes:
- Tubular gauze (stockinette)
- Cotton under-cast padding material (e.g., Webril)
- Casting material (rolls or strips)
- Water

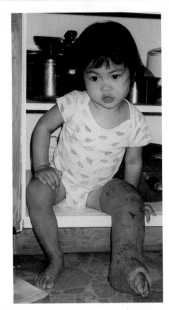

FIG 26-1   **Child in a synthetic cast.**

The tubular gauze is placed over the extremity to be casted, and the limb is held in the appropriate position. After applying a thin layer of under-cast padding and soaking the casting material in water, the physician or other trained staff applies the strips over the padding material, bringing the end of the padding material and stockinette over the end of the casting material and under the last casting strip to provide a smooth, padded edge. A chemical reaction between the casting material and the water causes a feeling of warmth as the cast is applied.

Traction

Effective immobilization may also be achieved with traction. Traction is a pull or force exerted on one part of the body; in treatment, traction may be applied to the spine, pelvis, or long bones of the upper and lower extremities. The angle formed by the placement of the pulley on the bed frame and the angle of the involved joint determine the direction of the pull or force.

Once the direction of the pull or force has been determined, the traction is directed along the long axis of the bone. Traction can be applied to the skin or the bone. Some forms of traction, such as halo femoral traction used for spinal problems, exert a force without the use of weights.

An opposing pull or force (countertraction) must be provided at the same time if the traction is to be effective. Countertraction results in a two-way pull that maintains alignment of the affected extremity. The child's weight is usually sufficient to provide the countertraction. If body weight is not sufficient, additional weights may be used. Depending on the age of the child, restraining devices may be needed to maintain countertraction.

The part of the bed that holds the traction apparatus is tilted or elevated, thereby assisting with countertraction. For example, if the leg were being placed in traction, the foot of the bed would be elevated. Otherwise, the child would slide in the direction of the traction, disrupting the alignment of the extremity and reducing the effectiveness of treatment. Also, the mattress should be firm and a foot board or foot plate may be necessary to keep the extremity in the correct position.

The disadvantages of traction include the need for hospitalization and prolonged immobility. Currently, early casting and percutaneous pinning are replacing the use of traction for some musculoskeletal conditions.

Traction can be described as either *continuous* or *intermittent*. Continuous traction exerts a constant pull and is used for fractures and dislocations. Intermittent traction provides a periodic pull or force and is used for contractures, low back pain, or muscle spasm. *The nurse should always assume that traction is continuous unless the physician states otherwise.* The removal of traction that was intended to be continuous could prove harmful to the child and result in poor healing. The nursing care plan should always reflect the frequency and amount of time intermittent traction may be removed. When removing the traction apparatus, the nurse must use the hands to maintain manual traction and pull on the body part.

Traction may also be described as *running* or *balanced*. Running, or straight, traction exerts a pull on the affected part without balanced support from a sling or splint. The child's weight provides the countertraction. Balanced, or suspension, traction also exerts a pull on the affected part, but the extremity is supported by a sling or splint. Countertraction is provided by weights and pulleys attached to the sling or splint. When balanced traction is applied, the pull remains constant, even when the child moves. The countertraction offsets any movement and results in fewer problems with immobility. Both balanced and running traction may be applied to either the skin or bone.

Skin Traction

Skin traction (Box 26-1) exerts force directly on the body surface. It is noninvasive and well tolerated and does not require anesthesia. Skin traction is most effective with children who weigh less than 30 lb or are younger than 2 to 3 years. It can be applied to the pelvis, spine, or extremities (usually the long bones). Skin traction is preferred for conditions in which invasive procedures are contraindicated, such as hemarthrosis (collection of blood in the joint) as a result of hemophilia. Foam rubber straps, adhesive moleskin, or cloth belts are applied to the skin and then attached to the weights and pulleys. Sometimes an elastic bandage is wrapped around the skin to hold the traction apparatus in place. If skin traction to the lower leg is needed, a foam rubber or fabric boot may be used; the fit should be secure.

The effectiveness of skin traction is determined by the amount of pull that can be placed on the extremity. For this reason, skin traction is not appropriate if the child has a skin infection, an open wound, or extensive tissue damage. Skin breakdown may also develop. Spraying the intact skin with tincture of benzoin before the traction is applied may protect against skin irritation.

If the traction has not been set up correctly, neurovascular impairment may occur. Hyperextension of the knee and elastic bandages that have been wrapped too tightly are the most common causes of this problem. A thorough assessment

| BOX 26-1 | **Types of Skin Traction** |

Buck's Extension

Purpose: Used to treat some fractures, hip disorders, contractures, and muscle spasms.

Description: Continuous or intermittent boot or circular wrap is applied to the skin. Traction is applied to boot or wrap. Rolled towels are placed on the external surface of the knee to prevent external rotation of the affected leg. Unless otherwise ordered, the mattress should be flexed at the knee (20 to 30 degrees) to maintain a neutral hip.*

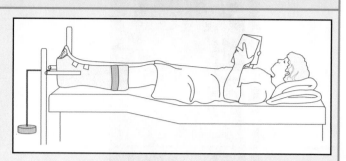

Russell Traction

Purpose: Used to stabilize fractured femurs until callus forms.

Description: Continuous traction. Knee slightly flexed and supported with sling. Trapeze overhead may be used by child for repositioning and upper extremity muscle integrity.

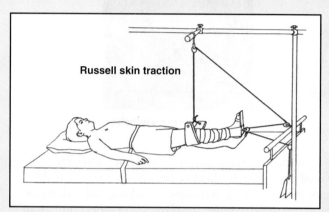

Russell skin traction

Cervical Traction

Purpose: Used to treat muscle or nerve irritation of shoulders and upper arms.

Description: May be continuous or intermittent. Maintains the head in extension by a halter: front straps fit under the chin, rear straps rest at base of skull. Spreader bar equalizes force of pull. Elevating the head of the bed 20 to 30 degrees helps maintain alignment.

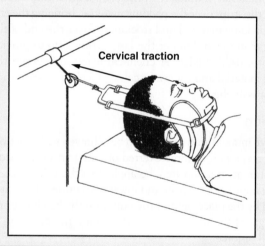

Cervical traction

*Byrne, T. (1999). The setup and care of a patient in Buck's traction. *Orthopaedic Nursing, 18*(2), 79-83.

of the traction apparatus and the extremity should be conducted at least once each shift as a preventive measure.

Skeletal Traction

Skeletal traction (Box 26-2 and Fig. 26-2) exerts greater force than skin traction and can be physiologically tolerated for longer periods. Traction is maintained by a metal device inserted into the bone. The fracture site determines the insertion site of the stainless steel wires, pins, or tongs. Common sites for skeletal traction include the skull, the proximal end of the ulna, and the distal end of the femur as well as the tibia and heel. Internal fixation is common in skeletal traction. It helps maintain correct alignment of the bony fragments and assists in proper healing. General anesthesia is required for internal fixation.

The most serious complication associated with skeletal traction is *osteomyelitis*, an infection involving the bone. Organisms gain access to the bone systemically or through the opening created by the metal pins or wires used for traction. Osteomyelitis may also occur with any open fracture. Clinical manifestations include localized pain, swelling, warmth, tenderness, or unusual odor. An elevated temperature may accompany the symptoms. To decrease the risk of infection at the pin sites, many facilities have an institutional protocol for frequent pin site care (once per day or more often). This procedure involves inspecting each site for signs of infection (e.g., tenting or pulling around the pin, redness at the site, purulent drainage), cleaning the skin around pin sites with one of various cleansing solutions (e.g., half-strength hydrogen peroxide, povidone-iodine solution, chlorhexidine

BOX 26-2	**Types of Skeletal Traction**

Halo Traction

Purpose: To stabilize fractures or displaced vertebrae in cervical and thoracic areas.

Description: The halo is fitted on with pins drilled directly into the skull. The halo is then attached by a rope to weights above the head or to a special vest connected to the halo with rods. When the halo is attached to weights, the center of the curved metal bar over the halo must extend along the same planes as the spinal cord. Traction pull is always along the axis of the spine. The child must maintain straight body alignment.

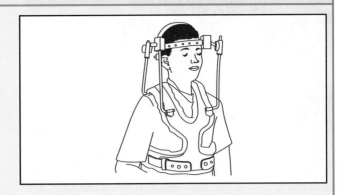

Balanced Suspension

Purpose: Suspends and immobilizes a leg without applying traction to the body.

Description: May be applied to a hip, tibia, fibula, or femur. The leg is supported by a Pearson attachment and a Thomas splint. A Thomas splint is a padded ring that fits around the upper leg; a Pearson attachment meets the Thomas splint at the knee and supports the lower leg. A canvas sling may be used to further support the lower leg.

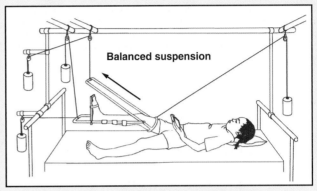

Balanced suspension

90/90 Femoral Traction

Purpose: Most commonly used traction for complicated fractures of the femur; most effective in children older than 6 years. Within 2 to 3 weeks, callus formation is sufficient to allow application of a spica cast.

Description: A pin or wire is inserted through the distal femur; the lower leg may be casted.

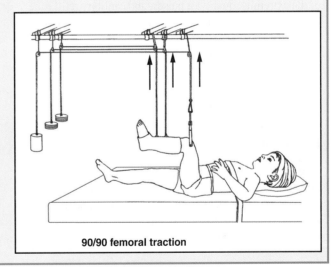

90/90 femoral traction

gluconate, plain normal saline, soap and water), and often applying an antibiotic ointment and a gauze pad.

Skeletal traction is always continuous. If the force of the traction were to be altered, the muscles would contract and fracture alignment would be disrupted. The tissues around the fracture could also be injured.

External Fixation Devices

External fixation devices, such as the Ilizarov external fixator (Fig. 26-3), consist of pins or wires inserted through skin, soft tissue, and bone and secured on the outer limb surface to a rigid metal frame. The external fixator provides distraction, keeping the bone ends separated and in alignment so healing can occur. In this way, the fixator acts like traction, except that, unlike traction, it allows the child to be somewhat mobile during the healing process. In fact, external fixation devices are becoming so common in the treatment of fractures that traction is now infrequently used. Because the screws of the external fixator pass through the skin to anchor in the bone, meticulous assessment of entry sites for signs of inflammation, infection, or loose pins is necessary. Pin care usually is recommended to prevent infection; in this instance, it is similar to pin care for children in traction. To prevent injury to the other limb or to others, sharp protrusions from the fixator need to be adequately covered. General anesthesia is necessary for removal of external fixation devices.

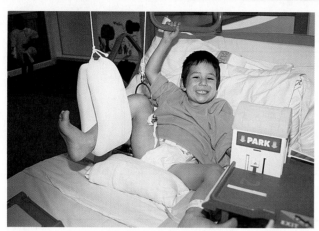

FIG 26-2 Skeletal traction is used to reduce and immobilize fractures and allows greater pull than would be possible with skin traction. Osteomyelitis may be a serious complication because skeletal traction is invasive. *(Courtesy Parkland Health and Hospital System, Dallas, TX.)*

CRITICAL TO REMEMBER
The Child in a Cast or Traction

Tissue ischemia and nerve damage are serious complications that may accompany immobilization in a cast or traction. Skin color and temperature, movement and sensation of the extremity, quality of pulses, and capillary refill time of the extremity are related to neurovascular status and should be carefully assessed; problems must be handled quickly to prevent permanent disabilities.

The five *P*'s of vascular impairment can be used as a guide when assessing neurovascular problems:

*P*ain
*P*allor
*P*ulselessness
*P*aresthesia
*P*aralysis

Pain or a burning sensation unrelieved by analgesia or nursing interventions may indicate tissue ischemia. Prompt intervention is crucial if neurovascular impairment is to be prevented. This type of symptom must be referred to the physician.

Nursing Considerations

Before application of an immobilizing device, assess the child's and parent's knowledge about the procedure. Also assess the child's skin and note the presence of any bruises or abrasions that may be covered by the device.

Neurovascular Status

After the device is applied, perform a neurovascular assessment (CSM—circulation, sensation, and motion) at least every 1 to 2 hours during the first 48 hours. Assess the strength of the pulse distal to the site, and compare it with the pulse in the uninvolved extremity. A sluggish capillary refill time usually indicates neurovascular impairment.

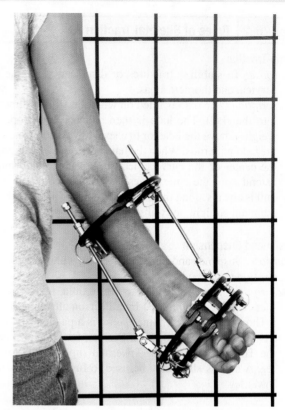

FIG 26-3 Ilizarov external fixator. *(Courtesy Shriners Hospitals for Children, Houston, TX.)*

Signs of circulatory impairment include coldness, pallor, blueness of the extremity, swelling, loss of motion, and numbness and tingling of the extremity. Touch the child's foot to assess temperature; ask the child to move the fingers or toes. Paresthesia, or numbness and tingling, can be assessed by touching the fingers or toes and noting any decrease or loss of feeling. Paresthesia is of serious concern because paralysis can result if the problem is not corrected. Report a child's complaints of a pins-and-needles sensation or of the extremity "feeling asleep."

Because young children are not always able to describe a feeling or sensation, avoid questions such as "Do you feel this?" Asking a child to wiggle the fingers or toes is an appropriate way to determine motor impairment.

Immobility

Children in immobilizing devices are subject to the consequences of immobility. Immobility can affect several body systems. Appropriate assessment and intervention can prevent adverse effects (Table 26-1).

Special Considerations for the Child in Traction

Children who are placed in traction are hospitalized from several days to weeks depending on the underlying condition. Effective traction prevents movement of the affected limb and maintains skeletal alignment during healing. The correct amount of weight is necessary to maintain bone position. After checking with the physician's order that the correct weight is applied, be sure that all weights are hanging

TABLE 26-1	Consequences of Immobility		
System Affected	**Assessment Criteria**	**Nursing Diagnosis**	**Intervention**
Integumentary	Red or irritated skin, presence of ulceration or drainage	Impaired Skin Integrity	Reposition the child every 2 hr and as needed; encourage the child in traction to use a trapeze to facilitate movement. Use an egg crate–type or sheepskin mattress under the back and lower legs; use water-filled gloves under the heels to prevent skin breakdown. Wash and thoroughly dry the areas twice a day; refrain from using lotion, powder, or talc, which can retain moisture. Change the untrained child's diapers frequently to prevent skin breakdown. Examine and record the child's skin condition once per shift.
Gastrointestinal	Decrease in number or consistency of bowel movements because of decreased gastrointestinal motility	Constipation	Monitor bowel sounds, abdominal distention, elimination pattern; be sure to know the child's normal pattern, usual stool consistency, and words used for defecation. Provide a diet high in roughage and fiber and increase fluid intake with foods and fluids the child likes. Position the child as upright as possible during defecation; administer stool softeners or mild laxatives if needed.
Respiratory	Decreased or altered respirations, shortness of breath, lying supine for prolonged periods, decreased breath sounds, adventitious breath sounds	Ineffective Breathing Pattern	Monitor respiratory status at least once per shift. Encourage coughing and deep breathing through the use of games, such as blowing bubbles, pinwheels, or magic tricks; older children can use an incentive spirometer. Reposition every 2 hr and as needed.
Genitourinary	Decreased urinary output from stasis or retention, concentrated or foul-smelling urine	Impaired Urinary Elimination	Maintain hydration levels that are age appropriate. Offer juices (cranberry, apple) and acid-ash foods (cereal, meats) that will acidify the urine. Monitor the child's urinary output.
Musculoskeletal	Reduced strength and joint mobility, loss of muscle tone and potential for increased muscle atrophy, limited range of motion	Impaired Physical Mobility	Test muscle strength and joint mobility every shift and as needed. Encourage active range-of-motion and stretching exercises of unaffected extremities as appropriate. Plan age-appropriate activities that require the use of unaffected extremities. Provide foods high in protein and calcium. Use elastic stockings or thromboembolitic disease hose to promote venous return and decrease circulatory stasis.
	Developmental regression, irritability, anxiety, excessive dependence on others, passive behavior	Powerlessness	Recognize the child's need to regress in response to the immobility; help child regain prior developmental stages when ready. Explain all routines and procedures to the child and parents and encourage them to participate in care. Provide the opportunity for therapeutic play—bean bags, foam balls, modeling clay, paints, remote-control toys (which give the feeling of mobility and control), puppet play, storytelling, role playing. Allow the child to use age-appropriate dishes and cups, clothing from home (may have to be adapted to fit over an immobilizing device), transitional object, night light. Determine and follow the child's usual routine. Encourage the school-age child and adolescent to keep up with schoolwork and keep in contact with peers. Frequently provide a change in environment—move the bed to take advantage of a different view; move the bed into the playroom. Allow the child some autonomy in decision making.

free and are not touching the floor or bed and that all ropes are appropriately on the pulleys. Elevate the head or foot of the bed as indicated to maintain countertraction. It may be necessary to draw a line on the child's bed sheet and ask the parents to keep the child above that line. An older child can pull on an overhead trapeze to maintain proper position and alignment.

Home Care

Most children are discharged home shortly after a cast application. Box 26-3 presents basic principles for caring for a child in a cast at home. Care for children discharged with an external fixator may involve frequent neurovascular assessments and possibly pin site care. Parents must be able to describe how to care for the cast or fixator, when they need to contact their physician, and how to contact any needed resources in the community (e.g., physical therapy, occupational therapy, school district personnel). The nurse can also help the parents select appropriate clothing and adaptive devices if appropriate. Encourage the parents to promote the child's self-care whenever possible.

LIMB DEFECTS

Limb defects are common in children and are a concern for parents. Most alterations of arms and legs are mild variations of normal posturing, but some are severe anomalies or abnormalities.

Etiology and Incidence

Limb defects result from birth anomalies and sometimes from trauma. These defects take many forms, including webbing (*syndactyly*) or extra digits (fingers or toes; *polydactyly*), congenital absence of all or part of an extremity, *genu valgum* ("knock knees") and *genu varum* (bowlegs); and clubfoot. Bowlegs are common in sturdily built infants and toddlers (Fig. 26-4). This condition is also associated with tibial torsion, a normal variation in toddlers. Knock knees are often seen in the preschool-age group. The structure and function of congenitally malformed limbs can be improved with therapy, but the affected limbs seldom become normal.

Trauma to or infection of an extremity may result in a variety of difficulties. Leg length discrepancy can be a result

---

| **BOX 26-3** | **PARENTS AND CHILD WANT TO KNOW** About Home Care for the Child in a Cast |

Check the Edges of the Cast as Follows:
- If they appear rough or are irritating the skin, "petal" the cast by overlapping moleskin or adhesive tape (1 to 2 inches in width; 3 to 4 inches in length with one rounded edge) around the cast edges.

To Assist With Drying the Cast, Do the Following:
- Place your child on a firm mattress.
- Support the cast and adjacent joints with pillows.
- For a plaster cast, reposition every 2 to 4 hours to ensure thorough drying.
- Lift the cast with the palms of your hands.
- You may direct a fan toward the cast to facilitate drying.
- Once dry, the cast should sound hollow and be cool to the touch.

Swelling Generally Peaks Within 24 to 48 Hours. To Prevent Problems, Do the Following:
- Apply bagged ice to the casted area (be sure to keep melting ice from touching the cast or leaking underneath).
- Elevate the extremity with pillows.
- Apply pressure to the nail bed of the child's casted extremity and count how long it takes for the color to return (it should take no longer than 2 seconds). Repeat every 2 to 3 hours for the first 24 to 48 hours.
- The casted extremity should be the same color and temperature as the other extremity.
- Check each finger or toe for sensation and movement several times each day for 2 days.

Protect the Cast as Follows:
- If the child is permitted to bathe or shower, be sure to cover the cast with plastic and waterproof tape to keep the cast dry.

- Do not put anything inside the cast. Keep small toys and sharp objects away from the cast. Supervise your child during mealtimes so the child does not get food underneath the cast.

Contact the Physician if any of the Following Occurs:
- The cast feels warm or hot or has an unusual smell.
- Any drainage or blood suddenly appears on the cast.
- Your child reports pain, burning, numbness, or tingling; the extremity changes color or temperature; or any swelling persists.
- Any fever above 101.5° F taken by mouth.

When Preparing to Remove the Cast, Do the Following:
- Explain the cast removal to your child. The cast cutter works by vibrations that create heat and a tickling feeling on the skin. It sometimes sounds loud, so you need to provide reassurance if your child is afraid of loud noises.
- Allow time for the child to adjust to the cast cutter. Ask the technician or physician if your child can examine the cast cutter and see how it works ahead of time. Sometimes children are allowed to remove a doll's cast with supervision.
- Once the cast is removed, the skin will be dry and flaky. Wash the area with warm water and soap.
- The extremity will be stiff for a while and will look smaller because the muscles have not been used. It may need to be supported with a sling. Normal movement will correct the stiffness.

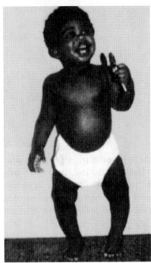
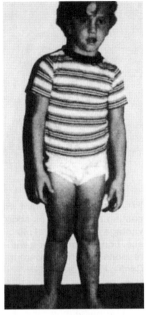

Bowlegs   **Knock knees**

FIG 26-4   **In the child with genu varum, or bowlegs, a persistent space is present between the knees when the ankles are together. Genu varum is a normal finding for 1 year after the child begins walking. In the child with genu valgum, or knock knees, a space is present between the ankles when the knees are together. To remember the terminology, link the r's and g's: genu va*r*um,—knees apa*r*t; genu val*g*um, knees to*g*ether.** *(From McKade, W. [1977]. Bowlegs and knock-knees. Pediatric Clinics of North America, 24[4], 831.)*

of trauma, infection, or radiation therapy (because the unaffected limb continues to grow).

Pathophysiology

Mild limb defects most frequently occur as a result of extrinsic pressure, such as in utero positioning, or the sitting and sleeping postures of young children. Heredity may also play a part in mild limb defects. These disorders are usually cosmetic, although occasionally function is altered as well. They tend to correct as the child grows.

Diagnostic Evaluation

Severe congenital defects are readily apparent at birth. Mild defects and deformities that develop over time are usually identified by parents or school nurses and are evaluated by specialized clinicians. Radiographs may be necessary to evaluate limb defects fully and assist with developing a treatment plan.

Therapeutic Management

Mild limb deformities often resolve without treatment. Exercises, splints, special shoes, or casts may be prescribed. Surgical intervention may be required for severe deformities to release tendons, reposition bones, reconstruct parts, retard growth of an extremity, or augment growth of a limb. In some situations, long-term immobility of an extremity is necessary by using casts or external fixation. Orthoses or physical therapy may be prescribed for specific needs.

Nursing Considerations

Nursing care varies with the defect and its treatment. Parents may need reassurance about the outcome of their child's therapy. The nurse should reinforce the principles of therapy, teach parents to carry out treatments at home, and encourage parents to persist with the treatment regimen even if the child does not like it. For example, exercises, special appliances, or braces may require daily use. Children in casts require specialized home care. Parents may be referred to an orthotist for construction of a device to assist with the child's function or mobility. Periodic follow-up is often necessary to reinforce correct use of appliances and care of the skin.

CLUBFOOT

Clubfoot is a congenital malformation of the lower extremity that affects the lower leg, ankle, and foot.

Etiology and Incidence

Clubfoot shows a genetic predisposition and a multifactorial etiology. Children with certain neuromuscular disorders, such as myelomeningocele, are especially at risk, as are children who have siblings with the disorder. The incidence of club foot in newborns is 1 in 1000 (Skinner, 2003). Boys are more commonly affected than girls by a 2:1 ratio. The prevalence is higher in Pacific Islanders (Cummings, Davidson, Armstrong, & Lehman, 2002).

Manifestations and Diagnostic Evaluation

The clinical manifestations of clubfoot include a plantar-flexed foot, with an inverted heel and adducted forefoot (Fig. 26-5), unilateral or bilateral defect, and a rigid limb that cannot be manipulated into a neutral position. Clubfoot is distinguished from *metatarsus adductus*, a nonrigid medial deviation of the forefoot. Clubfoot is readily apparent on clinical examination at birth. Radiographic imaging may be helpful for classifying the extent of the deformity.

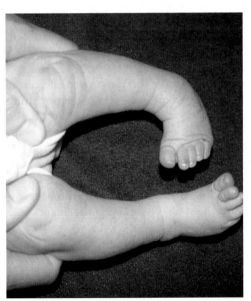

FIG 26-5   **An infant with left clubfoot. Note the positional difference between the two feet.**

Therapeutic Management

Treatment for clubfoot is started as soon after birth as possible and includes orthopedic and/or surgical approaches (Mary, Damsin, & Carlioz, 2004). The goal of treatment is to stretch tightened ligaments and tendons gently and return the foot to a maximal anatomic position. Serial stretching, manipulation, and casting are performed at least weekly. If sufficient correction is not achieved in 3 to 6 months, surgery followed by casting is usually indicated. Some malformations respond readily to treatment; other, more severe forms respond less well to even vigorous and prolonged therapy. Although early treatment may result in a foot that appears normal, recurrence is common. For this reason, long-term follow-up, until the child reaches skeletal maturity, is essential because further treatment may be indicated. Even with aggressive treatment, the foot is seldom completely normal.

Treatment for infants with metatarsus adductus, however, usually involves passive stretching exercises. Parents are instructed to perform these exercises several times a day in conjunction with some aspect of the infant's care routine, such as at each feeding or when diapers are changed. Occasionally a brace, a cast, or straight-last shoes may be needed. Many children outgrow this deformity with little treatment.

Nursing Considerations

Nursing interventions are related to the stage of treatment. Initially, parents need help understanding clubfoot and the possible treatments and outcomes. They also may need help acknowledging their disappointment in having a less-than-perfect baby. The nurse can encourage parents to discuss and recognize each other's unique strategies for coping. When physical therapy is used for treatment, the parents become trained, active participants in the child's stretching/taping program. The nurse should help the parent understand the significant time commitment involved (Richards, Johnston, & Wilson, 2005). Long-term casting with frequent cast changes also places great responsibility on the parents (Fig. 26-6). The nurse should assess the parents' ability to monitor the child adequately for complications and pursue long-term follow-up.

If surgery is needed, the nurse oversees pain management in the immediate postoperative period. Initially, an intravenous (IV) analgesic is used, with progression to an oral analgesic, such as codeine, and then to non-aspirin-containing, nonnarcotic analgesics. Elevate the child's feet postoperatively and apply ice bags to reduce swelling and pain. Assess the neurovascular status of the toes at least every 1 to 2 hours in the immediate postoperative period. Parents will need help positioning the infant for comfortable feeding.

The nurse also teaches parents how to keep the cast clean and dry at home. Parents should be taught how to bathe and diaper the infant without soiling or wetting the cast. When casts are changed on an outpatient basis, parents need to learn how to assess the child's neurovascular status and when to seek help.

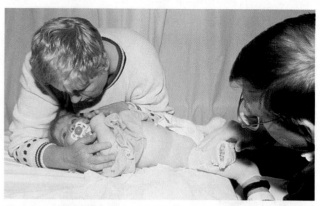

FIG 26-6   In the infant with clubfoot, serial manipulation and casting are started as soon after birth as possible to take advantage of the natural pliability of the neonate's connective tissue. Long-term casting with frequent cast changes places great responsibility on the parents.   *(Courtesy Cook Children's Medical Center, Fort Worth, TX.)*

The nurse may refer the family to the local visiting nurse agency. Because clubfoot can recur, all children with this condition require interval follow-up until they reach skeletal maturity.

DEVELOPMENTAL DYSPLASIA OF THE HIP

Developmental dysplasia of the hip (DDH) is a condition in which the head of the femur (ball) is improperly seated in the acetabulum (hip socket) of the pelvis. Hip dysplasia varies in severity from quite mild to severe dislocation. DDH can be present at birth (congenital), but in some children it develops after birth—hence the term *developmental*.

Etiology and Incidence

DDH appears to be multifactorial in origin. Genetic factors and prenatal and postnatal positioning seem to be implicated. Positive family history, laxity of the ligaments holding the femur head within the acetabulum, status as the first-born child, and breech deliveries are associated factors (Thompson, 2004). The incidence of DDH varies greatly among people of different races. It is less common in African-American and Asian infants and more common in Native Americans. There is a 9:1 female predominance (Thompson, 2004).

Manifestations

The manifestations of DDH vary according to age. In neonates, laxity of the ligaments around the hip allows the femoral head to be displaced from the acetabulum on manipulation. Infants beyond the newborn period exhibit asymmetry of the gluteal skinfolds when the infant is lying and the legs are extended against the examining table (or when the infant is held upright with the legs dangling). The affected hip has a limited range of motion, and asymmetric abduction is present when the child is placed supine with the knees and hips flexed. The femur on the affected side appears to be short. The walking child displays minimal to pronounced variations in gait, with lurching toward the affected side.

PATHOPHYSIOLOGY

DEVELOPMENTAL DYSPLASIA OF THE HIP

In the normal infant hip, the head of the femur is well seated in the acetabulum (hip socket) and is stable. Developmental dysplasia of the hip occurs in varying degrees, ranging from instability of the hip joint to frank dislocation, defined as the following:

- *Instability of the hip* is the appropriate term when the head of the femur is located in the acetabulum but may be subluxated (partially dislocated) or even dislocated with manual manipulation.

- *Subluxation of the hip* occurs when the head of the femur is positioned under the edge of the acetabulum. It is not well seated in the acetabulum, yet neither is it completely dislocated.

- *Dislocation of the hip* occurs when the head of the femur lies outside the acetabulum. It can occur as a late stage of developmental dysplasia of the hip, or it can occur in children with certain neuromuscular disorders.

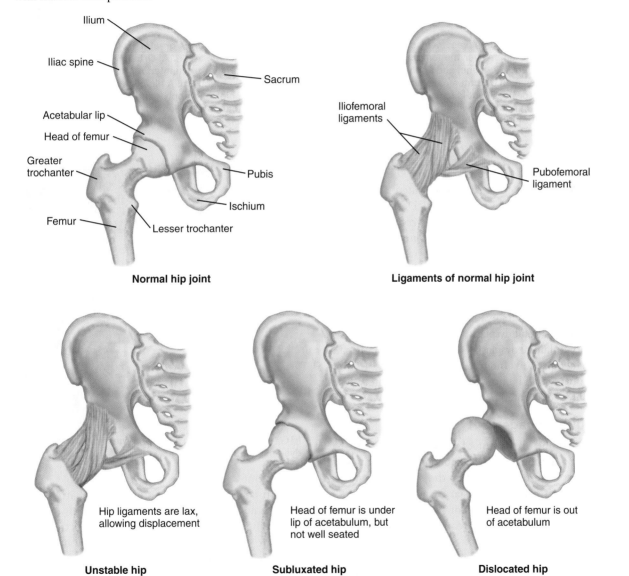

Normal hip joint

Ilium
Iliac spine
Sacrum
Acetabular lip
Head of femur
Greater trochanter
Pubis
Ischium
Femur
Lesser trochanter

Ligaments of normal hip joint

Iliofemoral ligaments
Pubofemoral ligament

Hip ligaments are lax, allowing displacement

Unstable hip

Head of femur is under lip of acetabulum, but not well seated

Subluxated hip

Head of femur is out of acetabulum

Dislocated hip

Diagnostic Evaluation

Because of the complexities of diagnosis, a well-trained nurse or physician should screen for developmental dysplasia at birth and during each routine infant well-child visit.

The diagnosis of DDH in the neonate can be difficult to make because the signs and symptoms may be quite subtle. In affected newborns, the hip joints appear lax rather than completely dislocated. Ortolani and Barlow tests (Fig. 26-7) can assess subluxation or laxity. Radiography is not useful in the neonate because bony ossification is not complete, but it can be diagnostic in an older infant. Ultrasonography, along with physical examination, seems to be the primary tool in the screening and diagnosis of DDH in infants (Dorn & Neumann, 2005). Computed tomography (CT)

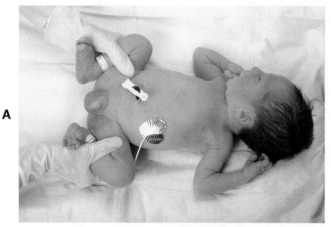

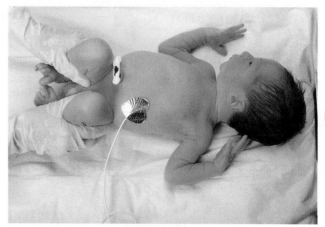

A

B

FIG 26-7   **Assessment of the hips. Place the fingers over the infant's greater trochanter and thumbs over the femur. Bend the knees and hips at a 90-degree angle. A, Ortolani's test. Abduct the thighs, and apply gentle pressure forward over the greater trochanter. A "clunking" sensation indicates a dislocated femoral head moving into the acetabulum. A hip click may be felt or heard but is usually normal. B, Barlow's test. Adduct the hips and apply gentle pressure down and back with the thumbs. In hip dysplasia, the examiner can feel the femoral head move out of the acetabulum.**   *(From Gorrie, T. M., McKinney, E. S., & Murray, S. S. [1998].* Foundations of maternal-newborn nursing *[2nd ed.]. Philadelphia: Saunders.)*

and magnetic resonance imaging (MRI) may be helpful in difficult cases, but use of these studies is limited.

In the older infant, the physical signs of DDH are different. The symptoms change from lax ligaments to contractures and stiffness in the affected hip joint or joints. Limited abduction on the affected side or sides is a major diagnostic sign. Any abnormalities in an older child's gait need to be carefully evaluated as possible signs of the condition. DDH, however, does not contribute to delayed walking, and delayed walking is not a usual reason for evaluation for DDH (Kamath & Bennet, 2004). Bilateral dysplasia is always more difficult to identify than unilateral dysplasia because no normal hip can be used for comparison. Interestingly, many unstable hips spontaneously resolve. If untreated, only approximately 20% will settle into a dislocated position.

Therapeutic Management

Early diagnosis and treatment of DDH are important to maximize the likelihood of a successful outcome. Treatment depends on the age of the child at the time of diagnosis and on the severity of the dysplasia. Because the neonate's musculoskeletal development is immature, early diagnosis and successful treatment of DDH can result in a normal or near-normal hip.

The primary goal of treatment in DDH, regardless of age, is to facilitate normal development of the femoral head and acetabulum. This is accomplished through approaches that provide anatomic reduction of the hip and maintenance of the reduction. In newborns and infants younger than 6 months, reduction of the hip joint by using several braces is the method of treatment (Bicimoglu, Agus, Omeroglu, & Tumer, 2003). Treatment involves splinting the hips with a Pavlik harness to maintain flexion and abduction and external rotation. The Pavlik harness consists of chest and shoulder straps and foot stirrups (Fig. 26-8). Initially, the harness

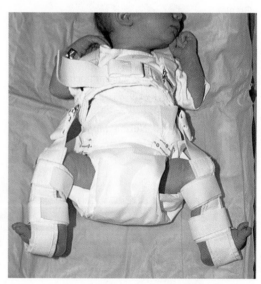

FIG 26-8   **An infant in a Pavlik harness to treat developmental dysplasia of the hip.**

is worn continuously. Positioning in the harness promotes development of a functional hip socket and a well-formed femoral head. This splinting may be the only treatment necessary to allow the hip to mold and grow normally. Hips that remain unstable become progressively deformed as the skeleton matures, resulting in functional disability. Parents must be taught the proper use of the harness because improper positioning of the infant's hip can cause interruption of the blood supply to the head of the femur, resulting in *avascular necrosis* (tissue damage caused by an inadequate blood supply). In addition, skin care, techniques for holding and feeding, and the importance of vigilant follow-up must be emphasized.

Treatment is more complicated when the condition is diagnosed after the newborn period. Traction or surgery to release muscles and tendons is usually necessary to allow adequate control of the hip joint. Positioning and immobilization in a spica cast follow the procedure. For profoundly affected children, traction is often followed by *osteotomy* (surgical cutting of the bone) and repositioning of the femur. After surgery, long-term immobilization in a spica cast is necessary until healing is achieved. Radiographs show the progress achieved with treatment. Follow-up monitoring is essential because the treatment may have to be modified.

NURSING CARE

The Child With Developmental Dysplasia of the Hip

Assessment
All infants should be assessed for DDH during routine neonatal and well-child visits to ensure prompt diagnosis and treatment. Assessment procedures are complex and vary with the age of the child. Once the diagnosis is established, nursing assessment is directed to the parents' knowledge level, their anxiety and coping abilities, and ensuring that the treatment regimen is followed.

> Because the needs of children with musculoskeletal disorders are often long term, parents usually have a good understanding of their child's progress. Questions such as "What concerns do you have about your child's progress today?" or "How are you doing at home?" acknowledge that the parents' feelings and ideas are valued and important. Information generated by such questions can become the focus for assessment and further intervention.

Monitor the skin integrity of an infant in a Pavlik harness or cast. When surgery becomes necessary, nursing priorities shift to an assessment of lower extremity circulation and pain.

Nursing Diagnosis and Planning
The nursing diagnoses and expected outcomes that may be appropriate for the child with DDH and the child's family include the following:

- Deficient Knowledge about the diagnosis of DDH and its treatment related to unfamiliarity with the child's condition.
  Expected Outcomes: The parents will demonstrate the therapeutic and safe use of a Pavlik harness. The parents will describe and demonstrate how to care for their child in a spica cast. The parents can describe adverse effects and complications of treatment.
- Anxiety (parental) related to having a less-than-perfect child and the need to provide complex care for an extended period.
  Expected Outcome: The parents will feel less anxious, as evidenced by being able to describe DDH and its treatment in lay terms to other family members; carry out treatment regimens, demonstrating increased self-confidence in the care of their child; treat the child as normally as possible;

and interact with health care providers and others in a calm and friendly manner.

- Risk for Impaired Skin Integrity related to skin chafing by the Pavlik harness or cast.
  Expected Outcomes: The child's skin will remain clear and free from lesions. On follow-up visits, the cast will be reasonably clean and dry and the child's skin will be clear and intact, without abrasions or sores.
- Ineffective Tissue Perfusion (lower extremities) related to impaired circulation as a result of surgery or casting.
  Expected Outcome: The circulation to the child's feet and toes will remain adequate as evidenced by capillary refill less than 2 seconds and toes that are pink and warm.
- Risk for Injury related to difficult positioning of a child in infant-carrying devices (infant seats, strollers, car seats).
  Expected Outcomes: The child will be safe from falls and will be adequately restrained when traveling in an automobile.
- Deficient Knowledge about home care related to depth of presented information.
  Expected Outcomes: The family will successfully manage treatment at home, as evidenced by correctly demonstrating harness or cast care, facilitating normal developmental milestones, and engaging in appropriate follow-up. The parents will describe age-appropriate home adaptations for the child.

Interventions
Teaching About the Pavlik Harness
Demonstrate and teach the parents the proper care and application of the Pavlik harness, including how to position and fasten the chest halter. Place the child's leg and foot into the stirrup and straps, and connect the straps to the halter. Because the requirements for harness use may change during therapy, teaching, demonstration, and return demonstration are essential at every visit. Harness straps should be secure enough to keep the child's hips flexed without being tight. The harness should be worn 23 hours per day and should be removed only according to the physician's recommendation. The hips and buttocks should be carefully supported if the infant is out of the harness. Encourage the parents to hold and cuddle the infant as much as possible. An infant in a Pavlik harness can be fed in the usual positions, with the parent carefully supporting the lower extremities during the feeding.

Teach the parents to protect the child's skin and legs under the harness. A long T-shirt ("onesie") under the halter reduces harness rubbing. The use of long socks and cotton padding (e.g., Webril) around the shoulder straps is helpful. The diaper should go on under the harness as well. Teach the parents to inspect the child's skin frequently for reddened or irritated areas and to reposition the child frequently.

Teaching About Spica Cast Care
Caring for a child in a spica cast is similar to caring for a child in any other type of cast (as previously discussed), with some additional adaptations. Because the cast covers the entire lower half of the child's body, with the exception of the perineal opening, managing the child's elimination is

Text continued on p. 849

Caring for Nicole, a Child in a Spica Cast

Four-year-old Nicole is immobilized in a spica cast after hip surgery. She receives IV morphine for pain. The therapies imposed by surgery and casting can lead to complications of respiration, elimination, skin breakdown, nutrition, and boredom. These potential complications, along with Nicole's growth and developmental needs, present challenges to her parents and the nurses caring for her.

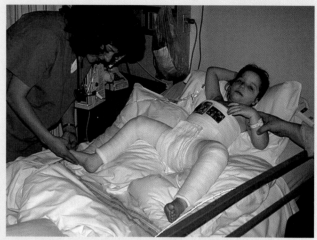

Nicole is positioned to her level of comfort with pillows at her back. A folded pillow under each leg keeps her heels from pressing against the mattress, thereby preventing pressure points. If Nicole were a few years younger, she would not be able to tell her caregivers where to place pillows for comfort or if her heels or toes were hurting or bent. Particular attention to potential pressure points is necessary with preverbal children.

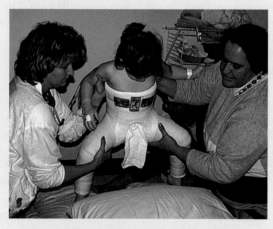

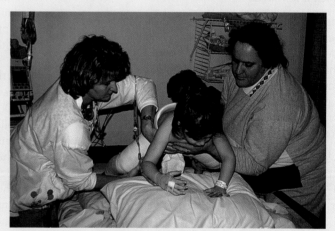

Three people are needed to turn Nicole: two to lift and turn her and a third to reposition pillows. Nicole is repositioned every 2 hours to prevent respiratory stasis. The crossbar between the legs of a spica cast (not present on this cast) should not be used as a handle when lifting the child. Once the child is feeling better and develops trust that she will not be dropped, repositioning is less frightening for her.

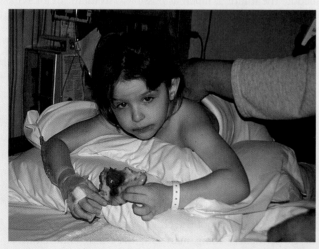

When prone, Nicole has a pillow under her chest to keep her face off the mattress and to allow her head mobility. A pillow under each leg keeps her feet and toes free. The prone position provides independence and increases Nicole's perception of control. To prevent aspiration, Nicole eats in a prone position. Because independence and autonomy are important to children, every opportunity to enhance the child's independence should be encouraged. Food should be served in bite-size pieces; finger foods may be preferred. Straws are used for liquids. The child should not be left unattended while eating.

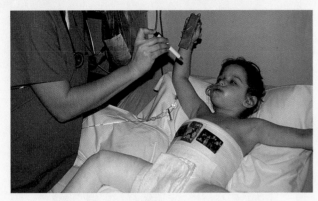

Respiratory assessment is performed at least every 8 hours. Deep breathing should be accomplished every 2 to 4 hours in the immediate postoperative period. Here the nurse asks Nicole to "blow out the light." Pinwheels, soap bubbles, and other tricks may be used to encourage deep breathing. In young children, crying provides the exercise of deep breathing.

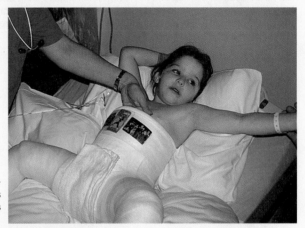

Nicole's nurse assesses her respiratory status. The cast must allow adequate room for respiratory excursion. Note that the nurse is able to fit several fingers under the edge of the cast around Nicole's chest.

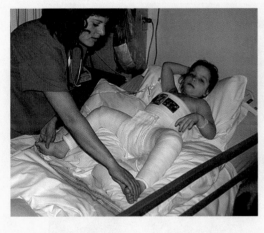

The nurse performs neurologic checks to ensure the adequacy of circulation and sensation in Nicole's feet. The nurse assesses bilaterally for color, temperature, sensation, swelling, and pulses.

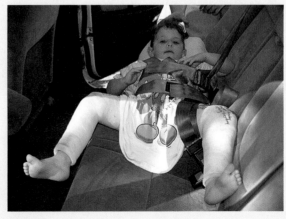

After Nicole is discharged from the hospital, her safety on the trip home is ensured by a special car seat restraint available for children in spica casts. Whenever she travels in the car, Nicole is secured safely with this restraint.

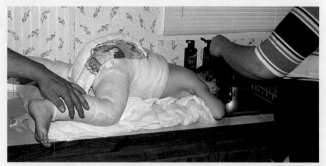

Before Nicole's discharge, her parents were instructed in body mechanics to prevent injury when lifting and turning Nicole in her heavy cast. At home, Nicole's mother washes her hair at the kitchen sink. Towels are used for comfort and to prevent water from running under the cast. Nicole is never left unattended on the kitchen counter or in other high places. To prevent burning Nicole, her mother is careful to check the water temperature.

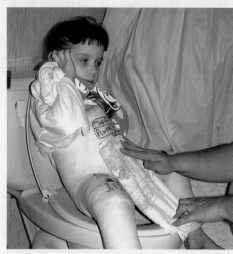

Nicole's mother has devised a system for using the toilet at home. Keeping Nicole in an upright position prevents soiling of the cast. Attention to bowel function is important because constipation is a potential problem. Increased dietary fiber and fluid intake, including prune juice, are usually adequate to promote regularity.

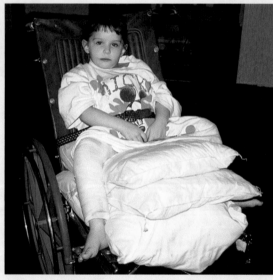

With pillows for positioning and comfort, Nicole uses a wheelchair for mobility. A younger child in a spica cast may be placed in a wagon padded with pillows. Children in wheelchairs and wagons should be strapped in to prevent falls. A child in a spica cast may also be placed on a blanket on the floor in an area of activity. This effort decreases the child's sense of isolation by increasing interactions with family members and friends.

Nicole is usually dressed in large T-shirts, which are soft, absorbent, and easy to put on and take off. Although Nicole is continent, a disposable diaper is taped under her perineal area in place of underpants. Clothing may be adapted with Velcro closures. Socks are used when needed to keep Nicole's feet warm.

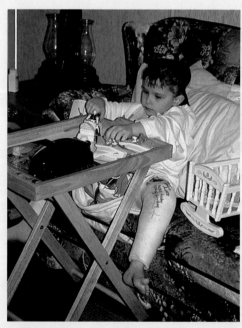

Age-appropriate activities help the immobilized child pass the time and can challenge and enhance development. Dolls, books, and coloring interest Nicole. At home, Nicole prefers to sit on the edge of the couch. She is never left alone and is old enough to request assistance if she feels herself sliding.

Photos courtesy of Judy Gross and Children's Hospital, Orthopediatric Unit, Medical University of South Carolina, Charleston, SC.

a challenge. Excess urine can trickle under the cast, irritating and macerating the skin, resisting drying, and becoming malodorous. Advise the family to tuck a disposable diaper underneath the cast edges at the circular perineal opening; advise parents not to use sheet plastic under the cast, which can cause pooling of urine beneath the cast and subsequent skin breakdown. Place sanitary napkins within the first diaper that is tucked under the cast edges, then cover the entire perineal opening and cast with a larger disposable diaper. Elevating the head of the bed helps urine and feces drain downward and away from the cast.

Monitor the child's neurovascular status frequently and teach the family the signs of neurovascular compromise. Fever, wound drainage, and discomfort may be signs of infection and should be reported promptly. Teach the family ways to provide environmental and developmental stimulation (e.g., by moving the child to different areas during the day, placing the child's bed near a window, placing appropriate toys within reach, providing age-appropriate activities). Teach the family to ensure that the extremities within the cast should always be supported, such as with pillows or rolled-up towels. "Bean bag" chairs also work very well for this purpose. Explain the importance of feeding the child a diet high in fluids, calories, calcium, protein, and fiber. Instruct the parents about ways to dress their child to accommodate climate, style, and other needs (e.g., by fitting socks over the toes of the cast, using Velcro closures on pants and shorts, using clothing made of stretch fabrics). Give the parents the name and telephone number of an easily accessible health care provider in case questions arise at home.

Alleviating Anxiety

Communicate information to parents in a clear, kind, and straightforward manner because complex or ambiguous messages raise anxiety. Adjust teaching to accommodate parents' need for information and support. Reduce waiting time during follow-up visits and express interest in the child and parents. Providing reliable, respectful, and empathetic care builds trust and reduces stress.

Preventing Injury

Assume a proactive role, and advise parents of the potential for injury and the importance of taking safety precautions. Most infant-carrying devices are not suitable or safe for infants in spica casts. Assist parents in identifying strategies for transporting their infant in a safe and comfortable manner, including the use of a car seat that can accommodate the wide leg spread caused by the spica cast. During waking hours, suggest placing the child on an open area of the floor that has been covered with a blanket as an alternative to an infant seat. Remind parents that the child must not be left unattended; infants and young children often develop a surprising ability to move despite the restrictions imposed by a cast.

Evaluation

- Do the parents demonstrate the use of the Pavlik harness or spica cast in a safe and therapeutic manner?
- Can the parents describe adverse effects or complications of treatment?

- Can the parents describe DDH and its treatment in lay terms to other family members, carry out the prescribed therapy to the greatest extent possible, and treat the child as a normal developing child?
- Do the parents and child appear calm and able to participate in care?
- Do the parents seek recommended health care and keep follow-up appointments?
- Is the child's skin clear and free of lesions or breakdown?
- Are the child's toes warm and pink, with capillary refill less than 2 seconds, and can the child move the toes freely?
- Does the child remain injury free?
- Can the parents describe home care adaptations, and are these appropriate for the child's developmental level?

LEGG-CALVÉ-PERTHES DISEASE

Legg-Calvé-Perthes disease, also known as *osteochondritis deformans juvenilis* or *coxa plana,* is a self-limiting disorder in which there is avascular necrosis of the femoral head. The child has a painful limp that is exacerbated by activities such as walking or running.

Etiology

Although the cause of Legg-Calvé-Perthes disease is unknown, it is widely accepted to be a disorder of growth. Children with Legg-Calvé-Perthes disease are usually of

---

PATHOPHYSIOLOGY

LEGG-CALVÉ-PERTHES DISEASE

A disturbance in the blood supply to the femoral epiphysis results in avascular necrosis of the femoral head. The most serious problem associated with Legg-Calvé-Perthes disease is the risk of permanent deformity. If the femoral head protrudes outside the acetabulum and the healing process within the femoral head is incomplete, over time the femoral head will flatten and take on a misshapen appearance. This could lead to later problems with arthritis.

The disorder is considered to be self-limiting and is classified by the extent of femoral head involvement and disease stage. The disorder usually progresses through five stages over a 1- to 2-year period.

During *stage 1,* the epiphysis begins to show the results of ischemia. Synovitis produces stiffness and pain. Necrosis begins; radiographs show a reduction in size and increased density of the femoral head. Once necrosis occurs *(stage 2),* the bone weakens and dies, causing collapse of the femoral head. *Stage 3* is the fragmentation stage, in which avascular bone is reabsorbed. Healing occurs as new bone is formed. During the reossification stage, *stage 4,* the femoral head and neck begin to re-form. *Stage 5,* or the stage of reconstitution, results in final healing.*

*Thompson, G. H. (2004). Bone and joint disorders. In R. Behrman, R. Kliegman, & H. Jenson (Eds.), *Nelson textbook of pediatrics* (17th ed., pp. 2251-2297). Philadelphia: Saunders.

shorter-than-average height; many of these children were low-birth-weight infants as well (<2.5 kg [5.5 lb]). Some children have demonstrated a deficiency in components of growth factor (Shah, 2002).

Incidence

The incidence of Legg-Calvé-Perthes disease is approximately 15 in 100,000. The ratio of affected boys to girls is 4:1, although involvement in girls appears to be more severe than in boys. Children 2 years to 12 years old are most susceptible to developing Legg-Calvé-Perthes disease, however most cases occur between 4 to 9 years of age (Dambro, 2005). Unilateral hip involvement is more common than bilateral involvement. This disease is rare in African Americans and Asians.

Manifestations

The most common symptom of Legg-Calvé-Perthes disease is persistent pain of the hip; patients may have a limp or limitation of motion. Other associated symptoms include thigh or knee soreness or stiffness; the pain may be intermittent. A painful limp, quadriceps muscle atrophy, and pain of insidious onset may also be present.

Diagnostic Evaluation

Laboratory studies, including studies of joint aspirate, are normal (Hay, Levin, Sondheimer, & Detarding, 2005). The diagnosis is made by radiographic examination. A bone scan or MRI study may reveal necrosis and irregularity of the femoral head. However, in the majority of cases, plain radiographs of the femoral head will disclose the condition.

Therapeutic Management

Treatment goals of Legg-Calvé-Perthes disease are to prevent deformity and incongruity of the hip and delay the onset of arthritis and degenerative joint disease that could occur in later adult life. Containment of the femoral head within the acetabulum, by either operative or nonoperative means, is the preferred method. Literature shows that later age at onset of disease has a poor prognosis because younger children have a greater growth potential of the femoral head and acetabulum (Grzegorzewski, Bowen, Guille, & Glutting, 2003). The femoral head is maintained in the acetabulum and protected from the stress of weight bearing during the healing process. This can be done by prolonged bed rest and traction, Petrie casts, or braces. In addition, synovitis should be reduced to improve range of motion. Some physicians, however, do not believe that weight bearing is harmful as long as the femur remains in the acetabulum.

Because Legg-Calvé-Perthes disease is first identified from the child's reports of a painful, stiff hip joint, the physician may recommend non-weight-bearing, range-of-motion exercises and bed rest. If improvement is not seen within 7 to 10 days and the child is still unable to abduct the hip, alternative methods of treatment are considered.

For children with severe necrosis, the femoral head is abducted and internally rotated in relation to the acetabulum through a type of containment device that uses the acetabulum to maintain the spherical shape of the femoral head. Containment prevents the acetabulum from rubbing against the weakened portion of the femoral head and creating a flat shape. Methods of containment usually include bracing or surgical intervention. Studies have shown that results of early surgery are better than late surgery (Joseph, Sreekumaran, Narasimha, Mulpuri, & Varghese, 2003).

The position of the femoral head is maintained in the acetabulum by abducting the leg. The child wears an abduction brace for approximately 18 months or until reossification is evident. Some abduction braces allow the child to be ambulatory without crutches.

Surgical procedures include an osteotomy, which places the femur more securely into the acetabulum, or an innominate osteotomy, which rotates the acetabulum to cover the femoral head completely. Many physicians recommend surgical intervention because it reduces treatment time and eliminates problems with adherence to treatment.

NURSING CARE

The Child With Legg-Calvé-Perthes Disease

Assessment

Assessment of a child with Legg-Calvé-Perthes disease reveals loss of internal hip rotation and limited abduction. The nurse should determine how long the child has been limping as well as the pattern, timing, and severity of the pain. The pain may be referred to the thigh or knee. The child will describe the pain as increasing with activity and decreasing with rest. Physical examination of the extremity may reveal muscle wasting of the thigh and buttock—a reflection of disuse. Shortening of the extremity on the affected side indicates collapse of the femoral head.

Nursing Diagnosis and Planning

The following nursing diagnoses and expected outcomes may be appropriate after assessment of the child with Legg-Calvé-Perthes disease:

- Impaired Physical Mobility related to the disease process and activity restrictions.

  Expected Outcomes: The child will maintain mobility and strength of all unaffected joints, tolerate activity restrictions, and cooperate with the treatment regimen.

- Risk for Impaired Skin Integrity related to skin contact with the brace.

  Expected Outcomes: The child's skin will remain free of chafing, redness, and irritation. The parents will describe and carry out appropriate skin care.

- Disturbed Body Image related to wearing a corrective brace.

  Expected Outcomes: The child will exhibit age-appropriate behaviors and adjustment to the altered mobility imposed by the brace. The child will appropriately express any frustrations or decrease in self-esteem.

- Deficient Knowledge about the condition and home management related to insufficient prior information.

 Expected Outcomes: The parents will provide safe home care, demonstrate the correct use of the brace or crutches, perform neurovascular assessments, and provide age-appropriate activities for their child.

Interventions

Facilitating Appropriate Activity

Activity restrictions are one of the most problematic areas in the care of a child with Legg-Calvé-Perthes disease. The child may become frustrated and angry when unable to meet the physical and social demands of peers. Initially, the child may appear to adjust to the lifestyle restrictions, but the nurse must be alert to subtle indicators of rebelliousness and uncooperative behavior. Other children will adapt quickly to the appliance they wear and demonstrate incredible activity levels. Do not construe a child's refusal to adhere to treatment regimens as maladaptive behavior. The demand to keep up with their peers is sometimes so great that children are simply unable to make cognitively appropriate choices regarding their health.

Returning to school with a brace poses unique problems as well. The school nurse and the child's teacher should be involved in the discharge planning because the child should participate in as many school-related activities as possible. Acknowledging the child's mobility limitations and working with school officials to identify appropriate alternatives will ensure a successful school reentry. Emphasizing hobbies and other creative activities provides ways for the child to excel and feel a sense of accomplishment.

Teaching Home Management

Because the child will receive the greater part of care as an outpatient, nursing care should focus on home care and management of the appliance selected for therapy. Parents will need information concerning the purpose, application, and care of the appliance. The family must clearly understand the issue of adherence and the role it will play in the healing process. Parents will need to learn how to perform neurovascular assessments. Also, the nurse should help parents identify safety issues regarding the child's mobility when wearing the brace. The physical therapist and occupational therapist are important resources for the parents.

The purpose of any brace used to treat Legg-Calvé-Perthes disease is to distribute the child's weight to the ischial tuberosities. Because of its design, the appliance places additional stress on the child's skin. Advise the parent to assess the child's skin condition frequently and identify any friction areas. Teach parents to check bony prominences; any reddened area on the skin that persists longer than 20 to 30 minutes demands immediate attention.

Mild soaps (e.g., Dove, Cetaphil) should be used during bathing. Do not use moisturizers on pressure areas; if lotion or moisturizers are used elsewhere on the skin, teach parents to wipe the excess off to prevent skin breakdown. Bony prominences should not be massaged. Place protective foam or transparent dressings over susceptible areas. If appropriate, protective cotton clothing may be worn under the brace, but keep the clothing as free from wrinkles as possible.

Evaluation

- Does the child exhibit normal joint and muscular integrity, and does the child cooperate with the treatment regimen?
- Is the child's skin intact, smooth, clear, and free from pressure areas?
- Can parents demonstrate skin care associated with an orthopedic appliance?
- Does the child participate in age-appropriate peer and school-related activities within activity limitations?
- Can the child appropriately express frustration or feelings about being different?
- Are the parents able to provide developmentally appropriate activities for their child?
- Can the parents describe and demonstrate brace care and neurovascular assessments?

SLIPPED CAPITAL FEMORAL EPIPHYSIS

Slipped capital femoral epiphysis (SCFE) is a condition that affects the upper (capital) femoral growth plate. It is a hip disorder related to times of rapid growth, particularly during adolescence.

Etiology and Incidence

The cause of slipped capital femoral epiphysis is unknown. Slippage appears to be related to increased stress on the proximal femur at a time when the epiphyseal plate is thinning in preparation for eventual closure. The weakness of the growth plate may be related to adolescent hormonal imbalance and is seen most frequently in adolescents who are short and heavy for their age but have not yet developed secondary sex characteristics. SCFE also can occur in adolescents who are tall and thin after a recent growth spurt (Thompson, 2004).

The incidence of SCFE is approximately 2 per 100,000 and occurs approximately two to three times more in young boys than young girls (Connecticut Children's Medical Center, 2005). Families may show an increased incidence. The majority of affected adolescents exceed the 95th percentile for weight and the 90th percentile for height. Although initially the condition is unilateral, approximately 25% become bilateral.

Pathophysiology

The epiphyseal plate begins to thin in response to hormonal influences during adolescence. Eventually the plate closes completely when the adolescent has reached skeletal maturity. Increased body weight and height place more stress on the epiphyses, causing a relative displacement (slip) of the femoral neck from the femoral head; the epiphyseal movement appears to be in a posterior and inferior direction. In most instances, the slippage occurs gradually.

Manifestations and Diagnostic Evaluation

The classic manifestations of SCFE include a limp, gait disturbance, and pain. The pain usually is in the groin, thigh, or knee; it is intermittent and worsens with activity. The leg often is externally rotated. Because the adolescent often has knee pain, hip involvement may be overlooked. Presenting symptoms along with characteristic growth signs suggest the diagnosis, so hip disease should be ruled out in adolescents with knee pain. Radiographs confirm the diagnosis. Radiographs are obtained with the legs in a frog-leg position.

Therapeutic Management and Nursing Considerations

Treatment is usually internal fixation: a pin or screw inserted across the growth plate secures the femoral head and prevents further slippage. More severe slips may require reconstruction of the femoral head, followed by pinning.

As soon as the diagnosis is made, the adolescent is admitted to the hospital and placed on bed rest to prevent exacerbation of the slip. Most orthopedic surgeons recommend reducing the slipped epiphysis and performing an osteotomy to decrease the risk of later degenerative arthritis (Song, Halliday, Reilly, & Keezel, 2004). Postoperatively, the adolescent uses crutches with partial weight bearing for 4 to 6 weeks. Depending on the severity of the slip and extent of the osteotomy, some adolescents may be required to be non-weight bearing for 4 to 6 weeks, with transfers to a wheelchair only. The screw or pin may be removed after several years.

The nurse should assess adolescents for slipped capital femoral epiphysis any time an adolescent reports knee or thigh pain. Interventions are similar to those for any child in traction or undergoing surgery. Postoperatively, the adolescent needs to be taught isometric exercises and crutch walking. Weight control may be an issue; the overweight adolescent needs to learn to develop good nutritional habits and avoid high-calorie foods. Referral to a dietitian may be helpful. Provide the adolescent and parent with written instructions before discharge.

CRITICAL THINKING EXERCISE 26-1

Children often come to the ambulatory care setting reporting hip or knee pain and walking with a limp. Compare and contrast the three common hip disorders in children.

FRACTURES

Although fractures are not always serious, they are important because they may lead to life-threatening complications. A fracture is a break or disruption in a bone's continuity. Generally fractures occur when excessive or traumatic force exceeds the strength of the bone.

Etiology

Fractures in children usually result from increased mobility and inadequate or immature motor and cognitive skills. They may result from trauma (e.g., falls, motor vehicle crashes, sports injuries, child abuse) or bone diseases that result in abnormally fragile bones (e.g., osteogenesis imperfecta).

An understanding of growth and development is helpful when assessing trauma in specific age groups. For example, fractures in infancy are generally rare because of the cartilaginous quality of the skeleton. Fractures in infants are usually the result of trauma during birth or nonaccidental trauma. Therefore fractures in infants warrant further investigation to rule out the possibility of child abuse.

Unintentional injury is the leading cause of death in children of all ages (see Chapter 1). Trauma, probably the most ominous threat to children today, frequently causes fractures. Traumatic musculoskeletal injuries are among the most frequently seen injuries in hospital emergency rooms (Walls, 2002).

The other major cause of children's fractures is falls. Because of protection reflexes, the outstretched arm often receives the full force of the fall (Fig. 26-9). This type of fall can affect every part of that outstretched arm (wrist, elbow, shoulder). A supracondylar humeral fracture, an elbow fracture commonly seen with this type of fall, is a serious injury because it may lead to circulatory impairment, cellular necrosis, and ischemic contracture (Volkmann's contracture).

A fractured clavicle can occur at any age. Lack of movement or a pseudoparalysis of the upper arm may be the only sign in an infant who has sustained a fractured clavicle during birth. An older child will report pain and show swelling on the clavicle at the point of the fracture.

Regardless of the cause of the fracture, a child with an uncomplicated fracture should not present with signs of shock. If shock is evident, more than likely a more serious problem exists and a thorough assessment is required.

Incidence

Because the daily actions of children include numerous gross motor activities that place them at risk for injuries, fractures are common during childhood and adolescence.

Children between ages 5 and 9 years are most likely to incur fractures, particularly of the hip and femur, related to motor vehicle crashes (see Chapter 10). The most common sites of fractures in children are the ulna, clavicle, tibia, and femur. Epiphyseal fractures are also common in children. A severe epiphyseal fracture can interfere with bone growth.

Manifestations

The signs and symptoms of a fracture vary with the location, type, and cause of the injury. General manifestations include pain or tenderness at the site, immobility or decreased range of motion, deformity of the extremity, and edema. Other signs and symptoms include crepitus, ecchymosis, erythema, muscle spasm, and inability to bear weight.

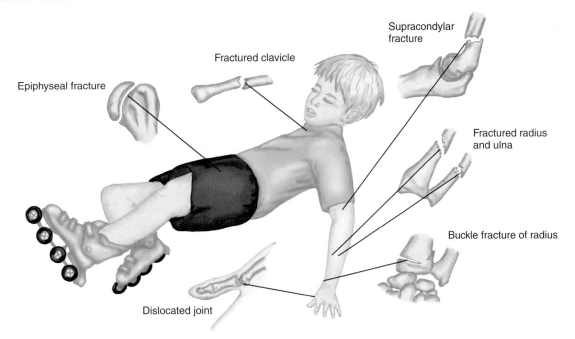

FIG 26-9   **Upper extremity fractures in children often occur when the child attempts to break a fall with an outstretched arm.**

Diagnostic Evaluation

Local signs and symptoms of a fracture are not always present, which may make assessment of a fracture difficult. Radiography of the skeleton is the most effective tool for determining the type and location of a fracture. Often a radiograph of the unaffected extremity is obtained for comparison purposes, especially when the physician is trying to determine whether a line on the radiograph represents a fracture or merely an epiphyseal line. Because the periosteum of children's bones is thicker and stronger than that of adults, it is less likely to displace at the fracture site. Consequently, the fracture may not be visible on radiographs until healing begins. Radiographs are also obtained after fracture reduction and during the healing process to assess progress.

Therapeutic Management

The key to healing is correct fracture reduction and retention. *Reduction* is the repositioning of the bone fragments into normal alignment. *Retention* entails the application of a device or mechanism that maintains alignment until healing occurs.

Reduction Methods

Fractures are treated by either closed or open reduction. Closed reduction is accomplished by manual alignment of the fragments followed by immobilization. Simple or closed fractures are treated by closed reduction. Hospitalization is seldom necessary for closed reduction, and most of these fractures heal without complications.

Open reduction entails the surgical insertion of internal fixation devices, such as rods, wires, or pins, that help maintain alignment while healing occurs. External fixation devices may also be used to lengthen bones and correct angular deformities that involve bone and soft tissue. External fixators allow periodic changes in alignment and length of the bone. When open reduction is used, hospitalization is required and the child is monitored for postoperative complications. Complications after open reduction include delayed healing and nonunion. Infections may also interfere with recovery. Close assessment by the health care team and strict adherence to sterile technique during dressing changes can decrease the risk of postoperative problems and promote healing.

Retention

Once the fracture is aligned, the fracture site must be protected and the position of the fragments maintained. This is accomplished through the application of a cast or, in certain situations, traction, which effectively immobilizes the area while healing occurs.

Nursing Considerations

Initial Trauma Assessment

Nursing assessment of the child with a traumatic fracture should begin with a thorough assessment of the child's airway, breathing, and circulation (see Chapter 10). Once this is done, obtain a history of the circumstances surrounding the fracture. Determining the cause of any fracture is important because nonaccidental trauma may be involved. Both a complete history of how the fracture occurred and physical findings are important if child abuse is suspected.

Examine the fracture site for bruising, skin lacerations, and swelling. Generally the child will favor the extremity, even to the point of cradling or supporting it. Often the child will report numbness and tingling distal to the fracture

PATHOPHYSIOLOGY

FRACTURES

When a fracture occurs, the break in the continuity of the bone results in bone fragmentation and injury to the surrounding tissues. Torn blood vessels cause bleeding from the bone and tissues around the bone fragments. As blood clots at the site, fibrin strands provide a network for healing. Osteoblasts begin forming in immense numbers almost immediately after the injury. This increased osteoblastic activity results in the formation of new bone matrix between the bone fragments. Calcium salts are deposited in the new bone matrix, forming a *callus*. The callus is responsible for stability and support of the fracture while healing occurs. Gradually the callus is formed into new bone. Remodeling, or correction of an injury at the fracture site through the buildup of callus, occurs more rapidly in growing children.

Fractures are referred to as *simple* or *compound*. A fracture that is *simple* (closed) is characterized as intact with no breaks in the skin. If wounds accompany a simple fracture, they are usually superficial or unrelated to the fracture. The nurse should never assume, however, that a simple fracture does not warrant close assessment. Other problems associated with the injury may exist. For example, if hemorrhage occurs, it would be internal.

A systemic risk associated with fractures, especially multiple fractures or femur fractures, is emboli. Emboli can form from postinjury bleeding with clotting or from

Pediatric fractures are seldom complete breaks. Rather, children's bones tend to bend or buckle because of increased flexibility. This flexibility is due to a thicker periosteum and increased amounts of immature bone.

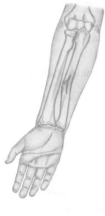

Greenstick

Break occurs through the periosteum on one side of the bone while only bowing or buckling on the other side. Seen most frequently in forearm.

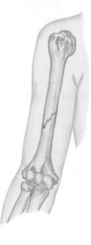

Spiral

Twisted or circular break that affects the length rather than the width. Seen frequently in child abuse.

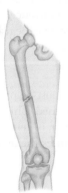

Oblique

Diagonal or slanting break that occurs between the horizontal and perpendicular planes of the bone.

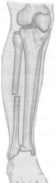

Transverse

Break or fracture line occurs at right angles to the long axis of the bone.

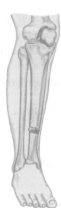

Comminuted

Bone is splintered into pieces. This is a rare occurrence in children.

site. Movement may be limited. The area of the fracture is important to determine because growth plate injuries are not always evident on radiographs.

Assessing and Managing Fat Embolism

A serious complication of orthopedic trauma is fat embolism, which occurs most often after traumatic injuries and fractures, especially of long bones and the hips (Gore & Lacey, 2005). Although the cause of fat embolism is unclear, particles of fat escape from the fracture site, are carried through the circulatory system, and lodge in the lung capillaries. Local inflammation increases capillary permeability, resulting in pulmonary edema that causes severe respiratory distress with hypoxemia and respiratory acidosis (Gore & Lacey, 2005). Rarely, fat emboli can lodge in the small capillaries in the brain or other vital organs. The complication of fat embolism occurs most commonly 21 to 72 hours after the injury (Gore & Lacey, 2005).

PATHOPHYSIOLOGY

FRACTURES—cont'd

fat droplets, shed from the fractured bone marrow (fat embolism), that enter the circulatory system and travel to the lungs or brain.

Fractures in which the skin, subcutaneous tissue, or muscle has been disrupted are called *compound* (open) fractures. Infection is a risk with this type of fracture because organisms can enter the fracture site through the wound. Children with compound fractures are at risk for blood loss as a result of external hemorrhage.

Epiphyseal injuries occur when a break or fracture occurs between the shaft of the bone and epiphyseal plate. In a growing bone, the region of least resistance to stress is the area between the metaphysis and the cartilaginous epiphyseal plate. The amount of growth arrest associated with an epiphyseal injury is determined by the extent of the damage to the epiphyseal plate. If the germinal cells remain with the epiphysis and appear uninjured, healing is rapid and growth is seldom affected. If the germinal layer is destroyed, however, growth disturbances will occur. The Salter-Harris classification system classifies epiphyseal growth plate injuries and their associated risk of growth disturbance.

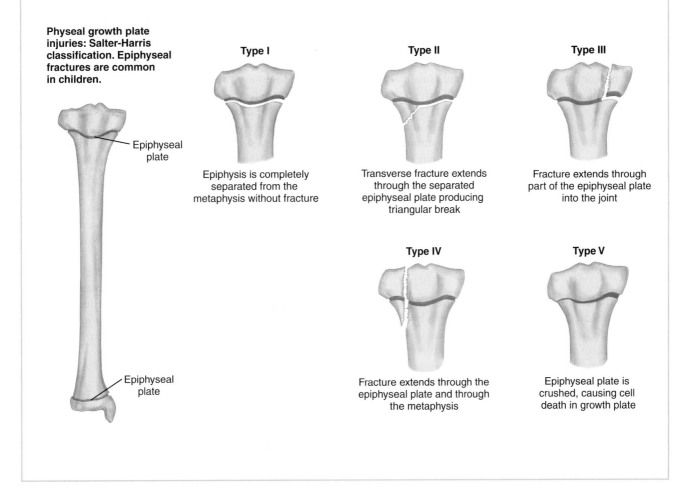

Physeal growth plate injuries: Salter-Harris classification. Epiphyseal fractures are common in children.

Epiphyseal plate

Epiphyseal plate

Type I
Epiphysis is completely separated from the metaphysis without fracture

Type II
Transverse fracture extends through the separated epiphyseal plate producing triangular break

Type III
Fracture extends through part of the epiphyseal plate into the joint

Type IV
Fracture extends through the epiphyseal plate and through the metaphysis

Type V
Epiphyseal plate is crushed, causing cell death in growth plate

Minimal movement of fractured extremities can prevent or lessen the effects of fat embolism. Treatment is primarily supportive and includes volume resuscitation, respiratory support, and adequate oxygenation.

Assessing and Managing Compartment Syndrome

Serious complications, such as nerve compression, circulatory impairment, or compartment syndrome, can result from swelling caused by trauma or an immobilizing device. The muscles and nerves of the upper and lower extremities are enclosed in compartments that are surrounded by tough, inelastic fascia. *Compartment syndrome* occurs when swelling causes pressure within this closed space to rise. The increased pressure compromises circulation to the muscles and nerves within the compartment and can result in paralysis and necrosis of tissues. Compartment syndrome is a true surgical emergency that requires prompt diagnosis and intervention (Newton & Walker, 2004).

Signs of compartment syndrome include severe pain, often unrelieved by analgesics, and signs of neurovascular impairment. Compartment syndrome is not uncommon in forearm fractures; therefore assess the quality of the radial pulse and the child's ability to extend the fingers. If extending the fingers produces pain, notify the physician. When assessing a report of pain, make a distinction between pain related to the fracture and burning sensations distal to the fracture. Pain associated with compartment syndrome usually is described as more intense than would be expected from the severity of the injury, and it does not remit with analgesics. In addition, assess for pallor, paresthesia, and pulselessness as previously described.

The diagnosis of compartment syndrome is made primarily on physical findings, but if physical findings provoke any question, measurement of the pressure within the affected compartment is necessary. An intracompartmental pressure measurement exceeding 30 to 35 mm Hg results in a definitive diagnosis (Skinner, 2003). If compartment syndrome is suspected, the nurse should immediately elevate the extremity only to the level of the child's heart, administer pain medication as ordered, and notify the physician (Walls, 2002).

Children who sustain fractures are treated with casts or traction. For this reason, nursing diagnoses, planning, intervention, and evaluation are the same as for any child in a cast or traction.

SOFT TISSUE INJURIES: SPRAINS, STRAINS, AND CONTUSIONS

Soft tissue injuries are common among children and are usually related to play or athletic activities.

Etiology

Sprains occur as a result of trauma to a joint in which ligaments are stretched or are partially or completely torn. Anterior cruciate ligament (ACL) tears are one of the most common types of knee injury, especially in athletes. *Strains*, also known as *pulls*, *tears*, or *ruptures*, result from an excessive stretch of muscle. *Contusions* occur when soft tissue, muscle, or subcutaneous tissues are damaged. Sprains and contusions frequently accompany each other. *Dislocations* occur when a joint is disrupted in such a way that articulating surfaces are no longer in contact.

Incidence

Sprains are not frequently seen in young children because of their poorly developed epiphyseal plate. A twisting or turning injury will more likely result in a fracture than a sprain because the epiphyseal plate is weaker. Sprains and strains are more common in adolescents and are frequently the result of athletic injuries. Sports-related trauma is a primary cause of orthopedic injury in adolescents (Conn, Annest, & Gilchrist, 2005). In general, sprains and contusions are more likely to occur with more physical or violent sports activities, such as basketball, football, cycling, gymnastics, and cheerleading (Conn et al., 2005).

Manifestations and Diagnostic Evaluation

Manifestations of soft tissue injuries include pain, swelling, localized tenderness, limited range of motion, poor weight bearing, and a pop or snapping sound (sprain). The diagnosis is made on the basis of the clinical picture. A radiographic examination, however, may be ordered to rule out a fracture. An MRI or arthroscopy may be necessary to diagnose knee ligament tears.

Therapeutic Management

Control of swelling and the prevention of further injury are paramount with sprains and contusions. Swelling can inhibit healing by keeping the ligament ends apart and increasing fibrous scarring. The earlier that treatment is initiated, the less severe the swelling and immobility become.

The injured area should be immediately wrapped with a thin layer of elastic bandage or elastic wrap to support the joint and control the swelling. To reduce the swelling, ice is applied to the injured area, with additional wrap used to secure the ice. Ice should be applied for no longer than 20 minutes every 1 to 4 hours, even though the effects of the ice can last as long as 5 to 6 hours. Ice is used for several days. Nonsteroidal antiinflammatory drugs (NSAIDs) alleviate pain and reduce inflammation.

For more severe soft tissue injury, the child should avoid weight bearing for 3 days; crutches may be necessary to ensure the child does not bear weight. An *air cast*, which is a plastic, air-filled pressure cuff, may be used over the elastic wrap to support the joint and reduce swelling; the child will use the air cast for several weeks while the joint is healing. When the swelling and pain have diminished, the child can begin stretching and isometric exercises to improve joint stability.

Immobilization of the injured joint and cold application are generally effective in the treatment of incomplete ligament tears. A complete rupture could require surgery to prevent excessive scar formation and long-term joint stability problems. Application of a cast or splint for 4 to 5 weeks may also be necessary, especially for knee injuries.

Nursing Considerations

One of the major nursing functions when assessing a sprain is to determine the severity of the injury. Assess the child for neurovascular impairment and for diminished range of motion. The initial examination may reveal localized tenderness over the injured joint as well as limited joint mobility.

Analgesics, such as ibuprofen or acetaminophen, are appropriate for pain management. Distraction as well as age-appropriate play activities can be effective in managing a child's pain.

The nurse needs to keep the extremity elevated above the heart. This position enhances venous return and aids in reducing the swelling. Pillows placed beneath the extremity provide support as well as comfort. When applying the elastic wrap, assess neurovascular status because wrap can be applied too tightly.

For the child who has undergone surgery for any type of knee ligament reconstruction, immediate postoperative use of a cold compression cuff and a *continuous passive motion (CPM) machine*—a machine that continuously moves the knee joint in flexion and extension—will likely be used. Nursing measures involve regular emptying and refilling of the cuff to maintain the cold temperature. The nurse must also check the settings on the CPM machine to ensure they match the ordered degree of flexion and extension. Pain control is most important.

Stretching and strengthening exercises are helpful in maintaining joint and muscle integrity. These exercises are done passively at first. As healing progresses, teach the child active stretching and strengthening exercises. Asking parents for a return demonstration helps evaluate the effectiveness of teaching. Physical therapy referrals may be helpful as well.

The amount of time needed for healing is determined by the severity of the injury. Weight bearing is gradually increased as the pain subsides. More severe injuries may require partial weight-bearing exercises, with full weight bearing introduced once the swelling has resolved. Sports activities may be restricted for 3 to 8 weeks.

Review the principles of rest, support, and the application of ice with the parents and child. If wraps, splints, or air casts are used, teach the parents and child how to assess neurovascular status. If crutches are required, review the principles of crutch walking with both the parents and the child. Make sure all family members understand activity and sports restrictions. Discuss follow-up appointments and the importance of adhering to activity restrictions until the injury has healed and the child has been cleared for sports.

CRITICAL TO REMEMBER
The Child With a Soft Tissue Injury

The first 6 to 12 hours after soft tissue injury are the most important in controlling swelling and reducing muscle damage. Treatment of soft tissue injuries is summarized in the acronyms *RICE* and *ICES:*

Rest	*Ice*
Ice	*Compression*
Compression	*Elevation*
Elevation	*Support*

OSGOOD-SCHLATTER DISEASE

The classic picture of Osgood-Schlatter disease is bilateral knee pain that is exacerbated by running, jumping, or climbing stairs in an active adolescent boy or girl who is involved in sports activities. The child will point to the tibial tubercle as the site of pain.

Etiology, Incidence, and Pathophysiology

The etiology of Osgood-Schlatter disease is believed to be related to repetitive stress from sports-related activities combined with overuse of immature muscles and tendons over an extended period and an imbalance in the strength of the quadriceps muscle during adolescent growth. Osgood-Schlatter disease occurs in boys and girls between ages 8 and 16 years, although it is more common in boys. Both knees are usually involved.

During the adolescent growth spurt, overuse trauma causes inflammation in the tibial tubercle at the tendon insertion site. This causes tendinitis of the distal infrapatellar tendon. Without treatment, the tubercle enlarges and can cause later functional and cosmetic problems.

Manifestations and Diagnostic Evaluation

Osgood-Schlatter disease is characterized by the insidious onset of knee pain and tenderness, followed by swelling of the tibial tubercle and difficulty with weight bearing. The diagnosis is made on the basis of the clinical picture and radiographic examination.

Therapeutic Management

Treatment is conservative because the disorder is usually self-limiting. The avoidance of activities such as kneeling, bicycling, and running provides adequate pain control. In some cases the physician may suggest wrapping the affected knee with elastic bandages. This limits knee flexion, reduces swelling, and provides time for healing. Physical therapy for quadriceps stretching and strengthening might be required.

In severe cases, ice, heat, and NSAIDs are helpful. A knee immobilizer or casting with the knee in full extension may be necessary to decrease pain in the child with severe pain. Activity may be restricted for 6 weeks or more. Improvement generally is seen within 6 to 8 weeks, and the problem disappears once growth stops.

Nursing Considerations

Because Osgood-Schlatter disease develops in response to repetitive stress from sports-related activities, the nurse should obtain a thorough history of the child's activities. Examine the knee for pain, tenderness, and swelling over the proximal tibia.

Pain that is aggravated by activities that require kneeling, running, or climbing stairs is an important feature of this disease. Inability to shift from a squatting position to a standing position without pain is highly significant. When asked to identify the area that hurts, the child will point to the tibial tubercle.

Nurses working with school-age children and adolescents should have a clear understanding of Osgood-Schlatter disease so that a simple report of knee pain is not overlooked or incorrectly diagnosed, resulting in more serious problems later. The restrictions placed on the child's activity may interfere with the healthy development of peer relationships and self-esteem. Missed school or sports-related activities, limited interactions with peers, or even the need for special arrangements to participate in a peer-related activity contribute to the child's sense of isolation and alienation. Continued contact with peers is important to help the child achieve age-appropriate developmental tasks.

Because prevention of sports-related injuries should be the primary concern among all those involved in youth athletic participation, the school nurse should provide injury prevention education to all children involved in athletics. The school nurse should work with teachers and coaches as well, giving them the information they need to recognize and prevent overuse syndromes.

Reassure parents that the child will outgrow this problem. Although Osgood-Schlatter disease is self-limiting, activity restrictions must be clearly understood by the parents. Before the child resumes athletics, the parents and child should discuss the advisability of such activities with their physician. Hamstring stretching exercises may be helpful, but physical therapy is frequently required. This can prove to be expensive.

OSTEOGENESIS IMPERFECTA
Etiology

Osteogenesis imperfecta, also known as *brittle bone disease*, is a disorder inherited through an autosomal dominant inheritance pattern and characterized by connective tissue and bone defects. The type of inheritance pattern determines the severity of the child's symptoms. Osteogenesis imperfecta affects 1 in 10,000 to 20,000 infants (Marini, 2004; Marlowe, 2002).

Manifestations

In the most common type of osteogenesis imperfecta (type 1), the child has osteoporosis, excessive bone fragility, blue sclerae, discolored teeth, and deafness by age 20 to 30 years as a result of problems with bony ear structures. The child's skin may appear transparent. Eventual adult height is shorter than average. By far, the most common sign is frequent fractures. Sometimes the excessive number of old fractures can cause health care personnel unfamiliar with the disease to suspect child abuse, but new genetic testing methods can accurately identify children with osteogenesis imperfecta.

Diagnostic Evaluation

Clinical evaluation is helpful in diagnosing osteogenesis imperfecta, with radiographs identifying current or healed fractures. Biochemical studies of collagen structure confirm the diagnosis; children with osteogenesis imperfecta may also demonstrate elevated alkaline phosphatase levels in infancy (Marini, 2004). Genetic testing may be ordered to rule out other hereditary problems as well as to advise the parents on the risk of the disease for other children. Level II ultrasound can diagnose severe osteogenesis prenatally (Marini, 2004).

PATHOPHYSIOLOGY

OSTEOGENESIS IMPERFECTA

In osteogenesis imperfecta, a biochemical defect exists in the synthesis of collagen. Because collagen is an essential component of connective tissue, the abnormal collagen results in the incomplete development of bones, teeth, ligaments, and sclerae. Bones are brittle and extremely fragile, and they fracture easily.

Therapeutic Management

Treatment goals include maintaining the integrity of the musculoskeletal system and preventing fractures. Various approaches, including traction, casting, fixation, and other orthopedic stabilizing methods, are used. Physical and occupational therapy are helpful adjuncts. Intravenous infusions of biphosphonate medications have demonstrated increased bone density, functional evaluation improvements, and decreased pain in most patients; however, new fractures have been know to occur during this therapy (Marni, Heeger, Lynch, & Decaro, 2003).

Nursing Considerations

The child with osteogenesis imperfecta has a history of multiple fractures and delayed growth. The extremities may have an angular deformity as a result of old fractures. On examination, the nurse may note deformities of the leg and kyphoscoliosis. The child appears short because of compression fractures of the spine, and joint mobility is unusual because of relaxed ligaments. The child's teeth may appear discolored because of abnormal enamel. Too often, because of the child's appearance, people assume that the child is cognitively impaired. Children with osteogenesis imperfecta have normal or above-normal intelligence.

Osteogenesis imperfecta has no cure; therefore providing care for a child with this disease requires attention to detail and the use of anticipatory guidance.

The identification of mobility issues that affect the child's functioning is important. Highest priority is given to preventing fractures and maintaining muscle and joint integrity. Gentle turning, passive range-of-motion exercises, daily skin care, and thorough assessment of high-stress areas of the body are necessary to protect the child from fractures and related complications. Many institutions have protocols for using precautions with patients with osteogenesis imperfecta, including using only manual blood pressure cuffs for obtaining blood pressure measurements. The automatic blood pressure cuffs can create too much pressure, causing a fracture.

Excessive weight gain can place undue stress on the musculoskeletal system. Maintaining optimal physiologic functioning is critical if the complications of osteogenesis imperfecta are to be avoided. Instruct parents about nutritional guidelines that support healthy growth and development, including emphasizing high-calcium foods. If necessary, calcium, magnesium, and vitamin supplements may be added to the diet.

Because each child is different, responses to the disease vary. Coping with a chronic illness (see Chapter 12) that involves repeated hospitalizations and restricted mobility places incredible stress on the child and family. Learning how to accept the illness and how to adapt to the demands of the disease while meeting the needs of the family stresses the parents' ability to cope. The nurse needs to become aware of family dynamics, determine how the illness is affecting the family system, and assess the effectiveness of current coping strategies. Once this is done, appropriate interventions should be developed to address problematic areas.

Parents may need assistance with dressing and bathing the child. Clothing may have to be altered to allow for ease in dressing and undressing. If the child is to be discharged with a cast, the nurse should review the principles of cast care and assessment of neurovascular status. Because of the risk of accidental fractures, the nurse should review the principles of safety during play and normal activities. A home referral may be appropriate to assist the family in the transition from hospital to home.

OSTEOMYELITIS

Osteomyelitis is a bacterial infection of the bone that involves the cortex or marrow cavity. It is classified as *acute* or *chronic*. Osteomyelitis is considered chronic if the infection persists longer than 1 month or does not respond to the initial antibiotic protocol. Regardless of advances in antibiotic treatment, osteomyelitis is a serious problem that can be difficult to diagnose and, if inadequately treated, results in high morbidity.

Etiology

Bacteria infiltrate the bone through endogenous routes (e.g., skin or respiratory infections, abscessed teeth, acute otitis media) or exogenous routes (e.g., injury, surgical procedures). The infection is usually the result of vascular spread of the bacteria. Osteomyelitis also may occur as a result of direct entry (open fracture) or injury to surrounding soft tissues (cellulitis). External fixation devices and skeletal traction can lead to osteomyelitis. Although strict adherence to aseptic techniques and frequent assessments of pin sites have greatly controlled this problem, the development of osteomyelitis can be a serious deterrent to successful healing.

The most common causative organism in all ages is *Staphylococcus aureus*. *Streptococcus pyogenes*, *Haemophilus influenzae* (in unimmunized infants), and *Escherichia coli* and group B streptococci (in neonates) also are responsible for osteomyelitis. In children older than 6 years, a *Pseudomonas aeruginosa* infection, which is associated with a puncture wound through an athletic shoe, is the most common cause (Lampe, 2004). The most common causative organism for osteomyelitis in children with sickle cell anemia is *Salmonella*.

Incidence

Osteomyelitis occurs in young children, most often children younger than 5 years. Boys are affected at least twice as often as girls (Lampe, 2004). Although osteomyelitis is more likely to occur during growth spurts, the age groups typically affected are preschoolers and adolescents.

Manifestations

The manifestations of osteomyelitis in infants can be vague and nonspecific, such as fever, irritability, and feeding difficulties. Some infants demonstrate signs of sepsis. In the older child the major signs and symptoms include pain, warmth, and tenderness localized over the site of infection; favoring of the affected extremity; erythema; limited range of motion; and systemic manifestations such as fever and lethargy. Pain,

---

PATHOPHYSIOLOGY

OSTEOMYELITIS

Osteomyelitis occurs most frequently in the metaphyseal region of the long bones, especially the femur or tibia. Bacteria enter the metaphysis by small capillaries, and the inflammatory process begins. A preceding trauma can cause rupture of these capillaries, providing a medium for bacterial growth. Pus forms, and because it cannot move from the metaphyseal area into a joint, it spreads toward the medullary canal as well as the cortex of the bone. Pus accumulates under the periosteum and displaces it, causing it to separate and form an abscess.*

The underlying blood supply is interrupted, which causes necrotic tissue to form *(sequestrum)*. New bone *(involucrum)* develops around the sequestrum, and the inflammatory process continues, causing further damage to surrounding bone tissue.†

Large sections of sequestrum may eventually become honeycombed with cavities or sinuses that contain infective material. These cavities are so effectively walled off that antibiotic therapy may not be successful. Thus osteomyelitis may become chronic.

*Lampe, R. (2004). Osteomyelitis and suppurative arthritis. In R. Behrman, R. Kliegman, & H. Jenson (Eds.), *Nelson textbook of pediatrics* (17th ed., pp. 2297-2302). Philadelphia: WB Saunders.
†Carroll, K. (2002). Alterations of musculoskeletal function in children. In K. McCance & S. Huether (Eds.), *Pathophysiology the biologic basis for disease in adults & children* (4th ed.; pp. 1419-1421). St. Louis: Mosby.

---

usually localized, can radiate to adjacent areas of the body; radiating pain to an adjacent joint necessitates an assessment for possible septic arthritis (Skinner, 2003).

Diagnostic Evaluation

Imaging studies such as radiography, ultrasonography, radionuclide bone scans, MRI, and CT scans diagnose and monitor the progress of osteomyelitis. Laboratory evidence of an infectious process, such as elevated erythrocyte sedimentation rate (ESR), elevated C-reactive protein (CRP) level, and an elevated white blood cell count, is usually present. The physician may choose to aspirate the affected area to obtain fluid for culture and sensitivity.

Therapeutic Management

Once a culture has been done and the organism's sensitivity to antibiotics determined, antibiotic treatment is initiated. Controversy exists regarding the length of time required for antibiotic therapy, the need for IV versus oral antibiotics, and the role of bactericidal antibiotics and therapeutic blood levels. Nevertheless, therapy for osteomyelitis generally requires high-dose parenteral therapy, preferably through a peripherally inserted central catheter (PICC). The organism involved dictates the type of antibiotic and the length of treatment. With some children, parenteral antibiotics can be changed to large-dose oral antibiotics after at least 1 week of therapy (Lampe, 2004).

Because the antibiotics are administered over an extended period and high-dose therapy may be necessary to obtain the desired outcome, assessment of the child's response to the antibiotics is an integral part of the treatment protocol. Peak and trough serum antibiotic levels are closely monitored. Renal and hepatic function should be monitored and blood cell counts measured frequently to determine bone marrow activity. Children receiving aminoglycosides should be periodically assessed for side effects such as ototoxicity and nephrotoxicity.

To limit the spread of infection and promote healing, the child is placed on complete bed rest. The extremity may be immobilized with a splint or bivalved cast. After several days of healing, physical therapy with passive range of motion exercises usually is indicated to prevent contractures (Lampe, 2004). Surgical intervention may be necessary if an abscess is present or if the infection does not respond to antibiotics. Invasive procedures include draining the abscess, debriding necrotic tissue, and performing a sequestrectomy (removal of the sequestrum). Osteomyelitis of the proximal femur generally requires some type of surgical decompression because septic arthritis of the hip may accompany this infection. Aseptic technique is critical after any type of orthopedic surgery because a secondary infection could inhibit the healing process.

NURSING CARE

The Child With Osteomyelitis

Assessment

Although the recollection of every injury their child has experienced is difficult for parents, a thorough history of recent falls or traumas is helpful in determining the source of the infection. The nurse should carefully examine the affected area and note any pain, tenderness, erythema, or swelling. Usually the child will appear to protect the extremity, even tensing adjacent muscles and demonstrating reluctance to straighten or move the extremity.

Nursing Diagnosis and Planning

The following nursing diagnoses and expected outcomes may be appropriate after assessment of the child with osteomyelitis:

- Risk for Injury related to complications of antibiotic therapy.

    Expected Outcomes: The parenteral insertion site will remain patent and free from signs of infection. The parents will properly store and administer the ordered antibiotics and properly dispose of IV equipment.

- Acute Pain related to the infectious process.

    Expected Outcome: The child will experience a decrease in pain, as evidenced by a decreased score on an appropriate pain assessment tool.

- Impaired Physical Mobility related to the infectious process and activity restrictions.

    Expected Outcomes: The child will exhibit full range of motion of the unaffected extremities and participate in self-care.

- Delayed Growth and Development related to immobility and activity restrictions.

    Expected Outcomes: The child will exhibit age-appropriate growth and developmental behavior. The parents will provide developmentally appropriate activities for their child.

- Deficient Knowledge about home management of long-term antibiotic therapy related to unfamiliarity with the procedures.

    Expected Outcomes: The parents will demonstrate the correct administration of antibiotics, verbalize reportable adverse effects, and identify any other concerns or issues regarding home care.

Interventions

Chart the child's neurovascular and pain status at least every 4 hours and more often if indicated. Because any movement of the involved extremity will be accompanied by discomfort, the extremity should be immobilized and supported with pillows. When moving or turning is necessary, ask the child what is the most comfortable way to achieve position changes. If the child is preverbal or not able to explain, the nurse should consult the parent. During the acute phase, the pain may be quite severe and the nurse should premedicate the child with an analgesic before any repositioning.

Administering Intravenous Antibiotics

Because a long-term IV site for antibiotic administration must be maintained, the nurse carefully and frequently monitors the site for signs of complications (see Chapter 14) and flushes the line according to facility protocol.

The nurse should have a thorough knowledge of the antibiotic being given. This includes calculating dosage on the basis of body weight or surface area, reviewing side effects and adverse effects, and determining if therapeutic blood levels are required. If the level of drug in the patient's blood exceeds the therapeutic range, the antibiotic should be withheld and the physician notified. Also notify the physician if the level is below the therapeutic level.

Because the child will probably receive multiple antibiotics, compatibility is important. Allergies and any problems the parent may have encountered during previous antibiotic administration should be noted. The nurse should periodically review current laboratory data to ensure adequate liver and kidney function. A complete blood cell count (CBC) and ESR should be measured on a regular basis to evaluate the child's response to treatment.

Providing Wound Care

Standard Precautions should be maintained at all times. Sterile technique and appropriate removal of soiled materials should be strictly enforced. Children with surgical wounds or drains need close monitoring. Drainage should be measured as accurately as possible and recorded at the end of the shift. The color and consistency of the drainage and any unusual odor should be noted in the nurses' notes. A description of the wound should also be included.

Maintaining Activity Limitations

Bed rest or non-weight bearing is important to prevent spread of the infection. The child's return to full weight bearing and self-care activities is determined by the his or her response to treatment and the physician's assessment of the healing process.

Actions to prevent consequences of immobility have been previously discussed. Immobility can diminish the child's appetite. Meeting the child's nutritional needs is essential to facilitate growth and development and assist with the healing process. The child should receive a diet high in calories and protein. Frequent small meals and food that has been brought from home are helpful in stimulating the child's appetite.

Teaching Home Management

If the child is to receive IV antibiotic therapy at home, teach the parent how to set up the medication and how to ensure the infusion is being safely administered. Plan the teaching to fit the parent's schedule, and pay particular attention to signs of frustration or anxiety. Repetitive questions, poor eye contact, and nervous gestures are indicators that anxiety may be interfering with the parent's ability to retain information. Allow the parent to express feelings of concern and give positive feedback as the parent learns procedures. A return demonstration is the most effective way to evaluate teaching effectiveness. Make a home care referral to assist the family with the IV infusions.

Children who have had a favorable clinical response to IV antibiotics will occasionally be discharged with a course of oral antibiotics. Adherence to the medication regimen must be discussed with the parent. Emphasize the importance of follow-up care. A referral to a home care agency would be appropriate.

Promoting Optimal Development

Developmental issues need to be addressed by the nurse. If the child is to remain at home with restricted activity, the family must clearly understand how the restrictions aid the healing process. Discuss age-appropriate activities that will maintain current developmental levels. If the child is exhibiting any residual fears or concerns related to hospitalization, therapeutic play activities may be needed. School-age children need to continue with their schoolwork and maintain contact with their friends. Advise and arrange for tutoring as soon as possible. Resources available to home-bound children should be explored with the parent.

Evaluation

- Is the peripheral insertion site free from redness or swelling, and does the antibiotic infuse well?
- Can the parent describe and demonstrate proper antibiotic administration and disposal of associated equipment?
- Does the child indicate decreased pain on an appropriate pain assessment scale?
- Can the child exhibit full range of motion of unaffected extremities?

- Does the child participate in self-care?
- Does the parent provide developmentally appropriate activities for the child within activity restrictions?
- Does the child exhibit any signs of developmental regression?
- Can the parent demonstrate all procedures needed for home care?

JUVENILE ARTHRITIS

Juvenile arthritis (JA), formerly known as *juvenile rheumatoid arthritis*, is an autoimmune inflammatory disease with no known cause. The term *juvenile rheumatoid arthritis* is misleading because it implies a positive rheumatoid factor (RF+), which is not always present in children with the disease. Because arthritis in children can appear in a number of different forms, each with a different treatment protocol and prognosis, the more accurate term is *juvenile arthritis*.

Regardless of which term is used, consensus is overwhelming that this is a multisystem disorder that affects the body's connective tissue. It is characterized by episodic exacerbations and remissions of joint swelling with limited range of motion accompanied by pain, tenderness, and inflammation, usually of multiple joints (Labyak, Bourguignon, & Docherty, 2003). For diagnostic purposes, the symptoms must be present for 6 weeks or more.

JA, one of the more common chronic diseases in children, is the leading cause of blindness and disability in children. JA is not a childhood version of rheumatoid arthritis. Rather, the onset and course of the disease are clearly defined. The prognosis is considered good, but success is influenced by how well the child's growth and developmental needs are integrated into the treatment plan.

PATHOPHYSIOLOGY

JUVENILE ARTHRITIS

The synovial joints are the primary structures involved in this rheumatic process. Normally synovial joints are movable and contain synovium, a highly vascular tissue that produces a clear, viscous synovial fluid that nourishes and lubricates articular cartilage. In juvenile arthritis, immune complexes in blood and synovial tissue initiate the inflammatory response, producing inflammatory cytokines. Phagocytosis and accumulation of immune complexes cause chronic inflammation and joint destruction.

As the synovium becomes inflamed, excessive fluid is produced. Unlike normal synovial fluid, this fluid is thin and watery. The synovium swells, and thickened villi and nodules protrude into the joint cavity. Pannus formation occurs over the articular cartilage.

Periarticular structures outside the joint may also become involved. With further deterioration, the articular cartilage and contiguous bone become eroded and are destroyed.

Etiology

Despite extensive research, the cause of JA remains unknown. Causes are cited as multifactorial, including genetic predisposition, abnormal immune response, and environmental triggering factors such as infection or trauma. Risk factors include human leukocyte antigens (HLAs) and positive rheumatoid factor. Presence of antinuclear antibody increases the associated risk of uveitis with JA (Dambro, 2005).

Incidence

JA affects 1.4 in 1000 children each year (Miller & Cassidy, 2004). It occurs before age 16 years, although in most cases the onset is between the toddler and the adolescent years. JA seldom occurs before age 6 months and is more than twice as likely to occur in girls than in boys. Approximately 45% of children with JA have moderate to severe functional limitations over the long term (Miller & Cassidy, 2004).

Manifestations

Intermittent joint pain that lasts longer than 6 weeks in one or more joints suggests JA. The joints may appear painful, stiff, swollen, warm to the touch (no redness), and with limited range of motion. Stiffness is worse in the morning or after a prolonged period of rest. This is referred to as the "gel phenomenon" because the joints seem to gel in place. Table 26-2 lists associated signs and symptoms of the JA subtypes. *Uveitis*, or inflammation of the eye structures in the uveal tract, can cause blindness.

Diagnostic Evaluation

The early diagnosis of JA relies on the recognition of the several modes of onset and incidence patterns. The character, frequency, and severity of the systemic and articular manifestations are also critical to the diagnosis. Rheumatoid factor (RF), antinuclear antibodies (ANA), an elevated ESR, and C-reactive protein (CRP) may or may not be present according to the type of JA. Certain types of JA are specific HLA antigen positive. Uveitis is diagnosed by slit lamp examination.

Therapeutic Management

Therapeutic management is supportive and directed toward preserving joint function, controlling the inflammatory process, minimizing deformity, and reducing the impact of the disease on the child's development. Drug therapy, physical and occupational therapy, family education regarding home care, and developmental interventions are the treatments of choice. None of these treatment modalities is curative. When they are used appropriately, however, synovitis can be reduced, mobility increased, and the child's growth and developmental needs appropriately addressed.

Drug Therapy

The major groups of drugs used to suppress the inflammatory process and control pain are the NSAIDs, such as ibuprofen, naproxen sodium (Naprosyn), tolmetin sodium (Tolectin), and aspirin. For children who do not respond well to NSAIDs and who have severe disease, the slower-acting antirheumatic drugs (SAARDs), such as hydroxychloroquine, gold salts, or penicillamine, can be given alone or in conjunction with the NSAIDs. Corticosteroid (e.g., prednisone) use is limited in the treatment of juvenile arthritis. Despite antiinflammatory properties, corticosteroid use neither cures JA nor prevents long-term joint damage. Moreover, the chronic side effects that frequently occur can be problematic for children (see Chapter 17). Indications for use are limited to life-threatening complications of JA, such as pericarditis, profound anemia, and vasculitis.

Immunosuppressive and cytotoxic agents (e.g., cyclophosphamides, chlorambucil) have been effective in the treatment of certain children with JA. Disease-modifying anti-rheumatic drugs (DMARDs) such as methotrexate, sulfasalazine, and etanercept are being used more frequently as second-line drugs because of their effectiveness and relatively few side effects (Ilowite, 2002; Miller & Cassidy, 2004).

Physical and Occupational Therapy

By controlling the synovitis of JA, drug therapy plays a role in preventing additional musculoskeletal problems. Preserving muscle integrity and joint mobility is equally important. JA places the child at risk for impaired mobility, contractures, and altered growth and development.

Rehabilitation is designed to prevent such problems from occurring. A program of rest, proper positioning, and exercises (strengthening, active and passive range of motion, resistive exercises) has been developed by occupational and physical therapists. To ensure cooperation when developing an exercise program, the therapist considers the child's interests as well as school and extracurricular activities.

To maximize the effectiveness of the exercise program, the strengths and limitations of the child's joints must be thoroughly evaluated. With this information, an individualized exercise program can be developed. Swimming is an excellent exercise for the child. The warmth of the water coupled with the mild resistance it provides make swimming the perfect medium for strengthening and range-of-motion exercises while protecting the joint.

Children are naturally active, and children with JA are no different. Activity helps maintain normal muscle and joint integrity. During remissions of the disease, the youthful activity level assists with maintaining muscle strength. During painful exacerbations of the disease, however, the child's natural reaction is to rest the painful joint. Inactivity could lead to muscle wasting and flexion deformity. Hot or cold packs, splinting, and positioning the affected joint in a neutral position help reduce the pain during painful episodes. Although resting the extremity is appropriate, simple isometric or tensing exercises should be begun as soon as the child is able. These exercises are appropriate during exacerbations of the disease because they do not involve joint movement.

Besides physical and occupational therapy, several other treatment modalities have proved effective. Ultrasound, cold, and electrical stimulation assist in controlling the child's pain and increasing joint mobility. Heat also helps reduce joint

TABLE 26-2 **Major Types of Juvenile Arthritis**

Type	Incidence	Gender Affected	Age	Joints Affected	Other Manifestations	Prognosis
Juvenile Rheumatoid Arthritis	50-100/100,000 children in general population*	Males and females equally affected	Any younger than 16 yr old; mean, 1-3 yr old	One or more joints	Gait disturbance, joint swelling, and morning stiffness	30% with severe, long-term functional limitations
Systemic	Approximately 10% of cases of juvenile arthritis	Females more than males	Any	One or more joints	Fever, joint pain, macular rash, and polyarthritis. Some children have pericarditis, hepatomegaly, splenomegaly, or lymphadenopathy.	Often remission occurs within 1 year
Pauciarticular	Approximately 40% of cases of juvenile arthritis	Females more than males	Onset approximately 2 years	Involves four or fewer joints, typically affects large joints such as knees, wrists, ankles, elbows	Most children limp or have a gait disturbance	Prognosis excellent; At risk for asymptomatic chronic iridocytes, which can lead to visual loss if untreated
Polyarticular	Approximately 50% of cases of juvenile arthritis	Primarily females	Early childhood, school age	Multiple symmetric involvement of joints or hands, feet, cervical spine, temporo-mandibular joint, and sternoclavicular joint.	May have short duration of systemic symptoms	Many children (approximately 50%-60%) do not have permanent joint disability

Modified from Graham, M. V., & Uphold, C. R. (2003). *Clinical guidelines in child health*, 3rd ed. (p. 693). Gainesville, FL: Barmarrae Books.
*Incidence taken from *www.nlm.nih.gov*, 2005.

stiffness and muscle spasm because the fibrous tissue found in joints and tendons yields better to stretching when it is heated. Examples of heat therapies are hot baths, whirlpools, Hydrocollator packs, and paraffin baths.

Surgical Treatment

Surgical intervention is considered when the child or adolescent is having problems with joint contractures and unequal growth of extremities. This type of treatment can range from diagnostic procedures, such as arthroscopic examination or open biopsy, to soft tissue release (*tenotomy*) for contractures. Surgery to correct leg length discrepancies as well as arthroplasty and joint replacement may also be necessary.

NURSING CARE

The Child With Juvenile Arthritis

Assessment

Most children with JA are managed successfully at home, and hospital admission is not needed. The nursing assessment focuses on the status of the affected joints, the physical restrictions placed on the child, the level and intensity of the pain, and the child's and family's response to the disease process.

Examine affected joints for warmth, tenderness, pain, and limited range of motion. Because children are not always able to identify the problem clearly, be alert for irritability, guarding of the painful joints, or refusal to bear weight. The child may limp or favor the extremity.

Pain is a major component of this disease. Attempt to determine the intensity and severity of the pain. Remember that the nonverbal child cannot report pain. The parent may describe the child as fussy and irritable in the morning. The young child may be reluctant to walk and want to be carried. Help the family determine what activities increase the pain and what the child does when the pain starts. Explore with the child methods that may relieve the pain and whether they are effective.

Assess joint stiffness, including the duration of the stiffness and the child's description of how difficult movement is after periods of inactivity. Assess the child for any indication of systemic involvement such as a history of temperature elevations, especially in the late afternoon or evening, and determine whether a rash occurs with the fever. Anorexia, weight loss, and failure to grow may be the first indicators that something is wrong. The parent may report that the child is not sleeping at night or may simply describe the child as irritable and fussy. Lethargy and malaise may also occur. Children with JA report poor sleep quality, daytime sleepiness, irritability, fatigue, and anxiety (Labyak et al., 2003).

During the physical examination, assess for lymphadenopathy, hepatosplenomegaly, and visual problems. Uveitis will be apparent only on slit lamp examination. Obtain an accurate height and weight and, if possible, plot past growth parameters on a growth chart to determine any alterations in growth. Cardiac and respiratory system assessments provide baseline information that will allow early detection of pericarditis and pleuritis.

Nursing Diagnosis and Planning

The following nursing diagnoses and expected outcomes may be appropriate to the child with juvenile arthritis and the child's family:

- Chronic Pain related to the inflammatory process.

  Expected Outcome: The child's pain will decrease, as evidenced by increased participation in usual activities and verbal report of decreased pain.

- Impaired Physical Mobility related to inflammation of the joint and associated muscle weakness.

  Expected Outcomes: As a result of appropriate activity and an ongoing exercise program, the child's joints will remain mobile. The child will correctly use any appropriate adaptive equipment to accomplish activities of daily living (ADLs) and participate in a regular exercise program. The child will show no signs of the hazards of immobility.

- Delayed Growth and Development related to activity intolerance.

  Expected Outcomes: The child will exhibit age-appropriate behaviors. The parents will support and maintain appropriate developmental activities for their child.

- Disturbed Body Image related to activity intolerance.

  Expected Outcomes: The child will maintain relationships with peers and participate in age-appropriate activities when able.

- Deficient Knowledge about the care and treatment of JA related to unfamiliarity with the condition.

  Expected Outcome: The parents will demonstrate safe home care and adherence to the treatment regimen and the prescribed exercise program.

Interventions

Managing Pain

Teach parents to identify both verbal and nonverbal pain indicators. Nonverbal cues are more difficult to recognize but may include restlessness, withdrawal, decreased attention span, increased crying, and decreased sleep. Maintaining a therapeutic blood level of pain medication is the most effective way to ensure maximal comfort. The nurse needs to teach parents the side effects of the prescribed medications and advise that most NSAIDs should be given with food or milk to prevent gastrointestinal irritation.

Because some medications used to treat juvenile arthritis cause immunosuppression, teach parents to recognize the signs of immunosuppression and notify the physician as appropriate. Some childhood immunizations may need to be postponed. Because the combination of aspirin and viral infection can predispose the child to Reye syndrome (see Chapter 28), aspirin should be discontinued if the child has a viral illness. As long as the child is not immunosuppressed, administer varicella and influenza vaccines to prevent these viral infections.

DRUG GUIDE

NAPROXEN, NAPROXEN SODIUM

Classification: NSAID.

Action: Unknown; reduces inflammation and fever, possibly by inhibiting prostaglandin synthesis.

Indication: JA.

Dosage and Route: 10 mg/kg per day orally in two divided doses; medication comes in tablet or liquid suspension (125 mg/5 mL).

Absorption: Absorbed rapidly from the gastrointestinal tract with peak action in 1 to 4 hours.

Excretion: Effects last approximately 7 hours; eliminated primarily by the kidneys.

Contraindications: Contraindicated in any child who has had an allergic reaction to this drug or similar drugs or in children with a syndrome of asthma, rhinitis, and nasal polyps; naproxen should not be administered concurrently with naproxen sodium.

Precautions: Can prolong bleeding time, alter liver functions, and contribute to renal toxicity. Use cautiously if the child is also taking methotrexate, aspirin, anticoagulants, probenecid, or steroids.

Adverse Reactions: Primarily gastrointestinal irritation (gastrointestinal ulceration with bleeding from prolonged use); edema; headache, drowsiness, or dizziness; tinnitus; pruritus or skin rash; risk for renal failure.

Nursing Considerations: Monitor closely for adverse reactions, particularly if the child is receiving long-term therapy. Advise the child to take the medication with food or milk to minimize gastrointestinal upset. Be aware that antiinflammatory medications can mask signs of infection. Teach the child and family signs of gastrointestinal bleeding.

Nonpharmacologic pain relief measures such as diversion, splinting, heat or cold application, imagery, and meditation can be useful for some children. Remind parents to continue encouraging isometric exercises.

Promoting Mobility

Teach positioning of inflamed joints, appropriate application of heat or cold, and how to support and protect the affected joints. Emphasize that isometric exercises and passive range-of-motion exercises will prevent contractures and deformities. Help the family identify when the child's condition has exacerbated.

Help the parents learn the exercise program. Be sure that the program is developmentally appropriate and fun for the child. Teach the parents how to assess joint mobility and maintain correct body alignment. The child may need elastic stockings if prolonged inactivity is expected.

Discuss with the parent and child age-appropriate play activities that involve the unaffected extremities; aerobic activities, such as swimming, will prevent stasis of respiratory secretions. The child will need more time than average to begin morning activities. Teach the parents to allow plenty of time for the child to awaken, take a warm shower or bath,

and relieve morning joint stiffness. Keeping the child's room or bed warm is important. Administering the medication with a snack first thing in the morning and allowing the medication to take effect before the child arises help reduce pain.

Facilitating Emotional and Social Development

Acknowledge the child's and family's anxiety and allow family members to express concerns. Encourage expressive therapeutic activities such as pounding boards, bean bag throws, clay, painting, story composing, and doll play. Therapeutic play provides a safe and effective mechanism for reducing the stress of immobility. The nurse should recognize that age, sex, and self-concept play a role in a child's adjustment to chronic illness. Use anticipatory guidance to help the child develop coping mechanisms that will foster the development of optimism and a sense of personal competence.

Communicate with the school nurse about scheduling necessary rest periods for the child during the school day. The child might enjoy a short period of quiet activity in the school health office if allowed to bring a friend. School nurses can help the child's daily transition to school by communicating with teachers about the child's needs.

Helping the child identify strengths and areas of accomplishments increases self-esteem. Identify creative hobbies or activities that will enhance the child's sense of self-worth.

Family Education

As part of the multidisciplinary approach, the nurse must take an active part in helping the parents and child learn how to cope with and adapt to the limitations of the disease. This includes referring them from the outset to sources of accurate information about the condition and its associated care. Information should be in a variety of media and appropriate for the child's developmental level. The Arthritis Foundation (see Evolve website) can provide information to parents and children. Parents also want to ensure that others in the community have an understanding of JA. Increased understanding by others in the child's environment will increase the affected child's ability to maintain a normal, developmentally appropriate lifestyle.

Because the greater part of the child's care takes place in the home, the success of the therapeutic plan will be determined by the parents. Planning begins as soon as possible in the course of the illness. The parents should be involved in as many nursing activities as possible. This will reduce their anxiety and increase their sense of control over a frightening situation. Provide verbal and written instructions and use return demonstrations to ensure parental understanding of procedures. Coordinate referrals and physical therapy with the child's and parents' routines and schedules.

Encourage the parents to provide a diet high in fiber, protein, and calcium and an adequate fluid intake. If the child has anorexia or pain while eating, consider smaller, more frequent high-calorie foods.

Emphasize regular visits to the ophthalmologist to prevent complications from uveitis. Children with JA should be referred to an ophthalmologist at diagnosis and for recommended periodic follow-ups (Graham & Uphold, 2003).

Evaluation

- Does the child experience pain control, as evidenced by report of decreased pain, increased sleep, decreased restlessness and irritability, and increased participation in age-appropriate activities?
- Is the child free from joint inflammation, and does the child demonstrate age-appropriate range of motion and muscle strength?
- During an exacerbation, is the child able to accept activity restrictions and participate in the exercise program?
- Is the child free from respiratory problems or other problems associated with immobility?
- Is the child able to perform age-appropriate self-care activities?
- Do the parents demonstrate the ability to facilitate the child's growth and development within the limitations posed by the child's disease?
- Does the child demonstrate age-appropriate behaviors, increased social interactions with friends, and appropriate adaptation to school?
- Are the parents able to articulate and demonstrate solutions to care for problems encountered in the home?

MUSCULAR DYSTROPHIES

Muscular dystrophies are a group of progressively degenerative, inherited diseases that affect the muscle cells of specific muscle groups, causing weakness and atrophy. They vary in pattern of inheritance and age at onset, but most are identified in early childhood and are characterized by progressive muscle weakness (Table 26-3). Duchenne muscular dystrophy is the most common of several forms of muscular dystrophy.

Etiology

Muscular dystrophies are inherited in various genetic patterns. Duchenne muscular dystrophy is a sex-linked recessive disorder; therefore it affects only males. Females are carriers and pass the defect on to their male children.

Incidence

Duchenne muscular dystrophy occurs in 1 in 3000 male children (MDA USA, 2003). Spontaneous mutations are responsible for 30% or more of those affected; therefore many of these children have no family history of the disorder. Other forms of muscular dystrophy are less common, with varying patterns of inheritance.

Pathophysiology

Over time, muscle fibers degenerate and are replaced by fat and connective tissue. Progressive weakness and wasting of symmetric groups of skeletal muscles result in increasing disability and deformity.

Manifestations

Progressive, symmetric muscle wasting and weakness without loss of sensation first appear after walking is achieved (usually 3 to 7 years). The child must use the Gowers' maneuver to rise from the floor (child puts hands on knees and moves the hands up legs until standing erect). The child has a waddling, wide-based gait. The muscles of the pelvis and shoulders are most often affected in Duchenne muscular dystrophy. The calf muscles are characteristically weak but hypertrophied. Increasing disability and deformities include hip and knee contractures, foot deformities, scoliosis, and lordosis; walking ability (in Duchenne muscular dystrophy) is lost by age 9 to 12 years. Associated signs and symptoms include moderate obesity, decreased intelligent quotient (IQ), cardiomyopathy, and shortened life span. Cardiopulmonary complications are the most common cause of death.

Diagnostic Evaluation

Children with a positive family history are especially at risk for muscular dystrophy and should be monitored for clinical symptoms, which generally do not appear until the preschool years. Serum creatine kinase (CK) levels are elevated in the early stages of the disease and then decrease as muscle bulk decreases. Electromyography and muscle biopsy may also assist with the diagnosis. The gene locus for Duchenne muscular dystrophy has been identified, which makes carrier status for women easier to determine.

Therapeutic Management

The therapeutic management of the child with a muscular dystrophy is aimed at maintaining ambulation and independence for as long as possible as muscle weakness progresses. Contractures further reduce mobility and independence. Surgery, bracing, and physical therapy contribute to keeping the child as mobile as possible. Later therapy is directed toward maximizing sitting capabilities, respiratory function, and self-care. The prevention of obesity to facilitate mobility and care is a priority. Prompt attention to infection, especially of the respiratory tract, is essential.

Nursing Considerations

When muscular dystrophy is present in the family history, infants and young children need to be monitored carefully for its occurrence. When a diagnosis is made, nursing interventions can become a major source of support for these children and their families. The family's ability to cope with chronic illness and the poor prognosis of muscular dystrophy need to be assessed. Over time, the child's mobility and self-care abilities should be monitored to ensure independence for as long as possible. The potential for weight gain and respiratory tract infection and the adequacy of support systems must be regularly assessed.

Nursing interventions for the child with muscular dystrophy include coordinating a variety of health care services. Anticipating the child's future needs requires a sensitive yet knowledgeable approach. Maintenance of activity and self-care functions is important to the child and the family, and independence must be fostered within the limits of safety. Activities such as swimming that promote range of motion and mobility for as long as possible are helpful. As the disease progresses and movement is increasingly restricted, the nurse

TABLE 26-3	**Muscular Dystrophies of Childhood**		
Type	**Onset and Progression**	**Inheritance and Incidence**	**Clinical Manifestations**
Duchenne	Onset: 1-4 yr Rapidly progressive; loss of walking by 9-10 yr; death in late teens from respiratory failure, heart failure, pneumonia	X-linked recessive Most common hereditary neuromuscular disease; affects all races Incidence: 1 in 3000 male infants	Progressive generalized weakness and muscle wasting affecting limb and trunk muscles first; calves often enlarged; waddling gait; lordosis; cardiomyopathy; Gowers' maneuver; mental retardation common
Myotonic (Steinert disease)	Onset: in severe neonatal form: weakness at birth, may have paralysis of diaphragm If child survives early weeks of life, steady improvement in motor function over the first decade, usually developing ability to walk; often survive to late adulthood	Autosomal dominant Incidence: 1 in 30,000 births	In the severe neonatal form, hypotonia and weakness are evident at birth; others may appear normal at birth; mild weakness in first few years, with progressive wasting of distal muscles; myotonia worsened by cold, fatigue, stress; mental retardation in approximately half of cases
Becker	Onset: 5-10 yr Slowly progressive; maintain walking past early teens; life span into third decade	X-linked recessive Incidence: 1 in 20,000 births	Almost identical to Duchenne but less severe; child is mobile until late teens; normal intelligence
Congenital	Onset: birth Typically slow but variable; many do not attain walking; shortened life span	Autosomal recessive Incidence: rare	Generalized muscle weakness with possible joint deformities; hypotonia; mental retardation and seizures common in types with central nervous system disease
Facioscapulohumeral (FSH, or Landouzy-Dejerine disease)	Onset: first decade Slowly progressive loss of walking in later life; variable life expectancy; disease may span many decades	Autosomal dominant or recessive Incidence: 3-10 per 1 million births	Earliest and most severe weakness occurs in facial and shoulder girdle muscles; may be unable to close eyes completely during sleep; progressive disability leading to inability to walk; may be mild, causing minimal disability
Scapuloperoneal or scapulohumeral (Emery-Dreifuss)	Onset: middle childhood to early teens Progression is quite slow; many survive to late adulthood	X-linked recessive Incidence: rare	Contractures of elbows and ankles develop early; shoulder muscles become wasted; slowly progressive, with eventual cardiac abnormality

can suggest activities that take less energy but keep the child involved with peers.

Because children in the late stages of muscular dystrophy have difficulty moving, the nurse and family should assist with position changes every 2 hours to prevent injury to the skin and other tissues from prolonged pressure. Adequate fluid intake must be encouraged to prevent urine stasis. A bowel regimen, including stool softeners or laxatives, may be necessary.

The home environment, including bathing and toileting facilities, may need to be modified to allow wheelchair mobility. Creative approaches to clothing can simplify dressing while meeting the needs of a child trying to fit in with peers.

Specific suggestions about dietary modifications to control weight may be necessary. The nurse can educate families about how to make dietary changes without making food a source of controversy. To reduce the chance of life-threatening respiratory infections, the child needs to be protected from children with respiratory and contagious diseases. As disability progresses, pulmonary hygiene and respiratory exercises are needed to maintain respiratory function.

Regular monitoring by a multidiscipline team helps meet the varying needs of the child and family as the child's condition changes. Therapy is individualized to address the specific needs of the child. Genetic screening and counseling are recommended for parents and siblings of children with muscular dystrophy.

Parents must be taught how to perform basic nursing tasks and be referred to agencies that can assist with home care and equipment, such as a motorized wheelchair. Extended family and support groups, such as the Muscular Dystrophy Association of America (see Evolve website), can provide needed emotional support and specific assistance as parental energies are exhausted. In addition, the needs of the grieving family should be addressed.

SCOLIOSIS

Although scoliosis is defined as lateral curvature of the spine, structural scoliosis is in fact a three-dimensional deformity involving rotation of the vertebral bodies. The forces of a curved spine on the structure of the body cause the rib cage to become misshapen. The body develops a compensatory curve to maintain posture and balance. Scoliotic curves are measured in degrees: a curve of 10 to 20 degrees is a slight curve; a curve of more than 40 degrees usually requires surgery; and a curve of more than 80 degrees compromises respiratory function and is considered severe. Nonstructural scoliosis, which does not involve rotational or muscular deformity, can result from poor posture, increased weight bearing on one shoulder (e.g., from carrying a heavy book bag), and other conditions that cause the child to lean in one direction. Nonstructural scoliosis is treated by correcting the underlying contributing factor.

Etiology

Most cases of scoliosis can be classified into three major categories, which offer some insight into the causes of the disorder. *Idiopathic scoliosis* is the predominant form of scoliosis. Although idiopathic scoliosis has no recognizable cause, the disease appears to have a genetic component. Most cases of idiopathic scoliosis occur in adolescent girls and tend to progress more rapidly during growth spurts, such as the period immediately preceding menarche. Idiopathic scoliosis can also occur in other age groups.

Congenital scoliosis is another major category of scoliosis. It is the result of vertebral abnormalities, such as hemivertebra or vertebral bars, and is associated with other congenital anomalies.

A third category of scoliosis is *neuromuscular scoliosis*. This type of scoliosis is relatively common in individuals with certain neuromuscular conditions, such as cerebral palsy, muscular dystrophy, paraplegia, or quadriplegia.

Scoliosis may also develop in children with certain other disorders, such as osteogenesis imperfecta, JA, and spinal cord tumors, and it may occur as a result of radiation therapy.

Incidence

The incidence of scoliosis varies with the cause. Idiopathic scoliosis is a common disorder, affecting approximately 10% of the population. Most cases of idiopathic scoliosis are of no clinical significance and go undetected. Idiopathic scoliosis is most common in girls and in families in which another member is affected. The incidence of congenital scoliosis is variable. It is believed to be caused by a variety of factors and is also associated with certain other congenital anomalies. Scoliosis is relatively common in children with neuromuscular disorders.

Manifestations

The clinical manifestations of scoliosis include a visible curve of the spine (Fig. 26-10), a rib hump when the child is bending forward, an asymmetric rib cage, uneven shoulder or pelvic heights, and prominence of the scapula or hip. A difference in

---

PATHOPHYSIOLOGY

SCOLIOSIS

Muscle weakness on one side of the spinal column results in shortening of the muscles and ligaments on the opposite side. These tight ligaments cause the spinal column to curve, compressing the vertebrae on that side into a concave curve. Spinal curvatures exacerbate most rapidly during the adolescent growth spurt and curves larger than 50 degrees result in spinal instability.* Spinal curvatures are measured in degrees through use of a procedure called the *Cobb method,* which measures the angle between two lines drawn from the top and bottom vertebrae on the curve. A *scoliometer* is a small screening device that approximates a spinal curve during screening.

* Carroll, K. (2002). Alterations of musculoskeletal function in children. In K. McCance & S. Huether (Eds.). *Pathophysiology the biologic basis for disease in adults & children* (4th ed.; pp. 1417-1418). St. Louis: Mosby.

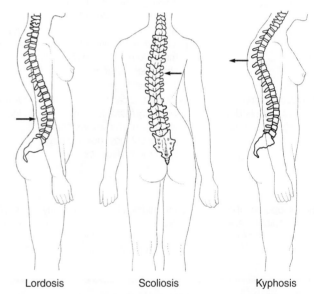

Lordosis   Scoliosis   Kyphosis

FIG 26-10   **Most spinal abnormalities in children are abnormal curvatures. In *scoliosis,* the spine curves laterally and the vertebrae rotate, pulling the ribs along. *Kyphosis* is a front-to-back rounding, usually of the thoracic spine; it is often accompanied by scoliosis. *Lordosis* is an exaggerated concave curvature of the spine, usually in the lumbar area.**   *(From Ignatavicius, D. D., Workman, M. L., & Mishler, M. A. [1995]. Medical surgical nursing: a nursing process approach [2nd ed., p. 1399]. Philadelphia: Saunders.)*

the space between the arms and the trunk is visible when the child is standing, as is an apparent leg length discrepancy. In severe cases the child's vital capacity is reduced (see Chapter 9 for a discussion of screening for scoliosis).

Diagnostic Evaluation

Scoliosis may be detected at any time during childhood or adolescence. It is often first discovered during routine screening for scoliosis either at school or a physician's office. Clinical manifestations should lead to more thorough assessment of the spine. Spinal curvatures are measured in degrees by the Cobb method. The Cobb angle measures the angle between two lines drawn from the top and bottom vertebrae in the curve. A scoliometer is a small screening device that approximates a spinal curve during screening (Hay et al., 2005). Radiographic examination of the thorax confirms the diagnosis and add information to be considered in planning treatment. In addition, children with disorders commonly associated with scoliosis should be monitored for the development of spinal deformity.

Therapeutic Management

The treatment of scoliosis is complex. Depending on the extent of the curve, the child's age and projected growth, and presence of associated complications, treatment options include regular and periodic observation with radiographic evaluation, bracing, or spinal fusion surgery. Although mild curvatures may never progress to the point that treatment is warranted, the curvature can become increasingly pronounced, which is why children must be examined regularly over the long term.

Bracing

In the past, bracing was used extensively in the treatment of scoliosis, and it may still be used today to stabilize some curves (those less than 40 degrees). Bracing will not resolve an existing curve, but theoretically it may reduce the progression of the curve during growth (Thompson, 2004). If used, the brace must be worn 18 to 23 hours per day. The child's skin needs to be meticulously monitored for signs of breakdown.

Surgery

Spinal fusion is used to treat severe scoliosis. Because fusion results in cessation of growth of the fused vertebrae, it is delayed for as long as possible to allow maximal skeletal growth. Many new surgical techniques have shown improved outcomes while decreasing the length of hospitalization. Most surgical techniques rely on some form of internal instrumentation—rods or wires—that corrects the deformity (curve) and holds the spine immobile during the long healing period. Operations are usually accomplished through incisions in the back (for posterior fusion); some surgeons prefer the anterior thoracic approach. An iliac bone graft can be used for the fusion.

Significant blood loss can occur during spinal fusion procedures, and replacement of blood is frequently necessary. Because spinal fusion for scoliosis is a planned procedure, children are often able to donate their own blood in the weeks preceding the surgery for use during surgery. Such autologous blood transfusions have become common in response to the human immunodeficiency virus (HIV) epidemic.

Prognosis

With close monitoring and follow-up, the treatment outcomes for idiopathic scoliosis are excellent. The older the child is at the time of surgery, the more successful the ultimate result is likely to be. The prognosis for congenital scoliosis is variable and depends on the underlying defect.

The treatment of scoliosis in children with neuromuscular disorders is a challenge, and outcomes are variable. These children must be monitored for an indefinite period for the possibility of curve progression.

Complications

A variety of complications can occur during treatment for scoliosis. Braces can cause skin irritation and even pressure sores. Neurologic damage can result from mechanical injury during surgery or from stretching of the spinal column during correction. Although electronic monitoring (somatosensory evoked potentials) during surgery helps reduce the possibility of spinal cord damage intraoperatively, postoperative sensation and motor function are the only definitive indicators of neurologic function.

Another complication in the surgical treatment of scoliosis is superior mesenteric artery syndrome. This disorder is caused by mechanical changes in the position of the patient's abdominal contents, resulting from lengthening of the body. It results in a syndrome of emesis and abdominal distention similar to that occurring with intestinal obstruction or paralytic ileus; therefore postoperative vomiting warrants attention. Fluid or electrolyte imbalances can also occur in the postoperative period, as can atelectasis and sluggish bowel function. Superficial or deep wound infection also is possible. The major long-term complication of spinal fusion is *pseudarthrosis*, or failure of one or more segments of the spine to fuse.

KYPHOSIS

Kyphosis is defined as a front-to-back rounding of the thoracic spine. Mild kyphosis occurs normally and in varying amounts. It may be a postural deviation related to self-consciousness that is manifested by round shoulders. Although kyphosis usually occurs in the thoracic area, it can occur in other areas of the spine, and it becomes especially problematic when it progresses uncontrollably and results in neurologic damage or reduced respiratory function. Kyphosis is often accompanied by scoliosis, although the reverse is not necessarily true.

Etiology and Incidence

Kyphosis can occur as a postural defect (idiopathic), as a result of structural abnormalities of the vertebral bodies of the spine, or as a result of certain neuromuscular disorders (e.g., myelomeningocele) or other factors (e.g., tumors, surgery, radiation therapy).

Postural kyphosis is found in about 4% of otherwise healthy adolescents. The incidence of kyphosis that occurs secondary to other conditions and disorders and that is severe enough to treat is variable.

Manifestations

The clinical manifestations of kyphosis include a visually appreciable humpback or convex deformity that predominantly affects the thoracic area but may involve a lower portion of the spine (see Fig. 26-10).

Text continued on p. 874

NURSING CARE PLAN

The Adolescent With Scoliosis in the Community Setting

Focused Assessment

Nurses are involved with routine screening of children and adolescents for scoliosis in acute care settings, outpatient settings, and schools. School nurses screen children for scoliosis, beginning in the fourth or fifth grade, although scoliosis usually does not become apparent until the adolescent growth spurt. For adolescents who have been diagnosed but are not undergoing treatment, periodic reassessment is necessary to monitor possible progression of the curve. For those undergoing treatment, assessment focuses on determining the adolescent's and parents' level of knowledge about scoliosis, any body image concerns, any anxiety about the various treatment modalities, and whether the adolescent is cooperative with prescribed treatments.

Examine the child or adolescent for any of the following: uneven scapulae, shoulders, and hips and other lack of symmetry in various postural positions (see Chapter 9). Ask about any family history of scoliosis. The school nurse should ensure that the family has followed up on any referral for medical evaluation of scoliosis and assess whether family members understand the course of treatment. Other assessment factors include whether the adolescent properly wears any corrective device and whether any body image concerns or concerns regarding appropriate activities exist.

NURSING DIAGNOSIS   Deficient Knowledge about natural history of scoliosis and the treatment modalities available.

EXPECTED OUTCOME   The adolescent and family will:
- Demonstrate knowledge acquisition, as evidenced by explaining what has been taught about scoliosis, including the reasons for therapy; demonstrating the skills taught (e.g., performance of prescribed exercise or brace care); asking appropriate questions that indicate a knowledge of scoliosis and its treatment (e.g., "Will I be able to play basketball?"); and following through with needed therapy at school and at home.

Intervention

1. Determine the adolescent's and family's knowledge level about scoliosis and treatment modalities.
2. Teach the adolescent and family about scoliosis, its signs and symptoms, progression, and treatment.
3. Identify the adolescent's and parents' areas of concern (e.g., activity restriction, outcomes of therapy).
4. Select instructional methods that are appropriate to the adolescent's developmental level (audiovisuals, pamphlets, talking with affected peers). Include the parents in the teaching.
5. Explain the reasons for the various interventions (e.g., exercise regimen, brace), and emphasize that adherence to the treatment will give the most desirable results.
6. Have the adolescent (or parents) demonstrate specific skills (e.g., brace application, skin care, daily exercises) (Box 26-4).

Rationale

1. Teaching needs to begin at the adolescent's level of understanding.
2. Knowledge and understanding increase motivation and adherence to treatment while reducing anxiety.
3. Teaching will be most effective if it is directed at the individual's needs.
4. Learning styles vary with individual interest, developmental level, and abilities. Including the parents in teaching increases their confidence level and improves consistency of care.
5. Adolescents are more cooperative in the treatment if they know the reason for interventions.

6. Demonstration allows the nurse to evaluate learning and encourages the adolescent to gain confidence in the ability to perform the appropriate skills.

Evaluation

- Can the adolescent and family describe the natural history of scoliosis and treatment prescribed?
- Can the adolescent and family demonstrate correct application of the brace (if required), proper skin care, or prescribed exercise regimen?

- Does the adolescent obtain information by asking appropriate questions of health care personnel?
- Does the adolescent follow the prescribed therapy?

NURSING CARE PLAN—cont'd

NURSING DIAGNOSIS Disturbed Body Image related to postural deformity, bracing, or any activity limitation.

EXPECTED OUTCOME The adolescent will:
- Demonstrate adjustment to changes in physical appearance or function, as evidenced by stated confidence in abilities (academic, physical, social) and willingness to try different strategies to enhance appearance.

Intervention	*Rationale*
1. Encourage the teen to talk about the diagnosis, treatment, and feelings about the experience.	1. This allows assessment of perceptions and provides opportunities to clarify misconceptions and vent feelings.
2. Engage the adolescent in conversation that focuses on body perception. For example, "Some girls I have known who have had to wear a brace have been anxious about whether they will be able to find attractive clothes to fit over the brace. If this is a concern of yours, maybe we can explore some strategies together."	2. This allows the nurse to provide emotional support and may ease anxiety.
3. Encourage the adolescent to discuss experiences with friends.	3. Friends are likely to be supportive and helpful if they share a knowledge of the disorder.
4. Provide information about the disorder and the treatment. Assist the adolescent to consider a school or recreational activity that can be mastered and create a sense of accomplishment.	4. This helps the adolescent gain a sense of control over the experience.
5. Provide privacy to the greatest extent possible for any adolescent who needs to adjust the brace or perform skin care during the school day.	5. Children and teens are quite modest.

Evaluation

- Does the adolescent express confidence in academic, physical, and social activities?
- Is the adolescent able to discuss creative strategies for dress or physical adaptations?

BOX 26-4	**ADOLESCENTS & PARENTS WANT TO KNOW** About Home Care for the Adolescent in an Orthoplast Jacket or Brace

- Follow your physician's directions about applying and wearing time for your brace. Different braces have different methods of application, but all should fit comfortably and snugly once applied. Be sure to ask whether the brace should be applied while in a lying or standing position. You may need a helper to get you into the brace. If you have had surgery, do not bend or twist while you are out of the brace.
- Always wear an all-cotton, preferably seamless, T-shirt under the brace to protect your skin, and be sure to pull down on the shirt to remove all wrinkles once the brace is applied. Your bra should be worn under the T-shirt unless the physician has directed otherwise; underpants and remaining clothes can go over the brace once it is on.
- Proper skin care is most important to prevent soreness or raw skin. Wash the skin that is covered by the brace once or twice a day, according to your physician's directions.

Before you wash your skin, examine it closely for pink or red areas. Notify the orthopedic nurse or physician if skin areas appear raw.
- After washing, dry the skin thoroughly and put on a clean T-shirt. Avoid using creams, lotions, or powders under the brace because they can soften the skin. If your skin is particularly dry, consult the orthopedic nurse or physician about approaches for this problem.
- Clean the inside and outside of the brace daily with mild soap and water; rinse and let dry for 20 to 30 minutes. Do not use a warm hair dryer or leave your brace anywhere warm because the plastic can soften and lose its shape.
- Notify your physician if any of the following occurs: signs of an infected incision (redness, drainage, fever) if you have had surgery; numbness or tingling of your arms, legs, or feet; cracks or breaks in the brace; skin problems; any respiratory problems.

Modified from *Brace Care* and from *Instructions for Wearing Your Boston Brace.* Children's Hospital, Boston, Division 10 Northwest and Orthopaedic Clinic.

NURSING CARE PLAN

The Adolescent Undergoing a Spinal Fusion

Focused Assessment

Preoperatively, adolescents can experience anxiety and fear about the surgical procedure, anticipated postoperative care, and the hospital experience. They are concerned about pain, the physical experience of the operative site, postoperative activity limitations, and altered appearance. In the immediate postoperative period, adolescents are closely assessed to determine the neurologic status of the lower extremities as well as to evaluate pain, fluid status, bleeding, and return of bowel function. Respiratory status must also be assessed, especially if the anterior/thoracic approach has been used and the adolescent has a chest tube. Most adolescents are able to be cared for on an orthopedic floor for 5 to 7 days; however, some may require one night in the ICU postoperatively.

As the adolescent stabilizes postoperatively, continue previous assessments along with wound healing, ease of mobility, and nutritional status. Before discharge, assess the adolescent's and family's understanding of home and follow-up care. A brace may be used postoperatively with some adolescents. Adolescents are sometimes discharged from the hospital by the fifth postoperative day. Because the treatment of scoliosis is a long-term process that can affect an adolescent for most of the growing years, close monitoring is important to ensure positive outcomes.

NURSING DIAGNOSIS   Anxiety (preoperative) related to impending surgery.

EXPECTED OUTCOME   The adolescent will:
- Reduce anxiety, as evidenced by seeking information about the surgery and postoperative care and by identifying and using effective coping mechanisms to address it.

Intervention	Rationale
1. Determine whether the adolescent is anxious about surgery.	1. The adolescent may not be anxious or may be hiding anxiety.
2. Initiate a conversation with the adolescent about what anxiety feels like and how anxiety is a normal response to anticipated surgery. For example, "Many girls facing surgery are nervous about what it will be like to have this operation. Perhaps you would like to know more about what it will be like."	2. The adolescent may need permission to discuss anxiety and may require assistance verbalizing feelings. Adolescents need to be assured that they are normal.
3. Assist the adolescent with identifying positive and effective means for resolving anxiety (e.g., talking with a friend, exercising or engaging in other activities, practicing relaxation techniques).	3. In role modeling for the adolescent and discussing various possibilities for coping, the nurse allows the adolescent to find a comfortable means for expressing feelings.
4. Identify and discourage negative behaviors associated with anxiety (e.g., verbal outbursts, physical aggression, withdrawal). Try telling the adolescent, "It's OK and normal to be anxious about surgery. This is hard for your parents, too. Let's talk about ways you might let your parents know how you are feeling."	4. The adolescent needs to understand that expressing feelings can be done in acceptable and unacceptable ways.
5. Reassure the adolescent about specific fears ("Can my parents be with me?" "Will I get a shot?" "Will I have a huge scar?").	5. Reassurance and conversation may help resolve some fears.
6. Determine the adolescent's need for specific information, particularly about postoperative care.	6. Fears about the unknown may be reduced by increasing knowledge.
7. Explain the reason for the various postoperative interventions: • Neurovascular checks every 1 to 2 hours for the first 24 hours and every 4 hours thereafter • Turning by log-rolling every 2 hours • Deep breathing and use of incentive spirometer (chest tube if anterior approach is used) • Wound dressing (if applicable) • Brace application and skin care	7. Adolescents are more cooperative in the postoperative period if they know the reason for interventions.

NURSING CARE PLAN—cont'd

8. Have the adolescent (or parents and adolescent) demonstrate specific skills (e.g., coughing, recumbent log-rolling).

8. This allows the nurse to evaluate learning and allows the adolescent to gain confidence in being able to perform the maneuver; confidence in managing care decreases anxiety.

9. Encourage the adolescent to ask questions and discuss concerns. Correct any inaccurate information.

9. Verbalizing concerns helps clarify misperceptions and decreases anxiety.

Evaluation

- Does the adolescent seek information about the surgery and its postoperative course?
- Is the adolescent able to talk about anxiety or fears with parents, friends, or the nurse?

- Can the adolescent use appropriate techniques to reduce anxiety?

NURSING DIAGNOSIS Acute Pain related to the operative procedure.

EXPECTED OUTCOMES The adolescent will:
- Indicate decreasing amounts of pain as measured on a pain scale.
- Appear calm and relaxed.
- Participate in postoperative activities.

Intervention

1. Frequently monitor the adolescent's pain level by using an appropriate pain rating scale in the postoperative period. (Statements of pain, anxiety, an inability to cough, hyperalertness, reluctance or refusal to move, and sweating may indicate pain.)
2. Provide prescribed analgesics in a timely manner (children usually receive patient-controlled analgesia [PCA] morphine or Dilaudid for several days).

3. Assist family members in understanding the adolescent's experience and interventions.
4. Explore alternative means for relieving pain (using anxiety-reducing techniques, dimming the room lights, reducing stimuli, playing music, receiving therapeutic touch).
5. Determine response to pain-relief measures and communicate with the physician about possible adjustments if needed. (See Chapter 15 for a thorough discussion of the nursing care of pain in children and teenagers.)

Rationale

1. Adolescents may be unable or unwilling to verbalize their pain.

2. Appropriate and timely use of analgesics provides optimal control of pain. Epidural analgesia provides more constant pain relief and prevents peaks and valleys of pain.
3. When parents understand and can participate in the adolescent's care, they can provide appropriate support.
4. Alternative therapy may be quite effective.

5. Adjustments may be necessary to achieve optimal pain relief.

Evaluation

- Can the adolescent use a pain scale to rate pain?
- Does the adolescent appear calm and relaxed?

- Is the adolescent able to participate in postoperative activities?

NURSING DIAGNOSIS Deficient Knowledge about home care related to unfamiliarity with information about spinal fusion.

EXPECTED OUTCOME The family and adolescent will:
- Successfully manage treatment at home, as evidenced by demonstrating procedures, accessing appropriate community resources, and keeping follow-up appointments.

Intervention

1. Teach the family and adolescent the correct technique for wound care (dressing or adhesive strips) and the signs of a wound infection (redness, swelling, drainage, fever). Discuss the importance of a well-balanced diet.

Rationale

1. Proper wound care and good nutrition promote healing and decrease the chance of infection.

Continued

NURSING CARE PLAN—cont'd

2. Discuss activity restrictions. (Usually these adolescents cannot ride a bike, use roller blades, ski, participate in sports or gym, mow the lawn, or lift more than 10 lb.) Show the adolescent how to perform activities without twisting or bending at the waist.

3. Instruct the family and child to be alert for unfavorable signs such as skin breakdown, pain, numbness or tingling in the extremities, or difficulty breathing, and inform them about problems that can be anticipated.

4. Provide the name and telephone number of an easily accessible health care provider if questions arise at home. Inform the family about community resources available, including resources for tutoring. Referral to national scoliosis associations (see Evolve website) may be helpful.

5. Before discharge, schedule a follow-up appointment. Emphasize the importance of keeping appointments.

2. Home care instructions for activity are important to reduce the possibility of complications. Activity restrictions are usually maintained for 6 to 9 months depending on the type of surgery and the physician.

3. Home care instructions reduce the possibility of complications.

4. Access to a health care provider and/or community resources decreases anxiety and improves adherence to treatment.

5. Periodic evaluation is important to recovery.

Evaluation

- Can the family demonstrate the procedures necessary to care for the adolescent at home?

- Is the family aware of sources of help if needed?
- Does the family keep follow-up appointments?

Diagnostic Evaluation

The diagnosis of kyphosis is relatively easy to establish from visual examination of the spine. It is often associated with other conditions, necessitating a comprehensive analysis of its cause.

Therapeutic Management and Nursing Considerations

Exercises may be recommended for mild postural curves. The treatment for severe kyphosis is similar to the treatment for scoliosis. Because the two conditions are often found in the same child, treatment is directed toward both conditions. In children who have not yet reached skeletal maturity and whose curves are flexible, casting or bracing may be attempted first. For complex progressive curves, spinal fusion frequently becomes necessary.

Nursing care of the child with kyphosis, including home care, is based on the same principles as outlined for scoliosis management.

LORDOSIS

Lordosis is an exaggerated concave curvature of the spine, usually in the lumbar area, where a mild concave curve is normal. Occasionally it occurs in other areas of the spine, in which case it is not considered normal because it can compress vital organs, such as the heart and lungs, and may require immediate intervention.

Etiology and Incidence

Lumbar lordosis by itself is usually not severe enough to cause concern. It may, however, occur as a result of other defects, such as hip flexion contracture, muscular dystrophy, obesity, or DDH. Lordosis is a frequent complication of myelomeningocele and several other neuromuscular disorders (see Chapter 28).

The incidence of lordosis is variable and depends on the presence of associated conditions.

Manifestations and Diagnostic Evaluation

The clinical manifestations of lordosis include an exaggerated concave curve in the lumbar area, pain in the lower back, and an accompanying defect such as DDH, hip flexion contracture, or obesity.

A diagnosis of lordosis is confirmed by physical examination and radiographic studies.

Therapeutic Management and Nursing Considerations

Treatment for lordosis depends on its cause, but treatment modalities are based on the principles outlined for scoliosis management.

The nursing care for children with lordosis, including home care, is similar to that outlined for children with scoliosis. In addition, accompanying disorders must be monitored and treated concurrently.

KEY CONCEPTS

- Musculoskeletal problems are frequently caused by trauma. Therefore nursing assessment should always begin with the child's airway, breathing, and circulation.

- The cause of the musculoskeletal injury must be determined because nonaccidental trauma or child abuse may be involved.

- The neurovascular assessment of a child in traction or a cast includes assessment of skin color, capillary refill time, temperature, and sensation in the extremity. The quality of the pulse distal to the site should also be evaluated and compared with that of the uninvolved extremity.

- When evaluating neurovascular status, remember to assess for the five Ps of ischemia—pain, pallor, pulselessness, paresthesia, and paralysis.

- Commonly seen musculoskeletal developmental disorders include clubfoot, DDH, Legg-Calvé-Perthes disease, and slipped capital femoral epiphysis. Each often requires splinting, traction, bracing, casting, or a combination.

- Treatment for Legg-Calvé-Perthes disease maintains the femoral head in the acetabulum and protects the hip from the stress of weight bearing during the healing process.

- Nursing outcomes for the child with Legg-Calvé-Perthes disease include adherence to activity restrictions, facilitating home care and management of the appliance selected for treatment, and promoting age-appropriate cognitive and emotional development.

- In an open fracture (marked by a wound or break in the skin), the possibility of infection is increased.

- Treatment of fractures involves repositioning the bone fragments (reduction) and applying a cast or traction to maintain alignment (retention) until healing occurs.

- Treatment for Osgood-Schlatter disease is conservative and involves limiting activities that require bending or kneeling. These restrictions may interfere with the achievement of developmental milestones and may result in isolation and alienation.

- Nursing care of the child with Osgood-Schlatter disease involves promoting adherence to treatment recommendations, reassuring the child that the problem is self-limiting, and assisting the child to achieve age-appropriate developmental tasks.

- Osteogenesis imperfecta places the child at risk for pathologic fractures, bony deformities caused by bending and bowing of softened bones, and kyphoscoliosis.

- Nursing outcomes for the child with osteogenesis imperfecta include avoidance of injury, the development of healthy coping behaviors, and the maintenance of developmental integrity.

- Nursing care of the child with osteomyelitis includes assessment and documentation of the child's status, support and immobilization of the extremity, administration of antibiotics without iatrogenic injury, and careful monitoring of the infusion equipment and IV site.

- Therapeutic management of JA is supportive and directed toward preserving joint function, controlling the inflammatory process, minimizing deformity, and reducing the impact of the disease on the child's development.

- Nursing outcomes for a child with JA include keeping the child free from injury, controlling pain, enhancing physical mobility, and promoting age-appropriate developmental behaviors.

- Nursing outcomes for a child with muscular dystrophy include maintaining physical activity, promoting respiratory function, managing weight, and reducing the impact of the disease on the child's development.

- Scoliosis, kyphosis, and lordosis are spinal abnormalities that require long-term assessment and management. Each has the potential for altering a child's body image, so nursing interventions must address emotional as well as physical consequences of these disorders.

ANSWERS TO
CRITICAL THINKING EXERCISE 26-1

The following summary compares the three common hip disorders.

	DDH	Legg-Calvé-Perthes Disease	Slipped Capital Femoral Epiphysis
Age at onset	Infancy, early childhood	Preschool, young school age	Adolescence
Manifestations	Hip instability, as evidenced by positive Barlow and/or Ortolani signs; limp or waddling gait in the older child; limited abduction on affected side	Presence of synovitis and necrosis on radiographs; limp; intermittent knee or hip soreness; child small for age; limited internal rotation and abduction on affected side	Radiographic demonstration of slippage; limp; intermittent knee or thigh pain that worsens with exercise; child large for age; external rotation of the affected leg

Joint synovitis, or septic hip, is a condition that can span age groups. Hip pain and joint limitation are prominent manifestations. Pain is of more acute onset and may be accompanied by fever and laboratory signs of inflammation.

REFERENCES AND READINGS

Bicimoglu, A., Agus, H., Omeroglu, H., & Tumer, Y. (2003). Six years of experience with a new surgical algorithm in developmental dysplasia of the hip in children under 18 months of age *Journal of Pediatric Orthopaedics, 23*(6), 693-698.

Conn, J., Annest, J., & Gilchrist, J. (2005). Sports and recreation related injuries in the U.S. population, 1997-1999. *Injury Prevention, 9*(2), 117-124.

Connecticut Children's Medical Center (2005). *Slipped capital femoral epiphysis;* Retrieved June 1, 2005, from *www.ccmckids.org.*

Cummings, J., Davidson, R., Armstrong, P., & Lehman, W. (2002). Congenital clubfoot. *Journal of Bone and Joint Surgery, 84*(2), 290-309.

Dambro, M. R. (2005). *Griffith's 5 minute consult,* 13th ed. Philadelphia: Lippincott, Williams, & Wilkins.

DiFazio, R. (2003). Creating a halo traction wheelchair resource manual: using the EBP approach. *Journal of Pediatric Nursing, 18*(2), 148-152.

Dorn, U., & Neumann, D. (2005). Ultrasound for screening developmental dysplasia of the hip: a European perspective. *Current Opinion in Pediatrics, 17(1),* 30-33.

Fort, C. W. (2002). Getting a fix on long-bone fracture. *Nursing, 32*(6), HN1-HN4.

Gore, T., & Lacey, S. (2005). Bone up on fat embolism syndrome. *Nursing, 35*(8), 32HN1 – 32HN4.

Graham, M. V., & Uphold, C. R. (2003). *Clinical guidelines in child health.* Gainesville, FL: Barmarrae Books.

Grzegorzewski, A., Bowen, J., Guille, J., & Glutting, J. (2003). Treatment of the collapsed femoral head by containment in Legg-Calvé-Perthes Disease. *Journal of Pediatric Orthopaedics, 23(1),* 15-19.

Hay, W. W., Levin, M. J, Sondheimer, J. M., & Detarding, R. R. (2005). *Current pediatric diagnosis & treatment,* 17th ed. New York: McGraw-Hill.

Ilowite, N. (2002). Current treatment of juvenile rheumatoid arthritis. *Pediatrics, 109*(1), 109-115.

Joseph, B., Sreekumaran, N. N., Narasimha, R. K., Mulpuri, K., & Varghese, G. (2003). Optimal timing for containment surgery for Perthes disease. *Journal of Pediatric Orthopaedics, 23*(5), 601-606.

Kamath, S., & Bennet, G. C. (2004). Does developmental dysplasia of the hip cause a delay in walking? *Journal of Pediatric Orthopaedics, 24*(3), 265.

Labyak, S. E., Bourguignon, C., & Docherty, S. (2003). Sleep quality in children with juvenile rheumatoid arthritis. *Holistic Nursing Practice, 17*(4), 193-200.

Lampe, R. (2004). Osteomyelitis and suppurative arthritis. In R. Behrman, R. Kliegman, & H. Jenson (Eds.), *Nelson textbook of pediatrics* (17th ed., pp. 2297-2302). Philadelphia: Saunders.

Macias, C., Bothner, J., & Wiebe, R. (1998). A comparison of supination/flexion to hyperpronation in the reduction of radial head subluxations. *Pediatrics, 102*(1), e10.

Marini, J. (2004). Osteogenesis imperfecta. In R. Behrman, R. Kliegman, & H. Jenson (Eds.), *Nelson textbook of pediatrics* (17th ed., pp. 2336-2338). Philadelphia, PA: Saunders.

Marlowe, A. (2002). Testing for osteogenesis imperfecta in cases of suspected non-accidental injury. *Journal of Medical Genetics, 39*(6), 382-387.

Marni, J. F., Heeger, S., Lynch, K. A., & Decaro, K. R. (2003). Intravenous biphosphate therapy in children with osteogenesis imperfecta. *Pediatrics 111*(3), 573-578.

Mary, P., Damsin, J.-P., & Carlioz, H. (2004). Correction of equines in clubfoot: the contribution of arthrography. *Journal of Pediatric Orthopaedics, 24*(3), 312-316.

MDA USA. (2003). *101 FAQs.* Retrieved June 1, 2005, *www.mda.org.*

Metzl, J. (2002). Expectations of pediatric sport participation among pediatricians, patients, and parents. *Pediatric Clinics of North America, 49,* 497-504.

Miller, M., & Cassidy, J. (2004). Juvenile rheumatoid arthritis. In R. Behrman, R. Kliegman, & H. Jenson (Eds.), *Nelson textbook of pediatrics* (17th ed., pp. 799-805). Philadelphia: Saunders.

Newton, M., & Walker, J. (2004). Acute quadriceps injury: a case study. *Emergency Nurse, 12*(8), 24-29.

Podeszwa, D., Mooney, J. F., Cramer, K. E., & Mendelow, M. (2004). Comparison of Pavlik harness application and immediate spica casting for femur fractures in infants. *Journal of Pediatric Orthopaedics, 24*(5), 460-462.

Richards, B., Johnston, C., & Wilson, H. (2005). Nonoperative clubfoot treatment using the French physical therapy method. *Journal of Pediatric Orthopedics, 25*(1), 98-102.

Sarnat, H. (2004). Neuromuscular disorders. In R. Behrman, R. Kliegman, & H. Jenson (Eds.), *Nelson textbook of pediatrics* (17th ed., pp. 2060-2064). Philadelphia: Saunders.

Shah, S. (2002). The hip. In F. Burg, J. Ingelfinger, R. Polin, & A. Gershon (Eds.), *Gellis & Kagan's current pediatric therapy* (17th ed., p. 844). Philadelphia: Saunders.

Shannon, E. G., Difazio, R., Kasser, J., Karlin, L., & Gerbino, P. (2005). Waterproof casts for immobilization of children's fractures and sprains. *Journal of Pediatric Orthopaedics, 25*(1), 56-59.

Skinner, H. B. (2003). *Current diagnosis and treatment in orthopedics,* 3rd ed. New York: McGraw-Hill.

Song, K. M., Halliday, S., Reilly, C., & Keezel, W. (2004). Gait abnormalities following slipped capital femoral epiphysis. *Journal of Pediatric Orthopaedics, 24*(2), 148-155.

Thompson, G. H. (2004). Bone and joint disorders. In R. Behrman, R. Kliegman, & H. Jenson (Eds.), *Nelson textbook of pediatrics* (17th ed., pp. 2251-2297). Philadelphia: Saunders.

Wall, M. (2002). Orthopedic trauma. *RN, 65*(7), 52-57.

Wilkinson, N., Jackson, G., & Gardner-Medwin, J. (2003). Biologic therapies for juvenile arthritis. *Archives of Disease in Childhood, 88*(3), 186-191.

CHAPTER 27

The Child With an Endocrine or Metabolic Alteration

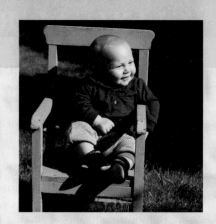

Learning Objectives

After studying this chapter, you should be able to:

- List the major hormones of the endocrine system.
- Describe negative feedback.
- Discuss nursing strategies to improve adherence with medication administration.
- Discuss and describe endocrine problems seen in the neonate.
- Describe the signs and symptoms of hypothyroidism versus hyperthyroidism.
- Compare and contrast diabetes insipidus and syndrome of inappropriate antidiuretic hormone as they relate to fluid and electrolyte balance.
- Describe the psychosocial issues concerning children with precocious puberty.
- Identify the role of insulin in the metabolism of carbohydrates, fats, and proteins in both the fasting and postprandial states.

- Compare and contrast type 1 diabetes mellitus and type 2 diabetes mellitus.
- Identify management goals and nursing implications of insulin therapy, diet therapy, exercise, self-monitoring of blood glucose, and urine ketone monitoring in the care of the child with type 1 diabetes.
- Describe the signs, symptoms, causes, and treatment of hypoglycemia and hyperglycemia in the child with diabetes.
- Identify the pathophysiology of diabetic ketoacidosis, and describe the management and nursing care of the child in diabetic ketoacidosis.
- Identify management goals and nursing implications of medication, diet therapy, exercise, and self-monitoring of blood glucose in the care of the child with type 2 diabetes.

Definitions

beta cells Specialized cells in the pancreas that manufacture and secrete insulin; thought to be the target of the autoimmune destructive process of type 1 diabetes mellitus.

diabetic ketoacidosis Metabolic consequence of severe insulin deficiency; marked by hyperglycemia, acidosis, and ketosis.

euthyroid Normal thyroid function.

gland An organ or structure that secretes a substance or hormone to be used in another part of the body.

glucagon A hormone produced by the alpha cells of the pancreas; counteracts the action of insulin by converting liver stores of glycogen to blood glucose, resulting in an elevation of the blood glucose concentration.

glucose The substrate of choice for cellular energy; the breakdown product of stored glycogen or dietary carbohydrate.

glycosuria Glucose in urine that occurs when the blood glucose level exceeds the renal threshold and glucose "spills" into the urine.

glycosylated hemoglobin A laboratory test used to evaluate long-term blood glucose control by measuring glycosylation (glucose attachment to a protein) of a portion of the hemoglobin molecule in red blood cells; offers a 3-month average of blood glucose control.

honeymoon phase An early stage of diabetes characterized by residual endogenous insulin production that results in a lower need for exogenous insulin to maintain normal blood glucose.

hormone A chemical substance produced by one gland or tissue and transported by the blood to other tissues or organs, where it causes a specific effect.

hyperglycemia Blood glucose in a diabetic child above the target range; in a nondiabetic child, fasting blood glucose of 110 mg/dL or higher.

hyperkalemia Elevated serum potassium level above the range for age.

hypoglycemia Blood glucose levels less than 70 mg/dL.

Continued

REVIEW OF THE ENDOCRINE SYSTEM

The endocrine system is composed of various tissues that produce and secrete chemicals called *hormones*. The hormones stimulate and regulate the actions of other tissues—the target tissues.

The endocrine system and the autonomic nervous system function in tandem to regulate growth, metabolism, and reproduction. The hypothalamic-pituitary axis controls their activities. The autonomic nervous system reacts to a stimulus, transmitting its message to the hypothalamus. In turn, the hypothalamus manufactures and secretes the appropriate hormonal factors. These are transmitted to the anterior pituitary gland, which then stimulates or inhibits the release of the involved hormones.

The principle of feedback control is involved in hormone production and secretion. In negative feedback, increasing levels of a specific hormone begin to inhibit the system responsible for releasing that hormone. As the hormonal secretion rises, the secretion and production of its stimulating hormone decrease. Conversely, when too little circulating hormone is present, the target gland is stimulated to secrete additional hormone.

The pituitary gland is composed of an anterior lobe and a posterior lobe. The anterior lobe secretes adrenocorticotropic hormone (ACTH), thyroid-stimulating hormone (TSH), follicle-stimulating hormone (FSH), luteinizing hormone (LH), growth hormone (GH), and prolactin. Four of these hormones (ACTH, TSH, LH, FSH) in turn stimulate their target glands to secrete the appropriate specific hormones. The posterior pituitary lobe stores and releases antidiuretic hormone (ADH) and oxytocin, which are synthesized by the hypothalamus.

Congenital malformations, infections, and neoplastic or autoimmune processes may disrupt normal endocrine function at the hypothalamus, pituitary gland, or target gland.

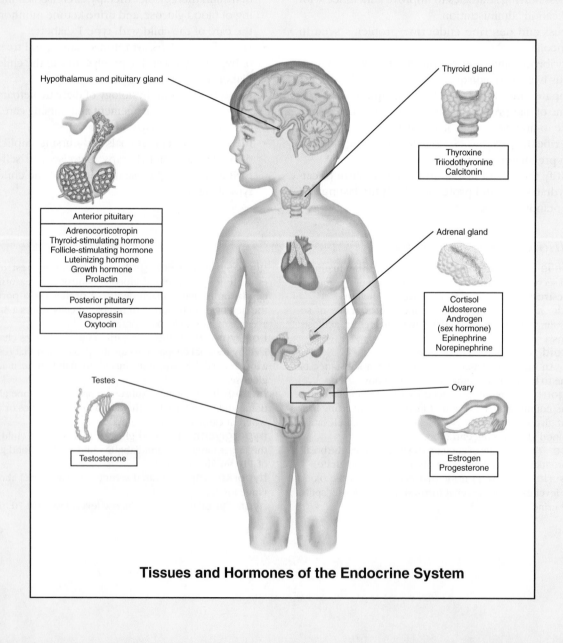

Tissues and Hormones of the Endocrine System

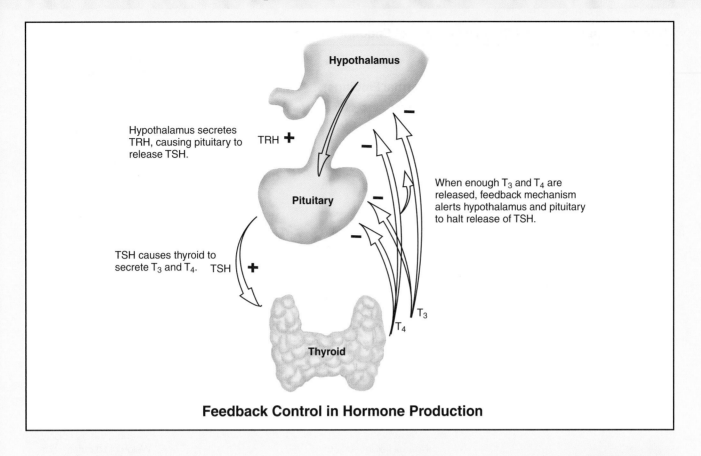

Hypothalamus

Hypothalamus secretes TRH, causing pituitary to release TSH.

TRH **+**

Pituitary

When enough T_3 and T_4 are released, feedback mechanism alerts hypothalamus and pituitary to halt release of TSH.

TSH causes thyroid to secrete T_3 and T_4. TSH **+**

T_3
T_4

Thyroid

Feedback Control in Hormone Production

PEDIATRIC DIFFERENCES IN THE ENDOCRINE SYSTEM

- The endocrine system is less developed at birth than any other body system.
- Hormonal control of many body functions is lacking until 12 to 18 months of age. As a result, infants may manifest imbalances in concentration of fluids, electrolytes, amino acids, glucose, and trace substances.

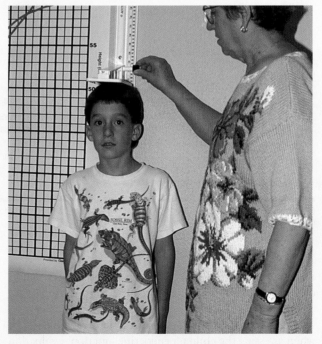

Fetal endocrine systems develop and function in utero. Portions of the endocrine system may be immature at birth but transition to more mature function after delivery.

DIAGNOSTIC TESTS AND PROCEDURES

Diagnosing endocrine dysfunction usually involves laboratory testing. Serum hormone levels are measured to determine if the amounts are adequate, deficient, or excessive. Laboratory screening is useful for diagnosing disease and monitoring children on hormone therapy.

Normal hormone levels are related to the child's age and stage of puberty. Because hormones are secreted at various times during the day or on a circadian rhythm, random blood samples may be difficult to interpret. Stimulation testing frequently demonstrates more accurate and definitive test results. With stimulation testing, a releasing factor or other agent is given to trigger the release or inhibition of a specific hormone. Serial blood sampling identifies the peak or trough

level of the hormone, aiding in more accurate interpretation. A list of the common stimulation studies is provided in the table.

Other diagnostic tests include radiography and imaging techniques. Bone age radiographs can determine bone maturation, and from this, growth potential can be determined. Computed tomography (CT) scans and magnetic resonance

Common Laboratory and Diagnostic Tests of Endocrine Function

Test	Description	Normal Findings	Indications	Preparation and Nursing Considerations
GH test	An agent (e.g., insulin, arginine, clonidine) is given to stimulate release of GH.	One or more peak levels of GH >7-10 ng/mL.	Evaluate GH production. Identify GH deficiency.	Time specific; specimens must be drawn accurately. NPO after midnight. Notify physician if hypoglycemia or hypotension develops.
Cortrosyn test	Cortrosyn (ACTH) is given after baseline laboratory values have been obtained and 1 hr later. Tests adrenal gland's ability to function.	Cortisol should rise at least double the baseline. Cortisol <18 μg/dL suggests adrenal insufficiency.	Evaluate adrenal production of cortisol. Identify infants with CAH.	Time specific; laboratory samples must be drawn before and 1 hr after Cortrosyn.
Factrel (gonadorelin) test	GnRH is administered IV or subcutaneously to test the pituitary-ovarian axis for central precocious puberty.	For IV test, <4-fold to 5-fold rise in LH is observed. For subcutaneous test, LH rises <8 ng/mL.	Evaluate for central precocious puberty. Identify premature thelarche.	Time specific; specimens must be drawn accurately. IV test with serial sampling of LH, FSH. Subcutaneous test with one laboratory sample drawn at 40 min.
Water-deprivation test	Child deprived of water and fluids for 7-8 hr.	Decreased urine output. Increased urine specific gravity. Normal serum sodium and osmolality.	Confirm diagnosis of diabetes insipidus.	Strict monitoring of serum sodium and serum and urine osmolality. Weigh child before, during, and after test. Stop test if significant weight loss or change in vital signs or neurologic status develops.
hCG test	Intramuscular hCG is administered serially to stimulate testicular production of testosterone. Allows test for conversion of testosterone to DHT. Tests function of undescended testes.	Low levels of testosterone and DHT in prelaboratory samples. Elevated levels of both testosterone and DHT—compare with known standards.	Confirm testicular insufficiency. Confirm 5-alpha-reductase deficiency. Undescended testes may descend.	Time specific; draw samples before and after hCG. Monitor for testicular descent and increase in phallic length.

GH, Growth hormone; *ACTH,* adrenocorticotropic hormone; *GnRH,* gonadotropin-releasing hormone; *LH,* leutinizing hormone; *FSH,* follicle stimulating hormone; *hCG,* Human chorionic gonadotropin; *DHT,* dihydrotestosterone.

imaging (MRI) are used to determine the presence of tumors or congenital malformations affecting the hypothalamus, pituitary, or target glands.

Accurate measurements of height and weight are essential when assessing the child for endocrine function. Evaluation of sexual development according to Tanner stages is also a part of the diagnostic workup (see Chapter 8). Developmental milestones and school performance should also be monitored because delays may be associated with endocrine disorders.

Definitions—cont'd

hypothalamus   Portion of the brain that secretes releasing factors to the pituitary gland for the maintenance of endocrine and metabolic activities.

idiopathic   For unknown reasons.

ketone, ketoacid   An acid produced in response to starvation (in the diabetic child, a result of insulin deficiency); produced from fat stores, which can be used for energy by some tissues when glucose is unavailable.

Kussmaul respiration   Deep, rapid respiration seen with diabetic ketoacidosis in which carbon dioxide is expelled as a respiratory compensation for acidosis; also described as "air hunger."

pituitary   An endocrine gland attached to the base of the brain that secretes numerous hormones, including thyroid-stimulating hormone, growth hormone, adrenocorticotropic hormone, antidiuretic hormone, prolactin, luteinizing hormone, and follicle-stimulating hormone.

Electronic Resources

Additional information related to the content in Chapter 27 can be found on:

the interactive companion CD-ROM

- Animation: Adrenal Function
- Audio Glossary
- NCLEX Review Questions

or the companion website at *evolve*
http://evolve.elsevier.com/james/ncoc

- Common Pediatric Laboratory Tests and Normal Values
- NCLEX Review Questions
- Resources for Health Care Providers and Families
- WebLinks

Pediatric endocrine disorders are generally managed in the outpatient setting. Most endocrine disorders are chronic conditions requiring long-term nursing management. The nurse assumes a role of both educator and advocate for the child. Also important for the care of children with chronic medical problems is a careful psychosocial evaluation on a regular basis.

NEONATAL HYPOGLYCEMIA

Hypoglycemia is an abnormally low level of glucose (sugar) in the blood. It can result from an excessive rate of removal of glucose from the blood or from decreased secretion of glucose into the blood. Hypoglycemia in the neonate is defined as a plasma glucose concentration of less than 40 mg/dL.

Etiology

Box 27-1 lists risk factors for hypoglycemia in the neonate. Hypoglycemia in some neonates results from hyperinsulinism, a genetic defect that affects beta-cell regulation of insulin secretion (Sperling, 2004). Postterm and large-for-gestational-age (LGA) neonates are at higher risk than the appropriate-for-gestational-age (AGA) term infant, but the neonates who are most likely to have hypoglycemia are premature infants and infants who are small for gestational age (SGA). The SGA infant has a higher risk for hypoglycemia because of lower glycogen stores, decreased muscle protein, and decreased body fat (Sperling, 2004).

Incidence

The incidence of hypoglycemia varies with the infant's gestational age at birth and appropriateness of growth. In general, the incidence is 1.3 to 3 in 1000 live births (Cranmer & Shannon, 2005). The incidence is much higher in SGA infants.

Manifestations

Many infants with hypoglycemia are asymptomatic and are diagnosed because risk factors in their history have prompted glucose monitoring. The symptomatic neonate may demonstrate jitteriness, poor feeding, lethargy, seizures, respiratory alterations including apnea, hypotonia, high-pitched cry, bradycardia, cyanosis, and temperature instability.

BOX 27-1	**Risk Factors for Hypoglycemia in the Neonate**

Transient Neonatal Hypoglycemia
Severe respiratory distress
Asphyxia or other birth stress
Prematurity
SGA Infant (<2,500 g)
Maternal toxemia
Infant with Rh incompatibility
Infant of a diabetic mother

Persistent Neonatal Hypoglycemia
Adrenal insufficiency
Hyperinsulinism
Family history of hypoglycemia
Pancreatic tumor

Underlying Disorders
Sepsis
Inborn errors of metabolism
Maternal propranolol use
Other maternal medication use (ritodrine, terbutaline)

Data from Cranmer, H., & Shannon, M. (2005). *Pediatrics, hypoglycemia.* Retrieved June 2, 2005, from *www.emedicine.com/emerg/topic384.htm.*

PATHOPHYSIOLOGY

NEONATAL HYPOGLYCEMIA

Glucose is the major source of energy for the fetus and is transported from the mother across the placenta to the fetus. This glucose is used to support the rapid growth taking place. In the last weeks of gestation, excess glucose is stored in the liver and skeletal muscle as glycogen or converted to fatty acids and then stored as triglycerides in fat cells. Insulin is not transported across the placenta, requiring the fetus to produce insulin.

At delivery, this glucose supply ceases, and infants must depend on their own hepatic glycogen stores and glucoregulatory mechanism to mobilize and use glucose. With the steady source of glucose stopped by the clamping of the umbilical cord, neonates undergo a decrease in glucose concentration, reaching a nadir (lowest level) at 1 to 3 hours of postnatal age.

The neonate's requirement for glucose is relatively high because of several factors. High energy needs postnatally result from increased metabolic and motor activity. The larger brain in proportion to body size requires glucose as its fuel source. Access to glucose is limited because of the neonate's immature liver enzyme system, including a decreased response to glucagon, the hormone that promotes the release of glucose from glycogen stores.

Diagnostic Evaluation

Neonates who demonstrate risk factors for hypoglycemia are screened. A blood glucose concentration can be determined by a laboratory chemical test. Although this method is the most accurate, it is lengthy. For this reason, screening tests are used in most nurseries even though the results can vary. A blood glucose monitor is used to test a drop of blood, which can be obtained by a heel stick. Severely low readings are often verified by laboratory determinations, but intervention is initiated before the results are available because of the potential for sequelae from prolonged hypoglycemia. Urinalysis may be performed to test for ketones, which are not present if the infant has hyperinsulinism. Other tests may be done to rule out underlying metabolic disorders.

Therapeutic Management

Infants who are hypoglycemic but asymptomatic may be fed breast milk, formula or dextrose 5% in water. Frequent glucose checks are needed to monitor response. Neonates who are lethargic and not interested in nipple feeding can be gavage fed. If the blood glucose level is less than 20 to 25 mg/dL, intravenous (IV) glucose is given, first by bolus (dextrose 10% in water, 2.5 mL/kg) and then by continuous drip. The goal is to maintain the blood glucose in the range of 50 mg/dL or greater (Cranmer & Shannon, 2005).

In some cases of intractable hypoglycemia, steroids may be used to stimulate gluconeogenesis from noncarbohydrate sources. Diazoxide may be given to suppress pancreatic insulin secretion in infants with hyperinsulinism.

Nursing Considerations

The assessment begins at the time of birth. Risk factors such as maternal diabetes, sepsis, shock, or perinatal asphyxia alert the caretaker that the infant may be at risk for hypoglycemia. Determination is also made of gestational age and appropriateness of growth. Delays in enteral feedings or in the initiation of IV fluids also place the infant at higher risk. Inappropriate behavior or changes in behavior, including commonly associated clinical signs and symptoms, are monitored.

The nurse monitors for signs and symptoms of hypoglycemia, keeping in mind that infants may be asymptomatic. Infants at risk should be identified by obtaining a complete perinatal history to identify factors such as maternal hypertension, maternal diabetes, fetal distress, intrauterine growth retardation, or perinatal asphyxia.

Because preterm, LGA, and SGA infants are at increased risk for hypoglycemia, a gestational-age assessment should be performed. The infant's weight, length, and head circumference should be plotted on a growth curve to determine appropriateness of growth.

If an infant is at risk, a blood glucose level should be obtained with a screening strip (e.g., Dextrostix, Chemstrip bG) by 2 hours of age. Clean the puncture site with an appropriate antiseptic solution and allow it to dry before the puncture (see Chapter 13). Blood glucose levels of less than 60 mg/dL should be reported.

Enteral feedings should be provided by nipple or gavage if required. The compromised infant may be unable to nipple feed safely as a result of respiratory distress or lethargy. Monitor IV sites for signs of infiltration and treat IV infiltrates with hyaluronidase because glucose infiltration can cause severe extravasation.

Because hypothermia increases glucose requirements, decrease the risk of hypoglycemia by providing the infant with a neutral thermal environment. If signs and symptoms persist, notify the physician according to nursery protocol. Persistent hypoglycemia requires extensive medical evaluation and treatment.

HYPOCALCEMIA

Hypocalcemia results from inadequate stores of calcium, ineffective calcium homeostasis because of immature hormonal control, the inability to mobilize calcium, or interference with calcium usage. Neonatal hypocalcemia is defined as total serum calcium concentration of less than 7.0 mg/dL. Neonatal hypocalcemia occurs most often in infants of diabetic mothers because maternal diabetes causes functional hypoparathyroidism in the neonate (Greenbaum, 2004). Other causes include birth asphyxia and SGA.

Neonates may experience twitching or tremors, irritability, jitteriness, electrocardiogram (ECG) changes and, rarely, seizures. Some infants are asymptomatic but are screened because of history.

Ionized serum calcium levels are measured. Normal levels for blood ionized calcium range from 4.8 to 5.2 mg/dL. Initiation of feedings is often the only treatment necessary to correct early hypocalcemia. In infants who are limited in their enteral intake or who have significant hypocalcemia, therapy includes both oral and parenteral calcium administration. Oral supplements are given with enteral feedings. IV supplementation may be given as bolus doses or continuous infusion with IV fluids. If oral calcium is ordered, give the medication with enteral feedings because it may cause gastric irritation. The IV site should be observed for signs of infiltration, and hyaluronidase is used to treat infiltrates. Extravasation of calcium-containing fluid can produce necrosis and ulceration. Many medications precipitate with calcium ions and should not be mixed together in IV lines. Do not mix calcium with sodium bicarbonate because this combination also will form a precipitate in IV fluids. Persistent hypocalcemia requires further diagnostic evaluation.

PHENYLKETONURIA

Phenylketonuria (PKU) is a genetic metabolic disorder that results in central nervous system (CNS) damage from toxic levels of phenylalanine in the blood. PKU is characterized by a deficiency of phenylalanine hydroxylase, the enzyme needed to convert phenylalanine to tyrosine.

Etiology

PKU is an autosomal recessive disorder and is manifested only in the homozygote (individual who inherited two identical genes for a specific trait). With both parents carrying the recessive gene, each pregnancy has a 25% chance that the child will have PKU.

Incidence

PKU occurs in approximately 1 in 15,000 births in the United States (Arnold, 2003). It is more prevalent in some European countries.

Manifestations

The underlying metabolic alterations begin to have an immediate effect on the infant, although signs may not be apparent until the infant is approximately 3 months old. The first sign may be digestive problems with vomiting. These infants also may have a musty or mousy odor to the urine, infantile eczema, hypertonia, and hyperactive behavior. Older children may have hypopigmentation of the hair, skin, and irises, and they are commonly blond with light blue eyes. Mental retardation is a long-term consequence of untreated PKU.

Diagnostic Evaluation

Routine neonatal screening for PKU is mandatory in all 50 states of the United States. With early postpartum discharge, screening is often performed at less than 2 days of age because of the concern that the infant will be lost to follow-up. Because the test depends on the accumulation of phenylalanine, screening done before the third day of life has a higher risk of a false-negative outcome. For this reason, testing should be done after the infant is 48 hours old or, if done earlier, the test should be repeated at several days of age. Small quantities of blood are collected on filter paper cards. Screening is done by bacterial inhibition (Guthrie test) or chromatographic or fluorometric assays. A positive result is not diagnostic but indicates which infants should be evaluated further. PKU is characterized by serum phenylalanine levels greater than 20 mg/dL (normal level <2 mg/dL) (Arnold, 2003).

Therapeutic Management

Treatment should be instituted as soon as the diagnosis is confirmed because the best results are obtained with early treatment. Infants and children with PKU are treated with a special diet that restricts phenylalanine intake. Phenylalanine tolerance varies according to the infant and the severity of the enzyme deficiency. The goal of therapy is to keep the serum phenylalanine level at 2 to 6 mg/dL in infants and young children and 2 to 15 mg/dL in children older than 12 years. Phenylalanine intake should be limited while providing enough to meet the body's growth requirement of this essential amino acid. Dietary management must be started early in neonatal life because the untreated infant will show evidence of CNS damage by several weeks of age. The age at which the diet may be discontinued is a point of controversy. Most health care facilities in the United States recommend lifelong continuation of the diet (Arnold, 2003).

Another consideration is women with the disorder who become pregnant. Adolescent girls require counseling about fetal risks, which can include mental deficiency, microcephaly, retarded growth, seizures, and an increased incidence of structural defects. The goal is to control phenylalanine levels before conception and maintain strict control during the pregnancy.

Nursing Considerations

Although a family history of PKU would alert the caregiver to an infant at risk, most infants with PKU are not identified at birth. Neonatal symptoms are usually not present. A screening test, part of the newborn screen done in all states, is the first diagnostic procedure. Newborn screenings usually include testing for PKU and congenital hypothyroidism as well as

---

> ### PATHOPHYSIOLOGY
>
> #### PHENYLKETONURIA
>
> Phenylketonuria (PKU) refers to a group of biochemical diseases associated with enzymatic blocks in the conversion of the essential amino acid *phenylalanine* to *tyrosine*. Classic PKU consists of the absence of the enzyme *phenylalanine hydroxylase*. This deficiency results in the toxic accumulation of phenylalanine in the bloodstream after the ingestion of protein containing phenylalanine. Phenylalanine can adversely affect the myelinization process in CNS development. Most of that process takes place during the first decade of life. Mental retardation occurs and progresses if treatment is not implemented.

any other screening tests mandated by local and state public health departments, such as sickle cell trait, galactosemia, and maple syrup urine disease. A positive screening result requires further diagnostic evaluation to verify the diagnosis.

A low-phenylalanine diet is begun immediately. The infant is fed with low-phenylalanine formula and, as foods are introduced, the child must follow a protein-restricted diet. The child must avoid high-protein foods such as meats, fish, eggs, cheese, milk, and legumes. Because protein is also present in grains, low-protein breads, cereals, and pastas are used. Dietary staples are vegetables, fruits, and starches. To avoid the consequences of insufficient protein for growth, children with PKU may take a phenylalanine-free protein supplement. The growth pattern and neurobehavior of the affected child must be followed.

Follow-up is provided for all infants if the initial screening result is abnormal. The nurse assists with referral to a genetic center that is capable of diagnosing and treating the infant. Phenylalanine requirements change rapidly in the first months of life. Encourage parental adherence to monitoring requirements for the infant diagnosed with PKU. Rigid regimens for diet control will not be successful unless the family accepts the changes required. Help the family deal with lifestyle changes by initiating referrals as needed (e.g., to social service agencies, registered dietitian, support groups). Online support groups and chat rooms provide helpful ideas for adapting recipes; specialized cookbooks are also available.

Encourage the parents to express their feelings about the infant's diagnosis and the risk of PKU in future children. Help family members recognize the problems caused by the disease and identify strategies for dealing with the stress of having a child with a chronic illness. Physical measurements and neurologic and intellectual development should be documented through standardized testing. If good control is established early, normal infant growth and development should occur.

INBORN ERRORS OF METABOLISM

Rarely, infants are born with other genetically transmitted metabolic diseases (Table 27-1). Nurses should create a climate in which parents can express their feelings about the lifelong care of their child as well as concerns for future pregnancies. Families with affected infants are referred to genetic counseling centers. Many of these infants are identified through universal newborn screening or screening specific for at-risk infants. Additional nursing care is related specifically to the disorder but is similar to that for the child with PKU.

TABLE 27-1   Inborn Errors of Metabolism

Condition	Description	Management
Galactosemia	A deficiency of galactose-1-phosphate uridyltransferase prevents the conversion of galactose to glucose in lactose digestion. Infants cannot properly digest milk or sugar. Although rare (1 in 40,000 to 60,000 live births), infants exhibit intrauterine growth retardation, hypotonia, liver damage, cataracts, and infections. The urine contains reducing substances. Vomiting and diarrhea occur after feedings.	The child is on a lifelong lactose-restricted diet and close monitoring for and treatment of infections. If untreated, the infant usually dies; infants who have been treated may have developmental or learning deficits. The condition is genetically transmitted through an autosomal recessive inheritance pattern; referral to a genetic counseling center is warranted.
Maple syrup urine disease	This is a very rare (1 in 250,000 to 300,000 live births) autosomal recessive inherited condition that affects metabolism of certain amino acids. Buildup of acids causes ketoacidosis, which appears 48-72 hr after birth. The infant is lethargic and can display poor feeding, vomiting, weight loss, seizures, and loss of reflexes. The urine smells like maple syrup.	Dialysis is needed to reduce accumulated acids. The child must be on a lifelong low-protein, limited–amino acid diet. If untreated, the child can die quickly; children who have been treated can have neurologic deficits. Referral to a genetic counseling center is warranted.
Tay-Sachs disease	A genetic condition that affects primarily infants in the Ashkenazi Jewish population. It is caused by an abnormal buildup of gangliosides (normal constituents in nerve synapse membrane) in the neurons. After a 6-mo period of relatively normal development, the infant begins to demonstrate developmental delay and progressive neurologic deterioration. The infant usually exhibits macrocephaly, seizures, blindness, and deafness; death occurs during early childhood.	Management is symptomatic and supportive to the child and family. Referral to a genetic counseling center is essential.

Modified from Behrman, R., Kliegman, R., & Jenson, H. (Eds.) (2004). *Nelson textbook of pediatrics* (17th ed., pp. 409-411; pp. 475-476; pp. 2030-2031). Philadelphia: Saunders.

CONGENITAL ADRENAL HYPERPLASIA

Congenital adrenal hyperplasia (CAH) is a group of disorders in which the adrenal gland is not able to manufacture adequate glucocorticoid and, while working to make glucocorticoid, produces excess androgens. CAH is caused by a defect in the enzymatic pathway of adrenal steroid production. Diminished glucocorticoid production prompts increased ACTH production, further increasing adrenal androgen excess.

Mineralocorticoid production may be normal or low. Infants with diminished mineralocorticoid production will waste salt through the kidneys, resulting in a "salt-wasting" crisis. Salt-wasting crisis results in hypovolemia, low serum sodium levels, and hyperkalemia. Several enzymatic defects have been identified, the most common being 21-hydroxylase deficiency. CAH is an autosomal recessive condition.

Manifestations

CAH is marked by ambiguous genitalia of the newborn female infant; postnatal virilization in both sexes; and salt-wasting crisis (in the first few weeks of life) with low serum sodium, high serum potassium, hypovolemia, and hypotensive crisis. Simple virilizing CAH is not associated with a salt-wasting crisis and presents with a muscular body, advanced bone age, and premature pubic hair. Typically this form presents later in infancy or early childhood. Untreated or poorly treated CAH can result in an advanced bone age with ultimate adult short stature. A milder form of CAH, 3-beta-hydroxysteroid dehydrogenase (3β-HSD), may present in childhood or adolescence with hirsutism, menstrual irregularities, or delayed menses.

Diagnostic Evaluation

The finding of ambiguous genitalia in the newborn infant should raise the possibility of CAH. The diagnosis is confirmed by elevated values of 17-hydroxyprogesterone, a glucocorticoid precursor. CAH is a part of newborn screening in many states. Appropriate evaluation including electrolytes, carbon dioxide level, and physical examination may avert a salt-wasting crisis. Serum sodium levels in the infant suspected of CAH will be low, with elevated serum potassium. Serum renin levels will be elevated, indicating mineralocorticoid deficiency. A karyotype to determine genetic sex may be indicated depending on the degree of genital ambiguity.

Therapeutic Management

Treatment for the child with CAH involves lifelong glucocorticoid therapy. Oral glucocorticoid (hydrocortisone acetate, cortisone acetate) dosage is prescribed on the basis of body size and is given two or three times per day in either liquid suspension or tablet form. For children with salt-wasting CAH, mineralocorticoid replacement is required. Fludrocortisone acetate (Florinef) is prescribed to be taken once or twice daily. Therapy is evaluated with serum electrolytes, 17-hydroxyprogesterone levels, and renin levels if mineralocorticoid replacement therapy is required. Special sick-day instructions should be provided to the family. The glucocorticoid dosage is usually doubled or tripled when the child is ill, has a broken bone, or is undergoing a surgical procedure. Bone age radiographs are performed yearly to assess skeletal maturity; poor adherence or undertreatment results in advanced bone age and will decrease final height.

Nursing Considerations

All newborn girls should be assessed for ambiguous genitalia: fused labia, enlarged clitoris, or migration of urethral opening. Infant boys with unexplained dehydration and low serum sodium levels should be considered to have adrenal insufficiency, which requires careful assessment of fluid and electrolyte status.

Infant girls with ambiguous genitalia might require reconstructive surgery. Depending on degree of virilization, surgical correction may be recommended in infancy or in early puberty. If appropriate, reassure parents that the infant has appropriate internal structures and that external structures can be corrected surgically. Allow them to express any concerns and encourage parent-infant attachment.

Assess older children receiving glucocorticoid replacement therapy for growth and signs of early puberty. Nonadherence can cause early virilization, increased growth velocity, diminished final adult height, and menstrual irregularities in girls. Blood pressure monitoring is important for children receiving mineralocorticoid replacement therapy.

CRITICAL TO REMEMBER
Congenital Adrenal Hyperplasia

- Children with salt-wasting congenital adrenal hyperplasia (CAH) require glucocorticoid replacement to survive.
- In the event of significant stress, such as fever, broken bone, or surgery, children with CAH will require "stress dose" medical therapy.
- If the child with CAH begins to vomit, the glucocorticoid must be administered parenterally.
- Mineralocorticoid therapy is required in salt-wasting CAH.
- Supplemental sodium occasionally may also be required.

Instruct parents about replacement hormone administration and the timing of medication. Develop a plan for sick-day dosage of medication. The infant with salt-wasting CAH may require salt supplements; the family needs instruction on preparation of the supplement.

Follow-up evaluations with the endocrinologist are scheduled every 2 to 3 months in infancy and every 4 to 6 months in the older child. Parents of the child with CAH should be referred to a genetics counselor if they plan more pregnancies because future children are at risk for CAH. In utero treatment is available to prevent virilization of the female fetus. This eliminates the need for surgical correction of ambiguous genitalia in the affected female infant.

Encourage the adolescent to assume increasing responsibility for medication administration. Emphasize the importance of adherence. Surgical genital reconstruction and vaginal dilation may be required in the adolescent years. Careful explanations of procedures reassure affected adolescents that they are "normal."

CONGENITAL HYPOTHYROIDISM

Congenital hypothyroidism is a condition in which the thyroid gland does not produce sufficient thyroid hormone to meet the body's metabolic needs. The condition is present from birth and, if not treated, can lead to mental retardation.

Etiology

Congenital hypothyroidism is caused by an absent (aplastic), underdeveloped, or ectopic thyroid gland. This group of congenital defects is referred to as *thyroid dysgenesis*. For unknown reasons, the fetal thyroid gland fails to develop properly or fails to migrate to the appropriate location. Other rare causes are hypothalamic or pituitary disorders in which TSH is insufficient to stimulate the thyroid gland. Biochemical defects in thyroid hormone production also cause congenital hypothyroidism. Maternal intake of medications such as propylthiouracil (PTU) during pregnancy to control maternal hyperthyroidism can cause transient hypothyroidism in the infant. Transfer of maternal antibodies to the fetus may also cause transient hypothyroidism (Bourgeois & Varma, 2004).

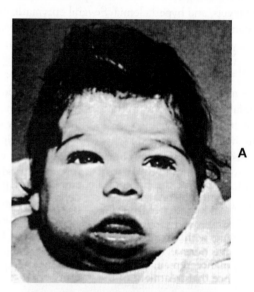

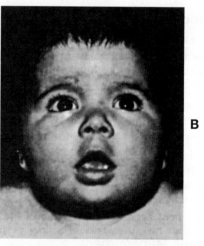

FIG 27-1   **A, This untreated 6-month-old infant with congenital hypothyroidism fed poorly and was constipated. She was lethargic and had no social smile or head control. Note her puffy face, large tongue, dull expression, and hirsute forehead. B, The same infant 4 months after treatment. Note the decreased facial puffiness, decreased hirsutism of the forehead, and an alert appearance. Newborn screening for hypothyroidism is important because treatment should begin in the first weeks of life to prevent mental retardation and other problems. Treatment consists of lifelong thyroid hormone replacement.**   *(From Behrman, R. E., Kliegman, R. M., & Jenson, H. B. [2004]. Nelson textbook of pediatrics [17th ed., p. 1876]. Philadelphia: Saunders.)*

PATHOPHYSIOLOGY

CONGENITAL HYPOTHYROIDISM

The thyroid gland is a butterfly-shaped gland located in front of the neck. TSH, secreted by the pituitary, induces the thyroid to produce T_4 and T_3. The thyroid traps iodine and produces T_4, which is essential for normal growth and development, especially brain development, in the first 2 years of life. Immediately after delivery, TSH increases dramatically, likely related to the stress of the birth process. Within the first week of life, the TSH level gradually falls.

Underdevelopment of the thyroid gland or a hypothalamic or pituitary disorder causes inadequate production of T_4, which is essential for brain development. If not treated, this can cause mental retardation in the developing child. An infant with congenital hypothyroidism has elevated TSH and low T_4 levels.

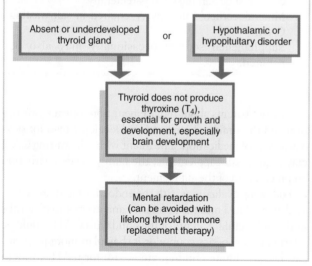

Incidence

The incidence of congenital hypothyroidism in the United States is approximately 1 in 4000 live births (Bourgeois & Varma, 2004). Because untreated hypothyroidism causes mental retardation, all states have mandatory newborn screening programs to diagnose hypothyroidism before symptoms occur. Early detection and treatment favor increased intellectual function. Most occurrences are spontaneous, with a smaller percentage having a genetic (autosomal recessive) inheritance that results in defective thyroxine synthesis (Bourgeois & Varma, 2004).

Manifestations

The infant with congenital hypothyroidism may display the following signs (Fig. 27-1): skin mottling, a large fontanel, a large tongue, hypotonia, slow reflexes, and a distended abdomen. Other signs and symptoms include prolonged jaundice, lethargy, constipation, feeding problems, coldness to touch, umbilical hernia, hoarse cry, and excessive sleeping. The infant with congenital hypothyroidism may have none of these signs or symptoms; screening is essential to recognize these infants.

Diagnostic Evaluation

Congenital hypothyroidism is usually diagnosed by newborn screening. Ideally, testing should be performed at 2 to 6 days of age. Tests performed sooner than 48 hours after delivery may be falsely interpreted because of the rise in TSH immediately after birth as part of the normal newborn transition.

Thyroid scans can identify any functioning thyroid tissue. Treatment should never be delayed while waiting for scan results.

Therapeutic Management

Treatment of children with congenital hypothyroidism consists of lifelong thyroid hormone replacement, usually in the form of levothyroxine. It is given as a single daily oral dose that varies with weight and age (Bourgeois & Varma, 2004). The dosage is titrated to maintain TSH and thyroxine (T_4) in a normal range.

NURSING CARE

The Infant With Congenital Hypothyroidism

Assessment

Nursing care of the infant with congenital hypothyroidism involves assessing growth and development and ensuring adherence to the prescribed medication regimen. Nurses can play a major role in recognizing the infant with hypothyroidism. Mental retardation caused by untreated hypothyroidism cannot be reversed, but it can be prevented through early identification and proper treatment. In general, infants with hypothyroidism are evaluated every 1 to 2 months for the first year of life and then every 3 to 6 months thereafter.

The nurse should obtain accurate measurements of height, weight, and head circumference at each visit. Frequent developmental assessments are also essential.

Nursing Diagnosis and Planning

The following nursing diagnoses and expected outcomes may be appropriate for the infant with congenital hypothyroidism and the infant's parents:

- Deficient Knowledge related to unfamiliarity with the congenital disorder.

  Expected Outcomes: The parents will demonstrate the ability to monitor their infant for signs and symptoms of hypothyroidism and hyperthyroidism; will verbalize an understanding of normal growth and developmental milestones; will give thyroid medication properly; and will discuss the child's lifelong needs and routine.

- Delayed Growth and Development related to disease process.

  Expected Outcome: As a result of appropriately managed disease, the infant will demonstrate growth and developmental milestones appropriate for age.

- Ineffective Thermoregulation related to decreased basal metabolic rate.

  Expected Outcome: As a result of disease management, the infant will maintain a temperature within normal range.

Interventions

Instruct family members on the importance of medication adherence. Emphasize that the medication is necessary for the child's growth, especially for the rapidly developing brain.

Teach the family how and when to administer the medication. Levothyroxine is given orally as a single daily dose. The medication can be dissolved in a small amount of water and given by syringe or placed into the nipple of a baby bottle along with a small amount of formula. Warn the caregiver not to dissolve the medication in a large amount of formula because, if the formula is unfinished, the infant will not receive the full dosage. When the infant is older, the medication can be given in a spoonful of cereal or baby food. Toddlers can usually chew tablets without difficulty. If the infant or child vomits within 1 hour of taking medication, the dose should be readministered. Frequently missed doses can lead to developmental delays and poor growth.

Also teach the parents the signs and symptoms of both hypothyroidism and hyperthyroidism and when to notify the physician if symptoms occur. Hyperthyroidism can develop in infants receiving too much medication. Parents need to be taught to count their child's pulse and notify their health care provider if the rate is greater than the recommended parameter.

Because hypothyroidism is a lifelong condition, school-age children and teenagers should be made aware of the importance of taking their medication and of keeping regular follow-up appointments with the physician.

CRITICAL TO REMEMBER
The Child With Congenital Hypothyroidism

- Untreated hypothyroidism leads to mental retardation.
- T_4 and TSH levels vary with age, but any infant with a low T_4 and an elevated TSH value, often rising to greater than 100 mU/L, is considered to have primary hypothyroidism until proven otherwise.*

*In R. Behrman, R. Kliegman, & H. Jenson (Eds.), *Nelson textbook of pediatrics* (17th ed., pp. 1875-1876). Philadelphia: Saunders.

Evaluation

- Have the parents demonstrated the ability to monitor the child's signs and symptoms, recognize growth and developmental problems, administer the medication, and discuss the child's lifelong needs and routines?
- Is the child developing appropriately for age according to growth charts and Denver Developmental Screening Test (DDST) scores?
- Does the child have normal results on thyroid function tests?
- Is the child's body temperature within normal limits?

ACQUIRED HYPOTHYROIDISM

Hypothyroidism is a condition in which the thyroid gland produces an inadequate amount of thyroid hormone to meet the body's metabolic needs.

Etiology

Hashimoto's thyroiditis, a common cause of acquired hypothyroidism, is usually associated with a goiter. It is the result of an autoimmune process. Other causes of acquired hypothyroidism include surgical thyroidectomy, radioactive iodine therapy for hyperthyroidism, radiation therapy for malignancies, and excessive iodine ingestion. Less frequently, decreased TSH secretion by the pituitary gland or decreased thyrotropin-releasing hormone (TRH) secretion by the hypothalamus causes hypothyroidism.

Autoimmune thyroiditis is the most common cause of acquired hypothyroidism in children and adolescents. It often occurs in families with a history of thyroid disease. Other family members may have positive thyroid antibodies. Thyroiditis is more common in girls, with as many as 10% of young girls exhibiting signs of autoimmune thyroid dysfunction, most often chronic lymphocytic thyroiditis (Straight & Bauer, 2003).

Pathophysiology

Circulating autoantibodies known as *thyroid-blocking immunoglobulins* decrease thyroid gland production of triiodothyronine (T_3) and T_4. These antibodies bind at the TSH receptor sites on the thyroid gland, resulting in decreased thyroid hormone production. The cause of antibody production is unknown.

In contrast to congenital hypothyroidism, adverse effects from hypothyroidism acquired after 2 to 3 years of age are often reversible. Goiter, an enlarged thyroid gland, occurs in response to increased TSH secretion, autoimmune attack of the thyroid gland, or goitrogens.

Manifestations

Clinical manifestations of hypothyroidism include goiter (one lobe frequently larger than the other); dry, thick skin; coarse, dull hair; fatigue; cold intolerance; constipation; weight gain; decreased linear growth; edema of face, eyes, and hands; and irregular or delayed menses.

Diagnostic Evaluation

Elevated TSH and low T_4 levels are diagnostic of hypothyroidism. Elevated TSH level is the most sensitive indicator of primary hypothyroidism.

Thyroiditis is diagnosed by the presence of circulating thyroid antibodies and is usually associated with a firm goiter. Initially TSH is elevated with normal T_4 levels, although T_4 decreases over time. With secondary or tertiary hypothyroidism TSH is not elevated; therefore thyroid-releasing hormone stimulation testing is usually required for diagnosis.

Therapeutic Management

Management of the child with hypothyroidism involves thyroid hormone replacement, usually with levothyroxine. Dosage varies according to the child's age and weight and is given as a single daily dose. The dose is titrated to maintain T_4 in the upper half of the normal range and to maintain TSH in the normal range for age.

NURSING CARE
The Child With Acquired Hypothyroidism

Assessment

Care of the child with acquired hypothyroidism includes assessing response to treatment and adherence to the medication regimen. With treatment, the goiter should decrease in size. Signs and symptoms of hypothyroidism should also resolve with adequate thyroid hormone replacement. Monitoring height, weight, and performance on the DDST at each visit assesses the child's growth and development. The nurse should monitor school performance as well and maintain contact with the school nurse.

Nursing Diagnosis and Planning

The following nursing diagnoses and expected outcomes may be appropriate for a child with acquired hypothyroidism:

- Constipation related to decreased basal metabolic rate as a result of hypothyroidism.

  Expected Outcome: The child will maintain regular bowel movements of normal consistency as basal metabolic rate improves.

- Activity Intolerance related to fatigue.

  Expected Outcome: The child will maintain normal energy levels for age, as evidenced by the ability to exercise at the same level as peers.

- Disturbed Body Image related to weight gain/obesity.

  Expected Outcomes: The child will verbalize feelings about body changes and will accept reassurances that changes will resolve with treatment.

- Ineffective Thermoregulation related to decreased basal metabolic rate secondary to hypothyroidism.

  Expected Outcome: As a result of appropriate disease management, the child will maintain normal body temperature.

Interventions

Parents and school-age children or older should be instructed on the correct dose and timing of thyroid medication. Thyroid hormone levels are usually checked every 3 to 6 months. Laboratory values within the normal range indicate good response to therapy. Instruct parents on the signs and symptoms of hypothyroidism and hyperthyroidism and to notify the physician if symptoms occur. Reassure the child that signs such as constipation, fatigue, and weight gain will resolve as the medication becomes effective.

Evaluation

- Has the child maintained regular bowel movements of normal consistency?
- Can the child tolerate exercise at the same level as peers?
- Does the child express feelings related to body changes and accept reassurances that problems will resolve?
- Has the child maintained normal body temperature?

HYPERTHYROIDISM (GRAVES DISEASE)

Graves disease is an autoimmune condition in which excessive thyroid hormones are produced by an enlarged thyroid gland. It is the most common cause of hyperthyroidism in children.

Incidence

The incidence of Graves disease in children is approximately 1 in 5000, with girls being five times more likely than boys to acquire the condition. Peak age for acquiring the condition is between 11 and 15 years (LaFranchi, 2004). Graves disease may also have a familial tendency. Children with autoimmune disease are at risk for other autoimmune disorders. Neonatal Graves disease is associated with maternal hyperthyroidism and is relatively uncommon.

Pathophysiology

Circulating autoantibodies known as *thyroid-stimulating immunoglobulins* (*TSIs*) stimulate the thyroid gland to make T_3 and T_4. These antibodies bind to the TSH receptor sites on the thyroid gland, resulting in excessive thyroid hormone production. The cause of antibody production is unknown. In newborns, maternal TSI is transferred through the placenta to the fetus. TSI binds to the TSH receptor, causing neonatal hyperthyroidism.

CRITICAL TO REMEMBER
Autoimmune Thyroid Disorders

- Treatment for Graves disease may be medical (antithyroid medications) or ablative (radioactive iodine or surgery).
- Adherence to medical therapy is problematic because of the requirement for twice-daily or three-times-daily dosing for protracted periods (2 to 3 years).
- Goiter may be present with either hypothyroidism or hyperthyroidism.
- Autoimmune thyroiditis resulting in either hypothyroidism or hyperthyroidism may be permanent or transient.

Manifestations

Goiter, increased appetite, weight loss, nervousness, diarrhea, increased perspiration, heat intolerance, increased heart rate, muscle weakness, palpitations, tremors, exophthalmos, poor attention span, and behavior or school problems are common in Graves disease (Box 27-2). In the neonate irritability, tachycardia, hypertension, voracious appetite with poor weight gain, flushing, prominent eyes, and thyroid enlargement are major signs. These are self-limiting signs, but cardiac failure and death can occur if the signs are unrecognized or poorly treated.

Diagnostic Evaluation

Elevated serum T_4 levels and suppressed TSH levels, associated with signs and symptoms of hyperthyroidism, suggest Graves disease. Autoantibodies to thyroid tissue usually are positive. Thyroid uptake of radioactive iodine is increased.

BOX 27-2	**Hypothyroidism Versus Hyperthyroidism**

Hypothyroidism	**Hyperthyroidism**
• Fatigue	• Nervousness, anxiety
• Constipation	• Diarrhea
• Cold intolerance	• Heat intolerance
• Weight gain	• Weight loss
• Dry, thick skin	• Smooth, velvety skin
• Edema of face, eyes, hands	• Prominent eyes
• Decreased growth	• Accelerated linear growth
• Decreased activity and energy	• Emotional lability
• Muscle hypertrophy (pseudodystrophy)	• Muscle weakness
• Decreased heart rate	• Increased heart rate
• Delayed skeletal maturation	• High blood pressure
• Delayed puberty	• Tremor
	• Increased appetite

Therapeutic Management

The three approaches to the management of Graves disease are antithyroid drug therapy, radioactive iodine, or surgery. Antithyroid drug therapy with propylthiouracil or methimazole is the treatment of choice for childhood hyperthyroidism. These drugs act by blocking thyroid hormone production by the thyroid gland (Yeung & Habra, 2005). The medications usually are given three times per day, and they lower thyroid hormone levels in several weeks. Minor adverse effects include arthralgia, skin rash, pruritus, and gastric intolerance. Major adverse effects may include neutropenia, hepatotoxicity, and hypothyroidism.

A second approach to management is oral radioactive iodine treatment. Radioactive iodine (^{131}I) is given as an oral solution. It is typically used in children older than 10 years. With this therapy, the radioactive iodine is absorbed and concentrated by the thyroid gland, destroying the thyroid tissue in approximately 6 to 18 weeks. Hyperthyroid symptoms may intensify briefly after treatment. Hypothyroidism can result once the thyroid gland is radiated, necessitating thyroid replacement therapy.

Subtotal or partial thyroidectomy, the surgical removal of thyroid gland tissue, is the third form of management. Lugol's solution (potassium iodide), given 10 to 14 days before surgery, decreases the gland's vascularity. Surgery carries the risk of injury to the parathyroid glands, resulting in hypocalcemia. Calcium levels are monitored after surgery.

Recurrence of hyperthyroidism is uncommon but possible. Affected children also have a 60% to 80% chance for developing hypothyroidism, which can be treated with thyroid replacement therapy.

Follow-up evaluations correlate with response to therapy. As thyroid functions normalize, follow-up endocrine evaluations are recommended once or twice per year.

NURSING CARE

The Child With Hyperthyroidism

Assessment

The treatment goals consist of normalizing thyroid hormone levels, alleviating symptoms of hyperthyroidism, and decreasing the goiter. The nurse should assess for adherence to medical therapy. Determine that the family understands that medical therapy might take several weeks to decrease thyroid hormone action. Propranolol, a beta-adrenergic blocker, may be prescribed to decrease adrenergic signs and symptoms (tachycardia, heat intolerance, tremor) until the antithyroid medication is effective. Monitor the child for adrenergic signs and symptoms.

A child being treated with propylthiouracil has an increased risk of neutropenia and hepatotoxicity; regular blood counts and liver function studies are done to assess these risks. Assess the child for fever, joint pain, edema, rash, or excessive bruising. A child who acquires a fever or sore throat while receiving propylthiouracil should be evaluated by a physician. A complete blood count should be obtained.

Nursing Diagnosis and Planning

The following nursing diagnoses and expected outcomes may be appropriate for a child with hyperthyroidism:

- Ineffective Therapeutic Regimen Management related to nonadherence to the medication regimen.
  Expected Outcome: The child will adhere to the medication regimen, as evidenced by normal thyroid hormone levels.
- Diarrhea related to increased basal metabolic rate secondary to hyperthyroidism.
  Expected Outcomes: The child will be euthyroid, as evidenced by normal results on thyroid function tests; the child will have normal bowel movements.
- Risk for Activity Intolerance related to loss of muscle mass from increased basal metabolic rate secondary to hyperthyroidism.
  Expected Outcome: The child will be able to exercise at the same level as peers as basal metabolic rate returns to normal.
- Disturbed Sleep Pattern related to increased basal metabolic rate secondary to hyperthyroidism.
  Expected Outcome: The child will gain appropriate amounts of sleep for age as basal metabolic rate returns to normal.
- Ineffective Thermoregulation related to increased basal metabolic rate secondary to hyperthyroidism.
  Expected Outcome: The child will regain normal body temperature as basal metabolic rate returns to normal.

Interventions

The antithyroid drugs *propylthiouracil* and *methimazole* are usually given two or three times per day. This regimen may be difficult for some children to follow. Advise the use of pill dispensers and a watch with an alarm to remind the child to take the medication at specific times. The endocrinologist should evaluate the child and monitor thyroid function every 2 to 4 months while the child is undergoing treatment. Normal values for thyroid function tests and alleviation of symptoms indicate appropriate response to therapy.

Once the child is euthyroid and asymptomatic, the child should be evaluated once or twice a year. Medical therapy may be tapered after 2 to 3 years to evaluate for remission. Contact sports should be limited while the child is being treated to decrease the possibility of damage to the liver. Collaboration with the school nurse to facilitate medication administration is an important nursing function.

Evaluation

- Does the child have normal results on thyroid function tests?
- Has the basal metabolic rate returned to normal?
- Does the child demonstrate normal bowel movements?
- Is the child able to exercise at an age-appropriate level?
- Does the child obtain an appropriate amount of sleep?
- Has the child maintained a normal body temperature?

DIABETES INSIPIDUS

Diabetes insipidus is an inability to concentrate urine because of a deficiency of vasopressin, also known as *antidiuretic hormone* (ADH).

Etiology

Diabetes insipidus frequently results from head trauma, tumors, or infection in the area of the hypothalamus. The most common type of tumor involving the hypothalamus that causes diabetes insipidus is craniopharyngioma.

Cranial radiation for treatment of tumors also may lead to ADH deficiency. Other causes include infections of the CNS, such as meningitis or encephalitis, and congenital malformations, such as septo-optic dysplasia or isolated pituitary malformation or ectopy. It may also be idiopathic.

Incidence

Diabetes insipidus is not common in the United States, occurring in 1 of every 25,000 individuals. Head trauma and cranial surgery account for the largest percentage of cases of

---

PATHOPHYSIOLOGY

DIABETES INSIPIDUS

ADH is produced in the hypothalamus, transported through the pituitary stalk, and stored in the posterior pituitary. It is carried through the blood to the kidneys, where it acts on the distal tubules and collecting ducts to increase reabsorption of free water, thereby concentrating urine and decreasing urinary output.

ADH is under the control of osmoreceptors in the anterior pituitary. These osmoreceptors operate on a negative-feedback system based on serum osmolality, particularly sodium concentration. When the osmolality is low, production of ADH decreases, causing increased urine output and normalizing osmolality; conversely, when osmolality is increased, ADH production increases, causing water retention and decreasing urine output. In diabetes insipidus, a deficiency of ADH makes the body unable to conserve water, which results in large volumes of dilute urine. Loss of free water leads to an increase in serum sodium concentration. If the child has an intact thirst center, increasing oral intake might compensate for the large fluid loss. If the thirst drive is not intact or the child is unable to drink enough, the child may become dehydrated and have a high serum sodium level.

A child with an intact thirst center is able to self-regulate fluid needs and intake. If the child is not able to recognize thirst because of head trauma or surgery, the physician may prescribe a 24-hour fluid requirement.

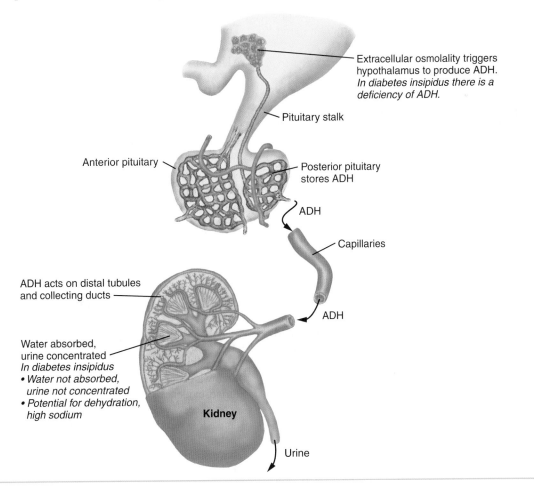

Extracellular osmolality triggers hypothalamus to produce ADH. *In diabetes insipidus there is a deficiency of ADH.*

Pituitary stalk

Anterior pituitary

Posterior pituitary stores ADH

ADH

Capillaries

ADH

ADH acts on distal tubules and collecting ducts

Water absorbed, urine concentrated
In diabetes insipidus
• *Water not absorbed, urine not concentrated*
• *Potential for dehydration, high sodium*

Kidney

Urine

diabetes insipidus. Thirty percent of cases are classified as idiopathic (Cooperman, 2003).

Manifestations

Increased urination (polyuria) and excessive thirst (polydipsia) are the classic manifestations of diabetes insipidus. Other signs and symptoms include nocturia and dehydration (Box 27-3).

Diagnostic Evaluation

Diagnostic criteria include polyuria with associated hypernatremia (>150 mEq/L) and low urine specific gravity (<1.005) in the absence of hyperglycemia. Urine should be checked for glucose to rule out hyperglycemia as a cause of increased urine output.

A water deprivation test may also be necessary to confirm the diagnosis. In this 7- to 8-hour procedure, the child is deprived of all fluid intake. A normal response is decreased urine output with a high urine specific gravity and no change in serum sodium. In diabetes insipidus, when fluid is restricted, the child continues to have large amounts of dilute urine, evidenced by low urine specific gravity. The serum sodium level also increases. To ensure the child's safety, this test is done in a hospital setting with frequent monitoring of serum sodium, hematocrit, and osmolality. Urine osmolality and output are also measured. The child is weighed at the beginning, middle, and conclusion of the water deprivation test. Water deprivation should be stopped if the child loses 3% to 5% of baseline body weight, becomes dehydrated, or demonstrates a significant change in vital signs or neurologic status.

Therapeutic Management

Treatment involves maintaining fluid balance and administering synthetic vasopressin (1-deamino-8-D-arginine vasopressin [DDAVP]). The dose of DDAVP ranges from 5 to 30 μg/day (intranasal) or 2-4 μg/day (IV/subcutaneous), divided into one to two doses. It is administered either intranasally, through a soft, flexible tube (rhinal tube) or metered spray, or by subcutaneous injection. The concentration of intranasal DDAVP is 100 μg/mL; the concentration of subcutaneous DDAVP is 4 μg/mL. The oral form of DDAVP is used primarily for nocturnal enuresis. It has also been used in the treatment of diabetes insipidus. Oral doses range from 25 to 300 μg every 8-12 hours (Breault & Majzoub, 2004).

Dosage is individualized on the basis of the child's age, size, urine output, and urine specific gravity. The duration of action varies from 8 to 24 hours. Doses are timed so that before the next dose, the child is allowed to have mildly increased urination. This helps prevent overtreatment and water retention. Parents are often taught to measure urine specific gravity at home to monitor effectiveness of treatment.

Nursing Considerations

Nursing care involves assessing the parents' and child's understanding of diabetes insipidus. Educate the family about the basic pathophysiology of water metabolism and the cause of diabetes insipidus. Include a description of signs and

---

> ## CRITICAL TO REMEMBER
> ### Diabetes Insipidus
> - Hypernatremia (sodium >150 mEq/L) and low urine specific gravity in the absence of hyperglycemia are diagnostic of diabetes insipidus.
> - DDAVP is the only therapy for central diabetes insipidus.
> - Overtreatment with DDAVP will result in fluid retention and dilutional hyponatremia. If the hyponatremia is severe enough, seizures may occur.

symptoms. Instruct the parents about signs and symptoms indicating the need for DDAVP (increased thirst, polyuria, dehydration) as well as signs and symptoms of excessive DDAVP (decreased urine output, headaches, water retention).

Teach the family the proper administration of DDAVP and observe a return demonstration of medication administration. If appropriate, instruct the family in using a refractometer to measure urine specific gravity. The child should wear a medical alert bracelet noting the diagnosis of diabetes insipidus. The child's teachers need to be aware of the diagnosis and must allow the child free access to water and toilet facilities. Advise the family to watch the child closely for signs of dehydration.

SYNDROME OF INAPPROPRIATE ANTIDIURETIC HORMONE

The syndrome of inappropriate antidiuretic hormone (SIADH) results from excessive production or release of ADH, or vasopressin.

Etiology

Childhood SIADH usually is caused by disorders affecting the CNS, including infections (e.g., meningitis), head trauma, and brain tumors (see Chapter 28). SIADH is rare in children and is usually related to an underlying cause. Surgery for brain tumors may cause the child to have transient SIADH. Often a triple response occurs after surgery. Initially the child has diabetes insipidus, then the child experiences temporary SIADH, and finally the child returns to diabetes insipidus (Breault & Majzoub, 2004). SIADH is usually transient and resolves when the underlying condition is corrected.

> ## PATHOPHYSIOLOGY
> ### SYNDROME OF INAPPROPRIATE ANTIDIURETIC HORMONE
> Excessive ADH results in the kidney reabsorbing too much free water. This causes decreased output of concentrated urine, evidenced by a high urine specific gravity (>1.030). The excess water also causes an expanded fluid volume and a low serum sodium level. Once the sodium level falls below 125 mEq/L, the child can become symptomatic and have anorexia, nausea, weakness, weight gain, confusion, irritability, and seizures.

Manifestations

Manifestations that occur with SIADH include decreased urine output, increased urine specific gravity, fluid retention, weight gain, hyponatremia, and increased urine osmolality (Box 27-3).

Diagnostic Evaluation

SIADH should be suspected in children with CNS involvement, such as infections or head trauma, who have decreased urine output despite adequate intake. Laboratory diagnosis includes evidence of hyponatremia, hypochloremia, and low serum osmolality. Urine osmolality is usually greater than serum osmolality. Urine specific gravity is more than 1.030. Adrenal, thyroid, and renal function studies can rule out other causes of hyponatremia.

Therapeutic Management

Initial treatment is correction of the underlying cause. The physician orders fluid restriction to correct hyponatremia (Greenbaum, 2004). A child with severe hyponatremia may need IV infusion of sodium chloride. Drug therapy usually is not indicated for transient SIADH. Medications such as lithium and demeclocycline block the action of ADH at the renal collecting tubules and have been used in the management of chronic SIADH.

Nursing Considerations

The nurse should assess the child with SIADH for signs and symptoms of fluid overload, including edema, weight gain, urine specific gravity more than 1.030, and dilutional hyponatremia. If the child is hyponatremic, monitor neuro-

BOX 27-3	Diabetes Insipidus versus SIADH
Diabetes Insipidus (High and Dry)	**SIADH (Low and Wet)**
• Increased urination	• Decreased urination
• Increased thirst	• Hypertension
• Nocturia	• Weight gain
• Dehydration	• Fluid retention
• Hypernatremia	• Hyponatremia
• Urine specific gravity <1.005	• Urine specific gravity >1.030
• Elevated serum osmolality (>300 mOsm/kg)	• Decreased serum osmolality (<280 mOsm/kg)
• Decreased urine osmolality	• Increased urine osmolality

BOX 27-4	Signs of Hyponatremia
Mild (Early)	**Moderate**	**Severe**
Anorexia	Confusion	Seizures
Nausea	Lethargy	Coma
Headache	Irritability	
Vomiting	Altered level of consciousness	

CRITICAL TO REMEMBER
SIADH
- SIADH is characterized by low serum sodium (<125 mEq/L) and high urine specific gravity as well as decreased serum osmolality and increased urine osmolality.
- Seizures may develop with hyponatremia.
- Treatment depends on strict fluid restriction to maintain serum sodium in a near-normal range. Strict measurements of intake and output are critical to evaluation and management of the child with SIADH.

---

logic status by assessing level of consciousness and observing for headache, irritability, or seizures (Box 27-4).

The child with fluid overload is at risk for injury related to seizures caused by hyponatremia. Interventions are directed toward maintaining fluid balance and preventing injury. Assess the child's hydration and neurologic status every 2 to 4 hours. Carefully maintain strict fluid restrictions and document intake and output. Weigh the child daily to monitor fluid retention.

The child may have difficulty adhering to the fluid restrictions. Explain to the child and parents the need for limited fluids and that the restriction is temporary. The nurse may give the child hard sugarless candies or apply wet washcloths to help keep mucous membranes moist.

Diet for the child with hyponatremia should include foods with high-sodium content because extra sodium can help correct this problem. Keep in mind, however, that salty foods such as chips may make the child thirsty.

Closely monitor serum electrolyte levels as ordered by the physician. Alert the physician immediately to any change in neurologic status. Because severe hyponatremia can cause seizures, initiate seizure precautions if the serum sodium level drops below 125 mEq/L.

Evaluation of the child with SIADH should address a balanced intake and output, stable weight, and normal serum sodium levels. Urine specific gravity should be maintained between 1.010 and 1.020.

PRECOCIOUS PUBERTY

Precocious puberty refers to early onset of puberty. Traditionally this has been viewed as the onset of puberty before 8 years of age in girls and before 9 years of age in boys. It is defined as the premature appearance of secondary sexual characteristics, accelerated growth rate, and advanced bone maturation. The major consequence of precocious puberty is rapid bone growth, which causes early growth-plate fusion and ultimately short stature in adulthood compared with genetic height potential.

Etiology

Central, or true, precocious puberty can be idiopathic or caused by CNS tumors (most commonly hamartomas), head trauma, or cranial radiation. Peripheral causes include abnormalities or tumors of the adrenal glands, ovaries, or testes. Congenital adrenal hyperplasia, a genetic disorder of the adrenal pathway, is the most common cause of peripheral precocious puberty. McCune-Albright syndrome may cause early puberty in girls and boys; the genetic disorder *familial testotoxicosis* causes early puberty in boys.

Incidence

Precocious puberty occurs more frequently in girls than in boys; approximately 70% of cases are idiopathic, although boys have a higher incidence of CNS lesions. Both boys and girls can have hypothalamic hamartomas.

PATHOPHYSIOLOGY

PRECOCIOUS PUBERTY

Puberty occurs when the hypothalamus releases GnRH. This stimulates the pituitary gland to release LH and FSH. In girls, FSH stimulates formation of ovarian follicles to produce estrogen. Estrogen is necessary for the development of secondary sexual characteristics, such as breast development and maturation of the vagina and labia. LH is involved in the process of ovulation. In boys, FSH triggers the testes to support the development of sperm. LH stimulates the production of testosterone, which is necessary for the development of sexual characteristics and sperm production. Puberty development is classified according to Tanner stages 1 through 5 (see Chapter 8). The adrenal glands produce the

hormone *dehydroepiandrosterone* (DHEA), which causes pubic and axillary hair growth. During puberty the growth rate increases, called a "growth spurt," in which a child grows an average of 4 to 6 inches per year.

In precocious puberty the sex hormones that accelerate growth also cause the bone plates to close early. Bone usually fuses at 14 years of age for girls and 17 years for boys. With true precocious puberty, children have hormonal changes that mimic the onset of normal puberty. These hormonal changes may be central, arising from the hypothalamus, or peripheral, arising from the ovaries, testes, or adrenal glands.

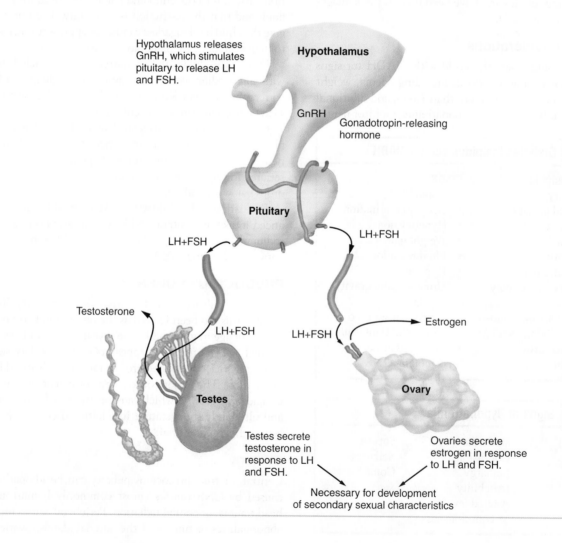

Manifestations

Manifestations of precocious puberty reflect gender differences:

Girls	Boys
Breast development	Testicular enlargement
Pubic hair	Penile enlargement
Axillary hair	Pubic hair
Enlargement of vagina, uterus, and ovaries	Facial hair
	Acne
Acne	Adult body odor
Growth spurt	Deepening of voice
Adult body odor	Moodiness
Onset of menstrual periods	
Moodiness	

Diagnostic Evaluation

Diagnosis of precocious puberty begins with a thorough history, including onset of sexual characteristics, and a physical examination. Blood tests are then necessary to evaluate for elevated levels of LH, FSH, testosterone, and estrogen. Unfortunately, because these hormones are released in small bursts during the day, random samples may not be adequate.

The gonadotropin-releasing hormone (GnRH) stimulation test is a definitive test to delineate between central (gonadotropin-dependent) and peripheral (gonadotropin-independent) causes of precocious puberty (Kakerla & Bradshaw, 2003). Synthetic GnRH is administered IV or subcutaneously to stimulate the release of LH and FSH from the pituitary gland. Serial samples of LH and FSH are then obtained over a 2-hour period after IV administration. With subcutaneous administration, a single sample of LH and FSH may be obtained with the use of an ultrasensitive assay. Before the onset of puberty, the FSH peak is higher than the LH peak. With the onset of puberty, the LH peak is higher than the FSH peak.

Radiographic studies also support the diagnosis of precocious puberty. Radiographs of the wrist determine bone age and maturation and can assist in predicting final adult height. Skull radiographs screen for CNS lesions, although CT scans and MRI are more accurate in visualizing tumors. Abdominal ultrasound and pelvic ultrasound are beneficial in diagnosing adrenal and ovarian tumors or cysts. Pelvic ultrasound also provides evidence of pubertal changes in the uterus and ovaries. Finally, isolated pubic hair development and elevated androgen hormone levels suggest an adrenal origin for premature sexual hair growth.

Therapeutic Management

Treatment of the child with precocious puberty aims to stop or reverse the development of secondary sexual characteristics and to maximize adult height. Current therapy for central precocious puberty involves administration of a GnRH agonist, or blocker. GnRH blockers inhibit the binding of GnRH to the pituitary gland, causing decreased production of the pubertal hormones and slowing or reversing sexual development.

Several commercially available GnRH agonists can be administered either intranasally or by a monthly intramuscular injection. Once therapy is initiated, GnRH secretion is suppressed within 2 to 4 weeks. The accelerated growth rate and bone maturation will slow, and some secondary sexual characteristics will regress within the first year of treatment. Nonadherence with medication therapy, such as missed or delayed administration of injections, can promote pubertal changes rather than suppress puberty.

No evidence suggests that GnRH agonist therapy interferes with the child's reproduction in the future. Once therapy is discontinued, pubertal progression resumes. For children with peripheral precocious puberty, treatment is aimed at correcting the underlying cause.

NURSING CARE

The Child With Precocious Puberty

Assessment

Nursing care of the child with precocious puberty addresses the physical and behavioral changes associated with puberty. A nurse working with these children may note that they feel more comfortable around older children rather than peers their own age. They often experience teasing about their bodies and may limit social activities, such as swimming. Boys often exhibit aggressive behavior. Children who go through early puberty appear older than their chronologic age and are often treated accordingly by adults. Because of their mature appearance, children with precocious puberty are at greater risk for sexual abuse.

CRITICAL TO REMEMBER
Precocious Puberty

- Children with precocious puberty appear older than their chronologic age. Although they tend to be treated as older children, they should be treated according to their chronologic age.
- Other children often tease children with precocious puberty.
- Children with precocious puberty are at increased risk of child abuse because of their more mature appearance.
- Precocious puberty may present in infancy or childhood.

If a child appears embarrassed or uncomfortable when being interviewed about sexual development, the nurse should explain to the child, "Everyone goes through body changes when growing up; it's just that these changes are happening to you sooner than most children. Can you tell me in your own words how you feel about your body?"

Nursing Diagnosis and Planning

The following nursing diagnoses and expected outcomes may be appropriate for the child with precocious puberty:

- Deficient Knowledge about medication administration related to inadequate understanding of intramuscular or intranasal GnRH agonist.

  Expected Outcomes: The parents will explain the need for the medication and will give an appropriate return demonstration of medication administration technique.

- Disturbed Body Image related to early sexual development.

  Expected Outcomes: The child will describe the relationship between early sexual development and the underlying condition, express feelings about early sexual development, and verbalize acceptance of body appearance.

- Impaired Social Interaction related to appearing older than chronologic age.

  Expected Outcome: The child will adjust socially to body changes, as evidenced by exhibiting age-appropriate behaviors and social interactions.

Interventions

Many parents may not be comfortable with their child's early development. The nurse explains the stages of puberty and each stage's associated behavioral changes. The nurse teaches parents that the child is experiencing normal changes at an earlier time than expected.

Explanations given to the child should be geared to the level of intellectual development. The nurse can direct the parent to books that explain sexual maturation in terms the child can understand. Psychological counseling might be necessary to help the family deal with the sensitive issues of sexuality.

The nurse also teaches the family about the prescribed medication regimen. In some instances, the parent is taught how to administer the injections. These might be stressful for the young child. The nurse demonstrates appropriate injection technique and teaches the child coping strategies to be used when the injection is given.

Evaluation

- Can the parents explain the need for the medication and demonstrate proper medication administration?
- Is the child able to relate the body changes to the underlying condition?
- Have the child and parents verbalized any concerns about the child's early sexual development?
- Is the child exhibiting age-appropriate social interactions?

GROWTH HORMONE DEFICIENCY

GH deficiency results from inadequate production or secretion of GH, causing poor growth and short stature. GH deficiency may also present as hypoglycemia.

Etiology

GH deficiency may be isolated or may be associated with an underlying cause. Such causes include hypopituitarism, congenital malformations of the pituitary gland, brain tumors (most commonly craniopharyngioma), and cranial irradiation. Other disorders associated with short stature that may respond to GH therapy include Turner syndrome, Prader-Willi syndrome, and chronic illnesses such as renal disease and inflammatory bowel disease.

Incidence

In the United States, approximately 4000 children are diagnosed with GH deficiency every year. Currently approximately 20,000 children receive GH therapy (Eledrisi, 2004).

Manifestations

Manifestations typical of GH deficiency include height less than fifth percentile for age and sex, diminished growth rate (less than two standard deviations from the mean for age and sex), immature or cherubic facies, delayed puberty, hypoglycemia, diminished muscle mass and relatively increased adiposity, and micropenis (associated with hypopituitarism).

Diagnostic Evaluation

Diagnosis of GH deficiency begins with careful measurements of growth over an extended period (usually 6 to 12 mo). Height should be measured on a consistent scale, preferably with a calibrated stadiometer.

PATHOPHYSIOLOGY

GROWTH HORMONE DEFICIENCY

GH, thyroxine, cortisol, and sex hormones all influence growth. The hypothalamus secretes GH-releasing factor, which stimulates the pituitary gland to release GH. This hormone is secreted in pulses, with increased secretion during the night. In the presence of hypoglycemia, GH is secreted to counteract insulin and raise the blood glucose level. Many children with GH deficiency may have hypoglycemia.

Most children with short stature have constitutional growth delay. Children with short stature or poor growth rates may also be deficient in other hormones. Normal thyroid function is essential for growth; therefore hypothyroidism may also present with short stature. Sex hormones are required for the growth spurt and sexual maturation that occurs with puberty. Children lacking more than one hormone produced by the pituitary gland are referred to as having *hypopituitarism*. Rate of growth and final adult height depend on factors such as family heights, nutrition, and general health. Any child growing less than 5 cm per year should be referred to an endocrinologist for further evaluation.

Initial screening involves thyroid function tests, electrolytes, blood urea nitrogen (BUN), creatinine, complete blood count, insulin-like growth factor 1 (IGF-1; formerly somatomedin-C) and IGF binding proteins (IGFBP-3) (indirect measures of GH production), and a bone age radiograph. Normal thyroid function is essential for adequate growth; thyroid studies are essential when evaluating for short stature. Complete blood count and other specific blood screening for any systemic or chronic illness should be done. Electrolytes and renal function studies eliminate primary kidney dysfunction as a cause of poor growth.

Because GH is normally secreted in pulses throughout the day and night, stimulation testing is necessary to confirm the diagnosis of GH deficiency. Agents used in provocative testing to stimulate GH production include insulin, arginine, clonidine, glucagon, and levodopa (L-dopa). Once the stimulating agent is given, serial GH levels are drawn. Although diagnostic criteria vary, most clinicians accept a GH level less than 10 ng/mL as indicative of GH deficiency. Generally, two positive tests are required for diagnosis.

Therapeutic Management

A child with GH deficiency requires replacement therapy. Synthetic GH comes in a powdered form that must be diluted for administration or a premixed liquid form. It is given as a subcutaneous injection six or seven times per week, usually at bedtime. An alternative form of administration is a subcutaneous deposition of time-release GH, designed to last 2 to 4 weeks. Dosage ranges from 0.18 to 0.3 mg/kg per week, depending on the child's age, pubertal stage, and response to therapy (Parks, 2004). Once diluted, GH must be stored at 36° to 46° F. Treatment is usually considered effective if the child exhibits a height increase of 2 cm/yr over the pretreatment growth rate. The earlier treatment is initiated, the greater the child's height potential. Treatment is continued until the child's growth plates close or the child reaches an acceptable height or predicted final height.

NURSING CARE

The Child With Growth Hormone Deficiency

Assessment

Nursing care of the child with GH deficiency includes assessment of family attitudes and perceptions. Parental attitudes regarding the child's size can influence the child's self-esteem. Assess the child's attitude about height. Are height and growth issues voiced more by the parent or by the child? If parents place excessive emphasis on height, the child may be more self-conscious or demonstrate low self-esteem. Height issues may affect a child's psychosocial adjustment, as demonstrated by poor school performance and lack of involvement in extracurricular activities. Often short children appear younger and are treated as such by adults, or they may be teased by their peers.

CRITICAL TO REMEMBER
Criteria for Suspecting Growth Hormone Deficiency
- Consistently poor growth (<5 cm/yr)
- Growth rate more than two standard deviations below the mean for age
- Downward deviation from the previous growth curve

When assessing a child with short stature, the nurse should ask the child if height causes any problems at school. For example, the nurse might ask, "Have you ever been teased or been in any fights at school because of your height?"

Once the child is receiving therapy, the nurse should assess adherence with the medication regimen, injection technique, and medication preparation and storage. These should be reviewed periodically and with each dosage change. As children with this problem mature, they might choose to learn to self-administer injections.

Nursing Diagnosis and Planning

The following nursing diagnoses and expected outcomes may be appropriate for the child with GH deficiency:
- Delayed Growth and Development related to GH deficiency.
  Expected Outcomes: The child will receive and respond to treatment, as evidenced by increased growth rate.
- Disturbed Body Image related to short stature.
  Expected Outcome: The child will demonstrate acceptance of body image, as evidenced by verbalization of acceptance of ultimate growth.
- Situational Low Self-Esteem related to short stature.
  Expected Outcome: The child will accept short stature, as evidenced by verbalizing appropriate feelings of self-esteem.
- Ineffective Family Therapeutic Regimen Management related to nonadherence with daily injection.
  Expected Outcome: The child and parents will adhere to the injection schedule, as evidenced by appropriate record keeping and the child's steady growth.

Interventions

The nurse reassures the child and parents that adherence to the injections will improve growth rate. Reminders that the injections are temporary and are helping them to grow are also helpful. Keeping a growth chart at home and needing larger clothing sizes are physical signs the child can use to monitor growth. These indicators also assist with adherence.

The nurse has an important role in educating children and families about the proper dilution and administration of the GH. Demonstrate injection technique to the caregiver and request a return demonstration.

Effectiveness of therapy is evaluated by growth rate. Children are evaluated approximately every 3 to 4 months by an endocrinologist. Accurate measurements of height are essential to evaluate efficacy. The use of a growth chart helps identify growth velocity. Therapy is continued until the child reaches an acceptable adult height or radiographic evidence shows growth-plate fusion.

Evaluation

- Has the child exhibited increased growth rate?
- Does the child verbalize feelings regarding body image and self-esteem?
- Do the child and family adhere to the injection schedule?

CRITICAL THINKING EXERCISE 27-1

Periodically, the media have drawn attention to the use of GH. Parents of young teenage boys often are concerned about their child's present and eventual height. Boys who are significantly shorter than their peers during early adolescence can experience altered self-esteem.

How should a nurse respond if parents ask whether giving GH to their short son will increase his eventual height?

DIABETES MELLITUS

Evidence has been accumulating that demonstrates a worldwide increase in the incidence of type 1 diabetes mellitus, with incidence rising specifically in areas where type 1 diabetes was previously low (Alemzadeh & Wyatt, 2004). Additionally, children are developing type 1 diabetes at an earlier age. The overall incidence of type 1 diabetes in 2010 is predicted to be approximately 40% higher than the incidence recorded in 1997 (Alemzadeh & Wyatt, 2004). The incidence of type 2 diabetes has also risen in children. Before 1990, only 5% of youth were classified as having type 2 diabetes; today, up to half of all diagnosed cases of diabetes in youth are classified as type 2 (Thomassian, 2004).

Type 1 Diabetes Mellitus

Type 1 diabetes mellitus results when the pancreas is unable to produce and secrete insulin. This form of diabetes, the most common childhood endocrine disorder, presents challenges in the areas of teaching, management, and adherence. Because of recent changes in the health care delivery system, meeting the needs associated with management of type 1 diabetes mellitus has become more complicated. Unless the newly diagnosed child is in diabetic ketoacidosis (DKA), the child may not be hospitalized. The nurse must develop a plan of care that involves family education, in either an inpatient or outpatient setting. Including the family in the child's care and support must be part of planning and implementation of nursing care. Type 1 and type 2 diabetes are chronic diseases; see Chapter 12 for a discussion of that aspect of care.

Etiology

Type 1 diabetes mellitus results from an autoimmune process that causes the destruction of the insulin-secreting cells of the pancreas. A genetic predisposition plus an environmental or viral trigger are thought to initiate the autoimmune destructive process. Current research focuses on identifying specific genes that may affect a person's susceptibility to type 1 diabetes mellitus and exploring methods of interrupting or preventing the autoimmune response in susceptible people (first-degree relatives of a diabetic person). At this time no prevention or cure is available; however, several different means of islet cell transplantation are being explored and are quite promising. Children with type 1 diabetes mellitus are prone to developing other autoimmune conditions, such as Grave disease, Hashimoto thyroiditis, and celiac disease (see Chapter 19), among others (ADA, 2006a).

Incidence

Thirteen million people in the United States are diagnosed with diabetes (American Diabetes Association, 2005). Approximately 210,000 people younger than 20 years have diabetes, 0.26% of all persons in this age group. Type 1 diabetes is diagnosed in approximately 1 of every 400 to 500 children and adolescents. The median age of onset is between 7 and 15 years (Alemzadeh & Wyatt, 2004).

Manifestations

The classic initial signs of hyperglycemia, known as the "three *P*'s," are *p*olyuria (or enuresis in a toilet-trained child), *p*olydipsia, and *p*olyphagia. The child's symptoms include weight loss (despite increased food intake), fatigue, and blurred vision.

If the condition progresses without intervention, the child can exhibit the following signs of DKA: nausea and vomiting, abdominal pain, acetone (fruity) odor to breath, dehydration, increasing lethargy, Kussmaul respirations, and coma.

Children who receive insulin for treatment of type 1 diabetes mellitus can have hypoglycemia. Table 27-3 compares hypoglycemia, hyperglycemia, and ketoacidosis.

Diagnostic Evaluation

Diagnosis of type 1 diabetes mellitus is made on the basis of a clinical picture of hyperglycemia (and acidosis if present) combined with the laboratory data of a fasting serum glucose exceeding 126 mg/dL and a random serum glucose of 200 mg/dL or greater (ADA, 2006a). Ketonuria, although not diagnostic, is a frequent finding, as is glycosuria. Glucose tolerance testing is rarely used in diagnosing type 1 diabetes mellitus. The glycosylated hemoglobin value is elevated in response to prolonged elevations of blood glucose.

Any child with severe fasting hyperglycemia, ketonemia, and metabolic abnormalities, whether diagnosed with type 1 or type 2 diabetes, will need insulin therapy to reverse the metabolic imbalances (Silverstein, Klingensmith, Copeland, Plotnick, Kaufman, & Laffel, 2005).

Therapeutic Management

Children diagnosed with type 1 diabetes will be started on insulin therapy. Approximately 30% of children, at the time of their initial type 1 diagnosis, also are in DKA. They

PATHOPHYSIOLOGY

TYPE 1 DIABETES MELLITUS

Glucose is the primary source of energy for body cells. Any extra glucose taken in by the body can be stored as glycogen in muscle or liver cells or the form of fatty tissues. Glucose can be extracted from glycogen for periods of fasting (e.g., overnight). Once glycogen stores have been depleted, new glucose (gluconeogenesis) is made from amino acids released from muscle into the bloodstream. The energy for gluconeogenesis is supplied by the breakdown of stored fats.

Insulin, a hormone, is secreted by the beta cells of the pancreas. Its main function is to regulate the blood glucose level by controlling the rate of glucose uptake by cells. Little or no insulin is secreted by the beta cells when a person is in the fasting state; greater quantities are secreted after the person has eaten a meal. In the fasting state, with relatively small quantities of available insulin, the body mobilizes fats and proteins to be used as fuel sources. The liver then converts the fats into ketoacids, or ketones. With the assistance of insulin, ketones are transported into the cells and are used as an alternative source of fuel for cellular energy. This process ensures an energy source during long periods of fasting. Not all cells in the body are capable of using ketone bodies and require glucose as their primary fuel (Table 27-2).

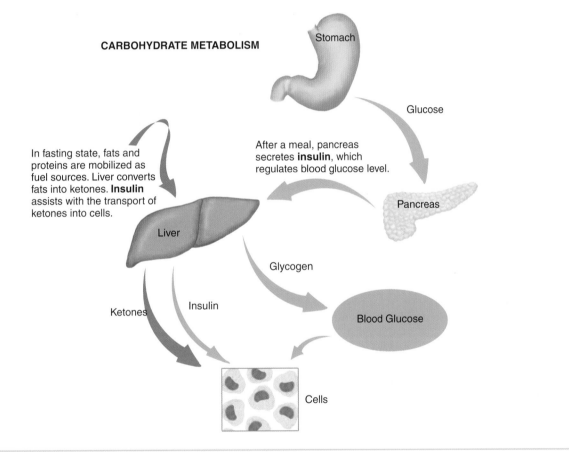

CARBOHYDRATE METABOLISM

Stomach

Glucose

After a meal, pancreas secretes **insulin**, which regulates blood glucose level.

In fasting state, fats and proteins are mobilized as fuel sources. Liver converts fats into ketones. **Insulin** assists with the transport of ketones into cells.

Pancreas

Liver

Glycogen

Blood Glucose

Ketones   Insulin

Cells

Continued

TABLE 27-2   Actions of Insulin

Anabolic Actions of Insulin	Catabolic Consequences of Insulin Deficit
Promotes glucose as a fuel source	Promotes fats and proteins as fuel sources
Promotes storage of glucose as glycogen	Allows glycogen stores to be broken down
Prevents breakdown of fat stores	Allows fat stores to be depleted
Increases protein synthesis	Allows protein breakdown into amino acids

PATHOPHYSIOLOGY

TYPE 1 DIABETES MELLITUS—cont'd

In the absence of insulin, the metabolism of fats, proteins, and carbohydrates is impaired. Glucose is unable to move into the intracellular space, resulting in hyperglycemia. As blood glucose levels exceed the renal threshold, glucose is "spilled" into the urine through osmotic diuresis, resulting in polyuria. Excessive thirst follows in response to fluid loss. Fatigue, hunger, and weight loss also accompany the onset of type 1 diabetes mellitus because cellular starvation continues in the absence of insulin.

Ketones (ketoacids), manufactured by the liver from adipose tissue, are produced in response to cellular starvation. In the absence of insulin, ketones are also unavailable to the cell for nourishment. Increasing blood levels of ketones (ketonemia) result in ketoacidosis.

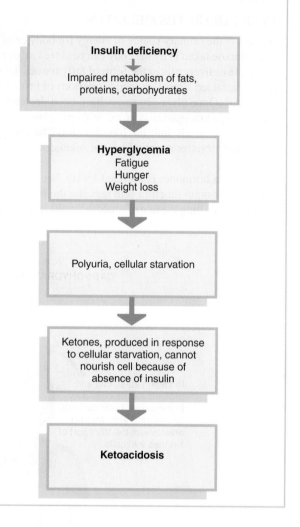

will require management in a pediatric intensive care unit (Silverstein et al., 2005).

The goals of diabetes management for children with type 1 diabetes mellitus include the following:

- Facilitating appropriate growth (height, weight)
- Maintaining an age-appropriate lifestyle
- Achieving near-normal glycosylated hemoglobin
- Preventing acute complications (hypoglycemia, hyperglycemia)

Insulin Therapy

The child with type 1 diabetes mellitus loses the ability to make insulin because of autoimmune destruction of the insulin-producing cells, the beta cells. Symptoms of hyperglycemia become evident when most of the beta cells are destroyed. After initiation of insulin therapy, the child may have a "honeymoon" phase characterized by hypoglycemia and a decreasing need for insulin. This may last from a few weeks to 1 year or longer. The nurse should prepare the child and family for the possibility of a honeymoon phase, both to avoid the misconception that the diabetes is "going away" and to provide instruction on recognition and treatment of hypoglycemia.

The goal of insulin therapy is to replace the insulin the child is no longer able to make. Synthetic human insulin, made by recombinant deoxyribonucleic acid (DNA) technology, is free of animal impurities and is recommended for children. Previously insulin was derived from bovine and porcine pancreatic extracts. Oral hypoglycemic agents, although useful in the treatment of type 2 diabetes, are not effective in the treatment of type 1 diabetes.

The choice of insulin types and schedule of injections is determined on the basis of the child's needs (Table 27-4). Daily self-monitoring of blood glucose aids in defining insulin requirements. The child in the honeymoon phase needs less insulin than the child who makes no endogenous insulin. The pubertal child requires larger insulin dosages.

Schedule. Insulin requirements are commonly based on age, body weight, and pubertal status. In general, children who are newly diagnosed with type 1 diabetes typically need an initial total daily dose of approximately 0.5 to 1.0 U/kg. Because dosages for infants and toddlers frequently are less than 1 U, the insulin is diluted with an approved diluent to increase the volume to be administered and improve accuracy in dosing (Silverstein et al., 2005). Most children

TABLE 27-3	Comparison of Hypoglycemia, Hyperglycemia, and Ketoacidosis		
Descriptor	**Hypoglycemia**	**Hyperglycemia**	**Ketoacidosis**
Onset	Rapid	Slow	Slow
Signs and symptoms	*Adrenergic signs:* Trembling Sweating Tachycardia Pallor Clammy skin	Increased urination Increased thirst Fatigue Weight loss (gradual, over several weeks) Blurred vision	*Hyperglycemia signs plus:* Abdominal pain Chest pain Kussmaul respirations Nausea and vomiting Acetone (fruity) breath odor *Signs and symptoms of dehydration:* Dry lips and mucous membranes Sunken eyes Sudden weight loss Decreased urination
Alterations in sensorium	Neuroglycopenic symptoms: Personality change Irritability Drunken behavior Slurred speech Decreased level of consciousness to total loss of consciousness Seizure activity	Emotional lability Headache Hunger	Increasing lethargy Decreasing level of consciousness Coma
Laboratory data	Blood glucose <70 mg/dL	Blood glucose >160 mg/dL	Blood glucose >300 mg/dL Urinary ketones positive Serum pH <7.25 Serum ketones positive
Causes	Too much insulin Excessive activity without eating extra carbohydrates Missed or delayed meal	Excessive intake of carbohydrate Little or no exercise Inadequate amount of insulin Increased stress, either emotional or physical	Inadequate amount of insulin Excessive stress
Treatment	15 g of carbohydrate *For loss of consciousness or seizure activity:* Glucagon subcutaneous or intramuscular IV glucose	Insulin Exercise Increased oral fluids	IV fluids IV insulin Electrolyte replacement Generalized supportive care

TABLE 27-4	Insulin Action by Type (Humulin)		
Type	**Onset**	**Peak**	**Duration**
Lispro/Aspart	10-15 min	30-90 min	3 hr
Regular	30-60 min	2-3 hr	3-6 hr
NPH or Lente	2-4 hr	4-10 hr	10-16 hr
Glargine	—	—	24 hr

are managed through administration of insulin by three or more injections a day of a combination long-acting basal and rapid-acting bolus (multiple daily injection [MDI]) given before meals and snacks or continuously by insulin pump (continuous subcutaneous insulin infusion [CSII]). The basal/bolus insulin regimen has demonstrated stable glycemic control (Silverstein et al., 2005). The injection schedule is individually prescribed according to the child's glycemic targets. The peak actions of these insulins are timed to correspond to the child's usual mealtimes and snack times to minimize the possibility of hypoglycemia. A recent option for the basal/bolus insulin regimen is a combination of rapid-acting analogs with a long-acting peakless insulin. Glargine (Lantus), a long-acting peakless analog, has been approved by the Food and Drug Administration (FDA) for children aged 6 years and older. Glargine, given in the evening as the basal insulin, and complemented during the day by a rapid-acting insulin (Lispro or Aspart) when the child eats carbohydrates, provides improved glycemic control (Fig. 27-2).

Administration. Because insulin is a protein and would be digested if taken orally, it is given parenterally. Insulin is administered by subcutaneous injection into the adipose tissue over large muscle masses: the back of the arms, the top and outer portion of the thighs, the abdomen, and the hip (Fig. 27-3). To avoid injecting into the muscle or vascular space, use a 45-degree angle of injection with a ½-inch needle or a 90-degree angle with a 5/16-inch needle. Rotation of injection sites helps prevent adipose hypertrophy (fatty lumps), which absorb insulin poorly. Various injection sites absorb insulin at slightly different rates. Absorption is also

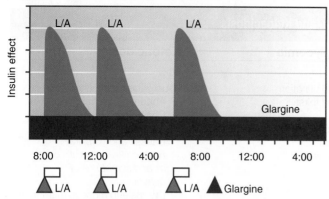

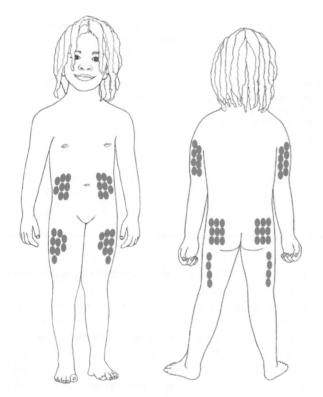

FIG 27-2   Peak action of insulin injections is timed to correspond with the child's usual meal and snack times to minimize the chance of hypoglycemia.   *(Data from Alemzadeh, R., & Wyatt, D. [2004]. Diabetes mellitus in children. In R. Behrman, R. Kliegmen, & H. Jenson [Eds.]. Nelson textbook of pediatrics [17th ed., p. 1956-1957]. Philadelphia: Saunders.)*

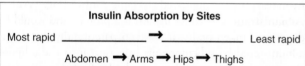

Insulin Absorption by Sites

Most rapid ⟶ Least rapid

Abdomen ⟶ Arms ⟶ Hips ⟶ Thighs

FIG 27-3   Subcutaneous insulin injection sites most commonly used are shown, although almost any area on the body may be used. Sites are rotated on a daily basis to help prevent the formation of fatty lumps, which absorb insulin poorly. However, because the rate of absorption varies by site (see chart), the child is advised to rotate sites within the same general area (e.g., arm, thigh) for a period of 2 to 3 weeks before changing to another area. This will help decrease variations in absorption from day to day.   *(Chart modified from Albisser, A. M., & Sperlich, M. [1993]. Adjusting insulins. Diabetes Educator, 18[3], 211-227.)*

affected by the amount of exercise the underlying muscle engages in and by body temperature. To help decrease day-to-day variations in absorption, the child should use one location within a major site for the morning injection, then rotate to another location within the site for the evening injection and a third location for the bedtime injection.

Insulin can be administered by an insulin syringe, air injector, or insulin pump. Disposable syringes are to be used only one time and then safely discarded (with the syringe placed in a puncture-resistant, opaque container before placing in the trash). The air injector uses compressed air to deposit the insulin within the fatty tissue without the use of a needle. The child or family must learn to use the device correctly: load insulin, adjust pressure settings to avoid intramuscular delivery, and clean properly.

The insulin pump is a battery-operated device that provides a continuous infusion of rapid-acting insulin. Use of the pump in the pediatric population continues to grow. Evidence suggests that the insulin pump provides tighter control of blood sugar and more flexibility in lifestyle (Weissberg-Benchell, Antisdel-Lomaglio, & Seshadri, 2003). The pump is a mechanical device, approximately the size of a pager, that is often worn on a belt or in a pocket. It delivers insulin to the body through an infusion set consisting of thin plastic tubing attached to a cannula or needle inserted into the thigh, abdomen, or buttocks. A continuous basal rate of insulin infusion is maintained, and bolus dosages are infused as determined by blood glucose testing.

The pump most closely mimics physiologic delivery of insulin and provides a more flexible lifestyle. This option may appeal to adolescents, but the candidate for insulin pump therapy must be willing to measure blood glucose meticulously (at least four glucose checks per day), be able to count carbohydrates and calculate appropriate insulin coverage, and have a supportive home environment. Caregivers can be the responsible person for the insulin pump when used by infants and toddlers. Dietary recommendations are different for children or adolescents using an insulin pump and are based on carbohydrate counting.

Nutrition Therapy

The goal of nutrition therapy is to promote normal growth, encourage healthy nutrition, prevent complications, and maintain near-normal blood glucose levels. Because the insulin dosage is balanced with food intake, the diet plan should stress a consistent intake, particularly of carbohydrate food products. The diet therapy chosen should be easy to understand and help the child and family learn to make healthy food choices. The meal plan is based on the child's diet history. The individualized meal plan should be tailored to food preferences, physical activity, cultural aspects, and schedules. As the child grows, the meal plan is tailored to meet changing dietary needs.

Physical Activity

Exercise is an important aspect of diabetes management. Exercise enhances the action of insulin in lowering blood glucose levels. In addition, exercise promotes a greater sense of well-being, improves physical and cardiovascular fitness, and

---

Managing the Child with Type 1 Diabetes Mellitus

Insulin
- Store insulin in a cool, dry place. Do not freeze or expose to excessive heat or agitation.
- Check the expiration date on the vial before using.
- Once opened, date the vial and discard as recommended.
- When mixing two different types of insulin, inject the appropriate amount of air into both vials and then withdraw the short-acting (clear) insulin first.

Nutrition
- Meals and snacks are balanced with insulin action.
- Both the timing of the meal or snack and the amount of food are important in avoiding hyperglycemia or hypoglycemia.
- Adherence to a daily schedule that maintains a consistent food intake combined with consistent insulin injections aids in achieving metabolic control.

Exercise
- Avoid exercising during insulin peak.
- Add extra 15- to 30-g carbohydrate snacks for each 45 to 60 minutes of exercise.

Blood Glucose Monitoring
- Record blood glucose results in a diary.
- A 3- to 4-day alteration in glucose levels requires an adjustment of insulin dose.

---

contributes to an improved lipid profile. The child with diabetes should be encouraged to participate in age-appropriate sports. Early enjoyment of a sport or activity can promote a lifelong active lifestyle. Because exercise lowers glucose levels, the child must be taught how to prevent hypoglycemia. The child should try to schedule activities to avoid exercising when an insulin dose is peaking. Maintaining proper hydration while exercising is important.

Teach the family to add extra snacks of 15 to 30 g carbohydrate for each 45 to 60 minutes of exercise. Coaches and teammates should be taught how to recognize and treat hypoglycemia. Delayed or nocturnal hypoglycemia can occur after strenuous activity. Additional carbohydrate might be required after exercise to maintain blood glucose levels. The child should always wear medical alert identification.

Blood Glucose Monitoring

Self-monitoring of blood glucose (SMBG) provides an objective tool to assist with diabetes control. Monitoring is recommended before meals and before the bedtime snack. More frequent monitoring may be used during prolonged exercise, during an illness, or if nighttime hypoglycemia is suspected.

Blood glucose goals must be tailored to the abilities of the family and the age of the child. Goals for the infant or toddler are usually liberalized to help prevent severe hypoglycemia. Preprandial blood glucose goals are as follows:
- Nondiabetic: 70 to 110 mg/dL
- Children with type 1 diabetes mellitus: 80 to 180 mg/dL

- Infants and toddlers with type 1 diabetes mellitus: 80 to 200 mg/dL

The identified goals are a target range; not all glucose levels fall in this range, even in the child with excellent diabetes control.

Glucose test results should be recorded in a glucose diary or record book. Patterns or trends in blood glucose levels outside the target range indicate a need to adjust the insulin dose. Three or four days of a consistent pattern of glucose values (e.g., 200 mg/dL before the evening meal for 3 consecutive days) indicate a need to increase the appropriate insulin. The health care team may provide the family with guidelines for increasing insulin dose on the basis of blood glucose patterns.

A majority of blood glucose meters can store multiple monitoring results so blood glucose patterns can be evaluated. Blood glucose meters are accurate only if used according to manufacturers' recommendations. Regardless of the brand selected, quality control procedures must be performed as recommended. Test supplies must be stored according to manufacturers' specifications and discarded when outdated.

Developmental Issues

Infant and Toddler. The infant or toddler with type 1 diabetes poses special challenges for diabetes management. The parents or primary caregivers must adapt to the diagnosis and master daily management of caring for their child with type 1 diabetes. Severe hypoglycemia tends to be highest in this age group. Achieving consistency in dietary intake with the infant can be quite difficult. Inconsistent intake, particularly of carbohydrates, contributes to blood glucose variability. Food control issues can easily become a battleground between the child and the parent. A diet strategy that stresses carbohydrate consistency rather than specific food groups offers more flexibility than a structured meal plan.

Allow the toddler to participate in making food choices (from perhaps two or three options) to offer the child a sense of control. The signs and symptoms of hypoglycemia are difficult to recognize in the infant or may be mistaken for the toddler's temper tantrum. The glucose goals for this age group are liberalized to avoid episodes of severe hypoglycemia.

Establishing rituals and routines helps the toddler feel more in control. Encourage a parent to have a specific place to perform the blood test and a special place to keep supplies. Toddlers feel more in control if they are able to predict and participate in diabetes activities (Table 27-5).

Preschooler. The preschool years are characterized by increasing motor maturity, a widening social circle, and magical thinking. The preschooler can understand simple explanations regarding diabetes. Such explanations help allay fears that the diabetes was caused by the child being "bad." Play therapy with dolls and diabetes equipment helps the preschooler express concerns regarding injections and finger sticks.

The preschooler has a more predictable appetite than the toddler and is frequently willing to try new foods. Nonetheless, supervision is necessary to ensure that meals and snacks are eaten, especially if the child is in a daycare setting with many distractions.

TABLE **27-5** Examples of Delegation of Diabetes Tasks (With Supervision)		
Developmental Characteristics	**Diabetes Task**	**Diet Task**
Toddler or Preschooler Likes rituals Finicky eater Not yet able to understand need for insulin	Chooses and cleans finger for puncture Helps by holding still for injection Identifies a word or phrase to describe a feeling of hypoglycemia	Helps by choosing foods
School-Age Child Present oriented Spends large amounts of time away from parents Begins to develop self-concept	Performs finger puncture and blood glucose test Chooses injection site according to rotation schedule Pushes plunger on insulin syringe after the needle is inserted by parent or gives own injection Performs ketone test	Recognizes need to eat on time to avoid hypoglycemia Knows treatment for hypoglycemia
Early Adolescent Looks to peer group for identity Needs to conform to peer-group norms Increased risk-taking behaviors	Records blood glucose values in diary Draws up insulin with supervision Performs insulin injection	Knows meal plan Can choose correct foods for snack Adds extra snack for increased activity
Middle or Late Adolescent Future oriented Wants to take charge of life Able to recognize consequences of behaviors and choices Emotional separation from parents	Draws up and injects insulin Looks for patterns in blood glucose values Recognizes when to test for ketones Initiates treatment for ketones (fluids)	Can plan meals and snacks based on meal plan Can choose appropriate foods at a party or when eating out

The preschooler may be able to identify the feelings associated with hypoglycemia. Use the child's description as a code word for the onset of hypoglycemia symptoms. Preschoolers' preference for high-energy activities puts them at risk for hypoglycemia. The caregiver should be prepared with readily available carbohydrate foods as well as emergency medications.

School-Age Child. The school-age child and family face the challenge of incorporating diabetes care within a busy school day. To avoid singling out the child, the diabetes care should be as unobtrusive as possible while still maintaining a safe environment for the child. Children with type 1 diabetes mellitus fall under the auspices of the Individuals with Disabilities Education Act and, as such, are entitled to services within the school setting. The child should have a diabetes management plan that specifically describes frequency of blood glucose testing, insulin doses, nutrition, and any other therapy or modifications associated with the diabetes (ADA, 2006a). The family should communicate with school personnel about the child's diabetes. A school nurse or health aide should be identified to supervise prelunch blood glucose monitoring, assist with insulin injections, and educate other school personnel in recognizing and treating hypoglycemia. Schools vary on the availability of nursing services. Parents may have to work with school personnel to identify appropriate staff to supervise their child's diabetes care.

Planning ahead for field trips, school parties, and athletic events allows the child with diabetes to participate safely in age-appropriate activities. For example, the child who has soccer practice three afternoons per week needs to plan how to prevent hypoglycemia during practice.

Adolescent. The adolescent's developmental milestones are often in conflict with the recommendations for achieving diabetes control. The young adolescent is concerned with body image and peer group acceptance and is moving away from the family for support and identity. Clothing, diet, lifestyle, and speech are areas in which the early adolescent strives to conform to peers.

The midadolescent is open to risk-taking behaviors and is more openly challenging of parental authority. By late adolescence, the person becomes more future-oriented, with behaviors based more on abstract morals and less on peer group demands.

These normally recognized milestones become dilemmas when diabetes control is affected. Missed injections, omitted blood tests, irregular meals, and dietary splurges are frequent complaints of parents of diabetic adolescents.

Parents and their adolescents must accept that diabetes responsibility increasingly shifts to the adolescent. Encourage parents to work as partners with the adolescent to achieve diabetes control. Identify what is important to the adolescent, and use that information as a tool to motivate adherence. The adolescent is not motivated by predictions

Text continued on p. 908

NURSING CARE PLAN

The Child With Type 1 Diabetes Mellitus in the Community Setting

Focused Assessment

Nursing assessment of the child diagnosed with type 1 diabetes mellitus begins with a careful history. Most children with diabetes are identified on a routine well visit, or the child may exhibit signs on a visit to the school nurse. Identify signs and symptoms of hyperglycemia—the three *P*'s (*p*olydipsia, *p*olyuria, and *p*olyphagia). Daytime polydipsia and polyuria may not worry a parent, but enuresis or accidents in the previously toilet-trained child and nighttime requests for water spark concern. New-onset diabetes is frequently overlooked in light of specific symptoms. A urinary tract infection may be suspected because of urinary frequency. An infective process frequently accompanies the onset of diabetes but is not the cause of the diabetes. The stress associated with an infection can compromise the function of the remaining insulin-secreting cells. A history of weight loss or fatigue is also a common parental observation. Nausea and vomiting are present in the child who is acidotic. Ask about other medications used. Glucocorticoids and some chemotherapeutic agents can cause hyperglycemia.

Physical assessment should include signs and symptoms of dehydration: dry mucous membranes, flushed skin, acute weight change, absence of tearing, or poor skin turgor. Identify the time of most recent voiding. Oliguria is a significant finding in the assessment of dehydration.

If the child is admitted to the hospital, assess for signs and symptoms of acidosis: abdominal pain, nausea and vomiting (which also contribute to dehydration), Kussmaul respirations coupled with a fruity breath odor, or decreasing level of consciousness (LOC). Ongoing assessment of the child in acidosis should include vital signs, LOC, and intake and output. Vital signs and LOC should be monitored frequently until stable.

Assess the family's knowledge of diabetes. For the newly diagnosed child, prepare the family to participate in a diabetes education program to learn home care skills. Encourage parents to arrange for time away from work and school to participate. Assess the family's ability to cope with the diagnosis of a chronic disease. Identify usual methods of coping with stress and usual support systems. Explore the availability of financial resources to meet the child's health care needs.

NURSING DIAGNOSIS   Deficient Knowledge related to unfamiliarity with home care needs of the child with type 1 diabetes mellitus.

EXPECTED OUTCOME   The child and family will:
- Be able to successfully manage diabetes, as evidenced by demonstration of skills and verbalization of concepts necessary for home care (Box 27-5).

Intervention

1. Identify barriers to learning that might hinder the family's ability to learn home care information. Barriers could include issues such as language fluency, literacy, employment pressures, and child care. These issues should be addressed before initiating education.
2. Identify learning objectives with the family.

3. Present information at a developmentally appropriate level for the child.

Rationale

1. Identifying and addressing these issues optimize the family's learning ability. For example, provide appropriate written materials for the person with low literacy skills or a different native language.

2. A written list of specific objectives helps the family prioritize education and provides a sense of accomplishment as learning objectives are met.
3. The child must cognitively understand diabetes. More advanced information can be presented as the child matures.

Evaluation

- Can the child and family successfully manage care, as evidenced by return demonstrations of skills necessary to provide home care?

- Are the child and family able to describe principles of diabetes management?

NURSING DIAGNOSIS   Interrupted Family Processes related to the chronic health care needs of a child with type 1 diabetes mellitus.

EXPECTED OUTCOME   The family will:
- Cope with caring for a child with diabetes, as evidenced by recognizing and identifying stresses and constructing strategies for dealing with the stress of a chronic disease.

Continued

NURSING CARE PLAN—cont'd

Intervention	Rationale
1. Help the family identify age-appropriate diabetes skills for the child's and the parent's responsibilities.	1. Delegation of responsibilities should occur as the child is both able to perform the skill and able to understand the implications of the skill. Parental support and supervision are essential for all children for successful home management of diabetes.
2. Help the child and family identify behaviors that the child recognizes as supportive; for example, all family members follow the child's meal plan, avoid having sweets in the home, offer to record blood glucose levels in the diary for the child, or recognize and praise the child's attempts at adherence.	2. Discussions of family support help involve all family members in the child's care, as well as give the child the opportunity to identify supportive behaviors. Adaptation is enhanced by focusing on the strengths of the child and family.
3. Identify community support systems available for the family, such as summer diabetes camp and age-specific support groups, parent support group, or participation in fund-raising activities in a local diabetes community group.	3. Community resources offer a variety of opportunities for support as well as an alternative to relying solely on family coping skills (see Evolve website). Activities for the diabetic child can build motivation and self-esteem.
4. Identify a "vacation" plan in which the major caregiver can take a break from diabetes responsibilities. This may include ongoing, day-to-day responsibility of diabetes management shared among parents, siblings, and others or temporarily sharing one aspect of the management.	4. Taking responsibility for diabetes control is very stressful and demanding. Sharing responsibilities among family members helps prevent burnout, discouragement, and frustration.

Evaluation

• Can the child and family verbalize a plan for sharing diabetes responsibility?

NURSING DIAGNOSIS Imbalanced Nutrition: Less Than Body Requirements related to insulin deficit.

EXPECTED OUTCOMES The family and child will:
   • Maximize nutritional status, as evidenced by demonstrating the ability to use insulin therapy, diet therapy, and glucose self-monitoring.
   The child will:
   • Be in nutritional balance, as evidenced by appropriate glucose levels and absence of hyperglycemia and hypoglycemia.

Intervention	Rationale
1. Teach the family the action of food (carbohydrates, fats, proteins) on blood glucose level: carbohydrates raise blood glucose levels; fats and proteins have minimal effects on glucose levels.	1. Understanding the relationship of food to blood glucose levels will help the family recognize the rationale for adhering to the diabetic diet.
2. Together with the family, develop an eating schedule that includes times for blood glucose testing, medication, meals, and snacks.	2. Consistency in timing of meals and snacks in relation to insulin injections is essential. Encouraging child and family input into this aspect of planning will impart a sense of control as well as promote adherence.
3. Ask the child to identify favorite foods and demonstrate how to incorporate these into the meal plan.	3. Most foods can be incorporated into the meal plan, even if only in small amounts. Allowing small amounts of favorite treats can encourage adherence.
4. Observe whether the child's hunger is satisfied on the prescribed diet. Instruct the child and parent to notify the dietitian if the meal plan forces the child to overeat or if the child is persistently hungry. Use an appropriate growth chart to track the child's height and weight with respect to age.	4. The meal plan is tailored to the child and the child's activity level. Nutritional needs vary with age as well as with variations in activity level. For example, a morning gym class may require that the child add a midmorning snack.

NURSING CARE PLAN—cont'd

5. Discuss the relationships of insulin, food (carbohydrate), and exercise. Identify ideal blood glucose goals for the child. Present a sample situation in which the blood glucose is out of the ideal range, and encourage the family to identify possible options using diet, insulin, and/or exercise to attain the blood glucose goal more closely.

6. Instruct the family to plan 3 or 4 days of menus based on the meal plan. Both the type of food and the amount of food should be included.

5. Diet, exercise, and insulin therapy are the tools of diabetes management. This exercise will develop problem-solving skills within the family and provide a sense of competency.

6. This exercise will help the family demonstrate understanding of the diet instructions.

Evaluation

- Do the child and family demonstrate appropriate insulin administration, diet therapy, and glucose monitoring?
- Are the child's height and weight appropriate for age compared with growth chart percentiles?

- Is the child free of episodes of severe hypoglycemia or hyperglycemia?

NURSING DIAGNOSIS   Risk for Injury related to hypoglycemia or hyperglycemia.

EXPECTED OUTCOMES   The child will:
- Remain injury free as a result of appropriate recognition and management of hypoglycemia or hyperglycemia.

Family members will:
- Demonstrate knowledge of the signs, symptoms, and treatment of hypoglycemia and hyperglycemia and will initiate appropriate treatment.

Intervention

For hypoglycemia (blood glucose level less than 70 mg/dL):

1. Teach the child and family to recognize the signs and symptoms of hypoglycemia (see Table 27-3). School personnel should also be involved in teaching. The school nurse, if available, can play a key role in the care of a child with diabetes.

2. Treat hypoglycemia promptly with 15 g of easily digested carbohydrate. If symptoms are not relieved (or blood glucose level is not higher than 80 mg/dL) in 15 minutes, repeat the treatment. If the hypoglycemia occurs during the night, treat with 30 g carbohydrate–15 g simple carbohydrate and 15 g complex carbohydrate–with protein. Examples of 15 g of carbohydrate include 4 oz of real fruit juice, 6 oz of regular soda, 6 Life Savers candy, or a commercial glucose product.

3. Help the child and family identify strategies to prevent hypoglycemia on the basis of its common causes: missed or delayed meal, excess insulin, or extra exercise without increasing carbohydrate intake. Encourage the family to teach the signs and symptoms of hypoglycemia and necessary treatment to school personnel and day care workers. Help the child prepare to explain hypoglycemia to friends. Compile a diabetes box for school and day care. The box should contain carbohydrates for treating hypoglycemia as well as written information. Instruct the child to wear medical alert identification at all times.

Rationale

1. Signs and symptoms of hypoglycemia should prompt the child or parent to test the blood glucose level. Some children do not display adrenergic signs of hypoglycemia. Neuroglycopenic signs (altered sensorium) may be the only clues to hypoglycemia in these children. These signs are quite hard for the child to recognize but can be observed by a parent or teacher. Blood glucose goals for this child may need to be modified to prevent hypoglycemic unawareness.

2. Prompt treatment reduces the possibility of a severe reaction. Candy bars, donuts, and cookies are poor treatment choices because of their high fat content, which can delay carbohydrate digestion. The child could also interpret these treats as a reward for hypoglycemia.

3. Many episodes of hypoglycemia can be avoided by careful planning and anticipating potential situations that could result in hypoglycemia. Instruction about the signs, symptoms, and treatment of hypoglycemia is essential information to be shared with people caring for the child. Hypoglycemia is a potential emergency that requires prompt recognition and treatment.

Continued

4. Teach the parents how to treat severe hypoglycemia. For the unconscious child or the child having a seizure, a small amount of glucose gel (cake frosting or honey will also work) can be rubbed on the inner cheek and gums. Avoid placing a large amount of gel in the mouth because the child could choke. Glucagon (available by prescription as Glucagon Emergency Kit from Eli Lilly Co.) can be injected subcutaneously or intramuscularly. Inject 1 mg for the child weighing more than 50 lb (22.75 kg) or 20 to 30 μg/kg for children weighing less than 50 lb (22.75 kg). The onset of action is 10 to 15 minutes. Position the unconscious child on the side. Once conscious, the child needs a large snack to replace lost glycogen stores.

4. The unconscious child or the child having a seizure requires prompt treatment. Glucagon is a pancreatic hormone that opposes the action of insulin and promotes the conversion of liver glycogen to blood glucose. The child is positioned on the side to prevent aspiration. Both severe hypoglycemia and glucagon administration can result in nausea with vomiting.

Intervention

For hyperglycemia (blood glucose level higher than target range):
1. Teach the family to recognize potential causes of hyperglycemia: inadequate insulin, increased dietary intake, decreased exercise, stress response (either emotional or physical stress [e.g., illness]).

2. Instruct family on sick-day diabetes management, including when and how to test for urine ketones. Identify a home treatment plan for ketones and identify precautions for vomiting (Box 27-6).

3. Identify strategies to prevent or treat hyperglycemia.

Rationale

1. Anticipating situations that could result in hyperglycemia can help the family plan for such events. The signs and symptoms of hypoglycemia and hyperglycemia can be difficult to distinguish from one another. Test blood glucose before treating to verify glucose level. If testing is impossible, treat for hypoglycemia.

2. Testing for ketones when ill or when blood glucose is 250 mg/dL or higher helps detect insulin deficit. Ketones are treated with (calorie-free) fluids and additional rapid-acting insulin as ordered by the physician. Nausea with vomiting leads to dehydration and cannot be treated with oral fluids. The physician must be notified if the child is vomiting.

3. Consistency in diet, exercise, and insulin injection times helps prevent hyperglycemia. Persistent hyperglycemia may indicate a need for an insulin dosage adjustment. The growing child needs periodic increases in baseline insulin dosages.

Evaluation

• Does the child remain injury free?

• Are the child and family able to recognize and correctly and promptly treat hypoglycemia and hyperglycemia?

of complications in the distant future. Rather, motivation should focus on issues important to the adolescent: personal appearance, athletic ability, strength and muscle mass, endurance, or ideal weight.

Delegating Diabetes Responsibilities

Children with diabetes are functionally able to perform diabetes skills far sooner than they can cognitively understand the implications of the activity or consequences of omitting the activity. Transfer of responsibility should be on a step-by-step basis, according to the child's cognitive understanding and functional abilities. Diabetes responsibilities shift from full parental responsibility to a partnership between parent and child and then to the acceptance of responsibility by the young adult. Delegating diabetes responsibility at an inap-

propriate age results in poor diabetes control and frequent bouts of DKA. The importance of ongoing parental support and supervision cannot be overemphasized.

DIABETIC KETOACIDOSIS

DKA is the metabolic consequence of a severe insulin deficit leading to hyperglycemia and presence of ketone bodies in the blood, followed by metabolic acidosis.

Etiology

DKA results from an absolute or relative insulin deficit. In the younger diabetic child, the most common cause is insulin resistance, such as a stress response initiated by an infection. In the adolescent, the most common cause is one or more missed insulin injections.

| BOX 27-5 | **FAMILIES WANT TO KNOW**   About Home Management of Type 1 Diabetes Mellitus |

The child and family are understandably overwhelmed with questions and fears about the diagnosis. Encourage all family members to participate. Choose a comfortable location subject to few interruptions. Provide appropriate literature and materials for family members. Videotapes, booklets, and pamphlets should be developmentally appropriate. Educational materials for the parents should also match the parents' literacy skills.

The following checklist of outcomes evaluates the family's understanding of the pertinent information:

- General information about type 1 diabetes mellitus
- How to administer and store insulin
- How to monitor blood glucose levels and use the equipment properly
- Signs and management of hypoglycemic episodes
- Signs and management of hyperglycemia
- Strategies for when the child is ill
- Nutrition and exercise principles
- Potential long-term complications
- Available resources for emotional and physical support

All family members should be given the opportunity to practice skills taught. Practicing procedures on themselves or each other helps allay fears and allows the child to supervise as a family member performs the procedure. Help develop problem-solving skills by using various scenarios that encourage decision making. Because education is an ongoing process, the family needs a contact person to whom they can turn for advice and support.

Outcomes

General Information

The child and family will be able to:

1. Describe the action of insulin in the body.
2. Describe the characteristics of type 1 versus type 2 diabetes.
3. Identify three factors that can be used to control blood glucose levels.

Medication Therapy

The child and family will be able to:

1. Name the child's insulin and identify the onset, peak, and duration of action.
2. State the storage recommendations for insulin.
3. State the recommended expiration date of the insulin.
4. Demonstrate accurate syringe preparation for a single type of insulin.
5. Demonstrate syringe preparation for two types of insulin.
6. Demonstrate subcutaneous insulin injection technique.
7. Identify insulin injection sites and describe a pattern of rotation.
8. Identify a plan for safe syringe disposal.
9. Identify recommended insulin dosages and injection times.

Home Glucose Monitoring

The child and family will be able to:

1. Identify nondiabetic blood glucose levels and target goals for good glucose control.
2. Demonstrate the use, calibration, control testing, and cleaning of the blood glucose monitor.
3. Identify a plan for recording blood glucose values.

Hypoglycemia

The child and family will be able to:

1. Identify the signs and symptoms of a hypoglycemic reaction.

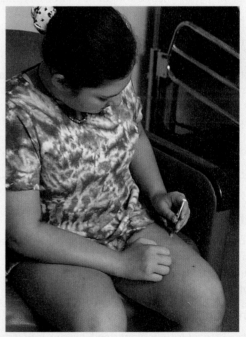

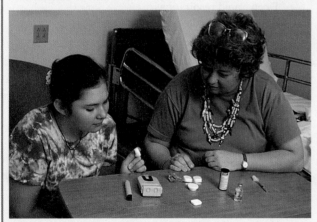

The school-age child is usually able to perform daily self-monitoring of blood glucose with parental help. However, the child should not be expected to adjust the insulin dose based on the reading. By early adolescence, the child can be in charge of recording blood glucose values in the diary.

When other parts of the treatment regimen have become familiar, the injections can be taught. Initially self-injecting insulin will be scary for the school-age child. A helpful start is having the parent insert the needle and the child push the plunger. The child can then progress to performing self-injection.

Continued

BOX 27-5 | **FAMILIES WANT TO KNOW**   About Home Management of Type 1 Diabetes Mellitus—cont'd

2. Describe appropriate treatment for both a mild and a severe hypoglycemic reaction.
3. Identify three potential causes of a hypoglycemic reaction.
4. Identify the importance of medical emergency identification.
5. Describe typical blood glucose trends during the honeymoon phase.

Hyperglycemia/Sick Day
The child and family will be able to:
1. Identify the signs and symptoms of hyperglycemia.
2. Identify strategies to control hyperglycemia.
3. Describe the possible effects of stress or illness on diabetes control.
4. Demonstrate the procedure for ketone (urine, serum) testing.
5. State when to test for ketones.
6. State basic treatment for ketones.
7. Describe the signs and symptoms requiring physician or other health care team contact.

Exercise
The child and family will be able to:
1. State the effect of exercise on blood glucose levels.
2. State the benefits and precautions for exercise.
3. Identify the correlation of diet, exercise, and insulin with blood glucose control.
4. Generate a home schedule that identifies mealtimes, blood test times, and insulin injection times.

Complications
The child and family will be able to:
1. Identify the role of glucose control in the prevention or delay of diabetes-related complications.
2. Identify appropriate health care follow-up for the child with diabetes.

Psychological Adjustment and Family Involvement
The child and family will be able to create a plan for the entire family to participate in diabetes care and management.

Community Resources
The child and family will be able to identify available community resources for ongoing diabetes education and support.

BOX 27-6 | **Sick-Day Rules for the Child with Type 1 Diabetes Mellitus**

1. Always give the insulin injection, even if the child does not have an appetite. If you believe that the child will become hypoglycemic with the usual dose, contact the physician or nurse educator for specific instructions. If ordered, use sliding-scale, rapid-acting insulin for hyperglycemia every 3 to 4 hours.
2. Test blood glucose level at least every 4 hours and more often for persistent hypoglycemia or hyperglycemia.
3. Test for urine ketones with each voiding. Notify the physician or nurse educator if moderate or large amounts of urine ketones are present. Additional regular insulin may be ordered.
4. Encourage calorie-free liquids. If ketones are present, liquids are essential to aid in clearing.

5. Follow the child's usual meal plan. If the child has a poor appetite, a sick-day diet consisting of simple carbohydrates can be substituted. Try to replace the usual grams of carbohydrate with simple carbohydrate foods.
6. Encourage rest, especially if urine ketones are present. Exercising while ketones are present results in increased ketone formation.
7. Notify the physician or nurse educator of the following:
   • Nausea and vomiting
   • Fruity odor to the breath
   • Deep, rapid respirations
   • Decreasing level of consciousness
   • Moderate or high urine ketones
   • Persistent hyperglycemia

Manifestations

Table 27-3 lists signs and symptoms of DKA, which include abdominal and chest pain, nausea and vomiting, fruity breath, decreased level of consciousness (LOC), Kussmaul respirations, and symptoms of dehydration.

Diagnostic Evaluation

Diabetic ketoacidosis is confirmed by the following test results:
• Blood glucose: elevated
• Arterial or venous pH: low
• Urine ketones: large

• Serum ketones (beta-hydroxybutyric acid, acetone): elevated
• Serum potassium: elevated, normal, or low
• Serum phosphorus: low
• White blood cell count (WBC): elevated as a result of stress demargination (higher with infection)
• Serum carbon dioxide: low

Therapeutic Management

The child in DKA usually is managed in an intensive care setting. Management includes hourly glucose monitoring, hourly vital and neurologic signs, strict and accurate intake

Text continued on p. 914

NURSING CARE PLAN

The Child in Diabetic Ketoacidosis

Focused Assessment

Assessment of the child in DKA includes assessing the child's level of consciousness, hydration status, respiratory status, and weight. If the child has a known history of type 1 diabetes mellitus, obtain the following data:

- Most recent blood glucose values
- History of urinary ketones and the steps taken to manage ketones at home

- Usual insulin dosages and the time and amount of the most recent injection
- Time of last meal and amount of food eaten
- Identification of the family member usually given the responsibility for injections and blood tests
- The family's understanding of the daily management of diabetes
- Usual sick-day management plan

NURSING DIAGNOSIS   Deficient Fluid Volume related to abnormal fluid losses through diuresis and emesis.

EXPECTED OUTCOME   The child will:
- Be safely rehydrated, as evidenced by normal weight, good skin turgor, appropriate urine output for age, and moist mucous membranes.

Intervention	*Rationale*
1. Determine the child's hydration status, evaluating weight, skin turgor, mucous membranes, and urine output.	1. This identifies baseline hydration status. A comparison of the child's usual weight with the admission weight provides an estimation of percent body fluid loss.
2. Encourage calorie-free fluids if the child is not nauseated. Initiate IV fluids as ordered. Normal saline is the initial fluid used, followed by half-normal saline.	2. Rehydration is the initial step in resolving DKA. If acidosis has resulted in nausea and vomiting, IV fluids are required. Fluid losses occur primarily from the osmotic diuresis occurring with hyperglycemia. Emesis can also contribute to fluid loss. Normal saline is the initial IV rehydration fluid. Although normally a hypertonic solution compared with blood, it is isotonic to hypotonic in states of dehydration.
3. Maintain strict intake and output monitoring.	3. Accurate intake and output records are essential in calculating rehydration status.
4. Observe for edema or pulmonary congestion during rehydration.	4. These signs indicate overhydration.
5. Weigh on arrival and frequently during rehydration (every 8 hr may be appropriate).	5. A comparison of the admission weight with the child's usual weight provides an indication of hydration status. Follow-up weights provide ongoing assessment.

Evaluation

- Is the child safely rehydrated, as evidenced by normal weight, urine output appropriate for age, good skin turgor, and moist mucous membranes?

NURSING DIAGNOSIS   Risk for Injury from altered acid-base balance leading to ketone production and acidosis related to lack of insulin.

EXPECTED OUTCOME   The child will:
- Have a resolution of ketosis and acidosis, as evidenced by laboratory results and clinical assessment.

Intervention	*Rationale*
1. Test all urine samples for the presence of ketones. Monitor the child's breath for acetone. Observe respirations to identify Kussmaul respirations.	1. The presence of urinary ketones indicates possible acidosis. Serum ketone analysis, or beta-hydroxybutyric acid, is a direct measurement of ketone activity. The liver produces three ketoacids: beta-hydroxybutyric acid, acetoacetate, and acetone. Acetone, the weakest of the acids, is expelled and can be assessed as a fruity smell to the child's breath. High acid levels trigger a rapid and deep respiration (Kussmaul respirations) in an effort to remove excessive acetone.

Continued

NURSING CARE PLAN—cont'd

2. Encourage calorie-free fluids if the child is able to drink. If ordered, begin IV fluids.

2. Fluids are essential in flushing ketones as well as in maintaining hydration. In severe dehydration, the osmotic pull of the blood glucose helps hold fluid in the bloodstream, thus preventing circulatory shock. Insulin is not given until rehydration has begun to diminish the risk of circulatory shock.

3. Initiate IV insulin therapy as ordered. Prime the IV tubing according to institution protocol.

3. Insulin therapy is initiated after rehydration has begun. A continuous IV infusion of regular insulin is titrated to keep blood glucose in a safe range while avoiding hypoglycemia. Insulin therapy inhibits the production of ketones. Subcutaneous insulin is not an appropriate therapy for the dehydrated child. With dehydration, peripheral vessels constrict, resulting in poor absorption and distribution of the insulin. Insulin adheres to the plastic of the IV bag and tubing, and it is not known whether this affects therapy. Some clinicians recommend priming the IV tubing with the insulin solution and flushing with a fresh solution before delivery. This technique saturates the binding sites of the plastic and provides nonfluctuating insulin delivery.

4. Monitor blood glucose frequently.

4. IV insulin acts rapidly. A continuous infusion of insulin could quickly result in hypoglycemia.

5. Provide glucose-containing IV fluids as ordered.

5. Insulin is needed to inhibit ketone formation. Even though blood glucose values may be in an acceptable range, the insulin infusion must continue until the serum ketones are cleared. To prevent hypoglycemia, glucose is added to the saline hydration solutions.

Evaluation

- Within 24 hours of admission, does the child display any evidence of ketosis (ketonuria, fruity breath, elevated blood glucose)?

NURSING DIAGNOSIS   Risk for Injury related to electrolyte imbalance from emesis and acidosis.

EXPECTED OUTCOME   The child will:
- Remain free from adverse consequences of electrolyte abnormalities, as evidenced by normal serum sodium and potassium values.

Intervention

1. Monitor potassium levels closely, looking for signs and symptoms of hyperkalemia, including bradycardia, muscle weakness, hyperreflexia, and respiratory arrest. Also monitor for symptoms of hypokalemia, including muscle weakness, fatigue, hypotension, and hyporeflexia.

Rationale

1. During acidosis, potassium moves out of the cell and into the intravascular spaces. Intravascular potassium is lost through diuresis. Initially, serum potassium levels may appear in an acceptable range, but this does not reflect the lost intracellular potassium. As rehydration and correction of acidosis begin, potassium moves back into the cells, resulting in lower serum levels. Serum potassium levels are obtained frequently (every 1 to 2 hr initially) during treatment of DKA to adequately assess potassium needs (see Chapter 18).

2. Use cardiac monitor to determine abnormal electrocardiogram resulting from altered potassium levels. Hypokalemia produces prolonged ST segment; notched, flat, or inverted T waves; and arrhythmias. Hyperkalemia produces flattened P wave or peaked T wave and ventricular fibrillation.

2. Hypokalemia or hyperkalemia can cause a medical emergency requiring rapid response.

3. After verifying urine output, initiate potassium therapy as ordered. If the child is anuric, notify the physician and do not give potassium.

3. Renal failure can result from severe dehydration. If the child is anuric, potassium is retained, causing abnormal serum levels. Replacement therapy must be done cautiously.

NURSING CARE PLAN—cont'd

Evaluation

- Does the child maintain a stable fluid and electrolyte balance, with serum sodium and potassium levels within normal limits?

NURSING DIAGNOSIS   Risk for Injury related to cerebral edema from resolving DKA.

EXPECTED OUTCOME   The child will:
- Remain free from adverse consequences of cerebral edema, as evidenced by appropriate level of consciousness, pupils equal and reacting to light, and absence of headache.

Intervention	*Rationale*
1. Observe the child frequently for signs of cerebral edema: reports of headache; decreasing level of consciousness; or unequal, fixed, or dilated pupils. Notify physician of any changes from the baseline assessment.	1. Cerebral edema is a complication of resolving DKA that can result in brain damage or death. The causes are unclear but may be related to overhydration; rapid fluid shifts, particularly into the cerebral intracellular space; and electrolyte imbalance. Frequent neurologic checks aid in prompt recognition and prevention of neurologic deficits.
2. Monitor blood glucose values frequently (hourly) when IV insulin is being infused.	2. Blood glucose values should not drop more than 50 to 100 mg/dL to prevent rapid osmotic shifts. As the serum glucose approaches the mid-200s, glucose will be added to the IV fluids. Blood glucose levels are maintained in the mid-200s for the duration of the IV insulin therapy.

Evaluation

- Is the child alert, with equal pupils and without reports of headache?

NURSING DIAGNOSIS   Deficient Knowledge related to unfamiliarity with home management during sick days.

EXPECTED OUTCOME   The family will:
- Demonstrate knowledge of home care, as evidenced by promptly recognizing and responding to situations requiring sick-day management.

Intervention	*Rationale*
1. Teach the family how and when to test for urine ketones; that is, when blood glucose level exceeds 250 mg/dL or when the child is ill.	1. Ketones are formed in response to insulin deficit. Either high glucose values or illness could be associated with insulin deficit.
2. Instruct family about sick-day management (see Box 27-6).	2. Stress, either from an infection or the environment, can cause hyperglycemia and uncontrolled diabetes. Early recognition and treatment of ketones can prevent acute complications.
3. Identify situations requiring the family to contact the diabetes health care team, including nausea with vomiting, high levels of urine ketones, procedures requiring NPO status, and signs of acidosis.	3. Early intervention is essential in preventing acidosis and its sequelae. The family can initiate outpatient management of ketones with direction from the diabetes team.
4. Provide the child and family with telephone numbers of appropriate health care professionals for questions on sick-day management.	4. The child and family should know whom to call and how to reach the appropriate health care professional for guidance during sick days.
5. Frequent bouts of DKA require evaluation of home care knowledge, adherence to recommended regimen, home supervision, and coping skills.	5. Frequent episodes of DKA may reflect poor adherence, poor understanding of home care needs, inappropriate or absent parental supervision, or depression. A team approach (including nurse educator, nutritionist, social worker, psychologist, physician) can address many of these issues.

Evaluation

- Does the child remain injury free?	- Are the child and family able to correctly recognize and promptly treat hypoglycemia and hyperglycemia?

and output measurements, frequent assessment of fluid and electrolyte status, IV fluid replacement, potassium replacement if needed, and provision of continuous insulin (Silverstein et al., 2005).

LONG-TERM HEALTH CARE NEEDS FOR THE CHILD WITH TYPE 1 DIABETES MELLITUS

Serious complications are associated with long-term diabetes: retinopathy, nephropathy, neuropathy, and cardiovascular disease. Studies have demonstrated that strict metabolic control of diabetes may decrease the onset or severity of complications. A team approach to diabetes management can best provide the tools to achieve metabolic control. The team includes the physician specialist, nurse educator, dietitian, and behavioral specialist. Regular checkups and telephone contact with the diabetes team are essential to address the needs of the growing child.

Routine health care for the child with diabetes should also include yearly dental and ophthalmologic evaluations as well as prophylactic interventions such as influenza vaccinations. Other referral sources should be used as specific needs are identified.

Diabetes research is aimed at preventing diabetes and finding a cure after diagnosis. Multiple immune intervention strategies are being identified and tested, and islet cell transplantation research holds promise for a cure.

TYPE 2 DIABETES MELLITUS

Type 2 diabetes is an emerging problem in the pediatric population. The rise in the incidence of overweight and obese children is directly related to the number of cases of type 2 diabetes in children (Martin, 2005; Thomassian, 2004). At the time of diagnosis, approximately 50% of the beta cells in a child with type 2 diabetes are still producing insulin. Children with type 2 diabetes mellitus have a combination of insulin resistance and decreased insulin secretion (ADA, 2006a). Current research suggests that adinopectin, a fat-derived protein, is related to diabetes, obesity, and poor lipid profiles, a clustering called the metabolic syndrome. Further research is needed to determine how adenopectin is related to the clustering of the syndrome (Martin, 2005).

Etiology

The majority of children with type 2 diabetes are obese or overweight at diagnosis and have glycosuria without ketonuria, absent or mild polydipsia and polyuria, and no or little recent weight loss. Type 2 diabetes is not caused by an autoimmune response (Thomassian, 2004). The pancreas still produces insulin, but in an amount insufficient to overcome the persistent hyperglycemia. Genetics and familial factors, maternal gestational diabetes, and intrauterine growth retardation, along with a lack of physical activity in childhood and adolescence, seem to be crucial in the development of type 2 diabetes in youth.

Incidence

Type 2 diabetes is on the rise among American Indian, Hispanic, and African American children and adolescents (ADA, 2006b). It commonly occurs in children who are overweight, in middle to late puberty, have a family history of type 2 diabetes, and are a member of these racial/ethnic groups.

Manifestations

Children with type 2 diabetes are typically overweight and have a velvety darkening of the skin around the neck (acanthosis nigricans). This may also be found on the inguinal folds, axillae, antecubital fossa, knees, or dorsum of the hand and is a marker for hyperinsulinism. Significant fluid and weight loss are not typical symptoms, but children with type 2 diabetes may have fatigue, yeast infections, blurry vision, or frequent urination. Hypertension, elevated triglyceride and low-density lipoprotein levels, and polycystic ovary syndrome may also be presenting signs.

Diagnostic Evaluation

Diagnosis of type 2 diabetes depends on careful physical examination, elevated endogenous insulin production, and no evidence of serum markers for autoimmunity. The fasting glucose level or a random serum glucose level is the same as for the diagnosis of type 1 diabetes in children.

Any child presenting with severe fasting hyperglycemia, ketonemia, and metabolic abnormalities, whether diagnosed with type 1 or type 2 diabetes, will need insulin therapy to reverse the metabolic imbalances (Silverstein et al., 2005).

Therapeutic Management

Children with type 2 diabetes may have been started on insulin while waiting for a definitive diagnosis. Once diagnosed, these children are managed with oral agents that decrease insulin resistance or augment endogenous insulin production. Blood glucose monitoring and diet management are important aspects of therapy. If these children lose weight, some can be managed with diet and exercise alone.

The goals of diabetes management for children with type 2 diabetes mellitus include the following:

- Achieving near-normal glycemic control (hemoglobin $A_{1c} < 7\%$)
- Facilitating reasonable weight for height
- Achieving normal blood glucose values
- Decreasing the frequency of microvascular complications of type 2 diabetes

Insulin Therapy

For the child with type 2 diabetes mellitus, oral hypoglycemic agents are used if the diabetes cannot be managed with diet and exercise. Pharmacologic management may include insulin, metformin (Glucophage), thiazolidinediones (TZDs), insulin secretagogues, and *a*-glucosidase inhibitors. At present, metformin is the only drug in the biguanide class and the only type 2 diabetes medication approved by the FDA for use in children aged 10 years and older. It is commonly prescribed as the initial oral hypoglycemic medication if severe hyperglycemia is not present. Reduced cholesterol levels and weight loss also are effects of metformin use.

TDZs (Avandia, Actos) increase insulin sensitivity and reverse insulin resistance. A reduction in visceral fat by TDZs can be beneficial if its associated weight gain can be addressed (Bloomgarden, 2004). Sulfonylureas such as glyburide (Micronase, Diabeta) and glipizide (Glucotrol) may also be used. These agents stimulate the pancreas to release more insulin into the blood. If monotherapy is unsuccessful in bringing down glucose levels, then combination therapy, insulin therapy, or both may be necessary. Currently in the United States, approximately 50% of children with type 2 diabetes receive insulin and approximately 50% take oral hypoglycemic agents.

Nutrition Therapy

Nutrition therapy goals for youths with type 2 diabetes are individualized, with emphasis on improved glycemic control and weight maintenance or loss. Improved glycemic control can be achieved through carbohydrate counting. Incorporating foods lower in saturated fat and higher in monounsaturated fat into the daily diet may help improve dyslipidemia (McKnight-Menci, Sababu, & Kelly, 2005). A diet with 60% to 70% of total calories from monounsaturated fat and carbohydrates is recommended for persons with diabetes. Participation of the entire family in a weight management program, which incorporates behavior modification strategies, is typically the key to success.

Physical Activity

For children with type 2 diabetes, participation for at least 60 minutes per day in a moderate to physical activity that the child likes is recommended. Watching television and engaging in sedentary activities should be limited to a maximum of 2 hours per day.

Blood Glucose Monitoring

The frequency of blood glucose testing for a child with type 2 diabetes is based on blood glucose goals as well as the willingness and ability to test.

KEY CONCEPTS

- The six major hormones of the endocrine system are ACTH, TSH, FSH, LH, GH, and prolactin.
- The pituitary gland stimulates target organs to produce specific hormones. When sufficient hormone is produced, the gland signals the pituitary to stop stimulation. This mechanism is referred to as *negative feedback.*
- To improve adherence to daily medications, the nurse may suggest pill dispensers or a watch with an alarm as a reminder to take medication at specific times.
- A variety of metabolic conditions, most of which are genetically transmitted, can affect newborns; many require

long-term dietary management and referral of the family to a genetic counseling center.
- CAH should be considered in any neonate with unusual-appearing genitalia.
- Signs and symptoms of hypothyroidism include fatigue; constipation; cold intolerance; weight gain; dry, thick skin; edema; and poor growth. Signs and symptoms of hyperthyroidism include nervousness; diarrhea; heat intolerance; weight loss; smooth, velvety skin; exophthalmos; and increased appetite.
- Diabetes insipidus is an inability to concentrate urine because of deficiency of ADH. Diabetes insipidus is characterized by polyuria, dehydration, increased serum sodium, and a low urine specific gravity. In comparison, SIADH results from excessive production of ADH. This is evidenced by decreased urine output, increased urine specific gravity, and decreased serum sodium.
- Psychosocial issues concerning children with precocious puberty include self-consciousness about their bodies, being treated as older than their chronologic age, and aggressive behavior by boys.
- In the absence of insulin, the metabolism of fats, proteins, and carbohydrates is impaired and glucose is unable to move into the intracellular space, resulting in hyperglycemia.
- Both type 1 diabetes mellitus and type 2 diabetes mellitus involve abnormal carbohydrate metabolism, but risks related to age of onset, body size, gender, ethnic background, and treatments differ for the two types of diabetes.
- The goals of diabetes management are to maintain appropriate height and weight, maintain an age-appropriate lifestyle, maintain near-normal glycosylated hemoglobin level, and prevent acute complications of hypoglycemia and hyperglycemia.
- Common nursing diagnoses associated with type 1 diabetes mellitus include Deficient Knowledge, Interrupted Family Processes, Imbalanced Nutrition: More or Less Than Body Requirements, and Risk for Injury related to hypoglycemia and hyperglycemia.
- Teaching needs associated with home management of type 1 diabetes mellitus are related to the disease process, medication, home glucose monitoring, hypoglycemia, hyperglycemia, exercise, complications, and support services.
- Hypoglycemia has adrenergic and neuroglycopenic clinical manifestations. Hypoglycemia should be treated with 15 g of easily digested carbohydrate.
- Hyperglycemia is caused by an inadequate amount of insulin, increased dietary intake, decreased amount of exercise, or a response to emotional or physical stress. Persistent hyperglycemia may indicate a need for an insulin dosage adjustment.
- Nursing diagnoses related to care of the child in DKA include Deficient Fluid Volume, Risk for Injury related to altered acid-base balance, Risk for Injury related to electrolyte imbalance, Risk for Injury related to cerebral edema, and Deficient Knowledge.

ANSWERS TO
CRITICAL THINKING EXERCISE 27-1

Signs of GH deficiency or another underlying disorder affecting growth are related to the rate of the child's growth, not to the height measurement itself. If, over a period of 6 to 12 months of careful growth measurement, the child demonstrates a marked downward deviation from a previous growth rate along with other signs of GH deficiency, the child needs to be referred for diagnostic evaluation.

Children grow and mature at varying rates depending on genetic and environmental factors. Many boys do not begin their growth spurts until the late teen years but still attain an adequate adult height. Some children have a familial tendency toward short stature not related to any underlying disorder. One way of estimating a child's eventual adult height (within 2 to 3 in) is to add the mother's and father's heights (in inches) and divide by 2. To this, add 2½ inches (for boys), or subtract 2½ inches (for girls). Emphasize to a worried parent that administration of GH will not help a child who does not have a true GH deficiency.

REFERENCES AND READINGS

Alemzadeh, R., & Wyatt, D. (2004). Diabetes mellitus in children. In R. Behrman, R. Kliegman, & H. Jenson (Eds.). *Nelson textbook of pediatrics* (17th ed., pp. 1947-1971). Philadelphia: Saunders.

American Diabetes Association. (2005). *National diabetes fact sheet.* Retrieved June 28, 2005, from *www.diabetes.org/uedocuments/NationalDiabetesFactSheetRev.pdf.*

American Diabetes Association. (2006a). Clinical practice recommendations 2006. *Diabetes Care, 29*(suppl 1).

American Diabetes Association (2006b). *Total prevalence of diabetes & pre-diabetes.* Retrieved September 19, 2006 from *www.diabetes.org/diabetes-statistics/prevalence.jsp.*

Anadiotis, G. A., & Berry, G. T. (2003). *Galactose-1-phosphate uridyltransferase deficiency (galactosemia).* Retrieved June 3, 2005, from *www.emedicine.com/PED/topic818.htm.*

Arnold, G. (2003). *Phenylketonuria.* Retrieved June 3, 2005, from *www.emedicine.com/PED/topic1787.htm.*

Bloomgarden, Z. (2004). Type 2 diabetes in the young: the evolving epidemic. *Diabetes Care, 27,* 999-1010.

Bourgeois, M. J., & Varma, S. (2004). *Congenital hypothyroidism.* Retrieved June 7, 2005, from *www.emedicine.com/ped/topic501.htm.*

Breault, D., & Majzoub, J. (2004). Diabetes insipidus. In R. Behrman, R. Kliegmen, & H. Jenson (Eds.). *Nelson textbook of pediatrics* (17th ed., pp. 1853-1855). Philadelphia: Saunders.

Bryant, K. G., Horns, K. M., Longo N., & Schiefelbein. J. (2004). A primer on newborn screening. *Advanced Neonatal Care, 4*(5), 306-317.

Caffrey, R. (2003). Diabetes under control: are all syringes created equal? *American Journal of Nursing, 103*(6), 46-49.

Cooperman, M. (2003). *Diabetes insipidus.* Retrieved June 7, 2005, from *www.emedicine.com/med/topic543.htm.*

Cranmer, H., & Shannon, M. (2005). *Pediatrics, hypoglycemia.* Retrieved June 2, 2005, from *www.emedicine.com/emerg/topic384.htm.*

Eledrisi, M. S. (2004). Growth hormone deficiency. Retrieved June 9, 2005, from *www.emedicine.com/med/topic930.htm.*

Greenbaum, L. A. (2004). Electrolyte and acid-base disorders. In R. Behrman, R. Kliegmen, & H. Jenson (Eds.). *Nelson textbook of pediatrics* (17th ed., pp. 191-242). Philadelphia: Saunders.

Kakarla, N., & Bradshaw, K. D. (2003). Disorders of pubertal development: precocious puberty. *Seminars on Reproductive Medicine, 21*(4):339-351.

LaFranchi, S. (2004). Disorders of the thyroid gland. In R. Behrman, R. Kliegmen, & H. Jenson (Eds.). *Nelson textbook of pediatrics* (17th ed., pp. 1870-1887). Philadelphia: Saunders.

Martin, L. (2005). Protecting the future: helping youth avoid diabetes. *Forefront, Winter/Spring,* 7-10.

McKnight-Menci, H., Sababu, S., & Kelly S. D. (2005). The care of children and adolescents with type 2 diabetes. *Journal of Pediatric Nursing, 20*(2), 1-15.

Olohan, K., & Zappitelli, D. (2003). The insulin pump. *American Journal of Nursing, 103*(4), 48-56.

Parks, J. (2004). Hypopituitarism. In R. Behrman, R. Kliegman, & H. Jenson (Eds.). *Nelson textbook of pediatrics* (17th ed., pp. 1847-1852). Philadelphia: Saunders.

Rezvani, I. (2000). An approach to inborn errors of metabolism. In R. Behrman, R. Kliegman, & H. Jenson (Eds.). *Nelson textbook of pediatrics* (17th ed., pp. 397-398). Philadelphia: Saunders.

Silverstein, J., Klingensmith, G., Copeland, K., Plotnick, L., Kaufman, F., Laffel, L., et al. (2005). Care of children and adolescents with type 1 diabetes: a statement of the American Diabetes Association. *Diabetes Care, 28*(1), 186-212.

Sperling, M. A. (2004). Hypoglycemia. In R. Behrman, R. Kliegman, & H. Jenson (Eds.). *Nelson textbook of pediatrics* (17th ed., pp. 505-518). Philadelphia: Saunders.

Straight, A. M., & Bauer, A. J. (2003). *Hypothyroidism.* Retrieved June 7, 2005, from *www.emedicine.com/ped/topic1141.htm.*

Sullivan-Bolyai, S., Deatrick, J., Gruppuso, P., Tamborlane, W., & Grey, M. (2003). Constant vigilance: mothers' work parenting young children with type I diabetes. *Journal of Pediatric Nursing, 18*(1), 21-29.

Thomassian, B. D. (2004). Type 2 diabetes among youth reaches epidemic proportions. *Nurse Week, November 29,* 27-29.

Weissberg-Benchell, J., Antisdel-Lomaglio, J., & Seshadri, R. (2003). Insulin pump therapy. *Diabetes Care, 26*(4), 1079-1087.

Wilson, T. A. (2005). *Congenital adrenal hyperplasia.* Retrieved May 17, 2005, from *www.emedicine.com/ped/topic48.htm.*

Wilson, T., et al. (2003). Update of guidelines for the use of growth hormone in children: the Lawson Wilkins Pediatric Society Drug and Therapeutics Committee. *Journal of Pediatrics, 143*(4), 415-421.

Yeung, S. J., & Habra, M. A. (2005). *Graves disease.* Retrieved June 7, 2005, from *www.emedicine.com/med/topic929.htm.*

CHAPTER 28

The Child With a Neurologic Alteration

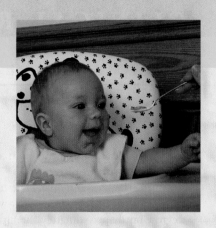

Learning Objectives

After studying this chapter, you should be able to:
- Describe the embryologic development of the nervous system.
- Describe the anatomy and physiology of the nervous system.
- Describe the normal compensatory mechanisms that keep intracranial pressure within a constant range.
- Identify the neurologic differences among the infant, child, and adult.
- Be able to perform a neurologic assessment of a child and record findings.
- Discuss the nursing implications of medications frequently used in the management of neurologic disorders.
- List the measures used to keep a child safe during a seizure.
- List the measures used to prevent or treat cerebral edema.
- Differentiate between abnormal flexion and extension and discuss the significance of each.
- List the compensatory mechanisms that affect intracranial blood flow and extravascular fluid volume if hydrocephalus develops.
- Describe teaching strategies that can be used for the child with neurologic problems and the child's family.

Definitions

Arnold-Chiari malformation Abnormalities of the fourth ventricle, lower cerebellum, and brainstem; often associated with myelomeningocele.

autoregulation The unique ability of the cerebral arteries to maintain a steady blood flow during changes in blood pressure and perfusion by adjusting their diameter in response to alterations in cerebral perfusion pressure.

basal ganglia A major communication and sorting area for messages to and from the cerebral hemispheres composed of masses of gray matter; controls movement and participates in emotion and cognition.

battle sign Bruising or hemorrhage over the mastoid.

blood-brain barrier The separation between brain tissue and blood; is quite selective and normally permeable only to glucose, water, carbon dioxide, and some chemicals and drugs.

brainstem Structure connected to the cerebral hemispheres by thick bunches of nerve fibers; all nerve fibers traverse through the brainstem from the hemispheres to the cerebellum and spinal cord.

cerebral cortex Gray matter of the cerebrum where the higher functions of thinking occur.

cerebral herniation Shift of brain tissue sideways, under the falx cerebri, or downward, causing severe neurologic dysfunction.

cerebral perfusion pressure The difference between mean arterial blood pressure and intracranial pressure.

Cushing's response Late sign of increased intracranial pressure; includes increased blood pressure, widened pulse pressure, decreased heart rate, and decreased or irregular respiratory rate.

extension (decerebrate) posture Abnormal extension of the upper extremities with internal rotation of the upper arms and wrists; lower extremities will extend with some internal rotation.

extrapyramidal tract Descending pathway of the motor neurons concerned with involuntary or unconscious skeletal muscle coordination and reflex control of coordination.

flexion (decorticate) posture Abnormal flexion of the upper extremities and extension of the lower extremities.

glia cells Cells composing the support tissue that nourishes and protects the neurons.

Monro-Kellie doctrine Theory describing the compensatory mechanism of the cranial contents to maintain a steady volume and pressure.

myelinization Formation of the proteolipid coating of the nerves that facilitates conduction of impulses.

papilledema Edema of the optic disc.

pyramidal tract Descending pathway of the upper motor neuron concerned with voluntary movement.

REVIEW OF THE CENTRAL NERVOUS SYSTEM
Embryologic Development

The nervous system is one of the first systems to form *in utero*. By the fourth week of gestation, the neural tube has closed at the anterior end to form the brain and at the posterior end to form the spinal cord.

During the second month of gestation the brain becomes the prominent body structure. It grows rapidly and continues to grow until approximately the fifth year of life. Two periods of rapid brain cell growth appear to occur during gestation. Between the fifteenth and twentieth weeks of gestation, the number of neurons increases significantly. At 30 weeks, the number of neurons increases again, continuing through 1 year of age. Appropriate prenatal care during periods of rapid neuronal increase can prevent developmental neurologic deficits.

The Myelin Sheath

Myelin is the fatty substance that surrounds the nerves of both the central and the peripheral nervous systems. The myelin begins to form at approximately the sixteenth week of gestation. Myelin insulates the nerves and helps conduct electrical impulses. Coordination of fine and gross motor skills progresses with the deposition of the myelin sheath. Nerve fibers can conduct impulses in the absence of myelin; however, the impulses travel more slowly. Gross motor skills develop before fine motor skills as coordination and control advance throughout childhood. The myelin sheath can be destroyed by disease, drugs, and the aging process.

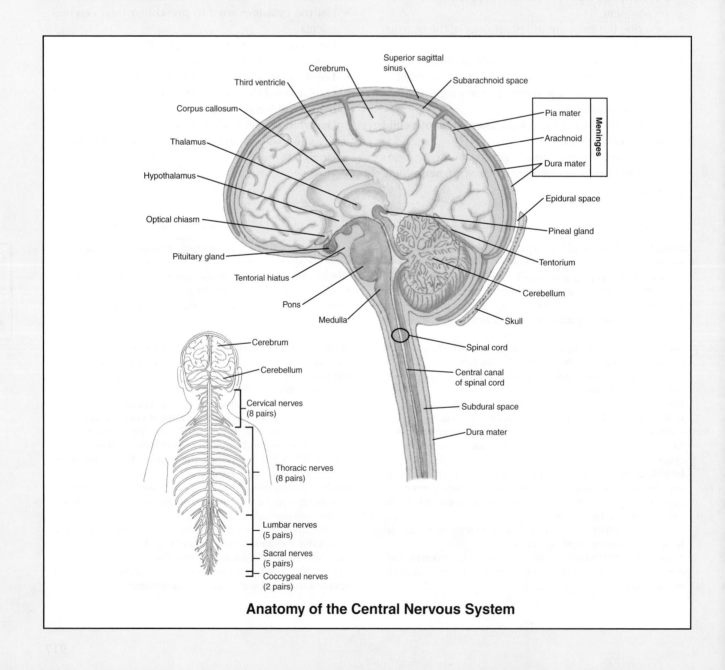

Anatomy of the Central Nervous System

PEDIATRIC DIFFERENCES IN THE CNS

- The brain constitutes 12% of a newborn's body weight compared with only 2% of an adult's body weight.
- The brain of a term infant is two thirds the weight of an adult's brain. By age 1 year, it weighs 80% as much as an adult's brain, and by age 6 years it weighs approximately 90% as much as an adult's brain.
- An infant has approximately 50 mL of CSF compared with 150 mL in an adult.
- The peripheral nerves are not completely myelinated by birth. As myelinization progresses, so do the child's coordination and fine muscle movements.
- The head circumference in a term infant is 34 to 35 cm. By age 6 months the head circumference is 44 cm, and by age 12 months it is 47 cm.
- Papilledema rarely occurs in infancy because of the open fontanels and sutures, which can expand with increased intracranial pressure.
- The primitive reflexes of Moro, grasp, and rooting, present at birth, disappear at various times during the first 5 months. These primitive reflexes may reappear with neurologic disease.

The Neural System

The neural system develops multiple connections among the areas of the brain that control specific functions, including vision, hearing, motor function, sensation, coordination, and speech. Each function is under the control of a specific area of the brain. The right half, or hemisphere, of the brain controls the left side of the body and is concerned with the social aspects of perception, intuition, and experience. The left hemisphere controls the right side of the body and is largely concerned with language acquisition and use and logical, verbal reasoning.

The neonate's neurologic system functions at a subcortical level. Spinal cord reflexes, such as sucking and cardiorespiratory functions, are present. Cortical functions, including memory and coordination, are only partially developed.

The Axial Skeleton

The axial skeleton protects the underlying structures of the central nervous system (CNS). For convenience of study, the bones of the skull and the vertebral column are divided into regions that form the wall of the cranial cavity and the spinal column. The frontal, occipital, temporal, and parietal bones form the cranial vault. The floor of the cranial vault is composed of three compartments, or fossae—the anterior, middle, and posterior fossae. The anterior fossa houses the frontal lobes of the brain, the middle fossa contains the upper brainstem and the pituitary gland, and the posterior fossa contains the lower brainstem. Blood vessels and cranial nerves enter and leave the skull through the foramina.

At birth, the skull plates are not fused but are separated by nonossified spaces called *fontanels*. The posterior fontanel usually fuses by age 2 months and the anterior fontanel by 16 to 18 months. The fontanels allow the cranium to expand in response to rapid brain growth. Before fusion of the fontanels and sutures, an increase in intracranial pressure (ICP) will produce an increase in head circumference.

Because brain growth is rapid during infancy, the long-term sequelae of neurologic insults that occur to infants are difficult to predict. Brain growth can be assessed by head circumference measurements. These measurements are an important part of the routine physical examination of children and should be plotted on a growth chart. Insufficient or excessive head and brain growth could indicate a potential neurologic problem. Premature closing of the fontanels or sutures can cause massive neurologic damage, and continued evaluation by the physician is needed.

The Meninges

The meninges are the membranes that surround the brain and spinal column. The outer layer is the dura mater, a fibrous connective tissue structure containing many blood vessels and fibroblastlike cells that secrete collagen to produce a tough, protective membrane (Martin, 2003). The dura mater consists of two layers having outer and inner meningeal components. Between the periosteum of the bone and the dura mater lies the epidural space. Sheets of dura also extend downward and inward to form partitions within the cranium. The falx cerebri separates the cerebral hemispheres, and the falx cerebelli separates the cerebellar hemispheres.

The *tentorium* is a tentlike structure that separates the cerebellum from the occipital lobe of the cerebrum. The large gap through which the brainstem passes is the tentorial hiatus.

The middle meningeal layer is the arachnoid, a delicate, avascular, weblike, serous membrane loosely covering the brain. Between the arachnoid and the dura lies the subdural space, which contains a small amount of fluid, just sufficient to prevent adhesion of the two membranes.

The innermost layer is the pia mater. It is a delicate, transparent membrane that adheres closely to the outer surface of the brain. The pia mater is a vascular membrane, consisting of arteries and veins.

Between the pia mater and the arachnoid is the subarachnoid space, which is filled with cerebrospinal fluid (CSF). The CSF acts as a cushion to reduce the force of trauma on the brain.

The Brain

The three sections of the brain are the cerebrum, the cerebellum, and the brainstem. The cerebrum is the largest component, filling the upper portion of the skull. It is divided into two hemispheres, right and left, which are separated by a longitudinal fissure. The two hemispheres are joined by a thin sheet of membrane called the *corpus callosum*. The cerebral hemispheres are further divided into lobes in relation to the cranial bones: frontal, parietal, temporal, and occipital. The cerebrum also includes part of the thalamus, hypothalamus, basal ganglia, and the olfactory and optic nerves.

The cerebellum is composed of white matter and gray matter. It is attached to the brainstem by paired bundles of

Animation: Brain Lobes

fibers. The brainstem consists of the midbrain, the pons, the medulla, the thalamus, and the third ventricle.

The Cranial Nerves

Twelve pairs of cranial nerves arise from the brain and brainstem, each with a specific function. Testing these nerves can indicate the location and degree of CNS injury (see Chapter 9).

The Spinal Cord

The spinal cord is described as segmented into the cervical, thoracic, lumbar, and sacral regions. The spinal nerves are named for their corresponding vertebral segments.

The spinal cord transmits signals to and from the brain and responds to local sensory information through automatic motor responses called *reflexes*. The simplest type of spinal cord response is the reflex arc. Sensation is transmitted to the spinal cord from a sensory nerve fiber. It synapses with a motor neuron in the same cord segment, causing a muscle or tendon contraction in the corresponding motor nerve. Deep tendon reflexes are examples of the reflex arc.

Sensory innervation occurs as sensory nerves carrying body sensations enter the spinal cord on the dorsal surface. Most sensory fibers for pain and temperature ascend to the brain by lateral spinal tracts. Sensory fibers for touch and pressure ascend through anterior tracts. Almost all sensory fibers pass through the thalamus, where the perceptions of touch, pressure, and temperature are interpreted. Perceptions of texture, size, and weight are interpreted in the cortex.

Motor nerves are stimulated to respond after the brain receives a signal from a sensory nerve. The motor nerves cross over to the *contralateral* (opposite) side of the spinal cord from which they originate and then exit on the ventral surface of the spinal cord. The side of the body contralateral to the injured side of the brain will be the side affected by injury.

Functional differences exist between the upper and lower motor neurons. The outcome of a spinal cord injury is affected by the site of the injury. An injury between the brain and the dendrites (the nerve fibers that carry impulses toward the cell body) will render the brain incapable of signaling the muscle cells to cease responding reflexively, and the muscle will become contracted, or spastic. If the injury is to a section of the nerve between the muscle and axons (the nerve fibers that carry impulses away from the cell body), the muscles will become incapable of responding reflexively, causing them to become flaccid.

CSF Analysis in Children: Normal Findings

Parameter	Neonate		Child Older than 6 Months
	Preterm	Term	
WBCs (per mm³)	≤25	≤7	≤5
Protein (mg/dL)	<150	<170	<40
Glucose (mg/dL)	>30	>60	>40
Red blood cells (per mm³)	>1000	<800	<5
Pressure (mm Hg)	50-80	50-80	100-280

CSF Analysis: Findings in Pathologic Conditions

Condition	Appearance	Pressure	Cells	Protein	Glucose/Other
Traumatic tap	Bloody; supernatant fluid clear	Normal	Any red blood cells	4 mg/dL rise per 5000 red cells	NA
Acute bacterial meningitis	Cloudy to milky or xanthochromatic	Usually elevated	Polymorphonuclear cells: ≥100/mm³	100-500 mg/dL	Decreased compared with blood
Viral meningitis	Clear	Normal or increased	Zero to a few hundred per mm³, mostly leukocytes	50-200 mg/dL	Normal
Encephalitis	Clear, colorless	Normal or slightly increased	Normal or increased	50-200 mg/dL	<40 mg/dL
Subdural hematoma	Yellow to clear, colorless	Increased	Normal	Normal or increased	Normal
Diabetic coma	Clear, colorless	Decreased	Normal	Normal or slightly increased	May be 200-300 mg/dL
GBS	Clear	Normal	<10 white blood cells	More than 2× normal	Normal

NA, Not applicable.

Cerebrospinal Fluid

CSF is a clear liquid produced in the choroid plexus of the ventricles. The CSF aids in protecting the brain, spinal cord, and meninges by acting as a watery cushion surrounding them to absorb the shocks to which they are exposed. It is reabsorbed through the arachnoid villi into the venous sinuses.

Cerebral Blood Flow

The internal carotid arteries supply blood to all parts of the brain. Approximately 17% of cardiac output and 20% of body oxygen are transported to the brain. The brain requires approximately 10 times the oxygen used by the rest of the body.

Common Diagnostic Tests and Procedures for Neurologic Disorders in Children

Test	Description	Purpose	Nursing Considerations
CT scan	Produces computer image of horizontal and vertical cross sections of brain at any axis.	Identifies abnormal tissue and structures, such as in brain tumor, bleeding, or hydrocephalus.	An IV line may need to be inserted if contrast medium is used. Notify the radiologist if the child is allergic to iodine. The child may be sedated if necessary.
Angiography	After IV contrast dye is injected, a clear image of the vessels is obtained because the computer eliminates all tissue that has not been infused by the contrast dye.	Shows vascular abnormalities.	May have nothing-by-mouth order. Notify the radiologist if the child is allergic to iodine. Obtain signed permission form. Some restrictions on activity necessary after the test.
Echoencephalography	Echoes from ultrasonic waves are recorded as they reflect off various surfaces of the skull.	Identifies abnormal structure, position, and function.	Painless procedure. No preparation.
EEG	Electrodes placed on the scalp conduct and amplify electrical activity; electrical potential of the brain is measured and recorded.	Identifies abnormal electrical brain discharges, such as in seizures.	Child may have regular diet or fluids but no caffeine or stimulants. Hair should be clean. May include sleep EEG; in this case, child should be sleep deprived the night before test. Tell the child the procedure is painless.
Long-term video EEG	Continuous EEG with video of physical symptoms. Process can last 24 hr to several days.	Clinical events can be recorded and played back for in-depth review as well as correlated with the presence of abnormal electrical activity.	Electrodes are secured with a skin glue. Electrode sites should be evaluated and documented every shift. Child will have to stay in a small area during testing. Age-appropriate toys and activities should be available for child.
Lumbar puncture	CSF pressure is measured and a specimen obtained as a needle is inserted into the subarachnoid space between L3 and L4.	Measures pressure, and analysis of CSF identifies infections. Procedure may be used to administer medications.	Obtain signed consent. Instruct the child to lie on the side with the knees up to chest. After the procedure, the child lies flat. If not fluid restricted, encourage fluids after the procedure.
MRI	Produces computer images of the brain by radiofrequency emissions from certain elements.	Demonstrates morphologic features of tissue and structures with degree of detail not achievable by other methods.	The procedure is painless, but the child may be sedated if necessary. Inform child that loud clicking noises will be heard. The child's head will be restrained.
Nuclear brain scan (single-photon emission computed tomography [SPECT])	A radioactive substance is injected IV (the amount of the substance is measured and recorded). Abnormal uptake indicates abnormal tissue or structure.	Identifies focal brain lesions and demonstrates CSF pathways.	The child needs to remain still during the test. An IV line is needed.

Cerebral blood flow (CBF) is controlled by *cerebral perfusion pressure* (CPP), which is the difference between the mean arterial blood pressure (MBP) and ICP.

Autoregulation, or self-regulation, is a unique physiologic ability. It allows cerebral arteries to change diameter in response to changes in the CPP. The cerebral vessels can maintain a steady blood flow to the brain during alterations in blood pressure and perfusion. However, autoregulation fails when the limits of cerebrovascular dilation are reached.

Autoregulation may be impaired as a result of trauma or ischemia. It is influenced significantly by changes in partial pressure of oxygen in arterial blood (PaO_2) and partial pressure of carbon dioxide in arterial blood ($PaCO_2$). An increase in $PaCO_2$ (above 40 mm Hg) produces cerebral vasodilation and an increase in CBF. A decrease in $PaCO_2$ (25 to 30 mm Hg) causes cerebral vasoconstriction and thus reduces blood flow to the brain. Alterations in PaO_2 between 80 and 100 mm Hg have little effect on CBF, although hypoxia will dramatically increase CBF.

TEACHING FOR A LUMBAR PUNCTURE

If the child is old enough to understand, explain the following:

- The child will need to lie on the side with body bent and knees and chin touching. Explain that you will help hold the child in that position by "hugging" the knees to the chin. If there is time, allow the child to practice the position. (An infant can be in a side-lying position or a sitting position with the infant facing you and your thumbs across the infant's scapulae; steady the infant's head against your body.)
- Tell the child that the physician will wash the back with a cool liquid. After that, the child might feel a "pinch" or "sting" as the needle is inserted. In some instances, a topical anesthetic may be used to decrease the pain caused by the needle. The child must remain still.

- Encourage the child to relax, sing, take deep breaths, or use guided imagery throughout the procedure to help decrease anxiety. The collection of CSF samples and pressure measurement usually takes several minutes. When the needle is withdrawn, the child will feel light pressure and the application of a small dressing.

Remember to do the following:

- Monitor the child's cardiorespiratory status throughout the procedure.
- Help the parents comfort the child during and after the procedure.

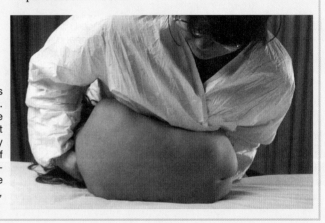

For the lumbar puncture: Place one hand farther down, under the child's neck. Your forearm moves behind the child's head to support the neck. Place the other arm farther under the child's upper thighs and curl the body by bringing the knees up to the head. Note that this nurse's weight is supported on the edge of the gurney, and the nurse leans slightly over the child, controlling the arms and legs. Because direct visibility of the child's respiratory status is limited in this position, a cardiorespiratory monitor must be on the child, or another nurse should be at the bedside. *(Photo courtesy Cook Children's Medical Center, Fort Worth, TX. © Bob Lukeman, photographer.)*

Electronic Resources

Additional information related to the content in Chapter 28 can be found on:

the interactive companion CD-ROM

- Animations: Brain Lobes
    Cranial Nerve Examination
    Seizure, Generalized
    Ventriculoperitoneal Shunt
- Audio Glossary
- NCLEX Review Questions
- Skills: Implementing Seizure Precautions
    Monitoring Neurovascular Status

or the companion website at *evolve*
http://evolve.elsevier.com/james/ncoc

- NCLEX Review Questions
- Resources for Health Care Providers and Families
- WebLinks

Care of the child with a neurologic problem requires knowledge of neuroanatomy, neurophysiology, and normal growth and development. The nurse plays an important role in the early recognition of pediatric neurologic problems, some of which have the potential for devastating long-term outcomes. The nurse assesses the child's condition by comparing the child's normal behavior with current behavior. The family is an invaluable source of information about the child's normal behavior and how current behavior deviates from that norm. The child and the family need support and understanding because the child's condition represents a crisis in their lives. The family's ability to respond and influence the child's coping mechanisms directly influences the recovery and adaptation process.

Many conditions of the nervous system share common assessment data, diagnoses, and interventions. Principles of nursing care for the child with a nervous system disorder can be applied to a variety of situations.

Text continued on p. 927

NURSING CARE PLAN

The Child With a Nervous System Disorder

Focused Assessment

Begin the neurologic assessment by testing the child's level of consciousness with the GCS modified for children, cerebral function, cerebellar function, and orientation. Note the child's mood and behavior. Compare the results with normal developmental milestones (see Chapters 5 through 8). Observe the child's interaction with the family and the environment for additional data. Note lethargy, drowsiness, hyperactivity, tremors, or jitteriness.

Assess balance, coordination, and motor skills by observing the child's behaviors, particularly while the child is dressing or playing. Coordination can be assessed by the finger-to-nose test or by observing the child throw a ball, handle a pencil, or use rapidly alternating movements. Observe the child's walking gait for hemiplegia, scissors gait, or an abnormally wide-spaced gait. Observe and record the child's muscle development, strength, and tone. Test deep tendon reflexes and range of motion of all joints. Check the sensory function of the face, trunk, arms, and legs. Test both sides of the child for vibration, superficial tactile sensation, superficial pain, and temperature.

NURSING DIAGNOSIS   Ineffective Tissue Perfusion (cerebral) related to alteration of arterial or venous blood flow, cerebral infarction, hemorrhage, hematoma, increased ICP, cerebral edema, seizures, hypoventilation, or increased cerebral metabolism.

EXPECTED OUTCOMES   The child will:
- Have improved cerebral perfusion, as evidenced by no cranial nerve deficits, improved or normal level of consciousness, vital signs in baseline normal, and GCS score within normal limits.
- Demonstrate appropriate behavior or thought patterns for age.

Intervention	*Rationale*
1. Determine the child's baseline age and developmental level.	1. Baseline age and developmental level will help the nurse gauge changes in neurologic status.
2. Perform a baseline neurologic and level of consciousness (LOC) assessment and measure vital signs on admission.	2. Changes in neurologic signs can indicate deterioration or improvement in status. Changes are compared with baseline.

Continued

NURSING CARE PLAN—cont'd

3. Monitor factors that may further increase cerebral edema and ICP (hypoxia, fever, seizures, hypotension, hypercapnia).
4. Maintain head of bed at a 30- to 45-degree angle.

5. Avoid the prone position, neck flexion, or hip flexion.

6. Organize nursing care around periods of low ICP.

7. Monitor pupil size and reactivity every hour as needed or as ordered.
8. Measure head circumference daily or as needed, and record on growth chart if age appropriate.
9. Palpate the anterior fontanel every shift if age appropriate.
10. Palpate the cranial suture lines every shift if age appropriate.
11. Observe the infant for irritability, lethargy, feeding intolerance, and decreasing GSC score.
12. Place emergency equipment (oxygen, suction, bag-valve-mask) near the child's room or at the bedside.

3. Monitoring these factors allows for correction of conditions that increase ICP and keeps cerebral metabolic needs to a minimum.
4. Venous outflow drainage of the brain is facilitated by gravity.
5. All these positions tend to increase ICP. Lying flat in bed increases ICP. Neck flexion kinks the jugular vein where venous drainage occurs. Hip flexion can increase intraabdominal or intrathoracic pressure, thus increasing ICP.
6. Nursing care, such as suctioning, bathing, and repositioning, increases ICP.
7. An increase in pupil size and inactivity may indicate an increase in ICP.
8. If fontanels are open, cranial expansion takes place when the CSF is under pressure.
9. An increase in fontanel size and tenseness may indicate an increase in CSF accumulation.
10. The cranial sutures may separate with an increase in CSF volume or pressure.
11. All are signs of increasing ICP and deteriorating neurologic status.
12. Increased ICP can cause apnea and may lead to cardiopulmonary arrest.

Evaluation

- Does the child demonstrate an improved LOC?
- Are vital signs within normal limits?

- Does the child show intact cranial nerve function, an optimum level on the GCS, and behavior and thought patterns appropriate for age?

NURSING DIAGNOSIS   Imbalanced Nutrition: Less Than Body Requirements related to restricted intake, neurologic impairment, swallowing or chewing difficulty, risk for aspiration, nausea, or vomiting.

EXPECTED OUTCOME   The child will:
- Have adequate nutritional intake, as evidenced by maintaining stable or normal weight for age and height; exhibiting normal serum proteins, moist mucous membranes, and adequate urine output; and being free of nausea and vomiting.

Intervention

1. Determine the child's LOC before giving liquids.

2. Weigh the child daily on the same scale, at the same time of day, and in the same clothes. Record on a growth chart.

3. Monitor skin turgor, mucous membranes, eye orbits, urine output, urine specific gravity, and serum and urine electrolyte values.
4. Consult a registered dietitian.

5. Position the child or infant upright after feedings. If the child is old enough and the ICP is not elevated, the head should be slightly flexed and facing forward. Arms should be positioned forward with feet placed on a firm surface.

Rationale

1. A decreased level of consciousness increases the risk of aspiration with swallowing.
2. Changes in weight indicate alterations in fluid balance and nutritional status. Being consistent with timing and type of clothing enhances accurate comparison. The nurse should weigh the child only if the procedure does not increase ICP.
3. These are indicators of fluid and electrolyte status.

4. The dietitian will advise how best to meet metabolic demands and plan the most efficient way to get calories.
5. Proper positioning will decrease the risk of aspiration, enhance comfort, prevent contractures, and provide for safety while feeding.

NURSING CARE PLAN—cont'd

6. Verify placement of any oral or nasogastric tube before tube feedings are initiated.
7. Provide a flexible feeding schedule with small feedings of favorite foods.
8. Minimize handling around feeding times.

9. If swallowing is impaired, assist the child with chewing by holding the child's chin and jaw.

10. Obtain order to medicate for nausea and vomiting if necessary.

6. Incorrect placement of a nasogastric tube will result in placing feedings into the lungs (see Chapter 13).
7. These techniques facilitate digestion and the ability to maintain adequate caloric intake.
8. Minimal handling during feeding decreases the likelihood of vomiting and aspiration.
9. Swallowing may be facilitated by this method, because it keeps the child's head stabilized in an appropriate anatomic position.
10. The child will be more likely to tolerate feedings when nausea is controlled.

Evaluation

- Does the child show normal growth for age, with no weight loss?
- Does the child have age-appropriate caloric intake daily?

- Does the child have proper hydration with moist mucous membranes and age-appropriate urine output for age?
- Is the child free from nausea and vomiting?

NURSING DIAGNOSIS Risk for Impaired Skin Integrity related to neuromuscular impairment, decreased level of consciousness, inadequate physical activity, immobility, or improper fluid or nutritional intake.

EXPECTED OUTCOME The child's skin will:
- Remain intact and free from pressure breakdown.

Intervention

1. Use pressure equalizing mattress or special flotation mattress to protect bony prominences. Reposition every 2 hr and as needed. Check for redness and pressure areas.
2. Observe skin condition every 2 hr with the repositioning of the child or infant.
3. Avoid putting temperature probes, cardiac monitor leads, or excessive tape over a shunt site.
4. Encourage parents or caregivers to participate in passive range-of-motion exercises for the child if appropriate.

5. If braces or splints are used, assess the skin before and after the splints or assistive devices are put on and taken off.
6. Implement a daily skin care regimen. Teach parents or family to check skin frequently.

Rationale

1. The child with a depressed LOC may not be active, and immobility can cause skin breakdown.

2. Prolonged pressure on the skin will quickly lead to its breakdown.
3. Irritation from adhesives will contribute to skin breakdown and possible infection.
4. Participating in the child's care enhances the parents' control and the child's sense of well-being. Passive range-of-motion exercises provide emotional and physical support for the child and increase the child's activity.
5. Correct application of braces will minimize pressure points and reduce skin breakdown.

6. Bathing, moisturizing, and inspecting the skin will preserve skin integrity.

Evaluation

- Does the child have intact, clean, dry skin without pressure areas or sores?

NURSING DIAGNOSIS Anxiety (parental) related to change in the child's health status, threat to self-concept, behavior changes, possible injury, social isolation, seizures, neurologic impairment, or lack of privacy.

EXPECTED OUTCOME The parents will:
- Demonstrate management of anxiety, as evidenced by maintaining social and personal relationships, verbalizing relaxation, verbalizing feelings about the child's neurologic impairment, and demonstrating effective coping skills.

Continued

NURSING CARE PLAN—cont'd

Intervention	*Rationale*
1. Keep the parents informed of the child's progress, prognosis, and plan of care. Encourage parents to talk about concerns and ask questions. Allow parents to make decisions when possible.	1. Control over any event in the child's care helps the parents feel they are part of the caregiving team and lessens their anxiety.
2. Encourage parents to participate actively in activities of daily living (e.g., oral hygiene, bathing, feeding).	2. Touching the child and actively participating in the child's care lower parental anxiety.
3. Orient the parents to hospital routine, and refer to clergy, social worker, and other team members.	3. A familiar environment is less threatening and will enable the family to deal with the child's condition and prognosis better.
4. Encourage rooming-in when possible.	4. Rooming-in will involve the parents more in the child's care, make them part of the health care team, and decrease the child's anxiety.
5. Assist with anxiety-reduction techniques, such as relaxation techniques, music, and guided imagery.	5. Such techniques facilitate coping and stress reduction.

Evaluation

- Are the parents able to discuss concerns and fears?
- Do the parents plan with the team for the child's future and participate in decision making?

- Are the parents able to state reduced feelings of anxiety?
- Do the parents demonstrate coping and problem-solving skills?

NURSING DIAGNOSIS   Deficient Knowledge related to unfamiliarity with infectious process, disease process, medication regimen, dietary or fluid needs, measures for prevention, or chronic illness of a child or infant.

EXPECTED OUTCOMES   The child and parents will:
- Verbalize and demonstrate an understanding of the child's disease process, as evidenced by stating age-appropriate, realistic factors about the child's condition, listing factors to decrease neurologic deficits and measures to prevent further occurrences of illness, and demonstrating medication administration and nutritional adaptations.

Intervention	*Rationale*
1. Allow time for teaching. If the child is to undergo surgery, provide preoperative teaching for the parents as well.	1. Teaching answers questions and reinforces information given to the parents by the physician. It includes the parents in the learning experience.
2. Determine the parents' understanding of the child's disability, including the child's need for physical, speech, or occupational therapy.	2. Parents need to understand the intellectual and physical abilities and disabilities of their child to give informed consent or reinforce the need for therapies.
3. Put parents in touch with community support groups.	3. Support can be gained by seeing or hearing how others coped with similar situations.
4. Supply the parents with telephone numbers to call for needed information once they are home.	4. Health care workers can help parents feel in touch and educate them at the same time by discussing the child's condition on the telephone.
5. Teach the parents important signs and symptoms of the child's condition, side effects of medications, and when to call the physician or nurse. Provide written instructions.	5. The parents need to state important signs and symptoms that indicate a change in the child's condition and be aware of when to seek medical attention. Anxiety reduces learning and attention span. A written copy of signs and symptoms provides an ongoing resource that can be referred to later.
6. Review the signs and symptoms of wound infection.	6. Until the surgical incision is healed, the risk of infection is present.
7. Review with the parents the signs and symptoms of urinary tract retention or infection.	7. Because of retention and reflux, the child may be at risk for urinary tract infections.

Evaluation

- Can the parents discuss the child's care appropriately?
- Are the parents able to list situations in which the child should be seen by the physician or nurse?

- Do the parents know how to contact community support?
- Can the parents demonstrate required adaptation?

INCREASED INTRACRANIAL PRESSURE

Increased ICP reflects the pressure exerted by the blood, brain, CSF, and any other space-occupying fluid or mass. Increased ICP results from a disturbance in autoregulation and is defined as pressure sustained at 20 mm Hg or higher.

Etiology

Alterations in the brain can result from a space-occupying lesion, such as a brain tumor or hematoma. The brain can swell as a result of head trauma, infection, or a hypoxic episode. Overproduction of fluid, malabsorption of fluid, or a communication problem within the system can disrupt CSF dynamics.

Manifestations

Signs and symptoms of increased ICP differ according to the child's developmental level (Box 28-1).

Level of Consciousness

Children with increased ICP often have an altered level of consciousness. The Glasgow Coma Scale (GCS) is a standardized scale that, in a modified form, is frequently used to assess level of consciousness in infants and children. It consists of a three-part assessment: eye opening, verbal response, and motor response (Table 28-1). Each level of response is assigned a number value. When the assessment of each response is complete, the scores are totaled, providing an objective measure of the child's level of consciousness. The total numeric scores range from 15, indicating no change in level of consciousness, to 3, indicating a deep coma and poor prognosis.

Behavior

Changes in the child's normal behavior pattern may be an important early sign of increased ICP. Parents often are the first to notice a change in the child's behavior; therefore a parent's comment that "he isn't acting like himself" should be taken seriously. The child who no longer recognizes parents, cannot follow commands, or has minimal response to pain is deteriorating. Decreased responsiveness to painful stimuli is a significant sign of alteration in level of consciousness.

PATHOPHYSIOLOGY

INCREASED ICP

The major pathophysiologic changes associated with increased ICP result from alterations in the brain, CSF dynamics, and CBF. To maintain cerebral pressure and volume within normal range, changes in one or more of the contents of the cranium must be compensated for by changes in the others; this is referred to as the *Monro-Kellie doctrine.*

Compensatory mechanisms include a reduction in CSF production, an increase in CSF absorption, and a reduction in cerebral mass as a result of fluid displacement. Once the limits of compensation are reached, any further increase in volume or pressure will cause a sudden increase in ICP and an associated decline in the child's clinical status.

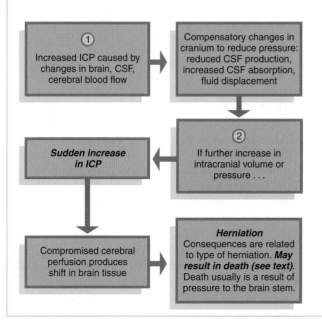

Ultimately, increased ICP will compromise cerebral perfusion and produce shifting of brain tissue, causing herniation. The consequences of herniation depend on its severity and location.

Herniation is classified into four types. *Transtentorial herniation* occurs when part of the brain herniates downward and around the tentorium cerebelli. It may be unilateral or bilateral and may involve anterior or posterior portions of the brain. If a large amount of tissue is involved, it may cause death because vital brain structures are compressed and become unable to perform their functions.

Temporal lobe herniation, or uncal herniation, refers to a shifting of the temporal lobe laterally across the tentorial notch. This produces compression of the third cranial nerve and ipsilateral pupil dilation. If pressure continues to rise, flaccid paralysis, pupil dilation, pupil fixation, and death will result.

Tonsillar herniation occurs when the cerebellar tonsils herniate through the foramen magnum. The child will develop nuchal rigidity, shoulder or arm numbness, and changes in heart and respiratory rates and patterns. Arnold-Chiari malformation, a condition sometimes associated with hydrocephalus, includes herniation of the cerebellar tonsils.

Brainstem herniation through the foramen magnum results in death as a result of compression of vital cardiorespiratory centers.

Infants are somewhat able to compensate for increasing ICP because their cranial sutures remain open. Craniosynostosis is premature closure of the cranial sutures. This abnormal skull development causes an abnormally shaped skull. In some cases, craniectomy is needed to manage the increased ICP.

BOX 28-1 | Developmental Manifestations of Increased ICP

Infant
- Poor feeding or vomiting
- Irritability or restlessness
- Lethargy
- Bulging fontanel
- High-pitched cry
- Increased head circumference
- Separation of cranial sutures
- Distended scalp veins
- Eyes deviated downward ("setting-sun" sign)
- Increased or decreased response to pain

Child
- Headache
- Diplopia
- Mood swings
- Slurred speech
- Papilledema (after 48 hr)
- Altered level of consciousness
- Nausea and vomiting, especially in the morning

TABLE 28-1   GCS Modified for Children

Child	Infant
Eyes	
4 = Opens eyes spontaneously	4 = Opens eyes spontaneously
3 = Opens eyes to speech	3 = Opens eyes to speech
2 = Opens eyes to pain	2 = Opens eyes to pain
1 = No response	**1 = No response**
_____ = Score (Eyes)	
Motor	
6 = Obeys commands	6 = Spontaneous movements
5 = Localizes	5 = Withdraws to touch
4 = Withdraws	4 = Withdraws to pain
3 = Flexion	3 = Flexion (decorticate)
2 = Extension	2 = Extension (decerebrate)
1 = No response	**1 = No response**
_____ = Score (Motor)	
Verbal	
5 = Oriented	5 = Coos and babbles
4 = Confused	4 = Irritable cry
3 = Inappropriate words	3 = Cries to pain
2 = Incomprehensible words	2 = Moans to pain
1 = No response	**1 = No response**
_____ = Score (Verbal)	

Total scores will range from 3 to 15.
Reprinted from James, H. E., Anas, N. G., & Perkin, R. M. (1985). *Brain insults in infants and children.* Orlando, FL: Grune & Stratton.

CRITICAL TO REMEMBER

Standard Terms for Level of Consciousness

Level of consciousness should be described by the nurse by using standard terminology:
- *Full consciousness:* awake, alert, oriented, interacts with environment
- *Confused:* lacks ability to think clearly and rapidly
- *Disoriented:* lacks ability to recognize place or person
- *Lethargic:* awakens easily but exhibits limited responsiveness
- *Obtunded:* sleeps unless aroused; once aroused has limited interaction with the environment
- *Stupor:* requires considerable stimulation to arouse
- *Coma:* vigorous stimulation produces no motor or verbal response

---

Pupil Evaluation

As ICP rises, compression of the third cranial nerve occurs, resulting in pupil dilation with sluggish or absent constriction in response to light. A fixed dilated pupil is an ominous sign in an unconscious child. This suggests a herniation of the center section of the brain (also known as a *transtentorial herniation*).

Motor Function

The child with increased ICP exhibits changes in motor function. Purposeful movement will decrease, and abnormal posturing may be observed. *Flexion,* or *decorticate, posturing* refers to flexion of the upper extremities (elbows, wrists) and extension of the lower extremities. Plantar flexion of the feet may also be observed. This type of posturing implies an injury to the cerebral hemispheres. *Extension,* or *decerebrate, posturing* involves extension of the upper extremities with internal rotation of the upper arm and wrist. The lower extremities will extend, with some internal rotation noted at the knees and feet. This type of posturing indicates damage to more areas of the brain, such as the diencephalon, midbrain, or pons. The progression from flexion to extension posturing usually indicates deteriorating neurologic function and warrants physician notification (Fig. 28-1). Flaccid paralysis indicates further deterioration in the child's condition.

Vital Signs

Temperature elevation may occur in children with increased ICP. *Cushing's response,* which consists of an increased systolic blood pressure with widening pulse pressure, bradycardia, and a change in respiratory rate and pattern, is usually apparent just before or at the time of brainstem herniation. This usually indicates an alteration in brainstem perfusion, with the body attempting to improve cerebral blood flow by increasing blood pressure. In children, Cushing's response is a late sign of increased ICP.

As ICP rises, the child's baseline respiratory pattern may change, exhibiting Cheyne-Stokes respiration, central neurogenic hyperventilation, or apneustic breathing. *Cheyne-Stokes respiration* refers to a pattern of breathing characterized by increasing rate and depth and then decreasing rate and depth with a pause of variable length. The cycle will be repeated

USING RESEARCH TO IMPROVE PRACTICE

The GCS (see Table 28-1) is one of the most widely used assessment tools for determining and monitoring changes in level of consciousness in people who have sustained neurologic insult. First introduced in the mid-1970s, its original purpose has been expanded in general use to include assessing diagnostic and prognostic criteria for individuals with traumatic brain injury (Fischer & Mathieson, 2001; Gabbe, Cameron, & Finch, 2003; Gill, Windemuth, Steele, & Green, 2005). Because the best verbal response of the GCS was particularly difficult to assess in preverbal infants and children, various modifications of the scale for use with this population have been presented in the literature.

Reliability and validity, however, for the modification to this scale have not been determined by research. In fact, research relating to reliability and validity of the original GCS has demonstrated varying results (Warrall, 2004). Because the GCS, or one of its modifications, is generally used when caring for children with neurologic insults, nurses in clinical practice should be certain the scale is used in a trustworthy manner and with high interrater reliability.

Several in-depth reviews of research on the GCS have suggested the following limitations that apply to clinical practice for nurses (Fischer & Mathieson, 2001; Gabbe et al., 2003; Gill et al., 2005; Warrall, 2004):

- Experienced personnel are more accurate and consistent in application of the scale criteria than are inexperienced personnel.
- Several conditions (e.g., sedation, endotracheal intubation, fractures) interfere with accurate observation of parts of the scale and therefore rely on individual clinician judgment for scoring.
- When assessing response to painful stimuli, nurses use a variety of methods to elicit the pain response, thus calling into question the consistency, accuracy, and reliability of the assessment.

What implications do these pieces of research have on clinical practice? The GCS is only one part of an overall neurologic assessment. Furthermore, because evidence suggests that experience increases accuracy, clinical agencies may want to consider first establishing a consistent and written procedure for assessing all components of the scale, then pairing inexperienced nurses with experienced nurses to ensure appropriate training and execution of the procedure. In addition, this is an area for interested nurse researchers to conduct studies establishing validity and interrater reliability for the GCS modified for preverbal children.

NURSING CARE PLAN

The Child With Increased ICP

Focused Assessment

Assessment of the child with increased ICP requires astute clinical observation. The assessment parameters are those common to all children with an underlying neurologic problem. The nurse should focus special attention on level of consciousness, behavior, pupil status, cranial nerve function, motor function, reflexes, and vital signs. Overt signs and symptoms may not occur until the ICP is significantly elevated and the child's condition is deteriorating rapidly.

Because the child's neurologic status directs nursing intervention, meticulous and ongoing assessment of neurologic status is required. The nurse should monitor and document a baseline level of consciousness with the modified GCS and observe the child's interactions with others. Pupils are evaluated to detect increasing ICP. Pupils are described according to size, equality, and reaction to light.

When evaluating pupils, be aware that some medications can affect pupillary reactions; for example, atropine will cause the pupils not to react to light.

Measure vital signs regularly, every 15 min to 2 hours, depending on the child's status. Particular attention should be given to careful measurement of blood pressure, pulse, and respiratory rate. Significant changes in vital signs should be reported immediately. Because elevated temperatures can increase ICP, initiating measures to decrease elevated temperatures (more than 40° C [104° F]) will be a priority in care.

Information about the child's normal behavior should be obtained from the parents or primary caregivers. Serial observations are made to assess changes in the child's condition. ICP monitoring devices may be used to measure pressure (see Box 28-2).

NURSING DIAGNOSIS   Risk for Infection related to invasive monitoring lines and procedures.

EXPECTED OUTCOME   The child will:
- Remain free from infection, as evidenced by being afebrile and having a normal WBC count, no evidence of meningitis or pneumonia, no CSF drainage or purulent drainage, and no urinary tract infection.

Continued

NURSING CARE PLAN—cont'd

Intervention	Rationale
1. Maintain strict asepsis when manipulating ventriculostomy drainage system.	1. Asepsis helps prevent an infection of the catheter site and CSF.
2. Monitor invasive sites for redness or drainage.	2. These are signs of infection.
3. Monitor temperature, WBC count, appearance on chest radiographs, and urinalysis results for signs of infection.	3. Steroids given to decrease ICP may mask infection and decrease immunity to infectious organisms.
4. Use aseptic technique with a Foley catheter.	4. Children on bed rest or who are immobilized are prone to urinary tract infection.

Evaluation

- Is the child's temperature within normal limits?
- Is the child free from other signs of infection?

NURSING DIAGNOSIS   Deficient Fluid Volume related to restricted intake, inability to swallow, and change in mental status.

EXPECTED OUTCOME   The child will:
- Maintain fluid and electrolyte balance, as evidenced by moist mucous membranes, serum osmolality and electrolyte values within normal limits for age, and intake and output normal for age.

Intervention	Rationale
1. Monitor intake and output and urine specific gravity. Notify physician of a urine output less than 1 mL/kg per hour or more than 2 mL/kg per hour.	1. SIADH or diabetes insipidus can occur with stress, surgery, brain dysfunction, or some medications. SIADH often occurs as a sequela to increased ICP (see Chapter 27).
2. Administer fluids within fluid restrictions.	2. Fluid restriction helps decrease extracellular fluid volume, which in turn decreases ICP.
3. Administer medications as ordered.	3. Osmotic and loop diuretics (mannitol, furosemide) will decrease cerebral edema by increasing fluid excretion.
4. Monitor serum sodium, electrolytes, and serum osmolality.	4. These levels indicate fluid status and help identify measures to take to keep electrolytes in balance. Hyponatremia will cause cerebral edema.

Evaluation

- Does the child demonstrate appropriate fluid balance and normal electrolyte levels?
- Is urinary output appropriate for age (see Chapter 18)?

BOX 28-2	**Instruments for Monitoring Increased ICP**

Subarachnoid Bolt

The end of the bolt is placed in the subarachnoid space. The top of the bolt is attached to a transducer to conduct a waveform to the monitor. The neurosurgeon adjusts the transducer to produce a waveform on the monitor.

Intraventricular Catheter

The catheter is placed in the lateral ventricle or subarachnoid space. The catheter provides a method for measuring pressure as well as a conduit to drain off extra fluid into the drainage bag. The manometer and drainage bag are part of a sterile closed system.

---

again and again. *Central neurogenic hyperventilation* is identified by a rapid rate despite normal arterial blood gas values. This type of breathing pattern usually indicates midbrain or pontine involvement. *Apneustic breathing* occurs when the child demonstrates prolonged inspiration and expiration. As Cushing's response occurs, the child will develop apnea.

Late signs of increased ICP include tachycardia that leads to bradycardia, apnea, systolic hypertension, widening pulse pressure, and flexion or extension posturing.

Diagnostic Evaluation and Therapeutic Management

Diagnostic tests for increased ICP include computed tomography (CT), magnetic resonance imaging (MRI), lumbar puncture, serum and urine electrolytes, arterial blood gas determinations, a complete blood count (CBC), electroencephalography (EEG), and radiography. Normal blood gas levels are PaO_2 greater than 80 mm Hg and $PaCO_2$ less than 45 mm Hg in a child with normal ICP. Passive hyperventilation

FlexionPosturing

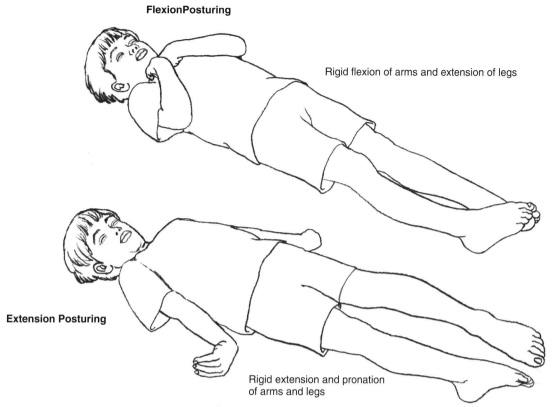

Rigid flexion of arms and extension of legs

Extension Posturing

Rigid extension and pronation
of arms and legs

FIG 28-1 **Flexion and extension posturing.**

may be an initial treatment for the child with increased ICP because it lowers the $PaCO_2$, causing cerebral vasoconstriction and decreased fluid. The goal of hyperventilation is to achieve a $PaCO_2$ between 30 and 35 mm Hg (Dias, 2004).

The management of increased ICP is directed toward treating its underlying cause, reducing the volume of the CSF, preserving cerebral metabolic function, and avoiding situations that increase ICP.

The head of the child's bed should be elevated 30 degrees. The child may be given an osmotic diuretic (e.g., mannitol) or dexamethasone.

SPINA BIFIDA

Spina bifida is a congenital neural tube defect characterized by incomplete closure of the vertebrae and neural tube during fetal development. Spina bifida is classified as spina bifida occulta and spina bifida cystica (Fig. 28-2). Spina bifida occulta usually occurs between the L5 and S1 vertebrae, with failure of the vertebrae to completely fuse. The child may have no sensory or motor defects. The only clinical manifestation that may appear is a dimple, a small tuft of hair, a hemangioma, or a lipoma in the lower lumbar or sacral area. These defects may be detected accidentally on routine radiographs.

Spina bifida cystica results in incomplete closure of the vertebrae and neural tube, evidenced by a saclike protrusion in the lumbar or sacral area with varying degrees of nervous tissue involvement. Spina bifida cystica is further described as meningocele, myelomeningocele, lipomeningocele, and lipomyelomeningocele. Meningocele is a saclike protrusion

filled with spinal fluid and meninges. The most severe form of meningocele is myelomeningocele, in which the sac is filled with spinal fluid, meninges, nerve roots, and spinal cord. Nearly 80% of infants with myelomeningocele develop hydrocephalus as a result of a type II Chiari malformation (Arnold-Chiari malformation) (Johnston & Kinsman, 2004).

Etiology and Incidence

The cause of spina bifida is unknown in most cases. Evidence suggests a possible genetic predisposition. Maternal folic acid deficiency has been strongly linked to neural tube defects. Daily consumption of 0.4 mg folic acid by all women of childbearing age is recommended. Evidence of a viral origin

---

PATHOPHYSIOLOGY

SPINA BIFIDA

Spina bifida occurs during the fourth week of gestation (days 24 to 28), when ventral induction of the neural tube fails to occur. The degree of impairment corresponds to the level of the defect on the spinal cord and the size of the defect. Ninety percent of spinal cord lesions are at or below the L2 vertebra. The lesion results in paralysis, partial paralysis, or varying sensory defects. Clubfeet, scoliosis, and contracture and dislocation of the hips may also be associated with the defect. Associated malformations include hydrocephalus and Arnold-Chiari malformation.

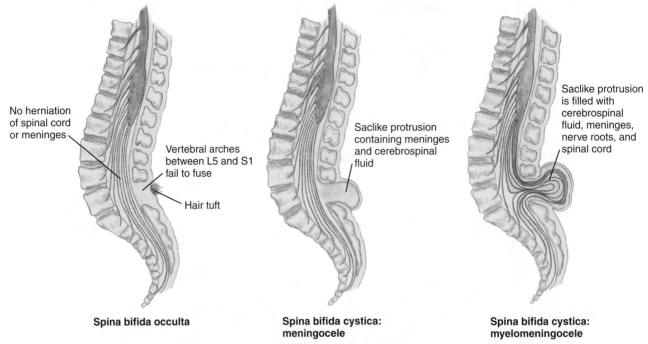

No herniation
of spinal cord
or meninges

Vertebral arches
between L5 and S1
fail to fuse

Hair tuft

Saclike protrusion
containing meninges
and cerebrospinal
fluid

Saclike protrusion
is filled with
cerebrospinal
fluid, meninges,
nerve roots, and
spinal cord

Spina bifida occulta

**Spina bifida cystica:
meningocele**

**Spina bifida cystica:
myelomeningocele**

FIG 28-2   Three forms of spina bifida.

has prompted research, but other than folic acid, no cause or preventive measures have been identified.

The incidence of myelomeningocele is 1 in 4000 live births. Geographic locations of incidence vary within the United States and worldwide (Johnston & Kinsman, 2004).

Manifestations

In addition to the appearance of the lesion, manifestations relate to the degree of deficit, which is determined by the level of the lesion (Fig. 28-3).

T12:	Flaccid lower extremities, decreased sensation, and bowel and bladder incontinence
L1 to L3:	Hip flexion, flail feet
L2 to L4:	Hip adduction
L3 to S2:	Hip adduction, hip extension, knee flexion
S3 and below:	No motor impairment
Sacral roots:	Plantar flexion

Children with spina bifida are at high risk for developing latex allergies because of frequent exposure to latex during catheterizations and multiple operations. Latex allergy is estimated to occur in approximately 50% of children with spina bifida (Elder, 2004). Allergic reactions can range from mild signs and symptoms to anaphylactic shock. Children should be tested for latex allergy, and precautions should be taken from birth to decrease exposures. The nurse should check equipment for latex and choose nonlatex alternatives.

Diagnostic Evaluation

Diagnostic tests include determining alpha-fetoprotein (AFP) levels in blood at 16 to 18 weeks of gestation. If the AFP screen is elevated, amniocentesis and fetal ultrasound are performed. After delivery, the infant may undergo a CT scan or myelography.

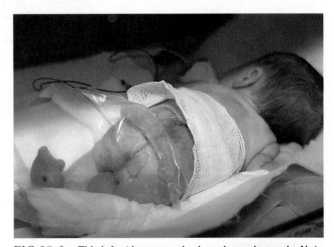

FIG 28-3   This infant has a repaired myelomeningocele. Note the left clubfoot. This deformity often accompanies the defect because normal intrauterine movement does not occur in the fetus with spina bifida, interfering with the development of the extremities. The legs are flaccid, and normal neonatal flexion is absent. The infant is also incontinent, dribbling stool and urine constantly. Hydrocephalus also commonly accompanies these neural tube defects.   *(Courtesy Parkland Health & Hospital System, Dallas, TX.)*

Therapeutic Management

Prenatal microsurgical closure of the myelomeningocele, performed at approximately 19 to 25 weeks' gestation, shows promise for reducing the severity of Chiari II malformations and incidence of hydrocephalus (Kaufman, 2004). Risks associated with antenatal surgery include premature birth, with its associated consequences and possible fetal death. Maternal risks (e.g., abruptio placenta, uterine rupture) are directly related to the hysterotomy (Kaufman, 2004).

Immediate surgical closure decreases the risk of infection, morbidity, and mortality. Other benefits are improved prognosis without further cord deterioration and earlier and easier physical handling and bonding.

The child will need lifelong management of neurologic, orthopedic, and urinary problems and is best managed in a multispecialty outpatient setting. Urodynamic studies are performed early, and a bladder-emptying program is initiated, with close monitoring of the child's infection status. In most instances, the child will require orthopedic bracing and possibly orthopedic surgery to maximize the child's mobility.

NURSING CARE PLAN

The Child With Spina Bifida

Focused Assessment

The saclike protrusion of the meningocele should be assessed and the lesion measured. The nurse should measure the infant's head circumference and regularly palpate the anterior fontanel for fullness.

Continuous baseline and neurologic assessment is necessary. Assess the infant's overall tone, taking special note of spontaneous movement of the extremities. The motor examination is performed with the infant at rest, using painful stimuli from the torso downward. Observe for voluntary movement below the level of the lesion.

The infant is at risk for infection before the sac is closed. Therefore the infant's temperature must be monitored every 1 to 2 hr. Note signs of infection along with irritability,

lethargy, or nuchal rigidity. A sterile saline dressing is placed over the sac to maintain the moisture of the sac and its contents. A risk of infection remains, however, and the dressing needs to be changed on a regular schedule or whenever soiled. Record the appearance of the sac and contents with each dressing change.

Other assessments and nursing care are similar to those discussed earlier for any child with a neurologic problem. Because children with spina bifida have multisystem, long-term problems, the nurse needs to do ongoing assessments of the child's emotional needs and coping skills. Communication with the school nurse may be required.

NURSING DIAGNOSIS   Risk for Infection related to the open sac and the operative procedure.

EXPECTED OUTCOMES   Preoperatively, the child will:
- Remain free of infection, as evidenced by the absence of drainage from the sac, normal WBC count, absence of signs of meningeal irritation, and normal temperature.
Postoperatively, the child will:
- Be free of infection, as evidenced by remaining afebrile; maintaining a WBC count within normal limits; and exhibiting no redness, swelling, or purulent drainage from the incision site.

Intervention	*Rationale*
1. Monitor vital signs and WBC count. Observe the sac or incision site for redness and clear or purulent drainage.	1. These are signs of infection that need to be documented and reported to the physician.
2. Perform regular neurologic checks, including palpating the fontanel.	2. Altered neurologic signs, irritability, and full fontanel are signs of meningeal infection.
3. Maintain sterile dressings over the sac or incision site.	3. Sterile dressings facilitate healing and decrease the risk of infection.

Evaluation

- Does the infant's sac remain intact preoperatively?
- Is the infant infection free (afebrile, normal WBC count, calm, able to eat)?
- Does the incision site appear intact and without redness or drainage?

NURSING DIAGNOSIS   Risk for Impaired Skin Integrity related to neurologic motor deficits.

EXPECTED OUTCOME   The child will:
- Have intact skin, as evidenced by absence of pressure areas or ulcerations.

Intervention	*Rationale*
1. Use a special mattress or pad for the infant's bed. Preoperatively, place the infant in a prone or side-lying position with a small blanket or diaper roll under the ankles and between the knees.	1. Special bedding can help alleviate pressure points caused by the required preoperative prone position. Blanket rolls help maintain anatomic position of the feet and hips.

Continued

NURSING CARE PLAN—cont'd

2. Assess the infant's skin and reposition frequently. Leave the diaper under the infant; do not fasten. Change a soiled diaper immediately and clean the diaper area when soiled.
3. Use stoma adhesive on each side of the sac to anchor the dressing; consult the stoma therapist if needed.

4. Teach the parents to check the child's skin routinely for pressure areas, particularly if the child requires bracing or other orthopedic support as the child grows.

2. Keeping the infant's diaper open facilitates frequent cleaning of the perineal area because oozing of stool and dribbling of urine may occur. Keeping the area clean and dry reduces skin breakdown.
3. Frequent dressing changes can irritate the skin, and the potential for irritation will be less if the tape is stuck to the stoma adhesive. The stoma therapist may make special recommendations for neonatal skin needs.
4. Because the child has sensory as well as motor deficits, the child may not be able to feel abnormal pressure. Pressure spots from orthopedic appliances can contribute to skin breakdown.

Evaluation

- Does the infant exhibit any signs of skin breakdown?
- Are the perineal area, incision site, and buttocks clean and dry?

- Do the parents and older child perform regular skin checks for abnormal pressure areas?

NURSING DIAGNOSIS   Impaired Physical Mobility related to neuromuscular impairment.

EXPECTED OUTCOMES   The child will:
- Maximize mobility by learning to use appropriate mobilization devices and by maximizing opportunities to be mobile.
- Achieve developmental milestones within the limits of the motor impairment.

The child and family will:
- Demonstrate proper application of any orthopedic devices.

Intervention

1. Determine and record physical impairments and abilities. Note the activities in which the child can participate and encourage as much activity as tolerated.
2. Maintain splints, braces, and casts. Use wheelchairs, walkers, and other assistive devices as needed. Teach parents how to apply the devices and perform routine skin care (see Chapter 26).
3. Ensure that the child attends physical therapy sessions and participates fully. Encourage self-care.
4. Refer the family to the Spina Bifida Association (see Evolve website).

Rationale

1. This documentation notes advances or regression in activities or the child's abilities. Activity maintains muscle tone.
2. These aids may be used for proper alignment and to decrease contractures. Other devices may increase independence and mobility.
3. Therapy and self-care help prevent contractures, encourage independence, and increase self-esteem.
4. Support groups can help families cope with the stresses of a chronic condition.

Evaluation

- Does the child enjoy mobility as desired and as allowed by impairments?
- Do the parents demonstrate proper use and application of orthopedic devices and encourage occupational and physical therapy?

- Do the parents facilitate the child's maximal development?

NURSING DIAGNOSIS   Impaired Urinary Elimination related to the neuromuscular deficit.

EXPECTED OUTCOME   The child will:
- Be free of urinary tract infections (UTIs), as evidenced by urine that is clear, odor free, and sterile.

Intervention

1. Observe urinary stream and teach the parents to observe for any dribbling of urine. Give the parents written instructions on how to administer any ordered medications (antispasmodics, antibiotics).
2. Offer adequate fluids.

Rationale

1. Urinary dribbling indicates interrupted innervation to the bladder. Antispasmodics act on the smooth muscle of the bladder, allowing for increased bladder capacity. Antibiotics are given to treat UTIs.
2. Good hydration helps prevent UTIs.

NURSING CARE PLAN—cont'd

3. Teach and maintain regular toilet habits. Teach the parents and child how to perform intermittent clean catheterization if necessary. Emphasize use of a latex-free catheter.

3. Regular toilet habits facilitate complete and regular emptying of the bladder and help prevent urine retention and UTIs. If catheterization is necessary, it is usually done every 2 to 4 hr while the child is awake. Children with spina bifida have a high incidence of allergies to latex and rubber products. Because of this only latex-free products should be used with these children.

4. Check urinary frequency, input and output, and specific gravity. Teach the parents to observe the color, clarity, and odor of the urine. Encourage follow-up with urine cultures if ordered.

4. These values may be initial indicators of urinary pattern alteration. The child will not experience urinary urgency or painful urination because of neurologic sensory deficits; observation of the urine is essential to recognize a developing UTI.

Evaluation

- Has the child established regular voiding or catheterization patterns?

- Are the urinalysis and urine cultures normal?

NURSING DIAGNOSIS Constipation related to sensory deficit and neurologic impairment.

EXPECTED OUTCOME The child will:
  - Be free of constipation or impaction, as evidenced by regular bowel movements and soft stool.

Intervention

1. Observe and record the infant's or child's anal tone and pattern of bowel movements.

2. Monitor for abdominal distention, vomiting, and poor feeding.

3. Develop a bowel program in cooperation with the parents; give a suppository before breakfast and have the child sit on toilet after breakfast. May need to stimulate the anal sphincter.

4. Consult a registered dietitian to be sure the diet provides adequate fluid and fiber.

Rationale

1. Absence of rectal sphincter tone indicates abnormal bowel function; noting the pattern will alert caregivers to implement a bowel program.

2. These signs may indicate constipation.

3. A bowel program ensures elimination needs are met.

4. Fluid and fiber facilitate softer stools and easier passage.

Evaluation

- Is the child free of constipation or impaction, as evidenced by regular bowel movements?

HYDROCEPHALUS

Hydrocephalus develops as a result of an imbalance between the production and absorption of CSF. As excess CSF accumulates in the ventricular system, the ventricles become dilated and the brain is compressed against the skull. This results in enlargement of the skull if the sutures are open; it results in signs and symptoms of increased ICP if the sutures are fused.

Etiology

Hydrocephalus may be congenital, acquired, or of unknown etiology. In infancy, hydrocephalus is most often congenital or related to prematurity. Congenital hydrocephalus results from developmental defects, such as Arnold-Chiari malformations, congenital arachnoid cysts, congenital tumors, or aqueductal stenosis. In premature infants, neonatal meningitis or subarachnoid hemorrhage may result in hydrocephalus.

Hydrocephalus is often associated with myelomeningocele. Intrauterine infection and perinatal hemorrhage cause hydrocephalus in some infants. In older children, hydrocephalus is usually acquired as a complication of meningitis, tumor, or hemorrhage.

Incidence

The incidence of hydrocephalus in infancy is 1.2 in 1000 births (Garton & Piatt, 2004). The incidence of hydrocephalus with spina bifida is considered to be 3 to 4 in 1000 births. Obstructive, or noncommunicating, hydrocephalus accounts for 99% of all cases of hydrocephalus in children.

Manifestations and Diagnostic Evaluation

Because of anatomic differences between infants and children, manifestations of hydrocephalus differ according to developmental stage (Table 28-2).

PATHOPHYSIOLOGY

HYDROCEPHALUS

CSF is produced primarily by the choroid plexus, which lines the lateral ventricles. CSF circulates through the ventricular system and flows into the subarachnoid space around the brain and the spinal cord. It is then reabsorbed within the subarachnoid spaces.

Hydrocephalus results when either of the following is present: (1) impaired absorption of CSF within the subarachnoid space *(communicating hydrocephalus)* or (2) obstruction of CSF flow within the ventricles that prevents CSF from circulating around the spinal cord and the subarachnoid space *(noncommunicating hydrocephalus)*. Hydrocephalus may rarely be caused by overproduction of CSF because of a tumor of the choroid plexus.

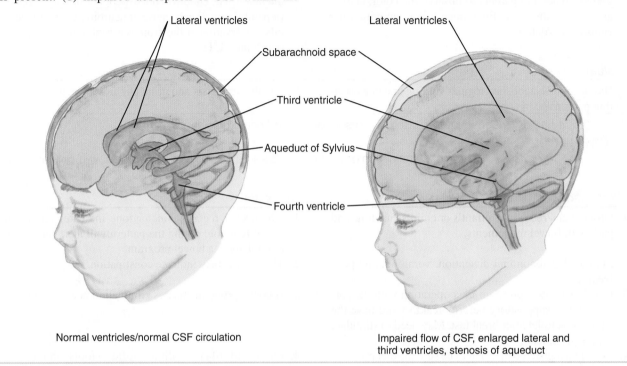

Normal ventricles/normal CSF circulation

Impaired flow of CSF, enlarged lateral and third ventricles, stenosis of aqueduct

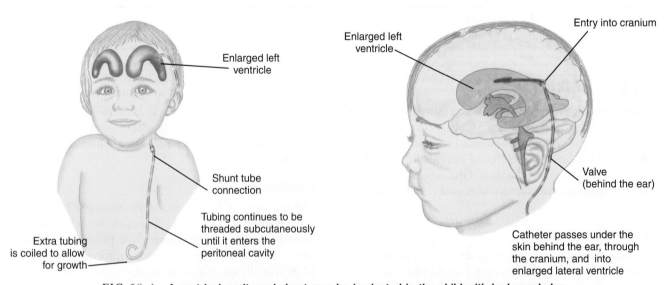

FIG 28-4 **A ventriculoperitoneal shunt may be implanted in the child with hydrocephalus to prevent excess accumulation of CSF in the ventricles. The tubing diverts the CSF from the ventricles into the peritoneal cavity, where it is reabsorbed. Nursing care of the child with a ventricular shunt includes monitoring for infection and pain, administering antibiotics and pain medications as ordered, and teaching the family how to change dressings and how to recognize shunt problems.**

TABLE 28-2 Early and Late Manifestations of Hydrocephalus	
Early	**Late**
Infant	
Rapid head growth—increase in head circumference above the normal growth curve	Setting-sun sign: sclera visible above the iris
Full, bulging anterior fontanel	Frontal bone enlargement or bossing
Irritability	Vomiting; difficulty swallowing or feeding
Poor feeding	Increased blood pressure, decreased heart rate
Distended, prominent scalp veins	Altered respiratory pattern
Widely separated cranial sutures	Shrill, high-pitched cry
	Sluggish or unequal pupillary response to light
Child	
Strabismus	Seizures
Frontal headache that occurs in the morning and is relieved by emesis or by sitting upright	Increased blood pressure
Nausea and vomiting that may be projectile	Decreased heart rate
Diplopia	Alteration in respiratory pattern
Restlessness	Blindness from herniation of the optic disc
Behavior or personality changes	Decerebrate rigidity
Ataxia	
Papilledema	
Irritability	
Sluggish and unequal pupillary response to light	
Confusion	
Changes in schoolwork	
Lethargy	

Diagnostic tests for hydrocephalus include serial measurements of head circumference, CT, MRI, and lumbar puncture.

Therapeutic Management

Therapy is aimed at preventing further CSF accumulation and reducing disability and death. The objective is to bypass the blockage and drain the fluid from the ventricles to an area where it may be reabsorbed into the circulation. A *ventriculoperitoneal shunt*, or tube leading from the ventricles out of the skull and passing under the skin to the peritoneal cavity, accomplishes this (Fig. 28-4). An alternative shunt, the *ventriculoatrial shunt*, which is used in older children, drains the fluid from the ventricles to the right atrium of the heart.

The shunt may need to be revised as the child grows. Long-term follow-up is essential. The child may exhibit mild learning challenges and may have accelerated pubertal development (Johnston & Kinsman, 2004).

A surgical procedure, endoscopic third ventriculostomy, has been used with increasing success in infants and children with obstructive hydrocephalus and, in many instances, is the initial treatment of choice (Fritsch & Mehdorn, 2002). For this procedure, the surgeon creates a small burr hole in the skull through which an endoscope is passed. The third ventricle is visualized and a small opening is created in its floor. This allows the CSF to bypass the fourth ventricle and return to circulation, where it is reabsorbed. The procedure is generally successful in children older than 2 years and in approximately 50% of infants with hydrocephalus (Fritsch & Mehdorn, 2002). The procedure delays or reduces the need for a permanent mechanical shunt.

NURSING CARE PLAN

The Child With Hydrocephalus

Focused Assessment

When an infant is born with hydrocephalus, signs may be apparent at birth or signs of an obstruction may appear over the next few months. The first sign may be an abnormal head circumference or a head circumference that is increasing at a rate greater than the expected percentile. The parent may notice and report increased irritability or other neurologic signs.

If the child is older, any change in level of consciousness, personality, interaction with the environment, or sleep patterns or any delays in developmental milestones need to be explored with the parents. Note reports of headache that may be relieved when the child sits upright and vomiting of unexplained origin. If the child has a history of vomiting, hydration status also should be assessed.

Continued

NURSING CARE PLAN—cont'd

Postoperatively, the infant's head circumference should be measured daily or more frequently, depending on the infant's condition, and should be recorded and plotted on a graph. To facilitate accuracy when different personnel take the measurement, make a pen mark on the scalp where the tape measure is placed. The tape measure is usually placed just above the top of the ears and around the head, around the midforehead and the most prominent portion of the occiput.

Palpate the infant's anterior fontanel for size, bulging, and tenseness and palpate the cranial sutures for separation. The fontanel is assessed with the baby sitting upright and quiet. It may bulge or pulsate if the infant is crying.

Observe the infant's behavior when the fontanel is full or tense. Ask the parent if the baby is irritable or lethargic or if any change in feeding behavior has been noticed. Ask if the infant has had any seizures. Vital signs are assessed to identify any changes from the infant's baseline measurements.

NURSING DIAGNOSIS   Risk for Infection related to surgical shunt placement.

EXPECTED OUTCOMES   The child will:
* Remain free of infection, as evidenced by a normal temperature; a clean, dry suture line; toleration of feedings; and no signs of increased ICP.

The parents will:
* Demonstrate infection control measures.

Intervention	Rationale
1. Monitor temperature every 1 to 2 hr and as needed. Observe for decreased level of consciousness and vomiting. Also monitor for swelling or redness along the shunt tract.	1. These are the first signs of an infection.
2. Observe head, abdominal, and chest dressings for drainage. Test drainage for glucose with a Dextrostix, or check for a halo sign on gauze.	2. Drainage could be CSF, indicating a route for infection to reach the brain. CSF contains glucose and makes a halo on gauze.
3. Position the child off the shunt site so that no weight is placed on the valve for the first 2 days.	3. Careful placement prevents skin breakdown and reduces the risk of infection.
4. Administer IV antibiotics as ordered and monitor serum levels to prevent subtherapeutic or toxic levels.	4. *Staphylococcus epidermidis* infection is the major complication of shunts.
5. Teach the parents the dressing change technique and show them how to recognize shunt infection.	5. Parents need to know how to care for their child at home and when to seek medical attention.

Evaluation

* Does the child have a normal body temperature?
* Does the child have a clean, dry suture site?

* Can the parent demonstrate dressing changes with aseptic technique and state the signs of infection?

NURSING DIAGNOSIS   Acute Pain related to operative procedure.

EXPECTED OUTCOME   The child will:
* Exhibit pain relief, as evidenced by stable vital signs, restful sleep, play when possible, and verbalization of decreased pain.

Intervention	Rationale
1. Determine the child's pain level, activity, and irritability and give pain medications as needed. Administer analgesics (e.g., codeine) as ordered if needed.	1. Pain relief will help decrease crying, ICP, and metabolic demands. Codeine does not interfere with the child's level of consciousness.
2. Hold, cuddle, and distract the child. Teach therapeutic play to family members and caregivers.	2. Nonpharmacologic methods of pain management also decrease ICP.

Evaluation

* Are the child's vital signs normal for age?
* Does the child smile and interact with the caregivers?

* Does the older child express pain relief or choose a lower value on a pain assessment scale?

NURSING DIAGNOSIS   Deficient Knowledge (parental) related to unfamiliarity with home care and signs and symptoms of shunt malfunction or complications.

EXPECTED OUTCOME   The parents will:
* Describe care of their child, as evidenced by an ability to demonstrate assessment of the child's level of consciousness, describe signs of infection, and discuss the shunt's purpose and function.

NURSING CARE PLAN—cont'd

Intervention	Rationale
1. Determine the parents' knowledge of changes in the child's level of consciousness. Begin teaching at their level of understanding.	1. Parents need to understand that shunt malfunction will cause increased ICP.
2. Teach the parents to observe the child for abdominal distention or discomfort.*	2. Underlying shunt infection may manifest as signs and symptoms of peritonitis.*
3. Teach the parents to observe for poor feeding, nausea or vomiting, elevated temperature, and skin redness or tenderness and report these to the physician.	3. These are all signs of an infection.
4. Teach parents safety measures for use in home care, playing, and the car (padded seats).	4. Anticipatory guidance for the growing child should be provided.
5. Emphasize the importance of neurosurgical follow-up care.	5. The shunt may need revision as the child grows.

Evaluation

• Can the parents describe how to assess level of consciousness and list signs of infection? • Can the parents discuss care of the child with a shunt?	• Are the parents able to describe signs of shunt malfunction?

*Garton, H., & Piatt, J. (2004). Hydrocephalus. *Pediatric Clinics of North America, 51*(2), 305-325.

CEREBRAL PALSY

Cerebral palsy, also known as *static encephalopathy*, is a chronic, nonprogressive disorder of posture and movement. It is characterized by difficulty in controlling the muscles because of an abnormality in the extrapyramidal or pyramidal motor system (motor cortex, basal ganglia, cerebellum).

Etiology and Incidence

The damage to the motor system can occur prenatally, perinatally, or postnatally (Box 28-3). The reported prevalence in children aged 3 to 10 years is 2 to 4 per 1000 children (Koman, Smith, & Shilt, 2004). The incidence and prevalence of cerebral palsy has slightly increased during the past 20 years both in the United States and in some European countries (Winter, Autry, Boyle, & Yeargin-Allsopp, 2002).

Increases in the incidence and prevalence of cerebral palsy in both lowest birth weight and normal weight infants may be related to improved diagnosis or documentation of cases by national registries (Winter et al., 2002). Lowest birth weight infants (less than 1000 g) may be at increased risk for cerebral palsy because of intracerebral hemorrhage or periventricular leukomalacia (Johnston, 2004).

Manifestations

The manifestations of cerebral palsy may vary, and one or more of the following may be observed in any one child: persistence of primitive reflexes, delayed gross motor development, and lack of progression through the developmental milestones. Abnormal posturing with inability to maintain normal posture and balance may be present, as well

---

BOX 28-3	Factors Associated With Cerebral Palsy

Prenatal
- Maternal diabetes
- Rh or ABO blood type incompatibility
- Rubella in the first trimester
- Genetic causes
- Intrauterine ischemic event
- Toxoplasmosis
- Cytomegalovirus
- Congenital brain abnormality

Perinatal
- Asphyxia
- Low birth weight
- Prematurity

- Precipitous delivery
- Pregnancy-induced hypertension
- Birth trauma
- Anoxia
- Prolonged labor
- Perinatal metabolic condition (diabetes)
- Intracranial hemorrhage

Postnatal
- Infections
- Trauma
- Stroke
- Poisoning

PATHOPHYSIOLOGY

CEREBRAL PALSY

A number of neuromuscular disabilities are associated with cerebral palsy. The alteration in voluntary muscular control is related to a cerebral insult. The area of the brain that has been injured determines the type of neuromuscular disability.

The five classifications of cerebral palsy are dyskinetic, spastic, ataxic, rigid, and mixed. *Dyskinetic (athetoid) palsy* refers to an injury in the basal ganglia. Slow, writhing, uncontrolled, involuntary movements involving all extremities characterize this type.

Spastic cerebral palsy is the most common type. The affected area of the brain is the cortex. Spastic cerebral palsy is characterized by increased deep tendon reflexes, hypertonia, flexion, and sometimes contractures. The child's muscles are very tense, and any stimulus may cause a sudden jerking movement. The child has to make a conscious effort to relax. Scissors gait, hip flexion with adduction and internal rotation, or toe walking because of tight heel cords may be present.

In *ataxic cerebral palsy,* the affected area of the brain is the cerebellum. This type of cerebral palsy is characterized by a loss of coordination, equilibrium, and kinesthetic sense. Overall, the child appears clumsy.

Rigid (tremor, atonic) cerebral palsy is relatively rare in children. The child has rigidity of both flexor and extensor muscles. In a child with tremors, the tremors are apparent both at rest and during movement. The prognosis for a child with this type of cerebral palsy is poor because of associated deformities and lack of active movement.

Approximately half of children with cerebral palsy have some degree of mental retardation and other disabilities. Other than epilepsy and mental retardation, learning problems, poor attention span, hyperactivity, hearing or visual loss, and emotional problems may be seen. Gastroesophageal reflux may be a problem (see Chapter 19). Intense movements cause a high expenditure of calories, and difficulty feeding leads to a calorie deficit.

as spasticity or uncontrollable movements in the extremities. Also documented are disturbances of gait (particularly ataxia and toe walking), seizures, attention deficit disorder, sensory impairment, failure of automatic reactions (equilibrium), and speech and swallowing impairments.

Diagnostic Evaluation and Therapeutic Management

Diagnostic tests include EEG, CT or MRI, electrolyte levels, metabolic workup, and a thorough neurologic examination. Persistent primitive reflexes are seen, as are abnormal muscle tone and posture and abnormal motor development.

The goal of managing the child with cerebral palsy is early recognition and intervention to maximize the child's abilities. Cerebral palsy often is not diagnosed before the child is 2 years old. Through repetition, new brain pathways develop through alternative receptor sites to achieve proper motor function. The child may be intellectually intact, but this may be overlooked because of the child's physical limitations. Intrathecal baclofen, a skeletal muscle relaxant, by an infusion pump can be used to treat severe spasticity in children with cerebral palsy. Close monitoring of the child for infection and the pump for malfunction is required (Johnston, 2004a).

A multidisciplinary health care team approach is necessary to meet the many needs of the child with cerebral palsy. The team includes the child and family, a pediatrician, neurologist, orthopedic surgeon, nurse, speech and hearing therapist, social worker, occupational therapist, physical therapist, and educators.

NURSING CARE PLAN

The Child With Cerebral Palsy in the Community Setting

Focused Assessment

The most important component of assessment is identifying the condition. The infant identified to be at risk is then monitored for irritability, feeding difficulties, delayed development, poor motor development, abnormal posturing, persistence of primitive reflexes, ataxic gait, and poor muscle tone. Assessing the child's response to therapy is important. Monitoring and documenting progress or lack of progress are just as important as identifying problems.

The nurse needs to be aware of normal growth and development, with special attention to developmental milestones, because delay in reaching these milestones may be a key indicator of cerebral palsy.

School and community nurses are in the best position to work with families and children with cerebral palsy. Many of these children will need both learning and physical adaptations as they enter school. For the most part, children with cerebral palsy are educated in the regular school program with assistive devices such as communication boards or computers. The school nurse regularly assesses these children because the nurse may be part of an educational team that develops an individual learning plan for the child.

NURSING CARE PLAN—cont'd

NURSING DIAGNOSIS Impaired Physical Mobility related to spasticity and muscle weakness.

EXPECTED OUTCOMES The child will:
- Maximize ability for movement, as evidenced by freedom from contractures or injuries and no complications from immobility.

The parents will:
- Demonstrate how to do the child's exercises and notify the school nurse if any changes are made in the child's plan.

Intervention	*Rationale*
1. Reinforce physical therapy exercises to strengthen and help coordination of muscles. These exercises may have to be performed in the school setting.	1. Early intervention and consistent therapy facilitate proper posture and circumvent the development of contractures.
2. Encourage parents to be active in the child's daily physical and occupational therapy.	2. Active involvement in the child's care empowers the parents.
3. Observe and record the child's response to physical therapy.	3. Changes in therapy may be made in a timely fashion for a higher degree of success.
4. Determine the need for special equipment for reading, writing, eating, and mobility. Convey this information to the school evaluation team.	4. The use of special equipment improves the chance for successful self-care. Incorporating this into the child's education plan will maximize learning potential.

Evaluation

- Have the child's joints remained mobile and free from contractures?
- Does the child demonstrate improved mobility and self-care?

- Can the parents demonstrate physical therapy techniques used for their child?
- Have the parents notified the school about any changes in the child's plan of care?

NURSING DIAGNOSIS Delayed Growth and Development related to neuromuscular impairment.

EXPECTED OUTCOME The child will:
- Maximize potential for meeting growth and development milestones, as evidenced by participation in family, social, and school activities.

Intervention	*Rationale*
1. Monitor the child's developmental level and intelligence. Administer the Denver Developmental Screening Test (see Chapter 4) if needed.	1. The child with cerebral palsy should be given opportunities to learn and should be exposed to new experiences to maximize developmental progress.
2. Encourage early intervention and participation in school programs. Refer for early intervention community programs.	2. Interventions by multidisciplinary groups will maximize the child's potential for learning.
3. Communicate and interact with the child at the child's functional level, not chronologic age.	3. A child with normal intelligence can understand age-appropriate communication and speech, but a child with decreased intelligence may have a different cognitive understanding than age would indicate.

Evaluation

- Do the parents encourage social and developmental activities that maximize the child's potential?
- Does the child attend public school and play with peers when possible?

- Does the child participate in physical, speech, and occupational therapy at school?

NURSING DIAGNOSIS Risk for Injury related to spasticity, uncontrolled muscle movements, or seizures.

EXPECTED OUTCOMES The child will:
- Have a safe environment, as evidenced by freedom from injuries.

The parents will:
- Describe ways to adapt the child's environment to maximize safety.

Intervention	*Rationale*
1. Teach the family principles for providing a safe environment (e.g., remove sharp objects and toys, pad sharp furniture edges).	1. A safe environment will reduce the risk of injury.

Continued

NURSING CARE PLAN—cont'd

2. Have the child wear a protective helmet and pads if the child falls frequently.
3. If the child is hospitalized, implement bedside seizure precautions. (Do not pad the rails with pillows.)

4. Provide safe toys that are appropriate for age and developmental level.

5. Position the child upright after meals.

2. A helmet protects against head injury.

3. Keeping suction, oxygen, and airway equipment at the bedside and padding the side rails help prevent injury and allow for resuscitation of the child if necessary. Pillows should not be used as pads because they may cause suffocation.
4. No sharp, very small, or easily shattered toys should be allowed for the child who may fall because of erratic movements.
5. An upright position prevents aspiration from gastro-esophageal reflux.

Evaluation

- Does the child remain free from injury?
- Do the parents demonstrate safety measures for the child?

- Have the parents adapted the child's environment to be safe and secure?

NURSING DIAGNOSIS   Impaired Verbal Communication related to neuromuscular impairment and difficulty with articulation.

EXPECTED OUTCOME   The child will:
- Maximize communication ability, as evidenced by appropriately expressing needs and developing methods for communicating with others.

Intervention

1. Use the child's usual mode of communicating, such as flash cards and talking boards, to facilitate communication.
2. Refer the child to a speech therapist.
3. Encourage and reinforce speech therapy techniques, nonverbal methods of communication, proper feeding techniques, and jaw control.
4. Encourage parents to convey in detail the child's communication techniques any time the child is in a new situation.

Rationale

1. Teaching aids help reinforce language and speech development and increase self-esteem.
2. Early intervention maximizes speech capabilities.
3. These techniques facilitate communication and decrease the child's frustration at not being understood. They also facilitate the goals of speech therapy.
4. Sharing the child's communication techniques helps the child adjust to new situations.

Evaluation

- Does the child participate in groups using appropriate communication?
- Does the child use various methods to communicate?

- Do the parents allow time for the child to respond to questions and conversations?
- Have the parents learned the same communication method that the child uses?

HEAD INJURY

Head injury refers to the pathologic result of any mechanical force to the scalp, skull, meninges, or brain.

Types of Head Injuries

Types of head injury include the following:
- *Closed head injury:* nonpenetrating injury to the head in which no break occurs in the integrity of the barrier between the outside environment and the intracranial cavity
- *Open head injury:* penetrating injury to the head in which there is a break in the integrity of the barrier (skull, meninges) between the outside environment and the intracranial cavity; infection is a major concern

- *Coup injury:* cerebral injury sustained directly below the site of impact
- *Contrecoup injury:* cerebral injury sustained in the region or pole opposite the site of impact; caused by the rapid movements of the semisolid brain within the cranial vault
- *Missile injury:* penetrating injury of the skull or brain, most often caused by a bullet
- *Impalement injury:* penetrating injury caused by a pierce to the scalp, skull, or brain with something sharp

Skull Fractures

Skull fractures include the following types:
- *Linear:* straight-line fracture; dura not involved

- *Depressed:* bone pressing downward, indented
- *Basilar:* fracture of the base of the skull; symptoms are Battle sign, raccoon eyes, rhinorrhea, otorrhea, and hemotympanum (blood behind the eardrum)
- *Comminuted:* fragmentation of the bone into many pieces or a multiple fracture line

Contusion

Contusions are petechial hemorrhages along the superficial aspects of the brain. They may occur at the site of impact or in association with a lesion remote from the site of direct impact.

Concussion

A concussion is a transient and reversible neuronal dysfunction, with instantaneous loss of awareness and responsiveness.

Intracranial Hemorrhage

Intracranial hemorrhages are defined as the following two types:

Epidural: blood accumulates between the dura and the skull; arterial damage is the usual type of injury, and the hemorrhage therefore develops rapidly.

Subdural: blood accumulates between the dura and the cerebrum; a subdural hemorrhage can be acute or chronic (Fig. 28-5).

Incidence

Multiple trauma is the leading cause of death in children beyond infancy. In the United States, more than 400,000 children between infancy and 14 years of age are seen in emergency departments for assessment and treatment of traumatic brain injury; falls and motor vehicle crashes are the primary cause of traumatic brain injury in this age group (National Center for Injury Prevention and Control [NCIPC], 2004). Other causes of head injuries include bicycle collisions, sports injuries, beatings, and gunshot wounds.

Manifestations

Head injuries are classified as minor, moderate, or severe as correlated with the GCS. Minor head injuries exhibit the following manifestations: possible change in level of consciousness, transient period of confusion, irritability, vomiting, somnolence, and headache. Moderate to severe head injuries are marked by altered mental states, changes in vital signs, signs of increased ICP, retinal hemorrhage, hemiparesis, and papilledema (Box 28-4).

Diagnostic Evaluation

A complete history of the event helps determine the mechanism of injury and whether the child lost consciousness. Spinal radiographs are obtained to ascertain any cervical spinal cord injury; radiographs are followed by a complete neurologic examination. Any indication of increased ICP

BOX 28-4	Classification of Severity of Head Injuries Based on Glasgow Coma Scale*

- Minimal head injury: GCS of 15 with no loss of consciousness or amnesia
- Mild head injury: GCS of 14 or 15 plus amnesia or brief (less than 5 min) loss of consciousness, or impaired alertness or memory

- Moderate head injury: GCS of 9-13 or a loss of consciousness of 5 min or more, or focal neurological deficit
- Severe head injury: GCS of 5-8
- Critical head injury: GCS of 3-4

*Stein, S., & Spettell, C. The Head Injury Severity Scale (HISS): a practical classification of closed head injury. *Brain Injury, 9*(5), 437-444.

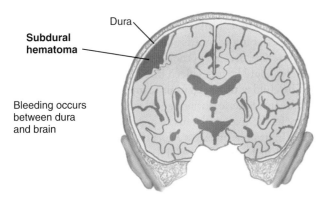

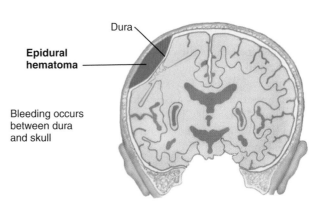

FIG 28-5   Subdural and epidural hematomas are the two most common cranial hematomas; one or the other occurs in 6% to 7% of head-injured children. A *subdural hematoma* is often caused when the head strikes an immovable object. However, in an infant a subdural hematoma may result from aggressive shaking (a form of child abuse); retinal hemorrhage is also a classic sign of shaking injury in infants. With *epidural hematoma,* a rapid decline in neurologic function may occur 4 to 8 hr after a brief period of lucidity. If untreated, the increased ICP can cause death in a short time.

PATHOPHYSIOLOGY

HEAD INJURY

The cranium is a rigid structure that contains blood, brain tissue, and CSF. The pressure exerted by these components on the cranium is between 4 and 15 mm Hg. According to the Monro-Kellie doctrine, an increase in one of these components must be accompanied by a decrease in one of the others to maintain ICP within normal range. Cerebral function depends on adequate delivery of nutrients, such as oxygen, glucose, and other substrates; an abnormal increase in ICP interferes with the balance and delivery of these nutrients.

Head injuries are either primary or secondary. *Primary head injuries* are those in which damage is sustained at the time of injury; *secondary head injuries* refer to the

consequences of the primary injury, particularly increased ICP. The severity of the injury depends on the amount of stress to the cranium and brain. Head injuries include concussions, contusions, lacerations, fractures, and hematomas.

Motor vehicle collisions, falls, sports injuries, and child abuse and neglect cause most head injuries in children. *Acceleration-deceleration* is the term used to describe the mechanism of injury. The shearing force of the initial impact moves the brain forward, followed by a countering, backward movement of the brain in the skull. The shearing force produces bruising, tearing, and bleeding. "Shaken baby syndrome," a type of child abuse, may result in epidural hematomas and retinal hemorrhages (see Chapter 29).

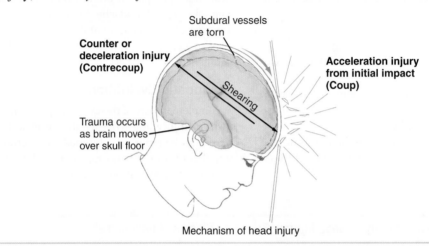

Mechanism of head injury

---

is quickly reported to the physician. CT or MRI is the most precise study with which to diagnose the specific kind of head injury sustained. A scalp hematoma in an infant suggests underlying skull fracture; skull radiography is recommended for these children (Dias, 2004).

Therapeutic Management

Initial management of the child with a head injury includes assessing ventilatory function, neurologic status, and any other injuries present (see Chapter 10). Interventions to maintain vital functions are provided until all injuries are determined. Increased ICP or seizures may develop in a child with a head injury. The long-term outcome of a head injury is related to the child's GCS score.

Nursing Considerations

Initial assessment of the child with a head injury includes the ABCs: evaluation of **a**irway, **b**reathing, and **c**irculation (see Chapter 10). The child's neck is immobilized because special attention is given to the cervical spine. Obtain and record baseline vital signs as well as further signs as indicated by the child's clinical condition. A complete history and comprehensive neurologic examination should be performed. Assess

the child's level of consciousness (with the GCS), pupil size, and pupil reactivity to light.

Test cranial nerve function to identify deficits resulting from the injury and monitor for increased ICP. The clinical signs and symptoms of increased ICP, with or without actual measurement of the ICP, determine both the child's clinical status and the medical and nursing interventions. Nasotracheal suctioning is contraindicated in a child with a basilar skull fracture; because of the nature of the injury, the suction catheter could be introduced into the brain.

The child with a head injury can have a postinjury alteration in antidiuretic hormone (ADH). Possibly as a result of injury to the hypothalamus or posterior pituitary, the child can exhibit signs of excess ADH (syndrome of inappropriate antidiuretic hormone [SIADH]) or deficit of ADH (diabetes insipidus) (see Chapter 27). Any child with a head injury needs to be assessed for fluid and electrolyte alteration.

Nursing care of the child with a head injury is similar to nursing care of any child with increased ICP, with the additional attention to fluid and electrolyte balance. The nurse carefully monitors any intravenous (IV) and oral fluid intake and determines and records hourly fluid output. If the child develops SIADH, fluids may be restricted to reduce the risk

---

BOX 28-5 | **PARENTS WANT TO KNOW** About Guidelines for the Child With a Head Injury

Apply ice to the child's head to prevent swelling. Clean any scrapes or cuts with soap and water. Encourage the child to rest and limit foods if the child is vomiting. You will need to watch the child carefully for 2 days. For 2 nights, awaken the child once at your bedtime and once 4 hours later. Check that the child becomes alert and can answer questions appropriately.

Call the physician immediately after the injury if the child demonstrates the following:
- Has bleeding that does not stop after pressure has been applied for 10 min
- Needs sutures
- Is younger than 1 year
- Had a seizure after the head injury
- Was unconscious or confused

- Has a severe headache or vomiting
- Has slurred speech or blurred vision
- Has blood or watery fluid coming from the ear or nose
- Has unequal pupils or crossed eyes
- Has difficulty walking or crawling or weakness in the arms
- Has other symptoms that concern you

Postconcussion Syndrome
Some children who have had a head injury can have an aftereffect called *postconcussion syndrome*. If your child has this condition, your child may be upset easily and may be irritable if tired or stressed. Memory problems are common, as are learning difficulties, double vision, dizziness, headaches, fatigue, and light sensitivity. These symptoms may last many months.

Data from Schmitt, B. D. (1999). *Instructions for pediatric patients* (2nd ed., p. 138). Philadelphia: Saunders.

---

of increasing ICP from cerebral edema. Fluid restriction is a nursing challenge because it involves the cooperation of parents and others involved in the child's care. Place a sign at the child's bedside to alert others of the restriction. Be sure to choose fluids the child likes and distribute the allocated amounts over the course of the child's waking hours.

If the child is discharged from the emergency department, written instructions should be given to parents (Box 28-5).

SPINAL CORD INJURY

Spinal cord injury can result from any trauma or injury to the spinal cord or its vascular supply or venous drainage.

Etiology

Spinal cord injuries in children are usually caused by motor vehicle crashes, falls, diving accidents, sports injuries, gunshot or knife wounds, or attempted suicide. In the infant, a common cause of spinal cord injury is intentional, aggressive shaking by an older person.

PATHOPHYSIOLOGY

SPINAL CORD INJURY

Spinal cord injuries occur in children when vertebral bodies are fractured or subluxation of the vertebra occurs. Subluxation results in malalignment of contiguous vertebrae so that the spinal cord is compressed. The cord may be crushed, stretched beyond tolerance, or completely divided. All neurons carrying sensations from those parts of the body below the lesion are unable to pass their message on to the brain. A severe cord injury will cause complete paralysis and complete loss of sensation below the severed level.

Flaccid paralysis of the affected limbs immediately follows a spinal cord injury. Paralysis is caused by spinal shock, which can last 3 weeks or more. The flaccidity changes to spasticity when the spinal shock resolves.

Incidence

Although spinal cord injuries are less common in children than in adults, 75% of spinal cord injuries in children occur in the cervical spine, between the occiput and C3. Young children are more susceptible to upper spinal cord injury because of the larger head size in relation to body size. As the child grows older, the site of the spinal cord injury moves distally.

Manifestations

Manifestations of spinal cord injury include loss of some or all movement or sensation below the level of injury, respiratory depression or apnea, hypotension and bradycardia, hypothermia, and neck pain.

Diagnostic Evaluation

After the nurse takes the history of the injury and performs a complete neurologic examination, the extent of the spinal cord injury is determined by radiography or MRI. The extent of the motor or sensory deficit may resolve somewhat as spinal shock resolves.

Therapeutic Management

Treatment includes steroid therapy, which may be administered within 8 hr of the injury as a bolus of 30 mg/kg followed by a continuous infusion of 5.4 mg/kg per hour for 23 hours. Until permanent surgical stabilization can be performed, other treatments such as halo traction (Fig. 28-6) and Gardner-Wells tongs, may be used as a temporary stabilization method.

NURSING CARE

The Child With a Spinal Cord Injury

Assessment

The spine must be immobilized before any attempt is made to move the child. The airway is assessed immediately, and

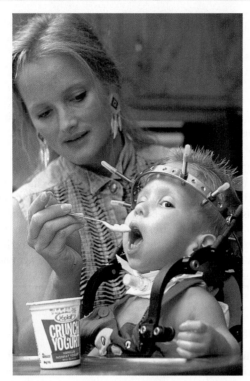

FIG 28-6 **Children who have injuries or birth defects that involve the upper spine may be placed in halo traction to stabilize the spine and prevent added nerve damage. Spinal cord injury is a catastrophic event for the child and family, who will need intense nursing support and education as well as referral to support groups.** *(Courtesy Cook Children's Medical Center, Fort Worth, TX.)*

if intubation is necessary it is done without hyperextending the neck (see Chapter 10). Next assess circulation, keeping in mind that hypotension may be a result of either hypovolemia or neurologic shock. Bradycardia and hypothermia may ensue. Attempt to maintain the body temperature and keep the child well oxygenated.

The neurologic assessment includes evaluating mobility, sensation, and reflexes. The injury may be complete or incomplete. In a complete spinal cord injury, the cord is completely severed and no spinal innervation is present below the injury. With an incomplete spinal cord injury, the cord has some function remaining. The neurologic assessment is ongoing and carefully documented so that changes can be dealt with in a timely fashion. The child is then assessed for trauma to other systems.

Nursing Diagnoses and Planning

The following nursing diagnoses and expected outcomes may be appropriate after assessment of the child with spinal cord injury:

- Ineffective Breathing Pattern related to weakness or paralysis of respiratory muscles after spinal cord injury.

  Expected Outcome: The child will not have respiratory distress, as evidenced by ABG values within normal limits, stable vital signs, and motor and sensory function.

- Risk for Impaired Skin Integrity related to immobility.

Expected Outcome: The child will maintain skin integrity, as evidenced by intact skin and absence of breakdown.

- Anxiety related to having a child with an acute condition.

  Expected Outcome: The child and parents will have decreased anxiety, as evidenced by an ability to verbalize what the spinal cord injury means to them.

- Interrupted Family Processes related to having a child with an acute and chronic injury.

  Expected Outcome: The parents will show signs of adapting to their child's injury, as evidenced by participating in the child's care and seeking appropriate support within the community.

- Impaired Physical Mobility related to neuromuscular impairment.

  Expected Outcome: The child will maximize potential for improvement of mobility, as evidenced by involvement in physical therapy and occupational therapy.

Interventions

The goal of nursing care is to minimize the potential for further injury, prevent the sequelae of immobility, and promote maximal spinal cord recovery. The spinal cord is immobilized with the use of tongs or halo traction. The child remains in traction for several weeks (see Chapter 26). The nurse is responsible for maintaining proper alignment by monitoring the status of the traction every 1 to 2 hr. Towels and rolls can be useful to help position the child. The nurse should perform a motor and sensory assessment after each change of position (see Chapter 9).

If the child's situation becomes unstable, surgical stabilization may become necessary. Progressive neurologic deterioration is the major indicator for surgery.

The child who is immobilized and neurologically impaired is at risk for respiratory complications as a result of muscle weakness and immobility. Respiratory status and pulse oximetry readings are assessed and recorded every 1 to 2 hr. Supplemental oxygen may be indicated. Nebulizer, incentive spirometry, and intermittent positive-pressure breathing (IPPB) may be ordered. Some children may need a tracheostomy and mechanical ventilation if the respiratory muscles are involved or if weaning from the ventilator is slow and difficult to accomplish.

The nurse assesses perfusion by monitoring vital signs, color, skin temperature, and intake and output. Because of bladder muscle weakness or paralysis, an indwelling urinary catheter facilitates bladder emptying and accurate measurement of intake and output, which is monitored hourly. If alterations in perfusion occur, the child receives crystalloids by bolus infusion. Vasopressors, such as dopamine and dobutamine, may also be used.

The child with a spinal cord injury may have a problem with body temperature control and so should be warmed or cooled as appropriate. If the child has an elevated temperature, samples of wound material and blood are obtained for culture. Sputum cultures may be necessary. Antipyretic and broad-spectrum antibiotic therapy is initiated after the specimens are sent to the laboratory.

The child may have a nasogastric tube in place. The nurse will maintain tube patency and monitor and record drainage. The pH of the gastric fluid may be tested and the child treated with antacids, sucralfate (Carafate), or histamine blockers. The child is at risk for stress ulcers and gastrointestinal hemorrhage. A bowel regimen is initiated and maintained to prevent impaction. Bowel training includes ingestion of a high-fiber diet (when the child is able to eat), the use of stool softeners, and increased water intake. While the indwelling catheter is in place, care is taken to prevent infection. Intermittent catheterization may eventually be initiated if necessary.

Inspect the child's skin frequently and administer skin care each time the child is repositioned. Pressure on the bony prominences is minimized with the use of special mattresses and padding.

Adequate nutrition is essential to the healing process. Caloric intake is monitored, and the child may receive nutrition by oral intake, tube feeding, or total parenteral nutrition. A good indicator of a favorable response to the nutrition is timely healing of wounds.

Spinal cord injury is a catastrophic event. The lives of the child and family have been suddenly and permanently altered. They will need intense assistance and support. These goals can be achieved through therapeutic play, promotion of independent functioning, referral to a multidisciplinary rehabilitation team, referral to support groups, and thorough discharge planning and home care teaching.

Evaluation

- Are body functions (respiration, elimination, muscle strength) maintained as normally as possible?
- Is the child's skin intact and free from breakdown?
- Do the child and parents verbalize feelings and emotions about the injury and the prognosis?
- Do the parents demonstrate ability to provide physical and emotional support for the child?
- Has the child's neurologic function improved?

SEIZURE DISORDERS

A seizure consists of brief paroxysmal behavior caused by excessive abnormal discharge of neurons. Epilepsy is marked by recurrent seizure activity that does not occur in association with an acute illness. The two types of seizures are partial (focal) and generalized. Partial seizures occur in one part of the brain and may or may not alter consciousness. Generalized seizures occur over the entire brain and do alter consciousness.

Etiology

Seizures are symptomatic of altered neuronal activity in the CNS. Seizures can occur for many reasons and are categorized as *primary* or *secondary*. Primary seizures occur in the absence of any underlying brain structural abnormality. Primary seizures are linked to genetic predisposition and include febrile seizures, absence seizures, and benign seizures of the newborn.

Secondary, or symptomatic, seizures are usually provoked by some temporary or permanent structural or metabolic abnormality. Cerebral lesions, malformations, metabolic disorders, acquired causes (e.g., anoxia, trauma, stroke), infections, degenerative disorders, and toxic disturbances are linked to secondary seizures. Approximately 50% of childhood seizures are idiopathic, meaning they have no known cause.

Incidence

Approximately 10% of all children younger than 18 years will have a seizure (Johnston, 2004b). An estimated 2% to 4% of children aged 6 months to 3 years will have a febrile seizure (Johnston, 2004b; Waruiru & Appleton, 2004). The majority of children with epilepsy experience the onset of seizures before 18 years of age. Because of the subtlety of neonatal seizures the incidence is difficult to determine; however, neonatal seizures occur primarily in preterm infants and mainly during the first week of life (Granelli & McGrath, 2004).

Pathophysiology

During a seizure excessive, self-limiting neuronal discharges occur. The result of these discharges is activation of associated motor or sensory organs. The extent of the seizure depends on the location and extent of the abnormal neuronal discharges. The brain consists of millions of nerve cells; electrical impulses are sent through many of these cells by neurotransmitters. When numerous nerve cells fire abnormally at the same time, a seizure may result.

Manifestations

Many types of seizures exist. The International Classification of Seizures is used to divide seizures into two major groups: generalized and partial. In addition, some other types of seizures are seen in children (unclassified seizures) (Box 28-6).

Febrile seizures are generally seen in young children. Although the risk of having a nonfebrile seizure is low in children who have had a febrile seizure (2% to 4%), febrile seizures are considered a risk factor for epilepsy (Waruiru & Appleton, 2004). The height and rapidity of temperature elevation seem to be factors in precipitating febrile seizures. The temperature is usually elevated above 38.8° C (102° F). The seizure activity occurs during the temperature rise rather than after prolonged elevation. Simple febrile seizures are familial and probably transmitted by autosomal dominant inheritance (Fenichel, 2005). Most febrile seizures occur as a result of fever caused by otitis media, pharyngitis, and adenitis. The family of a child who has a febrile seizure should be given information about these seizures and instructed what to do if another seizure occurs.

Neonatal seizures are usually caused by an underlying pathologic process. The most frequent cause of neonatal seizures is perinatal asphyxia leading to hypoxic-ischemic encephalopathy. The second major contributing factor is intracranial hemorrhage. Other causes include metabolic disturbances, intrauterine and perinatal infectious disorders,

BOX 28-6	**International Classification of Seizures**

Generalized Seizures

Onset starts at any age. Clinical features indicate involvement of both cerebral hemispheres. Consciousness is impaired.

Tonic, Clonic, and Tonic-Clonic Seizures

Formerly called *grand mal seizures,* tonic-clonic seizures cause an abrupt arrest of activity and impairment of consciousness. The *tonic phase* consists of a sustained, generalized stiffening of muscles, including the diaphragm, lasting a few seconds. The *clonic phase* is symmetric and rhythmic, consisting of alternating contraction and relaxation of major muscle groups. This phase usually ends spontaneously in less than 5 min. Respirations are irregular and the child may have stridor. Sphincter incontinence may or may not occur. The tonic-clonic seizure is followed by a variable period of confusion, lethargy, and sleep (postictal phase).

Atonic Seizures

Atonic seizures cause an abrupt loss of postural tone, impairment of consciousness, confusion, lethargy, and sleep.

Myoclonic Seizures

Myoclonic seizures are brief, random contractions of a muscle group, followed by loss of muscle tone and forward falling. They can occur on both sides of the body and may occur singly or in clusters. Impairment of consciousness may occur during myoclonic seizures. Onset can occur as early as age 2 months, but myoclonic seizures are more frequently seen in school-age children or adolescents than in very young children. Myoclonic seizures that occur during infancy are called *infantile spasms;* those that occur during adolescence are called *juvenile myoclonic epilepsy.*

Absence Seizures

Formerly called *petit mal seizures,* absence seizures are very brief episodes of altered consciousness. No muscle activity occurs except for eyelid fluttering, twitching, or head bobbing. The child has a blank facial expression. Absence seizures last only 5 to 10 sec, but they may occur repeatedly several times per day. The onset of absence seizures usually does not occur before age 5 years. Children usually outgrow absence seizures during adolescence.

Partial Seizures

Onset starts at any age. The clinical features suggest that only a limited functional area in one hemisphere of the brain is involved, and therefore symptoms are seen on only one side of the body. Partial seizures begin focally but may become generalized when the electrical impulses are passed across the corpus callosum to the other hemisphere. Partial seizures are further divided into those with or without change in level of consciousness.

Simple Partial Seizures

Simple partial seizures consist of motor, autonomic, or sensory symptoms. Level of consciousness does not change with simple partial seizures. Symptoms may include an odd taste in the mouth or odd smell, abdominal discomfort, unexplained feelings of fear or dread, or motor movements. This type of seizure may last 20 seconds to several minutes.

Complex Partial Seizures

Complex partial seizures may begin with or without an aura and with or without a simple partial seizure. Symptoms include impaired consciousness; transient staring; altered mental status; and feelings of fear, unreality, detachment, and disrupted memory. Distortions of perception or hallucinations, teeth grinding, lip smacking, chewing, swallowing, scratching, or pulling at shirt buttons may occur. Tonic-clonic movements of one side of the body may also be seen. The average duration of a complex partial seizure is 1 to 2 min. A complex partial seizure is followed by a variable period of confusion, lethargy, and sleep.

Unclassified Seizures

Seizures that do not fit into any of the previously described categories.

Modified from Johnston, M. (2004b). Seizures in childhood. In R. Behrman, R. Kliegman, & H. Jenson (Eds.). *Nelson textbook of pediatrics* (17th ed., pp. 1993-2009). Philadelphia: Saunders.

cerebral infarcts, drug withdrawal, hyperthermia, hypoglycemia, sodium and potassium imbalances, congenital anomalies of the CNS, and inherited syndromes (Graneli & McGrath, 2004).

The mechanism of neonatal seizures is not clearly understood. Possible explanations include an excess of excitatory neurotransmitter compared with inhibitory neurotransmitter, altered permeability of the neuronal membrane inhibiting sodium movement, and an imbalance between depolarization and repolarization of the neurons. Because of the overall anatomic and physiologic immaturity of the nervous system in the neonate, well-organized generalized seizures are rare.

Because of the lack of myelinization of fiber tracts, neonates do not have the same type of tonic-clonic seizure that an older child has. Seizures in neonates may produce subtle signs such as sustained eye opening, tonic horizontal deviation of the eyes, blinking or eyelid fluttering, sucking, smacking, drooling, tongue thrusting, pedaling movements of the legs, swimming movements of the arms, and apnea. These manifestations are more common in preterm infants and infants with hypoxic-ischemic encephalopathy. Neonatal seizures also can be focal, tonic, or myoclonic, with jerking movements of the extremities.

Diagnostic Evaluation

The child's health history and family history are important parts of the initial workup. A thorough description of the child's behavior before, during, and after the seizure activity is important to delineate the type of seizure. Video recording and EEG monitoring help identify the seizure. Serum electrolyte determinations, CBC, blood glucose determination, lumbar puncture, and other laboratory tests can help uncover metabolic causes. CT and MRI will indicate trauma, tumor, or congenital malformation. In neonates, several other laboratory tests may be included—such as *t*oxoplasmosis, *o*ther agents, *r*ubella, *c*ytomegalovirus, and *h*erpes simplex virus (TORCH) titers—to exclude congenital viral infections as well as amino acid and organic acid studies to exclude inborn errors of metabolism.

Therapeutic Management

The basic tenet of treatment for the child with seizures is to treat the whole child. The goals are to identify and correct the cause of the seizure, eliminate the seizure with a minimum of side effects and the least amount of medication, and normalize the child's and family's lives (Table 28-3).

Stimulating the vagal nerve via a device implanted in the chest wall has been found, in some cases, to reduce seizure occurrence through a currently unknown mechanism (Lee & Adelson, 2004). It has few side effects and can decrease the need for pharmacologic intervention.

Text continued on p. 952

TABLE 28-3   Common Seizure Medications

Drug Name	Seizure Type	Side Effects	Nursing Implications
Carbamazepine (Tegretol)	Partial or generalized	Sedation, cognitive deficits, behavior outbursts	Watch for change in behavior or decrease in school grades. Child should not be given erythromycin, which will cause an increase in drug level.
Felbamate (Felbatol)	Partial	Nausea and vomiting, weight loss, anorexia, agitation and aggression, aplastic anemia, liver failure	Shake oral suspension well.
Ethosuximide (Zarontin)	Generalized	Nausea and vomiting, lethargy	Observe for excessive drowsiness; take with food.
Lamotrigine (Lamictal)	Generalized or partial	Rash (increased risk of rash exists in children with previous reaction to any drug or to another antiepileptic drug), dizziness, headache, double vision, nausea and vomiting, ataxia	Not affected by food absorption.
Gabapentin (Neurontin)	Partial	Drowsiness, dizziness, nystagmus, nausea and vomiting, ataxia	Dosage must be adjusted for renal function.
Levetiracetam (Keppra)	Partial	Sleepiness, weakness, headache, infection	Monitor for side effects and frequency of seizures and renal dysfunction.
Phenobarbital	Generalized or partial	Sedation, cognitive deficits, behavior outbursts	Watch for excessive drowsiness, changes in school grades, and respiratory depression.
Phenytoin (Dilantin)	Partial, generalized, or status	Lethargy, nystagmus, ataxia, allergic reactions, hypertrophic gums, hirsutism	Teach meticulous oral care to decrease gum hypertrophy. IV form must be given in normal saline and filtered.
Topiramate (Topamax)	Partial	Fatigue, nervousness, decreased attention, anorexia, renal stones, tremor	Affects levels of other epilepsy medications. Keep children well-hydrated to decrease chances of renal stones.
Tiagabine (Gabitril)	Partial	Lethargy, sedation, double vision, ataxia	Monitor for generalized weakness.
Valproic acid (Depakene)	Generalized	Nausea and vomiting, tremor, weight gain, hair loss, thrombocytopenia, liver failure	Do not crush or cut pills/sprinkles; can cause stomach ulcers. Take with food.
Oxcarbazepine (Trileptal)	Partial	Fatigue, headache, dizziness, double vision, unsteadiness, nausea and vomiting	Interacts with other seizure medications. Levels of other medications should be monitored.

NURSING CARE PLAN

The Child With a Seizure Disorder in the Community Setting

Focused Assessment

A detailed history that includes the prenatal, perinatal, and neonatal periods is important in determining factors precipitating seizure activity. Pathologic precipitating factors include hypoxia, cerebral trauma, high fever, lead poisoning, metabolic disorders, brain tumors, birth trauma, and CNS infections. Nonpathologic factors include overhydration, oversedation, drug abuse, sleep deprivation, antihistamine drug use, alcohol intoxication, and family history.

Seizures often are not witnessed by the health care professional. Ask the parents about the child's age at onset of the seizure activity, time of onset, and precipitating events. Ask the parents to describe the seizures, including the child's behavior before, during, and after the seizure; how the seizure progresses; and how long it lasts.

The child is given a comprehensive physical examination with special emphasis on the neurologic system. Parameters include assessment of behavior, motor skills, and developmental level. The child's and family's emotional response to the seizure disorder is assessed at this time.

The school nurse may be called to a classroom to manage a child who is having a seizure. If the child is known to have had seizures in the past, the school nurse should have appropriate information in the child's record and communicate that information, if necessary, to the child's teacher. Accurate observation in the school setting can assist with seizure management.

NURSING DIAGNOSIS   Risk for Injury related to seizure activity.

EXPECTED OUTCOMES   The child will:
- Remain free from injury through the use of appropriate injury prevention strategies.

The parents and older child will:
- Discuss seizure prevention and demonstrate first aid for seizures.

Intervention	*Rationale*
1. If the child is hospitalized, institute seizure precautions: padded side rails, bed in low position, suction and airway at bedside. At home, place the child on a soft surface if not in bed. Remove sharp objects and keep furniture out of the way.	1. These actions make the environment safer for the child during the seizure.
2. Do not put anything into the child's mouth during a seizure.	2. Forcing something into the child's mouth may injure the child's mouth, gums, or teeth.
3. During a seizure, advise the parent or teacher to place the child on the side in a lateral position. Do not restrain the child. Loosen clothing around the child's neck.	3. Positioning the child on the side prevents aspiration because saliva will drain out the corner of the child's mouth. Restraints could cause injury to the child. The nurse or family may gently guide or protect the child's movements and may suction the child's mouth after the seizure is over if suction is available.
4. Record and advise the parent to record the time of seizures, precipitating factors, types of behavior observed during the seizure, bladder or bowel incontinence, and frequency of seizures.	4. These observations help pinpoint the focus of the seizure and help the physician treat the seizure correctly.
5. Stay with the child.	5. Staying with the child reduces the risk of injury and allows observation and documentation of the seizure.
6. If the seizure lasts longer than 5 min, notify a physician.	6. Medication may need to be administered to stop prolonged seizures. The main side effect of diazepam (Valium) and lorazepam (Ativan) is respiratory depression.

Evaluation

- Does the child remain injury free?
- Do the child and family implement injury-prevention strategies?

- Do the parents monitor the seizure and record vital information?
- Can the parents demonstrate first aid for seizures?

NURSING CARE PLAN—cont'd

NURSING DIAGNOSIS   Deficient Knowledge related to the need for information about how to manage a child with a seizure disorder.

EXPECTED OUTCOME   The child and parents will:
- Seek information about the child's management and describe how to meet the child's physical, emotional, and educational needs.

Intervention	*Rationale*
1. Determine the child's and parent's educational needs.	1. Determining educational needs provides baseline information to develop a teaching plan.
2. Provide an individual teaching plan for the child and parents for handling seizures.	2. An individualized teaching plan ensures that what is needed by the child and parents will be taught.
3. Explore actual and potential problems that may arise and interfere with treatment.	3. Exploring possible problems facilitates adjustment and normalizes life; it also provides anticipatory guidance.
4. Measure outcomes of education to ensure that learning has taken place and is facilitating acceptance.	4. Evaluation of teaching is an ongoing process to ensure continued learning.
5. Refer to an epilepsy support group. (See Evolve website for a list of resource organizations.)	5. Social support is helpful for some families and may promote adjustment to lifestyle changes.
6. Educate the child and parents about the medication regimen (see Box 28-7). Emphasize the importance of adhering to medical treatment.	6. The goal of pharmacologic management is to raise the seizure threshold, thus preventing seizures.
7. Identify the side effects of the medication and when medical attention should be sought.	7. Knowledge of what is expected and normal will facilitate proper use and adherence with medication.
8. Identify the hazards of nonadherence with medications. Encourage the parents and child not to discontinue medications even if the child is seizure free.	8. Nonadherence will affect the serum levels of anticonvulsants and may cause a seizure to occur.
9. Emphasize to the child and parents the importance of regular medical evaluation and follow-up, including measurement of blood levels of the medication and evaluating for toxicity or side effects.	9. Regular medical follow-up facilitates maintenance of appropriate therapeutic blood levels of anticonvulsants and identification of side effects of medication.
10. Inform the parent about the need for a medical alert bracelet for the child.	10. Medical alert bracelets alert others to the child's condition in an emergency. If the child has a seizure in a public place, the bracelet will inform passersby of what to do for the child.
11. Encourage the family to find alternative activities besides contact sports for the child. The child should avoid swimming or climbing alone. Identify the child's strengths—not what the child *cannot* do.	11. Appropriate activities reduce the risk of injury while promoting a positive self-image.
12. Encourage verbalization of fears and concerns about having seizures.	12. This therapeutic communication may identify issues that need to be addressed.
13. Teach the child and parent to educate other family members, friends, and teachers about seizures. Advise the family to provide necessary information to the school nurse.	13. Accurate information reduces the stigma associated with epilepsy.

Evaluation

- Does the child discuss having seizures, fears and concerns about seizures, and life with the condition?
- Does the child participate in the medical regimen by discussing medication side effects and dosage?

- Does the child demonstrate a positive self-image?
- Does the family administer anticonvulsants safely and appropriately and know when to call the physician?

| BOX 28-7 | PARENTS WANT TO KNOW   About Guidelines for the Child or Adolescent Taking Seizure Medication |

- Oral care is very important for children taking phenytoin (Dilantin) because phenytoin can cause gum problems. Your child should brush with a soft brush and floss after every meal. Take your child to the dentist every 3 to 6 months for a checkup and teeth cleaning.
- Once your child has started taking the medication, blood levels should be monitored to determine that the medication has reached and maintained a therapeutic level and to monitor for a toxic level. In addition, other blood tests may be needed to ensure the medication is not harming the liver or blood cells. Blood levels should be measured periodically as your physician recommends, if a seizure occurs, or if side effects are noticed.
- If your child is taking valproic acid, be alert for any signs of unusual bleeding or bruising. Valproic acid can affect the platelets (cells that help the blood clot) and cause the platelet counts to drop.

- Be sure your child does not suddenly stop taking antiepileptic medications without discussing it with a physician or nurse. Suddenly stopping medications can cause the child to have a seizure or status epilepticus.
- Some states require a driver to be seizure free for 6 to 12 months to obtain a driver's license. If your child is of driving age, discuss this with your health care provider.
- Birth control pills may be less effective while taking antiepileptic medications. If sexually active, your adolescent should consult a nurse or physician for additional forms of birth control.
- Cognitive and behavior changes may be seen with some of the antiepileptic medications. Attention spans, memory, and interpersonal interactions may become impaired.
- Alcohol, marijuana, and street drugs will lower the seizure threshold. These drugs should be avoided.

CRITICAL TO REMEMBER
Observations and Nursing Care During a Seizure

- As the seizure begins, look at your watch or a clock. You should be able to describe how long seizure activity lasts.
- Protect the child from injury by loosening clothing at the neck and turning the child gently onto the side. Do not restrain the child or insert any object into the child's mouth.
- Carefully observe where the seizure begins, its progression, and how it ends.
- Be able to describe any preceding or accompanying sensory or motor manifestations.
- When the seizure is over, allow the child to rest if she or he desires. Record the child's behavior before, during, and after the seizure and the approximate duration of the seizure.
- In neonates, if the movement can be initiated by a stimulus, such as touch, it is probably a tremor. If the movement cannot be stopped or controlled with gentle restraint or passive flexion, it is probably a seizure.

STATUS EPILEPTICUS

Status epilepticus is a pediatric emergency. It is marked by prolonged seizure activity, in the form of either a single seizure lasting 30 min or more or recurrent seizures lasting more than 30 min with no return to a normal level of consciousness between seizures. Any seizure lasting 10 min or more can suggest pending status and should be treated as such. The most common form of status epilepticus is generalized status, which has the highest potential for complications and possible death.

Etiology

The causes of status epilepticus are many. Acute CNS injury from head trauma, meningitis, or electrolyte imbalance frequently precipitates status epilepticus. The condition can also be caused by toxins and specific medications. Other causes are chronic CNS injury and sudden withdrawal from anticonvulsants.

Incidence

Status epilepticus occurs in 5% to 10% of children with epilepsy. The most common form in children younger than 3 years is febrile status epilepticus.

Pathophysiology

Status epilepticus is caused by the random discharge of large numbers of neurons firing abnormally. The discharges cause abnormal repetitive motor activity. In the CNS, the metabolic rate increases, glucose stores are depleted, and oxygen consumption increases. If cerebral metabolic demands are not met, these changes cause neuronal injury. Prolonged seizures cause lactic acidosis, an altered blood-brain barrier, and increased ICP.

Manifestations

See the International Classification of Seizures in Box 28-6.

Diagnostic Evaluation

Diagnostic laboratory tests should include blood glucose, arterial blood gases, electrolytes, anticonvulsant drug levels, a toxicology screen, and possibly lumbar puncture. Results may be similar to those of the child with increased ICP.

Therapeutic Management

Generalized tonic-clonic status epilepticus is a medical emergency. Treatment consists of maintaining optimal respiratory and hemodynamic function and identifying and treating the causes of the seizure activity. Diazepam (Valium) or lorazepam (Ativan) is given IV. If IV access cannot be obtained, medication can be given orally or rectally. Clorazepate dipotassium (Tranxene) can be given orally for cluster seizures. Fosphenytoin (Cerebyx) or phenobarbital may be given IV as a second round of drugs if diazepam or lorazepam does not stop the seizures. The intramuscular route is not used because it is unpredictable.

CRITICAL TO REMEMBER
Drug Therapy for Generalized Tonic-Clonic Status Epilepticus

Generalized tonic-clonic status epilepticus is a medical emergency. IV diazepam (Valium) or lorazepam (Ativan) is given. IV diazepam must be given directly into the vein (not the tubing, because it interacts with plastic) at a rate no greater than 1 mg/min. It should not be mixed with other drugs or solutions, and it can be diluted only with normal saline. Resuscitation equipment should be at the bedside and the child's respirations closely monitored during IV administration.

NURSING CARE
The Child With Status Epilepticus

Assessment
On arrival at the hospital, the child will exhibit seizure activity and have unstable vital signs. Along with general seizure precautions, this child requires rapid assessment and vigorous supportive therapy. Supportive measures include assessing and maintaining a patent airway and administering oxygen. IV hydration and drug therapy are initiated to arrest the seizure activity.

Nursing Diagnoses and Planning
The following nursing diagnoses and expected outcomes may apply to the child with status epilepticus:

- Impaired Gas Exchange related to decreased respirations associated with seizures.

  Expected Outcome: The child will remain free from respiratory distress, as evidenced by pulse oxygen saturation remaining at or above 95%.

- Ineffective Breathing Pattern related to loss of muscle control associated with seizures.

  Expected Outcome: The child will maintain a normal breathing pattern, as evidenced by pulse oxygen saturation remaining at or above 95% and respiratory rate within normal range.

- Ineffective Airway Clearance related to possible aspiration during seizure.

  Expected Outcome: The child's airways will be clear, as evidenced by clear breath sounds.

- Ineffective Cerebral Tissue Perfusion related to lactic acidosis with prolonged seizure activity.

  Expected Outcome: The child will reestablish tissue perfusion, as evidenced by a return to normal levels of consciousness.

Interventions and Evaluation
The child will initially require meticulous airway establishment and maintenance. Take frequent vital signs and perform neurologic checks. Once the child is stable, nursing interventions and evaluation are similar to those described for the child with epilepsy.

MENINGITIS

Meningitis is the most common infectious process affecting the CNS. It can occur as a primary disease or as a result of complications of neurosurgery, trauma, systemic infection, or sinus or ear infections. A wide variety of bacteria and viruses can be responsible for the primary infection. Earlier diagnosis and improved antibiotic therapy have reduced the mortality rate and incidence of complications from bacterial meningitis.

Etiology
The primary organisms responsible for causing bacterial meningitis vary according to age. Among children aged 2 months to 12 years, three pathogens seem to be the most prevalent; *Haemophilus influenzae* type B, *Neisseria meningitidis*, and *Streptococcus pneumoniae* cause 95% of cases of purulent meningitis in this age group. Tuberculous meningitis and *Borrelia burgdorferi* (Lyme disease) meningitis also are becoming more common in this age group. These types of meningitis usually result from extension of a localized infection, such as otitis media, sinusitis, pharyngitis, or pneumonia, into the CSF. The organisms primarily responsible for neonatal meningitis are group B streptococci and *Escherichia coli*.

Organisms also may be introduced directly after an injury in which the skin is broken and communication between skin, sinuses, and CSF occurs. Entry may occur in association with a lumbar puncture, skull fracture, or surgery.

Meningococcal meningitis caused by *Neisseria* usually occurs in older children and adolescents. Because it is transmitted primarily by droplet infection, the risk increases as the number of contacts increases.

Viral meningitis is associated with viruses such as mumps, paramyxoviruses, herpesviruses, and enteroviruses. In rare cases, protozoa or fungi are the infecting organisms. These types of meningitis are seen most frequently in children with acquired immunodeficiency syndrome (AIDS).

Incidence
Meningitis most commonly affects children between ages 1 month and 5 years, but it can occur at any age. Boys are affected more frequently than girls, and risk factors increase where individuals are in close contact with one another (e.g., day care centers, college dormitories, large families in small dwellings). Incidence is higher among African-American children than among white children. The incidence of *H. influenzae* type B infection related to meningitis has declined rapidly with the immunization of infants.

PATHOPHYSIOLOGY

MENINGITIS

Meningitis is an inflammation of the meninges of the brain that results from a pathogen entering the CNS and causing a toxic response. As the process continues, increased ICP develops along with subdural empyema. If the infection spreads to the ventricles, edema and tissue scarring around the ventricle cause obstruction of the CSF and subsequent hydrocephalus.

This process can happen quite rapidly; CSF is an excellent growth medium for bacteria because it contains nutrient substances such as protein and glucose. Leukocytes are unable to function as a defense mechanism in the fluid environment of the CSF. Leukocytes require a tissue surface to destroy bacteria, so there is little defense to stop the growth of bacteria, and they can multiply quickly.

As the infection spreads further into brain tissue, changes occur in the permeability of capillaries and blood vessels in the dura mater. These changes lead to increased passage of albumin and water into the subdural space, with a subsequent accumulation of protein and fluid. This results in an additional increase in ICP.

The most common neurologic sequelae of meningitis are hearing loss, mental retardation, seizures, visual impairment, and behavioral problems. Other complications include cranial nerve dysfunction, brain abscess, and SIADH. Meningococcemia, a fulminating manifestation of *Neisseria meningitides* infection that manifests with petechiae and purpura and signs of viral-type illness, can proceed in a matter of a few hours to adrenal insufficiency (Waterhouse-Friedrickson syndrome) and septic shock.*

*Woods, C. (2004). *Neisseria meningitides* (Meningococcus). In R. Behrman, R. Kliegman, & H. Jenson (Eds.). *Nelson textbook of pediatrics* (17th ed., pp. 896-899). Philadelphia: Saunders.

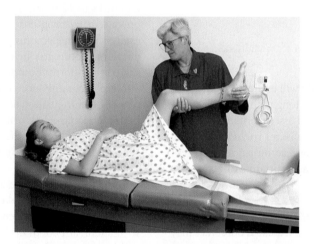

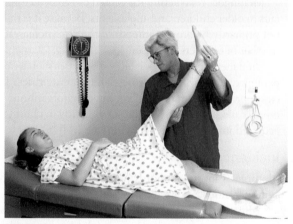

Kernig's Sign
The child can easily extend the leg when in the supine position. However, when the thigh is flexed toward the abdomen, pain prevents complete extension of the leg.

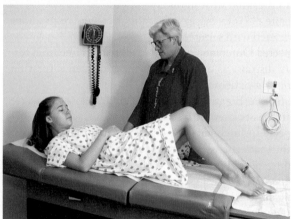

Brudzinski's Sign
In the supine position, the child bends her head toward her chest. (In a younger child, the nurse can bend the child's head.) This action usually produces involuntary hip and knee flexion in the child with meningitis.

FIG 28-7   As part of the assessment for meningitis, the nurse can attempt to elicit Kernig's sign and Brudzinski's sign. Both are early signs of meningitis in children and adolescents. *(Courtesy Parkland Health & Hospital System, Dallas, TX.)*

Manifestations

Signs and symptoms of meningitis vary according to the age of the child and the duration of the preceding illness. No single hallmark sign or symptom exists.

The clinical signs of meningitis in the neonate include poor feeding; poor sucking; vomiting; diarrhea; poor muscle tone; poor cry; hypothermia or hyperthermia; apnea; seizures; sepsis; disseminated intravascular coagulation (DIC); a full, tense, and bulging fontanel; and lethargy.

Clinical signs of meningitis in the infant and preschool age child include fever, poor feeding, vomiting, irritability, seizures, a high-pitched cry, a bulging anterior fontanel, and lethargy. In the neonate, infant, and young child, the symptoms of meningitis are frequently vague and nonspecific.

Early clinical signs of meningitis in children and adolescents include severe headache, photophobia, nuchal rigidity, fever, altered level of consciousness (lethargy, irritability), decreased appetite, vomiting, diarrhea, agitation, and drowsiness. Muscle or joint pain and purpura may be noted. Kernig's sign (pain with extension of leg and knee; Fig. 28-7) and Brudzinski's sign (flexion of head causing flexion of hips and knees; Fig. 28-7) are often exhibited. In addition, petechial or purpuric rash (meningococcal infection) may be observed.

Late clinical signs of meningitis in children and adolescents include changes in level of consciousness and seizures.

Diagnostic Evaluation

The diagnosis is made by testing CSF obtained by lumbar puncture. Findings usually include increased CSF pressure, cloudy CSF (in the case of bacterial meningitis), high protein concentration, and low glucose level. Blood cultures may be done, and nose and throat cultures are occasionally helpful if the CSF is negative.

Therapeutic Management

Acute bacterial meningitis is a medical emergency requiring early recognition and prompt, aggressive management. The child is placed in a private room on Droplet Transmission Precautions, and these are maintained for at least 24 hr after antibiotics are initiated. Prompt initiation and uninterrupted IV administration of appropriate antibiotics are essential in cases of suspected bacterial meningitis. Treatment is started before the causative organism is identified because cultures may take up to 3 days to yield results. Early use of antibiotics is vital because delay could be fatal. Antibiotic therapy is based on the age of the child, the pathogen most frequently encountered in that age group, and the initial appearance of the CSF. If IV access is difficult to achieve, the first dose of antibiotics should be administered intramuscularly.

Treatment for neonatal bacterial meningitis consists of ampicillin and an aminoglycoside or a third-generation cephalosporin. For older children and adolescents, the treatment of choice is ampicillin and penicillin G. The initial antibiotic must be a broad-spectrum drug to cover most of the suspected pathogens. When the culture and sensitivity test results are available, treatment regimens may have to be changed. The treatment for viral meningitis is symptomatic and supportive, usually with complete recovery. Current recommendations are that prospective college students receive meningococcal vaccine before college entry to prevent meningococcal meningitis.

NURSING CARE

The Child With Meningitis

Assessment

The information from the history and physical examination provides baseline data, along with a complete neurologic assessment that includes evaluating for the presence or absence of headaches, photophobia, hearing loss, seizure activity, changes in level of consciousness, changes in pupil reactions and size, nuchal rigidity, and muscle flaccidity. Personality changes and irritability may be noted. Any abnormal changes in food and fluid intake, nausea, vomiting, or loss of appetite are also important. The nurse should review the history for recent immunizations or recent illnesses, such as upper respiratory tract infections, otitis media, surgery, skull fracture, or previous lumbar puncture.

Early recognition and treatment of complications can substantially reduce morbidity and mortality rates. Thorough knowledge of the disease process is important, and assessments must be complete, frequent, and alert to any changes in the child's condition. Assessment of peak and trough antibiotic levels is important to prevent ototoxicity from aminoglycosides.

Nursing Diagnosis and Planning

Nursing diagnoses that apply to the child with meningitis include those common to other neurologic disorders. Care related to these nursing diagnoses is detailed on pp. 923-926. The following nursing diagnosis is specific to the child with meningitis and family:

- Deficient Knowledge related to seriousness of meningitis, possible residual neurologic deficits, home management, and prophylaxis.

Expected Outcome: The parent's level of understanding of meningitis will increase, as evidenced by an ability to discuss the disease process and possible sequelae, treatment, home management, and possible implications for spread of the disease.

Interventions

Discuss the disease process and prognosis with the parents after assessing their existing knowledge. Teach the family about the possible complications and sequelae of meningitis. Discuss the importance of follow-up care.

Prophylaxis for the ill child's close contacts is necessary. Ask the parents to identify others exposed to meningitis and refer them for treatment. Close contacts should not wait for signs of meningitis to develop but should seek prompt medical attention because they may be incubating the infection.

CRITICAL THINKING EXERCISE 28-1

Pediatric nurses in the community often are in a position to answer questions about childhood illnesses. Recently, parents of high school children received a notice from the school nurse that a male student had been diagnosed with meningococcal meningitis. The nurse recommended that parents should be watchful but not overly concerned. Her letter advised parents to watch their children for 2 weeks and call the physician at any sign of illness.

1. Is this course of action prudent?
2. If so, why? If not, why not?

CRITICAL TO REMEMBER
Guidelines for the Child With Meningitis

- The close contacts of the child with *Haemophilus influenzae* infection need prophylactic treatment with rifampin.
- Anyone who spent at least 4 hr with the child in the 5 to 7 days preceding the child's hospitalization with *H. influenzae* needs prophylactic treatment if not already immunized.
- All close contacts of children with *Neisseria meningitidis* need prophylactic treatment regardless of age or immunization status.
- Rifampin colors the urine and sweat red-orange and will stain contact lenses.

Instruct the parents about prescribed medications and treatments. Document instructions, and request a return demonstration by parents or caregiver. The parents will be anxious and grieving about the child's illness and outcome; learning will be difficult. To be sure the parents have learned, watch them perform the necessary procedures.

Complications of meningitis can include hydrocephalus, vision and hearing loss, delayed growth and development, seizures, subdural effusions, and cranial nerve palsy.

Evaluation

- Can the parents demonstrate the ability to administer the child's treatments and medications?
- Do the parents discuss the disease and treatments?
- Have the parents referred close contacts for treatment?

GUILLAIN-BARRÉ SYNDROME

Guillain-Barré syndrome (GBS) is characterized by rapidly progressing limb weakness and the loss of tendon reflexes. GBS is now the most common cause of acute, flaccid paralytic disease in developed countries now that poliomyelitis has been virtually eliminated. The illness may have originated as an upper respiratory infection, possibly viral in nature, such as rubella, enterovirus, Epstein-Barr virus, cytomegalovirus (CMV), mycoplasma, or varicella. The syndrome may also occur as a toxic response to immunizations. If the cause is

unknown, it may be related to an autoimmune or inflammatory response, which produces demyelinization of the motor and sometimes sensory nerves.

Incidence

GBS affects approximately 0.5 to 1.5 children in 100,000 per year worldwide (Sladky, 2004). It affects all ages, including infants. It occurs moderately more often in males.

Pathophysiology

The most prominent feature of the most frequently seen GBS type is the infiltration of lymphocytes in peripheral nerves, causing inflammation. Initially, the myelin sheath becomes edematous; as further inflammation takes place, segmental demyelinization occurs. This process takes place along the membrane surrounding the Schwann cells. As the inflammatory process continues, myelin loss increases and results in axonal degeneration.

Manifestations

- *Limb paresthesias and/or pain,* including numbness, tingling, and weakness of the lower extremities with an ascending loss of deep tendon reflexes leading to a flaccid paralysis.
- *Autonomic instability,* including blood pressure fluctuations, cardiac arrhythmias, postural hypotension, and urinary and bowel incontinence.
- *Cranial nerve dysfunction* may occur, such as facial nerve paralysis; dysphagia; and poor cough, gag, and swallow reflexes. If this occurs, respiratory function will be impaired.
- *Respiratory failure* results from the progressive motor paralysis of the intercostal and phrenic nerves. Respiratory failure may occur in 15% to 25% of patients with GBS.
- *Neuromuscular impairment* (bilateral ascending weakness or paralysis) usually progresses upward from the feet to the head and is reversed as healing takes place.

Diagnostic Evaluation

Bilateral ascending weakness or paralysis after an upper respiratory infection by 1 or 2 weeks is a diagnostic indication. The paralysis can affect the respiratory muscles quickly. The CSF may demonstrate high protein levels.

Therapeutic Management

Children with rapidly progressing paralysis are treated with high-dose IV immunoglobulin (IVIG) for several days. A recent randomized trial of IVIG suggests that no difference exists between a 2- and 5-day treatment of IVIG on the level of disability; however, IVIG (for either 2 or 5 days) may accelerate recovery (Korinthenberg, Schessl, Kirschner, & Monting, 2005). Medical management of the child with GBS is supportive, with attention given to the neurologic, respiratory, and cardiovascular systems. Special attention to respiratory support is needed because most deaths are attributed to respiratory failure. Plasmapheresis may be beneficial, as may steroids or immunosuppressive medications (Sladky, 2004).

NURSING CARE

The Child With Guillain-Barré Syndrome

Assessment

A complete history and physical examination are important to determine the presence of an antecedent viral illness and establish baseline clinical status. Special attention is given to the respiratory and neurologic systems. Respiratory assessment should take place frequently because of the risk of respiratory compromise and the need for prompt action if the child's respiratory status deteriorates. Major assessment parameters include respiratory rate, chest excursion, energy expended to breathe, and breath sounds. Pulse oximetry assesses adequate gas exchange. Daily pulmonary function testing may be necessary. The frequency of neurologic assessment depends on the child's clinical condition. Neurologic parameters include cranial nerve function, motor capabilities, sensory perception, and deep tendon reflexes.

Nursing Diagnosis and Planning

The following nursing diagnoses and expected outcomes may be appropriate after assessment of the child with GBS:

- Ineffective Breathing Pattern related to neuromuscular impairment.
  Expected Outcome: The child will remain free from respiratory distress, as evidenced by clear bilateral breath sounds, good chest expansion, and normal tidal volume.
- Decreased Cardiac Output related to autonomic instability.
  Expected Outcome: The child will maintain cardiac output, as evidenced by brisk capillary refill, normal urine output, good pulses in all extremities, and no arrhythmias.
- Risk for Impaired Skin Integrity related to immobility with paralysis.
  Expected Outcome: The child will maintain skin integrity, as evidenced by absence of skin breakdown or pressure sores.
- Impaired Verbal Communication related to neuromuscular impairment.
  Expected Outcome: The child will maintain ability to communicate, as evidenced by demonstration of new ways to communicate with available muscles, such as eye blinks or eye movements.
- Impaired Urinary Elimination related to paralysis.
  Expected Outcome: The child will have urinary elimination needs met, as evidenced by an empty bladder, no urinary tract infection or distention of the abdomen, and urine output within normal limits for age (see Chapter 20).
- Anxiety related to increasing ascending paralysis.
  Expected Outcome: The child will display decreased anxiety, as evidenced by an ability to interact calmly with caregivers and have decreased fretful periods and increased restful periods.
- Deficient Knowledge related to anxiety about disease progression and home care.

Expected Outcome: The child and parents will have increased knowledge of the disease and treatment, as evidenced by an ability to make plans about discharge care and discuss the illness and possible complications.

- Interrupted Family Processes related to having a child with a prolonged illness.
  Expected Outcome: The parents will use coping strategies to adjust to their child's illness, as evidenced by discussing support systems and changes in the family.

Interventions

The goals of nursing care for the child with GBS are to achieve optimal neurologic function with an emphasis on maintaining independence in activities of daily living and to facilitate a recovery without complication.

Treatment is largely supportive, with a focus on assessing and monitoring the child's clinical status and preventing or minimizing complications. The nurse must be able to recognize changes in the child's condition and intervene in a timely and effective manner.

Initially, the nurse must provide respiratory support if the respiratory system becomes compromised and muscles weaken and become flaccid. Resuscitation and ventilatory support may be needed; the appropriate emergency equipment and personnel should be at hand. Anticipate deterioration in respiratory status. Emergency equipment, such as a bag-valve-mask device, oxygen, suction, endotracheal tubes, laryngoscope, blade, and stylet, should be at the bedside.

Interruption in the autonomic nervous system reflexes can cause circulatory changes, resulting in arrhythmias, hypotension, dizziness, and night sweats. Early detection of neurologic changes is made by serial assessments, and prompt action should be taken to correct problems and prevent complications.

The child with GBS is at an increased risk for developing complications associated with immobility. Maintaining skin integrity is a priority. Frequent turning and repositioning, attention to pressure points, and use of special mattresses are all important steps to take to prevent skin breakdown. Managing incontinence also will help prevent skin breakdown. To prevent contractures, physical and occupational therapy must be initiated as part of the child's daily routine. Range of motion, self-help exercises, correct alignment, and application of splints and braces are part of the child's daily care.

Anticipate loss of motor function and initiate preventive nursing measures such as passive range of motion, turning, and repositioning at least every 2 hr. Chest physiotherapy should be done every 2 to 4 hr.

The risk of pulmonary embolus as a result of deep vein thrombosis is always a threat. Frequent turning and repositioning, with special attention to positioning the child's legs to alleviate pressure on the dorsal aspect of the knees, are essential. Anticoagulant therapy may be initiated; if so, the nurse should monitor clotting times and watch for any signs of bleeding.

As cranial nerve function is altered and interference with gag and swallow occurs, nutrition becomes an important issue. Adequate caloric intake is essential to prevent catabolism. Alternative methods of providing nutrition must be used. The physician may consider nasogastric, nasojejunostomy, or gastrostomy feedings. The nurse monitors the type and amount of feeding, tube placement and patency, and tolerance of feedings, as evidenced by residuals, abdominal distention, stools, and weight gain. Total parenteral nutrition is also an option. This is usually reserved for the acute or critical phase of the illness or for the child who does not tolerate alternative methods of nutritional support.

The progression of the disease is unpredictable, the loss of function is frightening, and the recovery time varies from months to years. The long-term implications for nursing care are easily identified. The child and family will require a great deal of emotional support. Full recovery from GBS is possible. The uncertainty of the progression of the disease can contribute to the child's and family's anxiety. Keep them well informed and answer their questions. Questions that the nurse cannot answer should be referred to the appropriate health care provider. Encourage verbalization of feelings concerning the illness and hospitalization, and support and validate the feelings of the family and child.

Foster the child's positive development during the illness by normalizing the situation as much as possible. As the child's clinical condition worsens and dependency on the parents increases, encourage control by offering choices and encouraging decision making when appropriate. Contact the child's teacher for continuation of studies and communication with school friends.

Support the role of the parent as the primary caregiver by facilitating parent participation. Help the parent support the child. If the child's clinical condition deteriorates enough to warrant transfer to a critical care unit, prepare the family for the move. Initiate telephone contact with the receiving nurse to establish a relationship before transfer to lessen the family's anxiety.

If possible, a physician or nurse orientation to the critical care unit will help the family deal with the stress of the transfer. Compassionate and competent health care team members can optimize the child's recovery.

Evaluation

- Does the child demonstrate normal respiratory function?
- Is the child able to communicate needs?
- Has the child's neurologic status returned to normal?
- Is the child's skin intact?
- Do the parents participate in and discuss the child's care?

NEUROLOGIC CONDITIONS REQUIRING CRITICAL CARE

A number of neurologic conditions, including encephalitis, Reye syndrome, botulism, and tetanus, require critical nursing care. Children with these conditions are frequently admitted to hospital critical care units where the care is specialized (Table 28-4).

HEADACHES

Headaches are a common disorder in children of all ages. Up to 82% of all children will suffer a significant headache before age 15 years (Connelly, 2003).

Etiology

The three primary sources of recurrent headache are vascular, tension, and increased ICP. Vascular headaches include migraine and headaches that occur as a result of arteriovenous malformations. Tension headache frequently is a sequela of stress. Contributing factors to increased ICP are a space-occupying lesion, hydrocephalus, and long-term lead poisoning. Sinusitis, eye disease, malocclusion of the teeth, and other systemic diseases can contribute to recurrent headache (Haslam, 2004).

Incidence

Migraine (vascular) headaches occur in close to 2% to 15% of children (Fleener & Holloway, 2004; Stafstrom, Rostasy, & Minster, 2002). Other frequent causes of headache in children include tension-type headaches and nonmigrainous headaches. Migraine in preadolescents is equally prevalent in males and females, but in adolescents the prevalence greatly increases for females. A family history of headache is noted in a majority of these cases.

Manifestations

Migraine

Symptoms range from mild episodes, in which case the child may continue with daily activities, to episodes that force the child to go to a quiet, dark room. In some cases, an aura may occur before the headache begins. The aura may include seeing flashing lights; smelling specific odors; blurry, double, or lost vision; and tingling in the arms or legs. Once the headache begins, the most common symptoms include throbbing pain, often on both sides of the head, nausea and vomiting, irritability, abdominal pain, photophobia, and phonophobia. The pain of a typical migraine lasts from 1 hr to more than 24 hr.

Tension-Type Headaches

The pain associated with tension-type headaches is usually more generalized than that of a migraine. The child may describe the pain as a bandlike tightness or pressure, tight neck muscles, or soreness of the scalp. Nausea is rare, but fatigue and dizziness are common. These headaches may last for days or weeks but usually do not interfere with the child's regular activities.

Diagnostic Evaluation

The International Headache Society published clinical criteria for diagnosing headaches in 1988, and this classification has been newly revised to identify clinical manifestations and diagnostic criteria more precisely for children with headache (International Headache Society, 2004). In addition to eliciting the signs and symptoms as described in the International Classification, the child's blood pressure should be evaluated,

TABLE 28-4 Neurologic Conditions Requiring Critical Care

Condition	Pathophysiology, Etiology, and Incidence	Manifestations	Therapeutic Management	Nursing Considerations
Encephalitis	Inflammation caused by infection or toxin and resulting in cerebral edema and neurologic dysfunction. Numerous agents are causative, such as St. Louis encephalitis and West Nile virus. Peak incidence is in middle to late childhood.	Headache, irritability, lethargy, altered level of consciousness, nuchal rigidity, seizures, fever, malaise, dizziness, nausea and vomiting, ataxia, sensory disturbances.	Diagnosed by lumbar puncture and CSF culture; EEG alterations are not unusual. Care includes hospitalization and monitoring for increased ICP. Medication: cephalosporin or acyclovir (depending on causative agent), anticonvulsants.	Care is similar to that for any child with increased ICP. Care also includes fever management with antipyretics and tepid baths; pharmacologic and nonpharmacologic headache relief measures; maintenance of fluid and electrolyte balance; support for anxious family members; assistance to the family with management of any long-term neurologic deficits; and facilitation of grieving for the family of a child with a poor prognosis.
Reye syndrome	Exposure to viral agent or toxin in at-risk children leads to liver cell damage with rising serum ammonia levels. The toxic serum ammonia levels result in cerebral dysfunction (encephalopathy, cerebral edema), fluid and electrolyte and acid-base imbalances, and coagulopathies. The average age at onset is 6-7 years. Reye syndrome may be related to administration of aspirin to children with viral disease.	Antecedent viral infection; malaise, nausea and vomiting, progressive neurologic deterioration. Laboratory tests: elevated serum ammonia levels, liver dysfunction on biopsy, hypoglycemia, altered coagulation times, increased ICP with respiratory dysfunction. Reye syndrome is clinically staged from I (lethargy) to V (coma with flaccidity/extension posturing) according to degree of altered consciousness.	Care includes hospitalization for monitoring of neurologic status, increasing ICP, hydration and acid-base balance, and cardiorespiratory status.	Care is similar to that for any child with increasing ICP, with the potential addition of mechanical respiratory support. Accurate, continuous monitoring of neurologic and cardiorespiratory status is essential because the child's condition can deteriorate suddenly. Fluid replacement is achieved with IV hypertonic solutions if ICP is not increased. Protect the child from coagulopathy-related injury.
Botulism	Food poisoning caused by *Clostridium botulinum* toxin. The source is honey (in infants) or improperly sterilized canned foods.	CNS symptoms 12-36 hr after ingestion: weakness, headache, double vision, vomiting, difficulty talking, respiratory paralysis, decreased deep tendon reflexes, impaired gag reflex.	Care is supportive and includes respiratory support and administering antitoxin. Recovery after treatment takes an average of 1 mo.	Advise parents not to give infants honey or syrup in their milk or water. Educate the public about proper food preparation techniques.
Tetanus (lockjaw)	Caused by endotoxin produced by the anaerobic, spore-forming, gram-positive bacillus *Clostridium tetani*. Entry sites include puncture wounds, burns, lacerations, and compound fractures. The incubation period is 3 days to 3 weeks.	Painful muscular rigidity of masseter and neck muscles, facial spasms, dysphagia, laryngospasm, severe pain, respiratory arrest.	Care includes ventilatory and respiratory support. Medication: diazepam (Valium) or lorazepam (Ativan) for seizures; tetanus immune globulin.	Assess the child's ventilatory and neurologic status and provide respiratory support as needed. Provide fluids and electrolytes, seizure precautions, quiet environment. Educate the child and family about immunizations.

and the child's head size should be measured (for evidence of chronically increased ICP). A detailed neurologic examination should be performed, with special attention given to auscultating for a bruit in the head (suggesting an arteriovenous malformation), assessing mental status, and examining both optic discs for papilledema. CT or MRI may be performed in children with chronic headaches or those with abnormalities found on the neurologic examination.

NURSING CARE

The Child With Headaches

Assessment

A detailed history of the child's headache and preheadache events is important to determine precipitating factors (e.g., poor diet, food sensitivities, altered sleep patterns, flashing lights). A social history of the child and family may identify triggering stressors (e.g., divorce; move to a new school; loss of a family member, friend, or pet). The child should receive a comprehensive physical examination with emphasis on the neurologic system.

Nursing Diagnosis and Planning

Nursing diagnoses that may apply to a child with a headache and the child's family include those common to other neurologic disorders, such as the following:

- Acute Pain or Chronic Pain related to underlying contributing factors.
  Expected Outcome: The child will have decreased pain related to headaches, as evidenced by an ability to identify triggering factors and demonstrate appropriate nonpharmacologic approaches.
- Deficient Knowledge related to unfamiliarity about management of a child with a headache and the child's medication regimen.
  Expected Outcome: The child and parents will discuss headaches and educational needs.
- Risk for Injury related to headache symptoms (change in vision, dizziness).
  Expected Outcome: The child will have risk for injury reduced, as evidenced by parents verbalizing a safety plan for the child during the headache and describing the medication regimen.

Interventions

Certain factors may trigger the onset of a headache. Triggers may include stress, food, menstruation, visual stimuli, fatigue, and certain medications. The child and family need to be educated about lifestyle changes that will lower stress and the avoidance of other triggers. Keeping a diary of the child's headaches and preheadache events will help identify the triggers specific for the child.

For mild or infrequent migraines and tension headaches, common analgesics, such as ibuprofen or acetaminophen, may be effective. For more severe migraine in adolescents, recommended treatment is nasal sumatriptan (Lewis et al.,

2004). If children have two or more severe migraine headaches per month, they may need daily prophylactic medication. Commonly used prophylactic medications include amitriptyline and propranolol. Psychological evaluation followed by relaxation therapy, counseling, and biofeedback therapy may be helpful for some children.

The nursing care for a child with headaches is acute and long term. Acute management includes placing the child in a dark, quiet environment and administering medication. Long-term management focuses on education about and elimination of trigger factors, stress relief measures, and medication administration.

Evaluation

- Can the child and parents describe the management of headache and the medication regimen?
- Do the child and parents understand the need for following a safety plan to prevent injury during headache and medication?
- Are the child and parents learning to eliminate headache trigger factors?
- Can the child demonstrate and benefit from relaxation therapy and biofeedback?

KEY CONCEPTS

- The CNS is composed of the brain and spinal cord, which are protected by bony coverings (skull, vertebral column). The skull has several bones that are not fused at birth and do not fuse until 12 to 18 months of life. The brain and spinal cord are also covered by the meninges, a fibrous connective tissue structure that contains many blood vessels.
- CSF surrounds the brain and spinal cord. The brain consists of the cerebrum, cerebellum, and brainstem.
- The peripheral nervous system consists of 12 pairs of cranial nerves and 31 pairs of spinal nerves. The autonomic nervous system consists of the sympathetic and parasympathetic systems, which are in control of the body's automatic functions.
- The physiologic process of autoregulation helps the body regulate blood flow. When autoregulation fails to change vascular diameter in response to changes in cerebral perfusion pressure, cerebrovascular dilation is impaired and cerebral blood flow decreases.
- Hypercapnia or hypoxia leads to cerebral dilation and increased ICP. Hypocapnia leads to cerebral arterial constriction and decreased ICP.
- An infant's brain is two thirds the size of an adult's brain. The brain grows to 80% of adult size by age 1 year.
- Head circumference can change in the infant and young child, but the head of the adolescent and adult is unyielding. This change has implications for head circumference measurement for growth and development in the infant and young child.

- The spinal cord, cranial nerves, and peripheral nerves get longer during childhood; the spinal cord terminates at L3 in the newborn and L1 to L2 in the adult.
- Myelinization of nerves begins in the third month of gestation and is completed in adolescence, as demonstrated by progressive development and coordination.
- Neurologic changes may be more subtle in the infant or child than in the adult and may be indicated by irritability or poor feeding behaviors.
- The neurologic examination assesses level of consciousness, pupil size and reaction to light, cranial nerve function, motor and sensory functions, respiratory status and function, vital signs, and head circumference.
- Different seizure types are treated with specific anticonvulsants to achieve optimal seizure control. Anticonvulsants have many side effects, which may include blood dyscrasias, liver damage, weight gain, abdominal discomfort, gum hypertrophy, cognitive, behavioral and cosmetic changes. The CBC and liver enzyme levels should be determined routinely.
- When anticonvulsants are given IV, the most common side effect is respiratory depression.
- Mannitol and furosemide (Lasix) are diuretics that are used to help decrease ICP. Their effect is monitored with serum electrolyte levels and serum osmolality.
- Cerebral edema is decreased by hyperoxygenating and hyperventilating the child, administering diuretics, elevating the head of the bed 30 to 45 degrees, keeping the child in good alignment so that venous drainage is not impaired, and reducing agitation and noxious stimuli.
- Abnormal posturing is an ominous neurologic sign. Flexion (decorticate) posturing refers to flexion of the upper extremities, arms, hands, and wrists. The child's legs are extended. Flexion indicates cortical damage. Extension (decerebrate) posturing refers to extended arms that are inwardly rotated and extended legs. Extension indicates damage to a greater area of the brain, theoretically extending to the brainstem.
- Impaired absorption of CSF in the arachnoid villi as a result of meningitis or subarachnoid hemorrhage is referred to as *communicating hydrocephalus*. Blockage of the flow of CSF through the ventricular system, most commonly related to tumor or developmental defect, is referred to as *noncommunicating hydrocephalus*. Changes in the brain include enlarged ventricles and increased ICP. If the cranial sutures are not ossified, the head circumference will be abnormally large.
- Teaching for the child with a neurologic deficit and the child's family is begun after the child's and family's needs have been assessed. The family's grieving may be verbalized; emotions and fears should be expressed and validated. The nurse reinforces information that has been supplied by other members of the health care team.
- The nurse encourages parents in their caregiving efforts when appropriate, assists the family in setting realistic goals for the child, and identifies support systems and refers to community agencies.

- The nurse has family members demonstrate skills necessary for home care and encourages therapeutic play, which can promote peer contact, when possible and appropriate. The nurse provides incentives for accomplishments and identifies the child's positive qualities and coping mechanisms.

ANSWERS TO CRITICAL THINKING EXERCISE 28-1

1. The course of action is a prudent one. Alerting large numbers of people at the same time while not creating panic is difficult. Although meningococcal meningitis can be serious in children, it is not so highly communicable that prophylaxis for the entire school would be required. For high school students prophylaxis is generally not required, even to classmates. The illness is transmitted through close or intimate contact and through contact with the ill person's oral secretions. Family members and other close personal contacts should receive rifampin or ceftriaxone prophylaxis.

2. If the student were in preschool or in a day care setting, the risk of coming in contact with oral secretions would be higher. Kissing or sharing eating utensils can transmit the illness, so prophylaxis should be considered for the teen's girlfriend. Also, if the ill teen is a member of a sports team, prophylaxis should be considered for the other members of the team because they share water bottles during practices and games. The parents of the other students should know the signs of meningitis and be given criteria for when to call their physician. Immunization against meningococcal meningitis is available. It should be considered for college-bound students.

REFERENCES AND READINGS

Baker E., Saulino M., Caristo, AM. (2002). A new age for childhood diseases: spina bifida. *RN, 65*(12), 33-39.

Betz, C. L., & Snowden, L. A. (2004). *Mosby's pediatric nursing reference.* St. Louis: Mosby.

Connelly, M. (2003). Recurrent pediatric headache: a comprehensive review. *Children's Health Care, 32*(3), 153-189.

Cross, C. (2004). Seizures: regaining control, *RN, 67*(12), 44-51.

Curley, M. A. Q., & Moloney-Harmon, P. A. (2001). *Critical care nursing of infants and children.* St. Louis: Mosby.

Dias, M. (2004). Traumatic brain and spinal cord injury. *Pediatric Clinics of North America, 51*(2), 271-304.

Dunbar, C. (2003). GBS—downward slide and uphill battle. *Nursing Spectrum, 15A*(October 20), 21.

Elder, J. (2004). Urologic disorders in infants and children. In R. Behrman, R. Kliegman, & H. Jenson (Eds.). *Nelson textbook of pediatrics* (17th ed., pp. 1807-1808). Philadelphia: Saunders.

Fenichel, G. M. (2005). *Clinical pediatric neurology: a signs and symptoms approach.* Philadelphia: Elsevier Saunders.

Finesilver, C. (2003). Use of standardized language in neuroscience nursing. *International Journal of Nursing Terminologies and Classification, 14*(suppl 4), 52.

Finnell, R. H., Gould, A., & Spiegelstein, O. (2003). Pathobiology and genetics of neural tube defects. *Epilepsia, 44*(Suppl 3), 14-23.

Fischer, J., & Mathieson, C. (2001). The history of the Glasgow Coma Scale: implications for practice. *Critical Care Nursing Quarterly, 23*(4), 52-58.

Fleener, V., & Holloway, B. (2004). Migraines, not just an adult problem. *The Nurse Practitioner, 29*(11), 27-39.

Fox, J. A. (2002). *Primary health care of infants, children, and adolescents.* St Louis: Mosby.

Frey, L., & Hauser, W. A. (2003). Epidemiology of neural tube defects. *Epilepsia, 44*(Suppl 3), 4-13.

Fritsch, M., & Mehdorn, M. (2002). Endoscopic intraventricular surgery for treatment of hydrocephalus and loculated CSF space in children less than one year of age. *Pediatric Neurology, 36*(4), 183-188.

Gabbe, B., Cameron, P., & Finch, C. (2003). The status of the Glasgow Coma Scale. *Emergency Medicine, 14,* 353-360.

Gambrell, M. (2004). Seizures 101. *Nursing, 34*(8), 36-42.

Garton, H., & Piatt, J. (2004). Hydrocephalus. *Pediatric Clinics of North America, 51*(2), 305-326.

Gill, M., Windemuth, R., Steele, R., & Green, S. (2005). A comparison of the Glasgow Coma Scale score to simplified alternative scores for the prediction of traumatic brain injury outcomes. *Annals of Emergency Medicine, 45,* 37-42.

Granelli, S., & McGrath, J. (2004). Neonatal seizures: diagnosis, pharmacologic interventions, and outcomes. *Journal of Perinatal Neonatal Nursing, 18*(3), 275-287.

Griffin, H. C., Fitch, C. L., & Griffen, L. N. (2004). The causal pathway model and CP. *Journal of Neonatal Nursing, 10*(3), 74.

Haslam, R. (2004). Headaches. In R. Behrman, R. Kliegman, & H. Jenson (Eds.), *Nelson textbook of pediatrics* (17th ed., pp. 2012-2015). Philadelphia: Saunders.

International Headache Society (2004). *The international classification of headache disorders* (2nd ed.). Oxford: Blackwell Publishing.

Jarrar, R. G., & Buchhalter, J. R. (2003). Therapeutics in pediatric epilepsy, part 1: the new antiepileptic drugs and the ketogenic diet. *Mayo Clinic Proceedings, 78*(3), 359-370.

Johnston, M. (2004a). Encephalopathies. In R. Behrman, R. Kliegman, & H. Jenson (Eds.). *Nelson textbook of pediatrics* (17th ed., pp. 2023-2028). Philadelphia: Saunders.

Johnston, M. (2004b). Seizures in childhood. In R. Behrman, R. Kliegman, & H. Jenson (Eds.). *Nelson textbook of pediatrics* (17th ed., pp. 1993-2009). Philadelphia: Saunders.

Johnston, M., & Kinsman, S. (2004). Congenital anomalies of the central nervous system. In R. Behrman, R. Kliegman, & H. Jenson (Eds.). *Nelson textbook of pediatrics* (17th ed, pp. 1983-1993). Philadelphia: Saunders.

Kamienski, M. (2003). Reye syndrome. *American Journal of Nursing, 103*(7), 54-57.

Kaufman, B. (2004). Neural tube defects. *Pediatric Clinics of North America, 51*(2), 389-420.

Kestle, J. R. W. (2003). Pediatric hydrocephalus: current management. *Neurologic Clinics 21*(4), 883-895.

Kneafsey, R., & Gawthorpe, D. (2004) Head injuries: long term consequences for patients and families and implications for nurses. *Journal of Clinical Nursing, 13*(5), 601-608.

Koman, L. A., Smith, B. P., & Shilt, J. S. (2004). Cerebral palsy. *Lancet, 363,* 1619-1631.

Korinthenberg, R., Schessl, J., Kirschner, J., & Monting, J. (2005). Intravenously administered immunoglobulin in the treatment of childhood Guillain-Barré Syndrome: a randomized trial. *Pediatrics, 116*(1), 8-14.

Lee, J., & Adelson, D. (2004). Neurosurgical management of pediatric epilepsy. *Pediatric Clinics of North America, 51*(2), 441-456.

Lewis, D. W. (2002). Headaches in children and adolescents. *American Family Physician, 65*(4), 625-632.

Lewis, D., Ashwal, S., Hershey, A., Hirtz, D., Yonker, M., & Silberstein, S. (2004). Practice parameter: pharmacological treatment of migraine headache in children and adolescents. Report of the American Academy of Neurology Quality Standards Subcommittee and the Practice Committee of the Child Neurology Society. *Neurology, 63,* 2215-2224.

Martin, J. H. (2003). *Neuroanatomy: text and atlas* (2nd ed.). Stamford, CT: Appleton & Lange.

National Center for Injury Prevention and Control Division of Injury and Disability Outcomes and Programs. (2004). *Traumatic brain injury in the United States: Emergency department visits, hospitalizations, and deaths.* Retrieved July 15, 2005, from *www.cdc.gov/Injury.*

Peate, I. (2004). Meningitis: An overview of meningitis signs, symptoms, treatment and support. *British Journal of Nursing, 13*(13), 796-801.

Pena, C. (2003). Emergency: seizure. *American Journal of Nursing, 103*(11), 73-81.

Reuter, D., & Brownstein, D. (2002). Common emergent pediatric neurologic problems. *Emergency Medical Clinics of North America, 20*(1), 155-176.

Selekman, J. (2003). Preventing meningitis. *Pediatric Nursing, 29*(6), 467-469.

Sladky, J. (2004). Guillain-Barré syndrome in children. *Journal of Child Neurology, 19*(3), 191-200.

Stafstrom, C. E., Rostasy, K., & Minster, A. (2002). The usefulness of children's drawings in the diagnosis of headaches. *Pediatrics, 109*(3), 460-472.

Stein, S., & Spettell, C. The Head Injury Severity Scale (HISS): a practical classification of closed head injury. *Brain Injury, 9*(5), 437-444.

Warrell, K. (2004). Use of the Glasgow coma scale in infants. *Paediatric Nursing, 16*(4), 45-49.

Waruiru, C., & Appleton, R. (2004). Febrile seizures: an update. *Archives of Disease in Childhood, 89,* 751-756.

Winter, S., Autry, A., Boyle, C., & Yeargin-Allsopp, M. (2002). Trends in the prevalence of cerebral palsy in a population-based study. *Pediatrics, 110*(6), 1220-1225.

CHAPTER 29

The Child With a Psychosocial Disorder

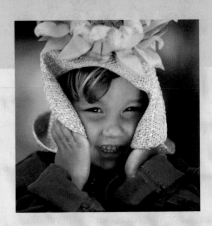

Learning Objectives

After studying this chapter, you should be able to:

- Identify common characteristics and behaviors of anxiety and depression, including separation anxiety.
- Identify the factors and behaviors that correlate with childhood depression, suicide, or suicide attempts.
- Develop a nursing care plan for a child at risk for suicide or for support of the family of a child who has committed suicide.
- Discuss the symptoms, causes, risk factors for, and psychologic dynamics associated with children with eating disorders and describe their nursing care.

- Identify the primary symptoms and manifestations of children with attention-deficit hyperactivity disorder and describe their nursing care.
- Identify signs and symptoms of various types of substance abuse.
- Describe family characteristics and social factors that contribute to physical, emotional, and sexual abuse of children.
- Identify the nurse's responsibilities for the safety and welfare of children relative to emotional, physical, and sexual abuse.
- Develop a nursing care plan for a child who has been abused and one who has failed to thrive.

Definitions

abuse Intentional physical injury or a nonaccidental act of omission by a parent or person responsible for the care of a child; may include physical injury, sexual molestation, neglect, or emotional injury.

comorbidity The simultaneous co-occurrence of two different but interactive conditions in a single individual.

double message A verbal message that contradicts the underlying tone or meaning of the message.

substance abuse Excessive or inappropriate use of medication or other potentially addicting substance to modify mood or behavior or in a manner that results in social, occupational, psychologic, or physical problems or in a situation that creates a physical hazard.

substance addiction Physical or psychologic dependence on a substance, with continued use even when it is known to impair cognitive or social functioning.

substance dependence A physical or psychologic craving for a chemical substance, the cessation of which causes withdrawal symptoms.

suicide Voluntary and intentional cessation of one's life.

suicide attempt Any actions taken by an individual toward self that will result in death if not interrupted.

suicide gesture A suicide attempt that is undertaken primarily to get attention rather than to actually take one's life; nonetheless, it is still considered a serious behavior.

suicide threat A statement or behavior that usually occurs before overt suicidal activity.

violence The use of extreme force or a destructive action that results in injury, discordance, or outrage; engaging in sudden intense activity to the point of loss of control.

Electronic Resources

Additional information related to the content in Chapter 29 can be found on:

the interactive companion CD-ROM

- Audio Glossary
- NCLEX Review Questions

or the companion website at *evolve*
http://evolve.elsevier.com/james/ncoc

- NCLEX Review Questions
- Resources for Health Care Providers and Families
- WebLinks

OVERVIEW OF CHILDHOOD PSYCHOPATHOLOGY

Neurobiologic, family, and sociocultural factors can contribute to the development of psychosocial disorders in children. Neurobiologic factors are briefly reviewed here; family, social, and cultural factors are discussed in the text in conjunction with the various disorders presented.

Neurobiologic Factors

For disorders with a psychologic basis, the primary organ involved is the brain, together with chemicals produced and used by the brain to initiate specific actions. These actions include memory, learning, attention and concentration, mood, and cognition. Because the brain develops throughout childhood, significant changes in the anatomy and physiology of the brain also occur. The most significant changes affecting psychosocial development include myelinization, growth of new tissue, and extension of the neural system throughout the brain. (See p. 919 for a review of brain anatomy and physiology.)

The brain increases in tissue mass and size throughout childhood and adolescence. The increase in the size of the brain results in an increased potential for memory and complex cognitive reasoning and the capacity to learn new skills and acquire new information. Cognitive development proceeds from the simple to the complex and from the concrete to the abstract.

The effect of brain damage depends on several factors. One of the most significant physical factors is the maturational stage of the brain at the time the damage occurs. Early damage spares more language functions but may cause changes in all subsequent areas of development related to the specific area of the brain that is injured. Another physiologic factor is the length of time the brain tissue is impaired (as a result of swelling, hemorrhage, or tissue destruction). Finally, the specific area of the brain that is damaged may determine the specific areas of deficit.

Other factors can influence behavior by indirectly affecting physiologic processes. Stress perception, such as post-traumatic stress disorder, and certain mood disorders, such as depression, are associated with increased cortisol levels over time. Unlike what was thought previously, these increased cortisol levels contribute to structural brain changes. Although an individual's behavior and perception of experiences affect future behavior by being encoded in the brain's memory system, the breakthrough of discovering actual structural changes with psychiatric disorders is revolutionary and drives the need for early and accurate treatment, as with any other physical manifestations.

Manifestations of Psychopathology

Psychosocial disorders are responses to stress and may be manifested as disturbances in feeling (e.g., depression, anxiety), in body functions (e.g., encopresis, enuresis), in behavior (e.g., conduct disturbance, school avoidance, passive-aggressive behaviors), or in performance (learning problems). The manner in which a child responds to stress depends on multiple factors.

Individual Responses to Stress

Factors that influence responses to stress include the following:
- Temperament and genetics
- Developmental level
- The nature and duration of the stress
- Past experiences
- Coping and adaptive abilities of the family

Diagnostic Evaluation

Diagnosing psychosocial disturbance in a child is difficult for several reasons. First, young children normally exhibit a wide range of emotional and social behaviors. Even through adolescence, the child is maturing and developing in terms of coping skills, attitudinal responses, and perspective. During childhood, behavioral responses to various situations are markedly inconsistent and unpredictable. Also, during examinations, both the child and the adolescent are distinctly affected by their relationship and level of comfort with the examiner and by the setting. Finally, children and adolescents are affected and shaped by their relationships with parents and other social figures. For a thorough assessment of psychosocial disorders, a structured mental status examination of the child must be completed. Various laboratory

---

PSYCHOSOCIAL DISORDERS TYPICALLY MANIFESTED IN CHILDHOOD

- Mental retardation (see Chapter 30)
- Pervasive developmental disorders, autistic disorder
- Learning disorders: reading, arithmetic, other skills
- Disruptive behavior disorders: attention-deficit hyperactivity disorder, conduct disorder, oppositional defiant disorder
- Anxiety disorders: separation anxiety disorder, PTSD, phobias, obsessive-compulsive disorder
- Mood disorders: depression, bipolar disorder
- Eating disorders: anorexia nervosa, bulimia nervosa, pica, obesity, rumination disorder of infancy
- Tic disorders: Tourette's disorder, chronic motor or vocal tics, transient tics
- Elimination disorders: functional encopresis, functional enuresis (see Chapters 19 and 20)
- Communication disorders: receptive or expressive language disorders, cluttering, stuttering, elective mutism

Data from American Psychiatric Association. (2000). *Diagnostic and statistical manual of mental disorders* (4th ed., text revision). Washington, DC: American Psychiatric Association.

and diagnostic tests may also be appropriate. The results of these tests will help determine whether pharmacologic and psychologic interventions may be effective. The literature on children's mental health issues describes several questionnaires that are used to assess emotional and behavioral problems in children and adolescents (McDonnell & Glod, 2003; Varley & Smith, 2003). A frequently used test that has proven reliability is the Child Behavior Checklist (CBCL), which is given to parents to complete; it assesses emotional and behavioral problems (McDonnell & Glod, 2003).

MENTAL STATUS EXAMINATION OF CHILDREN

- Appearance: dress, gestures, posture, tics, other repetitive movements; physical presentation, such as age, stature, race, age-appropriate behaviors
- Ability to attend to task
- Mood or affect: predominant feelings, mood fluctuations, mood congruence with verbalizations
- Manner of relating to the examiner: exploration of the child's understanding of the purpose of the interview, approach or avoidance behaviors, use of play materials available, verbalizations
- Intellectual skills: problem-solving abilities, conceptualization of causality, body image, memory, judgment, general fund of knowledge, insight (findings are compared with developmental norms)
- Capacity for imaginative thinking and play
- Sensorimotor development: fine and gross motor skills, symmetry and coordination of movement, hand and eye dominance, right-left discrimination
- Perceptions and thought content: presence or absence of suicidal-homicidal ideation, intent, plan; delusions or illusions; hallucinations
- Speech: fluency, tone, volume, age appropriateness

COMMON LABORATORY AND DIAGNOSTIC TESTS FOR PSYCHOSOCIAL DISORDERS IN CHILDREN AND ADOLESCENTS

- *Urine tests:* Used to assess specific drugs excreted by the kidneys
- *Blood and serum tests:* Used to assess the long-term effects of malnutrition, evidence of specific drugs or ingested chemicals, and the potency of selected pharmacotherapeutic agents prescribed for symptom reduction
- *Radiographs of the skull and long bones:* Frequently used to identify current and previous fractures, which are common signs of physical abuse
- *Genital and anal examinations:* Performed by a physician and used, together with slides of secretions, to help determine whether sexual abuse has occurred
- *Measurement of subcutaneous tissue:* May be ordered if physical neglect associated with malnutrition is suspected

---

Nurses caring for children encounter a number of disorders and conditions that are best viewed as psychosocial disorders because they involve primarily the way in which the child or adolescent relates to others and copes with stress. Most psychosocial disorders have a familial or biologic predisposition that may be triggered if the environment is demanding or unsupportive. Physical stressors, such as birth defects, physical injuries, and chronic illness, may produce psychosocial disorders. Emotional stressors, such as inconsistent or contradictory child-rearing practices, marital conflict, or neglect, may also contribute to psychiatric disorder development. Some psychosocial manifestations are associated with genetic syndromes, such as fragile X syndrome. Other disorders are related primarily to an inaccurate or inappropriate relationship between the child and significant others in the social environment. Research consistently shows that psychosocial disorders are caused by a combination of predisposing or inherent factors and environmental or interactional factors. Conditions discussed in this chapter are designed to describe some of the most frequently seen psychosocial disorders of childhood. For more in-depth discussion of any of these conditions, consult with a psychiatric nursing text.

ANXIETY AND MOOD DISORDERS

Although actually categorized in two different areas in the *Diagnostic and Statistical Manual of Mental Disorders*, anxiety disorders and mood disorders, such as depression and bipolar disorder, are difficult to differentiate in children for several reasons. In children and adolescents, the behavioral presentation of these disorders is similar. For example, the child who is anxious may be withdrawn, tearful, unwilling to engage in play, or prone to acting aggressively toward others. These same symptoms typically occur in children who are depressed. Moreover, it is often difficult to differentiate between normal mood changes that are the result of normal developmental maturation and adaptation and abnormal, persistent mood disturbances. Generally, however, mood disturbance is more intense and persistent and interferes with social relations and daily functioning. Finally, the child or adolescent can have both anxiety and a mood disorder.

Anxiety Disorders

Anxiety is one of the most common categories of psychopathology in childhood. Anxiety is expected and normal in children at specific times in development. For example, infants and children up to preschool age often show intense distress at times of separation from their parents or family members (see Chapter 11). It is not uncommon for young children to have short-lived fears related to darkness, storms, animals, and imaginary situations (see Chapters 6 and 7). Although school-age children typically express anxiety or fear of body harm or potentially real worries (e.g., thunder, lightning), adolescents may exhibit anxiety regarding social situations and acceptance (see Chapter 8). When worry and distress become overwhelming and begin to interfere with daily functioning, anxiety becomes pathologic and warrants serious intervention (Stafford, Boris, & Dalton, 2004).

Separation Anxiety

The essential hallmark of separation anxiety is disabling anxiety about being apart from one's parents or another significant person to whom the child is attached, or about being away from home. It may develop spontaneously or under stress (e.g., in temporary relation to a move or a death in the family) and may last for several years, waxing and waning. Children with separation anxiety frequently fear that if they are apart from their parents, harm will come to the parent or themselves. Separation anxiety occurs in approximately 4% of children and young adults (American Psychiatric Association, 2000) and in up to 3% of preschool age children (McDonnell & Glod, 2003).

School Refusal

School refusal is closely related to separation anxiety disorder in that separation from parents may cause the reluctance to attend school (Varley & Smith, 2003). Persistent reluctance or refusal to go to school or elsewhere may be the primary reason families seek intervention for separation anxiety disorder. Unlike truants, who are relatively fearless and avoid school to pursue other interests, children with separation anxiety stay home or attempt to remain with their parents. The child may complain of physical symptoms, cry, plead, or even exhibit panic symptoms shortly before the time for school approaches, but the symptoms subside after the child is allowed to stay home, only to reappear the next morning. Sometimes the child may simply refuse to leave the home. There may be other underlying contributing factors to school refusal, such as fear of bullying, fatigue, boredom, learning challenges, or upsetting incidents that occur in the school setting. (See Chapter 7 for an additional discussion of school refusal.)

School refusal may also be related to a *social phobia*, where children avoid social or performance situations to such a degree that their daily routine is affected (e.g., by refusing to participate in physical education exercises or by failing to raise their hands to ask a question in class). Social phobia can result in social isolation for the child who has difficulty establishing and maintaining peer relationships (Stafford et al., 2004).

Panic Disorder

Anxiety may be so intense that the child feels a sense of panic, in which case the disorder may be termed *panic disorder*. The onset of panic is more sudden than generalized anxiety,

and symptoms increase rapidly (Varley & Smith, 2003). Children have marked discomfort that includes cardiovascular (palpitations, chest pain) and respiratory (shortness of breath) symptoms and psychologic feelings of impending doom or fear that they are dying. Panic disorder is more frequently seen in adolescents (Stafford et al., 2004; Varley & Smith, 2003).

Posttraumatic Stress Disorder

One type of anxiety disorder that follows a specific and terrifying event is *posttraumatic stress disorder* (PTSD). Symptoms of this disorder include intense fear, helplessness, or horror, along with physiologic symptoms of increased arousal. The child demonstrates determined avoidance of stimuli associated with the traumatic event but may have persistent nightmares or flashbacks. Children also may re-enact the event during play. Symptoms interfere with the child's ability to concentrate, may contribute to sleep problems, and may cause the child to be hypervigilant or agitated. PTSD affects approximately 6% of children younger than 18 years (Stafford et al., 2004) and less than 1% of preschoolers (McDonnell & Glod, 2003). This disorder is frequently seen in children who have been sexually or physically abused (Varley & Smith, 2003), but it also occurs subsequent to other traumatic events, such as disasters or severe injury.

Obsessive-Compulsive Disorder

Affecting approximately 3% of children (Luo et al., 2004), obsessive-compulsive disorder (OCD) manifests as repetitive unwanted thoughts (obsessions) or ritualistic actions (compulsions), or both. Compulsions are designed to relieve the anxiety that the child usually realizes is irrational. Because young children cannot adequately describe their uncomfortable thoughts or concerns, severe temper tantrums, particularly when a ritual has been interrupted, may be the predominant symptom (Varley & Smith, 2003). Although OCD is generally considered to have a genetic component, a small subset of children with OCD is suspected to have pediatric autoimmune neuropsychiatric disorders (PANDAS) associated with streptococcal infection. These children have a more abrupt onset or exacerbation of symptoms of OCD after a group A beta-hemolytic streptococcal infection. Although this relationship has been described in various studies, evidence varies as to the strength of the relationship (Luo et al., 2004; Mell, Davis, & Owens, 2005).

Mood Disorders

Mood disorders are also varied and are specified according to the intensity or duration of depressive symptoms or the particular behaviors displayed by the child.

Depression

Depression during childhood and adolescence is being diagnosed more frequently, affecting approximately 1% of preschoolers, 2% to 3% of school-age children, and 5% or more of adolescents (Boris, Dalton & Forman, 2004; Elliott & Smiga, 2003; McDonnell & Glod, 2003; National Institute of Mental Health, 2001). Clinical signs of a depressive disorder include angry outbursts, irritability, loss of interest and enjoyment in usual activities, decreased energy, altered appetite, altered sleep patterns, decreased self-esteem, disengagement from family and friends, and thoughts of suicide. If the clinical presentation lasts at least 2 weeks (or longer), the child meets the criteria for *major depressive disorder*. Children or adolescents who exhibit a less severe but depressed or irritable mood for at least 1 year meet the criteria for *dysthymic disorder*. Depression appears to have a familial component. In young children, depression may be related to abuse or neglect or other situational stressors (Elliott & Smiga, 2003). After one depressive episode, there is increased risk for subsequent episodes. Depression often manifests in conjunction with substance abuse, so children and adolescents who abuse substances should be assessed for depression as well.

Bipolar Disorder

Bipolar disorder in children and adolescents may be difficult to recognize because of the normal mood swings that accompany certain developmental stages, particularly early adolescence. If the child has chronic, fluctuating, and extreme mood disturbances between depressive lows and manic highs for 1 year, bipolar mood disorder (*cyclothymic disorder*) may be diagnosed. The signs and symptoms of the depressive episode are similar to those discussed previously, and the child may exhibit psychosomatic complaints, such as headache and stomachache. The child or adolescent who is in a manic mood may be overly elated, easily distracted, irritable, and aggressive, and may also demonstrate increased risk-taking behavior, talk rapidly, and not be able to sleep (National Institute of Mental Health, 2000). Impaired social relationships are common.

In young children, bipolar disorder most often manifests in a rapid cycling form, which includes swiftly changing and extreme mood swings. The symptoms of irritability, anger, aggressive behavior, hyperactivity, and distractibility often can be confused with symptoms of attention deficit hyperactivity disorder, and children with these symptoms can be misdiagnosed (Boris et al., 2004). Bipolar mood disorders affect approximately 1% to 5% of adolescents (March & TADS Team, 2004; National Institute of Mental Health, 2000); although the prevalence in young children is not described, the diagnosis of bipolar disorder is being made more frequently (National Mental Health Association, 2005).

Psychophysiology

Research supports the view that both anxiety and mood disorders have biologic components that affect both brain structure and function in various complex ways. One focus of exploration (Oakley, 2005a, 2005b) is into neurotransmitters, primarily norepinephrine and serotonin, which chemically conduct electrical impulses across nerve synapses. Normally, these neurotransmitters are synthesized in a presynaptic nerve, released into the synaptic space, and bind to receptors in the postsynaptic nerve, where they excite, inhibit, or modify nerve action. The neurotransmitters are then released again by the postsynaptic nerve back into the synaptic space,

where they are either destroyed or taken back into the presynaptic nerve for future use (reuptake). In children with mood or anxiety disorders, available serotonin is decreased, either from decreased release or increased reuptake (Oakley, 2005a, 2005b); this particularly affects neurotransmitters in areas of the brain that regulate cognition, feelings and emotions, and motivation (prefrontal cortex and limbic system).

One other important area of exploration is into the hypothalamic-pituitary-adrenal axis, which regulates stress hormones. Theoretically, stress early in life can contribute to an exaggerated level of stress hormones with subsequent excessive stress response. The increase in stress hormones contributes to the symptoms seen particularly in children with anxiety disorders. In addition, children with OCD have heightened metabolic activity in areas of the brain associated with strong emotions (Takashi, 2002).

Etiology

Affective disorders have been shown to have a genetic basis. Having a first-degree relative with an anxiety or depressive disorder may predict an increased risk of the disorder in offspring. A family history of suicide or depression (particularly parental) is significant risk factor of approximately a 50% increase (Qin, 2003).

Psychosocial theories emphasize the importance of the interaction within the family system, behavioral patterns of the individual, and interpersonal factors in the development of depression. There is evidence that children and adolescents with a history of verbal, physical, or sexual abuse; frequent separation from or loss of loved ones; drug use; incarceration; lower socioeconomic status; homosexuality; chronic illness; behavioral disorders; and dysfunctional families are more likely than peers with healthy family patterns to have anxiety or depressive disorders (Sadock & Sadock, 2003).

Manifestations

The clinical manifestations of anxiety or depressive disorders have been described previously. Symptoms of anxiety and mood disorders can disrupt both the child and the family. Children with these disorders lose interest in usual play and school activities, the relationship with friends is impaired, and the child may exhibit learning deficits related to behavior in school or inability to concentrate on learning. Somatic complaints, such as recurrent abdominal pain or headaches with no physical cause, are common. Recurrent thoughts of death or suicide are sometimes reported. Hospitalization may be required.

Therapeutic Management

Antidepressants, particularly selective serotonin reuptake inhibitors, which inhibit the amount of serotonin that is removed from the nerve synapse, are frequently prescribed for anxiety and depressive disorders. The Food and Drug Administration (FDA) has issued a warning on the risk of increased suicidal thoughts in children who are being treated with antidepressants (U.S. Food and Drug Administration, 2005a). At this time, fluoxetine (Prozac) is the only antidepressant that is FDA approved for the treatment of depression in children and adolescents. Seretraline (Zoloft) is FDA approved for the treatment of anxiety, but not depression, in children and adolescents. It is not prohibited to use other antidepressants to treat these disorders in children or adolescents; however, it is advised to keep a close watch on initiating any type of medication treatment in this population. It is of importance to note that no suicides occurred in any of the studies that prompted this warning (U.S. Food and Drug Administration, 2005b). Use of selective serotonin uptake inhibitors medication management is still an appropriate and widely used treatment for depression and anxiety in children and adolescents.

Psychotherapy and cognitive behavioral therapy are also an effective treatment for children with these disorders. Many parents and clinicians may prefer to initiate psychotherapy before, and perhaps in lieu of, medications; however, the most effective treatment combines medication and the child's and family's exploration of situations and environmental factors that are related to the child's symptoms (March & TADS Team, 2004). Individual therapy and family therapy are essential for children with suicidal ideation or persistent mood disturbances.

It is common for both anxiety disorders and mood disorders to recur. Social skills training or group therapy may be most helpful for social anxiety. School phobia is treated by insisting that the child attend school, offering interventions during school time to reduce anxiety symptoms, and refusing to pick up the child from school, even if the child insists. This form of intervention is a type of desensitization therapy. Other strategies for decreasing anxiety or depressive symptoms include relaxation therapy, distraction strategies, self-talk, or cognitive strategies, as well as support from adults or friends who are safe and reassuring.

NURSING CARE

The Child With Anxiety or Depression

Assessment

A thorough history should be obtained from the child (if applicable) and the family. Initially it may be necessary to interview the child with the parents present, but once the child becomes more comfortable with the nurse, time alone with the child should be offered. The interview should cover both the child's moods and events related to those moods, physiologic symptoms, patterns of daily activities, identification of stressors, and information about the duration, frequency, and intensity of symptoms. Suicidal ideation or plans should be assessed by asking both direct and indirect questions (Elliott & Smiga, 2003).

Questions about the family environment should seek to identify those with whom the child relates most easily and to identify family interaction patterns. It is important to explore any family history of mood disturbance and other emotional problems or substance abuse problems. Ask the parent about any changes in the child's behaviors and when these changes began. Inquire about the child's ability to engage in routine activities or play, ability to interact with friends, and school progress. For a child suspected of having OCD, it is important to ask about observed compulsions or extreme reactions to changes in routine.

Several self-reporting instruments and interview schedules are available for the specific assessment of anxiety and depression. They are used to assess and quantify progress or regression of treatment.

Nursing Diagnosis and Planning

The nursing diagnoses and expected outcomes that apply to the child with anxiety or depression are as follows:

* Ineffective Coping related to loss of energy, sleep disturbance, biochemical imbalance, loss of control, or side effects of medication.
  Expected Outcome: The child will display adaptive ability, as evidenced by participation in and enjoyment of regular activities. The parent will describe any expected or unexpected side effects from the prescribed medication.
* Situational Low Self-Esteem related to cognitive distortions, inability to manage daily events, and a sense of hopelessness or guilt.
  Expected Outcome: The child will display increased self-esteem, as evidenced by verbalization of an increase in self-confidence and an increase in positive feelings about self.
* Risk for Self-Directed Violence related to suicidal ideation, guilt, or hopelessness.
  Expected Outcome: The child will demonstrate more positive moods and reduced anxiety levels and will talk to a responsible family member or professional about any thoughts of self-directed violence.
* Disturbed Sleep Pattern related to anxiety, depression, and inactivity.
  Expected Outcome: The child will exhibit appropriate sleep patterns, as evidenced by expressing feelings of being well rested, showing no signs of sleep deprivation (e.g., irritability, lethargy, restlessness), and showing no signs of excessive sleeping.
* Risk for altered growth and development related to poor concentration, fatigue, inability to participate in school
  Expected Outcome: The child will engage in appropriate play for developmental level, attend school, maintain educational progress, and continue positive relationship with peers.

Interventions

The nurse is part of a team that offers support for the entire family while exploring the factors that contribute to the emotional distress in the child. The nurse should identify specific changes in the environment and interaction patterns that could support a sense of control and positive regard for the child. Privacy and space for the child or family members to discuss their feelings as treatment progresses should be made available on a regular basis. The nurse teaches the family, and the child if appropriate, what to expect from any pharmacologic treatment and facilitates medication administration in the school setting.

If the child needs hospitalization, admission will generally be to a psychiatric unit where specialized nursing is available. Mood disturbances often are identified on pediatric units, in outpatient clinics, or in school systems. Educating parents and teachers about depression and anxiety and its treatment in childhood is an important service for nurses to provide to the community.

Evaluation
- Does the child exhibit an energy level that allows for interactions, play, and school?
- Does the child seem interested in people and events?
- Does the child communicate positive statements about self?
- Does the parent report that the child appears happier and more engaged?
- Does the child exhibit normal patterns of eating and sleeping?
- Can the parent describe the medication effects and side effects?

SUICIDE

Suicide is the third leading cause of death among adolescents between 15 and 19 years old and the seventh among children 5 to 14 years old (National Center for Health Statistics, 2004). Parents often underestimate the severity of warning signs, particularly depression, substance abuse, or other psychologic disorders, until a child actually attempts suicide or succeeds. Risk factors for suicide are depression, a family history of psychiatric disorders (especially depression and suicide), and previous attempts. Other significant risk factors are chronic medical illness, family violence, substance abuse, poor impulse control, poor school performance, homosexuality, and access to firearms in the household (Gould, Greenberg, Velting, & Shaffer, 2003).

Psychopathology

Most adolescent suicide attempts are impulsive; however, any verbalization or gesture of suicide should be taken very seriously. It is estimated that two thirds of adolescents who attempt suicide have high intent and a strong wish to die. The motive may be a desire to influence others, gain attention, communicate love or anger, or escape a difficult or painful situation.

The development of a concept of mortality and death follows the general principles of the development of cognitive and affective abilities, from the concrete to the abstract. Up to age 6 years, it is unlikely that a child has any realistic concept of death or looks for it in an active way. Children as young as 3 years, however, have tried to commit suicide and apparently understood what they were doing. Between ages 6 and 8 years, children abandon an egocentric view and discover that death is one of many events out of one's control. From age 9 years on, the child begins to view death as inevitable and universal.

> ### CRITICAL TO REMEMBER
> **Threats of Suicide**
>
> A suicide gesture or threat should *never* be ignored. The child should be encouraged to discuss the thought specifically to determine whether there is a plan and the lethality of the plan. Help should be obtained from qualified health professionals.

Etiology

Underlying depression, poor self-concept, and hopelessness appear to be the most significant factors contributing to suicide, regardless of age or sex. Long-standing family dysfunction is often present, with emotional detachment and isolation among family members. The suicide victim is typically a vulnerable individual who, under stress, seeks and finds a way to die. The individual is for some reason unable to elicit adequate adult support to stop the suicide process.

Incidence

Estimates of the prevalence of suicidal *ideation* are 12.8% in males and 21.3% in females. The prevalence of *suicide attempts* is 5.4% in males and 11.5% in females. Since 1991 the number of reported youths who planned suicide attempts decreased from 18.6% to 16.5% (Grunbaum et al., 2004). For completed suicides, the male-to-female ratio is 7:1. The higher incidence of completed suicides in males may be related to the more violent methods of suicide, such as the use of a gun, used by boys. It is also common for suicides to occur in a cluster within a community.

Of significant importance, gay and lesbian youths are two to seven times more likely to attempt suicide than are their heterosexual peers. This is not related to being homosexual but rather to the stigma and level of vulnerability and stress, such as lack of social and family support. Suicide is the leading cause of death in this group. Approximately 30% report at least one attempt (Frankowoski, 2004; O'Leary, 2004).

Manifestations and Risk Factors

The risk for suicide should be considered if the following are present:
- Previous suicide attempts
- Close family member who has committed suicide
- Past psychiatric hospitalization
- Recent losses: This may include the death of a relative, a family divorce, or a breakup with a girlfriend
- Suicidal clues, such as cryptic verbal messages, giving away personal items, and changes in expected patterns of behaviors (e.g., sudden calmness in a normally anxious teenager)
- Specific statements about suicide or self-harm
- Preoccupation with death, often manifested by an interest in death themes in literature and art
- Frequent risk-taking or self-abusive behaviors
- Use of alcohol or drugs to cope
- Overwhelming sense of guilt or shame

- Obsessional self-doubt
- Social isolation: The individual does not have social alternatives or skills to find alternatives to suicide
- Open signs of mental illness manifested as delusions or hallucinations
- Significant change or a major life event that is internally disruptive
- Exposure to violence in the home or the social environment: The individual sees violent behavior as a viable solution to life problems
- Handguns in the home, especially if loaded
- History of physical or sexual abuse
- Homosexuality, especially if the teen discovers same-sex orientation early in adolescence, experiences violence because of homosexual identity, or is rejected by family members as a result of sexual orientation

Therapeutic Management

Suicide prevention is viewed as the most significant mental health contribution and is promoted at local, state, and federal levels. Prevention is offered through multimedia educational presentations in schools, through support groups at local mental health centers, through community emphasis on stress reduction, through social affiliations, and through networking with support systems.

Screening for depression, both at school and in the health care system, is one of the most significant prevention strategies. Most children or adolescents who commit suicide have offered at least veiled information about their suicidal ideation or feelings of despair to classmates, teachers, or health care providers.

After a child's suicide, counseling services must be provided to family members and the child's immediate friends. It is important that these services be offered quickly, preferably within the first 24 hours after the suicide, and that counselors remain available for 1 year after the event. Grieving and emotional adjustments often take several months and may peak around the anniversary of the suicide event.

Children or adolescents with persistent suicidal ideation should undergo a thorough psychiatric evaluation by a mental health professional. The child may need pharmacotherapeutic agents, such as antidepressants or antipsychotic medications. The use of medications in children and adolescents at risk for suicide requires close monitoring and medications should be distributed in small doses because they could be used in a suicide attempt or act.

NURSING CARE

The Child or Adolescent at Risk for Suicide

Assessment

The risk of suicide is best assessed by a systematic approach to behaviors, attitudes, and risk factors. Several instruments have been developed to assess lethality and potentiality, which lessens the likelihood of overlooking contributing factors.

BOX 29-1	**Questions to Assess Suicide Potential**

1. Have you ever thought of trying to hurt yourself? How might you do this?
2. Have you ever thought of killing yourself? How might you do this?
3. Have you known anyone who has committed suicide? When did this occur? What was it like for you?
4. Do you have access to firearms or knives?
5. Do you ever do things to deliberately place yourself in danger, such as driving when you are drunk or playing Russian roulette with a gun?
6. Have you ever told anyone about wanting to kill yourself?
7. Have you ever been hospitalized for suicidal behavior?
8. Can you describe how you feel right now?

The instruments are similar and explore risk factors, stressors, lethality of method, coping mechanisms, and support systems. Subtle symptoms of depression or anxiety, such as decreased energy, persistent restlessness, or anger should also be considered. It is important to explore thought content and organization, awareness and expression of feelings, perceived level and types of stress, perceived availability of support resources, prior suicidal behaviors, and medical status (Box 29-1).

Nursing Diagnosis and Planning

The nursing diagnoses and expected outcomes that apply to the child or adolescent at risk for suicide and the family are as follows:

- Risk for Self-Directed Violence related to a desire to end emotional pain, to solicit the attention of others, or to avoid responsibility.

   Expected Outcome: The child or adolescent will indicate a decrease in the risk for self-directed violence, as evidenced by an ability to use effective communication techniques to express needs and feelings and verbalize that there are solutions to problems.

- Situational Low Self-Esteem or Chronic Low Self-Esteem related to a perception of failure and hopelessness about the ability to change self or circumstances.

   Expected Outcome: The child or adolescent will demonstrate increased self-esteem, as evidenced by verbalization of ability to change self or circumstances.

- Anxiety related to current or anticipated events.

   Expected Outcome: The child or adolescent will have decreased anxiety, as evidenced by recognizing and expressing anxiety and use of effective coping mechanisms to decrease anxiety.

- Interrupted Family Processes related to relational disturbance or possible abuse or neglect.

   Expected Outcome: The child or adolescent and family will access and mobilize appropriate support systems in an effective manner.

- Ineffective Coping related to a sense of despair or limited availability of support.

  Expected Outcome: The child or adolescent and family will work with professionals to begin to identify and express feelings and identify strengths, and to discuss appropriate actions when feelings become overwhelming

Interventions

The approach to therapy should be empathic and non-judgmental to decrease the child's or adolescent's sense of isolation and rejection. The nurse should adopt a voice and demeanor that are clear, direct, and supportive. Being emotionally and physically available, offering opportunities to discuss feelings and the suicidal event, and removing potentially harmful objects will help protect the youth from self-injury.

The nurse should suggest different coping strategies, such as choosing alternative activities when impulses arise and remaining near other people. The nurse can help the child identify specific feelings and effective ways to manage those feelings. It is important for the nurse to assess how closely a child needs to be monitored throughout the day, realizing that the potential for self-harm fluctuates.

To allow a balance between the need to explore personal issues and the need for social support, anticipatory guidance related to grieving for families of suicidal or potentially suicidal children is best provided on both an individual and a group basis. Grieving will occur even if the suicide attempt was unsuccessful. Individual and family therapy will also provide an opportunity to explore contributory factors that can be altered to reduce the suicide potential. Working with the parents, together with other therapeutic team members, will help the parents regain their ability to assist their child and manage the home environment. It is important to increase the adult-child interactions, thereby decreasing the risk of another suicide attempt.

Prevention of suicide is an essential role for the school nurse, especially for nurses at the middle or high school level. It is imperative that school nurses educate school personnel about recognizing the subtle signs of an impending suicide attempt so intervention can occur. Included in continuing education should be who to contact if a teacher or other school worker suspects a child is considering suicide, who will interview and evaluate the child, and what personnel will notify the family. Often, schools have professional teams that perform the evaluation and make appropriate referrals. Suicide prevention and incidence reduction are two of the national goals described in *Healthy People 2010* (U.S. DHHS, 2000).

Evaluation

- Is the child or adolescent able to identify times when suicidal potential is greatest and to seek help during these times?
- Does the child or adolescent participate in activities that reduce feelings of despair and hopelessness?

- Does the child or adolescent display evidence of positive self-esteem through positive self-statements or ability to describe how circumstances can be changed?
- Has the child or adolescent verbalized a decrease in anxiety?
- Is the family able to identify warning signs of suicidal risk?
- Do family members support one another, and can the family identify community resources to assist?
- Has the child or adolescent developed coping mechanisms and effective problem solving?
- Has the family developed a suicide prevention plan?

EATING DISORDERS: ANOREXIA NERVOSA AND BULIMIA NERVOSA

Eating disorder is a general term that encompasses anorexia nervosa, bulimia nervosa, pica, binge eating disorder, obesity (discussed in Chapter 7), and rumination disorders. Anorexia nervosa and bulimia nervosa are the two most frequently seen eating disorders in children. Anorexia and bulimia have overlapping features and similar underlying mechanisms, which supports viewing these disorders as a continuum.

Anorexia nervosa is characterized by a deliberate refusal to maintain adequate body weight, a distorted body image, and amenorrhea (in females). The term *anorexia* is a misnomer, because the individual rarely has a loss of appetite. Weight loss can be extremely dramatic. *Bulimia nervosa* is characterized by recurrent episodes of binge eating; a sense of lack of control over eating binges; self-induced vomiting or excessive use of laxatives, diuretics, or emetics to prevent weight gain; excessive exercise to prevent weight gain; and a persistent overconcern with body image, although body image is usually not distorted. Children and adolescents with eating disorders typically report shame and guilt about many life experiences, especially eating.

Individuals with severe eating disorders, particularly anorexia nervosa, have a mortality rate up to 20% from complications of the disorder or from suicide (Renfrew Center Foundation for Eating Disorders, 2003). Treatment resistance is very high in young people with anorexia and bulimia because all of their psychologic and sociologic experiences are framed by their body image and self-esteem and because of secondary gains such as attention, admiration, envy, and control over others through eating patterns. Unfortunately, in addition to the eating disorder, about 50% of these children and adolescents also meet criteria for other serious psychiatric disorders, such as major depression or a personality disorder.

Ritualistic behaviors are common in these children and adolescents, particularly around issues of food. For example, the child or adolescent may eat only at a particular time of day, eat foods only in a certain order, or insist on washing all foods before eating them. The rituals are often an attempt to control the portions, fat content, or nutrients ingested. The rituals also serve to enhance the individual's sense of control over food or dietary intake.

Children or adolescents with anorexia will go to extreme measures to prevent others from becoming aware of the weight loss or lack of food intake. They may ingest large amounts of water or insert heavy objects in the vaginal cavity before weighing to give the impression of weight gain. The child or adolescent with either anorexia or bulimia may eat in front of people and then go to the bathroom to purge after the meal.

Etiology

Disordered eating emerges from multiple risk factors including biologic, social, cultural, and psychologic factors. One of the most salient factors appears to be enmeshed family relationships in which the child is considered to be an extension of the parent or is viewed as a means of meeting the parent's needs rather than being allowed to develop as an autonomous individual. Family relationships may be chaotic and disordered (Phillips & Pratt, 2005). The disorder is more common among sisters and mothers of those with the disorder than in the general population, suggesting some familial predisposition.

The development and severity of the child's risk for eating disorders appear to be related to the child's response to biologic, psychologic, and social demands of maturation. Other significant risk factors are earlier pubertal development and higher body fat, depressive tendencies, concurrent psychologic disturbance, alterations in brain neurotransmitters, subsequent eating problems, cultural expectations to be thin, and the individual's pervasive sense of ineffective control of the environment (Sadock & Sadock, 2003; Sigman, 2003).

Children or adolescents with eating disorders often have a family history of affective disorders. The family dynamics for males with anorexia are reported to include poor father-son relationships, with the father typifying the strong, cultural image, and a mother who is overinvolved, overprotective, and overdependent on the mother-son relationship.

Incidence

In the United States, bulimia nervosa appears to be more prevalent than anorexia nervosa, with approximately 1% of the female adolescent population reporting symptoms; the prevalence of anorexia nervosa in girls is 0.5%. Eating disorders are rarer in boys; only 1 in 10 individuals with an eating disorder is male (American Academy of Pediatrics, 2003).

Manifestations

Anorexia Nervosa

The hallmark of anorexia nervosa is the refusal to maintain a body weight that exceeds the minimal weight recommended for height (15% below expected weight). Intense preoccupation with and unrelenting fear of obesity and a disturbed body image (weight, size, or shape) that is obviously contrary to reality (Fig. 29-1) are also observed. Other clinical manifestations in females include at least three missed menstrual periods (primary or secondary amenorrhea); a misperception of internal and external stimuli, particularly food-related cues such as hunger; overwhelming feelings of ineffectiveness and inadequacy; lanugo, dry or flaky skin, and dull, brittle hair; and fatigue and muscle wasting.

Boys with eating disorders demonstrate many behavior patterns similar to girls' behavior patterns, including weight loss through excessive dieting, compulsive activities, and purging, to get strong or to develop an athletic build (rather than to be thin, as reported by females).

Bulimia Nervosa

The clinical manifestations associated with bulimia nervosa include recurrent episodes of binge eating, a sense of lack of control over eating behaviors during binges, and strategies that prevent weight gain (self-induced vomiting; use of laxatives, diuretics, or emetics; fasting; vigorous and excessive exercise). A minimum of two binge eating episodes per week for at least 3 months and persistent overconcern with body shape and weight are also common factors. These children are also at increased risk for tooth erosion because of the effects of the acidic content on the teeth from the subsequent vomiting. Some children and adolescents with bulimia use excessive exercise along with bingeing and purging to control weight. Unlike children and adolescents with anorexia, those with bulimia are mostly within normal weight percentiles.

Diagnostic Evaluation

An electrocardiogram and a chest radiograph are typically obtained if symptoms of bradycardia, hypotension, or hypothermia are noted. Complete liver and renal function tests, thyroid function tests, and serum electrolyte studies are usually included in the medical workup.

Therapeutic Management

The treatment of eating disorders initially focuses on disrupting the cycle of the eating disorder and addressing the secondary effects of self-induced vomiting, excessive use of diuretics and laxatives, and insufficient nutrients to sustain the function of body systems. Treatment may take place in an outpatient setting or in the inpatient setting if the

---

> **PATHOPHYSIOLOGY**
>
> ### EATING DISORDERS
>
> Frequently, impaired carbohydrate metabolism in the hypothalamic-pituitary axis is noted in individuals with an eating disorder. The conversion of thyroxine (T_4) to triiodothyronine (T_3) is inadequate. Phosphate concentrations are inadequate, especially in patients with severe anorexia complicated by bulimic episodes. Individuals with eating disorders commonly have hypokalemia, hypochloremia, hyponatremia, alkalosis, dental enamel erosion, parotid and salivary gland enlargement, decreased transferrin levels, and malabsorption complications.

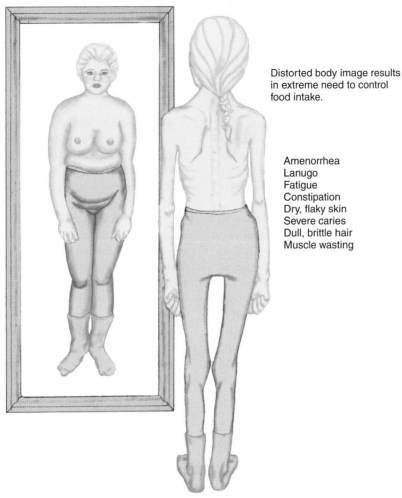

Distorted body image results
in extreme need to control
food intake.

Amenorrhea
Lanugo
Fatigue
Constipation
Dry, flaky skin
Severe caries
Dull, brittle hair
Muscle wasting

FIG 29-1   **In anorexia nervosa, the adolescent refuses to maintain adequate body weight, partly because of a distorted body image: she perceives herself as overweight when in fact she is below minimum weight.**

child's physical and emotional status requires more intensive treatment and monitoring (Sigman, 2003). Electrolyte levels and body chemistry values should be stabilized to prevent sustained damage to body systems, especially the cardiac, respiratory, and gastrointestinal systems. Adequate caloric intake is the next major goal of treatment and often requires strict monitoring to prevent sabotage of medical treatment. Continuing intensive and highly individualized therapy helps the adolescent cope with complex issues. Family intervention usually is necessary. Finally, alteration of misperceptions about body image and a reorientation to issues of control and self-management are necessary. Follow-up therapy for the individual and family is indicated for a period of several months to 3 years. A long-term consequence related to eating disorders is osteoporosis from interruption to bone density formation during adolescence (Sigman, 2003). Psychopharmacological treatment of children with anorexia nervosa has not been generally effective, although use of SSRIs may be helpful for adolescents with bulimia (Phillips & Pratt, 2005).

NURSING CARE

The Child or Adolescent With an Eating Disorder

Assessment

Children and adolescents with eating disorders typically have varying degrees of mistrust, ambivalence, and denial. It is generally better if the assessment is conducted in a structured and concrete manner (rather than as an open-ended exploration), with an emphasis placed on alliance building and periodic review of the assessment process for the child or adolescent. Determining motivations for changing behaviors is crucial, and motives should be assessed for each specific behavior (i.e., weight gain, induced vomiting, altered self-perception of body). A mental status examination should also be included because the side effects of restrictive dieting can impair cognitive functioning and perpetuate affective disturbances. Any history of self-injury should be noted. The nurse should assist the child or adolescent in gaining an understanding of impulse control problems and ritualistic and compulsive behaviors.

The medical history and physical assessment should be comprehensive, focusing on any medically based illness that mimics an eating disorder or exists concomitantly. Psychologic assessment of body image and identification of problems, substance abuse, and social support systems used by the child or adolescent are important components of the assessment. A family history of eating disorders or other psychiatric illnesses should be noted. Family dynamics, including the level or quality of interaction, support, discipline, and differentiation of members, should be explored in depth. Previous treatment attempts and coping strategies should also be identified.

School nurses or nurses in community settings are in an optimal position for recognizing children and adolescents with eating disorders. They become familiar with students they see on a regular basis and can readily assess changes in weight, emotional status, or behaviors. Once considered an adolescent problem, eating disorders are occurring in much younger children, so nurses in elementary schools need to be aware of the early signs. Awareness programs organized by school nurses often facilitate inquiries from children who might not normally speak about their eating problems or concerns about weight. Short screening tools are available to assist school nurses identify children at risk.

Nursing Diagnosis and Planning

The nursing diagnoses and expected outcomes that apply to the child or adolescent with an eating disorder follow:
- Imbalanced Nutrition: Less Than Body Requirements related to inadequate intake, malabsorption from extended periods of starvation, or distorted body image.
  Expected Outcome: The child or adolescent will meet daily nutritional requirements, as evidenced by sufficient weight gain or maintenance of an adequate weight to sustain systemic homeostasis and physiologic health.
- Anxiety, Fear, or Powerlessness related to weight gain, sense of inadequacy, and lack of control over body and self.
  Expected Outcome: The child or adolescent will display decreased anxiety, fear, and powerlessness, as evidenced by demonstration of the ability to seek help with anxiety management and demonstration of improved coping strategies, including open expression of feelings.
- Risk for Activity Intolerance or Disturbed Sleep Pattern related to fatigue, depression, and an excessive drive to exercise and expend energy.
  Expected Outcome: The child or adolescent will have adequate rest, as evidenced by an ability to establish improved sleeping and activity patterns with a corresponding improvement in affect, energy, and sense of well-being.
- Deficient Fluid Volume related to excessive use of diuretics or laxatives or inadequate fiber and fluid intake.
  Expected Outcome: The child or adolescent will maintain fluid and electrolyte balance, as evidenced by electrolyte levels within normal limits, normal skin turgor, and moist mucous membranes.

Interventions

Children and adolescents with severe eating disorders may need to be hospitalized to achieve physiologic stability. These children are then generally transferred to a day treatment program. Care focuses on restructuring cognitive perceptions, reducing opportunities to engage in ritualistic and self-injurious behaviors, and re-establishing physiologic homeostasis. The programs typically include interventions that enlist the adolescent's cooperation in a refeeding program. Nutritional consultation is provided to facilitate gradual weight gain. Intake and output, weight gain, vital signs, laboratory values, electrolyte status, and cardiac status are carefully monitored.

Support in exploring refeeding sensations of fullness, bloating, and delayed gastric emptying and help in tolerating these feelings and body sensations are important. The nurse and child or adolescent jointly participate in monitoring affect, mood, and potential for suicide. They also agree to a contract specifying necessary interventions to ensure safety and to monitor daily food intake and feelings. These interventions may take the form of interacting with the staff at regular intervals or agreeing to approach the staff if suicidal ideation is present. The nurse will need to validate the adolescent's feelings of ambivalence, fear, and powerlessness. If hyperalimentation or nasogastric tube feedings are needed for adequate nutritional intake, the nurse should support the child or adolescent and monitor feedings. Finally, the nurse should provide educational information about the short-term and long-term effects of starvation.

The nurse is likely to participate in providing or supporting psychologic treatments, such as individual, group, and family therapy sessions. Especially in the early phase of treatment, the child or adolescent may be very resistant to efforts to increase nutritional intake and may resort to denial, trickery, or manipulation to prevent a weight increase or thwart adherence to dietary regimens. It may be necessary to observe the child or adolescent after meals to prevent episodes of purging.

The family should be informed and involved in treatment goals and progress. Participation in family therapy is generally a required part of the treatment plan because the cause may be directly related to family interactional patterns. The nurse should support the family in voicing concerns while encouraging them to view the adolescent as having an independent identity and sense of control.

Evaluation

- Does the child or adolescent demonstrate an increase in food consumption adequate to sustain growth and developmental needs?
- Has the child or adolescent reduced bingeing or purging activities?
- Can the child or adolescent demonstrate a positive alteration in self-perceptions and body image, as evidenced by verbalizing an increased sense of self-control and decreased anxiety about the present and the future?

- Does the child or adolescent demonstrate a decrease in ambivalence and mistrust about self and significant others?
- Does the child or adolescent show increased energy and display appropriate affect?
- Are electrolyte levels within normal limits, and are mucous membranes moist?

ATTENTION-DEFICIT HYPERACTIVITY DISORDER

Attention-deficit hyperactivity disorder (ADHD) is the most common chronic behavioral disorder of children. ADHD is associated with significant problems in three areas: (1) attention and concentration, (2) impulse control, and (3) overactivity. Over the years, it has variously been called *postencephalitic behavior disorder, restlessness syndrome, hyperkinetic impulse disorder, minimal brain dysfunction,* and *hyperactive child syndrome.* There is evidence based on neuroimaging and on neurophysiologic and neurochemical data that developmental failure in brain circuitry underlies the impulsivity and hyperactivity or poor response regulation and inhibition (Meyers, Eisenhauer, & Ryan, 2003).

Referrals for ADHD may be made by parents or teachers. Of concern are not only the primary symptoms, which often result in frequent injuries, poor scholastic performance, and low performance motivation, but also the associated symptoms, which may include anxiety or depression, aggressiveness toward peers, and antisocial or oppositional defiance toward authority figures.

A single child affected with ADHD may exhibit wide variations in response to the environment. For example, a child with ADHD is likely to perform poorly on a highly complex task. If the structure is rigid or if behavior is severely restricted, the child with ADHD becomes increasingly frustrated and distinguishable from unaffected children. If instructions are repeated frequently or if the task is novel or unfamiliar, the child's performance tends to improve. Immediate reinforcement is very important because these children require much higher rates of reinforcement than their same-age peers. Fatigue may also affect the degree to which ADHD symptoms are exhibited.

Etiology

ADHD occurs more commonly in first-degree biologic relatives of people with the disorder than in the general population, which suggests a genetic predisposition for the disorder. Other central nervous system (CNS) abnormalities, such as the presence of neurotoxins and epilepsy, or other neurologic disorders are thought to be predisposing factors, although fewer than 5% of children with ADHD have definitive neurologic findings. Chaotic or abusive environments may predispose to the appearance of ADHD.

Incidence

Estimates of the incidence of ADHD range from 1% to 20%, but the general consensus is that 4% to 12% of children are affected with ADHD. Symptoms generally occur early in childhood, with the mean age at onset 3 or 4 years; however, medication treatment may not be started until the child is in a structured school setting (Sadock & Sadock, 2003). In epidemiologic studies, the male-to-female ratio is approximately 3:1 among nonreferred children displaying ADHD symptoms. Aggressive and antisocial behaviors are thought to explain the higher rate of referrals of boys.

Manifestations

Children with ADHD can typically exhibit clusters of signs and symptoms that are primarily inattentive, primarily impulsive/hyperactive, or a combination. Signs usually must be present for at least 6 months, have occurred before the age of 7 years, be present in two or more settings (e.g., home, school, recreation, church), not be associated with another mental or developmental disorder, and significantly impair at least one level of functioning (academic, social, occupational) (American Psychiatric Association, 2000). Although the American Psychiatric Association calls this disorder *ADHD,* not all children with the disorder exhibit hyperactivity, although most demonstrate a degree of impulsivity.

According to the American Psychiatric Association (2000), to be diagnosed with ADHD, a child must exhibit six or more of the hallmark behaviors included below under *inattention* and *impulsivity/hyperactivity:*

- *Inattention:* carelessness, inattention to details, difficulty attending to work or games, does not listen, poor follow-through with instructions or does not complete tasks, difficulty with organization skills, avoidance of tasks that require mental effort, misplaces equipment or supplies necessary to complete tasks, easily distracted, forgetful
- *Impulsivity/hyperactivity:* fidgets with hands, feet, or hair; unable to remain in a seat for extended periods; runs and climbs excessively in inappropriate settings; difficulty in engaging in quiet activities; mostly "on the go"; talks excessively; blurts out questions or answers; cannot await a turn; interrupts conversations

ADHD can also be associated with other disorders, such as motor disorders, oppositional defiant disorder, mood disorders, and anxiety disorders. Children with ADHD often have a diagnosed learning disability (Leslie, Weckerly, Plemmons, Landsverk, & Eastman, 2004).

PATHOPHYSIOLOGY

ATTENTION-DEFICIT HYPERACTIVITY DISORDER

Inconclusive but consistent evidence indicates that the basis of ADHD is a sluggish or underreactive neurologic, electrophysiologic response to stimulation. Prefrontal and limbic system connections in the brain are viewed as the likely locations for neurologic functional abnormalities. Hypotheses have been made that dopaminergic and noradrenergic function plays a central role because medications addressing these neurotransmitters are effective for treatment. This information suggests that higher levels of norepinephrine and lower levels of epinephrine activity seen in children with ADHD may play a role.

Diagnostic Evaluation

Although high-resolution magnetic resonance imaging and blood and urine studies of metabolites of brain neurotransmitters have been performed in individuals with ADHD, none of these tests have provided consistent diagnostic information. The diagnosis of ADHD is currently established on the basis of reports by the child, parent, and teacher. The behaviors and symptoms of ADHD must be present in two of three areas—home, school, or social situations—to support the diagnosis. These reports are coupled with psychologic assessments conducted while the child is completing tasks requiring vigilance, attention, and concentration and those involving delayed gratification. Clinical interviews may be coupled with clinical trials of psychopharmacologic agents to determine the child's behavioral response.

Therapeutic Management

The goal of therapeutic management is to reduce the frequency and intensity of unsocialized behaviors. This requires achieving a balance between the child's temperament and environmental demands, expectancies, and supports. Therefore, treatment interventions must be targeted at enhancing the child's capabilities and self-esteem. Expectations that may be appropriate for a child without ADHD—"he should be able to sit still in school for 40 minutes," or "she should be able to handle 1 hour of homework"—may need to be modified for the child with ADHD. In every case, the nurse should work with the parents to modify the environment and to develop strategies that foster competencies in the child. Most clinicians combine psychopharmacotherapy with behavior-oriented family therapy to achieve alterations in the child's internal functioning and external environment. Stimulant medications commonly used as part of the treatment plan include methylphenidate (Ritalin), dextroamphetamine (Dexedrine), and amphetamine/dextroamphetamine (Adderall). Newer timed-released formulas of methylphenidate (Concerta, Ritalin LA, and Metadate ER) and amphetamine/dextroamphetamine (Adderall XR) are advantageous for once-a-day

USING RESEARCH TO IMPROVE PRACTICE

Living with a child who has ADHD can be challenging for parents and other family members on a daily basis. Because of their sometimes disruptive or oppositional behavior, children with ADHD can interact negatively with others, even with family members, and family conflicts can become frequent. Often, parents of children with ADHD have difficulties themselves because their child's behavior offers fewer positive parenting experiences, decreases parenting self-confidence, and increases stress. These parenting outcomes can contribute to negative social, emotional, and educational outcomes in the child.

Kendall, Leo, Perrin, and Hatton (2005) wanted to explore the relationships among the behavior of the child with ADHD, maternal stress, and family conflict. They proposed to test a theoretic model that suggested that the child's sex (boy), age (older), and existence of other social or emotional problems would increase the child's behavior difficulties, maternal distress, and family conflict. They also theorized that both the child's behaviors and other sociodemographic factors, such as income and ethnicity, would directly affect family conflict as well.

This study was a descriptive, cross-sectional, and correlational design that explored the relationships among three main variables: the child's behavior problems (as measured by the CBCL), mother's distress (measured by subscales of the Brief Symptom Inventory), and family conflict (measured with the Family Environment Scale). Demographic information was obtained about the child and family characteristics. All measures used in this study had proven reliability; validity was not addressed by the authors.

The authors collected data from 157, ethnically diverse families (31% African American, 36% Latino, 33% white) having at least one child with ADHD and a mother in the home. This convenience sample came primarily from urban settings. The majority were single-parent families with income less than $40,000 per year.

Data were analyzed by using factor analysis and structural equation modeling to confirm the theoretic relationships. The results of this study are interesting and can be considered when planning nursing care for families who have a child with ADHD. Significant positive relationships were demonstrated between the presence of comorbidity and the child's behaviors, the level of the child's behavior problems and the mother's distress, the level of maternal stress and amount of family conflict, and the child's age and level of family conflict. Other results suggest that the higher the family income, the fewer behavior problems the child had; ethnicity was not shown to be a factor in either family conflict or the child's behavior, however, Latino families had fewer family conflicts compared with white families. The researchers acknowledge that limitations of the study include the nature of the cross-sectional design and the fact that data were collected from only one source and by one method. They also state that their sample size was less than ideal.

By far the most important finding of this study is the fact that the child's behavior problems do not directly affect the level of family conflict, but only indirectly by affecting the level of maternal stress. The researchers suggest that because mothers carry the primary responsibility for caring for the child, along with their other social and emotional responsibilities, and that the mother's distress level can affect family conflict, the mother's emotional health should receive important consideration.

Think about how these findings might be used in clinical practice. If, as the researchers suggest, nurses should intervene with mothers of children with ADHD, as well as the children themselves, what strategies might the nurse use to do this? In what setting should intervention take place?

Kendall, J., Leo, M., Perrin, N., & Hatton, D. (2005). Modeling ADHD child and family relationships. *Western Journal of Nursing Research, 27,* 500-518.

dosing, thereby eliminating midday trips to the nurse's office. Atomoxetine (Strattera), a nonstimulant medication, has also been used with success in the treatment of ADHD. Medication treatment is most effective when it is used in conjunction with behavior and psychosocial therapy. It is important to individually tailor the child's medication dosage to achieve maximum results with the fewest side effects. For this reason, medications usually are titrated over several weeks (Greydanus, Pratt, Sloane, & Rappley, 2003).

Some parents and professionals prefer more conservative approaches, such as dietary changes, to the treatment of ADHD. Although researchers continue to debate whether food additives and sugars have significant clinical influences on most children with ADHD, the general consensus is that they do not. Medication is typically administered during the school day, but it has become increasingly recognized that attention, concentration, and alertness are needed for any learning task, such as learning to play baseball or learning to drive a car. The side effects and potency of the medications used to treat ADHD often make parents and physicians hesitant to administer medications other than during critical learning periods.

NURSING CARE

The Child With Attention-Deficit Hyperactivity Disorder

Assessment

The nurse should document the parent's description of the typical behavior of the child playing alone and with other children, during mealtimes, and while the parent is on the telephone or occupied with chores. The length of time it takes the child to bathe or dress and how often the child becomes distracted during these tasks are also explored. These behaviors are then compared with those exhibited when the child is engaged in highly stimulating activities and activities with frequent feedback, such as video and computer games. The child's behavior is also compared during novel versus routine activities.

The child's developmental and family history are explored in detail, with the nurse noting the age at which the child began to exhibit independent behaviors, such as walking, getting out of bed alone, and exploring the environment. It is not uncommon for children with ADHD to explore the environment at an early age, with only limited need to return to the caregiver for support or approval. Family members diagnosed with ADHD or who exhibit similar behaviors are noted. Parents should be given self-report inventories, such as the CBCL, Conner's Teacher Rating Scale–Revised, or the Attention-Deficit/Hyperactivity Disorder Rating Scale, to complete and return to the appropriate professional.

Observation within the home or school setting is likely to generate the most valid information because the clinic environment may be unfamiliar and, by the nature of the disorder, may inhibit the child's natural tendency to explore, become distracted, or display limited motivation in task completion.

Nursing Diagnosis and Planning

The nursing diagnoses and expected outcomes that apply to the child with ADHD and the child's family are as follows:

- Impaired Social Interaction related to impulsivity, poor self-management skills, and aggressive behaviors.

 Expected Outcomes: The child will demonstrate an improvement in social interactions, as evidenced by improvement in impulse control and an ability to sustain attention on tasks. The child will relate in a more positive way with peers.

- Risk for Injury related to impulsivity, limited judgment skills, or excessive need for mobility and stimulation.

 Expected Outcome: The child will remain safe from injury, as evidenced by a decrease in injuries and implementation of a plan to prevent injuries.

- Compromised Family Coping or Disabled Family Coping related to the need for consistent and close supervision of the child, the child's hyperactivity, or social stigma of having a child with impulsive or aggressive behaviors.

 Expected Outcome: The family will mobilize coping strategies, as evidenced by an ability to discuss the child's needs and a plan to provide the needed support.

- Deficient Knowledge related to perceptions that the child is willfully defiant or disobedient in following directions or in testing limits.

 Expected Outcome: The family will increase knowledge related to their child's condition, as evidenced by a willingness to discuss the child's condition and display an understanding of the condition and its treatment.

Interventions

The primary nursing intervention for the child with ADHD is to teach the family about the disorder. Emphasis is placed on reducing the parents' blame and guilt about the child's problems and altering their perceptions that the child intentionally misbehaves or lacks motivation to learn or achieve. Teaching demonstrates ways to provide frequent positive reinforcement. Also, important for parents and the child is instruction about medications and the adaptations in environment that are needed to allow the child to practice new skills.

The nurse may facilitate communication between the family and the school about ways to accommodate the child's shortened attention span and increased need for mobility and frequent breaks. Often cognitive-behavioral therapy, provided by a specially trained professional, is helpful in identifying specific exercises that can reduce bothersome traits. Support groups for parents can help families cope with the child with ADHD and modify their interactions with and expectations of the child.

Ordinarily, positive effects of medication on the child's behavior are seen immediately; however, it may take several weeks to titrate the medication to the point that symptoms are controlled with the fewest side effects (Greydanus et al., 2003). It is common for the family to observe a rapid change in the child's behavior and to feel relief as manifestations subside. Continuing support is required because this disorder is life long and progress in self-control and behavioral patterns is usually slow. Parents and school nurses need to be actively involved in dispensing medication, even through adolescence, because children fluctuate in their willingness to adhere to therapy. Affected children also may have difficulty remembering to take the medication because of the attentional deficits characteristic of the disorder.

Evaluation

- Does the child adhere to the cognitive and pharmacologic strategies designed to increase self-control, as evidenced by a decrease in impulsivity and an increase in attention to task?
- Does the child complete school assignments in less time than formerly, with less distractibility?
- Does the child demonstrate increased skill in peer relations, as evidenced by fewer conflicts and more frequent positive statements to and about peers?
- Does the family provide a safe and supportive environment within the home, as evidenced by adequate supervision and opportunities for meeting the child's mobility needs in a safe manner?
- Does the family demonstrate acceptance of the child and the child's special needs?
- Does the family demonstrate an increased acceptance of the child's condition as a medical problem rather than a social or behavioral problem?
- Does the family adhere to the medication regimen?

SUBSTANCE ABUSE

Chemical agents that are typically abused by children and adolescents include alcohol, hallucinogens, sedatives, analgesics, anxiolytics, steroids, inhalants, and stimulants. The substance abused depends on its availability and cost and on social influences and parental behaviors or tolerance of drug use. Most professionals differentiate between *substance abuse* and *substance addiction*. However, the basic treatment concerns are similar. Substance abuse is generally considered to increase over time.

Etiology

Productive analysis of substance abuse considers risk factors, which include social, personal, and familial factors.

Substance abuse and substance dependence tend to cluster in families, with clinical evidence of genetic influences. For alcohol, as for most other drugs, there also is some evidence that substance abuse often represents the child's or adolescent's attempt to cope with anxiety generated by impaired social skills, low self-esteem, poor interpersonal relationships, or lack of adaptive behaviors. Some psychosocial disorders, such as ADHD, depression, and conduct disorder, are associated with an increased risk of substance abuse.

Incidence

Great variation exists in the types of substances abused across sexes and ages (Table 29-1). Typically, boys consume alcohol more than girls do. Female junior high school students are increasing their use of tobacco, whereas tobacco use by their male counterparts has remained consistent.

The National Institute on Drug Abuse has tracked illicit drug use and attitudes toward drug, alcohol, and cigarette among middle school and high school students nationwide since 1975. Each fall, the updated results of the Monitoring the Future Survey are released. According to the 2004 results, analysis from 2001 to 2004 revealed a 17% cumulative decline in drug use by eighth, tenth, and twelfth graders (National Institute of Drug Abuse, 2004).

Illicit drug use, including alcohol and tobacco, remains high despite reports of declining use among adolescents. In 2004, the percentage of teens using marijuana was between 11.8% and 34.3%, cocaine use was between 2% and 5.3%, and heroin use was at 1%. Nonmedical use of pain medication such as Vicodin (hydrocodone and acetaminophen) was between 5.2% and 9.3%, and alcohol use was 36.7% to 70.6%. The greatest concern in current trends of illicit use of drugs by teenagers is the increase in use of painkillers (Johnson, O'Malley, Bachman, & Schulenberg, 2005). It is estimated that 90% of adolescents have tried alcohol by the time they reach adulthood. The earlier an individual begins to use alcohol, the more likely dependence will develop (U.S. DHHS, 2000). Experimentation with marijuana, the most widely used illicit drug, is reported in nearly one fourth of eighth graders and approximately one half of twelfth graders. Research consistently supports the hypothesis that drug use progresses from beer or wine to cigarettes or hard liquor and then marijuana, followed by other illicit drugs. These substances are sometimes referred

---

CRITICAL TO REMEMBER
Risks for Substance Abuse

Family systems that are closed to outsiders, that have a history of psychiatric disturbance, including substance abuse, or that have poor communication skills are at risk for creating an environment in which substance abuse in youth occurs.

PATHOPHYSIOLOGY

SUBSTANCE ABUSE
The primary effect of substance abuse is on the brain and residually on the rest of the body. The actual action depends on the type of substance used because substances act in accordance with their specific chemical compositions. For example, alcohol affects the entire brain by decreasing its responsiveness.

TABLE 29-1	Commonly Abused Drugs and Their Effects

Drug	Expected Behaviors and Effects	Special Considerations
Tobacco	Chronic cough, wheezing, increased phlegm production, atherosclerosis	Considered a gateway drug; initial use usually begins in elementary school
Alcohol	Amount-related effects include euphoria followed by depression or hostility, decreased inhibitions, impaired judgment, uncoordination, and slurred speech	Considered a gateway drug; easily accessible
Marijuana	Relaxation, mild euphoria, loss of inhibition, decreased motivation, red eyes, dry mouth	Considered a gateway drug
Opiates	Euphoria, elation, pain relief, detachment and apathy, drowsiness, constricted pupils, constipation, slurred speech, impaired judgment	Long-term apathy about self, often leading to physical malnutrition and dehydration; criminal behaviors associated with obtaining drugs likely to occur; infections at injection sites common
Barbiturates	Similar to those associated with alcohol	Often used in conjunction with stimulants; may have a paradoxic effect of hyperactivity in children
Amphetamines	Euphoria, hyperactivity, agitation, irritability, insomnia, weight loss, tachycardia, hypertension	May have a paradoxic effect of depression in children
Cocaine	Euphoria, elation, agitation, hyperactivity, irritability, pressured speech, grandiosity, tachycardia, hypertension, diaphoresis, anorexia, weight loss, insomnia	Psychotic behavior possible if the dose is large; can be fatal if combined with other drugs
Hallucinogens (lysergic acid diethylamide [LSD], methylenedioxymeth-amphetamine ["ecstasy"])	Distorted perceptions, heightened awareness, hallucinations, illusions, depersonalization, dilated pupils, hypertension, increased salivation	Psychotic behaviors, panic flashbacks long after drug use ceases, self-destructive behaviors
Phencyclidine hydrochloride (PCP)	Euphoria, distorted perceptions, agitation, violence, antisocial behaviors, hypertension, increased salivation, increased pain response	Panic, irrational behaviors, psychosis

---

BOX 29-2	Phases of Substance Abuse

Phase 1: Experimentation
The drug is taken to see what it does or to appease peers.

Phase 2: Early Drug Use
A specific drug or various drugs are used with some regularity for their pleasurable effects or to reduce anxiety. Social use of drugs typically falls into this category.

Phase 3: True Drug Addiction
Drugs are used regularly, and physical dependence begins if it is characteristic of the drug. Social functioning revolves around a drug focus.

Phase 4: Severe Drug Addiction
The physical condition of the addicted child or adolescent deteriorates. All activities are related to obtaining or using the drug, with isolation from nondrug culture.

to as *gateway substances*. Substance use is strongly associated with other high-risk behaviors in adolescence, such as unintentional injuries and unprotected sexual encounters (Box 29-2).

Public awareness and emphasis on treatment and prevention seem to be working. Although these factors had very limited impact on teenagers in the 1990s, there is a promising indication of an increase in the belief that illicit drugs are harmful and increased numbers of teenagers disapprove of their use. Reducing substance abuse is a national health goal identified in *Healthy People 2010* (U.S. DHHS, 2000). An awareness of the possibility of substance abuse is the responsibility of the parent, teacher, and health professional. Knowing the clinical behavioral manifestations of substance abuse is essential, and much information is readily available to adults interested in prevention and early identification.

Manifestations

The clinical manifestations of substance abuse are marked by increased antisocial behavior as the desire for social conformity and acceptance decreases and the need for the substance increases. Behaviors that may indicate substance abuse problems include irregular school attendance, low grades or poor school performance, aggressive or rebellious behavior, excessive dependence on peer influence, and deterioration of relationships with family members or former friends. Rapid or extreme changes in behavior or mood and loss of interest in hobbies, sports, or other favorite activities are often observed. Lack of parental support and supervision and changes in eating or sleeping patterns that increase as manipulative behaviors increase, especially those that are related to the need to acquire desired substances, may also be involved.

CRITICAL TO REMEMBER
Relapse Among Substance Abusers
Substance abusers' rates of refusal to adhere to therapeutic recommendations, together with resulting relapses, are quite high. More than 60% of those completing a course of treatment continue to abuse substances throughout their lifetimes.

Therapeutic Management

Treatment in a center specifically designed for substance abuse is recommended and includes individual, group, and family therapy. Participation in Alcoholics Anonymous or Narcotics Anonymous is advocated. These organizations also offer support groups geared toward helping family members with programs that promote alterations in the family system to decrease the likelihood of relapse.

NURSING CARE

The Child or Adolescent With a Substance Abuse Problem

Assessment
Physical assessment should include evaluation of the child's or adolescent's respiratory rate, heart rate, blood pressure, activity level (hyperactive, hypoactive), mood, affect, judgment, speech, sensory responses, and memory. A thorough history of current and past drug use should be obtained. A family and social history, a medical history, and a legal history (e.g., past and current charges related to substance abuse) should be obtained.

Nursing Diagnosis and Planning
The nursing diagnoses and expected outcomes that apply to the child or adolescent with a substance abuse problem follow:
* Disturbed Thought Processes related to the specific effects of the particular substance involved.
  Expected Outcome: The child or adolescent will exhibit behaviors indicative of the absence of substance abuse, as evidenced by the ability to maintain orientation to time, place, and person.
* Disturbed Sensory Perception related to the specific effects of the particular substance involved.
  Expected Outcome: The child or adolescent will remain free from sensory changes, as evidenced by the absence of falls or other injuries.
* Anxiety related to a decrease in sense of control over self or the environment.

Expected Outcome: The child or adolescent will display decreased anxiety, as evidenced by verbalization of increased feelings of self-worth and the ability to change behavior.
* Ineffective Coping related to limited development of effective social interactions and problem-solving skills.
  Expected Outcome: The child or adolescent will increase ability to interact socially and to problem solve, as evidenced by an ability to identify current stressors leading to substance use or abuse.
* Impaired Social Interaction related to anxiety or limited social skills.
  Expected Outcome: The child or adolescent will begin to develop healthy social skills, as evidenced by an ability to identify alternative activities, people, and social situations that discourage substance abuse.
* Situational Low Self-Esteem or Chronic Low Self-Esteem related to limited social skills, ineffective coping skills, or a poor sense of self-management.
  Expected Outcome: The child or adolescent will increase self-esteem, as evidenced by replacing substance abuse with more appropriate social skills and developing meaningful relationships with nonabusing peers and family members.

Interventions
The nurse's responsibilities in caring for children or adolescents with substance abuse problems depend on the care setting, the severity of the abuse, and the treatment goals. Often, the use or abuse of substances in a child is reported to the school nurse by other students. In this instance, appropriate care and referral begins in the school setting and may include a thorough assessment and parent notification. The nurse can be a resource for parents and community members as to agencies within the community that can assist the child and family. Many school districts have a zero tolerance policy for tobacco, drugs, and alcohol; in some instances, the school resource officer or local police may need to be called. Often this decision is made by a crisis team within the school that includes the school nurse as a participating member. Most school districts actively incorporate alcohol and drug prevention programs in their curricula for students at various grade levels.

If the youth has been identified as a substance abuser and referred to a treatment facility, the nurse's primary responsibility will be to stabilize the child's or adolescent's physiologic status and support recommendations for treatment. Explaining the expectations and the types of services offered is important because most treatment programs increase child or adolescent and family responsibilities over time.

Initially, maintaining safety and an optimal level of physical comfort is necessary, especially if detoxification is required. This includes close observation, removal of any potentially dangerous items, and monitoring vital signs. Being readily available to discuss thoughts, concerns, and perceptions is important to create an emotional sense of safety. Additional interventions include educating the child or adolescent and family members about necessary laboratory tests and providing information about the nature of substance abuse.

Another significant nursing intervention is to assist the child or adolescent and family in developing social support systems and refer them to appropriate resources that can offer additional support as they make long-term changes in their social and emotional patterns of relating. It is also essential to help the youth assume responsibility for the substance abuse problem, rather than passing the blame on to others. Providing emotional support for the youth and family as they develop insight into their behaviors and the need for changes is important because these changes are often difficult to effect.

The relapse rate among youthful substance abusers is extremely high, and success in a short-term treatment program is not necessarily an indicator of long-term control. The incidence of relapse is generally reduced if the child and family maintain active, long-term involvement in support groups, such as Alcoholics Anonymous, Ala-Teen, Ala-Tot, and Narcotics Anonymous. Tough Love support groups for parents may also be beneficial in providing counsel and support.

Evaluation

- Has the child or adolescent remained substance free and been oriented to time and place?
- Has the child or adolescent remained injury free as a result of sensory or perceptual changes?
- Is the child or adolescent able to identify stressors and use appropriate coping mechanisms?
- Has the child or adolescent assumed responsibility for changing behaviors related to the substance abuse?
- Is the child or adolescent participating in daily activities?
- Does the child or adolescent show improvement in peer and family relationships?
- Does the child or adolescent demonstrate an increased sense of self-confidence?

INFANT WITH NEONATAL ABSTINENCE SYNDROME

Infants born to women who abuse drugs during their pregnancy may have withdrawal symptoms after birth and require nursing care on a pediatric unit or in a children's hospital. Neonatal abstinence syndrome refers to withdrawal symptoms in neonates caused by heroin or other opiates to which they have been exposed. Methadone exposure is a frequent cause of neonatal abstinence syndrome.

Incidence

Chemical dependence is one of the most frequently missed diagnoses in the management of pregnant women, increasing the risk for substance dependence in the neonate. Approximately 4% of pregnant women use illicit drugs, most often marijuana, at some time during their pregnancies. An equivalent number of pregnant women continue to use alcohol, and approximately 18% of pregnant women use tobacco (U.S. DHHS, Substance Abuse and Mental Health Services Administration, 2005). The true incidence of perinatal substance abuse is unknown because self-reporting of use is unreliable and toxicology screens usually detect use over only a short time frame. Approximately 10% to 20% of infants have prenatal substance exposure, and many of these display symptoms after birth (U.S. DHHS, Substance Abuse and Mental Health Services Administration National Clearinghouse for Alcohol and Drug Information, 2005).

Manifestations

The onset of withdrawal symptoms is variable. Symptoms may be present at birth or may not occur until 4 to 10 days after delivery. Infants born addicted to narcotics may exhibit withdrawal symptoms for 4 to 12 months. The majority of affected infants exhibit signs and symptoms described as follows:

- **W** = Wakefulness
- **I** = Irritability
- **T** = Tremulousness, temperature variation, tachypnea
- **H** = Hyperactivity, high-pitched persistent cry, hyperacusia, hyperreflexia, hypertonus
- **D** = Diarrhea, diaphoresis, dehydration, disorganized suck (uncoordinated and constant)
- **R** = Respiratory distress, rub marks, rhinorrhea
- **A** = Apnea, autonomic dysfunction
- **W** = Weight loss or failure to gain weight
- **A** = Alkalosis (respiratory)
- **L** = Lacrimation

In addition, the infant might exhibit an exaggerated Moro reflex and seizures.

Diagnostic Evaluation

When drug withdrawal has been identified or is suspected, obtaining urine and blood toxicology and drug screens on the mother and obtaining urine, blood, and meconium toxicology and drug screens on the infant can help confirm the diagnosis.

Therapeutic Management

Many infants undergoing withdrawal respond well to supportive measures. Sensory stimulation can be decreased by swaddling; a quiet, darkened environment; and comfort measures to prevent excessive crying. Frequent, small feedings of high-calorie formula help supply the additional caloric requirements.

More specific therapy may be required when withdrawal symptoms are severe. Infection, hypoglycemia, hypocalcemia, hypomagnesemia, hyperthyroidism, CNS hemorrhage, and anoxia must be excluded first as the etiology of the symptoms (American Academy of Pediatrics, 1998). Depending on the drug exposure involved, pharmacologic agents used in the treatment of withdrawal include tincture of opium, morphine, methadone, clonidine, diazepam (Valium), chlorpromazine (Thorazine), and phenobarbital. Because of the other addictive substances contained in paregoric, it should be used with particular caution (Johnson, Gerada, & Greenough, 2003). Polydrug exposure may require a combination of drugs.

Medication doses can be stabilized and then tapered once the infant sleeps well, eats effectively, and gains weight for 3 to 5 days. Failure to taper the dose may result in prolonged hospitalization. Treatment may last a few days or several weeks, depending on the severity of symptoms and the infant's response to treatment. Long-term follow-up of the infant's physical and mental development should be supervised by a physician who is knowledgeable about the symptoms and treatment of addicted infants and who is willing to communicate effectively with the parents. Although residual physical and psychosocial problems may persist in these infants, it is thought that they are less to do with the initial drug exposure than the subsequent social environment in which the child develops (American Academy of Pediatrics, 1998). Social workers are essential in determining the parents' ability to care for the infant after discharge.

Nursing Considerations

The nurse can help identify infants who are at risk for withdrawal by obtaining a social history from the parents and a detailed maternal drug history, including prescription and nonprescription drugs. The nurse should assess infants who are at risk for the presence of signs and symptoms of withdrawal. When drug withdrawal has been identified or is suspected, obtaining urine and blood toxicology and drug screens on the mother and urine, blood, and meconium toxicology and drug screens on the infant can help confirm the diagnosis. Nursing care is aimed at decreasing environmental stimuli, meeting the infant's nutritional needs, and promoting healthy parent-infant interaction. The infant's care is coordinated to limit the number of times the infant is disturbed. Noise and light levels in the nursery or home, especially in the infant's immediate vicinity, are maintained at minimal necessary levels. A light blanket can be placed over the top of the incubator to darken the area. Appropriate comfort measures are provided immediately when the infant exhibits irritability. These may include offering a pacifier, swaddling the infant, or rocking. The infant's ability to nipple-feed is assessed, and the infant is gavage-fed if necessary to provide adequate fluid and caloric intake. Weight gain is monitored daily, and length and head circumferences are monitored weekly to ensure that nutritional intake is sufficient for growth. Because these infants are usually irritable, providing their nursing care can be challenging and stressful. Parent-infant interaction is at an especially high risk in these cases, and special effort is made to involve the parents in the infant's care. Contact between parents and social services, such as child protection and community health agencies, is made before discharge in an effort to optimize the functioning of the family unit and the child's long-term psychological outcome.

CHILDHOOD PHYSICAL AND EMOTIONAL ABUSE AND CHILD NEGLECT

Child abuse includes emotional abuse, physical abuse, and sexual exploitation or molestation by caretakers or other individuals. Deliberate failure to provide for a child's physical, educational or emotional needs is considered to be neglect (U.S. DHHS Child Welfare Information Gateway, 2005). Although the federal definition of child abuse includes neglect, some states separately define neglect and each major type of abuse (U.S. DHHS Child Welfare Information Gateway, 2005).

Etiology

Family dysfunction underlies most forms of child abuse or neglect. The family profile varies with the type of abuse, although it is not uncommon for multiple types of abuse to exist in a single family. Generally, the dysfunctional family dynamics are multigenerational and involve both parents (Box 29-3).

Socioeconomic factors also appear to influence the incidence and etiology of child abuse, with increased physical abuse observed during periods of economic hardship or external stress. The typical perpetrator is a direct relative of the child, usually the parent (79.7%) or primary caretaker, younger than 40 years (43.8%), and female (58.2%) (U.S. DHHS Administration on Children, Youth, and Families, 2005).

In sexual abuse, the perpetrator is more likely to be a family friend or neighbor (75.9%) compared with a parent (2.7%) (U.S. DHHS Administration on Children, Youth, and Families, 2005). Often this individual has limited coping skills and was abused as a child or teenager (Mulryan, Cathers, & Fagin, 2004).

The typical profile of an abused child is more difficult to determine. Some research indicates that the child who is

---

BOX 29-3	**Characteristics of the Abusive Family**

- Isolation from community and social groups
- Intense competition for emotional resources within the family, such as affection, attention, and nurturing
- Low levels of differentiation among family members
- Low trust for outsiders and family members
- Unpredictable and unstable family environment
- Conflict resolution generally achieved through aggression or power struggle between family members
- Current focus and crisis-oriented actions for immediate gratification
- Communication often characterized by mixed or double messages, threats, or a focus on nonverbal communication rather than direct verbalization
- Family roles that are typically fixed and traditional, with rigid rules
- Frequent domination by a single family member who maintains control through manipulation, intimidation, deceit, and aggression

physically abused typically is younger than 5 years, often has mild physical abnormalities, is developmentally or physically delayed, has a difficult temperament, or reminds the abuser of someone else. A parent is far more likely to kill a stepchild than a biologic child. Victims of sexual abuse are usually between 6 and 9 years old at the onset of the abuse.

Incidence

Child abuse reports to child protective services have increased. This increase has been attributed to the public's, teachers', and clinicians' increased awareness and willingness to report rather than to an actual increase in prevalence. In 2003, 56.8% of reports to child protective services nationwide were made by professionals (U.S. DHHS Administration on Children, Youth, and Families, 2005).

In 2003, slightly fewer than 1 million children were identified as victims of substantiated physical or emotional abuse or neglect. Of those identified, 60.9% suffered from neglect, 18.9% were physically abused, and 5% were emotional maltreated. The national rate of victimization is 12.4 in 1000 children (U.S. DHHS Administration on Children, Youth, and Families, 2005).

Approximately 1500 children died from maltreatment in 2003. Seventy-nine percent of children killed were younger than 4 years and 43.6% were younger than 1 year when they died (U.S. DHHS Administration on Children, Youth, and Families, 2005).

Sexual Abuse

In 2003, 9.9% were victims of sexual abuse (U.S. DHHS Administration on Children, Youth, and Families, 2005). Girls outnumber boys as victims of sexual abuse, however, reported incidences of sexual abuse may represent less than the actual incidence in boys.

Manifestations

Physical Indicators of Physical Abuse

Physical indicators of physical abuse include unexplained bruises or welts that appear in various stages of healing, often in clustered patterns that reflect the shapes of the articles used to inflict injury, and unexplained burns, especially on the soles, palms, back, or buttocks; immersion burns may be seen (socklike, glovelike, or doughnut-shaped) on buttocks or genitalia (Fig. 29-2). Other signs may include infected burns, which indicate a delay in seeking treatment, and bald patches on the scalp. Unexplained fractures of the skull, nose, or facial structures or multiple or spiral fractures or dislocations, as well as numerous fractures in various stages of healing, are also significant (National Children's Advocacy Center, 2006; U.S. DHHS Child Welfare Information Gateway, 2006a).

Behavioral Indicators of Physical Abuse

Behavioral indicators of physical abuse include a child's wariness in response to adult contact, apprehension when others cry or lack of crying when approached by a stranger or examiner, and fear of parents or of going home. Extreme aggressiveness or withdrawal, vacant or frozen stares, monosyllabic responses to questions, and lying very still when surveying surroundings may be observed. Runaway behavior is not uncommon in abused adolescents. A capacity to engage only in superficial relationships and manipulative behaviors to get attention may also be reactions to abusive situations (National Children's Advocacy Center, 2006; U.S. DHHS Child Welfare Information Gateway, 2006a).

Physical Indicators of Neglect

Children experiencing neglect will most often show inadequate weight gain for age, poor growth pattern, and failure to thrive. They may exhibit constant hunger, poor hygiene, wasting of subcutaneous tissue, and bald patches on the scalp, and they may be dressed in clothes that are not seasonally suitable (e.g., no coat or shoes in winter). Reports of lack of supervision for long periods, permission to engage in unsafe activities, or abandonment may also accompany a neglected child (National Children's Advocacy Center, 2006; U.S. DHHS Child Welfare Information Gateway, 2006a).

Behavioral Indicators of Neglect

A child who begs or steals food, has inconsistent school attendance or comes very early and stays very late at school, or is constantly fatigued or listless in class may be exhibiting the effects of neglect. Other behavioral indicators of neglect include assuming adult responsibilities or roles, alcohol or substance abuse, and delinquency (National Children's Advocacy Center, 2006; U.S. DHHS Child Welfare Information Gateway, 2006a).

Physical Indicators of Emotional Abuse

Children who have been emotionally abused may exhibit speech disorders, lags in physical development, failure to thrive, or hyperactive and disruptive behaviors. (National Children's Advocacy Center, 2006; U.S. DHHS Child Welfare Information Gateway, 2006a).

Behavioral Indicators of Emotional Abuse

Behavioral indicators of emotional abuse may include habit disorders (sucking, biting, rocking), conduct or learning disorders, or overly adaptive or compliant behaviors (withdrawal, aggression). Neurotic traits, including sleep disorders, inhibition of play, and unusual fearfulness, as well as psychoneurotic reactions, such as hysteria, obsession, compulsions, phobias, and hypochondriasis, are also observed. Suicide attempts may also indicate emotional abuse (National Children's Advocacy Center, 2006; U.S. DHHS Child Welfare Information Gateway, 2006a).

Physical Indicators of Sexual Abuse

The sexually abused child may exhibit difficulty walking or sitting; torn, stained, or bloody underclothing; pain, swelling, or itching of genitalia; and pain on urination. Additional physical signs include bruises, bleeding, or lacerations involving the external genitalia, vagina, or anal

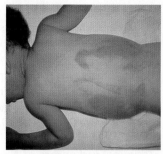
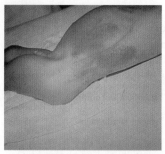

Nonaccidental distribution of bruises—All four surfaces of the midbody are involved, but there are no bruises on arms and legs.

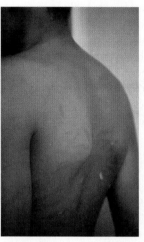
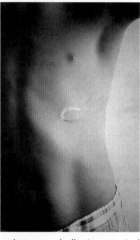
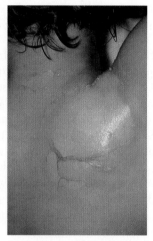

Pattern of injury—Linear scars of various ages indicate repeated abuse with a switch or a whip. The loop pattern on the boy's anterior torso is consistent with a looped electrical cord used as a whip.

Scald burn of shoulder and neck—The typical distribution of a scald burn in a toddler. This type of injury occurs when a toddler pulls a cup of coffee or pan of water off a stove.

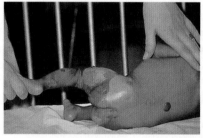

Nonaccidental immersion scald—Involvement of virtually the entire posterior surface of the legs indicates that the legs were held under scalding water; even an infant this young would flex the knees to avoid the hot water.

FIG 29-2   **Physical signs of child abuse. The nurse should be alert for the typical behavioral indicators of abuse.**   *(Courtesy Barbara Tenney, MD. From Henry, M. C., & Stapleton, E. R. [1992]. EMT: Prehospital care [p. 675]. Philadelphia: Saunders.)*

area and vaginal or penile discharge. Sexually transmissible disease, poor sphincter tone, and excessive masturbation may also be present (National Children's Advocacy Center, 2006; U.S. DHHS Child Welfare Information Gateway, 2006a).

Behavioral Indicators of Sexual Abuse
The sexually abused child may demonstrate an unwillingness to change clothes or participate in gym activities; withdrawal, fantasy, or infantile behavior; or bizarre, sophisticated, or unusual sexual behavior or knowledge. Promiscuity, poor peer relations, delinquency, running away, depression, or suicidal ideation, gestures, or attempts are often observed. These behaviors may coincide with aggression, a change in school performance, or sleep disturbances or nightmares. In addition, eating disturbances (obesity, anorexia, bulimia), self-destructive behaviors (substance abuse, self-mutilation), and sexual acting out toward a younger child are sometimes present (National Children's Advocacy Center, 2006; U.S. DHHS Child Welfare Information Gateway, 2006a).

In 1983 Summit (as cited in Giardino, 2006) described how children often cope with sexual victimization through an accommodation syndrome in which the coping mechanisms become the child's normal behaviors in response to an abnormal event. There is nothing the child can do to prevent the abuse. The initial strategy involves secrecy because the child realizes the situation lacks social acceptance. This awareness dominates the child's sense of self, and the child feels a great deal of guilt. The guilt may be intensified by the child's ambivalence about pleasure that may be experienced during the event. The secrecy is typically reinforced by threats that the child, the perpetrator, or another loved one will "get into trouble." (American Academy of Child and Adolescent Psychiatry, 2004; Giardino, 2006).

Other psychological mechanisms involved in the accommodation syndrome include (Summit, 1983 as cited in Giardino, 2006):

- Helplessness—Because the perpetrator may be a close friend or family member, the child feels as though there is no one to turn to. The child also feels isolated from peers because of shame and guilt. The child accommodates by pretending to be unaffected by the abuse.
- Entrapment—To cope with an enduring sense of having no way out of the abusive situation the child takes responsibility for the abuse. Almost universally, sexually abused children believe that the reason the abuse continues is because they are bad, rather than placing the responsibility on the perpetrator.
- Disclosure and retraction—Frequently the child will make veiled attempts at disclosure or will delay disclosure to keep the abuse secret and avoid the risk of alienating significant others. The child fears that the consequences of revealing the abuse will be worse than keeping the secret. In fact, most sexually abused children keep the abuse secret throughout their lives unless there is some intervention from outside the abusive system. Finally, the sexually abused child typically retracts the revelation of abuse once it has been made, out of fear of ridicule, retaliation, attending court, or losing contact with a loved one.

In addition to the preceding description of how the child may accommodate to sexual abuse, many sexually abused children, like other victims of severe child abuse, dissociate during the abuse to avoid feelings of physical pain. This dissociation is similar to that associated with post traumatic stress syndrome (Giardino, 2006).

CRITICAL TO REMEMBER
Denial of Abuse

It is common for the abuser, the noninvolved parent, and the child to deny the abuse. Each may deny the event, awareness of the event, impact of the event, or any responsibility for the event.

Other Specific Abusive Situations

Shaken Infant Syndrome. Shaken infant syndrome is a widely recognized form of physical child abuse that is caused by vigorous shaking of the infant while the child is held by the extremities or shoulders. This type of physical abuse leads to whiplash-induced intracranial and retinal bleeding. There is generally no external sign of head trauma, which makes this syndrome difficult to detect. The most common trigger of severe shaking is crying, especially if the child is colicky. Shaken infant syndrome should be considered in children with failure to thrive, seizures, apnea, respiratory irregularities, coma, or vomiting associated with drowsiness or lethargy (Giardino & Alexander, 2004).

Munchausen Syndrome by Proxy. Munchausen syndrome by proxy is the most difficult form of child abuse to diagnose. It is often inflicted by the mother or primary caretaker. The caretaker falsifies illness in the child through simulation or production of illness and then takes the child for medical care, claiming no knowledge of how the child became ill. The most common reasons these caretakers give for seeking medical treatment are bleeding, seizures, CNS depression, apnea, diarrhea, vomiting, fever, and rash. The long-term mortality rate in these cases is as high as 10% to 15%. Under the supervision of other adults, the child exhibits no symptoms and may appear normal and healthy. The parent's behavior reflects a serious disturbance that requires specialized psychiatric treatment and removal of the child from the parent's care. A multidisciplinary team is the best approach to diagnosing this disorder (Ragaisis, 2004).

CRITICAL THINKING EXERCISE 29-1

Matthew, age 2 years, is brought to the emergency department by his mother, Ms. Jackson, and her boyfriend. Ms. Jackson tells the nurse that Matthew has been crying and holding his arm since she picked him up at the babysitter's earlier in the evening. On further questioning, Ms. Jackson states that "Matthew is all boy. You have to watch him every minute or he is into something. He is constantly climbing and falling."

On examination, the nurse notes several bruises on Matthew's right leg and right arm. He also has a small abrasion on his nose. Ms. Jackson is holding Matthew and seems concerned, as does her boyfriend. Matthew quiets when his mother holds him and drifts off to sleep. Ms. Jackson's boyfriend leaves the room and returns with a snack for both Matthew and Ms. Jackson. He offers to hold Matthew.

1. What are some of the possible reasons Matthew is crying and holding his arm? Support your assumptions with rationales.
2. If the nurse suspects child abuse, what added assessments should be performed?
3. What legal responsibility does the nurse have in cases of suspected child abuse?

Text continued on p. 991

NURSING CARE PLAN

The Abused Child

Focused Assessment

The nurse should conduct a thorough assessment, which includes examination for skin integrity, especially examination of the scalp, bottoms of the hands and feet, front and back of the trunk, and genitalia. A baseline measurement of height and weight should be obtained, along with documentation of the birth weight for infants. An assessment of the child's anxiety level, ability to relate to the examiner, and emotional tone is also crucial. In addition, an assessment of the family support system, including patterns of interaction, belief systems, and social support systems, should be conducted.

During the physical assessment, information about bruises, injuries, and sexual abuse should be requested in a nonemotional, matter-of-fact manner with particular attention to the child's need for privacy and dignity. Comments made by the child should be written down verbatim because disclosure of abuse is often subtle and this information may be used in legal proceedings at a later time. Assessment should include an account of written or verbal contact with teachers, relatives (including both parents, siblings, and grandparents), and others who have been involved with the child over an extended period.

Trust may be enhanced by answering questions directly and specifically, assuming a nonjudgmental and supportive stance throughout all interactions, and acting as an advocate for the holistic care of the child and the family. Recognition of the child's low self-esteem, feelings of inadequacy, and fear will enable the nurse to relate in a manner that is supportive. The child will need encouragement to make self-care decisions and to discuss thoughts and feelings that may have been repressed to survive the trauma (Fig. 29-3). The child may also feel affection for the perpetrator and believe that the abuse is a necessary part of the relationship.

When sexual abuse is suspected, the child and parent should be interviewed in the same manner as described for physical abuse. The nurse should observe for clinical manifestations of sexual abuse in a manner that provides dignity and respect for both the child and the parent. Assessment tools are available that identify behaviors typical of the child who has been sexually abused. Nurses are considered to be mandated reporters and therefore *must* report any *suspected* child abuse to the appropriate authorities.

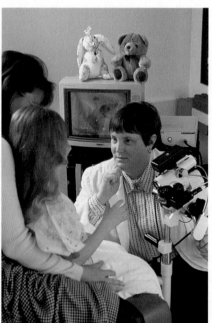

Drawings may help to identify the abused child and assist in therapy. Art can also help the child express what cannot be expressed in words.

Note the communication techniques designed to reassure the child and give the child some power. The little girl is not immediately positioned for a genital examination. The physician first sits to talk with the child at her eye level and makes eye contact with her.

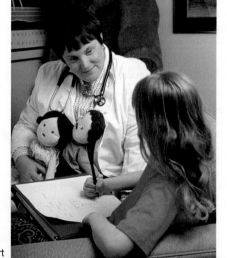

FIG 29-3   **Disclosure of abuse may be slow because the child often has difficulty trusting any adult. Identification of sexual abuse requires particular sensitivity because physical examination of the child's genitalia to detect signs of injury or sexually transmissible disease can be frightening for the child, who associates handling of the genitalia with pain or shame. Anatomically correct dolls are often used in the assessment of abuse within a family. These dolls help children express what they cannot express in words; young children in particular have a limited vocabulary to use when describing the events that have occurred.**   *(Courtesy Cook Children's Medical Center, Fort Worth, TX.)*

NURSING CARE PLAN—cont'd

NURSING DIAGNOSIS	Impaired Parenting related to immaturity, lack of knowledge, apathy on the part of parental caregivers, or limited or negative past parenting experience.
EXPECTED OUTCOME	The family will: • Exhibit appropriate parenting skills, as evidenced by describing the aspects of positive parenting models and responding to the child's needs in a timely and appropriate manner.

Intervention	Rationale
1. Elicit information about the parents' strengths and weaknesses, normal coping mechanisms, and the presence or absence of support systems. Special attention should be paid to: • Expectations with regard to the child • Comforting behaviors • Response to the child • General knowledge about the child	1. To provide optimal care for the child, involvement of the family is crucial. By understanding the needs of the family, the nurse can develop a plan of care, including referral to appropriate supportive agencies.
2. Discuss with the parents the parenting they received as children.	2. Parenting is a learned behavior.
3. Observe the parents' interactions with the child.	3. Although parents may verbalize a positive relationship with their child, observation of actual interactions provides a more realistic view of the parent-child relationship.
4. Provide an accepting environment.	4. Communication is encouraged by demonstrating acceptance.
5. Provide information for parents regarding normal growth and development.	5. Parents who are abusers often have unrealistic expectations of their children, in part because of their lack of knowledge regarding growth and development.
6. Include role modeling as a method of teaching parenting.	6. By observing the way the nurse touches and talks to the child in an affirming manner, the parents can observe firsthand the child's response to positive parenting-type skills.
7. Devote part of the time spent with the child and family to focusing on the child's positive attributes. You might say "I appreciate how quietly you have played with your toys while I have been talking with mommy," or "Look at how nicely you are talking to your doll."	7. Parents' negative perceptions of the child, which may be based on their own life experiences, can be altered by viewing the child through another's eyes.
8. Encourage the parents to participate in the child's care. Reinforce positive behaviors.	8. Strategies that encourage and reinforce positive parental participation in child care build self-esteem and confidence in parenting skills.

Evaluation

- Do the parents interact appropriately with the child through verbal, physical, and visual contact?
- Have the parents described features of normal growth and development?
- Do the parents make positive statements about the child?
- Do the parents bring the child in for follow-up visits?

NURSING DIAGNOSIS	Fear and/or Powerlessness related to the possible outcomes of disclosure, sense of shame, and possible loss of family.
EXPECTED OUTCOMES	The child will: • Verbalize the source of fear. • Express feelings related to shame and fear of loss of family.

Intervention	Rationale
1. Reassure the child in regard to personal safety.	1. Verbal reassurance can provide a sense of security.
2. Identify specific strategies the child can use to maintain a sense of stability (i.e., stay with a trusted adult, refuse to answer intrusive questions, limit exposure to adults who are not trusted).	2. By providing some viable options, the nurse can help the child begin to gain a sense of control over the experience.

Continued

NURSING CARE PLAN—cont'd

3. Acknowledge the child's fear.	3. Acknowledgment helps the child identify feelings and opens up new areas of communication.
4. Spend time with the child. Use both verbal and nonverbal forms of communication.	4. Actions of support provide comfort and encourage verbalization of feelings.
5. Offer choices, when available, regarding activities of daily living, recreation time, and time with other children and adults.	5. Being offered choices gives the child a sense of control and diminishes feelings of powerlessness.

Evaluation

- Does the child participate in play activities?
- Has the child verbalized specific fears related to abuse and disclosure?

- Has the child verbalized fears related to being removed from the family?

NURSING DIAGNOSIS   Deficient Knowledge about the child's realistic developmental abilities, how to access external support resources, or ways to manage internal and external stressors related to past inexperience with parenting.

EXPECTED OUTCOMES   The family will:
- Increase knowledge related to growth and development, as evidenced by verbalization of an understanding of the child's developmental and emotional needs in a framework that is oriented to the child's welfare.
- Identify support systems.

Intervention

Rationale

1. Determine the parents' knowledge of child growth and development.	1. A baseline assessment must be done to develop a plan of care.
2. Serve as a role model for positive parenting skills.	2. Learning can be enhanced through observing the application of parenting skills, which is more effective than listening to a lecture.
3. Assist the family in identifying stressors and the support systems and resources that may help decrease the parents' stress level.	3. If the parents' level of stress is decreased, the risk of abuse is decreased.
4. Refer the family to pertinent support groups, such as Parents Anonymous.	4. Lack of support and isolation are common among abusive families. A support group may decrease isolation.
5. Involve the parents in the care of the child.	5. Participation in care will provide opportunities for positive reinforcement, teaching, and increased emotional attachment to the child.
6. Provide education in the following areas: • Growth and development • Nutrition • Care related to activities of daily living • Routine well-child care • Manifestations of illness • Need for care and loving	6. Education in parenting skills may decrease unrealistic expectations, increase awareness of the needs of children, and increase the chances of positive parenting. Parents may not have had positive parenting role models as children.
7. Provide a consistent caregiver from among the nursing staff.	7. Consistency of care increases the child's feelings of trust and security and provides increased opportunities for the child to verbalize feelings.

Evaluation

- Can the parents describe normal child growth and development and developmental expectations?

- Have the parents joined a support group?

NURSING CARE PLAN—cont'd

NURSING DIAGNOSIS	Risk for Injury related to a family with a history of physical abuse, physical neglect, emotional abuse, or sexual abuse.
EXPECTED OUTCOME	Injury related to abuse will: • Cease, as evidenced by the child remaining free from physical or psychologic injury and neglect.

Intervention

1. Assess the child's physical and mental status.

2. Observe the interactions between child and family.

3. Obtain a thorough history.

4. Use a nonthreatening, nonjudgmental manner when interacting with the child's parents.

5. Report all cases in which abuse is suspected.

6. Assist in removing children from an unsafe environment.

7. Document the following:
   • Results of the child's physical assessment
   • Observations of interactions between the child and family and between the child and other adults and the child's reaction to hospitalization or the health care setting
   • Direct comments made by the child and the family that pertain to the child or the child's injury
   • Child's developmental level

8. If the child is removed from the home, provide the child and family with support and opportunities to verbalize feelings. Play therapy may be used effectively with children.

Rationale

1. All children should undergo a thorough physical assessment on presentation to the health care setting and should be assessed for bruises, burns, scars, and other signs of abuse. Children may enter the health care system for reasons other than injury.

2. Subtle signs of abuse may be detected in the way the child interacts with the abuser and other adults.

3. Frequent presentation of the child for injuries or signs of healed injuries may indicate a pattern of abuse.

4. By building a trusting relationship with the parents, the nurse can help the child. If the parents become suspicious or alienated, they may deny the child access to health care. They will become defensive and will not be open to teaching.

5. All 50 states require health care professionals to report all cases of suspected abuse.

6. Suspected abuse should be evaluated immediately so that the child can be removed to an environment that is safe, thereby preventing further injury.

7. Objective documentation is essential in all cases of suspected abuse.

8. Children who are removed from the custody of their parents will grieve their loss. Parents will need support in dealing with guilt and loss.

Evaluation

• Does the child remain free of inflicted injury?
• Has the child been placed in a safe environment?
• Has the child verbalized feelings regarding placement outside the home?

• Has the family sought psychologic counseling?

PATHOPHYSIOLOGY

FAILURE TO THRIVE

Three types of failure to thrive are typically described: organic, nonorganic, and mixed.

Organic failure to thrive is marked by failure to gain weight as a result of physical factors. These physical factors may be a specific physiologic impairment, such as a congenital heart defect, gastrointestinal disorder, or endocrine disorder. Alternatively, the physical factor may be a chronic infection, a CNS abnormality, a chromosomal disorder, or a metabolic disorder. Organic failure to thrive is a sign of possible human immunodeficiency virus infection in an infant (see Chapter 17).

Nonorganic failure to thrive is a diagnosis applied in the absence of a history contributing to, or physical or laboratory findings suggestive of, an organic disease capable of causing failure to gain weight. Generally, environmental factors influence a child's intake or use of calories. This form of the disorder is commonly believed to result from a complex interactive pattern between the infant and the primary caregivers.

Mixed failure to thrive is caused by a combination of organic and inorganic factors. The initial problem may be physical, such as respiratory distress, which limits effective suckling. This difficulty in turn interferes with the caregiver's sense of adequacy and ability to provide nurturing care to the infant. The infant becomes more irritable and difficult to manage, further increasing the caregiver's sense of inadequacy.

Persistent failure to gain weight is considered to originate with malnutrition. The long-term effects of undernutrition, regardless of the cause, may include secondary immune system dysfunction, deficiencies in micronutrients, and developmental delays in all major areas. Associated immune system dysfunctions include reductions in complement, secretory immunoglobulin A, and T cell function. Affected children may have repeated gastrointestinal or respiratory infections, with each episode raising the child's caloric needs and lowering intake, resulting in even greater vulnerability. Micronutrient deficiencies often complicate undernutrition by causing anemia and rickets. Iron and calcium deficiencies tend to increase lead absorption, which can lead to constipation, abdominal pain, or anorexia. Zinc deficiency impairs growth directly and can also interfere with taste bud function. Long-term undernutrition in the first 2 years of life can result in limited brain size, a reduction in neuronal number, and decreased synaptic complexity. Acquired microcephaly may persist even when somatic growth recovers.

Failure to thrive

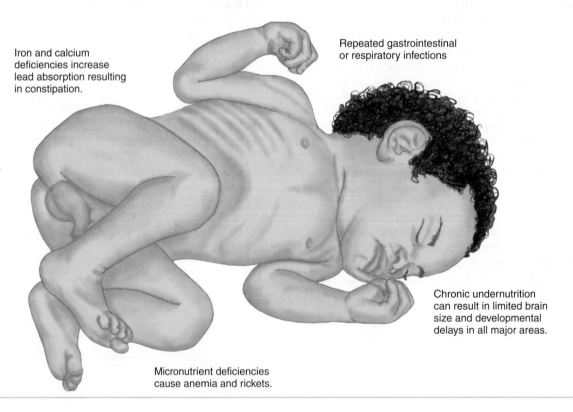

Iron and calcium deficiencies increase lead absorption resulting in constipation.

Repeated gastrointestinal or respiratory infections

Chronic undernutrition can result in limited brain size and developmental delays in all major areas.

Micronutrient deficiencies cause anemia and rickets.

FAILURE TO THRIVE

Most clinicians agree that failure to thrive is not an actual diagnosis but rather a term that describes a cluster of concurrent symptoms. In practice, if a child's weight falls below the 5th percentile or drops more than two major percentile groups or if the average daily growth gain in grams is less than normal values, the child is considered to be at risk for failure to thrive, and a more thorough evaluation is warranted.

Etiology

Failure to thrive can be organic, caused by an underlying physical problem, or nonorganic. The contributing factors to physical growth delay have been described in detail in previous chapters. Nonorganic failure to thrive is thought to be caused by multiple factors, including poverty, maternal depression, poor social support systems, poor bonding or maladaptive interactions between the child and mother, and an irritable, resistant-to-touch infant. A maladaptive parent-infant relationship, in which the parent displays impaired skills in reading or responding to the infant's cues, is the most commonly observed risk factor for nonorganic failure to thrive. The infant has difficulty eliciting attention and appropriate care, often becoming irritable or stiff, or exhibits feeding difficulties. These symptoms are difficult for new parents to manage, resulting in parental anxiety and difficulty in bonding emotionally with the infant (Sirotnak, 2003).

Incidence

From 1% to 5% of hospitalized infants are listed as being admitted for failure to thrive; however, these estimates of occurrence may be low. It is estimated that 10% of children seen in the primary care setting have symptoms of failure to thrive (Bassali & Benjamin, 2004). Although failure to thrive occurs in children of all social classes, a disproportionate number of these children are from low-income families.

Manifestations and Risk Factors

Physical Indicators

Physical indicators of failure to thrive include weight below the 5th percentile, a sudden or rapid deceleration in the growth curve, delay in reaching developmental milestones, and decreased muscle mass. Muscle hypotonia, abdominal distention, generalized weakness, and cachexia (general ill health and malnutrition) are additional signs.

Behavioral Indicators

Behavioral indicators of failure to thrive include avoidance of eye contact, avoidance of physical touch, intense watchfulness, and sleep disturbances. Lack of age-appropriate stranger anxiety, inappropriate lack of preference for one's own parents, and disturbed affect (e.g., apathy, extreme irritability, extreme compliance) may also be observed. Repetitive self-stimulating behaviors, such as rocking, head banging,

---

NURSING CARE PLAN

The Child Who Is Failing to Thrive

Focused Assessment

The initial assessment should include a complete history of the presenting problem, with an emphasis on age at onset, recent changes in the child's routines (e.g., travel out of the country), and attendance at large day care centers or shelter-type living environments. The nurse should also obtain information about any chronic nasal obstruction, episodes of bronchitis or wheezing, or other respiratory difficulties. Information about stool frequency, consistency, and any discomfort associated with excretion should be documented. A thorough dietary history should include all drinks, meals, and snacks consumed by the child and where, when, how, and by whom the child is typically fed. The nurse should explore possible reasons for low intake, such as recurrent infections or medical complications of earlier episodes of malnutrition (Box 29-4). Common dietary patterns may be overlooked if the dietary history is not carefully investigated.

The physical examination should focus especially on the skin, hair, nails, and mucous membranes of the child to identify signs of malnutrition. Also, the nurse should look for lesions that could interfere with eating, such as dental caries, tongue enlargement, mandibular

hypoplasia, unrecognized submucosal cleft palate, or tonsillar hypertrophy.

The nurse should complete a thorough psychosocial history that focuses on income, family (dis)organization, social isolation, stress factors, support systems, and family psychopathologic conditions, such as maternal depression, family violence, or alcoholism. It is important to ask about the availability of food, especially around the time of arrival of a paycheck or other forms of income. Finally, the psychosocial history should include questions about facilities for storing and preparing food.

Assessment of infant-parent interactions should focus on the ways in which the child is held and fed, how eye contact is initiated and maintained, and the facial expressions of both the child and the caregiver during interactions. Observations of various kinds of interactions are also important and should include play, talk, and touch by both the child and caregiver and the other's reaction to these attempts to engage in interaction. The nurse should note the responses of the caregiver to the child's cues, such as when the child cries, reaches out, or looks toward the caregiver. A feeling of synchrony or harmony should be sensed in the interaction.

Continued

NURSING CARE PLAN—cont'd

NURSING DIAGNOSIS   Imbalanced Nutrition: Less Than Body Requirements related to insufficient intake of calories, incomplete absorption of nutrients, impaired interactions with caregivers, or inadequate care by caregivers.

EXPECTED OUTCOME   The child's caloric intake will:
- Increase, as evidenced by an increase in physical growth.

Intervention	Rationale
1. Monitor the child's nutritional status: • Document physical alterations, especially changes in physical status during or after feedings. • Document the child's feeding patterns. • Document the nature of parent-child interactions, especially before, during, and after feedings.	1. Fatigue, colic, or respiratory distress may indicate an underlying cause of the disorder. Subtle deficits may have a significant bearing on nutritional intake. Psychologic components revealed in the context of interactions may be the most significant indicators of the cause for undernutrition.
2. Encourage the caregiver to discuss both positive and negative feelings about care, procedures, and interactions with the child.	2. The caregiver may be unaware of some of the underlying feelings that may be affecting the infant-caregiver relationship.
3. Increase the child's caloric intake by feeding the child on demand or increasing intake as tolerated, offering high-protein snacks between meals, offering small portions of a wide variety of food at mealtimes, teaching the child healthy mealtime behaviors (decrease distractions, make mealtime pleasurable), planning naps or rest periods, and intervening in the event of fretfulness or crying.	3. The child's intake must be greater than the caloric expenditure.
4. Monitor the child's intake and output.	4. Fluid loss may affect daily weight patterns.
5. Weight should be measured daily at the same time, with the same scales, and with the child dressed in the same amount of clothing each time.	5. This approach reduces the effect of various factors that influence weight measurements.
6. Provide a consistent caregiver from the nursing staff.	6. This strategy increases trust and provides the child with an adult who anticipates needs, thus decreasing the child's level of frustration.

Evaluation

- Is the child attaining developmental milestones?
- Does the child eat the food offered?
- Do the parents participate in feeding the child?
- Does the child's physical growth show an increase?

NURSING DIAGNOSIS   Deficient Knowledge related to lack of experience and of positive parenting training.

EXPECTED OUTCOME   Knowledge related to parenting will:
- Increase, as evidenced by caregiver holding and maintaining eye contact with the child and participating in feeding the child and by expression by the parents of realistic expectations of the child on the basis of the child's developmental needs.

Intervention	Rationale
1. Provide instruction in child care, being sure to model appropriate adult-child interactions. Include techniques for holding, touching, and feeding the child.	1. Instruction, coupled with modeling and practice, will facilitate integration of information.
2. Exhibit a positive attitude toward the parents.	2. Acceptance increases trust and fosters openness to learning.
3. Provide information regarding normal growth and development.	3. Parents may lack an understanding of normal growth and development and may have unrealistic expectations of the child.
4. Provide for rooming-in with the child.	4. This arrangement allows the nurse to observe parent-child interactions and provide further teaching if necessary.
5. Teach the parents ways to increase the child's caloric intake and to minimize the control issues associated with mealtimes (Box 29-5).	5. Lack of previous experience and knowledge may result in ineffective parenting skills.

NURSING CARE PLAN—cont'd

Evaluation

- Have the parents been observed interacting appropriately with the child during meals?
- Do the parents verbalize an openness to learning new techniques of feeding?

- Are the parents holding and touching the child?
- Have the parents asked appropriate questions related to parenting?

---

intense sucking, intense chewing on fingers or hands, and head rolling, are also seen.

Diagnostic Evaluation

The differential diagnosis is generally made by a multidisciplinary team whose initial task is to search for an organic cause of the growth failure. If no cause is identified, the approach is to diagnose by response. Nutrition and nurturing are provided in a consistent manner, and if the infant gains the expected weight, nonorganic failure to thrive is considered to be the appropriate diagnosis.

Therapeutic Management

Treatment provides nutritional therapy to increase the child's caloric intake. The goal is for the child to grow at two to three times the average rate for age. Daily multivitamin supplements with minerals are often prescribed to ensure that specific nutritional deficiencies do not occur in the course of rapid growth. Caloric enrichment of food is essential, and formula may be concentrated in titrated amounts up to 24 calories per ounce. Greater concentrations can lead to diarrhea and dehydration.

Family therapy may be indicated. Effective parenting classes can assist the parent to identify psychologic and physical factors that have contributed to the child's condition.

BOX 29-4 | Common Reasons for Inadequate Nutritional Intake in Infants and Children

- Overdilution of formula
- Large quantities of cereal or baby food in bottles
- Excessive intake of fluids other than formula or milk
- Selection of foods with inappropriate texture for infant's stage of development
- Infrequent feedings, especially in children who are temperamentally quiet or undemanding
- No set feeding times
- No highchair
- Frequent small sips from a bottle (grazing)
- Distractions during feedings (television, social interactions)
- Struggles over feeding between caregiver and child

BOX 29-5 | PARENTS WANT TO KNOW   About Effective Feeding Practices

Almost all children at one time or another do not eat as well as parents would like. If you are concerned about your child's eating, these guidelines may help:

- Children do well with schedules. Try to maintain consistent mealtimes and snack times each day.
- Children need to eat often, not constantly. Offer something every 2 to 3 hours, allowing three meals and two or three snacks per day.
- Make sure your child can easily reach the food served. Use a highchair or small table. Be certain the child is safely secured.
- Allow children to feed themselves. Try very small amounts at first. Offer seconds later. Expect messiness and prepare in advance for easy cleanup (use bibs, newspapers under the highchair, or whatever works for you). If you are worried that little food actually gets into the child's mouth, use two spoons: one for the baby to control and one for you to use for feeding.
- Do not force feed, bribe, or cajole! These approaches will backfire.
- Do not worry if your child wants to eat the same food every day; many children are like that. Variety is not

important to a toddler's nutrition. What matters is the total caloric and protein intake.
- At mealtimes, offer solids first. Liquids are filling and provide fewer calories.
- Limit the amount of juice, water, and carbonated drinks consumed. Offer milk or formula instead.
- Offer foods that are easy for your child to handle. Finger foods, such as Cheerios, French fries, slices of banana, and peas, are ideal. Make sure pieces are small to avoid the child's choking.
- For more calories per bite, add margarine, mayonnaise, gravies, and grated cheese to foods. For snacks, use peanut butter, cheese, pudding, bananas, or dried fruit.
- Limit the consumption of junk foods such as soda, chips, and candy. They take up valuable space in the stomach without providing nutrients.
- Eat with your child or allow your child to eat with others so that meals and snacks can be fun.
- Allow your child to participate in meal planning and preparation. Children enjoy eating foods that they make.

Modified from Frank, D. A., Silva, M., & Needlman, R. (1993, Feb.). Failure to thrive: Mystery, myth, and method. *Contemporary Pediatrics, 10,* 121.

KEY CONCEPTS

- In children and adolescents, the behavioral manifestations of anxiety and depression may be similar. Children with both diagnoses may be withdrawn, tearful, unwilling to engage in play, and aggressive toward others.
- It is difficult to differentiate between normal mood changes resulting from developmental maturation and abnormal, persistent mood disturbances.
- Separation anxiety and school avoidance need to be addressed if the problem becomes persistent or debilitating. Such anxiety is characterized by excessive fear, even panic, of being away from the parent or home.
- A suicide gesture or statement should never be ignored.
- Protecting a child or adolescent from inflicting harm to self involves being emotionally and physically available, offering opportunities to discuss feelings and the suicidal event, and removing potentially harmful objects.
- Support for grieving families of suicidal or potentially suicidal children or adolescents is best provided on both an individual and a group basis to allow exploration of personal issues and social support.
- Anorexia nervosa is characterized by a deliberate refusal to maintain adequate body weight, a distorted body image, and amenorrhea (in female patients).
- One common factor among children with an eating disorder is a family system in which the individual is considered to be an extension of the parent or serves as a means of meeting the parents' needs, rather than being allowed to develop as an autonomous individual The family is often disordered and chaotic, resulting in the child's sense of isolation.
- The focus of care for an adolescent with an eating disorder involves restructuring cognitive perceptions, reducing opportunities for engaging in ritualistic and self-injurious behaviors, and re-establishing physiologic homeostasis.
- During the early treatment phase of eating disorders, it may be necessary to observe the adolescent after meals to prevent episodes of purging.
- Attention-deficit hyperactivity disorder is a developmental disorder characterized by developmentally inappropriate degrees of inattention, overactivity, and impulsivity.
- Support groups are important in assisting families to cope with and modify expectations and interactions involving the child with ADHD.
- Educating the family about ADHD is a crucial component of caring for the child with this disorder.
- Low grades, irregular school attendance, aggressive or rebellious behavior, deteriorating relationships with family members or former friends, rapid or extreme changes in behaviors or mood, and loss of interest in hobbies, sports, or other activities are some common signs of substance abuse.
- A child or adolescent with a substance abuse problem, together with the family, should receive help in developing social support systems, with referral to appropriate resources that can offer additional support as they attempt to make long-term changes in their social and emotional patterns of relating.
- Physical child abuse tends to increase during times of economic hardship or external stress. Abusive families are often isolated, lack a support system, exhibit low levels of trust, resolve conflict through aggression, assume fixed and traditional roles within the family, and establish rigid rules.
- All suspected child abuse must be reported to the appropriate authorities.
- Abusive parents often have unrealistic expectations of their children, which may relate to lack of knowledge of normal growth and development.
- Role modeling positive parenting skills is an effective intervention in the care of the child who has been abused.
- The assessment of infant-parent interactions in cases of nonorganic failure to thrive should include observation of the ways in which the child is held and fed, how eye contact is initiated and maintained, and the facial expressions of both the child and the caregiver during interactions.

ANSWERS TO CRITICAL THINKING EXERCISE 29-1

1. Matthew may have fallen while at the baby-sitter's or even at home and either sprained or fractured his arm. Two-year-olds are curious and also like to climb. Children get frequent scrapes and bruises at this age. Because of the injured arm, bruises, and abrasion, physical abuse is also a possibility.

2. Matthew should be assessed for other bruises in various stages of healing or clustered in patterns reflecting the shape of a hand or an article that may have caused the bruise. The nurse must determine whether the injury matches the description of the cause. The nurse should also check for records of other emergency department visits for injuries or signs of old fractures on Matthew's radiographs. In addition, the nurse should gather information about the babysitter: Has any other injury occurred while Matthew was in the sitter's care? What explanation did the sitter give for Matthew's behavior when his mother picked him up? During the interview, the nurse should observe both Ms. Jackson and her boyfriend to assess their relationship with Matthew. Do they comfort him? Do they respond to his needs? Do they seem overly concerned about the injury? Matthew's behavior is not typical of an abused child. He seeks comfort from his parent and does not appear apathetic. If, at the end of the interview, history, assessment, and diagnostic testing, it is determined that an adult did not inflict the injury, the nurse should use the opportunity to explore ways that the injury could have been prevented. The roles of mother, babysitter, and boyfriend should be incorporated into the discussion.

3. If the nurse suspects child abuse, it must be reported to child protective services.

REFERENCES AND READINGS

American Academy of Child and Adolescent Psychiatry. (1998). Practice parameters for the assessment and treatment of children and adolescents with depressive disorders. *Journal of the American Academy of Child and Adolescent Psychiatry, 37*(Suppl. 10), 63S-83S.

American Academy of Child and Adolescent Psychiatry. (2004). Child sexual abuse. Retrieved September 23, 2006 from *www.aacap.org*.

American Academy of Pediatrics, Committee on Adolescence. (2003). Identifying and treating eating disorders [electronic version]. *Pediatrics, 111*, 204-211.

American Academy of Pediatrics, Committee on Drugs. (1998). *Policy statement neonatal drug withdrawal*. Retrieved November 11, 2005, from *www.aap.org*.

American Psychiatric Association. (2000). *Diagnostic and statistical manual of mental disorders* (4th ed., text revision.). Washington, DC: American Psychiatric Association.

Bassali, R., & Benjamin, J. (2004). *Failure to thrive*. Retrieved May 29, 2005, from *www.emedicine.com/ped/ topic738.htm*.

Boris, N., Dalton, R., & Forman, M. (2004). Mood disorders. In R. Behrman, R. Kliegman, & H. Jenson (Eds.). *Nelson textbook of pediatrics* (17th ed., 84-86). St. Louis: Elsevier Saunders.

Elliott, G., & Smiga, S. (2003). Depression in the child and adolescent. *Pediatric Clinics of North America, 50*, 1093-1106.

Frankowoski, B. (2004). Sexual orientation and adolescents. *Pediatrics, 113*, 1827-1832.

Giardino, A. P. (2006). *Child abuse & neglect: Sexual abuse*. Retrieved September 24, 2006 from *www.emedicine.com/PED/topic2649.htm*.

Giardino, A. P., & Alexander, R. (2004). *Child abuse: Quick reference for healthcare professionals, social services, and law enforcement*. St. Louis: G. W. Medical Publishing.

Gould, M. S., Greenberg, T., Velting, D. M., & Shaffer, D. (2003). Youth suicide risk and preventive interventions: A review of the past 10 years. *Journal of the American Academy of Child and Adolescent Psychiatry, 42*, 386-405.

Greydanus, D., Pratt, A., Sloane, M., Rappley, M. (2003). Attention-deficit/hyperactivity disorder in children and adolescents: Interventions for a complex, costly clinical conundrum. *Pediatric Clinics of North America, 50*, 1049-1092.

Grunbaum, J. A., et al. (2004). Youth risk behavior surveillance—United States, 2003. *Morbidity and Mortality Weekly Report Surveillance Summaries, 53*, 1-100.

Johnson, K., Gerada, C., & Greenough, A. (2003). *Treatment of neonatal abstinence syndrome*. Retrieved November 17, 2005, from *www.archdischild.com*.

Johnson, L. D., O'Malley, P. M., Bachman, J. G., & Schulenberg, J. E. (2005). *Monitoring the future national results on adolescent drug use: Overview of key findings, 2004*. Bethesda, MD: National Institute on Drug Abuse.

Kendall, J., Leo, M., Perrin, N., & Hatton, D. (2005). Modeling ADHD child and family relationships. *Western Journal of Nursing Research, 27*, 500-518.

Koschel, M. (2003). Is it child abuse? *American Journal of Nursing, 103*, 45-46.

Leslie, L., Weckerly, J., Plemmons, D., Landsverk, J., & Eastman, S. (2004). Implementing the American Academy of Pediatrics attention deficit/hyperactivity disorder diagnostic guidelines in primary care settings [electronic version]. *Pediatrics, 114*, 129-140.

Luo, F., Leckman, J., Katsovich, L. et al. (2004). Prospective longitudinal study of children with tic disorders and/or obsessive compulsive disorder: Relationship of symptom exacerbations to newly acquired streptococcal infections [electronic version]. *Pediatrics, 113*, e578-e585.

March, J., & Treatment for Adolescents with Depression Study Team. (2004). Fluoxetine, cognitive-behavioral therapy, and their combination for adolescents with depression [electronic version]. *Journal of the American Medical Association, 292*, 807-820.

McDonnell, A., & Glod, C. (2003). Prevalence of psychopathology in preschool age children. *Journal of Child and Adolescent Psychiatric Nursing, 16*, 141-152.

Mell, L., Davis, R., & Owens, D. (2005). Association between streptococcal infection and obsessive compulsive disorder, Tourette's syndrome, and tic disorder. *Pediatrics, 116*, 56-60.

Meyers, S., Eisenhauer, N., & Ryan, M. (2003). ADHD: It is real and it can be treated. *The Clinical Advisor: A Forum for Nurse Practitioners, 6*, 15-25.

Mulryan, K., Cathers, P., & Fagin, A. (2004). How to recognize and respond to child abuse. *Nursing 2004, 34*, 52-55.

Murthi, M., Servaty-Seib, H., & Elliott, A. (2005). Childhood sexual abuse and multiple dimensions of self-concept. *Journal of Interpersonal Violence, 21*, 982-999.

National Center for Health Statistics. (2004). *Health United States, 2004*. Retrieved October 22, 2005, from *www.cdc.gov*.

National Institute of Drug Abuse. (2004). *Monitoring the future study*. Retrieved May 1, 2005, from *www.nida.nih.gov*.

National Institute of Mental Health. (2000). *Child and adolescent bipolar disorder: An update from the National Institute of Mental Health*. Retrieved December 29, 2005, from *www.nimh.hih.gov*.

National Institute of Mental Health. (2001). *Let's talk about depression*. Retrieved December 29, 2005, from *www.nimh.nih.gov*.

National Mental Health Association. (2005). *Bipolar disorder and children*. Retrieved December 29, 2005, from *www.nmha.org*.

National Mental Health Association. (2005). *Depression and children*. Retrieved December 29, 2005, from *www.nmha.org*.

Oakley, L. (2005a). Neurobiology of nonpsychotic illnesses. In L. Copstead & J. Banasik, Eds. *Pathophysiology* (3rd ed., 1216-1220). St. Louis: Elsevier Saunders.

Oakley, L. (2005b). Neurobiology of psychotic illnesses. In L. Copstead & J. Banasik, Eds. *Pathophysiology* (3rd ed., 1203-1213). St. Louis: Elsevier Saunders.

O'Leary, D. (2004). Gay teens and attempted suicide. *National Association for Research and Therapy of Homosexuality*. Retrieved May 30, 2005, from *www.narth.com/docs/gayteens.html*.

Qin, P. (2003). The relationship of suicide risk to family history of suicide and psychiatric disorders. *Psychiatric Times, 20*. Retrieved April 14, 2005, from *www.psychiatrictimes.com/p031262.html*.

Phillips, E., & Pratt, H. (2005). Eating disorders in college. *Pediatric Clinics of North America, 52*, 85-96.

Ragaisis, K. (2004). When the system works: Rescuing a child from Munchausen's syndrome by proxy. *Journal of Child and Adolescent Psychiatric Nursing, 17*, 173-176.

Renfrew Center Foundation for Eating Disorders. (2003). Eating disorders 101 guide: A summary of issues, statistics and resources (revised). Retrieved May 30, 2005, from *http://www.renfrew.org*.

Rushton, J. L., Forcier, M., & Schectman, R. M. (2002). Epidemiology of depressive symptoms in the National Longitudinal Study of Adolescent Health. *Journal of the American Academy of Child and Adolescent Psychiatry, 41*, 199-205.

Sadock, B., & Sadock, V. A. (2003). *Kaplan and Sadock's synopsis of psychiatry: Behavioral sciences/clinical psychiatry* (9th ed.). Philadelphia: Lippincott Williams & Wilkins.

Sigman, G. (2003). Eating disorders in children and adolescents. *Pediatric Clinics of North America, 50*, 1139-1177.

Sirotnak, A. P. (2003). *Child abuse and neglect: Failure to thrive*. Retrieved April 15, 2005, from *www.emedicine.com/ped/topic2647.htm*.

Stafford, B., Boris, N., & Dalton, R. (2004). Anxiety disorders. In R. Behrman, R. Kliegman, & H. Jenson (Eds.). *Nelson textbook of pediatrics* (17th ed., pp. 81-84). St. Louis: Elsevier Saunders.

Takashi, L. (2002). Neurobiology of schizophrenia, mood disorders, and anxiety disorders. In K. McCance & S. Huether (Eds.). *Pathophysiology* (4th ed., pp. 555-563). St. Louis: Elsevier Mosby.

The National Children's Advocacy Center. (2006). *Physical and behavioral indicators of abuse*. Retrieved September 24, 2006 from *www.nationalcac.org*.

U.S. Department of Health and Human Services. (2000). *Healthy People 2010* (conference edition, in 2 volumes). Washington, DC: U.S. Department of Health and Human Services.

U.S. Department of Health and Human Services, Administration on Children, Youth and Families. (2005). *Child maltreatment 2003: Reports from the states to the national child abuse and neglect data system.* Washington, DC: U.S. Government Printing Office.

U.S. Department of Health and Human Services Child Welfare Information Gateway. (2005). *Definitions of child abuse and neglect.* Retrieved September 24, 2006 from *www.childwelfare.gov.*

U.S. Department of Health and Human Services Child Welfare Information Gateway. (2006a). *Long-term consequences of child abuse and neglect.* Retrieved September 24, 2006 from *www.childwelfare .gov.*

U.S. Department of Health and Human Services Child Welfare Information Gateway. (2006b). *Recognizing child abuse and neglect: Signs and symptoms.* Retrieved September 24, 2006 from *www .childwelfare.gov.*

U.S. Department of Health and Human Services, Substance Abuse and Mental Health Services Administration. (2005). *National survey on drug use and health. Substance use during pregnancy 2002 and 2003 update.* Retrieved November 11, 2005, from *http://oas.samhsa .gov.*

U.S. Department of Health and Human Services & Substance Abuse and Mental Health Services Administration National Clearinghouse for Alcohol and Drug Information. (2005). *Birth defects and adverse birth outcomes.* Retrieved December 29, 2005, from *www.ncadi .samhsa.gov.*

U.S. Food and Drug Administration. (2005a). *Fluoxetine hydrochloride information: Suicidal thoughts or actions in children and adults.* Retrieved December 29, 2005, from *www.fda.gov.*

U.S. Food and Drug Administration. (2005b). *Prozac—Warning.* Retrieved December 29, 2005, from *www.fda.gov.*

Varley, C., & Smith, C. (2003). Anxiety disorders in the child and teen. *Pediatric Clinics of North America, 50,* 1107-1138.

Walrath, C., Ybarra, M., Sheehan, A., Holden, E., & Burns, B. (2006). Impact of maltreatment on children served in community mental health programs [Electronic version]. *Journal of Emotional and Behavioral Disorders, 14,* 143-156.

CHAPTER 30

The Child With a Cognitive Impairment

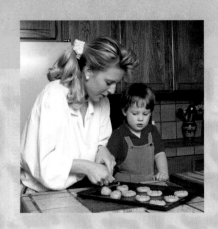

Learning Objectives

After studying this chapter, you should be able to:

- Define the concepts of cognitive impairment, mental retardation, and developmental disability.
- Identify the various causes of mental retardation.
- Identify specific tools used in assessing the presence and degree of mental retardation.
- Identify educational and support resources for families with a child who is mentally retarded or developmentally delayed.
- Develop appropriate nursing strategies for supporting the family and child with mental retardation or developmental delay.
- Develop nursing strategies for families caring for a child with Down syndrome.

- Identify behavioral characteristics and appropriate nursing actions when working with a child with fragile X syndrome.
- Identify characteristics and appropriate nursing interventions for an infant with fetal alcohol syndrome and for the child's family.
- Identify the basic diagnostic criteria for autism.
- Explain the ways autism differs from other types of pervasive developmental disorders.
- Identify the major considerations in working with the family of an autistic child.
- Develop home care interventions appropriate to the family's abilities and the developmental needs of a child with a cognitive disability.

Definitions

comorbidity The occurrence of two or more different disorders in the same individual; children with cognitive impairments often have coexisting psychiatric disorders.

echolalia Stereotyped repetition of another person's words or phrases.

functional age The age equivalent at which the child is actually able to perform specific self-care or relational tasks; for example, the child may be 6 years old chronologically but only able to perform skills representative of children 4 years old, and thus the child's functional age is 4 years.

intelligence The innate capacity of the individual; what individuals can do relative to learning, thinking, and problem solving; results obtained on intelligence tests that measure specific skills, such as verbal, nonverbal, or mechanical abilities.

mutation Variation in a gene that affects its function.

pervasive developmental disorders Infant and childhood disorders characterized by severe and pervasive impairment in several areas of development in a manner distinctly deviant from the individual's developmental level or mental age (American Psychiatric Association, 2000).

premutation Gene alteration that is generally not associated with symptoms, but could be inherited as a full mutation.

Electronic Resources

Additional information related to the content in Chapter 30 can be found on:

the interactive companion CD-ROM

- Audio Glossary
- NCLEX Review Questions

or the companion website at *evolve*
http://evolve.elsevier.com/james/ncoc

- NCLEX Review Questions
- Resources for Health Care Providers and Families
- WebLinks

Common Diagnostic Tests for Cognitive Disorders

Test	Description	Normal Findings	Indications	Nursing Implications
Vision test	Assessment of vision, ocular pressure, and structural defects	Normal vision, normal structures	Children with Down syndrome; 40%-45% have refractive errors, cataracts, or other visual problems.	Explain pupil dilation. Provide protective eyewear after examinations.
Hearing test	Assessment of perception of sound frequency and volume	Normal hearing range	Children with Down syndrome; 70%-80% have hearing defects. Children with autism and PDD often appear to have defective hearing despite normal hearing function, so hearing tests should be conducted.	Explain the test in simple terms. The test may require that the child wear a headphone, which may be difficult to tolerate.
Thyroid studies	Blood serum tests to determine thyroid levels — serum thyroxine	Ages 1-3 yr: 6.8-13.5 µg/dL Ages 3-10 yr: 5.5-12.8 µg/dL Puberty to adulthood: 4.2-13.0 µg/dL	Children with Down syndrome; slowed growth rates are common.	These studies should not be performed within 7 days of a radionuclide scan.
Adaptive behavior scales*	Assessment of language, motor, social, and self-care skills	Age-expected skills within 1 SD from mean	Children with suspected developmental delays.	Explain the test and how results will be interpreted.
IQ tests†	Assessment of cognitive abilities	Age-normal skills within 1½ SD from the mean	Children with suspected developmental delays.	Explain the test and how results will be interpreted.
Bone roentgenography	Assessment of bone plates and joint spaces	Age-expected bone age	Children with Down syndrome; decreased growth rate is common.	The child must be motionless during the study.
Brain sonography	Ultrasonogram of cranium	Normal position of brain's midline structures and normal blood flow velocity, no hemorrhages	Microcephaly or macrocephaly, misshapen cranium, family history of hydrocephaly.	The child must be supine. Any jewelry or metal objects should be removed from the child's head. The child may need sedation or may need to be restrained, because this procedure takes 1 hr to complete. Explain to the child that the test is not painful. Keep the child warm during the procedure.

Genetic analysis	Cytogenic bonding, culture media analysis	Normal findings for gene product analysis	Suspected genetic or neoplastic disorders.	Allow the child an opportunity to ask questions and express concerns about the possible results and implications of the testing.
Computed tomography	Special noninvasive radiographic technique that images brain tissue in very thin sections	No blood clots, tumors, or infections	Impaired development, such as microcephaly; family history of CNS malformations; possible tumors or subdural hematomas.	The child may need to be sedated or restrained and will need to assume supine position. Scans require the use of contrast medium so require informed consent.
Magnetic resonance imaging	Noninvasive method used to create images corresponding to density of tissue	Normal anatomy and physiology of the brain and spinal column	Same as for computed tomography.	The test requires informed consent. Remove metal or magnetic objects from the child before the study. Sedation of the child is usually required.
Positron emission tomography	Noninvasive means of comparing cerebral brain flow and metabolic changes; used to localize seizure foci, visualize brain hemodynamics, and study brain pharmacology using radioisotopes	Normal metabolism of glucose in brain, normal blood flow and electrical activity	Seizures, hydrocephaly, evidence of cerebral dysfunction.	The test requires informed consent. The child will need to be sedated. Liquids may be limited before the procedure. If not in diapers, the child will need to void before the procedure. Parents may be able to remain with the child during the procedure

SD, Standard deviation.

*Adaptive behavior scales include the AAMR test, the Minnesota Child Development Inventory Profile, the DDST-II, the Wechsler Preschool and Primary Scale of Intelligence (WPPSI), the Wechsler Intelligence Scale for Children (WISC-III), and the Wechsler Adult Intelligence Scale—Revised (WAIS-R).

†IQ tests include the Bayley Scales (birth to 3 yr), the Stanford-Binet Scale (2 yr and older), the WPPSI (3-6 yr), the WISC-III (6-16 yr), and the WAIS-R (16 yr and older).

Children with cognitive impairments have significant impairments in measured intelligence and adaptive behavior. Cognitive impairments can result from malformations of the brain and central nervous system (CNS), injury, infections, anoxia, poisoning, or prenatal alcohol use or the cause may be unknown. Specific disabilities are differentiated on the basis of an assessment of language, cognition, academic ability, self-help skills, social behaviors, and motor performance.

A cognitive impairment may be classified as a general delay, such as in mental retardation, or as a part of a larger constellation of failures in skill acquisition, such as in pervasive developmental disorders (PDDs). There is considerable overlap within several cognitive-related disorders. For example, children with autism, a specific disorder classified as a PDD, are often moderately or severely mentally retarded.

The family of a child with a cognitive impairment must cope with frequent and exceptionally high demands. The family is confronted with serious medical and environmental issues that rarely seem to be solved, only managed. Independence and self-management should be emphasized throughout childhood and adolescence so that, as the individual reaches adulthood, the possibility of independent living and gainful employment can be maximized.

The nurse is an integral part of the multidisciplinary team that manages the care of a child with a cognitive impairment. The nurse is involved in early assessment of the child, support of the family, assistance with self-care training and behavioral training, referral to support services, and providing the necessary nursing care for other disabilities the child may have. School and community nurses need a broad range of knowledge to support children who have multiple cognitive and physical disabilities.

TERMINOLOGY

The terminology associated with cognitive impairment differs according to the context of the setting in which the child is seen. Nurses encounter children with cognitive impairments in the hospital and community. The medical interpretation of cognitive impairment might differ from the legal interpretation; implications for nursing care will vary accordingly.

Cognitive Impairment

Cognitive impairment is a general term that denotes limitations in intellectual and functional abilities. Intelligence is a difficult concept, defined in a number of ways. The nurse needs to determine the meaning of the word as it is used by the professional and by the parent. Often, the child's intelligence quotient (IQ) has little meaning for the parent, so the nurse may need to explain its meaning and purpose. *Mental age* and *functional age* are terms often used to compare a child's mental ability with the expected mental or functional abilities of other children of the same chronologic age. Mental age gives some information about the level of cognitive understanding. For example, if an individual has a mental age of 5 years, the nurse's explanations need to be simple and specific, regardless of the individual's chronologic age. If the individual has a mental age of 12 years, however, the nurse's

explanations can provide more description and detail and can require some degree of inductive reasoning.

Functional age does not include the individual's life experience or functioning in adaptive skills. For example, an adult with a functional age of 12 years does not "have the mind of a 12-year-old" because that individual may have been affected by environmental experiences, such as job training and group living situations.

Mental Retardation

Mental retardation is a type of cognitive disability. The term mental retardation is often misunderstood because of the perception by some that mentally retarded people cannot learn self-care. Although mentally retarded children may have below-normal cognitive and adaptive functioning and may acquire self-care and intellectual skills more slowly than unaffected children, with support many can be educated, learn to hold a job, and independently accomplish some self-care activities (Centers for Disease Control and Prevention [CDC], 2004; National Dissemination Center for Children with Disabilities [NICHCY], 2004).

The American Association on Mental Retardation (AAMR), the leading professional organization in the area of mental retardation, has defined mental retardation as "a disability characterized by significant limitations both in intellectual functioning and in adaptive behavior as expressed in conceptual, social, and practical adaptive skills" (AAMR, 2002).

Mental retardation is not diagnosed unless the following conditions have been met (American Psychiatric Association, 2000):

- Manifests before age 18 years
- Includes significant subaverage general intellectual functioning
- Concurrent deficits in two or more adaptive areas, such as communication, home living, community use, health and safety, leisure, self-care, social skills, self-direction, functional academics, and work

Other terms used to describe individuals with mental retardation are *developmentally disabled*, *mentally handicapped*, and *mentally deficient*. The term applied usually reflects more the discipline of the professional assigning the diagnostic label rather than manifestations.

When standardized tests of intelligence are used, subaverage general intellectual functioning refers to an IQ score of 70 or below. Adaptive functioning refers to effective coping with common life demands, such as activities of daily living, communication skills, and social skills appropriate to others of the same age, sociocultural background, and community setting (NICHCY, 2004). Maximizing the child's identified strengths and supporting weak areas will allow the child to develop realistically to full potential (NICHCY, 2004).

Developmental Disability

Developmental disability is a term that has implications more for legal, administrative, and educational spheres than in medical or nursing diagnosis and treatment. The U.S.

government, in its attempt to provide equal rights for all disabled individuals, has defined a developmental disability as having the following components (Developmental Disabilities Assistance and Bill of Rights Act of 2000, 2000):

- Severe and chronic disability that is attributable to mental or physical impairment or a combination of both
- The impairment must be present before the individual turns 22 years old
- The impairment is likely to continue, reflecting the need for life-long individual services or support
- There must be substantial functional limitations in three or more areas, such as self-care, receptive and expressive language, learning, mobility, self-direction, capacity for independent living, or economic self-sufficiency

The definition of developmental disability encompasses children with mental retardation, sensory deficits (hearing, vision, and speech), orthopedic problems, and conditions such as cerebral palsy and PDDs.

Provisions in law that affect children with various disabilities have implications for nurses working in community or school settings. The Education for All Handicapped Children Act (PL 94-142) passed in 1975 required that states provide for all disabled children ages 3 to 21 years an education that is free and appropriate and in the least restrictive environment. Although the terminology has changed, this means that developmentally disabled children should be included in a regular classroom with their nondisabled peers. In 1990, this act was renamed the Individuals with Disabilities Education Act, and it was re-approved in 1997.

PL 99-457, signed into law in 1986, provided for early intervention for younger children. Early childhood intervention programs, such as Head Start, are ensured for any child with mental or physical disability from birth to age 3 years, at which time the public school system becomes involved.

As a result of these legislative efforts, each disabled child must have a written individualized education program (IEP) that outlines specialized instruction and services the school system will provide. The child's parents and school personnel design this after the school conducts an educational assessment. School nurses often sit on teams that design the IEP,

USING RESEARCH TO IMPROVE PRACTICE

Having a child who has either a physical or cognitive disability is challenging for parents, particularly if the child will require life-long care and support. Parents must not only adjust to the child's diagnosis but also to the long-term implications that their child's disability will have on social, emotional, and educational outcomes. Often referred to as the "burden of care," these parenting challenges involve generalized uncertainty about how to maximize the child's health and developmental outcomes within a climate of unpredictability (Lindblad, Rasmussen, & Sandman, 2005).

Nurses, both in community and acute care settings, can assist parents in various ways, through care, advocacy, and provision of support. Lindblad, Rasmussen, and Sandman (2005) suggest that providing support is an essential nursing intervention; however, in assessing what would constitute meaningful support, the nurse must first determine types of support parents believe they need. To this end, Lindblad, Rasmussen, and Sandman conducted a qualitative research study whose purpose was explore how parents of disabled children perceive receiving support from health professionals.

Unlike quantitative research, qualitative phenomenologic research explores a specific phenomenon in depth to gain a better understanding of its meaning to the participants. Lindblad, Rasmussen, and Sandman (2005) interviewed parents in 10 families and asked them to describe their experiences of being supported by health professionals. The authors recorded the interviews and later analyzed transcripts to identify relevant themes of support.

Overall, parents described increased support as that which assisted them with their daily burden and resulted in increased self-confidence in parenting a disabled child.

Conversely, they described decreased support as devaluing their child, minimizing their daily struggles, and decreasing their parenting self-confidence. Actions by health professionals that were seen by parents as disempowering included ignoring the parents' needs, minimizing their contributions to the child's care, focusing exclusively on the child's disability, viewing the child as being unworthy of assistance, and being unhelpful with the management of the daily burden (Lindblad et al., 2005). The authors suggest that unsupportive professionals can provoke confrontational and oppositional parenting strategies as the parents attempt to protect themselves and their child from perceived lack of caring.

Parents in this study described affirming issues such as recognizing the parents as individuals with their own needs and methods of coping, not just as being a parent of a disabled child; taking the time to establish and continue a trusting relationship; acknowledging parents as the experts in their child's care; being available and open for questions; assisting with referrals and information about legal rights; recognizing and valuing the child as a unique individual through effective communication with the child; and focusing on the child and not the disability. These constituted effective strategies of support that increased parents' self-confidence and empowered them.

After reading about this research on how parents perceive support, think about how you can improve the support you can provide to parents, whether you will practice in an acute care setting or in the community. What specific strategies might you use, for example, when admitting a child with a disability to a hospital unit or when communicating with parents in a school setting?

Lindblad, B., Rasmussen, B., & Sandman, P. (2005). Being invigorated in parenthood: Parents' experiences of being supported by professionals when having a disabled child. *Journal of Pediatric Nursing, 20,* 288-297.

giving expert advice about classroom adaptations or medical services needed for these children. When working with these families, the nurse may need to serve as a resource for helping families locate advocacy services for their children.

COGNITIVE IMPAIRMENT
Etiology

Cognitive impairment may be the result of congenital or early environmental factors such as maternal substance abuse or lack of stimulation in early childhood. It may also be the result of head injury, asphyxia, intracranial hemorrhage, infections, poisoning, or the presence or treatment of a brain tumor. Mental retardation has more than 350 known causes, but its specific cause is unknown in nearly half of all cases. New etiologies are being identified, and underlying mechanisms of known causes are becoming more clearly understood.

As medical technology advances, a medical basis for cognitive and adaptive impairments is found in an increasing proportion of cognitively impaired children. Often the cause is a subtle but nonetheless significant biologic factor, such as minor chromosomal abnormalities, rare genetic syndromes, subclinical lead intoxication, nutritional deficiencies, or exposure to numerous prenatal risks or trauma. Evidence suggests that early neurodevelopmental functioning and later neurologic integrity and intellectual ability are strongly associated. Low socioeconomic status and related factors have also been consistently reported as influencing cognitive function (Box 30-1).

Incidence

Cognitive impairments occur in 1% to 3% of the general population worldwide (World Health Organization, 2001). Among those diagnosed with mental retardation, 85% display only mild cognitive impairment, whereas only 0.3% to 0.5% exhibit signs of profound mental retardation (Shapiro & Batshaw, 2004). This distribution has clinical significance in that most families are able to care for mildly to moderately impaired children and adolescents at home.

Because a diagnosis of mental retardation and other developmental disabilities is based on adaptive behavior and intellectual functioning, the epidemiology varies throughout the life cycle. An increased incidence of retardation is reported in the early school years, and then the incidence declines in late adolescence as the children leave the formal education setting and are assimilated into the adult world. Most cognitively impaired individuals are able to marry (often to individuals with normal intellectual functioning), maintain employment, and have satisfying relationships.

Psychiatric comorbidity is common in people with cognitive impairment. For example, prevalence estimates for mental disorders and mental retardation are up to 60% to 70%, but the incidence is lower in children and adolescents compared with adults with mental retardation (Sadock & Sadock, 2003). Brain malfunctions that cause cognitive impairments frequently affect those areas of the brain that monitor emotional states. The most frequent accompanying diagnoses include disruptive behavioral disorders, depression, and atypical psychosis.

BOX 30-1	**Causes of Cognitive Impairment**

Hereditary Origin (5%)

Inborn errors of metabolism: galactosemia, Tay-Sachs disease, phenylketonuria

Hereditary syndromes: muscular dystrophy, tuberous sclerosis, neurofibromatosis

Chromosomal aberrations: Down syndrome, fragile X syndrome

Familial retardation of probable polygenic origin

Early Embryonic Alterations (30%–35%)

Sporadic chromosomal changes: Down syndrome

Multiple congenital anomalies: congenital hypothyroidism

Prenatal influence syndrome: intrauterine infections, drugs, alcohol, human immunodeficiency virus, unknown forces

Intrauterine infections: congenital rubella, toxoplasmosis, herpes

Early Intrauterine or Neonatal Alterations (10%–15%)

Fetal malnutrition: placental insufficiency, pregnancy-induced hypertension, drug addiction, maternal uterine cancer, multiple pregnancy

Neonatal conditions: prematurity, neonatal asphyxia, hyperbilirubinemia, hypoglycemia, CNS hemorrhage, ABO incompatibilities

Acquired Childhood Conditions or Diseases (3%–5%)

Complications of infections: meningitis, encephalitis, pertussis, varicella

Lead poisoning

Cranial trauma

Cerebral tumors

Cardiac arrest

Asphyxiation

Environmental Problems and Behavioral Syndromes (20%)

Psychosocial deprivation

Parental neurosis, psychosis, character disorder

Childhood psychosis, autism, other pervasive developmental disorders

Unknown Causes (30%–35%)

Data from American Psychiatric Association. (2000). *Diagnostic and statistical manual of mental disorders* (4th ed., text revision). Washington, DC: American Psychiatric Association; Mental retardation: A review of the past 10 years, part 1. (1997). *Journal of the American Academy of Child and Adolescent Psychiatry, 36,* 1656-1663.

There appears to be a significant relationship between developmental disabilities and child abuse. According to the Administration on Children, Youth, and Families, 6.5% of all reported child abuse case involved children with developmental disabilities (U.S. Department of Health and Human Services [DHHS], 2005). Possible reasons for this strong relationship are the intense stress experienced by families of disabled children, parental isolation, and unrealistic expectations for the child's performance because of a lack of knowledge about normal growth and development.

Evidence also suggests that abuse can result in developmental disabilities or physically disabling conditions.

Despite available funding and support groups, families of children with developmental delays often feel isolated from supportive services and report that professionals have limited understanding of their children's needs. These factors further perpetuate the sense of helplessness and lack of control in these family systems.

Manifestations

The cardinal sign of cognitive impairment or developmental disability is delayed achievement of developmental milestones. Specific congenital malformations often result in specific clinical manifestations. Also, the severity of the impairment affects the types and frequency of problem behaviors (Box 30-2).

In addition to general clinical manifestations based on the degree of impairment, many syndromes are characterized by particular features that are helpful in determining the cause of the cognitive impairment. Two genetic disorders in which cognitive impairment is a central feature are Down syndrome and fragile X syndrome. The infant with fetal alcohol syndrome (FAS) also has specific physical growth, facial, skeletal, and cardiac features.

Many disabilities associated with cognitive impairment can further limit a child's adaptive skills. These include cerebral palsy, visual deficits, seizure disorders, communication deficits, feeding problems, PDDs, failure to thrive, and attention deficit hyperactivity disorder. Speech and language development are often profoundly affected. Depending on the condition, seizure disorders frequently develop as the child matures.

Although children who are cognitively impaired can be generally healthy, the presence of associated disabilities may place these children at increased risk for illness (Fig. 30-1). For example, if a child who is cognitively impaired also has cerebral palsy, the risk for gastroesophageal reflux and aspiration pneumonia is high. Motor or swallowing problems may result in inadequate oral intake or insufficient weight gain.

Diagnostic Evaluation

Diagnostic evaluations may be performed in utero, during the neonatal period, or after the child fails to achieve expected developmental milestones. Tests may be general or specific

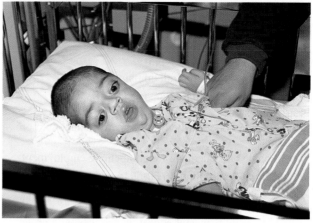

FIG 30-1 **Children with cognitive impairments may have other dysfunctions as well. The family of a child with a cognitive impairment often feels continual grief because the child does not meet their expectations. This child has Marshall-Smith syndrome, which does not appear to be hereditary. His bones ossified unusually early, necessitating a craniotomy to allow greater brain development. He has a tracheostomy because of respiratory difficulties associated with an abnormally developed larynx. A gastrostomy button facilitates his nutrition.** *(Courtesy Children's Medical Center, Dallas, TX.)*

for the neurologic or cognitive area in question. Several neuropsychologic tests assess the child's current level of functioning and help the clinician anticipate persistent cognitive impairments. These tests—which may involve pencil-and-paper tasks, motor tasks, sensory tasks, or some degree of cognitive processing—help determine both the severity and type of cognitive impairment (Box 30-3). Learning disabilities are often identified by using some of these same instruments, and many are available through the school system. Nurses also can learn to administer developmental screening tools, such as the Denver Developmental Screening Test II (DDST-II) (see Chapter 4 and Evolve website).

Often, a diagnosis of mental retardation is not made until the child enters school and has significant academic failure, prompting formal psychologic testing. Routine assessment of development during pediatric visits, however, is the best method of early detection.

Therapeutic Management

General Strategies

Medical strategies are directed toward preventing and treating infections, correcting structural deformities, and treating associated behaviors, such as aggressiveness. Corrective measures might include congenital heart surgery for malformations, inserting tympanostomy tubes, or placing splints on joints that are hypotonic and hyperextended. Frequently, antibiotics are given prophylactically to reduce the likelihood of infections. The treatment of behavioral difficulties and psychosocial disturbances may involve administration of medications.

Therapeutic management depends largely on community and educational resources. Obtaining services for these children, however, requires multidisciplinary efforts and strong advocacy on the part of both parents and professionals. Reduction in the occurrence of developmental disabilities is a national

BOX 30-2	Problems Related to Cognitive Impairment

Mild
Self-esteem issues related to presence or absence of physical features, largely determined by the cause of the cognitive disability
Social isolation and loneliness
Depression

Severe
Self-injury
Fecal smearing
Tearing of personal clothes and objects
Severe temper tantrums
Disrobing

Text continued on p. 1008

BOX 30-3	Expected Skills According to Intelligence Quotient Scores

Normal Intelligence (IQ 85-115)

Age-normal skills across all domains

Borderline Mental Retardation (IQ 71-84)

Early milestones achieved

Likely to be noticed when school performance is monitored

Vocational skills adequate for competitive employment

Mild Mental Retardation (IQ 50-55 to ≈70)

Slight delay in achieving developmental milestones

No alteration in sequence of skill acquisition

Likely to require special education services with an emphasis on vocational and self-maintenance skills

Able to form and maintain adult relationships

Moderate Mental Retardation (IQ 35-40 to 50-55)

Noticeable delay in motor and speech development

Early and persistent training in self-care required

Supervision required for complex activities or problem solving

Severe Mental Retardation (IQ 20-25 to 35-40)

Marked delay in all motor skills

Limited expressive speech even though some receptive language skills may be present

Constant supervision required

Profound Mental Retardation (IQ <20-25)

May be able to walk

May have primitive speech

Constant supervision required

Modified from American Psychiatric Association. (2000). *Diagnostic and statistical manual of mental disorders* (4th ed., text revision). Washington, DC: American Psychiatric Association; Batshaw, M. L. (2001). *When your child has a disability.* (2nd ed.). Baltimore: Paul H. Brookes Publishing.

priority identified in *Healthy People 2010* (U.S. DHHS, 2000). Adequate prenatal care is of primary importance. An additional priority related to children with disabilities is increasing the percentage of time children with disabilities spend in regular school programs (U.S. DHHS, 2000).

Safety Challenges

Children who are cognitively impaired are, by definition, less capable of managing environmental challenges than are their peers who are unimpaired. Because of impaired functioning, injuries are generally more common in these children than in same-age peers. Among preschool-age children, however, injuries are less common in those with cognitive impairment because the parents of these children are very protective and the children have less exposure to risk.

Table 30-1 presents some safety issues to be taught in the home and in the community. Although the learning needs of children who are cognitively impaired are similar to those of children without disabilities, children with cognitive impairments may need prolonged teaching, more demonstration during teaching, frequent verbal and visual reminders, and more practice.

CRITICAL TO REMEMBER

Safety for the Child With a Cognitive Impairment

Safety is a persistent concern of parents, teachers, and health professionals caring for children who are cognitively impaired. The child's maturation in anticipating danger, in problem solving, and in judgment is generally impaired across the life span. Children with motor disabilities are often unable to perform skills in ways that foster safety.

TABLE 30-1	Safety Concerns for Developmentally Delayed or Impaired Children	
Site of Concern	**Possible Injury**	**Education and Training Issues**
Home		
Kitchen	Burns Poisoning	*Preschool age:* preventive education (i.e., instruct not to touch hot stove, not to ingest toxic substances) *Elementary school age:* safe use of equipment, basic safety *High school age:* cooking safety, emergency precautions
Bathroom	Falls Burns Cuts	*Elementary school age:* tub safety, precautions on wet floors *High school age:* safe use of hair care equipment, shaving utensils, and similar objects
General		*Preschool and elementary school age:* avoidance of electrical outlets, safe passage around objects
Outdoors		
Yard or playground	Animal bites Poisoning Abduction	*Preschool age:* staying within boundaries, appropriate response to strange animals and people, safe use of equipment, avoidance of ingestion of berries *Elementary school age:* stranger safety, bicycle safety, traffic safety, water safety
Vehicles	Cuts Falls Serious injury	*Preschool and elementary school age:* seatbelt use, keeping hands in car *High school age:* traffic safety

NURSING CARE PLAN

The Child With a Cognitive Impairment in the Community Setting

Focused Assessment: The Child

Assess cognitive skills and level of adaptive functioning, keeping in mind age-expected abilities that can be used as a standard for comparison (see Chapters 5 through 8). Life experiences also affect a child's abilities. Children who have had limited exposure to social rules and limited opportunities for thinking about their experiences will talk and act differently from children who have had more practice in these areas. Alternating between questions and demonstrations may be helpful in maintaining the child's interest in the assessment.

Look directly at the child, and speak in a direct and simple yet noncondescending manner. Ask the child for as much of the necessary information as possible rather than relying solely on the parents to provide the information. As the child speaks, attend to the child's level of communication, skill in using words to communicate, and ability to follow one-step commands or more complicated requests.

Focused Assessment: The Family

Assess the family's level of functioning, particularly available coping skills and the family's awareness of and involvement in addressing the child's needs. The child may come from a home where the parents have below-average intellectual functioning, or the parents may be young and lack understanding of development, making them less aware of their child's abilities and functional deficits. Explore the family's social and financial resources in a manner that is informative but respectful of privacy. A matter-of-fact approach is helpful in assessing how the family meets the basic needs of each member and manages the exceptional medical, psychologic, educational, and social needs of the child who is cognitively impaired. This part of the assessment may be lengthy because it may be necessary to assist the family in seeking long-term assistance for meeting the child's needs.

The family's interaction patterns and situational coping skills should be assessed on a continuing basis. Families with developmentally disabled children feel grief much as do families of children with other chronic illnesses (see

Chapter 12), particularly when there is no known cause for the disability. During the grief process, the family becomes preoccupied with the child's disabilities and symptoms, and then the family begins to identify the child's strengths and resources and moves toward a sense of integration and homeostasis. This process is repeated with each new developmental stage or situational setback, such as surgery or illness.

An interdisciplinary approach is critical for the effective management of children with cognitive impairments. The team generally includes physicians, nurses, psychologists, speech and language pathologists, educational and recreational professionals, and possibly physical therapists and occupational therapists. In addition to nursing care, the family may be referred for genetic counseling and supportive psychotherapy. The assessment should identify the need for other team members or auxiliary services. Long-term services may include respite care, in-home services, parent training, and support groups.

NURSING DIAGNOSIS   Risk for Injury related to level of self-care skills and inability to anticipate danger.

EXPECTED OUTCOME   The parent and child will:
- Describe and avoid unsafe situations that lead to self-injury or unintentional injury.

Intervention	*Rationale*
1. Provide anticipatory guidance relative to the child's specific developmental abilities.	1. Parents may not be able to anticipate the child's cognitive or functional level accurately, particularly if the parents are inexperienced or have limited cognitive skills themselves.
2. Keep safety rails up on hospital beds and on the bed at home if the child is predisposed to falling or roaming at night. Provide child-size furniture, and select age- and skill-related play equipment.	2. These strategies help prevent accidental falls because these children are accident prone and have limited ability to assess the environment for safety.
3. Give simple explanations about unsafe areas in the environment. Use the child's cognitive level as a key to what the child can understand or the degree of unsupervised freedom that can safely be allowed.	3. Young or cognitively delayed individuals can understand concrete explanations.

Continued

NURSING CARE PLAN—cont'd

Evaluation

- Can the parent or child describe unsafe situations?
- Has the child remained safe and not sustained any injury?

NURSING DIAGNOSIS   Deficient Knowledge (family members) related to unfamiliarity with the cause and likely outcomes of the child's cognitive disabilities, available support systems, or information about sexuality, vocational options, leisure skills, and so on.

EXPECTED OUTCOMES   The family will:
- Describe and plan for the child's special needs.
- Access and use personal and community resources to increase the child's ability to develop personal skills for appropriate social, leisure, and vocational abilities.

Intervention	Rationale
1. Provide information that is simple, concrete, and solution focused.	1. Stress may impair the family's adaptive coping skills.
2. Explain any medical terms without assuming that the family knows the terminology. Give explanations to both the child and the parents. Use demonstrations and therapeutic play. If the child is hospitalized, communicate information about the child's cognitive and functional level to other team members.	2. The child may have a limited capacity to understand words but may be able to understand a demonstration.
3. Select skills that enhance self-care and socially appropriate behaviors. As the child reaches puberty, provide simple information about sexuality and physical changes. Support training in leisure skills.	3. Education that is practical and functional for the child's mental and chronologic age fosters self-esteem, compliance, and cooperation.
4. Identify for the parents local and national resources for care, education, and training of cognitively impaired children.	4. Additional services will be needed as the child grows or needs more specialized training. Families may have to find out-of-home placement if the child's disability is severe or destructive to the family.
5. Provide parents with anticipatory guidance about developmental milestones and anticipated skills, including safety, sexuality, skills that can be expected, and behavioral changes throughout the developmental process.	5. Parents may have unrealistic expectations or expect too little from the child.

Evaluation

- Has the family made progress in describing and planning for the child's special needs?
- Has the family used the resources available in the community to maximize the child's abilities?

NURSING DIAGNOSIS   Impaired Social Interaction related to an inability to initiate and maintain social relationships.

EXPECTED OUTCOMES   The child will:
- Develop positive relationships with family and peers.
- Have solitary leisure skills.

Intervention	Rationale
1. Encourage the parents to support the child in participating in group activities that promote peer interactions (e.g., Special Olympics, special camps) (Fig. 30-2). The family will arrange social activities with other children (e.g., visiting the park with friends, inviting friends to the home to play).	1. To accommodate to social expectations and demands, children who are cognitively impaired or developmentally disabled need to be exposed to children who are not impaired and to children with similar challenges.
2. Encourage the parents to participate in interactive activities, such as reading books and playing, on a regular basis.	2. Families are likely to limit interactions because the child offers reduced reinforcements in social situations.

NURSING CARE PLAN—cont'd

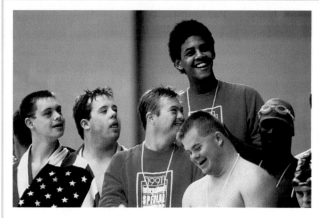

FIG 30-2 **Special Olympics International is the largest recreational program in the world for people with mental retardation. With more than 1 million athletes in 125 countries, Special Olympics offers opportunities for social interaction with peers and assists children who are mentally retarded in reaching their maximum potential.** *(Courtesy Special Olympics, Inc.)*

Evaluation

- Has the child demonstrated a sense of pleasure in social interactions with family members and with other individuals within the child's social sphere?

NURSING DIAGNOSIS Compromised Family Coping or Disabled Family Coping related to excessive emotional and financial strain on family members caring for a child who is cognitively impaired, lack of acceptance by society, or an extended grieving process associated with diagnosis of a child with a chronic disability.

EXPECTED OUTCOMES The family will:
- Integrate the child in the family system in a manner that facilitates maximum growth and maturity.
- Express self-satisfaction in their family management.
- Demonstrate social acceptance within the community.

Intervention

1. Provide anticipatory and continuing support for the grieving process. Parents should be told the diagnosis and be given needed information as quickly as possible. This information should be given when both parents or supportive family members are available. Information may need to be explained in different ways (orally, in writing, with videos) to help parents grasp the meaning of the diagnosis.

2. Assist in identifying appropriate resources for social interactions and social training (e.g., early intervention programs, special education programs, recreational programs for developmentally disabled children).

3. Identify and refer the family to appropriate community resources for both emotional support and family and child education. The nurse may need to act as an advocate and referral center (about support groups, education consultants, home health agencies).

4. Assist family members to identify realistic short- and long-term goals for the child and themselves. Encourage the family to express feelings and concerns; provide hope when appropriate.

Rationale

1. Families typically experience a cycle of grieving that is repeated when milestones are not reached or when the child has an illness or a change in behavior.

2. Individuals who are mildly or moderately impaired often feel loneliness and depression as a result of insufficient stimulation and social contact. Such programs can assist the child in reaching maximum potential.

3. The grieving process and the need to accommodate to the child's skill level are continuous; families often feel isolated and helpless in locating necessary resources.

4. Stress, grieving, and limited knowledge may impair the family's ability to set reasonable goals by itself.

Continued

NURSING CARE PLAN—cont'd

5. Educate the parents in monitoring the child for alterations in health status. Help the family recognize nonverbal signs of discomfort.

6. Assist family members in exploring their choices for home care, a group home, or a residential facility.

5. The child may be unable to verbalize pain typically associated with ear infections, colds, or major illnesses.

6. Families may hesitate to discuss care options out of fear of being perceived as uncaring or unable to provide home care.

Evaluation

• Does the family integrate the child in the family system in a manner that facilitates growth and maturity to the greatest degree possible?

• Does the family seek medical attention when needed and use several resources to meet the child's social, emotional, educational, and medical needs?

• Is the family able to meet financial responsibilities?
• Does the family participate in social activities outside the family?

DOWN SYNDROME

The genetic disorder most frequently seen as causing moderate to severe mental retardation is Down syndrome (trisomy 21). The assessment and nursing interventions for the child who is cognitively impaired are applicable to these individuals. Additional considerations, however, apply to those identified as having Down syndrome.

Depending on the severity of the symptoms, most parents raise the child at home until early adulthood, after which group home placement is an option. Supported employment is encouraged, and parents are typically advised to initiate vocational training in elementary school. The partnership of parents and professionals is vital in managing the symptoms and in providing the comprehensive services that are needed.

Services required throughout the life span include education and vocational training, transitional services, respite care, social services, financial supplements, psychotherapy, and preventive or corrective medical care (Box 30-4). This array of needed services may be overwhelming to the family, and the potential for frustration on the part of both the parents and the professional team is high. Communication and coordination of services are considered primary tasks for each team member (Fig. 30-3).

Etiology

Although the specific cause is unknown, late maternal age has been consistently identified as one of the most significant factors associated with Down syndrome. The risk of a 35-year-old woman bearing a child with trisomy 21 is 1 in 400; by age 40 years, the risk increases to 1 in 100. As a result of early screening for older women who are at high risk for having a child with Down syndrome, most of these children are now born to women younger than 35 years (80% of affected children) (March of Dimes, 2004).

Several chromosomal alterations that result in Down syndrome have been identified. In 97% of Down syndrome

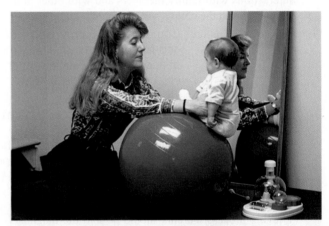

FIG 30-3 **Children with delayed motor or cognitive function, whether temporary or pervasive, benefit from early and vigorous therapy to help them reach their maximum development.** *(Courtesy Cook Children's Medical Center, Fort Worth, TX.)*

cases, *nondisjunction*, a failure of the chromosomes to separate normally during meiosis, occurs. The remaining 3% result from *translocation*, a fusion of two chromosomes, usually 21 and 15, resulting in a total of 46 chromosomes despite the extra chromosome 21. Translocator carrier parents are at increased risk for producing multiple offspring with Down syndrome (Cuckle, 2005).

Incidence

In the United States, more than 300,000 individuals have Down syndrome, with up to 10,000 new cases occurring each year. This syndrome accounts for one third of all cases of moderate to severe mental retardation. The prevalence of Down syndrome is 1 in 800 live births (Leshin, 2003). Affected boys outnumber affected girls. More than half the trisomy 21 pregnancies spontaneously abort early in the pregnancy (Hall, 2004).

| BOX 30-4 | **Medical Conditions Associated with Down Syndrome** |

Conditions Frequently Identified During the Neonatal Period

- Cardiac conditions:
  - —Endocardial cushion defect
  - —Tetralogy of Fallot
  - —Atrial septal defects
  - —Patent ductus arteriosus
  - —Ventricular septal defects
- Gastrointestinal conditions:
  - —Tracheoesophageal fistula
  - —Pyloric stenosis
  - —Imperforate anus
  - —Duodenal atresia
  - —Aganglionic megacolon (Hirschsprung's disease)
- Congenital cataracts
- Hypothyroidism
- Dysplastic hips
- Leukemia-like conditions

Conditions Frequently Identified During Childhood

- Endocrine disorders:
  - —Decreased growth
  - —Obesity resulting from overeating, underexercise, or undetected hypothyroidism
  - —Thyroid dysfunction
  - —Infertility (male)
  - —Alopecia
  - —Thin hair
- Sensitive skin and propensity for rashes
- Ophthalmic problems, such as myopia, strabismus, nystagmus, cataracts, blepharitis, and keratoconus
- Chronic serous otitis media
- Hematologic abnormalities:
  - —Subtle immune deficiencies
  - —Acute nonlymphoblastic leukemia
  - —Acute lymphoblastic leukemia
- Craniofacial defects:
  - —Malocclusions
  - —Delayed tooth eruption
  - —Periodontal disease and gingivitis
  - —Bruxism
  - —Sinusitis and rhinitis
  - —Sleep apnea as a result of cranial malformations
- Musculoskeletal abnormalities:
  - —Hypotonia
  - —Joint laxity and dislocations
  - —Atlantoaxial subluxation or dislocation
- Sensory deficits
- Seizure disorders
- Psychiatric disorders, particularly adjustment reaction disorders, anxiety disorders, depression, behavior disorders, dementia
- PDDs

PATHOPHYSIOLOGY

DOWN SYNDROME

Trisomy 21, or Down syndrome, occurs when three representatives of chromosome 21 are present instead of the usual two. There is some evidence that a particular region of chromosome 21 is responsible for the facial features, heart defects, mental retardation, and dermatologic changes. Many of the malformations in this disorder result from incomplete rather than abnormal embryogenesis. Examples include malformations of the atrioventricular canal, tracheoesophageal fistula, and imperforate anus. Alterations in neurotransmitters, particularly in the cholinergic system, are responsible for the premature aging and Alzheimer's-type dementia that are common in children with Down syndrome.

A number of medical problems in the newborn period can seriously compromise health and survival. If the child survives these complications, a number of less serious difficulties are generally encountered in childhood.

Manifestations

More than 100 signs describe Down syndrome, including altered facial and head features, such as brachycephaly (disproportionate shortness of the head); flat profile; upward slanted palpebral fissures; inner epicanthal folds; wide, flat, nasal bridge; narrow, high-arched palate; protruding tongue; small, short ears, which may be low-set; and delayed tooth eruption with poor alignment. In addition to facial and head features, certain body features also may be apparent in the child with Down syndrome. These include short stature; short, broad hands; simian line (single transverse palmar crease); broad, stubby feet with plantar crease; wide gap between first and second toes; short, broad neck; likelihood of umbilical hernia; dry skin with a tendency to crack and fissure; hyperextensibility of joints with hypotonicity of muscles; and atlantoaxial instability (i.e., at the first and second cervical vertebrae). Children with Down syndrome are more at risk for congenital cardiac defects, vision and hearing difficulties, and childhood leukemia.

In addition to the physical features of Down syndrome, children with Down syndrome have associated intellectual, language, and social dysfunctions, including mild to severe mental retardation; language development characterized by particular difficulty with grammar but general strength in social language (e.g., greeting others, carrying on a conversation in a give-and-take manner); social skills that exceed expected skills on the basis of intellectual capacity; limited ability to use the environmental cues available (i.e., infrequent scanning and use of only a few referential cues, such as eye contact with the primary caregiver, which often results in an inability to extract the information needed to draw conclusions); and blunted affect. As they age, people with Down syndrome have declining intellectual abilities, reduced social and adaptive skills, and the onset of Alzheimer's-type dementia.

Diagnostic Evaluation

Down syndrome is usually evident at birth because of the characteristic prominent features, although if the diagnosis is questionable, chromosomal analysis is conducted. Other diagnostic tests are conducted on the basis of the associated features, such as nasopharyngeal abnormalities or cardiac defects. Prenatal testing includes amniocentesis or chorionic villus sampling. An abnormal triple maternal serum screen value (low alpha-fetoprotein, low unconjugated estriol, and increased human gonadotropin levels) may prompt additional testing (Hall, 2004). More recently, ultrasonography can detect and measure neck folds along with characteristic cardiac or other abnormalities associated with Down syndrome (Hall, 2004).

To rule out associated disorders and to detect frequently encountered difficulties, clinicians recommend that the child be monitored frequently throughout the first 12 months of life, with an emphasis on gastrointestinal and cardiac symptoms. The diagnosis often requires a full cardiac workup initially and an electrocardiogram at the end of the first year. In the second to fourth years of life, the medical emphasis is on sleep and behavioral difficulties, along with annual thyroid screening and ophthalmologic assessment. Generally, the child is referred for dental assessments at 24 months and should be re-evaluated medically and behaviorally at least annually throughout childhood.

Therapeutic Management

The management of Down syndrome is manifestation specific because there is no cure for the disorder. Surgery to correct cardiac abnormalities, gastrointestinal malformations, and craniofacial deviations has been used to prolong life, alleviate discomfort, and decrease the likelihood of further medical complications. Neck radiography should be performed before the child participates in any sports because of the risk for children with Down syndrome to have atlantoaxial instability.

NURSING CARE

The Child With Down Syndrome

Assessment

Neonatal assessment is crucial in diagnosing Down syndrome on the basis of physiologic characteristics (see Chapter 5). Assessment for Down syndrome is based on family history, especially the mother's age. If Down syndrome is suspected or already confirmed on the basis of earlier genetic testing, serum alpha-fetoprotein levels, or amniotic fluid samples, an assessment is conducted to determine the severity of the manifestations and the family's ability to cope with and accommodate the needs of the infant. Assessment for mental retardation is also appropriate for the child with Down syndrome.

A thorough physical examination should be conducted, including hearing and vision examinations. Children with Down syndrome are at increased risk for hearing deficits and refractive errors or cataracts.

If a child with Down syndrome is hospitalized for surgical repair, infections, or injury, assess the child's typical coping patterns to support strategies already in place. Children with Down syndrome prefer routine and consistency, so an assessment of their daily routine is important; include times and habits related to mealtimes, bathing, and order of dressing. Assessing the child's understanding of language and ability to communicate is important to provide information that the child can understand. Knowing the child's words for specific body functions, such as voiding, defecating, or sleeping, will allow for greater comfort for the hospitalized child. It is important to assess the child's learning abilities before initiating any education or procedure-related play.

The child's motor skills are assessed to determine what procedures will be necessary to ensure the child's safety. Children with Down syndrome often are awkward and somewhat uncoordinated, which increases the likelihood of their falling. Self-stimulating behaviors (e.g., picking at the arm) need to be identified because they are often used as coping strategies but may also be self-injurious. Sensory deficits, such as vision or hearing difficulties, should be identified as part of the routine well assessment. Such deficits can be detected by closely observing as the child reaches for objects, by listening to conversation, or by speaking the child's name. The child with Down syndrome, however, may respond to sensory stimuli less noticeably than unimpaired children or may respond with dulled affect, even if hearing or vision deficits are not present.

> Health care professionals may forget the importance of discussing normal aspects of the child with parents. For example, the nurse may state, "Look how Billy's eyes light up when he sees someone he knows."

An environmental assessment will help determine whether it is conducive to safety and provides sufficient stimulation. Affected children frequently do not seek out stimulation and may need encouragement through colors, sound, and motion. An assessment of social behaviors is also important and should include play, social judgment skills, and social interest in the environment. The child may demonstrate inappropriate behaviors similar to those associated with severe mental retardation. Moreover, the child's natural curiosity may be diminished as a result of fear or frustration. Nursing care of the child with Down syndrome is similar to that for any child with a cognitive impairment with some specific additions.

Nursing Diagnosis and Planning

The nursing diagnoses and expected outcomes that are appropriate for the child with Down syndrome and the child's family are as follow:

- Impaired Parenting related to the child's delayed development, physical appearance, and medical complications.

  Expected Outcome: The family will demonstrate satisfying and supportive relationships that meet the physical and emotional needs of each family member.

- Self-Care Deficit (Bathing/Hygiene, Dressing/Grooming, Feeding, Toileting) related to cognitive immaturity.
  Expected Outcome: The child will demonstrate the ability to independently meet needs related to bathing/ hygiene, dressing/grooming, feeding, and toileting.
- Delayed Growth and Development related to poor sucking abilities or mouth deformities, flaccid facial muscles, or other abnormalities.
  Expected Outcomes: The child will maximize progress toward attaining developmental milestones and will demonstrate appropriate and measurable growth during childhood.

Interventions

When the child is a neonate, the parents will need assistance and support to accept the child's diagnosis and to appropriately plan for the child's care. The nurse assists the parents to identify positive features and behaviors in the child; looking at the child's strengths from the beginning reduces the likelihood that parents will see the child negatively as the child does not attain milestones along with others of the same chronologic age.

The nurse helps the parents explore options for fluid and calorie intake. Breastfeeding may not be possible if the child's muscle tone or sucking reflex is immature, although some children with Down syndrome can breastfeed adequately. As the child develops, special bottles or adaptive utensils may assist the child with feeding. Refer the parents for nutritional counseling as needed. Provide resources for behavioral training to encourage intake of new foods or the acquisition of new skills.

Children with Down syndrome like routine, and changes in routine often result in excessive frustration and decreased coping abilities. When the child is hospitalized, the nurse must try to keep the child's environment and routine as close to the home routine as possible; providing important details on the child's written care plan ensures consistency. Remember that the child's plan of care is based on the child's cognitive and adaptive abilities, rather than on chronologic age, and the child's skills may be age appropriate in some areas but markedly delayed in others. Parents must be encouraged to observe the child for signs of readiness to learn a new task (reaching for a cup, attempting to dress) and encourage self-care whenever possible. The child's level of coordination, muscle strength, and dexterity may not allow the child to zip, button, or feed self in the usual way, so adaptive tools may be needed.

As the child grows, advise the parents to encourage participation in recreational activities that the child can manage. Be sure to advise them that the child will need to have neck radiography before participating in any active sports program.

Evaluation

- Have the child and family demonstrated positive and mutually satisfying interactions?
- Are the parents able to identify the child's strengths and positive attributes?

- Do the parents state an interest and willingness to help the child learn new skills through demonstration, repetition, and much positive feedback?
- Does the child demonstrate continued development and a sense of competence in self-care skills?
- Does the child demonstrate steady progress toward attaining developmental milestones and appropriate measurable growth?

FRAGILE X SYNDROME

Fragile X syndrome is the most common inherited cause of mental retardation. The majority of boys who inherit this disorder are mentally retarded or have learning disabilities. The disorder usually does not manifest as mental retardation in females, but a female carrier normally passes the fragile X chromosome to her offspring. This syndrome has a unique profile of behavioral and cognitive patterns.

Etiology

The gene that causes fragile X syndrome is located on the X chromosome. Typically, a female child receiving the X chromosome that has a fragile site will become a carrier and will be mildly affected, if at all. The female may continue to pass on the abnormal X chromosome. A male, however, will usually exhibit the full effects if he receives the abnormal gene. Transmission occurs through carrier mothers and not through an unaffected "carrier" father.

Incidence

Fragile X syndrome affects approximately 1 in 4000 male children and 1 in 8000 female children (McBride & Choi, 2005). As many as 1 in 250 females and 1 in 1000 males carry the fragile X gene, either as a premutation or as a full mutation (Jewell, 2004). In general, only males exhibit the full effects of this X-linked recessive disorder because their single X chromosome has the abnormal gene. Approximately 50% to 70% of females with the full genetic mutation manifest cognitive impairments, usually with borderline to mild mental retardation.

Manifestations

Physical features associated with fragile X syndrome include facial dysmorphism, with large or prominent ears and a long, narrow face; a head circumference that may be disproportionate to height and weight; lowered epicanthal folds; and prominent nasal alae (cartilaginous flap on outer side of each

---

> **PATHOPHYSIOLOGY**
>
> **FRAGILE X SYNDROME**
>
> Fragile X syndrome is caused by an underlying single gene defect. There is an abnormality in the fragile X mental retardation (FMRI) gene in all affected individuals. There are excessive repetitions of the nucleotide CGG deoxyribonucleic acid (DNA) sequences in affected individuals.

nostril). In addition, the child may manifest enlarged testicles (postpubertal macro-orchidism), flat feet, lax ankles, hyperextensible fingers, soft and smooth skin, and mitral valve prolapse. There are intellectual, language, and social dysfunctions associated with fragile X syndrome, which include disruptive behaviors, such as temper tantrums; self-injurious behaviors; extreme agitation; autistic-like behaviors, such as gaze avoidance, hand flapping, echolalia, and abnormal speech patterns; hyperkinetic behaviors, including restlessness, agitation, and attention deficits; hand biting; and sensory motor integration deficits, such as poor coordination, motor planning deficits, and tactile defensiveness. Boys exhibit cognitive deficits in the moderate to severe range, with strengths in visual memory but weaknesses in auditory processing abilities and abstract reasoning, improved performance with simultaneous rather than sequential processing, language delays, perseveration, tangential speech, and other communicative disorders. Girls manifest only mild cognitive deficits, but with many variations. Many have progressive dementia.

Diagnostic Evaluation

Deoxyribonucleic acid testing is the definitive method of diagnosing fragile X syndrome. Identification of the *FMR1* gene mutation allows diagnosis in both carriers and those affected. Children with mental retardation of unknown cause or learning disabilities, together with manifestations of fragile X syndrome, should be considered for fragile X testing.

Therapeutic Management

Treatment is provided through various types of therapy. Special education, vocational programs, and behavioral management classes are important to overall development. Speech and language evaluation and therapy are generally prescribed during the first year of life and are made available on a continuing basis. Sensorimotor integration therapy may be offered to enhance motor planning, joint stability, coordination, and integration of visual, auditory, and tactile information. Sensorimotor therapy is considered to be the intervention of choice for these children with learning disabilities.

Nursing Considerations

The nursing care of individuals with fragile X syndrome is similar to care for any child with a cognitive impairment, but with specific attention to the behavioral and cognitive

---

PATHOPHYSIOLOGY

FETAL ALCOHOL SYNDROME

Alcohol and its metabolite (acetaldehyde) cross the placenta rapidly; therefore, the fetus has blood levels of alcohol equivalent to the maternal levels. Prenatal alcohol exposure is thought to affect protein synthesis, influencing growth and development of the brain and other tissues. This can result in decreased brain cell number, diminished intelligence, and brain malformation.

---

difficulties presented by the individual child. The plan should include a multidisciplinary team approach to assessment. Anticipatory guidance should be provided, with a review of the support groups and services available. Special education services will be necessary to address the child's specific cognitive and academic difficulties and to foster continued skill development and to reduce the stress created in the typical educational setting. Remediation services should include behavioral interventions specific to the child's needs, speech and language assistance, and possibly occupational and physical therapy to address visual-motor and motor skill deficits. Family members of children with fragile X syndrome should receive genetic counseling and testing.

Assessment for other related abnormalities, such as cleft palate, foot deformities, hip dislocations and other conditions involving joint hyperextensibility, hernias, and hypertonia, should also be performed. These children may have seizures, so medications and educating the family about seizure disorders may be warranted.

FETAL ALCOHOL SYNDROME

Fetal alcohol syndrome (FAS) is the most severe form of fetal alcohol spectrum disorder experienced by the infant exposed to alcohol in utero. FAS refers to the classic defects of persistent symmetric growth retardation, malformations of the face and skull, skeletal and cardiac malformation, and CNS functional abnormalities, including mental retardation.

Etiology and Incidence

Maternal alcohol consumption is the cause of FAS. No safe level of alcohol consumption during pregnancy has been established. The incidence of FAS is believed to be grossly underestimated because of lack of awareness in diagnosis and underreporting of alcohol intake during pregnancy. The incidence of FAS varies by country and ethnic group, but it is estimated to be 1 to 3 per 1000 live births in the United States (Chudney et al., 2005).

Manifestations

The infant with FAS exhibits prenatal and postnatal growth deficiency, microcephaly, joint anomalies, mild to moderate mental retardation, tremulousness in the neonatal period, and irritability; the child with FAS exhibits hyperactivity. Infants may have characteristic facial features, including short palpebral fissures, smooth philtrum (the vertical groove in the median portion of the upper lip), and thin upper lip. Other abnormalities, including altered palmar crease patterns, short distal phalanges, cervical vertebral malformations, ear anomalies, cleft lip and palate, severe cardiac defects, renal anomalies, strawberry hemangiomas, and genital anomalies, are associated with this syndrome.

Diagnostic Evaluation

The CDC convened a working group to explicitly define FAS and establish a consensus on diagnostic criteria for the syndrome (CDC, 2005). Alcohol exposure during pregnancy is established by self-report, reports by other reliable individuals, documented elevated blood alcohol level, alcohol treatment, or documentation of other known alcohol-related problems. The use of alcohol is not totally necessary, however, for a diagnosis of FAS (CDC, 2005). An infant or child can be diagnosed with FAS if the following criteria are present (CDC, 2005):

- Three facial abnormalities—smooth philtrum, thin vermillion border, small palpebral fissures
- Growth deficit—≤10th percentile for height, weight, or both
- CNS abnormalities—head circumference ≤10th percentile, brain abnormalities identified by imaging studies, motor deficits or seizures from no other identified cause, and cognitive/functional deficits below the expected range for the child's age, physical or psychosocial circumstances

FAS is diagnosed through physical examination and perinatal history, and a referral is often made to a geneticist. Families require counseling to help them cope with the diagnosis and to help them understand the risks involved in future pregnancies if lifestyle changes are not made.

NURSING CARE

The Infant With Fetal Alcohol Syndrome

Assessment

The family requires assistance in coping with the diagnosis and the difficulties associated with an irritable infant. Special attention must be given to involving the parents in the care of the infant. Early intervention maximizes the developmental potential.

When FAS is suspected, an extensive diagnostic workup is required. Microcephaly, hypotonia, tremulousness, and irritability can raise levels of suspicion. Feeding difficulties may be encountered as well.

Nursing Diagnosis and Planning

The nursing diagnoses and expected outcomes that apply to the infant with FAS and the family are as follow:

- Ineffective Infant Feeding Pattern related to congenital anomaly.
  Expected Outcome: The infant will establish appropriate sleep-wake and feeding patterns, as evidenced by appropriate weight gain and growth.
- Delayed Growth and Development related to FAS.
  Expected Outcome: The infant will develop to maximum potential, as evidenced by growth and development behaviors relative to age and potential.
- Deficient Knowledge (infant's anomalies and potential sequelae) related to lack of exposure to accurate information.
  Expected Outcome: Parents will increase knowledge related to the child's disorder, as evidenced by recognition of FAS and acknowledgment of the potential for future problems.
- Interrupted Family Processes related to birth of a disabled child.

Expected Outcome: The family will use coping strategies to care for the child, as evidenced by an ability to mobilize their energies toward caring for the infant with FAS.

Interventions

Daily weight gain is monitored, and intake and output are measured and documented. Various feeding strategies (e.g., varying the positioning of the infant; trying smaller, more frequent feedings; using different nipples) should be attempted until the infant is successful with nipple feedings or breastfeedings. Because parents may become frustrated or feel inadequate in dealing with a difficult feeder, it is important to assist the parents with feeding in a supportive manner. Promoting early parent-infant attachment will support the child's well-being. Encourage the family to visit frequently and involve parents in caretaking activities.

The infant with FAS is likely to have severe permanent neurologic and developmental sequelae. Discuss the infant's recognizable anomalies and the possible sequelae. Allow the parents to verbalize their concerns about their infant's future. Avoid encouraging unrealistic expectations; rather, acknowledge the infant's existing problems and suggest coping strategies.

The family is in a crisis situation, and the mother may feel guilt or may be blamed by other family members for the infant's disability. Encourage family members to verbalize their feelings. Initiate referrals to appropriate community resources. The needs of the high-risk family are significant and require long-term follow-up.

Evaluation

- Are the infant's sleep patterns appropriate for age?
- Is the infant gaining weight at a rate that is appropriate for age?
- Is the child able to attain appropriate growth and development milestones?
- Are the parents discussing the cause and prevention of FAS?
- Is the family able to identify its own strengths and weaknesses, coping skills, and support systems?
- Have referrals to community resources been made and implemented?

AUTISM

Autism is the most severe condition classified as a pervasive developmental disorder (PDD) by the American Psychiatric Association (2000). PDDs are disorders characterized by "severe and pervasive impairment in several areas of development: reciprocal social interaction skills, communication skills, or the presence of stereotyped behavior, interests, and activities" (American Psychiatric Association, 2000). Typically, these conditions are evident in the first 12 months of life, but they may be overlooked if gross motor skills are progressing normally. Frequently, they occur concurrently with a diverse group of other medical conditions. Other conditions included in this category are Asperger's disorder, Rett syndrome, and childhood thought disorders, formerly known as *childhood schizophrenia, symbiotic psychosis,* and *childhood psychosis.* Autism is the most severe of these disorders, but it is not the most frequently encountered disorder among PDDs.

There is no evidence that autism can be cured, so treatment is generally life long and is characterized by varying degrees of success. The earlier the disorder is diagnosed, the better the child's educational prognosis and other relevant outcomes.

Etiology

The cause of autism is unknown, but it is generally believed to be related to abnormal brain structures that are evidenced by brain scans comparing affected and unaffected children. Researchers theorize that the disorder can be caused by a wide range of prenatal, perinatal, and postnatal conditions, including maternal rubella, untreated phenylketonuria, tuberous sclerosis, anoxia during birth, encephalitis, seizures, and fragile X syndrome (Sadock & Sadock, 2003). It was once believed that family child-rearing practices and parental personality characteristics influenced the development of autism, but no controlled studies confirm this view. Because siblings are more likely to have the disorder than are children in the general population, genetic factors are believed to play a role. There have been theories of possible connections between autism and hazardous chemical exposures, including chemicals, such as thimerosal, in various vaccines administered during infancy and childhood. In an extensive review of epidemiologic studies looking at the relationship between the occurrence of autism and either the measles, mumps, rubella (MMR) vaccine or vaccines preserved with thimerosal, the Immunization Safety Review Committee of the Institute of Medicine has rejected any causal relationship between autism and either MMR or thimerosal (Immunization Safety Review Committee, 2004).

Incidence

A national prevalence for autism in the United States is unavailable. In a recent study by the CDC of the prevalence of autism in metropolitan Atlanta, autism was found to affect 3.4 in 1000 children (Yeargin-Allsopp et al., 2003). It is four to five times more common in boys than in girls. No differences in incidence have been correlated with race, socioeconomic level, or culture.

Manifestations

Autism is a severely incapacitating, life-long developmental disability that is characterized by a qualitative impairment in four developmental areas:

- Disturbance in the rate and appearance of physical, social, and language skills
- Abnormal responses of the body sensations
- Thinking capacity, but with absent or delayed speech and language
- Abnormal ways of relating to people, objects, and events

A child may have a vast vocabulary yet have no comprehension of the meaning of the words. Another child may be able to solve intricate mathematical problems but not be able to make change from a dollar. Children may seem oblivious to the sound of their own names but may come running into the room at the sound of a truck. Generally, they show a fixed, unchanging response to a particular stimulus. Self-stimulation is common and generally involves repetition of a particularly pleasing sensory stimulus, such as twirling a toy or rubbing the top of the head. The autistic child typically repeats an act, such as fingering an object or continuously spinning around, rather than responding to a new stimulus.

Apparently, interest is limited by nature, rather than by choice, to an extremely narrow range. The child with autism generally overreacts to any change within the environment. Often, autistic children do not have a typical sense of personal space and so may touch others on the face or stand face to face, with noses touching, even when encountering a total stranger.

Autism is usually apparent to parents before age 3 years, although a period of apparently normal development may be followed by rapid deterioration. There is a wide range in the degree of impairment produced. Autism shares some similarities with the characteristic presentation of what has been called *childhood schizophrenia* and *mental retardation* but with definitive differences. These differences are outlined in Table 30-2. Seventy-five percent of autistic children are cognitively impaired. A few children with autism also have an extremely developed skill in a particular area, such as music or mathematics. These individuals are sometimes known as *idiot savants* because they have both a severe cognitive impairment and an extraordinary cognitive skill or expertise.

The child with autism exhibits the following behaviors and characteristics (American Psychiatric Association, 2000).

Social
- Marked lack of awareness of the existence or feelings of others (e.g., individual ignores emotions of others)
- Lack of or abnormal amount of comfort-seeking at times of distress (e.g., individual does not show pain when hurt)
- Lack of or abnormal imitation of others' actions
- Lack of or abnormal social play (generally plays alone or involves others only as mere objects)
- Gross impairment in social peer relationships (appears not to want or need friends)

Language
- Lack of or impaired verbal communication and abnormalities in the production of speech (inappropriate volume, pitch, rate, rhythm, or intonation, such as a monotone voice or echolalia)
- Markedly abnormal nonverbal communication (i.e., the child uses no gestures or behavioral cues)
- Absence of imaginative play (no imitative or dramatic role playing)

TABLE 30-2	Differential Diagnosis of Autism, Mental Retardation, and Schizophrenia

Autism	**Mental Retardation**
Peaked skill profile	Flat skill profile
Lack of imitative skills	Imitation skills and gesturing
Nonsocial behaviors with little initiation	Social behavior, initiation of social contact
Abnormal communication and language	Limited language ability but sufficient for communication
Development of seizures possible during adolescence	Usually no seizures, Alzheimer's-type dementia in adulthood

Autism	**Schizophrenia**
Onset before age 30 mo	Onset during pubescence or adolescence
No remissions	Remissions and relapses
Hallucinations and delusions rare	Hallucinations and delusions common
Absence of thought disorder	Thought disorder
No family history of schizophrenia	Family history of schizophrenia
Self-stimulating behaviors	Odd behavior but no self-stimulating behaviors
Medications of limited use	Medications often helpful in reducing symptoms

- Impaired interactive speech and communication (the child does not allow for the normal give and take of conversation and tends to become preoccupied with a given subject or word out of context with the conversation)

Restricted Behavioral Repertoire

- Stereotyped body movements (e.g., spinning around, head banging, "flapping," rocking)
- Persistent preoccupation with characteristics of objects (smell, taste, texture) or an abnormal attachment to objects (e.g., piece of string, picture of a whale)
- Marked distress over a minor change in the environment (e.g., exhibiting tantrums when a light is turned on, refusing to look at a teacher who is wearing a new dress)
- Unreasonable insistence on routine (e.g., following a schedule exactly to the minute or second, refusal to attend an assembly during a scheduled mathematics class)
- Self-injurious behaviors (e.g., biting, picking at skin, scratching eyes)
- Marked restriction in range of interests (e.g., may repeatedly align objects and cannot be diverted from doing so)

Diagnostic Evaluation

A diagnosis of autism is usually established on the basis of manifestations. Often, the family is interviewed initially, followed by observation of the child alone, with the parent, and interacting with the examiner or others in the environment. Interviews are coupled with observations and the clinician's rating scales. The onset of characteristic delays or of abnormal functioning must occur before age 3 years.

Several screening tools are available to assist the clinician with a diagnosis of autism. They include the Childhood Autism Rating Scale (CARS) and the Checklist for Autism in Toddlers (CHAT). The CHAT, along with parental concern about the child's development, can assist with early

diagnosis (Beauchesne & Kelly, 2004; Dalton, Forman, & Boris, 2004).

Therapeutic Management

Early identification of autism is essential. Treatment generally entails creating an environment that facilitates interaction and promotes replacement of stereotypical behaviors with more normal behaviors. Behavioral methods are typically used. Autistic people have a normal life span; consequently, they require significant financial resources for treatment and supervision.

Because of the severity of the social impairment and the ineffectiveness of normal environmental interventions, affected children are usually referred to special programs designed to offer stimulation, modify stereotypical behaviors, or establish routines for teaching as soon as the disorder has been identified. Programs usually focus on safety precautions for self-injurious behaviors, such as head banging, and the promotion of communication. Facilitative communication through the use of picture boards or keyboards is controversial but has been used in many educational settings to help autistic children interact with the environment.

CRITICAL THINKING EXERCISE 30-1

You are a nurse working in a clinic and doing a health assessment on a 9-month-old infant. As you provide the parent with information about the MMR vaccine, which the baby would expect to receive at the 1-year well visit, the parent expresses concern that he has heard that the MMR vaccine causes autism.

1. What will be your response to this parent?
2. What kind of information can you give the parent to assist him evaluate information he reads or hears about through the lay media?

NURSING CARE
The Child With Autism

Assessment

Because there are no classic physical features that highlight autism, the nurse must assess the child with possible autism as if no physical or cognitive impairments are present. This is done before establishing a diagnosis. The primary characteristic of autism is lack of social interaction and awareness. For this reason, if the child is very young, the nurse who interacts only with the child's parents is unlikely to be aware of the child's degree of social disengagement. If the child has already been diagnosed as having autism and the purpose of assessment is to determine the severity of the disorder—or the assessment occurs before a procedure or hospitalization—it is performed in the same manner as with any normal child. The nurse, however, will quickly become aware of the child's social detachment or lack of language as the assessment continues.

A systematic exploration of the child's skills and comparison with developmental norms are essential. For the staff nurse or school nurse, this process may include evaluating the child's ability to feed self, dress, and toilet. The assessment should include the child's interactive patterns and verbalization skills. It is important to note the child's motor skills also because these have major implications for safety and self-care. For initial, generalized screening, the DDST-II may be helpful (see Chapter 4 and Evolve website). A family history of autism or other mental disorders, family coping skills, and available social support systems should also be assessed.

Nursing Diagnosis and Planning

The nursing diagnoses and expected outcomes that may be appropriate after assessment of the child with autism are as follow:

* Risk for Injury related to an inability to anticipate danger, a tendency for self-mutilation, and sensory perceptual deficits.
  Expected Outcome: The child's safety will be ensured, as evidenced by maintaining integrity of skin and avoiding self-injury or accidental injury.
* Impaired Social Interaction related to an inability to initiate and maintain social relationships and to limited verbal skills.
  Expected Outcomes: The child will demonstrate improvement in communication skills and will begin to show appropriate interaction with others.
* Disturbed Thought Processes related to an inability to perceive self or others accurately and to cognitive and perceptual dysfunction.
  Expected Outcomes: The child will show progress in developing an interest in surroundings and the ability to acknowledge others in the environment; will demonstrate orientation to person, place, and time; and will perform activities of daily living appropriate to this orientation.

Interventions

When working with autistic children in the hospital setting, the nurse needs to work closely with the family to determine the child's routines, habits, and preferences. The nurse should write down any specific cues that will help the child remain oriented to the environment and that will facilitate tolerance to change. For example, the nursing staff should be limited to as few individuals as possible. The child may need to perform toileting and self-care activities in a particular order. The child may need an environmental cue, such as stroking a favorite blanket, before being able to move from one activity to the next. The nurse can generally evaluate the child's tolerance of the situation by monitoring signs of anxiety or emotional comfort, as evidenced by such behaviors as attending or observing the nurse in the room or demonstrating a willingness to participate in self-care.

The nurse must work closely with the family to determine the specific ways in which the child communicates. The child may use sign language or pictures to specify needs if no verbal skills are developed. Children with autism are often reluctant to initiate or sustain direct eye contact, so the nurse may interpret this behavior as meaning that the child is not listening or is unaware of what is being said. In addition, the child may answer questions after several minutes' delay. The nurse should identify these behaviors, allow extra time, and be alert to differences in communication styles. Children with autism generally understand much more language than they are able to use expressively.

The child who demonstrates a tendency for head banging may need a helmet or side rolls. Meticulous observation may be necessary if the child is unable to remain in the bed at night. The nurse should help the parents understand and explain to their child any safety precautions that are unfamiliar to the child. The presence of a parent or older sibling is almost always necessary when an autistic child is hospitalized. Evaluating the child for safety is a continuing nursing function. Reducing the adjustment demands for the child may be necessary if the nurse recognizes behaviors indicating stress or anxiety.

Evaluation

* Has the child remained free of injury?
* Has the child developed a way to communicate needs?
* Does the child demonstrate an interest in surroundings?
* Does the child acknowledge the presence of others in the environment?
* Has the child developed the ability to perform activities of daily living?

CRITICAL TO REMEMBER
Maintaining Routine for the Child With Autism

Children with autism often are unable to tolerate even the slightest change in routine and may become withdrawn, self-abusive, or violent if their routines are altered.

KEY CONCEPTS

- Children with a cognitive deficit have limitations in social interactions, use of language for self-expression, and self-care abilities. If these limitations are severe, the child will need life-long care by mature, caring adults.

- Children with cognitive deficits have many normal needs, including the need for positive attention and opportunities for self-discovery and growth. The nurse needs to work closely with the family to identify the child's specific patterns of interacting with the environment. This is done by asking relevant, clear questions about how the child communicates and perceives experiences.

- The nurse should consider that families with a cognitively impaired child feel repeated stress and grief as the child continues to fail to reach developmental expectations.

- The nurse can be most helpful by offering family members an opportunity to discuss feelings and by identifying resources to help meet the child's needs. The nurse may act as an advocate for the parents in the school system and the community.

- Mental retardation may be the result of congenital or early environmental factors, or it may occur as the result of head injury, asphyxia, intracranial hemorrhage, infections, poisoning, prenatal alcohol use, or the presence of or treatment of a brain tumor.

- Developmental disability is a legal term that encompasses mental retardation and other cognitive impairments.

- Several neuropsychologic tests are available to assess levels of mental retardation. The best method of early detection is by assessing development during routine pediatric preventive care visits.

- Parents of children with cognitive deficits should be provided with anticipatory guidance relative to their child's developmental abilities.

- Changes in routine can frustrate the child with Down syndrome.

- The family of a child with Down syndrome may need assistance in identifying and obtaining adaptive tools for dressing, bathing, and eating.

- The family of a child with Down syndrome should be encouraged and assisted in helping the child learn new skills through demonstration, repetition, and positive feedback.

- Children with fragile X syndrome exhibit autistic-like behaviors, such as gaze avoidance, hand flapping, echolalia, and abnormal speech patterns. In addition, affected children have poor coordination, hyperkinetic behaviors, and cognitive deficits that are moderate to severe.

- Autism is characterized by an impairment in the rate and appearance of physical, social, and language skills; abnormal responses of the body sensations; thinking capacity, but with absent or delayed speech and language; and abnormal ways of relating to people, objects, and events.

- Autism shares similarities with childhood schizophrenia and mental retardation, but there are definitive differences.

- When working with children with autism, the nurse needs to work with the family to determine the child's routines, habits, and preferences.

ANSWERS TO CRITICAL THINKING EXERCISE 30-1

1. Both television and newspaper articles have suggested that MMR vaccine is related to the onset of autism. These reports were based on some nonepidemiologic studies done in Europe that reported inconsistent data. You can reassure the parent that the American Academy of Pediatrics convened a special panel to examine the available evidence and determined that the evidence does not support a causative relationship between MMR and autism.

2. It is important for the nurse to know how to advise parents and others about obtaining accurate information about health issues. Often, the media report on "newsworthy" issues on the basis of only one study or a piece of research that has not been appropriately peer reviewed. You can suggest to parents that they do the following:

- Look at whether the information comes from a reliable, peer-reviewed, scientific source and preferably from several sources finding the same results.

- Note whether the results have been found in humans and not just in animals.

- Assess whether the risk is large or small by putting the numbers in a format you understand (e.g., 1 in 100, 1%), and try to understand if the number given is a single number or if it is within a range of numbers.

- Look at the risk compared with other known risks.

- Access information from your health care provider, your local health department, government sources, libraries, and reputable Internet websites (websites of official organizations).

Data from Family Caregiver Alliance. (2004). Evaluating medical research findings and clinical trials. Retrieved May 30, 2005, from *www.caregiver.org/caregiver/jsp/content_node.jsp?nodeid=402*.

REFERENCES

American Association on Mental Retardation. (2002). *Fact sheet: What is mental retardation*. Retrieved May 29, 2005, from *www.aamr.org*.

American Psychiatric Association. (2000). *Diagnostic and statistical manual of mental disorders* (4th ed., text revision). Washington, DC: American Psychiatric Association.

Beauchesne, M., & Kelly, B. (2004). Evidence to support parental concerns as an early indicator of autism in children. *Pediatric Nursing, 30,* 57-66.

Centers for Disease Control and Prevention. (2004). *Mental retardation*. Retrieved December 1, 2005, from *www.cdc.gov*.

Centers for Disease Control and Prevention. (2005). Guidelines for identifying and referring persons with fetal alcohol syndrome. *MMWR Morbidity and Mortality Weekly Report, 54,* 1-11.

Chudney, A. E., Conry, J., Cook, J., Loock, C., Rosales, T., & LeBlanc, N. (2005). Fetal alcohol spectrum disorder: Canadian guidelines for diagnosis [Electronic version]. *Canadian Medical Association Journal, 172(5 Suppl.).* Retrieved May 30, 2005, from *www.cmaj.ca/cgi/content/full/172/5_suppl/S1.*

Cuckle, H. (2005). Primary prevention of Down's syndrome. *International Journal of Medical Science, 2,* 93-99.

Dalton, R., Forman, M., & Boris, N. (2004). Pervasive developmental disorders and childhood psychosis. In R. Behrman, R. Kliegman, & H. Jenson (Eds.). *Nelson textbook of pediatrics* (17th ed., pp. 93-95). St. Louis: Elsevier Saunders.

Developmental Disabilities Assistance and Bill of Rights Act of 2000 (PL 106-402). (2000). Passed by U.S. Congress on October 30, 2000.

Family Caregiver Alliance. (2004). *Evaluating medical research findings and clinical trials.* Retrieved May 30, 2005, from *www.caregiver.org/caregiver/jsp/content_node.jsp?nodeid=402.*

Hall, J. (2004). Chromosomal clinical abnormalities. In R. Behrman, R. Kliegman, & H. Jenson (Eds.). *Nelson textbook of pediatrics* (17th ed., pp. 382-386). Philadelphia: Elsevier Saunders.

Immunization Safety Review Committee. (2004). *Immunization safety review: Executive summary.* Retrieved December 15, 2005, from *www.nap.edu.*

Jewell, J. (2004). Fragile X syndrome. Retrieved May 29, 2005, from *www.emedicine.com/PED/topic800.htm#section.*

Leshin, L. (2003). *Down syndrome health issues: News and information for parents and health professionals.* Retrieved May 29, 2005, from *www.ds-health.com/.*

Lindblad, B., Rasmussen, B., & Sandman, P. (2005). Being invigorated in parenthood: Parents' experiences of being supported by professionals when having a disabled child. *Journal of Pediatric Nursing, 20,* 288-297.

March of Dimes. (2004). *Down syndrome.* Retrieved December 1, 2005, from *www.marchofdimes.com.*

McBride S., & Choi, C. (2005). Potential treatment for fragile X syndrome demonstrated in fruit fly model. *Science Daily.* Retrieved May 29, 2005, from *www.sciencedaily.com/releases/2005/03/050309131154.htm.*

National Dissemination Center for Children with Disabilities. (2004). *Mental retardation.* Retrieved December 1, 2005, from *www.nichcy.org.*

Sadock, B., & Sadock, V. A. (2003). *Kaplan and Sadock's synopsis of psychiatry: Behavioral sciences/clinical psychiatry* (9th ed.). Philadelphia: Lippincott Williams & Wilkins.

Shapiro, B., & Batshaw, M. (2004). Mental retardation. In R. Behrman, R. Kliegman, & H. Jenson (Eds.). *Nelson textbook of pediatrics* (17th ed., pp. 138-143). Philadelphia: Elsevier Saunders.

U.S. Department of Health and Human Services. (2000). *Healthy people 2010* (conference edition, in 2 volumes). Washington, DC: U.S. Department of Health and Human Services.

U.S. Department of Health and Human Services. (2005). Administration on Children, Youth, and Families. *Child maltreatment 2003.* Washington, DC: Government Printing Office. Retrieved May 29, 2005, from *www.acf.hhs.gov/programs/cb/publications/cm03.pdf.*

World Health Organization. (2001). *Mental and neurological disorders, fact sheet #265.* Retrieved December 1, 2005, from *www.who.int.*

Yeargin-Allsopp, M., Rice, C., Karapurkar, T., Docrnberg, N., Boyle, C., & Murphy, C. (2003). Prevalence of autism in a US metropolitan area. *JAMA, 289,* 49-55.

CHAPTER 31

The Child With a Sensory Alteration

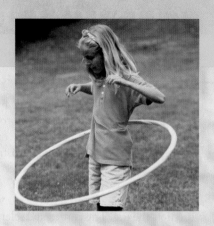

Learning Objectives

After studying this chapter, you should be able to:
- Describe the structure and function of the eye and ear.
- Describe the specific information required in a health history for a child with potential sensory alterations.
- Define the nurse's role in assessing for sensory alterations.
- Describe specific nursing care for children with health problems affecting the eye and ear.
- Describe how alterations in the sensory organs affect the child's ability to communicate.
- Identify potential growth and development interruptions that may occur with problems affecting the sensory organs.

Definitions

amblyopia Reduced visual acuity not correctable by refractive means and not attributable to structural or pathologic ocular anomalies.

astigmatism Abnormal curvature of the cornea or the lens.

cataract A loss of transparency of the crystalline lens or its capsule.

central hearing loss Result of damage to the conduction system between the brainstem and cerebral cortex.

concomitant strabismus Not of paralytic origin; remains constant for all directions of gaze.

conductive hearing loss Reversible loss caused by damage, inflammation, or obstruction to outer or middle ear; sound is prevented from progressing across middle ear.

congenital (infantile) glaucoma Increased intraocular fluid pressure that occurs during first 3 years of life because of a defect in the drainage network of the eye.

diplopia Double vision.

hyperopia Farsightedness; abnormal close vision.

hyphema A hemorrhage or sanguineous exudate in the anterior chamber of the eye.

mixed hearing loss Combination of conductive and sensorineural loss.

myopia Nearsightedness; abnormal distance vision.

nonconcomitant strabismus Angle of deviation varying with direction of gaze because of paralysis or paresis of one or more extraocular muscles.

nystagmus Involuntary eye movements that make the eyes appear to be darting back and forth.

ophthalmia neonatorum Conjunctivitis noted in the first few weeks of life; usually gonococcal or chlamydial.

refractive error Light rays passing through eye structures come into focus at an inappropriate location relative to the retina.

secondary glaucoma Increased intraocular fluid pressure that occurs after 3 years of age and may be the result of disease or surgery.

sensorineural hearing loss Result of damage or malformation of the middle ear or auditory nerve; hearing loss is usually permanent.

stereopsis Ability to see dimensions and perceive depth that results from convergence of visual images received by each eye.

strabismus "Squint," "cross-eyes"; a condition in which the eyes are not straight because of lack of coordination of the extraocular muscles; most often caused by muscle imbalance or paralysis of the extraocular muscles but may also result from conditions such as a brain tumor, myasthenia gravis, or infection.

subconjunctival hemorrhages Bleeding situated beneath the conjunctiva; in children, most frequent cause is trauma or severe coughing or sneezing episodes (Valsalva maneuvers); also caused by infection with *Streptococcus pneumoniae* or *Haemophilus influenzae*.

visual accommodation Ability to focus on distant and near objects.

visual acuity Clarity of vision; tested through use of vision charts, with results compared with what a person with normal vision can see at a distance of 10 or 20 feet.

REVIEW OF THE EYE
Structure and Function

The eye is attached to the skull by six accessory muscles. These are used to move the eye to achieve vision. Ciliary muscles function to alter the shape of the eye to provide focus and accommodation at various distances. Cranial nerves II, III, IV, V, and VI all affect the eye.

The orb, or eye, is made up of several parts. The cornea is the clear area located in the front of the eye, where light enters the eye. The cornea and sclera (white outer covering) make up the eye's outer layer. The middle layer is composed of the choroid (vascular lining), the lens (a clear structure that changes shape to allow accommodation of light on the retina), and the iris (the colored muscular ring located behind the cornea that expands or contracts to control the amount of light entering the eye). The inner layer of the eye is known as the *retina*. This area contains the rods and cones. These receive light impulses and transmit them through the optic nerve (cranial nerve II) to the brain. The macula contains the greatest concentration of nerve endings. The cornea and lens focus light onto the macula. The optic disc is the area where the optic nerve enters the eye.

Neonatal Development

The eyes begin to develop at approximately 22 days' gestation. The critical period for development is considered to be 22 to 50 days. Congenital abnormalities appear to be caused by either genetic or environmental factors or a combination. The eye is especially sensitive to teratogens, in particular infections such as cytomegalovirus and rubella.

REVIEW OF THE EAR
Structure and Function

The ear is divided into three parts: the outer ear, the middle ear, and the inner ear. The outer ear includes the auricle and external ear canal. It is separated from the middle ear by the tympanic membrane (eardrum). The tympanic membrane vibrates to conduct sound waves to the middle ear. The middle ear contains the bones of hearing—the malleus (hammer), incus (anvil), and stapes (stirrup). These bones conduct sound waves from the tympanic membrane to the inner ear. The inner ear contains the nerve endings that conduct sound impulses to the brain. These are located in a snail-shaped chamber (the cochlea) that is filled with fluid. The inner ear also controls balance. The eustachian tube connects the middle ear with the nasopharynx. It functions to allow fluids to drain into the nasopharynx and assist in equalizing pressure between the outer ear and the middle ear.

Neonatal Development

The ear begins to develop during the third week of gestation. The critical period for the development of the ear is between 4 and 6 weeks' gestation. Like the eye, the ear is quite sensitive to teratogens. It is innervated by the acoustic nerve (cranial nerve VIII). Congenital deafness largely appears to be the result of genetic factors.

SPEECH DEVELOPMENT

Because the fetus is capable of hearing during the second trimester of pregnancy and is able to hear voices and the mother's heartbeat, the infant is born with a sensitivity to variations of speech. Adequate hearing is essential for the development of speech. The infant begins to coo and vocalize quite early (birth to 4 months). Babbling begins at approximately 4 to 6 months. Babbling is followed by receptive language development (understanding words) and expressive language development (saying words; see Chapters 5 through 8 for specifics of speech development). Any hearing impairment can interfere with speech development, as can any alteration affecting the oral cavity.

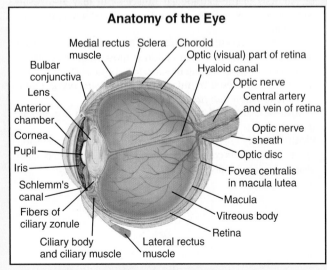

Anatomy of the Eye

Medial rectus muscle · Sclera · Choroid · Optic (visual) part of retina · Hyaloid canal · Optic nerve · Central artery and vein of retina · Optic nerve sheath · Optic disc · Fovea centralis in macula lutea · Macula · Vitreous body · Retina · Lateral rectus muscle · Ciliary body and ciliary muscle · Fibers of ciliary zonule · Schlemm's canal · Iris · Pupil · Cornea · Anterior chamber · Lens · Bulbar conjunctiva

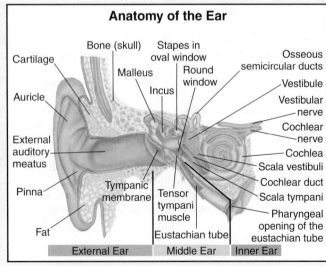

Anatomy of the Ear

Bone (skull) · Stapes in oval window · Osseous semicircular ducts · Malleus · Round window · Vestibule · Incus · Vestibular nerve · Cochlear nerve · Cochlea · Scala vestibuli · Cochlear duct · Scala tympani · Pharyngeal opening of the eustachian tube · Eustachian tube · Tensor tympani muscle · Tympanic membrane · Fat · Pinna · External auditory meatus · Auricle · Cartilage

External Ear | Middle Ear | Inner Ear

PEDIATRIC DIFFERENCES IN SENSORY FUNCTION

Vision

- Development of the eye is not complete at birth, but the newborn is able to fixate, follow an object to midline, and react to a change in intensity of light.
- By 3 months of age, the infant can follow moving objects; by 4 months of age, the infant can recognize familiar objects.
- Binocularity, the ability to fixate on one visual field with both eyes, is not present at birth but is established by 6 months of age. Frequent eye crossing after 6 months of age is abnormal and indicates strabismus.
- Visual acuity changes with age:

4 months	20/50 to 20/80
1 year	20/40 to 20/70
4 years	20/30 to 20/40
5 years	20/20 to 20/30

- Lacrimal glands are not fully developed at birth. Tears are not often present with crying until after 1 to 3 months. Temporary obstruction of lacrimal ducts may cause overflow of tears.
- The size of the orbits doubles by the time the child is 1 year of age and doubles again by 6 years. Eye growth is completed at 10 to 12 years of age.

Hearing

- Development of the ear begins during the third week of gestation and is complete by the third month of embryonic life. Infection or other insult to the fetus during this time can cause irreparable damage to the ear. Ear development occurs at the same time as kidney development, so malformation in one system may indicate problems in the other.
- An infant as young as 3 days is able to distinguish between familiar and unfamiliar sounds and can recognize the mother's voice. The infant can distinguish between frequently heard words and other words (nonsense language) by 1 year.
- Basic auditory skills are in place by 3 years of age. Hearing can be evaluated by audiometry testing by this age.
- Infants and young children have shorter, more horizontal, and more flaccid eustachian tubes, predisposing them to otitis media.

Speech and Language

- Infants can imitate sounds heard by 3 to 5 months of age.
- Verbal dialogue similar to an adult's is noted by approximately 6 months of age.

Electronic Resources

Additional information related to the content in Chapter 31 can be found on:

the interactive companion CD-ROM

- Audio Glossary
- NCLEX Review Questions

or the companion website at **evolve**
http://evolve.elsevier.com/james/ncoc

- NCLEX Review Questions
- Resources for Health Care Providers and Families
- WebLinks

Because a child learns so much through the senses, deficits in hearing and vision can have profound effects on development. Appropriate screening and early interventions are crucial. Early identification of vision and hearing deficits allows for early intervention—either correction or the provision of adaptive measures—so that the child's "normal" growth and development may be preserved. Because a child cannot report sensory deficits, nurses must carefully assess for alterations in vision or hearing.

U.S. legislation PL 94-142 (the Education for All Handicapped Children Act) was passed in 1975 and subsequently updated as the Individuals with Disabilities Education Act (see Chapter 30); it requires special education services for children with severe sensory deficits. The identification of children who might be eligible for special educational services at a young age is important so that their education can be maximized.

The health history of a child with a potential sensory deficit is essentially the same as for any child (see Chapter 9) but should include the following additional pieces of information:

- Thorough prenatal history
- Growth and developmental history
- History of any infections (including treatment because many medications can cause sensory deficits)
- Previous trauma to the eye or ear
- Changes noted in behavior (e.g., rubbing the eyes, turning up the volume on the television, decreased attention span)
- Changes in appearance (e.g., red, inflamed eyes; drainage from the eye or ear)
- Physical symptoms (e.g., reports of ear or eye pain, headache, nausea and vomiting)

After carefully reviewing the health history, the nurse performs a thorough physical examination with age-appropriate measures of vision and hearing acuity (see Chapter 9).

DISORDERS OF THE EYE

The nurse has an important role in the prevention and early detection of eye problems. All children should have vision screening performed at well visits and according to the following schedule (American Academy of Pediatrics [AAP], American Association of Certified Orthoptists, American Association for Pediatric Ophthalmology and Strabismus, & American Association of Ophthalmology, 2003; United States Preventive Services Task Force, 2005):

- *At birth:* external and internal appearance for structural abnormalities, red reflex, fixation.
- *Age 3 to 6 months:* fixation and ability to follow, alignment (cover/uncover test, corneal light reflex, photo screening).
- *Birth to 3 years:* all the above with ocular history.
- *Age 3 years and older:* all the above plus visual acuity using developmentally appropriate charts (HOTV, Lea symbols, "tumbling E") and ophthalmoscopy; stereopsis can be tested by using the random dot E test (see Chapter 9). Photoscreening, a process of photographing images of eye reflexes, can easily detect a variety of eye problems in young children. Photoscreening is particularly useful for detecting refractive errors, strabismus, and other conditions that contribute to amblyopia (AAP, 2002; AAP, American Association of Certified Orthoptists, American Association for Pediatric Ophthalmology and Strabismus,

& American Association of Ophthalmology, 2003). A variety of photoscreening techniques and equipment is available; a specialist must interpret the images obtained (Hartmann et al., 2000/2005).

Refer children who do not pass structural or vision screening for complete ophthalmologic evaluation. Careful attention to behavior and appearance changes as well as physical symptoms assists in the early detection and treatment of eye disorders (Box 31-1). Children who have any symptoms should be referred for further evaluation.

BOX 31-1	**Signs and Symptoms of Potential Vision Problems**

- Inability to fix both eyes on an object and follow the track of a moving object with both eyes
- Persistent discharge from one or both eyes, especially accompanied by redness of the sclera
- Excessive tearing, especially when accompanied by itchiness or pain
- Cloudiness or white areas in the pupil
- Deviation of the iris in an inward or outward direction (crossing)
- Head tilting or closing one eye to see
- Squinting
- Reports of headache or blurred or double vision
- The need to sit close to a television or blackboard to see
- Holding reading material close to the eyes
- Excessive fatigue with visual concentration

CRITICAL TO REMEMBER
Vision Screening

- Thoroughly explain the procedure to the child before beginning. If using a picture chart, show the child the pictures and ask the child to identify them. Children may have different names for the same picture. If using a machine to test the child's vision, demonstrate in advance how it works.
- Take the child to a quiet, nondistracting area that has been marked for the appropriate distance from the chart.
- Have the child cover one eye. Use a colorful, opaque cover that completely blocks the child's vision. The parent can help hold the cover in place.
- Point to a picture (letter, number) on a line that the child can probably see readily, and move to smaller lines. Vary the direction (left to right, right to left) to reduce the likelihood that the child is memorizing the symbols.
- Give positive feedback. Perform the test as quickly as possible because small children lose interest quickly.
- Test both eyes. Refer for further evaluation if is a discrepancy of two lines exists or if the child tests in the abnormal range on two successive screenings.

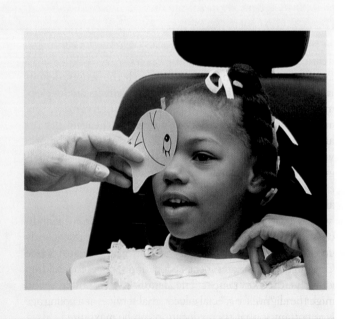

Nursing Considerations for the Child With Color Deficiency

Color "blindness," or color deficiency, occurs in 8% of the population and primarily affects males. It interferes with the ability to distinguish between colors within certain groups, such as red, blue, and green.

Testing should be done if the clinician suspects a problem (i.e., a suspected optic nerve or retinal dysfunction) or the family has a history of color deficiency. Testing is routine in preschool boys. The most common detection test is the pseudoisochromatic (color confusion) test, in which color plates include patterns that are hidden to a person with a color deficit. Pseudoisochromatic plates are also available for children who cannot yet read. If a problem is detected, more sophisticated testing may be necessary to determine the exact type of color deficiency. Although color deficiency has no cure, certain types of tints used in contact lenses and glasses can help the child discriminate color differences.

Because color deficiency cannot be cured, nursing care focuses on adaptive and supportive measures. Encourage parents to have children tested if the family has a history of color deficiency or if the nurse suspects the child is having trouble distinguishing colors.

Parent and child education is important for the child with color deficiency. Teaching should focus on alternative ways to discriminate the deficient colors. For the older child who can dress without assistance, clothes can be labeled or organized so that items can be easily coordinated.

Safety is a major concern for the color-deficient child. For example, the child who cannot distinguish red and green must learn another way to distinguish traffic signals and other warning lights. Finally, anticipatory guidance is sometimes related to appropriate career choices. For example, color deficiency might prohibit an adult from becoming a pilot, police officer, or firefighter.

Nursing Considerations for the Child With a Blocked Lacrimal Duct

A blocked lacrimal (tear) duct is characterized by excessive tearing (epiphora) and crusting on the eyelids on awakening. Parents may also note a small mass just below the inner aspect of the eye. Treatment usually consists of massaging the duct. If the duct remains blocked despite massaging or remains blocked after 1 year of age, surgical opening of the duct is indicated.

The nurse should carefully assess the mucoid drainage. In a noninfected duct, the drainage is usually white or clear. If the duct has become infected, however, the drainage may be green or yellow. If the drainage suggests an infected duct, treatment with antibiotic eye drops or ointment is indicated.

The nurse teaches the parent about the proper technique for lacrimal massage. This process involves washing hands thoroughly and placing the index finger over the lacrimal duct (at the inner aspect of the eye by the bridge of the nose) and "milking," or gently massaging, the duct in an upward motion. Emphasize that massaging down the nasal bone has very little effect on the duct because the lacrimal system is intraosseous and unaffected by massage over bone. Other teaching includes monitoring for signs and symptoms of infection.

Nursing Considerations for the Child With a Refractive Error

Refractive errors cause vision disturbances from alterations in the path of light rays through the eye. They usually result from an abnormally shaped orb; the orb may be flattened or elongated (Table 31-1). Refractive errors are often discovered when a child squints, frowns, or moves objects so they are more easily seen. Reports from the child or a teacher may also alert parents. *Legal blindness* is defined as a correction of 20/200 or worse in the better eye or a visual field of 20 degrees or less.

Nurses should assess children's vision at every well-child visit, particularly during the preschool years. Visual acuity can be reliably tested in a cooperative child as young as 3 years. When testing visual acuity, the nurse needs to remember that a vision discrepancy of two lines or more on the vision chart, even if one eye tests normal, is cause for referral. A child with this discrepancy could have *anisometropia*, or a large refractive discrepancy between eyes. If not corrected, this condition can lead to amblyopia.

School nurses routinely test children's vision and, in fact, annual vision screening is offered to children throughout the United States. Recent evidence-based research has examined the reliability and validity of various screening methods used to screen preschool and kindergarten-age children, and results suggest that the HOTV, Lea symbols, and the "tumbling E" test are all reliable and valid for screening children at this developmental level (Hartmann et al., 2000/2005).

School nurses have used various methods of notifying families of children who do not pass a school vision screening (e.g., telephone call to parents, letter brought home by the child, letter mailed home). However, the parent is responsible for follow-through with a visit to a specialist. Nurses need to be aware that some parents, for a variety of reasons, do not take the child for a follow-up comprehensive eye examination; for this reason, nurses in other settings must ask for details about the child's vision and previous vision testing.

To identify children at risk for altered vision at the earliest possible time, many states have revised the procedure for preschool and kindergarten vision screening (Arizona Department of Health Services, 2004; Commonwealth of Massachusetts Department of Public Health, 2005). Massachusetts, for example, requires that all children entering kindergarten must have passed an approved vision screening within the previous year or within 30 days of kindergarten entrance. Children who do not pass the vision screen must present evidence of a comprehensive eye examination performed by a licensed optometrist or ophthalmologist and recommendations for treatment and follow-up (Commonwealth of Massachusetts Department of Public Health, 2005).

TABLE 31-1 Types of Refractive Disorders			
Refractive Error	**Description**	**Clinical Manifestations**	**Treatment**
Myopia	Nearsightedness Ability to see close objects more clearly than those at a distance Caused by the image focusing in front of the retina	Difficulty seeing the blackboard or television clearly Decreased interest in activities requiring distance vision Squinting, head tilting, holding books close to eyes Decreased attention span, poor school performance	Treated with biconcave lenses New lenses may be required every 1-2 yr as the child grows
Hyperopia	Farsightedness Ability to see distant objects more clearly than those close up Caused by the image focusing beyond the retina	Most children are normally hyperopic until approximately 7 years of age but are able to accommodate to see clearly Strabismus or amblyopia may develop from prolonged hyperopia	Most young children with hyperopia need no correction If correction is required, convex lenses are used
Astigmatism	Unequal curvature of the cornea or the lens causing light rays to bend in different directions May coexist with myopia or hyperopia	Mild astigmatism may be asymptomatic Manifestations may be similar to myopia	Treated with special lenses to compensate for the unequal curvature of the cornea

Corrective lenses are used to improve the child's vision. Encourage the parent to look for impact-resistant eyeglasses with spring-loaded frames, which are less likely to bend or warp. Fitting glasses to an infant or young child can be challenging; the goal is to choose shatter-resistant lenses in a type of frame that can be closely fitted to prevent easy dislodging during activity. Infant frames often have elasticized straps to keep them properly positioned. Teach the parent, and child if appropriate, to always store the glasses in a case when not being used. Special directions for cleaning must be followed to avoid scratching the lenses. Special prescription sports goggles are available for athletes; protective eyewear should be selected according to the sport and the relative risk for injury (AAP & American Academy of Ophthalmology, 2004). Both gas-permeable and soft contact lenses provide an alternative for children old enough and responsible enough to care for contacts independently. The nurse needs to teach parents and children about appropriate care of corrective lenses and should educate parents and children about recognizing and intervening with vision problems early.

Nursing Considerations for the Child With Amblyopia

Amblyopia, or "lazy eye," one of the most common causes of diminished vision in children, results from a variety of eye alterations seen in children whose visual acuity is impaired (Quinn, 2004). Various reports state that the prevalence of amblyopia is between 2% and 5% of children and may be as high as 8% (Allison, 2005; American Academy of Ophthalmology, 2003; Lloyd, 2003). When both eyes are unable to focus simultaneously, the brain suppresses the image from the deviating eye to avoid double vision (diplopia). Amblyopia frequently accompanies strabismus as well as other eye conditions such as congenital cataract and severe refractive error. If the underlying eye condition is untreated in a child younger than 4 years (the critical period for development of the visual cortex), permanent loss of vision from amblyopia can result; amblyopia is not treatable in adolescents or adults (American Academy of Ophthalmology, 2002). Because the child loses binocular vision, depth perception may also be impaired. Early detection and treatment of strabismus or other underlying cause of amblyopia are essential to prevent loss of vision.

Two primary approaches are used to correct amblyopia, and each is designed to alter or obscure vision in the stronger eye to force the child to use the amblyopic eye. Atropine, which is a cycloplegic (paralyzes the ciliary muscles to dilate the eye), is used to blur the vision in the stronger eye. Recent studies with young children have demonstrated similar improvement in amblyopic children treated with 1% atropine drops and those treated with patching (Quinn, 2004). Eye drops appear to be a more acceptable method of treatment and may enhance adherence (American Academy of Ophthalmology, 2002; Quinn, 2004).

Patching is used primarily to correct amblyopia and is used mostly during the preschool years when the visual cortex is developing. In this treatment, the normal eye is patched so that the child is forced to use the weaker eye. The schedule for patching is individualized. Recent evidence suggests that for children with moderate amblyopia (20/40 to 20/100 vision in the affected eye), patching the eye for 2 hours a day is effective; for children with more severe amblyopia a 6 hour patching regimen yields effective results (Quinn, 2004). The patching regimen is prescribed by the ophthalmologist.

Cooperation with the patching regimen is essential. Teaching should explain the reasons for patching or corrective lenses, the expected results of wearing the patch or lens, correct placement of the patch, the number of hours per

BOX 31-2	**PARENTS WANT TO KNOW** Information about Eye Patching

- Your child will need to wear the eye patch for the exact time your physician has prescribed. Not adhering to the full wearing time could interfere with the treatment.
- Prescribed patching will not harm your child's stronger eye but will force the muscles of the weaker eye to be used.
- Apply the patch directly to your child's face, being sure to cover the whole eye. Do not leave any openings through which the child can peek.

- If your child wears eyeglasses as well, put the glasses on over the patch.
- It can be frustrating for the child to have to wear the patch. Try to be patient, understanding, and supportive. Patching must be nonnegotiable. Find decorative patches or put your own decoration on the patch. Praise your child frequently for cooperating with the treatment.

day the patch or lens is to be worn, and the expected length of treatment (Box 31-2). The child needs to understand that wearing the patch or lens is not negotiable. The nurse often must teach parents strategies for dealing with resistant behaviors.

Nursing Considerations for the Child With Strabismus

Strabismus is a condition in which the eyes are not aligned because of lack of coordination of the extraocular muscles. It is present in 2% to 4% of children younger than 4 years (Hartmann et al., 2000/2005). Strabismus is most often caused by muscle imbalance or paralysis of the extraocular muscles but may also result from conditions such as a brain tumor, myasthenia gravis, or infection. Infants and children with strabismus often have a close relative with the condition; other contributing factors include genetic abnormalities, neuromuscular disease, exposure to teratogens, and trauma (Ticho, 2003). The type of deviation noted defines strabismus (Box 31-3). When assessing infants for strabismus, the nurse needs to remember that strabismus is normal in the young infant but should not be present after approximately 3 months of age.

The corneal light reflex test, simultaneous red reflex test, cover-uncover test, and the alternate-cover test (see Chapter 9) are used in the diagnosis of strabismus. The nurse may suspect strabismus when the child reports frequent headaches, squints, or tilts the head to see. The parent may suspect something is wrong when a flash photograph of the child reveals unequal "red eye." Children who have family members with strabismus should be regularly assessed for development of the condition. Strabismus can contribute to amblyopia in the infant or young child.

Treatment of strabismus may include special corrective lenses, vision therapy, surgery, or pharmacologic therapy. If the deviation is caused by hyperopia, corrective lenses are indicated to correct vision. Eyeglasses with specially ground prism power may also be indicated. These glasses correct vision in the affected eye so that the brain receives the same image from both eyes.

Botulinum toxin (Botox) was approved in 1989 by the U.S. Food and Drug Administration as an alternative to surgery in some cases. The toxin is injected into the eye muscle and produces temporary paralysis. This condition allows the muscles opposite the paralyzed muscle to straighten the eye. With successful treatment, the correction remains after the medication wears off (in approximately 2 months). The most common side effect is a drooping eyelid (ptosis), which usually resolves spontaneously.

Surgery may be indicated to realign the weakened muscles in a child with strabismus. It is most often indicated when amblyopia is present and should be performed before the child is 2 years of age. The stronger eye may be patched before surgery to treat any existing amblyopia. Surgery may be required only on the weakened eye or on both eyes. More than one surgery may be necessary. During the surgery, small incisions are made and the weakened muscles are tightened or the stronger muscles are weakened and lengthened (Watkinson & Graham, 2005).

If the child is to have a surgical correction, the nurse should prepare the child and parents before surgery for what to expect after surgery and provide information about dressing changes, eye drops, corrective lenses, and any other postoperative treatments that may be required. Interventions are similar to those for any child having eye surgery (see pp. 1030-1031).

Nursing Considerations for the Child With Glaucoma

Glaucoma is a condition in which the intraocular fluid pressure of the eye is increased. This pressure increase, if left untreated, leads to atrophy of the optic disc and, ultimately, blindness. Children with congenital glaucoma comprise the largest sector of all children who are blind (Watkinson & Graham, 2005).

Several types of glaucoma occur in children. Congenital glaucoma and infantile glaucoma occur during the first 3 years of life and are caused by a defect in the drainage network of the eye. Primary congenital glaucoma has a genetic origin, with an autosomal recessive inheritance pattern. *Secondary glaucoma* refers to disease that occurs after 3 years of age and may be the result of inherited disease (juvenile glaucoma) or may be acquired from infection, trauma, or cataract removal (acquired glaucoma) (Kipp, 2003).

Clinical signs of glaucoma include excessive tearing, light sensitivity, blepharospasm (muscle spasm causing involuntary closing of the eyelid), and enlargement of the globe and cornea. Parents often note excessive tearing or corneal haziness

BOX 31-3	Types of Strabismus

Comitant strabismus: Most common type of strabismus in children. Constant deviation in all fields of gaze; not associated with eye muscle paralysis. All extraocular muscles function but are not coordinated. Child has difficulty seeing at close range and often squints. Accommodative nonparalytic strabismus may develop between 2 and 4 years of age as a result of a large refractive error.

Paralytic strabismus: Caused by a weakness or paralysis of one or more of the extraocular muscles. Usually involves dysfunction of one or more cranial nerves involved with ocular movement. The eye appears crossed when turned in the direction of the affected muscle. May cause headache and poor coordination. Diplopia may cause child to close one eye or tilt the head.

Esotropia (convergent): The eye turns inward; most common type of strabismus in infants. May occur with hyperopia as the eyes compensate for the refractive error by overconvergence.

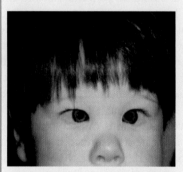

Child with early-onset esotropia. The deviation may not be apparent until age 3 or 4 months.

Exotropia (divergent): The eyes turn away from the midline; occurs most often when the child attempts to focus on a distant object. May be present at birth.

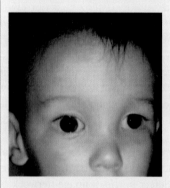

Child with left exotropia. Most exodeviations in childhood are intermittent.

Pseudostrabismus: Not true strabismus. The eyes appear to deviate inward but are actually in alignment. Facial features, such as epicanthal folds and a broad, flat nasal bridge, can give the appearance of misalignment.

Phoria: A tendency for the eye to deviate. More evident during times of stress, fatigue, or illness.

Tropia: A continuous or intermittent misalignment of the eye.

Photographs from Albert, D. M., & Jakobiec, F. A. (Eds.). (1994). *Principles and practice of ophthalmology* (pp. 2731, 2733). Philadelphia: Saunders.

caused by edema and bring the child in for clinical evaluation. The child may also be brought to the practitioner for what appears to be conjunctivitis ("pink eye").

Physical examination includes an assessment of visual acuity, measurement of intraocular pressure (tonometry), assessment of corneal diameter and clarity, and an examination of the retina to assess for optic nerve cupping. Any infant with a visible iris diameter greater than 10.5 mm should be evaluated. If retinal edema is present, the light reflex is diffuse. Because young children may not be able to cooperate during an examination, they are often sedated. Intraocular pressure should be measured only under light sedation, however, because deeper sedation may alter readings (either high or low, depending on the agent used).

The preferred treatment for childhood glaucoma is surgery. Medications to clear the cornea may be used before surgery to allow better visibility. Surgery should be performed as soon as possible after diagnosis to prevent loss (or further loss) of vision. The goal of surgery is to increase the outflow of the aqueous humor from the anterior chamber by correcting the structural abnormality causing the decreased outflow (goniotomy) or create a different route for the outflow (trabeculotomy) (Glaucoma Research Foundation, 2002). Medications such as cholinergic agents, beta-adrenergic blocking agents, or adrenergic agents may be indicated after surgery to maintain low intraocular pressure.

Prognosis varies from child to child. The earlier the glaucoma develops, the poorer the prognosis because infants and children with early-onset glaucoma usually have defects in the development of the anterior chamber of the eye that occurred during fetal development (Kipp, 2003). In general, with prompt treatment most children attain appropriate vision. Decreased vision may result from damage to the optic nerve, opacity of the cornea or lens, or amblyopia resulting from refractive errors. Children with glaucoma must be followed closely over the long term to identify any rise in intraocular pressure quickly.

Nursing interventions are similar to those for any child having eye surgery. Postoperative nursing care includes monitoring for signs and symptoms of increased intraocular pressure (pain, nausea and vomiting, increased inflammation) and administering any ordered medications, such as miotic eye drops (used to constrict the pupils) and antibiotic ointments or eye drops. If the child's eyes are patched, the nurse pays special attention to the resulting sensory deficits. The nurse also considers safety to be an issue when eyes are patched.

Parent education is essential to maintain the appropriate intraocular pressure and prevent complications (including blindness). Education includes the use of any prescribed medications, patching, and any other measures designed to correct refractive errors. The importance of returning for follow-up care should be emphasized. The child and caregivers should also be taught signs and symptoms of increasing intraocular pressure. Any signs of increasing intraocular pressure or infection should be immediately reported to the ophthalmologist. Referral for genetic counseling may be indicated (Watkinson & Graham, 2005).

Nursing Considerations for the Child With a Cataract

A cataract is an opacity, or loss of transparency, of the lens. Causes include an inherited tendency (usually an autosomal dominant trait), infection (e.g., rubella), trauma, or a metabolic imbalance; the cause of congenital cataracts is unknown (Watkinson & Graham, 2005). Cloudiness of the lens may be noted during examination in the newborn nursery (indicated by a white instead of red reflex) or by the parents. Ophthalmoscopy may reveal a dark spot in the lens. Parents may note that the infant exhibits visual inattentiveness and come in for an evaluation. Other clinical signs include nystagmus and strabismus.

The cataract alters vision because it does not allow a sharp, clear image to be formed on the retina. Early intervention (before 3 months of age) for the infant born with cataracts is crucial to allow vision to develop normally (Levin, 2003).

Treatment for cataracts is the surgical removal of the opaque lens. The resultant hyperopia is then dealt with by using a contact lens or an intraocular lens implant. Intraocular lens implants are being used more frequently, even for infants; the challenge is to assess the appropriate correction that will achieve maximal vision while allowing for the child's growth (Lloyd, 2003). Glasses may also be used to correct the resultant vision problem.

Amblyopia may be a consequence of congenital cataract. In this case, the normal eye may be patched after surgery to develop the weakened eye.

Postoperative interventions are directed toward avoiding increased intraocular pressure. Measures include preventing coughing, straining, vomiting, and touching the operative site. A patch and "hard shield" are usually in place after surgery to prevent injury to the operative site. To prevent edema and pressure on the site, the nurse should elevate the head of the bed slightly and position the child so that the affected eye is not in a dependent position. Monitor the child for signs and symptoms of infection (fever, drainage, redness). Medications, including antibiotics, mydriatics, and steroids, may be used after surgery.

Postoperative teaching includes how to insert, remove, and care for the child's contact lens. Parents need to be taught the signs and symptoms of infection and increasing intraocular pressure. To provide visual stimulation to the affected eye and prevent further loss of vision, the importance of adhering to the patching regimen should also be emphasized. Finally, the nurse teaches the importance of returning for follow-up visits to ensure that the lens fits correctly, the vision correction is appropriate, and no signs and symptoms of complications are present. Referral for genetic counseling for future pregnancies is indicated (Watkinson & Graham, 2005).

Nursing Considerations for the Child With an Eye Infection

Conjunctivitis

Conjunctivitis ("pink eye") is an inflammation of the conjunctiva (the clear, membranous lining of the lid and sclera). Signs and symptoms of conjunctivitis may include itching, burning, light sensitivity (photophobia), "scratchy" eyelids, redness, edema, and discharge. It is caused usually by either allergy or infection. Accurate diagnosis before treatment is important because inappropriate treatment can lead to complications.

Conjunctivitis noted in the first few weeks of life is called *ophthalmia neonatorum*. In infants, conjunctivitis occurring in the first 24 hours of life is usually caused by chemical irritation from infection prophylaxis administered soon after birth. Either infection or a blocked lacrimal duct can cause conjunctivitis that occurs after the first 24 hours. Infants acquire infection during birth (from passing through the birth canal) or after birth. *Chlamydia* is responsible for most eye infections noted in infants (Hammerschlag, 2004). Medical treatment should be directed at the cause of the infection. Antibiotic or antiviral eye drops or ointments are most often used to treat infectious conjunctivitis. If *Chlamydia* is the cause, however, systemic antibiotics (e.g., erythromycin) are also used to prevent pneumonia.

Conjunctivitis in older children may have a variety of causes, including bacteria, viruses, allergy, infection, and trauma. Organisms most frequently implicated in bacterial conjunctivitis include *Haemophilus influenzae* and *Streptococcus pneumoniae*, although with the introduction of *H. influenzae* type B (Hib) vaccine, *H. influenzae* has decreased as a major cause. As with the infant, treatment depends on the cause. The nurse obtains a detailed history to help determine the cause. Infection should be suspected if the child has recently been exposed to another person with conjunctivitis or has had an upper respiratory infection. Itching often identifies the cause as an allergic response. Although children with allergic conjunctivitis exhibit redness of the conjunctiva, they usually do not manifest the type of thick discharge seen in bacterial conjunctivitis.

Chlamydial conjunctivitis is rare in children older than 3 years. It may be suspected, however, in a sexually active adolescent with persistent conjunctivitis. A diagnosis of chlamydial conjunctivitis in an older child who is not sexually active should signal the health care provider to assess the child for possible sexual abuse.

Medical management depends on the cause of the conjunctivitis. If the cause is infection, antibiotic or antiviral eye drops or ointment may be prescribed. If allergies are suspected, antihistamines, either oral or in the form of eye drops, may be indicated. In severe cases of allergic conjunctivitis, steroid eye drops and cromolyn sodium eye drops may be helpful. The steroid eye drops are tapered over an approximately 7-day period. Because steroids can worsen the severity of many infections, they are used with caution and only for a short time. Used over the long term, steroids can exacerbate glaucoma and contribute to cataract development.

Teach parents to keep the child's eye clean and administer any prescribed medications (see Chapter 14). The parent can gently remove crusted material from the eye with a cotton ball soaked in warm water. Teach the parent to wipe the eye from the inner to the outer aspect and wash the hands and use a new cotton ball for the other eye. Because bacterial or viral conjunctivitis is extremely contagious, the nurse should teach infection control measures. These include good handwashing and not sharing towels and washcloths. Bottles of eye medication should never be shared with another person. The tip of the dropper or ointment tube should not touch the child's eye or eyelid during administration. The child should also be kept home from school or day care until 24 hours after antibiotics are started.

Preventing injury from rubbing the eye is also important. Mittens may be used for infants. These may be fashioned from bootie-type socks or may be commercially made. Distraction and constant reminding are recommended for toddlers and older children. If the child wears contact lenses, advise discontinuing them until the infection has completely cleared. Securing new contact lenses eliminates the chance of reinfection from contaminated contact lenses and also lessens the risk of a corneal ulceration. Eye makeup should also be discarded and replaced because the chance of reinfecting eyes from contaminated makeup is high. Mascara should be replaced routinely at least every 3 months.

If the conjunctivitis is allergic in origin, cool compresses and dark glasses may also help lessen the irritation and photophobia. If cromolyn sodium eye drops are prescribed, parents should be taught to begin using them *before* the allergy season because they need several weeks to reach full effectiveness. Ophthalmic nonsteroidal antiinflammatory preparations may also be helpful.

Orbital Cellulitis

Orbital cellulitis is caused by an infection of the soft tissues of the orbit. It may occur as a result of trauma or, more commonly, an infection of the ethmoid sinus. The usual infecting organisms are S. *aureus* and S. *pneumoniae*. Clinical signs and symptoms include severe eyelid edema, erythema, and an anteriorly displaced eye. Decreased or absent vision, increased intraocular pressure, and pain can complicate the child's condition. The child is febrile and has an elevated white blood cell count. Orbital cellulitis can be distinguished from periorbital cellulitis, inflammation of the tissue surrounding the orbit, which usually results from trauma (Sadovsky, 2003).

CT scanning of the eye and brain confirms the diagnosis and assists with developing the treatment plan (Coats, Carothers, Brady-McCreery, & Paysse, 2004). After cultures have been taken, the child is treated with intravenous administration of an antibiotic designed to act on the major causative organisms; the treatment is individualized when the culture results are available. If the area is painful, analgesics may also be prescribed. Children with orbital cellulitis need to be admitted to the hospital for observation and treatment because of the potential for rapid progression to systemic disease. Left untreated, the infection causing the orbital cellulitis can spread to the optic nerve and then directly to the brain, causing meningitis and blindness. Affected children need frequent vision assessments during treatment. Surgical intervention may be required.

Nursing care involves administering prescribed medications and monitoring the child receiving intravenous therapy. The child also should be carefully monitored for signs and symptoms that the infection is spreading. This includes a thorough neurologic assessment. Finally, the nurse frequently assesses the child's pain status. Hot packs four times a day and prescribed analgesics can relieve pain.

Corneal Ulcer

Corneal ulcers are usually caused by ocular infection as a result of trauma. Signs and symptoms include pain, tearing, purulent discharge, and blurred vision. Besides trauma, risk factors for corneal ulceration include extended wearing of soft contact lenses, surgical procedures, and viral infection in the eye (usually herpesvirus type 1). Corneal ulcerations may be a sign of underlying systemic disease. If not properly and aggressively treated, corneal ulcerations can cause corneal scarring and blindness.

Treatment includes aggressive topical antibiotic therapy with a broad-spectrum antibiotic until cultures return. Treatment is started with a potent new generation of fluoroquinolones: ciprofloxacin, ofloxacin, and norfloxacin. Topical antiviral preparations are used for ulcers caused by viral infection. Systemic acyclovir may decrease the risk of recurrence in those children with herpesvirus type 1 ocular infection (Coats et al., 2004; Hoyt & Haley, 2005)

The nurse teaches the parent about administration of any prescribed medications and the cause and prevention of future ulcerations. The parent needs to discourage the child from rubbing the eyes (which can worsen the injury). The child who wears contact lenses should avoid wearing them until the ulceration and infection are completely healed. Any lenses worn during the episode should be discarded.

Nursing Considerations for the Child With Eye Trauma

Corneal Abrasion

Corneal abrasions usually result from a scraping or tearing of the cornea by foreign bodies, contact lenses, paper, or fingernails. The child may present with light sensitivity, pain, excessive tearing, and decreased vision. The abrasion is diagnosed by instilling a fluorescein dye in the eye and examining the eye under a blue-filtered light (Wood's lamp) to highlight the injury. If foreign bodies remain in the eye, they should be removed.

If the abrasion is small, treatment consists only of the instillation of an appropriate antibiotic ointment or drops four times a day for 1 to 2 days with a follow-up evaluation to check healing. Larger abrasions require patching for 24 hours. Referral to an ophthalmologist should be considered with any eye injury, but particularly for a large abrasion or with the suspicion of a penetrating injury. Many authorities now recommend no patching unless the wound is large. If patched, the eye should be examined in 24 hours. Failure to treat an abrasion can result in loss of visual acuity or permanent scarring and opacity of the cornea.

Parent education is important in caring for the child with a corneal abrasion. Because an abrasion increases the risk of infection, parents should be taught the importance of administering ophthalmic antibiotics as prescribed. The child should not rub the eye because rubbing can worsen an abrasion. If the eye is patched, advise the parents not to remove the patch for 24 hours, even to instill ointment. Keeping the patch in place prevents further damage to the eye from blinking. The nurse also reinforces injury prevention, especially wearing safety goggles during sports and other activities, such as woodworking.

Hemorrhage

Subconjunctival hemorrhages present as red areas beneath the conjunctiva. They are often the result of Valsalva maneuvers, such as coughing, vomiting, or straining. Subconjunctival hemorrhages resolve on their own within 2 to 3 weeks and require no treatment. Although they often appear worse than they are, they may be associated with other ocular or physical problems and should be evaluated.

Because these hemorrhages resolve spontaneously, care is aimed at reassurance. Parents should be told that the hemorrhage will appear to grow larger in the first few days because of the effects of gravity.

Hemorrhages can occur with nonaccidental eye injury as well. In a child suspected of having shaken baby syndrome, for example, retinal hemorrhaging of various types can occur. The child will manifest abnormal findings on funduscopic examination and may exhibit retinal detachment (Lloyd, 2003). The infant or child who receives a direct blow to the eye will demonstrate bruising. Hyphema and damage to the eye structures are a consequence of this type of trauma.

Hyphema

A hyphema is a hemorrhage resulting from a blow or penetrating injury to the eye. Symptoms include a recent history of injury, pain, light sensitivity, decreased vision, the presence of floaters, and excessive tearing. The child is usually sleepy. If the child has no known history of injury, the child should be assessed for a bleeding disorder, anticoagulant therapy, renal or hepatic disease, retinoblastoma, or child abuse. Children with sickle cell disease are prone to hyphema. An examination of the eye reveals blood in the anterior chamber (between the cornea and iris) of the eye. Traumatic hyphema usually fills less than one third of the anterior chamber.

Recommendations for management vary. Any penetrating eye injury is an emergency, requiring rapid referral to an ophthalmologist and treatment to prevent blindness. At the scene of the injury, the eye should be immediately covered with a sterile dressing and an eye shield (manufactured rigid eye shield, Styrofoam or plastic cup); do not instill any type

of eye drops without orders from an ophthalmologist. Maintain minimal movement of the child's head and eye until the child is seen by a physician (Rodriguez, 2003).

Treatment for hyphema usually includes hospitalization, bed rest, sedation, and patching of both eyes. Because of the risk of a rebleed between the third and fifth days, bed rest and patching are often recommended (Hertle & Roy, 2002) for at least that length of time. Medications such as steroid eye drops, antifibrinolytic eye drops (tranexamic acid is best for pediatric use), antiglaucoma medications, and cycloplegic eye drops (atropine) may also be used.

Careful assessment is required for the child with a hyphema. Assess the eye frequently for a secondary hemorrhage, or rebleed. This condition is characterized by an increase in size of the hyphema, with bright-red "new" blood noted over the existing clot. Children who rebleed have a poorer long-term prognosis for vision because acute or chronic glaucoma can be a consequence. The child should also be monitored for signs and symptoms of increasing intraocular pressure (pain, nausea and vomiting, increased inflammation). The child should be closely monitored for side effects of medications, which will vary according to the prescribed therapy.

The child is usually restricted to bed rest with bathroom privileges. Elevating the head of the bed 30 to 40 degrees helps settle the hyphema in the inferior anterior chamber angle. Television viewing may or may not be allowed, and reading and other close-up activities are usually forbidden. Therefore boredom is a problem for most children. Offer diversional activities that do not involve reading or straining the eyes, such as music and books on tape. If both eyes are patched, the nurse orients the child to the environment and provides for safety.

Discharge teaching includes use of prescribed home medications, patching regimen (the eye is usually patched at night for 2 weeks after discharge), and prevention of further injury. The child's eye should be protected with a shield if an eye patch is worn at night. The child can usually return to all normal activities several weeks after the injury. Eye protection is recommended for all children who participate in sports or other high-risk activities, but lifelong use of protective eyewear is recommended for the child who has had hyphema. The nurse should also emphasize the importance of follow-up because the child is at risk for complications such as glaucoma and cataracts.

Teaching to prevent eye injury is an important nursing intervention (Box 31-4). Many school and recreational athletic organizations have policies regarding eye protection during

---

BOX 31-4 | **CHILDREN WANT TO KNOW** How to Prevent Eye Injuries While Participating in Sports

- High-risk sports include those in which no eye protection is worn, such as basketball, baseball/softball, paintball, and boxing.
- The highest percentage of injuries is seen in basketball and baseball.

- Wear certified protective eyewear—such as goggles, helmets and face shields—when possible.
- Wear sports goggles under helmets and with hockey masks.

Data from American Academy of Pediatrics & American Academy of Ophthalmology. (2004). Protective eyewear for young athletes. *Pediatrics, 113*(3), 619-622.

sports activities. Teens who attend vocational schools must wear protective eye covering in shops where eye injury is a risk. Of more concern is the potential for eye injury occurring during unsupervised play. For example, penetrating eye injuries occur more frequently in children who participate in paintball (Listman, 2004).

Splash Injury

Splash injury can occur any time infective, hot, or corrosive liquid splashes into a child's eye; burns of the eye constitute an ocular emergency. Burns may occur from any number of common household items, such as bleach, ammonia, drain opener, and oven cleaner.

NURSING CARE PLAN

The Child Having Eye Surgery

Focused Assessment

Assessment of the child and family begins with determining their understanding of the planned surgical procedure and why it is necessary. This includes assessing their knowledge of the care necessary after discharge as well as any changes to expect, including home schooling if both eyes are affected. The understanding of safety principles should also be addressed at admission and reinforced during the child's hospitalization. Finally, the nurse assesses understanding of any special adaptations for procedures and begins teaching at the time of admission.

NURSING DIAGNOSIS Disturbed Sensory Perception (visual impairment) related to eye patching or surgical procedure.

EXPECTED OUTCOMES The child and family will:
- Describe any anticipated temporary vision changes.
- Demonstrate familiarity with the surroundings and associated sights and sounds.

The child will:
- Remain alert and oriented to time and place.

Intervention	Rationale
1. Prepare the child and family before surgery for any changes expected in vision, including blurred vision or patched eyes.	1. Preoperative preparation allows the child and family to know what to expect, thus lessening anxiety.
2. Before surgery, orient the child and family to the surroundings, including the recovery room and hospital room. Describe any unfamiliar sounds the child may hear; have the child close the eyes and listen.	2. Preoperative orientation to surroundings allows the child a feeling of familiarity during the postoperative period.
3. Provide reality orientation (time, day) for the child during the postoperative period, especially if vision is impaired or eyes are patched.	3. Providing a sense of time passage and orienting to day and night prevent the child from becoming disoriented and confused.
4. Provide emotional support and allow expression of feelings of anger and frustration, possibly through play therapy and therapeutic communication.	4. Allowing the child and family to express their fears and frustrations provides an appropriate outlet and encourages the use of other senses.

Evaluation

- Can the child and family describe expected temporary postoperative vision changes?
- Can the child describe the hospital and room environment and its associated sounds?
- Does the child remain alert and oriented to time and place?

NURSING DIAGNOSIS Risk for Injury related to increased intraocular pressure resulting from bleeding, edema, hematoma, postoperative vomiting.

EXPECTED OUTCOME The child will:
- Remain free from injury (increased intraocular pressure, bleeding) through appropriate management of postoperative eye care, crying, nausea, and vomiting.

Intervention	Rationale
1. Fully orient the child to surroundings and ensure that unsafe objects are removed from the environment.	1. Orienting the child to the environment and ensuring that the environment is safe prevent falls and other injuries when the child is out of bed.
2. Ensure that the child wears eye patches or shields as ordered.	2. Eye patches and shields are often prescribed to prevent any further injury to the eye.

NURSING CARE PLAN—cont'd

3. Encourage the parents to remain with the child and prevent the child from rubbing the eyes. Restraints are used as a last resort to prevent injury. Encourage the parent to keep side rails up at all times.
4. Monitor for signs and symptoms of increased intraocular pressure. Give ordered antiemetics if the child is nauseated. Administer intravenous fluids until the child is stable.
5. Approach the child in a calm and soothing manner. Assign personnel whom the child has met and trusts. Encourage the parent to soothe the child who is crying.

3. Rubbing the eyes can damage the surgical site. If restraints are needed, elbow restraints provide protection without total restriction.
4. Increasing intraocular pressure can damage the eye and seriously impair vision. Vomiting can increase intraocular pressure.
5. Avoidance of crying postoperatively reduces the risk for increasing intraocular pressure. Assigning the child to a familiar nurse reduces fear and anxiety that may lead to crying.

Evaluation

- Does the child remain free of physical injury?
- Is the child's intraocular pressure within normal limits?

- Is the child free from crying, nausea, or vomiting?

NURSING DIAGNOSIS Risk for Infection related to surgical incision.

EXPECTED OUTCOME The child will:
- Remain free from infection, as evidenced by normal temperature and absence of discharge and excessive tearing or edema.

Intervention

1. Monitor the child for signs and symptoms of infection, including redness, drainage, fever, and excessive tearing or edema.
2. Administer antibiotic therapy as ordered.

Rationale

1. These are physical signs that a postoperative infection is developing in the eye.
2. Antibiotics may be used as prophylaxis against infection.

Evaluation

- Is the child free from fever, redness, edema, or excessive eye drainage?

NURSING DIAGNOSIS Acute Pain related to surgical procedure.

EXPECTED OUTCOME The child will:
- Experience minimal discomfort during the postoperative period, as evidenced by acceptable pain scale rating, normal vital signs, and participation in approved quiet activities.

Intervention

1. Monitor the child frequently (every 2 to 4 hr while awake) for pain by using a verbal age-appropriate pain scale. Use a preverbal pain scale, in addition to self-reported pain, to assess pain level in infants and young children whose eyes are occluded. Monitor physiologic signs of pain in the young child (increased pulse, restlessness, inability to sleep, inability to play).
2. Administer pain medications as ordered.

3. Provide nonpharmacologic pain-relief measures, such as ice pack and moist heat, as indicated. Use distraction techniques frequently (music, stories).

Rationale

1. Pain can increase anxiety and restlessness that could lead to increased intraocular pressure. The young child who would ordinarily use a visual scale to rate pain is unable to do so if eyes are patched.

2. Pain control decreases the child's need to rub or touch the eyes, which can cause trauma to the surgical site.
3. Nonpharmacologic pain-relief measures can replace or augment pharmacologic measures. Verbal distraction techniques can decrease pain and take the child's mind off the bandages.

Evaluation

- Does the child express relief of pain with an age-appropriate pain scale?

- Are the child's vital signs within normal limits, and can the child participate appropriately in approved quiet activities?

Initial care of the child with a splash injury to the eyes focuses on immediate irrigation with water or saline to prevent further injury. In a chemical splash, if the chemical is alkaline the irrigation may continue for several hours because the damaging action of alkaloids may be prolonged. If the burn is mild, irrigate for at least 30 minutes, using at least 2 L of irrigant; if the burn is severe, continue irrigating for 2 to 4 hours or with at least 10 L of irrigant (Olitsky & Nelson, 2004). The cornea may appear cloudy after an alkali burn. Irrigation of a frightened child's eyes can be difficult and painful. Helping the child lean over a water fountain that is spraying upward makes the task easier.

Further treatment may include referral to an ophthalmologist for topical steroids, medications to dilate the pupils and decrease the risk of adhesions, antibiotic ointment, and patching. Oral antibiotics and analgesics may also be indicated. Nursing care focuses on prescribed medical treatments, comfort measures, and injury prevention (particularly if both the child's eyes are patched).

Discharge teaching focuses on the prescribed medical treatments and the importance of adherence with long-term follow-up and injury prevention. Follow-up care includes monitoring visual acuity and for side effects such as increased intraocular pressure and cataracts.

CRITICAL TO REMEMBER
Working With a Child Who Has a Visual Impairment

- Orient the child to the hospital environment on admission. Orientation can be done by walking the child around the room and identifying objects such as the bed, bathroom, doorways, windows, and chairs.
- Never touch the child without identifying yourself and explaining what you plan to do.
- When describing objects or the environment to a child who is blind or visually impaired, use familiar terms. For example, if the child is older and recently blinded, you may be able to use color when describing objects. If the child has been blind since birth, color has no meaning. Describing how many steps away something is or the placement of eating utensils on a tray are both useful tactics. Remember that parents are often the best source for communication.
- Identify noises for the child because children who are visually impaired or blind often have difficulty establishing the source of a noise.
- Orient the child frequently to time and place. Confusion can be frightening.
- Keep all items in the room in the same location and order. Changing the order or spacing of objects may cause confusion or lead to injury.
- Provide detailed explanations and allow the child to progress through care in steps to learn the order.
- As with any child, allow as much control over the situation as possible.
- Supervise the child and counsel parents to supervise the child as needed.

EYE SURGERY

Several eye disorders seen in infancy and childhood require surgical correction. Any surgical procedure is stressful for the child and family. Eye surgery is particularly stressful because the child's visual fields or acuity may be greatly reduced or absent for a period. If both eyes are affected, the child's ability to maneuver and perform activities of daily living independently is also affected.

The nurse should pay special attention to education. If the child is going home with patches, drops, or any other procedure that must be performed, the family needs to know how to perform this care and should also know the safety precautions involved.

HEARING LOSS IN CHILDREN
Etiology

Damage to, or impairment of, any part of the ear can cause hearing loss. Four types of hearing loss have been identified: conductive, sensorineural, mixed, and central. Each has a different treatment regimen and response to intervention (Box 31-5). Hearing loss can be congenital or acquired. In infants with sensorineural hearing loss, an autosomal recessive inheritance pattern is the cause in more than 50% of cases. Infection and trauma from noise are the major causes of acquired hearing loss in children (Smith, Bale, & White, 2005).

Incidence

The incidence of newborns diagnosed with significant hearing loss is 1 to 6 in 1000 (Cunningham & Cox, 2003). As many as 15% of preschool and school-age children have

---

BOX 31-5	**Types and Etiology of Hearing Loss**

Conductive: Outer or middle ear affected by damage, inflammation, or obstruction. Sound conduction is prevented from progressing from the outer ear to the inner ear. May be the result of excessive cerumen (wax), foreign bodies, perforated tympanic membrane, or otitis media (with or without effusion). Hearing loss is often temporary and reversible.

Sensorineural: Result of damage or malformation of structures of the inner ear and/or auditory nerve. May be the result of heredity or environmental factors, such as infection (meningitis or intrauterine), exposure to loud noise, ototoxic medications, or prematurity. Meningitis is a significant cause of acquired sensorineural hearing loss in children. Hearing loss is usually permanent.

Mixed: Combination of conductive and sensorineural loss. Conductive loss is often reversible, whereas sensorineural loss is not.

Central: Result of damage to the conduction system between the auditory nervous system and cerebral cortex. May be the result of trauma, neurovascular changes, or brain tumors. May cause difficulty in differentiation of sounds, auditory memory.

PATHOPHYSIOLOGY

HEARING LOSS

Adequate hearing depends on intact auditory structures and quality of sound. Sound is described in terms that combine volume (expressed in decibels) and pitch, or frequencies (expressed in hertz). Normal speech ranges in volume between 10 and 60 dB. Normal hearing ranges from −10 to +15 dB at a variety of frequencies. Most people can hear frequencies between 10 and 20,000 Hz but are particularly sensitive to sounds between 1000 and 2000 Hz.* Hearing loss is categorized as follows:

Slight: failure to hear at 16 to 25 dB

Mild: failure to hear at 26 to 40 dB

Moderate: failure to hear at 41 to 55 dB

Moderately severe: failure to hear at 56 to 70 dB

Severe: failure to hear at 71 to 90 dB

Profound: failure to hear at more than 90 dB

A child with moderate hearing loss has difficulty hearing speech beyond a distance of 3 to 5 feet.* This deficit obviously poses problems for children who have not been identified as having a hearing loss and miss most of what a teacher says in a classroom.

Data from Smith, W., Bale, J., & White, K. (2005). Sensorineural hearing loss in children. *Lancet, 365,* 880.

*Nash, D., Schochat, E., Rozycki, A., & Musiek, F. (1997). When loud noises hurt. *Contemporary Pediatrics, 14*(6), 97-109.

BOX 31-6	**Risk Factors Indicating the Need for Hearing Screening**

Neonates (Birth to 28 Days)

- Family history of inherited permanent sensorineural hearing loss
- Exposure to intrauterine infections such as rubella, cytomegalovirus, and toxoplasmosis
- Presence of craniofacial abnormalities, including those of the outer ear
- NICU admission lasting more than 48 hours
- Any findings associated with a syndrome that includes hearing loss

Infants (29 Days to 2 Years) Developing Certain Conditions Associated With Hearing Loss

- Regardless of passing the newborn hearing screen, presence of parental concern about hearing, speech, language, or developmental delay
- History of exposure to intrauterine infection
- Acquired infections associated with sensorineural hearing loss
- Head trauma resulting in loss of consciousness or skull fracture
- Any findings associated with a syndrome or disorder that includes hearing loss, or syndromes that result in progressive hearing loss
- History of neonatal problems requiring intensive intervention
- Recurrent otitis media with effusion lasting at least 3 months

Data from Joint Committee on Infant Hearing. (2000). Year 2000 position statement: principles and guidelines for early hearing detection and intervention programs. *Pediatrics, 106*(4), 798-817.

---

slight hearing loss, which can adversely affect their academic performance (Smith et al., 2005).

Diagnostic Evaluation

Evidence suggests that infants with hearing loss who have been identified and treated before 6 months of age have a better prognosis than those for whom treatment has been delayed. The use of risk criteria for screening infants for hearing loss helps identify only approximately 50% of infants affected (Box 31-6). The Joint Committee on Infant Hearing (2000) has recommended that all infants be screened before 1 month of age, that hearing loss be identified before 3 months of age, and that intervention occur before 6 months of age. Many states have passed legislation making newborn hearing screening mandatory.

Hearing screening for infants is challenging because of their inability to give accurate behavioral cues indicating intact hearing. Historically, assessing hearing in the newborn or young infant often relied on eliciting a startle reflex with a loud noise. However, being certain that the response is actually caused by the sound itself is difficult. Two hearing screening tests can accurately identify infants with hearing deficits: the auditory brainstem response and the evoked otoacoustic emissions test (Box 31-7). Newer equipment has allowed these tests to be completed quickly and accurately in the hospital nursery. Both tests have a pass/refer option. If the infant does not pass after two tries (2 weeks apart), referral to an audiologist for more accurate testing is required. More sophisticated testing, such as visual reinforcement

audiometry or conditioned-play audiometry, is performed by audiologists.

Hearing testing in the older child (age 3 years and older) is done by play audiometry (e.g., the child performs a play activity when the sound is heard) or conventional audiometry (Cunningham & Cox, 2003). The child is presented tones of varying frequencies at a standard volume (usually 20 dB). A quick screening test performed in a physician's office with a hand-held audiometer tests frequencies of 500, 1000, 2000, and 4000 Hz. If the child does not pass the screening, particularly at lower frequencies and lower volume, a tympanogram may indicate middle ear effusion (see Chapter 21). The problem with office audiometric screening is that it can miss hearing loss at higher frequencies, which is usually sensorineural. When doing audiometric screening of children, the nurse should therefore perform the test in a quiet environment and determine ahead of time what signal the child will use to indicate hearing the tone.

Therapeutic Management

The goals of identification and management of infants and children with hearing loss are directed toward maximizing language development and preventing later problems with school performance and social interaction. Treatment of hearing loss depends on the type of loss. Conductive hearing loss is managed by medical or surgical correction of the underlying problem (otitis, cerumen).

Sensorineural hearing loss, which is seldom reversible, requires a different approach. Hearing aids are often recommended for these children. The type of aid chosen depends on the specific needs of the child. The aid should provide the best acoustics and be cosmetically appropriate. For example, an adolescent seldom chooses a body-type hearing aid if an ear-level aid (one inserted into the ear canal) suffices. The four types of hearing aids most commonly used for pediatric patients are the behind-the-ear, the ear-level (in the ear), the eyeglass (aids attached to the temples of eyeglass frames), and the body (a box with wires connected to an ear mold). Infants and young children often do better with ear-level hearing aids. Infants diagnosed with hearing loss need to begin wearing hearing aids as soon as possible to help facilitate language development.

Cochlear implants offer new options for children with sensorineural hearing loss, even those with some residual hearing. The implant is a small electronic device surgically implanted in the cochlea. It delivers electrical stimulation to the inner ear, causing nerve impulses to travel to the brain, where they are interpreted as normal sound. The implant improves communication, but commitment to rehabilitative efforts and proper use and maintenance of the device by the family and child are essential for success (Francis & Niparko, 2003). Cochlear implants are being used more frequently and successfully in infants younger than 12 months; the goal is to maximize hearing during the critical time for speech and language development (Waltzman & Roland, 2005).

Nursing Considerations for the Child With Hearing Loss

Assess the child's hearing at each well-child visit and with any report specific to ears, including otitis media (see Chapter 21). Note an infant's response to bells, rattles, clapping of hands, or horns held approximately 12 inches from the ear. Older children can be asked to repeat whispered words or phrases or listen for a ticking watch. Begin audiometry testing at 3 years of age or younger in a cooperative child.

Assess language skill development. Infants who are deaf babble like hearing infants until approximately 5 to 6 months of age, at which time babbling is noted to cease. The nurse also questions parents about the child's attention span, disruptive behavior, and other behaviors, such as increasing the volume on the television. If the child appears to have hearing loss or is lagging behind in developmental milestones, refer for further evaluation by an audiologist and ear, nose, and throat specialist.

When caring for a child who is hearing impaired, the nurse should do the following:

- If the child has a hearing aid, encourage its use. Make sure it is in place before beginning to speak.
- Look directly into the child's face. To enhance lip reading, have the child's complete attention before beginning to speak.
- Speak clearly. Slow speech slightly. Do not speak loudly.
- Eliminate background noise.
- Use visual aids to assist communication. These include pictures, hands, and written messages for older children.
- If the child uses American Sign Language to communicate, have a diagram of commonly used words readily available. Use an interpreter for more complex discussions.

An important nursing responsibility is to educate parents about preventable hearing loss. Mild sensorineural hearing loss can occur from exposure to loud noises, such as from firecrackers, firearms, loud infant squeak toys, outdoor yard equipment, boat and snowmobile motors, and rock music. People exposed to loud sounds over long periods need to wear protective ear coverings (e.g., ear plugs, mufflers). Advise teens to decrease exposure to loud rock music and to turn music volume down, especially when listening through earphones. Referral for genetic counseling, if the child has congenital sensorineural hearing loss, is important. Prevention also includes appropriate prevention and treatment of prenatal infection and infection during infancy and early

At the recommendation of the Joint Committee on Infant Hearing, most states and many areas of Canada have implemented mandatory newborn infant hearing screening programs. As part of these programs, newborns are screened before hospital discharge. Consider the advantages and disadvantages of this issue. Should nurses advocate that their states implement similar programs if they do not already exist?

childhood. Children with hearing loss may need speech therapy; referral to a speech therapist or early intervention program should occur as soon as possible.

LANGUAGE DISORDERS

Until 10 to 12 months of age, a child is considered prelingual. The sounds the child makes have no direct meaning or connection to future language. They are, instead, practice of a learned skill. Before approximately 6 months of age, infants make few sounds other than crying. At approximately 4 to 6 months of age, however, they enter the babbling phase. These are the cooing, happy sounds that an infant makes when content. The first words appear at approximately 10 to 12 months of age. First sentences appear at approximately

18 months of age. By 2 years of age, most children have at least a 50-word spoken vocabulary.

Girls have more rapid language development until approximately 3 years of age, when the difference disappears. By adolescence, however, girls again show superior verbal skills. Although a correlation exists between developmental delay and verbal skills, the relation between language development and intelligence is unclear. No scientific evidence seems to suggest that a child who talks early is brighter than one who does not. Children who talk quite early do appear, however, to be bright, whereas those who talk extremely late appear to have some developmental delay.

Language disorders in the child are usually of two types. The first is the inability to comprehend (receptive disorder). The second is a disorder in which the child cannot express thoughts through speech (expressive disorder). Receptive disorders result from some type of central nervous system failure or hearing deficit. This may be the result of trauma, a congenital malformation, persistent otitis media, autism, central nervous system disorder, or other failure of language development (Downey et al., 2002). This child cannot express symbols and abstract ideas in clearly spoken words or in a logical manner.

Expressive disorders are most often of three types. The first is a disorder of the voice. This is an alteration in the pitch and intonation that may result from a medical condition,

---

BOX 31-8 | **PARENTS WANT TO KNOW** How to Encourage Language Development

Talk

Talking to your child is necessary for language development. Because children usually imitate what they hear, how much you talk to your child, what you say, and how you say it affect how much and how well your child talks.

Look

Look directly at your child's face and wait until your child pays attention before you begin talking.

Control Distance

Be sure you are close to your child when you talk (no farther than 5 feet). The younger the child, the closer you should be.

Loudness

Talk slightly louder than you normally do. Remove background noise (e.g., turn off the radio, television, dishwasher).

Be a Good Speech Model

• Describe daily activities to your child as they occur.
• Expand what your child says. For example, if your child points and says "car," you say, "Oh, you want the car."
• Add new information. You might add, "That car is little."
• Build vocabulary. Make teaching new words and concepts a natural part of everyday activities. For example, use new words while shopping, taking a walk, or washing dishes.
• Repeat your child's words with adult pronunciation.

Play and Talk

Set aside times throughout each day for play time for just you and your child. Play can be looking at books, exploring toys, singing songs, coloring, and so on. Talk to your child during these activities, keeping the conversation at your child's level.

Read

Begin reading to your child at a young age (younger than 12 months). Ask a librarian for books that are right for your child's age. Reading can be a calming activity that promotes closeness between you and your child. Reading provides another opportunity to teach and review words and ideas. Some children enjoy looking at pictures in magazines and catalogs.

Do not Wait

Your child should have the following skills by these ages:

• 18 months: three-word vocabulary
• 2 years: 25- to 30-word vocabulary and several two-word sentences
• 2½ years: at least a 50-word vocabulary and two-word sentences consistently

If your child does not have these skills, tell your physician. A referral to an audiologist and speech pathologist may be indicated. Hearing and language testing may lead to a better understanding of your child's language development.

From Northern, J. L., & Downs, M. P. (1991). *Hearing in children* (4th ed., pp. 26-27). Baltimore: Williams & Wilkins.

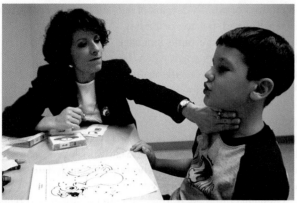

FIG 31-1   Expressive speech disorders include disorders of voice, articulation, and fluency. A speech therapist works with the child to help the child speak more clearly and be better understood. Early intervention is important to correct speech disorders The nurse should therefore assess speech patterns during each health screening. Referrals should be made for any problems noted.   *(Courtesy Cook Children's Medical Center, Fort Worth, TX.)*

such as a cleft palate. The second is a defect of articulation, or the way in which words are pronounced. This is the most common type of speech defect and may be related to neuromuscular disease or structural abnormalities of the nose, throat, and mouth. It may also be idiopathic. Finally, fluency disorders interrupt the flow of normal speech. Included in this category are lisping and stuttering. If stuttering persists after 5 years of age, the child should receive appropriate referrals for speech evaluation (Fig. 31-1). Some children have both expressive and receptive speech alterations (AAP, 2006).

As with screens for hearing loss, the nurse should assess the child's communication patterns with each well-child visit. Any problems should be noted and referrals made to provide appropriate intervention as soon as possible. Encourage parents to take measures to encourage speech and prevent speech problems.

KEY CONCEPTS

- Anything that alters a child's sensory perception can adversely affect growth and development.
- Sense organs develop quite early and are sensitive to teratogens. Any interference with development can result in later sensory alteration.
- Special care should be taken when caring for the child with sensory alterations. Orientation to a new environment is critical in preventing stress and possible injury.
- Most screenings for sensory alterations are noninvasive and relatively painless.
- Parent education and support are critical in assisting the child with sensory alteration to develop as normally as possible.
- Early intervention and special school supports for the child with sensory alterations allow for more normal growth and development.
- Health teaching should include injury prevention.

ANSWERS TO CRITICAL THINKING EXERCISE 31-1

With any new program, the cost/benefit ratio is important. The benefits of this program cannot be argued. The costs can be high, but the increased initial cost could decrease later costs associated with intervention, rehabilitation, and emotional stress for the child and family.

Advantages

- With this program, the approximately 1 to 4 in 1000 infants who are deaf at birth may be identified early enough to begin intervention.
- Deafness in the newborn is difficult to diagnose by behavior alone because responding to loud noises with a startle or blink may be related more to vibration than actual hearing.
- Delayed diagnosis compromises language development and future school performance.
- Only 50% of infants with deafness are identified under the risk referral criteria currently recommended.
- Diagnosis and intervention before the infant is 6 months old greatly improve outcomes.

Disadvantages

- Equipment to do valid testing on newborns is expensive.
- Not all institutions could afford to implement a program without some monetary assistance.
- Depending on the test used, additional personnel may be required.
- Follow-up by the parent cannot be mandated. Tracking those who do not follow up could require additional personnel and paperwork.

REFERENCES AND READINGS

Allegretti, C. (2002). The effects of a cochlear implant on the family of a hearing-impaired child. *Pediatric Nursing, 28*(6), 614-621.

Allison, C. (2005). Treatment options for non-refractive conditions. *Review of Optometry, 142*(5), 35-42.

American Academy of Pediatrics. (2002). Use of photoscreening for children's vision screening. *Pediatrics, 109*(3), 524-525.

American Academy of Pediatrics, American Association of Certified Orthoptists, American Association for Pediatric Ophthalmology and Strabismus, & American Academy of Ophthalmology. (2003). Eye examination in infants, children, and young adults by pediatricians. *Pediatrics, 111*(4), 902-907.

American Academy of Pediatrics & American Academy of Ophthalmology. (2004). Protective eyewear for young athletes. *Pediatrics, 113*(3), 619-622.

Arizona Department of Health Services. (2004). *Recommended vision screening guidelines.* Retrieved March 20, 2006, from *www.azdhs.gov/phs/owch/pdf/vision_screening_2004.pdf.*

Commonwealth of Massachusetts. (2005). *Massachusetts preschool age vision screening protocol.* Retrieved February 28, 2006, from *http://www.mass.gov/dph/fch/schoolhealth/preschool_vision_protocols.doc.*

Coats, D., Carothers, T., Brady-McCreery, K., & Paysse, E. (2004). Ocular infectious diseases. In R. Feigin, J. Cherry, G. Demmler, & S. Kaplan (Eds.). *Textbook of pediatric infectious disease* (5th ed., pp. 787-807). Philadelphia: Saunders.

Committee on Practice and Ambulatory Medicine. (2003). Eye examination in infants, children, and young adults by pediatricians. *Pediatrics, 111*(4), 902-907.

Cunningham, M., & Cox, E. (2003). Hearing assessment in infants and children: recommendations beyond neonatal screening. *Pediatrics, 111*(2), 436-441.

Curnyn, K., & Kaufman, L. (2003). The eye examination in the pediatrician's office. *Pediatric Clinics of North America, 50,* 25-40.

Downey, D., Mraz, R., Knott, J., Knutson, C., Holte, L., & Van Dyke, D. (2002). Diagnosis and evaluation of children who are not talking. *Infants & Young Children, 15*(1), 38-49.

Francis, H., & Niparko, J. (2003). Cochlear implantation update. *Pediatric Clinics of North America, 50,* 341-361.

Glaucoma Research Foundation. (2002). *Surgical treatments for pediatric glaucoma.* Retrieved March 16, 2006, from *www.glaucoma. org/treating/surgical_treatm.html.*

Greenwald, M. (2003). Refractive abnormalities in childhood. *Pediatric Clinics of North America, 50,* 197-212.

Hammerschlag, M. (2004). Chlamydia infections. In R. Feigin, J. Cherry., G. Demmler, & S. Kaplan (Eds.). *Textbook of pediatric infectious diseases* (5th ed., pp. 2482-2486). Philadelphia: Saunders.

Hartmann, et al. (2000, reaffirmed 2005). *Preschool vision screening: summary of a task force report.* Retrieved March 15, 2006, from *www.aap.org.*

Hertle, R., & Roy, C. (2002). Uveitis and hyphema. In F. Burg, J. Ingelfinger, R. Polin, & A, Gershon (Eds.). *Gellis & Kagan's current pediatric therapy* (17th ed., pp. 915-916). Philadelphia: Saunders.

Hoyt, S., & Haley, R. (2005). Innovations in advanced practice assessment and management of eye emergencies. *Topics in Emergency Medicine, 27*(2), 101-117.

Joint Committee on Infant Hearing. (1994). 1994 position statement. *ASHA, 36*(12), 38-41.

Joint Committee on Infant Hearing. (2000). Year 2000 position statement: principles and guidelines for early hearing detection and intervention programs. *Pediatrics, 106*(4), 798-817.

Kipp, M. (2003). Childhood glaucoma. *Pediatric Clinics of North America, 50,* 89-104.

Levin, A. (2003). Congenital eye anomalies. *Pediatric Clinics of North America, 50,* 55-76.

Listman, D. (2004). Paintball injuries in children: more than meets the eye. *Pediatrics, 113*(1), e15-e18.

Lloyd, C. (2003). Pediatric optometry; part II: pediatric eye disorders. *Optician, January 24,* 2. Retrieved March 14, 2006, from Health Reference Center Academic database.

Mittleman, D. (2003). Amblyopia. *Pediatric Clinics of North America, 50,* 189-196.

National Eye Institute. (2003). *Clinical studies database vision in preschoolers study (VIP Study).* Retrieved November 16, 2005, from *www.nei.nih.gov/neitrials/viewStudyWeb.aspx?id=*85.

Olitsky, S., & Nelson, L. (2004). Disorders of the eye. In R. Behrman, R. Kliegman, & H. Jenson (Eds.). *Nelson textbook of pediatrics* (17th ed., pp. 2083-2126). Philadelphia: Saunders.

Quinn, G. (2004). Recent advances in the treatment of amblyopia. *Pediatrics, 113*(6), 1800-1802.

Rodriguez, J. (2003). Prevention and treatment of common eye injuries in sports. *American Family Physician, 67*(7), 1481-1489.

Sadovsky, R. (2003). Distinguishing periorbital from orbital cellulites. *American Family Physician, 67*(6), 1349-1350.

Smith, R., Bale, J., & White, K. (2005). Sensorineural hearing loss in children. *Lancet, 365,* 879-890.

Thibodeau, L., & Johnson, C. (2005). Serving children with hearing loss in public school settings. *The ASHA Leader.* Retrieved March 14, 2006, from *www.asha.org.*

Ticho, B. (2003). Strabismus. *Pediatric Clinics of North America, 50,* 173-188.

United States Preventive Services Task Force. (2005). *Screening for visual impairment in children younger than five years: recommendation statement.* Retrieved March 14, 2006, from *www. aafp.org.*

United States Preventive Services Task Force. (2006). *Screening for speech and language delay in preschool children: recommendation statement.* Retrieved March 24, 2006, from *www.aap.org.*

Waltzman, S., & Roland, T. (2005). Cochlear implantation in children younger than 12 months. *Pediatrics, 116*(4), e487-e493.

Watkinson, S., & Graham, S. (2005). Visual impairment in children. *Nursing Standard, 19*(51), 58-65.

Recommendations for Preventive Pediatric Health Care

Recommendations for Preventive Pediatric Health Care (RE9535)

Committee on Practice and Ambulatory Medicine

Each child and family is unique; therefore, these **Recommendations for Preventive Health Care** are designed for the care of children who are receiving competent parenting, have no manifestations of any important health problems, and are growing and developing in satisfactory fashion. **Additional visits may become necessary** if circumstances suggest variations from normal.

These guidelines represent a consensus by the Committee on Practice and Ambulatory Medicine in consultation with national committees and sections of the American Academy of Pediatrics. The Committee emphasizes the great importance of **continuity of care** in comprehensive health supervision and the need to avoid **fragmentation of care.**

AGE[5]	PRENATAL[1]	NEWBORN[2]	2-4d[3]	By 1mo	2mo	4mo	6mo	9mo	12mo	15mo	18mo	24mo	3y	4y	5y	6y	8y	10y	11y	12y	13y	14y	15y	16y	17y	18y	19y	20y	21y
HISTORY Initial/Interval	●	●	●	●	●	●	●	●	●	●	●	●	●	●	●	●	●	●	●	●	●	●	●	●	●	●	●	●	●
MEASUREMENTS Height and Weight		●	●	●	●	●	●	●	●	●	●	●	●	●	●	●	●	●	●	●	●	●	●	●	●	●	●	●	●
Head Circumference		●	●	●	●	●	●	●	●	●	●	●																	
Blood Pressure												●	●	●	●	●	●	●	●	●	●	●	●	●	●	●	●	●	●
SENSORY SCREENING Vision		S	S	S	S	S	S	S	S	S	S	S	O[6]	O	O	O	O	O	S	S	S	S	O	S	S	O	S	S	S
Hearing		O[7]	S	S	S	S	S	S	S	S	S	S	S	O	O	O	O	O	S	S	S	S	S	S	S	O	S	S	S
DEVELOPMENTAL/ BEHAVIORAL ASSESSMENT[8]		●	●	●	●	●	●	●	●	●	●	●	●	●	●	●	●	●	●	●	●	●	●	●	●	●	●	●	●
PHYSICAL EXAMINATION[9]		●	●	●	●	●	●	●	●	●	●	●	●	●	●	●	●	●	●	●	●	●	●	●	●	●	●	●	●
PROCEDURES-GENERAL[10] Hereditary/Metabolic Screening[11]		←———●———→																											
Immunization[12]		●	●	●	●	●	●	←——●——→		←——●——→	●	●	●	←———————→				←——————————————————————————→											
Hematocrit or Hemoglobin[13]			●←——→●																←—————→										
Urinalysis															←———→													↓[20]	
PROCEDURES-PATIENTS AT RISK Lead Screening[16]							★		★			★	★	★	★	★	★	★	★	★	★	★	★	★	★	★	★	★	★
Tuberculin Test[17]									★		★	★	★	★	★	★	★	★	★	★	★	★	★	★	★	★	★	★	★
Cholesterol Screening[18]													★	★	★	★	★	★	★	★	★	★	★	★	★	★	★	★	★
STD Screening[19]																			★	★	★	★	★	★	★	★	★	★	★
Pelvic Exam[20]																			←————————————————————————————————————→										
ANTICIPATORY GUIDANCE[21] Injury Prevention[22]		●	●	●	●	●	●	●	●	●	●	●	●	●	●	●	●	●	●	●	●	●	●	●	●	●	●	●	●
Violence Prevention[23]		●	●	●	●	●	●	●	●	●	●	●	●	●	●	●	●	●	●	●	●	●	●	●	●	●	●	●	●
Sleep Positioning Counseling[24]	●	●	●	●	●	●	●																						
Nutrition Counseling[25]	●	●	●	●	●	●	●	●	●	●	●	●	●	●	●	●	●	●	●	●	●	●	●	●	●	●	●	●	●
DENTAL REFERRAL[26]														←———●———→															

Age groupings: INFANCY[*] (Prenatal–18mo) · EARLY CHILDHOOD[*] (15mo–4y) · MIDDLE CHILDHOOD[*] (5y–10y) · ADOLESCENCE[*] (11y–21y)

Key: ● = to be performed ★ = to be performed for patients at risk S = subjective, by history O = objective, by a standard testing method ←—→ = the range during which a service may be provided, with the dot indicating the preferred age.

1. A prenatal visit is recommended for parents who are at high risk, for first-time parents, and for those who request a conference. The prenatal visit should include anticipatory guidance, pertinent medical history, and a discussion of benefits of breastfeeding and planned method of feeding per AAP statement "The Prenatal Visit" (1996).
2. Every infant should have a newborn evaluation after birth. Breastfeeding should be encouraged and instruction and support offered. Every breastfeeding infant should have an evaluation 48-72 hours after discharge from the hospital to include weight, formal breastfeeding evaluation, encouragement, and instruction as recommended in the AAP statement "Breastfeeding and the Use of Human Milk" (1997).
3. For newborns discharged in less than 48 hours after delivery per AAP statement "Hospital Stay for Healthy Term Newborns" (1995).
4. Developmental, psychosocial, and chronic disease issues for children and adolescents may require frequent counseling and treatment visits separate from preventive care visits.
5. If a child comes under care for the first time at any point on the schedule, or if any items are not accomplished at the suggested age, the schedule should be brought up to date at the earliest possible time.
6. If the patient is uncooperative, rescreen within 6 months.
7. All newborns should be screened per the AAP Task Force on Newborn and Infant Hearing statement, "Newborn and Infant Hearing Loss Detection and Intervention" (1999).
8. By history and appropriate physical examination; if suspicious, by specific objective developmental testing. Parenting skills should be fostered at every visit.
9. At each visit, a complete physical examination is essential, with infant totally undressed, older child undressed and suitably draped.
10. These may be modified, depending upon entry point into schedule and individual need.
11. Metabolic screening (eg, thyroid, hemoglobinopathies, PKU, galactosemia) should be done according to state law.
12. Schedule(s) per the Committee on Infectious Diseases, published annually in the January edition of Pediatrics. Every visit should be an opportunity to update and complete a child's immunizations.
13. See AAP Pediatric Nutrition Handbook (1998) for a discussion of universal and selective screening options. Consider earlier screening for high-risk infants (eg, premature infants and low birth weight infants). See also "Recommendations to Prevent and Control Iron Deficiency in the United States. MMWR. 1998;47 (RR-3):1-29.
14. All menstruating adolescents should be screened annually.
15. Conduct dipstick urinalysis for leukocytes annually for sexually active male and female adolescents.
16. For children at risk of lead exposure consult the AAP statement "Screening for Elevated Blood Levels" (1998). Additionally, screening should be done in accordance with state law where applicable.
17. TB testing per recommendations of the Committee on Infectious Diseases, published in the current edition of Red Book: Report of the Committee on Infectious Diseases. Testing should be done upon recognition of high-risk factors.
18. Cholesterol screening for high-risk patients per AAP statement "Cholesterol in Childhood" (1998). If family history cannot be ascertained and other risk factors are present, screening should be at the discretion of the physician.
19. All sexually active patients should be screened for sexually transmitted diseases (STDs).
20. All sexually active females should have a pelvic examination. A pelvic examination and routine pap smear should be offered as part of preventive health maintenance between the ages of 18 and 21 years.
21. Age-appropriate discussion and counseling should be an integral part of each visit for care per the AAP Guidelines for Health Supervision III (1998).
22. From birth to age 12, refer to the AAP injury prevention program (TIPP*) as described in A Guide to Safety Counseling in Office Practice (1994).
23. Violence prevention and management for all patients per AAP statement "The Role of the Pediatrician in Youth Violence Prevention in Clinical Practice and at the Community Level" (1999).
24. Parents and caregivers should be advised to place healthy infants on their backs when putting them to sleep. Side positioning is a reasonable alternative but carries a slightly higher risk of SIDS. Consult the AAP statement "Positioning and Sudden Infant Death Syndrome (SIDS): Update" (1996).
25. Age-appropriate nutrition counseling should be an integral part of each visit per the AAP Handbook of Nutrition (1998).
26. Earlier initial dental examinations may be appropriate for some children. Subsequent examinations as prescribed by dentist.

NB: Special chemical, immunologic, and endocrine testing is usually carried out upon specific indications. Testing other than newborn (eg, inborn errors of metabolism, sickle disease, etc) is discretionary with the physician.

The recommendations in this statement do not indicate an exclusive course of treatment or standard of medical care. Variations, taking into account individual circumstances, may be appropriate. Copyright ©1999 by the American Academy of Pediatrics. No part of this statement may be reproduced in any form or by any means without prior written permission from the American Academy of Pediatrics except for one copy for personal use.

American Academy of Pediatrics

Growth Charts

Birth to 36 months: Girls
Length-for-age and Weight-for-age percentiles

NAME

RECORD #

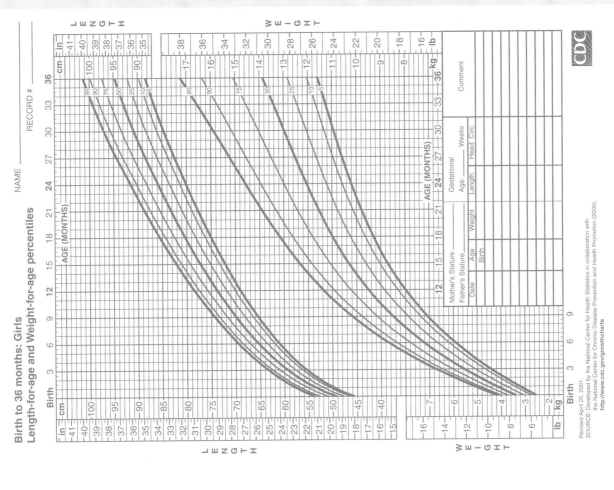

Revised April 20, 2001.
SOURCE: Developed by the National Center for Health Statistics in collaboration with
the National Center for Chronic Disease Prevention and Health Promotion (2000).
http://www.cdc.gov/growthcharts

Birth to 36 months: Boys
Length-for-age and Weight-for-age percentiles

NAME

RECORD #

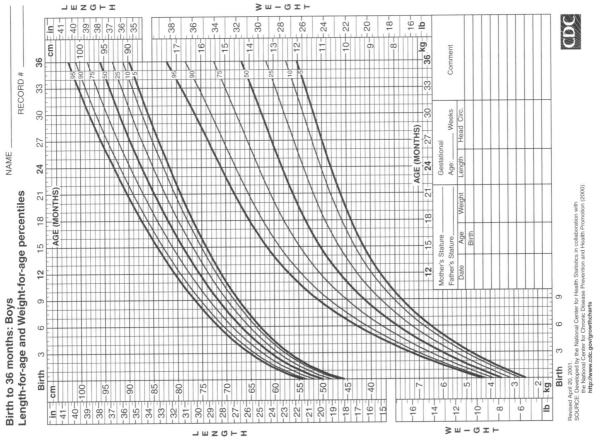

Revised April 20, 2001.
SOURCE: Developed by the National Center for Health Statistics in collaboration with
the National Center for Chronic Disease Prevention and Health Promotion (2000).
http://www.cdc.gov/growthcharts

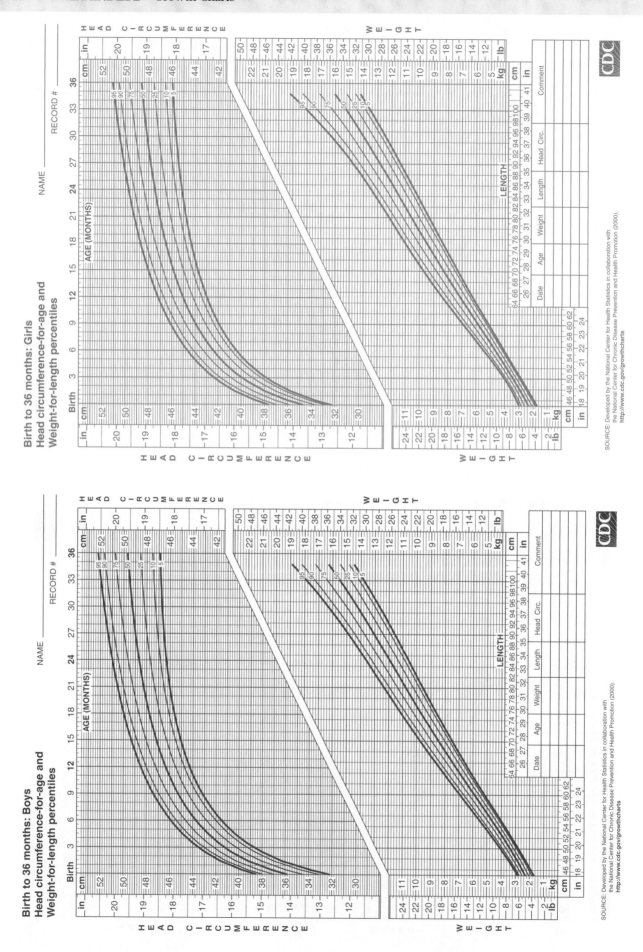

Birth to 36 months: Girls
Head circumference-for-age and
Weight-for-length percentiles

Birth to 36 months: Boys
Head circumference-for-age and
Weight-for-length percentiles

SOURCE: Developed by the National Center for Health Statistics in collaboration with
the National Center for Chronic Disease Prevention and Health Promotion (2000).
http://www.cdc.gov/growthcharts

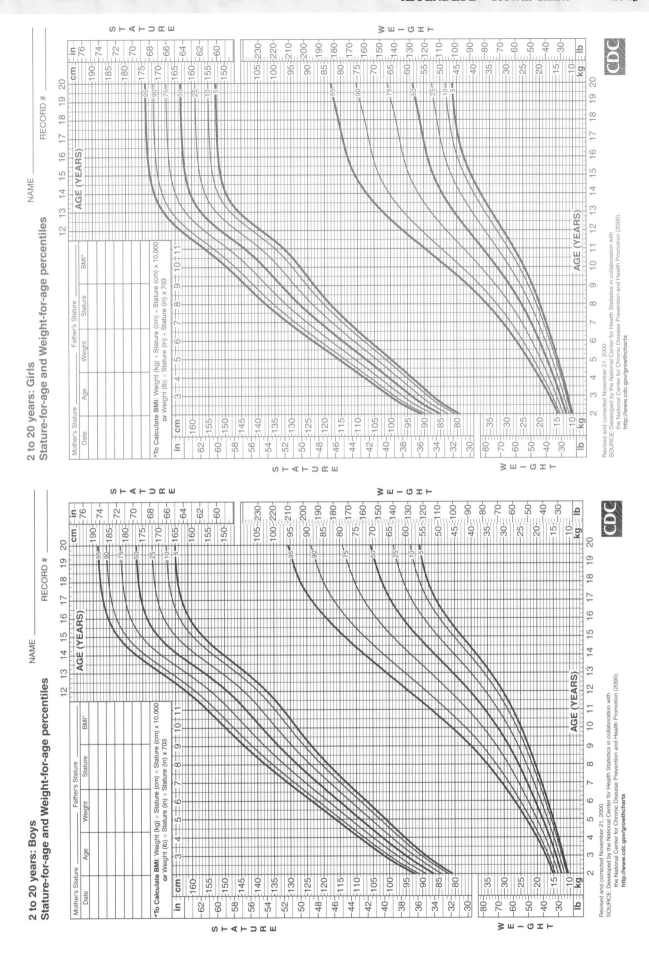

2 to 20 years: Boys
Stature-for-age and Weight-for-age percentiles

NAME

RECORD #

2 to 20 years: Girls
Stature-for-age and Weight-for-age percentiles

NAME

RECORD #

*To Calculate BMI: Weight (kg) ÷ Stature (cm) ÷ Stature (cm) × 10,000
or Weight (lb) ÷ Stature (in) ÷ Stature (in) × 703

Revised and corrected November 21, 2000.
SOURCE: Developed by the National Center for Health Statistics in collaboration with
the National Center for Chronic Disease Prevention and Health Promotion (2000).
http://www.cdc.gov/growthcharts

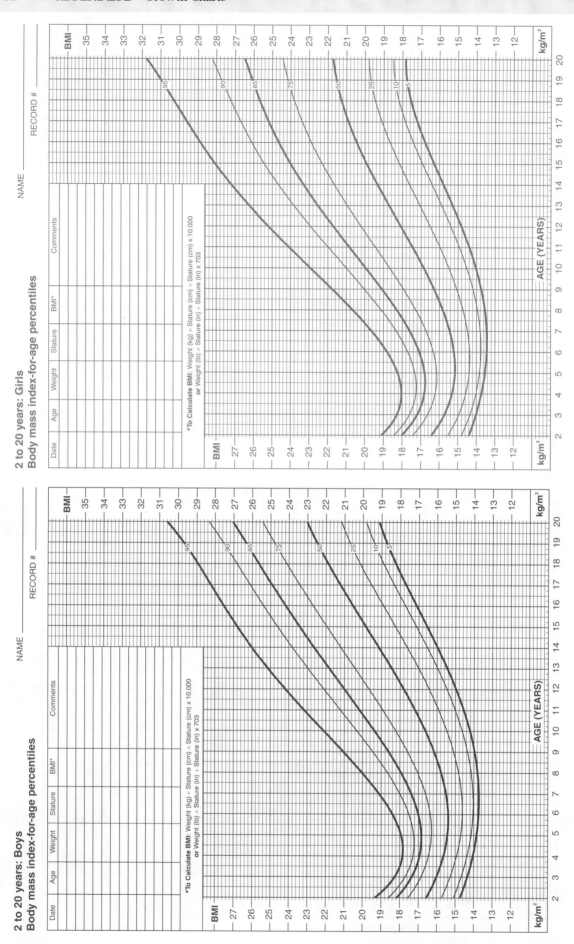

2 to 20 years: Boys
Body mass index-for-age percentiles

NAME _____

RECORD # _____

Date	Age	Weight	Stature	BMI*	Comments

*To Calculate BMI: Weight (kg) ÷ Stature (cm) ÷ Stature (cm) × 10,000
or Weight (lb) ÷ Stature (in) ÷ Stature (in) × 703

2 to 20 years: Girls
Body mass index-for-age percentiles

NAME _____

RECORD # _____

Date	Age	Weight	Stature	BMI*	Comments

*To Calculate BMI: Weight (kg) ÷ Stature (cm) ÷ Stature (cm) × 10,000
or Weight (lb) ÷ Stature (in) ÷ Stature (in) × 703

SOURCE: Developed by the National Center for Health Statistics in collaboration with
the National Center for Chronic Disease Prevention and Health Promotion (2000).
http://www.cdc.gov/growthcharts

SOURCE: Developed by the National Center for Health Statistics in collaboration with
the National Center for Chronic Disease Prevention and Health Promotion (2000).
http://www.cdc.gov/growthcharts

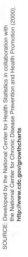

APPENDIX C

Blood Pressure Levels by Age and Height

TABLE 1   Blood Pressure Levels for Boys by Age and Height

Age, y	BP Percentile	SBP, mm Hg Percentile of Height							DBP, mm Hg Percentile of Height						
		5th	10th	25th	50th	75th	90th	95th	5th	10th	25th	50th	75th	90th	95th
1	50th	80	81	83	85	87	88	89	34	35	36	37	38	39	39
	90th	94	95	97	99	100	102	103	49	50	51	52	53	53	54
	95th	98	99	101	103	104	106	106	54	54	55	56	57	58	58
	99th	105	106	108	110	112	113	114	61	62	63	64	65	66	66
2	50th	84	85	87	88	90	92	92	39	40	41	42	43	44	44
	90th	97	99	100	102	104	105	106	54	55	56	57	58	58	59
	95th	101	102	104	106	108	109	110	59	59	60	61	62	63	63
	99th	109	110	111	113	115	117	117	66	67	68	69	70	71	71
3	50th	86	87	89	91	93	94	95	44	44	45	46	47	48	48
	90th	100	101	103	105	107	108	109	59	59	60	61	62	63	63
	95th	104	105	107	109	110	112	113	63	63	64	65	66	67	67
	99th	111	112	114	116	118	119	120	71	71	72	73	74	75	75
4	50th	88	89	91	93	95	96	97	47	48	49	50	51	51	52
	90th	102	103	105	107	109	110	111	62	63	64	65	66	66	67
	95th	106	107	109	111	112	114	115	66	67	68	69	70	71	71
	99th	113	114	116	118	120	121	122	74	75	76	77	78	78	79
5	50th	90	91	93	95	96	98	98	50	51	52	53	54	55	55
	90th	104	105	106	108	110	111	112	65	66	67	68	69	69	70
	95th	108	109	110	112	114	115	116	69	70	71	72	73	74	74
	99th	115	116	118	120	121	123	123	77	78	79	80	81	81	82
6	50th	91	92	94	96	98	99	100	53	53	54	55	56	57	57
	90th	105	106	108	110	111	113	113	68	68	69	70	71	72	72
	95th	109	110	112	114	115	117	117	72	72	73	74	75	76	76
	99th	116	117	119	121	123	124	125	80	80	81	82	83	84	84
7	50th	92	94	95	97	99	100	101	55	55	56	57	58	59	59
	90th	106	107	109	111	113	114	115	70	70	71	72	73	74	74
	95th	110	111	113	115	117	118	119	74	74	75	76	77	78	78
	99th	117	118	120	122	124	125	126	82	82	83	84	85	86	86
8	50th	94	95	97	99	100	102	102	56	57	58	59	60	60	61
	90th	107	109	110	112	114	115	116	71	72	72	73	74	75	76
	95th	111	112	114	116	118	119	120	75	76	77	78	79	79	80
	99th	119	120	122	123	125	127	127	83	84	85	86	87	87	88
9	50th	95	96	98	100	102	103	104	57	58	59	60	61	61	62
	90th	109	110	112	114	115	117	118	72	73	74	75	76	76	77
	95th	113	114	116	118	119	121	121	76	77	78	79	80	81	81
	99th	120	121	123	125	127	128	129	84	85	86	87	88	88	89

Continued

TABLE 1 Blood Pressure Levels for Boys by Age and Height—cont'd

Age, y	BP Percentile	SBP, mm Hg Percentile of Height							DBP, mm Hg Percentile of Height						
		5th	10th	25th	50th	75th	90th	95th	5th	10th	25th	50th	75th	90th	95th
10	50th	97	98	100	102	103	105	106	58	59	60	61	61	62	63
	90th	111	112	114	115	117	119	119	73	73	74	75	76	77	78
	95th	115	116	117	119	121	122	123	77	78	79	80	81	81	82
	99th	122	123	125	127	128	130	130	85	86	86	88	88	89	90
11	50th	99	100	102	104	105	107	107	59	59	60	61	62	63	63
	90th	113	114	115	117	119	120	121	74	74	75	76	77	78	78
	95th	117	118	119	121	123	124	125	78	78	79	80	81	82	82
	99th	124	125	127	129	130	132	132	86	86	87	88	89	90	90
12	50th	101	102	104	106	108	109	110	59	60	61	62	63	63	64
	90th	115	116	118	120	121	123	123	74	75	75	76	77	78	79
	95th	119	120	122	123	125	127	127	78	79	80	81	82	82	83
	99th	126	127	129	131	133	134	135	86	87	88	89	90	90	91
13	50th	104	105	106	108	110	111	112	60	60	61	62	63	64	64
	90th	117	118	120	122	124	125	126	75	75	76	77	78	79	79
	95th	121	122	124	126	128	129	130	79	79	80	81	82	83	83
	99th	128	130	131	133	135	136	137	87	87	88	89	90	91	91
14	50th	106	107	109	111	113	114	115	60	61	62	63	64	65	65
	90th	120	121	123	125	126	128	128	75	76	77	78	79	79	80
	95th	124	125	127	128	130	132	132	80	80	81	82	83	84	84
	99th	131	132	134	136	138	139	140	87	88	89	90	91	92	92
15	50th	109	110	112	113	115	117	117	61	62	63	64	65	66	66
	90th	122	124	125	127	129	130	131	76	77	78	79	80	80	81
	95th	126	127	129	131	133	134	135	81	81	82	83	84	85	85
	99th	134	135	136	138	140	142	142	88	89	90	91	92	93	93
16	50th	111	112	114	116	118	119	120	63	63	64	65	66	67	67
	90th	125	126	128	130	131	133	134	78	78	79	80	81	82	82
	95th	129	130	132	134	135	137	137	82	83	83	84	85	86	87
	99th	136	137	139	141	143	144	145	90	90	91	92	93	94	94
17	50th	114	115	116	118	120	121	122	65	66	66	67	68	69	70
	90th	127	128	130	132	134	135	136	80	80	81	82	83	84	84
	95th	131	132	134	136	138	139	140	84	85	86	87	87	88	89
	99th	139	140	141	143	145	146	147	92	93	93	94	95	96	97

From the National High Blood Pressure Education Program Working Group on High Blood Pressure in Children and Adolescents (2004). The fourth report on the diagnosis, evaluation, and treatment of high blood pressure in children and adolescents. *Pediatrics, 114,* 558.

TABLE 2 Blood Pressure Levels for Girls by Age and Height

Age, y	BP Percentile	SBP, mm Hg Percentile of Height							DBP, mm Hg Percentile of Height						
		5th	10th	25th	50th	75th	90th	95th	5th	10th	25th	50th	75th	90th	95th
1	50th	83	84	85	86	88	89	90	38	39	39	40	41	41	42
	90th	97	97	98	100	101	102	103	52	53	53	54	55	55	56
	95th	100	101	102	104	105	106	107	56	57	57	58	59	59	60
	99th	108	108	109	111	112	113	114	64	64	65	65	66	67	67
2	50th	85	85	87	88	89	91	91	43	44	44	45	46	46	47
	90th	98	99	100	101	103	104	105	57	58	58	59	60	61	61
	95th	102	103	104	105	107	108	109	61	62	62	63	64	65	65
	99th	109	110	111	112	114	115	116	69	69	70	70	71	72	72
3	50th	86	87	88	89	91	92	93	47	48	48	49	50	50	51
	90th	100	100	102	103	104	106	106	61	62	62	63	64	64	65
	95th	104	104	105	107	108	109	110	65	66	66	67	68	68	69
	99th	111	111	113	114	115	116	117	73	73	74	74	75	76	76
4	50th	88	88	90	91	92	94	94	50	50	51	52	52	53	54
	90th	101	102	103	104	106	107	108	64	64	65	66	67	67	68
	95th	105	106	107	108	110	111	112	68	68	69	70	71	71	72
	99th	112	113	114	115	117	118	119	76	76	76	77	78	79	79

TABLE 2   Blood Pressure Levels for Girls by Age and Height—cont'd

Age, y	BP Percentile	SBP, mm Hg Percentile of Height							DBP, mm Hg Percentile of Height						
		5th	10th	25th	50th	75th	90th	95th	5th	10th	25th	50th	75th	90th	95th
5	50th	89	90	91	93	94	95	96	52	53	53	54	55	55	56
	90th	103	103	105	106	107	109	109	66	67	67	68	69	69	70
	95th	107	107	108	110	111	112	113	70	71	71	72	73	73	74
	99th	114	114	116	117	118	120	120	78	78	79	79	80	81	81
6	50th	91	92	93	94	96	97	98	54	54	55	56	56	57	58
	90th	104	105	106	108	109	110	111	68	68	69	70	70	71	72
	95th	108	109	110	111	113	114	115	72	72	73	74	74	75	76
	99th	115	116	117	119	120	121	122	80	80	80	81	82	83	83
7	50th	93	93	95	96	97	99	99	55	56	56	57	58	58	59
	90th	106	107	108	109	111	112	113	69	70	70	71	72	72	73
	95th	110	111	112	113	115	116	116	73	74	74	75	76	76	77
	99th	117	118	119	120	122	123	124	81	81	82	82	83	84	84
8	50th	95	95	96	98	99	100	101	57	57	57	58	59	60	60
	90th	108	109	110	111	113	114	114	71	71	71	72	73	74	74
	95th	112	112	114	115	116	118	118	75	75	75	76	77	78	78
	99th	119	120	121	122	123	125	125	82	82	83	83	84	85	86
9	50th	96	97	98	100	101	102	103	58	58	58	59	60	61	61
	90th	110	110	112	113	114	116	116	72	72	72	73	74	75	75
	95th	114	114	115	117	118	119	120	76	76	76	77	78	79	79
	99th	121	121	123	124	125	127	127	83	83	84	84	85	86	87
10	50th	98	99	100	102	103	104	105	59	59	59	60	61	62	62
	90th	112	112	114	115	116	118	118	73	73	73	74	75	76	76
	95th	116	116	117	119	120	121	122	77	77	77	78	79	80	80
	99th	123	123	125	126	127	129	129	84	84	85	86	86	87	88
11	50th	100	101	102	103	105	106	107	60	60	60	61	62	63	63
	90th	114	114	116	117	118	119	120	74	74	74	75	76	77	77
	95th	118	118	119	121	122	123	124	78	78	78	79	80	81	81
	99th	125	125	126	128	129	130	131	85	85	86	87	87	88	89
12	50th	102	103	104	105	107	108	109	61	61	61	62	63	64	64
	90th	116	116	117	119	120	121	122	75	75	75	76	77	78	78
	95th	119	120	121	123	124	125	126	79	79	79	80	81	82	82
	99th	127	127	128	130	131	132	133	86	86	87	88	88	89	90
13	50th	104	105	106	107	109	110	110	62	62	62	63	64	65	65
	90th	117	118	119	121	122	123	124	76	76	76	77	78	79	79
	95th	121	122	123	124	126	127	128	80	80	80	81	82	83	83
	99th	128	129	130	132	133	134	135	87	87	88	89	89	90	91
14	50th	106	106	107	109	110	111	112	63	63	63	64	65	66	66
	90th	119	120	121	122	124	125	125	77	77	77	78	79	80	80
	95th	123	123	125	126	127	129	129	81	81	81	82	83	84	84
	99th	130	131	132	133	135	136	136	88	88	89	90	90	91	92
15	50th	107	108	109	110	111	113	113	64	64	64	65	66	67	67
	90th	120	121	122	123	125	126	127	78	78	78	79	80	81	81
	95th	124	125	126	127	129	130	131	82	82	82	83	84	85	85
	99th	131	132	133	134	136	137	138	89	89	90	91	91	92	93
16	50th	108	108	110	111	112	114	114	64	64	65	66	66	67	68
	90th	121	122	123	124	126	127	128	78	78	79	80	81	81	82
	95th	125	126	127	128	130	131	132	82	82	83	84	85	85	86
	99th	132	133	134	135	137	138	139	90	90	90	91	92	93	93
17	50th	108	109	110	111	113	114	115	64	65	65	66	67	67	68
	90th	122	122	123	25	126	127	128	78	79	79	80	81	81	82
	95th	125	126	127	129	130	131	132	82	83	83	84	85	85	86
	99th	133	133	134	136	137	138	139	90	90	91	91	92	93	93

From the National High Blood Pressure Education Program Working Group on High Blood Pressure in Children and Adolescents (2004). The fourth report on the diagnosis, evaluation, and treatment of high blood pressure in children and adolescents. *Pediatrics, 114,* 559.